ANTIBIOTIC AND CHEMOTHERAPY

Commissioning Editor: Sue Hodgson
Development Editor: Nani Clansey
Editorial Assistant: Poppy Garraway/Rachael Harrison
Project Manager: Jess Thompson
Design: Charles Gray
Illustration Manager: Bruce Hogarth
Illustrator: Merlyn Harvey
Marketing Manager (USA): Helena Mutak

ANTIBIOTIC AND CHEMOTHERAPY

ANTI-INFECTIVE AGENTS AND THEIR USE IN THERAPY

NINTH EDITION

Roger G. Finch
MB BS FRCP FRCP(Ed) FRCPath FFPM
Professor of Infectious Diseases, School of Molecular Medical Sciences,
Division of Microbiology and Infectious Diseases, University of Nottingham and
Nottingham University Hospitals, The City Hospital,
Nottingham, UK

David Greenwood
PhD DSc FRCPath
Emeritus Professor of Antimicrobial Science, University of Nottingham Medical School,
Nottingham, UK

S. Ragnar Norrby
MD PhD FRCP
Professor, The Swedish Institute for Infectious Disease Control, Stockholm, Sweden

Richard J. Whitley
MD
Distinguished Professor Loeb Scholar in Pediatrics, Professor of Pediatrics, Microbiology,
Medicine and Neurosurgery, The University of Alabama at Birmingham, Birmingham,
Alabama, USA

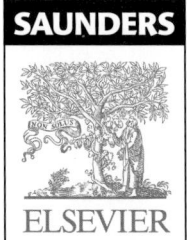

SAUNDERS

ELSEVIER

Edinburgh London New York Philadelphia St Louis Sydney Toronto 2010

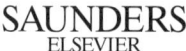

SAUNDERS
ELSEVIER

SAUNDERS an imprint of Elsevier Limited

First edition 1963
Second edition 1968
Third edition 1971
Fourth edition 1973
Fifth edition 1981
Sixth edition 1992
Seventh edition 1997
Eighth edition 2003

Notices

Knowledge and best practice in this field are constantly changing. As new research and experience broaden our understanding, changes in research methods, professional practices, or medical treatment may become necessary. Practitioners and researchers must always rely on their own experience and knowledge in evaluating and using any information, methods, compounds, or experiments described herein. In using such information or methods they should be mindful of their own safety and the safety of others, including parties for whom they have a professional responsibility.

With respect to any drug or pharmaceutical products identified, readers are advised to check the most current information provided (i) on procedures featured or (ii) by the manufacturer of each product to be administered, to verify the recommended dose or formula, the method and duration of administration, and contraindications. It is the responsibility of practitioners, relying on their own experience and knowledge of their patients, to make diagnoses, to determine dosages and the best treatment for each individual patient, and to take all appropriate safety precautions.

To the fullest extent of the law, neither the Publisher nor the authors, contributors, or editors, assume any liability for any injury and/or damage to persons or property as a matter of products liability, negligence or otherwise, or from any use or operation of any methods, products, instructions, or ideas contained in the material herein.

ISBN: 978-0-7020-4064-1

British Library Cataloguing in Publication Data
A catalogue record for this book is available from the British Library

Library of Congress Cataloging in Publication Data
A catalog record for this book is available from the Library of Congress

Printed in China

Last digit is the print number: 9 8 7 6 5 4 3 2 1

Contents

Preface

The first edition of this book was published almost half a century ago. Subsequent editions have generally been published in response to the steady flow of novel antibacterial compounds or the marketing of derivatives of existing classes of agents exhibiting advantages, sometimes questionable, over their parent compound. In producing the ninth edition of this book the rationale has been not so much in response to the availability of new antibacterial compounds, but to capture advances in antiviral and, to a lesser extent, antifungal chemotherapy and also to highlight a number of changing therapeutic approaches to selected infections. For example, the recognition that combination therapy has an expanded role in preventing the emergence of drug resistance; traditionally applied to the treatment of tuberculosis, it is now being used in the management of HIV, hepatitis B and C virus infections and, most notably, malaria among the protozoal infections.

The impact of antibiotic resistance has reached critical levels. Multidrug-resistant pathogens are now commonplace in hospitals and not only affect therapeutic choice, but also, in the seriously ill, can be life threatening. While methicillin-resistant *Staphylococcus aureus* (MRSA) has been taxing healthcare systems and achieved prominence in the media, resistance among Gram-negative bacillary pathogens is probably of considerably greater importance. More specifically, resistance based on extended spectrum β-lactamase production has reached epidemic proportions in some hospitals and has also been recognized, somewhat belatedly, as a cause of much community infection. There are also emerging links with overseas travel and possibly with the food chain. The dearth of novel compounds to treat resistant Gram-negative bacillary infections is particularly worrying. What is clear is that the appropriate use of antimicrobial drugs in the management of human and animal disease has never been more important.

As in the past, the aim of this book is to provide an international repository of information on the properties of antimicrobial drugs and authoritative advice on their clinical application. The structure of the book remains unchanged, being divided into three parts. Section 1 addresses the general aspects of antimicrobial chemotherapy while Section 2 provides a detailed description of the agents, either by group and their respective compounds, or by target microorganisms as in the case of non-antibacterial agents. Section 3 deals with the treatment of all major infections by site, disease or target pathogens as appropriate. Some new chapters have been introduced and others deleted. The *recommended International Non-proprietary Names (rINN)* with minor exceptions has once again been adopted to reflect the international relevance of the guidance provided.

Our thanks go to our international panel of authors who have been selected for their expertise and who have shown patience with our deadlines and accommodated our revisions. We also thank those who have contributed to earlier editions and whose legacy lives on in some areas of the text. Here we wish to specifically thank both Francis O'Grady and Harold Lambert who edited this book for many years and did much to establish its international reputation. Their continued support and encouragement is gratefully acknowledged. We also welcome and thank Tim Hill for his pharmacy expertise in ensuring the accuracy of the information contained in the *Preparation and Dosages* boxes and elsewhere in the text. Finally, we thank the Editorial Team at Elsevier Science for their efficiency and professionalism in the production of this new edition.

Roger Finch, David Greenwood, Ragnar Norrby, Richard Whitley
Nottingham, UK; Stockholm, Sweden; Birmingham, USA.

February 2010

List of Contributors

Peter C. Appelbaum, MD PhD
Professor of Pathology and Director of Clinical
    Microbiology
Penn State Hershey Medical Center
Hershey, PA, USA

Stephen P. Barrett, BA MSc MD PhD FRCPath DipHIC
Consultant Medical Microbiologist
Microbiology Department
Southend Hospital
Westcliff-on-Sea
Essex, UK

Mark Boyd, MD FRACP
Clinical Project Leader, Therapeutic and
    Vaccine Research Program
National Centre in HIV Epidemiology and Clinical
    Research and
Senior Lecturer, University of New South Wales;
Clinical Academic in Infectious Diseases and HIV Medicine
St Vincent's Hospital
Darlinghurst
Sydney, Australia

Eimear Brannigan, MB MRCPI
Consultant in Infectious Diseases
Infection Prevention and Control
Charing Cross Hospital
London, UK

Derek Brown, BSc PhD FRCPath
Consultant Microbiologist
Peterborough, UK

André Bryskier, MD
Consultant in Anti-Infective Therapies
Le Mesnil le Roi, France

Karen Bush, PhD
Adjunct Professor
Biology Department
Indiana University Bloomington
Bloomington, Indiana, USA

Christopher C. Butler, BA MBChB DCH FRCGP MD CCH
HonFFPHM
Professor of Primary Care Medicine, Cardiff University
Head of Department of Primary Care and Public Health
    and Vice Dean (Research)
Cardiff University Clinical Epidemiology Interdisciplinary
    Research Group
School of Medicine, Cardiff University
Cardiff, UK

Kevin A. Cassady, MD
Assistant Professor of Pediatrics
Division of Infectious Diseases
Department of Pediatrics
University of Alabama at Birmingham
Children's Harbor Research Center
Birmingham, Alabama, USA

Peter L. Chiodini, BSc MBBS PhD MRCS FRCP FRCPath
FFTMRCPS(Glas)
Honorary Professor, Infectious and Tropical Diseases
The London School of Hygiene and Tropical Medicine;
Consultant Parasitologist, Department of Clinical Parasitology
Hospital for Tropical Diseases
London, UK

Ian Chopra, BA MA PhD DSc MD(Honorary)
Professor of Microbiology and Director of the
    Antimicrobial Research Centre
Division of Microbiology, Institute of Molecular and
    Cellular Biology
University of Leeds
Leeds, UK

George A. Conder, PhD
Director and Therapeutic Area Head
Antiparasitics Discovery Research
Veterinary Medicine Research and Development
Pfizer Animal Health
Pfizer Inc
Kalamazoo, MI, USA

David A. Cooper, MD DSc
Professor of Medicine
Consultant Immunologist
Faculty of Medicine
University of New South Wales
St Vincent's Hospital
National Centre in HIV Epidemiology and Clinical Research
Darlinghurst
Sydney, Australia

Simon L. Croft, PhD
Professor of Parasitology
Head of Department of Infectious and Tropical Diseases
London School of Hygiene and Tropical Medicine
London, UK

Carmel M. Curtis, PhD MRCP
Microbiology Specialist Registrar
Department of Parasitology
The Hospital for Tropical Diseases
London, UK

Robert Davidson, MD FRCP DTM&H
Consultant Physician, Honorary Senior Lecturer
Department of Infectious and Tropical Diseases
Northwick Park Hospital
Harrow, Middlesex, UK

Peter G. Davey, MD FRCP
Professor in Pharmacoeconomics and
    Consultant in Infectious Diseases
Ninewells Hospital and Medical School
University of Dundee
Dundee, UK

Olivier Denis, MD PhD
Scientific Advice Unit
European Centre for Disease
Prevention and Control
Stockholm, Sweden

Linda Ficker, BSc FRCS FRCOphth EBOD
Consultant Ophthalmologist
Moorfield Eye Hospital
London, UK

**Roger G. Finch, MB BS FRCP FRCP(Ed)
FRCPath FFPM**
Professor of Infectious Diseases
School of Molecular Medical Sciences
Division of Microbiology and Infectious
    Diseases
University of Nottingham and Nottingham
    University Hospitals
The City Hospital
Nottingham, UK

Arne Forsgren, MD PhD
Professor of Clinical Bacteriology
Department of Laboratory Medicine
Medical Microbiology
Lund University
Malmö University Hospital
Malmö, Sweden

Adam P. Fraise, MB BS FRCPath
Consultant Microbiologist
University Hospital Birmingham
Microbiology Department
Queen's Elizabeth Hospital
Birmingham, UK

**Nicholas A. Francis, BA MD PG Dip
(Epidemiology) PhD MRCGP**
Clinical Lecturer
South East Wales Trials Unit
Department of Primary Care and Public Health
School of Medicine, Cardiff University
Cardiff, UK

Kate Gould, MB BS FRCPath
Consultant in Medical Microbiology
Honorary Professor in Medical Microbiology
Regional Microbiologist, Health Protection
    Agency
Department of Microbiology
Freeman Hospital
Newcastle upon Tyne, UK

John M. Grange, MSc MD
Visiting Professor
Centre for Infectious Diseases and International
    Health
Royal Free and University College Medical
    School
Windeyer Institute for Medical Sciences
London, UK

David Greenwood, PhD DSc FRCPath
Emeritus Professor of Antimicrobial Science
University of Nottingham Medical School
Nottingham, UK

Phillip Hay, MD
Senior Lecturer in Genitourinary Medicine
Courtyard Clinic
St George's Hospital
London, UK

Roderick J. Hay
Honorary Professor, Clinical Research Unit
London School of Hygiene and Tropical Medicine
Consultant Dermatologist
Infectious Disease Clinic Dermatology Department
King's College Hospital
Chairman
International Foundation for Dermatology
London, UK

Tim Hills, BPharm MRPharmS
Lead Pharmacist Antimicrobials and Infection
    Control
Pharmacy Department
Nottingham University Hospitals NHS Trust
    Queens Campus
Nottingham, UK

Peter J. Jenks, PhD MRCP FRCPath
Director of Infection Prevention and Control
Department of Microbiology
Plymouth Hospitals NHS Trust
Derriford Hospital
Plymouth, UK

Gunnar Kahlmeter, MD PhD
Professor of Clinical Bacteriology
Head of Department of Clinical Microbiology
Central Hospital
Växjö, Sweden

Chris C. Kibbler, MA FRCP FRCPath
Professor of Medical Microbiology
Centre for Medical Microbiology
University College London
Clinical Lead
Department of Medical Microbiology
Royal Free Hospital NHS Trust
London, UK

Sheena Kakar, MBBS Grad Dip Med (STD/HIV)
Research Fellow/Registrar
Sexually Transmitted Infections Research
    Centre (STIRC)
Westmead Hospital
Westmead, Australia

Donna M. Kraus, PharmD
Associate Professor of Pharmacy Practice and
    Pediatrics
Colleges of Pharmacy and Medicine
University of Illinois at Chicago
Chicago, USA

**Lucy Lamb, MA (Cantab)
MRCP DTM&H**
Specialist Registrar Infectious Diseases and
    General Medicine
Northwick Park Hospital
Middlesex, UK

Saba Lambert, MBChB
Doctor
London, UK

Giancarlo Lancini, PhD
Consultant Microbial Chemistry
Lecturer in Microbial Biotechnology
University Varese
Gerenzano (VA), Italy

David Leaper, MD ChM FRCS FACS
Visiting Professor
Cardiff University
Department of Wound Healing
Cardiff Medicentre
Cardiff, UK

Diana Lockwood, BSc MD FRCP
Professor of Tropical Medicine
London School of Hygiene and Tropical
    Medicine
Consultant Physician and Leprologist
Hospital for Tropical Diseases
Department of Infectious and Tropical
    Diseases, Clinical Research Unit
London School of Hygiene and Tropical Medicine
London, UK

Andrew M. Lovering, BSc PhD
Consultant Clinical Scientist
Department of Medical Microbiology
Southmead Hospital
Westbury on Trym
Bristol, UK

**Alasdair P. MacGowan, BMedBiol MD
FRCP(Ed) FRCPath**
Professor of Clinical Microbiology and
    Antimicrobial Therapeutics
Department of Medical Microbiology
Bristol Centre for Antimicrobial Research and
    Evaluation
North Bristol NHS Trust
Southmead Hospital
Bristol, UK

Janice Main, MB ChB FRCP (Edin & Lond)
Reader and Consultant Physician in Infectious
    Diseases and General Medicine
Department of Medicine
Imperial College
St Mary's Hospital
London, UK

Lionel A. Mandell, MD FRCPC FRCP (Lond)
Professor, Division of Infectious Diseases
Director, International Health and Tropical
    Diseases Clinic at Hamilton Health
    Sciences
Member, IDSA Practice Guidelines
    Committee
Chairman, Community Acquired Pneumonia
    Guideline Committee of IDSA and
    Canadian Infectious Disease Society
McMasters University
Hamilton, ON, Canada

Sharon Marlowe, MB ChB MRCP DTM&H
Clinical Research Fellow
Clinical Research Unit, Infectious and Tropical
    Diseases Dept
London School of Hygiene and Tropical
    Medicine
London, UK

Michael Millar, MB ChB MD MA FRCPath
Consultant Microbiologist
Division of Infection
Barts and the London NHS Trust
London, UK

Adrian Mindel, MD FRCP FRACP
Professor of Sexual Health Medicine,
    University of Sydney
Director, Sexually Transmitted Infections
    Research Centre (STIRC)
Westmead Hospital
Westmead, Australia

Peter Moss, MD FRCP DTMH
Consultant in Infectious Diseases and
    Honorary Senior Lecturer in Medicine
Department of Infection and Tropical Medicine
Hull and East Yorkshire Hospitals NHS Trust
Castle Hill Hospital
Cottingham, East Riding of Yorkshire, UK

Johan W. Mouton, MD PhD
Consultant-Medical Microbiologist
Department Medical Microbiology and
    Infectious Diseases
Canisius Wilhelmina Hospital and Department
    of Microbiology
Radboud University
Nijmegen Medical Centre
Nijmegen, The Netherlands

**Dilip Nathwani, MB DTM&H FRCP
(Edin, Glas, Lond)**
Consultant Physician and Honorary Professor
    of Infection
Infection Unit
Ninewells Hospital and Medical School
University of Dundee
Dundee, UK

S. Ragnar Norrby, MD PhD FRCP
Professor
The Swedish Institute for Infectious
    Disease Control
Stockholm, Sweden

Anna Norrby-Teglund, PhD
Professor of Medical Microbial Pathogenesis
Karolinska Institute
Center for Infectious Medicine,
Karolinska University Hospital Huddinge
Stockholm, Sweden

**Tim O'Dempsey, MB ChB FRCP DObS DCH
DTCH DTM&H**
Senior Lecturer in Clinical Tropical Medicine
Liverpool School of Tropical Medicine
Pembroke Place
Liverpool, UK

**L. Peter Ormerod, BSc(Hons) MBChB(Hons)
MD DSc(Med) FRCP**
Consultant Respiratory and General Physician
Professor of Respiratory Medicine
Chest Clinic
Blackburn Royal Infirmary
Lancashire, UK

Peter G. Pappas, MD FACP
Professor of Medicine
Principal Investigator, Mycoses Study Group
Division of Infectious Diseases
University of Alabama at Birmingham
Birmingham, Alabama, USA

Francesco Parenti, PhD
Director
Newron Pharmaceuticals
Bresso, Italy

Rüdiger Pittrof, MRCOG
Specialist Registrar
St George's Hospital
London, UK

Anton Pozniak, MD FRCP
Consultant Physician and Director of HIV Services;
Executive Director of HIV Research
Department of HIV and Genitourinary Medicine
Chelsea and Westminster Hospital
London, UK

Parisa Ravanfar, MD
Clinical Research Fellow
Center for Clinical Studies
Webster, USA

Robert C. Read
Professor of Infectious Diseases
University of Sheffield Medical School
Sheffield, UK

David S. Reeves, MD FRCPath
Honorary Consultant Medical Microbiologist
North Bristol NHS Trust
Honorary Professor of Medical Microbiology
University of Bristol
Bristol, UK

Una Ni Riain, FRCPath
Consultant Medical Microbiologist
Department of Medical Microbiology
University College Hospital
Galway, Ireland

Kristian Riesbeck, MD PhD
Professor of Clinical Bacteriology
Head, Department of Laboratory Medicine
Medical Microbiology, Lund University
Malmö University Hospital
Malmö, Sweden

Keith A. Rodvold, PharmD FCCP FIDSA
Professor of Pharmacy Practice and
    Medicine
Colleges of Pharmacy and Medicine
University of Illinois at Chicago
Chicago, USA

Hector Rodriguez-Villalobos, MD
Clinical Microbiologist
Laboratory of Medical Microbiology
Erasme University Hospital
Universite Libre de Bruxelles
Brussels, Belgium

Ethan Rubinstein, MD LLb
Sellers Professor and Head
Section of Infectious Diseases
Faculty of Medicine
University of Manitoba
Winnipeg, Canada

Anita K. Satyaprakash, MD
Clinical Research Fellow
Center for Clinical Studies
Webster, USA

W. Michael Scheld, MD
Bayer-Gerald L Mandell Professor of Infectious
    Diseases
Professor of Neurosurgery
Director, Pfizer Initiative in International
    Health
University of Virginia Health System
Charlottesville, USA

**David V. Seal, MD FRCOphth FRCPath MIBiol
Dip Bact**
Retired Medical Microbiologist
Anzère, Switzerland

Paula S. Seal, MD MPH
Fellow
Department of Infectious Diseases
The University of Alabama at Birmingham
Birmingham, Alabama, USA

Karin Seifert, Mag. pharm. Dr.rer.nat
Lecturer
Department of Infectious and Tropical Diseases
London School of Hygiene and Tropical
    Medicine
London, UK

Francisco Soriano, MD PhD
Professor of Medical Microbiology
Department of Medical Microbiology and
    Antimicrobial Chemotherapy
Fundacion Jiminez Diaz-Capio
Madrid, Spain

Stephen J. Streat, BSc MB ChB FRACP
Special Intensivist, Department
    of Critical Care Medicine, Auckland
    City Hospital
Clinical Associate Professor
Department of Surgery
University of Auckland
Auckland, New Zealand

Marc J. Struelens, MD PhD FSHEA
Professor of Clinical Microbiology
Head, Department of Microbiology
Erasme University Hospital
Universite Libre de Bruxelles
Brussels, Belgium

Lars Sundström, PhD
Associate Professor in Microbiology
Department of Medical Biochemistry and
    Microbiology
IMBIM, Uppsala University
Uppsala, Sweden

Göte Swedberg, PhD
Associate Professor in Microbiology
Department of Medical Biochemistry and
    Microbiology
Biomedical Centre, Uppsala University
Uppsala, Sweden

Jeffrey Tessier, MD FACP
Assistant Professor of Research
Division of Infectious Diseases and International
    Health
University of Virginia
Charlottesville, USA

Howard C. Thomas, BSc MB BS PhD
FRCP(Lond & Glas) FRCPath FMedSci
Professor of Medicine
Department of Medicine
Imperial College School of Medicine
St Mary's Hospital
London, UK

Mark G. Thomas, MBChB MD FRACP
Associate Professor in Infectious Diseases
Department of Molecular Medicine and
    Pathology
Faculty of Medical and Health Sciences
The University of Auckland
Auckland, New Zealand

Carl Johan Treutiger, MD PhD
Consultant in Infectious Diseases
Department of Infectious Diseases
Karolinska University Hospital, Huddinge
Stockholm, Sweden

Stephen K. Tyring, MD PhD
Medical Director, Center for Clinical Studies
Professor of Dermatology, Microbiology/
    Molecular Genetics and Internal
    Medicine
Department of Dermatology
University of Texas Health Science Center
Houston, USA

David Wareham, MB BS MSc PhD MRCP
FRCPath
Senior Clinical Lecturer (Honorary Consultant)
    in Microbiology
Queen Mary University London
Centre for Infectious Disease
London, UK

David W. Warnock, PhD
Director, Division of Foodborne, Bacterial and
    Mycotic Diseases
National Center for Zoonotic, Vector-borne
    and Enteric Diseases
Centers for Disease Control and Prevention
Atlanta, USA

Emmanuel Wey, MB BS MRCPCH MSc
DLSHTM
Specialist Registrar Microbiology and Virology
Royal Free Hospital NHS Trust
London, UK

Nicholas J. White, OBE DSc MD FRCP
FMedSci FRS
Professor of Tropical Medicine, Mahidol
    University and Oxford University
Faculty of Tropical Medicine
Mahidol University
Bangkok, Thailand

Richard J. Whitley, MD
Distinguished Professor Loeb Scholar in Pediatrics
Professor of Pediatrics, Microbiology, Medicine
    and Neurosurgery
The University of Alabama at Birmingham
Birmingham, Alabama, USA

Mark H. Wilcox, BMedSci BM BS MD FRCPath
Consultant/Clinical Director of Microbiology/
    Pathology
Professor of Medical Microbiology
University of Leeds
Department of Microbiology
Old Medical School
Leeds General Infirmary
Leeds, UK

Peng Wong, MB ChB MD MRCS
Surgical Specialist Registrar
Sunderland Royal Hospital
Billingham
Cleveland, UK

Neil Woodford, BSc PhD FRCPath
Consultant Clinical Scientist
Antibiotic Resistance Monitoring & Reference
    Laboratory
Health Protection Agency – Centre for Infections
London, UK

Werner Zimmerli, MD
Professor of Internal Medicine and Infectious
    Diseases
Medical University Clinic
Kantonsspital
Liestal, Switzerland

General aspects

1 Historical introduction

David Greenwood

The first part of this chapter was written by Professor Lawrence Paul Garrod (1895–1979), co-author of the first five editions of *Antibiotic and Chemotherapy*. Garrod, after serving as a surgeon probationer in the Navy during the 1914–18 war, then qualified and practiced clinical medicine before specializing in bacteriology, later achieving world recognition as the foremost authority on antimicrobial chemotherapy. He witnessed, and studied profoundly, the whole development of modern chemotherapy. A selection of over 300 leading articles written by him (but published anonymously) for the *British Medical Journal* between 1933 and 1979, was reprinted in a supplement to the *Journal of Antimicrobial Chemotherapy* in 1985.* These articles themselves provide a remarkable insight into the history of antimicrobial chemotherapy as it happened.

Garrod's original historical introduction was written in 1968 for the second edition of *Antibiotic and Chemotherapy* and updated for the fifth edition just before his death in 1979. It is reproduced here as a tribute to his memory. The development of antimicrobial chemotherapy is summarized so well, and with such characteristic lucidity, that to add anything seems superfluous, but a brief summary of events that have occurred since about 1975 has been added to complete the historical perspective.

THE EVOLUTION OF ANTIMICROBIC DRUGS

No one recently qualified, even with the liveliest imagination, can picture the ravages of bacterial infection which continued until rather less than 40 years ago. To take only two examples, lobar pneumonia was a common cause of death even in young and vigorous patients, and puerperal septicaemia and other forms of acute streptococcal sepsis had a high mortality, little affected by any treatment then available. One purpose of this introduction is therefore to place the subject of this book in historical perspective.

This subject is chemotherapy, which may be defined as the administration of a substance with a systemic antimicrobic action. Some would confine the term to synthetic drugs, and the distinction is recognized in the title of this book, but since some all-embracing term is needed, this one might with advantage be understood also to include substances of natural origin. Several antibiotics can now be synthesized, and it would be ludicrous if their use should qualify for description as chemotherapy only because they happened to be prepared in this way. The essence of the term is that the effect must be systemic, the substance being absorbed, whether from the alimentary tract or a site of injection, and reaching the infected area by way of the blood stream. 'Local chemotherapy' is in this sense a contradiction in terms: any application to a surface, even of something capable of exerting a systemic effect, is better described as antisepsis.

THE THREE ERAS OF CHEMOTHERAPY

There are three distinct periods in the history of this subject. In the first, which is of great antiquity, the only substances capable of curing an infection by systemic action were natural plant products. The second was the era of synthesis, and in the third we return to natural plant products, although from plants of a much lower order; the moulds and bacteria forming antibiotics.

1. Alkaloids. This era may be dated from 1619, since it is from this year that the first record is derived of the successful treatment of malaria with an extract of cinchona bark, the patient being the wife of the Spanish governor of Peru.† Another South American discovery was the efficacy of ipecacuanha root in amoebic dysentery. Until the early years of this century these extracts, and in more recent times the alkaloids, quinine and emetine, derived from them, provided the only curative chemotherapy known.

---

*Waterworth PM (ed.) L.P. Garrod on antibiotics. *Journal of Antimicrobial Chemotherapy* 1985; 15 (Suppl. B)

† Garrod was mistaken in perpetuating this legend, which is now discounted by medical historians.

2. Synthetic compounds. Therapeutic progress in this field, which initially and for many years after was due almost entirely to research in Germany, dates from the discovery of salvarsan by Ehrlich in 1909. His successors produced germanin for trypanosomiasis and other drugs effective in protozoal infections. A common view at that time was that protozoa were susceptible to chemotherapeutic attack, but that bacteria were not: the treponemata, which had been shown to be susceptible to organic arsenicals, are no ordinary bacteria, and were regarded as a class apart.

The belief that bacteria are by nature insusceptible to any drug which is not also prohibitively toxic to the human body was finally destroyed by the discovery of Prontosil. This, the forerunner of the sulphonamides, was again a product of German research, and its discovery was publicly announced in 1935. All the work with which this book is concerned is subsequent to this year: it saw the beginning of the effective treatment of bacterial infections.

Progress in the synthesis of antimicrobic drugs has continued to the present day. Apart from many new sulphonamides, perhaps the most notable additions have been the synthetic compounds used in the treatment of tuberculosis.

3. Antibiotics. The therapeutic revolution produced by the sulphonamides, which included the conquest of haemolytic streptococcal and pneumococcal infections and of gonorrhoea and cerebrospinal fever, was still in progress and even causing some bewilderment when the first report appeared of a study which was to have even wider consequences. This was not the discovery of penicillin – that had been made by Fleming in 1929 – but the demonstration by Florey and his colleagues that it was a chemotherapeutic agent of unexampled potency. The first announcement of this, made in 1940, was the beginning of the antibiotic era, and the unimagined developments from it are still in progress. We little knew at the time that penicillin, besides providing a remedy for infections insusceptible to sulphonamide treatment, was also a necessary second line of defence against those fully susceptible to it. During the early 1940s, resistance to sulphonamides appeared successively in gonococci, haemolytic streptococci and pneumococci: nearly 20 years later it has appeared also in meningococci. But for the advent of the antibiotics, all the benefits stemming from Domagk's discovery might by now have been lost, and bacterial infections have regained their pre-1935 prevalence and mortality.

The earlier history of two of these discoveries calls for further description.

SULPHONAMIDES

Prontosil, or sulphonamido-chrysoidin, was first synthesized by Klarer and Mietzsch in 1932, and was one of a series of azo dyes examined by Domagk for possible effects on haemolytic streptococcal infection. When a curative effect in mice had been demonstrated, cautious trials in erysipelas and other human infections were undertaken, and not until the evidence afforded by these was conclusive did the discoverers make their announcement. Domagk (1935) published the original claims, and the same information was communicated by Hörlein (1935) to a notable meeting in London.‡

These claims, which initially concerned only the treatment of haemolytic streptococcal infections, were soon confirmed in other countries, and one of the most notable early studies was that of Colebrook and Kenny (1936) in England, who demonstrated the efficacy of the drug in puerperal fever. This infection had until then been taking a steady toll of about 1000 young lives per annum in England and Wales, despite every effort to prevent it by hygiene measures and futile efforts to overcome it by serotherapy. The immediate effect of the adoption of this treatment can be seen in Figure 1.1: a steep fall in mortality began in 1935, and continued as the treatment became universal and better understood, and as more potent sulphonamides were introduced, until the present-day low level had almost been reached *before penicillin became generally available.* The effect of penicillin between 1945 and 1950 is perhaps more evident on incidence: its widespread use tends completely to banish haemolytic streptococci from the environment. The apparent rise in incidence after 1950 is due to the redefinition of puerperal pyrexia as any rise of temperature to 38°C, whereas previously the term was only applied when the temperature was maintained for 24 h or recurred. Needless to say, fever so defined is frequently not of uterine origin.

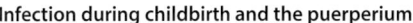

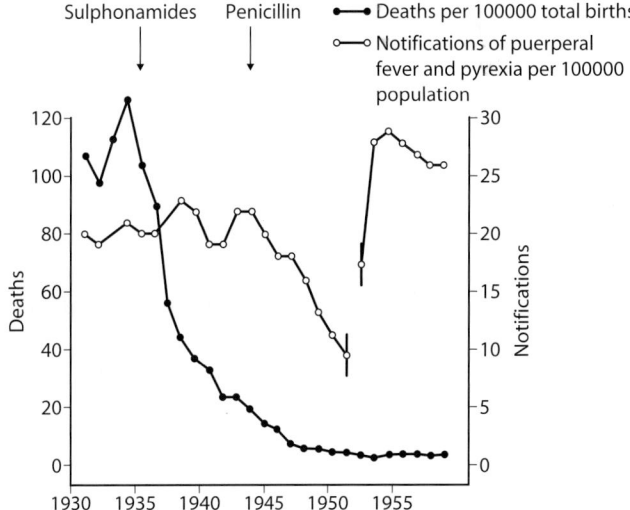

Fig. 1.1 Puerperal pyrexia. Deaths per 100 000 total births and incidence per 100 000 population in England and Wales, 1930–1957. N.B. The apparent rise in incidence in 1950 is due to the fact that the definition of puerperal pyrexia was changed in this year (*see text*). (Reproduced with permission from Barber 1960 *Journal of Obstetrics and Gynaecology* 67:727 by kind permission of the editor.)

---

‡ A meeting at which Garrod was present.

Prontosil had no antibacterial action in vitro, and it was soon suggested by workers in Paris (Tréfouël et al 1935) that it owed its activity to the liberation from it in the body of *p*-aminobenzene sulphonamide (sulphanilamide); that this compound is so formed was subsequently proved by Fuller (1937). Sulphanilamide had a demonstrable inhibitory action on streptococci in vitro, much dependent on the medium and particularly on the size of the inoculum, facts which are readily understandable in the light of modern knowledge. This explanation of the therapeutic action of Prontosil was hotly contested by Domagk. It must be remembered that it relegated the chrysoidin component to an inert role, whereas the affinity of dyes for bacteria had been a basis of German research since the time of Ehrlich, and was the doctrine underlying the choice of this series of compounds for examination. German workers also took the attitude that there must be something mysterious about the action of a true chemotherapeutic agent: an effect easily demonstrable in a test tube by any tyro was too banal altogether to explain it. Finally, they felt justifiable resentment that sulphanilamide, as a compound which had been described many years earlier, could be freely manufactured by anyone.

Every enterprising pharmaceutical house in the world was soon making this drug, and at one time it was on the market under at least 70 different proprietary names. What was more important, chemists were soon busy modifying the molecule to improve its performance. Early advances so secured were of two kinds, the first being higher activity against a wider range of bacteria: sulphapyridine (M and B 693), discovered in 1938, was the greatest single advance, since it was the first drug to be effective in pneumococcal pneumonia. The next stage, the introduction of sulphathiazole and sulphadiazine, while retaining and enhancing antibacterial activity, eliminated the frequent nausea and cyanosis caused by earlier drugs. Further developments, mainly in the direction of altered pharmacokinetic properties, have continued to the present day and are described in Chapter 1 (*now Ch. 29*).

ANTIBIOTICS

'Out of the earth shall come thy salvation.' – S.A. Waksman

 ## DEFINITION

Of many definitions of the term antibiotic which have been proposed, the narrower seem preferable. It is true that the word 'antibiosis' was coined by Vuillemin in 1889 to denote antagonism between living creatures in general, but the noun 'antibiotic' was first used by Waksman in 1942 (Waksman & Lechevalier 1962), which gives him a right to re-define it, and definition confines it to substances produced by

micro-organisms antagonistic to the growth or life of others in high dilution (the last clause being necessary to exclude such metabolic products as organic acids, hydrogen peroxide and alcohol). To define an antibiotic simply as an antibacterial substance from a living source would embrace gastric juice, antibodies and lysozyme from man, essential oils and alkaloids from plants, and such oddities as the substance in the faeces of blowfly larvae which exerts an antiseptic effect in wounds. All substances known as antibiotics which are in clinical use and capable of exerting systemic effect are in fact products of micro-organisms.

 ## EARLY HISTORY

The study of intermicrobic antagonism is almost as old as microbiology itself: several instances of it were described, one by Pasteur himself, in the seventies of the last century.[§] Therapeutic applications followed, some employing actual living cultures, others extracts of bacteria or moulds which had been found active. One of the best known products was an extract of *Pseudomonas aeruginosa*, first used as a local application by Czech workers, Honl and Bukovsky, in 1899: this was commercially available as 'pyocyanase' on the continent for many years. Other investigators used extracts of species of *Penicillium* and *Aspergillus* which probably or certainly contained antibiotics, but in too low a concentration to exert more than a local and transient effect. Florey (1945) gave a revealing account of these early developments in a lecture with the intriguing title 'The Use of Micro-organisms as Therapeutic Agents': this was amplified in a later publication (Florey 1949).

The systemic search, by an ingenious method, for an organism which could attack pyogenic cocci, conducted by Dubos (1939) in New York, led to the discovery of tyrothricin (gramicidin + tyrocidine), formed by *Bacillus brevis*, a substance which, although too toxic for systemic use in man, had in fact a systemic curative effect in mice. This work exerted a strong influence in inducing Florey and his colleagues to embark on a study of naturally formed antibacterial substances, and penicillin was the second on their list.

 ## PENICILLIN

The present antibiotic era may be said to date from 1940, when the first account of the properties of an extract of cultures of *Penicillium notatum* appeared from Oxford (Chain et al 1940): a fuller account followed, with impressive clinical evidence (Abraham et al 1941). It had been necessary to find means of extracting a very labile substance from culture fluids, to examine its action on a wide range of bacteria, to examine its toxicity by a variety of methods, to establish a unit of its activity, to study its distribution and excretion when

---

[§] i.e. the nineteenth century.

administered to animals, and finally to prove its systemic efficacy in mouse infections. There then remained the gigantic task, seemingly impossible except on a factory scale, of producing in the School of Pathology at Oxford enough of a substance, which was known to be excreted with unexampled rapidity, for the treatment of human disease. One means of maintaining supplies was extraction from the patients' urine and re-administration.

It was several years before penicillin was fully purified, its structure ascertained, and its large-scale commercial production achieved. That this was of necessity first entrusted to manufacturers in the USA gave them a lead in a highly profitable industry which was not to be overtaken for many years.

 ## LATER ANTIBIOTICS

The dates of discovery and sources of the principal antibiotics are given chronologically in Table 1.1. This is far from being a complete list, but subsequently discovered antibiotics have been closely related to others already known, such as aminoglycosides and macrolides. A few, including penicillin, were chance discoveries, but 'stretching out suppliant Petri dishes' (Florey 1945) in the hope of catching a new antibiotic-producing organism was not to lead anywhere. Most further discoveries resulted from soil surveys, a process from which a large annual outlay might or might not be repaid a hundred-fold, a gamble against much longer odds than most oil prospecting. Soil contains a profuse and very mixed flora varying with climate, vegetation, mineral content and other factors, and is a medium in which antibiotic formation may well play a part in the competition for nutriment. A soil survey consists of obtaining samples from as many and as varied sources as possible, cultivating them on plates, subcultivating all colonies of promising organisms such as actinomycetes and examining each for antibacterial activity. Alternatively, the primary plate culture may be inoculated by spraying or by agar layering with suitable bacteria, the growth of which may then be seen to be inhibited in a zone surrounding some of the original colonies. This is only a beginning: many thousands of successive colonies so examined are found to form an antibiotic already known or useless by reason of toxicity.

Antibiotics have been derived from some odd sources other than soil. Although the original strain of *P. notatum* apparently floated into Fleming's laboratory at St. Mary's from one on another floor of the building in which moulds were being studied, that of *Penicillium chrysogenum* now used for penicillin production was derived from a mouldy Canteloupe melon in the market at Peoria, Illinois. Perhaps the strangest derivation was that of helenine, an antibiotic with some antiviral activity, isolated by Shope (1953) from *Penicillium funiculosum* growing on 'the isinglass cover of a photograph of my wife, Helen, on Guam, near the end of the war in 1945'.

Table 1.1 Date of discovery and source of natural antibiotics

Name	Date of discovery	Microbe
Penicillin	1929–40	*Penicillium notatum*
Tyrothricin {Gramicidin / Tyrocidine}	1939	*Bacillus brevis*
Griseofulvin	1939	*Penicillium griseofulvum Dierckx*
	1945	*Penicillium janczewski*
Streptomycin	1944	*Streptomyces griseus*
Bacitracin	1945	*Bacillus licheniformis*
Chloramphenicol	1947	*Streptomyces venezuelae*
Polymyxin	1947	*Bacillus polymyxa*
Framycetin	1947–53	*Streptomyces lavendulae*
Chlortetracycline	1948	*Streptomyces aureofaciens*
Cephalosporin C, N and P	1948	*Cephalosporium* sp.
Neomycin	1949	*Streptomyces fradiae*
Oxytetracycline	1950	*Streptomyces rimosus*
Nystatin	1950	*Streptomyces noursei*
Erythromycin	1952	*Streptomyces erythreus*
Oleandomycin	1954	*Streptomyces antibioticus*
Spiramycin	1954	*Streptomyces ambofaciens*
Novobiocin	1955	*Streptomyces spheroides Streptomyces niveus*
Cycloserine	1955	*Streptomyces orchidaceus Streptomyces gaeryphalus*
Vancomycin	1956	*Streptomyces orientalis*
Rifamycin	1957	*Streptomyces mediterranei*
Kanamycin	1957	*Streptomyces kanamyceticus*
Nebramycins	1958	*Streptomyces tenebraeus*
Paromomycin	1959	*Streptomyces rimosus*
Fusidic acid	1960	*Fusidium coccineum*
Spectinomycin	1961–62	*Streptomyces flavopersicus*
Lincomycin	1962	*Streptomyces lincolnensis*
Gentamicin	1963	*Micromonospora purpurea*
Josamycin	1964	*Streptomyces narvonensis* var. *josamyceticus*
Tobramycin	1968	*Streptomyces tenebraeus*
Ribostamycin	1970	*Streptomyces ribosidificus*
Butirosin	1970	*Bacillus circulans*
Sissomicin	1970	*Micromonospora myosensis*
Rosaramicin	1972	*Micromonospora rosaria*

He proceeds to explain that he chose the name because it was non-descriptive, non-committal and not pre-empted, 'but largely out of recognition of the good taste shown by the mould … in locating on the picture of my wife'.

Those antibiotics out of thousands now discovered which have qualified for therapeutic use are described in chapters which follow.

FUTURE PROSPECTS

All successful chemotherapeutic agents have certain properties in common. They must exert an antimicrobic action, whether inhibitory or lethal, in high dilution, and in the complex chemical environment which they encounter in the body. Secondly, since they are brought into contact with every tissue in the body, they must so far as possible be without harmful effect on the function of any organ. To these two essential qualities may be added others which are highly desirable, although sometimes lacking in useful drugs: stability, free solubility, a slow rate of excretion, and diffusibility into remote areas.

If a drug is toxic to bacteria but not to mammalian cells the probability is that it interferes with some structure or function peculiar to bacteria. When the mode of action of sulphanilamide was elucidated by Woods and Fildes, and the theory was put forward of bacterial inhibition by metabolite analogues, the way seemed open for devising further antibacterial drugs on a rational basis. Immense subsequent advances in knowledge of the anatomy, chemical composition and metabolism of the bacterial cell should have encouraged such hopes still further. This new knowledge has been helpful in explaining what drugs do to bacteria, but not in devising new ones. Discoveries have continued to result only from random trials, purely empirical in the antibiotic field, although sometimes based on reasonable theoretical expectation in the synthetic.

Not only is the action of any new drug on individual bacteria still unpredictable on a theoretical basis, but so are its effects on the body itself. Most of the toxic effects of antibiotics have come to light only after extensive use, and even now no one can explain their affinity for some of the organs attacked. Some new observations in this field have contributed something to the present climate of suspicion about new drugs generally, which is insisting on far more searching tests of toxicity, and delaying the release of drugs for therapeutic use, particularly in the USA.

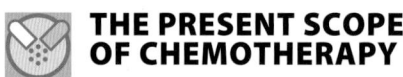

THE PRESENT SCOPE OF CHEMOTHERAPY

Successive discoveries have added to the list of infections amenable to chemotherapy until nothing remains altogether untouched except the viruses. On the other hand, however, some of the drugs which it is necessary to use are far from ideal, whether because of toxicity or of unsatisfactory pharmacokinetic properties, and some forms of treatment are consequently less often successful than others. Moreover, microbic resistance is a constant threat to the future usefulness of almost any drug. It seems unlikely that any totally new antibiotic remains to be discovered, since those of recent origin have similar properties to others already known. It therefore will be wise to husband our resources, and employ them in such a way as to preserve them. The problems of drug resistance and policies for preventing it are discussed in Chapters 13 and 14.

ADAPTATION OF EXISTING DRUGS

A line of advance other than the discovery of new drugs is the adaptation of old ones. An outstanding example of what can be achieved in this way is presented by the sulphonamides. Similar attention has naturally been directed to the antibiotics, with fruitful results of two different kinds. One is simply an alteration for the better in pharmacokinetic properties. Thus procaine penicillin, because less soluble, is longer acting than potassium penicillin; the esterification of macrolides improves absorption; chloramphenicol palmitate is palatable, and other variants so produced are more stable, more soluble and less irritant. Secondly, synthetic modification may also enhance antimicrobic properties. Sometimes both types of change can be achieved together; thus rifampicin is not only well absorbed after oral administration, whereas rifamycin, from which it is derived, is not, but antibacterially much more active. The most varied achievements of these kinds have been among the penicillins, overcoming to varying degrees three defects in benzylpenicillin: its susceptibility to destruction by gastric acid and by staphylococcal penicillinase, and the relative insusceptibility to it of many species of Gram-negative bacilli. Similar developments have provided many new derivatives of cephalosporin C, although the majority differ from their prototypes much less than the penicillins.

One effect of these developments, of which it may seem captious to complain, is that a quite bewildering variety of products is now available for the same purposes. There are still many sulphonamides, about 10 tetracyclines, more than 20 semisynthetic penicillins, and a rapidly extending list of cephalosporins, and a confident choice between them for any given purpose is one which few prescribers are qualified to make – indeed no one may be, since there is often no significant difference between the effects to be expected. Manufacturers whose costly research laboratories have produced some new derivative with a marginal advantage over others are entitled to make the most of their discovery. But if an antibiotic in a new form has a substantial advantage over that from which it was derived and no countervailing disadvantages, could not its predecessor sometimes simply be dropped? This rarely seems to happen, and there are doubtless good reasons for it, but the only foreseeable opportunity for simplifying the pre-scriber's choice has thus been missed.

 ## References

Abraham EP, Chain E, Fletcher CM, et al. *Lancet*. 1941;ii:177–189.

Chain E, Florey HW, Gardner AD, et al. *Lancet*. 1940;ii:226–228.

Colebrook L, Kenny M. *Lancet*. 1936;i:1279–1286.

Domagk G. *Dtsch Med Wochenschr*. 1935;61:250–253.

Dubos RJ. *J Exp Med*. 1939;70:1–10.

Florey HW. *Br Med J*. 1945;2:635–642.

Florey HW. *Antibiotics*. London: Oxford University Press; 1949 [chapter 1].

Fuller AT. *Lancet*. 1937;i:194–198.

Honl J, Bukovsky J. *Zentralbl Bakteriol Parasitenkd Infektionskr Hyg*. Abteilung. 1899;126:305 [see Florey 1949].

Hörlein H. *Proc R Soc Med*. 1935;29:313–324.

Shope RE. *J Exp Med*. 1953;97:601–626.

Tréfouël J, Tréfouël J, Nitti F, Bovet D. *C R Séances Soc Biol Fil (Paris)*. 1935;120:756–758.

Waksman SA, Lechevalier HA. In: *The Actinomycetes*. Vol 3. London: Baillière; 1962.

LATER DEVELOPMENTS IN ANTIMICROBIAL CHEMOTHERAPY

ANTIBACTERIAL AGENTS

At the time of Garrod's death, penicillins and cephalosporins were still in the ascendancy: apart from the aminoglycoside, amikacin, the latest advances in antimicrobial therapy to reach the formulary in the late 1970s were the antipseudomonal penicillins, azlocillin, mezlocillin and piperacillin, the amidi-nopenicillin mecillinam (amdinocillin), and the β-lactamase-stable cephalosporins cefuroxime and cefoxitin. The latter compounds emerged in response to the growing importance of enterobacterial β-lactamases, which were the subject of intense scrutiny around this time. Discovery of other novel, enzyme-resistant, β-lactam molecules elaborated by micro-organisms, including clavams, carbapenems and monobactams (*see* Ch. 15) were to follow, reminding us that Mother Nature still has some antimicrobial surprises up her copious sleeves.

The appearance of cefuroxime (first described in 1976) was soon followed by the synthesis of cefotaxime, a meth-oximino-cephalosporin that was not only β-lactamase stable but also exhibited a vast improvement in intrinsic activity. This compound stimulated a wave of commercial interest in cephalosporins with similar properties, and the early 1980s were dominated by the appearance of several variations on the cefotaxime theme (ceftizoxime, ceftriaxone, cefmenoxime, ceftazidime and the oxa-cephem, latamoxef). Although they have not been equally successful, these compounds argu-ably represent the high point in a continuing development of cephalosporins from 1964, when cephaloridine and cephalo-thin were first introduced.

The dominance of the cephalosporins among β-lactam agents began to decline in the late 1980s as novel derivatives such as the monobactam aztreonam and the carbapenem imi-penem came on stream. The contrasting properties of these two compounds reflected a still unresolved debate about the relative merits of narrow-spectrum targeted therapy and ultra-broad spectrum cover. Meanwhile, research emphasis among β-lactam antibiotics turned to the development of orally absorbed cephalosporins that exhibited the favorable properties of the expanded-spectrum parenteral compounds; formulations that sought to emulate the successful combina-tion of amoxicillin with the β-lactamase inhibitor, clavulanic acid; and variations on the carbapenem theme pioneered by imipenem.

Interest in most other antimicrobial drug families lan-guished during the 1970s. Among the aminoglycosides the search for new derivatives petered out in most countries after the development of netilmicin in 1976. However, in Japan, where amikacin was first synthesized in 1972 in response to concerns about aminoglycoside resistance, several novel aminoglycosides that are not exploited elsewhere appeared on the market. A number of macrolides with rather undistin-guished properties also appeared during the 1980s in Japan and some other countries, but not in the UK or the USA. Wider interest in new macrolides had to await the emergence of compounds that claimed pharmacological advantages over erythromycin (*see* Ch. 22); two, azithromycin and clarithro-mycin, reached the UK market in 1991 and others became available elsewhere.

Quinolone antibacterial agents enjoyed a renaissance when it was realized that fluorinated, piperazine-substituted derivatives exhibited much enhanced potency and a broader spectrum of activity than earlier congeners (*see* Ch. 26). Norfloxacin, first described in 1980, was the forerunner of this revival and other fluoroquinolones quickly followed. Soon manufacturers of the new fluoroquinolones such as ciprofloxacin, enoxacin and ofloxacin began to struggle for market dominance in Europe, the USA and elsewhere, and competing claims of activity and toxicity began to circulate. The commercial appeal of the respiratory tract infection mar-ket also ensured a sustained interest in derivatives that reli-ably included the pneumococcus in their spectrum of activity. Several quinolones of this type subsequently appeared on the market, though enthusiasm has been muted to some extent by unexpected problems of serious toxicity: several were with-drawn soon after they were launched because of unacceptable adverse reactions.

As the 20th century drew to a close, investment in new antibacterial agents in the pharmaceutical houses underwent a spectacular decline. Ironically, the period coincided with a dawning awareness of the fragility of conventional resources in light of the spread of antimicrobial drug resistance. Indeed, such new drugs that have appeared on the market have arisen from concerns about the development and spread of resis-tance to traditional agents, particularly, but not exclusively, methicillin-resistant *Staphylococcus aureus*. Most have been developed by small biotech companies, often on licence from the multinational firms.

Further progress on antibacterial compounds in the 21st century has been spasmodic at best, though some compounds in trial at the time of writing, notably the glycopeptide orita-vancin and ceftobiprole, a cephalosporin with activity against methicillin-resistant *Staph. aureus,* have aroused considerable interest.

OTHER ANTIMICROBIAL AGENTS

ANTIVIRAL AGENTS

The massive intellectual and financial investment that was brought to bear in the wake of the HIV pandemic began to pay off in the last decade of the 20th century. In the late 1980s only a handful of antiviral agents was available to the prescriber, whereas about 40 are available today (*see* Chs 36 and 37). Discovery of new approaches to the attack on HIV opened the way to effective combination therapy (*see* Chs 36 and 43). In addition, new compounds for the prevention and treatment of influenza and cytomegalovirus infection emerged (*see* Ch. 37).

ANTIFUNGAL AGENTS

Many of the new antifungal drugs that appeared in the late 20th century (*see* Chs 32, 59 and 60) were variations on older themes: antifungal azoles and safer formulations of ampho-tericin B. They included useful new triazoles (fluconazole and itraconazole) that are effective when given systemically and a novel allylamine compound, terbinafine, which offers a welcome alternative to griseofulvin in recalcitrant dermato-phyte infections. Investigation of antibiotics of the echinocan-din class bore fruit in the development of caspofungin and micafungin. The emergence of *Pneumocystis jirovecii* (former-ly *Pneumocystis carinii*; long a taxonomic orphan, but now accepted as a fungus) as an important pathogen in HIV-infected persons stimulated the investigation of new therapies, leading to the introduction of trimetrexate and atovaquone for cases unresponsive to older drugs.

ANTIPARASITIC AGENTS

The most serious effects of parasitic infections are borne by the economically poor countries of the world, and research into agents for the treatment of human parasitic disease has always received low priority. Nevertheless, some use-ful new antimalarial compounds have found their way into therapeutic use. These include mefloquine and halofan-trine, which originally emerged in the early 1980s from the extensive antimalarial research program undertaken by the Walter Reed Army Institute of Research in Washington, and the hydroxynaphthoquinone, atovaquone, which is used in

antimalarial prophylaxis in combination with proguanil. Derivatives of artemisinin, the active principle of the Chinese herbal remedy qinghaosu, also became accepted as valuable additions to the antimalarial armamentarium. These devel-opments have been slow, but very welcome in view of the inexorable spread of resistance to standard antimalarial drugs in *Plasmodium falciparum*, which continues unabated (*see* Ch. 62).

There have been few noteworthy developments in the treatment of other protozoan diseases, but one, eflornithine (difluoromethylornithine), provides a long-awaited alterna-tive to arsenicals in the West African form of trypanosomia-sis. Unfortunately, long-term availability of the drug remains insecure. Although a commercial use for a topical formu-lation has emerged (for removal of unwanted facial hair), manufacture of an injectable preparation is uneconomic. For the present it remains available through a humanitarian arrangement between the manufacturer and the World Health Organization.

On the helminth front, the late 20th century witnessed a revolution in the reliability of treatment. Three agents – albendazole, praziquantel and ivermectin – emerged, which between them cover most of the important causes of human intestinal and systemic worm infections (*see* Chs 34 and 64). Most anthelmintic compounds enter the human anti-infective formulary by the veterinary route, underlying the melancholy fact that animal husbandry is of relatively greater economic importance than the well-being of the approximately 1.5 bil-lion people who harbor parasitic worms.

THE PRESENT SCOPE OF ANTIMICROBIAL CHEMOTHERAPY

Science, with a little help from Lady Luck, has provided for-midable resources for the treatment of infectious disease dur-ing the last 75 years. Given the enormous cost of development of new drugs, and the already crowded market for antimicro-bial compounds, it is not surprising that anti-infective research in the pharmaceutical houses has turned to more lucrative fields. Meanwhile, antimicrobial drug resistance continues to increase inexorably. Although most bacterial infection remains amenable to therapy with common, well-established drugs, the prospect of untreatable infection is already becoming an occasional reality, especially among seriously ill patients in high-dependency units where there is intense selective pres-sure created by widespread use of potent, broad-spectrum agents. On a global scale, multiple drug resistance in a num-ber of different organisms, including those that cause typhoid fever, tuberculosis and malaria, is an unsolved problem. These are life-threatening infections for which treatment options are limited, even when fully sensitive organisms are involved.

Garrod, surveying the scope of chemotherapy in 1968 (in the second edition of this book), warned of the threat of microbial resistance and the need to husband our resources. That threat and that need have not diminished. The challenge for the future is to preserve the precious assets that we have acquired by sensible regulation of the availability of antimicrobial drugs in countries in which controls are presently inadequate; by strict adherence to control of infection procedures in hospitals and other healthcare institutions; and by informed and cautious prescribing everywhere.

 Further information

Bud R. *Penicillin. Triumph and tragedy.* Oxford: Oxford University Press; 2007.
Greenwood D. *Antimicrobial drugs. Chronicle of a twentieth century medical triumph.* Oxford: Oxford University Press; 2008.
Lesch JE. *The first miracle drugs. How the sulfa drugs transformed medicine.* Oxford: Oxford University Press; 2007.
Wainwright M. *Miracle cure. The story of antibiotics.* Oxford: Basil Blackwell Ltd; 1990.

2 Modes of action

Ian Chopra

Selective toxicity is the central concept of antimicrobial chemotherapy, i.e. the infecting organism is killed, or its growth prevented, without damage to the host. The necessary selectivity can be achieved in several ways: targets within the pathogen may be absent from the cells of the host or, alternatively, the analogous targets within the host cells may be sufficiently different, or at least sufficiently inaccessible, for selective attack to be possible. With agents like the polymyxins, the organic arsenicals used in trypanosomiasis, the antifungal polyenes and some antiviral compounds, the gap between toxicity to the pathogen and to the host is small, but in most cases antimicrobial drugs are able to exploit fundamental differences in structure and function within the infecting organism, and host toxicity generally results from unexpected secondary effects.

ANTIBACTERIAL AGENTS

Bacteria are structurally and metabolically very different from mammalian cells and, in theory, there are numerous ways in which bacteria can be selectively killed or disabled. In the event, it turns out that only the bacterial cell wall is structurally unique; other subcellular structures, including the cytoplasmic membrane, ribosomes and DNA, are built on the same pattern as those of mammalian cells, although sufficient differences in construction and organization do exist at these sites to make exploitation of the selective toxicity principle feasible.

The most successful antibacterial agents are those that interfere with the construction of the bacterial cell wall, the synthesis of protein, or the replication and transcription of DNA. Indeed, relatively few clinically useful agents act at the level of the cell membrane, or by interfering with specific metabolic processes within the bacterial cell (Table 2.1).

Unless the target is located on the outside of the bacterial cell, antimicrobial agents must be able to penetrate to the site of action. Access through the cytoplasmic membrane is usually achieved by passive diffusion, or occasionally by active transport processes. In the case of Gram-negative organisms,

Table 2.1 Sites of action of antibacterial agents

Site	Agent	Principal target
Cell wall	Penicillins	Transpeptidase
	Cephalosporins	Transpeptidase
	Bacitracin, ramoplanin	Isoprenylphosphate
	Vancomycin, teicoplanin	Acyl-D-alanyl-D-alanine
	Telavancin	Acyl-D-alanyl-D-alanine (and the cell membrane)
	Cycloserine	Alanine racemase/ligase
	Fosfomycin	Pyruvyl transferase
	Isoniazid	Mycolic acid synthesis
	Ethambutol	Arabinosyl transferases
Ribosome	Chloramphenicol	Peptidyl transferase
	Tetracyclines	Ribosomal A site
	Aminoglycosides	Initiation complex/translation
	Macrolides	Ribosomal 50S subunit
	Lincosamides	Ribosomal A and P sites
	Fusidic acid	Elongation factor G
	Linezolid	Ribosomal A site
	Pleuromutilins	Ribosomal A site
tRNA charging	Mupirocin	Isoleucyl-tRNA synthetase
Nucleic acid	Quinolones	DNA gyrase (α subunit)/topoisomerase IV
	Novobiocin	DNA gyrase (β subunit)
	Rifampicin	RNA polymerase
	5-Nitroimidazoles	DNA strands
	Nitrofurans	DNA strands
Cell membrane	Polymyxins	Phospholipids
	Daptomycin	Phospholipids
Folate synthesis	Sulfonamides	Pteroate synthetase
	Diaminopyrimidines	Dihydrofolate reductase

the antibacterial drug must also cross the outer membrane (Figure 2.1). This contains a lipopolysaccharide-rich outer bilayer, which may prevent a drug from reaching an otherwise sensitive intracellular target. However, the outer membrane contains aqueous transmembrane channels (porins), which does allow passage of hydrophilic molecules, including drugs, depending on their molecular size and ionic charge. Many antibacterial agents use porins to gain access to Gram-negative organisms, although other pathways are also exploited.[1]

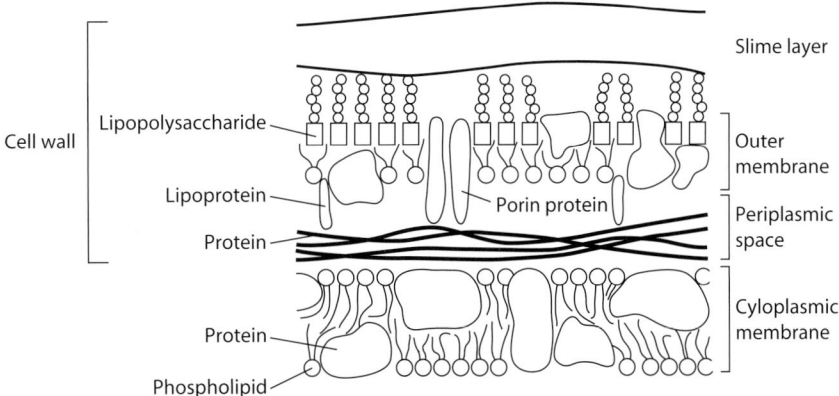

Fig. 2.1 Diagrammatic representation of the Gram-negative cell envelope. The periplasmic space contains the peptidoglycan and some enzymes. (Reproduced with permission from Russell AD, Quesnel LB (eds) *Antibiotics: assessment of antimicrobial activity and resistance. The Society for Applied Bacteriology Technical Series no. 18.* London: Academic Press; p.62, with permission of Elsevier.)

INHIBITORS OF BACTERIAL CELL WALL SYNTHESIS

Peptidoglycan forms the rigid, shape-maintaining layer of most medically important bacteria. Its structure is similar in Gram-positive and Gram-negative organisms, although there are important differences. In both types of organism the basic macromolecular chain is *N*-acetylglucosamine alternating with its lactyl ether, *N*-acetylmuramic acid. Each muramic acid unit carries a pentapeptide, the third amino acid of which is L-lysine in most Gram-positive cocci and *meso*-diaminopimelic acid in Gram-negative bacilli. The cell wall is given its rigidity by cross-links between this amino acid and the penultimate amino acid (which is always D-alanine)

of adjacent chains, with loss of the terminal amino acid (also D-alanine) (Figure 2.2). Gram-negative bacilli have a very thin peptidoglycan layer, which is loosely cross-linked; Gram-positive cocci, in contrast, possess a very thick peptidoglycan coat, which is tightly cross-linked through interpeptide bridges. The walls of Gram-positive bacteria also differ in containing considerable amounts of polymeric sugar alcohol phosphates (teichoic and teichuronic acids), while Gram-negative bacteria possess an outer membrane as described above.

A number of antibacterial agents selectively inhibit different stages in the construction of the peptidoglycan (Figure 2.3). In addition, the unusual structure of the mycobacterial cell wall is exploited by several antituberculosis agents.

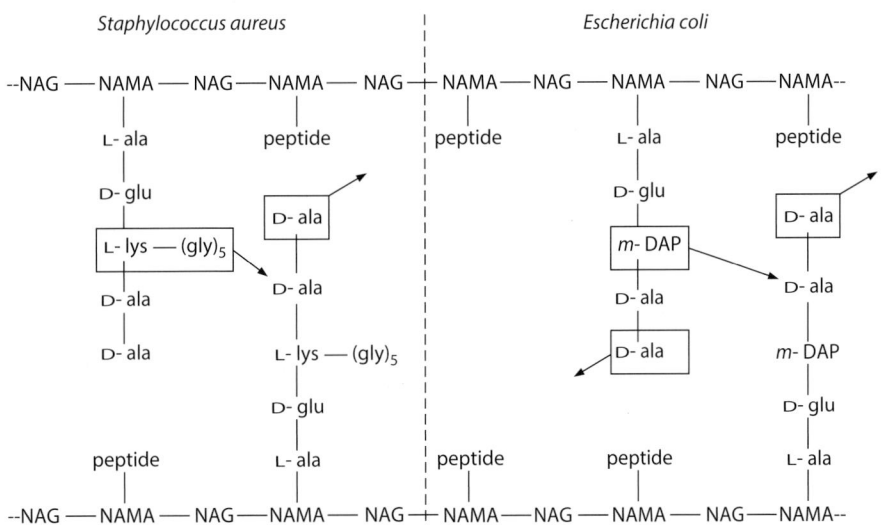

Fig. 2.2 Schematic representations of the terminal stages of cell wall synthesis in Gram-positive (*Staphylococcus aureus*) and Gram-negative (*Escherichia coli*) bacteria. See text for explanation. Arrows indicate formation of cross-links, with loss of terminal D-alanine; in Gram-negative bacilli many D-alanine residues are not involved in cross-linking and are removed by D-alanine carboxypeptidase. NAG, *N*-acetylglucosamine; NAMA, *N*-acetylmuramic acid; ala, alanine; glu, glutamic acid; lys, lysine; gly, glycine; *m*-DAP, *meso*-diaminopimelic acid.

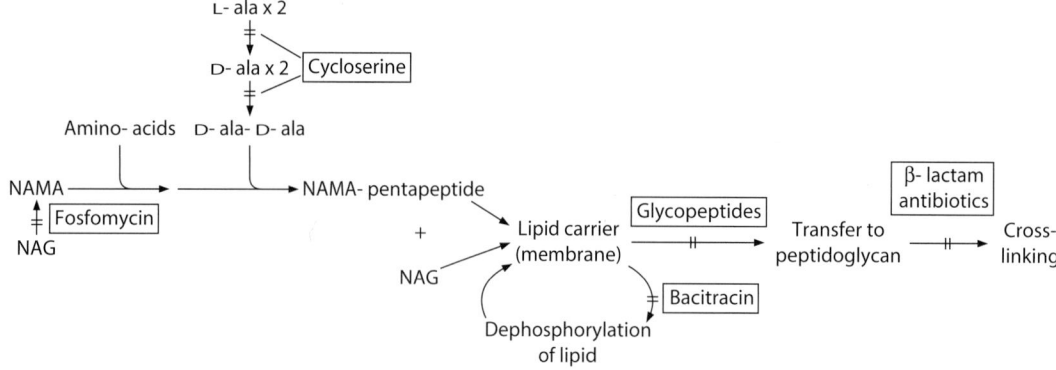

Fig. 2.3 Simplified scheme of bacterial cell wall synthesis, showing the sites of action of cell wall active antibiotics. NAG, *N*-acetylglucosamine; NAMA, *N*-acetylmuramic acid. (Reproduced with permission from Greenwood D, Ogilvie MM, Antimicrobial Agents. In: Greenwood D, Slack RCB, Peutherer JF (eds). *Medical Microbiology* 16th edn. 2002, Edinburgh: Churchill Livingstone, with permission of Elsevier.)

 ## FOSFOMYCIN

The *N*-acetylmuramic acid component of the bacterial cell wall is derived from *N*-acetylglucosamine by the addition of a lactic acid substituent derived from phosphoenolpyruvate. Fosfomycin blocks this reaction by inhibiting the pyruvyl transferase enzyme involved. The antibiotic enters bacteria by utilizing active transport mechanisms for α-glycerophosphate and glucose-6-phosphate. Glucose-6-phosphate induces the hexose phosphate transport pathway in some organisms (notably *Escherichia coli*) and potentiates the activity of fosfomycin against these bacteria.[2]

 ## CYCLOSERINE

The first three amino acids of the pentapeptide chain of muramic acid are added sequentially, but the terminal D-alanyl-D-alanine is added as a dipeptide unit (*see* Figure 2.3). To form this unit the natural form of the amino acid, L-alanine, is first racemized to D-alanine and two molecules are then joined by D-alanyl-D-alanine ligase. Both of these reactions are blocked by the antibiotic cycloserine, which is a structural analog of D-alanine.

 ## VANCOMYCIN, TEICOPLANIN AND TELAVANCIN

Once the muramylpentapeptide is formed in the cell cytoplasm, an *N*-acetylglucosamine unit is added, together with any amino acids needed for the interpeptide bridge of Gram-positive organisms. It is then passed to a lipid carrier molecule, which transfers the whole unit across the cell membrane to be added to the growing end of the peptidoglycan macromolecule (*see* Figure 2.3). Addition of the new building block (transglycosylation) is prevented by vancomycin (a glycopeptide antibiotic) and teicoplanin (a lipoglycopeptide antibiotic) which bind to the acyl-D-alanyl-D-alanine tail of the muramylpentapeptide. Telavancin (a lipoglycopeptide derivative of vancomycin) also prevents transglycosylation by binding to the acyl-D-alanyl-D-alanine tail of the muramylpentapeptide. However, telavancin appears to have an additional mechanism of action since it also increases the permeability of the cytoplasmic membrane, leading to loss of adenosine triphosphate (ATP) and potassium from the cell and membrane depolarization.[3] Because these antibiotics are large polar molecules, they cannot penetrate the outer membrane of Gram-negative organisms, which explains their restricted spectrum of activity.

 ## BACITRACIN AND RAMOPLANIN

The lipid carrier involved in transporting the cell wall building block across the membrane is a C_{55} isoprenyl phosphate. The lipid acquires an additional phosphate group in the transport process and must be dephosphorylated in order to regenerate the native compound for another round of transfer. The cyclic peptide antibiotics bacitracin and ramoplanin both bind to the C_{55} lipid carrier Bacitracin inhibits its dephosphorylation and ramoplanin prevents it from participating in transglycosylation. Consequently both antibiotics disrupt the lipid carrier cycle (*see* Figure 2.3).

 ## β-LACTAM ANTIBIOTICS

The final cross-linking reaction that gives the bacterial cell wall its characteristic rigidity was pinpointed many years ago as the primary target of penicillin and other β-lactam agents. These compounds were postulated to inhibit formation of the transpeptide bond by virtue of their structural resemblance to the terminal D-alanyl-D-alanine unit that participates in the transpeptidation reaction. This knowledge had to be reconciled with various concentration-dependent morphological responses that Gram-negative bacilli undergo on exposure to penicillin and other β-lactam compounds: filamentation (caused by inhibition of division rather than growth of the bacteria) at low concentrations, and the formation of osmotically fragile spheroplasts (peptidoglycan-deficient forms that have lost their bacillary shape) at high concentrations.

Three observations suggested that these morphological events could be dissociated:

- The oral cephalosporin cefalexin (and some other β-lactam agents, including cefradine, temocillin and the monobactam, aztreonam) causes the filamentation response alone over an extremely wide range of concentrations.
- Mecillinam (amdinocillin) does not inhibit division (and hence does not cause filamentation in Gram-negative bacilli), but has a generalized effect on the bacterial cell wall.
- Combining cefalexin and mecillinam evokes the 'typical' spheroplast response in *Esch. coli* that neither agent induces when acting alone.[4]

It was subsequently shown that isolated membranes of bacteria contain a number of proteins that bind penicillin and other β-lactam antibiotics. These penicillin-binding proteins (PBPs) are numbered in descending order of their molecular weight.[5] The number found in bacterial cells varies from species to species: *Esch. coli* has at least seven and *Staphylococcus aureus* four. β-Lactam agents that induce filamentation in Gram-negative bacilli bind to PBP 3; similarly, mecillinam binds exclusively to PBP 2. Most β-lactam antibiotics, when present in sufficient concentration, bind to both these sites and to others (PBP 1a and PBP 1b) that participate in the rapidly lytic response of Gram-negative bacilli to many penicillins and cephalosporins.

The low-molecular-weight PBPs (4, 5 and 6) of *Esch. coli* are carboxypeptidases, which may operate to control the extent of cross-linking in the cell wall. Mutants lacking these enzymes grow normally and have thus been ruled out as targets for the inhibitory or lethal actions of β-lactam antibiotics. The PBPs with higher molecular weights (PBPs 1a, 1b, 2 and 3) possess transpeptidase activity, and it seems that these PBPs represent different forms of the transpeptidase enzyme necessary to arrange the complicated architecture of the cylindrical or spherical bacterial cell during growth, septation and division.

The nature of the lethal event

The mechanism by which inhibition of penicillin-binding proteins by β-lactam agents causes bacterial lysis and death has been investigated for decades. Normal cell growth and division require the coordinated participation of both peptidoglycan synthetic enzymes and those with autolytic activity (murein, or peptidoglycan hydrolases; autolysins). To prevent widespread hydrolysis of the peptidoglycan it appears that the autolysins are normally restricted in their access to peptidoglycan. Possibly, as a secondary consequence of β-lactam action, there are changes in cell envelope structure (e.g. the

formation of protein channels in the cytoplasmic membrane) that allow autolysins to more readily reach their peptidoglycan substrate and thereby promote destruction of the cell wall.[6]

 ## ANTIMYCOBACTERIAL AGENTS

Agents acting specifically against *Mycobacterium tuberculosis* and other mycobacteria have been less well characterized than other antimicrobial drugs. Nevertheless, it is believed that several of them owe their activity to selective effects on the biosynthesis of unique components in the mycobacterial cell envelope.[7] Thus isoniazid and ethionamide inhibit mycolic acid synthesis and ethambutol prevents arabinogalactan synthesis.[8] The mode of action of pyrazinamide, a synthetic derivative of nicotinamide, is more controversial. Pyrazinamide is a prodrug which is converted into pyrazinoic acid (the active form of pyrazinamide) by mycobacterial pyrazinamidase. Some evidence suggests that pyrazinoic acid inhibits mycobacterial fatty acid synthesis,[8] whereas other data support a mode of action involving disruption of membrane energization.[9]

INHIBITORS OF BACTERIAL PROTEIN SYNTHESIS

The process by which the information encoded by DNA is translated into proteins is universal in living systems. In prokaryotic, as in eukaryotic cells, the workbench is the ribosome, composed of two distinct subunits, each a complex of ribosomal RNA (rRNA) and numerous proteins. However, bacterial ribosomes are open to selective attack by drugs because they differ from their mammalian counterparts in both protein and RNA structure. Indeed, the two types can be readily distinguished in the ultracentrifuge: bacterial ribosomes exhibit a sedimentation coefficient of 70S (composed of 30S and 50S subunits), whereas mammalian ribosomes display a coefficient of 80S (composed of 40S and 60S subunits). Nevertheless, bacterial and mitochondrial ribosomes are much more closely related and it is evident that some of the adverse side effects associated with the therapeutic use of protein synthesis inhibitors as antibacterial agents results from inhibition of mitochondrial protein synthesis.[10]

In the first stage of bacterial protein synthesis, messenger RNA (mRNA), transcribed from a structural gene, binds to the smaller ribosomal subunit and attracts *N*-formylmethionyl transfer RNA (fMet-tRNA) to the initiator codon AUG. The larger subunit is then added to form a complete initiation complex. fMet-tRNA occupies the P (peptidyl donor) site; adjacent to it is the A (aminoacyl acceptor) site aligned with the next trinucleotide codon of the mRNA. Transfer RNA (tRNA) bearing the appropriate anticodon, and its specific amino acid, enters the A site assisted by elongation factor Tu. Peptidyl transferase activity joins *N*-formylmethionine to the new amino acid with loss of the tRNA in the P site, via the exit

(E) site. The first peptide bond of the protein has therefore been formed. A translocation event, assisted by elongation factor G, then moves the remaining tRNA with its dipeptide to the P site and concomitantly aligns the next triplet codon of mRNA with the now vacant A site. The appropriate aminoacyl-tRNA enters the A site and the transfer process and subsequent translocation are repeated. In this way, the peptide chain is synthesized in precise fashion, faithful to the original DNA blueprint, until a termination codon is encountered on the mRNA that signals completion of the peptide chain and release of the protein product. The mRNA disengages from the ribosome, which dissociates into its component subunits, ready to form a new initiation complex. Within bacterial cells, many ribosomes are engaged in protein synthesis during active growth, and a single strand of mRNA may interact with many ribosomes along its length to form a polysome.

Several antibacterial agents interfere with the process of protein synthesis by binding to the ribosome (Figure 2.4). In addition, the charging of isoleucyl tRNA, i.e. one of the steps in protein synthesis preceding ribosomal involvement, is subject to inhibition by the antibiotic mupirocin. Therapeutically useful inhibitors of protein synthesis acting on the ribosome include many of the naturally occurring antibiotics, such as chloramphenicol, tetracyclines, aminoglycosides, fusidic acid, macrolides, lincosamides and streptogramins. Linezolid, a newer synthetic drug, also selectively inhibits bacterial protein synthesis by binding to the ribosome. In recent years considerable insight into the mode of action of agents that inhibit bacterial protein synthesis has been gained from structural studies on the nature of drug binding sites in the ribosome.[11–14]

 CHLORAMPHENICOL

The molecular target for chloramphenicol is the peptidyl transferase center of the ribosome located in the 50S subunit. Peptidyl transferase activity is required to link amino acids in the growing peptide chain. Consequently, chloramphenicol prevents the process of chain elongation, bringing bacterial growth to a halt. The process is reversible, and hence chloramphenicol is fundamentally a bacteristatic agent. Structural studies reveal that chloramphenicol binds exclusively to specific nucleotides within the 23S rRNA of the 50S subunit and has no direct interaction with ribosomal proteins.[11] The structural data suggest that chloramphenicol could inhibit the formation of transition state intermediates that are required for the completion of peptide bond synthesis.

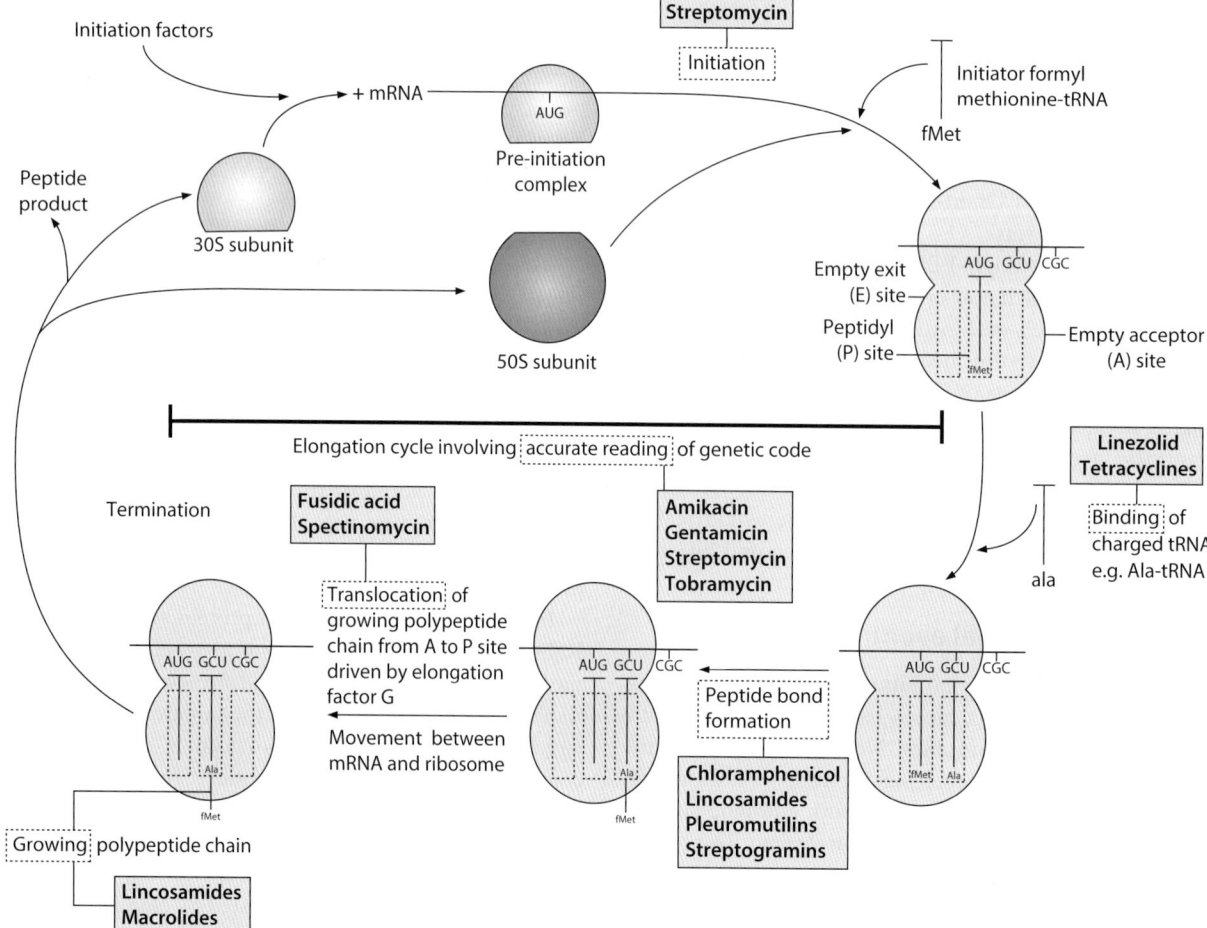

Fig. 2.4 The process of protein synthesis and the steps inhibited by various antibacterial agents.

TETRACYCLINES

Antibiotics of the tetracycline group interact with 30S ribosomal subunits and prevent the binding of incoming aminoacyl-tRNA to the A site.[12] However, this appears to occur after the initial binding of the elongation factor Tu–aminoacyl-tRNA complex to the ribosome, which is not directly affected by tetracyclines. Inhibition of A-site occupation prevents polypeptide chain elongation and, like chloramphenicol, these antibiotics are predominantly bacteristatic. Structural analysis reveals several binding sites for tetracycline in the 30S subunit which account for the ability of the antibiotic to cause physical blockage of tRNA binding in the A site.[12]

Tetracyclines also penetrate into mammalian cells (indeed, the effect on Chlamydiae depends on this) and can interfere with protein synthesis on eukaryotic ribosomes. Fortunately, cytoplasmic ribosomes are not affected at the concentrations achieved during therapy, although mitochondrial ribosomes are. The selective toxicity of tetracyclines thus presents something of a puzzle, the solution to which is presumably that these antibiotics are not actively concentrated by mitochondria as they are by bacteria, and concentrations reached are insufficient to deplete respiratory chain enzymes.[15]

AMINOGLYCOSIDES

Much of the literature on the mode of action of aminoglycosides has concentrated on streptomycin. However, the action of gentamicin and other deoxystreptamine-containing aminoglycosides is clearly not identical, since single-step, high-level resistance to streptomycin, which is due to a change in a specific protein (S12) of the 30S ribosomal subunit, does not extend to other aminoglycosides.

Elucidation of the mode of action of aminoglycosides has been complicated by the need to reconcile a variety of enigmatic observations:

- Streptomycin and other aminoglycosides cause misreading of mRNA on the ribosome while paradoxically halting protein synthesis completely by interfering with the formation of functional initiation complexes.
- Inhibition of protein synthesis by aminoglycosides leads not just to bacteristasis as with, for example, tetracycline or chloramphenicol, but also to rapid cell death.
- Susceptible bacteria (but not those with resistant ribosomes) quickly become leaky to small molecules on exposure to the drug, apparently because of an effect on the cell membrane.

A complete understanding of these phenomena has not yet been achieved, but the situation is slowly becoming clearer. The two effects of aminoglycosides on initiation and misreading may be explained by a concentration-dependent effect on ribosomes engaged in the formation of the initiation complex and those in the process of chain elongation:[16] in the presence of a sufficiently high concentration of drug, protein synthesis is completely halted once the mRNA is run off because re-initiation is blocked; under these circumstances there is little or no opportunity for misreading to occur. However, at concentrations at which only a proportion of the ribosomes can be blocked at initiation, some protein synthesis will take place and the opportunity for misreading will be provided.

The mechanism of misreading has been clarified by recent structural information on the interaction of streptomycin with the ribosome.[13] Streptomycin binds near to the A site through strong interactions with four nucleotides in 16S rRNA and one residue in protein S12. This tight binding promotes a conformational change which stabilizes the so-called *ram* state in the ribosome which reduces the fidelity of translation by allowing non-cognate aminoacyl-tRNAs to bind easily to the A site.

The effects of aminoglycosides on membrane permeability, and the potent bactericidal activity of these compounds, remain enigmatic. However, the two phenomena may be related.[17] The synthesis and subsequent insertion of misread proteins into the cytoplasmic membrane may lead to membrane leakiness and cell death.[18]

Spectinomycin

The aminocyclitol antibiotic spectinomycin, often considered alongside the aminoglycosides, binds in reversible fashion (hence the bacteristatic activity) to the 16S rRNA of the ribosomal 30S subunit. There it interrupts the translocation event that occurs as the next codon of mRNA is aligned with the A site in readiness for the incoming aminoacyl-tRNA. Structural studies reveal that the antibiotic binds to an area of the 30S subunit known as the head region which needs to move during translocation. Binding of the rigid spectinomycin molecule appears to prevent the movement required for translocation.[13]

MACROLIDES, KETOLIDES, LINCOSAMIDES, STREPTOGRAMINS

These antibiotic groups are structurally very different, but bind to closely related sites on the 50S ribosomal subunit of bacteria. One consequence of this is that a single mutation in adenine 2058 of the 23S rRNA can confer cross-resistance to macrolides, lincosamides and streptogramin B antibiotics (MLS_B resistance).

Crystallographic studies indicate that, although the binding sites for macrolides and lincosamides differ, both drug classes interact with some of the same nucleotides in 23S rRNA.[11] Neither of the drug classes binds directly to ribosomal proteins. Although streptogramin B antibiotics have not been co-crystallized with ribosomes, it is assumed that parts of their binding sites overlap with those of macrolides and lincosamides (see above). The structural studies support a model whereby macrolides block the entrance to a channel that directs nascent peptides away from the peptidyl transferase center. Lincosamides also affect the exit path of the nascent polypeptide chain but in addition disrupt the binding of aminoacyl-tRNA and peptidyl-tRNA to the ribosomal A and P sites.

The streptogramins are composed of two interacting components designated A and B. The type A molecules bind to 50S ribosomal subunits and appear, like lincosamides, to affect both the A and P sites of the peptidyl transferase center, thereby preventing peptide bond formation. Type B streptogramins occupy an adjacent site on the ribosome and also prevent formation of the peptide bond; in addition, premature release of incomplete polypeptides also occurs.[19] Type A molecules bind to free ribosomes, but not to polysomes engaged in protein synthesis, whereas type B can prevent further synthesis during active processing of the mRNA. The bactericidal synergy between the two components arises mainly from conformational changes induced by type A molecules that improve the binding affinity of type B compounds.[20]

Ketolides, such as telithromycin, which are semisynthetic derivatives of the macrolide erythromycin, appear to block the entrance to the tunnel in the large ribosomal subunit through which the nacent polypeptide exits from the ribosome.[21] However, the binding of ketolides must differ from those of the macrolides, lincosamides or streptogramin B antibiotics because the ketolides are not subject to the MLS$_B$-based resistance mechanism.[21]

PLEUROMUTILINS

Pleuromutilins such as tiamulin and valnemulin have been used for some time in veterinary medicine to treat swine infections.[22] More recently a semisynthetic pleuromutilin, retapamulin, has been introduced as a topical treatment for Gram-positive infections in humans.[23] Pleuromutilins inhibit the peptidyl transferase activity of the bacterial 50S ribosomal subunit by binding to the A site.[22,24]

FUSIDIC ACID

Fusidic acid forms a stable complex with an elongation factor (EF-G) involved in translocation and with guanosine triphosphate (GTP), which provides energy for the translocation process. One round of translocation occurs, with hydrolysis of GTP, but the fusidic acid–EF-G–GDP complex cannot dissociate from the ribosome, thereby blocking further chain elongation and leaving peptidyl-tRNA in the P site.[25]

Although protein synthesis in Gram-negative bacilli – and, indeed, mammalian cells – is susceptible to fusidic acid, the antibiotic penetrates poorly into these cells and the spectrum of action is virtually restricted to Gram-positive bacteria, notably staphylococci.[25]

LINEZOLID

Linezolid is a synthetic bacteristatic agent that inhibits bacterial protein synthesis. It was previously believed that the drug prevented the formation of 70S initiation complexes. However, more recent analysis suggests that the drug interferes with the binding, or correct positioning, of aminoacyl-tRNA in the A site.[14]

MUPIROCIN

Mupirocin has a unique mode of action. The epoxide-containing monic acid tail of the molecule is an analog of isoleucine and, as such, is a competitive inhibitor of isoleucyl-tRNA synthetase in bacterial cells.[25-27] The corresponding mammalian enzyme is unaffected.

INHIBITORS OF NUCLEIC ACID SYNTHESIS

Compounds that bind directly to the double helix are generally highly toxic to mammalian cells and only a few – those that interfere with DNA-associated enzymic processes – exhibit sufficient selectivity for systemic use as antibacterial agents. These compounds include antibacterial quinolones, novobiocin and rifampicin (rifampin). Diaminopyrimidines, sulfonamides, 5-nitroimidazoles and (probably) nitrofurans also affect DNA synthesis and will be considered under this heading.

QUINOLONES

The problem of packaging the enormous circular chromosome of bacteria (>1 mm long) into the cell requires it to be twisted into a condensed 'supercoiled' state – a process aided by the natural strain imposed on a covalently closed double helix. The twists are introduced in the opposite sense to those of the double helix itself and the molecule is said to be negatively supercoiled. During the process of DNA replication, the DNA helicase and DNA polymerase enzyme complexes introduce positive supercoils into the DNA to allow progression of the replication fork. Re-introduction of negative supercoils involves precisely regulated nicking and resealing of the DNA strands, accomplished by enzymes called topoisomerases. One topoisomerase, DNA gyrase, is a tetramer composed of two pairs of α and β subunits, and the primary target of the action of nalidixic acid and other quinolones is the α subunit of DNA gyrase, although another enzyme, topoisomerase IV, is also affected.[28] Indeed, in Gram-positive bacteria, topoisomerase IV seems to be the main target.[29] This enzyme does not have supercoiling activity; it appears to be involved in relaxation of the DNA chain and chromosomal segregation.

Although DNA gyrase and topoisomerase IV are the primary determinants of quinolone action, it is believed that the drugs bind to enzyme–DNA complexes and stabilize intermediates with double-stranded DNA cuts introduced by the enzymes. The bactericidal activity of the quinolones is believed to result from accumulation of these drug stabilized covalently cleaved intermediates which are not subject to rescue by DNA repair mechanisms in the cell.[30]

The coumarin antibiotic novobiocin acts in a complementary fashion to quinolones by binding specifically to the β subunit of DNA gyrase.[31]

RIFAMPICIN (RIFAMPIN)

Rifampicin and other compounds of the ansamycin group specifically inhibit DNA-dependent RNA polymerase; that is, they prevent the transcription of RNA species from the DNA template. Rifampicin is an extremely efficient inhibitor of the bacterial enzyme, but fortunately eukaryotic RNA polymerase is not affected. RNA polymerase consists of a core enzyme made up of four polypeptide subunits, and rifampicin specifically binds to the β subunit where it blocks initiation of RNA synthesis, but is without effect on RNA polymerase elongation complexes. The structural mechanism for inhibition of bacterial RNA polymerase by rifampicin has recently been elucidated.[32] The antibiotic binds to the β subunit in a pocket which directly blocks the path of the elongating RNA chain when it is two to three nucleotides in length. During initiation the transcription complex is particularly unstable and the binding of rifampicin promotes dissociation of short unstable RNA–DNA hybrids from the enzyme complex. The binding pocket for rifampicin, which is absent in mammalian RNA polymerases, is some 12 Å away from the active site.

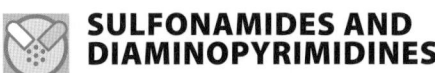

SULFONAMIDES AND DIAMINOPYRIMIDINES

These agents act at separate stages in the pathway of folic acid synthesis and thus act indirectly on DNA synthesis, since the reduced form of folic acid, tetrahydrofolic acid, serves as an essential co-factor in the synthesis of thymidylic acid.[33]

Sulfonamides are analogs of *p*-aminobenzoic acid. They competitively inhibit dihydropteroate synthetase, the enzyme that condenses *p*-aminobenzoic acid with dihydropteroic acid in the early stages of folic acid synthesis. Most bacteria need to synthesize folic acid and cannot use exogenous sources of the vitamin. Mammalian cells, in contrast, require preformed folate and this is the basis of the selective action of sulfonamides. The antileprotic sulfone dapsone, and the antituberculosis drug *p*-aminosalicylic acid, act in a similar way; the basis for their restricted spectrum may reside in differences of affinity for variant forms of dihydropteroate synthetase in the bacteria against which they act.

Diaminopyrimidines act later in the pathway of folate synthesis. These compounds inhibit dihydrofolate reductase, the enzyme that generates the active form of the co-factor tetrahydrofolic acid. In the biosynthesis of thymidylic acid, tetrahydrofolate acts as hydrogen donor as well as a methyl group carrier and is thus oxidized to dihydrofolic acid in the process. Dihydrofolate reductase is therefore crucial in recycling tetrahydrofolate, and diaminopyrimidines act relatively quickly to halt bacterial growth. Sulfonamides, in contrast, cut off the supply of folic acid at source and act slowly, since the existing folate pool can satisfy the needs of the cell for several generations.

The selective toxicity of diaminopyrimidines comes about because of differential affinity of these compounds for dihydrofolate reductase from various sources. Thus trimethoprim has a vastly greater affinity for the bacterial enzyme than for its mammalian counterpart, pyrimethamine exhibits a particularly high affinity for the plasmodial version of the enzyme and, in keeping with its anticancer activity, methotrexate has high affinity for the enzyme found in mammalian cells.

5-NITROIMIDAZOLES

The most intensively investigated compound in this group is metronidazole, but other 5-nitroimidazoles are thought to act in a similar manner. Metronidazole removes electrons from ferredoxin (or other electron transfer proteins with low redox potential) causing the nitro group of the drug to be reduced. It is this reduced and highly reactive intermediate that is responsible for the antimicrobial effect, probably by binding to DNA, which undergoes strand breakage.[34] The requirement for interaction with low redox systems restricts the activity largely to anaerobic bacteria and certain protozoa that exhibit anaerobic metabolism. The basis for activity against microaerophilic species such as *Helicobacter pylori* and *Gardnerella vaginalis* remains speculative, though a novel nitroreductase, which is altered in metronidazole-resistant strains, is implicated in *H. pylori*.[35]

NITROFURANS

As with nitroimidazoles, the reduction of the nitro group of nitrofurantoin and other nitrofurans is a prerequisite for antibacterial activity. Micro-organisms with appropriate nitroreductases act on nitrofurans to produce a highly reactive electrophilic intermediate and this is postulated to affect DNA as the reduced intermediates of nitroimidazoles do. Other evidence suggests that the reduced nitrofurans bind to bacterial ribosomes and prevent protein synthesis.[36] An effect on DNA has the virtue of explaining the known mutagenicity of these compounds in vitro and any revised mechanism relating to inhibition of protein synthesis needs to be reconciled with this property.

AGENTS AFFECTING MEMBRANE PERMEABILITY

Agents acting on cell membranes do not normally discriminate between microbial and mammalian membranes, although the fungal cell membrane has proved more amenable to selective attack (*see below*). The only membrane-active antibacterial agents to be administered systemically in human medicine are polymyxin, the closely related compound colistin (polymyxin E) and the recently introduced cyclic lipopeptide daptomycin. The former have spectra of activity restricted to Gram-negative bacteria whereas daptomycin is active against Gram-positive bacteria, but inactive against Gram-negative species.

Polymyxin and colistin appear to act like cationic detergents, i.e. they disrupt the Gram-negative bacterial cytoplasmic membrane, probably by attacking the exposed phosphate groups of the membrane phospholipid. However, initial interaction with the cell appears to depend upon recognition by lipopolysaccharides in the outer membrane followed by translocation from the outer membrane to the cytoplasmic membrane.[37] The end result is leakage of cytoplasmic contents and death of the cell. Various factors, including growth phase and incubation temperature, alter the balance of fatty acids within the bacterial cell membrane, and this can concomitantly affect the response to polymyxins.[38]

The cyclic lipopeptide daptomycin exhibits calcium-dependent insertion into the cytoplasmic membrane of Gram-positive bacteria, interacting preferentially with anionic phospholipids such as phosphatidyl glycerol.[39] It distorts membrane structure and causes leakage of potassium, magnesium and ATP from the cell together with membrane depolarization (Figure 2.5).[40-42] Collectively these events lead to inhibition of macromolecular synthesis and bacterial cell death.[41,42] Daptomycin is inactive against Gram-negative bacteria because it fails to penetrate the outer membrane. However, the basis of selective toxicity against the cytoplasmic membrane of Gram-positive bacteria as opposed to eukaryotic membranes is currently unclear.

ANTIFUNGAL AGENTS

The antifungal agents in current clinical use can be divided into the antifungal antibiotics (griseofulvin and polyenes) and a variety of synthetic agents including flucytosine, the azoles (e.g. miconazole, ketoconazole, fluconazole, itraconazole, voriconazole, posaconazole), the allylamines (terbinafine) and echinocandins (caspofungin, micafungin, anidulafungin).[43-45]

In view of the scarcity of antibacterial agents acting on the cytoplasmic membrane, it is surprising to find that some of the most successful groups of antifungal agents – the polyenes, azoles and allylamines – all achieve their effects in this way.[43-45] However, the echinocandins, the most recent antifungals introduced into clinical practice,[46] differ in affecting the synthesis of the fungal cell wall.[45,47]

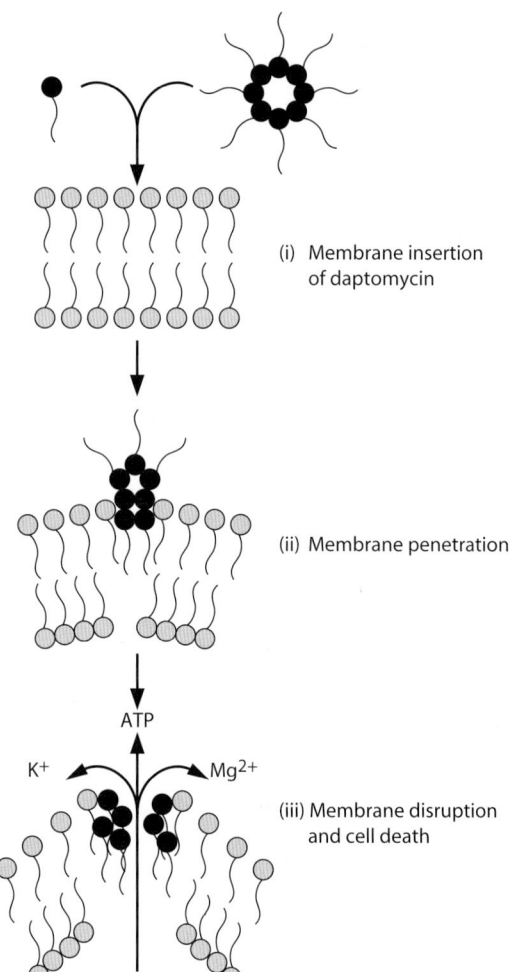

Fig. 2.5 A model for the mode of action of daptomycin in Gram-positive bacteria. (i) Daptomycin, in the presence of Ca^{2+}, inserts into the cytoplasmic membrane either as an aggregate or as individual molecules that aggregate once within the membrane. (ii) Daptomycin penetrates the membrane and causes membrane curvature. (iii) Extensive membrane curvature and strain results in membrane disruption leading to leakage of intracellular components, membrane depolarization, loss of biosynthetic activity and cell death. Daptomycin (black-filled circles); phospholipids (gray-filled circles).

(i) Membrane insertion of daptomycin

(ii) Membrane penetration

ATP

K^+ Mg^{2+}

(iii) Membrane disruption and cell death

GRISEOFULVIN

The mechanism of action of the antidermatophyte antibiotic griseofulvin is not fully understood.[45] There are at least two possibilities:

- Inhibition of synthesis of the fungal cell wall component chitin
- Antimitotic activity exerted by the binding of drug to the microtubules of the mitotic spindle, interfering with their assembly and function.

POLYENES

The polyene antibiotics (nystatin and amphotericin B) bind only to membranes containing sterols; ergosterol, the predominant sterol of fungal membranes, appears to be particularly susceptible.[45,47] The drugs form pores in the fungal membrane which makes the membrane leaky, leading to loss of normal membrane function. Unfortunately, mammalian cell membranes also contain sterols, and polyenes consequently exhibit a relatively low therapeutic index.

AZOLES

In contrast to the polyenes, whose action depends upon the presence of ergosterol in the fungal membrane, the antifungal azoles prevent the synthesis of this membrane sterol. These compounds block ergosterol synthesis by interfering with the demethylation of its precursor, lanosterol.[45,48] Lanosterol demethylase is a cytochrome P_{450} enzyme and, although azole antifungals have much less influence on analogous mammalian systems, some of the side effects of these drugs are attributable to such action.

Antifungal azole derivatives are predominantly fungistatic but some compounds at higher concentrations, notably miconazole and clotrimazole, kill fungi apparently by causing direct membrane damage. Other, less well characterized, effects of azoles on fungal respiration have also been described.[49]

ALLYLAMINES

The antifungal allylamine derivatives terbinafine and naftifine inhibit squalene epoxidase, another enzyme involved in the biosynthesis of ergosterol.[50] Fungicidal effects may be due to the accumulation of squalene in the membrane leading to its rupture, rather than a deficiency of ergosterol. In *Candida albicans* the drugs are primarily fungistatic and the yeast form is less susceptible than is mycelial growth. In this species there is less accumulation of squalene than in dermatophytes, and ergosterol deficiency may be the limiting factor.[51]

ECHINOCANDINS

Caspofungin and related compounds inhibit the formation of glucan, an essential polysaccharide of the cell wall of many fungi, including *Pneumocystis jirovecii* (formerly *Pneumocystis carinii*). The vulnerable enzyme is β-1,3-glucan synthase, which is located in the cell membrane.[47,52]

FLUCYTOSINE (5-FLUOROCYTOSINE)

The spectrum of activity of flucytosine (5-fluorocytosine) is virtually restricted to yeasts. In these fungi flucytosine is transported into the cell by a cytosine permease; a cytosine deaminase then converts flucytosine to 5-fluorouracil, which is incorporated into RNA in place of uracil, leading to the formation of abnormal proteins.[45] There is also an effect on DNA synthesis through inhibition of thymidylate synthetase.[53] The absence of major side effects in humans can be attributed to the lack of cytosine deaminase in mammalian cells.[45]

ANTIPROTOZOAL AGENTS

The actions of some antiprotozoal drugs overlap with, or are analogous to, those seen with the antibacterial and antifungal agents already discussed. Thus, the activity of 5-nitroimidazoles such as metronidazole extends to those protozoa that exhibit an essentially anaerobic metabolism; the antimalarial agents pyrimethamine and cycloguanil (the metabolic product of proguanil), like trimethoprim, inhibit dihydrofolate reductase.

A number of antibacterial agents also have antiprotozoal activity. For instance the sulfonamides, tetracyclines, lincosamides and macrolides all display antimalarial activity, although they are most frequently used in combination with specific antimalarial agents. Some antifungal polyenes and antifungal azoles also display sufficient activity against *Leishmania* and certain other protozoa for them to have received attention as potential therapeutic agents.

There is considerable uncertainty about the mechanism of action of other antiprotozoal agents. Various sites of action have been ascribed to many of them and, with a few notable exceptions, the literature reveals only partial attempts to define the primary target.

ANTIMALARIAL AGENTS

QUINOLINE ANTIMALARIALS

Quinine and the various quinoline antimalarials were once thought to achieve their effect by intercalation with plasmodial DNA after concentration in parasitized erythrocytes. However, these effects occur only at concentrations in excess of those achieved in vivo.[54] Moreover, a non-specific effect on DNA does not explain the selective action of these compounds at precise points in the plasmodial life cycle or the differential activity of antimalarial quinolines.

Clarification of the mode of action of these compounds has proved elusive, but it now seems likely that chloroquine and related compounds act primarily by binding to ferriprotoporphyrin IX, preventing its polymerization by the parasite.[54,55] Ferriprotoporphyrin IX, produced from hemoglobin in the food vacuole of the parasites, is a toxic metabolite which is normally rendered innocuous by polymerization.

Chloroquine achieves a very high concentration within the food vacuole of the parasite and this greatly aids its activity. However, quinine and mefloquine are not concentrated to the same extent, and have much less effect on ferriproto-porphyrin IX polymerization, raising the possibility that other (possibly multiple) targets are involved in the action of these compounds.[56,57]

8-Aminoquinolines like primaquine, which, at therapeutically useful concentrations exhibit selective activity against liver-stage parasites and gametocytes, possibly inhibit mitochondrial enzyme systems by poorly defined mechanisms. Furthermore, whether this action is due directly to the 8-aminoquinolines, or their metabolites, is unknown.[54]

 ## ARTEMISININ

Artemisinin, the active principle of the Chinese herbal remedy qinghaosu, and three derivatives of artemisinin are widely used antimalarial drugs.[54] These drugs are all converted in vivo to dihydroartemisinin which has a chemically reactive peroxide bridge.[54] This is cleaved in the presence of heme or free iron within the parasitized red cell to form a short-lived, but highly reactive, free radical that irreversibly alkylates malaria proteins.[58,59] However, artemisinin may have other mechanisms of action, including modulation of the host's immune response.[59]

 ## ATOVAQUONE

The hydroxynaphthoquinone atovaquone, which exhibits antimalarial and anti-*Pneumocystis* activity, is an electron transport inhibitor that causes depletion of the ATP pool. The primary effect is on the iron flavoprotein dihydro-orotate dehydrogenase, an essential enzyme in the production of pyrimidines. Mammalian cells are able to avoid undue toxicity by use of preformed pyrimidines.[60] Dihydro-orotate dehydrogenase from *Plasmodium falciparum* is inhibited by concentrations of atovaquone that are very much lower than those needed to inhibit the *Pneumocystis* enzyme, raising the possibility that the antimicrobial consequences might differ in the two organisms.[61] Although atovaquone was originally developed as a monotherapy for malaria, high level resistance readily emerges in *Plasmodium falciparum* when the drug is used alone.[54] Consequently, atovaquone is now combined with proguanil.

OTHER ANTIPROTOZOAL AGENTS

Arsenical compounds, which are still the mainstay of treatment of African sleeping sickness, appear to poison trypanosomes by affecting carbohydrate metabolism through inhibition of glycerol-3-phosphate, pyruvate kinase, phosphofructokinase and fructose-2,6,-biphosphatase.[62,63] This is achieved through binding to essential thiol groups in the enzymes. This mechanism of action accounts for the poor selective toxicity of the arsenicals, since they also inhibit many mammalian enzymes through the same mechanism.[62]

The actions of other agents with antitrypanosomal activity, including suramin and pentamidine, are also poorly characterized.[62,64] Various cell processes, mainly those involved in glycolysis within the specialized glycosomes of protozoa of the trypanosome family, have been implicated in the action of suramin.[65] However, a variety of other unrelated biochemical processes are also inhibited.[62,63] Consequently, the mode of action of suramin remains obscure. However, suramin appears to be more effectively accumulated by trypanosomes compared to mammalian cells and this may account for the selective toxicity of the drug.[62]

Pentamidine and other diamidines disrupt the trypanosomal kinetoplast, a specialized DNA-containing organelle, probably by binding to DNA, though they also interfere with polyamine synthesis and have been reported to inhibit RNA editing in trypanosomes.[61,62,65,66]

Laboratory studies of *Leishmania* are hampered by the fact that in-vitro culture yields promastigotes that are morphologically and metabolically different from the amastigotes involved in disease. Such evidence as is available suggests that the pentavalent antimonials commonly used for treatment inhibit ATP synthesis in the parasite.[67] Whether this is due to a direct effect of the antimonials or conversion to trivalent metabolites is uncertain.[67] Antifungal azoles take advantage of similarities in sterol biosynthesis among fungi and leishmanial amastigotes.[68]

Eflornithine (difluoromethylornithine) is a selective inhibitor of ornithine decarboxylase and achieves its effect by depleting the biosynthesis of polyamines such as spermidine, a precursor of trypanothione.[62,69] The corresponding mammalian enzyme has a much shorter half-life than its trypanosomal counterpart, and this may account for the apparent selectivity of action.[62] The preferential activity against *Trypanosoma brucei gambiense* rather than the related *rhodesiense* form may be due to reduced drug uptake or differences in polyamine metabolism in the latter subspecies.[70]

Several of the drugs used in amebiasis, including the plant alkaloid emetine and diloxanide furoate appear to interfere with protein synthesis within amebic trophozoites or cysts.[71]

ANTHELMINTIC AGENTS

Just as the cell wall of bacteria is a prime target for selective agents and the cell membrane is peculiarly vulnerable in fungi, so the neuromuscular system appears to be the Achilles' heel of parasitic worms. Several anthelmintic agents work by paralyzing the neuromusculature. The most important agents are those of the avermectin/milbemycin class of anthelmintics including ivermectin, milbemycin oxime, moxidectin and selamectin.[72] These drugs bind to, and activate, glutamate-gated chloride channels in nerve cells, leading to inhibition of neuronal transmission and paralysis of somatic muscles in the parasite, particularly in the pharyngeal pump.[72,73]

The benzimidazole derivatives, including mebendazole and albendazole, act by a different mechanism. These broad-spectrum anthelmintic drugs seem to have at least two effects on adult worms and larvae: inhibition of the uptake of the chief energy source, glucose; and binding to tubulin, the structural protein of microtubules.[74,75]

The basis of the activity of the antifilarial drug diethylcarbamazine has long been a puzzle, since the drug has no effect on microfilaria in vitro. Consequently it seems likely that the effect of the drug observed in vivo is due to alterations in the surface coat of the microfilariae, making them more responsive to immunological processes from which they are normally protected.[76,77] This may be mediated through inhibition of arachidonic acid synthesis, a polyunsaturated fatty acid, present in phospholipids.[77]

ANTIVIRAL AGENTS

The prospects for the development of selectively toxic antiviral agents were long thought to be poor, since the life cycle of the virus is so closely bound to normal cellular processes. However, closer scrutiny of the relationship of the virus to the cell reveals several points at which the viral cycle might be interrupted.[78] These include:

- Adsorption to and penetration of the cell
- Uncoating of the viral nucleic acid
- The various stages of nucleic acid replication
- Assembly of the new viral particles
- Release of infectious virions (if the cell is not destroyed).

NUCLEOSIDE ANALOGS

In the event, it is the process of viral replication (which is extremely rapid relative to most mammalian cells) that has proved to be the most vulnerable point of attack, and most clinically useful antiviral agents are nucleoside analogs. Aciclovir (acycloguanosine) and penciclovir (the active product of the oral agent famciclovir), which are successful for the treatment of herpes simplex, achieve their antiviral effect by conversion within the cell to the triphosphate derivative. In the case of aciclovir and penciclovir, the initial phosphorylation, yielding aciclovir or penciclovir monophosphate, is accomplished by a thymidine kinase coded for by the virus itself. The corresponding cellular thymidine kinase phosphorylates these compounds very inefficiently and thus only cells harboring the virus are affected. Moreover, the triphosphates of aciclovir and penciclovir inhibit viral DNA polymerase more efficiently than the cellular enzyme; this is another feature of their selective activity. As well as inhibiting viral DNA polymerase, aciclovir and penciclovir triphosphates are incorporated into the growing DNA chain and cause premature termination of DNA synthesis.[79]

Other nucleoside analogs – including the anti-HIV agents zidovudine, didanosine, zalcitabine, stavudine, lamivudine, abacavir and emtricitabine, and the anti-cytomegalovirus agents ganciclovir and valganciclovir are phosphorylated by cellular enzymes to form triphosphate derivatives.[79,80] In their triphosphate forms the anti-HIV compounds are recognized by

viral reverse transcriptase and are incorporated as monophosphates at the 3' end of the viral DNA chain, causing premature chain termination during the process of DNA transcription from the single-stranded RNA template.[79,80] Consequently, the triphosphate derivatives of the anti-HIV compounds act both as competitors of the normal deoxynucleoside substrates and as alternative substrates being incorporated into the DNA chain a deoxynucleoside monophosphates. Similarly, ganciclovir acts as a chain terminator during the synthesis of cytomegalovirus DNA.[79] Since these compounds lack a hydroxyl group on the deoxyribose ring, they are unable to form phosphodiester linkages in the viral DNA chain.[79-81] Ribavirin is also a nucleoside analog with activity against orthomyxoviruses (influenza A and B) and paramyxoviruses (measles, respiratory syncytial virus). In its 5' monophosphate form ribavirin inhibits inosine monophosphate dehydrogenase, an enzyme required for the synthesis of GTP and dGTP, and in its 5' triphosphate form it can prevent transcription of the influenza RNA genome.[79] In vitro, ribavirin antagonizes the action of zidovudine, probably by feedback inhibition of thymidine kinase, so that the zidovudine is not phosphorylated.[82]

NON-NUCLEOSIDE REVERSE TRANSCRIPTASE INHIBITORS

Although they are structurally unrelated, the non-nucleoside reverse transcriptase inhibitors nevirapine, delavirdine and efavirenz all bind to HIV-1 reverse transcriptase in a non-competitive fashion.[79,80]

PROTEASE INHIBITORS

An alternative tactic to disable HIV is to inhibit the enzyme that cleaves the polypeptide precursor of several essential viral proteins. Such protease inhibitors in therapeutic use include saquinavir, ritonavir, indinavir, nelfinavir, amprenavir, lopinavir and atazanavir.[79,80]

NUCLEOTIDE ANALOGS

The nucleotide analog cidofovir is licensed for the treatment of cytomegalovirus disease in AIDS patients.[79] It is phosphorylated by cellular kinases to the triphosphate derivative, which then becomes a competitive inhibitor of DNA polymerase.

PHOSPHONIC ACID DERIVATIVES

The simple phosphonoformate salt foscarnet and its close analog phosphonoacetic acid inhibit DNA polymerase activity of herpes viruses by preventing pyrophosphate exchange.[79] The action is selective in that the corresponding mammalian polymerase is much less susceptible to inhibition.

AMANTADINE AND RIMANTIDINE

The anti-influenza A compound amantadine and its close relative rimantadine act by blocking the M2 ion channel which is required for uptake of protons into the interior of the virus to permit acid-promoted viral uncoating (decapsidation).[79,83]

NEURAMINIDASE INHIBITORS

Two drugs target the neuraminidase of influenza A and B viruses: zanamivir and oseltamivir. Both bind directly to the neuraminidase enzyme and prevent the formation of infectious progeny virions.[79,83]

ANTISENSE DRUGS

Fomivirsen is the only licensed antisense oligonucleotide for the treatment of cytomegalovirus retinitis. The nucleotide sequence of fomivirsen is complementary to a sequence in the messenger RNA transcript of the major immediate early region 2 of cytomegalovirus, which is essential for production of infectious virus.[79]

CONCLUSION

The modes of action of the majority of antibacterial, antifungal and antiviral drugs are well understood, reflecting our sophisticated knowledge of the life cycles of these organisms and the availability of numerous biochemical and molecular microbiological techniques for studying drug interactions in these microbial groups. In contrast, there are many gaps in our understanding of the mechanisms of action of antiprotozoal and anthelmintic agents, reflecting the more complex nature of these organisms and the technical difficulties of studying them.

 References

1. Denyer SP, Maillard JY. Cellular impermeability and uptake of biocides and antibiotics in gram-negative bacteria. *J Appl Microbiol.* 2002;92(suppl):35S–45S.
2. Kahan FM, Kahan JS, Cassidy PJ, et al. The mechanism of action of fosfomycin (phosphonomycin). *Ann N Y Acad Sci.* 1974;235:364–386.
3. Higgins DL, Chang R, Debabov DM, et al. Telavancin, a multifunctional lipoglycopeptide, disrupts both cell wall synthesis and cell membrane integrity in methicillin-resistant *Staphylococcus aureus. Antimicrob Agents Chemother.* 2005;49:1127–1134.
4. Greenwood D, O'Grady F. The two sites of penicillin action in Escherichia coli. *J Infect Dis.* 1973;128:791–794.
5. Massova I, Mobashery S. Kinship and diversification of bacterial penicillin-binding proteins and β-lactamases. *Antimicrob Agents Chemother.* 1998;42:1–17.
6. Bayles KW. The bactericidal action of penicillin: new clues to an unsolved mystery. *Trends Microbiol.* 2000;8:274–278.
7. Brennan PJ, Nikaido H. The envelope of mycobacteria. *Annu Rev Biochem.* 1995;64:29–63.
8. Kremer L, Besra GS. Current status and future development of antitubercular chemotherapy. *Expert Opin Investig Drugs.* 2002;11:1033–1049.
9. Zhang Y, Wade MM, Scorpio A, et al. Mode of action of pyrazinamide: disruption of *Mycobacterium tuberculosis* membrane transport and energetics by pyrazinoic acid. *J Antimicrob Chemother.* 2003;52:790–795.
10. Bottger EC. Antimicrobial agents targeting the ribosome: the issue of selectivity and toxicity – lessons to be learned. *Cell Mol Life Sci.* 2007;64:791–795.
11. Schlunzen F, Zarivach R, Harms J, et al. Structural basis for the interaction of antibiotics with the peptidyl transferase centre in eubacteria. *Nature.* 2001;413:814–821.
12. Pioletti M, Schlunzen F, Harms J, et al. Crystal structures of complexes of the small ribosomal subunit with tetracycline, edeine and IF3. *EMBO J.* 2001;20:1829–1839.
13. Carter AP, Clemons WM, Broderson RJ, et al. Functional insights from the structure of the 30S ribosomal subunit and its interaction with antibiotics. *Nature.* 2000;407:340–348.
14. Leach KL, Swaney SM, Colca JR, et al. The site of action of oxazolidinone antibiotics in living bacteria and in human mitochondria. *Mol Cell.* 2007;26:393–402.
15. Chopra I, Hawkey PM, Hinton M. Tetracyclines, molecular and clinical aspects. *J Antimicrob Chemother.* 1992;29:245–277.
16. Tai PC, Davis BD. The actions of antibiotics on the ribosome. In: Greenwood D, O'Grady F, eds. *The scientific basis of antimicrobial chemotherapy.* Cambridge: Cambridge University Press; 1985:41–68.
17. Davis BD. The lethal action of aminoglycosides. *J Antimicrob Chemother.* 1988;22:1–3.
18. Davis BD. Mechanism of bactericidal action of aminoglycosides. *Microbiol Rev.* 1987;51:341–350.
19. Cocito C, Di Giambattista M, Nyssen E, Vannuffel P. Inhibition of protein synthesis by streptogramins and related antibiotics. *J Antimicrob Chemother.* 1997;39(suppl A):7–13.
20. Vannuffel P, Cocito C. Mechanism of action of streptogramins and macrolides. *Drugs.* 1996;51(suppl 1):20–30.
21. Bryskier A. Ketolides. In: Bryskier A, ed. *Antimicrobial agents.* Washington, DC: American Society for Microbiology Press; 2005:527–569.
22. Hunt E. Pleuromutilin antibiotics. *Drugs of the Future.* 2001;25:1163–1168.
23. Yang LP, Keam SJ. Spotlight on retapamulin in impetigo and other uncomplicated superficial skin infections. *Am J Clin Dermatol.* 2008;9:411–413.
24. Bryskier A. Mutilins. In: Bryskier A, ed. *Antimicrobial agents.* Washington, DC: American Society for Microbiology Press; 2005:1239–1241.
25. Bryskier A. Fusidic acid. In: Bryskier A, ed. *Antimicrobial agents.* Washington, DC: American Society for Microbiology Press; 2005:631–641.
26. Bryskier A. Mupirocin. In: Bryskier A, ed. *Antimicrobial agents.* Washington, DC: American Society for Microbiology Press; 2005:964–971.
27. Hurdle JG, O'Neill AJ, Chopra I. Prospects for aminoacyl-tRNA synthetase inhibitors as new antimicrobial agents. *Antimicrob Agents Chemother.* 2005;49:4821–4833.
28. Hooper DC. Quinolone mode of action. *Drugs.* 1995;49(suppl 2):10–15.
29. Ng EYW, Trucksis M, Hooper DC. Quinolone resistance mutations in topoisomerase IV: relationship to the *fiqA* locus and genetic evidence that topoisomerase IV is the primary target and DNA gyrase is the secondary target of fluoroquinolones in Staphylococcus aureus. *Antimicrob Agents Chemother.* 1996;40:1881–1888.
30. Drlica K. Mechanisms of fluoroquinolone action. *Curr Opin Microbiol.* 1999;2:504–508.
31. Bryskier A, Klich M. Coumarin antibiotics: novobiocin, coumermycin and clorobiocin. In: Bryskier A, ed. *Antimicrobial agents.* Washington, DC: American Society for Microbiology Press; 2005:816–825.
32. Campbell EA, Korzheva N, Mustaev A, et al. Structural mechanism for rifampicin inhibition of bacterial RNA polymerase. *Cell.* 2001;104:901–912.
33. Veyssier P, Bryskier A. Dihydrofolate reductase inhibitors, nitroheterocycles (furans), and 8-hydroxyquinolines. In: Bryskier A, ed. *Antimicrobial agents.* Washington, DC: American Society for Microbiology Press; 2005:941–963.
34. Edwards DI. Nitroimidazole drugs – action and resistance mechanisms. I. Mechanisms of action. *J Antimicrob Chemother.* 1993;31:9–20.
35. Goodwin A, Kersulyte D, Sisson G, et al. Metronidazole resistance in *Helicobacter pylori* is due to null mutations in a gene (*rdxA*) that encodes the oxygen-insensitive NADPH nitroreductase. *Mol Microbiol.* 1998;28:383–393.

36. McOsker CC, Fitzpatrick PM. Nitrofurantoin: mechanism of action and implications for resistance development in common uropathogens. *J Antimicrob Chemother*. 1994;33(suppl. A):23–30.

37. Hancock RE, Chapple DS. Peptide antibiotics. *Antimicrob Agents Chemother*. 1999;43:1317–1323.

38. Gilleland HE, Champlin FR, Conrad RS. Chemical alterations in cell envelopes of *Pseudomonas aeruginosa* upon exposure to polymyxin: a possible mechanism to explain adaptive resistance to polymyxin. *Can J Microbiol*. 1984;20:869–873.

39. Hachmann A-B, Angert ER, Helmann JD. Genetic analysis of factors affecting susceptibility of *Bacillus subtilis* to daptomycin. *Antimicrob Agents Chemother*. 2009;53:1598–1609.

40. Straus SK, Hancock RE. Mode of action of the new antibiotic for Gram-positive pathogens daptomycin: comparison with cationic antimicrobial peptides and lipopeptides. *Biochim Biophys Acta*. 2006;1758:1215–1223.

41. Silverman JA, Perlmutter NG, Shapiro HM. Correlation of daptomycin bactericidal activity and membrane depolarization in *Staphylococcus aureus*. *Antimicrob Agents Chemother*. 2003;47:2538–2544.

42. Hobbs JK, Miller K, O'Neill AJ, et al. Consequences of daptomycin-mediated membrane damage in Staphylococcus aureus. *J Antimicrob Chemother*. 2008;62:1003–1008.

43. Elewski BE. Mechanisms of action of systemic antifungal agents. *J Am Acad Dermatol*. 1993;28:S28–S34.

44. Ghannoum MA, Rice LB. Antifungal agents: mode of action, mechanisms of resistance, and correlation of these mechanisms with bacterial resistance. *Clin Microbiol Rev*. 1999;12:501–517.

45. Grillot R, Lebeau B. Systemic antifungal agents. In: Bryskier A, ed. *Antimicrobial agents*. Washington, DC: American Society for Microbiology Press; 2005:1260–1287.

46. Kauffman CA. Clinical efficacy of new antifungal agents. *Curr Opin Microbiol*. 2006;9:483–488.

47. Bowman SM, Free SJ. The structure and synthesis of the fungal cell wall. *Bioessays*. 2006;28:799–808.

48. Borgers M. Antifungal azole derivatives. In: Greenwood D, O'Grady F, eds. *The scientific basis of antimicrobial chemotherapy*. Cambridge: Cambridge University Press; 1985:133–153.

49. Fromtling RA. Overview of medically important antifungal azole derivatives. *Clin Microbiol Rev*. 1988;1:187–217.

50. Stütz A. Allylamine derivatives – inhibitors of fungal squalene epoxidase. In: Borowski E, Shugar D, eds. *Molecular aspects of chemotherapy*. New York: Pergamon; 1990:205–213.

51. Ryder NS. The mode of action of terbinafine. *Clin Exp Dermatol*. 1989;14:98–100.

52. Georgopapadakou NH. Update on antifungals targeted to the cell wall: focus on beta-1,3-glucan synthase inhibitors. *Expert Opin Investig Drugs*. 2001;10:269–280.

53. Odds FC. *Candida and candidosis*. London: Baillière Tindall; 1988.

54. White NJ. Malaria. In: Cook GC, Zumla AI, eds. *Manson's tropical diseases*. 21st ed. Edinburgh: Saunders; 2003:1205–1295.

55. Slater AFG, Cerami A. Inhibition by chloroquine of a novel haem polymerase enzyme activity in malaria trophozoites. *Nature*. 1992;355:167–169.

56. Foote SJ, Cowman AF. The mode of action and the mechanism of resistance to antimalarial drugs. *Acta Trop*. 1994;56:157–171.

57. Foley M, Tilley L. Quinoline antimalarials: mechanisms of action and resistance and prospects for new agents. *Pharmacol Ther*. 1998;79:55–87.

58. Meshnick SR, Taylor TE, Kamchonwongpaison S. Artemisinin and the antimalarial endoperoxides: from herbal remedy to targeted chemotherapy. *Microbiol Rev*. 1996;60:301–315.

59. Keiser J, Utzinger J. Artemisinins and synthetic trioxolanes in the treatment of helminth infections. *Curr Opin Infect Dis*. 2007;20:605–612.

60. Artymowicz RJ, James VE. Atovaquone: a new antipneumocystis agent. *Clin Pharm*. 1993;12:563–569.

61. Ittarat I, Asawamahasakada W, Bartlett MS, et al. Effects of atovaquone and other inhibitors on *Pneumocystis carinii* dihydroorotate dehydrogenase. *Antimicrob Agents Chemother*. 1995;39:325–328.

62. Burri C, Brun R. Human African trypanosomiasis. In: Cook GC, Zumla AI, eds. *Manson's tropical diseases*. 21st ed. Edinburgh: Saunders; 2003:1303–1323.

63. Nok AJ. Arsenicals (melarsoprol), pentamidine and suramin in the treatment of human African trypanosomiasis. *Parasitol Res*. 2003;90:71–79.

64. Denise H, Barrett MP. Uptake and mode of action of drugs used against sleeping sickness. *Biochem Pharmacol*. 2001;61:1–5.

65. Voogd TE, Vansterkenburg ELM, Wilting J, et al. Recent research on the biological activity of suramin. *Pharmacol Rev*. 1993;45:177–203.

66. Sands M, Kron MA, Brown RB. Pentamidine: a review. *Rev Infect Dis*. 1985;7:625–635.

67. Dedet JP, Pratlong F. Leishmaniasis. In: Cook GC, Zumla AI, eds. *Manson's tropical diseases*. 21st ed. Edinburgh: Saunders; 2003:1339–1364.

68. Berman JD. Chemotherapy for leishmaniasis: biochemical mechanisms, clinical efficacy and future strategies. *Clin Infect Dis*. 1988;10:560–586.

69. McCann PP, Bacchi CJ, Clarkson AB, et al. Inhibition of polyamine biosynthesis by α-difluoromethylornithine in African trypanosomes and *Pneumocystis carinii* as a basis for chemotherapy: biochemical and clinical aspects. *Am J Trop Med Hyg*. 1986;35:1153–1156.

70. Bacchi CJ. Resistance to clinical drugs in African trypanosomes. *Parasitol Today*. 1993;9:190–193.

71. Khaw M, Panosian CB. Human antiprotozoal therapy: past, present and future. *Clin Microbiol Rev*. 1995;8:427–439.

72. Yates DM, Wolstenholme AJ. An ivermectin-sensitive glutamate-gated chloride channel subunit from *Dirofilaria immitis*. *Int J Parasitol*. 2004;34:1075–1081.

73. Omura S, Crump A. The life and times of ivermectin. *Nat Rev Microbiol*. 2004;2:984–989.

74. Lacey E. The mode of action of benzimidazoles. *Parasitol Today*. 1990;6:112–115.

75. McKellar QA, Jackson F. Veterinary anthelmintics: old and new. *Trends Parasitol*. 2004;20:456–461.

76. Hawking F. Chemotherapy for filariasis. *Antibiot Chemother*. 1981;30:135–162.

77. Maizels RM, Denham DA. Diethylcarbamazine (DEC): immunopharmacological interactions of an anti-filarial drug. *Parasitology*. 1992;105(suppl):S49–S60.

78. Crumpacker CS. Molecular targets of antiviral therapy. *N Engl J Med*. 1989;321:163–172.

79. De Clercq E. Antiviral drugs in current clinical use. *J Clin Virol*. 2004;30:115–133.

80. De Clercq E. Anti-HIV drugs: 25 compounds approved within 25 years after the discovery of HIV. *Int J Antimicrob Agents*. 2009;33:307–320.

81. Lipsky JJ. Zalcitabine and didanosine. *Lancet*. 1993;341:30–32.

82. Vogt MW, Hartshom KL, Furman PA, et al. Ribavirin antagonizes the effect of azidothymidine on HIV replication. *Science*. 1987;235:1376–1379.

83. De Clercq E. Antiviral agents active against influenza A viruses. *Nat Rev Drug Discov*. 2006;5:1015–1025.

 Further information

Detailed information on the mode of action of anti-infective agents can be found in the following sources:

Bryskier A, ed. *Antimicrobial agents: antibacterials and antifungals*. Washington, DC: American Society for Microbiology; 2005.

Cook GC, Zumla AI, eds. *Manson's tropical diseases*. 21st ed. Edinburgh: Saunders; 2003.

Franklin TJ, Snow GA. *Biochemistry and molecular biology of antimicrobial drug action*. 6th ed. New York: Springer; 2005.

Gale EF, Cundliffe E, Reynolds PE, Richmond MH, Waring MJ. *The molecular basis of antibiotic action*. 2nd ed. Chichester: Wiley; 1981.

Greenwood D. *Antimicrobial chemotherapy*. Oxford and New York: Oxford University Press; 2007.

Hooper DC, Rubinstein E, eds. *Quinolone antimicrobial agents*. 3rd ed. Washington, DC: American Society for Microbiology; 2003.

Frayha GJ, Smyth JD, Gobert JG, Savel J. The mechanism of action of antiprotozoal an anthelmintic drugs in man. *Gen Pharmacol*. 1997;28:273–299.

James DH, Gilles HM. *Human antiparasitic drugs: Pharmacology and usage*. Chichester: Wiley; 1985.

Mascaretti OA. *Bacteria versus antibacterial agents, an integrated approach*. Washington, DC: American Society for Microbiology; 2003.

Rosenthal PJ, ed. *Antimalarial chemotherapy: mechanisms of action, resistance, and new directions*. Totowa, NJ: Humana Press; 2001.

Scholar EM, Pratt WB. *The antimicrobial drugs*. 2nd ed. Oxford: Oxford University Press; 2000.

Walsh C. *Antibiotics: actions, origins, resistance*. Washington, DC: American Society for Microbiology; 2003.

The problem of resistance

Olivier Denis, Hector Rodriguez-Villalobos and Marc J. Struelens

Antibiotic resistance is increasing worldwide at an accelerating pace, reducing the efficacy of therapy for many infections, fuelling transmission of pathogens and majoring health costs, morbidity and mortality related to infectious diseases.[1] This public-health threat has been recognized as a priority for intervention by health agencies at national and international level.[2,3] In this chapter we will address the definition of resistance, its biochemical mechanisms, genetic basis, prevalence in major human pathogens, epidemiology and strategies for control.

DEFINITION OF RESISTANCE

Antibiotic resistance definitions are based on in-vitro quantitative testing of bacterial susceptibility to antibacterial agents. This is typically achieved by determination of the minimal inhibitory concentration (MIC) of a drug; that is, the lowest concentration that inhibits visible growth of a standard inoculum of bacteria in a defined medium within a defined period of incubation (usually 18–24 h) in a suitable atmosphere (see Ch. 9). There is no universal consensus definition of bacterial resistance to antibiotics. This is related to two issues: first, the resistance may be defined either from a biological or from a clinical standpoint; secondly, different 'critical breakpoint' values for categorization of bacteria as resistant or susceptible were selected by national reference committees. In recent years, major advances toward international harmonization of resistance breakpoints have been made thanks to the consensus achieved within the European Committee for Antimicrobial Susceptibility Testing (EUCAST).[4]

According to the Clinical Laboratory Standards Institute (CLSI), formerly known as the US National Committee for Clinical and Laboratory Standards (NCCLS), infecting bacteria are considered *susceptible* when they can be inhibited by achievable serum or tissue concentration using a dose of the antimicrobial agent recommended for that type of infection and pathogen.[4] This 'target concentration' will not only depend on pharmacokinetic and pharmacodynamic properties of the

drug (*see* Ch. 4), but also on recommended dose, which may vary by country. EUCAST[5] developed distinct definitions for microbiological and clinical resistance. The *microbiological definition* of *wild type* (or naturally susceptible) bacteria includes those that belong to the most susceptible subpopulations and lack acquired or mutational mechanisms of resistance. The *definition* of *clinically susceptible* bacteria is those that are susceptible by a level of in-vitro antimicrobial activity associated with a high likelihood of success with a standard therapeutic regimen of the drug. In the absence of this clinical information, the definition is based on a consensus interpretation of the antibiotic's pharmacodynamic and pharmacokinetic properties. The clinically susceptible category may include fully susceptible and borderline susceptible, or moderately susceptible, bacteria which may have acquired low-level resistance mechanism(s) (Figure 3.1).

Clinical resistance is defined by EUCAST as a level of antimicrobial activity associated with a high likelihood of therapeutic failure even with high dosage of a given antibiotic. EUCAST defines as *microbiologically resistant* bacteria that possess any resistance mechanism demonstrated either phenotypically or genotypically. These may be defined statistically by an MIC higher than the 'epidemiological cut-off value' that separates the normal distribution of wild type versus non-wild type bacterial strains, irrespective of source or test method.[4–6]

The *clinically intermediate* (EUCAST) or *intermediate* (CLSI) category is used for bacteria with an MIC that lies between the breakpoints for clinically susceptible and clinically resistant. These strains are inhibited by concentrations of the antimicrobial that are close to either the usually or the maximally achievable blood or tissue level and for which the therapeutic response rate is less predictable than for infection with susceptible strains.[6] This category also provides a technical buffer zone that should limit the probability of misclassification of bacteria in susceptible or resistant categories.

Some strains of species that are naturally susceptible to an antibiotic may *acquire* resistance to the drug. This phenomenon commonly arises when populations of bacteria have grown in the presence of the antibiotic which selects mutant

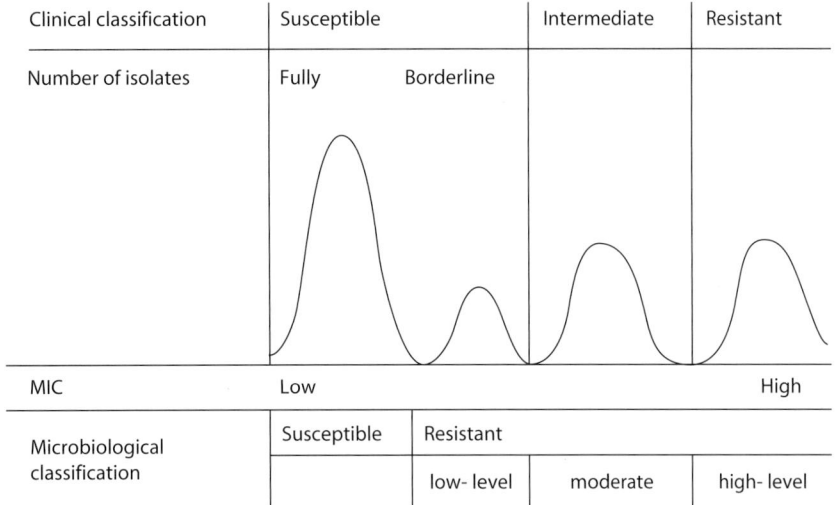

Clinical classification	Susceptible		Intermediate	Resistant
Number of isolates	Fully	Borderline		

MIC — Low ... High

Microbiological classification	Susceptible	Resistant		
		low-level	moderate	high-level

Fig. 3.1 Hypothetical distribution of MICs among clinical isolates of bacteria, classified clinically and microbiologically as susceptible or resistant. Adapted from European Committee for Antimicrobial Susceptibility Testing (EUCAST). Terminology relating to methods for the determination of susceptibility of bacteria to antimicrobial agents. **Clin Microbiol Infect.** 2000;6:503–508.[6]

strains that have increased their MIC by various adaptive mechanisms (*see below*). It may also result from horizontal gene transmission and acquisition of a resistance determinant, for example a β-lactamase, from a bacterial donor (*see below*). The range of MIC distribution of 'clinically susceptible' isolates of a given species may include 'microbiologically resistant' strains based on standard breakpoints, although revisions of breakpoints toward lower values have recently been made so as to minimize the probability of this occurring.[7] In such cases it is important to demonstrate that the isolates have an acquired resistance mechanism (*see below*) not present in others. This is particularly crucial if clinical studies demonstrate that such 'low-level resistant' strains are associated with an increased probability of treatment failure, as shown for bacteremia caused by *Escherichia coli* and *Klebsiella pneumoniae* strains producing extended-spectrum β-lactamase treated with cephalosporins.[8]

Unfortunately, definitions that relate clinical response to microbiological susceptibility are less useful than might be expected because of the many confounding factors that may be present in patients. These range from relative differences of drug susceptibility dependent on the inoculum size and physiological state of bacteria grown in logarithmic phase in vitro versus those of biofilm-associated, stationary phase bacteria at the infecting site, limited distribution or reduced activity of the antibiotic in the infected site due to low pH or high protein binding, competence of phagocytic and immune response to the pathogen, presence of foreign body or undrained collections, to misidentification of the infective agent and straightforward sampling or testing error.

From an early stage in the development of antibacterial agents it became clear that a knowledge of antibiotic pharmacokinetics and pharmacodynamics could be used to bolster the inadequate information gained from clinical use (*see* Ch. 4). It is assumed that if an antibiotic reaches a

concentration at the site of infection higher than the MIC for the infecting agent, the infection is likely to respond. Depending on the antibiotic class, maximal antibacterial activity, including the killing rate, may be related either to the peak drug concentration over MIC ratio (as with the aminoglycosides) or to the proportion of the time interval between two doses when concentration is above the MIC (as with the β-lactams). Assays of antibiotics in sites of infection are complex and serum assays have been widely used as a proxy, even though there may be substantial intra- and interindividual variation depending on the patient's pathophysiological conditions.

Different breakpoint committees have used different pharmacokinetic parameters in their correlations with pharmacodynamic characteristics. The approach of the CLSI has been based on wide consultation, and includes strong input from the antibiotic manufacturers. In Europe, EUCAST has harmonized antimicrobial MIC breakpoints and set those for new agents by consensus of professional experts from national committees. EUCAST clinical breakpoints are published together with supporting scientific rationale documentation.[4] Clearly, international consensus on susceptibility breakpoints is progressing, thereby reducing the confusion created by a given strain to be labeled antibiotic susceptible in some countries and resistant in others.

MECHANISMS OF RESISTANCE

For an antimicrobial agent to be effective against a given micro-organism, two conditions must be met: a vital target susceptible to a low concentration of the antibiotic must exist in the micro-organism, and the antibiotic must penetrate the bacterial envelope and reach the target in sufficient quantity.

There are six main mechanisms by which bacteria may circumvent the actions of antimicrobial agents:

- Specific enzymes may inactivate the drug before or after it enters the bacterial cell.
- The bacterial cell envelope may be modified so that it becomes less permeable to the antibiotic.
- The drug may be actively expelled from the cell by transmembrane efflux systems.
- The target may be modified so that it binds less avidly with the antibiotic.
- The target may be bypassed by acquisition of a novel metabolic pathway.
- The target may be protected by production of protein which prevents the antibiotic reaching it.

However, these resistance mechanisms do not exist in isolation, and two or more distinct mechanisms may interact to determine the actual level of resistance of a micro-organism to an antibiotic. Likewise, *multidrug resistance* is increasingly common in bacterial pathogens. It may be defined as resistance to two or more drugs or drug classes that are of therapeutic relevance. More recently, the terms *extensive drug resistance* and *pan-drug resistance* have been introduced to describe strains that have only very limited or no susceptibility to any approved and available antimicrobial agent.[9] Classically, *cross-resistance* is the term used for resistance to multiple drugs sharing the same mechanism of action or, more strictly, belonging to the same chemical class, whereas *co-resistance* describes resistance to multiple antibiotics associated with multiple mechanisms.

DRUG-MODIFYING ENZYMES

 ### β-LACTAMASES

The most important mechanism of resistance to β-lactam antibiotics is the production of specific enzymes (β-lactamases).[10] These diverse enzymes bind to β-lactam antibiotics and the cyclic amide bonds of the β-lactam rings are hydrolyzed. The open ring forms of β-lactams cannot bind to their target sites and thus have no antimicrobial activity. The ester linkage of the residual β-lactamase acylenzyme complex is readily hydrolyzed by water, regenerating the active enzyme. These enzymes have been classified based on functional and structural characteristics (*see* Table 15.1).[11]

Among Gram-positive cocci, the staphylococcal β-lactamases hydrolyze benzylpenicillin, ampicillin and related compounds, but are much less active against the antistaphylococcal penicillins and cephalosporins. Among Gram-negative bacilli the situation is complex, as these organisms produce many different β-lactamases with different spectra of activity. All β-lactam drugs, including the latest carbapenems, are degraded by some of these enzymes, many of which have recently evolved through stepwise mutations selected in patients treated with cephalosporins. Several of these β-lactamases are increasing in prevalence among Gram-negative pathogens in many parts of the world. The most widely dispersed are the group 2be extended-spectrum β-lactamases (ESBLs) that include those derived by mutational modifications from TEM and SHV enzymes as well as the CTX-M enzymes that originate from *Kluyvera* spp. ESBLs can hydrolyze most penicillins and all cephalosporins except the cephamycins. These enzymes are plasmid-mediated in Enterobacteriaceae, notably in *Esch. coli* isolates from both community and hospital settings, and *K. pneumoniae* strains from hospital epidemics in all continents.[12] Another group of problematic β-lactamases is the group 1, which includes both the AmpC type, chromosomal, inducible cephalosporinases in *Enterobacter*, *Serratia*, *Citrobacter* and *Pseudomonas aeruginosa* and similar plasmid-mediated enzymes that are now spreading among Enterobacteriaceae such as *Esch. coli* and *K. pneumoniae*.[13] Both hyperproduction of the chromosomal enzyme and high-copy number plasmid encoded enzymes are causing an increasing prevalence of resistance to all β-lactam drugs except some carbapenems (*see* Chs 13 and 15). A third group of β-lactamases of emerging importance is the group 3 metalloenzymes that can hydrolyze all β-lactam drugs except monobactams.[14] These β-lactamases, also called metallo-carbapenemases, include both diverse chromosomal enzymes found in aquatic bacteria such as *Stenotrophomonas maltophilia* and *Aeromonas hydrophila* and plasmid-mediated enzymes increasingly reported in clinical isolates of *Ps. aeruginosa*, *Acinetobacter* and Enterobacteriaceae in Asia, America and Europe.[4,14] A group of β-lactamases that now constitute a major threat to available drug treatments is the class A, group 2f carbapenemases, of which KPC enzymes produced by *K. pneumoniae* have become widespread in parts of the USA and Europe.[15] Likewise, many anaerobic bacteria also produce β-lactamases, and this is the major mechanism of β-lactam antibiotic resistance in this group. The classification and properties of β-lactamases are described more fully in Chapter 15.

 ## AMINOGLYCOSIDE-MODIFYING ENZYMES

Much of the resistance to aminoglycoside antibiotics observed in clinical isolates of Gram-negative bacilli and Gram-positive cocci is due to transferable plasmid-mediated enzymes that modify the amino groups or hydroxyl groups of the aminoglycoside molecule (*see* Ch. 12). The modified antibiotic molecules are unable to bind to the target protein in the ribosome. The genes encoding these enzymes are often transposable to the chromosome. These enzymes include many different types of acetyltransferases, phosphotransferases and nucleotidyl transferases, which vary greatly in their spectrum of activity and in the degree to which they inactivate different aminoglycosides (*see* Ch. 12).[16] Based on phylogenetic analysis, their origin is believed to be aminoglycoside-producing *Streptomyces* species. In recent years, the amikacin-modifying 6'-acetyltransferase tended to predominate and multidrug-resistant pathogens acquired multiple modifying enzymes, often combined with mechanisms of resistance such as decreased uptake and active efflux (*see below*), rendering them resistant to all of the available aminoglycosides.

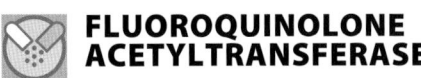
FLUOROQUINOLONE ACETYLTRANSFERASE

A plasmid-mediated mechanism of resistance to quinolones has been related to a unique allele of the aminoglycoside acetyltransferase gene designated as *aac*(6′)-*Ib*-cr. Two amino acid substitutions in the AAC(6′)-Ib-cr protein are associated with the capacity to *N*-acetylate ciprofloxacin at the amino nitrogen on its piperazinyl substituent, thereby increasing the MIC of ciprofloxacin and norfloxacin.[17]

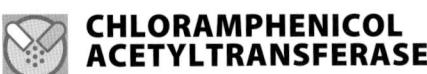
CHLORAMPHENICOL ACETYLTRANSFERASE

The major mechanism of resistance to chloramphenicol is the production of a chloramphenicol acetyltransferase which converts the drug to either the monoacetate or the diacetate. These derivatives are unable to bind to the bacterial 50S ribosomal subunit and thus cannot inhibit peptidyl transferase activity. The chloramphenicol acetyltransferase (CAT) gene is usually encoded on a plasmid or transposon and may transpose to the chromosome. Surprisingly, in view of the very limited use of chloramphenicol, resistance is not uncommon, even in *Esch. coli*, although it is most frequently seen in organisms that are multiresistant.

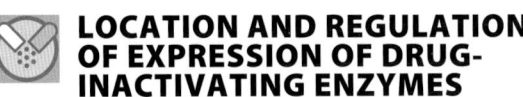
LOCATION AND REGULATION OF EXPRESSION OF DRUG-INACTIVATING ENZYMES

In Gram-positive bacteria β-lactam antibiotics enter the cell easily because of the permeable cell wall, and β-lactamase is released freely from the cell. In *Staphylococcus aureus*, resistance to benzylpenicillin is caused by the release of β-lactamase into the extracellular environment, where it reduces the concentration of the drug. This is a population phenomenon: a large inoculum of organisms is much more resistant than a small one. Furthermore, staphylococcal penicillinase is an inducible enzyme unless deletions or mutations in the regulatory genes lead to its constitutive expression.

In Gram-negative bacteria the outer membrane retards entry of penicillins and cephalosporins into the cell. The β-lactamase needs only to inactivate molecules of drug that penetrate within the periplasmic space between the cytoplasmic membrane and the cell wall. Each cell is thus responsible for its own protection – a more efficient mechanism than the external excretion of β-lactamase seen in Gram-positive bacteria. Enzymes are often produced constitutively (i.e. even when the antibiotic is not present) and a small inoculum of bacteria may be almost as resistant as a large one. A similar functional organization is exhibited by the aminoglycoside-modifying enzymes. These enzymes are located at the surface of the cytoplasmic membrane and only those molecules of aminoglycoside that are in the process of being transported across the membrane are modified.

ALTERATIONS TO THE PERMEABILITY OF THE BACTERIAL CELL ENVELOPE

The bacterial cell envelope consists of a capsule, a cell wall and a cytoplasmic membrane. This structure allows the passage of bacterial nutrients and excreted products, while acting as a barrier to harmful substances such as antibiotics. The capsule, composed mainly of polysaccharides, is not a major barrier to the passage of antibiotics. The Gram-positive cell wall is relatively thick but simple in structure, being made up of a network of cross-linked peptidoglycan complexed with teichoic and lipoteichoic acids. It is readily permeable to most antibiotics. The cell wall of Gram-negative bacteria is more complex, comprising an outer membrane of lipopolysaccharide, protein and phospholipid, attached to a thin layer of peptidoglycan. The lipopolysaccharide molecules cover the surface of the cell, with their hydrophilic portions pointing outwards. Their inner lipophilic regions interact with the fatty acid chains of the phospholipid monolayer of the inner surface of the outer membrane and are stabilized by divalent cation bridges. The phospholipid and lipopolysaccharide of the outer membrane form a classic lipid bilayer, which acts as a barrier to both hydrophobic and hydrophilic drug molecules. Natural permeability varies among different Gram-negative species and generally correlates with innate resistance. For example, the cell walls of *Neisseria* species and *Haemophilus influenzae* are more permeable than those of *Esch. coli*, while the walls of *Pseudomonas aeruginosa* and *Stenotrophomonas maltophilia* are markedly less permeable.

Hydrophobic antibiotics can enter the Gram-negative cell by direct solubilization through the lipid layer of the outer membrane, but the dense lipopolysaccharide cover may physically block this pathway. Changes in surface lipopolysaccharides may increase or decrease permeability resistance. However, most antibiotics are hydrophilic and cross through the outer membrane of Gram-negative cells via water-filled channels created by membrane proteins called porins. The rate of diffusion across these channels depends on size and physicochemical structure, small hydrophilic molecules with a zwitterionic charge showing the faster penetration. Some antimicrobial resistance in Gram-negative bacteria is due to reduced drug entry caused by decreased amounts of specific porin proteins, usually in combination with either overexpression of efflux pumps or β-lactamase production. This phenomenon is associated with significant β-lactam resistance, such as low-level resistance to imipenem in strains of *Ps. aeruginosa* and *Enterobacter* spp. that are hyperproducing chromosomal cephalosporinase and deficient in porins.[18,19] Porin-deficient mutant strains emerge sporadically during therapy and were thought to be unfit to spread. However, multidrug-resistant, porin-deficient strains of *Ps. aeruginosa* have caused nosocomial outbreaks.[20]

The target molecules of antibiotics that inhibit cell wall synthesis, such as the β-lactam antibiotics and the glycopeptides, are located outside the cytoplasmic membrane, and it is not necessary for these drugs to pass through this membrane to exert their effect. Most other antibiotics must cross the membrane to reach their intracellular sites of action. The cytoplasmic membrane is freely permeable to lipophilic agents such as minocycline, chloramphenicol, trimethoprim, fluoroquinolones and rifampicin (rifampin), but poses a significant barrier to hydrophilic agents such as aminoglycosides, erythromycin, clindamycin and the sulfonamides. These drugs are actively transported across the membrane by carrier proteins, and some resistances have been associated with various changes in these transporters. Resistance to aminoglycosides in both Gram-positive and Gram-negative bacteria may be mediated by defective uptake due to the mutational inactivation of proton motive force-driven cytoplasmic pump systems, a defect which is associated with slow growth rate and production of 'small colony variants'.

RESISTANCE DUE TO DRUG EFFLUX

Single drug and multidrug efflux pumps have been recognized to be ubiquitous systems in micro-organisms, and have been found in all bacterial genomes.[21] These systems are involved in the natural resistance phenotype of many bacteria. Furthermore, they may produce clinically significant acquired resistance by mutational modification of the structural gene, overexpression due to mutation in regulatory genes or horizontal transfer of genetic elements. Most of the bacterial efflux pumps belong to the class of secondary transporters

that mediate the extrusion of toxic compounds from the cytoplasm in a coupled exchange with protons.

Multidrug pumps can be subdivided into several superfamilies, including the major facilitator superfamily (MFS), small multidrug-resistance family (SMR), resistance-nodulation-cell division family (RND) and multidrug and toxic compound extrusion family (MATE) (Table 3.1). RND and MATE systems appear to function as detoxifying systems and transport heavy metals, solvents, detergents and bile salts, whereas MFS pumps are closely related to specific efflux pumps and appear to function as major Na^+/H^+ transporters. MFS and SMR pumps are mostly found in Gram-positive bacteria, whereas RND pumps are mostly found in Gram-negative bacteria, in which they function in association with special outer membrane channel proteins and periplasmic membrane fusion proteins, forming a tripartite transport system spanning both the inner and outer membranes (Table 3.1 and Figure 3.2). This allows the pumps to expel their substrates directly from the inner membrane or cytoplasm into the extracellular space. Although these pumps confer resistance mostly to a range of lipophilic and amphiphilic drugs (including β-lactams, fluoroquinolones, tetracyclines, macrolides and chloramphenicol) some pumps, such as MexY of Ps. aeruginosa, also transport aminoglycosides.

Among the best studied systems are the AcrB system of Esch. coli and the MexB system of Ps. aeruginosa. The AcrB pump is controlled by the Mar regulon, which is widespread among enteric bacteria. The MarA global activator, which can be derepressed by tetracycline or chloramphenicol, simultaneously upregulates the AcrAB-TolC transport complex and downregulates the synthesis of the larger porin OmpF, thereby acting in a synergistic manner to block the drug penetration

Table 3.1   Selected multidrug efflux systems determining multiple antibiotic resistance in pathogenic and commensal bacteria

Transporter		Associated proteins				
Class	Pump	Periplasmic	OM Channel	Regulator(s)	Organism	Antibiotic resistance profile
MFS	NorA	–	–	–	Staphylococcus aureus	Fluoroquinolones, chloramphenicol
MATE	NorM	–	–	–	Vibrio parahaemolyticus	Fluoroquinolones, aminoglycosides
RND	AcrB	AcrA	TolC	AcrR, MarA	Escherichia coli	β-Lactams, tetracyclines, macrolides, fluoroquinolones, chloramphenicol
RND	MexB	MexA	OprM	MexR	Pseudomonas aeruginosa	β-Lactams, tetracyclines, macrolides, fluoroquinolones, chloramphenicol
RND	MexD	MexC	OprJ	MexS	Ps. aeruginosa	Group 6 cephalosporins, tetracyclines, fluoroquinolones, chloramphenicol
RND	MexF	MexE	OprN	MexT	Ps. aeruginosa	Fluoroquinolones, chloramphenicol
RND	MexY	MexX	OprM	MexZ	Ps. aeruginosa	Macrolides, tetracyclines, aminoglycosides
RND	MtrD	MtrC	MtrE	MtrR	Neisseria gonorrhoeae	β-Lactams, macrolides, tetracyclines, chloramphenicol

MATE, multiple drug and toxic compound extrusion; MFS, major facilitator superfamily; OM, outer membrane; RND, resistance-nodulation-cell division.
Adapted from Nikaido & Zgwiskaya.[21]

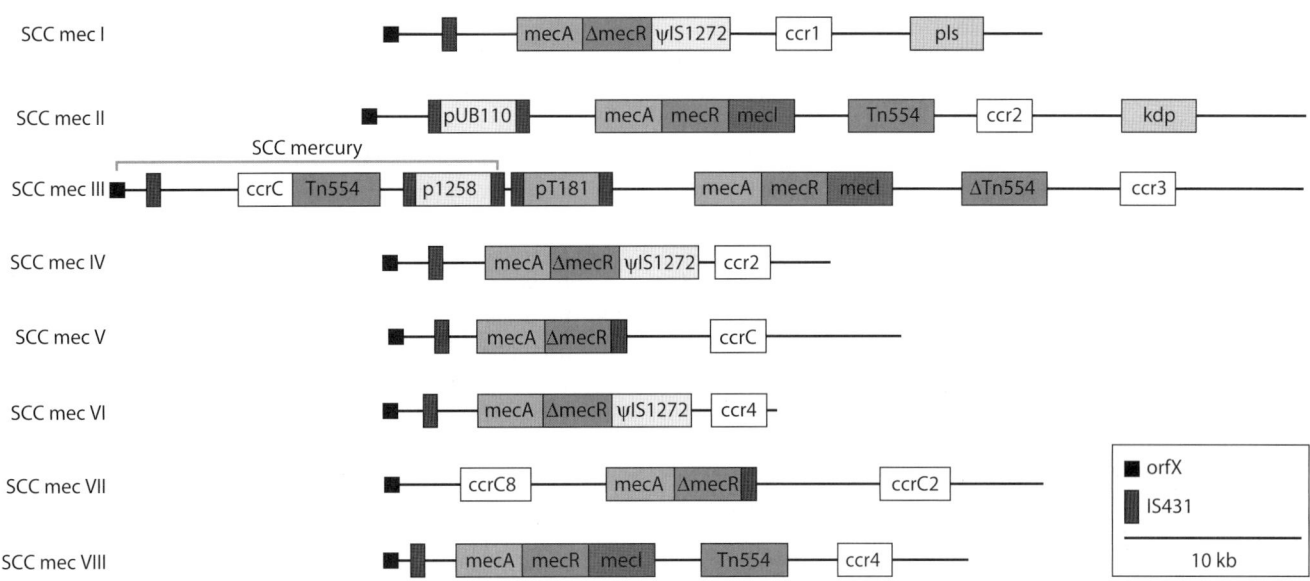

Fig. 3.2 Structure of different types of staphylococcal chromosome cassette (SCC) *mec* described in *Staphylococcus aureus.*

into the cell. Constitutive overexpression of AcrAB is present in most ciprofloxacin-resistant *Esch. coli* clinical isolates.[22] In *Ps. aeruginosa*, overexpression of the MexAB-OprM transport complex occurs commonly during β-lactam therapy by selection of mutants with altered specific repressor gene *mexR*. This increased efflux determines resistance to fluoroquinolones, penicillins, cephalosporins and meropenem. Another cause for concern is the selection of multidrug pumps by disinfectants such as triclosan, which is increasingly used in housekeeping products.

Active efflux of the drug from the bacterial cell is one of the major resistance mechanisms to tetracyclines, the second being 30S ribosome protection by elongation factor G-like proteins.[23] Efflux can be mediated either by tetracycline-specific efflux pumps or by multidrug transporter systems. Specific pumps of the TetA-E and TetG-H families are widespread in Gram-negative bacteria, whereas the specific pumps TetK and TetL are common in Gram-positive bacteria. These determinants are often encoded by genes located on plasmids or transposons. These specific pumps are single proteins located on the inner membrane that export the drug into the periplasm, in contrast with multidrug transporter systems that extrude tetracyclines from the cytoplasm directly outside the cell.

Specific efflux proteins have been shown to play a major role in macrolide resistance, including the Mef(A) transporters of the MFS that determine resistance to 14-C macrolides in pneumococci, β-hemolytic and oral streptococci and enterococci, and the Msr(A) ATP-binding transporters that confer resistance to erythromycin and streptogramin B in staphylococci.[24] The *mef* genes are located on conjugative elements that readily transfer across Gram-positive genera and species.

Finally, a plasmid-mediated QepA efflux pump belonging to the MFS transporters was recently shown to be capable of extruding hydrophilic fluoroquinolones and conferring low-level resistance to these drugs.[25]

RESISTANCE DUE TO ALTERATIONS IN TARGET MOLECULES

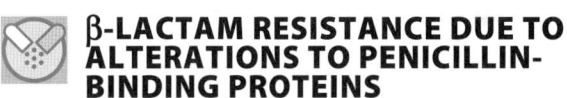 β-LACTAM RESISTANCE DUE TO ALTERATIONS TO PENICILLIN-BINDING PROTEINS

These proteins are associated with the bacterial cell envelope and are the target sites for β-lactam antibiotics. Each bacterial cell has several penicillin-binding proteins (PBPs), which vary with the species. PBPs are transpeptidases, carboxypeptidases and endopeptidases that are required for cell-wall synthesis and remodeling during growth and septation. Some, but not all, PBPs are essential for cell survival (*see* Ch. 2). PBPs are related to β-lactamases, which also bind β-lactam antibiotics. However, unlike β-lactamases, PBPs form stable complexes with β-lactams and are themselves inactivated. β-Lactam antibiotics thus inactivate PBPs, preventing proper cell growth and division, and producing cell-wall defects that lead to death by osmolysis. Alterations in PBPs, leading to decreased binding affinity with β-lactam antibiotics, are important causes of β-lactam resistance in a number of species, most commonly Gram-positive bacteria.

Penicillin-resistant strains of *Streptococcus pneumoniae* produce one or more altered PBPs that have reduced ability to bind penicillin. Stepwise acquisition of multiple changes in the genes encoding these PBPs produce various levels of penicillin resistance.[26] The genetic sequences encoding normal PBPs in sensitive strains of *Str. pneumoniae* are highly conserved; the genes in resistant strains are said to be 'mosaics' since they consist of blocks of conserved sequences interspersed with blocks of variant sequences. As more variant blocks are introduced into the mosaic, the more penicillin resistant the recipient strain tends to become. These gene sequences have probably been derived by transformation from oral streptococcal species such as *Str. mitis* and *Str. oralis*.[27] Whereas high-level resistance to penicillin involves changes in at least PBP 1a, PBP 2x and PBP 2a that require multiple transformation events, resistance to group 4 cephalosporins (*see* Ch. 13) can result from a single transformation event through co-transformation of the closely linked genes encoding PBP 1a and PBP 2x.

The relative penicillin resistance of enterococci is due to the normal production of PBPs with low binding affinity. The higher levels of penicillin and ampicillin resistance often seen in *Enterococcus faecium* are the result of overexpression of PBP 5 (which exhibits a lower affinity for penicillin than other PBPs), which can be further decreased by point mutations in the very high level resistant strains. Other species showing β-lactam resistance due to altered PBPs include group B *Streptococcus*, *Neisseria gonorrhoeae*, *N. meningitidis* and *Haemophilus influenzae*. The genes encoding altered PBPs in both *Neisseria* species appear to be mosaics, and the variant blocks may have been derived from *N. flavescens* and other commensal *Neisseria*.

Methicillin resistance in *Staph. aureus* and in coagulase-negative staphylococci is caused by an acquired chromosomal gene (*mecA*) which results in the synthesis of a fifth penicillin-binding protein (PBP 2a), with decreased affinity for methicillin and other β-lactam agents, in addition to the intrinsic PBP 1 to 4.[28] Many methicillin-resistant *Staph. aureus* (MRSA) strains exhibit heterogeneity in the expression of resistance, with only a small proportion of the total cell population expressing high-level resistance. The proportion of resistant cells is dependent on environmental conditions such as temperature and osmolality. This phenomenon is related to the presence of the regulatory loci *mecI* and *mecR1* upstream of *mecA*, which exhibit significant sequence and functional homology with the β-lactamase regulators *blaI-blaR1*. Deletion of these elements produces homogeneous expression of methicillin resistance. The *mecA* gene is located on an antibiotic resistance island, called the staphylococcal cassette chromosome *mec* (SCC*mec*), a mobile element driven by site-specific recombinases.[29]

GLYCOPEPTIDE RESISTANCE DUE TO METABOLIC BYPASS

Glycopeptides are large hexapeptides that inhibit bacterial peptidoglycan synthesis by binding the carboxy-terminal D-alanyl-D-alanine dipeptide residue of the muramyl pentapeptide precursor, thereby blocking access to three key steps in the peptidoglycan polymerization: transglycosylation, transpeptidation and carboxypeptidation (*see* Ch. 2). Most clinically important Gram-positive bacteria build their peptidoglycan from this conserved pentapeptide precursor and are naturally sensitive to the glycopeptides vancomycin and teicoplanin. Acquired glycopeptide resistance was described in enterococci in 1986 and in coagulase-negative staphylococci in 1987. Decreased susceptibility and resistance to

vancomycin were reported in *Staph. aureus* in 1997 and 2003, respectively.

In enterococci, seven different glycopeptide resistance genotypes are now recognized:[30]

1. VanA, inducible high-level transferable resistance to both vancomycin and teicoplanin; usually seen in *E. faecium*, sometimes in *E. faecalis* and rarely in *E. avium*, *E. hirae*, *E. casseliflavus*, *E. mundtii* and *E. durans*.
2. VanB, inducible low-level transferable resistance, usually to vancomycin alone; found in *E. faecium*, sometimes in *E. faecalis*.
3. VanC, constitutive low-level vancomycin resistance, seen in *E. gallinarum*, *E. casseliflavus* and *E. flavescens*.
4. VanD, constitutive or inducible moderate-level resistance, usually to vancomycin alone; rarely acquired in *E. faecium*.
5–7. VanE, VanG and VanL, low-level resistance to vancomycin alone; rarely acquired in *E. faecalis*.

Enterococcal resistance to glycopeptides is due to multienzymatic metabolic bypass, mediated by replacement of the normal D-alanyl-D-alanine termini of peptidoglycan precursors by abnormal precursors with D-alanyl-D-lactate, or D-alanyl-D-serine termini, none of which can bind glycopeptides. The *vanA* gene cluster is carried by a 10.8 kb transposon (Tn*1546*) that contains nine functionally related genes encoding mobilization of the element (resolvase and transposase) and coordinated replacement of muramyl pentapeptides.[30] The *vanA* gene encodes an abnormal D-alanine-D-alanine ligase that synthesizes the D-alanine-D-lactate dipeptide. The *vanH* gene codes for a dehydrogenase that generates D-lactate. The *vanX* and *vanY* genes encode two enzymes that hydrolyze normal precursors: VanX, a D, D-dipeptidase that hydrolyzes D-alanyl-D-alanine dipeptides and VanY, a D, D-carboxypeptidase that cleaves terminal alanine from normal precursors. The *vanR* and *vanS* genes regulate the expression of the *vanHAX* operon through a two-component sensor system for glycopeptides. The *vanB* gene cluster has a similar organization, albeit with more heterogeneity, and is located on a large conjugative transposon (Tn*1547*) that is usually integrated in the chromosome and occasionally plasmid borne.

Over the past decade, the prevalence of glycopeptide resistance has increased markedly in clinical isolates of enterococci, particularly *E. faecium*, as a result of nosocomial spread of transposons, plasmids and multiresistant clones. In the USA, the *vanA* and *vanB* genotypes are widespread in many hospitals and frequently cause nosocomial infection but are rarely found in the community. In Europe, the *vanA* genotype was initially predominant in the healthy population and in farm animals due to the widespread use of avoparcin (a glycopeptide related to vancomycin) as a growth promoter between 1970 and 1998. The *vanA* gene cluster has been transferred experimentally to other Gram-positive bacteria where it is expressed.[31] It has been found in clinical isolates of *Staph. aureus*, *Bacillus circulans*, *Oerskovia turbata*, and *Arcanobacterium haemolyticum*.

Glycopeptide resistance in *Staph. aureus* could be classified into low-level and high-level resistance. Since their first description in 1997 from Japan,[32] vancomycin-intermediate *Staph. aureus* (VISA) isolates have been reported worldwide.[30,33] These isolates were recovered in chronically ill patients failing prolonged glycopeptide therapy of infections with indwelling devices or undrained collections. In addition to VISA, other strains, named hetero-VISA, appear to be susceptible to vancomycin (MIC <4 mg/L) but exhibit low-level subpopulations (10^{-6} cells) able to grow at concentrations of 4–8 mg/L. Those strains could represent first-step mutants that develop into VISA strains under selective pressure. Recently, the CLSI lowered vancomycin breakpoints for staphylococci and many of these hetero-VISA isolates would now be accordingly reclassified as VISA.

Low-level resistance to glycopeptides in VISA strains has been associated with stepwise mutations in several loci, including global regulator systems, such as *agr*, *vra* and *gra*, and genes encoding proteins of the cell wall and membrane biosynthesis pathways.[30] Phenotypic abnormalities reported in VISA strains include increased cell-wall thickness, reduced autolytic activity, increased production of glutamine non-amidated muropeptides and D-Ala-D-Ala residues, and reduced peptidoglycan cross-linking.[33] These abnormalities suggest that the increased production of dipeptides acts as false targets which trap the antibiotic away from its lethal target site of cell-wall synthesis adjacent to the membrane. In addition, VISA strains show decreased susceptibility to daptomycin, despite its different mechanisms of action.

The experimental transfer of the *vanA* operon from *E. faecalis* to *Staph. aureus* by conjugation was reported in 1992. In 2002, the first clinical vancomycin-resistant *Staph. aureus* (VRSA) strain was isolated in the USA.[34] Since then, eight other cases have been confirmed in the USA.[34] All isolates carried the *vanA* gene on Tn*1546*-like elements integrated into staphylococcal plasmids and had an MIC to vancomycin ranging from 32 to 1024 mg/L. All patients with VRSA had a history of MRSA and vancomycin-resistant enterococci (VRE) co-colonization or infection; underlying conditions included chronic skin ulcers, diabetes, chronic renal failure and obesity.[35] Most had received vancomycin. No secondary transmission was observed after implementation of infection control measures.[35]

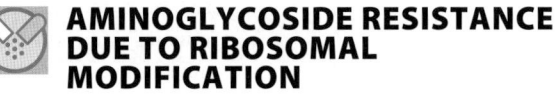

AMINOGLYCOSIDE RESISTANCE DUE TO RIBOSOMAL MODIFICATION

Aminoglycoside resistance may be produced by alterations in specific ribosomal binding proteins or ribosomal RNA, although this is still uncommon in clinical isolates. Recently, plasmid-mediated 16S rRNA methylases that exert methylation of the G1405 residue of 16S rRNA have been reported to confer broad aminoglycoside co-resistance in Gram-negative bacilli due to loss of affinity for these drugs.[36] These determinants, especially ArmA, are commonly found in association with CTX-M ESBL production.

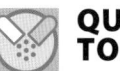

QUINOLONE RESISTANCE DUE TO ALTERED TOPOISOMERASES

The main targets for quinolones are the type II topoisomerase DNA gyrase and type IV topoisomerase, both of which are essential enzymes involved in chromosomal DNA replication and segregation (*see* Ch. 2). Fluoroquinolones exert their bactericidal action by trapping topoisomerase–DNA complexes, thereby blocking the replication fork. Both of these structurally related target enzymes are tetrameric. DNA gyrase is composed of two pairs of GyrA and GyrB subunits while topoisomerase type IV is composed of two pairs of the homologous ParC and ParE subunits.

Bacterial resistance to fluoroquinolones is generally mediated by chromosomal mutations leading either to reduced affinity of DNA gyrase and/or topoisomerase IV, or to overexpression of endogenous MDR efflux systems (*see above*).[37] Plasmid-mediated resistance was first reported in *K. pneumoniae*.[38] The commonest target-resistance modifications arise from spontaneous mutations, occurring at a frequency of 1 in 10^6 to 1 in 10^9 cells, that substitute amino acids in specific domains of GyrA and ParC subunits and less frequently in GyrB and ParE. These regions of the enzymes, called the quinolone resistance-determining regions, either contain the active site, a tyrosine that covalently binds to DNA, or constitute parts of quinolone binding sites.

Fluoroquinolones have different potencies of antibacterial activity against different bacteria, a variance which is to a large part related to the different potency against their enzyme targets. The more sensitive of the two enzymes is the primary target. In general, DNA gyrase is the primary target in Gram-negative bacteria and topoisomerase IV is the primary target in Gram-positive bacteria. Resistance develops progressively by stepwise mutations. The first step in increasing resistance level results from amino acid change in the primary target and is followed by second-step mutational modifications of amino acid in the secondary target. The higher the difference in drug potency against the two enzymes, the higher the MIC increase provided by first-step mutation. Fluoroquinolones with a low therapeutic index (defined as the drug concentration at the infected site divided by the MIC of that drug) are more likely to select first-step mutants. This explains why resistance to quinolones has emerged rapidly after the introduction of ciprofloxacin and ofloxacin for human therapeutics in two species, *Ps. aeruginosa* and *Staph. aureus*, which develop significant resistance after only a single mutation in *gyrA*. In *Staph. aureus*, fluoroquinolone resistance quickly became associated with methicillin resistance. This was the consequence of two factors: increased likelihood of exposure of multiresistant strains to therapy with these drugs, leading to multiple mutations and high-level resistance; and the further selective advantage for nosocomial spread conferred by this resistance.[39] In organisms in which multiple mutational changes are required to reach clinical resistance to these drugs, such as *Esch. coli*, *Campylobacter jejuni* and *N. gonorrhoeae*, it appeared later and was accelerated by other epidemiological factors. For *C. jejuni*, this was related to the massive use of the cross-selecting fluoroquinolone enrofloxacin in the poultry industry followed by food-borne transmission to humans.[40] For *N. gonorrhoeae*, the emergence of fluoroquinolone resistance was soon followed by outbreaks of person-to-person transmission.

MLS AND LINEZOLID RESISTANCE DUE TO RIBOSOMAL MODIFICATION

Macrolides inhibit protein synthesis by dissociation of the peptidyl-tRNA molecule from the 50S ribosomal subunit. Macrolides bind to a ribosomal site that overlaps with the binding site of the structurally unrelated lincosamide and streptogramin B antibiotics. The most common type of acquired resistance to erythromycin and clindamycin (and other macrolides and lincosamides) is seen in streptococci, enterococci and staphylococci, and is called macrolide–lincosamide–streptogramin B (MLS$_B$) resistance. This is due to the production of enzymes that methylate a specific adenine residue in 23S rRNA, resulting in reduced ribosomal binding of the three antibiotic classes.[24] Low concentrations of erythromycin induce resistance to all the macrolides and lincosamides (so-called 'dissociated' resistance), but some strains may produce the methylase constitutively following mutations or deletions in the regulatory genes. More than 20 *erm* genes encode MLS$_B$ resistance. Most are located on conjugative and non-conjugative transposons that predominantly insert in the chromosome and are occasionally plasmid borne. They are frequently associated with other resistance genes, particularly those encoding tetracycline resistance by ribosomal protection. Increased use of macrolides has been related to spread of MLS$_B$ resistance in group A β-hemolytic streptococci and pneumococci.[41]

Linezolid is an oxazolidinone which acts on Gram-positive bacteria by ribosome inhibition following fixation on a 23S rRNA residue which is specific to the attachment of *N*-formylmethionyl transfer RNA (fMet-tRNA). In staphylococci, linezolid resistance can be mediated by mutations of the target 23S rRNA gene or by horizontal acquisition of the *cfr* gene which encodes an rRNA methyltransferase. Mutations in the domain V region of 23S rDNA, particularly G2447T, T2500A and G2576T, have been associated with resistance to linezolid.[42] The level of linezolid resistance correlates with the number of 23S rRNA genes carrying the point mutations. The *cfr* gene encodes for a 23S rRNA methyltransferase which confers cross-resistance to oxazolidinones, lincosamides, streptogramin A, phenicols and pleuromutilins but not to macrolides. This enzyme involves methylation of 23S rRNA at position A2503.[43] The *cfr* gene is carried on plasmids in *Staph. aureus* and coagulase-negative staphylococci (CNS). In enterococci, linezolid resistance is conferred by mutation of the domain V region (mutation G2576T) of 23S rRNA.

In bacteria with a low copy number of ribosomal operons, such as the mycobacteria and *C. jejuni* and *Helicobacter pylori*, macrolide resistance is commonly caused by mutational modification of the 23S rRNA peptidyl transferase region at the same adenine that is modified by *erm* methylases or adjacent nucleotides (A2057 to A2059). In most other bacteria, such mutations are recessive due to multicopy rRNA genes.

RIFAMPICIN (RIFAMPIN) RESISTANCE DUE TO MODIFICATION OF RNA POLYMERASE

Rifampicin resistance is commonly the result of a mutation that alters the β-subunit of RNA polymerase, reducing its binding affinity for rifampicin. Mutation usually produces high-level resistance in a single step, but intermediate resistance is sometimes seen. Mutational resistance occurs relatively frequently, and for this reason rifampicin is combined with other agents for the treatment of tuberculosis and staphylococcal infection. Meningococcal carriers treated with rifampicin alone have readily shown the emergence of rifampicin resistance.

MUPIROCIN RESISTANCE DUE TO METABOLIC BYPASS

Mupirocin (pseudomonic acid) is widely used for topical treatment of Gram-positive skin infections and the clearance of nasal carriers of methicillin-sensitive and methicillin-resistant *Staph. aureus*. It acts by inhibiting bacterial isoleucyl-tRNA synthetase, and resistance is mediated by the production of modified enzymes. Isolates showing low-level resistance have a single chromosomally encoded synthetase modified by point mutation, while those with high-level resistance have a second enzyme that cannot bind the drug and is encoded on a transferable plasmid.[44]

SULFONAMIDE AND TRIMETHOPRIM RESISTANCE DUE TO METABOLIC BYPASS

Acquired sulfonamide resistance is usually due to the production of an altered dihydropteroate synthetase that has reduced affinity for sulfonamides. Resistance is encoded on transferable plasmids and associated with transposons. Trimethoprim resistance occurs much less commonly. It is usually due to plasmid-mediated synthesis of new dihydrofolate reductases, which are much less susceptible to trimethoprim than the natural ones. The resistance genes are again associated with transposons.

FUSIDIC ACID RESISTANCE DUE TO MODIFICATION OF ELONGATION FACTOR G

Fusidic acid acts by inhibiting protein synthesis by interfering with ribosome translation. Mutation alteration of the target molecule, the elongation factor G (EF-G), confers resistance by decreasing the affinity of fusidic acid to its target.[45] This occurs at high frequency in *Staph. aureus* in vitro, and therefore it is recommended that fusidic acid should not be used alone to treat staphylococcal infections. Resistance to fusidic acid can also result from the horizontal acquisition of the *fusB* gene which encodes an EF-G binding protein that protects the translation from inhibition by fusidic acid.[45]

FAILURE TO METABOLIZE THE DRUG TO THE ACTIVE FORM

Both metronidazole and nitrofurantoin must be converted to an active form within the bacterium before they can have any effect. Resistance arises if the pathogen cannot effect this conversion. Aerobic organisms cannot reduce metronidazole to its active form and are therefore inherently resistant, but resistance in anaerobic organisms is very uncommon. Resistant strains of *Bacteroides fragilis* that have been investigated have reduced levels of pyruvate dehydrogenase; the enzyme necessary for the reduction of metronidazole to the active intermediate. Nitrofurantoin must be reduced to an active intermediate by nicotinamide adenine dinucleotide (NADH) or nicotinamide adenine dinucleotide phosphate (NADPH) reductases. Resistance to nitrofurans is uncommon, since such strains must lose more than one reductase to become resistant.

TARGET PROTECTION

In 1998, the plasmid-encoded Qnr protein was discovered in *K. pneumoniae* and shown to increase fluoroquinolone MICs eight-fold to 64-fold below the level of the clinical resistance breakpoint.[38] Since then, four types of *qnr* gene have been described: *qnrA* (six variants), *qnrB* (19 variants), *qnrC* and *qnrD* (one variant each), and *qnrS* (three variants). Qnr proteins are capable of binding and protecting DNA gyrase and type IV topoisomerase from quinolone inhibition. They show a global distribution across a variety of plasmids and bacterial genera. Recent homology data suggest that they have originated from environmental bacteria.[46] Their prevalence is unknown but can exceed 20% among ESBL-producing Enterobacteriaceae, mostly in association with CTX-M and CMY enzymes.[17]

GENETIC BASIS OF RESISTANCE

INTRINSIC RESISTANCE

Resistance of bacteria to antimicrobial agents may be intrinsic or acquired. Intrinsic resistance to some antibiotics is the natural resistance possessed by most strains of a bacterial species and is part of their genetic make-up, encoded on the chromosome. Intrinsic multiresistance is characteristic of free-living organisms, which may have evolved because of metabolic polyvalence and exposure to natural antibiotics and other toxic compounds in the environment. Multiresistance is due mostly to decreased antibiotic uptake by highly selective outer membrane porins and multiple efflux systems. Although these organisms have low virulence, their multiresistance allows them to persist in hospital environments and cause nosocomial infections. An example of a free-living opportunistic pathogen with a high degree of intrinsic resistance is *Ps. aeruginosa*.

MUTATIONAL RESISTANCE

Acquired resistance may be due to mutations affecting genes on the bacterial chromosome, to acquisition of mobile foreign genes or to mutation in acquired mobile genes. Mutations usually involve deletion, substitution or addition of one or a few base pairs, causing substitution of one or a few amino acids in a crucial peptide. Mutational resistance can affect the structural gene coding for the antibiotic target. This usually results in a gene product with reduced affinity for the antibiotic. An example is fluoroquinolone resistance from alterations in DNA topoisomerases. Mutational resistance can also involve regulatory loci, leading to overproduction of detoxifying systems such as the multiple resistance expressed by the MexAB-OprD efflux pump overproducing mutants of *Ps. aeruginosa*.

Although the basal rate of mutation is low in bacterial genomes, it is not constant but varies by a factor of 10 000 according to a number of intrinsic and external factors.[5] Among these factors are the sequence of the gene, with some hypermutable loci associated with short tandem repeats that are prone to deletions and duplications by slipped-strand mispairing; the mutator phenotype associated with a defective mismatch repair system; and stress-induced mutagenesis, including exposure to antibiotics and host defenses. Once a resistant mutant has been selected during exposure to the antibiotic, it usually shows a decreased fitness for competing with the wild-type ancestor, defined as the competitive efficiency of multiplication in the absence of the antibiotic. This deficiency is called the biological cost of resistance. It has been observed, however, that this reduction in fitness may be compensated by secondary mutations in other chromosomal loci, thereby ensuring the persistence of the mutant. The probability that antibiotic treatment will select a resistant mutant depends on a complex network of factors including the drug, its concentration, the organism, its resistance mutation rate, inoculum size, physiological state and structure of the bacterial population.[47]

TRANSFERABLE RESISTANCE

Horizontal spread of a resistance gene from organism to organism occurs by conjugation (intercellular passage of plasmid or transposon), transduction (DNA transfer via bacteriophage) or transformation (uptake of naked DNA). The acquisition of resistance by transduction is rare in nature (the most important example is the transfer of the penicillinase plasmid in *Staph. aureus*). Transformation of resistance factors is an important mechanism in the few bacterial species that are readily transformable during part of their life cycle and are said to be naturally competent. These organisms, which include *Str. pneumoniae, H. influenzae, Helicobacter, Acinetobacter, Neisseria* and *Moraxella* spp., show extensive genetic variation resulting from natural transformation. They may also acquire chromosomally encoded antimicrobial resistance. Examples, as discussed above, include penicillin- or ampicillin-resistant *Str. pneumoniae* and *N. meningitidis* that acquired mosaic genes for the production of altered PBPs by transformation and site-specific recombination from phylogenetically related, co-resident commensal bacteria.

PLASMIDS

These are molecules of DNA that replicate independently from the bacterial chromosome. 'R-plasmids' carry one or more genetic determinants for drug resistance. This type of resistance is due to a dominant gene, usually one resulting in production of a drug-inactivating or drug-modifying enzyme.

Conjugation is the most common method of resistance transfer in clinically important bacteria.[48] Conjugative plasmids, which are capable of self-transmission to other bacterial hosts, are common in Gram-negative enteric bacilli, whereas non-conjugative plasmids are common in Gram-positive cocci, *H. influenzae, N. gonorrhoeae* and *Bacillus fragilis*. Non-conjugative plasmids can transfer to other bacteria if they are mobilized by conjugative plasmids present in the same cell, or by transduction or transformation. Large plasmids are usually present at one or two copies per cell, and their replication is closely linked to replication of the bacterial chromosome. Small plasmids may be present at more than 30 copies per cell, and their distribution to progeny during cell division is ensured by the large number present.

Plasmids tend to have a restricted host range: for example, those from Gram-negative bacteria cannot generally transfer to or maintain themselves in Gram-positive organisms, and vice versa. Conjugative transfer of plasmids has been observed, however, between these distant bacterial groups and even between bacteria and eukaryotic cells such as yeasts.

TRANSPOSONS

These are discrete sequences of DNA, capable of translocation from one replicon (plasmid or chromosome) to another – hence the epithet 'jumping gene'. They may encode genes for resistance to a wide variety of antibiotics, as well as many other metabolic properties. They are circular segments of double-stranded DNA, 4–25 kb in length, and usually consist of a functional central region flanked by long terminal repeats, usually inverted repeats. Complex transposons also carry genes for the transposition enzymes transposase and resolvase and their repressors. They need not share extensive regions of homology with the replicon into which they insert, as is required in classic genetic recombination. Depending upon the transposon involved, they may transpose into a replicon randomly or into favored sites, and they may insert at only a few or at many different places.

A special type of element, called a conjugative transposon, can transfer directly between the chromosome of one strain to the chromosome of another without a plasmid intermediate. Antibiotics can function as pheromones that are capable of inducing conjugation of conjugative transposons that in turn mobilize the transfer of co-resident R-plasmids. These transposons are less restrictive than plasmids in the host range. A well-studied example is Tn*416*, which has spread the *tetM* gene from Gram-positive cocci to diverse bacteria such as *Neisseria, Mycoplasma* and *Clostridium*.[49]

Other important genetic elements by which transposons and plasmids acquire multiple antibiotic resistance determinants are called integrons. These are site-specific recombination systems that recognize and capture antibiotic resistance gene cassettes in a high-efficiency expression site.[48,50] The structure of class 1 integrons (Figure 3.3) includes an integrase gene (*int*), an adjacent integration site (*att1*) that can contain one or more gene cassettes, and one or more promoters. Class 1 integrons, the most frequently observed type, also contain a 3′ conserved segment that includes the genes encoding resistance to quaternary ammonium compounds (*qacEΔ*) and sulfonamides (*sul1*). The integrase is capable of excision and integration of up to five gene cassettes, each of which is associated with a related 59 bp palindromic element that acts as a recombination hotspot. Gene cassettes include determinants of β-lactamases, aminoglycoside-modifying enzymes, chloramphenicol acetyltransferase and trimethoprim-resistant DFR enzymes. Integrons are widespread among antibiotic-resistant clinical isolates of diverse Gram-negative species and have also been reported in Gram-positive bacteria. The genetic linkage of resistance to sulfonamides and to newer antibiotics in these integrons may explain the persistence of sulfonamide resistance in *Esch. coli* in spite of a huge decrease in sulfonamide use.[51] Likewise, mercury released from dental amalgams has been suggest to select for antibiotic resistance in the oral and intestinal flora of humans because of the physical linkage between integron

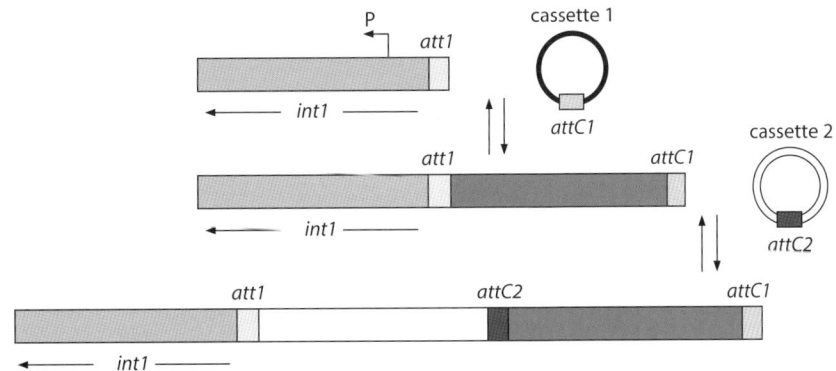

Fig. 3.3 Integron structure and gene cassette movement. The *int1* gene encodes the integrase that mediates site-specific integration of circular gene cassettes between the *att1* and *attC* sites. P denotes the common promoter. Adapted from Ploy MC, Lambert T, Couty JP et al. Integrons: an antibiotic resistance gene capture and expression system. **Clin Chem Lab Med.** 2000;38:483–487.[50]

and mercury resistance in the ubiquitous Tn*21*-like transposons.[52] Clearly, transposons and integrons are responsible for much of the diversity observed among plasmids, and play a major role in the evolution and dissemination of antibiotic resistance among bacteria.[49,52]

STAPHYLOCOCCAL CASSETTE CHROMOSOME

Staphylococcal cassette chromosome (SCC) elements are always inserted in one copy into a specific region of the *Staph. aureus* genome, the attBssc at the 3′ end of the *orfX* gene, near the origin of replication. They carry recombinase (*ccr*) genes that catalyze excision and integration of the element. The mechanism of horizontal transfer of SCC elements between staphylococci is unknown. The SCC elements may encode antibiotic resistance genes such as the SCC*mec* and SCC*far* for methicillin and fusidic acid resistance, respectively.

The SCC*mec* elements have been grouped into types I–VIII, which range in size from 20.9 kb to 66.9 kb (Figure 3.2)[53,54] They are classified according to the combination of *ccr* genes and *mec* complex that they carry. Five major *mec* complexes (A–E) have been described but only three (A–C) have been identified in *Staph. aureus*. The *mec* complexes differ by integration of IS*1272* and IS*431* elements and by deletion of *mecI* and a part of *mecR*. The *ccr* genes are classified into five allotypes which have been designated ccrAB1, ccrAB2, ccrAB3, ccrAB4 and ccrC. The SCC*mec* type III prototype is a composite element that consists of the recombination of two SCC elements, i.e. SCC*mec* type III and SCC*mercury*. The SCC*mec* complexes often carry plasmids (e.g. pUB110, pI258 and pT181) and transposons (e.g. Tn*554* and ΨTn*554*) integrated into them.

The SCC*mec* elements also comprise three junkyard (J) regions. The variations in the J regions within the same *mec* and *ccr* combination define the SCC*mec* subtypes within a type.

CURRENT THERAPEUTIC PROBLEMS WITH RESISTANCE

STAPHYLOCOCCUS AUREUS

Approximately 85% of *Staph. aureus* are resistant to penicillin by plasmid-mediated β-lactamase. During the 1950s, large epidemics of hospital infection were caused by 'the hospital staphylococcus', a virulent strain of *Staph. aureus* resistant to penicillin, tetracycline, erythromycin, chloramphenicol and other drugs. After the introduction of the penicillinase-stable penicillins, the incidence of hospital infection with multiresistant staphylococci gradually declined during the 1960s and 1970s. Although strains of methicillin-resistant *Staph. aureus* (MRSA) were seen as early as 1961, gentamicin-resistant MRSA emerged later as a major pathogen of hospital infection in the 1980s. Since then, MRSA has continued to increase in prevalence in several countries, including the USA, UK and countries in Southern and Eastern Europe, but was well contained in others such as Scandinavian countries and the Netherlands (Figure 3.4). Epidemic strains of MRSA have been associated with large nosocomial outbreaks spreading to whole regions by interhospital transfer of colonized patients or staff.[55,56] Deep-seated MRSA infections have been associated with increased mortality compared with oxacillin-susceptible *Staph. aureus* infection in some settings.[57] After becoming endemic in many acute care hospitals in the 1980s and 1990s, MRSA strains have disseminated into long-term care facilities which have become a reservoir of carriers. In the 1990s, community-acquired (CA-) MRSA infections have been reported from Australia, the USA and Europe in populations lacking previous contact with healthcare facilities.[58] CA-MRSA strains are unrelated to nosocomial strains and frequently produce the Panton–Valentine leukocidin (PVL) exotoxin. Recently, MRSA carriage has been reported with unexpected high prevalence among livestock animals, farmers and veterinarians in Europe and the USA.[59] These MRSA strains appear clonal and unrelated to either nosocomial or CA-MRSA clones.

Proportion of MRSA isolates in participating countries in 2008
(c) EARSS

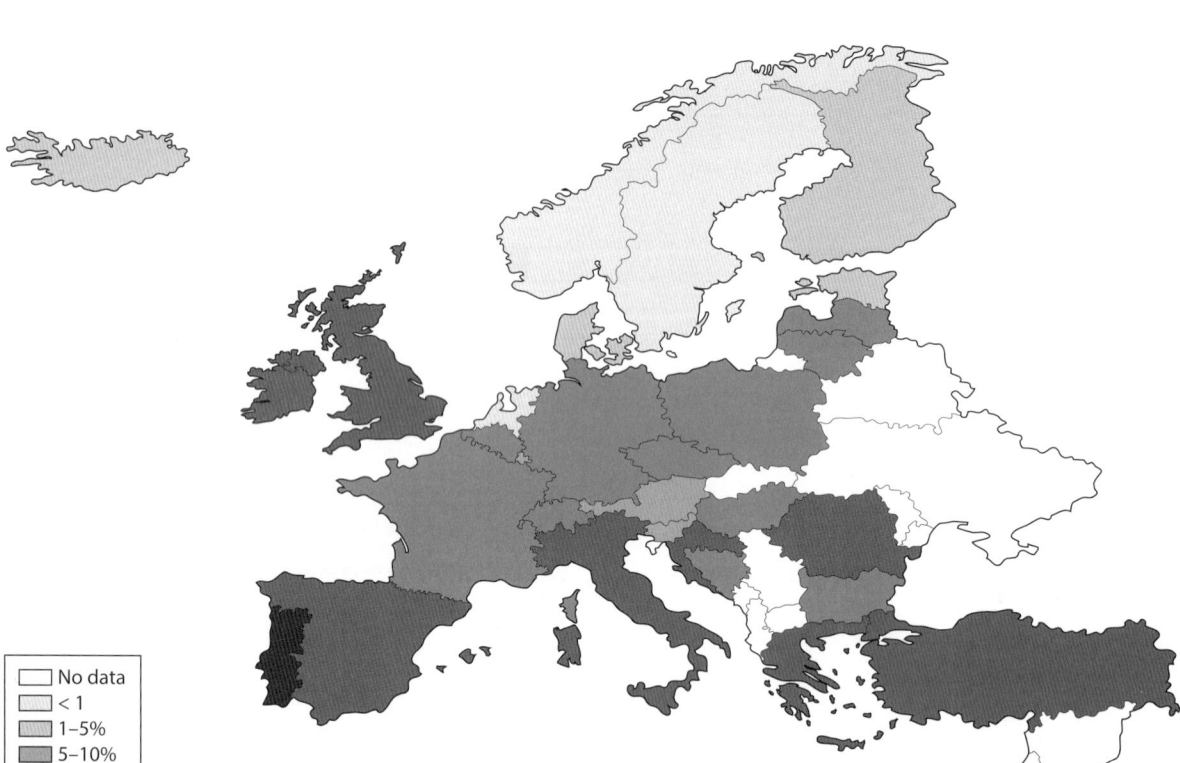

No data
< 1
1–5%
5–10%
10–25%
25–50%
> 50%

Fig. 3.4 Proportion of methicillin-resistant *Staph. aureus* isolates from bloodstream infections, EARSS participating countries, 2008. Available at http://www.earss.rivm.nl.

MRSA strains have become multiresistant by a number of mechanisms. The chromosomal DNA region harboring the *mecA* gene, the staphylococcal cassette chromosome *mec*, contains a number of insertion sites. These permit the accumulation of multiple mobile genetic elements encoding resistance to other classes of antibiotics such as macrolides, lincosamides, streptogramins, sulfonamides and tetracyclines. In addition, MRSA may acquire other resistances encoded on plasmids and transposons, including β-lactamase production and resistance to trimethoprim and the aminoglycosides. Aminoglycoside resistance is mediated by at least six aminoglycoside-modifying enzymes. Following the rapid emergence of mutational resistance to quinolones and to other drugs such as rifampicin and mupirocin, fuelled by clonal spread,[59] many strains of MRSA remain sensitive only to the glycopeptides vancomycin and teicoplanin. The recent recognition of MRSA strains with reduced susceptibility or high resistance to glycopeptides (*see above*) is likely to further complicate therapy of serious staphylococcal infection. Among the recently available antistaphylococcal antibiotics, such as linezolid, quinupristin–dalfopristin, tigecycline and daptomycin, partial or full resistance by mutational mechanisms has already been reported in clinical isolates.

COAGULASE-NEGATIVE STAPHYLOCOCCI

These organisms are important causes of nosocomial infections associated with prosthetic and indwelling devices. In the community, people are normally colonized by relatively sensitive strains of *Staph. epidermidis*; after admission to hospital and treatment with antibiotics, patients often become colonized with more resistant strains of *Staph. epidermidis* or *Staph. haemolyticus*. A majority of coagulase-negative staphylococci isolated in hospitals show multiple antibiotic resistance, including resistance to methicillin (and other β-lactams), gentamicin and quinolones. *Staph. haemolyticus* frequently shows low-level, inducible, teicoplanin resistance.[60] Multiresistant strains may act as a reservoir of resistance genes that can be transferred to *Staph. aureus* and enterococci.

ENTEROCOCCI

The enterococci are naturally sensitive to ampicillin, but are intrinsically relatively resistant to other β-lactams such as cloxacillin, the cephalosporins and the carbapenems. They are also usually resistant to trimethoprim and the sulfon-amides, quinolones and aminoglycosides. These organisms have a remarkable ability to acquire new resistances to ampicillin, vancomycin and teicoplanin, chloramphenicol, erythromycin, tetracyclines, high levels of aminoglycosides and clindamycin.[61]

E. faecalis is the most common enterococcal species to be isolated from clinical specimens, but *E. faecium* is increasing in frequency. *E. faecium* is inherently more resistant to penicillin and ampicillin than *E. faecalis*, and hospital isolates tend to show increasing high-level resistance due to altered PBPs (*see above*). The production of β-lactamase and the overproduction or alteration of penicillin-binding proteins has been reported in ampicillin-resistant *E. faecalis* strains that have caused large hospital outbreaks in the USA.[62]

In the USA, acquired vancomycin resistance increased more than 40-fold among nosocomial isolates of enterococci, from 0.3% in 1989 to over 70% in 2007.[63] This rise followed an increase by more than 100-fold in the use of vancomycin in hospitals in the last 20 years. Initially, clonal epidemics of vancomycin-resistant enterococci broke out in intensive care units and later in whole hospitals. This was followed by spread of resistance plasmids and transposons among multiple strains of *E. faecium* and *E. faecalis*.[61] In Europe, the incidence of nosocomial infection caused by VRE varies widely from <1% to >40%.[30] Outbreaks have also been reported in Europe, especially in hematological, transplant and intensive care units. Transmission occurs by cross-contamination via the hands of healthcare personnel and the environment, and is enhanced by exposure to therapy with glycopeptides, cephalosporins and drugs with anti-anaerobic activity.[64] The phylogenic analysis of a large collection of *E. faecium* isolates from humans and animals showed the worldwide expansion of complex-17 lineage causing hospital outbreaks and characterized by ampicillin resistance and specific virulence factors.[65]

In the USA, most of the vancomycin-resistant strains are resistant to all other available antimicrobials, making therapy extremely difficult and requiring combinations of drugs or the use of new drugs such as quinupristin–dalfopristin, daptomycin and linezolid.[63] Resistance to these new antimicrobials has already been reported in clinical isolates. As the consumption of linezolid increased, several outbreaks of linezolid- and vancomycin-resistant *E. faecium* have been reported in hematological and transplant wards in Europe and the USA.[66] In a meta-analysis of enterococcal bloodstream infection, the mortality attributable to the infection was independently associated with vancomycin resistance, although the specific impact of antibiotic therapy is difficult to ascertain because of the severity of the underlying disease.[67]

STREPTOCOCCUS PNEUMONIAE

Acquired multidrug resistance in *Str. pneumoniae* has become a worldwide health problem, with increasing incidence of resistance to β-lactams, macrolides, lincosamides and tetracyclines

in most parts of the world in the last three decades.[68–71] The MIC of penicillin for sensitive strains of pneumococci is <0.01 mg/L; the first penicillin-resistant isolates, reported in 1967 from Papua New Guinea, showed 'low-level' resistance with MICs of up to 1 mg/L, but in 1977 pneumococci were isolated in South Africa showing 'high-level' resistance with penicillin MICs of >1 mg/L. High-level penicillin resistance has so far been confined to a few serotypes, whereas low-level resistance is now found in nearly all the common serotypes. There is a wide geographical variation in the prevalence of penicillin-resistant pneumococci, even between regions of a particular country.

There is conclusive evidence of international spread of multiresistant clones, such as the Spanish serotype 23F clone that was apparently 'exported' from Spain to the USA.[72] Several serotypes, showing multiresistance, significantly decreased in incidence after the introduction of the 7-valent conjugate vaccine in both the USA and Europe.[69] These strains were replaced by non-vaccine serotypes such as the multidrug-resistant serotype 19A in the USA and Europe.[70] According to two recent worldwide surveys and Europe-wide surveillance data (http://www.earss.rivm.nl), in some countries, such as in Northern Europe, only a few percent of pneumococcal isolates show low-level penicillin resistance and high-level resistance is rare; however, in other countries such as France, Poland, Turkey, Israel and the USA, 25% or more of isolates are penicillin resistant, of which up to 15% of isolates are high-level resistant.[71] In recent surveys, resistance to third-generation cephalosporins varied between <1% and 15%.[70,71]

A high prevalence (from 10% to >50%) of macrolide resistance among *Str. pneumoniae* strains is reported from all continents. The predominant mechanisms of resistance to macrolides are ribosomal methylation conferred by the *erm*B gene, followed by drug efflux pump encoded by the *mef*A gene.[73] In North America, macrolide resistance is more frequently caused by MefA, which does not affect lincosamides. However, the proportion of isolates positive for both ErmB and MefA is increasing. In Europe and the Asia–Pacific regions the predominant mechanism of resistance is ErmB conferring the MLS_B phenotype. There is a strong association of co-resistance to penicillin, macrolides, lincosamides, chloramphenicol, tetracycline and co-trimoxazole.

The resistance of *Str. pneumoniae* to fluoroquinolones is due to chromosomal mutations in the DNA gyrase (*gyrA* and *gyrB*) and topoisomerase IV (*parC* and *parE*) and/or active efflux. Both mechanisms have so far been reported at low prevalence (<1%) in a majority of countries but with higher frequency in China (4–14%), Japan (0.5–6%) and Italy (6%).[74] This is a cause for concern, given the usefulness of newer generation fluoroquinolones for the treatment of lower respiratory tract infections.

Respiratory and bloodstream infections with strains of pneumococci showing low- to moderate-level penicillin resistance (MIC <4.0 mg/L) can be treated with high doses of penicillin, amoxicillin or cephalosporins as there is no firm evidence that this level of penicillin resistance is associated with increased risk of treatment failure. On the other hand, meningitis treatment failures have been documented in infections with even low-level penicillin-resistant strains. Therefore, initial treatment of meningitis in areas with high levels of penicillin and cephalosporin resistance includes high-dose cefotaxime or ceftriaxone in association with vancomycin. Both drugs should be continued in case of infection with cefotaxime-intermediate resistant pneumococci (MIC of 1.0 mg/L), and rifampicin should be added if the cefotaxime MIC is ≥2 mg/L (*see* Ch. 50).

HAEMOPHILUS INFLUENZAE

Ampicillin resistance due to plasmid-mediated TEM-1 β-lactamase production was first noted in 1972, and is now widespread, ranging from 3% in Germany to 65% in South Korea in lower respiratory and blood specimens. The prevalence of β-lactamase-producing strains rose in the 1990s, followed by a subsequent decline in the 2000s in the USA, Canada, Japan and Spain.[75] In 1981, Rubin et al. reported a novel β-lactamase in *H. influenzae*, later called ROB-1.[76] The recent prevalence of this enzyme varies greatly (from 4% to 30%) and was found with the highest frequency in Mexico and USA.[73]

β-Lactamase-negative, ampicillin-resistant (BLNAR) strains are associated with changes in penicillin-binding proteins, especially PBP 3. This form of ampicillin resistance appears to be globally rare (<0.5%) but was reported locally at much higher rates (10–40%) in recent surveys from Europe and Japan, possibly due to differences in the methods and definitions used.[75] Cephalosporins and amoxicillin–clavulanate remain very active (>99% sensitivity), as are fluoroquinolones, tetracyclines, rifampicin and chloramphenicol. Rates of chloramphenicol resistance in excess of 10% were occasionally found in some Latin American and Asian countries. Co-trimoxazole resistance rates vary markedly by region, with the highest rates reported from Latin America, the Middle East and Spain (about 30%), followed by Eastern Europe and North America (10–20%).

NEISSERIA MENINGITIDIS

The emergence of sulfonamide resistance in *N. meningitidis*, due to mutational or recombinational modification of the target dihydropteroate synthase, emerged in the early 1960s and is now widespread. Of greater concern today is the emergence of penicillin resistance. The MIC of penicillin for meningococci is usually <0.08 mg/L, but this may be increased in moderately susceptible isolates up to 0.5 mg/L. These strains were first reported in the 1960s but have increased in frequency in some countries, especially in Spain. This low-level penicillin resistance is due to alterations in PBP 2, with a mosaic gene structure arising as a result of transformation from commensal *Neisseria* species. In the 1990s, Spain suffered a clonal epidemic associated with a moderately susceptible penicillin strain that accounted for more than 60% of invasive serogroup C isolates. There are only scant clinical data indicating that meningitis with the moderately susceptible meningococcal strains may be associated with penicillin treatment failures. Third-generation cephalosporins remain very active on these strains. In addition, β-lactamase production by meningococci has been reported in four cases and appears to be encoded on a gonococcal plasmid. Chloramphenicol resistance has been reported recently from Vietnam and was determined by a *catP* gene located on a defective transposon from *Clostridium perfringens*. Although up to 10% of carriers treated with rifampicin are subsequently found to harbor rifampicin-resistant meningococci, caused by a point mutation in the *rpoB* gene, such strains remain extremely rare in invasive disease. Four cases of meningococcal disease caused by ciprofloxacin-resistant *N. meningitidis* serogroup B have been reported in the USA.[77] They were caused by the same strain which revealed a *gyrA* mutation that was possibly acquired by horizontal gene transfer from the commensal *N. lactamica*.[77]

NEISSERIA GONORRHOEAE

Low-level resistance to benzylpenicillin (MIC 0.1–2 mg/L) has been increasing in strains of *N. gonorrhoeae* for several decades, and is now very common. This type of resistance is due to mutational alterations in the penicillin-binding proteins PBP 1 and PBP 2 and to impermeability associated with alteration of PI porin. Alterations in *penA* genes conferring decreased susceptibility to third-generation oral cephalosporins has been documented in Japan, Hong Kong and the Western Pacific Region.[78] Since 1976, a high-level plasmid-mediated type of resistance to penicillin, caused by production of TEM-1 β-lactamase, appeared in South East Asia and West Africa and spread to Western countries.[79] These penicillinase-producing strains of *N. gonorrhoeae* remain common (30–65%) in many developing countries, but account for only 5–10% of gonococcal isolates in the West. Low-level resistance to tetracyclines is often associated with multiple resistance to penicillin, erythromycin and fusidic acid. It is caused by mutational derepression of the MtrRCDE efflux system.[21] Plasmid-mediated high-level resistance to all tetracyclines, including doxycycline, determined by the ribosomal protection protein TetM carried on a transposon, emerged in 1985. It has reached a high prevalence, which unfortunately reduces the clinical utility of this group of drugs for the treatment of dual infection with gonococci and chlamydia.[80] Spectinomycin resistance, due to mutational alteration of the 30S ribosomal subunit, remains rare. Resistance to fluoroquinolones, due to GyrA and/or ParC mutational alteration, emerged in several countries during the 1990s and increased globally by clonal spread to reach prevalence rates up to 94% in South East Asia and more than 50% in some European countries.[80] This dramatic increase in resistance has markedly reduced the value of fluoroquinolones for empirical treatment of urethritis.

ESCHERICHIA COLI

Acquired resistance to ampicillin is conferred to *Esch. coli* by a plasmid-encoded, Tn*3*-associated TEM-1 β-lactamase. First described in 1965, this mobile gene has spread so extensively throughout the world that 40–60% of both hospital and community strains are now resistant by this mechanism. Up to 50% of these ampicillin-resistant organisms are also resistant to the combination of amoxicillin with clavulanic acid, either because of hyperproduction of TEM-1 β-lactamase or by production of a mutant, inhibitor-resistant TEM enzyme. Other plasmid-encoded β-lactamases are seen in *Esch. coli* with increasing frequency, including extended-spectrum β-lactamases of the TEM, SHV and AmpC families. Fluoroquinolone resistance in *Esch. coli* is an increasingly common problem in Europe and has reached prevalence rates as high as 50% in Turkey, and 40% in Hong Kong. Intestinal carriage was found in 25% of healthy individuals in Spain.[81] Fluoroquinolone-resistant *Esch. coli* is particularly common in patients with complicated urinary tract infections and in neutropenic patients developing bacteremia during fluoroquinolone prophylaxis.

Esch. coli has been recognized as the major source of ESBLs with a higher increase in prevalence in the community than in the hospital setting.[12] This increase was initially due to the spread of multiple clones harboring different CTX-M enzymes into diverse genetics elements (integrons and transposons). These enzymes show higher hydrolyzing activity against cefotaxime than ceftazidime. They display high homology with chromosomal β-lactamases from *Kluyvera* species. The insertion sequences IS*Ecp1* and Orf*513* contribute to their mobilization. Among the CTX-M, CTX-M-15 is the predominant enzyme found in the community and in long-term care facilities. This enzyme harbors the Asp240Gly substitution that confers an eight-fold higher level of resistance to ceftazidime than its parental CTX-M-3 enzyme. CTX-M-15 *Esch. coli* has emerged globally by acquisition of epidemic plasmids into highly virulent strains of the B2 phylogenetic subgroup, sequence type ST131, serogroup O25:H4.[82] Co-resistance to fluoroquinolones is frequently mediated by *qnr* genes and *aac* (6′)-*Ib*-cr in these ESBL-producing strains.

In addition to ESBL, new variants of cephalosporinases called extended-spectrum AmpC (ESAC) β-lactamases, which confer resistance against oxyimino-cephalosporins including cefepime and cefpirome, have been described since 1995 in *Ent. cloacae*, *Serratia marcescens* and *Esch. coli*.[83] Plasmid-encoded AmpC enzymes conferring resistance to third-generation cephalosporins (such as CMY-2) have become frequent in the USA but remain rare in Europe. Resistance to carbapenems by metallo-β-lactamase production (VIM-1) has been reported sporadically in clinical *Esch. coli* isolates from Spain and Greece.

KLEBSIELLA, ENTEROBACTER AND SERRATIA SPP

These organisms are intrinsically resistant to ampicillin, and *Enterobacter* and *Serratia* spp. are resistant to older cephalosporins. They all have the ability to cause hospital outbreaks of opportunistic infection, and they often exchange plasmid-borne resistances. *K. pneumoniae* is the most common nosocomial pathogen of the three, and appears to have the greatest ability to receive and disseminate multiresistance plasmids. The ampicillin resistance of *K. pneumoniae* is mediated by chromosomal SHV-1 β-lactamase. In the 1970s, organisms carrying plasmid-borne aminoglycoside resistance often caused large outbreaks of hospital infection and sometimes disseminated their resistances to *Enterobacter*, *Serratia* and other enterobacterial species. These outbreaks diminished when the newer cephalosporins and aminoglycosides became available.

Starting in the mid-1980s in Europe and Latin America and in the 1990s in the USA, hospital outbreaks due to *K. pneumoniae* with resistance to third-generation cephalosporins by plasmid-borne production of extended-spectrum β-lactamases (ESBL) were reported, particularly in intensive care units (ICUs). ESBL-encoding plasmids were also transferred to *K. oxytoca*, *Citrobacter* spp., *Esch. coli*, *Proteus mirabilis* and *Enterobacter* spp. Pan-European surveys in ICUs showed that the proportion of ESBL-producing klebsiellae varies markedly by hospital and by country, from 3% in Sweden to 60% in Turkey.[84] Co-resistance to aminoglycosides, co-trimoxazole, tetracyclines and fluoroquinolones is common.

Resistance to carbapenems has been reported increasingly in *K. pneumoniae* (Figure 3.5). In the majority of cases, this was related to the spread of plasmid-encoded class A carbapenemases (KPC) and class B carbapenemases (VIM), especially in *K. pneumoniae*.[15] Less commonly, carbapenem-resistant Enterobacteriaceae were due to high-level production of cephalosporinase- or oxacillinase-mediated resistance combined with other β-lactamases and porin mutation.[85] The *K. pneumoniae* carbapenemase (KPC) was initially reported in North Carolina in 1996 and subsequently worldwide.[15] Six variants of the *bla*$_{KPC1/2}$ gene have been reported. Although these enzymes confer decreased susceptibility to all β-lactams, impaired outer membrane permeability is often required to achieve full resistance to carbapenems. The *bla*$_{KPC}$ genes have been identified within a Tn*3*-type transposon (Tn*4001*) in large transferable plasmids. These plasmids frequently carry aminoglycoside determinants and have been associated with ESBL (CTX-M-15) and the quinolone-resistance proteins QnrA and QnrB. Co-resistance to other non-β-lactam antibiotics limits therapeutic options for these strains. The *bla*$_{KPC}$ genes have been reported in other Enterobacteriaceae (*Enterobacter* spp., *Esch. coli*, *K. oxytoca*, *C. freundii*, *P. mirabilis*, *Salmonella* spp. and *S. marcescens*) and at chromosomal and plasmid locations in *Ps. aeruginosa*.

**Proportion of carbapenems-resistant *K. pneumoniae* isolates in participating countries in 2008
(c) EARSS**

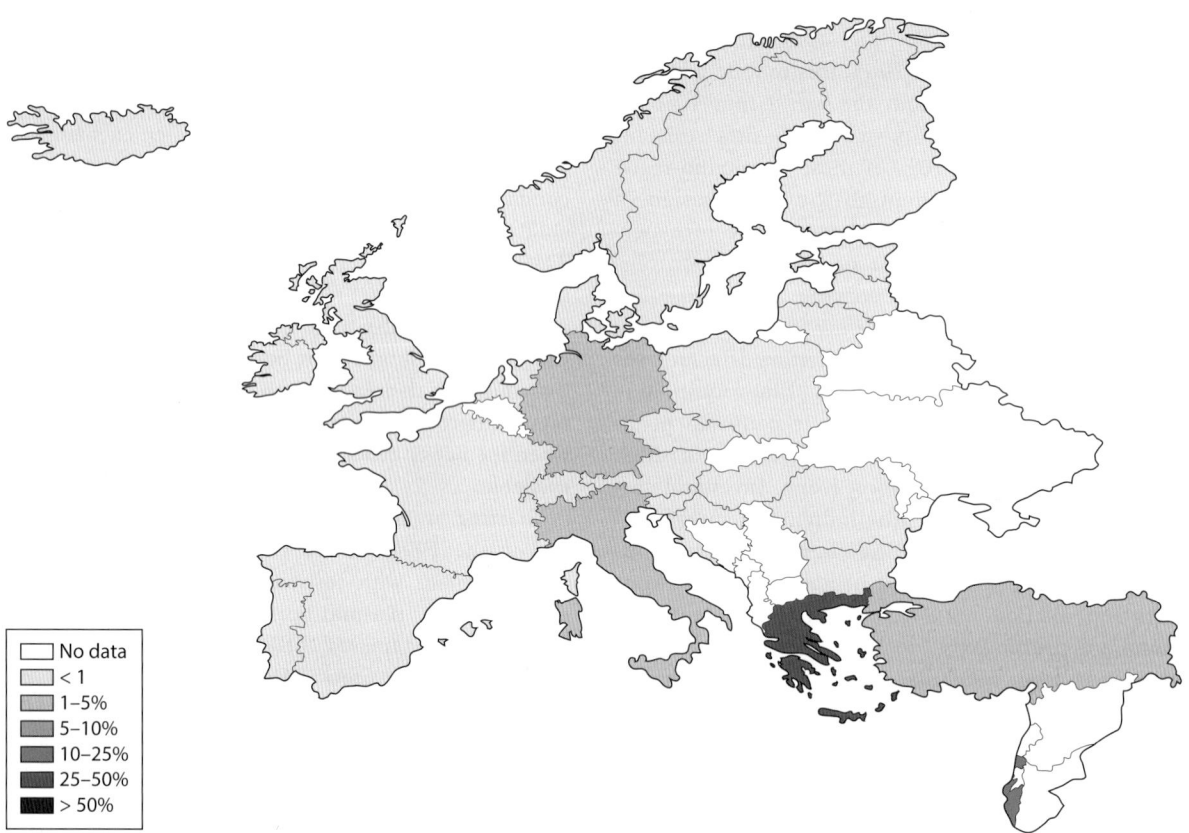

No data
< 1
1–5%
5–10%
10–25%
25–50%
> 50%

Fig. 3.5   Proportion of carbapenem-resistant *K. pneumoniae* isolates from bloodstream infections, EARSS participating countries, 2008. Available at http://www.earss.rivm.nl.

The KPC-producing bacteria are widespread in the USA, Israel, China, Latin America and Greece, but remain rare in western and northern Europe.[15] Since 2001 sporadic isolates and small outbreaks of multiresistant VIM-producing *K. pneumoniae* have been reported in some European countries (France, Spain, Italy, Greece, Turkey and Belgium). In several cases these strains were traced back to patient transfer from hospitals in Greece, where the proportion of resistance to imipenem increased from <1% in 2001 to >70% in isolates from ICUs and to >20% in isolates from hospital wards from 2001 to 2007 (http://www.earss.rivm.nl). Co-resistance to colistin has been reported in some of these strains, leaving very few active therapeutic options.

About 30% of hospital isolates of *Enterobacter* spp. show cephalosporinase hyperproduction.[84] In the 1990s, ESBL-producing (mostly TEM-24), multiresistant *Ent. aerogenes* strains emerged as a common cause of nosocomial infection in France, Spain and Belgium. Epidemic strains were first reported in ICUs and have since disseminated hospital-wide to cause large regional epidemics.[86] Many of these ESBL-producing strains remain susceptible only to carbapenems, which are the drugs of choice for treatment of serious infection with these organisms. In *Enterobacter* strains with high-level cephalosporinase combined with ESBL production,

however, emergence of porin-resistant mutants during imipenem therapy may lead to treatment failure, requiring the use of colistin or doxycycline for infections with strains resistant to all β-lactams and fluoroquinolones.[87] The resistance to carbapenems by enzymes of class A (SME, IMI, NMC, GES) and Class B (IMP, VIM, SPM) in species such as *Ent. cloacae*, *K. oxytoca*, *Citrobacter* spp., *P. mirabilis*, *Providencia stuartii* and *S. marcescens* is a growing problem worldwide.[14]

SHIGELLA

Shigellae were among the first organisms to be shown in the 1950s to harbor transferable antibiotic resistance determinants on conjugative plasmids. In developing countries, rates of multiple resistance are high, with >50% of isolates resistant to ampicillin, chloramphenicol, tetracycline, co-trimoxazole or nalidixic acid. In the last few years, fluoroquinolone resistance in *Shigella* spp. increased in the Indian subcontinent as a result of both *gyrA* and *parC* mutations,[88] compromising the use of fluoroquinolones as the first line of treatment for dysentery in that region. Multiresistance is most common in *Shigella dysenteriae*, followed by *Shigella flexneri* and *Shigella sonnei*. In developed countries rates of resistance are higher in shigellosis patients with a history of travel abroad.

SALMONELLA

Salmonella enterica serotype Typhi has developed multiple resistance to first-line antibiotics in many developing countries. In the 1970s, strains with plasmid-mediated resistance to ampicillin and chloramphenicol caused epidemics in Latin America. In the 1980s, strains with plasmid-mediated resistance to ampicillin, chloramphenicol and co-trimoxazole emerged in South East Asia and have since become widespread in Asia and Latin America, where rates of 30–70% multiresistant *Salmonella* Typhi were reported in the 1990s. Fluoroquinolone resistance is now emerging in MDR strains and has been associated with recent outbreaks of typhoid fever in Tajikistan, Vietnam and the Indian subcontinent. The proportion of *Salmonella* Typhi with low-level resistance to ciprofloxacin showed a rapid increase to more than 20% in 1999 in the UK, and was mostly seen in travelers returning from the Indian subcontinent.[89]

In the 1990s, multiple resistance also rose rapidly in nontyphoidal salmonellae in Europe and in the USA. There is conclusive evidence that antibiotics used in animal husbandry have contributed to antibiotic resistance in human isolates. In the UK and other European countries, the incidence of human infections with multiresistant *Salmonella* ser. Typhimurium DT104 resistant to ampicillin, chloramphenicol, streptomycin, co-trimoxazole and tetracycline increased markedly during the period 1990–1996, at a time when penicillin and tetracycline were commonly used in cattle feed. In Denmark, an outbreak of food-borne salmonellosis caused by a multidrug and low-level fluoroquinolone-resistant *Salmonella* ser. Typhimurium was traced to an infected swine herd. This strain was nalidixic acid resistant and showed increased ciprofloxacin MIC (0.06–0.12 mg/L). Although this level of susceptibility is categorized as sensitive by current breakpoints, patients treated with fluoroquinolones showed poor clinical response.[90]

Soon after the introduction of enrofloxacin for veterinary use in the UK in 1993, human *Salmonella* isolates with decreased susceptibility to ciprofloxacin increased 10-fold from 1994 to 1997. In 1999, soon after the introduction of codes of good practice for the prophylactic use of fluoroquinolones in animal husbandry in the UK, there was a 75% decline in isolations of multiresistant *Salmonella* ser. Typhimurium DT104 from clinical specimens, which may indicate a favorable impact of more prudent antibiotic use.[91] The extended-spectrum β-lactamases have appeared in some *Salmonella* strains, possibly as a result of plasmid transfer from commensal enterobacteria in the human gut. ESBL-producing salmonellae caused epidemics in Greece and spread to other European countries in the 1990s.[92] The first case of infection by ceftriaxone-resistant *Salmonella* reported in the USA was linked to contact with infected cattle treated with cephalosporins on a Nebraska farm.[93]

CAMPYLOBACTER

Campylobacter spp. have also shown increasing antimicrobial resistance in the past decade, and again much of this resistance appears related to the veterinary use of antibiotics. Although there is considerable geographic variation, macrolide resistance in *C. jejuni*, which is mainly due to mutational alteration of domain V of 23S rRNA, is increasing worldwide, including in Europe and the USA.[94] *C. coli* shows higher erythromycin resistance rates (4–50%) than *C. jejuni* (0–20%). The proportion of isolates resistant to fluoroquinolones, which is caused by stepwise mutations in *gyrA* and/or *parC* genes, has increased dramatically around the world over the last 20 years (from 0% to over 80% in some areas). There is consistent evidence that this is a result of the addition of quinolones to chicken feed.[40,95] In every country where this has been investigated, quinolone resistance in human *Campylobacter* isolates increased in frequency soon after the introduction of these drugs in animal husbandry, but long after their licensing in human medicine. In the USA, domestic chickens were determined by epidemiological and molecular investigations as the predominant source of quinolone-resistant *C. jejuni* infection in the years after these drugs were licensed for use in poultry in 1995.[95] In South Africa, Thailand and Taiwan, very high rates of multiple resistance to quinolones, macrolides, tetracyclines and ampicillin often leave no effective antimicrobial treatment for *Campylobacter* enteritis.[96]

HELICOBACTER PYLORI

Peptic ulcer disease caused by *H. pylori* infection is treated by associations of antibiotics, which may include amoxicillin, tetracyclines, clarithromycin and metronidazole. Eradication fails, however, in 10–30% of cases. This is in part due to primary or secondary resistance to one or more of these drugs, most commonly to metronidazole or clarithromycin.[97] Development of secondary resistance may occur in over 50% of cases with suboptimal regimens. Nitroimidazole resistance is mostly related to mutational inactivation of the *rdxA* gene encoding an oxygen-sensitive NADPH nitroreductase. The cure rate with most combination regimens drops by about 50% in case of nitroimidazole resistance. The prevalence of this resistance is rising and currently ranges from 10% to 40% of isolates in the West and from 50% to 80% in developing countries. Resistance to clarithromycin is caused by a mutation at position 2142 or 2143 in 23S rRNA. Its impact on cure rate appears similar to that of nitroimidazole resistance for most treatment regimens. The prevalence of primary macrolide resistance varies by region between 3% and 25% and is increasing. Standardization of resistance detection methods for this pathogen is much needed to assess the efficacy of treatment regimens based on primary resistance patterns and to guide local recommendations based on surveillance data.[98] The prevalence of resistance to amoxicillin and to tetracycline is very low (<1%) in *H. pylori* except in a few countries like South Korea. In contrast, resistance to fluoroquinolones, mainly caused by mutation in the *gyrA* gene, shows a higher prevalence (9–20%).

PSEUDOMONAS AERUGINOSA

Ps. aeruginosa is a leading cause of nosocomial infection in critically ill patients and is associated with the highest attributable mortality among opportunistic Gram-negative bacteria. It is intrinsically resistant to most β-lactam antibiotics, tetracyclines, chloramphenicol, sulfonamides and nalidixic acid, due to the interplay of impermeability with multidrug efflux, principally mediated by MexAB-OprM.[99] Acquired resistance to anti-pseudomonal antibiotics develops rapidly in more than 10% of patients during treatment. This occurs most commonly with imipenem and ciprofloxacin.[100] Multiple types of acquired β-lactam resistance are expressed by this adaptable organism, often in combination: hyperproduction of AmpC cephalosporinase, acquisition of transposon and plasmid-mediated ESBLs, oxacillinases or carbapenemases; mutational loss of porins or upregulation of efflux pumps.[18]

Three types of aminoglycoside resistance are seen: high-level, plasmid-mediated resistance to one or two aminoglycosides, due to the production of aminoglycoside-modifying enzymes, and broad-spectrum resistance to all the aminoglycosides, due to a reduction in the permeability of the cell envelope and/or overexpression of an efflux pump. Fluoroquinolone resistance is mediated by topoisomerase gene mutations, decreased permeability and efflux overexpression. Surveys of clinical isolates of *Ps. aeruginosa* from ICUs have indicated resistance rates >10% to all drugs in European countries.[84] Resistance rates varied by region, with Latin America showing the highest prevalence, followed by Europe with high β-lactam resistance (>25% to ceftazidime) and fluoroquinolone resistance rates (>30% to ciprofloxacin), particularly in Southern Europe. Multidrug-resistant strains were found in 1% of isolates from the USA, 5% from Europe and 8% from Latin America, and their distribution by participating center suggested local outbreaks.

Only 10 years after the first description of VIM-1 in a *Ps. aeruginosa* isolate in 1997, the VIM-2 variant has become the most widespread metallo-β-lactamase (MBL) among *Ps. aeruginosa* strains.[101] VIM-producing strains have caused hospital outbreaks worldwide. IMP enzymes have also been reported in this organism. The bla_{IMP} and bla_{VIM} genes are inserted into class 1 integrons. Other mobile genes encoding MBL enzymes were reported in *Ps. aeruginosa*, including the SMP (endemic in Brazil) and GIM (reported in Germany) enzymes.[101] These carbapenemase-producing *Ps. aeruginosa* strains are multiresistant and on many occasions susceptible to colistin only. Class A β-lactamases such as VEB have been described with increasing frequency in this organism, whereas the GES and KPC enzymes were found in Latin America.[101] Multiresistant *Ps. aeruginosa* is becoming one of the most problematic nosocomial pathogens, particularly in view of the

lack of new antimicrobial classes in clinical development that are active on this organism.

ACINETOBACTER SPP

Acinetobacters are free-living, non-fermenting organisms that often colonize human skin and cause opportunistic infections. Furthermore, these organisms are able to survive for prolonged periods in inanimate environments. The most frequently isolated species, and one most likely to acquire multiple antibiotic resistance, is *Acinetobacter baumannii*. In the early 1970s, acinetobacters were usually sensitive to many common antimicrobial agents but many hospital strains are now resistant to most available agents, including co-trimoxazole, aminoglycosides, cephalosporins, quinolones and, to a lesser extent, carbapenems. The mechanisms and genetics of resistance in this species are complex, but they involve several plasmid-borne β-lactamases and aminoglycoside-modifying enzymes, as well as alterations in membrane permeability and penicillin-binding proteins. The acquisition of these multiple mechanisms may be due to the fact that this group of organisms is physiologically competent and can acquire DNA by transformation in vivo.

Multiresistant *A. baumannii* strains have caused epidemics in several countries and nosocomial infections with these strains have been associated with excess mortality. Although not exclusively, many MDR *A. baumannii* strains are associated with epidemic lineages (EU clones I, II and III) that were found to spread in many European countries.

A. baumannii naturally harbor a carbapenem-hydrolyzing oxacillinase (OXA-51/69 variants) which, when overexpressed, confers a decreased susceptibility to carbapenem. Class D (OXA-type) β-lactamases conferring resistance to carbapenems have been widely reported in *A. baumannii*. These enzymes belong to three unrelated groups (represented by OXA-23, OXA-24 and OXA-58) that can be either plasmid (OXA-23 and OXA-58) or chromosomally encoded. OXA-23- and OXA-58-producing *Acinetobacter* have been associated with outbreaks in several countries such as the UK, China, Brazil and France.[101] Class B metallo-β-lactamases (VIM, IMP, SIM) that confer resistance to all β-lactams except aztreonam have been reported worldwide in *Acinetobacter* strains, especially in Asia and Western Europe. Other mechanisms of carbapenem resistance in this organism include the reduced expression of several outer membrane proteins (porins) such as CarO.[102] Active efflux of carbapenems may be associated.

Colistin, sulbactam and tigecycline may be the only active drugs available to treat infections caused by multiresistant strains. The activity of sulbactam against carbapenem-resistant isolates is decreasing. Clinical reports support the effectiveness of colistin for treating infection with multiresistant acinetobacters whereas clinical evidence with tigecycline is still scarce in spite of its good antimicrobial activity. High-level resistance to tigecycline mediated by upregulation of chromosomally encoded efflux pumps has been reported among MDR strains. Strains resistant to all available antimicrobial agents have been reported.[103]

OTHER NON-FERMENTING ORGANISMS

Sten. maltophilia and *Burkholderia cepacia* are intrinsically resistant to many of the antimicrobial agents used for infection with Gram-negative organisms, including the aminoglycosides and cephalosporins, and often acquire further resistance to co-trimoxazole and fluoroquinolones. Because of this, and despite their relatively low virulence, they are seen with increasing frequency in areas of high antibiotic usage such as ICUs. *Sten. maltophilia* is intrinsically resistant to all the aminoglycosides, to imipenem and most β-lactams, and up to 30% of isolates have acquired resistance to co-trimoxazole and tetracyclines. It has considerable ability to develop further multiple resistances by several mechanisms, including decrease in outer membrane permeability, active efflux and the production of inducible broad-spectrum β-lactamases. Bacteria of the *B. cepacia* complex are also generally resistant to the aminoglycosides and most β-lactam antibiotics, but sensitive to ciprofloxacin, temocillin and meropenem. However, acquired multiple resistance was found in epidemic strains that are associated with rapid deterioration in infected cystic fibrosis patients.

MYCOBACTERIUM TUBERCULOSIS

M. tuberculosis has limited susceptibility to standard antimicrobial agents, but can be treated by combinations of antituberculosis drugs, of which the common first-line agents are rifampicin, isoniazid, ethambutol and pyrazinamide (*see* Chs 33 and 58). Resistance is the result of spontaneous chromosomal mutations at various loci. Mutational resistance occurs at the rate of about 1 in 10^8 for rifampicin, 1 in 10^8 to 1 in 10^9 for isoniazid, 1 in 10^6 for ethambutol and 1 in 10^5 for streptomycin. Since a cavitating lung lesion contains up to 10^9 organisms, mutational resistance appears quite frequently when these drugs are used singly for treatment, but is uncommon if three or more are used simultaneously.

The action of isoniazid against *M. tuberculosis* may involve multiple mechanisms, including transport and activation of the drug by mechanisms involving catalase-peroxidase, pigment precursors, nicotinamide adenine dinucleotide (NAD) and peroxide; generation of reactive oxygen radicals; and inhibition of mycolic acid biosynthesis. Mutations at several loci might be involved in decreased susceptibility to isoniazid, including the *katG* gene that encodes catalase-peroxidase activity, the *inhA* gene which is involved in mycolic acid synthesis, and the *aphC* gene which encodes alkylhydroxyperoxide reductase.[104] Likewise, resistance to ethambutol may result from diverse mutations in the *embCAB* operon, which is involved in the biosynthesis of cell-wall arabinan, or in other genes.

Resistance to rifampicin, fluoroquinolones and streptomycin appears to be caused in *M. tuberculosis* by mechanisms similar to those seen in other species, as the result of mutations in the *rpoB* gene that encodes the β-subunit of RNA polymerase, the *gyrA* gene encoding the A subunit of DNA gyrase and either the *rrs* gene encoding 16S rRNA or the *rpsL* gene encoding the S12 ribosomal protein, respectively. Resistance to pyrazinamide, however, does not appear to be due to altered target but to inactivation of the *pncA* gene encoding pyrazinamidase, an enzyme which is necessary for transformation of the prodrug into active pyrazinic acid.[104] An open access database of putative and well-established tuberculosis resistance mutations is available.[104]

In 2007, *M. tuberculosis* caused 9.27 million new cases of tuberculosis and 1.78 million deaths according to the World Health Organization (WHO). The main factors for the appearance of tuberculosis drug resistance are the emergence of drug-resistant mutants from wild-type susceptible strains during treatment (acquired resistance), increasing development of resistance in drug-resistant strains because of inappropriate treatment (amplified resistance) and direct transmission of drug-resistant strains (transmitted resistance). Multidrug-resistant tuberculosis (MDR-TB) implies resistance to at least two of the first-line antituberculosis drugs: rifampicin and isoniazid. These two drugs are essential for initial or short-course treatment regimens, and strains of *M. tuberculosis* resistant to them soon develop resistance to other drugs. Patients with MDR-TB thus fail to respond to standard therapy and disseminate resistant strains to their contacts (including healthcare workers), both before and after the resistance is discovered. MDR-TB emerged in the 1990s and today represents a major problem in several parts of the world, such as some countries from the former Soviet Union and in China.[105,106] Although the median worldwide prevalence of MDR-TB among new cases of tuberculosis is 1%, these rates can reach 22% in some areas of Eastern Europe, Russia, Iran and China.[106] A higher prevalence of drug resistance is also seen in immigrants to Western countries.

Extensively drug-resistant *M. tuberculosis* (XDR-TB), which is defined as bacteria resistant to at least isoniazid and rifampicin, any fluoroquinolone, and at least one of three injectable second-line drugs (amikacin, capreomycin or kanamycin), has recently emerged as a major public health threat.[106] By the end of 2008, 55 countries reported at least one case of XDR-TB. Five countries from the former Soviet Union documented 25 cases or more with a prevalence of XDR-TB ranging from 7% to 24% among MDR-TB.[106]

MDR-TB is difficult and expensive to treat and is associated with high mortality rates in immunocompromised patients, especially in people infected with HIV, which is a common association. Large nosocomial and community outbreaks of MDR-TB were seen in some American cities in the early 1990s, and later reported in Europe, Asia and Brazil.[107] The clinical outcome of patients infected with XDR-TB is even poorer than with MDR-TB. The mortality rate of XDR-TB is particularly high in patients co-infected with

HIV.[106] Epidemic and clinically highly virulent MDR- and XDR-TB strains are associated with successful clones such as Beijing/W and KwaZulu-Natal genotypes which have accumulated resistance to second-line drugs. Factors that contribute to this situation include insufficient public health services directed towards control of tuberculosis; inadequate training of healthcare workers in the diagnosis, treatment and control of tuberculosis; laboratory delays in the detection and sensitivity testing of *M. tuberculosis*; admission to hospitals unprepared for control of airborne transmission of pathogens; addition of single drugs to failing treatment regimens; an increase in the number and promiscuity of individuals at high-risk of acquiring and disseminating tuberculosis, including those infected with HIV, the poor and the homeless; and increasing migration of people from areas where tuberculosis is common.[107] The single most important factor in the prevention and successful control of further emergence of MDR/XDR-TB is probably the re-introduction of supervised observed therapy. In addition, substantial commitment of resources, healthcare planning, surveillance of drug resistance and the use of appropriate hospital isolation facilities have brought nosocomial MDR-TB under control.[107]

EPIDEMIOLOGY OF ANTIBIOTIC RESISTANCE

Epidemiological and biological studies have shown that the rise of antibiotic resistance among human pathogenic bacteria is a global phenomenon which is related to the interplay of several factors in different ecosystems (Figure 3.6).[1] These factors include the development of environmental and human reservoirs of antibiotic resistance genes and resistant bacteria, patterns of antibiotic use in medicine and agriculture that select for and amplify these reservoirs, and socioeconomic changes that influence the transmission of pathogens. The genetic

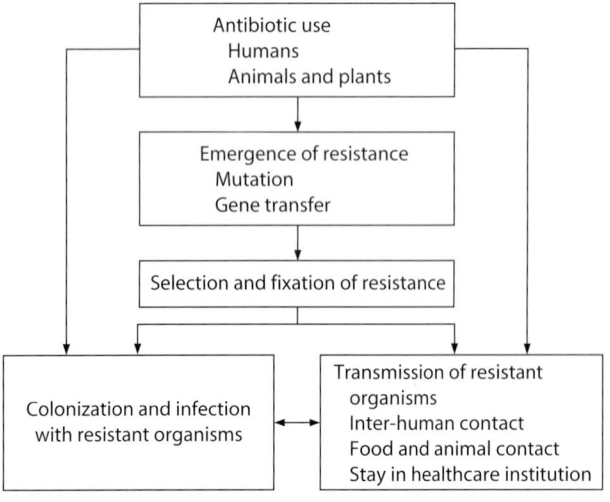

Fig. 3.6 Factors contributing to the emergence and spread of antibiotic resistance in interconnected ecosystems.

mechanisms that confer antibiotic resistance on bacteria must have existed long before the antibiotic era. Conjugative plasmids devoid of resistant genes were detected in clinical isolates of bacteria collected before the 1940s. Many resistance genes have presumably evolved from detoxifying mechanisms in antibiotic-producing fungi and streptomycetes living in soil and water and were later mobilized by genetic transfer to commensal and pathogenic bacteria.[48] Whatever the origins of resistance genes, there has clearly been a major increase in their prevalence during the past 60 years. This can be closely correlated with the use of antibiotics in humans and animals, and it is clear that resistance has eventually emerged to each new agent.

Antibiotic use is the driving force that promotes the selection, persistence and spread of resistant organisms. The phenomenon is common to hospitals, which have seen the emergence of a range of multidrug-resistant pathogens,[108] to the community at large, where respiratory and gut pathogens have become resistant to often freely available antibiotics,[109] and to animal husbandry, where the use of antibiotics for growth promotion and for mass therapy has promoted resistance in *Salmonella* and *Campylobacter*,[94] and created a reservoir of glycopeptide-resistant enterococci that can be transmitted to humans.[30]

In the community, where about 80–90% of human antibiotic consumption takes place, a large proportion of antibiotics is inappropriately prescribed for upper respiratory infections. Patients' misperceptions about the utility of antibiotics in self-resolving viral infections, commercial promotion, poor compliance with prescriptions and over-the-counter sales of antibiotics in some countries are contributing to this misuse of antimicrobials.[109] The factors relating prescription patterns to increasing resistance are only incompletely understood. Low dosage and prolonged administration have been associated with increased risk of development of β-lactam resistance in pneumococci.[110] Finnish surveillance data show that macrolide resistance in *Str. pyogenes* has increased as the national use has increased – and, conversely, has declined as a result of the much diminished use of erythromycin.[41] There are wide variations in per capita antibiotic consumption in Europe, with lowest levels of consumption in the Nordic countries correlating with a much lower prevalence of resistance in most bacterial pathogens than in the other parts of Europe (*see* Figure 3.4). Socioeconomic changes are also powerful drivers of the resurgence of infectious diseases and drug resistance.[1,3] The impoverishment of large sections of the population and disruption of the healthcare system in the former Soviet Union has had a clear impact on the spread of MDR-TB. Globalization is stimulating international circulation of goods and people, and plays a role in accelerating the dissemination of pathogens, including resistant strains.

The hospital, particularly the intensive care unit, is a major breeding ground for antibiotic-resistant bacteria. Here, a high-density population of patients with compromised host defenses is exposed to a usage of antibiotics that is about 100 times more concentrated than in the community, and frequent contact with healthcare personnel creates cease-less opportunities for cross-infection.[108] Most new drugs and injectable agents are first administered to hospital patients. Topical antibiotics are particularly likely to select for resistance, as illustrated by the emergence of gentamicin-resistant *Ps. aeruginosa* and fusidic acid- or mupirocin-resistant *Staph. aureus* that has often followed heavy topical use of gentamicin in burns and fusidic acid or mupirocin in dermatological patients. Multiple drug resistance can be encouraged by the use of a single agent, since this may select for plasmids conferring resistance to multiple antibiotics.

Selection of resistance during antibiotic therapy in infecting or colonizing bacteria is enhanced by factors related to the patient: immune suppression, presence of a large bacterial inoculum, and biofilm-associated infection of foreign bodies which impede local host defenses.[47] Other resistance-predisposing factors relate to the modalities of treatment: drug underdosing or inappropriate route of administration which causes failure to achieve bactericidal drug levels at the site of infection.[111] Alteration of the endogenous microflora during antibiotic therapy also enhances replacement of susceptible organisms by resistant strains from the hospital microflora.

Nosocomial transmission of MDR bacteria occurs most commonly by indirect contact between patients (via the contaminated hands of healthcare personnel) and, less commonly, by contaminated fomites. Patient factors predisposing to this transmission include the severity of underlying illness, length of stay in hospital, intensity and duration of exposure to broad-spectrum antibiotics, and use of invasive devices (such as intravenous catheters) or procedures.[108] Hospital patients and staff colonized with resistant bacteria, especially in the feces or on the skin, further disseminate these organisms both within the hospital and into the community. Cost containment in hospitals has resulted in chronic understaffing, increased patient turnover and inter-institutional transfer, factors which have been well documented to enhance nosocomial transmission of MDR bacteria such as MRSA and ESBL-producing Gram-negative bacteria.[108]

About 30% of the patients in acute care hospitals receive antibiotics for therapy or prophylaxis. Although antibiotics are essential for modern hospital care, many studies have shown that up to 50% of these prescriptions may be unnecessary or inappropriate. Insufficient training in antibiotic therapy, difficulty of selecting the appropriate anti-infective drugs empirically, underuse of microbiological testing, drug promotion by pharmaceutical companies and fear of litigation are some of the factors that are stimulating the use of broad-spectrum drugs.

PUBLIC HEALTH AND ECONOMIC IMPACT

Antibiotic resistance places an increasing burden on society in terms of increased morbidity, mortality and costs. In spite of the methodological complexities in studying the impact of antibiotic resistance on clinical outcomes, it is recognized that, for many diseases, individuals infected with resistant pathogens are more likely to receive ineffective therapy, to more frequently require hospital care, to stay in for longer, to develop complications and to die of the disease.[1,2] The cost of care is also increased for such patients, due to the need for more costly second-line drugs, longer duration of hospital stay, increased need for intensive care and diagnostic testing, higher incidence of complications, and expenses incurred by use of isolation precautions. There are also longer-term costs for society related to patient disability from the increased incidence of acute infectious diseases and their sequelae.

CONTROL AND PREVENTION

Learned societies and expert panels have published guidelines for optimizing antibiotic use and curtailing antibiotic resistance in hospitals.[112–118] Key components of these guidelines include:

- better undergraduate and postgraduate training in healthcare;
- establishment of hospital antimicrobial stewardship programs, involving multidisciplinary cooperation between hospital administrators, clinicians, infectious disease specialists, infection control team, microbiologists and hospital pharmacists;
- formulary-based local guidelines on anti-infective therapy and prophylaxis, education and regulation of prescriptions by consultant specialists, monitoring and auditing drug use, surveillance and reporting of resistance patterns of the hospital flora;
- surveillance and early detection of outbreaks by molecular typing, detection and notification of patients colonized with communicable resistant bacteria to the infection control team when useful for patient isolation and/or decolonization;
- promotion and monitoring of basic hospital infection control practices such as hand hygiene.

These guidelines are mostly based on local experience and on the results of before–after and analytic studies.[112–117] Few strategies have been formally tested for cost-effectiveness in controlled intervention studies. Mathematical modeling provides interesting insights into the prediction of epidemiological factors that are the most vulnerable to effective interventions.[55,64] Because each hospital has its own ecosystem and micro-society where determinants of antibiotic resistance are quite specific and evolve rapidly, effective solutions should be tailored to local circumstances and resources. On the other hand, early coordination of policies at regional or national level has been successful in controlling the transmission of emerging MDR nosocomial pathogens.[115]

In the past few years, antibiotic resistance has been universally identified as a public health priority and action plans to combat resistance have been developed by several national health agencies and international organizations such as the US Centers for Disease Control and Prevention (CDC), the WHO and the European Union (EU).[2,3,118] These strategic plans call for:

- public and professional education toward rational use of antimicrobials;
- coordination of surveillance of antibiotic resistance and antibiotic use in human and animal health sectors;
- refined regulation of antibiotic registration for use in both sectors;
- development and evaluation of improved diagnostic methods;
- promotion and evaluation of medical and veterinary practice guidelines;
- restriction of antibiotic use as growth promoters in food animals;
- promotion of infection control practice in healthcare institutions;
- development of novel antimicrobial drugs and vaccines;
- closer international cooperation.

A number of national action plans and international surveillance systems are now in development to implement these strategies and provide early warning of the emergence of threatening antibiotic-resistant bacteria to guide timely interventions.

Physicians can no longer avoid their responsibilities as antibiotic prescribers and their impact on the global ecosystem of microbial pathogens. If we want to prove wrong the prediction of an impending post-antibiotic era, we must strive to continuously improve our antibiotic prescribing and infection control practices and develop new strategies for controlling resistance.

 References

1. Cohen ML. Epidemiology of drug resistance: implications for a post-antimicrobial era. *Science.* 1992;257:1050–1055.
2. US Interagency Task Force on Antimicrobial Drug Resistance. Public health action plan to combat antimicrobial drug resistance. 2001; Online. Available at http://www.cdc.gov/drugresistance/actionplan.
3. WHO. Global strategy for containment of antimicrobial resistance Geneva. 2001; Online. Available http://who.int/emc/amr.html.
4. Kahlmeter G, Brown DF, Goldstein FW, et al. European Committee on Antimicrobial Susceptibility Testing (EUCAST) Technical Notes on antimicrobial susceptibility testing. *Clin Microbiol Infect.* 2006;12:501–503.
5. Clinical Laboratory Standard Institute. *Methods for dilution antimicrobial susceptibility testing for bacteria that grow aerobically.* 9th ed. Approved Standard M7-A9. Wayne, PA: CLSI; 2009.
6. European Committee for Antimicrobial Susceptibility Testing (EUCAST). Terminology relating to methods for the determination of susceptibility of bacteria to antimicrobial agents. *Clin Microbiol Infect.* 2000;6:503–508.
7. European Committee for Antimicrobial Susceptibility Testing (EUCAST). Determination of antimicrobial susceptibility test breakpoints. *Clin Microbiol Infect.* 2000;6:570–572.
8. Paterson DL, Ko WC, Von Gottberg A, et al. Outcome of cephalosporin treatment for serious infections due to apparently susceptible organisms producing extended-spectrum beta-lactamases: implications for the clinical microbiology laboratory. *J Clin Microbiol.* 2001;39:2206–2212.
9. Falagas ME, Karageorgopoulos DE. Pandrug resistance (PDR), extensive drug resistance (XDR), and multidrug resistance (MDR) among Gram-negative bacilli: need for international harmonization in terminology. *Clin Infect Dis.* 2008;46:1121–1122.
10. Bush K. New beta-lactamases in Gram-negative bacteria: diversity and impact on the selection of antimicrobial therapy. *Clin Infect Dis.* 2001;32:1085–1089.
11. Bush K, Jacoby GA, Medeiros AA. A functional classification scheme for beta-lactamases and its correlation with molecular structure. *Antimicrob Agents Chemother.* 1995;39:1211–1233.
12. Pitout JD, Laupland KB. Extended-spectrum beta-lactamase-producing Enterobacteriaceae: an emerging public-health concern. *Lancet Infect Dis.* 2008;8:159–166.
13. Jacoby GA. AmpC beta-lactamases. *Clin Microbiol Rev.* 2009;22:161–182.
14. Queenan AM, Bush K. Carbapenemases: the versatile beta-lactamases. *Clin Microbiol Rev.* 2007;20:440–458.
15. Nordmann P, Cuzon G, Naas T. The real threat of *Klebsiella pneumoniae* carbapenemase-producing bacteria. *Lancet Infect Dis.* 2009;9:228–236.
16. Mingeot-Leclercq MP, Glupczynski Y, Tulkens PM. Aminoglycosides: activity and resistance. *Antimicrob Agents Chemother.* 1999;43:727–737.
17. Robicsek A, Jacoby GA, Hooper DC. The worldwide emergence of plasmid-mediated quinolone resistance. *Lancet Infect Dis.* 2006;6:629–640.
18. Livermore DM. Of *Pseudomonas*, porins, pumps and carbapenems. *J Antimicrob Chemother.* 2001;47:247–250.
19. Deplano A, Denis O, Poirel L, et al. Molecular characterization of an epidemic clone of panantibiotic-resistant *Pseudomonas aeruginosa*. *J Clin Microbiol.* 2005;43:1198–1204.
20. Charrel RN, Pages JM, De Micco P, et al. Prevalence of outer membrane porin alteration in beta-lactam-antibiotic-resistant *Enterobacter aerogenes*. *Antimicrob Agents Chemother.* 1996;40:2854–2858.
21. Nikaido H, Zgwiskaya HI. Antibiotic efflux mechanisms. *Curr Opin Infect Dis.* 1999;12:529–536.
22. Mazzariol A, Tokue Y, Kanegawa TM, et al. High-level fluoroquinolone-resistant clinical isolates of *Escherichia coli* overproduce multidrug efflux protein AcrA. *Antimicrob Agents Chemother.* 2000;44:3441–3443.
23. Chopra I, Roberts M. Tetracycline antibiotics: mode of action, applications, molecular biology, and epidemiology of bacterial resistance. *Microbiol Mol Biol Rev.* 2001;65:232–260.
24. Roberts MC, Sutcliffe J, Courvalin P, et al. Nomenclature for macrolide and macrolide-lincosamide-streptogramin B resistance determinants. *Antimicrob Agents Chemother.* 1999;43:2823–2830.
25. Perichon B, Courvalin P, Galimand M. Transferable resistance to aminoglycosides by methylation of G1405 in 16S rRNA and to hydrophilic fluoroquinolones by QepA-mediated efflux in *Escherichia coli*. *Antimicrob Agents Chemother.* 2007;51:2464–2469.
26. Hakenbeck R, Kaminski K, Konig A, et al. Penicillin-binding proteins in beta-lactam-resistant *Streptococcus pneumoniae*. *Microb Drug Resist.* 1999;5:91–99.
27. Dowson CG, Coffey TJ, Kell C, et al. Evolution of penicillin resistance in *Streptococcus pneumoniae*, the role of *Streptococcus mitis* in the formation of a low affinity PBP2B in *S. pneumoniae*. *Mol Microbiol.* 1993;9:635–643.
28. Chambers HF. Methicillin resistance in staphylococci: molecular and biochemical basis and clinical implications. *Clin Microbiol Rev.* 1997;10:781–791.
29. Katayama Y, Ito T, Hiramatsu K. A new class of genetic element, *Staphylococcus* Cassette Chromosome *mec*, encodes methicillin resistance in *Staphylococcus aureus*. *Antimicrob Agents Chemother.* 2000;44:1549–1555.
30. Werner G, Strommenger B, Witte W. Acquired vancomycin resistance in clinically relevant pathogens. *Future Microbiology.* 2008;3:547–562.
31. Noble WC, Virani Z, Cree RGA. Co-transfer of vancomycin and other resistance genes from *Enterococcus faecalis* NCTC12201 to *Staphylococcus aureus*. *FEMS Microbiol Lett.* 1992;93:195–198.
32. Hiramatsu K, Aritaka N, Hanaki H, et al. Dissemination in Japanese hospitals of strains of *Staphylococcus aureus* heterogeneously resistant to vancomycin [see comments]. *Lancet.* 1997;350:1670–1673.
33. Sakoulas G, Moellering Jr RC. Increasing antibiotic resistance among methicillin-resistant *Staphylococcus aureus* strains. *Clin Infect Dis.* 2008;46(suppl 5):S360–S367.
34. Chang S, Sievert DM, Hageman JC, et al. Infection with vancomycin-resistant *Staphylococcus aureus* containing the *vanA* resistance gene. *N Engl J Med.* 2003;348:1342–1347.
35. Sievert DM, Rudrik JT, Patel JB, et al. Vancomycin-resistant *Staphylococcus aureus* in the United States, 2002–2006. *Clin Infect Dis.* 2008;46:668–674.
36. Liou GF, Yoshizawa S, Courvalin P, et al. Aminoglycoside resistance by ArmA-mediated ribosomal 16S methylation in human bacterial pathogens. *J Mol Biol.* 2006;359:358–364.
37. Hooper DC. Emerging mechanisms of fluoroquinolone resistance. *Emerg Infect Dis.* 2001;7:337–341.

38. Martinez-Martinez L, Pascual A, Jacoby GA. Quinolone resistance from a transferable plasmid. *Lancet*. 1998;351:797–799.

39. Deplano A, Zekhnini A, Allali N, et al. Association of mutations in *grlA* and *gyrA* topoisomerase genes with resistance to ciprofloxacin in epidemic and sporadic isolates of methicillin-resistant *Staphylococcus aureus*. *Antimicrob Agents Chemother*. 1997;41:2023–2025.

40. Endtz HP, Ruijs GJ, van Klingeren B, et al. Quinolone resistance in campylobacter isolated from man and poultry following the introduction of fluoroquinolones in veterinary medicine. *Antimicrob Agents Chemother*. 1991;27:199–208.

41. Seppala H, Klaukka T, Vuopio-Varkila J, et al. The effect of changes in the consumption of macrolide antibiotics on erythromycin resistance in group A streptococci in Finland. Finnish Study Group for Antimicrobial Resistance. *N Engl J Med*. 1997;337:441–446.

42. Tsiodras S, Gold HS, Sakoulas G, et al. Linezolid resistance in a clinical isolate of *Staphylococcus aureus*. *Lancet*. 2001;358:207–208.

43. Toh SM, Xiong L, Arias CA, et al. Acquisition of a natural resistance gene renders a clinical strain of methicillin-resistant *Staphylococcus aureus* resistant to the synthetic antibiotic linezolid. *Mol Microbiol*. 2007;64:1506–1514.

44. Gilbart J, Perry CR, Slocombe B. High-level mupirocin resistance in *Staphylococcus aureus*: evidence for two distinct isoleucyl-tRNA synthetases. *Antimicrob Agents Chemother*. 1993;37:32–38.

45. O'Neill AJ, McLaws F, Kahlmeter G, et al. Genetic basis of resistance to fusidic acid in staphylococci. *Antimicrob Agents Chemother*. 2007;51:1737–1740.

46. Poirel L, Rodriguez-Martinez JM, Mammeri H, et al. Origin of plasmid-mediated quinolone resistance determinant QnrA. *Antimicrob Agents Chemother*. 2005;49:3523–3525.

47. Lewis K. Riddle of biofilm resistance. *Antimicrob Agents Chemother*. 2001;45:999–1007.

48. Davies J. Inactivation of antibiotics and the dissemination of resistance genes. *Science*. 1994;264:375–382.

49. Salyers AA, Amabilc-Cuevas CF. Why are antibiotic resistance genes so resistant to elimination? *Antimicrob Agents Chemother*. 1997;41:2321–2325.

50. Ploy MC, Lambert T, Couty JP, et al. Integrons: an antibiotic resistance gene capture and expression system. *Clin Chem Lab Med*. 2000;38:483–487.

51. Enne VI, Livermore DM, Stephens P, et al. Persistence of sulphonamide resistance in *Escherichia coli* in the UK despite national prescribing restriction. *Lancet*. 2001;357:1325–1328.

52. Liebert CA, Hall RM, Summers AO. Transposon Tn*21*, flagship of the floating genome. *Microbiol Mol Biol Rev*. 1999;63:507–522.

53. Chongtrakool P, Ito T, Ma XX, et al. Staphylococcal cassette chromosome *mec* (SCC*mec*) typing of methicillin-resistant *Staphylococcus aureus* strains isolated in 11 Asian countries: a proposal for a new nomenclature for SCC*mec* elements. *Antimicrob Agents Chemother*. 2006;50:1001–1012.

54. Zhang K, McClure JA, Elsayed S, et al. Novel staphylococcal cassette chromosome mec type, tentatively designated type VIII, harboring class A *mec* and type 4 *ccr* gene complexes in a Canadian epidemic strain of methicillin-resistant *Staphylococcus aureus*. *Antimicrob Agents Chemother*. 2009;53:531–540.

55. Austin DJ, Anderson RM. Transmission dynamics of epidemic methicillin-resistant *Staphylococcus aureus* and vancomycin-resistant enterococci in England and Wales. *J Infect Dis*. 1999;179:883–891.

56. Deplano A, Witte W, van Leeuwen WJ, et al. Clonal dissemination of epidemic methicillin-resistant *Staphylococcus aureus* in Belgium and neighboring countries. *Clin Microbiol Infect*. 2000;6:239–245.

57. Mekontso-Dessap A, Kirsch M, Brun-Buisson C, et al. Poststernotomy mediastinitis due to *Staphylococcus aureus*: comparison of methicillin-resistant and methicillin-susceptible cases. *Clin Infect Dis*. 2001;32:877–883.

58. Tristan A, Bes M, Meugnier H, et al. Global distribution of Panton–Valentine leukocidin-positive methicillin-resistant *Staphylococcus aureus*, 2006. *Emerg Infect Dis*. 2007;13:594–600.

59. Voss A, Loeffen F, Bakker J, et al. Methicillin-resistant *Staphylococcus aureus* in pig farming. *Emerg Infect Dis*. 2005;11:1965–1966.

60. Sieradzki K, Villari P, Tomasz A. Decreased susceptibilities to teicoplanin and vancomycin among coagulase-negative methicillin-resistant clinical isolates of staphylococci. *Antimicrob Agents Chemother*. 1998;42:100–107.

61. Murray BE. Vancomycin-resistant enterococcal infections. *N Engl J Med*. 2000;342:710–721.

62. Ono S, Muratani T, Matsumoto T. Mechanisms of resistance to imipenem and ampicillin in *Enterococcus faecalis*. *Antimicrob Agents Chemother*. 2005;49:2954–2958.

63. Hidron AI, Edwards JR, Patel J, et al. NHSN annual update: antimicrobial-resistant pathogens associated with healthcare-associated infections: annual summary of data reported to the National Healthcare Safety Network at the Centers for Disease Control and Prevention, 2006–2007. *Infect Control Hosp Epidemiol*. 2008;29:996–1011.

64. Austin DJ, Bonten MJ, Weinstein RA, et al. Vancomycin-resistant enterococci in intensive-care hospital settings: transmission dynamics, persistence, and the impact of infection control programs. *Proc Natl Acad Sci U S A*. 1999;96:6908–6913.

65. Willems RJ, Top J, van Santen M, et al. Global spread of vancomycin-resistant *Enterococcus faecium* from distinct nosocomial genetic complex. *Emerg Infect Dis*. 2005;11:821–828.

66. Herrero IA, Issa NC, Patel R. Nosocomial spread of linezolid-resistant, vancomycin-resistant *Enterococcus faecium*. *N Engl J Med*. 2002;346:867–869.

67. DiazGranados CA, Zimmer SM, Klein M, et al. Comparison of mortality associated with vancomycin-resistant and vancomycin-susceptible enterococcal bloodstream infections: a meta-analysis. *Clin Infect Dis*. 2005;41:327–333.

68. Klugman KP. Pneumococcal resistance to antibiotics. *Clin Microbiol Rev*. 1990;3:171–196.

69. Richter SS, Heilmann KP, Dohrn CL, et al. Changing epidemiology of antimicrobial-resistant *Streptococcus pneumoniae* in the United States, 2004–2005. *Clin Infect Dis*. 2009;48:e23–e33.

70. Moore MR, Gertz Jr RE, Woodbury RL, et al. Population snapshot of emergent *Streptococcus pneumoniae* serotype 19A in the United States, 2005. *J Infect Dis*. 2008;197:1016–1027.

71. Reinert RR, Reinert S, van der LM, et al. Antimicrobial susceptibility of *Streptococcus pneumoniae* in eight European countries from 2001 to 2003. *Antimicrob Agents Chemother*. 2005;49:2903–2913.

72. Munoz R, Coffey TJ, Daniels M, et al. Intercontinental spread of a multi-resistant clone of serotype 23F *Streptococcus pneumoniae*. *J Infect Dis*. 1991;164:302–306.

73. Farrell DJ, Couturier C, Hryniewicz W. Distribution and antibacterial susceptibility of macrolide resistance genotypes in *Streptococcus pneumoniae*: PROTEKT Year 5 (2003–2004). *Int J Antimicrob Agents*. 2008;31:245–249.

74. Van Bambeke F, Reinert RR, Appelbaum PC, et al. Multidrug-resistant *Streptococcus pneumoniae* infections: current and future therapeutic options. *Drugs*. 2007;67:2355–2382.

75. Tristram S, Jacobs MR, Appelbaum PC. Antimicrobial resistance in *Haemophilus influenzae*. *Clin Microbiol Rev*. 2007;20:368–389.

76. Rubin LG, Medeiros AA, Yolken H, Moxon ER. Ampicillin treatment failure of apparently beta-lactamase-negative *Haemophilus influenzae* type b meningitis due to novel beta-lactamase. *Lancet*. 1981;ii:1008–1010.

77. Wu HM, Harcourt BH, Hatcher CP, et al. Emergence of ciprofloxacin-resistant *Neisseria meningitidis* in North America. *N Engl J Med*. 2009;360:886–892.

78. Ito M, Deguchi T, Mizutani KS, et al. Emergence and spread of *Neisseria gonorrhoeae* clinical isolates harboring mosaic-like structure of penicillin-binding protein 2 in Central Japan. *Antimicrob Agents Chemother*. 2005;49:137–143.

79. Phillips I. Beta-lactamase-producing, penicillin-resistant gonococcus. *Lancet*. 1976;ii:656–657.

80. Newman LM, Moran JS, Workowski KA. Update on the management of gonorrhea in adults in the United States. *Clin Infect Dis*. 2007;44(suppl 3):S84–S101.

81. Garau J, Xercavins M, Rodriguez-Carballeira M, et al. Emergence and dissemination of quinolone-resistant *Escherichia coli* in the community. *Antimicrob Agents Chemother*. 1999;43:2736–2741.

82. Clermont O, Lavollay M, Vimont S, et al. The CTX-M-15-producing *Escherichia coli* diffusing clone belongs to a highly virulent B2 phylogenetic subgroup. *J Antimicrob Chemother*. 2008;61:1024–1028.

83. Barnaud G, Labia R, Raskine L, et al. Extension of resistance to cefepime and cefpirome associated to a six amino acid deletion in the H-10 helix of the cephalosporinase of an *Enterobacter cloacae* clinical isolate. *FEMS Microbiol Lett*. 2001;195:185–190.

84. Hanberger H, Gareia-Rodriguez JA, Gobernado M, et al. Antibiotic susceptibility among aerobic gram-negative bacilli in intensive care units in 5 European countries. French and Portuguese ICU Study Groups. *J Am Med Assoc*. 1999;281:67–71.

85. Cuzon G, Naas T, Demachy MC, et al. Plasmid-mediated carbapenem-hydrolyzing beta-lactamase KPC-2 in *Klebsiella pneumoniae* isolate from Greece. *Antimicrob Agents Chemother*. 2008;52:796–797.

86. De Gheldre Y, Struelens MJ, Glupczynski Y, et al. National epidemiologic surveys of *Enterobacter aerogenes* in Belgian hospitals from 1996 to 1998. *J Clin Microbiol*. 2001;39:889–896.

87. De Gheldre Y, Maes N, Rost F, et al. Molecular epidemiology of an outbreak of multidrug-resistant *Enterobacter aerogenes* infections and in vivo emergence of imipenem resistance. *J Clin Microbiol*. 1997;35:152–160.

88. Talukder KA, Khajanchi BK, Islam MA, et al. Fluoroquinolone resistance linked to both *gyrA* and *parC* mutations in the quinolone resistance-determining region of *Shigella dysenteriae* type 1. *Curr Microbiol*. 2006;52:108–111.

89. Threlfall EJ, Ward LR. Decreased susceptibility to ciprofloxacin in *Salmonella enterica* serotype Typhi, United Kingdom. *Emerg Infect Dis*. 2001;7:448–450.

90. Molbak K, Baggesen DL, Aarestrup FM, et al. An outbreak of multidrug-resistant, quinolone-resistant, *Salmonella enterica* serotype typhimurium DT104. *N Engl J Med*. 1999;341:1420–1425.

91. Threlfall EJ, Ward LR, Skinner JA, Graham A. Antimicrobial drug resistance in non-typhoidal salmonellas from humans in England and Wales in 1999: decrease in multiple resistance in *Salmonella enterica* serotypes Typhimurium, Virchow, and Hadar. *Microb Drug Resist*. 2000;6:319–325.

92. Tassios PT, Gazouli M, Tzelepi E, et al. Spread of a *Salmonella typhimurium* clone resistant to expanded-spectrum cephalosporins in three European countries. *J Clin Microbiol*. 1999;37:3774–3777.

93. Fey PD, Safranek TJ, Rupp ME, et al. Ceftriaxone-resistant salmonella infection acquired by a child from cattle. *N Engl J Med*. 2000;342:1242–1249.

94. Gibreel A, Taylor DE. Macrolide resistance in *Campylobacter jejuni* and *Campylobacter coli*. *J Antimicrob Chemother*. 2006;58:243–255.

95. Smith KE, Besser JM, Hedberg CW, et al. Quinolone-resistant *Campylobacter jejuni* infections in Minnesota, 1992–1998. Investigation Team. *N Engl J Med*. 1999;340:1525–1532.

96. Moore JE, Barton MD, Blair IS, et al. The epidemiology of antibiotic resistance in Campylobacter. *Microbes Infect*. 2006;8:1955–1966.

97. Houben MH, Van Der BD, Hensen EF, et al. A systematic review of *Helicobacter pylori* eradication therapy – the impact of antimicrobial resistance on eradication rates. *Aliment Pharmacol Ther*. 1999;13:1047–1055.

98. Megraud F, Lehours P. *Helicobacter pylori* detection and antimicrobial susceptibility testing. *Clin Microbiol Rev*. 2007;20:280–322.

99. Li XZ, Nikaido H, Poole K. Role of mexA-mexB-oprM in antibiotic efflux in *Pseudomonas aeruginosa*. *Antimicrob Agents Chemother*. 1995;39:1948–1953.

100. Carmeli Y, Troillet N, Eliopoulos GM, et al. Emergence of antibiotic-resistant *Pseudomonas aeruginosa*: comparison of risks associated with different antipseudomonal agents. *Antimicrob Agents Chemother*. 1999;43:1379–1382.

101. Walsh TR. Clinically significant carbapenemases: an update. *Curr Opin Infect Dis*. 2008;21:367–371.

102. Mussi MA, Limansky AS, Viale AM. Acquisition of resistance to carbapenems in multidrug-resistant clinical strains of *Acinetobacter baumannii*: natural insertional inactivation of a gene encoding a member of a novel family of beta-barrel outer membrane proteins. *Antimicrob Agents Chemother*. 2005;49:1432–1440.

103. Gales AC, Jones RN, Sader HS. Global assessment of the antimicrobial activity of polymyxin B against 54 731 clinical isolates of Gram-negative bacilli: report from the SENTRY antimicrobial surveillance programme (2001–2004). *Clin Microbiol Infect*. 2006;12:315–321.

104. Sandgren A, Strong M, Muthukrishnan P, et al. Tuberculosis drug resistance mutation database. *PLoS Med*. 2009;6:e2.

105. Wright A, Zignol M, Van Deun A, et al. Epidemiology of antituberculosis drug resistance 2002–07: an updated analysis of the Global Project on Anti-Tuberculosis Drug Resistance Surveillance. *Lancet*. 2009;373:1861–1873.

106. Jassal M, Bishai WR. Extensively drug-resistant tuberculosis. *Lancet Infect Dis*. 2009;9:19–30.

107. Nolan CM. Nosocomial multidrug-resistant tuberculosis – global spread of the third epidemic. *J Infect Dis*. 1997;176:748–751.

108. Struelens MJ. The epidemiology of antimicrobial resistance in hospital acquired infections: problems and possible solutions. *Br Med J*. 1998;317:652–654.

109. Okeke IN, Lamikanra A, Edelman R. Socioeconomic and behavioral factors leading to acquired bacterial resistance to antibiotics in developing countries. *Emerg Infect Dis*. 1999;5:18–27.

110. Guillemot D, Carbon C, Balkau B, et al. Low dosage and long treatment duration of beta-lactam: risk factors for carriage of penicillin-resistant *Streptococcus pneumoniae*. *J Am Med Assoc*. 1998;279:365–370.

111. Richard P, Le Floch R, Chamoux C, et al. *Pseudomonas aeruginosa* outbreak in a burn unit: role of antimicrobials in the emergence of multiply resistant strains. *J Infect Dis*. 1994;170:377–383.

112. Goldmann DA, Weinstein RA, Wenzel RP, et al. Strategies to prevent and control the emergence and spread of antimicrobial-resistant microorganisms in hospitals. A challenge to hospital leadership. *J Am Med Assoc*. 1996;275:234–240.

113. Lucet JC, Decre D, Fichelle A, et al. Control of a prolonged outbreak of extended-spectrum beta-lactamase-producing enterobacteriaceae in a university hospital. *Clin Infect Dis*. 1999;29:1411–1418.

114. Chaix C, Durand-Zaleski I, Alberti C, et al. Control of endemic methicillin-resistant *Staphylococcus aureus*: a cost–benefit analysis in an intensive care unit. *J Am Med Assoc*. 1999;282:1745–1751.

115. Ostrowsky BE, Trick WE, Sohn AH, et al. Control of vancomycin-resistant enterococcus in health care facilities in a region. *N Engl J Med*. 2001;344:1427–1433.

116. Struelens MJ. Multidisciplinary antimicrobial management teams: the way forward to control antimicrobial resistance in hospitals. *Curr Opin Infect Dis*. 2003;16:305–307.

117. Dellit TH, Owens RC, McGowan Jr JE, et al. Infectious Diseases Society of America and the Society for Healthcare Epidemiology of America guidelines for developing an institutional program to enhance antimicrobial stewardship. *Clin Infect Dis*. 2007;44:159–177.

118. Bronzwaer S, Lönnroth A, Haigh R. The European Community strategy against antimicrobial resistance. *Euro Surveill*. 2004;9:30–34.

4

Pharmacodynamics of anti-infective agents: target delineation and susceptibility breakpoint selection

Johan W. Mouton

The goal of anti-infective chemotherapy is to administer the drug in such a way that it will generate the highest probability of a good therapeutic outcome while at the same time having the lowest probability of a drug-related toxicity event that is related to the time–concentration profile of the drug. In order to reach that goal, it is therefore necessary to determine the concentration–effect relationship of the drug over time, determine which concentration profile ensures this to become true and design dosing regimens that bring about this concentration profile. This approach applies to all anti-infectives, whether they are antibacterials, antivirals, antifungals or antiparasitic agents. In this chapter the discussion and examples are mainly taken from the antibacterial scene, but it should be emphasized that the concepts can be applied to all anti-infective agents.

One of the unique features of anti-infectives is that the target of the drug – the receptor of the molecule – is located on the micro-organism rather than in humans. This stands out against virtually all other drugs where the receptor of the drug is located in humans themselves. Unfortunately, for some anti-infectives there are also receptors in humans, resulting in toxicity, and for some drug classes this is a major limitation to their use. Since the receptor of the anti-infective is on the microbe, it is relatively easy to study the effect of antimicrobials in model systems, both in in-vitro systems as well as in in-vivo infection models. The downside is that, because there are as many different receptors as there are different species, exposure–response relationships cannot always be generalized and need to be studied in detail for various drug–micro-organism combinations. The primary focus of this chapter is to describe the approach to determine exposure–response relationships of anti-infectives and to translate these to optimal dosing regimens and the choice of anti-infective.

PHARMACODYNAMIC TARGETS AND TARGET DELINEATION

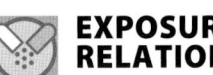 ### EXPOSURE–RESPONSE RELATIONSHIPS IN VIVO

Figure 4.1A shows a diagram of the concentration–time curve of an anti-infective agent. Two major pharmacokinetic parameters describe this profile: the peak concentration (C_{max}) and the area under the concentration–time curve (AUC). These in turn are the result of the pharmacokinetic properties of the drug, clearance and volume of distribution. However, a pharmacokinetic description as such does not convey any information with respect to the activity of the drug in vivo. One way to do this is to use the relationship between the exposure of the anti-infective and the activity (or potency) of the drug as determined in an in-vitro system such as minimum inhibitory concentration (MIC) testing. Other measures of potency include the half maximal effective concentration (EC_{50}) in vitro for antivirals and some antifungals. Figure 4.1B shows the same diagram as in Figure 4.1A but includes the MIC of a micro-organism. Instead of two pharmacokinetic parameters there are now three pharmacodynamic indices (PIs) that can be recognized: the AUC and the C_{max}, both relative to the MIC, and in addition the time the concentration of the drug remains above the MIC ($T_{>MIC}$). The latter is usually expressed as the $\%T_{>MIC}$ of the dosing interval. These three PI values – AUC/MIC, C_{max}/MIC and $\%T_{>MIC}$ – thus describe the relationship between exposure of the anti-infective over a

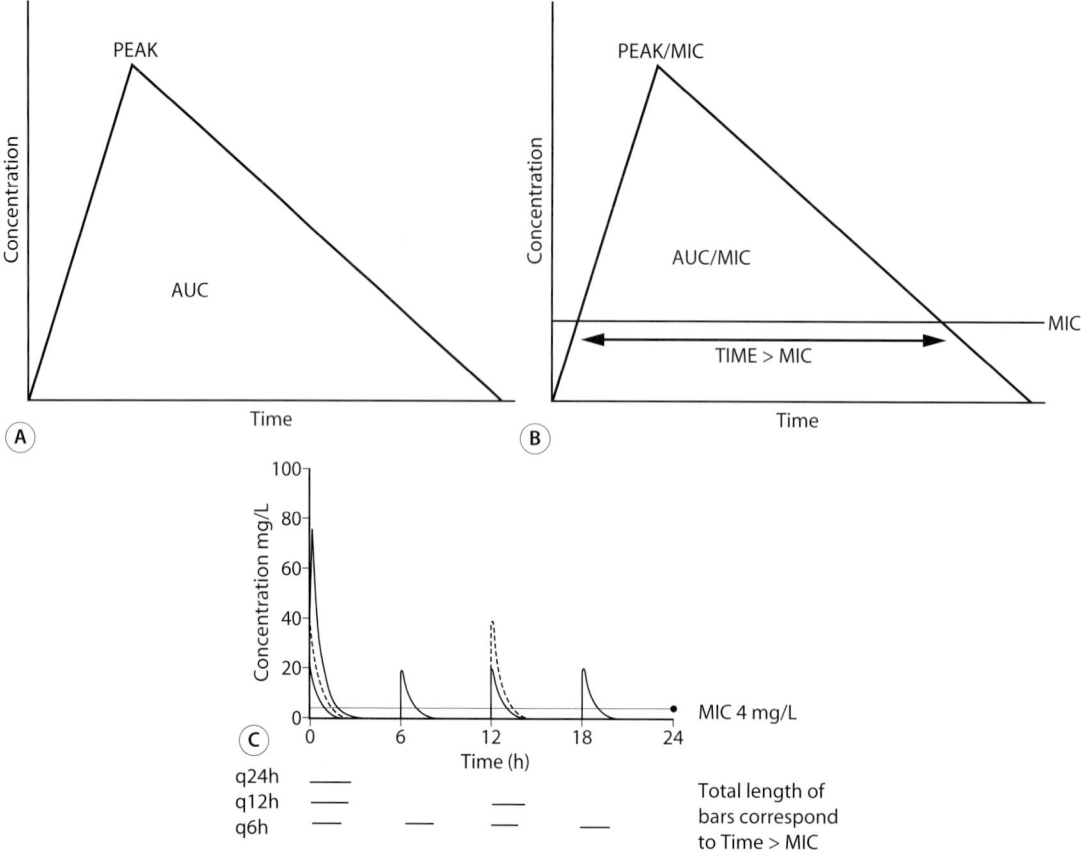

Fig. 4.1 (A) Diagram of a concentration–time curve showing the pharmacokinetic parameters Peak (or C_{max}) and AUC. (B) The PK/PD indices are derived by relating the pharmacokinetic parameter to the MIC: AUC/MIC, C_{max}/MIC and $T_{>MIC}$. (C) Diagram showing that the $T_{>MIC}$ increases if daily doses are divided. The length of the bars beneath Figure 4.1C correspond to the $T_{>MIC}$.

defined time interval in relation to the potency of the antimicrobial as defined by the MIC. For the AUC/MIC and the C_{max}/MIC, it follows that the value of the PI is proportional to the AUC and C_{max}. Since the pharmacokinetic profile for most antimicrobials is proportional to dose in a linear fashion, it follows that: (1) doubling the dose usually results in a doubling of AUC/MIC and C_{max}/MIC, and (2) administration of the dose twice will double the AUC/MIC while the C_{max} will not change. For the %$T_{>MIC}$, dividing the same dose over multiple smaller doses will result in an increased %$T_{>MIC}$ while retaining the same AUC/MIC (Figure 4.1C).

Using different dosing regimens in animal models of infection by varying both the frequency and the dose of the drug, and thereby different exposures and corresponding PIs, it has been shown that there is a clear relationship between a pharmacokinetic/pharmacodynamic (PK/PD) index and efficacy.[1] Figure 4.2 shows the relationship for two drugs belonging to different classes of antimicrobials, the quinolones and the β-lactams. In general, for concentration-dependent drugs there is a clear relationship between AUC:MIC ratio and/or C_{max}:MIC ratio and efficacy, while for time-dependent drugs it is the %$T_{>MIC}$ that is best correlated with effect.

CURVE–EFFECT DESCRIPTION AND PHARMACODYNAMIC TARGETS IN ANIMAL MODELS

In most cases, the relationship between exposure and effect can be described by a sigmoid curve. The E_{max} model with varying slope, or Hill equation, is most commonly used to describe this sigmoid relationship. An example is shown in Figure 4.3, displaying the relationship between AUC/MIC ratio and effect. The effect here is the number of colony forming units (CFU) after 24 h of treatment with different dosing regimens of levofloxacin. Apart from the parameter estimates that describe the curve, such as the EC_{50} and the E_{max}, there are other parameters related to the curve, the most important of which is the net static effect. This is the dose or exposure resulting in the measure of effect being unchanged from baseline to the time of evaluation (e.g. the number of CFU at t = 0 h [baseline, start of treatment] and t = 24 h [time of sampling]). The use of the term 'static' does not imply that no changes have occurred during the period of reference; indeed kill and regrowth may have occurred (repeatedly) during this period.[4] Other characteristics include exposures that result in the E_{max}, 90% of the E_{max}, or a 2 log drop. The PI value that

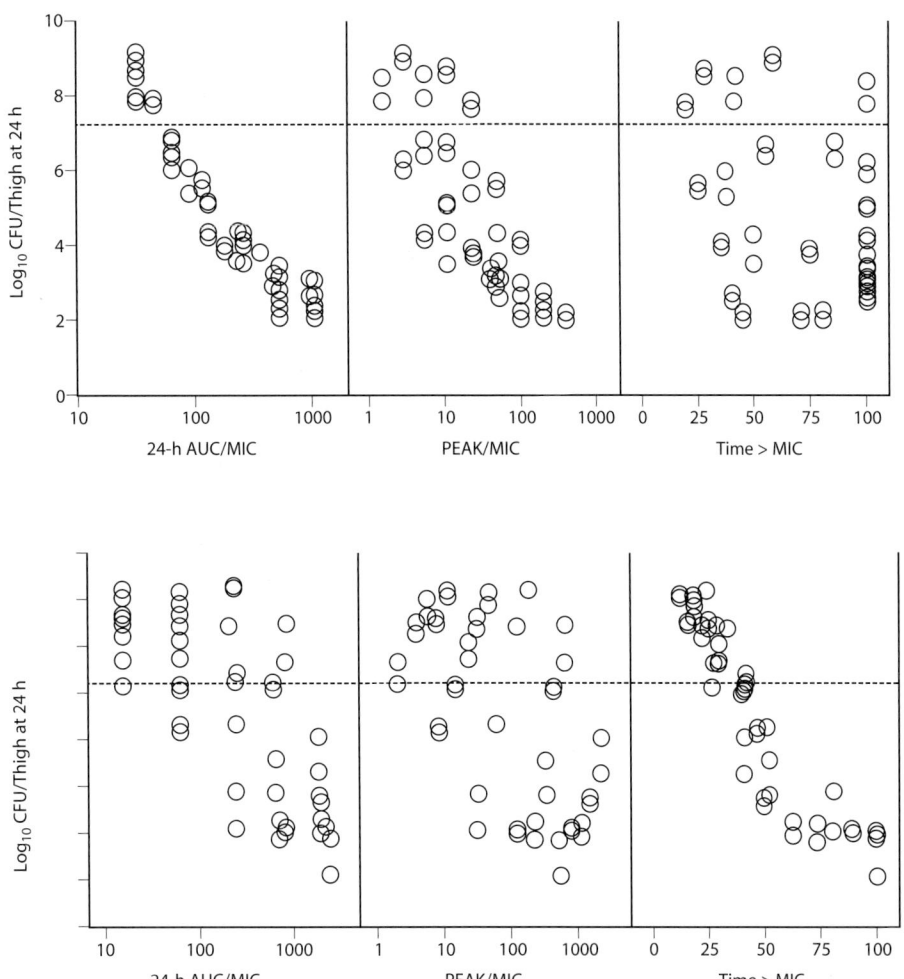

Fig. 4.2 Relationship between $T_{>MIC}$, AUC and peak of levofloxacin (upper) and ceftazidime (lower) in a mouse model of infection with *Streptococcus pneumoniae* as obtained by various dosing regimens and efficacy expressed as colony forming units (CFU). The best relationship is obtained with the AUC for levofloxacin and $T_{>MIC}$ for ceftazidime; the curve drawn represents a model fit of the Hill equation with variable slope to the data. Reproduced from Andes D, Craig WA. Animal model pharmacokinetics and pharmacodynamics: a critical review. **Int J Antimicrob Agents.** 2002;19(4):261–268, with permission of Elsevier.[2]

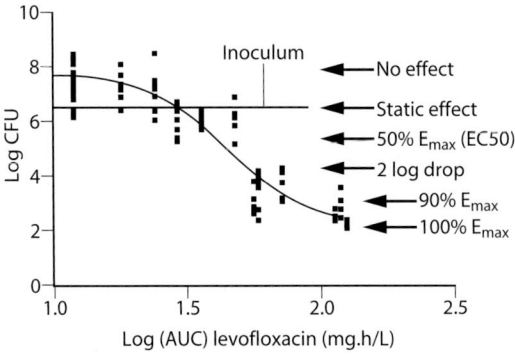

Fig. 4.3 Diagram showing various characteristic effect levels of a sigmoid dose–response relationship, in this example levofloxacin. From F. Scaglione, J.W. Mouton, R. Mattina and F. Fraschini, Pharmacodynamics of levofloxacin and ciprofloxacin in a murine pneumonia model: peak concentration/MIC versus area under the curve/MIC ratios. **Antimicrob Agents Chemother.** 47 (2003), pp. 2749–2755. Copyright © 2003, American Society for Microbiology.[3]

will result in one of the effects described and is desired is also called the pharmacodynamic target (PT). Pharmacodynamic targets have been described for many micro-organism–anti-infective combinations and in general show a good concordance with survival and clinical cure (*see below*), in particular for the free, non-protein bound fraction of the drug. In the following, the prefix *f* indicates that the parameters or indices apply to the fraction unbound (*see also* 'Exposure in first compartment', below).

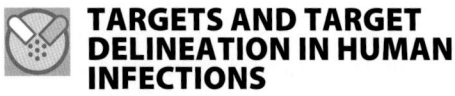

TARGETS AND TARGET DELINEATION IN HUMAN INFECTIONS

The relationship between PI and effect is increasingly being studied in humans. There are two major differences with animal models that need consideration and have, or may have, a significant effect on conclusions. The first is that the outcome parameter is usually binomial instead of (semi) continuous. That is, instead of colony forming units, outcome is determined as cure versus no cure, persistence of colonization versus elimination, or mortality versus survival, and therefore the statistical and/or mathematical models that describe the relationship between PI and effect differ as well.

Binomial outcome

If outcome is measured at a single point in time, for instance clinical cure 28 days after the start of antimicrobial treatment, univariate or multivariate logistic regression is the analysis tool primarily used. Alternatively, if outcome is determined over time, such as time to defervescence or time to pathogen clearance, a Kaplan–Meier analysis can be applied and/or Cox regression. The advantage of determining outcome over time is that in general it is much more powerful to show differences between groups – if present – and therefore fewer patients are needed to determine differences in effects. This was shown in a study by Ambrose and colleagues, studying the effect of levofloxacin in maxillary sinusitis and taking serial sinus aspirates.[5]

While these methods do indicate differences between groups if present, and the models can also be used to estimate the parameters that determine outcome, they do not answer the question as to which *value* of the PI makes the difference between a high probability of cure and a low probability of cure. To that purpose, classification and regression tree analysis (CART) has been used increasingly. This tool uses exploratory non-parametric statistical algorithms that can accommodate continuous numerical data, as well as categorical data, as either independent or dependent variables. For a dependent variable that is categorical such as clinical response, it can be used to identify threshold values in an independent continuous variable such as an AUC:MIC ratio that separates groups with a high probability of cure from those with a low probability of cure. The results can subsequently be used to test for significance in univariate or multivariate logistic regression analyses.

One of the first exposure–response analyses of clinical data that utilized this approach was by Forrest et al.[6] Intravenous ciprofloxacin was studied in critically ill patients with pneumonia involving predominantly Enterobacteriaceae and *Pseudomonas aeruginosa*. Multivariate logistic regression analyses identified the AUC_{0-24}:MIC ratio as being predictive of clinical and microbiological response ($p <0.003$). Recursive partitioning identified a threshold AUC_{0-24}:MIC ratio value of 125. Patients who had an AUC_{0-24}:MIC ratio of 125 or greater had a significantly higher probability of a positive therapeutic response than those patients in whom lesser exposures were attained. Another example is provided in Figure 4.4 showing a jitter plot of the relationship between the $fAUC_{0-24}$:MIC ratio of five quinolones and microbiological response. CART analysis indicates that patients with an AUC:MIC ratio above 34 (cure rate 92.6%) had a significantly ($p = 0.01$) increased probability of cure compared to those that had not (cure rate 66.7%).[7]

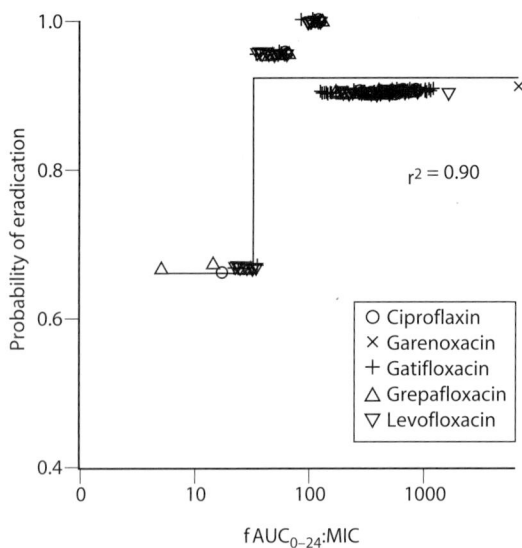

Fig. 4.4 Jitter plot of the relationship between the ratio of free drug area under the concentration–time curve at 24 h to the MIC ($fAUC_{0-24}$:MIC) for five quinolones (ciprofloxacin, garenoxacin, gatifloxacin, grepafloxacin and levofloxacin) and microbiological response in 121 patients with respiratory tract infection pneumonia, acute exacerbation of chronic bronchitis or acute maxillary sinusitis associated with *Streptococcus pneumoniae*. Reproduced from Rodriguez-Tudela JL, Almirante B, Rodriguez-Pardo D, et al. Correlation of the MIC and Dose/MIC ratio of fluconazole to the therapeutic response of patients with mucosal candidiasis and candidaemia. **Antimicrob Agents Chemother.** 2007;51(10):3599–3604. Copyright © 2007, American Society for Microbiology.[7]

(Semi)-continuous outcome

There are an increasing number of studies that have strived to look for outcome data that are continuous or semi-continuous. These have the advantage that they are much more informative, and therefore fewer subjects are needed to show an exposure–response relationship. In addition, E_{max} models can be fit to the data to show exposure–response relationships in a more meaningful manner than binomial data.

An approach for a semi-continuous outcome was the exposure–response relationship of fluconazole for the treatment of oropharyngeal candidiasis (Figure 4.5). Patients were treated with various doses of fluconazole and outcome recorded, while MICs were determined from cultures taken before and after treatment. Because of the variation in doses and MICs, a large number of groups could be distinguished, with each group designated by a specific dose:MIC ratio or AUC:MIC ratio. The percentage cure per group was plotted, and the E_{max} model fitted to the data. This resulted in a clear exposure–response relationship. The authors concluded that the pharmacodynamic target would be an AUC:MIC ratio of near 100, corresponding to the near maximum effect in this study.

It is, however, not easy to find an outcome variable that is continuous in humans that is meaningful. One example is the use of the relative increase in FEV1 (the forced volume of expiration during the first second) after a specified period of treatment

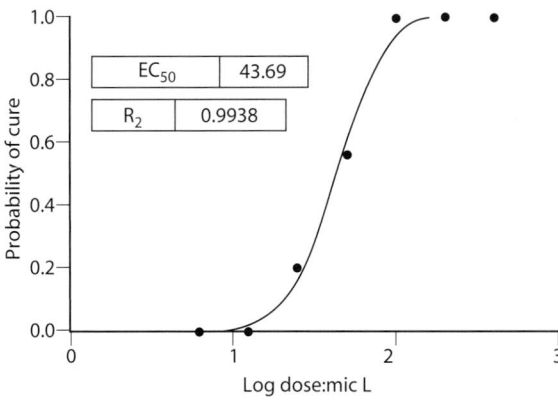

Fig. 4.5 Dose/MIC–response relationship for fluconazole in patients with oropharyngeal candidiasis. The dose:AUC ratio for fluconazole is 1, thus the plot for AUC/MIC is similar. Reproduced from Rodriguez-Tudela JL, Almirante B, Rodriguez-Pardo D, et al. Correlation of the MIC and Dose/MIC ratio of fluconazole to the therapeutic response of patients with mucosal candidiasis and candidaemia. **Antimicrob Agents Chemother.** 2007;51(10):3599–3604. Copyright © 2007, American Society for Microbiology.[8]

with antipseudomonal therapy in patients with cystic fibrosis as shown in Figure 4.6. An E_{max} model fitted the data well, and by using a continuous variable instead of a dichotomous one, the authors could show an exposure–response relationship in a limited number of patients, indicating the significant increase in power if a continuous outcome variable is used.

Variance in exposure

The second major difference between human studies and animal models, or in-vitro pharmacokinetic models, is the variance in exposure. With some exceptions, such as the relationship between fluconazole exposure and effect (*see* Figure 4.5), only one or two different dosing regimens can be analyzed, resulting in a significant correlation between the various

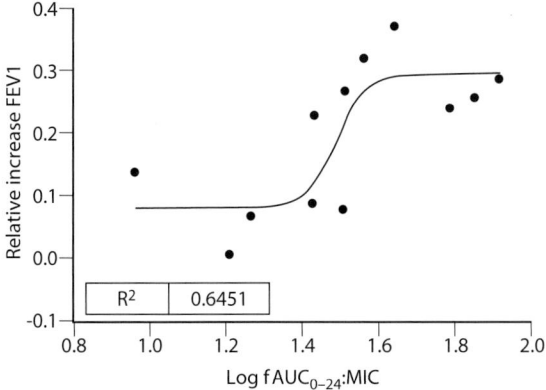

Fig. 4.6 Relationship between $fAUC_{0-24}$:MIC ratio of tobramycin as a measure of exposure and relative increase in FEV1 as a measure of effect in patients with cystic fibrosis. Reproduced from Preston SL, Drusano GL, Berman AL, et al. Pharmacodynamics of levofloxacin: a new paradigm for early clinical trials [see comments]. **Journal American Medical Association.** 1998;279(2):125–129.[9]

PIs. While this does not affect the estimate of the pharmacodynamic target if the PI that drives the effect is known, this co-linearity makes it almost impossible to determine the PI that drives outcome. This information thus needs to be derived from other sources. Alternatively, if different drugs from the same class with the same mechanism of action are analyzed simultaneously, this will result in the variety of exposures being sought. A clear example is the study of Ambrose and colleagues who looked at the exposure–response relationship of various quinolones as discussed above (*see* Figure 4.4).

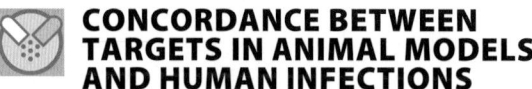

CONCORDANCE BETWEEN TARGETS IN ANIMAL MODELS AND HUMAN INFECTIONS

In general, there is a rather good concordance between PK/PD animal studies and data from infected patients, as shown by Ambrose and colleagues[10] in Table 4.1. With the exception of telithromycin, the magnitudes of the PK/PD measure necessary for clinical effectiveness were similar to those identified from animal data across drug classes and across multiple clinical indications. As illustrated in Table 4.1, the magnitude of exposure identified for a 2 log unit reduction in bacterial burden in immunocompromised animals was similar to the exposure threshold associated with good clinical outcomes for patients with hospital-acquired pneumonia associated with Gram-negative bacilli treated with ciprofloxacin or levofloxacin. For instance, Drusano and colleagues (Jumbe et al.[11]) demonstrated that for levofloxacin and *Ps. aeruginosa*, a total drug AUC_{0-24}:MIC ratio of 88 in immunosuppressed mice was associated with a 99% reduction in bacterial burden, while Craig.[12] showed that for fluoroquinolones and primarily Gram-negative bacilli in immunosuppressed animals, the AUC_{0-24}:MIC ratio was predictive of survival. Thus, it can be inferred that the exposure target in immunocompromised animals predictive of an adequate response in humans with such pneumonias is a minimum 2 log unit reduction in bacterial burden. This means that, in the circumstance where human exposure–response data are unavailable, as is the case in newly developed anti-infectives, we can use the PT in animals to predict clinical effectiveness in humans.

OPTIMIZING DOSING REGIMENS: TRANSLATING PHARMACODYNAMIC TARGETS TO OPTIMIZING THERAPY

In the first part of the chapter the relationship between exposure and response was discussed, both in models of infection as well as in the treatment of human infections. Using those relationships, PI values were derived that could differentiate between the probability of a good outcome versus a worse outcome, and these are pharmacodynamic targets one aims to attain in patients. Once this PT is known, a dosing regimen to optimally treat infections can be determined by optimizing the exposure of the drug to the micro-organism in the patient. Since the value of the PT is dependent on both the

Table 4.1 Pharmacodynamic targets derived from animal infection models and clinical data

Disease state	Drug	Clinically derived PK/PD target	Animal infection model; organism studied	Animal-derived PK/PD target
Hospital-acquired pneumonia	Quinolones	$fAUC_{0-24}$:MIC ratio: 62–75	Neutropenic mouse thigh; Gram-negative bacilli	$fAUC_{0-24}$:MIC ratio: 70–90 for 90% animal survival or 2 log-unit kill
Community-acquired respiratory tract infections	Quinolones	$fAUC_{0-24}$:MIC ratio: 34	Immunocompetent mouse thigh; *Streptococcus pneumoniae*	$fAUC_{0-24}$:MIC ratio: 25–34 for 90% animal survival or 2 log-unit kill
	β-Lactams	$T_{>MIC}$: 40% of the dosing interval	Immunocompetent mouse thigh; *Str. pneumoniae*	$T_{>MIC}$: 30–40% of the dosing interval for 90% animal survival
	Telithromycin	AUC_{0-24}:MIC ratio: 3.375	Neutropenic mouse thigh; *Str. pneumoniae*	AUC_{0-24}:MIC ratio: 1000 for stasis
Bacteremia	Oritavancin	$fT_{>MIC}$: 22% of the dosing interval for *Staphylococcus aureus*	Neutropenic mouse thigh; *Staph. aureus*	$fT_{>MIC}$: 20% of the dosing interval for a 0.5 log-unit kill
	Linezolid	AUC_{0-24}:MIC ratio: 85 for *Staph. aureus* or *Enterrococcus faecium*	Neutropenic mouse thigh; *Staph. aureus*	AUC_{0-24}:MIC ratio: 83 for stasis
Complicated skin and skin structure infections	Tigecycline	AUC_{0-24}:MIC ratio: 17.9	Neutropenic mouse thigh; *Staph. aureus*	AUC_{0-24}:MIC ratio: 20 for stasis
	Linezolid	AUC_{0-24}:MIC ratio: 110	Neutropenic mouse thigh; *Staph. aureus*	AUC_{0-24}:MIC ratio: 83 for stasis

From Ambrose et al.[10]

exposure as such, as well as the MIC of the micro-organism, it follows that the pharmacokinetic profile has to be optimized accordingly.

TARGET ATTAINMENT

The simplest method to determine the dosing regimen required to obtain a certain exposure or PT is to tabulate or plot the PI as a function of MIC for a number of dosing regimens. Pharmacokinetic parameters are used to calculate the pharmacokinetic profiles using standard equations and the PI calculated for a range of MICs. An example is provided in Figure 4.7, showing the $T_{>MIC}$ for amoxicillin–clavulanic acid.[13] If the MICs that need to be covered are known, MICs that can supposedly be covered with a certain dosing regimen can be read directly from the figure for a certain PT. Although there are other factors that need to be considered to optimize dosing regimens, this approach yields a straightforward comparison of exposures of various dosing regimens (or drugs within the same class; see for instance Mouton et al.[14]).

PROBABILITY OF TARGET ATTAINMENT

When a specific pharmacodynamic index value is used as a pharmacodynamic target to predict the probability of successful treatment, this should be true not only for the population mean, but also for each individual within the population. Since the pharmacokinetic behavior differs for each individual, the PK part of the PI differs as well. An example

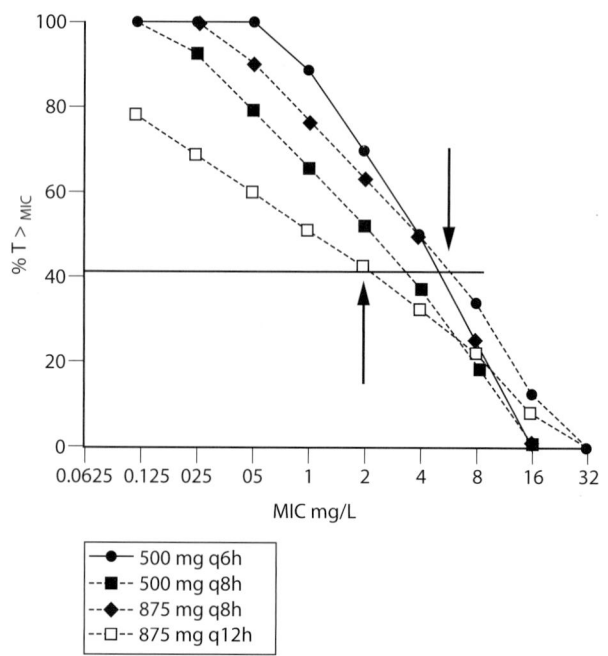

Fig. 4.7 Diagram showing the relationship between $T_{>MIC}$ and MIC of amoxicillin for four different dosing regimens of amoxicillin–clavulanic acid to demonstrate that the clinical breakpoint is dependent on the dosing regimen. Assuming that 40% $T_{>MIC}$ is the time of the dosing regimen needed for effect, the breakpoint for the 875 mg every 12 h is 2 mg/L while for the dosing regimen of 500 mg every 6 h it is 8 mg/L. Based on Mouton JW, Punt N. Use of the T>MIC to choose between different dosing regimens of beta-lactam antibiotics. **J Antimicrob Chemother.** 2001;47(4):500–501. © 2001 The British Society for Antimicrobial Chemotherapy.[13]

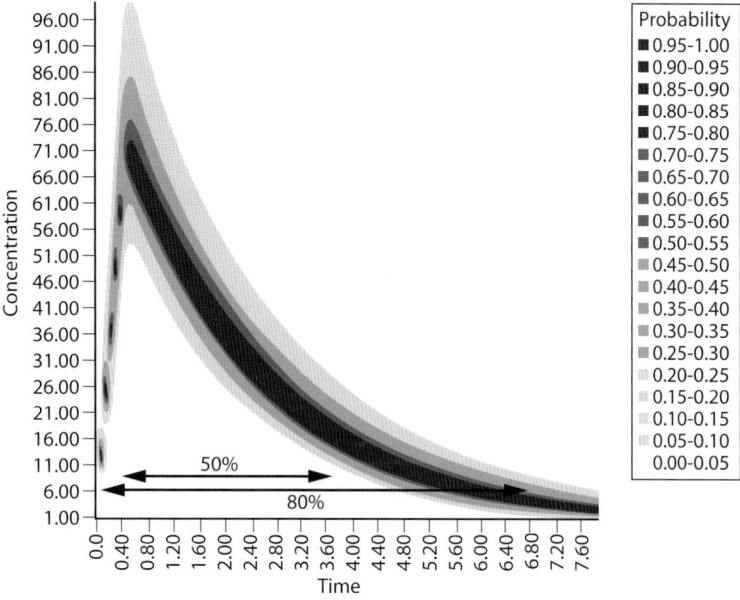

Fig. 4.8 Simulation of ceftazidime after a 1 g dose. The grayscale indicates the probability of presence of a certain concentration. Due to interindividual variability, some individuals in the population will have a T$_{>MIC}$ of 50%, while others will have a value of 80%. The population mean is in the middle of the black area. Reproduced from Mouton JW. Impact of pharmacodynamics on breakpoint selection for susceptibility testing. **Infect Dis Clin North Am.** 2003;17(3):579–598, with permission of Elsevier.[15]

is given in Figure 4.8. The figure shows the proportion of the population reaching a certain concentration of ceftazidime after a 1 g dose. It is apparent from Figure 4.8 that there are individuals with a T$_{>MIC}$ of 50%, while others have, with the same dosing regimen, a T$_{>MIC}$ of more than 80%. Thus, when designing the dosing regimen that should result in a certain pharmacodynamic target, this interindividual variation should be taken into consideration.

The most popular method to do this is to use Monte Carlo simulations (MCS). This approach was first used by Drusano et al. who presented an integrated approach of population pharmacokinetics and microbiological susceptibility information to the US Food and Drug Administration (FDA) Anti-infectives Product Advisory Committee.[16,17] The first step in that approach is to obtain estimates of the pharmacokinetic parameters of the population, using population pharmacokinetic analysis. Importantly, not only the estimates of the parameters are obtained, but also estimates of dispersion. These are then applied to simulate multiple concentration–time curves by performing Monte Carlo simulation. This is a method which takes the variability in the input variables into consideration in the simulations.[18] For each of the pharmacokinetic curves generated, all of which are slightly different because the input parameters vary to a degree in relation to the variance of the parameters, the value of the PK/PD index is determined for a range of MICs. For each MIC value, the proportion of the population that will reach a specific pharmacodynamic target is displayed in tabular or graphical form. As an example, Table 4.2 displays the probability of target attainment (PTA) for various targets for a 1 g dose of ceftazidime. The optimal dosing regimen follows from the PT that one considers necessary and the MIC range that needs to be

Table 4.2 Probability of target attainment for various pharmacodynamic targets for ceftazidime given three times daily

MIC (mg/L)	% Time > MIC			
	30	40	50	60
0.5	100	100	100	100
1	100	100	100	100
2	100	100	100	100
4	100	100	100	100
8	100	99	84	42
16	54	10	1	0
32	0	0	0	0

From Mouton JW, Punt N, Vinks AA. A retrospective analysis using Monte Carlo simulation to evaluate recommended ceftazidime dosing regimens in healthy volunteers, patients with cystic fibrosis, and patients in the intensive care unit. **Clin Ther.** 2005;27(6):762–772, with permission of Elsevier.[19]

covered. Vice versa, existing dosing regimens can be evaluated bearing this in mind.

Another approach was presented at the Clinical and Laboratory Standards Institute (CLSI) in 2004 by the European Committee on Antimicrobial Susceptibility Testing (EUCAST)[20] as part of the method being used to evaluate susceptibility breakpoints. It has the advantage that it shows the total probability function irrespective of the target and therefore provides a more complete picture of the data.[19] An example is shown in Figure 4.9. In the figure, the $fT_{>MIC}$ of ceftazidime is displayed as a function of MIC for a 1 g dose. The middle line represents the values for the mean of the

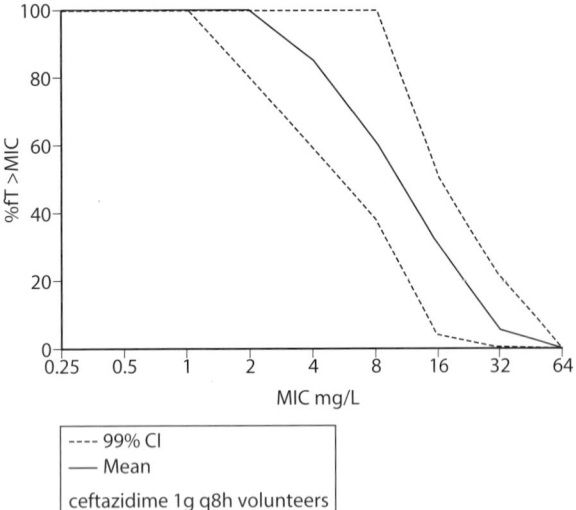

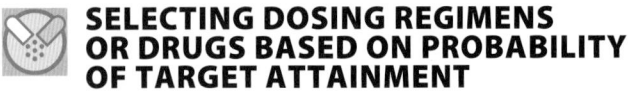

Fig. 4.9 Means and 99% confidence interval estimates using Monte Carlo simulation for %$fT_{>MIC}$ of ceftazidime, based on the population pharmacokinetic parameter estimates. Reproduced from Mouton JW, Punt N, Vinks AA. A retrospective analysis using Monte Carlo simulation to evaluate recommended ceftazidime dosing regimens in healthy volunteers, patients with cystic fibrosis, and patients in the intensive care unit. **Clin Ther.** 2005;27(6):762-772, with permission of Elsevier.[19]

population, similar to Figure 4.7. The lines on both sides represent the confidence interval estimations of the mean values. MICs that can supposedly be covered with the dosing regimen can be read directly from the figure at the intersection of the horizontal line concurring with the pharmacodynamic target and the lower confidence interval. Alternatively, the effect of choosing a different PT can be observed directly.

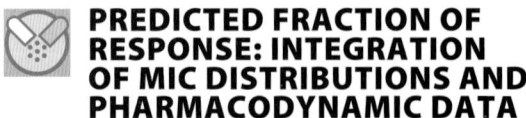

SELECTING DOSING REGIMENS OR DRUGS BASED ON PROBABILITY OF TARGET ATTAINMENT

With the information obtained by MCS, dosing regimens or drugs can be compared and selected (*see above*), but now taking the population variability into account. In drug development, this information can be used to select dosing regimens. An example is shown in Table 4.3 for two dosing regimens of ceftobiprole (BAL9141), a cephalosporin with anti-methicillin-resistant *Staphylococcus aureus* (MRSA) activity recently under clinical investigation. The PTA for two simulated dosing regimens, 250 mg every 12 h and 750 mg every 12 h, is displayed for several values of $T_{>MIC}$. Since the frequency distributions of the target pathogens indicate that the highest MIC is 2 mg/L for most species and only rare isolates of 4 mg/L, the dosing regimen of 250 mg every 12 h is clearly insufficient to obtain target attainment ratios nearing 100% for %$T_{>MIC}$ as low as 30%. Of the two regimens compared here, it is recommended that the 750 mg every 12 h course of therapy is followed up in clinical trials.

Table 4.3 Probability of target attainment (%) for two dosing regimens of ceftobiprole using data from human volunteers. PTAs are displayed for 30, 40, 50 and 60% $fT_{>MIC}$

Dosing regimen MIC (mg/L)	250 mg every 12 h (%)				750 mg every 12 h (%)			
	30	40	50	60	30	40	50	60
0.5			100	100				
1		100	99	71				100
2	100	59	3	0			100	99
4	0	0	0		100	100	78	15
8					69	3	0	0
16					0	0		
32								
PTA 100%	2	1	0.5	0.5	4	4	2	1

Modified from Mouton JW, Schmitt-Hoffmann A, Shapiro S, Nashed N, Punt NC. Use of Monte Carlo Simulations To Select Therapeutic Doses and Provisional Breakpoints of BAL9141. **Antimicrob Agents Chemother.** 2004;48(5):1713–1718. Copyright © 2004, American Society for Microbiology.[21]

Similar comparisons can be made for drugs within the same class to determine the optimal drug choice. The choice will also depend on the MIC distribution of the species to be covered. For instance, the PTA for ciprofloxacin is inferior to other quinolones for the treatment of pneumococci but superior for *Ps. aeruginosa* infections.

PREDICTED FRACTION OF RESPONSE: INTEGRATION OF MIC DISTRIBUTIONS AND PHARMACODYNAMIC DATA

The approach can be taken one step further by incorporating the frequency distribution of MIC values of the target pathogen. By multiplying the PTA and the relative frequency of the target pathogen, the fraction of target attainment is obtained at each MIC; by cumulating these, the cumulative fraction of target attainment is obtained. In this fashion, not only the variability in pharmacokinetic parameters is considered, but also the variance in susceptibility in the target pathogen population. The major drawback of this approach is that the MIC frequency distribution of the target micro-organism population has to be unbiased and this is almost never the case. The cumulative frequency of target attainment can be very useful, however, in the development phase of a drug to determine whether the response is sufficiently adequate for further follow-up. For instance, Drusano and colleagues showed that the cumulative fraction of target attainment for a 6 mg/kg dose of everninomicin would be 34% given the priors in the simulations and thereby concluded that further development of the drug was not justified.[17]

BREAKPOINTS

In choosing an antibiotic, the clinician is guided by reports from the microbiology laboratory. In the report, classifications of 'susceptible' (S) and 'resistant' (R) are used to indicate whether the use of an antimicrobial will have a reasonable probability of success or failure, respectively.[20,22]

Ideally, when an anti-infective drug is developed, the pharmacodynamic target is determined in various models of infection. This provides the estimates of exposure required to treat infectious micro-organisms. Phase I trials provide information on pharmacokinetic parameters of the drug in humans. Using the derived population pharmacokinetic parameters and measures of dispersion, Monte Carlo simulations can subsequently be used to determine the dosing regimens needed to obtain the exposures required at a range of MICs. Then, the MICs that need to be covered – based on the indications of the antimicrobial and micro-organisms causing the infection – need to be established. Finally, the dosing regimen resulting in an exposure in a significant part of the patient population – using a diagram such as Figure 4.9 or Table 4.3 – can be derived that will cover the relevant wild-type (WT) distribution. This dosing regimen is then validated in phase II and phase III trials. It follows, therefore, that the clinical breakpoint of the species to be covered is at the right-end of the WT distribution. In other words, the breakpoint is the MIC for which the PTA was considered to choose the adequate dose.

Unfortunately, most of the anti-infective drugs that are available today were developed before this whole approach became feasible because the knowledge was not available at the time. Breakpoints derived in the past are therefore more the result of practical use, appropriate or less appropriate comparative trials, assumptions of efficacy in vivo and local history. A full discussion regarding this subject can be found in Mouton et al.[23] The essential difference with the procedure described above is that dosing regimens have been established for years and sometimes decennia ago without the pharmacokinetic/pharmacodynamic information that is presently available. Two clear examples are the evaluation of piperacillin breakpoints[24] and cefepime breakpoints.[25] In a retrospective analysis looking at mortality after 30 and 28 days, respectively, it was shown that current CLSI breakpoints are too high with respect to the dosing regimens commonly applied, and those breakpoints do not distinguish between a high and a lower probability of cure. This clearly indicates that periodic re-evaluation of breakpoints is necessary as science evolves.

SOME OTHER FACTORS TO BE CONSIDERED WHEN DEFINING OPTIMAL EXPOSURES

TARGET DELINEATION

The pharmacodynamic target to select a dosing regimen and a susceptibility breakpoint is based on the information that we have (*see above*), but the true value is unknown. For instance, the target value for the AUC is usually taken as 100–125 for Gram-negatives, because that value has been found to be discriminative between groups of patients responding to therapy and those who did not. However, there are several reports that in some cases higher values are clearly necessary, while lower values have also been described. In the study published by Forrest et al.,[4] 125 (notably, total drug) was the cut-off value below which the probability of cure was distinctly lower, but values above 250 resulted in a faster cure rate. Thus, although the final effect was more or less equal for patients with AUC/MIC values of 125 and above, the rate at which the effect was achieved differed. Similarly, although the current assumption is that the PK/PD index value necessary for (bacteriological) cure is similar for most infections, this is not necessarily the case. For instance, it has been shown that PK/PD index values needed to reach a maximum effect in sustained abscesses is higher.[26] Thus, the target value may be different by micro-organism as well as by clinical indication.

EMERGENCE OF RESISTANCE

While the above discussion was focused on efficacy, and pharmacodynamic targets based on cure (either clinical or microbiological), other factors should also be considered. One of the most important factors is emergence of resistance. While hardly any data existed before the millennium change, it becomes increasingly clear that emergence of resistance is also dependent on exposure. Although space prohibits a full discussion, it must be noted that several authors have shown that the PT to prevent emergence of resistance has a different value from the one for efficacy. Most often it is higher and it may even be different from the PI best predicting efficacy.[27]

POPULATION TO BE TREATED

The output of MCS is directly dependent on the pharmacokinetic parameter values and their measures of dispersion used for input. Thus, if pharmacokinetic parameter estimates are used from a small group of healthy young male volunteers obtained in phase I or phase II studies, the simulations will be biased towards relatively low PTAs, because the elimination rate of most drugs is higher in volunteers than in the average patient. On the other hand, there are patient groups such as patients with cystic fibrosis known to have higher clearances for most drugs, and specific analyses have been made for such specific patient groups.[19] Comparing the results of Monte Carlo simulations of ceftazidime for three different populations – healthy volunteers, patients with cystic fibrosis and intensive care unit patients – significant differences in PTA were shown, in particular at the extremes of the distribution.[19]

EXPOSURE IN FIRST COMPARTMENT (SERUM) AS OPPOSED TO CONCENTRATIONS AT THE SITE OF INFECTION

While most of the exposure–response relationships have been drawn from concentrations in serum, these are – except for bacteremias – used as a surrogate for concentrations at the actual receptor site. While these relationships show a marked consistency, it has to be borne in mind that the actual concentration–effect relationships at the site of infection are usually unknown. However, most bacterial infections are located in the extracellular compartment and it is those concentrations that are of primary interest. Most antibiotics have been shown to reach the extracellular fluid rapidly, with concentrations in extracellular fluid comparable to the non-protein-bound concentration in serum or plasma,[28] although there seem to be some exceptions such as cerebrospinal fluid (CSF) and epithelial lining fluid (ELF) concentrations.[29] Nowadays, microdialysis techniques which only measure unbound drug concentrations are increasingly being used to obtain concentration–time profiles in interstitial fluid.[30] Thus, the strong relationship between unbound drug concentrations in serum or plasma with those in extracellular fluid explains the good correlation found between unbound serum concentrations and in-vivo effects. Using data obtained from in-vitro time kill curves, we have shown that the predicted $fT_{>MIC}$ for a static

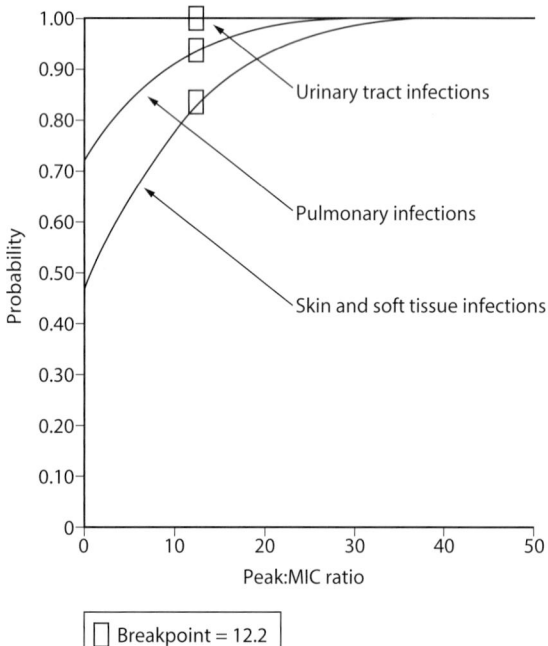

effect in an animal model of infection was between 35% and 40%, substantiating the paradigm that effects in vivo can be predicted by exposures in serum.[31]

There are, however, differences that should be considered. The equilibrium and the type of infection do matter. There are several papers which clearly show that the exposure–response relationship differs by type and site of infection, in particular pulmonary infections.[32,33] An example is shown in Figure 4.10.

TOXICITY

The approach to pharmacodynamic targets for toxicity is essentially similar to that for efficacy as described above, in that the exposure–response description is sought for, and PTAs are determined. The conclusions from this relationship, however, are fundamentally different in that the PT is at the minimum part of the curve instead of the maximum. For some drugs, optimizing the PT for efficacy and toxicity results are clearly at odds with each other and a compromise then needs to be sought in a conflict. An excellent paper discussing this issue is focused on optimizing aminoglycoside therapy.[34]

CONCLUSION

As our understanding of the processes underlying antimicrobial activity evolves and more information becomes available it allows for improved antimicrobial treatment. The major advances over the last two decades have been to describe exposure–response relationships for anti-infectives in a meaningful manner. This has resulted in a more rational approach to the design of dosing regimens and it applies, as indicated at the start of the chapter, to all anti-infective agents. It has also changed the way we look at antimicrobial breakpoints and how antimicrobials can be developed. While the main focus of target delineation has been on efficacy of antimicrobials, the primary challenge during the present era is to uncover pharmacodynamic targets that prevent emergence of resistance. This is a fast developing field that needs continuous attention.

Fig. 4.10 Exposure–response relationship for different sites of infection. Reproduced from Preston SL, Drusano GL, Berman AL, et al. Pharmacodynamics of levofloxacin: a new paradigm for early clinical trials [see comments]. **Journal American Medical Association.** 1998;279(2):125–129.[33]

References

1. Craig WA. Pharmacokinetic/pharmacodynamic parameters: rationale for antibacterial dosing of mice and men. *Clin Infect Dis.* 1998;26(1):1–10 quiz 1–2.
2. Andes D, Craig WA. Animal model pharmacokinetics and pharmacodynamics: a critical review. *Int J Antimicrob Agents.* 2002;19(4):261–268.
3. Scaglione F, Mouton JW, Mattina R, eds. *Pharmacodynamics of levofloxacin in a murine pneumonia model: importance of peak to MIC ratio versus AUC.* Interscience Conference on Antimicrobial Agents and Chemotherapy, San Fransisco. Washington, DC: American Society for Microbiology; 1999.
4. Mouton JW, Dudley MN, Cars O, Derendorf H, Drusano GL. Standardization of pharmacokinetic/pharmacodynamic (PK/PD) terminology for anti-infective drugs: an update. *J Antimicrob Chemother.* 2005;55(5):601–607.
5. Ambrose PG, Anon JB, Bhavnani SM, et al. Use of pharmacodynamic endpoints for the evaluation of levofloxacin for the treatment of acute maxillary sinusitis. *Diagn Microbiol Infect Dis.* 2008;61(1):13–20.

6. Forrest A, Nix DE, Ballow CH, Goss TF, Birmingham MC, Schentag JJ. Pharmacodynamics of intravenous ciprofloxacin in seriously ill patients. *Diagn Microbiol Infect Dis*. 1993;37(5):1073–1081.

7. Ambrose PG, Bhavnani SM, Owens Jr RC. Clinical pharmacodynamics of quinolones. *Infect Dis Clin North Am*. 2003;17(3):529–543.

8. Rodriguez-Tudela JL, Almirante B, Rodriguez-Pardo D, et al. Correlation of the MIC and dose/MIC ratio of fluconazole to the therapeutic response of patients with mucosal candidiasis and candidaemia. *Diagn Microbiol Infect Dis*. 2007;51(10):3599–3604.

9. Mouton JW, Jacobs N, Tiddens H, Horrevorts AM. Pharmacodynamics of tobramycin in patients with cystic fibrosis. *Diagn Microbiol Infect Dis*. 2005;52(2):123–127.

10. Ambrose PG, Bhavnani SM, Rubino CM, et al. Pharmacokinetics–pharmacodynamics of antimicrobial therapy: it's not just for mice anymore. *Clin Infect Dis*. 2007;44(1):79–86.

11. Jumbe N, Louie A, Leary R, et al. Application of a mathematical model to prevent in vivo amplification of antibiotic-resistant bacterial populations during therapy. *J Clin Invest*. 2003;112(2):275–285.

12. Craig WA. 2002: Pharmacodynamics of antimicrobials: general concepts and applications. In: Nightingale CH TM, Ambrose PG, eds. *Antimicrobial pharmacodynamics in theory and clinical practice*. New York: Marcel Dekker.

13. Mouton JW, Punt N. Use of the $T_{>MIC}$ to choose between different dosing regimens of beta-lactam antibiotics. *J Antimicrob Chemother*. 2001;47(4):500–501.

14. Mouton JW, Touzw DJ, Horrevorts AM, Vinks AA. Comparative pharmacokinetics of the carbapenems: clinical implications. *Clin Pharmacokinet*. 2000;39(3):185–201.

15. Mouton JW. Impact of pharmacodynamics on breakpoint selection for susceptibility testing. *Infect Dis Clin North Am*. 2003;17(3):579–598.

16. Drusano GL, D'Argenio DZ, Preston SL, et al. Use of drug effect interaction modeling with Monte Carlo simulation to examine the impact of dosing interval on the projected antiviral activity of the combination of abacavir and amprenavir. *Diagn Microbiol Infect Dis*. 2000;44(6):1655–1659.

17. Drusano GL, Preston SL, Hardalo C, et al. Use of preclinical data for selection of a phase II/III dose for evernimicin and identification of a preclinical MIC breakpoint. *Diagn Microbiol Infect Dis*. 2001;45(1):13–22.

18. Bonate PL. A brief introduction to Monte Carlo simulation. *Clin Pharmacokinet*. 2001;40:15–22.

19. Mouton JW, Punt N, Vinks AA. A retrospective analysis using Monte Carlo simulation to evaluate recommended ceftazidime dosing regimens in healthy volunteers, patients with cystic fibrosis, and patients in the intensive care unit. *Clin Ther*. 2005;27(6):762–772.

20. Kahlmeter G, Brown DF, Goldstein FW, et al. European harmonization of MIC breakpoints for antimicrobial susceptibility testing of bacteria. *J Antimicrob Chemother*. 2003;52(2):145–148.

21. Mouton JW, Schmitt-Hoffmann A, Shapiro S, Nashed N, Punt NC. Use of Monte Carlo simulations to select therapeutic doses and provisional breakpoints of BAL9141. *Diagn Microbiol Infect Dis*. 2004;48(5):1713–1718.

22. ISO, Organisation IS. ISO 20776-1. *Clinical laboratory testing and in vitro diagnostic tet systems – susceptibility testing of infectious agents and evaluation of performance of antimicrobial susceptibility testing devices – Part 1*. Geneva: International Standards Organisation; 2006.

23. Mouton JW, Ambrose PG, Kahlmeter G, Wikler M, Craig WA. Applying pharmacodynamics for susceptibility breakpoint selection and susceptibility testing. In: Nightingale C, Ambrose PG, Drusano GL, Mukisawa T, eds. *Antimicrobial pharmacodynamics in theory and clinical practice*. New York: Informa Health Care; 2007:21–44.

24. Tam VH, Gamez EA, Weston JS, et al. Outcomes of bacteremia due to *Pseudomonas aeruginosa* with reduced susceptibility to piperacillin–tazobactam: implications on the appropriateness of the resistance breakpoint. *Clin Infect Dis*. 2008;46(6):862–867.

25. Bhat SV, Peleg AY, Lodise Jr TP, et al. Failure of current cefepime breakpoints to predict clinical outcomes of bacteremia caused by Gram-negative organisms. *Diagn Microbiol Infect Dis*. 2007;51(12):4390–4395.

26. Stearne LE, Buijk SL, Mouton JW, Gyssens IC. Effect of a single percutaneous abscess drainage puncture and imipenem therapy, alone or in combination, in treatment of mixed-infection abscesses in mice. *Diagn Microbiol Infect Dis*. 2002;46(12):3712–3718.

27. Goessens WH, Mouton JW, Ten Kate MT, Bijl AJ, Ott A, Bakker-Woudenberg IA. Role of ceftazidime dose regimen on the selection of resistant *Enterobacter cloacae* in the intestinal flora of rats treated for an experimental pulmonary infection. *J Antimicrob Chemother*. 2007;59(3):507–516.

28. Craig WA, Suh B. Theory and practical impact of binding of antimicrobials to serum proteins and tissue. *Scand J Infect Dis Suppl*. 1978;14:92–99.

29. Drusano GL, Preston SL, Gotfried MH, Danziger LH, Rodvold KA. Levofloxacin penetration into epithelial lining fluid as determined by population pharmacokinetic modeling and Monte Carlo simulation. *Diagn Microbiol Infect Dis*. 2002;46(2):586–589.

30. Muller M, Haag O, Burgdorff T, et al. Characterization of peripheral-compartment kinetics of antibiotics by in vivo microdialysis in humans. *Diagn Microbiol Infect Dis*. 1996;40(12):2703–2709.

31. Mouton JW, Punt N, Vinks AA. Concentration–effect relationship of ceftazidime explains why the time above the MIC is 40 percent for a static effect in vivo. *Diagn Microbiol Infect Dis*. 2007;51(9):3449–3451.

32. Rayner CR, Forrest A, Meagher AK, Birmingham MC, Schentag JJ. Clinical pharmacodynamics of linezolid in seriously ill patients treated in a compassionate use programme. *Clin Pharmacokinet*. 2003;42(15):1411–1423.

33. Preston SL, Drusano GL, Berman AL, et al. Pharmacodynamics of levofloxacin: a new paradigm for early clinical trials [see comments]. *J Am Med Assoc*. 1998;279(2):125–129.

34. Drusano GL, Ambrose PG, Bhavnani SM, Bertino JS, Nafziger AN, Louie A. Back to the future: using aminoglycosides again and how to dose them optimally. *Clin Infect Dis*. 2007;45(6):753–760.

5 Antimicrobial agents and the kidneys

S. Ragnar Norrby

Antimicrobial drugs may interact with the kidneys in several ways. Decreased renal function often results in slower excretion of drugs or their metabolites. In the extreme situation the patient lacks renal function and is treated with hemodialysis, peritoneal dialysis or hemofiltration; since most antimicrobial drugs are low-molecular-weight compounds they are often readily eliminated from blood by such treatments. However, more and more drugs (e.g. the fluoroquinolones and many of the macrolides) are so widely distributed in tissue compartments and/or so highly protein bound that only a small fraction is available for elimination from the blood. Moreover, many antimicrobials are eliminated by liver metabolism and can be administered at full doses, irrespective of renal function, provided their metabolites are not toxic.

Another type of interaction between drugs and the kidneys is nephrotoxicity. Some of the most commonly used antimicrobial drugs (e.g. the aminoglycosides and amphotericin B) are also nephrotoxic when used in normal doses relative to the patient's renal function.

This chapter deals with general aspects on interactions between antimicrobial drugs and the kidneys. The readers are referred to section 2 for details about dosing in patients with reduced renal function.

RENAL FUNCTION AND AGE

The prematurely born child has reduced renal function. Thereafter the glomerular filtration rate (GFR) is higher than in the adult. The young, healthy adult has a GFR of about 120 mL/min. Creatinine clearance overestimates GFR by 8–10%. With increasing age GFR becomes markedly reduced and in the very old (>85 years) is often lower than 30 mL/min, even if there are no signs of renal disease. For drugs that are excreted only by glomerular filtration, which are not metabolized and which have low protein binding (e.g. the aminoglycosides and many of the cephalosporins), the renal clearances are normally directly proportional to the GFR. As shown in Figure 5.1,[1] the elimination time (the plasma half-life) of the drug increases slowly in the range from normal GFR to markedly reduced GFR but then increases drastically. Clinically this means that the drug will not accumulate markedly until renal function is profoundly decreased. However, when that is the case, only very slight further reductions of renal function will result in a marked increase in the elimination time and an obvious risk of accumulation to toxic levels.

Measurement of GFR is difficult because it requires precise collection and volume measurement of urine over time for determination of creatinine clearance or repeated plasma samples when ^{51}Cr clearance or inulin clearance are studied. For ^{51}Cr clearance there is also a need to administer and handle an isotope, and none of these methods is suitable for routine clinical use. The most frequently used way to measure renal function is by serum creatinine assay, which in the last decades has replaced blood urea nitrogen. However, serum creatinine depends on renal function and muscle mass. Therefore, in a very old person with reduced muscle mass, serum creatinine may be within normal values despite the fact that GFR is <25 mL/min. As a consequence, serum creatinine must be related to age, sex and weight (or preferably lean body mass). Two widely used routine methods are available: the Cockroft and Gault formula (Figure 5.2)[2] and a nomogram (Figure 5.3).[3]

ELIMINATION OF ANTIMICROBIAL DRUGS IN RENAL FAILURE

GENERAL ASPECTS

Only water-soluble drugs are eliminated via the kidneys: liver metabolism normally aims at producing water-soluble metabolites that can be excreted renally. In the kidneys water-soluble compounds that are not bound to protein are eliminated by glomerular filtration, tubular secretion or both of these mechanisms. For protein-bound drugs, only the free fraction is available for glomerular filtration. Following glomerular filtration some drugs (e.g. the aminoglycosides) are reabsorbed into, and sometimes accumulate in, proximal tubular cells.

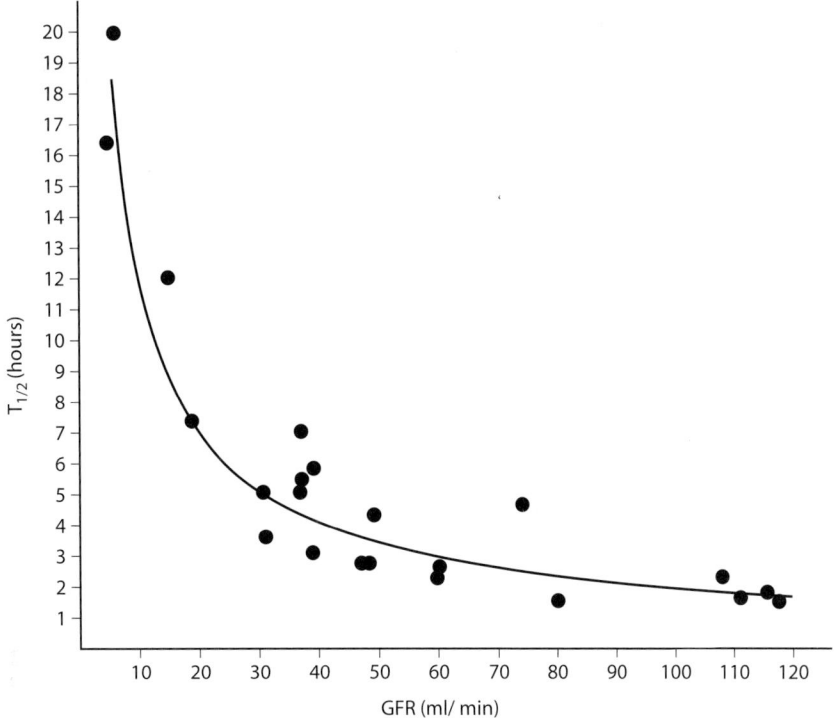

Fig. 5.1 Correlation between glomerular filtration rate (GFR) and serum half-life (t$_{1/2}$) of ceftazidime. After Alestig et al. Ceftazidime and renal function. *Journal of Antimicrobial Chemotherapy* 1989; 13: 177–181 with permission of Oxford University Press.

In renal failure glomerular filtration is reduced while tubular secretion is often maintained. The effect of renal failure depends to a large degree on whether the drug is also metabolized or eliminated through the bile. For example, among the cephalosporins, cefuroxime has low protein binding and is not metabolized; its plasma clearance will be virtually identical to creatinine clearance. Ceftriaxone, on the other hand, has a relatively high protein binding and is eliminated via the bile; in patients with renal failure the elimination half-life of ceftriaxone will not increase markedly because the proportion of drug eliminated by biliary excretion will increase. Another example is imipenem, which is excreted by glomerular filtration but which also has a (non-hepatic) metabolism that is constant over time. In renal failure the plasma half-life of imipenem will increase, but only to about 3 h in the anuric patient (compared with 1 h in an individual with normal renal function). In contrast, cilastatin, the enzyme inhibitor administered with imipenem, has relatively little metabolism and low protein binding, and its half-life will increase from about 1 h to more than 10 h in severe renal failure.

$$\text{Creatinine clearance (mL/min)} = \frac{f \times (140 - \text{age (years)} \times \text{Body weight (kg)}}{\text{Serum creatinine (} \mu \text{mol/L)}}$$

f = 1.23 for men and 1.04 for women

Fig. 5.2 Cockroft and Gault[2] formula for estimation of creatinine clearance.

It is essential to know the mode of elimination of all antimicrobial drugs used as well as the effects on elimination time of renal failure. Many compounds are toxic if given in overdose, and failure to correct dosages in patients with markedly reduced renal function may result in serious adverse effects.

ANTIMICROBIAL DRUGS THAT ARE INDEPENDENT OF RENAL FUNCTION FOR THEIR ELIMINATION

Some antimicrobial drugs can be given at full doses even to patients with severe renal failure (Table 5.1). However, also in such patients elimination by hemodialysis or hemofiltration should be considered. A relatively simple rule of thumb is that drugs that are highly protein bound (≥90%) and drugs that have a large volume of distribution tend not to be eliminated. Alternatively, for most drugs with low protein binding and/or low volume of distribution, a further dose should be considered after peritoneal dialysis, hemodialysis or hemofiltration.

ANTIMICROBIAL DRUGS THAT SHOULD BE AVOIDED IN SEVERE RENAL FAILURE

Nephrotoxic drugs should not be used in patients with renal failure unless they are anephric. When using formulations that are combinations of two drugs, it should be noted that the pharmacokinetics of the two components in renal failure

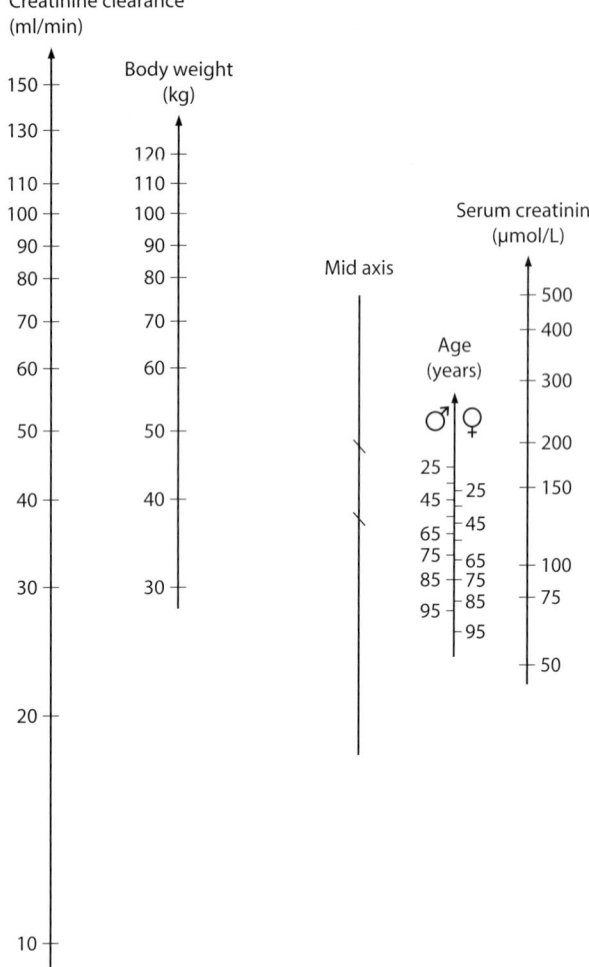

Fig. 5.3 Nomogram for calculation of creatinine clearance. Connect body weight and age with a ruler and mark the crossing on the mid axis. Connect the crossing with the serum creatinine value and read the estimated creatinine clearance. After Siersbaek-Nielsen K, Mølholm Hansen J, Kampmann J, Kristensen M. Rapid evaluation of creatinine clearance. **Lancet**. 1971;i:1333–1334.

Table 5.1 Antimicrobial drugs that can be given at full doses to patients with severe renal failure

Drug	Comments
Anidulafungin	
Atazanavir	
Azithromycin	
Caspofungin	
Ceftriaxone	The manufacturer recommends a maximum daily dose of 2 g if glomerular filtration rate is <10 mL/min
Chloramphenicol	
Clarithromycin	
Clindamycin	
Darunavir	
Doxycycline	Other tetracyclines should not be used in renal failure
Efavirenz	
Erythromycin	It has been proposed that the risk of toxicity should increase in patients with renal failure
Ethambutol	
Fosamprenavir	Limited data
Indinavir	No data but minimal renal excretion
Itraconazole	
Ketoconazole	
Linezolid	Exposure to two main metabolites increases 10 times at a glomerular filtration rate of <30 mL/min
Lopinavir	Limited data for anuric patients
Mebendazole	
Mefloquine	
Metronidazole	
Mezlocillin	Liver metabolism
Posaconazole	
Praziquantel	
Primaquine	
Pyrazinamide	
Quinine	
Rifampicin	
Ritonavir	No data but minimal renal excretion
Saquinavir	No data but minimal renal excretion
Sulfonamides	
Tigecycline	
Tinidazole	
Tipranavir	
Voriconazole	
Zanamivir	

may differ from those in patients with normal kidney function. Examples are imipenem–cilastatin and piperacillin–tazobactam: the elimination times of cilastatin and tazobactam increase far more drastically than those of imipenem and piperacillin, which both undergo substantial metabolism.

PERITONEAL DIALYSIS

Modern medicine offers several replacement treatments of severe renal failure: hemodialysis, continuous ambulatory peritoneal dialysis (CAPD), continuous arteriovenous hemofiltration (CAVHF), continuous venovenous hemofiltration (CVVHF) and continuous venovenous hemodiafiltration (CVVHDF). The degrees of elimination of individual antimicrobial drugs by these methods vary and are sometimes incompletely studied.

In terms of reproducibility of the elimination rate, CAPD is likely to be the least reproducible, both with the same patient and between patients. The main reason for this is that, with time, a person undergoing CAPD is likely to develop fibrin adherence, which limits the peritoneal surface area available for dialysis. The efficacy of the dialysis may also vary with the position of the patient and the amount of dialysis fluid administered during a specified time. Other factors limiting elimination of drugs with CAPD are protein binding and molecular size. There is often limited information about rate of elimination of an antimicrobial agent in patients using CAPD. For renally eliminated antibiotics, the most common recommendation is to give the dose normally administered to a patient with a GFR <10 mL/min. When aminoglycosides are given to patients on CAPD, about 50% of the dose given is found in the dialysate fluid but regular serum concentration assays are recommended (*see below*).

In patients undergoing CAPD, antibiotics are also frequently used as additives to peritoneal dialysate fluid to treat peritonitis, a common complication in these patients. Since the most common agent causing these infections is coagulase-negative staphylococci that are often methicillin resistant, vancomycin is most frequently used. In such treatment varying but generally quite high plasma concentrations are achieved as a result of passage of the antibiotic from the dialysate fluid to plasma. This is especially important to note if the patient is also on systemic antibiotic treatment.

HEMODIALYSIS

In hemodialysis toxic substances are cleared from blood through passive diffusion across a membrane. Drug elimination via hemodialysis depends on molecular size of the drug, protein binding and volume of distribution (drugs with a molecular weight <500 Da normally pass through the dialysis filter easily if they are not protein bound). Factors of the dialysis technique that influence drug elimination are dialysis time, blood and dialysate flow rates, and dialysis membrane permeability, pore size and surface area. Elimination of molecules of 500–5000 Da will depend largely on the type of filter used; some of the modern filters also allow passage of relatively large molecules.

For most antibiotics, the effect of hemodialysis on elimination is known, although information is more limited on antifungal, antiparasitic and antiviral drugs (Tables 5.2 and 5.3). With drugs that are readily eliminated during hemodialysis it is necessary to give a new dose directly after hemodialysis; no dose corrections are needed for those that are not significantly eliminated.

Table 5.2 Antimicrobial drugs which are removed during hemodialysis

Drug	Dose recommendation
Abacavir	The manufacturer does not recommend the use of abacavir in patients with severe renal insufficiency
Aciclovir	Maximal oral dose 800 mg every 12 h. New parenteral dose after dialysis and then half normal dose every 24 h
Adefovir dipivoxil	One dose weekly
Amikacin	Two-thirds of normal dose after dialysis. Monitor serum concentrations
Amoxicillin	New dose after dialysis
Amoxicillin–clavulanic acid	New dose after dialysis
Ampicillin	New dose after dialysis
Aztreonam	Half normal dose after dialysis and one-quarter of normal dose between dialyses
Cefaclor	New dose after dialysis
Cefadroxil	New dose after dialysis
Cefalexin	New dose after dialysis
Cefamandole	New dose after dialysis
Cefapirin	New dose after dialysis
Cefazolin	New dose (maximum 1 g) after dialysis
Cefdinir	New dose after dialysis
Cefepime	0.5 g per day. New dose (maximum 1 g) after dialysis
Cefixime	New dose after dialysis
Cefoperazone	New dose after dialysis
Cefotaxime	New dose (maximum 1 g) after dialysis
Cefotetan	New dose (maximum 1 g) after dialysis
Cefpodoxime	New dose after dialysis
Cefprozil	250 mg after dialysis
Cefradine	New dose after dialysis
Ceftazidime	New dose (maximum 1 g) after dialysis
Cefuroxime	New dose after dialysis
Clarithromycin	New dose after dialysis
Daptomycin	Insufficient data to allow dosage recommendations

Didanosine	New dose after dialysis and then once daily
Doripenem	Insufficient data to allow dosage recommendations
Emtricitabine	New dose every 96 h
Entecavir	0.1 mg every 24 h or 0.5 mg every 72 h
Ertapenem	Insufficient data to allow dosage recommendations
Famciclovir	New dose after dialysis and then every 48 h
Fluconazole	New dose after dialysis
Flucytosine	New dose after dialysis. Monitor serum concentrations
Ganciclovir	Half dose after dialysis and then 0.625 mg/kg three times/week
Gentamicin	Two-thirds normal dose after dialysis. Monitor serum concentrations
Imipenem–cilastatin	New dose after dialysis and then 0.5 g every 12 h
Lamivudine	25 mg once daily
Levofloxacin	125 mg per day
Mecillinam	New dose after dialysis
Meropenem	New dose after dialysis
Metronidazole	New dose after dialysis
Netilmicin	Two-thirds normal dose after dialysis. Monitor serum concentrations
Ofloxacin	100 mg every 12 h
Paludrine	50 mg every week
Penicillin V and G	New dose after dialysis
Piperacillin	1 g after dialysis and then 2 g every 8 h
Piperacillin–tazobactam	2 g (of piperacillin) after dialysis and then 4 g (of piperacillin) every 12 h
Stavudine	New dose after dialysis and then once daily
Sulfamethoxazole	New dose after dialysis
Sulfisoxazole	New dose after dialysis
Teicoplanin	Dose for GFR <10 mL/min. Monitor serum concentrations
Telbivudine	New dose every 96 h
Tenofovir disoproxil	New dose once weekly
Ticarcillin	New dose after dialysis
Tobramycin	Two-thirds normal dose after dialysis. Monitor serum concentrations
Trimethoprim	New dose after dialysis
Valaciclovir	Maximal dose 1 g once daily
Valganciclovir	Insufficient data to allow dosage recommendations
Vancomycin	Dose for GFR <10 mL/min. Monitor serum concentrations

Doses, when specified, are for adults. GFR, glomerular filtration rate.
Data are partly taken from Livornese et al.[4]

No information has been found on elimination of the following in patients on hemodialysis: abacavir, artemether plus lumefantrine, daptomycin, doripenem, ertapenem, foscarnet, indinavir, itraconazole, ketoconazole, mefloquine, moxifloxacin, polymyxin B (colistin), ritonavir, saquinavir, sparfloxacin, trovafloxacin, zalcitabine and zidovudine. The manufacturer of isoniazid states that it is eliminated during hemodialysis but gives no dosage recommendations. The combination of atovaquone and proguanil (Malarone) for malaria prophylaxis should not be used in patients with severe renal dysfunction.

HEMOFILTRATION AND HEMODIAFILTRATION

There is far less information on elimination of drugs in patients on hemofiltration than there is for those on hemodialysis. The principle of removal of compounds by hemofiltration is convection of the compound in solution in plasma water over a filter, while hemodialysis involves diffusion against a dialysis fluid. In hemofiltration the drug is removed by drag of plasma

Table 5.3 Antimicrobial drugs that are not removed by hemodialysis

Drug	Comments
Amphotericin B	Large molecular weight
Azithromycin	Large molecule; very large volume of distribution
Ceftriaxone	High protein binding; alternative biliary excretion
Chloramphenicol	Large volume of distribution
Chloroquine	Large volume of distribution
Ciprofloxacin	Large volume of distribution
Clindamycin	Large volume of distribution; high protein binding
Cloxacillin	High protein binding
Dicloxacillin	High protein binding
Doxycycline	High protein binding; large volume of distribution
Erythromycin	Large molecule; large volume of distribution
Fusidic acid	High protein binding
Mefloquine	High protein binding
Minocycline	High protein binding; large volume of distribution
Nafcillin	High protein binding
Quinine	Large volume of distribution
Quinupristin–dalfopristin	Large volumes of distribution; large molecules
Rifabutin	Large volume of distribution; high protein binding
Rifampicin	Large volume of distribution
Spectinomycin	Always single dose
Tetracycline	High protein binding; large volume of distribution

Table 5.4 Comparison of meropenem pharmacokinetics in patients treated with continuous venovenous hemofiltration (CVVHF) or hemodiafiltration (CVVHDF)

Parameter (mean ± pL SD)	CVVHF	CVVHDF (1 L/h)	CVVHDF (2 L/h)
Meropenem half-life (h)	7.5 ± pL 2.0	5.6 ± pL 1.4[a]	4.8 ± pL 1.2[a,b]
Meropenem clearance (L/h)	3.3 ± pL 2.3	4.7 ± pL 2.7[a]	5.7 ± pL 3.6[a]

[a] Significantly ($p < 0.05$) different from the CVVHF.
[b] Significantly ($p < 0.05$) different from the CVVHDF (1 L/h) phase.
Data from Valtonen et al.[5]

water. Only free drug can be removed by this process and protein binding is a major factor restricting elimination. Large molecular size is also a restrictive factor. The efficiency with which a drug is removed is measured as the *sieving coefficient*; a drug with a sieving coefficient of 1 will cross the filter freely; one with a coefficient of 0 is unable to cross. Amikacin has a sieving coefficient of 0.9, amphotericin B (which has a high molecular weight) 0.3 and oxacillin (which has a very high protein binding) 0.02.

Hemofiltration is generally less efficient than hemodialysis in eliminating drugs from plasma. The most common recommendation for drugs which are normally given in a full dose after each intermittent hemodialysis is to give the dose used in patients with moderate renal failure (GFR 10–50 mL/min) during CVVHF or CAVHF. In patients treated with aminoglycosides or glycopeptides, serum concentrations should be monitored to avoid toxic reactions.

Another way of treating patients with acute renal failure is to use continuous venovenous hemodiafiltration (CVVHDF), which combines hemofiltration and hemodialysis. This technique is more efficient in eliminating filterable and dialyzable drugs. Table 5.4 gives a comparison of CVVHF and CVVHDF when used in patients treated with meropenem.

NEPHROTOXICITY OF ANTIMICROBIAL DRUGS

Some antimicrobial drugs – such as the aminoglycosides, vancomycin and amphotericin B – are also nephrotoxic when dosed correctly in relation to the renal function of the patients. Others (e.g. cefaloridine; no longer available) are nephrotoxic

if overdosed while a large number of drugs, especially the penicillins and rifampicin (rifampin), have been reported to cause interstitial nephritis in a very low frequency of patients treated. Some antimicrobial agents (e.g. older sulfonamides, quinolones and indinavir) may cause urolithiasis as a consequence of precipitation in the renal pelvis.

AMINOGLYCOSIDE NEPHROTOXICITY

This subject has been excellently reviewed by Mingeot-Leclercq and Tulkens.[6] Following glomerular filtration, approximately 5% of an aminoglycoside dose is reabsorbed in the proximal tubular cells of the kidneys. This process is assumed to be, at least partially, the result of adsorptive endocytosis and most of the reabsorbed aminoglycoside is found in endosomal and lysosomal vacuoles. However, part of the reabsorbed drug is found in the Golgi complex. The tubular reabsorption of aminoglycosides results in accumulation of drug in the proximal tubular cells since the release from the cells is far slower than the rate of uptake. Important for the discussion below of optimal dosing of aminoglycosides is the fact that the uptake into the tubular cells seems to be saturable.

At normal aminoglycoside doses, signs of nephrotoxicity can be observed after a few days, manifest as release of brush border and lysosomal enzymes and increased excretion of potassium, magnesium, calcium, glucose and phospholipids. After prolonged treatment (>7 days) serum creatinine increases as a consequence of reduced GFR. At the subcellular level, accumulation of polar lipids into so-called 'myeloid bodies' is seen. There is some evidence that generation of toxic oxygen metabolites (hydrogen peroxide) plays an important role in this pathological process.[7] If these early changes are overlooked and if the patient is overdosed, the end result will be tubular necrosis and renal failure.

The best way to reduce the effects of aminoglycoside nephrotoxicity is to adjust doses in order to avoid overdosing and subsequent risks for serious nephrotoxicity and for ototoxicity. This can be achieved by regular monitoring of serum concentrations of the aminoglycoside used (*see later*).

The pharmacodynamics of aminoglycosides are characterized by a direct correlation between antibacterial efficacy and the area under the serum concentration curve, i.e. the higher

Table 5.5 Results of a meta-analysis of single versus multiple daily dosing of aminoglycosides

Parameter	Mean difference[a]	95% confidence interval
Overall clinical response	3.06% (p = 0.04)	0.17–5.95%
Overall microbiological response	1.25% (not significant)	−0.40 to 2.89%
Nephrotoxicity	−0.18% (not significant)	−2.17 to 1.81%
Ototoxicity	1.38% (not significant)	−0.99 to 3.75%
Vestibular toxicity	−3.05% (not significant)	−10.7 to 4.59%

[a]A positive result for response or a negative result for toxicity favors single daily dose regimens.
Data modified from Ali & Goetz.[8]

the individual dose the more bactericidal the aminoglycoside. This speaks in favor of using few doses per time unit. Fortunately, several studies show there to be no increase in toxicity of aminoglycosides when once-a-day regimens have been used rather than regimens with two or three daily doses. Table 5.5 shows the results of a meta-analysis of studies comparing single and multiple daily dosing of aminoglycosides. From the results of that study (and others) it seems clear that aminoglycosides should be administered once daily. This has been questioned for neutropenic patients in whom there may be a reduced post-antibiotic effect of the aminoglycoside. However, studies have indicated no reduction in efficacy or safety of aminoglycosides when single and multiple daily dosing have been compared in neutropenic patients.

GLYCOPEPTIDE NEPHROTOXICITY

Both vancomycin and teicoplanin are nephrotoxic but the latter appears to be less so.[9] The mechanism by which these antibiotics are nephrotoxic is not completely known. It has been postulated that glycopeptides accumulate in proximal tubular cells as a result of passage from the blood rather than by tubular reabsorption.

The risk of developing nephrotoxicity seems to vary with certain risk factors. In one study cisplatin administration, high APACHE scores and administration of carboplatin, cyclophosphamide or non-steroidal anti-inflammatory drugs correlated to increased nephrotoxicity of vancomycin in cancer patients.[10] High individual doses (high area under the serum concentration curve) and prolonged treatment seem to increase the risk of nephrotoxicity.[11]

Nephrotoxicity of glycopeptides seems to be reversible in most cases. However, vancomycin therapy should be monitored with serum concentration assays (*see below*). Teicoplanin concentrations should also be monitored but this is more to achieve therapeutic levels (e.g. in a patient with endocarditis) than to prevent nephrotoxicity.

NEPHROTOXICITY OF β-LACTAM ANTIBIOTICS

Cefaloridine (no longer available for therapeutic use) was the first cephalosporin with marked dose-related nephrotoxicity. Cefaloridine accumulates in proximal renal tubular cell, probably by active anionic transport. Thus, probenecid, which blocks such transport, eliminates the nephrotoxicity of cephaloridine.

Nephrotoxicity of the cefaloridine type has been seen with imipenem given intravenously to rabbits. That toxicity is completely blocked if imipenem is administered as a 1:1 combination with cilastatin, an inhibitor of the brush border renal enzyme (dehydropeptidase-I) which metabolizes imipenem and which also has a probenecid-like effect.

Ceftazidime, which has a mode of elimination and renal handling very similar to that of cefaloridine, has shown slight nephrotoxicity in overdose.

Dicloxacillin, when used as prophylaxis in orthopedic surgery, increases serum creatinine. So far no explanation has been offered as to why single doses of dicloxacillin (with or without single dose of gentamicin) should result in increased serum creatinine.

NEPHROTOXICITY OF POLYMYXIN B (COLISTIN)

Colistin is an antibiotic which is being used more commonly now than when it was introduced because of its activity against multiresistant Gram-negative bacteria, especially *Acinetobacter baumanii* and Enterobacteriaceae producing extended spectrum β-lactamases. It had a bad reputation due to reports of neurotoxicity and nephrotoxicity. Recent studies have shown lower rates of nephrotoxicity than previously reported.[12,13] However, in one of these reports,[12] 7/42 patients with high serum creatinine values prior to colistin treatment developed renal failure.

AMPHOTERICIN B NEPHROTOXICITY

Amphotericin B acts by binding to ergosterol in the cytoplasmic membrane of the fungal cell. It is fungicidal and, for systemic treatment of several clinically important mycoses, is often the only therapeutic choice. Unfortunately, amphotericin B also binds to ergosterol in the human cell and in particular the proximal tubular cells of the kidney. Thus, treatment of mycoses such as aspergillosis and disseminated candidiasis with normal doses of amphotericin B results in reduced renal function manifested by loss of potassium, loss of magnesium, signs of tubular necrosis and decreased GFR. Factors of importance for how long treatment can continue are total dose given and renal function at the start of treatment.

The nephrotoxicity of amphotericin B can be reduced considerably, but not eliminated, by administration of the drug as a lipid formulation. Several variants of such formulations (e.g. incorporation of amphotericin B in liposomes and complex binding to phospholipids) have been developed (*see* Ch. 32).

ACUTE INTERSTITIAL NEPHRITIS AND ANTIMICROBIAL DRUGS

The following antimicrobial drugs have been reported to cause acute nephritis: aciclovir, cephalosporins, chloramphenicol, erythromycin, ethambutol, fluoroquinolones (ciprofloxacin and norfloxacin), gentamicin, minocycline, penicillins, rifampicin, sulfonamides, trimethoprim and vancomycin.[14] Typically, the patient develops hematuria and proteinuria after more than 10 days of treatment. Other common symptoms are fever and rash, often with eosinophilia. These conditions are normally rapidly reversible if treatment is stopped.

UROLITHIASIS CAUSED BY ANTIMICROBIAL DRUGS

Sometimes a drug may precipitate in the kidney as a result of poor solubility in urine. Important factors in the risk of formation of precipitates are urine volume, urine pH and drug solubility. Drugs with a high tendency to precipitate and cause symptoms of urolithiasis include the older sulfonamides and indinavir, an HIV protease inhibitor. For ciprofloxacin and some other fluoroquinolones, the solubility is very poor at alkaline pH. Thus, a patient with a renal infection caused by *Proteus* spp. may be at risk of clinically significant precipitation of the quinolone.

MONITORING OF SERUM CONCENTRATIONS OF ANTIMICROBIAL DRUGS

Serum concentration assays have two purposes: to avoid exceeding drug levels known to increase the risk of toxicity and to ensure that the dose given is sufficient to achieve therapeutic activity. For most antimicrobial drugs, serum concentration assays are not meaningful because there are no defined limits for toxicity or therapeutic efficacy. With some antibiotics (e.g. imipenem) concentration assays should be avoided because the drug is very unstable and transportation of the sample may lead to degradation of imipenem and falsely low concentrations in the assay. However, for some antimicrobial agents serum concentration assays are clinically indicated (Table 5.6).

Table 5.6 Antimicrobial drugs for which serum concentration monitoring is indicated

Drug	Comments
Aminoglycosides	High trough levels clearly related to nephrotoxicity and ototoxicity; low peak levels related to increased risk of therapeutic failure
Flucytosine	Concentrations <25 mg/L increase risk of emergence of resistance; concentrations >100 mg/L may result in toxicity
Glycopeptides	High trough levels related to nephrotoxicity and ototoxicity; low peak levels related to increased risk of therapeutic failure
Isoniazid	Concentration assay helps in identifying fast and slow acetylators; concentrations may be too low in the former and toxic in the latter

 References

1. Alestig K, Trollfors B, Andersson R, Olaison L, Suurküla M, Norrby SR. Ceftazidime and renal function. *J Antimicrob Chemother*. 1984;13:177–181.
2. Cockroft DW, Gault MH. Prediction of creatinine clearance from serum creatinine. *Nephron*. 1976;16:31–41.
3. Siersbaek-Nielsen K, Mølholm Hansen J, Kampmann J, Kristensen M. Rapid evaluation of creatinine clearance. *Lancet*. 1971;i:1333–1334.
4. Livornese LL, Slavin D, Benz RL, Ingerman MJ, Santoro J. Use of antibacterial agents in renal failure. *Infect Dis Clin North Am*. 2000;14:371–390.
5. Valtonen M, Tiula E, Backman JT, Neuvonen PJ. Elimination of meropenem during continuous veno-venous haemofiltration and haemodiafiltration in patients with acute renal failure. *J Antimicrob Chemother*. 2000;45:701–704.
6. Mingeot-Leclercq MP, Tulkens PM. Aminoglycosides: nephrotoxicity. *Antimicrob Agents Chemother*. 1999;43:1003–1012.
7. Walker PD, Barry Y, Shah SV. Oxidant mechanisms in gentamicin nephrotoxicity. *Ren Fail*. 1999;21:433–442.
8. Ali MZ, Goetz B. Meta-analysis of the relative efficacy and toxicity of single daily dosing versus multiple daily dosing of aminoglycosides. *Clin Infect Dis*. 1997;24:796–809.
9. Wood MJ. The comparative efficacy and safety of teicoplanin and vancomycin. *J Antimicrob Chemother*. 1996;37:209–222.
10. Elting LS, Rubenstein EB, Kurtin D, et al. Mississippi mud in the 1990s. Risks and outcomes of vancomycin-associated toxicity in general oncology praxis. *Cancer*. 1998;15:2597–2607.
11. Lodise TP, Lomaestro B, Graves J, Drusano GL. Larger vancomycin doses (at least four grams per day) are associated with an increased incidence of nephrotoxicity. *Antimicrob Agents Chemother*. 2008;52:1330–1336.
12. Ouderkirk JP, Nord JA, Turett GS, Kislak JW. Polymyxin B nephrotoxicity and efficacy against nosocomial infections caused by multiresistant Gram-negative bacteria. *Antimicrob Agents Chemother*. 2003;47:2659–2662.
13. Falagas ME, Kasiakou SK. Toxicity of polymyxins: a systematic review of the evidence from old and recent studies. *Crit Care*. 2006;10:R27.
14. Alexopulos E. Drug-induced acute interstitial nephritis. *Ren Fail*. 1998;20:809–819.

 Further information

Alestig K, Trollfors B, Andersson R, Olaison L, Suurkula M, Norrby SR. Ceftazidime and renal function. *J Antimicrob Chemother*. 1984;13:177–181.
Bailey TC, Little JR, Littenberg B, Reichley RM, Dunagan WC. A meta-analysis of extended-interval dosing versus multiple daily dosing of aminoglycosides. *Clin Infect Dis*. 1995;24:786–795.
Baliga R, Ueda N, Walker PD, Shah SV. Oxidant mechanisms in toxic acute renal failure. *Drug Metab Rev*. 1999;31:971–997.

Beauchamps D, Laurent G, Grenier L, et al. Attenuation of gentamicin-induced nephrotoxicity in rats by fleroxacin. *Antimicrob Agents Chemother.* 1997;41:1237–1245.

Brown NM, Reeves DS, McMullin CM. The pharmacokinetics and protein-binding of fusidic acid in patients with severe renal failure requiring either haemodialysis or continuous ambulatory peritoneal dialysis. *J Antimicrob Chemother.* 1997;39:803–809.

Chow AW, Azar RW. Glycopeptides and nephrotoxicity. *Intensive Care Med.* 1994;20:523–529.

De Vriese AS, Robbrecht DL, Vanholder RC, Vogelaers DP, Lamiere NH. Rifampicin-associated acute renal failure: pathophysiologic, immunologic, and clinical features. *Am J Kidney Dis.* 1998;31:108–115.

DelDot ME, Lipman J, Tett SE. Vancomycin pharmacokinetics in critically ill patients receiving continuous haemodiafiltration. *Br J Clin Pharmacol.* 2004;58:259–268.

Fanos V, Cataldo L. Antibacterial-induced nephrotoxicity in the newborn. *Drug Saf.* 1999;20:245–267.

Gilbert DN, Lee BL, Dworkin RJ, et al. A randomized comparison of the safety of once-daily or thrice-daily gentamicin combination with ticarcillin–clavulanate. *Am J Med.* 1998;105:182–191.

Hatal R, Dinh TT, Cook DJ. Single daily dosing of aminoglycosides in immunocompromised adults: a systematic review. *Clin Infect Dis.* 1997;24:810–815.

Krueger WA, Schroeder TH, Hutchison M, et al. Pharmacokinetics of meropenem in critically ill patients with acute renal failure treated with continuous hemodiafiltration. *Antimicrob Agents Chemother.* 1998;42:2421–2424.

Murray KR, McKinnon PS, Mitrzyk B, Rybak MJ. Pharmacodynamic characterization of nephrotoxicity associated with once-daily aminoglycoside. *Pharmacotherapy.* 1999;19:1252–1260.

Norrby SR. Carbapenems: imipenem/cilastatin and meropenem. *Antibiotics for Clinicians.* 1998;2:25–33.

Nucci M, Loureiro M, Silveira F, et al. Comparison of the toxicity of amphotericin B in 5% dextrose with that of amphotericin B in fat emulsion in a randomized trial with cancer patients. *Antimicrob Agents Chemother.* 1999;43:1445–1448.

Rohde B, Werner U, Hickstein H, Ehmcke H, Drewelow B. Pharmacokinetics of mezlocillin and sulbactam under continuous veno-venous hemodialysis (CVVHD) in intensive care patients with acute renal failure. *Eur J Clin Pharmacol.* 1997;53:111–115.

Rougier F, Claude D, Maurin M, et al. Aminoglycoside nephrotoxicity: modeling, simulation, and control. *Antimicrob Agents Chemother.* 2003;47:1010–1016.

Ryback MJ, Abate BJ, Kang SL, Ruffing MJ, Lerner SA, Drusano GL. Prospective evaluation of the effect of an aminoglycoside dosing regimen on rates of observed nephrotoxicity and ototoxicity. *Antimicrob Agents Chemother.* 1999;43:1549–1555.

Sànches Alcaraz A, Vargas A, Quintana MB, et al. Therapeutic drug monitoring of tobramycin: once-daily versus twice-daily dosage schedules. *J Clin Pharm Ther.* 1998;23:367–373.

Solgaard T, Tuxoe JI, Mafi M, Due Olofsen S, Toftgaard Jensen T. Nephrotoxicity by dicloxacillin and gentamicin in 163 patients with trochanteric hip fractures. *Orthopedics International.* 2000;24:155–157.

Staatz CE, Byrne C, Thomson AH. Population pharmacokinetic modeling of gentamicin and vancomycin in patients with unstable renal function following cardiothoracic surgery. *Br J Clin Pharmacol.* 2006;28:3382–3388.

Swan SK. Aminoglycoside nephrotoxicity. *Semin Nephrol.* 1997;17:27–33.

Takeda M, Tojo A, Sekine T, Hosoyamada M, Kanai Y, Endou H. Role of organic anion transporter 1 in cephaloridine (CER)-induced nephrotoxicity. *Kidney Int.* 1999;56:2128–2136.

Tegeder FI, Neumann F, Bremer F, Brune K, Lötsch J, Geisslinger G. Pharmacokinetics of meropenem in critically ill patients with acute renal failure undergoing continuous venovenous hemofiltration. *Clin Pharmacol Ther.* 1999;65:50–57.

Van der Verf TS, Mulder POM, Zijlstra JG, Uges DRA, Stegeman CA. Pharmacokinetics of piperacillin and tazobactam in critically ill patients with renal failure, treated with continuous veno-venous hemofiltration (CVVH). *Intensive Care Med.* 1997;23:873–877.

Van der Verf TS, Fijen JW, Van de Merbel NC, et al. Pharmacokinetics of cefpirome in critically ill patients with renal failure treated by continuous veno-venous hemofiltration. *Intensive Care Med.* 1999;25:1427–1431.

Warkentin D, Ippoliti C, Bruton J, Van Besien K, Champlin R. Toxicity of single daily dose of gentamicin in stem cell transplantation. *Bone Marrow Transplant.* 1999;24:57–61.

Wingard JR, Kabilkis P, Lee L, et al. Clinical significance of nephrotoxicity in patients treated with amphotericin B for suspected or proven aspergillosis. *Clin Infect Dis.* 1999;29:1402–1407.

Wingard JR, White HM, Anaisse E, Raffalli J, Goodman J, Arrieta A. A randomized, double-blind comparative trial evaluating the safety of liposomal amphotericin B versus an amphotericin B lipid complex in the empirical treatment of febrile neutropenia. L Amph/ABLC Collaborative Study Group. *Clin Infect Dis.* 2000;31:1155–1163.

6 Drug interactions involving anti-infective agents

Keith A. Rodvold and Donna M. Kraus

The medical treatment of common causes of infectious diseases (e.g. HIV, fungi, tuberculosis, and resistant Gram-negative or Gram-positive bacteria) has continued to evolve. The standard of care for these infections often requires patients to receive combinations of anti-infective agents as well as other medications to treat other diseases or clinical conditions. The medication profiles of individual patients in the infectious diseases clinic or hospital services have become increasingly more complex and are associated with higher probabilities of drug–drug interactions and adverse drug reactions.

Recent regulatory actions by the US Food and Drug Administration (FDA) remind us that important drug–drug interactions with anti-infective agents can result in withdrawal of drugs from the marketplace, termination of clinical development and restrictive dosage recommendations. Examples of these consequences include the withdrawal of terfenadine, astemizole and cisapride in the 1990s after patients experienced serious cardiac toxicity when taking these antihistamine or prokinetic drugs in combination with macrolide antibiotics or azole antifungals.[1] The antiviral agent, pleconaril, was not recommended for FDA approval for the treatment of the common cold in 2002 because of the potential for drug–drug interactions.[2] Pleconaril, a known cytochrome P_{450} (CYP) inducer, can potentially lower the plasma drug concentrations of CYP3A substrates and reduce their effectiveness, including oral contraceptive steroids such as ethinyl estradiol. Finally, the product package insert of the CCR5 co-receptor antagonist, maraviroc, is an example of the FDA restricting the dosing recommendations (Table 6.1) because of potential drug–drug interactions with potent CYP3A inhibitors or inducers during combination therapy.[3] Both the pharmaceutical industry and regulatory agencies have issued guidance papers on the methodologies of in-vitro and in-vivo pharmacokinetic drug–drug interaction studies because of the increasing concern about drug–drug interactions.[4] In addition, labeling of product package inserts has recently been revised and various sections describe relevant information about metabolic enzymes, drug transporters and drug–drug interactions.

Drug–drug interactions in the field of infectious diseases continue to expand as old and new agents requiring metabolic enzymes and transporters are commonly used, treatment recommendations for co-infections are revised, and the use of multiple medications (e.g. polypharmacy) proliferates in an aging population.[5–7] In addition, commonly prescribed medications with known drug–drug interactions are more likely to cause serious adverse health outcomes in elderly patients admitted to the hospital. Juurlink et al. recently performed a case-control study to determine the odds ratio (OR) for association between hospital admission of elderly patients with digoxin toxicity and use of clarithromycin within the previous week.[6] A total of 1051 patients admitted to the hospital for digoxin toxicity were compared to a control group (n = 51 896) without toxicity. The patients with digoxin toxicity were 13 times more likely to have received prior clarithromycin therapy (OR, 13.6; confidence interval [CI] 8.8–20.8). In comparison, no significant association (OR, 2.0; CI, 0.6–6.4) was found between patients with digoxin toxicity and prior use of cefuroxime within 1 week of hospital admission. This evidence is further supported by a large retrospective study that demonstrated a five-fold increased in the rate of cardiac-related sudden death in patients who were co-administered CYP3A inhibitors and erythromycin compared to patients who did not receive a CYP3A inhibitor or anti-infective agent.[7] These studies illustrate that many of the known drug–drug interactions are avoidable and that clinicians must consider alternative therapy when appropriate.

This chapter provides an overview of the principles and mechanisms of drug–drug interactions and uses extensive tables to summarize pharmacokinetic–pharmacodynamic interactions commonly associated with each anti-infective class. Physicochemical and in-vitro antimicrobial activity (e.g. additive, synergistic or antagonistic) interactions will not be discussed. This review was based on information available in the product package inserts, primary literature retrieval from PubMed, computer databases of Micromedex Drugdex® System, and current issues of the following textbooks: Piscitelli and Rodvold's *Drug Interactions in Infectious Diseases*,[8] Hansten and Horn's *Drug Interactions Analysis and Management*,[9] Tatro's *Drug Interaction Facts*[10] and *Stockley's Drug Interactions*.[11] In addition, *Stockley's Herbal Medicine Interactions*[12] is a recently published textbook that provides a comprehensive review of drug interactions with herbal medicines, dietary supplements and nutraceuticals. The reader is referred to these resources as well as to the primary literature and online websites for detailed information and reference lists about drug–drug interactions associated with a specific anti-infective agent. The reference list at the end of this chapter is mainly limited to secondary literature because of the publication space restrictions.

Table 6.1 Dosing recommendations for maraviroc associated with drug–drug interactions

Maraviroc dosage	Dosing recommendation for interacting drugs
300 mg every 12 h	Standard dose of maraviroc with no concomitant administration of cytochrome P$_{450}$ (CYP) 3A inhibitors or inducers; recommended dosage of maraviroc with concomitant administration of tipranavir–ritonavir or nevirapine
150 mg every 12 h	Reduced dose of maraviroc with concomitant administration of CYP3A4 inhibitors (with or without a CYP3A inducer) including protease inhibitors (exception: tipranavir–ritonavir [see above dosage recommendation]), delavirdine, ketoconazole, itraconazole, clarithromycin (including with etravirine plus ritonavir-boosted protease inhibitors or with efavirenz plus either lopinavir–ritonavir or saquinavir–ritonavir), and other strong CYP3A inhibitors (e.g. nefazodone, telithromycin)
600 mg every 12 h	Increased dose of maraviroc with CYP3A inducers (without a CYP3A inhibitor) including rifampicin, carbamazepine, phenytoin, phenobarbital, efavirenz and etravirine

PHARMACOKINETIC AND PHARMACODYNAMIC DRUG–DRUG INTERACTIONS

A drug–drug interaction is defined as the change in efficacy or toxicity of one drug by prior or concomitant administration of a second drug. In general, drug–drug interactions involve two drugs: the interacting drug (e.g. precipitant, perpetrator) is the agent that causes a change to occur upon another drug (e.g. substrate, object, victim). Alterations in the pharmacokinetic or pharmacodynamic characteristics of the object drug are the two commonly used mechanisms for categorizing drug–drug interactions.[13]

Pharmacokinetic interactions are those associated with alterations in the processes of absorption, distribution, metabolism or elimination of a medication. The consequences of this type of drug–drug interaction include increased or decreased concentrations of a drug in the blood, body fluids and/or tissues, which may in turn alter the efficacy or toxicity of the object drug. The most commonly measured pharmacokinetic parameters used to describe and assess these changes include maximum drug concentration (C_{max}), area under the concentration–time curve (AUC), apparent drug clearance (CL), half-life ($t_{1/2}$) or total amount of drug excreted in the urine (Ae).

Absorption interactions generally involve orally administered drugs and occur in the mucous membranes of the gastrointestinal (GI) tract. Common causes for drug–drug interactions involving absorption include: (1) alterations in GI pH; (2) adsorption, chelation or other complexing mechanisms; (3) changes in GI motility; (4) induction or inhibition of drug transporter proteins or intestinal CYP isoenzymes; (5) malabsorption caused by drugs; and (6) alteration to the normal GI flora.[11] Oral anti-infective agents such cefpodoxime

proxetil, ketoconazole, itraconazole, delavirdine and atazanavir have dissolution and absorption that is pH dependent and can be affected by antacids, proton pump inhibitors and histamine$_2$ (H$_2$) antagonists.[11,14] Antacids, vitamin/mineral supplements or other therapeutic agents containing divalent and trivalent cations, such as aluminum, magnesium, calcium or iron, chelate tetracycline and fluoroquinolones, resulting in markedly reduced oral GI absorption, lower systemic drug concentrations and lower anti-infective efficacy.[15]

The oral bioavailability of digoxin can be increased or decreased by agents such as clarithromycin and rifampicin (rifampin), respectively. These effects are most likely explained by alterations to P-glycoprotein (P-gp).[16] This efflux transporter can reduce drug absorption from the GI tract, as well as promote drug removal or decrease drug entry at various sites of distribution and elimination. Rifampicin is an inducer of P-gp which leads to decreased oral absorption of medications while macrolides such as erythromycin and clarithromycin are inhibitors of intestinal and renal P-gp of digoxin. Oral neomycin can impair the absorption of digoxin by causing a malabsorption syndrome similar to non-tropical sprue.[11] Antibiotics can also alter the normal GI flora and thus affect the metabolism and absorption of medications such as warfarin and estrogen-containing products (e.g. oral contraceptive agents).

Pharmacokinetic drug–drug interactions can be related to protein binding and distribution characteristics of medications. Drug–drug interactions associated with protein binding could be clinically significant if the drug being displaced has a narrow therapeutic index, small volume of distribution, high extraction ratio, and is highly protein bound (>90%) at therapeutic concentrations. Displacement interactions have often been associated with drugs that are highly protein bound (e.g. warfarin, phenytoin). However, these agents have a low extraction ratio and drug concentrations are independent of protein binding changes since they can effectively clear any increase in the unbound fraction of the drug. The significance of drug–drug interactions involving protein binding and drug displacement is less than what was once thought since steady-state unbound (free) drug concentrations often redistribute and remain unaltered.[17] In addition, some drug–drug interactions once thought to be associated with protein binding and drug displacement have been shown to be associated with other interaction mechanisms. For example, the increased anticoagulant activity associated with warfarin when administered with trimethoprim–sulfamethoxazole is more likely caused by the inhibition of S-warfarin metabolism (e.g. CYP2C9) than from warfarin being displaced from its protein-binding sites.[15]

There are several transport proteins which play a role in mediating tissue-specific distribution as well as absorption and excretion of drugs.[18–21] The two major gene superfamilies responsible for the transport of drugs are ABC (**A**TP **b**inding **c**assette) and SLC (**sol**ute **c**arrier). P-glycoprotein (P-gp, also termed *MDR*1) is one of the most studied transporters from the ABC superfamily. P-gp and other transport proteins are located throughout the body in tissues and can control exposure of drugs at target organs. It has also been shown P-gp and **o**rganic **a**nion **t**ransporting **p**olypeptide (OATP) and **o**rganic **a**nion **t**ransporter (OAT) families are involved with efflux transport in the blood–brain barrier and blood–cerebrospinal fluid (CSF) barrier. The organic transport systems are particularly important in the distribution of β-lactam agents. Membrane transporters and drug response is a growing field of research and should further clarify drug–drug interactions associated with the distribution of anti-infective agents.

Drug metabolism serves as the major mechanism of many pharmacokinetic drug–drug interactions.[13,22] Drugs are mainly metabolized by enzymes in the liver, GI tract, skin, lungs and blood. Drug-metabolizing enzymes are found in the endoplasmic reticulum of these sites and are classified as microsomal enzymes. There are two major types of drug metabolizing reaction: phase I, which increases the polarity of drugs predominantly through oxidation, reduction or hydrolysis; and phase II, which catalyzes drugs and/or metabolites to inactive products by glucuronidation, sulfation or acetylation. Phase II reactions are most commonly mediated by sulfotransferase (SULT), uridine diphosphate glucuronosyltransferase (UGT), glutathione-S-transferase (GST), *N*-acetyltransferase (NAT) and thiopurine methyltransferase (TPMT) (Figure 6.1). Many of the enzymes involved in phase II are still being further defined, and drug–drug interactions are being further investigated.

The majority of phase I reactions are catalyzed by cytochrome P$_{450}$ enzymes in the liver and small intestine, which are heme-containing, membrane-bound proteins. Cytochrome P$_{450}$ is a superfamily of enzymes divided into families (designated by CYP followed by a number, e.g. CYP2), subfamilies (designated by a capital letter, e.g. CYP2C), and individual members (designated by a number, e.g. CYP2C19) based on amino acid sequence homology. The most common individual members of enzyme subfamilies responsible for the majority of phase I metabolic reactions are CYP3A4, CYP2D6, CYP1A2, CYP2C9 and CYP2C19 (Figure 6.2).[13,22]

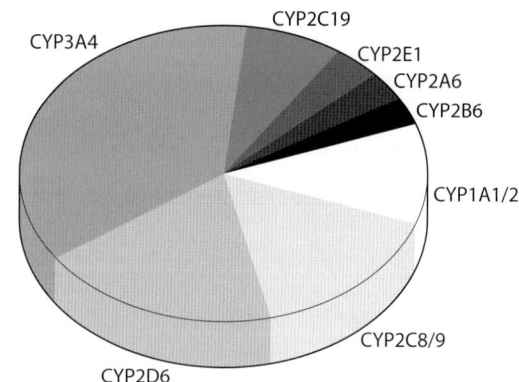

Fig. 6.2 The relative proportions of clinically used drugs metabolized by phase I (cytochrome P$_{450}$ [CYP]) enzymes.

More than 50% of all drugs on the market are metabolized by CYP3A4.[13,22] CYP3A4 is the major CYP isoform found in the adult liver and accounts for 28% of total hepatic CYP enzymes. In addition, CYP3A4 is also found in the GI tract and has effects on bioavailability. There is significant overlapping activity between P-gp and CYP3A4 at both of these sites, and a drug causing an effect on P-gp will also have the same effect on CYP3A4. Many drug–drug interactions previously thought to be due to only CYP3A4 may actually involve the additive effects of both P-gp and CYP3A4. Phase I reactions can also involve other CYP-independent enzymes such as monoamine oxidases and epoxide hydrolases.

Drug–drug interactions involving CYP isoenzymes are often the result of either enzyme inhibition or induction.[13] A drug that is an inhibitor of a specific drug-metabolizing enzyme will decrease the rate of metabolism and increase plasma concentrations of an object drug. Increased drug accumulation can result in enhanced therapeutic effects or adverse effects, especially if the object drug has a narrow therapeutic range or index. A greater increase in the AUC or C$_{max}$ of the object drug would be predicted to occur when the specific drug-metabolizing enzyme is the primary elimination pathway compared to substrates with multiple elimination pathways of which the enzyme plays only a minor role. Inhibition of metabolic pathways can also lead to decreased formation of an active metabolite of the object drug and this may result in decreased therapeutic efficacy of the drug.

Inhibition of CYP3A4 is a common cause of drug–drug interactions with anti-infective agents. Table 6.2 provides examples of some of the serious and/or life-threatening drug–drug interactions known to occur between substrates of CYP3A4 and anti-infective agents known to be potent inhibitors of CYP3A4. The co-administration any CYP3A4 inhibitors should be avoided or only undertaken with extreme precautions (e.g. dosage adjustments or use of less potent inhibitors) with the listed substrates due to the serious clinical consequences. Anti-infective agents that are moderate to strong inhibitors of CYP3A4 include protease inhibitors, delavirdine, azole antifungal agents, clarithromycin, erythromycin and telithromycin.

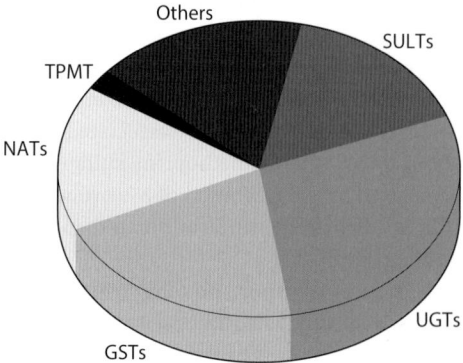

Fig. 6.1 The relative proportions of clinically used drugs metabolized by phase II enzymes. GST, glutathione-S-transferase; NAT, *N*-acetyltransferase; TPMT, thiopurine methyltransferase; SULT, sulfotransferase; UGT, uridine diphosphate glucuronosyltransferase.

Table 6.2 Substrates of CYP3A4 with major or life-threatening interactions when co-administered with a CYP3A inhibitor[1]

CYP3A4 substrate	Pharmacological effect	Management recommendation
Astemizole,[2] terfenadine,[2] cisapride,[2] bepridil,[2] pimozide	QTc interval prolongation, arrhythmias, sudden death, torsade de pointes	Contraindicated
Ciclosporin, sirolimus, tacrolimus	Increased serum concentrations and immunosuppression	Monitor immunosuppressive agent serum concentrations; adjust dose as needed
Ergot alkaloids	Ergotism, peripheral ischemia	Contraindicated
Lovastatin, simvastatin	Risk of rhabdomyolysis	Use other HMG-CoA reductase inhibitors such as pravastatin or fluvastatin
Midazolam, triazolam	Excessive sedation	Use other benzodiazepines such as lorazepam, oxazepam or temazepam
Rifabutin	Uveitis, neutropenia, flu-like syndrome	Reduce dose of rifabutin
Sildenafil, tadalafil, vardenafil	Hypotension, priapism	Reduce dose or avoid use entirely
Vincristine, vinblastine	Neurotoxicity	Reduce dose and monitor for vinca toxicity

[1]Examples of anti-infective agents that are potent cytochrome P_{450} (CYP) 3A4 inhibitors include clarithromycin, erythromycin, telithromycin, protease inhibitors, delavirdine, ketoconazole, itraconazole and voriconazole.
[2]Drugs not longer commercially available in the USA.
HMG-CoA, hydroxymethylglutaryl-coenzyme A.

Inhibition of a specific drug-metabolizing enzyme can be either competitive or non-competitive. Competitive inhibition occurs when two drugs are substrates for the same drug-metabolizing enzyme. Binding of one agent to the enzyme prevents binding by the other, thereby decreasing the rate of metabolism and increasing systemic exposure and/or pharmacological effects of the drug with lower enzyme-binding affinity. In contrast, non-competitive inhibition occurs when one drug is an inhibitor of a specific drug-metabolizing enzyme (e.g. CYP3A4) and can substantially reduce the metabolism of an object drug of that enzyme. However, the inhibitor is metabolized by a different drug-metabolizing enzyme (e.g. CYP2D6) than the object drug being inhibited. The onset and dissipation of drug–drug interactions involving inhibition is rapid and occurs within the first few days after co-administration.

Phase I and II reactions can also be induced. Enzyme induction occurs when the precipitant drug induces the synthesis of the drug-metabolizing enzyme. Drugs that induce cytochrome P_{450} isoenzymes cause increased drug clearance and decreased plasma concentrations of substrate drugs. Rifampicin is one of the most potent inducers and has effects on both CYP enzymes and P-gp.[22–24] Rifampicin can also induce phase II enzymes such as UGT as well as other relevant transporter proteins. Because of this broad and potent range of induction activity, numerous drug–drug interactions have been reported between rifampicin and various therapeutic classes of drugs, including anti-infective agents (Table 6.3).[23] Because induction requires creation of new enzymes, the time course of the onset and dissipation of induction is slow and can take weeks to occur. When rifampicin induces the metabolism of an object drug, serum drug concentrations are gradually decreased and the full effect may not be seen for 2 weeks.

Many of the commonly used anti-infective agents are substrates, inhibitors and/or inducers of the clinically significant CYP isoenzymes, P-gp and UGT (Table 6.4). In addition, an updated list of drugs from various therapeutic classes and their designation as substrates, inhibitors or inducers of specific CYP isoenzymes can be found on the website http://medicine.iupui.edu/clinpharm/ddis. These tables can assist in the semi-quantitative prediction of potential drug–drug interactions, particularly when no published studies are available. It is important to appreciate that a drug can be a substrate of more than one CYP isoenzyme and that the same drug may serve as an inhibitor or inducer of a different CYP isoenzyme than the one being metabolized by it.

Factors that play an important role in determining the magnitude of changes in substrate metabolism include single or multiple substrate elimination pathways, existence of dominant elimination isoforms and the inhibitory-induction potency. Simultaneous therapy with both inducers and inhibitors of CYP isoforms may have unpredictable effects. There are no dosage guidelines that address these competing effects. It is suggested that close monitoring for toxicity or alternative agents that do not interact be used.

The clinical significance of the potential pharmacokinetic drug–drug interaction is supratherapeutic drug concentrations resulting in an exaggerated clinical response, toxicity, or both, or subtherapeutic drug concentrations resulting in loss of efficacy, the development of resistance, or both. For inhibition, the clinical consequences may be amplification of known adverse effects or the occurrence of a concentration-related toxicity. The therapeutic index, type of concentration-dependent toxicity and the dosage that the patient is receiving when the enzyme inhibitor is added to the treatment regimen are all important considerations.

Table 6.3   Drug–drug interactions of rifampicin (rifampin)

Interacting drug	Comments and management strategy
Anti-infective agents	
Atovaquone	Monitor clinical response; increase dose if needed; consider alternative agent
Caspofungin	Monitor clinical response; increase dose to 70 mg per day
Chloramphenicol	Monitor chloramphenicol serum concentrations; increase dose if needed
Clarithromycin	Monitor clinical and microbiological response; increase dose if needed
Dapsone	Monitor clinical response and hematological toxic effects
Delavirdine	Avoid rifampicin; use rifabutin or alternative agent and monitor viral response
Doxycycline	Monitor clinical and microbiological response; increase dose if needed
Efavirenz	Monitor viral response; increase dose if needed (e.g. 800 mg if >60 kg)
Etravirine	Avoid rifampicin; use rifabutin or alternative agent and monitor viral response
Fluconazole	Monitor clinical and microbiological response; increase dose if needed
Itraconazole, voriconazole	Avoid rifampicin; if used, increase dose of azole and monitor response
Maraviroc	Monitor viral response; appropriate dosing with inducers and inhibitors (see Table 6.1)
Mefloquine	Consider avoiding combination; larger study needed
Metronidazole	Monitor clinical and microbiological response; increase dose if needed
Nevirapine	Avoid rifampicin; use rifabutin or alternative agent and monitor viral response
Praziquantel	Consider alternative agent if possible; monitor clinical response
Protease inhibitors	Avoid rifampicin; use rifabutin or alternative agent and monitor viral response
Quinine	Monitor clinical response; consider alternative agent if possible
Raltegravir	Consider using rifabutin; if rifampicin is used, monitor viral response
TMP–SMX	Monitor clinical and microbiological response; increase dose if needed
Analgesics	
Codeine	Monitor pain control and clinical response
COX-2 inhibitors[1]	Monitor clinical response; increase dose if needed
Fentanyl	Monitor pain control; increase dose if needed
Methadone	Increase methadone dose; monitor and control withdrawal symptoms
Morphine	Monitor pain control and clinical response
Anticonvulsants	
Phenytoin	Monitor phenytoin serum concentrations and seizure activity; increase dose if needed
Antidiabetic agents	
Sulfonylureas[2]	Monitor blood glucose levels; adjust dose based on blood glucose control
Meglitidinides[3]	Monitor blood glucose levels; adjust dose based on blood glucose control
Thiazolidinediones[4]	Monitor blood glucose levels; adjust dose based on blood glucose control
Anticoagulants (oral)	Monitor INR; increase anticoagulant dose as needed
Cardiovascular drugs	
Beta-blocking agents	Monitor clinical response; increase propranolol or metoprolol dose if needed
Digitoxin	Monitor clinical response and/or arrhythmia control, monitor digitoxin serum concentrations
Digoxin (oral)	Monitor clinical response and/or arrhythmia control, monitor digitoxin serum concentrations
Diltiazem	Use alternative agent; monitor patient for clinical response
Disopyramide	Monitor arrhythmia control; increase dose if needed
Losartan	Monitor clinical response; increase dose if needed
Nifedipine	Consider alternative agents; if used, monitor clinical response; increase dose if needed
Nilvadipine	Monitor clinical response; increase dose if needed
Propafenone	Monitor clinical response; increase dose if needed; consider alternative agent
Quinidine	Monitor quinidine serum concentrations and arrhythmia control; increase dose if needed
Tocainide	Monitor arrhythmia control; increase dose if needed
Verapamil	Use alternative agent; monitor patient for clinical response
Contraceptives (oral)	Use alternative form(s) of birth control; counsel patient and document
Glucocorticoids	Increase dose of glucocorticoid two- to three-fold
HMG-CoA reductase inhibitors[5]	Monitor lipid panel; increase dose if needed (likely for simvastatin)
Immunosuppressants	
Ciclosporin	Monitor ciclosporin serum concentrations; increased dose if needed
Tacrolimus	Monitor tacrolimus serum concentrations; increase dose if needed
Everolimus	Monitor everolimus serum concentrations; increase dose if needed
Psychotropic agents	
Buspirone	Monitor clinical response; increased dose likely needed; use alternative agent if possible

(Continued)

Table 6.3 Drug–drug interactions of rifampicin (rifampin)—cont'd

Interacting drug	Comments and management strategy
Clozapine	Monitor clinical response; increase dose if needed or use alternative agent if possible
Haloperidol	Monitor clinical response; increase dose if needed
Nortriptyline	Monitor clinical response and nortriptyline serum concentrations
Sertraline	Monitor clinical response; increase dose if needed
Others	
5-HT$_3$ antiemetics[6]	Monitor clinical response; increase dose if needed; use alternative agent if needed
Diazepam	Monitor clinical response; increase dose if needed
Gefitinib	Avoid combination; if must use, increase dose
Imatinib	Avoid combination; if must use, increase dose
Levothyroxine	Monitor thyroid stimulating hormone; increased dose likely needed
Lorazepam	Monitor clinical response; increase dose if needed
Midazolam	Avoid combination; use alternative agent if possible
Tamoxifen, toremifene	Monitor clinical response; increased dose likely needed
Theophylline	Monitor theophylline serum concentrations; increase dose if needed
Triazolam	Avoid combination; use alternative agent if possible
Zolpidem	Monitor clinical response; increase dose if needed or use alternative agent if possible

[1]Examples include celecoxib and rofecoxib (no longer available).
[2]Examples include tolbutamide, chlorpropamide, gliclazide and glimepiride.
[3]Examples include repaglinide and nateglinide.
[4]Examples include rosiglitazone and pioglitazone.
[5]Examples include simvastatin, atorvastatin and pravastatin.
[6]Examples include ondansetron and dolasetron.
5-HT$_3$, 5-hydroxytryptamine 3; HMG-CoA, hydroxymethylglutaryl-coenzyme A; TMP–SMX, trimethoprim–sulfamethoxazole.

With this knowledge, one can decide whether the drug–drug interaction makes co-administration potentially hazardous. For induction, a hypothetical clinical consequence may be loss of anti-infective activity or possible development of resistance. In both of these examples, co-administration would not be advisable. Alternatively, these interactions may be overcome with higher doses. However, higher doses have often not been studied in most cases and unless recommended in the product monograph this is not advisable. Suggested dosage adjustment recommendations are based on mean changes in substrate clearance, and in most in-vivo dosage interaction trials, doses used were less than currently recommended. It is often unknown whether product monograph dosage adjustment recommendations will result in safe and therapeutic substrate concentrations.

Regulatory agencies such as the FDA have placed greater emphasis on in-vitro and in-vivo drug–drug interaction assessment.[1,21] Information on the likely potential of drug–drug interactions involving CYP enzymes and drug transporter proteins is included in the product package inserts of recently approved medications. For example, the product insert for daptomycin states that metabolic drug–drug interactions are unlikely since in-vitro studies have shown that daptomycin neither induces nor inhibits CYP isoforms 1A2, 2A6, 2C9, 2C19, 2D6, 2E1 and 3A4.[25] Similar to CYP isoforms, further information about metabolism and potential drug–drug interactions of phase II reactions are being included in product package information. The product insert for raltegravir states that this agent is mainly eliminated by metabolism via a UGT1A1-mediated glucuronidation pathway and is not a substrate of CYP enzymes.[26] Drugs known to inhibit (e.g. atazanavir) and induce (e.g. rifampicin) UGT1A1 have been shown in vivo to increase and decrease plasma concentrations of raltegravir, respectively.

There is significant interindividual variability in the outcomes of drug–drug interactions. This variability is often associated with patient-specific factors such as disease states, other concomitant medications and genetics. Genetic polymorphism has been identified with CYP2D6, CYP2C9 and CYP2C19, as well as many of the phase II enzymes. Clinically significant polymorphisms can contribute to ethnic differences in metabolism as well as drug safety and efficacy.[27] For CYP2D6, the prevalence of poor metabolizers is 5–8% in Caucasians and <1% in Asians. In comparison, the incidence of CYP2C19 poor metabolizers is 2–6% of Caucasians and 18–20% of Asians. The magnitude that drug–drug interactions will have is dependent in part on whether the initial enzyme activity is at a high or a low level. Inhibition of a drug-metabolizing enzyme in extensive or rapid metabolizers may result in more significant effects than in slow metabolizers. Thus, drug–drug interactions involving polymorphisms must be assessed for clinical relevance to an individual patient.

Pharmacokinetic drug–drug interactions can also occur during renal excretion. These interactions are rapid and occur competitively. The mechanisms for drug–drug interactions of renal elimination involve glomerular filtration, tubular secretion, tubular reabsorption, and drug transporter proteins (e.g. P-gp and OATs).[13,18,19] Tubular secretion is the most common site of renal interactions since drugs often compete with each other for the same active transport system in the renal tubules. The classic anti-infective example is probenecid reducing the renal excretion of penicillin to increase anti-infective serum concentrations for therapeutic benefit. It has more recently been appreciated that organic anion transport (OAT) proteins are primarily located in the kidneys and facilitate the active renal secretion of several anti-infective agents including cidofovir, adefovir, aciclovir (acyclovir), ganciclovir, zidovudine and β-lactam antibiotics.[18,19] Probenecid,

Table 6.4 Examples of anti-infective agents as substrates, inhibitors and inducers of CYP enzymes, UGT and P-gp

Enzymes or transporter	Substrates	Inhibitors	Inducers
CYP1A2	Ritonavir	Erythromycin, clarithromycin, ciprofloxacin, norfloxacin, ritonavir	Ritonavir, rifampicin
CYP2C9	Nelfinavir, ritonavir, fluconazole, voriconazole, dapsone	Erythromycin, metronidazole, sulfamethoxazole, trimethoprim–sulfamethoxazole, fluconazole, miconazole, voriconazole, isoniazid	Rifampicin, rifapentine
CYP2C19	Chloramphenicol, nelfinavir, ritonavir, fluconazole, voriconazole	Chloramphenicol, ritonavir, fluconazole, ketoconazole, voriconazole	Rifampicin
CYP2D6	Ritonavir	Primaquine, ritonavir	Rifampicin
CYP2E1	Ritonavir, isoniazid, dapsone	Ritonavir, isoniazid	Isoniazid
CYP3A4	Erythromycin, clarithromycin, telithromycin, clindamycin, protease inhibitors, delavirdine, nevirapine, NNRTIs, maraviroc, miconazole, ketoconazole, itraconazole, fluconazole, voriconazole, posaconazole, dapsone, quinine	Chloramphenicol, erythromycin, clarithromycin, telithromycin, norfloxacin, ciprofloxacin, amprenavir, nelfinavir, lopinavir–ritonavir, ritonavir, saquinavir, indinavir, delavirdine, efavirenz, quinupristin–dalfopristin, clotrimazole, miconazole, itraconazole, ketoconazole, fluconazole, voriconazole, posaconazole	Efavirenz, nevirapine, rifampicin, rifabutin, rifapentine, ritonavir
UGT	Posaconazole, zidovudine, raltegravir	Ketoconazole, fluconazole, atazanavir	Rifampicin
P-gp	Clarithromycin, erythromycin, indinavir, nelfinavir, ritonavir, saquinavir, maraviroc, ketoconazole, itraconazole, fluconazole, posaconazole,	Clarithromycin, erythromycin, ketoconazole, itraconazole, indinavir, nelfinavir, ritonavir, saquinavir	Rifampicin, ritonavir

CYP, cytochrome P_{450}; NNRTIs, non-nucleoside reverse transcriptase inhibitors; P-gp, P-glycoprotein; UGT, uridine diphosphate glucuronosyltransferase.

a known OAT1 inhibitor, blocks the tubular transport of the nucleotide cidofovir and reduces its renal clearance to the rate of glomerular filtration. Concomitant use of probenecid decreases the risk of nephrotoxicity associated with cidofovir and is considered a beneficial drug–drug interaction. Although cidofovir does not affect the disposition of other agents, the concurrent administration of probenecid can inhibit renal tubular secretion of other commonly administered agents such as reverse transcriptase inhibitors (e.g. zidovudine, zalcitabine), β-lactams, methotrexate and non-steroidal anti-inflammatory drugs (NSAIDs). Various anti-infective agents (e.g. clarithromycin, itraconazole), as well as probenecid, have been shown to inhibit P-gp in the kidney. As with liver metabolism, significant overlapping activity exists between P-gp and other transport mechanisms involved with renal excretion.

In addition to pharmacokinetic drug–drug interactions, pharmacodynamic interactions can also occur.[13,15] Pharmacodynamic drug–drug interactions are associated with a change in the pharmacological response (e.g. efficacy or toxicity) of the object drug, with or without changes in pharmacokinetics. Pharmacodynamic interactions can be categorized as:

- *additive*: two agents leads to enhanced pharmacological effect (e.g. increased bone marrow suppression with concurrent use of zidovudine and ganciclovir);
- *synergistic*: use of two or more agents results in drug effect greater than (e.g. exponential vs additive) the addition of all of the drugs together (e.g. combined effect with

concurrent use of indinavir, lamivudine, and zidovudine than the sum of their individual effects); or
- *antagonistic*: the pharmacological effect of one agent is reduced due to concurrent therapy with another agent (e.g. concurrent use of zidovudine and stavudine reduces antiviral effect).

Some of the common additive or overlapping adverse effects associated with anti-infective agents include ototoxicity, nephrotoxicity, bone marrow suppression and prolongation of the QTc interval. Concurrent administration of aminoglycoside antibiotics and other nephrotoxic agents such as amphotericin B, cisplatin, ciclosporin or vancomycin would be examples of additive risk for developing nephrotoxicity.[15] Pharmacodynamic drug–drug interactions are less predictive a priori than pharmacokinetic interactions, and fewer reports exist in the literature.

IDENTIFICATION OF CLINICALLY SIGNIFICANT DRUG–DRUG INTERACTIONS

The prescribing of safe and effective anti-infective therapy has becoming increasingly important as issues of resistance and treatment failure constantly challenge our anti-infective armamentarium. In addition, anti-infective drug regimens have become more complex because of the expansion of different drug classes; increased number of agents per anti-infective class; the availability of more agents as substrates, inhibitors and/or inducers of metabolism or transporter systems; and multiple different drug therapies being required to prevent or treat acute and chronic conditions or diseases due to both infectious and non-infectious causes. Awareness of clinically significant drug–drug interactions and appropriate inventions to minimize their occurrence are essential as anti-infective regimens become more complex.

Strategies for avoiding drug–drug interactions when selecting agents for use include:[28]

- obtaining a detailed medication history before prescribing anti-infective agents;
- avoiding adding a drug with high drug–drug interaction potential;
- delaying initiation of an interacting drug until anti-infective therapy is completed;
- reviewing and considering concomitant diseases states that influence drug disposition and interactions;
- selecting specific agents with the least potential for known drug–drug interactions;
- avoiding agents associated with serious adverse effects or toxicities;
- avoiding concurrent administration of drugs with overlapping or additive adverse effects;
- using the lowest effective drug doses; and
- not underestimating the ability of patients to adhere to the recommended drug dosage regimens.

Many of the drug–drug interactions involving absorption can be simply avoided by separating or spacing the times of concurrent drug administration. While not all drug–drug interactions are avoidable, many can be better managed with dosage adjustments, selection of alternative agents with lower interaction probabilities, and therapeutic drug monitoring.

Infectious disease clinicians are often forced to assess of the possibility of a potential drug–drug interaction in patients already receiving multiple medications from different drug classes. Clues that should prompt careful evaluation of pre-existing drug regimens for potential drug–drug interactions include:[28]

- drugs with well-documented drug–drug interaction potential;
- drugs with known, relatively narrow therapeutic ranges or indices;
- drugs with well-described pharmacodynamic determinants of efficacy or toxicity;
- drugs associated with serious adverse effects or toxicities; and
- the presence of extensive medication profiles in patients who cannot be easily monitored for drug efficacy and toxicity.

In addition, the drug interaction probability scale (DIPS) is a new tool that may be of assistance in providing a guide to evaluating drug–drug interaction causation in a specific patient.[29] Consultation with other infectious diseases physicians, pharmacists or drug-information specialists may also be valuable when multiple interactions are encountered.[30]

Computer programs are a practical and potentially effective method for detecting drug–drug interactions.[5,30] The intention of most of these programs is to alert the prescriber or dispensing pharmacist of a potential drug–drug interaction based on the information available in the patient medication profile. However, the level of concordance, specificity and sensitivity varies between programs, including those used in the community and hospital setting. In addition, many software programs and/or order entry systems have differing limitations such as accuracy in the classification or the lack of evidence for specific drug–drug interactions. Most programs do not provide timely updates as new information becomes available. Several studies have shown that users often override many of the different types of alerts and warnings being flagged. This often results in 'alert fatigue', which causes clinicians to ignore critical drug–drug interaction warnings which may require further information to determine the clinical relevance of the interaction and the individual patient being treated.

ANTIBACTERIAL AGENTS (Table 6.5)

Nearly all mechanisms of drug–drug interactions are represented by antibacterial agents.[15,31–33] Several different types of absorption drug–drug interaction occur with different antibacterial agents:

- alterations in gastric pH caused by antacids, H_2-receptor antagonists or proton pump inhibitors (e.g. oral cephalosporins);
- inhibition of a transport pump such as intestinal P-gp (e.g. effect of clarithromycin on plasma digoxin concentrations);
- alterations of gut flora (e.g. decreased effectiveness of oral contraceptives or augmentation of effects of warfarin); and
- chelation of drug (e.g. tetracyclines or fluoroquinolones) by co-administration of divalent or trivalent cations such as calcium, magnesium, aluminum or iron. Common products containing multivalent cations include antacids, laxatives, antidiarrheals, multivitamins, sucralfate, didanosine tablets or powder, molindone, and quinapril tablets.

Sulfonamides can potentially displace sulfonylurea hypoglycemics and methotrexate from plasma protein binding sites, resulting in hypoglycemia and severe bone marrow depression, respectively.

Significant drug–drug interactions involving CYP3A4 and P-gp have been well documented for macrolide and ketolide agents (e.g. erythromycin, clarithromycin, telithromycin) since many of these drug–drug interactions are associated with serious or life-threatening adverse events (see Table 6.2).[15,33] In addition, several classes of antibacterial agent are selective inhibitors of CYP2C8 and CYP2C9 (trimethoprim and sulfamethoxazole, respectively) and CYP3A4 (e.g. quinupristin–dalfopristin). Carbapenems can significantly decrease (e.g. by 40–80%) the serum concentrations of valproic acid by inhibiting the

Table 6.5 Drug–drug interactions of antibacterial agents

Antibacterial agent	Interacting drug	Interaction and management strategy
Oral cephalosporin prodrugs[1]	H[2] antagonists or antacids	Decreased absorption of cephalosporin; space administration by at least 2 h
Penicillins, cephalosporins and carbapenems[2]	Probenecid	Increased serum concentrations of β-lactam agent; avoid concomitant use when higher concentrations are not desirable or increased risk in toxicity (e.g. CNS) may occur
Ampicillin or amoxicillin	Allopurinol	Increased risk (three-fold higher) for rash; monitor for rash; consider alternative agent if possible
Carbapenems[3]	Valproic acid	Decreased serum concentrations of valproic acid; monitor serum valproic acid concentrations and seizure activity; increase dose of valproic acid if needed or avoid concomitant use
Imipenem	Ganciclovir or ciclosporin	Increased risk for CNS toxicity; concomitant use of these agents is not recommended
Erythromycin, clarithromycin or telithromycin	Substrates of CYP3A4	See Table 6.2
	Antiarrhythmic agents[4]	Increased serum concentrations of antiarrhythmic agents leading to the risk of QTc prolongation, torsades de pointes and death; alternative agents should be considered
	Calcium channel blockers[5]	Increased serum concentrations of calcium channel blocker; monitor for hypotension, tachycardia, edema, flushing and dizziness; increased risk of sudden cardiac death (diltiazem, verapamil); consider alternative agent if possible
	Colchicine	Increased toxicity and mortality; avoid concurrent administration
	Digoxin	Increased digoxin serum concentrations and risk of toxicity; monitor serum digoxin concentrations and toxicity; decrease dose of digoxin as needed
	Theophylline	Increased theophylline serum concentrations and risk of toxicity; monitor serum theophylline concentrations and toxicity; decrease dose of theophylline as needed
	Tricyclic antidepressants and antipsychotic agents[6]	Increased serum concentrations of antidepressant or antipsychotic agent; risk of QTc prolongation and torsades de pointes; alternative agents should be considered
	Warfarin	Enhanced anticoagulation; monitor PT/INR and adjust warfarin dose appropriately
Fluoroquinolones[7]	Multivalent cations[8]	Decreased absorption of fluoroquinolone; space administration by at least 2–4 h
	Class la and IIIa antiarrhythmic agents	Increased risk of QTc prolongation and torsades de pointes; alternative agents should be considered in patients who at risk (e.g. history QTc prolongation or uncorrected electrolyte abnormalities)
	Theophylline	Ciprofloxacin or norfloxacin can increased theophylline serum concentrations and risk of toxicity; monitor serum theophylline concentrations and toxicity; decrease dose of theophylline as needed
	Tizanidine	Ciprofloxacin can increased tizanidine serum concentrations and risk of hypotensive effects; use alternative agents such a fluoroquinolones without CYP1A2 inhibition (e.g. levofloxacin or moxifloxacin)
Aminoglycosides,[9] polymyxin, colistin	Nephrotoxic agents[10]	Direct or additive injury to the renal tubule; concomitant therapy should be avoided or used with caution and includes monitoring of renal function and dosage adjustment based on body weight, creatinine clearance estimation and/or serum aminoglycoside concentrations
	Ototoxic agents[11]	Increased risk of ototoxicity; concomitant therapy should be avoided or used with caution at the lowest possible dose; consider alternative agent if possible
	Neuromuscular blocking agents[12]	Increased respiratory suppression produced by neuromuscular agent; concomitant therapy should be avoided or used with caution and includes monitoring for respiratory depression
Vancomycin	Aminoglycosides	Direct or additive injury to the renal tubule; concomitant therapy should be used with caution and includes monitoring of renal function and dosage adjustment based on body weight, creatinine clearance estimation and/or serum aminoglycoside and vancomycin concentrations
Daptomycin	HMG-CoA reductase inhibitors[13]	May increase creatinine phosphokinase concentrations or cause rhabdomyolysis; monitor for signs and symptoms and consider temporarily discontinuation of HMG-CoA reductase inhibitor during daptomycin therapy
Linezolid	Selective serotonin reuptake inhibitors (SSRIs)[14]	Increased serotonin concentrations and development of serotonin syndrome (hyperpyrexia, cognitive dysfunction); concomitant therapy should be avoided or used with caution and includes monitoring for serotonin syndrome
	Sympathomimetic agents[15]	Enhance pharmacological (e.g. enhanced vasopressor effect); concomitant therapy should be avoided or used with caution; counsel patients regarding choice of OTC products

(Continued)

Table 6.5 Drug–drug interactions of antibacterial agents—cont'd

Antibacterial agent	Interacting drug	Interaction and management strategy
Quinupristin–dalfopristin	Substrates of CYP3A4	See Table 6.2
Tigecycline	Warfarin	Potential decreased clearance of warfarin; monitor PT/INR and adjust warfarin dose appropriately
Tetracyclines	Multivalent cations,[8] colestipol, kaolin–pectin, activated charcoal, and sodium bicarbonate	Decreased absorption of tetracyclines; space administration by at least 2 h
	Atovaquone	Decreased atovaquone concentrations; parasitemia should be closely monitored; consider alternative agent if possible
	Digoxin	Increased digoxin serum concentrations and toxicity; monitor digoxin serum concentrations and adjust dose appropriately
	Ergotamine tartrate	Increased ergotism; monitor for ergotism and use alternative therapy when possible
	Isotretinoin, acitretin	Additive effects of pseudotumor cerebri (benign intracranial hypertension); avoid concurrent use
	Lithium	Increased lithium serum concentrations and toxicity; monitor lithium serum concentrations and adjust dose appropriately
	Methotrexate	Increased methotrexate serum concentrations and toxicity; monitor methotrexate serum concentrations and use leucovorin rescue as needed
	Quinine	Increased quinine serum concentrations; monitor for quinine toxicity
	Theophylline	Increased theophylline serum concentrations; monitor toxicity and theophylline serum concentrations, and adjust dose appropriately
	Warfarin	Enhanced anticoagulation; monitor PT/INR and adjust warfarin dose appropriately
Doxycycline	Barbiturates, chronic ethanol ingestion, carbamazepine, phenytoin, fosphenytoin, rifampicin, rifabutin	Decreased doxycycline serum concentrations; use other tetracycline product or alternative agent if possible
Metronidazole	Ethanol, OTC and prescription products containing ethanol or propylene glycol[16]	Produces a disulfiram-like reaction (e.g. flushing, palpitation, tachycardia, nausea, vomiting); avoid concomitant therapy within 2 or 3 days of taking metronidazole; counsel patients about these potential side effects
	5-Fluorouracil	Increased toxicity; avoid concomitant use
	Lithium, busulfan, ciclosporin, tacrolimus, phenytoin, carbamazepine	Increased serum concentrations of interacting drugs; monitor toxicity and serum drug concentrations; adjust dose appropriately
	Phenobarbital, phenytoin, rifampicin, prednisone	Decreased metronidazole serum concentrations; monitor efficacy; doses of metronidazole may need to be increased
	Warfarin	Enhanced anticoagulation; monitor PT/INR and adjust warfarin dose appropriately
Chloramphenicol	Paracetamol	Equivocal changes to chloramphenicol serum concentrations; monitor chloramphenicol serum concentrations and adjust dose appropriately; use other analgesic or antipyretic agents
	Cyclophosphamide	Decreased effectiveness of cyclophosphamide; avoid concomitant use
	Cimetidine	Bone marrow suppression and increased risk for aplastic anemia; avoid concomitant use and consider use of other antiulcer medications
	Folic acid, iron, cyanocobalamin	Delayed response of anemias; avoid concomitant use
	Ciclosporin, tacrolimus, phenobarbital, phenytoin	Increased serum drug concentrations of the interacting drug; monitor toxicity and serum drug concentrations; adjust dose appropriately
	Phenobarbital, phenytoin, rifampicin	Decreased chloramphenicol serum concentrations; monitor efficacy and chloramphenicol serum concentrations; adjust dose appropriately
	Sulfonylurea hypoglycemic[17]	Enhanced hypoglycemia; monitor efficacy and blood glucose concentrations
	Warfarin	Enhanced anticoagulation; monitor PT/INR and adjust warfarin dose appropriately

(Continued)

Table 6.5 Drug–drug interactions of antibacterial agents—cont'd

Antibacterial agent	Interacting drug	Interaction and management strategy
Trimethoprim–sulfamethoxazole	Amantadine, dapsone, digoxin, dofetilide, lamivudine, methotrexate, phenytoin, fosphenytoin, procainamide, zidovudine	Increased serum drug concentrations of the interacting drug; monitor for toxicity, drug concentrations (e.g. digoxin, procainamide and its metabolite, NAPA) or appropriate laboratory test (dapsone: methemoglobin level; zidovudine: CBC) and adjust dose appropriately; avoid concomitant use (e.g. dofetilide, methotrexate) if possible
	Azathioprine	Increased leucopenia; monitor CBC
	Ciclosporin	Decreased ciclosporin serum concentrations and azotemia; monitor ciclosporin serum concentrations and renal function; adjust dose appropriately
	Enalapril (ACE inhibitors), potassium, potassium-sparing diuretics	Hyperkalemia; monitor serum potassium level
	Methenamine	Crystallization of sulfonamides in urine; avoid concomitant use
	Metronidazole	Disulfiram reaction (ethanol in intravenous TMP–SMX product); use alternative therapy when possible
	Procaine, tetracaine	Decreased effect of sulfonamides; use alternative therapy when possible
	Pyrimethamine	Megaloblastic anemia and pancytopenia; monitor CBC and consider adding leucovorin rescue; avoid concomitant use
	Repaglinide, rosiglitazone, sulfonylurea hypoglycemic[17]	Increased serum concentrations of interacting drug and increased hypoglycemic effect; monitor serum glucose concentrations and adverse effects
	Rifabutin	Increased sulfamethoxazole hydroxylamine concentrations; monitor for SMX toxicity
	Rifampicin	Increased rifampicin concentrations and decreased TMP–SMX concentrations; monitor TMP–SMX efficacy
	Thiazide diuretics	Hyponatremia; monitor serum sodium level
	Warfarin	Enhanced anticoagulation; monitor PT/INR and adjust warfarin dose appropriately

[1]Oral cephalosporin prodrugs such as cefpodoxime proxetil, cefuroxime axetil and cefditoren pivoxil.
[2]Inhibition of tubular secretion of most renally eliminated β-lactam agents.
[3]Imipenem, meropenem, ertapenem and doripenem.
[4]Examples include quinidine, ibutilide, sotalol, dofetilide, amiodarone and bretylium.
[5]Examples include nifedipine, felodipine, diltiazem and verapamil.
[6]Examples include amitriptyline, haloperidol, risperidone and quetiapine.
[7]Norfloxacin, ciprofloxacin, levofloxacin and moxifloxacin.
[8]Examples include antacids (containing aluminum or magnesium or calcium), iron, zinc, bismuth subsalicylate, multivitamin products, laxatives, sucralfate, didanosine, sevelamer and quinapril.
[9]Gentamicin, tobramycin, amikacin.
[10]Examples include amphotericin B, cisplatin, ciclosporin, vancomycin, foscarnet, intravenous pentamidine, cidofovir, polymyxin B, colistin, radio contrast and aminoglycosides.
[11]Examples include ethacrynic acid, furosemide, urea, mannitol and cisplatin.[11]
[12]Examples include succinylcholine, d-tubocurarine, vecuronium, pancuronium and atracurium
[13]Hydroxymethylglutaryl-coenzyme A (HMG-CoA) reductase inhibitors (or the 'statins'), such as simvastatin, lovastatin, pravastatin and fluvastatin.
[14]Examples include sertraline, paroxetine, citalopram and fluoxetine.
[15]Examples include dopamine, epinephrine, and OTC cough and cold preparations that contain pseudoephedrine or phenylpropanolamine.
[16]Examples include oral (cough and cold OTC preparations, ritonavir solution) and intravenous products (diazepam, nitroglycerin, phenytoin, TMP–SMX). Amprenavir oral solution has a high content of propylene glycol.
[17]Examples include tolbutamide, chlorpropamide, glipizide and glibenclamide (glyburide).
ACE, angiotensin converting enzyme; CBC, complete blood count; CNS, central nervous system; CYP, cytochrome P_{450}; OTC, over-the-counter; PT/INR, prothrombin time/international normalized ratio; TMP–SMX, trimethoprim–sulfamethoxazole.

hydrolysis process between the glucuronide metabolite and valproic acid.[31,34] Chloramphenicol has recently been shown to be a potent inhibitor of CYP2C19 and CYP3A4 and a weak inhibitor of CYP2D6 in human liver microsomes. In contrast, newer agents such daptomycin, linezolid and tigecycline do not have significant activity to inhibit common human CYP isoforms (1A2, 2C9, 2C19, 2D6 and 3A4).[15,25,33]

Probenecid inhibits OAT1 and renal tubular secretion of most β-lactams eliminated by the kidney.[18,19] The product package insert states that doripenem and probenecid should not be co-administered.[34] Other agents with the potential to inhibit tubular secretion of β-lactams include methotrexate, aspirin and indometacin. Trimethoprim is a potent inhibitor of renal tubular secretion and can increase plasma concentrations of amantadine, dapsone, digoxin, dofetilide, lamivudine, methotrexate, procainamide and zidovudine. Trimethoprim can also inhibit sodium channels of the renal distal tubules and can potentially cause hyperkalemia with angiotensin converting enzyme (ACE) inhibitors, potassium supplements and potassium-sparing diuretics. In addition, hyponatremia has been associated with thiazide diuretics and trimethoprim therapy.

Several classes of antibacterial agent are associated with pharmacodynamic drug–drug interactions involving over-lapping and/or additive toxicity.[15,33] Numerous reports have documented the increased risk of developing nephrotoxicity with the concurrent administration of aminoglycosides with amphotericin B, cisplatin, ciclosporin (cyclosporine), vancomycin or indometacin (in neonates with patent ductus arteriosus). In addition, aminoglycosides should be avoided or used with caution with the above agents as well as other known nephrotoxic agents such as foscarnet, intravenous pentamidine, cidofovir, polymyxin B and colistin. An increased risk of ototoxicity has been reported with the co-administration of aminoglycosides and loop diuretics. Ethacrynic acid has been reported to cause hearing loss when administered alone and in conjunction with aminoglycosides such as kanamycin and streptomycin. Furosemide has also been identified as an additive risk factor for increased rates of nephrotoxicity and ototoxicity with aminoglycosides. Ethacrynic acid, furosemide, urea and mannitol should be used cautiously at the lowest possible doses in patients receiving concurrent aminoglycoside therapy. Aminoglycosides and clindamycin may enhance the effects of neuromuscular blocking agents (e.g. d-tubocurarine, pancuronium, vecuronium) and result in a prolonged duration of neuromuscular blockade.

Additive inhibition of dihydrofolate reductase to azathioprine, methotrexate or pyrimethamine contributes, in part, to the increased risk of myelotoxicity, pancytopenia and/or megaloblastic anemia when these agents are combined with trimethoprim and/or sulfamethoxazole.[15,33,35] The combining of cimetidine with chloramphenicol has been associated with additive bone marrow suppression and increased risk for aplastic anemia. Tetracycline may potentiate the toxicities of lithium, methotrexate, methoxyflurane and ergotamine tartrate. The combination of tetracyclines or tigecycline with retinoids (e.g. acitretin, isotretinoin) is not recommended due to the potential additive effects of pseudotumor cerebri (benign intracranial hypertension).

Metronidazole produces a disulfiram-like reaction (e.g. flushing, palpitations, tachycardia, nausea, vomiting) in some patients who drink ethanol while taking the drug.[15] Careful selection of over-the-counter and prescription medication is necessary since several oral (e.g. cough and cold preparations, ritonavir solution) and intravenous (e.g. diazepam, nitroglycerin, phenytoin, trimethoprim–sulfamethoxazole) products contain ethanol. Metronidazole and medications with a high content of propylene glycol should also be avoided or used with caution since metronidazole inhibits the alcohol and aldehyde dehydrogenase pathway that metabolizes propylene glycol.

Several case reports have been published regarding the temporal drug–drug interaction relationship between linezolid and selective serotonin reuptake inhibitors (SSRIs) such as sertraline, paroxetine, citalopram and fluoxetine.[15,33] The reversible monoamine oxidase inhibitor (MAOI) activity of linezolid also has the potential for drug–drug interactions involving over-the-counter cough and cold preparations containing adrenergic agents such as pseudoephedrine and phenylpropanolamine.

ANTIFUNGAL AGENTS (Table 6.6)

Amphotericin B and flucytosine are eliminated by renal excretion and are associated with significant adverse effects. Drug–drug interactions of amphotericin B and flucytosine involve overlapping or additive pharmacodynamic adverse effects (e.g. increased risks for myelosuppression or nephrotoxicity).[36] Amphotericin B-associated nephrotoxicity can cause fluid and electrolyte imbalances (e.g. hypokalemia) and these changes result in additive effects with diuretics, aminoglycosides or corticosteroids, or enhanced pharmacological effects with digoxin. However, combination therapy of amphotericin B and flucytosine may have synergistic antifungal effects and can be beneficial in the treatment of cryptococcal meningitis.

Azole antifungal agents are associated with numerous pharmacokinetic drug–drug interactions involving both induction and inhibition of CYP isoenzymes.[36–39]

- Ketoconazole is a substrate and strong inhibitor of CYP3A4.
- Fluconazole is an inhibitor of CYP3A4, CYP2C9 and CYP2C19. It is also a substrate of P-gp and inhibitor of UGT. Fluconazole is a much less potent inhibitor of CYP3A4 than itraconazole and ketoconazole; however, it is a stronger inhibitor of CYP2C9 than voriconazole. Unlike other azole agents, fluconazole is mainly renally eliminated (e.g. 80%) and only 11% is metabolized to two inactive metabolites.
- Itraconazole is a substrate and potent inhibitor of CYP3A4 (hepatic and intestinal) and P-gp.
- Voriconazole is a substrate and an inhibitor of CYP2C19, CYP3A4 and CYP2C9.
- Posaconazole is metabolized by phase II biotransformation using UGT and is an inhibitor of CYP3A4.
- Miconazole is a potent inhibitor of CYP2C9 and has been associated with drug–drug interactions (e.g. warfarin), even though miconazole is most commonly administered as a topical or oral gel.

Examples of clinically significant pharmacokinetic azole–drug interactions include induction (e.g. reduced plasma concentration of the azole by rifamycins), inhibition of CYP2C9 (e.g. warfarin and voriconazole), inhibition of CYP and breast cancer resistance protein (e.g. lovastatin and itraconazole), inhibition of CYP and P-gp (e.g. quinidine and itraconazole), inhibition of P-gp (e.g. digoxin and itraconazole), inhibition of UGT (e.g. zidovudine and fluconazole), and two-way interactions (e.g. induction of CYP or UGT by phenytoin and inhibition of CYP3A4 by azole). In addition, ketoconazole and itraconazole may have altered gastric absorption because

Table 6.6 Drug–drug interactions of antifungal agents

Antifungal agent	Interacting drug	Interaction and management strategy
Amphotericin B	Flucytosine	May increase myelosuppression; monitor CBC, renal function and flucytosine serum concentrations; initiate flucytosine at a low dosage (e.g. 75–100 mg/kg) and adjust dose as needed
	Nephrotoxic agents[1]	Direct or additive injury to the renal tubule; concomitant therapy should be avoided or used with caution and includes monitoring of renal function and dosage adjustment based on toxicity, body weight and creatinine clearance estimation
	Zidovudine, ganciclovir	May increase bone marrow toxicity; monitor CBC weekly
Flucytosine	Amphotericin B	May increase myelosuppression; monitor CBC, renal function and flucytosine serum concentrations; initiate flucytosine at a low dosage (e.g. 75–100 mg/kg) and adjust dose as needed
	Cytarabine	Antagonizes the antifungal activity of flucytosine; avoid concomitant use
	Zidovudine, ganciclovir	May increase bone marrow toxicity; monitor CBC weekly
Fluconazole	Substrates of CYP3A4	See Table 6.2; fluconazole is contraindicated for concomitant use with ergot alkaloids and drugs (e.g. astemizole, terfenadine, cisapride, quinidine, pimozide, mesoridazine, bepridil, thioridazine, levomethadyl, ziprasidone) that are CYP3A4 substrates and prolong the QTc interval
	Ciclosporin, tacrolimus, sirolimus, everolimus	Increased ciclosporin, tacrolimus, sirolimus or everolimus serum concentrations; monitor toxicity and serum drug concentrations, adjust dose as needed
	Phenytoin, fosphenytoin	Increased phenytoin serum concentrations and phenytoin toxicity; monitor toxicity and phenytoin serum concentrations and adjust dose as needed
	Rifampicin, rifapentine	Decreased fluconazole serum concentrations; monitor efficacy and increase dose as needed
	Sulfonylurea hypoglycemic[2]	Enhanced hypoglycemia; monitor efficacy and blood glucose concentrations
	Theophylline	Increased theophylline serum concentrations and risk of toxicity; monitor serum theophylline concentrations and toxicity; decrease dose of theophylline as needed
	Warfarin	Enhanced anticoagulation; monitor prothrombin time/international normalized ratio (PT/INR) and adjust warfarin dose appropriately
	Zidovudine	Increased zidovudine serum concentrations; monitor for toxicity and adjust dose as needed
Itraconazole	Substrates of CYP3A4	See Table 6.2; itraconazole is contraindicated for concomitant use with ergot alkaloids, HMG-CoA reductase inhibitors metabolize by CYP3A4 (lovastatin, simvastatin), oral midazolam, triazolam, alprazolam, astemizole, terfenadine, cisapride, quinidine, pimozide, dofetilide, levomethadyl, silodosin, eplerenone, nisoldipine, ranolazine, alfuzosin or conivaptan
	Antacids, H₂ antagonist (e.g. famotidine), proton pump inhibitor (e.g. omeprazole), didanosine (buffered formulation)	Decreased itraconazole absorption and serum concentrations; loss of antimycotic efficacy; alternative antifungal agent or interacting drug should be considerate; space antacid administration by at least 2 h; administer itraconazole with a cola beverage if receiving H₂ antagonist; use new didanosine formulation with buffer
	Buspirone, haloperidol, risperidone, diazepam	Increased serum concentrations of interacting agents; monitor toxicity and adjust dose as needed
	Busulfan, docetaxel	Increased serum concentrations of interacting drugs and toxicity; monitor toxicity and complete blood count; adjust dose appropriately
	Calcium channel blockers[3]	Increased serum concentrations of calcium channel blocking agents; monitor toxicity and adjust dose as needed
	Ciclosporin, tacrolimus, sirolimus, everolimus	Increased ciclosporin, tacrolimus, sirolimus or everolimus serum concentrations; monitor toxicity and serum drug concentrations; adjust dose as needed
	Digoxin	Increased digoxin serum concentrations and toxicity; monitor digoxin serum concentrations and adjust dose appropriately
	Loperamide	Increased loperamide serum concentrations; monitor for increased loperamide toxicity (e.g. nausea, vomiting, dry mouth, dizziness or drowsiness)
	Protease inhibitors (indinavir, ritonavir, saquinavir)	Increased serum concentrations of protease inhibitors and/or itraconazole; monitor toxicity and adjust dose as needed
	Rifampicin, rifabutin, isoniazid, carbamazepine, phenobarbital, efavirenz, nevirapine, St John's wort	Decreased itraconazole serum concentrations and loss of antimycotic efficacy; alternative antifungal agent or interacting drug should be considerate
	Warfarin	Enhanced anticoagulation; monitor PT/INR and adjust warfarin dose appropriately

(Continued)

Table 6.6 Drug–drug interactions of antifungal agents—cont'd

Antifungal agent	Interacting drug	Interaction and management strategy
Posaconazole	Substrates of CYP3A4	See Table 6.2; posaconazole is contraindicated for concomitant use with ergot alkaloids, sirolimus and drugs (e.g. astemizole, terfenadine, cisapride, quinidine, pimozide, halofantrine) that are CYP3A4 substrates and prolong the QTc interval
	Cimetidine	Decreased posaconazole serum concentrations; avoid concomitant use and consider use of other antiulcer medications
	Ciclosporin, tacrolimus	Increased ciclosporin or tacrolimus serum concentrations; reduce dose of ciclosporin (by 25%) or tacrolimus (by 66%), monitor toxicity and ciclosporin or tacrolimus serum concentrations, and adjust dose as needed
	Phenytoin, fosphenytoin	Decreased posaconazole serum concentrations and increased phenytoin serum concentrations; avoid concomitant use; if concomitant use required, monitor efficacy, toxicity and phenytoin serum concentrations, and adjust dose as needed
Voriconazole	Substrates of CYP3A4	See Table 6.2; voriconazole is contraindicated for concomitant use with ergot alkaloids, ritonavir (400 mg every 12 h), sirolimus and drugs (e.g. astemizole, terfenadine, cisapride, quinidine, pimozide, ranolazine) that are CYP3A4 substrates and prolong the QTc interval
	Ciclosporin, tacrolimus	Increased ciclosporin or tacrolimus serum concentrations; reduce dose of ciclosporin or tacrolimus by 33–50%, monitor toxicity and ciclosporin or tacrolimus serum concentrations, and adjust dose as needed
	Methadone	Increased *R*-methadone concentrations and risk of toxicity (e.g. QTc prolongation, respiratory depression); monitor for toxicity and adjust dose as needed
	Omeprazole	Increased omeprazole serum concentrations; reduce omeprazole dose in half
	Phenytoin, fosphenytoin	Decreased voriconazole serum concentrations and increased phenytoin serum concentrations; increase voriconazole dose to 400 mg every 12 h (oral) or 5 mg/kg every 12 h (intravenous), monitor efficacy, toxicity and phenytoin serum concentrations and adjust dose as needed
	Rifampicin, rifabutin, carbamazepine, phenobarbital, mephobarbital, efavirenz, St John's wort	Decreased voriconazole serum concentrations; voriconazole is contraindicated for concomitant use with these interacting drugs
	Warfarin	Enhanced anticoagulation; monitor PT/INR and adjust warfarin dose appropriately
Anidulafungin	Ciclosporin	Slight increase in anidulafungin serum concentrations; no dose adjustment required
Caspofungin	Ciclosporin	Increased caspofungin serum concentrations and transient elevations in liver enzymes (e.g. ALT and AST); monitor for toxicity and liver enzymes
	Rifampicin (and potentially other potent inducers)	Decreased serum concentrations of caspofungin; monitor clinical response and increase caspofungin maintenance dose to 70 mg per day if needed
	Tacrolimus	Increased tacrolimus blood concentrations; monitor tacrolimus blood concentrations and adjust as needed
Micafungin	Ciclosporin	Decreased oral clearance and increased half-life of ciclosporin; monitor ciclosporin serum concentrations and adjust dose as needed
	Nifedipine	Increased nifedipine serum concentrations; monitor for nifedipine toxicity and reduce dose if needed

[1]Examples include amphotericin B, cisplatin, ciclosporin, vancomycin, foscarnet, intravenous pentamidine, cidofovir, polymyxin B, colistin, radio contrast and aminoglycosides.
[2]Examples include tolbutamide, chlorpropamide, glipizide and glibenclamide (glyburide).
[3]Examples include nifedipine, felodipine, diltiazem and verapamil.
ALT, alanine aminotransferase; AST, aspartate aminotransferase; CYP, cytochrome P_{450}; HMG-CoA, hydroxymethylglutaryl-coenzyme A; PT/INR, prothrombin time/international normalized ratio.

of alteration in gastric pH or binding drug–drug interactions. Fluconazole, ketoconazole and voriconazole can also be associated with pharmacodynamic drug–drug interactions involving QTc prolongation.

Echinocandin antifungal agents are not commonly associated with drug–drug interactions.[36] Anidulafungin and micafungin are not clinically important substrates, inducers or inhibitors of CYP isoenzymes or P-gp. Caspofungin is a poor substrate for CYP isoenzymes and is not a substrate for P-gp. Co-administration of rifampicin decreases serum concentrations of caspofungin. Caution is recommended when other potent drug inducers (e.g. carbamazepine, phenytoin, efavirenz, nevirapine, dexamethasone) are administered with caspofungin.

ANTIRETROVIRAL AGENTS

Some of the most challenging drug–drug interactions are associated with antiretroviral agents, particularly with non-nucleoside reverse transcriptase inhibitors, protease inhibitors and chemokine receptor antagonists.[35,40,41] The increased knowledge about how these agents are metabolized and eliminated from the body has been helpful in predicting and managing many of the clinically significant drug–drug interactions. The reader should refer to the most recent report by the Panel on Antiretroviral Guidelines for Adults and Adolescents: A Working Group of the Office of AIDS Research Advisory Council (http://www.aidsinfo.nih.gov) for up-to-date guidelines on prescribing and monitoring antiretroviral agents, including important drug–drug interactions. In addition, there are several websites (e.g. http://hivinsite.ucsf.edu; http://www.hiv-druginteractions.org) that are readily available and contain updated information about drug–drug, drug–food and drug–herbal interactions with antiretroviral agents.

NUCLEOSIDE AND NUCLEOTIDE REVERSE TRANSCRIPTASE INHIBITORS (NRTIs) (Table 6.7)

Nucleoside and nucleotide reverse transcriptase inhibitors do not undergo metabolism or inhibition by common human CYP isoforms.[35,40] The majority of drug–drug interactions associated with NRTIs involve drug absorption (e.g. didanosine), antagonism of intracellular phosphorylation (e.g. stavudine and zidovudine) or increased/additive toxicity. Mechanisms of many of these drug–drug interactions of NRTIs remain unclear.

NON-NUCLEOSIDE REVERSE TRANSCRIPTASE INHIBITORS (NNRTIs) (Table 6.8)

The possibility of drug–drug interactions should be carefully considered and monitored in all patients prescribed NNRTIs.[35,40] All NNRTIs are metabolized in the liver by

Table 6.7 Drug–drug interactions of nucleoside and nucleotide reverse transcriptase inhibitors (NRTIs)

Antiviral agent	Interacting drug	Interaction and management strategy
Abacavir	Methadone	Decreased methadone serum concentrations; monitor for methadone withdrawal and titrate methadone dose as needed
	Tipranavir–ritonavir	Decreased abacavir serum concentrations; monitor for abacavir efficacy; appropriate dose for this combination is not established
Didanosine	Ganciclovir, valganciclovir (oral)	Increased didanosine serum concentrations and decreased ganciclovir serum concentrations after oral administration; monitor ganciclovir efficacy and didanosine toxicity
	Ribavirin	Increased didanosine intracellular concentrations; contraindicated for co-administration
	Hydroxyurea	Peripheral neuropathy, lactic acidosis and pancreatitis have been seen with this combination (with or without stavudine); avoid co-administration if possible
	Stavudine	Peripheral neuropathy, lactic acidosis and pancreatitis have been seen with this combination (with or without hydroxyurea); avoid co-administration if possible
	Allopurinol	Increased didanosine serum concentrations and increased risk for toxicity (pancreatitis, neuropathy); contraindicated for co-administration
	Atazanavir	Decreased didanosine serum concentrations with simultaneous co-administration; space administration by 2 h before or 1 h after didanosine
	Tipranavir–ritonavir	Decreased didanosine and tipranavir serum concentrations; space administration by at least 2 h
	Indinavir	Decreased indinavir serum concentrations after pediatric solution; space administration by at least 1 h
	Delavirdine	Decreased delavirdine serum concentrations after didanosine pediatric solution; space administration by at least 1 h
	Tenofovir	Increased didanosine serum concentrations; decrease didanosine dose (e.g. delayed-release capsules: if CL_{CR}>60 mL/min: 250 mg per day if patient weighs >60 kg; 200 mg if patient weighs <60 kg)
	Methadone	Decreased didanosine serum concentrations with didanosine pediatric solution; monitor didanosine efficacy
	Fluoroquinolones	Decreased fluoroquinolone serum concentrations with simultaneous co-administration of didanosine pediatric solution but not delayed-release capsules; space administration by at least 2–6 h
	Tetracyclines	Decreased tetracycline serum concentrations with simultaneous co-administration of didanosine pediatric solution; space administration by at least 1–2 h
	Itraconazole	Decreased itraconazole serum concentrations with concurrent administration of didanosine pediatric solution; space administration by at least 2 h

(Continued)

Table 6.7   Drug–drug interactions of nucleoside and nucleotide reverse transcriptase inhibitors (NRTIs)—cont'd

Antiviral agent	Interacting drug	Interaction and management strategy
Emtricitabine	No major interactions	–
Lamivudine	Trimethoprim–sulfamethoxazole	Increased lamivudine serum concentrations; monitor lamivudine toxicities
Stavudine	Zidovudine	Antagonism may occur; competitive inhibition of intracellular phosphorylation of stavudine by zidovudine; avoid concomitant administration
	Methadone	Decreased stavudine serum concentrations; monitor stavudine efficacy
	Didanosine	Peripheral neuropathy, lactic acidosis and pancreatitis have been seen with this combination (with or without hydroxyurea); avoid co-administration if possible
Tenofovir	Didanosine	Increased didanosine serum concentrations; decrease didanosine dose (e.g. delayed-release capsules: if CL_{CR} >60 mL/min: 250 mg per day if patient weighs >60 kg; 200 mg if patient weighs <60 kg)
	Atazanavir–ritonavir	Decreased atazanavir serum concentrations and increased tenofovir serum concentrations; recommended dosage regimen: atazanavir 300 mg, ritonavir 100 mg, tenofovir 300 mg given once daily with food; monitor for tenofovir toxicities; avoid concomitant administration without ritonavir
	Darunavir–ritonavir	Increased tenofovir serum concentrations; monitor tenofovir toxicities
	Lopinavir–ritonavir	Increased tenofovir serum concentrations; monitor tenofovir toxicities
	Tipranavir–ritonavir	Decreased tenofovir serum concentrations; monitor tenofovir efficacy
Zidovudine	Stavudine	Antagonism may occur; competitive inhibition of intracellular phosphorylation of stavudine by zidovudine; avoid concomitant administration
	Ganciclovir, valganciclovir	Increased risk of hematological toxicity (e.g. anemia, neutropenia, pancytopenia) and GI toxicity; concomitant therapy should be avoided or used with caution with careful monitoring of hematological function and at the lowest possible dose; consider alternative antiretroviral agent
	Aciclovir	Increased risk of neurotoxicity (e.g. drowsiness, lethargy); monitor for adverse events
	Ribavirin	Ribavirin inhibits intracellular phosphorylation of zidovudine; avoid concomitant administration; if administered together, monitor virological efficacy and hematological toxicities
	Methadone	Increased zidovudine serum concentrations; monitor zidovudine toxicities
	Atazanavir	Decreased zidovudine serum concentrations; monitor zidovudine efficacy
	Tipranavir–ritonavir	Decreased zidovudine and tipranavir serum concentrations; monitor virological efficacy
	Atovaquone	Increased zidovudine serum concentrations; monitor zidovudine toxicities
	Probenecid	Increased zidovudine serum concentrations; monitor zidovudine toxicities
	Cidofovir	Manufacturer recommends that on days of cidofovir plus probenecid (*see* Table 6-10) co-administration, zidovudine should be temporarily discontinued or given at a 50% reduced dose
	Fluconazole	Increased zidovudine serum concentrations; monitor zidovudine toxicities
	Valproic acid	Decreased zidovudine serum concentrations; monitor virological efficacy

CL_{CR}, creatinine clearance; GI, gastrointestinal.

the cytochrome P_{450} system. Delavirdine is a substrate and a potent inhibitor of CYP3A4. Delavirdine is also a weak inhibitor of CYP2C9, CYP2D6 and CYP2C19 in vitro. The concurrent administration of drugs outlined in Table 6.2 should be avoided or used with extreme caution in patients receiving delavirdine. In addition, strong inducers and inhibitors of CYP3A4 will significantly decrease and increase plasma concentrations of delavirdine, respectively.

Nevirapine is metabolized by CYP3A4 and CYP2B6. Nevirapine is a moderate inducer of CYP3A4 and will lower the plasma concentrations of CYP3A4 substrates.

The metabolism of efavirenz is mainly by CYP2B6 but also to a lesser extent by CYP3A4. Efavirenz is a moderate inducer of CYP3A4 but also an inhibitor of CYP3A4, CYP2C9 and CYP2C19. The impact that nevirapine and efavirenz may have on substrates of CYP3A4 by lowering plasma concentrations must be carefully considered. In addition, potent inducers of CYP3A4 (e.g. rifampicin, anticonvulsants, St John's wort) can lower the plasma concentrations of nevirapine and efavirenz, and appropriate dosing guidelines or alternative agents (e.g. rifabutin) need to be considered.

Etravirine is the newest NNRTI and is metabolized by CYP3A4, CYP2C9, CYP2C19 as well as glucuronidation (minor).[41] Etravirine is a moderate inducer of CYP3A4 and acyl glucuronides, and an inhibitor of CYP2C9 and CYP2C19. It is recommended that other inducers such as nevirapine, efavirenz and rifampicin not be given in combination with etravirine. In addition, clarithromycin, unboosted protease inhibitors, tipranavir–ritonavir, fosamprenavir–ritonavir and atazanavir–ritonavir should not be co-administered with etravirine. It is recommended that the dose of phosphodiesterase 5 inhibitors (e.g. sildenafil) be increased and titrated to the desired effect when administered with etravirine.

Table 6.8 Drug–drug interactions of non-nucleoside reverse transcriptase inhibitors (NNRTIs)

NNRTI	Interacting drug	Interaction and management strategy
Delavirdine	Substrates of CYP3A4	See Table 6.2; delavirdine is contraindicated for concomitant use with ergot alkaloids, drugs (e.g. astemizole, terfenadine, cisapride, pimozide, bepridil) that are CYP3A4 substrates and prolong the QTc interval, simvastatin, lovastatin, rifampicin, rifapentine, rifabutin, alprazolam, oral midazolam, triazolam, St John's wort, fosamprenavir, carbamazepine, phenobarbital and phenytoin
	Antacids–didanosine	Decreased delavirdine concentrations; space administration by at least 1 h
	Clarithromycin	Increased clarithromycin and delavirdine concentrations; reduce clarithromycin dose by 50% if CL_{CR} 30–60 mL/min and by 75% if CL_{CR} <30 mL/min
	Benzodiazepines: alprazolam, diazepam	Avoid concomitant use; consider alternative agent (e.g. lorazepam)
	Hormonal contraceptives	Consider using additional methods
	Atorvastatin	Use lowest possible dose; use alternative lipid-lowering agent
	Protease inhibitors	See Table 6.9
	Maraviroc	Increased maraviroc serum concentrations; use lower maraviroc dose (e.g. 150 mg every 12 h)
	Methadone	Monitor for methadone toxicity; adjust dose as needed
	Warfarin	Monitor PT/INR; adjust dose as needed
Efavirenz	Itraconazole, posaconazole	Decreased itraconazole, OH-itraconazole and posaconazole serum concentrations; adjust dose as needed
	Voriconazole	Contraindicated at standard dose; use voriconazole 400 mg every 12 h and efavirenz 300 mg per day
	Carbamazepine, phenobarbital, phenytoin	Decreased carbamazepine concentrations; monitor anticonvulsant serum concentrations; adjust dose as needed or use alternative anticonvulsant
	Clarithromycin	Decreased clarithromycin serum concentrations; monitor efficacy or use alternative agent
	Rifabutin	Decreased rifabutin serum concentrations; increase dose
	Rifampicin	Decreased rifampicin serum concentrations; increase dose
	Oral midazolam	Do not administer with oral midazolam
	St John's wort	Avoid combination
	Hormonal contraceptives	Use alternative or additional methods
	Atorvastatin	Adjust atorvastatin dose according to lipid response
	Lovastatin, simvastatin	Adjust statin dose according to lipid response
	Pravastatin, rosuvastatin	Adjust statin dose according to lipid response
	Protease inhibitors	See Table 6.9
	Methadone	Decreased methadone serum concentrations; adjust dose as needed; monitor for withdrawal
	Warfarin	Monitor PT/INR; adjust dose as needed

(Continued)

Table 6.8 Drug–drug interactions of non-nucleoside reverse transcriptase inhibitors (NNRTIs)—cont'd

NNRTI	Interacting drug	Interaction and management strategy
Etravirine	Antiarrhythmic agents	Decreased antiarrhythmic serum concentrations; use with caution, monitor antiarrhythmic serum concentrations and adjust dose as needed
	Dexamethasone	Decreased etravirine serum concentrations; use with caution or consider alternative corticosteroid for long-term use
	Itraconazole	Decreased itraconazole and increased etravirine serum concentrations; adjust dose as needed
	Voriconazole	Decreased itraconazole and etravirine serum concentrations; adjust voriconazole dose as needed
	Carbamazepine, phenobarbital, phenytoin	Do not co-administer; consider alternative anticonvulsant
	Clarithromycin	Decreased clarithromycin and increased OH-clarithromycin serum concentrations; increased etravirine serum concentrations; consider alternative agent
	Rifabutin	Use alternative agent or adjust dose appropriately
	Rifampicin	Do not co-administer
	Diazepam	Increased diazepam serum concentrations; decrease dose
	St John's wort	Avoid combination
	Hormonal contraceptives	Increased ethinyl estradiol serum concentrations; no dosage adjustment needed
	Atorvastatin, fluvastatin	Increased atorvastatin serum concentrations; standard dose; adjust dose according to response
	Lovastatin, simvastatin	Decreased statin serum concentrations; adjust dose according to response
	Sildenafil	Decreased sildenafil serum concentrations; may need to increase sildenafil dose based on clinical effect
	Protease inhibitors	See Table 6.9
	Warfarin	Monitor PT/INR; adjust dose as needed
Nevirapine	Fluconazole	Increased nevirapine serum concentrations and hepatotoxicity; monitor hepatotoxicity
	Carbamazepine, phenytoin, phenobarbital	Decreased nevirapine serum concentrations; contraindicated; do not co-administer
	Clarithromycin	Increased nevirapine and decreased clarithromycin serum concentrations; monitor efficacy or use alternative agent
	Rifampicin	Decreased nevirapine concentrations; do not co-administer
	St John's wort	Avoid combination
	Protease inhibitors	See Table 6.9
	Methadone	Decreased methadone serum concentrations; monitor for opiate withdrawal and increased methadone dose as needed
	Warfarin	Monitor PT/INR; adjust dose as needed

CL_{CR}, creatinine clearance; CYP, cytochrome P_{450}; PT/INR, prothrombin time/international normalized ratio.

PROTEASE INHIBITORS (Table 6.9)

Protease inhibitors are major substrates of CYP3A4.[40,41] The only exception is nelfinavir which is a major substrate of CYP2C19 and only a minor substrate of CYP3A4. The active metabolite of nelfinavir (M8) is a major substrate of CYP3A4. Ritonavir is also a substrate of CYP2C9 and CYP2D6. Protease inhibitors can be affected by potent inhibitors or inducers of these substrates and, in selected cases, co-administration should be avoided (e.g. rifampicin or St John's wort).

Protease inhibitors can cause significant drug–drug interactions with other antiretroviral agents, antibacterial agents, ergot derivatives, sedatives/hypnotics, phosphodiesterase inhibitors and HMG Co-A reductase inhibitors because of inhibition of CYP3A4 and/or P-gp (Tables 6.1, 6.2 and 6.9).[40,41]

Table 6.9 Drug–drug interactions of protease inhibitors[1]

Protease inhibitor	Interacting drug	Interaction and management strategy
Atazanavir	Substrates of CYP3A4	See Table 6.2; atazanavir is contraindicated for concomitant use with ergot alkaloids, drugs (e.g. astemizole, terfenadine, cisapride, pimozide, bepridil) that are CYP3A4 substrates and prolong the QTc interval, simvastatin, lovastatin, rifampicin, rifapentine, oral midazolam, triazolam, St John's wort and fluticasone
	Antacids	Decreased atazanavir concentrations; space administration by 2 h before or 1 h after antacid
	Didanosine	Decreased didanosine serum concentrations with simultaneous co-administration; space administration by 2 h before or 1 h after didanosine
	H_2-receptor antagonist	Decreased atazanavir concentrations; three dosing recommendations: • H_2-receptor antagonist dose should not exceed a dose equivalent to famotidine 40 mg every 12 h in treatment-naive patients or 20 mg every 12 h in treatment-experienced patients • Atazanavir 300 mg plus ritonavir 100 mg should be administered simultaneously with and/or $\geq$10 h after the H_2-receptor antagonist • In treatment-experienced patients, if tenofovir is used with H_2-receptor antagonists, atazanavir 400 mg plus ritonavir 100 mg should be used
	Proton pump inhibitors	Decreased atazanavir concentrations; proton pump inhibitors are not recommended in patients receiving unboosted atazanavir or in treatment-experienced patients For atazanivir plus ritonavir, proton pump inhibitors should not exceed a dose equivalent to omeprazole 20 mg per day in treatment-naive patients; proton pump inhibitor should be administered $\geq$12 h prior to atazanavir plus ritonavir
	Itraconazole	Potential bi-directional inhibition between itraconazole and atazanavir plus ritonavir; high-dose itraconazole (>200 mg per day) is not recommended; monitor itraconazole serum concentrations if possible
	Voriconazole	Atazanavir plus ritonavir 100–200 mg: decreased voriconazole serum concentrations; concomitant administration is not recommended; atazanavir plus ritonavir 400 mg every 12 h or higher is contraindicated
	Carbamazepine, phenytoin, phenobarbital	Monitor anticonvulsant and atazanavir serum concentrations and virological response; consider alternative anticonvulsant and ritonavir-boosting regimen
	Clarithromycin	Increased clarithromycin serum concentrations may prolong QTc; reduce clarithromycin dose by 50%; consider alternative therapy
	Rifabutin	Increased rifabutin serum concentrations; rifabutin dose of 150 mg every other day or three times per week
	Benzodiazepines: alprazolam, diazepam	Avoid concomitant use; consider alternative agent (e.g. lorazepam, oxazepam or temazepam)
	Calcium channel blockers: dihydropyridine, diltiazem	Caution: dose titration with ECG monitoring. Increased diltiazem serum concentrations with atazanavir plus ritonavir; decrease diltiazem dose by 50%; ECG monitoring recommended
	Hormonal contraceptives	*Boosted regimen*: decreased ethinyl estradiol and increased progestin serum concentrations; oral contraceptive should contain at least 35 mcg of ethinyl estradiol; consider using alternative or additional methods *Unboosted regimen*: increased ethinyl estradiol serum concentrations; oral contraceptive should contain at least 30 mcg of ethinyl estradiol; consider using alternative or additional methods
	Atorvastatin, rosuvastatin	Use lowest possible dose with careful monitoring; use alternative lipid-lowering agent
	Indinavir	Co-administration is not recommended because of potential additive hyperbilirubinemia
	Efavirenz	Decreased atazanavir serum concentrations; in treatment-naive patients: atazanavir 400 mg plus ritonavir 100 mg plus standard dose of efavirenz. Do not co-administer in treatment-experienced patients
	Etravirine	Decreased atazanavir and increased etravirine serum concentrations; do not co-administer with boosted or unboosted atazanavir regimens
	Maraviroc	Increased maraviroc serum concentrations; use lower maraviroc dose (e.g. 150 mg every 12 h)
	Methadone	*Boosted regimen*: decreased methadone serum concentrations; monitor for methadone withdrawal; adjust dose as needed
	Warfarin	Monitor PT/INR; adjust dose as needed

(Continued)

Table 6.9 Drug–drug interactions of protease inhibitors—cont'd

Protease inhibitor	Interacting drug	Interaction and management strategy
Darunavir	Substrates of CYP3A4	See Table 6.2; darunavir is contraindicated for concomitant use with ergot alkaloids, drugs (e.g. astemizole, terfenadine, cisapride, pimozide) that are CYP3A4 substrates and prolong the QTc interval, simvastatin, lovastatin, rifampicin, rifapentine, oral midazolam, triazolam, St John's wort, fluticasone, carbamazepine, phenytoin and phenobarbital
	Itraconazole	Potential bi-directional inhibition between itraconazole and darunavir plus ritonavir; high-dose itraconazole (>200 mg per day) is not recommended; monitor itraconazole serum concentrations if possible
	Voriconazole	Darunavir plus ritonavir 100–200 mg: decreased voriconazole serum concentrations; concomitant administration is not recommended; darunavir plus ritonavir 400 mg every 12 h or higher is contraindicated
	Clarithromycin	Increased clarithromycin serum concentrations; reduce clarithromycin dose by 50% if CL_{CR} 30–60 mL/min; reduce clarithromycin dose by 75% if CL_{CR} <30 mL/min; consider alternative therapy
	Rifabutin	Increased rifabutin serum concentrations; rifabutin dose of 150 mg every other day or three times per week
	Benzodiazepines: alprazolam, diazepam	Avoid concomitant use; consider alternative agent (e.g. lorazepam, oxazepam or temazepam)
	Hormonal contraceptives	Consider using alternative or additional methods
	Atorvastatin, pravastatin, rosuvastatin	Use lowest possible dose with careful monitoring; use alternative lipid-lowering agent
	Paroxetine, sertraline	Decreased paroxetine and sertraline serum concentrations; monitor efficacy and titrate dose as needed
	Lopinavir–ritonavir, saquinavir	Decreased darunavir and increased lopinavir serum concentrations; co-administration is not recommended because dosing is not established
	Efavirenz	Decreased darunavir and increased efavirenz serum concentrations; use standard doses and monitor virological response
	Etravirine	Decreased etravirine serum concentrations; use standard doses and monitor virological response
	Nevirapine	Increased nevirapine serum concentrations; use standard doses and monitor virological response
	Maraviroc	Increased maraviroc serum concentrations; use lower maraviroc dose (e.g. 150 mg every 12 h)
	Methadone	*Boosted regimen*: decreased methadone serum concentrations; monitor for methadone withdrawal; adjust dose as needed
	Warfarin	Monitor PT/INR; adjust dose as needed
Fosamprenavir	Substrates of CYP3A4	See Table 6.2; fosamprenavir is contraindicated for concomitant use with ergot alkaloids, drugs (e.g. astemizole, terfenadine, cisapride, pimozide, bepridil) that are CYP3A4 substrates and prolong the QTc interval, simvastatin, lovastatin, rifampicin, rifapentine, oral midazolam, triazolam, St John's wort, fluticasone, delavirdine and oral contraceptives
	Antacids	Decreased amprenavir concentrations; space administration by 2 h before or 1 h after antacid
	Didanosine	Decreased didanosine serum concentrations with simultaneous co-administration; space administration by 2 h before or 1 h after didanosine
	H$_2$-receptor antagonist	Decreased amprenavir serum concentrations in unboosted regimen; separate administration if co-administration is necessary; consider boosting with ritonavir
	Itraconazole	Potential bi-directional inhibition between itraconazole and fosamprenavir plus ritonavir; high-dose itraconazole (>200 mg per day) is not recommended; monitor itraconazole serum concentrations if possible
	Voriconazole	Fosamprenavir plus ritonavir 100–200 mg: decreased voriconazole serum concentrations; co-administration is not recommended; fosamprenavir plus ritonavir 400 mg every 12 h or higher is contraindicated
	Carbamazepine, phenytoin, phenobarbital	*Unboosted regimen*: potential bi-directional inhibition; monitor for toxicities *Boosted regimen*: decreased phenytoin and increased amprenavir serum concentrations; monitor anticonvulsant serum concentrations and adjust dose as needed
	Rifabutin	*Unboosted regimen*: increased amprenavir serum concentrations; no dosage adjustment *Boosted regimen*: increased rifabutin serum concentrations; rifabutin dose of 150 mg every other day or three times per week *Unboosted regimen*: increased rifabutin serum concentrations; rifabutin dose of 150 mg every other day or 300 mg three times per week
	Benzodiazepines: alprazolam, diazepam	Avoid concomitant use; consider alternative agent (e.g. lorazepam, oxazepam or temazepam)

(Continued)

Table 6.9 Drug–drug interactions of protease inhibitors—cont'd

Protease inhibitor	Interacting drug	Interaction and management strategy
	Hormonal contraceptives	*Boosted regimen*: decreased ethinyl estradiol and norethindrone serum concentrations; use alternative or additional methods *Unboosted regimen*: increased ethinyl estradiol, norethindrone and amprenavir serum concentrations; use alternative or additional methods
	Atorvastatin, rosuvastatin	Use lowest possible dose with careful monitoring; use alternative lipid-lowering agent
	Delavirdine	Increased amprenavir and delavirdine serum concentrations; avoid concomitant administration
	Efavirenz	Decreased amprenavir serum concentrations; fosamprenavir dose of 1400 mg plus ritonavir 300 mg per day, or fosamprenavir 700 mg plus ritonavir 100 mg every 12 h plus standard dose of efavirenz
	Etravirine	Increased amprenavir serum concentrations; do not co-administer with boosted or unboosted atazanavir regimens
	Maraviroc	Use lower maraviroc dose (e.g. 150 mg every 12 h)
	Methadone	Decreased methadone serum concentrations; monitor for methadone withdrawal; adjust dose as needed
	Warfarin	Monitor PT/INR; adjust dose as needed
Indinavir	Substrates of CYP3A4	See Table 6.2; indinavir is contraindicated for concomitant use with ergot alkaloids, drugs (e.g. astemizole, terfenadine, cisapride, pimozide, amiodarone) that are CYP3A4 substrates and prolong the QTc interval, simvastatin, lovastatin, rifampicin, rifapentine, oral midazolam, triazolam, St John's wort and atazanavir
	Itraconazole	Potential bi-directional inhibition between itraconazole and indinavir plus ritonavir; high-dose itraconazole (>200 mg per day) is not recommended; monitor itraconazole serum concentrations if possible *Unboosted regimen*: indinavir 600 mg every 8 h; do not exceed 200 mg itraconazole every 12 h
	Voriconazole	Indinavir plus ritonavir 100–200 mg: decreased voriconazole serum concentrations; concomitant administration is not recommended; indinavir plus ritonavir 400 mg every 12 h or higher is contraindicated
	Carbamazepine, phenytoin, phenobarbital	Monitor anticonvulsant and indinavir serum concentrations and virological response; consider alternative anticonvulsant- and ritonavir-boosting regimen
	Clarithromycin	Increased clarithromycin serum concentrations; reduce clarithromycin dose by 50% if CL_{CR} 30–60 mL/min; reduce clarithromycin dose by 75% if CL_{CR} <30 mL/min; consider alternative therapy
	Rifabutin	*Boosted regimen*: increased rifabutin serum concentrations; rifabutin dose of 150 mg every other day or three times per week *Unboosted regimen*: increased rifabutin and decreased indinavir serum concentrations; rifabutin 150 mg per day or 300 mg three time weekly plus indinavir 1000 mg every 8 h or consider ritonavir boosting
	Benzodiazepines: alprazolam, diazepam	Avoid concomitant use; consider alternative agent (e.g. lorazepam, oxazepam or temazepam)
	Calcium channel blockers: dihydropyridine	Caution: dose titration with ECG monitoring. Increased amlodipine serum concentrations with indinavir plus ritonavir
	Hormonal contraceptives	*Ritonavir-boosted regimen*: consider using alternative or additional methods *Unboosted regimen*: increased ethinyl estradiol and indinavir serum concentrations; no dose adjustments needed
	Atorvastatin, rosuvastatin	Use lowest possible dose with careful monitoring; use alternative lipid-lowering agent
	Atazanavir	Co-administration is not recommended because of potential additive hyperbilirubinemia
	Delavirdine	Increased indinavir serum concentrations; indinavir dose of 600 mg every 8 h; standard dose for delavirdine
	Efavirenz	Decreased indinavir serum concentrations; indinavir dose of 1000 mg every 8 h; consider boosting regimen; standard efavirenz dose
	Nevirapine	Decreased indinavir serum concentrations; indinavir dose of 1000 mg every 8 h; consider boosting regimen; standard nevirapine dose
	Maraviroc	Possibly increased maraviroc serum concentrations; use lower maraviroc dose (e.g. 150 mg every 12 h)
	Methadone	For ritonavir-boosted regimen: decreased methadone serum concentrations; monitor for methadone withdrawal; adjust dose as needed
	Warfarin	Monitor PT/INR; adjust dose as needed

(Continued)

Table 6.9 Drug–drug interactions of protease inhibitors—cont'd

Protease inhibitor	Interacting drug	Interaction and management strategy
Lopinavir–ritonavir	Substrates of CYP3A4	See Table 6.2; Lopinavir–ritonavir is contraindicated for concomitant use with ergot alkaloids, drugs (e.g. astemizole, terfenadine, cisapride, pimozide, flecainide, propafenone) that are CYP3A4 substrates and prolong the QTc interval, simvastatin, lovastatin, rifampicin, rifapentine, oral midazolam, triazolam, St John's wort and fluticasone
	Itraconazole	Increased itraconazole serum concentrations; do not exceed 200 mg per day; monitor itraconazole serum concentrations if possible
	Voriconazole	Atazanavir plus ritonavir 100–200 mg: decreased voriconazole serum concentrations; concomitant administration is not recommended; atazanavir plus ritonavir 400 mg every 12 h or higher is contraindicated
	Carbamazepine, phenytoin, phenobarbital	Increased carbamazepine and decreased phenytoin, phenobarbital and lopinavir serum concentrations; monitor anticonvulsant and lopinavir serum concentrations and virological response; consider alternative anticonvulsant
	Clarithromycin	Increased clarithromycin serum concentrations; reduce clarithromycin dose by 50% if CL_{CR} 30–60 mL/min; reduce clarithromycin dose by 75% if CL_{CR} <30 mL/min; consider alternative therapy
	Rifabutin	Increased rifabutin serum concentrations; rifabutin dose of 150 mg every other day or three times per week
	Benzodiazepines: alprazolam, diazepam	Avoid concomitant use; consider alternative agent (e.g. lorazepam, oxazepam or temazepam)
	Calcium channel blockers: dihydropyridine	Increased amlodipine serum concentrations; caution is warranted and clinical monitoring is required
	Hormonal contraceptives	Decreased ethinyl estradiol; use alternative or additional methods
	Atorvastatin, rosuvastatin	Use lowest possible dose with careful monitoring; use alternative lipid-lowering agent
	Ritonavir	Additional ritonavir is not recommended
	Tipranavir	Decreased lopinavir serum concentrations; avoid co-administration
	Maraviroc	Increased maraviroc serum concentrations; use lower maraviroc dose (e.g. 150 mg every 12 h)
	Methadone	For ritonavir-boosted regimen: decreased methadone serum concentrations; monitor for methadone withdrawal; adjust dose as needed
	Warfarin	Monitor PT/INR; adjust dose as needed
Nelfinavir	Substrates of CYP3A4	See Table 6.2; nelfinavir is contraindicated for concomitant use with ergot alkaloids, drugs (e.g. astemizole, terfenadine, cisapride, pimozide) that are CYP3A4 substrates and prolong the QTc interval, simvastatin, lovastatin, rifampicin, rifapentine, oral midazolam, triazolam and St John's wort
	Proton pump inhibitors	Decreased nelfinavir and metabolite (M8) concentrations; avoid concomitant administration of proton pump inhibitors and nelfinavir
	Itraconazole	Potential bi-directional inhibition between itraconazole and nelfinavir plus ritonavir; high-dose itraconazole (>200 mg per day) is not recommended; monitor itraconazole serum concentrations if possible
	Voriconazole	Nelfinavir plus ritonavir 100–200 mg: decreased voriconazole serum concentrations; concomitant administration is not recommended; nelfinavir plus ritonavir 400 mg every 12 h or higher is contraindicated
	Carbamazepine, phenytoin, phenobarbital	Monitor anticonvulsant and nelfinavir serum concentrations and virological response; consider alternative anticonvulsant and ritonavir-boosting regimen
	Rifabutin	Increased rifabutin and decreased nelfinavir concentrations; rifabutin dose of 150 mg per day or 300 mg three times per week
	Benzodiazepines: alprazolam, diazepam	Avoid concomitant use; consider alternative agent (e.g. lorazepam, oxazepam or temazepam)
	Hormonal contraceptives	*Boosted regimen*: decreased ethinyl estradiol and progestin serum concentrations; use alternative or additional methods *Unboosted regimen*: decreased ethinyl estradiol and norethindrone serum concentrations; use alternative or additional methods
	Atorvastatin, rosuvastatin	Use lowest possible dose with careful monitoring; use alternative lipid-lowering agent

(Continued)

Table 6.9 Drug–drug interactions of protease inhibitors—cont'd

Protease inhibitor	Interacting drug	Interaction and management strategy
	Delavirdine	Decreased delavirdine and increased nelfinavir serum concentrations; monitor delavirdine virological efficacy and nelfinavir toxicities
	Efavirenz	Increased nelfinavir serum concentrations; use standard doses of each agent
	Nevirapine	Increased nelfinavir serum concentrations; use standard doses of each agent
	Maraviroc	Use lower maraviroc dose (e.g. 150 mg every 12 h)
	Methadone	Decreased methadone serum concentrations; monitor for methadone withdrawal; adjust dose as needed
	Warfarin	Monitor PT/INR; adjust dose as needed
Ritonavir[2]	Substrates of CYP3A4	See Table 6.2; ritonavir is contraindicated for concomitant use with ergot alkaloids, drugs (e.g. astemizole, terfenadine, cisapride, pimozide, bepridil, amiodarone, flecainide, propafenone, quinidine) that are CYP3A4 substrates and prolong the QTc interval, simvastatin, lovastatin, rifampicin, rifapentine, oral midazolam, triazolam, St John's wort, fluticasone, alfuzosin and voriconazole (with ritonavir $\geq$400 mg every 12 h)
	Desipramine	Increased desipramine serum concentrations; reduce desipramine dose and monitor toxicities
	Trazodone	Increased trazodone serum concentrations; use lowest dose of trazodone and monitor CNS and cardiovascular toxicities
	Theophylline	Decreased theophylline serum concentrations; monitor theophylline serum concentrations and adjust dose as needed
	Hormonal contraceptives	Use alternative or additional methods
	Delavirdine	Increased ritonavir serum concentrations; no data on dosing recommendations
	Efavirenz	Increased ritonavir and efavirenz serum concentrations; use standard doses
	Nevirapine	Decreased ritonavir serum concentrations; use standard doses
	Maraviroc	Increased maraviroc serum concentrations; use lower maraviroc dose (e.g. 150 mg every 12 h)
Saquinavir	Substrates of CYP3A4	See Table 6.2; saquinavir–ritonavir is contraindicated for concomitant use with ergot alkaloids, drugs (e.g. astemizole, terfenadine, cisapride, pimozide) that are CYP3A4 substrates and prolong the QTc interval, simvastatin, lovastatin, rifampicin, rifapentine, oral midazolam, triazolam, St John's wort and fluticasone
	Proton pump inhibitors	*Boosted regimen*: increased saquinavir serum concentrations; monitor for toxicities
	Itraconazole	Potential bi-directional inhibition between itraconazole and saquinavir plus ritonavir; use lower doses of itraconazole; monitor itraconazole serum concentrations if possible
	Voriconazole	Saquinavir plus ritonavir 100–200 mg: decreased voriconazole serum concentrations; concomitant administration is not recommended; atazanavir plus ritonavir 400 mg every 12 h or higher is contraindicated
	Carbamazepine, phenytoin, phenobarbital	Monitor anticonvulsant and saquinavir serum concentrations and virological response; consider alternative anticonvulsant and ritonavir-boosting regimen
	Clarithromycin	Increased clarithromycin serum concentrations; reduce clarithromycin dose by 50% if CL_{CR} 30–60 mL/min; reduce clarithromycin dose by 75% if CL_{CR} <30 mL/min; consider alternative therapy
	Rifabutin	Increased rifabutin serum concentrations; rifabutin dose of 150 mg every other day or three times per week
	Benzodiazepines: alprazolam, diazepam	Avoid concomitant use; consider alternative agent (e.g. lorazepam, oxazepam or temazepam)
	Calcium channel blockers: dihydropyridine, diltiazem	Caution: dose titration with ECG monitoring. Increased diltiazem serum concentrations with atazanavir plus ritonavir; decrease diltiazem dose by 50%; ECG monitoring recommended
	Hormonal contraceptives	*Boosted regimen*: decreased ethinyl estradiol serum concentrations; use alternative or additional methods
	Atorvastatin, rosuvastatin	Use lowest possible dose with careful monitoring; use alternative lipid-lowering agent
	Delavirdine	Increased saquinavir serum concentrations; recommended dose: saquinavir–ritonavir 1000 mg/100 mg every 12 h

(Continued)

Table 6.9 Drug–drug interactions of protease inhibitors—cont'd

Protease inhibitor	Interacting drug	Interaction and management strategy
	Efavirenz	Decreased saquinavir and efavirenz serum concentrations; recommended dose: saquinavir–ritonavir 1000 mg/100 mg every 12 h
	Etravirine	Decreased saquinavir and etravirine serum concentrations; recommended dose: saquinavir–ritonavir 1000 mg/100 mg every 12 h
	Maraviroc	Increased maraviroc serum concentrations; use lower maraviroc dose (e.g. 150 mg every 12 h)
	Methadone	For ritonavir-boosted regimen: decreased methadone serum concentrations; monitor for methadone withdrawal; adjust dose as needed
	Warfarin	Monitor PT/INR; adjust dose as needed
Tipranavir–ritonavir	Substrates of CYP3A4	See Table 6.2; tipranavir–ritonavir is contraindicated for concomitant use with ergot alkaloids, drugs (e.g. astemizole, terfenadine, cisapride, pimozide, bepridil, amiodarone, flecainide, propafenone, quinidine) that are CYP3A4 substrates and prolong the QTc interval, simvastatin, lovastatin, rifampicin, rifapentine, oral midazolam, triazolam, St John's wort and fluticasone
	Antacids	Decreased tipranavir concentrations; space administration by 2 h before or 1 h after antacid
	Proton pump inhibitors	Decreased omeprazole serum concentrations; may need to increase the dose of omeprazole
	Itraconazole	Potential bi-directional inhibition between itraconazole and tipranavir plus ritonavir; high-dose itraconazole (>200 mg per day) is not recommended; monitor itraconazole serum concentrations if possible
	Voriconazole	Tipranavir plus ritonavir 100–200 mg: decreased voriconazole serum concentrations; concomitant administration is not recommended; atazanavir plus ritonavir 400 mg every 12 h or higher is contraindicated
	Carbamazepine, phenytoin, phenobarbital	Monitor anticonvulsant and tipranavir serum concentrations and virological response; consider alternative anticonvulsant and ritonavir-boosting regimen
	Clarithromycin	Increased clarithromycin serum concentrations; reduce clarithromycin dose by 50% if CL_{CR} 30–60 mL/min; reduce clarithromycin dose by 75% if CL_{CR} <30 mL/min; consider alternative therapy
	Rifabutin	Increased rifabutin serum concentrations; rifabutin dose of 150 mg every other day or three times per week
	Benzodiazepines: alprazolam, diazepam	Avoid concomitant use; consider alternative agent (e.g. lorazepam, oxazepam or temazepam)
	Hormonal contraceptives	*Boosted regimen*: decreased ethinyl estradiol serum concentrations; use alternative or additional methods
	Atorvastatin, rosuvastatin	Use lowest possible dose with careful monitoring; use alternative lipid-lowering agent
	Efavirenz	Decreased or no change in tipranavir serum concentrations; use standard doses
	Etravirine	Decreased etravirine and increased tipranavir serum concentrations; avoid co-administration
	Maraviroc	Use standard doses of maraviroc (e.g. 300 mg every 12 h)
	Methadone	For ritonavir-boosted regimen: decreased methadone serum concentrations; monitor for methadone withdrawal; adjust dose as needed
	Warfarin	Monitor PT/INR; adjust dose as needed

[1] Adapted from: Panel on Antiretroviral Guidelines for Adults and Adolescents: A Working Group of the Office of AIDS Research Advisory Council (OARAC), Department of Health and Human Services. Guidelines for the use of antiretroviral agents in HIV-1-infected adults and adolescents. November 3, 2008. (Please refer the product package insert and literature for complete details and potential list of both studied and theoretical drug–drug interactions.)
[2] Ritonavir is used at low doses (e.g. 100–200 mg) to increase serum concentrations of most protease inhibitors so review other protease inhibitor recommendations; over 200 drugs used in HIV-infected patients have been investigated for potential drug–drug interactions; please review the product package insert and literature for complete details and potential list of both studied and theoretical drug–drug interactions.
CL_{CR}, creatinine clearance; CNS, central nervous system; CYP, cytochrome P_{450}; ECG, electrocardiograph; PT/INR, prothrombin time/international normalized ratio.

Several drugs are contraindicated while administering protease inhibitors because of the potential for serious or life-threatening adverse events. In addition, some protease inhibitors are also inducers (e.g. ritonavir, lopinavir, tipranavir, darunavir) of CYP3A4 and/or P-gp, resulting in decreased concentrations and effectiveness of drugs such as oral contraceptives and SSRIs (e.g. sertraline). Drug–drug interactions are less predictable and quite variable when a protease inhibitor or the combination of two protease inhibitors (e.g. tipranavir–ritonavir) has both inhibition and induction properties to a CYP isoform.

Ritonavir and nelfinavir can also induce glucuronyl transferase, CYP2C9 and CYP2C19. Lopinavir induces glucuronidation and can lower plasma concentrations of NRTIs such as zidovudine and abacavir (*see* Table 6.7). In contrast, atazanavir inhibits the phase II glucuronidation enzyme, UGT1A1. Because of the magnitude of inhibition or induction differs among the protease inhibitors, careful evaluation of potential drug–drug interaction with protease inhibitors is critical.

The current use of ritonavir is commonly at low doses (e.g. 100 or 200 mg) for its inhibitory effect on the CYP3A4 metabolism of other protease inhibitors. The co-administration of ritonavir is recommended with saquinavir, lopinavir, tipranavir and darunavir. This beneficial drug–drug interaction is used to increase and sustain the plasma drug concentrations of other protease inhibitors (booster effect). Benefits from booster ritonavir dosing with other protease inhibitors includes higher minimum (trough) serum concentrations, reduced development of drug resistance by increasing drug exposure, less frequent dosing, and enhance adherence by reducing the pill burden and simplifying the dosing regimen. Current drug–drug interaction reports with protease inhibitors must be carefully reviewed with regard to whether or not boosted ritonavir dosing was used and what dose of each protease inhibitor was administered.

OTHER ANTIRETROVIRAL AGENTS

The CCR5 co-receptor antagonist, maraviroc, is a substrate of CYP3A4 enzymes and the P-gp transport system.[3,41] Maraviroc is neither an inhibitor nor an inducer of CYP3A4 or P-gp. Plasma concentrations of maraviroc are significantly decreased by potent CYP3A inducers and increased by potent CYP3A inhibitors. Table 6.1 outlines the dosage guidelines of maraviroc when administered with and without inducers and inhibitors.

Raltegravir is an HIV-1 integrase strand transfer inhibitor and is neither an inhibitor nor an inducer of CYP enzymes or P-gp.[26,41] Raltegravir is primarily eliminated by glucuronidation (e.g. UGT1A1). Strong inducers of UGT1A1 (e.g. rifampicin) can reduce the plasma concentrations of raltegravir and these combinations should be carefully monitored and used with caution. The recommended dosage of raltegravir is 800 mg every 12 h during co-administration with rifampicin. Other drug–drug interactions associated with reduced plasma concentrations of raltegravir include efavirenz, etravirine and tipranavir–ritonavir, whereas increased plasma concentrations of raltegravir were associated with co-administration of atazanavir, atazanavir–ritonavir and omeprazole. No adjustments to the dosage of raltegravir have been recommended with these drug–drug interactions.

Enfuvirtide is an infusion inhibitor that undergoes catabolism of its amino acid constituent. Enfuvirtide is not associated with clinically significant drug–drug interactions.

ANTIVIRAL AGENTS (NON-RETROVIRAL)

The following section will review the drug–drug interactions associated with antiviral agents that are systemically administered for non-human immunodeficiency virus (non-HIV) infections. The individual drugs have been grouped according to their most common clinical use as antiviral agents.[15]

ANTIHERPESVIRUS AGENTS (Table 6.10)

The majority of drug–drug interactions with aciclovir, ganciclovir and foscarnet involve the risk of overlapping and/or additive myelosuppressive, central nervous system (CNS) toxicity or nephrotoxicity.[15,35] In addition, probenecid inhibits renal tubular secretion of the nucleoside analogs, resulting in an increased AUC and reduced renal clearance of each agent. Cautious use and close monitoring for blood dyscrasias are recommended when ganciclovir is combined with agents such as antineoplastics, amphotericin B, dapsone, flucytosine, intravenous pentamidine, primaquine, pyrimethamine, trimethoprim–sulfamethoxazole and trimetrexate. The combined use of ganciclovir and zidovudine should be avoided whenever possible. In a controlled trial of patients receiving zidovudine and ganciclovir, approximately 80% of patients required a dosage reduction because of hematological (anemia or neutropenia) or gastrointestinal toxicity. Caution is also recommended in the use of ganciclovir, foscarnet or high-dose intravenous aciclovir with other nephrotoxic agents (e.g. aminoglycosides, amphotericin B, cidofovir, foscarnet, ciclosporin, intravenous pentamidine) because of the additive potential of nephrotoxicity. Case reports have suggested dosage adjustments may be needed for phenytoin, valproic acid or theophylline (e.g. agents with a narrow therapeutic index) when co-administered with aciclovir. However, no clinically significant drug–drug interactions and only minor alterations in pharmacokinetic parameter values have been observed with the co-administration of famciclovir with digoxin, cimetidine, allopurinol, theophylline or zidovudine. Severe symptomatic hypocalcemia can be increased when foscarnet is combined with intravenous pentamidine. Serum electrolyte, calcium and magnesium should be carefully monitored in all patients to minimize adverse effects.

Cidofovir-associated nephrotoxicity is a result of renal cellular uptake via OAT1 and drug accumulation in the renal proximal tubules.[15,18,35] To minimize the risk of nephrotoxicity, intravenous cidofovir is administered with high-dose probenecid (2 g 3 h before, and 1 g 2 and 8 h after, cidofovir infusion). The use of other nephrotoxic agents (e.g. aminoglycosides, amphotericin B, foscarnet, intravenous pentamidine, NSAIDs, contrast dye) are contraindicated during cidofovir therapy, and the manufacturer recommends waiting at least 7 days between exposure of these agents and administration of cidofovir.

Table 6.10 Drug–drug interactions of antiherpesvirus agents

Antiviral agent	Interacting drug	Interaction and management strategy
Aciclovir, valaciclovir, famciclovir	Cimetidine	Increased serum concentrations of antiviral agents; avoid concomitant use when high-dose aciclovir or patients who require a dose adjustment because of renal impairment or current adverse effects; monitor for adverse events
	Mycophenolate	Increased serum concentrations of antiviral agent and glucuronide metabolite of mycophenolate; monitor for adverse events and CBC
	Probenecid	Increased serum concentrations of antiviral agents; avoid concomitant use when high-dose aciclovir or patients who require a dose adjustment because of renal impairment or current adverse effects; monitor for adverse events
Aciclovir	Phenytoin, fosphenytoin, valproic acid	Increased risk of seizures; monitor seizure activity and serum concentrations of the anticonvulsant agents; adjust dose as needed
	Theophylline	Increased theophylline serum concentrations and risk of toxicity; monitor theophylline serum concentrations and toxicity; decrease dose of theophylline as needed
	Tizanidine	Increased tizanidine serum concentrations and risk of toxicity (e.g. hypotension, sedation); concomitant therapy should be avoided; consider alternative agent for managing spasticity
	Zidovudine	Increased risk of neurotoxicity (e.g. drowsiness, lethargy); monitor for adverse events
Ganciclovir, valganciclovir	Didanosine	Increased didanosine and slightly decreased ganciclovir serum concentrations; monitor for didanosine toxicity
	Imipenem–cilastatin	Increased risk of seizures; monitor adverse events and consider alternative antibacterial agent
	Myelosuppressive agents[1]	Increased risk of blood dyscrasias; concomitant therapy should be avoided or used with caution at the lowest possible dose; consider alternative agent if possible
	Nephrotoxic agents[2]	Additive injury to the renal tubule; concomitant therapy should be avoided or used with caution and includes monitoring of renal function and dosage adjustment based on creatinine clearance estimation
	Probenecid	Increased ganciclovir serum concentrations; monitor for ganciclovir toxicity
	Zidovudine	Increased risk of hematological toxicity (e.g. anemia, neutropenia, pancytopenia) and GI toxicity; concomitant therapy should be avoided or used with caution with careful monitoring of hematological function and at the lowest possible dose; consider alternative antiretroviral agent
Foscarnet	Nephrotoxic agents[2]	Direct or additive injury to the renal tubule; concomitant therapy should be avoided or used with caution and includes monitoring of renal function and dosage adjustment based on creatinine clearance estimation
	Pentamidine (intravenous)	Increased risk for severe symptomatic hypocalcemia; monitor electrolytes, calcium and magnesium to minimize adverse events
	Saquinavir and/or ritonavir	Increased risk of abnormal renal function; monitor renal function and consider alternative antiretroviral agents
Cidofovir	Nephrotoxic agents[2]	Concomitant administration of cidofovir with potentially nephrotoxic drugs is contraindicated, and the manufacturer recommends waiting at least 7 days between exposure to these agents and administration of cidofovir
	Probenecid	Concomitant probenecid is used to decrease the risk of renal toxicity of cidofovir by decreasing its concentrations within proximal tubular cells; careful monitoring for other drug–drug interactions of probenecid and dose adjust as needed

[1]Examples include antineoplastics, amphotericin B, flucytosine, dapsone, trimethoprim–sulfamethoxazole, intravenous pentamidine, primaquine and pyrimethamine.
[2]Examples include amphotericin B, cisplatin, ciclosporin, vancomycin, foscarnet, intravenous pentamidine, cidofovir, polymyxin B, colistin, radio contrast and aminoglycosides.
CBC, complete blood count; GI, gastrointestinal.

AGENTS FOR INFLUENZA (Table 6.11)

Additive anticholinergic effects and/or increased CNS adverse effects of amantadine can potentially occur with the concomitant administration of anticholinergic agents (e.g. benzatropine, biperiden, trihexyphenidyl), sedating antihistamines (e.g. chlorphenamine [chlorpheniramine], phenylpropanolamine) and buproprion.[15] If any of above combinations is used, patients need to be monitored for CNS reactions and dosage adjustment may be required. Triamterene–hydrochlorothiazide, quinidine, quinine and trimethoprim (alone or in combination with sulfamethoxazole) can reduce

Table 6.11 Drug–drug interactions of anti-influenza agents

Antiviral agent	Interacting drug	Interaction and management strategy
Amantadine	Anticholinergic agents[1] or antihistamines[2]	Increased central nervous system (CNS) adverse effects (e.g. additive anticholinergic effects); avoid combination or use lowest possible dose or alternative agent
	Bupropion	Increased risk of neurotoxicity (e.g. restlessness, agitation, gait disturbances, dizziness); avoid combination or use alternative agent
	Triamterene–hydrochlorothiazide, quinidine, quinine or trimethoprim (alone or in combination with sulfamethoxazole)	Increased amantadine serum concentrations and CNS toxicities; avoid combination or use lowest possible dose or alternative agent
Rimantadine	No major interactions	–
Oseltamivir	Probenecid	Increased oseltamivir carboxylate metabolite serum concentrations; no dose adjustment or monitoring is recommended because of wide margin of safety
Zanamivir	No major interactions	–

[1] Examples include benzatropine, biperiden and trihexyphenidyl.
[2] Examples include chlorphenamine (chlorpheniramine) and phenylpropanolamine.

the renal tubular secretion of amantadine and may cause increased plasma drug concentrations and CNS toxicities. The reported drug–drug interactions for rimantadine have only been minor alterations in pharmacokinetic parameters which are unlikely to be clinically important.

In-vitro studies demonstrate that oseltamivir and zanamivir are not substrates and do not affect any of the common human CYP isoenzymes.[15] No clinically significant metabolic drug–drug interactions have been reported with either agent. The co-administration of probenecid completely reduces the anionic tubular secretion of oseltamivir carboxylate and results in a 50% decrease in renal clearance, a 1.9-fold increase in C_{max} and a 2.5-fold increase in the AUC of oseltamivir carboxylate. Despite these changes, no dosage adjustment is recommended due to the wide margin of safety associated with the active metabolite.

AGENTS FOR TUBERCULOSIS (Table 6.12)

Rifampicin as well as other rifamycins such as rifabutin and rifapentine are potent inducers of oxidative metabolic systems such as the CYP isoenzyme system.[23,24,42–44] In addition, rifampicin can induce transmembrane efflux pumps such as P-gp and conjugative enzyme systems such as UGT and sulfonyltransferases. Consequently, there exists an extensive drug–drug interaction profile with the use of rifampicin

(*see* Table 6.3). Substitution of rifabutin for rifampicin is often used clinically, especially when used concomitantly in patients with HIV receiving highly active antiretroviral therapy (HAART). Similarly, isoniazid inhibits CYP isoenzyme systems and monoamine oxidase and is associated with some drug–drug interactions. For example, inhibition of CYP2C9, CYP2C19 and CYP3A4 by isoniazid is considered the mechanism of interaction with phenytoin, carbamazepine, diazepam and warfarin.[42,43] The potential for this interaction is greater in slow acetylators, which comprise 30–50% of Caucasians and African–Americans. In contrast, a limited number of drug–drug interactions have been reported for other first-line agents such as ethambutol and pyrazinamide, as well as second-line agents such as aminosalicylic acid, capreomycin, cycloserine and ethionamide.[42,43] It is important to note that a few interaction studies have incorporated the effect of combination antituberculosis agents, for example the inhibitory effect of isoniazid on CYP may be negated or overinfluenced by the induction of this system by rifampicin. Consequently, therapeutic drug monitoring and thoughtful consideration of the adverse event profile of concomitantly used agents is critical.

ANTIMALARIAL AGENTS (Table 6.13)

Various drug classes are used as antimalarial agents.[44–47] Most of the agents are metabolized in the liver and are substrates of CYP3A4 or CYP2C isoforms. The combination product artemether–lumefantrine has recently been approved for use by the FDA. A limited number of drug–drug interactions have been reported so far (Table 6.13) but in-vitro and/or clinical studies are desperately needed to assess the effects of co-administered CYP3A4 inducers or inhibitors as well as specific anti-infective classes (e.g. rifampicin, NNRTIs, protease inhibitors) that would likely be used concurrently in patients with malaria.[44–48] Mefloquine, ketoconazole and lopinavir–ritonavir have been shown to alter the AUC of artemether and/or lumefantrine; however, the clinical significance of these changes is unknown.[48]

The plasma AUC of atovaquone is decreased by potent inducers of CYP-mediated drug metabolism (e.g. rifampicin, rifabutin, ritonavir), as well as by tetracycline and metoclopramide.[11,35,46] Concomitant administration of rifampicin and atovaquone is not recommended. The plasma AUC of didanosine and zidovudine can be decreased with concurrent administration of atovaquone, whereas the systemic exposure of rifampicin and etoposide is increased. Alteration in binding to plasma proteins has also been suggested as a mechanism of drug–drug interactions for atovaquone. Proguanil, which is combined with atovaquone, is mainly metabolized by CYP2C19 and CYP3A4 to an active metabolite, cycloguanil. Further studies are needed to identify and understand the clinical significance of drug–drug interactions with proguanil and/or cycloguanil, particularly in patients on combination therapy or with various genetic polymorphisms (slow versus fast metabolizers).

In-vitro studies have suggested that chloroquine is an inhibitor of CYP2D6, although less in-vivo evidence is available to

Table 6.12 Drug–drug interactions of antituberculosis agents

Antituberculosis agent	Interacting drug	Interaction and management strategy
Aminosalicylic acid	Probenecid	Increased aminosalicylic acid serum concentrations (transiently); monitor for toxicity
	Diphenhydramine	Decreased absorption of aminosalicylic acid; avoid concomitant use
	Digoxin	Increased digoxin serum concentrations and toxicity; monitor digoxin serum concentrations and adjust dose appropriately
	Warfarin	Enhanced anticoagulation; monitor PT/INR and adjust warfarin dose appropriately
	Ammonium chloride	Increased probability of crystalluria; avoid concomitant use
Capreomycin	Nephrotoxic agents[1]	Direct or additive injury to the renal tubule; concomitant therapy should be avoided or used with caution and includes monitoring of renal function and dosage adjustment based on body weight and creatinine clearance estimation
	Ototoxic agents[2]	Increased risk of ototoxicity; concomitant therapy should be avoided or used with caution at the lowest possible dose; consider alternative agent if possible
	Neuromuscular blocking agents[3]	Increased respiratory suppression produced by neuromuscular blocking agent; concomitant therapy should be avoided or used with caution and includes monitoring for respiratory depression
Cycloserine	Isoniazid	Increased CNS adverse effects (e.g. dizziness, drowsiness) when both drugs are used concurrently; monitor toxicity
	Ethionamide	Increased CNS adverse effects (e.g. seizures) when both drugs are used concurrently; monitor toxicity
	Phenytoin, fosphenytoin	Increased phenytoin serum concentrations; monitor toxicity and phenytoin serum concentrations, and adjust dose as needed
Ethambutol	Antacids	Decreased ethambutol serum concentrations with aluminum-containing antacids; space administration by at least 4 h
	Ethionamide	Increased adverse effects (e.g. GI distress, headache, confusion, neuritis, hepatotoxicity) when both drugs are used concurrently; monitor toxicity and avoid concomitant use when possible
Ethionamide	Aminosalicylic acid, ethambutol, isoniazid, pyrazinamide, rifampicin	Potentiates the adverse effects of other antituberculosis agents (hepatotoxicity, peripheral neuritis, GI distress, headache, confusion, neuritis, seizures, encephalopathy); monitor toxicity
	Excessive alcohol	Increased psychotic reactions; avoid concomitant use
	Isoniazid	Increased isoniazid serum concentrations (temporarily); monitor for toxicity
Isoniazid	Cycloserine, ethionamide	Increased CNS adverse effects; monitor toxicity
	Carbamazepine	Increased carbamazepine serum concentrations and toxicity (e.g. ataxia, headache, blurred vision, drowsiness, confusion); monitor toxicity and carbamazepine serum concentrations; decrease dose if needed
	Phenytoin, fosphenytoin	Increased phenytoin serum concentrations and toxicity; monitor toxicity and phenytoin serum concentrations; decrease dose if needed
	Primidone	Increased primidone serum concentrations; monitor toxicity and primidone serum concentrations; adjust dose if needed
	Meperidine	Increased toxicity (e.g. serotonin syndrome); monitor toxicity and adjust dose if needed
	Itraconazole	Decreased itraconazole serum concentrations and loss of antimycotic efficacy; alternative antifungal agent or interacting drug should be considered
	Warfarin	Enhanced anticoagulation; monitor PT/INR and adjust warfarin dose appropriately
	Disulfiram	Increased CNS changes (e.g. coordination difficulties, mood or behavioral changes); monitor toxicity and consider dose reduction or discontinuation of disulfiram
	Paracetamol	Increased risk for hepatotoxicity; avoid concomitant use or limit use of paracetamol
	Diazepam	Increased diazepam serum concentrations; monitor toxicity and adjust dose if needed
	Levodopa	Increased toxicity (e.g. flushing, palpitations, hypertension); monitor toxicity and adjust dose if needed
	Aluminum hydroxide	Decreased isoniazid serum concentrations; space administration by at least 1 h

(Continued)

Table 6.12   Drug–drug interactions of antituberculosis agents—cont'd

Antituberculosis agent	Interacting drug	Interaction and management strategy
Pyrazinamide	Ethionamide or rifampicin	Increased hepatotoxicity; monitor liver enzymes and toxicity
	Ciclosporin	Decreased ciclosporin serum concentrations; monitor clinical response and ciclosporin serum concentrations; adjust dose as needed
	Zidovudine	Decreased pyrazinamide serum concentrations and efficacy; consider alternative antituberculosis agent if possible
	Probenecid	Decreased efficacy of probenecid (e.g. increased serum uric acid levels, worsening symptoms of gout); monitor serum uric acid levels and adjust probenecid dose as needed
Rifabutin	Ritonavir-boosted protease inhibitors (ATV/r, FPV/r, DRV/r, IDV/r, LPV/r, SQV/r, TPV/r)	Increased rifabutin serum concentrations; rifabutin dosing to 150 mg every other day or three times weekly; monitor viral response and CBC
	Fosamprenavir	Increased rifabutin serum concentrations; rifabutin dosing to 150 mg per day or 300 mg three times weekly; monitor viral response and CBC
	Indinavir	Increased rifabutin and decreased indinavir serum concentrations; rifabutin dosing to 150 mg per day or 300 mg three times weekly; indinavir 1000 mg every 8 h or consider ritonavir boosting; monitor viral response and CBC
	Nelfinavir	Increased rifabutin and decreased nelfinavir serum concentrations; rifabutin dosing to 150 mg per day or 300 mg three times weekly; monitor viral response and CBC
	Delavirdine	Increased rifabutin and decreased delavirdine serum concentrations; co-administration is not recommended
	Efavirenz	Decreased rifabutin serum concentrations; dose rifabutin 450–600 mg per day or 600 mg three times weekly if efavirenz is not co-administered with a protease inhibitor; monitor viral response and CBC
	Etravirine	Decreased rifabutin and metabolite serum concentrations and decreased etravirine serum concentrations; dose rifabutin 300 mg per day if not co-administered with a ritonavir-boosted protease inhibitor; if co-administered with lopinavir plus ritonavir, dose rifabutin 150 mg per day or three times weekly
	Nevirapine	Increased rifabutin and decreased nevirapine serum concentrations; dosage adjustment is not recommended; monitor viral response and CBC
	Maraviroc	Maraviroc dose of 300 mg every 12 h if used without a strong CYP3A inducer or inhibitor; maraviroc dose of 150 mg every 12 h if used with a strong CYP3A inhibitor; monitor viral response
	Fluconazole	Increased rifabutin serum concentrations and potential rifabutin toxicity (uveitis, ocular pain, photophobia, visual disturbances); monitor toxicity and CBC
	Itraconazole, voriconazole, posaconazole	Increased rifabutin serum concentrations and potential rifabutin toxicity (uveitis, ocular pain, photophobia, visual disturbances); decreased azole serum concentrations and/or loss of antimycotic efficacy; alternative antifungal agent should be considered
	Clarithromycin	Decreased clarithromycin serum concentrations and increased risk of rifabutin toxicity (rash, GI disturbances, hematological abnormalities); monitor efficacy, toxicity and CBC
	Ciclosporin	Decreased ciclosporin serum concentrations; monitor clinical response and ciclosporin serum concentrations; adjust dose as needed
	Warfarin	Decreased anticoagulation; monitor PT/INR and adjust warfarin dose appropriately
	Oral contraceptives	Use alternative form(s) of birth control; counsel patient and document
Rifampicin	See Table 6.3	

CBC, complete blood count; CNS, central nervous system; GI, gastrointestinal; PT/INR, prothrombin time/international normalized ratio.

Table 6.13 Drug–drug interactions involving antimalarial agents

Antimalarial drug	Interacting drug	Mechanism/effects	Management recommendations
Artemether–lumefantrine (co-artemether)	Ketoconazole	↑ artemether AUC by 132%, ↑ dihydroartemisinin AUC by 51%, and ↑ lumefantrine AUC by 61%	Clinical significance unknown; no dosage adjustment recommended
	Lopinavir–ritonavir	↓ artemether AUC by 34%, ↓ dihydroartemisinin AUC by 45%, and ↑ lumefantrine AUC by 230%	Clinical significance unknown; no dosage adjustment recommended
	Mefloquine	↓ lumefantrine AUC by 30–41% and C_{max} by 29%	Clinical significance unknown
	Quinine	Increased risk for QTc prolongation; ↓ quinine AUC by 46%	Monitor for toxicity and clinically significant lengthening of the QTc interval
Atovaquone	Didanosine	↓ didanosine AUC by 24%	Not clinically significant; administer didanosine without food and atovaquone with food
	Etoposide	↑ etoposide AUC by 8.6% and ↑ catechol metabolite AUC by 28.4%	Separate administration by 1–2 days and use caution with concurrent substrates of CYP3A4 or P-glycoprotein
	Indinavir	↑ atovaquone AUC by 13% and ↓ indinavir AUC by 5–9%	Clinical significance unknown; monitor effectiveness of indinavir
	Metoclopramide	↓ atovaquone concentrations	Caution in concomitant administration; if used, monitor effectiveness of atovaquone
	Rifabutin	↓ atovaquone AUC by 34% and ↓ rifabutin AUC by 19%	Caution in concomitant administration; if used, monitor effectiveness of atovaquone
	Rifampicin	↓ atovaquone AUC by 50% and ↑ rifampicin AUC by 30%	Avoid concomitant administration; if used, monitor effectiveness of atovaquone
	Ritonavir	↓ atovaquone concentrations (predicted)	Monitor effectiveness of atovaquone; may need to increase atovaquone dose
	Tetracycline	↓ atovaquone concentrations by 40%	Monitor effectiveness of atovaquone
	Zidovudine	↑ zidovudine AUC by 30% and ↓ CL by 25%; inhibition of zidovudine glucuronidation	Clinical significance unknown; monitor for zidovudine toxicity
Chloroquine	Ampicillin	↓ ampicillin absorption from 29% to 19%	Separate administration by at least 2 h; use other antibacterial agent
	Antacid (magnesium trisilicate)	↓ chloroquine AUC by 18%	Separate administration by 2–3 h
	Chlorpromazine	↑ chlorpromazine concentrations by 1.7- to 4.3-fold; increased sedation	Monitor toxicity; decrease dose of chlorpromazine
	Colestyramine	↓ chloroquine AUC by 30%	Separate administration either 1 h before or 4–6 after chloroquine
	Cimetidine	↓ chloroquine CL by 50%; prolonged $t_{\frac{1}{2}\beta}$ from 3.1 to 4.6 h	Use other H_2-receptor antagonists (e.g. ranitidine) that do not have this drug–drug interaction
	Ciprofloxacin	↓ ciprofloxacin AUC by 43% and C_{max} by 18%	Monitor efficacy; increase ciprofloxacin dose for systemic infections
	Ciclosporin	↑ ciclosporin serum concentrations and nephrotoxicity	Monitor ciclosporin concentrations and renal function; adjust dose as needed
	Digoxin	↑ digoxin serum concentrations by 70%	Monitor digoxin concentrations; adjust dose as needed
	Halofantrine	Warning: the combination may cause prolongation of the QTc interval	Avoid concurrent administration; if used, monitor for toxicity and clinically significant lengthening of the QTc interval
	Insulin	↓ insulin requirement by 25%	Monitor blood glucose and adjust insulin dose as needed
	Kaolin	↓ chloroquine AUC by 28%	Separate administration by 2–3 h

(Continued)

Table 6.13 Drug–drug interactions involving antimalarial agents—cont'd

Antimalarial drug	Interacting drug	Mechanism/effects	Management recommendations
	Methotrexate	↓ methotrexate AUC by 28% and C_{max} by 17–20%; ↑ methotrexate AUC by 52% with hydroxychloroquine	Monitor for efficacy and methotrexate serum concentrations; adjust methotrexate dose as needed
	Methylthioninium chloride (methylene blue)	↓ chloroquine AUC by 20% and desethylchloroquine (metabolite) AUC by 35%	Clinical significance unknown
	Metoprolol	Hydroxychloroquine ↑ metoprolol AUC by 65% and C_{max} by 72% in extensive CYP2D6 metabolizers	Not clinically significant; monitor for toxicity
	Penicillamine	↑ penicillamine AUC by 34% and C_{max} by 55%	Monitor toxicity (e.g. serious hematological effects)
	Praziquantel	↓ praziquantel AUC by 65% and C_{max} by 59%	Monitor for efficacy; ↑ dose of praziquantel for systemic infection
	Proguanil	1.5-fold ↑ in mouth ulcers and 1.33-fold ↑ in diarrhea	Monitor toxicity and treat as needed
	Promethazine	↑ chloroquine AUC and metabolite by 85%	Monitor toxicity; consider other agents
Mefloquine	Ampicillin	↑ mefloquine AUC by 34% and C_{max} by 49%	Clinical significance unknown
	Anticonvulsants	Increased risk of seizures	Avoid concurrent administration
	Artemether	↓ mefloquine AUC by 27%; cure rates similar	Clinical significance unknown
	Artesunate	↓ mefloquine AUC by 27% and ↑ CL by 2.6-fold; lower cure rates	Administer mefloquine 24 h after artesunate
	Cardioactive drugs[1]	Warning: mefloquine plus one of these agents contribute to the prolongation of the QTc interval, but do not contraindicate the use of mefloquine with these agents	Avoid concurrent administration (contraindicated with halofantrine); if used, monitor for toxicity and clinically significant lengthening of the QTc interval
	Cimetidine	↑ mefloquine AUC by 0–34% and C_{max} by 20–42% and ↓ CL by 40%; prolonged $t_{\frac{1}{2}\beta}$ from 9.6 to 14.4 days	Clinical significance unknown; use other H_2-receptor antagonists that do not have this drug–drug interaction
	Co-artemether	↓ lumefantrine AUC by 30–41% and C_{max} by 29%	Clinical significance unknown
	Hypoglycemic agents	Reduced blood glucose levels and hypoglycemia	Monitor blood glucose and adjust dose as needed
	Ketoconazole	↑ mefloquine AUC by 79%, C_{max} by 64% and $t_{\frac{1}{2}\beta}$ by 34%	Monitor toxicity
	Metoclopramide	↓ mefloquine absorption $t_{\frac{1}{2}}$ from 3.2 to 2.4 h and ↑ C_{max} by 31%; reduced GI adverse effects	Clinical significance unknown; however, less mefloquine toxicity
	Quinine (and related drugs [e.g. chloroquine])	Increased risk for QTc prolongation and seizures	Avoid concurrent administration; if used, delay mefloquine administration until at least 12 h after the last dose of quinine; monitor for toxicity and clinically significant lengthening of the QTc interval
	Quinolones	Increased risk for QTc prolongation and seizures	Avoid concurrent administration; if used, monitor for toxicity and clinically significant lengthening of the QTc interval
	Rifampicin	↓ mefloquine AUC by 68% and C_{max} by 19%	Avoid concurrent administration; if used, monitor for efficacy
	Ritonavir	↓ ritonavir AUC by 31% and C_{max} by 36% after multiple dosing	Clinical significance unknown
	Tetracycline	↑ mefloquine AUC by 30% and C_{max} by 38%, and ↓ $t_{\frac{1}{2}\beta}$ from 19.3 to 14.4 days	Not clinically significant
	Typhoid vaccine (oral)	Reduced efficacy of oral vaccine	Separate administration by 12 h (does not apply to capsular polysaccharide typhoid vaccine for injection)
Primaquine	Quinacrine	Increased toxicity	Avoid concomitant use (contraindicated)

(Continued)

Table 6.13 Drug–drug interactions involving antimalarial agents—cont'd

Antimalarial drug	Interacting drug	Mechanism/effects	Management recommendations
Proguanil	Antacid (magnesium trisilicate)	↓ proguanil AUC by 65%	Separate administration by 2–3 h
	Chloroquine	1.5-fold ↑ in mouth ulcers and 1.33-fold ↑ in diarrhea	Monitor toxicity and treat as needed
	Cimetidine	↑ proguanil AUC and $t_{\frac{1}{2}\beta}$; ↑ C_{max} by 89%; ↓ concentrations of active metabolite, cycloguanil	Clinical significance unknown; use other H_2-receptor antagonists that do not have this drug–drug interaction
	Cloxacillin	↓ cloxacillin bioavailability	Clinical significance unknown
	Ethinyl estradiol–levonorgestrel (hormonal contraceptives)	↓ concentrations of active metabolite, cycloguanil, by 34% in extensive metabolizer via CYP2C19	Clinical significance unknown
	Fluvoxamine	↓ CL of proguanil by 40%, cycloguanil by 85%, and 4-chlorophenylbiguanide by 89% in extensive metabolizer via CYP2C19	Clinical significance unknown; monitor efficacy
	Omeprazole	↓ AUC of active metabolite, cycloguanil, by 50% in extensive metabolizer via CYP2C19	Clinical significance unknown
Quinine sulfate	Amantadine	↓ renal CL of amantadine by 30% and ↑ plasma concentrations; ↓ CL of quinine by 50%	Clinical significance unknown
	Astemizole	↑ astemizole (and desmethyl metabolite) AUC and C_{max} by three-fold after a single 430 mg dose of quinine; increased risk for QTc prolongation and cardiac arrhythmias	Avoid concurrent administration (contraindicated by manufacturer); use a different antihistamine product
	Co-artemether	Increased risk for QTc prolongation; ↓ quinine AUC by 46%	Monitor for toxicity and clinically significant lengthening of the QTc interval
	Carbamazepine	↑ carbamazepine AUC by 104% and C_{max} by 81%	Monitor efficacy and carbamazepine plasma concentrations; adjust dose as needed
	Cimetidine	↑ quinine AUC by 42%, ↓ CL by 27%, and ↑ $t_{\frac{1}{2}\beta}$ from 7.6 to 11.3 h	Use other H_2-receptor antagonists (e.g. ranitidine) that do not have this drug–drug interaction
	Desipramine	↓ urinary excretion of 2-hydroxydesipramine by 56% in rapid hydroxylators	Monitor for toxicity (including QTc prolongation) and desipramine plasma concentrations; adjust dose as needed
	Digoxin	↑ digoxin plasma concentrations by 11–92%; ↓ CL by 26% and ↓ renal CL by 20%	Monitor for toxicity and digoxin plasma concentrations; adjust dose as needed
	Flecainide	↑ flecainide AUC by 21% and ↓ CL by 16.5%; increased PR and QRS prolongation on electrocardiogram	Monitor for toxicity; adjust dose as needed
	Halofantrine	Warning: combination may cause prolongation of the QTc interval	Avoid concurrent administration; if used, monitor for toxicity and clinically significant lengthening of the QTc interval
	Ketoconazole	↓ quinine CL by 31% and AUC of 3-hydroxyquinine by 30%	Clinical significance unknown
	Mefloquine	Increased risk for QTc prolongation and seizures	Avoid concurrent administration; if used, delay mefloquine administration until at least 12 h after the last dose of quinine; monitor for toxicity and clinically significant lengthening of the QTc interval
	Phenobarbital	↑ phenobarbital AUC by 57% and C_{max} by 53%	Monitor efficacy and phenobarbital plasma concentrations; adjust dose as needed
	Phenytoin (fosphenytoin)	↓ quinine plasma concentrations	Limited data; monitor efficacy of quinine
	Rifampicin	↓ quinine plasma concentrations; ↑ quinine CL by six-fold and ↓ $t_{\frac{1}{2}\beta}$ from 11 to 5.5 h	Monitor efficacy of quinine and increase dose as needed
	Tetracycline	↑ quinine plasma concentrations by two-fold	Increased efficacy; no drug–drug interaction with doxycycline
	Urine alkalinizers[2]	↓ excretion of unchanged quinine	Clinical significance unknown

(Continued)

Table 6.13 Drug–drug interactions involving antimalarial agents—cont'd

Antimalarial drug	Interacting drug	Mechanism/effects	Management recommendations
Sulfadoxine and pyrimethamine	Artemether	↑ pyrimethamine C_{max} by 44%	Clinical significance unknown
	Chlorpromazine	↑ chlorpromazine 3-h plasma concentrations by four-fold and ↑ hydroxyl metabolite plasma concentrations	Monitor toxicity; decrease dose of chlorpromazine
	Halofantrine	↑ halofantrine AUC_{0-6} and C_{max} by 60%	Monitor for toxicity and clinically significant lengthening of the QTc interval
	Trimethoprim–sulfamethoxazole or sulfonamides	Increased risk of myelosuppression; serious pancytopenia and megaloblastic anemia when given with pyrimethamine	Monitor whole blood cell count and toxicity; avoid concomitant therapy with other folate antagonists; administer leucovorin as needed
	Zidovudine	Increased risk of myelosuppression	Monitor whole blood cell count and toxicity; administer leucovorin as needed

[1]Examples of cardioactive drugs include antiarrhythmics (e.g. class Ic and III), beta-blockers (e.g. propranolol), calcium channel blockers, antihistamines (e.g. astemizole and terfenadine), phenothiazines, related antimalarials (e.g. quinine), halofantrine and ziprasidone.
[2]Examples of urine alkalinizers include sodium bicarbonate and acetazolamide.
AUC, area under the plasma concentration–time curve; CL, clearance; C_{max}, maximum plasma drug concentration; CYP, cytochrome P_{450}; GI, gastrointestinal; $t_{1/2\beta}$, elimination half-life.

support this effect.[11,46] A fair number of drug–drug interactions have been reported with chloroquine use and the great majority are easily managed.

Mefloquine is completely metabolized in the liver to a carboxy metabolite, probably by CYP3A4.[11,46] Potent inhibitors (e.g. ketoconazole) and inducers (e.g. rifampicin) of CYP3A4 have increased and decreased the systemic exposure of mefloquine, respectively. Mefloquine has the potential to be associated with clinically significant pharmacodynamic drug–drug interactions and overlapping toxicities such as QTc prolongation, neuropsychiatric disturbances and seizures. Concurrent administration of quinine, quinidine, chloroquine and fluoroquinolones should be avoided. The administration of oral typhoid vaccine and mefloquine should be separated by 12 h to ensure adequate immunization from the vaccine.

Quinine is extensively metabolized in the liver to several metabolites, including biologically active 3-hydroxyquinine.[11,46] The metabolism of quinine is a result of CYP3A (major) and CYP2C19 (minor). In contrast, quinidine is metabolized by intestinal and liver CYP3A4 and is a potent inhibitor of CYP2D6. Cimetidine, ketoconazole, tetracycline and urine alkalinizers can increase the systemic exposure or decrease the renal clearance of quinine or 3-hydroxyquinine. Both quinine and quinidine can increase the plasma concentrations of digoxin. Drugs that prolong the QTc interval should be avoided or used with caution and monitored for toxicity.

The antifolate agents such sulfadiazine and pyrimethamine are not associated with major pharmacokinetic drug–drug interactions.[11,35] Overlapping adverse hematological toxicity (e.g. neutropenia, anemia, thrombocytopenia) may occur with concurrent use of trimethoprim–sulfamethoxazole or other sulfonamides, zidovudine or ganciclovir. Close monitoring and/or use of alternative therapies are recommended when possible.

ANTIPROTOZOAL AND ANTHELMINTIC AGENTS (Table 6.14)

A variety of different drug classes are used to treat protozoal and parasitic infections.[11,35] Agents that can be used for these infections, as well as an antibacterial agent (e.g. metronidazole, clindamycin or trimethoprim–sulfamethoxazole), have been discussed in a previous section (e.g. Antibacterial agents; see Table 6.5) in this chapter.

Interactions involving antiprotozoal and anthelmintic agents may occur secondary to pharmacokinetic and/or pharmacodynamic mechanisms.[11] Drug–drug interactions involving albendazole, mebendazole and praziquantel mainly involve enzyme induction or inhibition. Agents reported in these drug–drug interactions have included anticonvulsants (e.g. phenytoin, carbamazepine, phenobarbital or valproic acid), rifampicin, dexamethasone and cimetidine. Tiabendazole (thiabendazole) appears to inhibit CYP1A2, and has significantly (e.g. >50%) increased the plasma concentrations of xanthine derivatives such as theophylline and caffeine. Renal excretion of diethylcarbamazine can be increased or decreased with concurrent administration of urinary acidifiers or alkalinizers, respectively.

Furazolidone is an MAOI and must be used with caution when other drugs (e.g. sympathomimetic amines) as well as food or drink containing tyramine are concurrently administered during or before therapy.[11] Disulfiram-like reactions have been associated with concurrent administration of alcohol and furazolidone or levamisole. The common adverse effects associated with pentamidine (e.g. bone marrow suppression, nephrotoxicity, pancreatitis or hypocalcemia) can result in additive toxicity when used in conjunction with antiviral and antiretroviral agents.

Table 6.14 Drug–drug interactions involving antiprotozoal and anthelmintic agents

Drug	Interacting drug	Mechanism/effects	Management recommendations
Albendazole	Carbamazepine, phenobarbital, phenytoin (fosphenytoin)	↓ (+)-albendazole sulfoxide AUC by 49% (carbamazepine), 61% (phenobarbital), and 66% (phenytoin) and ↓ (+)-albendazole sulfoxide C_{max} by 50–63%	Monitor efficacy of systemic infections and increase dose of albendazole as needed
	Cimetidine	↑ albendazole sulfoxide plasma concentrations and ↑ $t_{1/2\beta}$ from 7.4 to 19 h	Clinical significance unknown; increased efficacy observed
	Dexamethasone	↑ albendazole sulfoxide plasma concentrations by 50%	Clinical significance unknown
	Levamisole	↓ albendazole sulfoxide AUC by 75%	Caution with concomitant use; monitor efficacy of systemic infections
Atovaquone	See Table 6.13		
Diethylcarbamazepine	Ammonium chloride	Increased urinary excretion	Clinical significance unknown
	Sodium bicarbonate	Decreased urinary excretion	Clinical significance unknown
Furazolidone	Alcohol	Disulfiram-like reaction	Avoid alcohol during and shortly after therapy with furazolidone
	Omeprazole	↓ furazolidone AUC by 30%	Monitor efficacy; increase dose if needed
	Sympathomimetics[1] (indirectly acting)	MAOI activity and pressor responses to tyramine, dextroamfetamine or pargyline	Avoid concomitant sympathomimetic drugs or tyramine-containing foods or drinks that may have non-selective MAOI effects; warn patients about prohibiting the use of these agents
Ivermectin	Alcohol	↑ ivermectin plasma concentrations by 51–66%	Monitor for toxicity (e.g. ataxia and postural hypotension)
	Levamisole	↑ ivermectin AUC by two-fold	Monitor for toxicity
Levamisole	Albendazole	↓ albendazole sulfoxide AUC by 75%	Caution with concomitant use; monitor efficacy of systemic infections
	Alcohol	Disulfiram-like reaction	Avoid alcohol during and shortly after therapy with levamisole
	Ivermectin	↑ ivermectin AUC by two-fold	Monitor for toxicity
Mebendazole	Carbamazepine, phenytoin (fosphenytoin)	↓ mebendazole serum concentrations	Monitor efficacy of systemic infections and increase dose of mebendazole as needed
	Cimetidine	↑ mebendazole C_{max} by 48%	Clinical significance unknown; increased efficacy observed
	Metronidazole	Increased risk of Stevens–Johnson syndrome/toxic epidermal necrolysis	Avoid concomitant administration
	Valproic acid	↑ mebendazole serum concentrations	Clinical significance unknown; monitor for toxicity
Pentamidine	Foscarnet	Additive hypocalcemia	Monitor serum calcium levels and toxicity
	Nephrotoxic agents[2]	Direct or additive injury to the renal tubule	Concomitant therapy should be avoided or used with caution and includes monitoring renal function and dosage adjustments based on toxicity, body weight and creatinine clearance estimation
	Zalcitabine, stavudine, didanosine	Additive pancreatic toxicity	Avoid concurrent administration; if used, zalcitabine therapy should be interrupted while receiving pentamidine
	Zidovudine	Additive bone marrow suppression	Monitor WBC and toxicity
Piperazine	Pyrantel	Piperazine opposes anthelmintic action of pyrantel	Avoid concomitant administration

(Continued)

Table 6.14 Drug–drug interactions involving antiprotozoal and anthelmintic agents—cont'd

Drug	Interacting drug	Mechanism/effects	Management recommendations
Praziquantel	Carbamazepine, phenobarbital, phenytoin (fosphenytoin)	↓ praziquantel AUC by 90% (carbamazepine) and 74% (phenytoin); ↓ praziquantel plasma concentrations with phenobarbital	Monitor efficacy of systemic infections and increase dose of praziquantel as needed
	Chloroquine	↓ praziquantel AUC by 65% and C_{max} by 59%	Monitor efficacy; ↑ dose of praziquantel for systemic infection
	Cimetidine	↑ praziquantel AUC and plasma concentrations by two-fold	May improve efficacy or reverse drug–drug interactions that ↓ praziquantel AUC (e.g. anticonvulsants, steroids)
	Dexamethasone	↓ praziquantel plasma steady-state concentrations by 50%	Monitor efficacy of systemic infections and increase dose of praziquantel as needed
	Rifampicin	↓ praziquantel plasma steady-state concentrations by 85–100%	Avoid concomitant administration
Pyrantel	Piperazine	Piperazine opposes anthelmintic action of pyrantel	Avoid concomitant administration
Tiabendazole	Aminophylline, theophylline	↑ theophylline plasma concentrations via inhibition of CYP1A2	Reduce theophylline dosage by 50% or stop theophylline while on tiabendazole; consider using albendazole or mebendazole (not associated with this drug interaction); if used concurrently, monitor toxicity and plasma theophylline concentrations, and adjust dose as needed
	Caffeine	↑ caffeine AUC by 57%, ↑ $t_{½β}$ by 140% and ↓ CL by 66%	Monitor and inform patient of adverse effects of caffeine

[1]Examples of indirectly acting sympathomimetic amines include amfetamines, phenylpropanolamine and ephedrine.
[2]Examples include amphotericin B, cisplatin, ciclosporin, vancomycin, foscarnet, intravenous pentamidine, cidofovir, tenofovir, polymyxin B, colistin, radio contrast and aminoglycosides.
AUC, area under the plasma concentration–time curve; CL, clearance; C_{max}, maximum plasma drug concentration; MAOI, monoamine oxidase inhibitor; $t_{½β}$, elimination half-life; WBC, white blood cell count.

References

1. Lasser KE, Allen PD, Woolhandler SJ, Himmelstain DU, Wolfe SM, Bor DH. Timing of new black box warnings and withdrawals for prescription medications. *J Am Med Assoc.* 2002;287:2215–2220.
2. Fleischer R, Laessig K. Safety and efficacy evaluation of pleconaril for treatment of the common cold. *Clin Infect Dis.* 2003;37:1722.
3. MacArthur RD, Novak RM. Maraviroc: the first of a new class of antiretroviral agents. *Clin Infect Dis.* 2008;47:236–241.
4. Reynolds KS. Drug interactions: regulatory perspective. In: Piscitelli SC, Rodvold KA, eds. *Drug Interactions in Infectious Diseases.* 2nd ed. Totowa: Humana Press; 2005:83–99.
5. Seden K, Back D, Khoo S. Antiretroviral drug interactions: often unrecognized, frequently unavoidable, sometimes unmanageable. *J Antimicrob Chemother.* 2009;64:5–8.
6. Juurlink DN, Mamdani M, Kopp A, Laupacis A, Redelmeier DA. Drug–drug interactions among elderly patients hospitalized for drug toxicity. *J Am Med Assoc.* 2003;289:1652–1658.
7. Ray WA, Murray KT, Meredith S, Narsimhulu SS, Hall K, Stain CM. Oral erythromycin and the risk of sudden death from cardiac causes. *N Engl J Med.* 2004;351:1089–1096.
8. Piscitelli SC, Rodvold KA, eds. *Drug Interactions in Infectious Diseases.* 2nd ed. Totowa: Humana Press; 2005.
9. Hansten PD, Horn JR. *Drug Interactions Analysis and Management 2008.* St Louis: Wolters Kluwer Health; 2008.
10. Tatro DS. *Drug Interaction Facts 2009: The Authority on Drug Interactions.* St Louis: Wolters Kluwer Health; 2009.
11. Baxter K, ed. *Stockley's Drug Interactions.* 8th ed. London: Pharmaceutical Press; 2008.
12. Williamson E, Driver S, Baxter K, eds. *Stockley's Herbal Medicines Interactions.* London: Pharmaceutical Press; 2009.
13. Kashuba ADM, Bertino JS. Mechanisms of drug interactions I. In: Piscitelli SC, Rodvold KA, eds. *Drug Interactions in Infectious Diseases.* 2nd ed. Totowa: Humana Press; 2005:13–39.
14. Falcon RW, Kakuda TN. Drug interactions between HIV protease inhibitors and acid-reducing agents. *Clin Pharmacokinet.* 2008;47:75–89.
15. Pai MP, Momary KM, Rodvold KA. Antibiotic drug interactions. *Med Clin North Am.* 2006;90:1223–1255.
16. Fenner KS, Troutman MD, Kempshall S, et al. Drug–drug interactions mediated through P-glycoprotein: clinical relevance and in vitro–in vivo correlation using digoxin as a probe drug. *Clin Pharmacol Ther.* 2009;85:173–181.
17. Rolan PE. Plasma protein binding displacement interactions; why are they still regarded as clinically important? *Br J Clin Pharmacol.* 1994;37:125–128.
18. Giacomini KM, Sugiyama Y. Membrane transporters and drug response. In: Brunton LL, Lazo JS, Parker KL, eds. *Goodman & Gilman's The Pharmacological Basis of Therapeutics.* 11th ed. New York: McGraw-Hill; 2009:41–70.
19. Penzak SR. Mechanisms of drug interactions II: transport proteins. In: Piscitelli SC, Rodvold KA, eds. *Drug Interactions in Infectious Diseases.* 2nd ed. Totowa: Humana Press; 2005:41–82.
20. Tsuji A. Impact of transporter-mediated drug absorption, distribution, elimination and drug interactions in antimicrobial chemotherapy. *J Infect Chemother.* 2006;12:241–250.
21. Zhang L, Strong JM, Qui W, Lesko LJ, Huang S-M. Scientific perspectives on drug transporters and their role in drug interactions. *Mol Pharm.* 2006;3:62–69.
22. Gonzalez FJ, Tukey RH. Drug metabolism. In: Brunton LL, Lazo JS, Parker KL, eds. *Goodman & Gilman's The Pharmacological Basis of Therapeutics.* 11th ed. New York: McGraw-Hill; 2009:71–91.

23. Baciewicz AM, Chrisman CR, Finch CK, Self TH. Update on rifampin and rifabutin drug interactions. *Am J Med Sci*. 2008;335:126–136.

24. Niemi M, Backman JT, Fromm MF, Neuvoene PJ, Kivisto KT. Pharmacokinetic interactions with rifampicin: clinical relevance. *Clin Pharmacokinet*. 2003;42:819–850.

25. Schriever CA, Fernandez C, Rodvold KA, Danziger LH. Daptomycin: a novel cyclic lipopeptide antimicrobial. *Am J Health Syst Pharm*. 2005;62:1145–1158.

26. Hicks C, Gulick RM. Raltegravir: the first HIV type 1 integrase inhibitor. *Clin Infect Dis*. 2009;48:931–939.

27. Phillips KA, Veenstra DL, Oren E, Lee JK, Sadee W. Potential role of pharmacogenomics in reducing adverse drug reactions: a systematic review. *J Am Med Assoc*. 2001;286:2270–2279.

28. Fish DN. Circumventing drug interactions. In: Piscitelli SC, Rodvold KA, eds. *Drug Interactions in Infectious Diseases*. 2nd ed.Totowa: Humana Press; 2005:463–481.

29. Horn JR, Hansten PD, Chan L-N. Proposal for a new tool to evaluate drug interactions cases. *Ann Pharmacother*. 2007;41:674–680.

30. Pham FA. Drug–drug interaction programs in clinical practice. *Clin Pharmacol Ther*. 2008;83:396–397.

31. Neuhauser MM, Danziger LH. β-lactam antibiotics. In: Piscitelli SC, Rodvold KA, eds. *Drug Interactions in Infectious Diseases*. 2nd ed.Totowa: Humana Press; 2005:225–287.

32. Guay DRP. Quinolones. In: Piscitelli SC, Rodvold KA, eds. *Drug Interactions in Infectious Diseases*. 2nd ed.Totowa: Humana Press; 2005:215–254.

33. Susla GM. Miscellaneous antibiotics. In: Piscitelli SC, Rodvold KA, eds. *Drug Interactions in Infectious Diseases*. 2nd ed.Totowa: Humana Press; 2005:339–381.

34. Paterson DL, Depestel DD. Doripenem. *Clin Infect Dis*. 2009;49:291–298.

35. Tseng A. Drugs for HIV-related opportunistic infections. In: Piscitelli SC, Rodvold KA, eds. *Drug Interactions in Infectious Diseases*. 2nd ed.Totowa: Humana Press; 2005:137–189.

36. Gubbins PO, McConnell SA, Amsden JR. Antifungal agents. In: Piscitelli SC, Rodvold KA, eds. *Drug Interactions in Infectious Diseases*. 2nd ed.Totowa: Humana Press; 2005:289–337.

37. Bruggemann RJM, Alffenaar J-WC, Blijlevens NMA, et al. Clinical relevance of the pharmacokinetic interactions of azole antifungal drugs with other coadministered agents. *Clin Infect Dis*. 2009;48:1441–1458.

38. Nivoix Y, Leveque D, Herbrecht R, Koffel J-C, Beretz L, Ubeaud-Sequier G. The enzymatic basis of drug–drug interactions with systemic triazole antifungals. *Clin Pharmacokinet*. 2008;47:779–792.

39. Andes D, Pascual A, Marchetti O. Antifungal therapeutic drug monitoring: established and emerging indications. *Antimicrob Agents Chemother*. 2009;53:24–34.

40. Struble KA, Piscitelli SC. Drug interactions with antiretrovirals for HIV infection. In: Piscitelli SC, Rodvold KA, eds. *Drug Interactions in Infectious Diseases*. 2nd ed. Totowa: Humana Press; 101–136.

41. Brown KC, Paul S, Kashuba ADM. Drug interactions with new and investigational antiretrovirals. *Clin Pharmacokinet*. 2009;48:211–241.

42. Yew WW. Clinically significant interactions with drugs used in the treatment of tuberculosis. *Drug Saf*. 2002;25:111–133.

43. Namdar R, Ebert SC, Peloquin CA. Drugs for tuberculosis. In: Piscitelli SC, Rodvold KA, eds. *Drug Interactions in Infectious Diseases*. 2nd ed.Totowa: Humana Press; 2005:191–213.

44. Sousa M, Pozniak A, Boffito M. Pharmacokinetics and pharmacodynamics of drug interactions involving rifampicin, rifabutin, and antimalarial drugs. *J Antimicrob Chemother*. 2008;62:872–878.

45. German PI, Aweeka FT. Clinical pharmacology of artemisinin-based combination therapies. *Clin Pharmacokinet*. 2008;47:91–102.

46. Giao PT, de Vries PJ. Pharmacokinetic interactions of antimalarial agents. *Clin Pharmacokinet*. 2001;40:343–373.

47. Koo S, Back D, Winstanley P. The potential for interactions between antimalarial and antiretroviral drugs. *AIDS*. 2005;19:995–1005.

48. German P, Parikh S, Lawrence J, et al. Lopinavir/ritonavir affects pharmacokinetic exposure of artemether/lumefantrine in HIV-uninfected healthy volunteers. *J Acquir Immune Defic Syndr*. 2009;51:424–429.

7 Antibiotics and the immune system

Arne Forsgren and Kristian Riesbeck

Numerous reports on the effect of antibacterial agents on the immune system have accumulated in recent years. However, immune capacity is difficult to examine, and different results, sometimes conflicting, will be obtained depending on the derivative, incubation time, cell type, analysis method or experimental animal used. In this chapter, selected current literature is reviewed.

Comprehensive reviews on the effects of antibiotics on the immune response have been published over the last three decades. Hauser and Remington in 1983 concluded that a potential for immunosuppression exists for several antibiotics,[1] although the clinical relevance of the experimental observations remained to be elucidated. Milatovic characterized the published results on phagocytosis to a large extent as controversial, thus rendering the evaluation rather difficult.[2] Labro's review of the therapeutic relevance of the observed effects on phagocyte functions and future research prospects raises more questions than answers.[3] Extensive reviews on the immuno-modulatory effects of quinolones have been published by Riesbeck[4] and Dalhoff and Shalit.[5]

During an infection, antibiotics interfere with both the infecting bacterium and the host in a complicated fashion (Figure 7.1). In addition to the conventional effects of an antibiotic, i.e. bacteristatic and bactericidal activity (A), some antibiotics act directly on important components in the host defense such as granulocytes and lymphocytes (B). Antibiotics can alter the susceptibility of bacteria to host defenses and alter release of toxins and inflammatory products, with secondary effects on the host (C). Phagocytic or other host cells can also protect bacteria against antibiotics (D).

CHEMOTAXIS

Most studies on the direct effect of antibiotics on phagocytic cells concern chemotaxis. The effect of 20 different antibiotics on chemotaxis in vitro towards an *Escherichia coli* filtrate was studied by an agarose technique.[6] Human leukocytes preincubated with clinically obtainable concentrations of rifampicin (rifampin) and sodium fusidate showed markedly depressed directional migration and, at concentrations slightly above those clinically achievable, doxycycline also inhibited chemotaxis. The clinical implications of these results must, however, be questioned as the experiments were performed in a low-protein tissue culture suspension, and fusidic acid particularly is heavily protein bound. In patients and healthy volunteers given doxycycline, leukocyte migration was studied ex vivo with the agarose technique and in vivo with a skin window technique. The very high dose 600 mg doxycycline administered intravenously had only an insignificant effect, while controls given non-steroidal anti-inflammatory drugs (NSAIDs) had significantly reduced values both ex and in vivo (A Scheja, A Forsgren, unpublished results). Aminoglycosides, β-lactams, macrolides, clindamycin, sulfamethoxazole, trimethoprim and also fluoroquinolones have shown no interactions with agarose chemotaxis. In contrast to those results, it has been reported that macrolides potentiate human neutrophil locomotion in vitro by inhibition of leukoattractant-activated superoxide generation and auto-oxidation. In addition, aminoglycosides have been reported to inhibit chemotaxis. The effects of macrolides and aminoglycosides have not been confirmed in in-vivo studies. The anti-inflammatory activities of quinolones were investigated with an in-vitro model of transendothelial migration

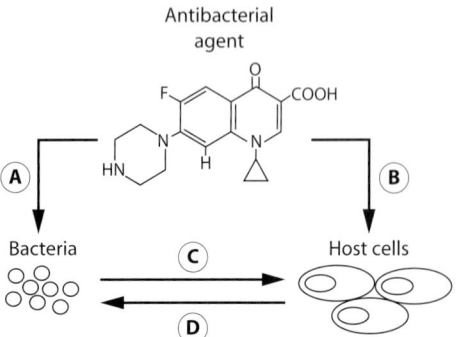

Antibacterial
agent

Fig. 7.1 Schematic drawing demonstrating host–cell interactions and different levels of intervention by antibacterial agents. See text for details.

(TEM). Human umbilical vein endothelial cells (HUVEC) infected with *Chlamydophila* (formerly *Chlamydia*) *pneumoniae* or stimulated with tumor neurosis factor alpha (TNF-α), as well as neutrophils and monocytes, were preincubated with quinolones. A significantly decreased neutrophil and monocyte migration and interleukin-8 (IL-8) production compared to antibiotic-free controls was detected. It was speculated that the decreased migration was due to decreased IL-8 levels.[7]

PHAGOCYTOSIS AND KILLING

Studies of the direct influence of antibiotics on other phagocytic cell functions such as engulfment, killing and metabolic responses are more scarce. In-vitro experiments by a number of investigators have shown that, at clinical concentrations slightly above those levels obtained in vivo, tetracyclines inhibit the uptake of different bacteria, yeast and particles. Furthermore, leukocytes harvested from healthy volunteers after ingestion of tetracycline also demonstrated decreased phagocytic capacity for yeasts, although results are conflicting. For aminoglycosides, decreased, increased or no effect on uptake has been reported. Other antibiotics have not been studied or have not shown effect on phagocyte engulfment or killing functions. At clinically achievable concentrations, for example, fluoroquinolones in general do not affect phagocyte functions.

INTRACELLULAR EFFECTS

Intracellular effects of antibiotics cannot be predicted on the simple basis of cellular drug accumulation and minimum inhibitory concentration (MIC) in broth. In most cases, intracellular activity is actually lower than extracellular activity, despite the fact that all antibiotics reach intracellular concentrations that are at least equal to, and more often higher than, the extracellular concentrations. This discrepancy may result from impairment of the expression of antibiotic activity or a change in bacterial responsiveness inside the cells. It therefore appears important to evaluate the intracellular activity of antibiotics in appropriate models.[8]

The penetration of antibiotics into human cells has been addressed by different methods, often including radiolabeled drugs. Again results vary with experimental conditions; for example, using different media with (or without) albumin considerably affects the outcome.[9] Penicillins, cephalosporins and aminoglycosides have, in general, been shown to have limited access to the intracellular space with a cellular/extracellular ratio (C/E) less than 1, whereas quinolones, tetracyclines, ethambutol and rifampicin are enriched intracellularly. Azithromycin, clarithromycin, clindamycin, erythromycin, roxithromycin and telithromycin, as well as teicoplanin, demonstrate a C/E of 10:1 to 100:1 or higher. There are also large differences between host cells regarding their capacity to accumulate antibiotics intracellularly. Most

authors have reported a lack of intracellular accumulation of β-lactams in phagocytic cells. However, during longer incubations, β-lactam antibiotics diffuse through membranes into the cell cytosol. Macrophages and also fibroblasts incubated with aminoglycosides for several days accumulate these drugs to an apparent C/E of 2 to 4. Macrophages take up penicillins and aminoglycosides by pinocytosis, in contrast to granulocytes that lack this uptake mechanism. In macrophages actively ingesting bacteria and also in resting macrophages obtained from smokers, there is an increased rate of penetration of the drugs. The intracellular distribution of antibiotics will influence their ultimate biological activity. A prerequisite for a beneficial intracellular antibacterial effect is the localization of the antibiotic and the pathogen in the same intracellular compartment. Thus, intracellular bioactivity is not a common property among antibacterial agents, even though they are accumulated intracellularly.

Bacteria are internalized by both phagocytic and non-professional phagocytic cells in which they may not only survive but also multiply. The ability of bacteria to enter non-phagocytic host cells such as epithelial cells, endothelial cells and fibroblasts requires specific uptake mechanisms including invasins, which interact with specific host cell receptors or bacterial proteins, triggering membrane ruffling and concomitant bacterial uptake. Although the molecular details in the uptake mechanism of phagocytic cells differ among intracellular bacteria, the first event following the specific interaction between the bacterial cell and the phagocyte is always the formation of a primary phagosome. After being taken up, most extracellular bacteria are quickly or more slowly inactivated by the subsequent generation of reactive oxygen intermediates and nitrogen oxide, together with lytic enzymes supplied by the lysosomes. However, it is widely recognized that intracellular survival or even multiplication of many bacteria, traditionally referred to as extracellular parasites, play a significant role in the pathogenesis of the disease these organisms cause. This is evident in infections caused by *Staphylococcus aureus* but is also seen in the case of *Haemophilus influenzae*, pneumococci and streptococci. In order to escape these hostile conditions in the phagosome, intracellular bacteria have invented two different strategies either to modify the phagosomal compartment in a variety of ways to prevent the bactericidal attack or to escape from the primary phagosome into the cytosol of the host cell. The first strategy is used by *Salmonella* spp., *Mycobacterium tuberculosis*, *Legionella pneumophila* and *Chlamydia* spp. In contrast, *Listeria*, *Shigella* and *Rickettsia* spp. escape from the primary phagosome into the host cytosol, where they continue replicating.

The activity of antibiotics against intracellular bacteria was reviewed by van den Broek who commented on the difficulties in comparing data generated by different laboratories.[10] Most antibiotics have not been tested in vitro for intracellular effect against microbes with different locations. Intracellular *Staph. aureus* have been shown to present a problem in antibiotic therapy and staphylococci phagocytosed by granulocytes have often been used as a model. Although there are discrepancies in the literature on the ability of antibiotics to kill intracellular *Staph. aureus*, most studies have shown a good intraphagocytic activity for rifampicin. In contrast, studies on the intracellular accumulation and activity of ciprofloxacin, levofloxacin and moxifloxacin using different cellular models of *Staph. aureus*-infected phagocytes, have reported a bacteristatic rather than a bactericidal effect of fluoroquinolones despite a many-fold accumulation of the drugs. These concordant data clearly indicate that as yet unknown factors must be at work to decrease the intracellular antibiotic efficiency of fluoroquinolones.[11] Macrolides, clindamycin, vancomycin and teicoplanin giving high intracellular levels have shown inability to kill intracellular *Staph. aureus*. This may be due to the fact that clindamycin (and also erythromycin) is mainly associated with the cytosol fraction and less with the lysosomal fraction where the staphylococci are found. In addition, macrolides and clindamycin are negatively affected by acidic pH in the lysosomal fraction. In most studies, β-lactam antibiotics and aminoglycosides have not shown reduction of *Staph. aureus* within neutrophils. However, in contrast, phenoxymethylpenicillin, cloxacillin, flucloxacillin and aminoglycosides have been shown to exert some activity against staphylococci within macrophages. It is widely believed that aminoglycosides only affect extracellular bacteria. However, as pointed out above, aminoglycosides enter macrophages and accumulate slowly. The activity of aminoglycosides against intracellular *M. tuberculosis* has been confirmed in classic macrophage studies. The activity of rifampicin against intracellular *Legionella pneumophilia* and *M. tuberculosis* is well accepted. In addition, the intraphagocytic bactericidal effects of erythromycin on *Legionella* and *Chlamydia* spp. seem well established. This may, however, vary due to the cell type in question, as infection with *C. pneumoniae* in circulating human monocytes is refractory to antibiotic treatment with azithromycin and rifampicin.[12]

Extracellular respiratory tract pathogens such as *H. influenzae*, pneumococci and streptococci can enter epithelial cells and macrophages and survive intracellularly. When the activity of azithromycin, gentamicin, levofloxacin, moxifloxacin, penicillin G, rifampicin, telithromycin and trovafloxacin were tested against intracellular pneumococci, moxifloxacin, trovafloxacin and telithromycin were most active. Telithromycin killed all intracellular organisms.[13]

STRUCTURAL CHANGES IN BACTERIA EXPOSED TO ANTIBIOTICS

Altered uptake and killing of bacteria exposed to antibiotics has been clearly documented as reviewed by Gemmel and Lorian.[14,15] Bacteria exposed to various antibiotics including β-lactam antibiotics, vancomycin, macrolides and quinolones have been reported to be more easily phagocytosed and killed. In contrast to those drugs, tetracycline and gentamicin have been reported to decrease phagocytosis. The reason for the improved killing varies but some bacteria exposed to low concentrations of antibiotics, i.e. below MIC (sub-MIC), often show increased killing. Structural changes can be one reason for changed uptake and killing. β-Lactam antibiotics produce the most dramatic alteration of the bacterial morphology. The functional role of penicillin binding proteins (PBPs) in bacterial growth and morphological integrity provides the biochemical base for most of the alterations occurring in the presence of β-lactam antibiotics. Each β-lactam antibiotic has a characteristic binding activity for each PBP and at sub-MIC the antibiotic binds to that PBP for which it has the highest affinity, resulting in antibiotic-dependent specific changes (e.g. filaments or oval cells). However, all β-lactam antibiotics have similar morphological effects on staphylococci and other Gram-positive cocci due to little variation in PBP affinity in these bacteria. Fosfomycin and vancomycin, which inhibit earlier stages of cell wall synthesis, produce similar morphological alterations in Gram-positive cocci. Sub-MICs of antibiotics with targets other than cell-wall synthesis induce different morphological changes. Exposure of staphylococci to chloramphenicol, tetracycline, rifampicin and also synercid results in bacteria with multiple layers of cell wall. In Gram-negative bacteria, ciprofloxacin and trimethoprim leads to production of filaments.

Antibiotics may also inhibit the synthesis of key surface molecules. The enhanced phagocytosis and killing of clindamycin-exposed *Bacteroides* spp. appear to be due to the disappearance of capsule from the bacterial surface. Similarly, clindamycin and linezolid reduce the amount of protein A on the surface of *Staph. aureus* and M protein on group A streptococci: consequently these bacteria become more susceptible to phagocytic uptake and killing. In addition, these two antibiotics impair coagulase and hemolysin production of *Staph. aureus* as well as streptolysin and DNase of group A streptococci. Ceftriaxone and monobactams reduce the antiphagocytic antigen of *Esch. coli*. In parallel, ampicillin and chloramphenicol alter the antiphagocytic capsule of *H. influenzae* type b, resulting in increased uptake.

ENDOTOXIN AND EXOTOXIN RELEASE

As early as 1960, Hinton and Orr observed that α-hemolysin production by *Staph. aureus* is inhibited by streptomycin or bacitracin at concentrations below those interfering with bacterial growth. Confirmation of these findings was performed using other antibiotics (tetracyclines, clindamycin, chloramphenicol and erythromycin). Specific inhibition of, for example, toxic shock syndrome toxin is possible with sub-MIC levels of clindamycin. Treatment of several other species (e.g. *Clostridium difficile*, *Pseudomonas aeruginosa*, group A streptococci and *Esch. coli*) with mainly protein synthesis inhibitors reduces both toxin synthesis and the production of other virulence factors.[14] Clindamycin has recently been used as an important supplement to, for example, benzylpenicillin to lower exotoxin levels in the treatment of patients suffering from infections with β-hemolytic group A streptococci.

An effect of great importance of antibacterial agents would be their potential ability to limit release of endotoxin (lipopolysaccharide; LPS), the major constituent of the outer membrane of Gram-negative bacteria, in the critically ill patient.

In-vitro and animal experiments as well as some clinical studies have shown that endotoxin concentrations increase after antibiotic treatment of Gram-negative infections. Antibiotics differ in their capacity to cause endotoxin release depending on their mode of action. β-Lactam antibiotics, acting on the cell wall, lead to a higher endotoxin release than aminoglycosides and other groups of antibiotics, affecting bacterial protein synthesis. Among the β-lactam antibiotics, there are also differences in capacity to liberate endotoxin depending on their affinities for the various PBPs. Furthermore, affinities for PBPs have been shown to be dose dependent. Ceftazidime has been demonstrated to bind to PBP 3 at low doses, leading to the formation of long filamentous structures with an increased endotoxin production before lysis. With increasing doses, ceftazidime also has a high affinity for PBP 1, leading to rapid lysis without elongation and with less endotoxin release.

In a randomized, multicenter, double-blind study, no differences in the levels of proinflammatory cytokines were detected in patients with Gram-negative urosepsis treated with either imipenem or ceftazidime.[16] Thus, well-controlled clinical investigations are required to shed light on complicated biological phenomena. Reduced endotoxin shedding has been reported when β-lactam antibiotics have been combined with clindamycin and tobramycin.[17]

CELL PROLIFERATION AND CYTOKINE PRODUCTION

Effects of antibiotics on lymphoid cells or cells of other origins have been described for most antibiotics that accumulate intracellularly. Fluoroquinolones reach concentrations in human leukocytes 3–20 times the extracellular concentration.[4,5] Importantly, these drugs are not associated with any specific cellular organelle and do not require cell viability for accumulation. At concentrations slightly above those clinically achievable, the effects of fluoroquinolones on the immune system have been thoroughly investigated by us and others. We have used ciprofloxacin as a model drug for this large group of derivatives. Ciprofloxacin (range 5–80 μg/mL), and to a lower degree other fluoroquinolones, superinduces IL-2 synthesis by mitogen-activated peripheral blood lymphocytes.[18-20] Experiments with T-cell lines and primary T lymphocytes transiently transfected with a plasmid containing the IL-2 promoter region, show ciprofloxacin to enhance IL-2 gene activation. In parallel with these observations, under certain in-vitro conditions, ciprofloxacin (20–80 μg/mL) counteracts the effect of the immunosuppressive agent ciclosporin (cyclosporine) that normally inhibits the phosphatase activity of calcineurin inhibiting NFAT-1 activity. Ciprofloxacin thus interferes with a regulative pathway common to several cytokines.

Indeed, analysis of cytokine mRNAs in ciprofloxacin-treated peripheral blood lymphocytes revealed that not only is IL-2 mRNA enhanced, but also an array of other cytokine mRNAs including interferon gamma (IFN-γ) and IL-4 (Figure 7.2A). An earlier and stronger ciprofloxacin-dependent activation of the transcriptional regulation factors NFAT-1 and activator protein-1 (AP-1) has been observed in T-cells explaining the upregulated mRNA transcription (Figure 7.2B). These data suggest a program commonly observed in mammalian stress responses. In fact, when microarray analysis was done on ciprofloxacin-treated T lymphocytes, several gene transcripts ($n = 104$) were upregulated in cells treated with ciprofloxacin, whereas 98 transcripts were downregulated out of 847 total genes included on the microarray.[21] The increased mRNAs were distributed between major gene programs, including interleukins (36.5%), signal-transduction molecules (13.5%), adhesion molecules (10.6%), tumor necrosis factor and transforming growth factor superfamilies (10.6%), cell-cycle regulators (9.6%) and apoptosis-related molecules (8.7%). In parallel with this hypothesis, ciprofloxacin and trovafloxacin at experimental concentrations potentiate IL-8 and E-selectin (CD62E) synthesis in stimulated endothelial cells.[22] However, the fluoroquinolone moxifloxacin (MXF) inhibits nuclear factor kappa B (NF-κB) activation, mitogen-activated protein kinase activation and synthesis of the proinflammatory cytokines IL-8, TNF-α and IL-1β in activated human monocytic cells.[23] It also had a protective anti-inflammatory effect in vivo in a model of *Candida albicans* pneumonia in immune suppressed animals, resulting in enhanced survival and reduction in IL-8 and TNF-α in lung homogenates.

Several reports exist on ciprofloxacin-dependent immunomodulation in vivo, strongly indicating that the observed cytokine upregulation is not an in-vitro artefact.[4,5] It is thus clear that the fluoroquinolone ciprofloxacin stimulates bone marrow regeneration in both transplanted and sublethally irradiated mice by interfering with IL-3 and granulocyte–macrophage colony-stimulating factor (GM-CSF) synthesis. The treated mice demonstrated a higher number of white blood cells and myeloid progenitor cells in bone marrow and spleen on days 4 and 8 post-irradiation as compared to saline-treated animals. Despite brilliant results in mouse models, only one successful study exists on this phenomenon in human subjects. In contrast to specific effects on the bacteria, fluoroquinolones (7% and 50% for trovafloxacin and tosufloxacin, respectively) protected mice from LPS-dependent mortality when animals were injected with lethal doses.[24] IL-6 and TNF-α serum concentrations were significantly reduced in fluoroquinolone-treated animals compared to drug-free controls. In parallel, numerous studies have shown that fluoroquinolones inhibit monokine production by LPS-activated monocytic cell, albeit at drug concentrations higher than the ones achieved in serum.

Macrolides including erythromycin, clarithromycin and roxithromycin have been analyzed in several cell systems using various stimulatory compounds such as cytokines and

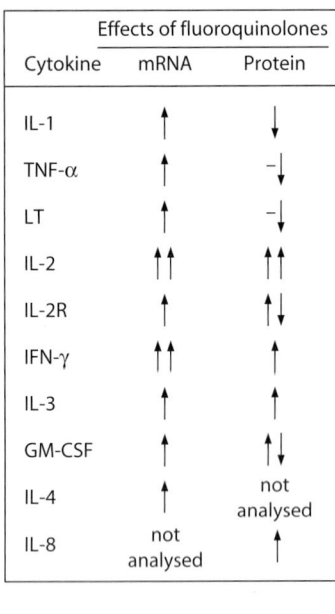

Effects of fluoroquinolones		
Cytokine	mRNA	Protein
IL-1	↑	↓
TNF-α	↑	–↓
LT	↑	–↓
IL-2	↑↑	↑↑
IL-2R	↑	↑↓
IFN-γ	↑↑	↑
IL-3	↑	
GM-CSF	↑	↑↓
IL-4	↑	not analysed
IL-8	not analysed	↑

(A)

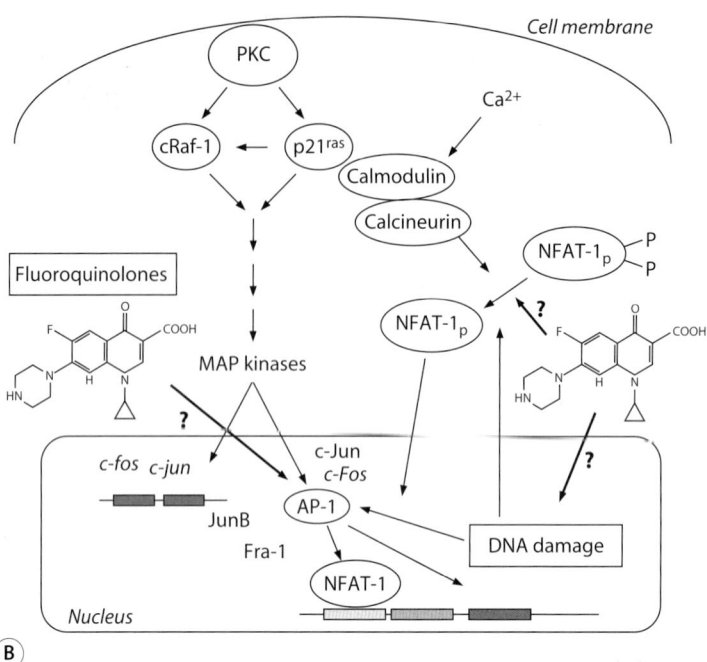

(B)

Fig. 7.2 Immunomodulatory effects of the representative fluoroquinolone ciprofloxacin and its putative site(s) of action in a schematically drawn T lymphocyte. (A) Fluoroquinolones upregulate virtually all examined mRNA transcripts in mitogen-activated peripheral blood lymphocytes (4,5,21) or monocytes (IL-8) (23), whereas mainly T helper 1 and 2 cytokines are paralleled by an increased protein synthesis. (B) delineates the signaling events in a T lymphocyte stimulated through the T-cell receptor/CD3 complex resulting in protein kinase C (PKC) activation followed by triggering of the MAP kinase cascade on one hand and the increased Ca²⁺ mobilization on the other causing, dephosphorylation of the pre-existing nuclear factor of activated T cells-1 (NFAT-1p). It is not completely clear, however, whether ciprofloxacin directly interferes with the transcriptional regulation factors activator protein-1 (AP-1) or NFAT-1, or inhibits the DNA topoisomerase II resulting in DNA damage and genotoxic stress, leading to a secondary activation of the transcription factors (as indicated by the question marks).

endotoxins. Since macrolides are strongly accumulated intracellularly (>10- to 200-fold), this group of antibiotics consequently has the prerequisite to interfere with eukaryotic cell activities. The molecular target for macrolides as tested with erythromycin seems to be the nuclear transcription factor NF-κB or a target upstream.[25] A common feature of the macrolides in in-vitro experimental systems is to inhibit production of proinflammatory cytokines, such as IL-6, TNF-α and IL-8. The effects by the macrolides are similar on epithelial and monocytic cells. Macrolides also interfere directly with eosinophils (i.e. inhibited IL-8 synthesis) and neutrophils (decreased superoxide anion production) suggesting that, together with available data on inhibitory effects on proinflammatory cytokines, macrolides may inhibit the inflammatory response on different levels.[26]

Tetracycline derivatives, and in particular doxycycline, have repeatedly been reported to interfere with the components of the immune system. For example, doxycycline inhibits proliferation of mitogen-activated peripheral blood lymphocytes,[6] and minocycline has been shown to decrease T-helper cell cytokines such as IL-2 and IFN-γ. The primary target for tetracyclines may be mitochondria as tetracyclines inhibit mitochondrial protein synthesis, leading to a reduced mitochondrial mass and consequently a decreased oxidative phosphorylation and energy supply.[27]

Fusidic acid at clinically achievable concentrations in low protein tissue culture suspension significantly inhibits mitogen-activated peripheral blood lymphocytes.[5] Nitrofurantoin also interferes with lymphocyte proliferation, whereas penicillins, cephalosporins, aminoglycosides and trimethoprim do not appear to exert any specific effects on lymphocyte immune functions.

Rifampicin modifies several aspects of the immune response;[1] it interferes with lymphocyte proliferation as demonstrated by a decreased thymidine incorporation,[6] and significantly prolongs graft survival up to 40% when examined in a split-heart allograft transplantation model. The mechanism responsible for this has not yet been thoroughly elucidated, but it is most likely that the drug inhibits the cellular immune response to the transplanted tissue. Interestingly, cytokine-activated monocytes incubated with rifampicin show an increased CD1b expression,[3] a phenomenon that might be beneficial in tuberculosis patients on rifampicin therapy since CD1b plays a role in presentation of non-peptide antigens.

Cephalosporins do not in general potentiate or modify the immune system. The results obtained in several studies on cefodizime are contradictory and the precise mechanisms have not yet been defined, although the effects of cefodizime have been summarized by Bergeron et al.[28] The drug has been reported to exert negative, neutral or positive effects on polymorphonuclear chemotaxis; to have no effect or positive effects on phagocytosis; to downregulate TNF-α, IL-1 and IL-6 released by stimulated human monocytes; to have no effect on IL-1 release; and to upregulate IL-8 release and GM-CSF from monocytes and bronchial epithelial cells, respectively. Ex vivo, cefodizime shows either neutral or positive effects on chemotaxis and phagocytosis. In vivo, cefodizime restores IL-1 and interferon production in immunocompromised hosts, and enhances phagocytosis and survival of mice infected with cefodizime-resistant pathogens. The drug decreases TNF-α synthesis and inflammation in mice infected by *Streptococcus pneumoniae*, whereas TNF-α production is increased in cefodizime-treated mice administered heat-killed *Klebsiella pneumoniae*.

CONCLUSION

Since the field of immunology expanded in the early 1980s, many studies have been performed in order to elucidate the effects of clinically useful antibiotics on different immune functions. Several antibiotics (e.g. certain fluoroquinolones, macrolides, tetracyclines and rifampicin) significantly interfere with the immune response; however, despite much effort, only a few of the precise mechanisms behind the immunomodulatory capacities have been elucidated. The term *biological response modifiers* has been coined for some drugs, but an antibiotic that is solely chosen for its immunomodulatory activity in lieu of others is not yet available. We are still awaiting drug derivatives with defined antibacterial activities in addition to well-clarified chemical structures that superinduce or inhibit specific immune functions. The field is still in its infancy; structural chemistry followed by high-throughput screening and modern molecular immunology should point us towards new drugs.

 References

1. Hauser WE, Remington JS. Effect of antibiotics on the immune response. *Am J Med.* 1982;72:711–716.
2. Milatovic D. Antibiotics and phagocytosis. *Eur J Clin Microbiol.* 1983;2:414–425.
3. Labro MT. Interference of antibacterial agents with phagocyte functions: immunomodulation or 'immuno-fairy tales'?. *Clin Microbiol Rev.* 2000;13:615–650.
4. Riesbeck K. Immunomodulating activity of quinolones: Review. *J Chemother.* 2002;14(1):3–12.
5. Dalhoff A, Shalit I. Immunomodulatory effects of quinolones. *Lancet Infect Dis.* 2003;3:359–371.
6. Forsgren A, Banck G, Beckman H, Bellahsène A. Antibiotic-host defence interactions in vitro and in vivo. *Scand J Infect Dis.* 1980;(suppl 24):195–203.
7. Uriarte SM, Molestina RE, Miller RD, et al. Effects of fluoroquinolones on the migration of human phagocytes through *Chlamydia pneumoniae*-infected and tumor necrosis factor alpha-stimulated endothelial cells. *Antimicrob Agents Chemother.* 2004;48(7):2538–2543.
8. Van Bambeke F, Barcia-Macay M, Lemaire S, Tulkens PM. Cellular pharmacodynamics and pharmacokinetics of antibiotics: current views and perspectives. *Curr Opin Drug Discov Devel.* 2006;9(2):218–230.
9. Tulkens PM. Intracellular distribution and activity of antibiotics. *Eur J Clin Microbiol Infect Dis.* 1991;10:100–106.
10. van den Broeck PJ. Antimicrobial drugs, microorganisms and phagocytes. *Rev Infect Dis.* 1989;11:213–245.
11. Nguyen HA, Denis O, Vergison A, Tulkens PM, Struelens MJ, Van Bambeke F. Intracellular activity of antibiotics in a model of human THP-1 macrophages infected by a *Staphylococcus aureus* small colony variant isolated from a cystic fibrosis patient: 2. Study of antibiotic combinations. *Antimicrob Agents Chemother.* 2009;53(4):1443–1449.
12. Gieffers J, Fullgraf H, Jahn J, et al. *Chlamydia pneumoniae* infection in circulating human monocytes is refractory to antibiotic treatment. *Circulation.* 2001;103:351–356. ·
13. Mandell GL, Coleman EJ. Activities of antimicrobial agents against intracellular pneumococci. *Antimicrob Agents Chemother.* 2000;44:2561–2563.
14. Gemmell CG, Lorian V. Effects of low concentrations of antibiotics on ultrastructure, virulence, and susceptibility to immunodefenses: clinical significance. In: Lorian V, ed. *Antibiotics in laboratory medicine.* Baltimore: Williams and Wilkins; 1996:397–452.
15. Gemmel CG, Ford CW. Virulence factor expression by Gram-positive cocci exposed to subinhibitory concentrations of linezolid. *J Antimicrob Chemother.* 2002;50:665–672.
16. Luchi M, Morrison DC, Opal S, et al. A comparative trial of imipenem versus ceftazidime in the release of endotoxin and cytokine generation in patients with gram-negative urosepsis. Urosepsis Study Group. *J Endotoxin Res.* 2000;6:25–31.
17. Goscinski G, Tano E, Löwdin E, Sjölin J. Propensity to release endotoxin after two repeated doses of cefuroxime in an in vitro kinetic model: higher release after the second dose. *J Antimicrob Chemother.* 2007;60:328–333.
18. Riesbeck K, Andersson J, Gullberg M, Forsgren A. Fluorinated 4-quinolones induce hyper-production of interleukin-2. *Proc Natl Acad Sci U S A.* 1989;86:2809–2813.
19. Riesbeck K, Forsgren A, Henriksson A, Bredberg A. Ciprofloxacin induces an immunomodulatory stress response in human T lymphocytes. *Antimicrob Agents Chemother.* 1998;42:1923–1930.
20. Shalit I. Immunological aspects of new quinolones. *Eur J Clin Microbiol Infect Dis.* 1991;10:262–266.
21. Eriksson E, Forsgren A, Riesbeck K. Several gene programs are induced in ciprofloxacin-treated human lymphocytes as revealed by microarray analysis. *J Leukoc Biol.* 2003;74:456–463.
22. Galley HF, Nelson SJ, Dubbels AM, Webster NR. Effect of ciprofloxacin on the accumulation of interleukin-6, interleukin-8, and nitrite from a human endothelial cell model of sepsis. *Crit Care Med.* 1997;25:1392–1395.
23. Fabian I, Reuveni D, Levitov A, Halperin D, Priel E, Shalit I. Moxifloxacin enhances antiproliferative and apoptotic effects of etoposide but inhibits its proinflammatory effects in THP-1 and Jurkat cells. *Br J Cancer.* 2006;95:1038–1046.
24. Khan AA, Slifer TR, Araujo FG, Suzuki Y, Remington JS. Protection against lipopolysaccharide-induced death by fluoroquinolones. *Antimicrob Agents Chemother.* 2000;44:3169–3173.
25. Aoki Y, Kao PN. Erythromycin inhibits transcriptional activation of NF-kappaB, but not NFAT, through calcineurin-independent signaling in T cells. *Antimicrob Agents Chemother.* 1999;43:2678–2684.
26. Amsden GW. Anti-inflammatory effects of macrolides – an under-appreciated benefit in the treatment of community acquired respiratory tract infections and chronic inflammatory pulmonary condition? *J Antimicrob Chemother.* 2005;55:10–21.
27. Riesbeck K, Bredberg A, Forsgren A. Ciprofloxacin does not inhibit mitochondrial functions but other antibiotics do. *Antimicrob Agents Chemother.* 1990;34:167–169.
28. Bergeron Y, Deslauriers AM, Ouellet N, Gauthier MC, Bergeron MG. Influence of cefodizime on pulmonary inflammatory response to heat-killed *Klebsiella pneumoniae* in mice. *Antimicrob Agents Chemother.* 1999;43:2291–2294.

8 General principles of antimicrobial chemotherapy

Roger G. Finch

Antimicrobial agents have had a major impact on the practice of medicine for almost three-quarters of a century. They remain life-saving for many severe infections, such as meningitis, pneumonia and bloodstream infections. However, their use has also controlled many non-life-threatening infections, for example, those affecting the skin, respiratory and urinary tracts, thereby alleviating suffering and controlling the social and economic impact of infectious disease.

Their widespread use in surgical prophylaxis (*see* Ch. 10) has greatly reduced the infectious complications of surgical operations and made possible transplant surgery and the treatment of malignant disease, notably those requiring profound immunosuppression and cytotoxic chemotherapy for their control.

The very success of antibiotics has led to their widespread use and, indeed, misuse through overprescribing, prolonged treatment courses and for unproven indications. This, in part, has been due to the general acceptance by the public and prescribing professionals of the benefits and relative safety of these agents. Indeed, in many countries, antibiotics may be purchased without prescription from pharmacy stores, thereby adding further to their use.

Among therapeutic agents, antimicrobial drugs have several unique properties. Their use is not directed at particular host-derived disease or pathological processes, but at an infecting micro-organism(s). In general, they are used for short periods (single dose to a few days) rather than for prolonged periods of time as with many other drugs. However, of greater importance is their vulnerability to antimicrobial resistance mechanisms as a result of genetic mutation among target pathogens. Such resistance mechanisms are not only diverse, complex and continuously increasing, but also are readily transmitted both vertically and horizontally among bacterial species and across genera.

This continuous erosion of efficacy through drug resistance has been of professional concern for many years. More recently it has entered the public domain and given rise to political concern. Many countries have introduced a variety of initiatives which are attempting to stem the tide of drug resistance and encourage the development of new agents.

The clinical impact of drug resistance has been to steadily limit therapeutic choice and modify recommendations for managing many common infections (Table 8.1). More recently, multidrug-resistant pathogens have emerged and spread locally, nationally and, in some cases, globally. Reports of formerly sensitive, but now 'untreatable' pathogens are beginning to emerge.

Table 8.1 Impact of antibiotic resistance on prescribing choice

Target organisms	Agents formerly reliably active but for which sensitivity testing is now required
Staphylococcus aureus	Penicillin, methicillin, mupirocin
Streptococcus pneumoniae	Penicillin, tetracycline, erythromycin
Streptococcus pyogenes	Erythromycin, tetracycline
Enterococci	Ampicillin, teicoplanin, vancomycin
Neisseria gonorrhoeae	Penicillin, tetracycline, ciprofloxacin, cephalosporins
Neisseria meningitidis	Sulfonamides
Haemophilus influenzae	Ampicillin, chloramphenicol
Enterobacteriaceae	Ampicillin, cephalosporins, trimethoprim, ciprofloxacin
Salmonella spp.	Ampicillin, sulfonamides, chloramphenicol, ciprofloxacin
Shigella spp.	Ampicillin, tetracycline, sulfonamides
Pseudomonas aeruginosa	Gentamicin, ceftazidime

Drug resistance is by no means exclusive to bacteria. In the few years in which effective chemotherapy has become available to treat HIV infection, drug resistance (phenotypic as well as genotypic) has been the major reason for disease progression. Among fungi, primary and acquired resistance to azole antifungals is increasingly recognized, particularly among *Candida* spp. Worldwide resistance of *Plasmodium falciparum* to chloroquine and other drugs is a major cause of failure of therapeutic and prophylactic control of malaria.

For all the above reasons, a set of prescribing principles has evolved to guide prescribing practice of antimicrobial drugs in the management of infectious disease.[1] The basis for these principles is not only to ensure effective and safe management of infection, but also to reduce the risk of drug resistance emerging. Antibiotic prescribing can also have an ecological impact that may not only affect the recipient of the medication but also has the potential to spread either locally (within the hospital) or more widely in the community. International travel has added a global dimension to such dissemination.

THE PRINCIPLES OF ANITMICROBIAL PRESCRIBING

DEFINING THE TARGET INFECTION

Fundamental to all antimicrobial prescribing is the need to establish the presence and nature of a particular target infection and to decide whether it is an antibiotic responsive or non-responsive condition. Ideally, such a diagnosis should be supported by microbiological evidence that confirms the nature of the infection. This is only possible where there is ready access to laboratory facilities as in hospital practice, or where reliable near-patient testing is available.

Very few infectious diseases present clinically in a manner that is pathognomonic and for which the microbiological diagnosis can be inferred. Examples include erysipelas caused by *Streptococcus pyogenes*, meningococcal septicemia with rash (*Neisseria meningitidis*) and varicella complicated by a primary pneumonia. The majority of infections do not permit such accurate diagnosis. Syndromes such as pneumonia, meningitis and pyelonephritis are the result of infection by diverse organisms. Microbiological investigations are of limited value in defining a microbial etiology. Initial management, where early microbiological information is unavailable or laboratory facilities do not exist, must therefore be based on a clinical assessment and a presumptive consideration of the likely or possible causal organisms. Such empirical prescribing governs the majority of infections managed in primary care and also reflects the initial management of infectious conditions admitted to hospital, especially where these are life-threatening.

ANTIBIOTIC SELECTION

Knowledge of the likely pathogens responsible for a particular target disease (e.g. urinary tract infection, meningitis, community-acquired pneumonia) is important in making an appropriate choice of agent. This can be greatly enhanced when it is based on local knowledge of the usual repertoire of pathogens and their current susceptibility to therapeutic agents.

Dosage regimens for specific indications are based on clinical trial data, accumulated experience and appropriate dose modification for the patient's age and, where relevant, excretory organ dysfunction, in order to reduce the risk from toxic effects. Dose adjustment may be necessary for pathogens causing 'site protected infections', such as pneumococcal meningitis for which much higher doses of penicillin G are required to produce therapeutic concentrations in the cerebrospinal fluid in comparison with the dosage regimen to treat pneumococcal pneumonia.

Antimicrobial agents, like other drugs, are bound to circulating plasma proteins, mostly albumen. Although microbiologically inactive in the bound state, there is rapid dissociation to the unbound state at the site of infection. The degree of protein binding varies widely, being high for flucloxacillin

(95%) and less marked for ciprofloxacin (30%) and amoxicillin (20%). Highly protein bound agents can perform less satisfactorily against pathogens of borderline susceptibility or in situations where drug concentrations at the site of infection are marginal. In general, the degree of protein binding has little impact on the treatment of infections.

PHARMACOKINETIC AND PHARMACODYNAMIC CONSIDERATIONS

In the past decade or so, pharmacokinetic/pharmacodynamic (PK/PD) modeling, which is derived from the pharmacokinetic behavior of a drug in comparison with the susceptibility of particular target pathogens, has had a major impact on dosage selection, dosage intervals and, more recently, in providing supporting evidence of clinical efficacy. This PK/PD approach plays a major part in new drug development and has been applied not only to antibacterial agents, but also to antiretroviral and antifungal drugs. In some instances, data from such PK/PD modeling have resulted in modification of dosage regimens post-licensing (*see* Ch. 4). PK/PD modeling has also been investigated for its ability to guide dosage regimens less likely to result in the emergence of drug resistance, by defining the 'mutant preventing concentration' of an agent.

ROUTE OF ADMINISTRATION

Antimicrobial agents can be administered systemically (parenterally or orally) or topically to the skin, eyes and external auditory meati. Other routes include aerosol administration to the lungs in the treatment of lower respiratory tract infections complicating cystic fibrosis and, very rarely, intrathecally or intraventricularly in the specialist management of central nervous system (CNS) infections. In the latter situation, the risk of drug toxicity is considerable and requires particular caution in dose selection and drug administration and, in general, is best avoided.

Drugs with high degrees of bioavailability, such as the fluoroquinolones, produce therapeutic blood and tissue concentrations following oral administration such that parenteral use can often be avoided. This approach is less costly, avoids the complications of vascular access and also supports early step-down therapy from intravenous to oral administration.

DURATION OF TREATMENT

The duration of therapy is poorly defined for many target diseases and is in general based on custom and practice and licensed data. For some diseases, the duration of treatment has been determined scientifically – for example, standard 6-month regimens of combination therapy in the treatment of pulmonary tuberculosis. Another example is the treatment of streptococcal endocarditis, where the species and, more particularly, the in-vitro susceptibility of the target pathogen, permit short-course therapy (2–4 weeks) for highly sensitive viridans streptococci and prolonged courses (6 weeks) for less susceptible strains, notably enterococcal species.

For many common infections, the licensed duration of treatment has often been 1–2 weeks. In recent years and increasingly based on clinical trial data, 5–7 days is widely accepted for a variety of uncomplicated diseases, including lower respiratory tract infections. Likewise, uncomplicated urinary tract infections generally respond to 3 days' treatment. Many of the clinical features of infection are the result of the host inflammatory response, which often takes a few days to subside after the infecting micro-organism is eliminated. Short-course therapy has much to commend it in terms of compliance, lowered ecological impact, adverse drug effects and cost.

ADVERSE DRUG REACTIONS

No drug is free from side effects. Good prescribing practice must balance the potential benefits of treatment against the known repertoire of adverse effects and likelihood of these occurring in a particular patient. Some are predictable, while others are not. Drug hypersensitivity is particularly common with some agents, notably the β-lactams. Hence it is always important to enquire after any previous adverse reaction from past drug exposure. The known cross-hypersensitivity between the penicillins and cephalosporins precludes substitution of the latter, where an accelerated hypersensitivity reaction (anaphylaxis) has occurred. In contrast, the cautious use of a cephalosporin is often possible where the previous reaction to penicillin was that of delayed hypersensitivity.

Dose-related toxicity is a particular issue for agents dependent upon renal excretion. Where renal function is impaired, drug accumulation can arise. The most notable example is in the use of the aminoglycosides. Dose-related nephrotoxicity and ototoxicity are issues that require constant vigilance and careful monitoring. Therapeutic drug monitoring of gentamicin by timed assays has greatly increased safety in use by ensuring therapeutic, non-toxic serum concentrations linked to careful dose adjustment.

PLACE OF SINGLE AND COMBINED DRUG THERAPY

Whenever possible, single-agent therapy is preferred and is widely adopted in the management of community infections. It has the advantage of simplicity, cost, limits the risks of drug interactions and restricts the risk of adverse reactions to those of the single agent.

Combining agents has benefits in selected patients – for example, in the severely ill septic patient where prompt empirical treatment is necessary. This is usually in response to infections for which a range of pathogens may be responsible,

notably intra-abdominal or lower respiratory tract infections. Combined drug regimens ensure that the potential range of organisms is effectively covered whilst awaiting microbiological confirmation as to the nature of the infection. Once obtained, treatment can often be adjusted to a single agent. Recommendations and evidence-based guidelines now support the management of specific infections with combined drug therapy in the severely affected. The initial empirical management of severe community-acquired pneumonia is one such condition.

In the treatment of tuberculosis, HIV and malaria, combination therapy is now the standard approach but for another reason, namely to limit the risk of selecting drug-resistant strains. In the case of tuberculosis, low frequency primary drug resistance to isoniazid or rifampicin (rifampin) is an ever-present risk. By using combination treatment (e.g. isoniazid plus rifampicin plus ethambutol/pyrazinamide) as the initial regimen, the selection and emergence of drug-resistant disease is greatly limited.

BACTERICIDAL VERSUS BACTERISTATIC PROPERTIES

Another issue of importance in treating infection in severely immunocompromised patients is the need to select a bactericidal drug regimen. This is of particular importance in profoundly neutropenic patients, such as transplant recipients and those receiving cytotoxic chemotherapy for malignant disease. Regimens based on bactericidal agents such as the β-lactams and aminoglycosides are used in preference to bacteristatic agents, notably tetracyclines and antifolate drugs, which rely on an intact phagocytic cell system to eliminate the pathogens. Another example is the use of bactericidal regimens when treating bacterial endocarditis, since the target pathogens are embedded within the cardiac vegetations which is, in essence, an immunologically protected site into which phagocytic cells penetrate poorly.

PROPHYLACTIC USE

Antibiotics have been used extensively in surgical practice to prevent postoperative wound infections. Such prophylactic use has resulted in significant reductions in infectious morbidity and mortality complicating a range of operative procedures (*see* Ch. 10). For example, the infectious complications of colectomy have been reduced from approximately 40% to 5%. Implant surgery has also benefited, notably joint replacement and cardiac valve surgery.

The rationale for selection of a particular drug regimen for prophylactic use is based on the known risk of an infectious complication, predictable and normally susceptible target organism(s), and a regimen that has been shown to be safe and well tolerated. The latter is important in practice since prophylaxis will be administered to large numbers of patients, for some of whom the risk of infection will be absent. By limiting such prophylaxis to short-course (usually single dose) perioperative use, concerns over adverse reactions, drug resistance and superinfections are greatly reduced.

Antibiotic prophylaxis also has applications in medical practice to prevent infection in at-risk individuals or, in the case of transmissible infections, to reduce spread to close contacts. For example, those with anatomical or functional asplenia are vulnerable to severe sepsis by *Str. pneumoniae* and other pathogens. Long-term penicillin (erythromycin for those hypersensitive to penicillin) is recommended, especially for those under the age of 16 years. Likewise, rifampicin, ceftriaxone or ciprofloxacin as single dose or short-course therapy is given to close contacts of patients with meningococcal meningitis or septicemia to prevent secondary cases.

FAILURE OF ANTIBIOTIC THERAPY

Despite adhering to the above principles of prescribing, some infections fail to respond to treatment. Hence, it is important to monitor progress in an individual patient.

Failure to respond to antibiotic treatment may be the result of a variety of factors. The nature of the original diagnosis may have been incorrect or may have been more complex than originally conceived (e.g. cellulitis complicated by underlying osteomyelitis). The microbiological nature of the infection should also be reassessed – for example, an atypical pneumonia unresponsive to β-lactams, or a mixed aerobic/anaerobic intra-abdominal infection, while drug-resistant pathogens are increasingly recognized.

Other important causes of failure of treatment include infection related to implanted medical devices (e.g. intravascular catheters), prosthetic devices and retained surgical sutures or pus that requires drainage. Micro-organisms adhere to foreign materials, form biofilms and are then relatively protected from conventional antibiotic therapy. Likewise, antibiotics may be either inactivated or fail to penetrate collections of purulent material which require incision and drainage for their resolution.

THE ROLE OF THE LABORATORY IN DIAGNOSIS AND TREATMENT

In clinical practice it is often impossible to determine the identity let alone the drug susceptibility of the causal agent, hence the importance of sound microbiological practice and good communication between the clinician and the laboratory. Nevertheless, even where laboratory services are not available, by employing the principles of antibiotic use it is often possible to make a logical and successful choice of agent. Laboratory investigations range from simple to sophisticated fully automated methods. Much valuable rapid diagnostic information can be gleaned from reliably performed Gram stains and Ziehl–Neelsen stains of cerebrospinal fluid (CSF) or pus, as well as microscopic analysis of urine and CSF.

It is important that all relevant specimens be collected before treatment is started (an occasional exception is the need sometimes to begin treatment in acute meningitis before lumbar puncture is done) and that these be handled properly and expeditiously. The responsibility for this stage in diagnosis, falling as it does between clinician and laboratory, may, if badly executed, result in missed opportunities for diagnosis. The proper collection, handling and examination of specimens in the diagnosis and management of infection are paramount.

Culture-based laboratory methods remain important in the management of bacterial infections. The growth, isolation and subsequent identification of the pathogen(s) from a clinical specimen add precision to the clinical diagnosis and furthermore guide therapeutic management as a result of antibiotic susceptibility testing. This is of increasing importance as drug-resistant pathogens become dominant and is of particular importance in the management of infections caused by methicillin-resistant *Staphylococcus aureus* (MRSA) and other staphylococci, glycopeptide-resistant enterococci and multidrug-resistant Enterobacteriaceae, *Acinetobacter* and *Pseudomonas* spp. Such pathogens are increasingly isolated from hospitalized patients in high dependency and transplant units.

Drug resistance is no longer restricted to bacteria and is increasing among fungi (notably *Candida* spp. to antifungals) and viruses where it has had a major impact on the management of HIV/AIDS with antiretroviral drugs. Laboratory testing for susceptibility to such agents is of increasing importance.

The occasional consequences of antibiotic use also include the selection of fungi and *C. difficile* which in turn may result in secondary infection. Here, laboratory investigations are key to their recognition and management.

ANTIBIOTIC FORMULARIES AND POLICIES (SEE CH. 11)

Antibiotic formularies are in widespread use. In their simplest form they are a listing of the classes and drugs available or licensed. These may be produced locally (to indicate what agents are stocked), nationally (e.g. *British National Formulary*) or internationally as, for example, the World Health Organization's *Model Lists of Essential Medicines*.[2] Formularies increasingly contain guidance on the indications, dosage regimens, adverse drug reactions and other information linked to usage.

In order to support good prescribing practice, avoid unnecessary use and to counter the threat from antibiotic resistance, prescribing guidance has evolved into policies with increasing levels of prescribing support and audit. Again, these may be developed locally, by institutional Drug and Therapeutics Committees or their equivalent, or be developed nationally. These increasingly provide detailed prescribing recommendations for specific diseases and conditions. Such recommendations are increasingly based on guidance derived from an evidence-based assessment of published studies for specific target diseases. They may be produced by professional societies, international collaborations of experts and national agencies, such as the National Institute of Health and Clinical Excellence (NICE) in the UK.

Antibiotic prescribing is increasingly subject to monitoring and audit. Antibiotic usage data collection varies in sophistication from a simple quantitative assessment of drug purchased or prescribed, to more detailed monitoring of primary care prescriptions as in the UK; this identifies prescribing patterns by individual practices or practitioners. International comparisons of prescribing rates are published annually by the European Surveillance of Antimicrobial Consumption,[3] where the unit of prescribing is based on the defined daily dose (DDD) per 1000 inhabitants. Such surveillance systems are helpful in informing local and, indeed, national strategies to improve or modify prescribing practice. However, they fail to provide day-to-day support for the prescriber. Here, online IT systems are essential – but not universally available. By linking prescribing to the medical record and patient-specific laboratory information, a much more sophisticated support system can be created. Prescribing guidance by diagnosis can also support good clinical practice and permits audit of a variety of management and clinical outcomes.

 ## References

1. Finch R. Antimicrobial therapy: principles of use. *Medicine.* 2009;37(10):545–550.
2. World Health Organization. *Model Lists of Essential Medicines.* 15th ed. WHO, Geneva. Online. Available at http://www.who.int/medicines/publications/essentialmedicines/en/; 2007.
3. *European Surveillance of Antimicrobial Consumption.* Online. Available at http://app.esac.ua.ac.be/public.

9 Laboratory control of antimicrobial therapy

Gunnar Kahlmeter and Derek Brown

Most antimicrobial therapy is empirical. However, empirical therapy is based on scientific evaluation of the outcome of clinical trials in which the results of drug therapy have been related to laboratory tests of the antimicrobial susceptibility of the causative micro-organisms and on clinical experience built up during the years following registration of a new antibiotic. The scientific proof of the effectiveness of a drug against certain micro-organisms in specific clinical situations is usually based on results with micro-organisms that lack resistance mechanisms because acquired or mutational resistance (i.e. resistance caused by a genetic alteration) is rare when the drug is new or because organisms with resistance to the drug are excluded by the clinical trials protocol. If factors determining therapeutic success (indications for therapy, drug formulation and dosing, target micro-organisms and antimicrobial susceptibility of target micro-organisms) were constant over time, antimicrobial susceptibility testing in the routine microbiological laboratory would be unnecessary. However, due to the worldwide rapid increase in antimicrobial resistance, empirical therapy becomes more and more uncertain and the foundation for empirical therapy needs constant re-evaluation. Due to sometimes major local differences in the occurrence of resistance, this re-evaluation has to be based on local resistance frequencies.

WHY SUSCEPTIBILITY TESTING?

Susceptibility testing is performed:

- to predict the outcome of antimicrobial chemotherapy in individual patients, i.e. as an instrument for directing antimicrobial chemotherapy;
- to predict the outcome of antimicrobial chemotherapy in future patients, i.e. for continuous evaluation of the basis for empirical therapy;
- to permit epidemiological intervention through:
  - the early detection of bacteria with certain resistance mechanisms in the hospital, e.g. methicillin-resistant *Staphylococcus aureus* (MRSA), glycopeptide non-susceptible enterococci or staphylococci, extended spectrum β-lactamase

(ESBL)-producing Gram-negative bacteria, and in the community, e.g. multiresistant *Mycobacterium tuberculosis*, multiresistant *Salmonella enterica* serotype Typhimurium, penicillin and multiresistant *Streptococcus pneumoniae*;
  - the early detection of trends in resistance frequencies and the identification of factors affecting the dynamics of such trends, such as consumption of antibiotics, infection control, associated resistance to other antibiotics or other substances, overcrowded conditions in hospitals and in society at large, etc.

Knowledge obtained in this way forms the basis for national and local antibiotic policies and interventions, and affects national and international legislation (e.g. the prohibition of the use of some antimicrobials as growth promoters in animal husbandry).

THE CATEGORIZATION OF ANTIMICROBIAL SUSCEPTIBILITY

The antimicrobial susceptibility of bacteria and fungi is traditionally categorized with the letters S for *Susceptible* or *Sensitive*, I for *Intermediate* or *Indeterminate* and R for *Resistant*. There is some variation in the definitions of the different categories of susceptibility which can lead to confusion, particularly with the intermediate category. The International Organization for Standardization (ISO)[1] has defined susceptibility categories as follows:

- *Susceptible*: A bacterial strain inhibited in vitro by a concentration of an antimicrobial agent that is associated with a high likelihood of therapeutic success.
- *Resistant*: A bacterial strain inhibited in vitro by a concentration of an antimicrobial agent that is associated with a high likelihood of therapeutic failure.
- *Intermediate*: A bacterial strain inhibited in vitro by a concentration of an antimicrobial agent that is associated with uncertain therapeutic effect.

The 'uncertain effect' in the intermediate category implies that an infection due to the isolate can be appropriately treated in body sites where the drugs are physiologically concentrated (e.g. lower urinary tract) or when a high dosage of drug can be used. It may be taken as a signal from the microbiologist to the clinician that the bacterium is now compromised (i.e. has acquired some degree of resistance) and that the interpretation is difficult in the individual patient and/or that a higher dosage than that normally used may be required. There is also a long tradition for breakpoint committees to use the I category as a 'buffer zone' to prevent small, uncontrolled technical factors from causing major discrepancies in interpretation of in-vitro tests.

Differences in breakpoints recommended by different national or international breakpoint committees can be significant. For example, a comparison of breakpoints from the European Committee on Antimicrobial Susceptibility Testing (EUCAST; http://www.eucast.org) and the USA Clinical and Laboratory Standards Institute (CLSI; http://www.clsi.org) shows that, of 36 breakpoints for drugs used to treat infections caused by Enterobacteriaceae, not a single set of breakpoints (S/R) is currently the same. The corresponding numbers for staphylococci are 4/31, streptococci 2/25, *Str. pneumoniae* 3/29, enterococci 0/14, *Haemophilus influenzae* 0/27, *Pseudomonas* 1/18 and *Acinetobacter* 1/11. Some of the differences in minimum inhibitory concentration (MIC) breakpoints are quite pronounced and should be resolved.

A useful supplement to the classic clinical definitions of susceptibility categories was the introduction by EUCAST of the 'epidemiological MIC cut-off values' (or 'microbiological breakpoints') designed to delineate the 'wild type' of each species and to provide a means of early detection and sensitive quantitative description of the emergence of resistance. Clinical breakpoints should be based on the correlation between MICs and clinical outcome of therapy, where doses and duration of therapy are selected on the basis of pharmacological and pharmacodynamic data. The epidemiological cut-off values should be based on the correlation between MICs and the presence and absence of resistance mechanisms to the drug, or class of drug, in question. Epidemiological breakpoints can be used for epidemiological surveillance, for determining factors important for resistance development, and for planning and measuring the effects of interventions to counteract resistance development.

DETECTION OF ANTIMICROBIAL RESISTANCE

The detection of resistance can be phenotypic or genotypic. Phenotypic methods include disk diffusion and automated systems, which are in some way related to the MIC of the organism, and methods detecting a resistance mechanism, such as the detection of β-lactamases or of PBP 2a (indicating methicillin resistance in staphylococci). Genotypic methods detect a defined gene(s), such as *mecA* coding for methicillin

resistance in staphylococci or the *van* genes coding for glycopeptide resistance in enterococci. Genotypic tests tend to be 'either/or', i.e. if positive, the organism is considered resistant to the drug or class of drug. All susceptibility tests require both methodological standardization to ensure reproducibility and appropriate interpretive criteria to ensure that results are clinically or epidemiologically meaningful.

THE MINIMUM INHIBITORY CONCENTRATION (MIC)

In MIC tests the micro-organisms are subjected to a range of antibiotic concentrations, conventionally two-fold, in solid or liquid medium, in a defined atmosphere, at a defined temperature and for a defined period of time. The macroscopic inhibition of growth is measured as the absence or near absence of growth on a solid medium or as the absence of turbidity in a liquid medium. The MIC is defined as the lowest concentration which clearly inhibits the growth of the micro-organisms. The MIC is traditionally the antimicrobial susceptibility testing standard against which other methods are assessed. Performance of the methods is affected by technical factors including medium, additives, pH, ion content, incubation time, temperature, atmosphere, etc. Hence methods need to be standardized.

 ## BREAKPOINT METHODS

Most models for susceptibility testing use two MIC breakpoints to divide bacteria into the three susceptibility categories S, I and R defined above. In some susceptibility testing techniques only the breakpoint concentrations are incorporated in solid or liquid media, in which case only two plates or two tubes/microdilution plate wells are needed. Growth at neither the low nor the high concentration indicates that the organism is susceptible, growth at the lower but not the higher concentration indicates intermediate susceptibility and growth at both concentrations is interpreted as resistance. Breakpoint methods are more difficult to control than full MIC determinations or agar disk diffusion because MIC values for control strains are often not close to tested concentrations. Hence the controls may fail to detect significant changes in test concentrations.

 ## AUTOMATED SYSTEMS

A number of automated or semi-automated systems on the market utilize the breakpoint principle, some including additional dilutions around the breakpoints. With additional dilutions a restricted range MIC value for the isolate can be given, together with the corresponding interpretation. With the one- or two-concentration breakpoint system only the interpretation is given. Automated systems are widely used and have some advantages over manual systems in the standardization of methodology, labor saving and data handling.

 ## GRADIENT METHODS

Gradient methods such as the Etest® (BioMérieux) or MICE® (Oxoid) are a variation on MIC determination. A series of two-fold dilutions of an antibiotic are incorporated on a plastic carrier strip from which the antibiotic diffuses freely into the agar, creating a diffusion gradient along the length of the strip. After incubation overnight, the MIC is read as the point where the growth inhibition ellipse intersects the MIC scale on the strip. Recommendations are provided by the manufacturers for standardization of the inoculum, type of medium to be used for different organisms and reading of the tests. Gradient tests have brought MIC determination to those clinical laboratories that did not previously have the facilities or expertise to do the rather elaborate work needed to set up a standard MIC test in solid or liquid medium.

 ## AGAR DISK DIFFUSION

The diameter of the zone of growth inhibition which forms during incubation of the agar plate constitutes a measure of the susceptibility of the bacterium to the antibiotic. Zone diameters are traditionally correlated with MICs through a regression analysis performed on the parallel MIC and disk diffusion test results obtained with collections of isolates with a range of susceptibilities. The MIC breakpoints are then transformed into corresponding zone diameter breakpoints through the regression line. In the classic Kirby–Bauer[2] and Ericsson and Sherris[3] regression analyses, a collection of bacteria was analyzed in a regression analysis involving many different species and all species received common MIC and zone diameter breakpoints. To be able to characterize the slope of the regression line, it is often necessary to include species inherently insensitive to the drug, which may be poorly representative of bacteria with acquired resistance. Thus, multi-species regression lines may not reflect the relationship between MIC and zone diameter for future isolates with acquired resistance and may not be valid for some species. Species-related zone diameter breakpoints are now usually set in line with species-related MIC breakpoints, and zone diameter breakpoints are more commonly set by adjusting breakpoints so that errors in reporting are as low as possible (the 'error-minimization' approach).

Disk diffusion methods are versatile, economic and remain the most widely used approach to routine susceptibility testing in many countries. The Kirby–Bauer method[2] is the basis of the recommendations of the CLSI in the USA, with Mueller–Hinton agar as the only approved medium and an inoculum of confluent growth. Standardized methods in Europe have been based on the recommendations in the Ericsson and Sherris[3] International Collaborative Study (ICS) report, with either Mueller–Hinton agar or other defined media and semi-confluent inoculum, with which it is easier to see when the correct inoculum is not obtained.

Agar disk diffusion as a screening test

In situations where resistance is rare but clinically or epidemiologically important, and provided the zone diameter breakpoints are specific to the species and set very close to the wild-type population, a standard disk diffusion test can be used as a test to screen for suspicious isolates for further testing (e.g. methicillin resistance in *Staph. aureus*, penicillin resistance in *Str. pneumoniae*, fluoroquinolone resistance in Enterobacteriaceae). In some cases the next step is a confirmatory test such as a polymerase chain reaction (PCR) test for the detection of the specific gene responsible for a known resistance mechanism (e.g. *mecA* gene indicating methicillin resistance in staphylococci). In other cases a follow-up MIC test provides a means for laboratories to define more closely the degree of reduced susceptibility (e.g. *Str. pneumoniae* with penicillin).

 ## MIC AND ZONE DIAMETER BREAKPOINTS

To decide on national MIC and zone diameter breakpoints, and in some instances to describe national methods and standards for susceptibility testing, several countries have breakpoint committees or antibiotic reference groups (*see below*) consisting of clinical microbiologists and infectious disease specialists, and sometimes pediatricians, general practitioners, clinical pharmacologists and representatives of the pharmaceutical industries. Several of these groups in Europe have combined and harmonized their breakpoints as part of the European Committee on Antimicrobial Susceptibility Testing (EUCAST).

The MIC and zone diameter breakpoints published during the 1960s and 1970s were, with a few exceptions (*Neisseria gonorrhoeae*, *M. tuberculosis*), common for all bacterial species and for all clinical situations. The Swedish Reference Group for Antibiotics (SRGA) was first systematically to collect large species-defined parallel databases of MIC values and zone diameter distributions for bacteria lacking resistance mechanisms. Their original database of MIC and disk diffusion zone diameter distributions was later enlarged considerably under the auspices of EUCAST and is now in the public domain on the internet: http://www.eucast.org. The database now consists of over 20 000 MIC distributions and some distributions include as many as 120 000 MIC values. The collated distributions include contributions from many sources, including individual investigators, resistance surveillance programs and companies from all over the world. The species-defined database underlined two particular points:

- Unimodal distributions of MICs or zone diameters for any organism with a particular antibiotic were identical irrespective of where in the world and when the isolates were collected, and in non-unimodal distributions only that part of the wild-type distribution consisting of non-wild-type strains was affected (Figure 9.1). Furthermore, it was evident that distributions of MICs or inhibition zone diameter values for a species were identical

irrespective of whether the isolates were from humans or animals. This is illustrated for tigecycline in *Escherichia coli* in Figure 9.2.[7] Distributions based on isolates from different individuals and on data from repeat testing of the same isolate were very similar (Figure 9.2), indicating limited biological variation among wild-type individuals of a species in their susceptibility to an antimicrobial agent.

- Breakpoints common to all species often failed in one of two principal ways. Either the breakpoints would divide biologically homogenous populations of a species in such

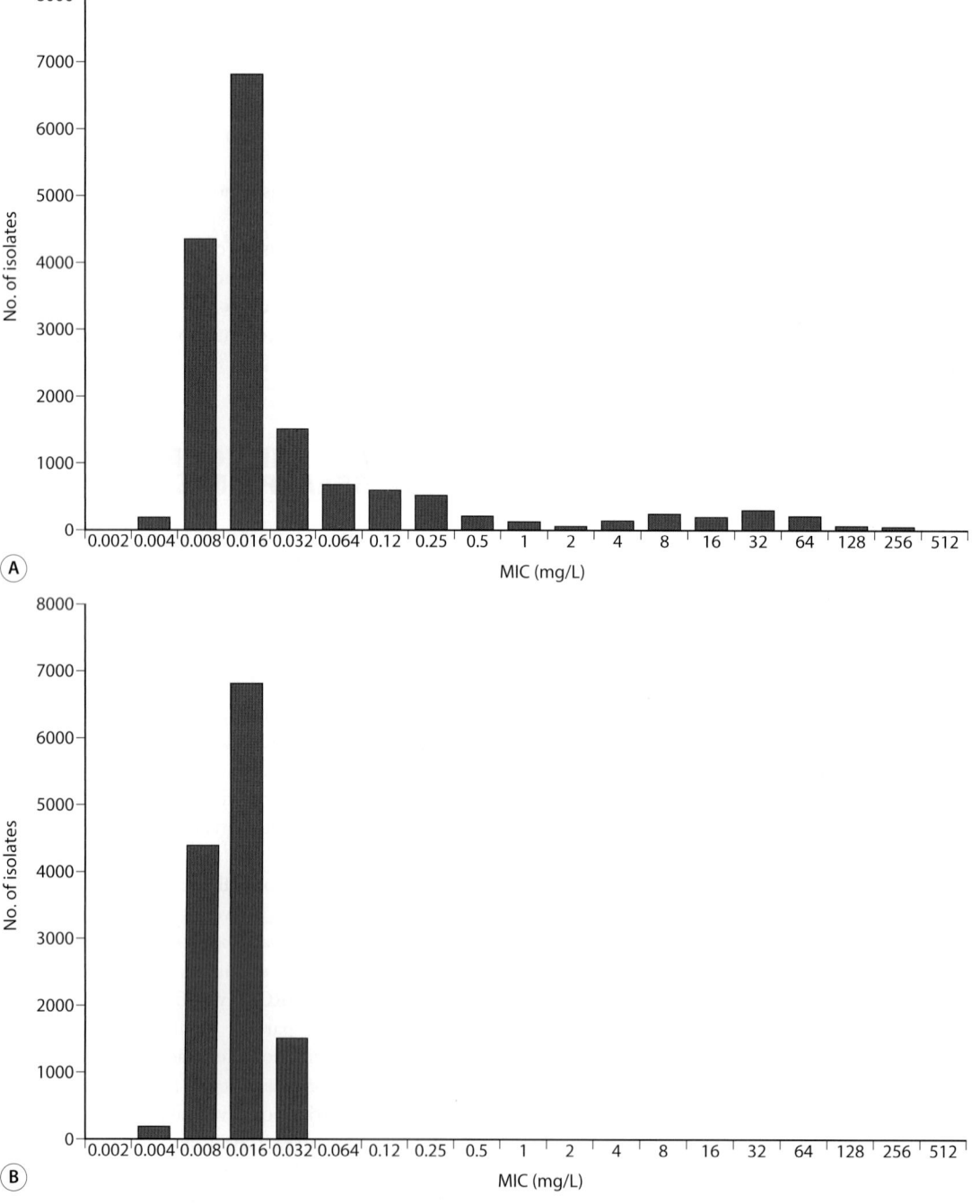

Fig. 9.1 *Escherichia coli* ciprofloxacin MIC (mg/L) distributions from the EUCAST website (http://www.eucast.org) where graph A shows all available data on 16 247 isolates from 81 data sources and graph B shows data on the 12 836 isolates (same data sources) considered devoid of fluoroquinolone resistance mechanisms. The highest MIC value for isolates devoid of resistance mechanisms has been designated by EUCAST the 'epidemiological cut-off value' or ECOFF (for *Esch. coli* against ciprofloxacin, the ECOFF is 0.032 mg/L).

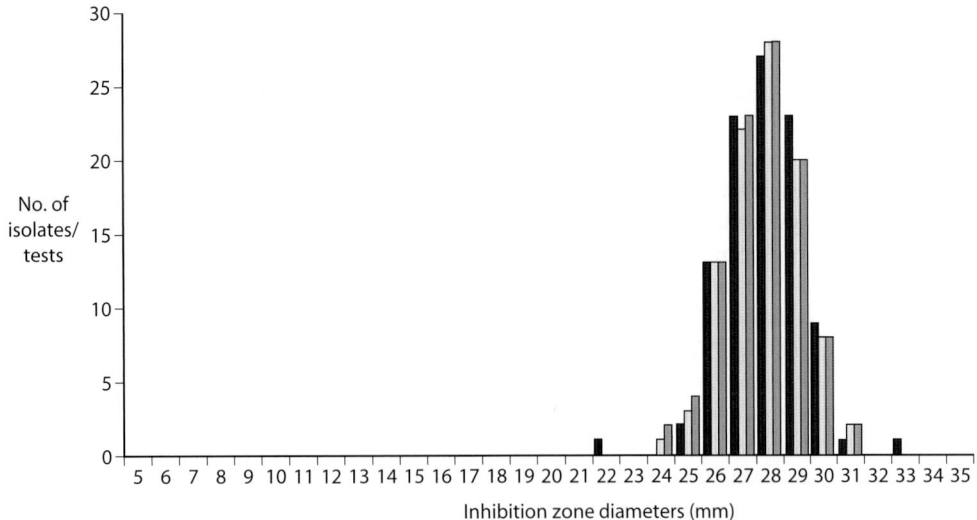

Fig. 9.2 Tigecycline activity (inhibition zone diameters in disk diffusion testing on Mueller–Hinton agar) against *Escherichia coli* from human bloodstream infections (100 consecutive patient isolates, black bars), the gut of 99 arctic non-migrating gulls from three widely separate arctic areas (white bars) and against type strain *Esch. coli* ATCC 25922 (repeat testing of the same strain; gray bars). (Adapted from Sjölund M, Bengtsson S, Bonnedahl J, Hernandez J, Olsen B, Kahlmeter G. **Clin Microbiol Infect.** 2009;15(5):461–465. Epub 2009 Mar 2, with permission from Wiley.[7])

a way that organisms without biological difference in their relationship to the drug in question would be classified as being different (this is not only unhelpful from a clinical point of view but also detrimental to the reproducibility of susceptibility results) or, because the drug was very active against a certain species (e.g. fluoroquinolones and *Neisseria* or *Haemophilus* spp.), the common breakpoint was so generous that resistance development would go undetected. This is especially true for broad-spectrum antimicrobials considered active against both Gram-positive and Gram-negative bacteria. The solution to this problem is to make species-related adjustments to breakpoints to avoid dividing wild-type populations. This need is now recognized by most breakpoint committees and is one of the guiding principles for setting breakpoints by EUCAST.

ANTIBIOTIC BREAKPOINT COMMITTEES AND/OR REFERENCE GROUPS FOR ANTIBIOTICS

Many countries have their own antibiotic breakpoint committees and/or reference groups for antibiotics, e.g.:

- **BSAC** (British Society for Antimicrobial Chemotherapy, UK; http://www.bsac.org.uk)
- **CA-SFM** (Comité de l'ántibiogramme de la Société Française de Microbiologie, France; http://www.sfm.asso.fr)
- **CLSI** (Clinical and Laboratory Standards Institute, USA; http://www.clsi.org)
- **CRG** (Commissie Richtlijnen Gevoeligheids-bepalingen, The Netherlands)

- **DIN** (Deutsches Institut für Normung, Germany; http://www.din.de)
- **NWGA** (Norwegian Working Group on Antibiotics, Norway; http://www.unn.no/category10274.html)
- **SRGA** and **SRGA-M** (Swedish Reference Group for Antibiotics and its subcommittee on methodology, Sweden; http://www.srga.org).

Many of the reference groups are more than just breakpoint committees. Several publish guidelines on methodology, on quality assurance and on the use of reference strains. Some undertake education of laboratory personnel, surveillance of antimicrobial resistance and liaison with regulatory bodies, the medical profession and the pharmaceutical industry.

In 2002, the national reference groups in Europe and the European Society of Clinical Microbiology and Infectious Diseases (ESCMID; http://www.escmid.org) co-organized a joint committee, EUCAST, with the principal purpose of achieving harmonized MIC breakpoints and methods in Europe. EUCAST is funded by the European Centre for Disease Prevention and Control (ECDC), ESCMID and the national committees. EUCAST has specialist subcommittees on antifungal susceptibility testing, expert rules and anaerobes. In 2009 the process of harmonization of MIC breakpoints for all commonly used agents was completed. MIC breakpoints for new agents are now set by EUCAST as part of the licensing process for new agents through the European Medicines Agency (EMEA). Reference MIC methods have been described and a disk diffusion method calibrated to EUCAST MIC breakpoints has been developed. Full details of the EUCAST structure and organization are given on the EUCAST website at http://www.eucast.org.

TESTS FOR β-LACTAMASE

Various methods are available for detection of β-lactamase activity (http://www.bsac.org.uk/_db/_documents/Chapter_6. pdf). An increasing array of PCR methods for specific detection or typing of β-lactamases is available but these are rarely used for routine purposes. The most commonly used routine test is the nitrocefin test, which is commercially available in various formats. Nitrocefin is a β-lactam molecule that changes color when hydrolyzed by a β-lactamase. The color change is often rapid but can take up to 60 min. The nitrocefin test works well with *H. influenzae*, *Moraxella catarrhalis*, *N. gonorrhoeae*, *N. meningitidis* and *Enterococcus faecalis* (β-lactamase production in the last two is very rare). The method is less reliable with *Staph. aureus*, where induction with penicillin or oxacillin may be required and, because of false-positive reactions, the nitrocefin test should not be used for *Staph. saprophyticus*. Alternative methods are the 'clover leaf' test, the acidometric method and the iodometric method.

Enterobacteriaceae exhibit a multitude of β-lactamases, most of which are cell bound and not reliably detected in conventional β-lactamase tests unless induced and extracted. The phenotypic resistance conferred by β-lactamases depends on the level of expression, the substrate profile of the particular enzyme or combination of enzymes, and the presence of other complementary resistance mechanisms, such as permeability/efflux. For this reason the detection of β-lactamase-mediated resistance in the clinical laboratory is based on phenotypic susceptibility testing of penicillins (with and without β-lactamase inhibitors) and cephalosporins.

Detection of resistance mediated by extended-spectrum β-lactamases (ESBLs) is usually based on detection of resistance to specific indicator β-lactams – for example, cefotaxime (or ceftriaxone) plus ceftazidime, or cefpodoxime alone. Provided breakpoints are set close to the wild-type populations (epidemiological cut-off values) of relevant species of Enterobacteriaceae, the susceptibility test will detect most ESBL-mediated resistance. Confirmation of ESBL production is usually based on detection of β-lactamase inhibition by clavulanate.

AmpC enzymes are mostly chromosomal and are inducible in most *Enterobacter* spp., *Citrobacter freundii*, *Serratia* spp., *Morganella morganii*, *Providencia* spp. and *P. aeruginosa*. With *Enterobacter* spp. and *C. freundii*, induction by cefoxitin antagonizes the activity of third-generation cephalosporins, which do not induce enzyme production. Resistance is usually obvious in strains with mutation to derepressed production of AmpC enzymes. The presence of AmpC enzymes may be indicated in tests with boronic acid, which inhibits AmpC activity.

Detection of resistance mediated by carbapenemases can be challenging as carbapenem MICs may be low. As with ESBLs, if breakpoints are set close to the wild-type populations (epidemiological cut-off values) of relevant species, the susceptibility test will detect most carbapenemase-mediated resistance, particularly with ertapenem. The clover leaf test is a particularly sensitive method for detection of carbapenemases and the presence of metallo-enzymes can be indicated in tests based on detection of β-lactamase inhibition by EDTA, although false positives have been reported for both these methods.

DETECTION OF RESISTANCE GENES WITH MOLECULAR TECHNIQUES

Many different genotypic tests have been described for the detection of resistance genes or organisms carrying resistance genes.[4] PCR methods can be used for the detection of most resistance mechanisms – for example, methicillin resistance in staphylococci (MRSA, MRSE) where detection of the *mecA* gene coding for PBP 2a classifies the organism as resistant to all currently marketed β-lactam antibiotics except ceftobiprole; and glycopeptide resistance mediated by the *van* genes in enterococci. PCR techniques for the detection of genes coding for β-lactamases, aminoglycoside-inactivating enzymes, macrolide resistance and others have also been described. Molecular methods might be used to detect resistant organisms directly in clinical specimens, although mixtures with normal flora that may contain resistance genes are a problem. This problem has been largely overcome in one method for direct detection of MRSA where the PCR target identifies both *Staph. aureus* and the SCC*mec* elements that include the *mecA* gene. Where resistance is sometimes equivocal in phenotypic tests, such as with MRSA or glycopeptide-resistant enterococci, PCR is a very useful confirmatory tool, especially in low-prevalence areas where epidemiological intervention in the form of sometimes cumbersome activities may be undertaken to prevent dissemination of resistance. Molecular tests are also valuable in epidemiological studies of the spread of particular resistance genes and may be used as the reference method in evaluation of susceptibility tests for some resistances. However, it is not yet practical routinely to detect the very wide range of genes that might confer resistance. Furthermore, molecular techniques will detect only the genes included in the particular tests, so new resistance genes or mutations in existing genes may be missed, and they give no indication of the level of expression or the effects of combinations of genes, which may significantly affect phenotypic susceptibility. Therefore, phenotypic susceptibility tests are most commonly used to discriminate between resistant and susceptible isolates.

QUALITY ASSURANCE

All susceptibility testing needs effective control to ensure the quality of results. The manufacturers of media, antibiotic disks, gradient strips, microdilution plates with ready-made antibiotic concentrations, etc., and the producers of automated or semi-automated systems, have a responsibility to ensure that their products are of adequate quality. The laboratory has a responsibility to ensure that the reagents and systems are used correctly and to include control tests to detect problems in performance of the tests.

INTERNAL QUALITY CONTROL

Quality control must be part of the daily routine in the laboratory. Well-defined strains representing non-fastidious and fastidious Gram-negative and Gram-positive bacteria can be obtained from type culture collections (e.g. ATCC, NCTC, CCUG) and from some national antibiotic reference groups. Most standardized methods recommend type strains of *Esch. coli*, *Ps. aeruginosa*, *Staph. aureus*, *E. faecalis*, *Str. pneumoniae*, *H. influenzae* and *N. gonorrhoeae* and that they should be tested daily (some methods permit less frequent testing when daily testing has shown the method to be in control) against the panels of antibiotics used in the daily routine. Control strains should be handled exactly as patient isolates. The MICs or the zone diameters should be recorded and may be plotted in a Shewhart diagram to facilitate visual inspection. Target values and/or control limits for control strains are published for all national guidelines and defined action should be taken if results fall outside these limits.

EXTERNAL QUALITY ASSESSMENT

In external quality assessment (EQA), organisms of known but undisclosed susceptibility are distributed by a central laboratory; participants test the organisms by their routine procedures and send the results back to the central laboratory. The expected results based on reference methods and a summary of the results of all participants are sent to participants so they can evaluate their performance in relation to the expected result and other participants' results. Most EQA programs distribute micro-organisms with defined resistance mechanisms as well as fully susceptible isolates. The international external quality assessment scheme for clinical microbiology organized from the UK (UK NEQAS; http://www.ukneqas.org.uk) has a wide coverage, with laboratories from all over Europe and many other parts of the world as subscribers. As well as detecting poor-performing laboratories, which are offered guidance where appropriate, the UK NEQAS scheme has highlighted inadequate performance in some areas of susceptibility testing, such as penicillin resistance in *Str. pneumoniae*, low-level glycopeptide resistance in enterococci and β-lactamase-negative ampicillin resistance in *H. influenzae*. Associations have also been demonstrated between laboratory performance and methods used.[5]

External quality assessment programs have been criticized for distributing strains that are not challenging as susceptibility is too obvious, but strains with borderline susceptibility or difficult resistances are now commonly distributed, and a small proportion of laboratories fail even when strains are obviously resistant or susceptible. In some countries participation in EQA is not mandatory and it may be that laboratories subscribing to EQA programs are more proficient than those that do not. National efforts, including accreditation requirements, to encourage laboratories to take part in EQA programs, are needed.

ANTIBIOTIC ASSAY

Assays of antibiotic concentrations in serum and other body fluids were developed with the introduction of the modern aminoglycosides during the 1960s and 1970s. A vast number of articles described various assay methods and nomograms for ensuring therapeutic and non-toxic concentrations of gentamicin, tobramycin, amikacin and netilmicin. At the same time the first serious attempts were made to measure and describe antimicrobial tissue concentrations and their relation to therapeutic effect. Pharmacokinetic and eventually pharmacodynamic modeling also depended on the development of assays for measuring the concentration of antimicrobial drugs.

The monitoring of antimicrobial drug therapy is undertaken for four main reasons:

- To ensure therapeutic concentrations – especially where the therapeutic margin is narrow (aminoglycosides, vancomycin) or where there are wide individual variations in the pharmacokinetics of the drug (e.g. rifampicin [rifampin], isoniazid).
- To avoid potentially toxic concentrations (e.g. aminoglycosides, vancomycin).
- To prevent accumulation of drug (aminoglycosides, fluoroquinolones in the elderly) – most often caused by deteriorating renal function.
- To ensure compliance and bioavailability in long-term oral therapy.

Apart from the listed reasons, it is preferable to optimize drug therapy in very sick patients on multidrug therapy in whom drug interactions, failing renal function, dialysis and other factors affecting pharmacokinetics may make dosing difficult even at the best of times.

Clinical laboratories that take on drug monitoring should be prepared to measure and advise on the serum concentrations of at least one aminoglycoside and vancomycin. For both these classes of drugs clinicians trying to avoid potentially toxic serum levels run the risk of underdosing the patient. On the other hand, aminoglycoside therapy administered as part of intensive care or over longer periods is always accompanied by some degree of renal function deterioration (i.e. the drug negatively affects its own major pathway of elimination). Toxic effects such as further damage to the proximal tubular cells and ototoxicity due to accumulation of drug, common when therapy goes beyond 3–5 days, can be counteracted by monitoring pre-dose levels. Vancomycin serum levels are measured mainly to ensure that therapeutic levels are attained but high levels of vancomycin should be avoided. The reader is referred to the excellent publication *Clinical Antimicrobial Assays*[6] for more detailed information on assay of antimicrobial drugs.

References

1. International Organization for Standardization (ISO). *Clinical laboratory testing and in vitro diagnostic test systems – susceptibility testing of infectious agents and evaluation of performance of antimicrobial susceptibility test devices – Part 1: Reference method for testing the in vitro activity of antimicrobial agents against rapidly growing aerobic bacteria involved in infectious diseases.* International Standard 20776-1. Geneva: ISO; 2006.
2. Bauer AW, Kirby W, Sherris J, Turck M. Antibiotic susceptibility testing by a standardized single disk method. *Am J Clin Pathol.* 1966;45:493–496.
3. Ericsson HM, Sherris JC. Antibiotic sensitivity testing. Report of an international collaborative study. *Acta Pathol Microbiol Scand [B].* 1971;(suppl 217):1–90.
4. Rasheed JK, Cockerill F, Tenover FC. Detection and characterization of antimicrobial resistance genes in pathogenic bacteria. In: Murray PR, Baron EJ, Jorgensen JH, Landry ML, Pfaller MA, eds. *Manual of Clinical Microbiology.* 9th ed. Washington, DC: American Society for Microbiology; 2007:1248–1267.
5. Snell JJ, Brown DF. External quality assessment of antimicrobial susceptibility testing in Europe. *J Antimicrob Chemother.* 2001;47:801–810.
6. Reeves DS, Wise R, Andrews JM, White LO. *Clinical Antimicrobial Assays.* Oxford: Oxford University Press; 1999.
7. Sjölund M, Bengtsson S, Bonnedahl J, Hernandez J, Olsen B, Kahlmeter G. Antimicrobial susceptibility in *Escherichia coli* of human and avian origin – a comparison of wild-type distributions. *Clin Microbiol Infec.* 2009;15(5):461–465.

10 Principles of chemoprophylaxis

S. Ragnar Norrby

Chemoprophylaxis aims at preventing clinical infections and should be separated from early treatment. Prophylactic use of antimicrobial drugs has been established in several types of surgery to prevent postoperative infections. In patients with certain heart disorders antibiotic treatment is recommended to prevent endocarditis following invasive procedures that may lead to bacteremia (e.g. dental treatment and urogenital surgery). Patients who are neutropenic or otherwise immunocompromised often receive prophylactic antibiotics and/or antifungal or antiviral agents to prevent infections.

These are all examples of primary prophylaxis; the aim is to prevent infections occurring. Other examples include prophylactic use of anti-malarial drugs in travelers (see Ch. 62) and prophylaxis against *Pneumocystis jirovecii* pneumonia in HIV-infected patients with low CD4 lymphocyte counts. Following certain infections in immuno-compromised patients (e.g. those with AIDS who have had *P. jirovecii* pneumonia or *Cryptococcus neoformans* meningitis) secondary chemoprophylaxis is used to prevent recurrences of the infections for as long as the patient remains immunodeficient.

SURGICAL PROPHYLAXIS

Several surgical procedures (such as abdominal surgery with enterotomies, transvaginal surgery and lung surgery) will result in spillage of material that contains the normal bacterial flora. In other types of surgery the risk of postoperative infection is increased by the use of foreign material, such as hip and knee prostheses. Prophylactic use of antibiotics has been found to reduce the incidence of postoperative bacterial infections in these procedures. In other types of surgery in which spillage is not a major problem and where foreign bodies are not implanted, advantages of prophylaxis cannot be proven and its use is often doubtful. Table 10.1 gives examples of types of surgery where antibiotic prophylaxis has been proven to be beneficial, where it is routinely used but with no solid documentation of efficacy and where it has been proven not to reduce the incidence of postoperative infections.[1]

Correct timing of antibiotic prophylaxis in surgery is essential. Treatment should aim at obtaining high antibiotic concentration in tissue and tissue fluids during the surgical procedure, and in particular when there is a high risk of contamination (e.g. when an enterotomy is performed). One study demonstrated that if antibiotics with short plasma half-lives were used, administration more than 2 h before or 3 h after surgery resulted in poor prophylactic effect.[2] Today it is agreed that surgical prophylaxis should be perioperative, i.e. it should be administered during surgery and terminated when the wound is closed.[3–7] Prolonged antibiotic prophylaxis is costly, gives no further benefits and increases the risk of selection of antibiotic-resistant bacteria.

An alternative to systemic antibiotic prophylaxis might be topical application of antibiotics, which has been proven to be effective when chloramphenicol was compared to placebo in 'high risk' wounds.[8]

ENDOCARDITIS PROPHYLAXIS

It is generally recommended that patients who have had endocarditis or known cardiac valvular defects and/or prostheses should be considered for antibiotic prophylaxis when subjected to certain procedures, including extensive dental surgery and treatment, and genitourinary, gastrointestinal and respiratory tract surgery (i.e. medical interventions which increase the risk of bacteremia and the number of bacteria in bacteremia).[9] However, the scientific background for using antibiotic prophylaxis has recently been questioned.[10]

The choice of antibiotics in endocarditis prophylaxis has been modified in the latest recommendations from the American Heart Association.[9] For example, the standard regimen before dental and respiratory procedures is today 2 g amoxicillin 1 h before dental treatment or surgery; in patients hypersensitive to penicillin, erythromycin has been replaced by clindamycin or azithromycin. The use of amoxicillin is further supported by a study in which placebo, amoxicillin,

Table 10.1 Need for antibiotic prophylaxis in various surgical procedures

Procedures for which antibiotic prophylaxis is documented and indicated
- Esophageal, gastric and duodenal surgery
- Intestinal surgery (including appendectomy)
- Acute laparotomy
- Inguinal hernia repair
- Transurethral or transvesical prostatectomy
- Total hysterectomy
- Cesarean section
- Surgical legal abortion
- Amputations
- Reconstructive vascular surgery (not surgery on the carotid arteries) with or without the use of grafts
- Cardiac surgery
- Pulmonary surgery

Procedures for which antibiotic prophylaxis is often used but with incompletely documented efficacy
- Pancreatic surgery
- Liver surgery (resection)
- Urological surgery with enteric substitutes
- Implanted urological prostheses
- Transrectal prostate biopsy
- Hemiplastic surgery in patients with cervical hip fractures
- Back surgery with metal implantation
- Aortic graft-stents
- Neck surgery

Procedures for which antibiotic prophylaxis is not documented or indicated
- Biliary tract surgery in patients with normal bile ducts and no stents
- Endoscopic examination of the urinary tract
- Reconstructive urethral surgery
- Arthroscopic procedures

From the Swedish-Norwegian Consensus Group. Antibiotic prophylaxis in surgery: summary of a Swedish-Norwegian consensus conference. **Scand J Infect Dis.** 1998;30:547–557.[1]

clindamycin or moxifloxacin was given to patients undergoing dental extractions.[11] The frequencies of bacteremia were 96%, 46%, 85% and 57%, respectively.

PREVENTION OF TRAVELERS' DIARRHEA

Up to 50% of travelers to tropical and subtropical countries will develop travelers' diarrhea. The most common pathogens causing this condition are strains of *Escherichia coli* producing enterotoxin (ETEC), *Campylobacter* spp., *Vibrio parahaemolyticus*, *Vibrio cholerae*, *Salmonella enterica* serotypes and *Shigella* spp. In addition, diarrhea may be the result of food poisoning with bacterial toxins produced by *Staphylococcus aureus*, *Bacillus cereus* or *Clostridium perfringens*. Vaccines are available only against *V. cholerae* (one of the cholera vaccines may also give short-term protection against ETEC) and *Salmonella* Typhi.

Chemoprophylaxis using trimethoprim–sulfamethoxazole, doxycycline, fluoroquinolones or other antibiotics effectively decreases the incidence of travelers' diarrhea. Arguments against such use of antibiotics are the risks of adverse effects and of emergence of resistance. However, prophylaxis should be considered in individuals with underlying diseases that may be complicated by acute diarrhea (e.g. people with diabetes mellitus, reactive arthritis or inflammatory bowel disease). Patients treated with drugs that reduce the gastric acidity should also be considered for prophylaxis because they are at increased risk of developing diarrhea due to a defective acidic barrier.

PROPHYLAXIS AGAINST MENINGOCOCCAL DISEASE

It is well known that individuals who have had close contact with a patient with meningococcal disease are at increased risk of developing the disease. Two types of prophylaxis have been used. The most common one is to use ciprofloxacin or rifampicin (rifampin) in order to eradicate carriage of *Neisseria meningitidis*. Another approach, commonly used in Norway, is to treat contacts of a patient with meningococcal disease with penicillin V for 7 days. Such a regimen will prevent disease but will not eradicate carriage. For further details, see Chapter 50.

CHEMOPROPHYLAXIS IN PATIENTS WITH IMMUNE DEFICIENCIES

Prophylactic antibiotics and antiviral drugs are commonly used in patients with various types of immune deficiency and are summarized in Table 10.2. The use of primary and secondary prophylaxis against *P. jirovecii* pneumonia with trimethoprim–sulfamethoxazole (which also seems to prevent *Toxoplasma*

Table 10.2 Primary chemoprophylaxis in immunodeficient patients

Type of immune deficiency	Prophylaxis against	Drugs used
Organ transplantation (Chapter 40)	*Pneumocystis jirovecii* Herpes simplex Cytomegalovirus *Candida* infections	Trimethoprim–sulfamethoxazole Aciclovir Ganciclovir, aciclovir Azole antifungals
Neutropenia (Chapter 40)	Bacterial infections *Candida* infections	Various Azole antifungals
Asplenia	Pneumococcal infections	Penicillin V
HIV infection (Chapter 43)	*P. jirovecii* *Toxoplasma gondii* Atypical mycobacteria Neonatal transmission	Trimethoprim–sulfamethoxazole Trimethoprim–sulfamethoxazole Various Antiretroviral drugs

gondii encephalitis) and secondary prophylaxis against *C. neoformans* meningitis have been proven to be effective. Primary prophylaxis against fungal infections, especially those caused by *Candida* spp. in HIV-positive patients, seems more doubtful since the time during which prophylaxis is used by necessity must be long and might result in selection of resistant strains, especially when oral treatment with an azole antifungal agent such as fluconazole or itraconazole is used. Importantly, it has been demonstrated that during effective, so-called 'highly active' antiretroviral treatment (HAART), pneumocystis prophylaxis can be discontinued without negative effects.[12]

Another type of prophylaxis in HIV-infected patients that has been proven to be effective is the administration of antiretroviral drugs to pregnant women and to their newborn children in order to prevent intrauterine and neonatal transmission of HIV.

 ## References

1. Swedish-Norwegian Consensus Group. Antibiotic prophylaxis in surgery: summary of a Swedish-Norwegian consensus conference. *Scand J Infect Dis.* 1998;30:547–557.
2. Classen DC, Evans RS, Pestotnik SL, Horn SD, Menlove RL, Burke JP. The timing of prophylactic administration of antibiotics and the risk of surgical wound infections. *N Engl J Med.* 1992;326:161–169.
3. Waddell TK, Rotstein OD. Antimicrobial prophylaxis in surgery. *Can Med Assoc J.* 1994;151:925–931.
4. Page CP, Bohnen JMA, Fletcher JR, McManus AT, Solomkin JS, Wittman DH. Antimicrobial prophylaxis for surgical wounds. *Arch Surg.* 1993;128:79–88.
5. Norrby SR. Cost-effective prophylaxis in surgical infections. *Pharmacoeconomics.* 1996;10:129–140.
6. Bucknell SJ, Mohajeri M, Low J, McDonald M, Hill DG. Single-versus multiple-dose antibiotic prophylaxis for cardiac surgery. *Aust N Z J Surg.* 2000;70:409–411.
7. Zelenitsky SA, Ariano RE, Harding GKM, Silverman RE. Antibiotic pharmacodynamics in surgical prophylaxis: an association between intraoperative antibiotic concentrations and efficacy. *Antimicrob Agents Chemother.* 2002;46:3026–3030.
8. Heal CF, Buettner PG, Cruickshank R, et al. Does single application of topical chloramphenicol to high risk sutured wounds reduce incidence of wound infections? Prospective randomised placebo controlled double blind trial. *Br Med J.* 2009;338:a2812.
9. Dajani AS, Taubert KA, Wilson W, et al. Prevention of bacterial endocarditis: recommendations by the American Heart Association. *Clin Infect Dis.* 1997;25:1448–1458.
10. Strom BL, Abrutyn E, Berlin JA, et al. Dental and cardiac risk factors for infective endocarditis. A population-based, case-control study. *Ann Intern Med.* 1998;129:761–769.
11. Dios PD, Carmona T, Posse PJ, et al. Comparative efficacies of amoxicillin, clindamycin, and moxifloxacin in prevention of bacteremia following dental extractions. *Antimicrob Agents Chemother.* 2006;50:2996–3002.
12. Furrer H, Egger M, Opravil M, et al. Discontinuation of primary prophylaxis against *Pneumocystis carinii* pneumonia in HIV-1-infected adults treated with combination antiretroviral therapy. Swiss HIV Cohort Study. *N Engl J Med.* 1999;340:1301–1306.

 ## Further information

Benson CA, Williams PL, Cohn DL, et al. Clarithromycin or rifabutin alone or in combination for primary prophylaxis of *Mycobacterium avium* complex disease in patients with AIDS: a randomized, double-blind, placebo-controlled trial. The AIDS Clinical Trials Group 196/Terry Beirn Community Programs for Clinical Research on AIDS 009 Protocol Team. *J Infect Dis.* 2000;181:1289–1297.

Boeckh M, Kim HW, Flowers MED, Bowden RA. Long-term acyclovir for prevention of varicella zoster virus disease after allogeneic hematopoietic cell transplantation – a randomized double-blind placebo-controlled study. *Blood.* 2006;107:1800–1805.

Cornley OA, Böhme A, Buchheidt D, et al. Primary prophylaxis of invasive fungal infections in patients with hematologic malignancies. Recommendations of the Infectious Diseases Working Party of the German Society for Haematology and Oncology. *Haematologica.* 2009;94:113–122.

Danchin N, Duval X, Leport C. Prophylaxis of infective endocarditis: French recommendations 2002. *Heart.* 2005;91:715–718.

Dobay KJ, Freier DT, Albear P. The absent role of prophylactic antibiotics in low-risk patients undergoing laparoscopic cholecystectomy. *Am Surg.* 1999;65:226–228.

Fleschner SM, Avery RK, Fisher R, et al. A randomized prospective controlled trial of oral acyclovir versus oral ganciclovir for cytomegalovirus prophylaxis in high-risk kidney transplant recipients. *Transplantation.* 1998;66:1682–1688.

Kasatpibal N, Nørgaard M, Sørensen HT, Schøheyder HC, Jamulitra S, Chongsuvivatwong V. Risk of surgical infection and efficacy of antibiotic prophylaxis: a cohort study of appendectomy patients in Thailand. *BMC Infect Dis.* 2006;6:2334–2336.

Kreter B, Woods M. Antibiotic prophylaxis for cardiothoracic operations. Meta-analysis of thirty years of clinical trials. *J Thorac Cardiovasc Surg.* 1992;13:606–608.

Lallemant M, Jourdian G, Le Coeur S, et al. A trial of shortened zidovudine regimens to prevent mother-to-child transmission of human immunodeficiency virus type 1. Perinatal HIV Prevention Trial (Thailand) Investigators. *N Engl J Med.* 2000;343:1036–1037.

Meijer E, Boland GJ, Verdonck LF. Prevention of cytomegalovirus disease in recipients of allogeneic stem cell transplants. *Clin Microbiol Rev.* 2003;16:647–657.

Mittendorf R, Aronson MP, Berry RE, et al. Avoiding serious infections associated with abdominal hysterectomy; a meta-analysis of antibiotic prophylaxis. *Am J Obstet Gynecol.* 1993;142:1119–1124.

Nucci M, Biasoli I, Aiti T, et al. A double-blind, randomized, placebo-controlled trial of itraconazole capsules as antifungal prophylaxis for neutropenic patients. *Clin Infect Dis.* 2000;30:300–305.

Salminen US, Viljanen TU, Valtonen W, Ikonen TE, Sahlman AE, Harjula AL. Ceftriaxone versus vancomycin prophylaxis in cardiovascular surgery. *J Antimicrob Chemother.* 1999;44:287–290.

Sawaya GF, Grady D, Kerlikowske K, Grimes DA. Antibiotics at the time of induced abortions: the case for universal antibiotic prophylaxis based on a meta-analysis. *Obstet Gynecol.* 1996;87:884–890.

Wiström J, Norrby SR. Fluoroquinolones and bacterial enteritis. *J Antimicrob Chemother.* 1995;36:23–40.

Yerdel MA, Akin MB, Dolalan S, et al. Effect of single-dose prophylactic ampicillin and sulbactam on wound infection after tension-free inguinal hernia repair with polypropylene mesh. The randomized, double-blind, prospective trial. *Ann Surg.* 2001;233:26–33.

11 Antibiotic policies

Peter G. Davey, Dilip Nathwani and Ethan Rubinstein

Antibiotic resistance is a global public health problem.[1,2] In Europe in 2008 16 countries had developed a national strategy to contain antimicrobial resistance and nine countries had an action plan.[3] A core component of most of these strategies is antimicrobial stewardship, which has been defined as a set of measures delivered by a multidisciplinary team working in healthcare institutions to optimize antimicrobial use amongst patients in order to improve patient outcomes, ensure cost-effective therapy and reduce adverse sequelae of antimicrobial use, including ecological effects such as resistance and *Clostridium difficile* infections.[4,5] Targets for antimicrobial stewardship include appropriate antibiotic selection, dosing, route, and duration of therapy. Antimicrobial stewardship combined with infection prevention measures will limit the emergence and transmission of antimicrobial resistance.[6]

Antibiotic policies are an integral component of antimicrobial stewardship programs. The terms 'guidelines', 'formularies' and 'policies' are often used interchangeably but they are separate, complementary components of a strategy for prudent antimicrobial use.

- *Guidelines* provide advice about what drug should be prescribed for a specific clinical condition. They may take the form of a care pathway or flow chart outlining processes of care, including investigations and therapies other than just antimicrobial compounds (e.g. oxygenation in a pneumonia guideline). National guidelines have been published as templates for local consultation and adaptation.[7,8]

- A *formulary* is a limited list of drugs available for prescription. It may include information about available dosing instructions and advice about safety or interactions but it does not include detailed guidance for use.

- An *antimicrobial policy* contains guidelines about treatment of specific conditions. This can also include a limited list of antimicrobial agents that are generally available to all prescribers – in other words an antimicrobial formulary. In addition to guidance, antimicrobial policies may include enforcement strategies such as compulsory order forms for restricted drugs.

- An *antimicrobial management team* is a multidisciplinary team in which each member is given specific roles and which collectively takes responsibility for implementation of local policies (see Figure 11.1). To be effective the team must have full support from hospital leadership, work closely with infection control teams and provide regular feedback to individual clinicians and clinical teams about their compliance with policies.

There is considerable variation in the use of antibiotic policies and control measures in European hospitals.[9] Consequently, efforts to coordinate and standardize antimicrobial stewardship programs across multiple hospitals and primary care organizations have been initiated by countries (e.g. Scotland,[10] Sweden[11]) or networks such as the European Union antibiotic stewardship program (ABS International[12]).

Antibiotic policies have been used since the 1950s and have evolved in complexity over time.[13] In 1990 the *Drug and Therapeutics Bulletin* concluded that local prescribing policies are worth the time and money they take to produce, improve the quality of prescribing and reduce overall costs in hospitals and in general practice.[14] Nonetheless, in 1994 only 62% of 427 UK hospitals had a policy for antibiotic therapy and 75% had an antibiotic formulary.[15] In 2001 the House of Lords Select Committee on Science and Technology again had to urge the Department of Health to pursue any hospitals that did not have a formal prescribing policy.[1] A further survey of acute healthcare trusts in England in 2004/5 revealed that an antimicrobial policy was in place in 89% of responding trusts (109/123).[16] This is clearly an improvement on the previous survey result but it is disappointing that 11% of responding hospitals had not taken the essential first step of writing an antibiotic policy. In the USA 100% of 47 hospitals surveyed in 2000 had an antibiotic formulary.[17] However, only 47% had written policies for surgical prophylaxis, a key area of antibiotic misuse.[18]

The problems of antibiotic resistance linked to widespread prescribing of antibiotics are even more pressing in developing countries. In India and Sri Lanka 66% of community prescriptions include an antimicrobial; in Bangladesh and Egypt antibiotic use accounts for 54% and 61%, respectively, of all hospital prescribing.[19] The potential value of antibiotic policies in such countries and their current role have recently been reviewed.[20]

In this chapter we review the aims of antibiotic policies, the methods for policy implementation and the evidence that policies achieve their aims.

STIMULI FOR THE INTRODUCTION OF ANTIBIOTIC POLICIES

Many of the stimuli for antibiotic policies are common to policies for other drug groups, but some are unique to antibiotics (Table 11.1). The general advantages of defining a core list of drugs that are used regularly have been recognized for many years by the World Health Organization.[21] The aim is to encourage rational prescribing, which is based on knowledge of pharmacology, efficacy, safety and cost. Drug resistance amongst microbes is a unique stimulus to control of antibiotic prescribing.

Table 11.1 General and specific advantages of an antibiotic policy

Category	Benefits
Knowledge	*General* Promotes awareness of benefits, risks and cost of prescribing Facilitates educational and training programs within the healthcare setting Reduces the impact of aggressive marketing by the pharmaceutical industry Encourages rational choice between drugs based on analysis of pharmacology, clinical effectiveness, safety and cost *Specific to antimicrobials* Provides education about local epidemiology of pathogens and their susceptibility to antimicrobials Promotes awareness of the importance of infection control

Attitudes	*General*
	Acceptance by clinicians of the importance of setting standards of care and prescribing
	Acceptance of peer review and audit of prescribing
	Specific to antimicrobials
	Recognition of the complex issues underlying antimicrobial chemotherapy
	Recognition of the importance of the special expertise required for full evaluation of antimicrobial chemotherapy:
	   Diagnostic microbiology
	   Epidemiology and infection control
	   Clinical diagnosis and recognition of other diseases mimicking infection
	   Pharmacokinetics and pharmacodynamics

Behavior	*General* Increased compliance with guidelines and treatment policies Reduction of medical practice variation *Specific to antimicrobials* Improved liaison between clinicians, pharmacists, microbiologists and the infection control team
Outcome	*General* Standardization and reduction in practice variation are key strategies for improving the quality of healthcare Improved efficiency of prescribing by increasing sensitivity (patients who can benefit receive treatment) and specificity (treatment is not prescribed to patients who will not benefit) Improved clinical outcome Reduces medicolegal liability *Specific to antimicrobials* Limit collateral damage (emergence and spread of drug-resistant strains or superinfection by *Clostridium difficile,* other bacteria or fungi)

PRACTICAL ADVANTAGES OF LIMITING THE RANGE OF ANTIMICROBIALS PRESCRIBED

In the hospital, the prescription of an antimicrobial by a clinician has implications for nurses, pharmacists and microbiologists who will all be involved in preparation, administration and monitoring of the prescribed drug. Limiting the range of drugs used allows the team to become familiar with the necessary processes.[22] Many of the staff who take responsibility for these processes will rotate through several departments in the hospital or will provide cross cover outside working hours. Having common policies within and between clinical directorates reduces the need for time-consuming retraining of staff as they move between clinical units. The need for national guidance about antibiotic prescribing in primary care has also been recognized[7] in response to earlier evidence of considerable variation in content and quality across policies in primary care.[23]

Providers of healthcare are increasingly being asked for evidence about quality assurance. Auditing practice is only possible if standards of care have been defined. The narrower the range of drugs, the easier it is to write and audit detailed standards of care. It is also likely that staff will find it easier to comply with policies that cover a limited range of drugs.

COST

Antibiotics account for 3–25% of all prescriptions and up to 30% of the drug budget in a hospital.[24] New drugs are inevitably more expensive than old drugs and new drugs will be heavily promoted by pharmaceutical companies. One of the aims of antibiotic policies is to encourage prescribers to continue to use older, more familiar drugs unless there are good reasons not to. Intravenous antibiotics are usually about 10-fold more expensive than equivalent oral formulations and intravenous administration requires additional consumables and staff time.[25] Policies that include specific recommendations about route of administration may reduce costs considerably.[4] Limiting the range of drugs also reduces the range of stock that is sitting on the pharmacy shelves.

QUALITY AND SAFETY OF PRESCRIBING

Prescribing drugs that do not benefit the patient exposes them to unnecessary risk and one study found that 26% of all adverse drug reactions in a hospital were caused by drugs that were prescribed unnecessarily.[26] Unnecessary prescribing of antimicrobials carries additional risks for the patient (increased risk of cross infection by resistant organisms or *C. difficile*) and the environment (selection of drug-resistant bacteria, e.g. *Enterococcus faecalis*). Therefore, assessment of the quality of prescribing must consider several elements, including the risks and benefits of introducing another drug and of intravenous versus oral administration. In practice it is very difficult to assess the appropriateness of an entire course of treatment, particularly in hospital. What is appropriate on one day may be inappropriate the next. This problem has been recognized in a practical system for reviewing each day of an antibiotic prescription and then computing the proportion of inappropriate days.[27] The term 'inappropriate' covers a multitude of sins and encompasses both undertreatment and unnecessary overtreatment. Judgment of appropriateness is therefore complex and it is worrying that the few studies of interrater reliability show very poor agreement.[28] Use of computerized case vignettes may provide a more reliable system of assessing inpatient antimicrobial appropriateness.[29]

Monitoring of community prescribing is challenging, especially where drugs are freely available over the counter. Self-medication rates reported include 51% in Ecuador, 70% in Thailand, 75% in Brazil, 82% in Ethiopia and 92% in the Philippines.[19] There are undoubtedly some potential advantages to increasing the availability of antibacterials without prescription, such as convenience for the patient, faster initiation of treatment and reduction in primary care workload.[30] However, in the European Union[2] and in North America,[31] the risks of increasing access to antibacterials are thought to outweigh these benefits.

In the second half of the 20th century there was an inexorable increase in the number of prescriptions for antibiotics in the community in developed countries.[32] More recently this trend has reversed and several countries have reported a significant reduction in antibiotic prescribing in primary care.[11,33–35] Nonetheless, there is still plenty of room for improvement. For example, although the Netherlands has the lowest overall use of antibiotics in Europe,[36] a detailed investigation suggested that 75% of prescriptions for otitis media in primary care might be unnecessary.[37] Longitudinal analysis that combines quantitative and qualitative methods is required to understand how socioeconomic factors and changes in the delivery of care might influence antibiotic use.[38,39]

Educational training and support is an important component of improving the quality and safety of prescribing. The skills and competencies required are both technical and non-technical.[40] These skills are applicable to all professional prescribers.[41] Some of this knowledge can be acquired through the use of a range of high-quality educational web-based resources.[42] The British Society for Antimicrobial Chemotherapy (BSAC) and the European Society for Clinical Microbiology and Infectious Diseases (ESCMID) are collaborating on a teaching resource that uses common clinical infection vignettes as a means of learning about infection management and use of local policies.[43]

COLLATERAL DAMAGE FROM ANTIBIOTIC USE: RESISTANCE AND CROSS-INFECTION

The mechanisms and epidemiology of drug resistance are described in Chapter 3. Control of antibiotic resistance has always been a strong stimulus to the development of antibiotic policies.[13] Antibiotic use stimulates the emergence of resistance but the spread of resistance mainly occurs through cross-infection of resistant strains from one patient to another. The epidemiology of resistance shows that the probability of infection with resistant bacteria is related to both the previous intensity of antibiotic use in the environment or population and the exposure of individual patients who enter the environment or population. Previous use facilitates the emergence of resistance in the environment or population, while exposure of individual patients facilitates persistence of resistant strains.[44] Because acquisition of resistant strains is almost always determined by cross-infection, infection control must be integrated with antimicrobial stewardship (Figure 11.1).

In addition to antimicrobial resistance, collateral damage from antibiotic use includes infection by *Clostridium difficile* and by fungi. The same principles apply to these infections; antimicrobial stewardship will only work if it is combined with infection control (Figure 11.1).

WHAT INTERVENTIONS CHANGE ANTIBIOTIC PRESCRIBING?

The evidence base for antibiotic policies is the subject of two Cochrane Systematic Reviews, one of interventions for patients in ambulatory care[45] and one of interventions for hospital inpatients.[46] A variety of resources linked to the hospital inpatients review can be accessed from the BSAC website (http://www.bsac.org.uk), including all publications, additional details of included studies with microbial outcomes and slide sets with explanatory notes.[47]

The majority of interventions in both reviews were successful: 81 (76%) of 106 interventions on prescribing to hospital inpatients[46] and 30 (75%) of 40 interventions on prescribing in ambulatory care[45] were associated with statistically significant improvements in the primary outcome. However, these two reviews reveal important differences between ambulatory and hospital care in the targets for intervention, the types of intervention and the outcomes that have been measured (Table 11.2).

TARGET FOR THE INTERVENTION

In hospitals, 19 (18%) of the interventions aimed to increase the intensity of antibiotic treatment (Table 11.2). Examples include ensuring that antibiotics were received by patients who would benefit from them[48] or reducing time from admission to start of antibiotic treatment for patients with pneumonia.[49] In contrast, none of the interventions in ambulatory care aimed to increase the intensity of antibiotic treatment (Table 11.2). In hospitals, the commonest target for intervention was the choice of drug (80%), whereas in ambulatory care only 45% of the interventions targeted the choice of drug (Table 11.2). In ambulatory care the commonest target for interventions was the decision to

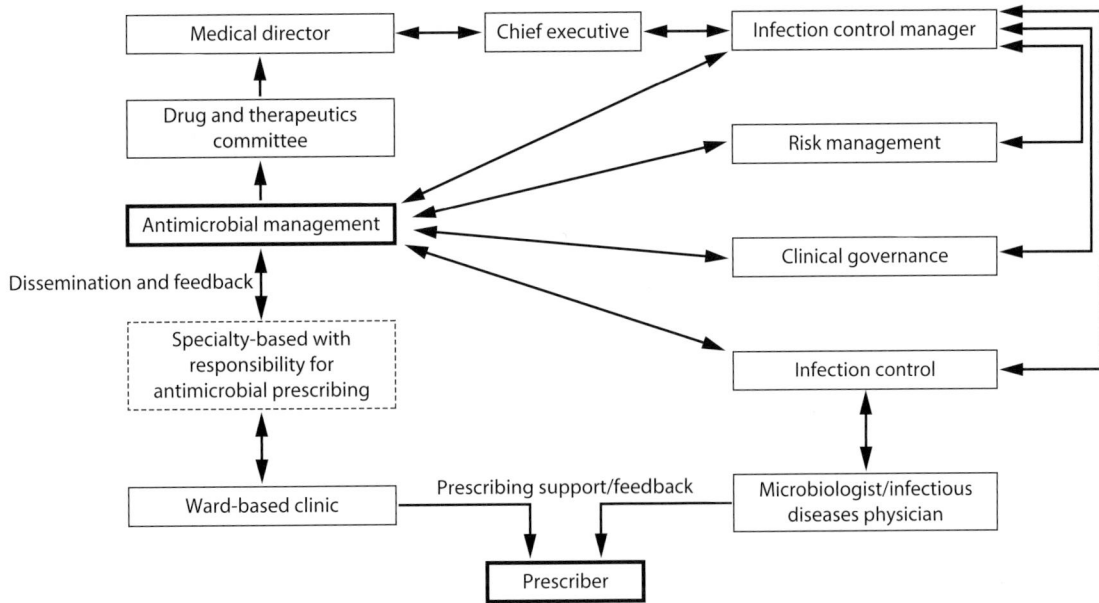

Fig. 11.1   Model pathway for implementing improvements in antimicrobial prescribing practice in hospitals. The antimicrobial management team has a central coordinating role in feedback of information to individual prescribers, clinical teams and senior management. (From Nathwani D. Antimicrobial prescribing policy and practice in Scotland: recommendations for good antimicrobial practice in acute hospitals. **J Antimicrob Chemother.** 2006;57:1189–1196, by permission of Oxford University Press.[10])

prescribe an antibiotic, with 26 (65%) of the studies aiming to reduce the proportion of patients who received an antibiotic (Table 11.2). In contrast, in secondary care, only 8 (8%) of the studies targeted the decision to prescribe and in three of these the aim was to increase the proportion of patients who received effective antibiotic therapy so that only 5 (5%) of the studies on hospital inpatients aimed to reduce the proportion of patients who received an antibiotic. Computerized decision support is a promising method for reducing the number of patients who receive unnecessary antibiotics[50] and one study has clearly shown the potential for this approach in hospital care.[51]

TYPE OF INTERVENTION

In hospital, 47 (44%) of the interventions included a restrictive component, which limited the choice of professionals (Table 11.3). In contrast, in ambulatory care all but two of the interventions were persuasive, the two exceptions being a restrictive primary care formulary that limited the use of fluoroquinolones and an intervention to change the reimbursement and organization of services in primary care.[45] The two commonest persuasive interventions used in hospitals were distribution of educational materials and reminders, whereas in ambulatory care they were educational meetings and educational outreach visits (Table 11.3). Only 10% of interventions in either setting used audit and feedback (Table 11.3). Patient-based interventions were only used in ambulatory care (Table 11.3). These were either patient information sheets or delayed prescriptions, which allowed patients

to obtain an antibiotic without reconsulting the doctor if they had persistent symptoms (Table 11.3).

DESIGN OF EVALUATION OF INTERVENTIONS

The commonest method for evaluation of interventions was an interrupted time series (ITS) in hospitals (55% of studies) whereas in primary care it was a randomized controlled trial (RCT, 63% of studies, *see* Table 11.2). The Cochrane Effective Practice and Organisation of Care Group have recently updated their criteria for assessing risk of bias in studies.[52] These criteria have been applied to the 106 studies in the review of interventions to improve antibiotic use for hospital inpatients (Table 11.4). ITS was the evaluation design that had the lowest risk of bias and was the only design with <50% of studies at high risk of bias (Table 11.4). In contrast, 67% of RCTs were at high risk of bias and only one RCT had a low risk of bias (Table 11.4). The reason is that it is virtually impossible to conceal allocation and avoid contamination in a trial in which professionals are randomly assigned to receive an intervention in a hospital. This can only realistically be achieved in a large RCT that involves multiple hospitals.[53] In contrast, in an ITS study, the control and intervention periods are separated and studies will have a low risk of bias provided that they have reliable primary outcome measures and enough data to show that the intervention effect is likely to be independent of seasonal variation. Consequently, ITS is usually the best design for evaluation of the impact of an antibiotic policy in a single hospital. For research, the strengths of ITS and RCT can be combined in a design called a stepped wedge.[54]

Table 11.2   Comparison of evaluations of interventions to improve antimicrobial prescribing for hospital inpatients and in ambulatory care

Comparison	Hospital inpatients		Ambulatory care	
	Number	%[1]	Number	%[1]
Design				
Controlled before and after study	15	14	12	30
Controlled clinical trial	3	3	1	3
Randomized clinical trial	30	28	25	63
Interrupted time series	58	55	2	5
Target				
Undertreatment of infection	19	18	0	0
Decision to prescribe	8	8	26	65
Choice of drug	89	84	18	45
Timing	9	8	0	0
Duration of treatment	17	16	4	10
Intervention				
Persuasive, professional	56	53	40	100
Restrictive, healthcare system	47	44	2	5
Structural	7	7	0	0
Single component	63	59	32	80
Multifaceted	44	42	8	20
Outcome				
Antimicrobial use	88	83	38	95
Financial savings	33	31	3	8
Clinical outcome	32	30	2	5
Microbial outcomes	31	29	4	10
Cost of design and implementation of the intervention	13	12	0	0
Total studies	106		40	

[1]Some studies had more than one target or outcome.

SUMMARY: WHAT INTERVENTIONS CHANGE ANTIBIOTIC PRESCRIBING?

These two reviews of interventions in hospital and ambulatory care reinforce the message that there are 'No magic bullets', meaning that it is not possible to provide general guidance about the most appropriate method for improving professional practice in any context.[55] Both reviews provide further evidence that the most successful interventions are those which involve the professionals who are the targets for change in both the development and dissemination phases, and provide concurrent feedback of information about implementation.[55–57]

However, this approach requires considerable investment of time by professionals, plus information systems that are capable of providing concurrent feedback. Simply providing prescribers with educational information may be relatively unsuccessful; however, as it requires much less in the way of resources, it could be a more cost-effective method for achieving change. As in most areas of medicine, the most complex and effective intervention available is not necessarily the most appropriate and it makes sense to test interventions in order of complexity, starting with the simplest.[56]

In hospitals restrictive interventions were associated with a greater immediate impact than persuasive interventions.[46] However, the impact of persuasive and restrictive

Table 11.3 Types of intervention used to influence antibiotic prescribing

Intervention	Description	Hospital inpatients		Ambulatory care	
		Number	%	Number	%
Persuasive professional interventions					
Distribution of educational materials	Distribution of published or printed recommendations for clinical care, including clinical practice guidelines, audiovisual materials and electronic publications. The materials may have been delivered personally or through mass mailings	56	53	4	10
Educational meetings	Healthcare providers participating in conferences, lectures, workshops or traineeships	14	13	10	25
Educational outreach visits	Use of a trained person who meets with providers in their practice settings to give information with the intent of changing the providers' practices. The information given may have included feedback on the performance of the provider(s)	4	4	8	20
Local opinion leaders	Use of providers nominated by their colleagues as 'educationally influential'. The investigators must have explicitly stated that their colleagues identified the opinion leaders	2	2	0	0
Patient-mediated interventions	New clinical information (not previously available) collected directly from patients and given to the provider	0	0	5	13
Audit and feedback	Any summary of clinical performance of healthcare over a specified period of time. The summary may also have included recommendations for clinical action. The information may have been obtained from medical records, computerized databases or observations from patients	11	10	4	10
Reminders	Patient or encounter-specific information provided verbally, on paper or on a computer screen, which is designed or intended to prompt a health professional to recall information. This would usually be encountered through their general education, in the medical records or through interactions with peers, and so remind them to perform or avoid some action to aid individual patient care. Computer-aided decision support and drug dosage are included	44	42	3	8
Other types of intervention					
Healthcare system	Restriction of professional choice through removal of drugs from stock, compulsory order forms that limit drugs to specific conditions, requiring signed approval by another professional, therapeutic substitution of the physician's original choice of antibiotic by another professional, automatic stop order after a fixed duration of treatment or prophylaxis. Changes in methods of physician remuneration	47	44	2	5
Structural	Inclusion of equipment where technology in question is used in a wide range of problems and is not disease specific (e.g. rapid laboratory testing or therapeutic drug monitoring)	8	8	0	0

interventions was similar after 6 months and after 12 months there was a suggestion that persuasive interventions had greater impact.

In ambulatory care all five studies that included patient-based interventions (information sheets or delayed antibiotic prescriptions) resulted in a statistically significant reduction in antibiotic use. The review authors concluded that in ambulatory care multifaceted interventions combining physician, patient and public education in a variety of venues and formats were the most successful in reducing antibiotic prescribing for inappropriate indications.[45] However, in hospitals multifaceted interventions were not associated with greater impact than single component interventions.[46]

TO WHAT EXTENT DO ANTIBIOTIC POLICIES ACHIEVE THEIR SECONDARY AIMS?

CAN ANTIBIOTIC POLICIES REDUCE HEALTHCARE COSTS?

The literature is full of claims that implementation of antibiotic policies reduces healthcare costs, in hospital or in the community. However, the Cochrane Systematic Reviews revealed significant gaps in the evidence base. In hospital care 31% of studies estimated the financial savings from reduction in use of the target drugs but only 12% of studies included

Table 11.4 Rigorous designs for evaluation of interventions to change practice and organization of care*

Design	Criteria for assessment of quality	Description	Total	Risk of bias					
				Low		Medium		High	
				N	%	N	%	N	%
Studies with a separate control group	Was the allocation sequence adequately generated? Was the allocation adequately concealed? Were baseline outcome measurements similar? Were baseline characteristics similar? Were incomplete outcome data adequately addressed? Was knowledge of the allocated interventions adequately prevented during the study? Was the study adequately protected against contamination? Was the study free from selective outcome reporting? Was the study free from other risks of bias?	*Randomized controlled trial* Participants (patients, doctors, healthcare teams, etc.) were assigned by random allocation (e.g. random number generation, coin flips)	30	1	3	9	30	20	67
		Controlled clinical trial Participants (patients, doctors, healthcare teams, etc.) were assigned by quasi-random allocation method (e.g. alternation, date of birth, patient identifier)	3	0		0		3	100
		Controlled before and after study Involvement of intervention and control groups other than by random process, and inclusion of baseline period of assessment of main outcomes	15	0		1	7	14	93
Interrupted time series	Was the intervention independent of other changes? Was the shape of the intervention effect pre-specified? Was the intervention unlikely to affect data collection? Was knowledge of the allocated interventions adequately prevented during the study? Were incomplete outcome data adequately addressed? Was the study free from selective outcome reporting? Was the study free from other risks of bias?	A change in trend attributable to the intervention, with repeated measures of the main outcomes before and after the intervention.	58	25	24	31	29	50	47

*Includes criteria for assessment of quality and the risk of bias in 106 studies of interventions to improve antibiotic prescribing in hospitals. The minimum criteria for any design are objective measurement of performance, behavior or health outcomes in a clinical, not test, situation and relevant and interpretable data presented or obtainable.

information about the cost of design and implementation of the intervention, which is essential to the overall assessment of cost-effectiveness.[46]

In ambulatory care only three (7.5%) of the studies reported the impact of the intervention on total antibiotic costs and none reported the impact on other costs (e.g. number of practice visits). None of the ambulatory care studies reported the cost of designing, disseminating or implementing the intervention.

CAN ANTIBIOTIC POLICIES CONTROL COLLATERAL DAMAGE?

In hospitals 31 (29%) of the studies provided reliable data about microbial outcomes and 24 interventions were associated with significant improvement. Studies with microbial outcomes are subject to additional risks of bias.[58] Nonetheless, there are examples of studies with medium or low risk of bias that demonstrate sustained reduction in the prevalence of antimicrobial-resistant bacteria and *C. difficile* infections associated with change in antibiotic policy (Figure 11.2). Unfortunately, some published studies use inappropriate statistical methods and report unreliable conclusions about the impact of antibiotic policies[58,60] – for example, changes in a hospital formulary were made to limit an outbreak of vancomycin-resistant enterococci.[61] In the published report, the effect of this formulary change on other resistant pathogens was analyzed with parametric statistics, which are not appropriate for microbial outcomes.[60] Segmented regression analysis shows that the change in antibiotic policy was associated with a small but not statistically significant decrease in ceftazidime-resistant *Klebsiella pneumoniae* and methicillin-resistant *Staphylococcus aureus* (MRSA), whereas there was a statistically significant increase in cefotaxime-resistant *Acinetobacter* spp. (Figure 11.3).

In ambulatory care four studies in the systematic review included microbial outcomes (one macrolide-resistant streptococci and three penicillin-resistant pneumococci).[45] Only one of these studies showed that reduction in antibiotic use

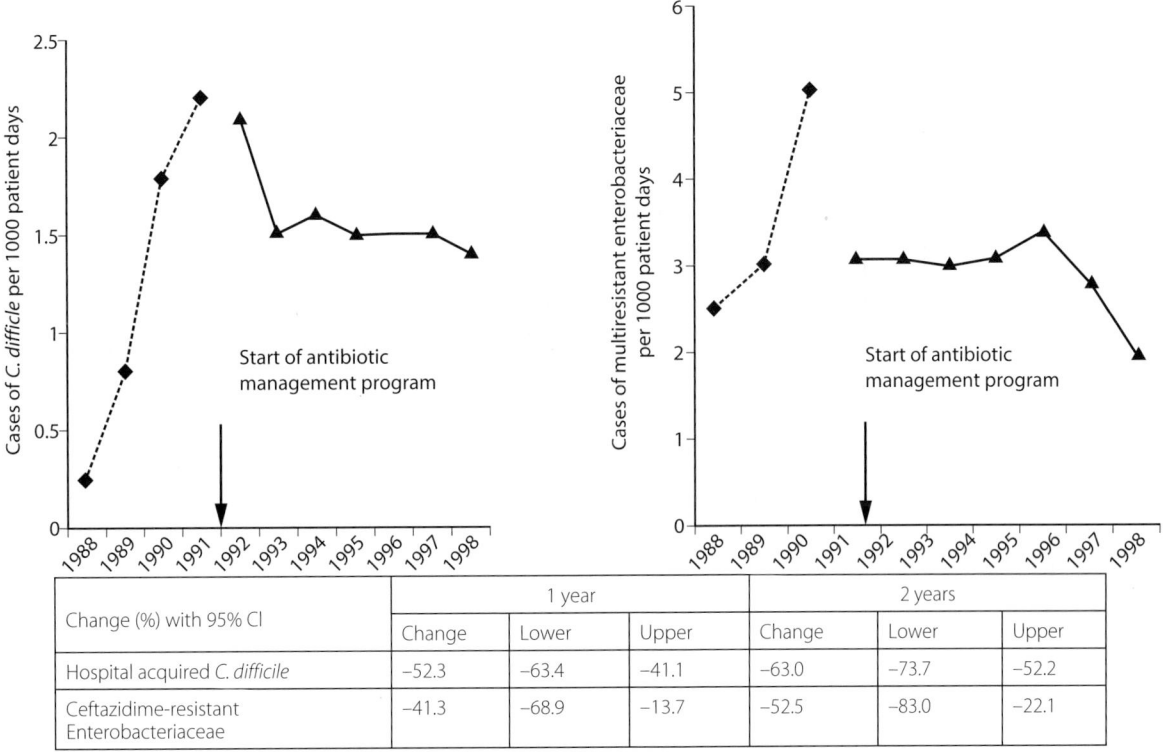

Change (%) with 95% CI	1 year			2 years		
	Change	Lower	Upper	Change	Lower	Upper
Hospital acquired *C. difficile*	−52.3	−63.4	−41.1	−63.0	−73.7	−52.2
Ceftazidime-resistant Enterobacteriaceae	−41.3	−68.9	−13.7	−52.5	−83.0	−22.1

Fig. 11.2 Examples of interrupted time series analysis of the impact of antibiotic policy change on the prevalence of *Clostridium difficile* infection and infections with ceftazidime-resistant Enterobacteriaceae per 1000 patient days.[59] The segmented regressions analysis of the effect size was performed for a systematic review of interventions to change antibiotic prescribing in hospitals.[46] (Redrawn from data from Carling P, Fung T, Killion A et al. Favorable impact of a multidisciplinary antibiotic management program conducted during 7 years. **Infection Control and Hospital Epidemiology.** 2003;24:699–706.[59])

was associated with a significant reduction in resistance.[62] There are two possible explanations:

1. Duration of follow-up: the successful study had 4 years of post-intervention data whereas the other three studies all had no more than 1 year.
2. Antibiotic resistance in Gram-positive bacteria is not associated with much fitness cost, meaning that there is little survival advantage for sensitive bacteria even in the absence of antibiotic pressure.[63,64]

In support of this second explanation, a recent study from Israel showed that a national restriction of ciprofloxacin use was associated with an immediate marked reduction in ciprofloxacin resistance in Gram-negative bacteria isolated from urine.[65] In contrast with Gram-positive bacteria, resistance to quinolones in Gram-negative bacteria is associated with considerable fitness cost.[66]

WHAT IMPACT DO ANTIBIOTIC POLICIES HAVE ON CLINICAL OUTCOME?

In hospitals, 32 (30%) of the studies included reliable data about clinical outcomes. However, in 12 of these studies the intervention was either wholly ($n = 8$) or partially ($n = 4$) designed to increase the intensity of antibiotic treatment. Clinical outcomes were measured in only 20 (23%) of 87

studies that aimed solely to reduce the intensity of antibiotic treatment. These studies do provide some reassurance that there were no unintended adverse clinical consequences.

In ambulatory care only two (5%) of 40 studies included reliable data about clinical outcome: one showed that delayed antibiotic prescription for otitis media was associated with a 1.1-day increase in the duration of symptoms (95% CI; from 0.5 to 1.5-day increase);[67] the other showed that reduction in antibiotic prescribing for the common cold had no significant impact on symptom score.[68] Additional reassurance was provided by a third study, which showed that a reduction in the use of antibiotics for acute bronchitis was not associated with any significant increase in repeat office visits or in hospitalizations for respiratory tract infection.[69]

DEVELOPMENT, DISSEMINATION AND IMPLEMENTATION OF ANTIBIOTIC POLICIES

Development of policies should be informed by the wide variety of resources and information available on the world wide web.[42] A great deal of information can be captured within a simple flow chart, providing an easily accessible reminder to prescribers on the walls of a treatment room, in a pocket-sized antibiotic policy or available on the hospital intranet and world wide web.[70]

A simple but effective model for improvement[71] is based on three questions:

1. What are we trying to accomplish?
2. How will we know that change is an improvement?
3. What changes can we make that will result in improvement?

In order to answer the first question the team must define a consensus goal for improvement. The second question requires measurement of process or outcome. The third question requires tests of change. These should be small, rapid and repeated.[48]

It is clear that measurement and improvement are intertwined; it is impossible to make improvements without measurement.[56] There are eight key principles to the use of data to improve daily clinical practice:[56]

1. Seek usefulness, not perfection in the measurement.
2. Use a balanced set of process, outcome and cost measures.
3. Keep measurement simple (think big, start small).
4. Use qualitative and quantitative data.
5. Write down the operational definition of measures.
6. Measure small, representative samples.
7. Build measurement into daily work.
8. Develop a measurement team.

Inclusion of targets for audit of implementation (Box 11.1) is a key component of the assessment of evidence-based guidelines.[72]

HOW SHOULD COMPLIANCE WITH ANTIBIOTIC POLICIES BE MONITORED?

Hospitals fortunate enough to have sophisticated information systems may be able to use these to monitor compliance with policies.[73] However, this remains the exception rather than the rule. Less sophisticated information systems can still provide valuable information but there is often no substitute for collection of data by hand.[74] This is not necessarily

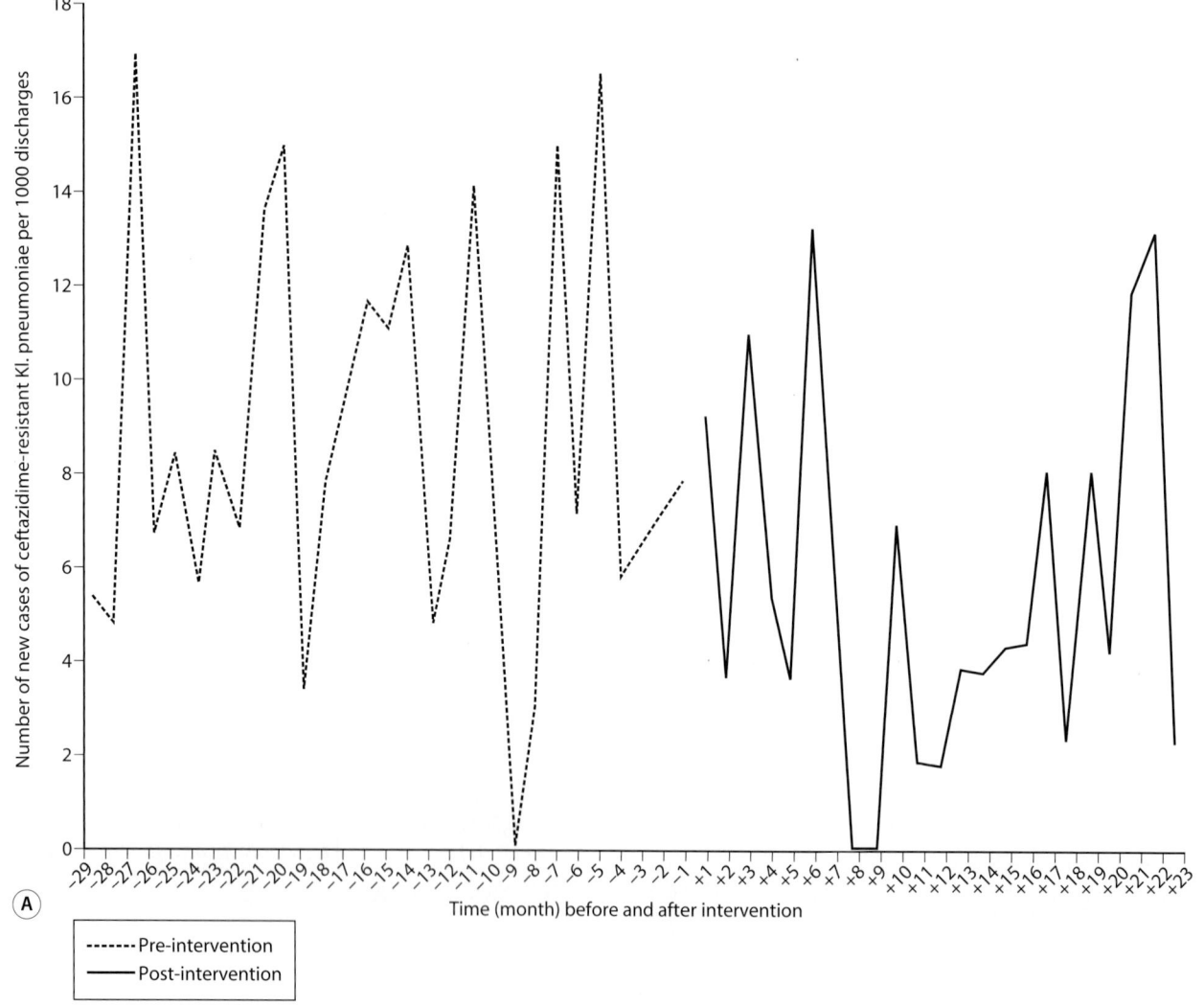

Fig. 11.3 Examples of interrupted time series analysis of the impact of antibiotic policy change on the prevalence of resistant bacteria.[61] The segmented regression analysis of the effect size was performed for a systematic review of interventions to change antibiotic prescribing in hospitals.[46] (A) New cases of ceftazidime-resistant *Klebsiella pneumoniae* per 1000 discharges.

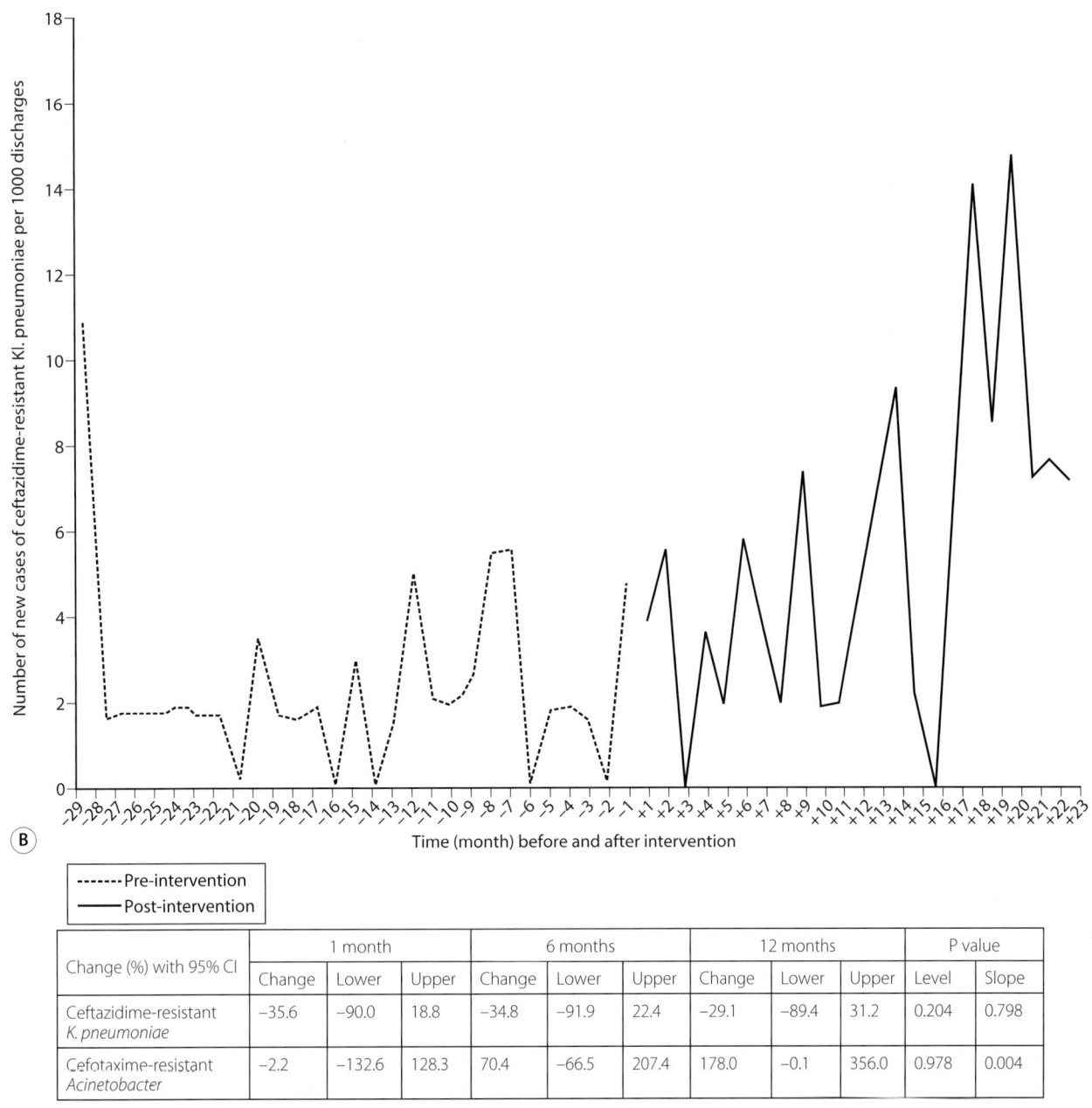

Change (%) with 95% CI	1 month			6 months			12 months			P value	
	Change	Lower	Upper	Change	Lower	Upper	Change	Lower	Upper	Level	Slope
Ceftazidime-resistant *K. pneumoniae*	−35.6	−90.0	18.8	−34.8	−91.9	22.4	−29.1	−89.4	31.2	0.204	0.798
Cefotaxime-resistant *Acinetobacter*	−2.2	−132.6	128.3	70.4	−66.5	207.4	178.0	−0.1	356.0	0.978	0.004

Fig. 11.3—cont'd (B) New cases of cefotaxime-resistant *Acinetobacter* spp. per 1000 discharges. (C) Segmented regression analysis of data from Figures 11.3A and 11.3B. (Redrawn from data from Landman D, Chockalingam M, Quale JM. Reduction in the incidence of methicillin-resistant Staphylococcus aureus and ceftazidime-resistant Klebsiella pneumoniae following changes in a hospital antibiotic formulary. **Clinical Infectious Diseases.** 1999;28:1062–1066, The University of Chicago Press.[61])

as daunting as it may seem; a 1-day prevalence survey of an entire hospital can be achieved in a few hours and may be a useful tool to detect deviations from guidelines and provide physicians with educational feedback. The European Surveillance of Antimicrobial Consumption (ESAC) project has adapted a web-based tool for antibiotic surveillance developed in Sweden[75] and successfully used this for comparative surveillance of hospitals in 20 European countries.[76] A variety of staff can be involved in auditing policies, including trainee nurses, pharmacists, doctors and medical students.[77] Participation in data collection is an educational

experience and the information can be used to agree care bundles of three or four essential processes of care that must be completed and documented for every patient to monitor antibiotic compliance and review infection management.[78] In hospitals bacteremia provides a manageable focus for attention. Review of patients with bacteremia identifies patients who are being overtreated, including those with contaminated blood cultures. However, about one-third of patients reviewed will have inadequate treatment because of delay in starting and selection of the wrong drug, dose or route of administration.[79–81]

Box 11.1   Core indicators for audit from a national guideline on surgical prophylaxis[18] From Scottish Intercollegiate Guidelines Network (SIGN). Antibiotic Prophylaxis in Surgery. Edinburgh Royal College of Physicians of Edinburgh 2008 http://www.sign.ac.uk/pdf/sign104.pdf (15th August 2009, date last accessed).

Process measures

Was prophylaxis given for an operation included in local guidelines?

If prophylaxis was given for an operation not included in local guidelines, was a clinical justification for prophylaxis recorded in the case notes?

Was the first dose of prophylaxis given within 30 min of the start of surgery?

Was the prescription written in the 'once-only' section of the drug prescription chart?

Was the duration of prophylaxis greater than 24 h?

Outcome measures

Surgical site infection (SSI) rate = number of SSIs occurring postoperatively/total number of operative procedures.

Rate of SSIs occurring postoperatively in patients who receive inappropriate prophylaxis (as defined in guideline) compared with rate of this infection in patients who receive appropriate prophylaxis, expressed as a ratio.

Rate of *Clostridium difficile* infections occurring postoperatively in patients who receive inappropriate prophylaxis (as defined in guideline) compared with rate of this infection in patients who receive appropriate prophylaxis, expressed as a ratio.

Minimum data set for surgical antibiotic prophylaxis

Date

Operation performed

Classification of operation (clean/clean-contaminated/contaminated)

Elective or emergency

Patient weight (especially children)

Any previous adverse reactions/allergies to antibiotics

Justification for prophylaxis (e.g. evidence of high risk of SSI) if prophylaxis is given for an operation that is not one of the indications for routine prophylaxis

Time of antibiotic administration

Name of antibiotic

Dosage of antibiotic

Route of administration

Time of surgical incision

Duration of operation

Second dosage indicated?

Second dosage given?

Postoperative antibiotic prophylaxis indicated?

Postoperative antibiotic prophylaxis given?

Antibiotic prophylaxis continued for >24 h

Documentation recorded appropriately (in correct place, clarity)

Name of anaesthetist

Name of surgeon

Designation of surgeon

In primary care routine data about antibiotic prescribing are more generally available and can be used to measure the impact of prescribing interventions.[82] More sophisticated data systems that include diagnosis may be required to monitor the impact of targeted interventions – for example, to reduce prescribing for bronchitis.[69] However, as in hospitals, hand collection of data may be the only practical method available.

Community pharmacists have an important potential role in the audit of antibiotic prescribing in primary care.[83]

Data about measures of professional practice or clinical outcomes are best displayed as run charts or statistical process control charts (Figure 11.4) as these clearly demonstrate progress over time. Small amounts of data collected regularly can be very informative. The statistical process control charts in Figure 11.4 only have one patient observation for every data point so each chart only includes data from 17 patients, yet the charts clearly show the impact of the intervention. Resources for testing change (such as Plan Do Study Act cycles), designing and using measures for improvement are publicly available on clinical effectiveness websites.[84] For infrequent events (e.g. number of new MRSA or *C. difficile* infections) the time since the last new infection is a powerful method for displaying information.[85] Posting of 'days since last infection' data allows staff to see at a glance the importance and status of critical infections. In this way, positive feedback is provided as infection-free days accrue, and analysis of cause occurs when the days go back to zero.[85]

LEGAL IMPLICATIONS OF ANTIBIOTIC POLICIES

Having considered the advantages of antibiotic policies, it is important to be aware of their legal implications. It is not unusual for audits to show that only a minority of professionals' practice is fully consistent with antibiotic policies. In that case, are the majority of professionals guilty of negligence? Moreover, is the organization in which the professionals practice also guilty of negligence unless it takes action and achieves 100% adherence to policies? Although interventions can improve adherence to policies, the changes are often small.[45,46] Even when the best methods for development, dissemination and implementation are used, a majority of professionals may still not adhere to the policy.[86] The reasons include lack of knowledge, awareness, familiarity, agreement, outcome expectancy and ability to overcome the inertia of previous practice.[87] Guidelines by their very nature consider common problems in typical patients and may fail to adequately address the needs of individual patients, particularly the elderly and the patient with a complicated course.[86] Guidelines frequently lack objective parameters, lack graded recommendations and do not favor a multidisciplinary approach.[88] As has already been noted, a major flaw of much of the literature on the implementation of antibiotic policies is the failure to include measures of clinical outcome (*see* Table 11.2). For all of these reasons 100% concordance between clinical practice and guidelines is neither desirable nor achievable.

Written policies and practice guidelines have a major impact on courts of law, particularly if they are endorsed by national societies or other professional bodies. As a legal standard, their testimonial relevance, or 'weight' in that respect, is just below regulations issued by the primary or secondary lawmaker. The legal implication of this position is that presentation of a policy or guideline in court may overcome expert opinion, results

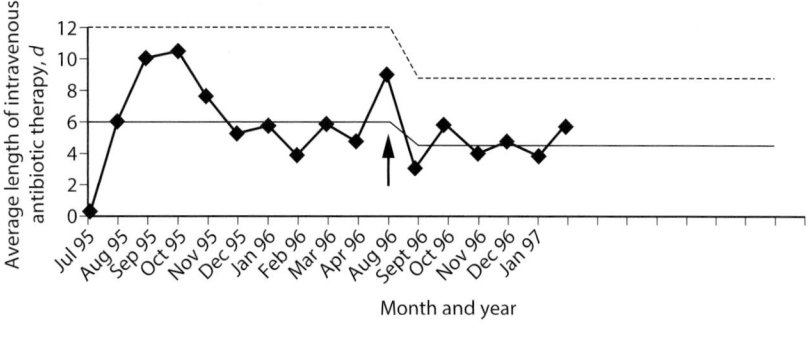

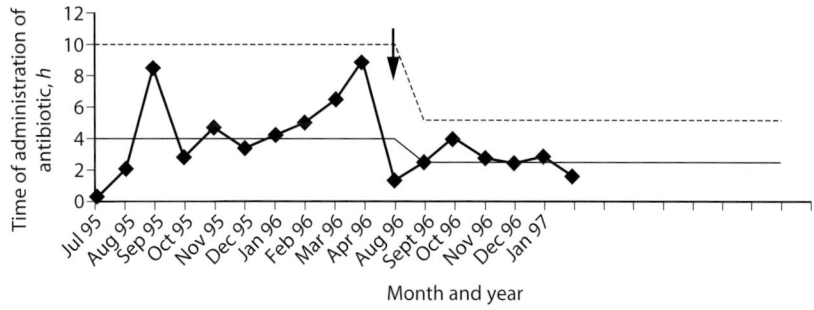

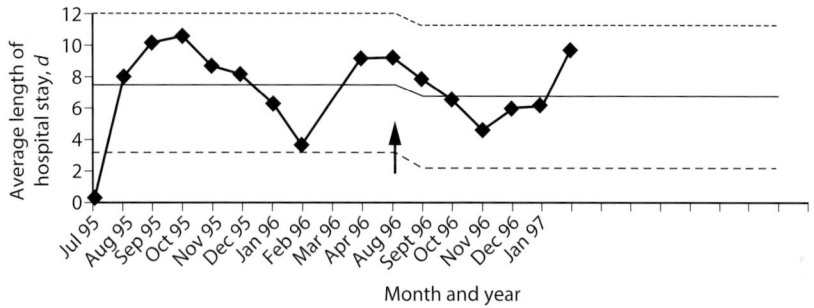

Fig. 11.4 Instrument panel of three statistical process control charts for hospitalized patients with community-acquired pneumonia. Duration of intravenous antibiotic therapy, time to administration of antibiotic therapy and average length of hospital stay were thought to be key measures that the pneumonia care team wanted to follow over time. The solid lines represent the mean values plotted over time. The dotted lines represent the upper and lower control limits or natural process limits for the measured variables (lower limits in the top and middle panels were less than zero and are not shown). The arrows indicate the points at which changes were implemented. The upper and lower natural process limits were computed by using the following formula: mean ⊥ 2.66 (average point-to-point variation, also called the moving range). This formula is recommended for calculation of process limits when the size of the subgroup is 1; it was chosen because each data point is a measurement from a single patient. From Nelson EC, Splaine ME, Batalden PB et al. Building measurement and data collection into medical practice. Annals of internal medicine 1998;128:460–466, by permission of the American college of Physicians.[56])

of well-conducted studies and even meta-analysis (particularly if published after the guideline was written). Most courts will assign a written policy/guideline a burden of evidence far beyond the importance assigned to the policy/guideline by those who wrote it or use it. Writers of guidelines, such as the Scottish Intercollegiate Guidelines Network, often clearly state that the intention is to provide guidance rather than to impose stiff regulations. Nonetheless, courts of law may still interpret guidelines as minimum standards of care.

Conversely, a court can even declare a policy or guideline as insufficient or unacceptable; the court is sovereign to decide upon the standard according to its own legal policies – which are usually aimed at improving the health of the public.

Thus, if the court finds a certain policy, even if approved by official bodies, to be insufficient, it can declare it as a non-standard and set its own standard. The following quote is from the book *International Medical Malpractice Law*: 'A common practice (regardless if founded on guidelines) simply may not be good enough to fulfill the standard required by the law.'[89] In 1993 the supreme court of Canada expressed the view that 'conformity with standard practice (based on policy or guidelines) in a profession does not necessarily insulate a doctor from negligence where the standard of practice itself is negligent'.[90] In the UK, the House of Lords has stated the view that the court can, in rare cases, reach a conclusion that a professional standard is not based on a rational analysis, and that the experts express views that are not logical or responsible.[91] These judgments have important implications for antibiotic policy makers. Concerns about antibiotic resistance may be used to justify restriction of antibiotics even when there is compelling evidence to suggest that this is not in the interests of the individual patient.[92] However, a court may not agree with this decision; indeed the court is likely to decide that a doctor's primary duty is care of the individual patient. The problem of antibiotic resistance confronts prescribers and the healthcare organizations in which they work with two conflicting ethical duties: one is their duty of fidelity to the individual patient; the other is their duty of stewardship for the resources that have been entrusted to them.[93] Rigid enforcement of the duty of fidelity would result in prescription of antibiotics to any patient who might conceivably have infection and selection of an empirical regimen that covers all possible pathogens. Such a policy is clearly not in the long-term interests of the public. However, would a court of law support a healthcare organization that put the long-term interests of the public before the interests of the individual patient?[94]

Antibiotic restriction policy has been implied in farm husbandry in view of human infections with resistant mutants (e.g. fluoroquinolone-resistant *C. jejunii* originating in fluoroquinolone-fed chickens). A quantitative risk assessment model of microbiological risks suggests that these outcomes may be more than coincidental: prudent use of animal antibiotics may actually improve human health, while total bans on animal antibiotics, intended to be precautionary, inadvertently may harm human health. Moreover, the ban of fluoroquinolones as food additives to chicken in the USA and some other jurisdictions was not associated with a decrease in fluoroquinolone resistance among other human pathogens, lessening the impact of antibiotic restrictive policies in agriculture on human disease. A court, when coming to decide on a case in which non-human use of antibiotics was associated with human harm (except for the case of *C. jejunii*), will confront great difficulties in obtaining direct evidence for this association and may thus have uncertainty in its final decision.

Legislation should also be considered as an instrument for helping to achieve the aims of antibiotic policies. Once antimicrobial drug resistance has been recognized as a concern by public health authorities they will ask for legal as well as scientific analysis of the problem, and international organizations such as the European Union and the World Health Organization will also seek legal solutions.[95] However, cooperative initiatives may be more practical and speedy than legislation, at least in the first instance.[95] Similarly, at the national level, it has been recognized that development of local solutions may be more productive than imposing national legislation.[95] Nonetheless, Fidler provides several practical proposals for introducing legislation to help to control antimicrobial prescribing:[95]

1. International legal harmonization of principles for prudent antimicrobial drug use will have to include monitoring and enforcement, as well as financial,

technical and legal assistance by industrialized countries to developing countries.

2. In the USA, Congress could regulate use of antimicrobial drugs by monitoring interstate commerce in these products. Congress probably does not have the authority to regulate antimicrobial prescription practices directly; such authority rests with the states.

3. Perhaps the most powerful US federal strategy would be to make implementation of state policies to curb the misuse of antimicrobial drugs mandatory before states receive federal funds earmarked for public health. In countries where governments subsidize the purchase of antimicrobial drugs, legislative or regulatory changes in these subsidies could lead to a decline in the use of the drugs.

4. Fulfillment of legal duties often hinges on sufficient resources. In many developing countries public health systems may be inadequate. Thus, financial and technical leadership is needed from national governments towards local authorities and from international organizations towards developing countries. A precedent can be found in the proposed Convention on the Provision of Telecommunication Resources for Disaster Mitigation and Relief Operations, which obligates the parties, where possible, to lower or remove regulatory barriers for using telecommunication resources during disasters.

5. Lessons from international environmental efforts suggest that international law must play a major role in setting international standards for implementation domestically and creating the political, technical and financial conditions necessary to integrate international and national law.

KEY QUESTIONS ABOUT ANTIBIOTIC POLICIES AND ANTIMICROBIAL STEWARDSHIP

WHAT IS THE MOST COST-EFFECTIVE METHOD FOR IMPLEMENTING POLICIES?

It is probably unrealistic to expect a definitive answer to this question because of the influence of context as well as the knowledge, attitudes and beliefs of both the professionals who are the targets for change and the patients that they serve.[96] However, even a partial answer to the question requires more basic information about the cost of development, testing and implementation of antibiotic policies and other interventions (*see* Table 11.2). In particular, it would be very helpful to have more information about the added value of audit and feedback for implementation of antibiotic policies (*see* Table 11.3). Only 10% of studies in ambulatory or hospital care used this, yet the quality improvement literature suggests that measurement and feedback are integral to the implementation of change.[56]

WHEN SHOULD RESTRICTIVE STRATEGIES BE USED TO IMPLEMENT ANTIBIOTIC POLICIES?

Restrictive strategies are perceived as dictatorial or punitive and are likely to be less appealing to clinicians.[97] It is generally acknowledged that practice guidelines achieve their greatest good by expanding medical knowledge, which may not be achieved by punitive measures.[98] In hospitals the evidence suggests that restrictive interventions have greater short-term effects but that persuasive interventions may have greater long-term effects. More data would be helpful but we believe that the available evidence already suggests that a case should be made for urgency in order to justify restrictive antibiotic policies.

WHAT BALANCING MEASURES SHOULD BE USED TO EVALUATE ANTIBIOTIC POLICIES?

Now that the evidence base on beneficial effects of antibiotic policies is growing, the research and policy agenda needs to pay more attention to reassuring the public and professionals about unintended consequences of antibiotic policies. The few studies that include balancing measures clearly show that unintended consequences can happen (*see* Figure 11.3B).

 References

1. House of Lords Select Committee on Science and Technology. In: *Resistance to Antibiotics*. London: The Stationery Office; 2001:1–34.
2. European Union. The Copenhagen Recommendations. Report from the Invitational EU Conference on The Microbial Threat. In: Rosdahl VK, Pedersen KB, eds. Copenhagen, Denmark: Ministry of Health, Ministry of Food, Agriculture and Fisheries; 1998:1–52. http://www.sum.dk/.
3. Monnet D, Kristinsson K. Turning the tide of antimicrobial resistance: Europe shows the way. *Euro Surveill*. 2008;13(46).
4. MacDougall C, Polk RE. Antimicrobial stewardship programs in health care systems. *Clin Microbiol Rev*. 2005;18:638–656.
5. Rice LB.. The Maxwell Finland Lecture: For the duration – rational antibiotic administration in an era of antimicrobial resistance and *Clostridium difficile*. *Clin Infect Dis*. 2008;46:491–496.
6. Dellit TH, Owens RC, McGowan Jr JE, et al. Infectious Diseases Society of America and the Society for Healthcare Epidemiology of America guidelines for developing an institutional program to enhance antimicrobial stewardship. *Clin Infect Dis*. 2007;44:159–177.
7. Health Protection Agency. *Management of infection guidance for primary care for consultation and local adaptation*. London: HPA. Online. Available athttp://www.hpa.org.uk/web/HPAwebFile/HPAweb_C/1194947340160.
8. Specialist Advisory Committee on Antimicrobial resistance (SACAR). *UK template for hospital antimicrobial guidelines*. London: SACAR; 2005. Online Available at http://www.bsac.org.uk/_db/_documents/Template_for_hospital_antimicrobial_guidelines_May_2005.doc.
9. MacKenzie FM, Struelens MJ, Towner KJ, et al. Report of the Consensus Conference on Antibiotic Resistance; Prevention and Control (ARPAC). *Clin Microbiol Infect*. 2005;11:938–954.
10. Nathwani D. Antimicrobial prescribing policy and practice in Scotland: recommendations for good antimicrobial practice in acute hospitals. *J Antimicrob Chemother*. 2006;57:1189–1196.
11. Molstad S, Erntell M, Hanberger H, et al. Sustained reduction of antibiotic use and low bacterial resistance: 10-year follow-up of the Swedish Strama programme. *Lancet Infect Dis*. 2008;8:125–132.
12. Allerberger F, Lechner A, Wechsler-Fordos A, et al. Optimization of antibiotic use in hospitals – antimicrobial stewardship and the EU project ABS international. *Chemotherapy*. 2008;54:260–267.
13. Kunin CM, Tupasi T, Craig WA. Use of antibiotics. A brief exposition of the problem and some tentative solutions. *Ann Inter Med*. 1973;79:555–560.
14. Anonymous. Implementing a local prescribing policy. *Drug Ther Bull*. 1990;28:93–95.
15. Working Party of the British Society of Antimicrobial Chemotherapy. Working Party Report: Hospital antibiotic control measures in the UK. *J Antimicrob Chemother*. 1994;34:21–42.
16. Wickens HJ, Jacklin A. Impact of the Hospital Pharmacy Initiative for promoting prudent use of antibiotics in hospitals in England. *J Antimicrob Chemother*. 2006;58:1230–1237.
17. Lawton RM, Fridkin SK, Gaynes RP, et al. Practices to improve antimicrobial use at 47 US hospitals: the status of the 1997 SHEA/IDSA position paper recommendations. *Infect Control Hosp Epidemiol*. 2000;21:256–259.
18. Scottish Intercollegiate Guidelines Network (SIGN). *Antibiotic prophylaxis in surgery: a national clinical guideline*. Edinburgh: Royal College of Physicians of Edinburgh; 2008. Online Available at http://www.sign.ac.uk/pdf/sign104.pdf.
19. Bapna JS, Tripathi CD, Tekur U. Drug utilisation patterns in the third world. *Pharmacoeconomics*. 1996;9:286–294.
20. Sosa A. Antibiotic policies in developing countries. In: Gould I, Van der Meer NJ, eds. *Antibiotic policies: theory and practice*. New York: Kluwer Academic/Plenum Publishers; 2005:593–616.
21. Hogerzeil HV. Promoting rational prescribing: an international perspective. *Br J Clin Pharmacol*. 1995;39:1–6.
22. Barber N. Improving quality of drug use through hospital directorates. *Qual Health Care*. 1993;2:3–4.
23. Wiffen PJ, Mayon White RT. Encouraging good antimicrobial prescribing practice: a review of antibiotic prescribing policies used in the South East Region of England. *BMC Public Health*. 2001;1:4.
24. von Gunten V, Reymond JP, Boubaker K, et al. Antibiotic use: is appropriateness expensive? *J Hosp Infect*. 2009;71:108–111.
25. Parker SE, Davey PG. Pharmacoeconomics of intravenous drug administration. *Pharmacoeconomics*. 1992;1:103–115.
26. Ponge T, Cottin S, Fruneau P, et al. Iatrogenic disease. Prospective study, relation to drug consumption. *Therapie*. 1989;44(1):63–66.
27. Dunagan WC, Woodward RS, Medoff G, et al. Antibiotic misuse in two clinical situations: positive blood culture and administration of aminoglycosides. *Rev Infect Dis*. 1991;13:405–412.
28. Marwick C, Watts E, Evans J, et al. Quality of care in sepsis management: development and testing of measures for improvement. *J Antimicrob Chemother*. 2007;60:694–697.
29. Schwartz DN, Wu US, Lyles RD, et al. Lost in translation? Reliability of assessing inpatient antimicrobial appropriateness with use of computerized case vignettes. *Infect Control Hosp Epidemiol*. 2009;30:163–171.
30. Reeves DS, Finch RG, Bax RP, et al. Self-medication of antibacterials without prescription (also called 'over-the-counter' use). A report of a Working Party of the British Society for Antimicrobial Chemotherapy [In Process Citation]. *J Antimicrob Chemother*. 1999;44:163–177.
31. Wenzel RP, Kunin CM. Should oral antimicrobial drugs be available over the counter? *J Infect Dis*. 1994;170:1256–1259.
32. Davey PG, Bax RP, Newey J, et al. Growth in the use of antibiotics in the community in England and Scotland in 1980–1993. *Br Med J*. 1996;312:613.
33. Goossens H, Guillemot D, Ferech M, et al. National campaigns to improve antibiotic use. *Eur J Clin Pharmacol*. 2006;62:373–379.
34. Bauraind I, Lopez-Lozano JM, Beyaert A, et al. Association between antibiotic sales and public campaigns for their appropriate use. *JAMA*. 2004;292:2468–2470.
35. L'Assurance Maladie SS. *Programme Antibiotiques: un premier cap est franchi, la mobilisation pour le bon usage doit se poursuivre*. Online. Available athttp://www.ameli.fr/fileadmin/user_upload/documents/DP_Antibiotiques_10-01-2008.pdf.
36. Goossens H, Ferech M, Vander SR, et al. Outpatient antibiotic use in Europe and association with resistance: a cross-national database study. *Lancet*. 2005;365:579–587.

37. Damoiseaux RA, de Melker RA, Ausems MJ, et al. Reasons for non-guideline-based antibiotic prescriptions for acute otitis media in The Netherlands. *Fam Pract*. 1999;16:50–53.

38. Deschepper R, Grigoryan L, Lundborg CS, et al. Are cultural dimensions relevant for explaining cross-national differences in antibiotic use in Europe?. *BMC Health Serv Res*. 2008;8:123.

39. Davey P, Ferech M, Ansari F, et al. Outpatient antibiotic use in the four administrations of the UK: cross-sectional and longitudinal analysis. *J Antimicrob Chemother*. 2008;62:1441–11147.

40. Flin R, Maran N. Identifying and training non-technical skills for teams in acute medicine. *Qual Saf Health Care*. 2004;13(suppl 1):i80–i84.

41. Davey P, Garner S, on behalf of the Professional Education Subgroup of SACAR. Professional education on antimicrobial prescribing: a report from the Specialist Advisory Committee on Antimicrobial Resistance (SACAR) Professional Education Subgroup. *J Antimicrob Chemother*. 2007;60:i27–i32.

42. Pagani L, Gyssens IC, Huttner B, et al. Navigating the Web in search of resources on antimicrobial stewardship in health care institutions. *Clin Infect Dis*. 2009;48:626–632.

43. British Society for Antimicrobial Chemotherapy. *Prudent antibiotic user (PAUSE)* http://www.pause-online.org.uk.

44. Lipsitch M. The rise and fall of antimicrobial resistance. *Trends Microbiol*. 2001;9:438–444.

45. Arnold SR, Straus SE. Interventions to improve antibiotic prescribing practices in ambulatory care. *Cochrane Database Syst Rev*. 2005; CD003539.pub2.

46. Davey P, Brown E, Fenelon L, et al. Interventions to improve antibiotic prescribing practices for hospital inpatients. *Cochrane Database Syst Rev*. 2005; CD003543.

47. British Society for Antimicrobial Chemotherapy. *Resource Library, Cochrane Review: Interventions to improve antibiotic prescribing practices for hospital inpatients*. Online. Available at http://www.bsac.org.uk/resource:library. cfm?cit_id=571&FAArea1=customWidgets.content_view_1&usecache=false.

48. Weinberg M, Fuentes JM, Ruiz AI, et al. Reducing infections among women undergoing cesarean section in Colombia by means of continuous quality improvement methods. *Arch Intern Med*. 2001;161:2357–2365.

49. Barlow G, Nathwani D, Williams F, et al. Reducing door-to-antibiotic time in community-acquired pneumonia: controlled before-and-after evaluation and cost-effectiveness analysis. *Thorax*. 2007;62:67–74.

50. Sintchenko V, Coiera E, Gilbert GL. Decision support systems for antibiotic prescribing. *Curr Opin Infect Dis*. 2008;21:573–579.

51. Paul M, Andreassen S, Tacconelli E, et al. Improving empirical antibiotic treatment using TREAT, a computerized decision support system: cluster randomized trial. *J Antimicrob Chemother*. 2006;58:1238–1245.

52. Cochrane Effective Practice and Organisation of Care (EPOC) Group. *EPOC resources for review authors*. Online. Available at http://www.epoc.cochrane. org/en/handsearchers.html.

53. Franz AR, Bauer K, Schalk A, et al. Measurement of interleukin 8 in combination with C-reactive protein reduced unnecessary antibiotic therapy in newborn infants: a multicenter, randomized, controlled trial. *Pediatrics*. 2004;114:1–8.

54. Brown C, Lilford R. The stepped wedge trial design: a systematic review. *BMC Med Res Methodol*. 2006;6:54.

55. Oxman A, Thomson M, Davis D, et al. No magic bullets: a systematic review of 102 trials of interventions to improve professional practice. *Canadian Medical Journal*. 1995;153:1423–1431.

56. Nelson EC, Splaine ME, Batalden PB, et al. Building measurement and data collection into medical practice. *Ann Intern Med*. 1998;128:460–466.

57. Grimshaw JM, Thomas RE, MacLennan G, et al. Effectiveness and efficiency of guideline dissemination and implementation strategies. *Health Technol Assess*. 2004;8:iii–72.

58. Davey P, Brown E, Fenelon L, et al. Systematic review of antimicrobial drug prescribing in hospitals. *Emerg Infect Dis*. 2006;12:211–216.

59. Carling P, Fung T, Killion A, et al. Favorable impact of a multidisciplinary antibiotic management program conducted during 7 years. *Infect Control Hosp Epidemiol*. 2003;24:699–706.

60. Stone SP, Cooper BS, Kibbler CC, et al. The ORION statement: guidelines for transparent reporting of outbreak reports and intervention studies of nosocomial infection. *J Antimicrob Chemother*. 2007;59:833–840.

61. Landman D, Chockalingam M, Quale JM. Reduction in the incidence of methicillin-resistant *Staphylococcus aureus* and ceftazidime-resistant *Klebsiella pneumoniae* following changes in a hospital antibiotic formulary. *Clin Infect Dis*. 1999;28:1062–1066.

62. Seppala H, Klaukka T, Vuopio-Varkila J, et al. The effect of changes in the consumption of macrolide antibiotics on erythromycin resistance in group A streptococci in Finland. *N Engl J Med*. 1997;337:441–446.

63. Gustafsson I, Cars O, Andersson DI. Fitness of antibiotic resistant *Staphylococcus epidermidis* assessed by competition on the skin of human volunteers. *J Antimicrob Chemother*. 2003;52:258–263.

64. Rozen DE, McGee L, Levin BR, et al. Fitness costs of fluoroquinolone resistance in *Streptococcus pneumoniae*. *Antimicrob Agents Chemother*. 2007;51:412–416.

65. Gottesman BS, Carmeli Y, Shitrit P, et al. The impact of quinolone restriction on resistance patterns of *Escherichia coli* isolated from urine cultures in a community setting. *Clin Infect Dis*. 2009;49:869–875.

66. Komp Lindgren P, Marcusson LL, Sandvang D, et al. Biological cost of single and multiple norfloxacin resistance mutations in *Escherichia coli* implicated in urinary tract infections. *Antimicrob Agents Chemother*. 2005;49:2343–2351.

67. Little P, Gould C, Williamson I, et al. Pragmatic randomised controlled trial of two prescribing strategies for childhood acute otitis media. *Br Med J*. 2001;322:336–342.

68. Arroll B, Kenealy T, Kerse N. Do delayed prescriptions reduce the use of antibiotics for the common cold? A single-blind controlled trial. *J Fam Pract*. 2002;51:324–328.

69. Gonzales R, Steiner JF, Lum A, et al. Decreasing antibiotic use in ambulatory practice: impact of a multidimensional intervention on the treatment of uncomplicated acute bronchitis in adults. *JAMA*. 1999;281:1512–1519.

70. Tayside NHS. *Adult empirical treatment of infection guidelines*. Dundee: NHS Tayside. Online. Available at http://www.nhstaysideadtc.scot.nhs.uk/TAPG%20html/MAIN/Front%20page.htm.

71. Langley GL, Nolan KM, Nolan TW, et al. *The improvement guide: a practical approach to enhancing organizational performance*. San Francisco: Jossey-Bass; 1996.

72. Scottish Intercollegiate Guidelines Network (SIGN). SIGN 50. *A guideline developer's handbook*. Scotland: Edinburgh Scottish Intercollegiate Guidelines Network, NHS Quality Improvement; 2008. Online Available at http://www. sign.ac.uk/guidelines/fulltext/50/index.html.

73. Pestotnik SL, Classen DC, Scott Evans R, et al. Implementing antibiotic practice guidelines through computer-assisted decision support: clinical and financial outcomes. *Ann Intern Med*. 1996;124:884–890.

74. Cooke DM, Salter AJ, Phillips I. The impact of antibiotic policy on prescribing in a London Teaching Hospital. A one-day prevalence survey as an indicator of antibiotic use. *J Antimicrob Chemother*. 1983;11:447–453.

75. Erntell M. *The STRAMA Point Prevalence Survey 2003 and 2004 on hospital antibiotic use. Stockholm STRAMA (Swedish Strategic Programme against Antibiotic Resistance)*. 2004. Online Available at http://en.strama.se/dyn//,86,5.html.

76. Ansari F, Goossens H, Erntell M, et al. The European Surveillance of Antimicrobial Consumption (ESAC) point prevalence survey of antibacterial use in 20 European hospitals in 2006. *Clin Infect Dis*. 2009;49:1507–1515.

77. Nathwani D, Davey PG. Strategies to rationalize sepsis management – a review of 4 years' experience in Dundee. *J Infect*. 1998;37:10–17.

78. Pulcini C, Defres S, Aggarwal I, et al. Design of a 'day 3 bundle' to improve the reassessment of inpatient empirical antibiotic prescriptions. *J Antimicrob Chemother*. 2008;61:1384–1388.

79. Horn DL, Opal SM. Computerized clinical practice guidelines for review of antibiotic therapy for bacteremia. *Infectious Diseases in Clinical Practice*. 1992;1:169–173.

80. Nathwani D, Davey PG, France AJ, et al. Impact of an infection consultation service for bacteraemia on clinical management and use of resources. *Q J Med*. 1996;89:789–797.

81. Minton J, Clayton J, Sandoe J, et al. Improving early management of bloodstream infection: a quality improvement project. *Br Med J*. 2008;336:440–443.

82. Baquero F. Evolving resistance patterns of *Streptococcus pneumoniae*: a link with long-acting macrolide consumption? *J Chemother*. 1999;11 (suppl 1):35–43.

83. Costello I, Wong IC, Nunn AJ. A literature review to identify interventions to improve the use of medicines in children. *Child Care Health Dev*. 2004;30:647–665.

84. NHS Scotland Educational Resources Clinical Governance. *Managing clinical effectiveness*. Scotland, Edinburgh: NHS Quality Improvement. Online. Available at http://www.clinicalgovernance.scot.nhs.uk/section2/inpractice. asp.

85. Stockwell JA. Nosocomial infections in the pediatric intensive care unit: affecting the impact on safety and outcome. *Pediatr Crit Care Med*. 2007;8:S21–S37.

86. Halm EA, Atlas SJ, Borowsky LH, et al. Understanding physician adherence with a pneumonia practice guideline: effects of patient, system, and physician factors. *Arch Intern Med*. 2000;160:98–104.

87. Cabana MD, Rand CS, Powe NR, et al. Why don't physicians follow clinical practice guidelines? A framework for improvement. *JAMA*. 1999;282:1458–1465.

88. Grilli R, Magrini N, Penna A, et al. Practice guidelines developed by specialty societies: the need for a critical appraisal. *Lancet*. 2000;355:103–106.

89. Giesen D. *International medical malpractice law*. Dordrecht, The Netherlands: Kluwer; 1988.

90. Dominion Law Reports. *ter Neuzen v. Korn*. Ontario, Canada: Canada Law Book; 2001.

91. House of Lords Judgments – Bolitho v. *City and Hackney Health Authority*. London: London Judicial Office, House of Lords; 1997. Online Available at http://www.parliament.the-stationery-office.co.uk/pa/ld199798/ldjudgmt/jd971113/boli01.htm.

92. Pauker SG, Rothberg M. Commentary: resist jumping to conclusions. *Br M J*. 1999;318:1616–1617.

93. Sabin JE. Fairness as a problem of love and the heart: a clinician's perspective on priority setting. *Br Med J*. 1998;317:1002–1004.

94. Leibovici L, Shraga I, Andreassen S. How do you choose antibiotic treatment? *Br Med J*. 1999;318:1614–1618.

95. Fidler DP. Legal issues associated with antimicrobial drug resistance. *Emerg Infect Dis*. 1998;4:169–177.

96. Campbell NC, Murray E, Darbyshire J, et al. Designing and evaluating complex interventions to improve health care. *Br Med J*. 2007;334:455–459.

97. Murray MD, Kohler RB, McCarthy MC, et al. Attitudes of house physicians concerning various antibiotic-use control programs. *Am J Hosp Pharm*. 1988;45:584–588.

98. Woolf SH. Practice guidelines: a new reality in medicine. *Arch Intern Med*. 1993;153:2646–2655.

Agents

Introduction to Section 2

The number and variety of antimicrobial agents has expanded inexorably since the appearance of the first edition of this book nearly 50 years ago and organization of the information on individual agents in a way that helps the reader to make sense of the profusion is a continuing challenge. Once again we have tried to present the information in a uniform, accessible and succinct manner. The authorship reflects the most recent revision based, in most cases, on pre-existing text written by different hands for the various editions of the book that have appeared over the years.

As always, the aim has been to be as inclusive and up to date as possible and we have sought to include all but the most obscure compounds that are available worldwide. Compounds used exclusively in veterinary medicine are mentioned by name if appropriate, but are not otherwise dealt with.

The amount of detail provided for older or less important drugs has been reduced to a short summary of their most important properties. For the rest we have tried to present the most important information in a standard and logical manner, tabulating such information as could be easily accommodated in this form. For large groups of agents, such as the penicillins, cephalosporins, macrolides, aminoglycosides and quinolones, the individual drug monographs are preceded by a general account of the group and its classification.

For the individual monographs, the following conventions have been adopted:

Drug names: The recommended International Non-proprietary Name (rINN) is used throughout, with the United States Adopted Name (USAN) and any other commonly used alternative name given at the beginning of each monograph. An exception has been made for methicillin (rINN: meticillin), since this antibiotic is no longer generally available and the original spelling is commonly used in the context of 'methicillin-resistant *Staphylococcus aureus*'.

Structures: Simple two-dimensional structures of the most important compounds are given, together with the molecular weights and those of appropriate salts.

Antimicrobial activity: For antibacterial agents, minimum inhibitory concentration (MIC) values for the most common Gram-positive and Gram-negative pathogens are tabulated with members of the same drug group appearing in the same Table. Since published MIC values differ, sometimes quite widely, depending on the methodology used and the source of the micro-organisms tested, those given are representative ones, usually based on fully susceptible strains. Activity against other relevant pathogens is described in the text. Nomenclature of micro-organisms follows current recommendations (e.g. all clinically important salmonellae are described as *Salmonella enterica* serotypes rather than individual species).

Acquired resistance: Common mechanisms of acquired resistance and its general prevalence are described.

Pharmacokinetics: Basic pharmacokinetic parameters are tabulated: oral absorption (if relevant); maximum plasma concentration (C_{max}) for common dosage forms; plasma half-life; volume of distribution (usually in liters or, preferably, L/kg); and plasma protein binding. Values given normally refer to data from healthy adult volunteers and may be altered in disease or at the extremes of age. Unless otherwise stated, the plasma half-life is the β-phase value; when the terminal half-life differs substantially, this is described in the accompanying text. A more extensive account of absorption, distribution, metabolism and excretion characteristics is added for the more important compounds.

Interactions: Some important interactions are described, but a more extensive account is provided in Section 1 (Ch. 6).

Toxicity and side effects: The most important adverse reactions are given. For compounds for which class effects are prominent, this information is to be found in the section on general properties of the class earlier in the chapter.

Clinical use: The most common uses are listed. Information on the mode of use in different clinical settings is dealt with in appropriate chapters of Section 3.

Preparations and dosage: Common proprietary names are given, but others may be used in individual markets, especially for older compounds with many generic forms. Dosages are commonly accepted regimens for adults and children. Since recommended dosage regimens sometimes vary in different countries, the information may differ from that found in local formularies.

Further information: No in-text references are provided, but appropriate up-to-date sources of information are listed. Extensive monographs on many anti-infective drugs can be found in *Therapeutic Drugs*, 2nd edn (Dollery, C. ed.), Churchill Livingstone, Edinburgh, 1999.

12 Aminoglycosides and aminocyclitols

Andrew M. Lovering and David S. Reeves

The aminoglycoside antibiotics comprise a large group of naturally occurring or semisynthetic polycationic compounds. The therapeutically important members of the group have amino sugars glycosidically linked to aminocyclitols – cyclic alcohols that are also substituted with amino functions. Most are bactericidal agents and share the same general range of antibacterial activity, pharmacokinetic behavior, a tendency to damage one or both branches of the eighth nerve, and a propensity to cause renal damage. The degree and nature of toxicity varies among compounds, and for some it is so great as to preclude systemic use.

Streptomycin was the first aminoglycoside, identified in 1944 by Waksman's group as a natural product of a soil bacterium, *Streptomyces griseus*. This was followed by the discovery of neomycin by the same group in 1949 and of kanamycin by Umezawa and his colleagues in 1957. Gentamicin, the most important aminoglycoside in use today, was first reported in 1963. Thereafter there followed an era in which research on new aminoglycosides concentrated on the chemical modification of known compounds, largely in response to developing resistance.

CLASSIFICATION

In most aminoglycosides in regular clinical use, the aminocyclitol moiety is 2-deoxystreptamine; these compounds can be subdivided into the neomycin group, in which there are carbohydrate substitutions at positions 4 and 5 of 2-deoxystreptamine, and the kanamycin and gentamicin groups, in which the aminocyclitol is 4,6-disubstituted. In streptomycin the aminocyclitol ring is another derivative of streptamine, streptidine. Several less important compounds exhibit other structural variations on the aminoglycoside–aminocyclitol theme.

2-Deoxystreptamine-containing aminoglycosides

Gentamicin group	Kanamycin group	Neomycin group	Other aminoglycosides/ aminocyclitols
Gentamicin	Amikacin	Neomycin	Astromicin
Isepamicin	Arbekacin	Paromomycin	Spectinomycin
Micronomicin	Dibekacin		Streptomycin
Netilmicin	Kanamycin		
Sisomicin	Tobramycin		

The nomenclature of the aminoglycoside structure is illustrated by that of kanamycin B:

The carbon atoms in the 2-deoxystreptamine ring are labeled 1 to 6; those in the amino sugar substituted at position 4 are labeled 1′ to 6′ and those in the 6-position amino sugar 1″ to 6″.

Some natural aminoglycosides consist of mixtures of closely related compounds. For example, there are four principal gentamicins, three kanamycins and two neomycins, often with interbatch variability in the ratio of these within pharmaceutical preparations. Moreover, there are close relationships between some of the differently named compounds.

For example, tobramycin is 3'-deoxykanamycin B and the substitution of an amino for a hydroxyl group in paromomycin I gives neomycin B. The chemical differences are particularly important in determining sensitivity of the compounds to inactivation by bacterial aminoglycoside-modifying enzymes.

ANTIMICROBIAL ACTIVITY

The activity of the more important aminoglycosides against common pathogens is summarized in Table 12.1. They are active to different degrees against *Staphylococcus aureus*, coagulase-negative staphylococci and *Corynebacterium* spp., but the activity against many other Gram-positive bacteria, including streptococci, is generally limited. However, they interact synergistically with antibiotics such as penicillin against streptococci, enterococci and some other organisms, and this combination is used as first-line therapy in enterococcal endocarditis (p. 591).

As a group, they are widely active against the Enterobacteriaceae and other aerobic Gram-negative bacilli including, for some compounds, *Pseudomonas aeruginosa*. Several, including streptomycin, are active against *Mycobacterium tuberculosis* and some other mycobacteria. Aminoglycosides require a threshold membrane potential to cross the bacterial cell membrane and, as this is diminished under anaerobic conditions, aminoglycosides are not active against anaerobic bacteria.

They are generally bactericidal in concentrations close to the minimum inhibitory concentration (MIC) and the rate of killing increases directly with the concentration, up to about 10 times the MIC value. Activity is increased by low Mg^{2+} and Ca^{2+} concentrations and diminished under anaerobic or hypercapnic conditions.

AMINOGLYCOSIDE TRANSPORT

Diffusion of such highly polar cationic compounds across the bacterial cell membrane is very limited and intracellular accumulation of the drugs is brought about by active transport, which occurs in three phases:

- Initial energy-independent binding of the compounds to the exterior of the cell, which is inhibited by Ca^{2+} and Mg^{2+} ions.
- Energy-dependent phase I (so called because it is abolished by molecules that inhibit energy metabolism), in which the aminoglycosides are driven across the cytoplasmic membrane by the negative electrical potential difference across the membrane.
- A faster, energy-dependent phase II, which starts after aminoglycosides have bound to ribosomes and seems to be an effect, rather than a cause, of their action on the cell.

Uptake is adversely affected by low pH and reduced oxygen tension as they affect the membrane potential. Consequently, activity of the drugs in vitro is reduced in acid media or anaerobic conditions and by the presence of divalent cations; the susceptibility of *Ps. aeruginosa* is particularly sensitive to the cation concentration. Because of the effects of pH on activity, it is hard to be sure that the relatively high MICs seen for organisms that require carbon dioxide truly reflect their degree of resistance.

Table 12.1 Median MICs (mg/L) of aminoglycosides for common pathogenic bacteria

Bacterium	Gentamicin	Netilmicin	Tobramycin	Amikacin	Kanamycin	Neomycin	Streptomycin	Spectinomycin
Staphylococcus aureus	0.25	0.25	0.25	1	1	0.5	4	64
Coagulase-negative staphylococci	0.03	0.03	0.03	0.25	0.5	0.06	2	32
Streptococcus pyogenes	4	4	16	32	32	16	8	32
Str. pneumoniae	4	8	16	64	64	128	32	8
Enterococcus faecalis	16	8	16	128	64	32	128	64
Neisseria meningitidis	16	16	16	32	32	4		8
N. gonorrhoeae	4	4	4	16	16	16	8	16
Haemophilus influenzae	0.5	0.5	1	1	1	2	2	4
Escherichia coli	0.5	0.5	1	2	4	1	8	8
Klebsiella pneumoniae	0.5	0.5	0.5	2	2	1	4	16
Bacteroides fragilis	R	R	R	R	R	R	R	R
Mycobacterium tuberculosis	R		R	1	8	0.5	0.5	
M. avium	4			8	4		2	

R, resistant; no useful activity at clinically achievable concentrations.

ACQUIRED RESISTANCE

Resistance in many organisms originally susceptible to the older compounds, such as streptomycin and kanamycin, is now widespread. Resistance to the more clinically important agents such as gentamicin has also increased, but there are marked differences even within countries depending on antibiotic use policies. Resistance rates for gentamicin in North America and Europe have so far generally remained low. However, many strains with plasmid-encoded extended-spectrum β-lactamases (p. 228–231) and other resistances are also aminoglycoside resistant, so outbreaks of infection with such strains may result in an increase in aminoglycoside resistance rates.

Bacterial resistance to the aminoglycosides is usually mediated through one, or more, of the three main mechanisms:
- Alteration in the ribosomal binding of the drug
- Reduced uptake
- Inactivation by specific aminoglycoside-modifying enzymes.

RIBOSOMAL RESISTANCE

Strains of bacteria with ribosomes that have a diminished affinity for streptomycin may emerge during therapy with streptomycin and the MIC is often in excess of 1000 mg/L. Such resistance results from alteration of a single ribosomal protein or rRNA, usually in the *rpsL* gene, and occurs at a natural mutational rate of 10^{-5} per generation in *Escherichia coli*. In contrast, ribosomal resistance to other clinically useful amino-glycosides is not encountered during therapy, as resistance usually requires mutations at two or three ribosomal binding sites. Ribosomal alterations confer high-level resistance to the aminoglycoside against which they were selected (and closely related ones), but not other aminoglycosides. Such resistance is not transferable to other bacteria.

REDUCED UPTAKE

Resistance resulting from a diminished ability to accumulate aminoglycosides occurs as a result of changes in energy metabolism or outer membrane structure, and may be clinically significant. Such resistance is caused by selection of chromosomal mutations at several loci during exposure to the drug and may lead to cross-resistance to other aminoglycosides, including those resistant to aminoglycoside-modifying enzymes. Reversion to wild type occurs rapidly in coliforms in the absence of selective pressure. The isolates often show altered ability to couple oxidative phosphorylation to electron transport and the level of resistance conferred is generally modest; they are frequently slow growing and are of reduced pathogenicity. However, in *Pseudomonas* isolates the changes are relatively stable and generally due to changes in the MexXY multidrug efflux system. Such isolates are relatively common and are frequently found in isolates from cystic fibrosis patients.

AMINOGLYCOSIDE-MODIFYING ENZYMES

Production of modifying enzymes usually confers a high degree of resistance and is the most common mechanism of resistance. The enzymes are usually plasmid encoded and the resistance conferred is frequently transferable. As with β-lactamase production, the organisms owe their survival to the inactivation of the agent to which they remain intrinsically susceptible and a large number of enzymes have been identified from different bacterial species.

There are three classes of aminoglycoside-modifying enzyme, which differ in the nature of the sites modified:
- *N*-acetyltransferases (AAC) modify amino groups
- *O*-phosphotransferases (APH) modify hydroxyl groups
- *O*-nucleotidyltransferases (ANT) modify hydroxyl groups.

The sites of attack of these enzymes on gentamicin are shown below:

Gentamicin C1a

The position of the group attacked and the ring that carries it are indicated by the number of the enzyme: thus AAC(3) is the acetyltransferase that modifies the amino group in the 3-position on the aminocyclitol ring while ANT(2″) modifies the hydroxyl group at the 2″-position on an aminosugar. If two enzymes act at the same position on the molecule, but differ in the aminoglycosides modified, they are distinguished by roman numerals. For example, AAC(3)-I confers resistance to gentamicin alone, whereas AAC(3)-II confers resistance to tobramycin and netilmicin as well as to gentamicin and so on (Table 12.2). Many aminoglycoside-modifying enzymes that are apparently identical in terms of resistance profile have different amino acid sequences. Lower case letters after the roman numeral are used to designate the different subgroups: thus, AAC(6′)-Ia and AAC(6′)-Ib are two unique proteins conferring identical resistance profiles. Finally, lower case italicized letters are used to indicate the gene responsible, so that the gene coding for the AAC(6′)-Ia enzyme is *aac(6′)Ia*.

Table 12.2 Range of activity of enzymes that modify 2-deoxystreptamine-containing aminoglycosides

Enzyme	Kanamycin A	Neomycin	Amikacin	Tobramycin	Gentamicin	Netilmicin	Sisomicin
APH(3')-I, II, IV, VII	+	+	–	0	0	0	0
APH(3')-III & VI	+	+	+	0	0	0	0
APH(3')-V	–	+	–	0	0	0	0
APH(2″)	+	0	–	+	+	–	0
ANT(4')	+	+	+	+	0	0	0
ANT(2″)	+	0	–	+	+	–	0
AAC(3)-I & VI	–	–	–	–	+	–	–
AAC(3)-II	±	–	–	+	+	+	–
AAC(3)-III	+	+	–	+	+	–	–
AAC(3)-IV	±	+	–	+	+	+	+
AAC(2')	0	+	0	+	+	+	0
AAC(6')-I	+	+	+	+	Variable[a]	+	0
AAC(6')-II	+	–	–	+	+	+	0

[a]Gentamicin C$_{1a}$, C$_2$ and sisomicin +, gentamicin C$_1$ ±/–.
+, Modified; ±, poorly modified; –, not modified; 0, substituent necessary for modification absent.

Resistance to aminoglycosides results from the interplay between the rate of drug inactivation by the modifying enzyme and the rate of drug transport. Thus the resistance phenotype of a particular isolate depends on the enzyme kinetics, best defined by the ratio of V_{max} to K_m for a given substrate, and the rate of drug uptake. Consequently, enzymes that poorly inactivate some aminoglycosides, and fail to confer resistance to them, may confer clinically relevant resistance when associated with a change in cell permeability.

The discovery that AAC(6')-Ib-cr can acetylate fluoroquinolones with a piperazinyl moiety (e.g. ciprofloxacin; *see* Ch. 26) and confer resistance to them has led to the identification of further bifunctional enzymes and is helping to shed light upon the ecological origins of this large family of enzymes, over 50 different types of which are currently known.

DISTRIBUTION OF MODIFYING ENZYMES

Most aminoglycoside-modifying enzymes are encoded by transposable elements in resistant bacteria; however, some are chromosomally determined with the presence of the gene, if not its expression in terms of resistance profile, characteristic of the species. The most notable examples are:

- *aac(2')-Ia*; characteristic of *Providencia stuartii*
- *aac(6')-Ic*; characteristic of *Serratia marcescens*
- *aac(6')-Ii*; present in all *Enterococcus faecium* strains.

The expression of these genes appears to be tightly regulated. Thus, although the chromosomal *aac(6')-Ic* gene is found in all *Ser. marcescens* strains, most are aminoglycoside susceptible with little or no *aac(6')-Ic* mRNA detectable.

Certain enzymes may be found in a restricted host range, but most are widely distributed throughout clinically important bacterial genera. The prevalence of the individual enzymes within an individual geographic area usually reflects the selective pressure exerted by the aminoglycoside usage there. In many instances there is linkage with other resistance determinants; for example, most gentamicin resistance seen in *Staph. aureus* relates to methicillin-resistant *Staph. aureus* (MRSA) and is a reflection of the transmissibility of these strains rather than the use of gentamicin.

Since the prevalence of the enzymes differs widely with geographic area and over relatively short time periods, reflecting antibiotic prescribing habits and the opportunities for resistant organisms to spread, it is imperative that the local prevalence of resistance to individual agents be established when choosing between aminoglycosides. This is particularly important for the treatment of severe sepsis of undetermined origin. Identification of aminoglycoside-modifying enzymes can often be deduced with varying degrees of confidence from the resistance patterns of the organisms. However, molecular diagnostic products that can be used to identify the most prevalent enzymes are becoming available and it is likely that more accurate identification will soon be within the capacity of many laboratories. Moreover, most of the gene sequences have been published, and departments with appropriate expertise can develop polymerase chain reaction (PCR)-based diagnostic tests for locally troublesome enzymes.

Genome sequences have identified several putative aminoglycoside resistance genes, even in organisms known to be sensitive to these drugs, suggesting a complex evolutionary history for these enzymes. Most of the genes that have been characterized in vitro do not code for bona fide resistance enzymes, but a substantial reservoir of potential aminoglycoside resistance genes may exist within bacterial genomes.

PHARMACOKINETICS

Aminoglycosides are highly polar molecules that carry a net positive charge. Less than 1% of an oral dose is absorbed from the gut, but this may be clinically significant in the presence of renal failure or where gut inflammation leads to increased uptake. Absorption is rapid from intramuscular sites and serous cavities. Plasma protein binding is low (<10%), and aminoglycosides are distributed into the extracellular water and some serous fluids (ascites, pleural fluid), with volumes of distribution of about 0.25 L/kg. Intracellular penetration is low, as is penetration into cerebrospinal fluid (CSF) and aqueous humor, although concentration in these fluids may be higher when inflammation is present. There is extensive binding to tissues, principally renal, which accounts for initial incomplete excretion of aminoglycosides and prolonged excretion after dosing is terminated. The plasma half-lives are typically about 2 h, but this varies between individuals and particularly when renal function is impaired. Excretion is almost entirely as unchanged drug by glomerular filtration, which gives high concentration of active antibiotic in the urine with normal dosages, and no clinically relevant metabolites are known. When renal function is impaired, aminoglycoside excretion is reduced and accumulation can occur.

Because of their low protein binding, relatively small volumes of distribution and small molecular size, aminoglycosides are readily removed by hemodialysis, during which their half-life is reduced to about 4 h from the 50 h typically seen in end-stage renal failure. Some 50% of the drug is removed during a 3–4 h hemodialysis session. Removal by peritoneal dialysis is much less efficient, the half-life being around 36 h.

Aminoglycosides are inactivated by many β-lactam antibiotics with which they combine chemically. This is clinically relevant if the antibiotics are mixed for infusion or, possibly, in renal failure, where the long half-life of both antibiotics may allow time for this interaction.

BLOOD CONCENTRATIONS AND DOSAGE ADJUSTMENTS

Aminoglycosides cause exposure-dependent ototoxicity and nephrotoxicity, with the risk of toxicity increasing with the exposure and, in particular, with sustained rather than transiently high concentrations. Consequently, therapeutic drug monitoring to ensure exposure does not exceed target levels should be used in all patients receiving more than 48 h of systemic therapy. Monitoring is often driven by concerns of toxicity rather than by the need to ensure that adequate exposure is attained. This is slightly curious, as it has been an improved understanding of the pharmacodynamics of aminoglycosides and the factors driving outcome that has led to the widespread adoption of once daily administration. However, at present almost all approaches to therapeutic drug monitoring of gentamicin are based on detection of elevated concentrations in the pre-dose sample and none adequately detects subtherapeutic concentrations in such a sample.

In both in-vitro and animal models, the measure that most strongly correlates with outcome is the ratio of the maximum serum concentration (C_{max}) to the MIC, with enhanced killing seen up to C_{max}:MIC ratios of 8–10. There is evidence to suggest that the ratio of the area under the time–concentration curve (AUC) to MIC also affects outcome and is important (see Ch. 4). For the assessment of therapeutic concentrations, a post-dose sample is needed, with a satisfactory peak concentration defined as a concentration of 10× the MIC. Although it might be expected that a therapeutic concentration should be achieved in most patients, and post dose monitoring is not needed in practice it is often not attained, particularly in critically ill patients with severe sepsis. In such patients, volumes of distribution are increased, due to capillary leakage and fluid loading, and the peak concentration is lowered. Monitoring of post-dose concentrations in this patient group may help to identify subtherapeutic concentrations.

Since aminoglycosides penetrate poorly into adipose tissue, dosage based on total body weight can give excessive plasma concentrations in obese patients. Appropriate dosage adjustment should be made in patients who are 30% or more over ideal body weight. Likewise, in patients with an abnormally low percentage of fat, increased volumes of distribution, and lower peak concentrations, may be seen. These effects occur in children and to a lesser extent in patients with cystic fibrosis, where volumes of distribution may be increased by 50% or more due to body morphology. As a result, peak gentamicin concentrations may be depressed in patients with a high lean body weight and the assay of post-dose samples is helpful in identifying significant underdosing.

Although high clearance leading to low AUC exposure is a known issue in patients with burns, and cystic fibrosis, where abnormally high renal clearances and volume of distribution changes often require increased doses, it is rarely considered in other patient populations. Consequently, in patients with high renal clearances, such as the young and previously fit, lower than expected drug exposure may occur. Unfortunately, the use of a peak sample will fail to identify such patients, as a concentration of 10× the MIC will usually be attained, and the only reliable way to identify them is by the use of two post-dose samples, one taken at 1 h post and the other taken 6–14 h post dose.

Alteration in the pharmacokinetics of these drugs requiring dose adjustment may also be anticipated in patients with physiologically (e.g. newborns and the elderly) or pathologically (e.g. patients with oliguria or systemic hypotension) impaired renal function. In children a number of distinct physiological processes occur. At birth, aminoglycoside volumes of distribution approximate to the volume of the extracellular water at 0.5–0.8 L/kg, and decrease over the first 3 months of life to a value of about 0.4 L/kg during childhood and to a value the same as adults by late childhood (12 years). Similarly, renal function at birth is low at 40 mL/min/1.73 m² but increases rapidly over the first 2 weeks of life and then more slowly to reach, or exceed, adult values of 100 mL/min/1.73 m² by the age of 3 months. Although renal function is much lower in preterm infants, there is considerable interpatient variability, and measures based solely on gestational age often poorly predict actual renal function.

Since patients receiving a course of an aminoglycoside must be subject to blood monitoring, access to a rapid and reliable assay service is essential. Although nomograms have been recommended for initial dosage calculation before and during therapy, because of interindividual variation, continuing therapy needs to be monitored. The size and exact time of all doses must be recorded, as must the exact time of blood samples for assays, since this information is essential to the correct interpretation of the assay results. A laboratory method should be used that gives accurate and rapid (<1 h) results.

TOXICITY AND SIDE EFFECTS

A wide range of adverse effects can occur following the administration of aminoglycosides, ototoxicity and nephrotoxicity being the most important. There are differences in the absolute and relative frequencies of these adverse effects between the various aminoglycosides.

OTOTOXICITY

Aminoglycosides are potentially ototoxic to both the cochlear and vestibular functions of the eighth cranial nerve, with such damage usually being permanent. To damage the hair cells, which are the sensory cells involved, the aminoglycoside must accumulate in the endolymph and possibly the perilymph. Accumulation is caused by persisting and high plasma concentrations, which prevent aminoglycoside from diffusing back into plasma. Consequently, ototoxicity has been associated with impaired renal function. Once damage to the hair cells has occurred it may continue to increase in severity for up to 4 weeks after the drug has been stopped. Vestibulotoxicity is manifest by vertigo, especially on rising out of bed, ataxia and oscillopsia. Cochleotoxicity presents as deafness, particularly to high tones. Ototoxicity is potentiated by previous aminoglycoside exposure, and concomitant exposure to loop diuretics and other drugs, and to noise.

Although ototoxicity can occur in all patients receiving amino-glycosides, an enhanced susceptibility to cochlear toxicity has been linked to an A–G substitution in location 1555 of the mitochondrial ribosomal ribonucleic acid (RNA); a second mutation involving a thymidine deletion in the 12S ribosomal RNA gene can predispose patients to auditory toxicity. These patients may experience ototoxicity at relatively normal drug exposures. Genetic testing may be useful in prospectively identifying them before starting therapy, but it may be more valuable in the subsequent review of patients who develop ototoxicity.

NEPHROTOXICITY

Aminoglycosides accumulate in the renal cortex to cause nephrotoxicity. The frequency with which this occurs depends on many factors related to the clinical state of the patient, the agent itself, and the way it is administered. Unlike ototoxicity, which is largely specific to aminoglycosides, the diagnosis of nephrotoxicity is made uncertain because of the many causes of diminished renal function.

Nephrotoxicity is associated with poorer outcomes and it is important to detect the onset as soon as practicable in order to decide on the clinical value of continuing aminoglycoside therapy. Serial measurement of plasma creatinine should be made daily or not less than every 3 days, depending on the clinical state of the patient. Since the plasma concentration of creatinine can vary from day to day, measuring the clearance of the aminoglycoside itself may give an earlier indication of the onset of nephrotoxicity. Other indicators of renal damage, such as urinary phospholipid, renal enzymes or β₂-microglobulin, are currently not in widespread routine use.

Rates of nephrotoxicity vary greatly, but may reach 60% in patients on intensive care. A longer dosage interval lowers the rate by allowing more time for the drug to clear from renal tissue between doses. The problem is more frequently associated with treatment for more than 7 days. Simultaneous exposure to other potentially nephrotoxic drugs, such as vancomycin, amphotericin B, cephalosporins, angiotensin-converting enzyme inhibitors and non-steroidal anti-inflammatory agents, increases the likelihood of nephrotoxicity. Iodinated contrast media have also been implicated. Patient factors increasing the frequency of nephrotoxicity include hypotension, shock, hypovolemia and diabetes.

Renal damage is produced to very different degrees by the various aminoglycosides and is related to the accumulation of high concentrations in the renal cortex. The frequency of nephrotoxicity after systematic administration differs markedly, from around 2% to 60% depending on the patient population, dosage and criteria of renal damage. Gentamicin is generally regarded as more nephrotoxic than netilmicin because of its lower excretion rate and higher degree of net reabsorption. The abnormal persistence of aminoglycosides in the plasma between doses may be the earliest and most sensitive indication of the onset of renal impairment.

If acute tubular necrosis develops it usually does so towards the end of the first week of treatment, while the drugs are accumulated at tissue binding sites. The appearance of brush border membrane fragments in the urine or new cylindruria are strongly correlated with decline of renal function. Restoration of function usually occurs if the drug is discontinued.

Risk factors include dosage and duration of therapy, plasma concentration and renal function. Age has emerged in some studies as the dominant or even sole independent determinant of toxicity risk. Renal damage is probably more likely and more severe with simultaneous use of other agents that act on the kidney, including some diuretics and cisplatin.

NEUROMUSCULAR BLOCKADE

Aminoglycosides can produce neuromuscular blockade, probably by functioning as membrane stabilizers in the same way as curare. The effect is relatively feeble, and is rarely seen in those with normal neuromuscular function. However, antibiotics are customarily given in much larger amounts than curare, and patients who are also receiving muscle relaxants or anesthetics, or who are suffering from myasthenia gravis, are at special risk. Analogous effects, which can be reversed by calcium, have been described on the gut and uterus.

CLINICAL USE

Aminoglycosides are the mainstay of the treatment of severe sepsis caused by enterobacteria and some other Gram-negative aerobic bacilli. For the treatment of severe sepsis of undetermined cause they are often administered in combination with agents active against Gram-positive or anaerobic bacteria as appropriate. Some are also used for a number of specialized infections, including endocarditis, respiratory infections and tuberculosis.

Gentamicin, tobramycin or amikacin are most commonly used. There is no clear choice on the grounds of toxicity because differences between the various members of the group are of no proven clinical relevance. Differences in invitro activity depend largely on the local prevalence of particular resistance mechanisms.

Gentamicin is a sensible choice for the treatment of suspected or confirmed infections caused by Gram-negative bacilli unless resistance is a major problem. It is often used as first-choice therapy for patients without renal functional deficit. Tobramycin may have some advantage for proven *Ps. aeruginosa* or *Acinetobacter* infections. Amikacin is preferred if there is resistance to other aminoglycosides. These drugs can be combined with a β-lactam antibiotic and metronidazole as appropriate for microbiologically undiagnosed severe infection, unless microbiological or epidemiological evidence indicates a high probability of resistance in any individual case. However, aminoglycoside monotherapy appears to be as effective as combination therapy in areas with a low prevalence of resistance.

 Further information

Al-Hasan MN, Lahr BD, Eckel-Passow JE, Baddour LM. Antimicrobial resistance trends of *Escherichia coli* bloodstream isolates: a population-based study, 1998–2007. *J Antimicrob Chemother*. 2009;64:169–174.

Anaizi N. Once-daily dosing of aminoglycosides. A consensus document. *Int J Clin Pharmacol Ther*. 1997;35:223–226.

Barclay ML. Experience of once-daily aminoglycoside dosing using a target area under the concentration–time curve. *Aust N Z J Med*. 1995;25:230–235.

Barclay ML, Begg EJ. Aminoglycoside toxicity and relation to dose regimen. *Adverse Drug React Toxicol Rev*. 1994;13:207–234.

Batchelor M, Hopkins KL, Liebana E, et al. Development of a miniaturised microarray-based assay for the rapid identification of antimicrobial resistance genes in Gram-negative bacteria. *Int J Antimicrob Agents*. 2008;31:440–451.

De Broe ME, Verbist L, Verpooten GA. Influence of dosage schedule on renal cortical accumulation of amikacin and tobramycin in man. *J Antimicrob Chemother*. 1991;27(suppl C):41–47.

Drusano GL, Ambrose PG, Bhavnani SM, Bertino JS, Nafziger AN, Louie A. Back to the future: using aminoglycosides again and how to dose them optimally. *Clin Infect Dis*. 2007;45:753–760.

Edson RS, Terrell CL. The aminoglycosides. *Mayo Clin Proc*. 1999;74:519–528.

Hawkey PM, Jones AM. The changing epidemiology of resistance. *J Antimicrob Chemother*. 64(suppl 1):i3–i10.

Kirkpatrick CMJ, Duffull SB, Begg EJ, Frampton C. The use of a change in gentamicin clearance as an early predictor of gentamicin-induced nephrotoxicity. *Ther Drug Monit*. 2003;25:623–630.

Li H, Steyger PS. Synergistic ototoxicity due to noise exposure and aminoglycoside antibiotics. *Noise Health*. 2009;11:26–32.

Mattie H, Craig WA, Pechère JC. Determinants of efficacy and toxicity of aminoglycosides. *J Antimicrob Chemother*. 1989;24:281–293.

Nicasio AM, Kuti JL, Nicolau DP. The current state of multidrug-resistant gram-negative bacilli in North America. *Pharmacotherapy*. 2008;28:235–249.

Oliveira JF, Silva CA, Barbieri CD, Oliveira GM, Zanetta DM, Burdmann EA. Prevalence and risk factors for aminoglycoside nephrotoxicity in intensive care units. *Antimicrob Agents Chemother*. 2009;53:2887–2891.

Pacifici GM. Clinical pharmacokinetics of aminoglycosides in the neonate: a review. *Eur J Clin Pharmacol*. 2009;65:419–427.

Qian Y, Guan MX. Interaction of aminoglycosides with human mitochondrial 12S rRNA carrying the deafness-associated mutation. *Antimicrob Agents Chemother*. 2009;53(11):4612–4618.

Rea RS, Capitano B. Optimizing use of aminoglycosides in the critically ill. *Semin Respir Crit Care Med*. 2007;28:596–603.

Rea RS, Capitano B, Bies R, Bigos KL, Smith R, Lee H. Suboptimal aminoglycoside dosing in critically ill patients. *Ther Drug Monit*. 2008;30:674–681.

Rizzi MD, Hirose K. Aminoglycoside ototoxicity. *Curr Opin Otolaryngol Head Neck Surg*. 2007;15:352–357.

Rybak ML, Abate BJ, Kang SL, Ruffing MJ, Lerner SA, Drusano GL. Prospective evaluation of the effect of an aminoglycoside dosing regimen on rates of observed nephrotoxicity and ototoxicity. *Antimicrob Agents Chemother*. 1999;43:1549–1555.

Selimoglu E. Aminoglycoside-induced ototoxicity. *Curr Pharm Des*. 2007;13:119–126.

Shaw KJ, Rather PN, Hare RS, Miller GH. Molecular genetics of aminoglycoside resistance genes and familial relationships of the aminoglycoside-modifying enzymes. *Microbiol Rev*. 1993;57:138–163.

Touw DJ, Westerman EM, Sprij AJ. Therapeutic drug monitoring of aminoglycosides in neonates. *Clin Pharmacokinet*. 2009;48:71–88.

Triggs E, Charles B. Pharmacokinetics and therapeutic drug monitoring of gentamicin in the elderly. *Clin Pharmacokinet*. 1999;37:331–341.

Wright GD, Berghuis AM, Mobashery S. Aminoglycoside antibiotics: structures, functions, and resistance. *Adv Exp Med Biol*. 1998;456:27–69.

GENTAMICIN GROUP

GENTAMICIN

A mixture of fermentation products of *Micromonospora purpurea* supplied as the sulfate. In the commercial product gentamicins C_1, C_{1a}, C_2 and C_{2a} make up the bulk of the antimicrobial activity and are required to be present in certain proportions for therapeutic use. Minute amounts of gentamicin C_{2b} (micronomicin) are also present.

Gentamicin	R_1	R_2	Mol. wt.
C_1	CH_3	CH_3	477.6
C_2	CH_3	H	463.58
C_{1a}	H	H	449.55

ANTIMICROBIAL ACTIVITY

Activity against common pathogenic bacteria is shown in Table 12.1 (p. 146). It is active against staphylococci, but streptococci are at least moderately resistant. Gram-positive bacilli, including *Actinomyces* and *Listeria* spp., are moderately susceptible, but clostridia and other obligate anaerobes are resistant. There is no clinically useful activity against mycobacteria. It is active against most enterobacteria, including *Citrobacter*, *Enterobacter*, *Proteus*, *Serratia* and *Yersinia* spp., and against some other aerobic Gram-negative bacilli including *Acinetobacter*, *Brucella*, *Francisella* and *Legionella* spp., although its in-vitro activity against intracellular parasites such as *Brucella* spp. is of doubtful usefulness. It is active against *Ps. aeruginosa* and other members of the fluorescens group, but other pseudomonads are often resistant and *Flavobacterium* spp. are always resistant.

The MIC for susceptible strains of *Ps. aeruginosa* can vary more than 300-fold with the Mg^{2+} content of the medium. Activity against *Ps. aeruginosa* is also significantly lower in serum or sputum than in ion-depleted broth, as a result both of binding (more in sputum than in serum) and antagonism by ions.

The action is bactericidal and increases with pH, but to different degrees against different bacterial species. Marked bactericidal synergy is commonly demonstrable with β-lactam antibiotics, notably with ampicillin or benzylpenicillin against *E. faecalis*, and with vancomycin against streptococci and staphylococci. Bactericidal synergy with β-lactam antibiotics can also be demonstrated in vitro against many Gram-negative rods, including *Ps. aeruginosa*. Antagonism with chloramphenicol occurs in vitro, but this is of doubtful clinical significance.

Like other aminoglycosides, gentamicin is degraded in the presence of high concentrations of some β-lactam agents.

ACQUIRED RESISTANCE

Resistant strains of staphylococci, enterobacteria, *Pseudomonas* and *Acinetobacter* spp. have been reported from many centers, often from burns and intensive care units where the agent has been used extensively. Overall prevalence rates of resistance in various countries range from 3% to around 50% for Gram-negative organisms. Countries in which control of the prescription of antibiotics is lax often have very high rates.

Acquired resistance in Gram-negative organisms is usually caused by aminoglycoside-modifying enzymes. The prevalence of the different enzymes varies geographically. ANT(2″) is most common in the USA, but in Europe various forms of AAC(3), particularly AAC(3)-II, are common. ANT(2″) is also common in the Far East, usually accompanied by AAC(6′). Strains that owe their resistance to a non-specific decrease in uptake of aminoglycosides have been involved in outbreaks of hospital-acquired infection, and are cross-resistant to all aminoglycosides.

Resistance in staphylococci and high-level resistance in enterococci is usually caused by the bifunctional APH(2″)-AAC(6′) enzyme. Other aminoglycoside-modifying enzymes do not contribute greatly to gentamicin resistance. Gentamicin-resistant staphylococci began to emerge in the mid-1970s. Rates of resistance in the UK are around 2.5% in methicillin-sensitive *Staph. aureus*, 9% in MRSA and 23–73% in coagulase-negative staphylococci depending on methicillin susceptibility.

High-level resistance to gentamicin (MIC >2000 mg/L) in *E. faecalis* is widespread, accounting for around one-third of blood culture isolates in some places. Penicillin does not exert synergistic bactericidal activity against such strains, although the combination of penicillin with streptomycin may remain active. High-level gentamicin resistance in *E. faecium* is much less common, but has been reported in the UK, the USA and Asia.

PHARMACOKINETICS

C_{max} 1 mg/kg intramuscular	4–7.6 mg/L after 0.5–1 h
80 mg intramuscular	4–12 mg/L after 0.5–2 h
5 mg/kg infusion	>10 mg/L after 1 h
Plasma half-life (mean)	2 h
Volume of distribution	0.25 L/kg
Plasma protein binding	<10%

Absorption

Gentamicin is almost unabsorbed from the alimentary tract, but well absorbed after intramuscular injection.

Wide variations are observed in the peak plasma concentrations and half-lives of the drug after similar doses, but individual patients tend to behave consistently. Some patients with normal renal function develop unexpectedly high, or unexpectedly low, peak values on conventional doses. Severe sepsis appears to be a significant factor in reducing the peak concentration, and anemia is a significant factor in raising it. The mechanisms involved in these effects seem to be principally related to volume of distribution changes.

Intravenous infusion over 20–30 min achieves concentrations similar to those after intramuscular injection. The peak plasma concentration increases proportionally with dose and there is dose linearity in the AUC. Despite the very high bronchial concentrations achieved, nebulised administration does not give rise to detectable plasma concentrations.

There is a marked effect of age: in children up to 5 years the peak plasma concentration is about half, and for children between 5 and 10 years about two-thirds, of the concentration produced by the same dose per kg in adults. This difference can be eliminated to a large extent by calculating dosage not on the basis of weight but on surface area, which is more closely related to the volume of the extracellular fluid in which gentamicin is distributed.

Some febrile neutropenic patients do not differ from normal subjects in their pharmacokinetics, but in others, as in patients with cystic fibrosis, gentamicin clearance is enhanced and dosage adjustment is necessary.

Absorption of around half the dose is achieved by addition to the dialysate in patients on continuous ambulatory peritoneal dialysis (CAPD).

Distribution

Gentamicin does not enter cells so intracellular organisms are protected from its action. Fat contains less extracellular fluid than other tissues and pharmacokinetic comparisons indicate that the volume of distribution in obese patients approximates to the lean body mass plus 40% of the adipose mass.

Sputum

Access to the lower respiratory tract is limited. Rapid intravenous infusion produces high but short-lived intrabronchial concentrations, while intramuscular injection produces lower but more sustained concentrations.

CSF

It does not reach the CSF in useful concentrations after systemic administration. In patients receiving 3.5 mg/kg per day plus 4 mg intrathecally, CSF concentrations of 20–25 mg/L have been found. Formulations specifically designed for intrathecal use should be used, owing to issues with the excipients present.

Serous fluids and exudates

Concentrations in pleural, pericardial and synovial fluids are less than half the simultaneous plasma concentrations but may rise in the presence of inflammation. In cirrhotic patients with bacterial peritonitis treated with 3–5 mg/kg per day, concentrations of 4.2 mg/L were found in the peritoneal fluid with a fluid to serum ratio of 0.68. The maximum concentration in inflammatory exudate is less than that in the plasma, partly because it is reversibly bound in purulent exudates, but it persists much longer.

Other tissues

Concentrations in skin and muscle, as judged from assay of decubitus ulcers excised 150 min after patients had received 80 mg intramuscularly, were 5.8 and 6.5 mg/kg, respectively, the serum concentrations at that time being 5.1 and 5.4 mg/L.

Peak concentrations in bone exceed 5 mg/L and closely mirror the pharmacokinetic profile in blood. Penetration varies from 28% to 47% depending on the method used.

Concentrations in fetal blood are about one-third of that in the maternal blood.

Excretion

The initial plasma half-life is about 2 h, but a significant proportion is eliminated much more slowly, the terminal half-life being of the order of 12 days. There is much individual variation.

Gentamicin accumulates in the renal cortical cells, and over the first day or two of treatment only about 40% of the dose is recovered. The renal clearance is around 60 mL/min. Subsequently it is excreted virtually unchanged in the urine, principally by glomerular filtration. In severely oliguric patients some extrarenal elimination by unidentified routes evidently occurs. Urinary concentrations of 16–125 mg/L are found in patients with normal renal function receiving 1.5 mg/kg per day. In the presence of severe renal impairment, urinary concentrations as high as 1000 mg/L may be found. The clearance of the drug is linearly related to that of creatinine, and this relationship is used as the basis of the modified dosage schedules that are required in patients with impaired renal function in order to avoid accumulation of the drug. Concentrations in bile are less than half the simultaneous plasma concentration.

Hemodialysis can remove the drug at about 60% of the rate at which creatinine is cleared, but the efficiency of different dialyzers varies markedly. Peritoneal dialysis removes about 20% of the administered dose over 36 h – a rate that does not add materially to normal elimination (*see* Ch. 5).

 ## TOXICITY AND SIDE EFFECTS

Ototoxicity

Vestibular function is usually affected, but labyrinthine damage has been reported in about 2% of patients, usually in those with peak plasma concentrations in excess of 8 mg/L. Symptoms range from acute Ménière's disease to tinnitus and are usually permanent. Deafness is unusual but may occur in patients treated with other potentially ototoxic agents. In an extensive study, the overall incidence of ototoxicity was 2%. Vestibular damage accounted for two-thirds of this and impaired renal function was the main determinant.

Nephrotoxicity

Some degree of renal toxicity has been observed in 5–10% of patients. Among 97 patients receiving 102 courses of the drug in dosages adjusted in relation to renal function, nephrotoxicity was described as definite in 9.8% and possible in 7.8%. In patients treated for 39–48 days, serum creatinine increased initially, but renal function recovered after 3–4 weeks despite continuing treatment. However, many patients are treated for severe sepsis associated with shock or disseminated intravascular coagulopathy, or from other disorders that are themselves associated with renal failure. In critically ill patients with severe sepsis, treatment has been complicated by nephrotoxicity in 23–37%.

Autoradiographic localization indicates that gentamicin is very selectively localized in the proximal convoluted tubules, and a specific effect on potassium excretion may both indicate the site of toxicity and provide an early indication of renal damage. Accumulation of the drug and excretion of proximal tubular enzymes may precede any rise in the serum creatinine.

Alanine aminopeptidase excretion is an unreliable predictor of renal damage. β_2-Microglobulin excretion may indicate decreased tubular function both before and during treatment. Excretion of the protein has also been shown to parallel increases in elimination half-life in patients on well-controlled therapy in whom reduction of creatinine clearance occurred, although the serum creatinine concentration remained within normal limits.

Other effects

Neuromuscular blockade is possible but unlikely in view of the small amounts of the drug administered. Intrathecal injection may result in radiculitis, fever and persistent pleocytosis. Significant hypomagnesemia may occur, particularly in patients also receiving cytotoxic agents.

CLINICAL USE

In severe sepsis of unknown origin, gentamicin has been traditionally combined with other agents. However, monotherapy has been shown to be as effective as combination therapy. In systemic *Ps. aeruginosa* infections it is advisable to combine gentamicin with an antipseudomonal penicillin or cephalosporin, owing to likelihood of gentamicin resistance.

Suspected or documented Gram-negative septicemia, particularly when shock or hypotension is present

Enterococcal endocarditis (with a penicillin)

Respiratory tract infection caused by Gram-negative bacilli

Urinary tract infection

Bone and soft-tissue infections, including peritonitis, burns complicated by sepsis and infected surgical and traumatic wounds

Serious staphylococcal infection when other conventional antimicrobial therapy is inappropriate

---

Gentamicin drops are used for conjunctival infections and for infections of the external ear. The drug is also used in orthopedic surgery in bone cements. In these applications systemic concentrations achieved are negligible and toxicities are restricted to local effects.

In the elderly and those with renal impairment the dosage must be suitably modified.

Preparations and dosage

Proprietary names: Genticin, Cidomycin.

Preparations: Injection, various topical.

Dosage: Adult: i.m., i.v. infusion 3–5 mg/kg per day in three divided doses or 5–7 mg/kg infusion in a single dose once daily. 1 mg/kg every 8 h when used with a β-lactam antibiotic in the treatment of endocarditis.

Neonate: i.v. infusion, <32 weeks postmenstrual age, 4–5 mg/kg as a single dose every 36 h; ≥32 weeks postmenstrual age, 4–5 mg/kg as a single dose every 24 h; *or* <29 weeks postmenstrual age, 2.5 mg/kg every 24 h; 29–35 weeks postmenstrual age, 2.5 mg/kg every 18 h; >35 weeks postmenstrual age, 2.5 mg/kg every 12 h.

Child: 1 month–18 years, 7 mg/kg as a single daily dose and adjust dose on the basis of serum concentrations; *or* 1 month–12 years, 2.5 mg/kg every 8 h; 12–18 years 2 mg/kg every 8 h.

Widely available.

Further information

Aran JM, Erre JP, Lima da Costa D, Debbarh I, Dulon D. Acute and chronic effects of aminoglycosides on cochlear hair cells. *Ann N Y Acad Sci.* 1999;884:60–68.

Begg EJ, Vella-Brincat JW, Robertshawe B, McMurtrie MJ, Kirkpatrick CM, Darlow B. Eight years' experience of an extended-interval dosing protocol for gentamicin in neonates. *J Antimicrob Chemother.* 2009;63:1043–1049.

Bianco TM, Dwyer PN, Bertino JS. Gentamicin pharmacokinetics, nephrotoxicity and prediction of mortality in febrile neutropenic patients. *Antimicrob Agents Chemother.* 1989;33:1890–1895.

Freeman CD, Nicolau DP, Belliveau PP, Nightingale CH. Once-daily dosing of aminoglycosides: review and recommendations for clinical practice. *J Antimicrob Chemother.* 1997;39:677–686.

Meunier F, Van der Auwera P, Schmitt H, de Maertelaer V, Klastersky J. Pharmacokinetics of gentamicin after i.v. infusion or i.v. bolus. *J Antimicrob Chemother.* 1987;19:225–231.

Nielsen EI, Sandström M, Honoré PH, Ewald U, Friberg LE. Developmental pharmacokinetics of gentamicin in preterm and term neonates: population modelling of a prospective study. *Clin Pharmacokinet.* 2009;48:253–263.

Rao SC, Ahmed M, Hagan R. One dose per day compared to multiple doses per day of gentamicin for treatment of suspected or proven sepsis in neonates. *Cochrane Database Syst Rev.* 2006;(1) CD005091.

Smyth AR, Bhatt J. Once-daily versus multiple-daily dosing with intravenous aminoglycosides for cystic fibrosis. *Cochrane Database Syst Rev.* 2006;(3) CD002009.

Triggs E, Charles B. Pharmacokinetics and therapeutic drug monitoring of gentamicin in the elderly. *Clin Pharmacokinet.* 1999;37:331–341.

NETILMICIN

Molecular weight (free base): 475.58.

The semisynthetic 1-*N*-ethyl derivative of sisomicin supplied as the sulfate salt.

ANTIMICROBIAL ACTIVITY

The susceptibility of common pathogenic bacteria is shown in Table 12.1 (p. 146). It is active against a wide range of enterobacteria as well as many *Acinetobacter*, *Pseudomonas*, *Citrobacter*, *Proteus* and *Serratia* spp. Staphylococci, including methicillin-resistant and coagulase-negative strains, are usually susceptible. Nocardiae are inhibited by 0.04–1 mg/L. *Providencia* spp. and anaerobic bacteria are generally resistant.

It is active against some gentamicin-resistant strains, particularly those that synthesize ANT(2″) or AAC(3)-I. It exhibits typical aminoglycoside properties: bactericidal activity at or close to the MIC; greater activity at alkaline pH; depression of activity against *Pseudomonas* by divalent cations; and synergy with β-lactam antibiotics. Bactericidal synergy can be demonstrated regularly with benzylpenicillin against viridans streptococci and *E. faecalis*, but seldom against *E. faecium*, which characteristically synthesizes AAC(6′), to which netilmicin is susceptible.

ACQUIRED RESISTANCE

It is resistant to ANT(2″), AAC(3)-I and AAC(3)-III, but sensitive to AAC(6′) (Table 12.2, p. 148). AAC(3)-II confers resistance, but generally to a lesser degree than to gentamicin.

Resistance rates are generally about the same as, or a little lower than, those for gentamicin.

PHARMACOKINETICS

C$_{max}$ 1 mg/kg intramuscular	4–6 mg/L after 0.5–1 h
2 mg/kg intravenous 30-min infusion	c. 12 mg/L end infusion
5 mg/kg	>10 mg/L after 1 h
Plasma half-life	2–2.5 h
Volume of distribution	0.25 L/kg
Plasma protein binding	<10%

The pharmacokinetics are similar to those of gentamicin. In patients receiving 200 mg (2.2–3.6 mg/kg) intramuscularly every 8 h for 10 days, a mean peak plasma concentration of around 14 mg/L was found. Peak concentrations of about 10 mg/L were found in children with pyelonephritis treated with 5 mg/kg per day, compared with peaks of about 5 mg/L in children given 2 mg/kg every 8 h. The serum half-life is linearly inversely related to creatinine clearance in patients with renal impairment. Plasma concentrations decreased by 63% during hemodialysis. In older patients with a mean creatinine clearance of 63 mL/min, the half-life was 6.2 h after a dose of 2 mg/kg.

In the newborn, intramuscular injection of 2.5 mg/kg produced peak plasma concentrations of 1–5 mg/L 1 h after the dose, with a plasma half-life of 4 h. In newborns given 6 mg/kg per day, plasma concentrations were 7.4–13.2 mg/L after 2 h. Half-lives were greater (mean 6.7 h) than in those of >36 weeks postmenstrual age (mean 4.6 h), and pre-dose concentrations were 2.1 and 1.6 mg/L, respectively, suggesting that a lower daily dose (4.5 mg/kg) may be appropriate. Children with cystic fibrosis had a higher total body clearance.

Distribution

Netilmicin is distributed in the extracellular water and in patients with cystic fibrosis the apparent volume of distribution seems not to be increased.

Very little reaches the CSF even in the presence of inflammation. Concentrations of 0.13–0.45 mg/L were found in patients without meningeal inflammation following an intravenous dose of 400 mg. In patients with meningitis, the drug was undetectable, although concentrations of 0.2–5 mg/L could be found later in the course of treatment in some cases.

Excretion

It is excreted unchanged in the urine in the glomerular filtrate, with some tubular reabsorption. Over the first 6 h, about 50% and by 24 h about 80% of the dose appears. No metabolites are known and it is likely that this represents binding to tissues. Clearance on hemodialysis is similar to that reported for gentamicin.

TOXICITY AND SIDE EFFECTS

It is considered to be less nephrotoxic than gentamicin, a difference not easily explained since the renal clearance and renal and medullary concentrations of the drugs appear to be similar. Both vestibular and cochlear toxicity appear to be low and vestibular toxicity without audiometric abnormality is rare. In some patients, plasma concentrations up to 30 mg/L over periods exceeding 1 week have not resulted in ototoxicity. Evidence of some renal toxicity in the excretion of granular casts has occurred fairly frequently in patients receiving 7.5 mg/kg per day, and is more likely to occur in the elderly and in those receiving higher doses or longer courses. In patients treated for an average of 35 days with 2.4–6.9 mg/kg per day, there was no effect on initially normal renal function, even in the elderly. Long-term treatment led to an increase in elimination half-life from 1.5 to 1.9 h. Nephrotoxicity has been observed in some diabetic patients. Overall estimates of the frequency of nephrotoxicity have ranged from 1% to 18%. Increases in serum transaminase and alkaline phosphatase concentrations have been seen in some patients without other evidence of hepatic impairment.

Once-daily dosing is thought to be safer than twice or three times daily dosing.

 ## CLINICAL USE

Severe infections (including septicemia, lower respiratory tract infections, urinary tract infections, peritonitis, endometritis) caused by susceptible strains of Gram-negative bacilli and staphylococci

 ## Preparations and dosage

Proprietary names: Netromycin.

Preparation: Injection.

Dosage: Adults: i.m., i.v., i.v. infusion 4–6 mg/kg per day in a single dose or divided doses every 8–12 h. In severe infections up to 7.5 mg/kg per day in divided doses every 8 h, reduced as soon as is clinically indicated, usually within 48 h.

Children: 6–7.5 mg/kg per day, divided into three equal doses and administered every 8 h. This should be reduced to 6 mg/kg per day as soon as clinically indicated.

Infants and neonates (>1 week of age): 7.5–9 mg/kg per day, divided into three equal doses and administered every 8 h. Premature and full-term neonates (<1 week of age): 6 or 4.5 mg/kg per day, as a single daily dose or divided into two equal doses every 12 h.

No longer widely available.

 ## Further information

Craig WA, Gudmundsson S, Reich RM. Netilmicin sulfate: a comparative evaluation of antimicrobial activity, pharmacokinetics, adverse reaction and clinical efficacy. *Pharmacotherapy.* 1983;3:305–315.

Ettlinger JJ, Bedford KA, Lovering AM, Reeves DS, Speidel BD, MacGowan AP. Pharmacokinetics of once-a-day netilmicin (6 mg/kg) in neonates. *J Antimicrob Chemother.* 1996;38:499–505.

Dahlager JI. The effect of netilmicin and other aminoglycosides on renal function. A survey of the literature on the nephrotoxicity of netilmicin. *Scand J Infect Dis.* 1980;23(suppl):96–102.

Manoharan A, Lalitha MK, Jesudason MV. In vitro activity of netilmicin against clinical isolates of methicillin resistant and susceptible *Staphylococcus aureus*. *Natl Med J India.* 1997;10:61–62.

OTHER GENTAMICIN GROUP AMINOGLYCOSIDES

 ## ISEPAMICIN

Hydroxyamino propionyl gentamicin B. A semisynthetic derivative of gentamicin B, modified to render it more resistant to microbial inactivation.

In-vitro activity is comparable to or slightly greater than amikacin against *Staph. aureus* and most enterobacteria; it is much more active against *Ser. marcescens*, *Enterobacter* spp. and *Klebsiebella pneumoniae*. It is also active in vitro against the *Mycobacterium avium* complex and *Nocardia asteroides*. It is less susceptible than amikacin or gentamicin to inactivation by β-lactam antibiotics. It retains activity against some strains resistant to most other aminoglycosides.

Pharmacokinetics in neonatal, pediatric, adult, elderly and renally impaired patients are similar to those of other aminoglycosides. In adult volunteers the plasma half-life was 2.1 h. Clearance is reduced in neonates and the elderly. A 7.5 mg/kg once-daily dosage is recommended for children less than 16 days old. No dosage adjustment is required for the elderly unless renal function is impaired. Clearance is proportional to creatinine clearance in patients with chronic renal impairment, and it is eliminated by hemodialysis.

It has been used in respiratory tract infections, urinary tract infections and intra-abdominal infections, in adults and children. It appears to be as effective and well tolerated as amikacin. It is available in Japan.

 ## MICRONOMICIN (SAGAMICIN; GENTAMICIN C$_{2b}$)

Antibacterial and pharmacokinetic properties are similar to those of its precursor gentamicin C$_{1a}$ but it is more resistant to AAC(6′). Dosage is similar to that for gentamicin, and should be controlled by blood level determinations. It is available in Japan.

 ## SISOMICIN (SISSOMICIN; RICKAMICIN)

A fermentation product of *Micromonospora inyoensis*. A dehydro derivative of gentamicin C$_{1a}$, supplied as the sulfate salt.

It is virtually identical to gentamicin in activity and pharmacokinetic behavior. An intramuscular dose of 1–1.5 mg/kg achieves a peak plasma concentration of 1.5–9.0 mg/L after 0.5–1 h. It is widely distributed in body water, but concentrations in CSF are low, even in the presence of inflammation. The plasma half-life is 2.5 h and protein binding is <10%.

It is eliminated almost completely over 24 h in the glomerular filtrate. Excretion decreases proportionately with renal impairment and because of the virtual identity of the behavior of the two compounds, a gentamicin nomogram can be used to adjust dosage. About 40% of the dose is eliminated during a 6-h dialysis period, during which the elimination half-life falls to about 8 h.

Mild and reversible impairment of renal function occurs in about 5% of patients. Nephrotoxicity is more likely to be seen in those with pre-existing renal disease or treated concurrently with other potentially nephrotoxic drugs. Ototoxicity mainly affecting vestibular function has been found in about 1% of patients. Neuromuscular blockade and other effects common to aminoglycosides including rashes, paresthesiae, eosinophilia and abnormal liver function tests have been described.

Its uses are identical to those of gentamicin, which it closely resembles. It is of limited availability.

KANAMYCIN GROUP

AMIKACIN

Molecular weight: 585.61 (free base); 683.68 (sulfate).

A semisynthetic derivative of kanamycin A, in which the 1-amino group of the deoxystreptamine moiety is replaced by a hydroxyaminobutyric acid group. Supplied as the sulfate.

ANTIMICROBIAL ACTIVITY

The activity against common pathogenic bacteria is shown in Table 12.1 (p. 146). Among other organisms, *Acinetobacter*, *Alkaligenes*, *Campylobacter*, *Citrobacter*, *Hafnia*, *Legionella*, *Pasteurella*, *Providencia*, *Serratia* and *Yersinia* spp. are usually susceptible in vitro. *Stenotrophomonas maltophilia*, many non-aeruginosa pseudomonads and *Flavobacterium* spp. are resistant. *M. tuberculosis* (including most streptomycin-resistant strains) and some other mycobacteria (including *M. fortuitum* and the *M. avium* complex) are susceptible; most other mycobacteria, including *M. kansasii*, are resistant. *Nocardia asteroides* is susceptible.

It exhibits typical aminoglycoside characteristics, including an effect of divalent cations on its activity against *Ps. aeruginosa* analogous to that seen with gentamicin and synergy with β-lactam antibiotics.

ACQUIRED RESISTANCE

Amikacin is unaffected by many of the modifying enzymes that inactivate gentamicin and tobramycin (Table 12.2, p. 148) and is consequently active against staphylococci, enterobacteria and *Pseudomonas* that owe their resistance to the production of those enzymes. However, AAC(6′), ANT(4′) and some forms of APH(3′) can confer resistance; because these enzymes generally do not confer gentamicin resistance, amikacin-resistant strains can be missed in routine susceptibility tests when gentamicin is used as the representative aminoglycoside.

There have been reports of resistance arising during treatment of infections due to *Serratia* spp. and *Ps. aeruginosa*. Outbreaks of infection with multiresistant strains of enterobacteria and *Ps. aeruginosa* have occurred after extensive use, particularly in burns units. Bacteria that owe their resistance to the expression of ANT(4′) have been described in *Staph. aureus*, coagulase-negative staphylococci, *Esch. coli*, *Klebsiella* spp. and *Ps. aeruginosa*. In *E. faecalis*, resistance to penicillin–aminoglycoside synergy has been associated with plasmid-mediated APH(3′). Resistance in Gram-negative organisms is usually caused by either reduced accumulation of the drug or, more commonly, by the aminoglycoside-modifying enzymes AAC(6′) or AAC(3)-VI. The latter enzyme is usually found in *Acinetobacter* spp., but has also been found, encoded by a transposon, in *Prov. stuartii*. One type of AAC(6) is chromosomally encoded by *Ser. marcescens*, though not usually expressed.

The prevalence of resistance to amikacin remains low (<5%) in many countries but can change rapidly with increased usage of the drug. However, the spread of extended spectrum β-lactamases belonging to the TEM and SHV families may result in an increase in amikacin resistance that is not associated with use, since most strains that produce such enzymes also produce AAC(6′).

PHARMACOKINETICS

C_{max} 7.5 mg/kg intramuscular	c. 30 mg/L after 1 h
500 mg 30-min infusion	35–50 mg/L end infusion
15 mg/kg 30-min infusion	>50 mg/L after 1 h
Plasma half-life	2.2 h
Volume of distribution	0.25–0.3 L/kg
Plasma protein binding	3–11%

It is readily absorbed after intramuscular administration. Rapid intravenous injection of 7.5 mg/kg produced concentrations in excess of 60 mg/L shortly after injection.

Most pharmacokinetic parameters follow an almost linear correlation when the once-daily doses (15 mg/kg) are compared with the traditional 7.5 mg/kg twice daily. In patients on CAPD, there was no difference in mean peak plasma concentration or volume of distribution whether the drug was given intravenously or intraperitoneally. However, in patients with significant burn injuries, doses should be increased to 20 mg/kg.

In infants receiving 7.5 mg/kg by intravenous injection, peak plasma concentrations were 17–20 mg/L. No accumulation occurred on 12 mg/kg per day for 5–7 days. There was little change in the plasma concentration or the half-life (1.7 and 1.9 h) on the third and seventh days of a period over which 150 mg/m² was infused over 30 min every 6 h. When the dose was raised to 200 mg/m² the concentration never fell below 8 mg/L. The plasma half-life was longer in babies of lower birth weight and was still 5–5.5 h in babies aged 1 week or older. The importance of dosage control in the neonate is emphasized by the findings that there is an inverse relationship between post-conception age and plasma elimination half-life, though in extremely premature babies the weight of the child is also a significant predictor of half-life.

Distribution

The apparent volume of distribution indicates distribution throughout the extracellular water. Following an intravenous bolus of 0.5 g, peak concentrations in blister fluid were around 12 mg/L, with a mean elimination half-life of 2.3 h. In patients with impaired renal function, penetration and peak concentration increased linearly with decrease in creatinine clearance.

In patients with purulent sputum, a loading dose of 4 mg/kg intravenously plus 8 h infusions of 7–12 mg/kg produced sputum concentrations around 2 mg/L, with a mean sputum:serum ratio of 0.15. With brief infusions over 10 min for 7 days, sputum concentrations of around 9% of the simultaneous serum values have been found.

Concentrations in the CSF of adult volunteers receiving 7.5 mg/kg intramuscularly were less than 0.5 mg/L and virtually the same in patients with meningitis. Rather higher, but variable, concentrations up to 3.8 mg/L have been found in neonatal meningitis.

Amikacin crosses the placenta, and concentrations of 0.5–6 mg/L have been found in the cord blood of women receiving 7.5 mg/kg in labor. Concentrations of 8 mg/L and 16.8 mg/L were reached in the fetal lung and kidney, respectively, after a standard dose of 7.5 mg/kg given to healthy women before therapeutic abortion.

Excretion

Only 1–2% of the administered dose is excreted in the bile, with the remainder excreted in the urine, producing urinary concentrations of 150–3000 mg/L. Renal clearance is 70–84 mL/min, and this, with the ratio of amikacin to creatinine clearance (around 0.7), indicates that it is filtered and tubular reabsorption is insignificant. Accumulation occurs in proportion to reduction in renal function, although there may be some extrarenal elimination in anephric patients. The mean plasma half-life in patients on hemodialysis was around 4 h, while that on peritoneal dialysis was 28 h.

In patients receiving 500 mg/kg preoperatively, concentrations in gallbladder wall reached 34 mg/L and in bile 7.5 mg/L

in some patients. In patients given 500 mg intravenously 12 h before surgery and 12 hourly for four doses thereafter, the mean bile:serum ratio 1 h after the dose was around 0.4.

TOXICITY AND SIDE EFFECTS

Ototoxicity

Neurosensory hearing loss (mainly high-tone deafness) and labyrinthine injury have been detected, but have seldom been severe. High-frequency hearing loss and vestibular impairment have been described in about 5% of patients and conversational loss in about 0.5%; more in patients monitored audiometrically (29%) and by caloric testing (19%).

Patients with high-tone hearing loss have generally received more drug and for longer than patients without; in patients receiving long-term treatment for tuberculosis no other factors were associated with the development of ototoxicity. On multiple daily dosing, over half the patients with peak serum concentrations exceeding 30 mg/L or trough concentrations exceeding 10 mg/L developed cochlear damage; here, the main contributory factor was previous treatment with other aminoglycosides.

Nephrotoxicity

Impairment of renal function, usually mild or transient, has been observed in 3–13% of patients, notably in the elderly or those with pre-existing renal disorders or treated concurrently or previously with other potentially nephrotoxic agents.

Other reactions

Adverse effects common to aminoglycosides occur, including hypersensitivity, gastrointestinal disturbances, headache, drug fever, peripheral nervous manifestations, eosinophilia, mild hematological abnormalities and disturbed liver function tests without other evidence of hepatic derangement.

CLINICAL USES

Severe infection (including septicemia, neonatal sepsis, osteomyelitis, septic arthritis, respiratory tract, urinary tract, intra-abdominal, peritoneal and soft tissue infections) caused by susceptible micro-organisms

Sepsis of unknown origin (combined with a β-lactam or anti-anaerobe agent as appropriate).

Mycobacterial infection

Amikacin is principally used for the treatment of infections caused by organisms resistant to other aminoglycosides because of their ability to degrade them. Peak concentrations on 15 mg/kg once daily administration should exceed 45 mg/L, and trough concentration of <5 mg/L should be maintained to achieve therapeutic effects.

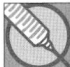

Preparations and dosage

Proprietary name: Amikin.

Preparation: Injection.

Dosage: Adults i.m., i.v., i.v. infusion 15 mg/kg per day in a single dose or in two divided doses.

Neonate: 15 mg/kg per day. Alternatively, an initial loading dose of 10 mg/kg followed by 15 mg/kg per day in two divided doses.

Child: 1 month–18 years, 7.5 mg/kg every 12 h. Alternatively, 1 month–12 years, 7.5 mg/kg every 12 h or 12–18 years, 7.5 mg/kg every 12 h, increasing to every 8 h in serious sepsis. Maximum accumulated dose 15 g. The dosage must be reduced if renal function is impaired, and in elderly patients.

Widely available.

Further information

Conil JM, Georges B, Breden A, et al. Increased amikacin dosage requirements in burn patients receiving a once-daily regimen. *Int J Antimicrob Agents.* 2006;28:226–230.

Edson RS, Terrel CL. The aminoglycosides. *Mayo Clin Proc.* 1999;74:519–528.

Fujimura S, Tokue Y, Takahashi H, et al. Novel arbekacin- and amikacin-modifying enzymes of methicillin-resistant *Staphylococcus aureus. FEMS Microbiol Lett.* 2000;190:299–303.

Gonzalez LS, Spencer JP. Aminoglycosides: a practical review. *Am Fam Physician.* 1998;58:1811–1820.

Guggenheim M, Zbinden R, Handschin AE, Gohritz A, Altintas MA, Giovanoli P. Changes in bacterial isolates from burn wounds and their antibiograms: a 20-year study (1986–2005). *Burns.* 2009;35:553–560.

Kenyon CF, Knoppert DC, Lee SK, Vandenberghe HM, Chance GW. Amikacin pharmacokinetics and suggested dosage modifications for the preterm infant. *Antimicrob Agents Chemother.* 1990;34:265–268.

Lima Da Costa D, Erre JP, Pehourq F, Aran JM. Aminoglycoside ototoxicity and the medial efferent system: II. comparison of acute effects of different antibiotics. *Audiology.* 1998;37:162–173.

KANAMYCIN

Kanamycin	R	Mol. wt.
A	OH	484.5
B	NH$_2$	483.5

A fermentation product of *Streptomyces kanamyceticus* formulated as the sulfate. Commercial preparations contain a mixture of kanamycins A, B and C, predominantly kanamycin A; the content of kanamycin B is required to be less than 3% (BP) or less than 5% (USP).

ANTIMICROBIAL ACTIVITY

The susceptibility of common pathogenic bacteria is shown in Table 12.1 (p. 146). It is active against staphylococci, including methicillin-resistant strains. Other aerobic and anaerobic Gram-positive cocci and most Gram-positive rods are resistant, but *M. tuberculosis* is susceptible. It is widely active against most aerobic Gram-negative rods, except *Burkholderia cepacia* and *Sten. maltophilia. Treponema pallidum, Leptospira* and *Mycoplasma* spp. are all resistant.

ACQUIRED RESISTANCE

Resistance is usually plasmid borne and due to enzymatic inactivation of the drug by enzymes that also inactivate gentamicin or tobramycin (Table 12.2, p. 148). Resistance due to reduced permeability is also encountered.

PHARMACOKINETICS

C_{max} 500 mg intramuscular	c. 15–20 mg/L after 1 h
Plasma half-life	2.5 h
Volume of distribution	0.3 L/kg
Plasma protein binding	Low

Absorption and distribution

Very little is absorbed from the intestinal tract. The peak plasma concentration in the neonate is dose related: concentrations of 8–30 mg/L (mean 18 mg/L) have been found 1 h after a 10 mg/kg dose. The drug is confined to the extracellular fluid. The concentration in serous fluids is said to equal that in the plasma, but it does not enter the CSF in therapeutically useful concentrations even in the presence of meningeal inflammation.

Excretion

It is excreted almost entirely by the kidneys, almost exclusively in the glomerular filtrate. Up to 80% of the dose appears unchanged in the urine over the first 24 h, producing concentrations around 100–500 mg/L. It is retained in proportion to reduction in renal function. Less than 1% of the dose appears in the bile. In patients receiving 500 mg intramuscularly preoperatively, concentrations of 2–23 mg/L have been found in bile and 8–14 mg/kg in gallbladder wall.

TOXICITY AND SIDE EFFECTS

Intramuscular injections are moderately painful, and minor side effects similar to those encountered with streptomycin have been described. Eosinophilia in the absence of other manifestations of allergy occurs in up to 10% of patients. Other manifestations of hypersensitivity are rare.

As with other aminoglycosides, the most important toxic effects are on the eighth nerve and much less frequently on the kidney. Renal damage is seen principally in patients with pre-existing renal disease or treated concurrently or sequentially with other potentially nephrotoxic agents. The drug accumulates in the renal cortex, producing cloudy swelling, which may progress to acute necrosis of proximal tubular cells with oliguric renal failure. Less dramatic deterioration of renal function, particularly exaggeration of the potential nephrotoxicity of other drugs or of existing renal disease, is of principal importance because it increases the likelihood of ototoxicity.

Vestibular damage is uncommon but may be severe and prolonged. Hearing damage is usually bilateral, and typically affects frequencies above the conversational range. Acute toxicity is most likely in patients in whom the plasma concentration exceeds 30 mg/L, but chronic toxicity may be seen in patients treated with the drug over long periods. Auditory toxicity may be potentiated by concurrent treatment with potent diuretics like ethacrynic acid. If tinnitus – which usually heralds the onset of auditory injury – develops, the drug should be withdrawn.

Neuromuscular blockade is seen particularly in patients receiving other muscle relaxants or suffering from myasthenia gravis and may be reversed by neostigmine.

 ## CLINICAL USE

Formerly used for severe infection with susceptible organisms, it has largely been superseded by other aminoglycosides.

Preparations and dosage

Proprietary name: Kantrex.

Preparations: Injection, ophthalmic, capsules.

Dosage: Adults, i.m. injection 250 mg every 6 h, or 500 mg every 12 h. Adults and children, i.v. infusion, 15–30 mg/kg per day in 2–4 divided doses. The dosage should be reduced in renal impairment.

Widely available. No longer available in the UK.

 ### Further information

Davis RR, Brummett RE, Bendrick TW, Himes DL. Dissociation of maximum concentration of kanamycin in plasma and perilymph from ototoxic effect. *J Antimicrob Chemother.* 1984;14:291–302.

TOBRAMYCIN

Nebramycin factor 6; 3′-deoxy kanamycin B. Molecular weight (free base): 467.52.

A natural fermentation product of *Streptomyces tenebraeus*, supplied as the sulfate in various preparations.

 ## ANTIMICROBIAL ACTIVITY

The susceptibility of common pathogenic organisms is shown in Table 12.1 (p. 146). In-vitro activity against *Ps. aeruginosa* is usually somewhat greater than that of gentamicin; against other organisms activity is similar or a little lower. Other *Pseudomonas* species are generally resistant, as are streptococci and most anaerobic bacteria. Other organisms usually susceptible in vitro include *Acinetobacter*, *Legionella* and *Yersinia* spp. *Alkaligenes*, *Flavobacterium* spp. and *Mycobacterium* spp. are resistant. It exhibits bactericidal activity at concentrations close to the MIC and bactericidal synergy typical of aminoglycosides in combination with penicillins or cephalosporins.

ACQUIRED RESISTANCE

It is inactivated by many aminoglycoside-modifying enzymes that inactivate gentamicin (Table 12.2, p. 148). However, AAC(3′)-I does not confer tobramycin resistance and AAC(3′)-II confers a lower degree of tobramycin resistance than of gentamicin resistance. Conversely, ANT(4′) confers tobramycin but not gentamicin resistance, as do some types of AAC(6′). Overproduction of APH(3′), conferring a low degree of resistance to tobramycin (MIC 8 mg/L), but not gentamicin (MIC 2 mg/L), was ascribed to 'trapping' rather than phosphorylation.

Resistance rates are generally similar to those of gentamicin, although they may vary locally because of the prevalence of particular enzyme types.

 ## PHARMACOKINETICS

C_{max} 80 mg intramuscular	3–4 mg/L after 30 min
1 mg/kg intravenous	6–7 mg/L after 30 min
5 mg/kg	>10 mg/L after 1 h
Plasma half-life	1.5–3 h
Volume of distribution	c. 0.25 L/kg
Plasma protein binding	<30%

The pharmacokinetic behavior after systemic administration closely resembles that of gentamicin. In patients treated for prolonged periods with 2.5 mg/kg intravenously every 12 h, average peak steady-state values were 6.5 mg/L after 30 weeks and 7.1 mg/L after 40 weeks. Continuous intravenous infusion of 6.6 mg/h and 30 mg/h produced steady-state concentrations of 1 and 3.5–4.5 mg/L, respectively. Higher concentrations (10–12 mg/L) have been obtained by bolus injection over about 3 min. Peak concentrations of around 50 mg/L have been reported in cystic fibrosis patients given 9 mg/kg once daily. Ten minutes after a 300 mg dose of tobramycin solution for inhalation, mean concentration of drug in the sputum of cystic fibrosis patients was 1.2 mg/g and ranged from 0.04 to 1.4 mg/g. The systemic availability of nebulized drug is very variable (6–27%). In general, the concentration found in the sputum of cystic fibrosis patients is high when administered by inhalation, but varies widely depending on individual airway pathology and nebulizer efficiency.

In the neonate, peak plasma concentrations of 4–6 mg/L have been found 0.5–1 h after doses of 2 mg/kg. Mean plasma elimination half-lives of 4.6–8.7 h were inversely proportional to the birth weight and creatinine clearance. The half-life was found to be initially extremely variable (3–17 h) in infants weighing 2.5 kg at birth, but considerably more stable (4–8 h) at the end of therapy 6–9 days later.

β-Lactam inactivation

In common with other aminoglycosides, tobramycin interacts with certain β-lactam agents, but is said to be stable in the presence of ceftazidime, imipenem and aztreonam. Of the penicillins tested, piperacillin caused least inactivation in vitro.

Distribution

The volume of distribution slightly exceeds the extracellular water volume; it increases in patients with ascites, and is relatively smaller in morbidly obese patients. In tracheostomized or intubated patients given a loading dose of 1 mg/kg and then intravenous infusions every 8 h of 2–3.5 mg/kg, average concentrations in the bronchial secretions were 0.7 mg/L with a mean secretion:serum ratio of 0.18. In patients with cystic fibrosis receiving 10 mg/kg of the drug per day, the bronchial secretions may contain 2 mg/L or more.

Concentrations are low in peritoneal fluid but can rise to 60% of the plasma concentration in peritonitis and in synovial fluid. Tobramycin crosses the placenta, and concentrations of 0.5 mg/L have been found in the fetal serum when the mother was receiving a dose of 2 mg/kg. Penetration into the CSF resembles that of gentamicin.

Excretion

It is eliminated in the glomerular filtrate and is unaffected by probenecid. Renal clearance is 90 mL/min. About 60% of the administered dose is recovered from the urine over the first 10 h, producing urinary concentrations after a dose of 80 mg of 90–500 mg/L over the first 3 h. The nature of the extra-renal disposal of the remaining 40% of the drug has not been established. The total body clearance is increased in patients with cystic fibrosis and the plasma half-life is shorter, which may necessitate higher dosage (15 mg/kg per day) for optimum blood concentrations. Renal clearance is increased in younger burn patients. In patients with impaired renal function, urinary concentrations of the drug are depressed and the plasma half-life prolonged in proportion to the rise in serum creatinine, reaching 6–8 h at a creatinine concentration of 350 µmol/L. Dosage in patients with impaired renal function may be based on the procedures used for gentamicin since behavior of the two drugs is virtually identical. About 70% of the drug is removed by hemodialysis over 12 h, but the efficiency of different dialyzers varies markedly.

 # TOXICITY AND SIDE EFFECTS

Ototoxicity

The effect is predominantly on the auditory branch of the eighth nerve; vestibular function is seldom affected. Experimental evidence suggests that comparable effects on cochlear electrophysiology and histology require doses about twice those of gentamicin. In patients, electrocochleography has shown an immediate and dramatic reduction of cochlear activity when the serum tobramycin concentration exceeded 8–10 mg/L, but there were no associated symptoms and function recovered fully as the drug was eliminated. Clinical ototoxicity is rare and most likely to be seen in patients with renal impairment, or treated concurrently or sequentially with other potentially ototoxic agents.

Nephrotoxicity

Renal impairment with proteinuria, excretion of granular casts, oliguria and rise of serum creatinine have been noted in 1–2% of patients. Some evidence of nephrotoxicity has been found in about 10% of patients, depending on the sensitivity of the tests employed. In patients treated with a 120 mg loading dose and 80 mg every 8 h, renal enzyme excretion increased and there was a small but significant reduction in chrome-EDTA clearance even when the clinical condition improved. It has been suggested that intermittent dosage with large but infrequent plasma peaks may be less toxic than, and as efficacious as, continuous dosing. Tobramycin appears to be less nephrotoxic than gentamicin in critically ill patients.

The likelihood of toxicity is thought to increase with pre-existing renal impairment and higher or more prolonged dosage, but in a comparison of patients treated with 8 mg/kg per day for *Pseudomonas* endocarditis with those treated with 3 mg/kg per day for Gram-negative sepsis there was no evidence of renal impairment in either group. Although there was audiological evidence of high-frequency loss in some patients receiving the higher dosage, there was no sustained loss of conversational hearing. There seems to be no significant effect of age: in patients aged 20–39 years the mean elimination half-life of the drug at the end of treatment was 2.3 h while in those aged 60–79 years it was 2.4 h. Evidence of renal toxicity may be found in 20% of severely ill patients.

Other reactions

Other toxic manifestations are rare. Local reactions sometimes occur at the site of injection. Rashes and eosinophilia in the absence of other allergic manifestations are seen. Voice alterations and tinnitus were rare in cystic fibrosis patients receiving tobramycin by inhalation. Increased transaminase levels may occur in the absence of other evidence of hepatic derangement.

CLINICAL USE

> Severe infections caused by susceptible micro-organisms
>
> *Ps. aeruginosa* infections, including chronic pulmonary infections in cystic fibrosis (administration by injection or nebulizer)

For practical purposes use is identical to that of gentamicin, except possibly for *Pseudomonas* infection, where it has somewhat greater activity against gentamicin-susceptible and some gentamicin-resistant strains. Its value as a substitute for gentamicin in the speculative treatment of severe undiagnosed infection is offset by its lower activity against other organisms that may be implicated.

It has been used extensively to treat *Ps. aeruginosa* infections in patients with cystic fibrosis.

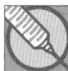

Preparations and dosage

Proprietary names: Nebcin, Tobradex, Tobrex, TOBI.

Preparations: Injections, topical and inhalation formulations.

Dosage: Adults i.m., i.v. 5 mg/kg per day in a single dose or in three divided doses.

Neonate: i.v. infusion, <32 weeks postmenstrual age, 4–5 mg/kg as a single dose every 36 h; ≥32 weeks postmenstrual age, 4–5 mg/kg as a single dose every 24 h. Alternatively, if <7 days old, 2 mg/kg every 12 h; if 7–28 days old, 2–2.5 mg/kg every 8 h.

Child: 1 month–18 years, 7 mg/kg as a single daily dose and adjust dose on the basis of serum concentrations. Alternatively, 1 month–12 years, 2–2.5 mg/kg every 8 h, *or* 12–18 years, 1 mg/kg (5 mg/kg in severe cases) every 8 h.

Cystic fibrosis: adults and children, 300 mg inhaled twice daily.

Widely available.

The dosage should be reduced in renal impairment. Dosage should be controlled in all patients by blood level determinations; these should be done at least weekly in patients on long-term treatment.

Further information

Bonsignore CL. Inhaled tobramycin (TOBI). *Pediatr Nurs.* 1998;24:258–259.

Burdette SD, Limkemann AJ, Slaughter JB, Beam WB, Markert RL. Serum concentrations of aerosolised tobramycin in medical, surgical and trauma patients. *Antimicrob Agents Chemother.* 2009;53:4568.

Geller EG, Pitlick WH, Nardella PA, Tracewell WG, Ramsey BW. Pharmacokinetics and bioavailability of aerosolized tobramycin in cystic fibrosis. *Chest.* 2002;122:219–226.

Jacoby GA, Blaser MJ, Santanam P, et al. Appearance of amikacin and tobramycin resistance due to 4′-aminoglycoside nucleotidyltransferase [ANT(4′)-II] in Gram-negative pathogens. *Antimicrob Agents Chemother.* 1990;34:2381–2386.

Lima da Costa L, Erre JP, Pehourq F, Aran JM. Aminoglycoside ototoxicity and the medial efferent system: II. Comparison of acute effects of different antibiotics. *Audiology.* 1998;37:162–173.

Mann HJ, Canafax DM, Cipolle RJ, et al. Increased dosage requirements of tobramycin and gentamicin for treating *Pseudomonas aeruginosa* pneumonia in patients with cystic fibrosis. *Pediatr Pulmonol.* 1985;1:238–243.

Robinson P. Cystic fibrosis. *Thorax.* 2001;56:237–241.

Winslade NE, Adelman MH, Evans EJ, Schentag JJ. Single-dose accumulation pharmacokinetics of tobramycin and netilmicin in normal volunteers. *Antimicrob Agents Chemother.* 1987;31:605–609.

OTHER KANAMYCIN GROUP AMINOGLYCOSIDES

ARBEKACIN (HABEKACIN)

The 1-*N*-(4-amino-2-hydroxybutyryl) derivative of dibekacin, to which it bears the same relation as amikacin bears to kanamycin A. Supplied as the sulfate.

Activity and stability to aminoglycoside-modifying enzymes are comparable with those of amikacin. It is active against many strains of methicillin-resistant *Staph. aureus*, either alone or in combination with β-lactam or other agents. Synergy with ampicillin has been observed for high-level gentamicin- and vancomycin-resistant enterococci.

A 3 mg/kg intravenous dose achieved a peak concentration of *c.* 8 mg/L after 1 h. The plasma half-life is about 2 h and protein binding 3–12%.

About 85% of the dose can be recovered from urine over 48 h. It is retained in renal failure, but moderately well removed by hemodialysis with a plasma half-life of 2–4 h. Peak concentrations of 10.9 mg/L and trough concentrations of 1.7 mg/L have been reported in patients treated for MRSA infection where C_{max}:MIC ratios of >25 and AUC:MIC ratios of >186 were associated with improved cure rates, and both C_{min} and AUC were associated with the incidence of nephrotoxicity.

Toxicity and side effects are typical of the aminoglycoside class. It is used in severe infection cause by susceptible micro-organisms, but is not widely available.

Further information

Fukuoka N, Aibiki M. Recommended dose of arbekacin, an aminoglycoside against methicillin-resistant *Staphylococcus aureus*, does not achieve desired serum concentration in critically ill patients with lowered creatinine clearance. *J Clin Pharm Ther.* 2008;33:521–527.

Sato R, Tanigawara Y, Kaku M, Aikawa N, Shimizu K. Pharmacokinetic–pharmacodynamic relationship of arbekacin for treatment of patients infected with methicillin-resistant *Staphylococcus aureus*. Antimicrob Agents Chemother. 50:3763–3769.

Tanigawara Y, Sat R, Morita K, Kaku M, Aikawa N, Shimizu K. Population pharmacokinetics of arbekacin in patients infected with methicillin-resistant *Staphylococcus aureus*. Antimicrob Agents Chemother. 2006;50:3754–3762.

 ## DIBEKACIN

3′,4′-Dideoxy kanamycin B. A semisynthetic aminoglycoside closely related to the natural compound tobramycin (3′-deoxy kanamycin B). Supplied as the sulfate.

It is active against staphylococci including methicillin-resistant strains, a wide range of enterobacteria, *Acinetobacter* and *Pseudomonas* spp. It is also active against *M. tuberculosis* and the *M. avium* complex (MICs 4–16 mg/L). It exhibits the usual aminoglycoside properties of bactericidal activity at concentrations close to the MIC and bactericidal synergy with selected β-lactam antibiotics.

Absence of hydroxyl groups present in the parent kanamycin B renders dibekacin resistant to phosphorylation by APH(3′). It is also resistant to some forms of ANT(4′). However, the type of this enzyme, ANT(4′), found in some Gram-positive organisms modifies dibekacin at the 2″-hydroxyl group; nevertheless dibekacin has much greater activity than tobramycin against organisms that produce the enzyme.

A 1 mg/kg intravenous bolus dose achieves a peak plasma concentration of around 5 mg/L. The plasma half-life is 2.3 h. Protein binding is 3–12%. It is eliminated principally by the renal route, 75–80% of the dose appearing in the urine in the first 24 h. Elimination is inversely related to renal function. In patients maintained on chronic hemodialysis, the half-life rises to 54 h between dialyses and falls to 6–7 h on dialysis.

Toxic effects are those typical of aminoglycosides with a frequency similar to or less than those of gentamicin.

It is used for severe infections caused by susceptible microorganisms, especially those resistant to established aminoglycosides, but availability is limited.

 ## BEKANAMYCIN (KANAMYCIN B; KANENDOMYCIN)

A component of the mixture of kanamycins produced by *Streptomyces kanamyceticus*. It is approximately twice as active as kanamycin A and is twice as toxic. It is not active against amikacin-resistant strains of MRSA. It is poorly active against *Ps. aeruginosa*.

The pharmacokinetics and uses are similar to those of kanamycin. A 0.5% ophthalmic solution has been used to treat gonococcal ophthalmia neonatorum. It is available in Japan.

NEOMYCIN GROUP

NEOMYCIN

Fradiomycin. Molecular weight (sulfate): 711.7; (free base): 614.7.

Neomycins A, B and C are fermentation products of *Streptomyces fradii*. The product marketed as 'neomycin' is a mixture of neomycin B and its isomer, neomycin C, supplied as the sulfates. Neomycin B is available alone under the name framycetin for topical use. It is required to contain not more than 3% neomycin C and not more than 1% neomycin A. Buffered aqueous solutions (pH 7) are stable at room temperature.

 ## ANTIMICROBIAL ACTIVITY

The susceptibility of common pathogenic bacteria is shown in Table 12.1 (p. 146). Among other organisms susceptible in vitro (MIC 4–8 mg/L) are *Pasteurella*, *Vibrio*, *Borrelia* and *Leptospira* spp. It is active against *M. tuberculosis*, including streptomycin-resistant strains. Synergy has been reported with polymyxin B. The bactericidal effect is enhanced at alkaline pH.

 ## ACQUIRED RESISTANCE

Resistance is acquired in a stepwise fashion and staphylococci may become resistant as a result of prolonged topical use. The use of neomycin–bacitracin–polymyxin mixtures may contribute to this, as many strains resistant to neomycin are also resistant to bacitracin. Resistant enterobacteria may appear in the feces of patients treated orally and in those treated for prolonged periods; most have been found to possess multiple transferable antibiotic resistance. Cross-resistance with kanamycin is often due to the synthesis of APH(3′), although AAC(6′) some forms of AAC(3) and ANT(4′) also modify both neomycin and kanamycin. Resistant strains of *Staph. aureus* are usually more resistant to kanamycin than to neomycin. The rare enzyme AAC(1) confers resistance to neomycin and paromomycin, but not to other aminoglycosides.

PHARMACOKINETICS

C_{max} 0.5 g intramuscular	20 mg/L after 1 h
Plasma half-life	2–3 h
Volume of distribution	0.25–0.35 L/kg
Plasma protein binding	Low

Very little is absorbed after oral administration and more than 95% is eliminated unchanged in the feces. Peak plasma concentrations of less than 4 mg/L have been found after an oral dose of 3 g. Distribution and excretion resemble that of streptomycin, but the toxicity of neomycin precludes systemic administration except in the most extreme cases.

TOXICITY AND SIDE EFFECTS

Neomycin is the most likely of all the aminoglycosides to damage the kidneys and the auditory branch of the eighth nerve (Table 12.3). This has almost entirely restricted it to topical and oral use.

Irreversible deafness may develop even if the drug is stopped at the first sign of damage. Loss of hearing may occur as a result of topical applications to wounds or other denuded areas, particularly if renal excretion is impaired. Instillation of ear drops containing neomycin can result in deafness. This generally develops in the second week of treatment and is usually reversible.

Rashes have been described in 6–8% of patients treated topically and these patients may be rendered allergic to other aminoglycosides. Nausea and protracted diarrhea may follow oral administration. Sufficient drug may be absorbed from the gut on prolonged oral administration to produce deafness but not renal damage. Intestinal malabsorption and superinfection have been seen in patients receiving 4–9 g per day and may develop in patients receiving as little as 3 g of the drug per day. Precipitation of bile salts by the drug may impair the hydrolysis of long-chain triglycerides. Large doses instilled into the peritoneal cavity at operation may be absorbed, with resultant systemic toxicity, and patients concurrently exposed to anesthetics and muscle relaxants are liable to suffer neuromuscular blockade, which is reversible by neostigmine.

CLINICAL USE

Superficial infections with staphylococci and Gram-negative bacilli (topical; alone or in combination with bacitracin, chlorhexidine or polymyxin)

Treatment of staphylococcal nasal carriers (topical, in combination with chlorhexidine or bacitracin)

Eye infections (topical; alone or in combination)

Otitis externa (alone or with a corticosteroid)

Gut decontamination before abdominal surgery (oral)

Prophylaxis after urinary tract instrumentation (instillation)

Use is discouraged because of the possibility of promoting the appearance of aminoglycoside-resistant strains, and because of the risk of absorption with the consequent danger of systemic toxicity or neuromuscular blockade.

Preparations and dosage

Neomycin

Proprietary names: Mycifradin, Nivemycin.

Preparations: Tablets, elixir, topical.

Dosage: Adults, oral, 1 g every 4 h for a maximum of 72 h.
Children 6–12 years, 250–500 mg every 4 h.

Widely available.

Framycetin (neomycin B)

Proprietary name: Soframycin.

Preparations: Tablets, topical ophthalmic, aural.

Dosage: Adult, oral, 2–4 g per day in divided doses.

Widely available in topical preparations.

Table 12.3 Relative toxicity index[a] of aminoglycosides

	Vestibular	Auditory	Renal
Streptomycin	4	1	<1
Neomycin	1	4	4
Kanamycin	1	2	1
Gentamicin	3	2	2
Tobramycin	2	2	2

[a]1–4: least to most toxic.
Based on Price KE, Godfrey JC, Kawaguchi H 1974 *Advances in Applied Microbiology* 18: 191–307.

Further information

Langman AW. Neomycin ototoxicity. *Otolaryngol Head Neck Surg.* 1994;110:441–444.

Lima da Costa L, Erre JP, Pehourq F, Aran JM. Aminoglycoside ototoxicity and the medial efferent system: II. Comparison of acute effects of different antibiotics. *Audiology.* 1998;37:162–173.

Tempera G, Mangiafico A, Genovese C, et al. In vitro evaluation of the synergistic activity of neomycin–polymyxin B association against pathogens responsible for otitis externa. *Int J Immunopathol Pharmacol.* 2009;22:299–302.

PAROMOMYCIN

Aminosidine, catenulin, crestomycin, hydroxymycin, estomycin, monomycin A, neomycin E, paucimycin. Molecular weight (free base): 615.63.

A fermentation product of *Streptomyces rimosus* var. *paromomycinus*, supplied as the sulfate. The commercial product is a mixture of the two isomeric paromomycins I and II, which are closely related to neomycin.

The antibacterial activity is almost identical to that of neomycin. Since it differs from neomycin in having a hydroxyl rather than an amino group at the 6′-position it is not sensitive to AAC(6′) modifying enzymes. It is active against *M. tuberculosis*, including multidrug-resistant strains, and the *M. avium* complex.

Unlike other aminoglycosides, paromomycin is active against some protozoa, including *Entamoeba histolytica*, *Cryptosporidium parvum*, *Leishmania* spp., *Giardia lamblia* and *Trichomonas vaginalis*. It also exhibits activity against the tapeworms *Taenia saginata*, *Taenia solium*, *Diphyllobothrium latum* and *Hymenolepis nana*.

It closely resembles neomycin in pharmacokinetic behavior and liability to produce deafness and intestinal malabsorption.

CLINICAL USE

Intestinal amebiasis (oral)

Cutaneous leishmaniasis (topical) and visceral leishmaniasis (intramuscular)

Nitroimidazole-resistant trichomoniasis (topical)

Its antiprotozoal activity has attracted some attention, but it has largely been superseded by more active and less toxic compounds. Success in treating nitroimidazole-resistant trichomoniasis with topical paromomycin has been reported. Trials in India and East Africa of parenteral paromomycin alone, or in combination with sodium stibogluconate, for treatment of visceral leishmaniasis have shown promising results.

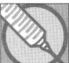

Preparations and dosage

Proprietary names: Gabbroral.

Preparations: Capsules, syrup, topical.

Dosage: Adult, oral dosage, 25–35 mg/kg per day in three divided doses with meals for 5–10 days; adult, i.m. dosage, 16–20 mg/kg per day for 21 days.

Limited availability. Available in the USA and continental Europe, but not in the UK.

📖 Further information

Chappuis F, Sundar S, Hailu A, et al. Visceral leishmaniasis: what are the needs for diagnosis, treatment and control? *Nat Rev Microbiol.* 2007;5:873–882.

Donald PR, Sirgel FA, Kanyok TP, et al. Early bactericidal activity of paromomycin (aminosidine) in patients with smear-positive pulmonary tuberculosis. *Antimicrob Agents Chemother.* 2000;44:3285–3287.

Kayok TP, Reddy MV, Chinnaswamy J, Danziger LH, Gangadharam PR. Activity of aminosidine (paromomycin) for *Mycobacterium tuberculosis* and *Mycobacterium avium*. *J Antimicrob Chemother.* 1994;33:323–327.

Murray HW. Treatment of visceral leishmaniasis (kala-azar): a decade of progress and future approaches. *Int J Infect Dis.* 2000;4:158–177.

Nyirjesy P, Sobel JD, Weitz MV, Leaman DJ, Gelone SP. Difficult-to-treat trichomoniasis: results with paromomycin cream. *Clin Infect Dis.* 1998;26:986–988.

OTHER AMINOGLYCOSIDES AND AMINOCYCLITOLS

STREPTOMYCIN

Molecular weight (free base): 581.58.

A fermentation product of *Streptomyces griseus*. It is available in some countries as the calcium chloride or as the hydrochloride, but usually supplied as the sulfate. Solutions are stable for long periods if refrigerated.

ANTIMICROBIAL ACTIVITY

Activity against common bacterial pathogens is shown in Table 12.1 (p. 146). It is less active than gentamicin group compounds against most micro-organisms within the spectrum, but it is particularly active against mycobacteria, including *M. kansasii* and most strains of *M. ulcerans*. *Brucella* (MIC 0.5 mg/L), *Francisella*, *Pasteurella* spp. and *Yersinia pestis* are susceptible.

It is actively bactericidal, the speed of killing increasing progressively with concentration. The antibacterial activity is greatest in a slightly alkaline medium (pH 7.8) and is considerably reduced below pH 6.0. It is so sensitive to the effect of pH that the natural acidity of a solution of streptomycin sulfate may be sufficient to depress its antibacterial activity.

 ## ACQUIRED RESISTANCE

In contrast to most other aminoglycosides, high level resistance can result from a single-step mutation in the gene encoding ribosomal protein S12 (*rpsL*), which alters the protein so that binding is reduced. Resistance in some clinical isolates of *M. tuberculosis* is associated either with missense mutations in the *rpsL* gene, or with base substitutions at position 904 in the 16S rRNA.

Resistance can also be caused by aminoglycoside-modifying enzymes: phosphotransferases that modify the 3″-hydroxyl group in both Gram-negative and Gram-positive organisms; a phosphotransferase that modifies the 6-hydroxyl group in *Pseudomonas* spp.; and a nucleotidyl-transferase that modifies the 3″-hydroxyl group in Gram-negative organisms.

Increase in resistance often occurs within a few days (for *M. tuberculosis* a few weeks) of the beginning of treatment, and resistance of many species is now common. Primary streptomycin resistance in *M. tuberculosis* is much more common in the Far East and less developed countries than in the UK and USA. However, several clusters of multidrug-resistant tuberculosis have been identified among hospital patients with AIDS in the USA.

Strains of streptococci and enterococci showing moderate resistance (MIC 6–500 mg/L) exhibit synergy with penicillin, but strains showing high levels of resistance (MIC >500 mg/L) have ribosomes that are resistant to streptomycin and simultaneous treatment with penicillin is without effect.

It is not uncommon to find strains of bacteria, including *M. tuberculosis*, that are actually favored by the presence of the antibiotic or completely dependent on it. Isolated ribosomes from streptomycin-dependent *Esch. coli* show a change in the same single ribosomal protein that determines resistance and synthesize peptides only in the presence of the drug.

Streptomycin-resistant bacteria usually remain sensitive to other aminoglycosides. Enterococci with high-level resistance to gentamicin, and consequent resistance to gentamicin–β-lactam synergy, may show synergy between the β-lactam and streptomycin.

 ## PHARMACOKINETICS

C_{max} 1 g intramuscular	26–58 mg/L after 0.5–1.5 h
Plasma half-life	2.4–2.7 h
Volume of distribution	0.3 L/kg
Plasma protein binding	35%

Absorption

Absorption from the intestinal tract is negligible. In patients treated for tuberculosis considerable interindividual variability of C_{max} has been observed following both intramuscular and intravenous administration due to differences in distribution volume and, in the case of intramuscular administration, rate of absorption. In patients over the age of 40 years, excretion is delayed and in older subjects commonly incomplete at 24 h. In such patients a dose of 0.75 g intramuscularly produces peak plasma concentrations around 25–60 mg/L with a half-life up to 9 h.

Distribution

Streptomycin diffuses fairly rapidly into most body tissues, but is distributed only in the extracellular fluid. It appears in the peritoneal fluid in concentrations of about one-quarter to one-half those present in the blood, and in pleural fluid the concentrations may equal those in the blood. It does not penetrate into the CSF or thick-walled abscesses, but significant amounts are usually present in tuberculous cavities. Concentrations in cord blood are similar to those in maternal blood.

Excretion

It is rapidly excreted by glomerular filtration and is unaffected by agents that block tubular secretion. The renal clearance is 1.8–4.2 L/h and 30–90% of the dose is usually excreted in the first 24 h. Concentrations in the urine often reach 400 mg/L after doses of 0.5 g. In oliguria, the plasma half-life is prolonged and dosage must be reduced if toxic concentrations are to be avoided. Plasma half-life during hemodialysis approaches that in normal renal function.

 ## TOXICITY AND SIDE EFFECTS

Pain and irritation at the site of injection are common, and sterile inflammatory reactions or peripheral neuritis from direct involvement of a nerve sometimes occur. Many patients experience circumoral paresthesia, vertigo and ataxia, headaches, lassitude and 'muzziness in the head'. Renal dysfunction is rare but has been described in patients receiving 3–4 g per day.

Ototoxicity

The most common serious toxic effect is vestibular disturbance, which is related to total dosage and excessive blood concentrations, and hence to the age of the patient and the state of renal function. In older patients the risk of damage is higher and compensation is less than in young patients. Persistence of the drug in the perilymph after the plasma concentration has fallen may play an important part in such ototoxicity. There is no significant relation between incidence of dizziness and peak streptomycin concentration, but a highly significant relation to plasma concentrations exceeding 5 mg/L at 24 h. The risk to hearing is much less, but damage sometimes occurs after only a few doses. Congenital hearing loss or abnormalities in the caloric test or audiogram have been described several times in children born to women treated with streptomycin in pregnancy. There is considerable individual variation in susceptibility to its toxic effects, which may be partly genetically determined.

Allergy

In addition to eosinophilia unassociated with other allergic manifestations, rashes and drug fever occur in about 5% of treated patients. These are usually trivial and respond to antihistamine treatment, so that in most cases therapy can be continued, although this should be done with caution, since occasionally severe and even fatal exfoliative dermatitis may develop. Skin sensitization is also common in nurses and dispensers who handle streptomycin and may lead to severe dermatitis, sometimes associated with periorbital swelling and conjunctivitis. Reactions most frequently develop between 4 and 6 weeks, but may appear after the first dose or after 6 months' treatment. Patients who develop hypersensitivity during prolonged therapy can generally be desensitized by giving 20 mg prednisolone daily plus 10 daily increments from 0.1 to 1.0 g streptomycin when normal dosage will usually be tolerated, or by giving increased doses of streptomycin every 6 h.

Neuromuscular blockade

It is rare for neuromuscular blockade to develop in those whose neuromuscular mechanisms are normal, but patients who are also receiving muscle relaxants or anesthetics, or are suffering from myasthenia gravis are at special risk.

Other effects

Rare neurological manifestations include peripheral neuritis and optic neuritis with scotoma. Other rare effects have been aplastic anemia, agranulocytosis, hemolytic anemia, thrombocytopenia, hypocalcemia and severe bleeding associated with a circulating factor V antagonist.

 ## CLINICAL USE

> Tuberculosis (in combination with other antituberculosis drugs)
>
> Infections caused by *M. kansasii* (in combination with other antimycobacterial agents)
>
> Plague and tularemia, including tularemia pneumonia
>
> Bacterial endocarditis (in combination with a penicillin)
>
> Brucellosis
>
> Whipple's disease (in combination with other antibiotics)

The most important use of streptomycin is in the treatment of tuberculosis (*see* Ch. 58). Depression of vestibular function by streptomycin has been used in the treatment of patients suffering from Ménière's disease.

 ### Preparations and dosage

Proprietary names: Many generic forms.

Preparation: Injection.

Dosage: Tuberculosis: Adults, i.m., 1 g per day (750 mg per day for adults >40 years of age or <50 kg body weight). Children, i.m., 15 mg/kg per day (maximum 1 g). Can also be given intravenously.

Widely available.

 ### Further information

Akaho E, Maekawa T, Uchinashi M, Kanamori R. A study of streptomycin blood level information of patients undergoing hemodialysis. *Biopharm Drug Dispos.* 2002;23:47–52.

Bagger-Sjoback D. Effect of streptomycin and gentamicin on the inner ear. *Ann N Y Acad Sci.* 1997;830:120–129.

de Jager P, van Altena R. Hearing loss and nephrotoxicity in long-term aminoglycoside treatment in patients with tuberculosis. *Int J Tuberc Lung Dis.* 2002;6:622–627.

Gill V, Cunha BA. Tularemia pneumonia. *Semin Respir Infec.* 1997;12:61–67.

Honore N, Cole ST. Streptomycin resistance in mycobacteria. *Antimicrob Agents Chemother.* 1994;38:238–242.

Peloquin CA, Berning SE, Nitta AT, et al. Aminoglycoside toxicity: daily versus thrice-weekly dosing for treatment of mycobacterial diseases. *Clin Infect Dis.* 2004;38:1538–1544.

Shea JJ. The role of dexamethasone or streptomycin perfusion in the treatment of Ménière's disease. *Otolaryngol Clin North Am.* 1997;30:1051–1059.

Zhu M, Burman WJ, Jaresko GS, et al. Population pharmacokinetics of intravenous and intramuscular streptomycin in patients with tuberculosis. *Pharmacotherapy.* 2001;21:1037–1054.

SPECTINOMYCIN

Aminospectacin; actinospectacin. Molecular weight (free base): 332.35.

An aminocyclitol that lacks an aminoglycosidic function and which is a fermentation product of *Streptomyces spectabilis* and *Streptomyces flavopersicus*. It is supplied as the dihydrochloride and the sulfate.

ANTIMICROBIAL ACTIVITY

Its activity is modest (Table 12.1, p. 146) and markedly affected by medium composition and pH. It exerts only moderate activity against Gram-positive organisms. It is widely active against enterobacteria, but *Providencia* spp. are resistant. Anaerobic bacteria are also resistant.

Of particular interest is its activity against *N. gonorrhoeae*, including β-lactamase-producing strains. Among other sexually acquired organisms, *Ureaplasma urealyticum* is susceptible, but *Chlamydia trachomatis* and *T. pallidum* are resistant.

For most organisms, the minimum bactericidal concentration (MBC) is at least four times the MIC and it is regarded as essentially bacteristatic. In contrast, it is bactericidal for gonococci at concentrations close to the MIC, which is of the order of 2–16 mg/L for both penicillin-susceptible and resistant strains.

ACQUIRED RESISTANCE

N. gonorrhoeae strains resistant to spectinomycin have emerged in South East Asia, the USA and the UK; the resistance of UK isolates was not attributable to aminoglycoside-modifying enzymes. In most countries where its use remains low the prevalence of resistance in gonorrhea is also low.

Acquired resistance in enterobacteria, enterococci and staphylococci can be caused by nucleotidyltransferases that modify the drug at position 9. The enzyme from Gram-negative organisms ANT(3″) (9) also modifies streptomycin at position 3″, thus conferring cross-resistance to the two drugs. There is no enzymatic cross-resistance with 2-deoxystreptamine-containing aminoglycosides.

PHARMACOKINETICS

C_{max} 25 mg/kg intramuscular	60–80 mg/L after 1 h
Plasma half-life	2–3 h
Volume of distribution	10–13.4 L
Plasma protein binding	<10%

It is poorly absorbed on oral administration. It is almost completely excreted unchanged in the urine over 48 h, concentrations on conventional dosage reaching 1 g/L. Excretion is prolonged in renal impairment, and is unaffected by probenecid.

TOXICITY AND SIDE EFFECTS

Transient headache, dizziness, pain at the site of injection and occasional fever have been described. No evidence of ototoxicity or renal toxicity has been found in volunteers receiving doses of 2 g every 6 h for 3 weeks, amounts much in excess of those used therapeutically.

CLINICAL USE

Gonorrhea in penicillin-allergic patients or due to penicillin-resistant strains (single-dose treatment)

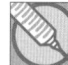

Preparations and dosage

Proprietary names: Trobicin, Trobicine.
Preparation: Injection.
Dosage: Deep i.m. injection adults, 2 g as a single dose, or 4 g in two separate i.m. sites in those difficult to treat and in areas of resistance. Children, i.m., 40 mg/kg as a single dose (maximum dose, 2 g per day). Widely available.

Further information

Farhi D, Hotz C, Poupet H, et al. *Neisseria gonorrhoeae* antibiotic resistance in Paris, 2005 to 2007: implications for treatment guidelines. *Acta Derm Venereol.* 2009;89:484–487.

Ison CA. Antimicrobial agents and gonorrhoea: therapeutic choice, resistance and susceptibility testing. *Genitourin Med.* 1996;72:253–257.

Moran JS, Levine WC. Drugs of choice for the treatment of uncomplicated gonococcal infections. *Clin Infect Dis.* 1995;20(suppl 1):S47–S65.

ASTROMICIN

A pseudodisaccharide aminoglycoside produced by *Micromonospora olivoasterospora*. Formulated as the sulfate.

Intrinsic activity is similar to that of amikacin for most groups of organisms, but activity against *Ps. aeruginosa* is relatively poor. It is resistant to many aminoglycoside-modifying enzymes, but is sensitive to AAC(3) and the APH(2″)/AAC(6′) bifunctional enzyme.

Peak concentrations of 10–12 mg/L were found in the blood following 200 mg intravenous or intramuscular administration to volunteers. The plasma half-life was 1.5–2 h. Over 85% of the drug was recovered in urine during the 8 h following administration.

Toxicity and side effects are similar to those observed with other aminoglycosides. Where the drug is available it is used instead of amikacin in the treatment of infections caused by susceptible organisms.

 Further information

Matsuhashi Y, Yoshida T, Hara T, Kazuno Y, Inouye S. In vitro and in vivo antibacterial activities of dactimicin, a novel pseudodisaccharide aminoglycoside, compared with those of other aminoglycoside antibiotics. *Antimicrob Agents Chemother*. 1985;27:589–594.

Nakashima M, Takiguchi Y, Inoue A, Kobayashi S.A, phase I. study on intravenous drip infusion of astromicin. *Jpn J Antibiot*. 1986;39:1543–1572.

13 β-Lactam antibiotics: cephalosporins

David Greenwood

All cephalosporins are based on cephalosporin C, which was discovered by Edward Abraham and his colleagues in Oxford as a minor component of the antibiotic complex produced by *Cephalosporium acremonium*, a mold cultivated from a Sardinian sewage outfall by Giuseppe Brotzu in 1948. Interest in cephalosporin C was fuelled by its stability to staphylococcal β-lactamase (shared by all subsequent cephalosporins), which was causing concern at the time, and they probably owe their continued development to this property. Over 100 semisynthetic cephalosporins have since been marketed, although not all have survived into present-day use.

In all cephalosporins the β-lactam ring is fused to a six-membered dihydrothiazine ring in place of the five-membered thiazolidine ring of penicillins (*see* pp. 226–227). The basic 7-aminocephalosporanic acid skeleton can be modified at a number of positions.

- Alterations at the C-3 position tend to affect the pharmacokinetic and metabolic properties.
- Introduction of a methoxy group at C-7 yields a cephamycin with enhanced stability to β-lactamases, including the cephalosporinases of certain *Bacteroides* spp.
- Changes at the 7-amino position alter, in general, the antibacterial activity or β-lactamase stability or both.

Other compounds conveniently considered alongside the cephalosporins, since their properties are very similar, include:

- the oxacephems, in which the sulfur of the dihydrothiazine ring is replaced by oxygen
- the carbacephems, in which the sulfur is replaced by carbon.

CLASSIFICATION

As new cephalosporins have become available they have been loosely classified into 'generations', but these descriptions are too simplistic, and are to be discouraged. The following grouping is adopted here:

- *Group 1*: Parenteral compounds of moderate antimicrobial activity and susceptible to hydrolysis by a wide variety of enterobacterial β-lactamases.
- *Group 2*: Oral compounds of moderate antimicrobial activity and moderately resistant to some enterobacterial β-lactamases.
- *Group 3*: Parenteral compounds of moderate antimicrobial activity resistant to a wide range of β-lactamases. Some are available as esters for oral administration.
- *Group 4*: Parenteral compounds with potent antimicrobial activity and resistance to a wide range of β-lactamases.
- *Group 5*: Oral compounds (often achieved by esterification) resistant to a wide range of β-lactamases. Most exhibit potent activity against enterobacteria; activity against Gram-positive cocci is variable.
- *Group 6*: Parenteral compounds with activity against *Pseudomonas aeruginosa*. They vary widely in their spectrum of activity against other bacterial species.
- *Group 7*: Compounds characterized by activity against methicillin-resistant staphylococci.

Although the 'generation' categories often used are imprecise, 'first-generation' compounds roughly correspond to Groups 1 and 2; 'second-generation' to group 3; 'third-generation' to groups 4–6. Certain group 6 and 7 compounds are sometimes allocated to so-called 'fourth and fifth generations'.

Some cephalosporins, including cefalonium and cefaloram (group 1) and cefquinone and ceftiofur (group 4) are used only in veterinary medicine and are not discussed further here.

Group 1	Group 2	Group 3	Group 4	Group 5	Group 6	Group 7
Cefacetrile	Cefaclor	Cefbuperazone*	Cefmenoxime	Cefcapene	Cefepime	Ceftaroline
Cefaloridine	Cefadroxil	Cefmetazole*	Cefodizime	Cefdinir	Cefoperazone	Ceftobiprole
Cefalotin	Cefalexin	Cefminox*	Cefotaxime	Cefditoren	Cefozopran	
Cefamandole	Cefatrizine	Cefotetan*	Ceftizoxime	Cefetamet	Cefpimizole	
Cefapirin	Cefprozil	Cefotiam	Ceftriaxone	Cefixime	Cefpiramide	
Cefazolin	Cefradine	Cefoxitin*	Flomoxef†	Cefpodoxime	Cefpirome	
Cefonicid	Cefroxadine	Cefuroxime	Latamoxef†	Cefteram	Cefsulodin	
Ceforanide	Loracarbef‡			Ceftibuten	Ceftazidime	

*7-Methoxycephalosporin (cephamycin).
†7-Methoxyoxacephem.
‡1-Carbacephem.

ANTIMICROBIAL ACTIVITY

Most cephalosporins are active against staphylococci other than methicillin-resistant strains, including those producing β-lactamase. The degree of activity varies among different members of the group. Streptococci, including pneumococci, are susceptible but *Enterococcus faecalis*, *Ent. faecium* and *L. monocytogenes* are virtually completely resistant. *Streptococcus pneumoniae* strains with reduced susceptibility to penicillins are also less susceptible to the cephalosporins. Many Gram-negative species including neisseriae, *Haemophilus influenzae*, *Escherichia coli*, salmonellae, some klebsiellae and *Proteus mirabilis* are sensitive to varying degrees. Inoculum-related effects are common, particularly when compounds of groups 1 and 2 are tested against Gram-negative bacilli. *Ps. aeruginosa* is sensitive only to group 6 compounds. Except for cephamycins, activity against many anaerobes is unreliable. Mycobacteria, mycoplasmas, chlamydiae and fungi are resistant.

Cephalosporins are usually bactericidal at concentrations above the minimum inhibitory concentration (MIC) and bactericidal synergy is commonly demonstrable with aminoglycosides and a number of other agents.

ACQUIRED RESISTANCE

The most important form of resistance is that due to the elaboration of β-lactamases (pp. 228–231). All cephalosporins are relatively stable to staphylococcal β-lactamase, but resistance among Gram-negative genera is a good deal more complicated. The chromosomal β-lactamase of *Esch. coli*, which has virtually no hydrolytic activity against ampicillin, slowly degrades some group 1 cephalosporins and is responsible for the inoculum effect observed with *Esch. coli*. Chromosomal β-lactamases of *Bacteroides fragilis* are also more active against cephalosporins than against penicillins, but cephamycins and oxacephems are unusual in their stability to these enzymes. Cephalosporins exhibit considerable variation in stability to the enzymes of genera with an inducible, or derepressible, chromosomal β-lactamase and to plasmid-mediated enzymes of Gram-negative bacilli (pp. 230–231).

The resistance of Gram-negative bacilli does not depend solely on β-lactamase formation. It varies also with the extent to which the antibiotic can penetrate the outer cell membrane and reach the site of enzyme formation. This property, known as crypticity, can be measured by comparing the enzyme activity of intact and disrupted cells. Resistance may also result from a change in the biochemical target of the antibiotic (i.e. the penicillin-binding proteins).

PHARMACOKINETICS

Group 2 agents are well absorbed, with bioavailability often exceeding 85%. The bioavailability of some of the agents in other groups is enhanced by prodrug formulation. These agents tend to have improved absorption following food, whereas food has little or a deleterious effect on the absorption of group 2 compounds.

Cephalosporins are usually well distributed, achieving high concentrations in the interstitial fluid of tissues and in serous cavities. Penetration into the eye and the cerebrospinal fluid (CSF) is poor, though some cephalosporins achieve adequate levels in the CSF in the presence of meningeal inflammation. They cross the placenta.

Compounds that carry an acetoxymethyl group at C-3, such as cefalotin and cefotaxime, are susceptible to mammalian esterases that remove the acetyl group to form the corresponding hydroxymethyl derivative with reduced antibacterial activity. The relevance (if any) of deacetylation to therapy has not been established.

Cephalosporins are generally excreted into urine by glomerular filtration and tubular secretion; elimination is depressed by probenecid and renal failure. Most are rapidly eliminated with plasma half-lives of 1–2 h but some are more persistent. The less active metabolites resulting from removal of acetoxymethyl groups at C-3 are also excreted in the urine. Some excretion is via the bile, and certain compounds, notably cefoperazone and cefpiramide, are preferentially excreted by this route.

TOXICITY AND SIDE EFFECTS

HYPERSENSITIVITY

Hypersensitivity occurs in 0.5–10% of patients, mostly in the form of rashes, eosinophilia, drug fever and serum sickness. In addition to immediate reactions, a maculopapular rash with or without fever, lymphadenopathy and eosinophilia may appear after several days' treatment. As with penicillins, allergy to cephalosporins is probably based on major and minor antigenic determinants, but they are less well characterized than with penicillins. Clinical reactions to cephalosporins in penicillin-allergic patients are uncommon and severe reactions are very rare. About 10% of such reactions are said to occur, generally in patients who react to a variety of drugs. Nonetheless, the generally accepted advice is that cephalosporins should not be given to patients who have previously suffered a well-documented severe reaction to penicillins. Specific allergy to cephalosporins also occurs, but there is no evidence that the compounds differ markedly in allergenicity.

HEMATOLOGIC TOXICITY

Rare reversible abnormalities of platelet function and coagulation resulting from several different mechanisms have been described. Thrombocytopenia and neutropenia are occasionally seen.

Although penicillins have long been associated with clotting abnormalities, it was cephalosporins that brought bleeding associated with β-lactam antibiotics into prominence when cefamandole, cefoperazone, latamoxef and other compounds with a methylthiotetrazole side chain at the C-3 position were found to induce severe hypoprothrombinemia, especially in patients who were malnourished, had renal failure or were treated for prolonged periods. The deficiency is readily reversed by vitamin K_1.

OTHER ADVERSE REACTIONS

Pain at the site of intramuscular injection and phlebitis at the site of intravenous administration is fairly common. *Candida* overgrowth with vaginitis has been a feature of some studies.

Diarrhea occurs in about 5% of patients and pseudomembranous colitis has been described. Changes in bowel flora, accompanied by emergence of resistant organisms, including *Clostridium difficile*, are particularly likely with those agents

which are extensively excreted in the bile and because of their non-absorption achieve substantial fecal concentrations.

Rare disturbances of renal function appear to have the direct toxic or allergic origins described for penicillins. Claims that the nephrotoxicity of cephalosporins is potentiated by aminoglycosides have been disputed.

As with other β-lactam antibiotics, central nervous system (CNS) disturbances may occur if they are given in excessive doses, particularly to patients with renal failure. Transient abnormalities of liver function tests without other evidence of hepatotoxicity and gastrointestinal disturbances also occur.

In addition to hypoprothrombinemia (*see above*) cephalosporins with a methylthiotetrazole side chain may cause a disulfiram-like reaction, evidently due to inhibition of aldehyde dehydrogenase. Patients should be advised to avoid alcohol during and 3 days after treatment with these agents.

CLINICAL USE

GROUP 1

Group 1 cephalosporins are no longer widely used. They are not reliable for the treatment of severe respiratory tract infection, severe undiagnosed sepsis or meningitis. They should be avoided in the treatment of diseases where *H. influenzae* or enterococci may be implicated.

GROUP 2

The older oral agents have had widespread use for the treatment of upper respiratory, urinary, soft tissue and various other infections. They are possible alternatives to benzylpenicillin in allergic patients for the treatment of streptococcal, pneumococcal and staphylococcal infections.

GROUPS 3 AND 4

The properties of the β-lactamase-stable cephalosporins strongly commend them for the treatment of severe sepsis of unknown or mixed bacterial origin. It is not established that the superior activity in vitro of group 4 over group 3 compounds is reflected in greater clinical efficacy. Despite the difference in potency, it is customary to give similar doses of compounds in both groups, partly because the very high activity seen against enterobacteria is not exhibited against staphylococci. They have been successfully used in hospital-acquired pneumonia, particularly that due to enterobacteria. They are inactive against *Legionella pneumophila*, *Mycoplasma pneumoniae* and *Coxiella burnetii*.

Group 4 agents now have an established place in the treatment of meningitis due to many enterobacteria, β-lactamase-producing *H. influenzae* and penicillin-resistant pneumococci. They are not effective in the treatment of meningitis due to

L. monocytogenes, Enterobacter, Ps. aeruginosa or *Serratia* spp. Despite their in-vitro potency, they do not appear to offer any advantage over established therapy in the treatment of meningitis due to *Neisseria meningitidis*. Their activity and resistance to β-lactamases has led to their successful use for the treatment of infection due to β-lactamase-producing gonococci.

GROUP 5

Those oral compounds may replace the group 2 agents if resistance to the earlier compounds becomes significant. The relatively lower activity of cefixime and ceftibuten against Gram-positive cocci suggests they should be used with caution in infections with these organisms.

GROUPS 6 AND 7

Ceftazidime has been widely used in serious infection due to *Ps. aeruginosa*. Cefsulodin and cefoperazone are indicated only in proven or highly suspected pseudomonas infection and in combination with an appropriate aminoglycoside. Other group 6 compounds are appropriate for use in patients with severe infections caused by bacteria with plasmid and chromosomally mediated β-lactamases. Their main use is in hospital-acquired infections or in serious problems in the neutropenic patient.

The newer group 7 compounds have been specifically developed for their action against methicillin-resistant staphylococci.

Further information

Asbel LE, Levison ME. Cephalosporins, carbapenems, and monobactams. *Infect Dis Clin North Am.* 2000;14:435–437.

Marshall WF, Blair JE. The cephalosporins. *Mayo Clin Proc.* 1999;74:187–195.

Moreno E, Macías E, Dávila I, Laffond E, Ruiz A, Lorente F. Hypersensitivity reactions to cephalosporins. *Expert Opin Drug Saf.* 2008;7:295–304.

Nathwani D. Place of parenteral cephalosporins in the ambulatory setting: clinical evidence. *Drugs.* 2000;59(suppl 3):37–46.

Pichichero ME. A review of evidence supporting the American Academy of Pediatrics recommendation for prescribing cephalosporin antibiotics for penicillin-allergic patients. *Pediatrics.* 2005;115:1048–1057.

Wise R. Antibacterial agents: oral cephalosporins. *Prescribers Journal.* 1994;34:110–115.

GROUP 1 CEPHALOSPORINS

CEFALOTIN

Cephalothin. Molecular weight (sodium salt): 418.4.

A semisynthetic cephalosporin supplied as the sodium salt.

ANTIMICROBIAL ACTIVITY

Its activity against common pathogenic bacteria is shown in Table 13.1. Cefalotin is active against staphylococci, including β-lactamase-producing strains. Streptococci, including penicillin-sensitive pneumococci, but not enterococci, are highly susceptible. It is active against a range of enterobacteria, but is hydrolyzed by many enterobacterial β-lactamases. *Pasteurella* and *Vibrio* spp., *H. influenzae*, *Bordetella* and *Brucella* spp. are moderately resistant. *Campylobacter*, *Citrobacter*, *Enterobacter*, *Pseudomonas* and *Listeria* spp. are resistant. Most anaerobes, with the exception of *B. fragilis*, are susceptible: *Treponema pallidum* and *Leptospira* spp. are susceptible, but mycobacteria and mycoplasma are resistant.

PHARMACOKINETICS

C$_{max}$ 1 g intravenous	30 mg/L after 15 min
1 g intramuscular	15–20 mg/L after 0.5–1 h
Plasma half-life	*c.* 0.8 h
Volume of distribution	0.26 L
Plasma protein binding	60–70%

Distribution

Intramuscular administration is commonly painful and it is normally given intravenously. Continuous infusion of 12 g per day produces steady-state plasma levels of 10–30 mg/L. Penetration into the CSF is very poor, rising in the presence of inflammation to less than 2 mg/L after a 2 g intravenous dose.

Table 13.1 Activity of group 1 cephalosporins against common pathogenic bacteria: MIC (mg/L)

	Cefamandole	Cefalotin	Cefazolin
Staphylococcus aureus	0.5–1	0.25–0.5	0.25–0.5
Streptococcus pyogenes	0.06–1	0.1	0.1–0.25
Str. pneumoniae	0.06–16	0.06–0.1	0.1
Enterococcus faecalis	32–R	32	R
Neisseria gonorrhoeae	0.06	0.25–2	0.1–0.5
N. meningitidis	0.1–0.5	0.5	
Haemophilus influenzae	0.25–2	4–8	2–8
Escherichia coli	0.5–4	4–8	0.5–4
Klebsiella pneumoniae	0.5–2	4	1–4
Pseudomonas aeruginosa	R	R	R
Bacteroides fragilis	R	32–64	16–32
R, resistant (MIC >64 mg/L).			

Concentrations in sputum are 10–25% of the corresponding serum levels. An intravenous dose of 1 g produces a concentration in bone around 4 mg/kg.

Metabolism and excretion

It is deacetylated by hepatic esterases. The metabolite has about 20% of the activity of the parent compound and accounts for 20–30% of concentrations in serum and urine.

Urinary concentrations of 500–2000 mg/L are achieved during the first 6 h after a 1 g dose. Excretion is depressed by probenecid, indicating significant tubular secretion, and by renal failure although, because of metabolism, the plasma half-life of the drug is only moderately prolonged to about 3 h, while that of the principal metabolite rises to 12 h or more. Impaired tubular secretion is responsible for the elevated levels of the drug found in newborn and premature infants. Biliary excretion is trivial and liver disease has little effect on its half-life or plasma protein binding.

 ## TOXICITY AND SIDE EFFECTS

In volunteers receiving very large doses (8 g per day for 2–4 weeks) a serum-sickness-like illness developed. Positive Coombs' reactions associated with red cell agglutination, but very seldom with hemolysis, are common. Thrombocytopenia and leukopenia have been described. Coagulopathy with prolonged prothrombin time has been encountered in patients with renal failure or very high plasma levels resulting from excessive dosage. Evidence has been cited of exaggeration of pre-existing renal disease or renal damage, perhaps enhanced by simultaneous administration of aminoglycosides or furosemide (frusemide), in which direct tubular injury or allergic nephritis may have been involved.

 ## CLINICAL USE

It has been used in staphylococcal and streptococcal infections in penicillin-allergic patients, but is no longer recommended.

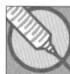 ### Preparations and dosage

Proprietary name: Keflin.

Preparation: Injection.

Dosage: Adults, i.m., i.v., 0.5–1 g every 4–6 h; up to 12 g per day in severe infections. Children, 50–150 mg/kg per day in divided doses.

No longer widely available.

 ## Further information

Anonymous. Cephalothin (sodium). In: Dollery C, ed. *Therapeutic Drugs.* 2nd ed. Edinburgh: Churchill Livingstone; 1999:C147–C149.

CEFAZOLIN

Cephazolin. Molecular weight (sodium salt): 476.5.

A semisynthetic cephalosporin supplied as the sodium salt.

 ## ANTIMICROBIAL ACTIVITY

Activity against common pathogenic bacteria is shown in Table 13.1. *Enterobacter, Klebsiella, Providencia, Serratia* spp. and *Pr. vulgaris* are all resistant. *B. fragilis* is resistant, but other anaerobes are susceptible.

 ## PHARMACOKINETICS

C_{max} 1 g intramuscular	65–70 mg/L at 1 h
1 g intravenous bolus	180–200 mg/L end infusion
Plasma half-life	1.5–2.0 h
Volume of distribution	c. 10 L
Plasma protein binding	75–85%

Distribution

The volume of distribution is the smallest of the cephalosporins in group 1, perhaps an indication of relative confinement to the plasma space. It crosses inflamed synovial membranes, but the levels achieved are well below those of the simultaneous serum levels and entry to the CSF is poor. In patients receiving 10 mg/kg by intravenous bolus, mean concentrations in cancellous bone were 3.0 mg/kg when the mean serum concentration was 33 mg/L, giving a bone:serum ratio of 0.09. Some crosses the placenta, but the concentrations found in the fetus and membranes are low.

Metabolism and excretion

It is not metabolized. Around 60% of the dose is excreted in the urine within the first 6 h, producing concentrations in excess of 1 g/L. Excretion is depressed by probenecid. The renal clearance is around 65 mL/min and declines in renal failure, when the half-life may rise to 40 h, although levels in the urine sufficient to inhibit most urinary pathogens are still found. It is moderately well removed by hemodialysis and less well by peritoneal dialysis.

Levels sufficient to inhibit a number of enteric organisms likely to infect the biliary tract are found in T-tube bile (17–31 mg/L after a 1 g intravenous dose), but this is principally due to the high serum levels of the drug and the total amounts excreted via the bile are small.

TOXICITY AND SIDE EFFECTS

Side effects are those common to other cephalosporins (p. 172), including rare bleeding disorders and encephalopathy in patients in whom impaired excretion or direct instillation leads to very high CSF levels. Neutropenia has been described and hypoprothrombinemic bleeding has been attributed to the side chain.

CLINICAL USE

Cefazolin has been widely used in surgical prophylaxis, especially in biliary tract (because of the moderately high concentrations achieved in bile), orthopedic, cardiac and gynecological surgery.

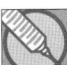

Preparations and dosage

Proprietary name: Kefzol.

Preparation: Injection.

Dosage: Adults, i.m., i.v., i.v. infusion 0.5–2 g every 6–12 h, up to 12 g per day in severe infections. Children, 25 mg/kg per day in divided doses, increasing to 100 mg/kg per day in severe infection.

Widely available.

Further information

Anonymous. Cefazolin (sodium). In: Dollery C, ed. *Therapeutic Drugs*. 2nd ed. Edinburgh: Churchill Livingstone; 1999:C89–C93.

Ortiz A, Martin-Llonch N, Garron MP, et al. Cefazolin-induced encephalopathy in uremic patients. *Rev Infect Dis*. 1991;13:772–774.

Periti P, Mazzei T, Orlandini F, et al. Comparison of the antimicrobial prophylactic efficacy of cefotaxime and cephazolin in obstetric and gynaecological surgery: a randomised multicentre study. *Drugs*. 1988;35:133–138.

Thompson JR, Garber R, Ayers J, Oki J. Cefazolin-associated neutropenia. *Clin Pharm*. 1987;6:811–814.

OTHER GROUP 1 CEPHALOSPORINS

CEFACETRILE

Its spectrum resembles that of cefalotin. Following an intramuscular dose of 1 g, a peak plasma concentration around 15 mg/L is achieved at 1 h. About 25% is bound to plasma protein. Penetration into the CSF is limited. About 80% of the drug is excreted in the urine, producing concentrations in excess of 1 g/L, 25% of which is in the desacetylated form. Clearance is depressed by probenecid and in renal failure. Little is excreted in the bile.

Manifestations of hypersensitivity in patients not known to be allergic to β-lactam antibiotics are common. It is no longer used.

CEFALORIDINE (CEPHALORIDINE)

Its activity and spectrum are similar to those of cefalotin. A 1 g intramuscular dose produces peak plasma levels of 20–40 mg/L at 1 h. The plasma half-life is 1.5 h. It is about 20% bound to plasma protein. In the presence of inflammation, CSF concentrations are around 25% of simultaneous plasma levels.

It is excreted unchanged in the urine, mainly in the glomerular filtrate. Moderate doses produce many hyaline casts in the urine and large doses sometimes cause proximal tubular necrosis, occasionally leading to oliguria and renal failure. Renal toxicity is enhanced by furosemide and ethacrynic acid. It is no longer used.

CEFAMANDOLE

A semisynthetic cephalosporin supplied as the nafate, an antibacterially inactive ester hydrolyzed in the body to cefamandole. It is active against common pathogenic bacteria (Table 13.1), but there is considerable strain variation in susceptibility. It is somewhat more stable than other group 1 agents to enterobacterial β-lactamases. *Acinetobacter*, *Serratia* and *Pseudomonas* spp. are often resistant. Some anaerobic Gram-negative rods are susceptible but *B. fragilis* is resistant.

A 1 g intramuscular dose achieves a plasma concentration of 20–35 mg/L after 1 h. It is widely distributed in body tissues. CSF levels are poor in the absence of meningeal inflammation. Therapeutically effective concentrations (c. 9 mg/kg) are found in bone after an intravenous dose of 2 g. Protein binding is 65–80%.

Renal excretion with a plasma half-life of around 50 min is mainly by both glomerular and tubular routes. A small amount is excreted in the bile and concentrations around 150–250 mg/L are found in T-tube bile following a 1 g intravenous dose. Only about 5% is removed by hemodialysis.

Cefamandole is one of the analogs containing the methylthiotetrazole side chain associated with bleeding (p. 172). Rare renal damage or enhancement of existing renal damage has been described. Thrombophlebitis on intravenous administration is relatively common.

Experience in the treatment of a variety of infections and for surgical prophylaxis has been mixed and it is no longer recommended.

Further information

Anonymous. Cefamandole (nafate). In: Dollery C, ed. *Therapeutic Drugs*. 2nd ed. Edinburgh: Churchill Livingstone; 1999:C86–C88.

CEFAPIRIN

Its antibacterial spectrum is almost identical to that of cefalotin, but it is more labile to staphylococcal β-lactamase. Intramuscular injections can be painful. A peak plasma concentration of 15–25 mg/L is obtained 0.5 h after intramuscular injection of 1 g. The plasma half-life is 0.4–0.8 h. It is *c*. 50% plasma protein bound and metabolized to the desacetyl form. The metabolite accounts for almost half the drug in the urine. Less than 1% of the dose appears in the bile.

A serum-sickness-like illness analogous to that seen with cefalotin has been observed. It is no longer used.

CEFONICID

Activity against Gram-positive and Gram-negative organisms in vitro is depressed by the presence of 50% serum. It is highly bound to plasma protein (98%) and has an extended plasma half-life of 4.5–5 h. A 1 g intramuscular dose achieves a mean peak plasma concentration of around 83 mg/L. Following a 1 g intravenous bolus dose, mean peak plasma concentrations of 130–300 mg/L have been reported. In patients treated for community-acquired pneumonia, concentrations of 2–4 mg/L have been found in sputum.

It is predominantly excreted by renal secretion, 83–89% being recovered unchanged in the urine over 24 h. Plasma half-life is linearly related to creatinine clearance. As a result of its high protein binding it is not removed by hemodialysis.

It is generally well tolerated; pain on injection, rash and positive Coombs' test are reported in some patients. It has been used to treat respiratory, soft tissue and urinary infections. Available in Italy.

Further information

Saltier E, Brogden RN. Cefonicid. A review of its antibacterial activity, pharmacological properties and therapeutic use. *Drugs*. 1986;32:222–259.

CEFORANIDE

A semisynthetic parenteral cephalosporin with activity broadly similar to that of cefalotin. Its activity in vitro is significantly reduced in the presence of serum. A 1 g intravenous dose achieves a concentration of *c*. 135 mg/L at the end of infusion. The response after 0.25, 0.5 and 1 g intravenous doses is essentially linear. A 1 g intramuscular dose produces mean peak values of around 70 mg/L. Plasma protein binding is around 85%.

It is almost entirely eliminated in the urine with a half-life of about 2.5 h, 80–95% being recovered in the first 12 h. The half-life is inversely related to renal function, rising to around 20 h when the creatinine clearance falls below 5 mL/min. About half the dose is removed by hemodialysis over 6 h.

It is generally well tolerated; phlebitis and pain at the site of injection are reported in some patients with occasional transient neutropenia and increased transaminase levels. It has been used principally for the treatment of infections due to Gram-positive cocci, including staphylococcal and streptococcal soft-tissue infections, but is no longer widely available.

Further information

Campoli-Richards DM, Lackner TE, Monk JP. Ceforanide. A review of its antibacterial activity, pharmacokinetic properties and clinical efficacy. *Drugs*. 1987;34:411–437.

GROUP 2 CEPHALOSPORINS

CEFACLOR

Molecular weight (monohydrate): 385.8.

A semisynthetic oral cephalosporin available as the monohydrate. Aqueous solutions are stable at room temperature and 4°C for 72 h at pH 2.5 but rapidly lose activity at pH 7. A delayed-release formulation is available.

ANTIMICROBIAL ACTIVITY

Its activity against common pathogenic bacteria is shown in Table 13.2. It is less resistant than other group 2 cephalosporins to staphylococcal β-lactamase. It is active against *N. gonorrhoeae* and *H. influenzae* and against most enterobacteria, but it is susceptible to common enterobacterial β-lactamases. *Pr. vulgaris* and *Providencia*, *Acinetobacter* and *Serratia* spp. are resistant. *B. fragilis* and clostridia are resistant but other anaerobes are commonly susceptible.

Table 13.2 Activity of group 2 cephalosporins against common pathogenic bacteria: MIC (mg/L)

	Cefaclor	Cefadroxil	Cefatrizine	Cefalexin[a]	Cefprozil	Loracarbef
Staphylococcus aureus	2–4	2–4	0.5–1	2–4	0.25–4	1–8
Streptococcus pyogenes	0.25	0.1–0.5	0.03–0.1	0.5–2	0.06–0.25	0.12–1
Str. pneumoniae	0.5–1	1	0.25–0.5	2	0.06–0.25	0.5–2
Enterococcus faecalis	R	R	R	R	16	R
Neisseria gonorrhoeae	0.1–0.5	4	0.25–0.5	0.5–4	0.12–0.25	0.004–1
Haemophilus influenzae	1–2	16–32	2–8	8–32	0.006–8	0.5–2
Escherichia coli	2–8	8–16	2–8	8	1–4	1–2
Klebsiella pneumoniae	4–8	8–16	8	8	1–64	1–8
Pseudomonas aeruginosa	R	R	R	R	R	R
Bacteroides fragilis	R	R	R	R	R	R

[a]Cefradine and cefroxadine have almost identical activity. R, resistant (MIC >64 mg/L).

PHARMACOKINETICS

Oral absorption	*c.* 90%
C_{max} 250 mg oral	*c.* 6–7 mg/L after 50 min
Plasma half-life	0.5–1 h
Volume of distribution	0.37 L
Plasma protein binding	25%

Absorption

Food intake increases the time taken to reach peak plasma levels and reduces the peak by 25–50%. The actual amount absorbed is unaffected. In children receiving 15 mg/kg per day (maximum daily dose 1 g) the mean peak serum level was 16.8 mg/L at 0.5–1 h. There is no accumulation of the drug during repeated administration.

Distribution

In patients receiving 500 mg every 8 h for 10 days, concentrations were 0–1.7 (mean 0.5) mg/L in mucoid sputum and 0–2.8 (mean 1.0) mg/L in purulent sputum. In children with chronic serous otitis media receiving 15 mg/kg per day, the mean peak concentration in middle ear secretion was 3.8 mg/L within 30 min of the dose when the mean simultaneous serum concentration was 12.8 mg/L.

Metabolism and excretion

No metabolites have been identified, but the drug probably chemically degrades in serum. About half of the dose is recovered from the urine in the first 6 h and 70% in 24 h. Probenecid prolongs the plasma levels but in renal insufficiency the plasma half-life is only moderately increased. In patients with creatinine clearance values of 5–15 mL/min the mean plasma elimination half-life rose to 2.3 h and the 24 h urinary excretion fell to less than 10%. In patients requiring intermittent hemodialysis and receiving 500 mg every 8 h for 10 days, the half-life rose to 2.9 h. Dialysis removed 34% of the dose.

TOXICITY AND SIDE EFFECTS

Apart from mild gastrointestinal disturbance, the drug is well tolerated. Transiently increased transaminase levels and symptomatic vaginal candidosis have been noted. Clusters of a serum sickness-like illness have been described in children.

CLINICAL USE

Uses are similar to those of other group 2 cephalosporins. It is among the few suitable for use in respiratory infections because of its activity against *H. influenzae*.

Preparations and dosage

Proprietary name: Distaclor.

Preparations: Tablets, suspension, capsules.

Dosage: Adults, oral, 250–500 mg every 8 h, depending on severity of infection (maximum dose, 4 g per day). Children >1 month, 20 mg/kg per day in divided doses every 8 h. In more severe infections, 40 mg/kg per day in divided doses (maximum dose, 1 g per day).

Widely available.

Further information

Anonymous. Cefaclor. In: Dollery C, ed. *Therapeutic Drugs*. 2nd ed. Edinburgh: Churchill Livingstone; 1999:C83–C86.

Meyers BR. Cefaclor revisited. *Clin Ther*. 2000;22:154–166.

Verhoef J. Cefaclor in the treatment of skin, soft tissue and urinary tract infections: a review. *Clin Ther*. 1988;11(suppl A):71–82.

CEFADROXIL

Molecular weight (monohydrate): 381.4.

p-Hydroxycephalexin, available as the mono- and trihydrate.

 ## ANTIMICROBIAL ACTIVITY

Resembles closely that of cefalexin (Table 13.2).

 ## PHARMACOKINETICS

Oral absorption	>90%
C$_{max}$ 250 mg oral	*c.* 9 mg/L after 1.2 h
500 mg oral	*c.* 18 mg/L after 1.2 h
Plasma half-life	1–1.5 h
Plasma protein binding	20%

Absorption is little affected by administration with food. Distribution is similar to that of cefalexin. It is eliminated unchanged by glomerular filtration and tubular secretion; 90% of the dose appears in the urine over 24 h, most in the first 6 h, producing concentrations exceeding 500 mg/L.

 ## TOXICITY AND SIDE EFFECTS

Side effects described are those common to oral cephalosporins.

 ## CLINICAL USE

It has been used for various community-acquired infections for which oral cephalosporins are appropriate.

 ### Preparations and dosage

Proprietary name: Baxan.

Preparations: Capsules, suspension, tablets.

Dosage: Adults, oral, ≥40 kg, 0.5–1 g every 12 h. Children <1 year, 25 mg/kg per day in divided doses; children 1–6 years, 250 mg every 12 h; children >6 years, 500 mg every 12 h.

Widely available.

 ### Further information

Miller LM, Mooney CJ, Hansbrough JF. Comparative evaluation of cefaclor versus cefadroxil in the treatment of skin and skin structure infections. *Curr Ther Res.* 1989;46:405–410.

Tanrisever B, Santella PJ. Cefadroxil. A review of its antibacterial, pharmacokinetic and therapeutic properties in comparison with cephalexin and cephradine. *Drugs.* 1986;32(suppl 3):1–16.

CEFALEXIN

Cephalexin. Molecular weight (monohydrate): 365.4.

 ## ANTIMICROBIAL ACTIVITY

Activity against common pathogens is shown in Table 13.2. It is resistant to staphylococcal β-lactamase. Gram-positive rods and fastidious Gram-negative bacilli, such as *Bordetella* spp. and *H. influenzae*, are relatively resistant. It is active against a range of enterobacteria, but it is degraded by many enterobacterial β-lactamases. *Citrobacter, Edwardsiella, Enterobacter, Hafnia, Providencia* and *Serratia* spp. are all resistant. Gram-negative anaerobes other than *B. fragilis* are susceptible. Because of its mode of action (p. 13) it is only slowly bactericidal to Gram-negative bacilli.

 ## PHARMACOKINETICS

Oral absorption	>90%
C$_{max}$ 500 mg oral	*c.* 10–20 mg/L after 1 h
Plasma half-life	0.5–1 h
Volume of distribution	15 L
Plasma protein binding	10–15%

Absorption and distribution

It is almost completely absorbed when given by mouth, the peak concentration being delayed by food. Intramuscular preparations are not available: injection is painful and produces delayed peak plasma concentrations considerably lower than those obtained by oral administration.

In synovial fluid, levels of 6–38 mg/L have been described after a 4 g oral dose, but penetration into the CSF is poor. Useful levels are achieved in bone (9–44 mg/kg after 1 g orally) and in purulent sputum. Concentrations of 10–20 mg/L have been found in breast milk. Concentrations in cord blood following a maternal oral dose of 0.25 g were minimal.

Metabolism and excretion

It is not metabolized. Almost all the dose is recoverable from the urine within the first 6 h, producing urinary concentrations exceeding 1 g/L. The involvement of tubular secretion is indicated by the increased plasma peak concentration and reduced urinary excretion produced by probenecid. Renal clearance is around 200 mL/min and is depressed in renal failure, although a therapeutic concentration is still obtained in the urine. It is removed by peritoneal and hemodialysis. Some is excreted in the bile, in which therapeutic concentrations may be achieved.

 ## TOXICITY AND SIDE EFFECTS

Nausea, vomiting and abdominal discomfort are relatively common. Pseudomembranous colitis has been described and overgrowth of *Candida* with vaginitis may be troublesome. Otherwise, mild hypersensitivity reactions and biochemical changes common to cephalosporins occur. Very rare neurological disturbances have been described, particularly in patients in whom very high plasma levels have been achieved. There are rare reports of Stevens–Johnson syndrome and toxic epidermal necrolysis.

 ## CLINICAL USE

As for group 2 cephalosporins (p. 172). It should not be used in infections in which *H. influenzae* is, or is likely to be, implicated. It should not be used as an alternative to penicillin in syphilis.

 ### Preparations and dosage

Proprietary names: Keflex, Ceporex.

Preparations: Capsules, tablets, suspension.

Dosage: Adults, oral, 1–2 g per day in divided doses; for severe infections, increase dose to 1 g every 8 h or 3 g every 12 h. Children, 25–50 mg/kg per day in 2–3 divided doses, for severe infection increase dose to 100 mg/kg per day in 4 divided doses (maximum dose, 4 g per day).

Widely available.

 ### Further information

Anonymous. Cephalexin. In: Dollery C, ed. *Therapeutic Drugs.* 2nd ed. Edinburgh: Churchill Livingstone; 1999:C144–C146.

Speight TM, Brogden RN, Avery GS. Cephalexin: a review of its antibacterial, pharmacological and therapeutic properties. *Drugs.* 1972;3:9–76.

CEFPROZIL

Molecular weight (monohydrate): 407.5.

A semisynthetic oral cephalosporin formulated as the monohydrate.

 ## ANTIMICROBIAL ACTIVITY

Activity against Gram-positive cocci and Gram-negative bacilli is better than that of cefadroxil (which it structurally resembles) but is not as good as that of group 5 agents (Tables 13.2 and 13.5). It is moderately stable to hydrolysis by the common plasmid-mediated β-lactamases, but is hydrolyzed by the chromosomal enzymes of Gram-negative bacilli (p. 230).

PHARMACOKINETICS

Oral absorption	>90%
C_{max} 250 mg oral	5–7 mg/L after 1 h
500 mg oral	10 mg/L after 1
Plasma half-life	1–1.4 h
Volume of distribution	15–20 l
Plasma protein binding	35–45%

Absorption and distribution

It is almost completely absorbed and well distributed, penetrating well into tonsillar and other tissues and inflammatory exudate. Absorption is unaffected by food or antacids and there is no accumulation on multiple dosing regimens.

Metabolism and excretion

Most of the dose is excreted unchanged in urine, though about 20% is found in feces. Urinary concentrations after a 500 mg oral dose usually exceed 1 g/L. The elimination half-life is prolonged in patients with renal impairment, reaching 6 h in anuric patients. About half the drug is removed in 3 h by hemodialysis.

 ## TOXICITY AND SIDE EFFECTS

It is well tolerated. Diarrhea and gastrointestinal discomfort may occur. There have been a few reports of pseudomembranous colitis and serum sickness-like reactions.

CLINICAL USE

It has been used for various infections for which oral cephalosporins are appropriate.

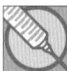 ## Preparations and dosage

Proprietary name: Cefzil.

Preparations: Tablets, suspension.

Dosage: Adults, oral, 250–500 mg every 12–24 h depending on infection being treated. Children, 7.5–15 mg/kg every 12 h.

Available in the UK, USA and continental Europe.

 ## Further information

Anonymous. Cefprozil (monohydrate). In: Dollery C, ed. *Therapeutic Drugs*. 2nd ed. Edinburgh: Churchill Livingstone; 1999:C118–C120.

Barriere SL. Review of in vitro activity, pharmacokinetic characteristics, safety, and clinical efficacy of cefprozil, a new oral cephalosporin. *Ann Pharmacother*. 1993;27:1082–1089.

Wise R. Comparative microbiological activity and pharmacokinetics of cefprozil. *Eur J Clin Microbiol Infect Dis*. 1994;13:839–845.

Wiseman LR, Benfield P. Cefprozil. A review of its antibacterial activity, pharmacokinetic properties, and therapeutic potential. *Drugs*. 1993;45:295–317.

OTHER GROUP 2 CEPHALOSPORINS

 ## CEFATRIZINE

A semisynthetic cephalosporin formulated for oral use. The spectrum is similar to that of cefalexin but it is more active against *H. influenzae* (Table 13.2). Wide strain variations in susceptibility have been reported.

It is only partially absorbed when given by mouth. A 500 mg oral dose achieves a concentration of *c.* 6 mg/L after 1–2 h. The normal half-life of 2.5 h is extended to 5.5 h in end-stage renal failure. Distribution resembles that of cefalexin. It crosses the placenta readily. Plasma protein binding is 40–60%.

Urinary recovery in 6 h is 35% of an oral dose, producing urinary levels of 50–1500 mg/L. It is presumed that the remainder is metabolized, but no metabolites have been identified.

Apart from some mild diarrhea, it is well tolerated. It is available in Japan.

 ## Further information

Pfeffer M, Gaver RC, Ximinez J. Human intravenous pharmacokinetics and absolute oral bioavailability of cefatrizine. *Antimicrob Agents Chemother*. 1983;24:915–920.

Santella PJ, Tanrisever B. Cefatrizine: a clinical overview. *Drugs Exp Clin Res*. 1985;11:441–445.

 ## CEFRADINE

Cephradine. A semisynthetic cephalosporin available in both oral and injectable forms. The antibacterial spectrum and susceptibility to β-lactamases are almost identical to those of cefalexin (Table 13.2).

It is almost completely absorbed when given by mouth. A 500 mg oral dose achieves a concentration of about 18–20 mg/L after 1 h. The peak is delayed and reduced by food, but the half-life is not altered. Intramuscular administration of 1 g results a plasma concentration of 10–12 mg/L within 2 h. The plasma half-life is around 1 h and protein binding low.

Concentrations of up to 40% of those simultaneously found in the serum have been demonstrated in lung tissue. Penetration into the CSF is poor. Levels in sputum were about 20% of those simultaneously present in the plasma following a 1 g oral dose and similar levels have been found in bone. Breast milk concentrations approaching 1 mg/L have been found after 500 mg orally every 6 h and similar concentrations have been found in amniotic fluid. Cord blood concentration is said to be similar to that in the maternal blood.

It is excreted unchanged in the urine mostly in the first 6 h, achieving concentrations exceeding 1 g/L. Probenecid markedly increases the plasma concentration and delays the peak. There is some biliary excretion.

The parenteral forms may give rise to local pain or thrombophlebitis. Other side effects common to cephalosporins have been described. In some patients *Candida* vaginitis has been troublesome.

Clinical use is similar to that of cefalexin, but it has been largely superseded by later cephalosporins.

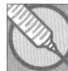 ## Preparations and dosage

Proprietary name: Velosef.

Preparations: Capsules, syrup, injection.

Dosage: Adults, oral, 250–500 mg every 6 h, or 0.5–1 g every 12 h (maximum dose, 4 g per day). Children, 25–100 mg/kg per day in 2–4 divided doses.

Adults, i.m., i.v., 2–8 g per day in divided doses depending on severity of infection. Children, 50–100 mg/kg per day in four divided doses; more serious illnesses may require 200–300 mg/kg per day.

Widely available.

 ## Further information

Anonymous. Cephradine. In: Dollery C, ed. *Therapeutic Drugs*. 2nd ed. Edinburgh: Churchill Livingstone; 1999:C150–C152.

 ## CEFROXADINE

Cefroxadine is closely related to cefradine, the structure differing only by the presence of a methoxy group replacing methyl at the C-3 position. The antimicrobial spectrum is identical to that of cefradine and cefalexin (Table 13.2). A dose of 1 g as film-coated tablets produced mean peak plasma levels of 25 mg/L at 1 h. Absorption is depressed and delayed by administration with food. The plasma elimination half-life is 0.8 h, rising to 40 h in end-stage renal failure and falling to 3.4 h during hemodialysis. Around 85% of an oral dose is excreted unchanged in the urine. It is available in Japan.

Further information

Gerardin A, Lecaillon JB, Schoeller JP, Humbert G, Guibert J. Pharmacokinetics of cefroxadine (CGP 9000) in man. *J Pharmacokinet Biopharm.* 1982;10:15–26.
Lecaillon JB, Hirtz JL, Schoeller JP, Humbert G, Vischer W. Pharmacokinetic comparison of cefroxadine (CGP 9000) and cephalexin by simultaneous administration to humans. *Antimicrob Agents Chemother.* 1980;18:656–660.

LORACARBEF

An oral carbacephem, with carbon replacing sulfur in the fused ring structure. Its structure and properties are otherwise closely related to those of cefaclor, but it has improved chemical stability. Activity and stability to β-lactamases correspond closely to those of cefaclor (Table 13.2).

It is almost completely absorbed by the oral route, but food delays absorption. A 500 mg oral dose achieves a serum concentration of around 16 mg/L after 1.3 h. Adequate concentrations are achieved for the treatment of upper respiratory tract infection. Sputum concentrations have been found to be around 2% of the corresponding plasma level. The plasma half-life is about 1 h and protein binding is 25%.

Most of the dose is excreted unchanged in the urine, 60% within 12 h. The elimination half-life is increased in patients with impaired renal function. Probenecid delays excretion.

Diarrhea is the most prominent side effect, occurring in about 4% of patients. Other gastrointestinal upsets are also reported. It has been used for the oral treatment of upper respiratory tract infection, skin and soft-tissue infections, and uncomplicated urinary tract infection caused by sensitive organisms, but is not widely available.

Further information

Anonymous. Loracarbef. In: Dollery C, ed. *Therapeutic Drugs.* 2nd ed.Edinburgh: Churchill Livingstone; 1999:L89–L95.
Brogden RN, McTavish D. Loracarbef: a review of its antimicrobial activity, pharmacokinetic properties and therapeutic efficacy. *Drugs.* 1993;45:716–736.

GROUP 3 CEPHALOSPORINS

CEFOXITIN

Molecular weight (sodium salt): 449.4.

A semisynthetic cephamycin available as the sodium salt for intramuscular or intravenous injection.

ANTIMICROBIAL ACTIVITY

Its activity against common pathogenic bacteria is shown in Table 13.3. Most Gram-positive bacilli are susceptible, but

Table 13.3 Activity of group 3 cephalosporins against common pathogenic bacteria: MIC (mg/L)

	Cefbuperazone	Cefmetazole	Cefminox	Cefotetan	Cefotiam	Cefoxitin	Cefuroxime
Staphylococcus aureus	8	1	8–16	8–16	1	2–8	1–4
Streptococcus pyogenes	2–8	0.5	4–8	1	0.03	0.25–1	0.03–0.1
Str. pneumoniae	2–4	0.5	0.5–2	2	0.25	1–2	0.03–0.1
Enterococcus faecalis	R	R	R	R	R	R	R
Neisseria gonorrhoeae		0.5	0.5–1	0.5–1	0.1	0.1–0.5	0.06–0.1
N. meningitidis		0.25		0.1	0.06	0.25	0.06
Haemophilus influenzae	1	4–8	0.25–2	1–4	0.5	2–4	0.5
Escherichia coli	0.25	1–2	0.25–2	0.1–0.5	0.1	2–8	1–4
Klebsiella pneumoniae	0.5	1–2	0.5–1	0.1–0.5	0.5	2–8	2–4
Pseudomonas aeruginosa	R	R	R	R	R	R	R
Bacteroides fragilis	2	4–R	0.5–4	4–32	R	4–32	4–64

R, resistant (MIC >64 mg/L).

L. monocytogenes is resistant. It is resistant to many Gram-negative β-lactamases and is active against organisms elaborating them, including some *Citrobacter*, *Providencia*, *Serratia* and *Acinetobacter* spp. *Enterobacter* spp. are resistant. It is moderately active against *Bacteroides* spp., but considerable strain variation in susceptibility occurs.

ACQUIRED RESISTANCE

Resistant strains of *Bacteroides*, some of which produce β-lactamases that hydrolyze cefoxitin, have been described. Resistance may be transferable to other *Bacteroides* spp. It is a potent inducer of chromosomal cephalosporinases of certain Gram-negative bacilli (p. 230) and can antagonize the effect of cefotaxime and other β-lactam agents.

PHARMACOKINETICS

C_{max} 500 mg intramuscular	11 mg/L after 20 min
1 g intravenous	*c.* 150 mg/L end injection
Plasma half-life	0.7–1 h
Volume of distribution	*c.* 10 L
Plasma protein binding	65–80%

Absorption

It is not absorbed when given orally, but is very rapidly absorbed from intramuscular sites. Doubling the dose approximately doubles the plasma level. It is absorbed from suppositories to varying degrees depending on the adjuvants: peak serum levels around 9.8 mg/L have been obtained after a dose of 1 g, giving a bioavailability of around 20%. In infants and children treated with 150 mg/kg per day, mean serum concentrations 15 min after intravenous and intramuscular administration were 81.9 and 68.5 mg/L, with elimination half-lives of 0.70 and 0.67 h, respectively.

Distribution

About 20% of the corresponding serum levels are found in sputum. In patients given 1 g by intravenous bolus preoperatively, concentrations in lung tissue at 1 h were around 13 mg/g. Penetration into normal CSF is very poor; even in patients with purulent meningitis CSF concentrations seldom exceed 6 mg/L. In children with meningitis receiving 75 mg/kg every 6 h, peak concentrations of 5–6 mg/L were found around 1 h after the dose. In patients receiving 2 g intravenously before surgery, the mean penetrance into peritoneal fluid was 86%. In patients receiving 2 g intramuscularly before hysterectomy, mean concentrations in pelvic tissue were 7.8 mg/g. Breast milk contained 5–6 mg/L after a 1 g intravenous dose. Concentrations up to 230 mg/L have been found in bile after 2 g intravenously.

Metabolism and excretion

Less than 5% of the drug is desacetylated and in a few subjects deacylation of 1 or 2% of the dose to the antibacterially inactive descarbamyl form also occurs.

It is almost entirely excreted in the urine by both glomerular filtration and tubular secretion, 80–90% being found in the first 12 h after a parenteral dose, producing concentrations in excess of 1 g/L. Furosemide, in doses of 40–160 mg, had no effect on the elimination half-life of doses of 1 or 2 g. Probenecid delays the plasma peak and decreases the renal clearance and urine concentration. The renal clearance has been calculated variously to lie between 225 and 330 mL/min. The plasma half-life increases inversely with creatinine clearance to reach 24 h in oliguric patients, with corresponding reduction in total body clearance. In patients on peritoneal dialysis, peritoneal clearance accounted for only 7.5% of mean plasma clearance and the mean plasma half-life during 6 h dialysis was 7.8 h.

TOXICITY AND SIDE EFFECTS

Reactions are those common to cephalosporins. Pain on intramuscular, and thrombophlebitis on intravenous, injection occur. Substantial changes can occur in the fecal flora, with virtual eradication of susceptible enterobacteria and non-*fragilis* *Bacteroides*, and appearance of, or increase in, yeasts, enterococci and other resistant bacteria including *C. difficile*. Development of meningitis due to *H. influenzae* and *Str. pneumoniae* in patients treated for other infections has been observed.

CLINICAL USE

As for other group 3 cephalosporins, with particular emphasis on mixed infections including anaerobes, notably abdominal and pelvic sepsis. In considering its use, its low activity against aerobic Gram-positive cocci should be noted.

Preparations and dosage

Proprietary name: Mefoxin.

Preparation: Injection.

Dosage: Adults, i.m., i.v., 1–2 g every 6–8 h (maximum dose, 12 g per day in 4–6 divided doses). Children <1 week, 20–40 mg/kg every 12 h; children 1–4 weeks, 20–40 mg/kg every 8 h; children >1 month, 20–40 mg/kg every 6–8h (maximum dose, 200 mg/kg per day).

Widely available.

Further information

Anonymous. Cefoxitin. In: Dollery C, ed. *Therapeutic Drugs*. 2nd ed. Edinburgh: Churchill Livingstone; 1999:C106–C109.

Brogden RN, Heel RC, Speight TM, Avery GS. Cefoxitin: a review of its antibacterial activity, pharmacological properties and therapeutic use. *Drugs.* 1979;17:1–37.
Goodwin CS. Cefoxitin 20 years on: is it still useful? *Rev Med Microbiol.* 1995;6:146–153.

CEFUROXIME

Molecular weight (sodium salt): 446.4.

A semisynthetic cephalosporin supplied as the sodium salt, or as the acetoxyethyl ester (cefuroxime axetil).

ANTIMICROBIAL ACTIVITY

Activity against common pathogenic bacteria is shown in Table 13.3. The methoximino side chain provides stability to most Gram-negative β-lactamases and it is active against most enterobacteria, including many multiresistant strains. *Acinetobacter* spp., *S. marcescens* and *Ps. aeruginosa* are resistant, although some *Burkholderia cepacia* strains are susceptible. Some anaerobic Gram-negative rods are susceptible, but *B. fragilis* is resistant. The minimum immobilizing concentration for the Nichol's strain of *T. pallidum* is 0.01 mg/L.

PHARMACOKINETICS

Oral absorption (axetil)	40–50%
C_max 500 mg intramuscular	c. 18–25 mg/L after 0.5–1 h
0.75 g intravenous infusion	c. 50 mg/L end infusion
500 mg oral (axetil)	6–9 mg/L after 1.8–2.5 h
Plasma half-life	1.1–1.4 h
Volume of distribution	11–15 L
Plasma protein binding	30%

Absorption

The acetoxyethyl ester (cefuroxime axetil) is rapidly hydrolyzed on passage through the intestinal mucosa and in the portal circulation to liberate cefuroxime, acetaldehyde and acetic acid. No unchanged ester is detectable in the systemic circulation. Absorption is independent of dose in the range 0.25–1 g, and there is no accumulation on repeated dosing.

Bioavailability is improved after food to around 50%. In elderly subjects receiving doses of 500 mg every 8–12 h, peak plasma levels were 5.5 mg/L after 1.5–2 h in the fasting state, rising to 7.6 mg/L after 20 min when the dose was administered with food.

Distribution

In patients with severe meningeal inflammation, the mean CSF concentration after a 1.5 g intravenous dose was in the range 1.5–3.7 mg/L. In about one-third of patients with normal CSF, no drug could be detected and in the remainder concentrations were 0.2–1 mg/L. In children treated for meningitis with 50 or 75 mg/kg, the CSF:serum ratios were 0.07 and 0.10, respectively. Concentrations in pleural drain fluid after thoracic surgery approximated to serum levels at 2 h after doses of 1 or 1.5 g and exceeded serum levels at 4 h, when they were still around 10 mg/L. Levels in pericardial fluid were similar, with fluid:serum ratios of 0.44 between 0.5 and 2 h. In patients receiving 1.5 g by intravenous bolus preoperatively, concentrations around 22 mg/g were found in subcutaneous tissue at about 5 h with an elimination half-life of about 1.5 h.

Mean bone:serum ratios in the femoral head after 750 mg intramuscular and 1.5 g intravenous bolus injections were 0.14 and 0.23, respectively. In patients with chronic otitis media treated with 0.75 g every 8 h for 6–8 days, peak concentrations in the middle ear of 0.7–1.7 mg/L were reached about 2 h after the dose. In patients given 750 mg intramuscularly on five consecutive days the mean sputum concentration rose from 0.57 mg/L on the first day to 1.15 mg/L on the third.

Excretion

The drug is excreted unchanged in the urine mostly within 6 h of administration, producing concentrations exceeding 1 g/L. About 45–55% of the drug is excreted by tubular secretion, so that the administration of probenecid increases the serum peak and prolongs the plasma half-life. Renal clearance is slightly affected by the route of administration but lies between 95 and 180 L/min. The plasma half-life is prolonged in the elderly up to 2.4 h.

TOXICITY AND SIDE EFFECTS

It is well tolerated with little pain or phlebitis on injection. Minor hypersensitivity reactions and biochemical changes common to cephalosporins are described.

The axetil ester may cause diarrhea and, in some cases, vomiting. Changes in the bowel flora, sometimes with the appearance of *C. difficile*, have been reported in about 15% of patients. Vaginitis is reported in about 2% of female patients.

CLINICAL USE

It has been used successfully to treat urinary, soft-tissue and pulmonary infections, as well as septicemia, and as a single-dose treatment (with probenecid) of gonorrhea due to β-lactamase-producing strains. It has been widely used for surgical prophylaxis.

Preparations and dosage

Cefuroxime

Proprietary name: Zinacef.

Preparation: Injection.

Dosage: Adults, i.m., i.v., 750 mg every 6–8h; 1.5 g every 6–8h in severe infections. Children, 30–100 mg/kg per day in 3–4 divided doses; 50–60 mg/kg every 8 h for severe infections. Neonates, 30–100 mg/kg per day in 2–3 divided doses.

Widely available.

Cefuroxime axetil

Proprietary name: Zinnat.

Preparations: Tablets, suspension, sachets.

Dosage: Adults, oral, 250–500 mg every 12 h depending on severity of infection. Children 3 months to 2 years, 10 mg/kg (maximum 125 mg) twice daily; >2 years 15 mg/kg (maximum 250 mg) twice daily.

Widely available.

Further information

Anonymous. Cefuroxime (sodium and axetil). In: Dollery C, ed. *Therapeutic Drugs.* 2nd ed. Edinburgh: Churchill Livingstone; 1999:C135–C140.

Brogden RN, Heel RC, Speight TM, Avery GS. Cefuroxime: a review of its antibacterial activity, pharmacological properties and therapeutic use. *Drugs.* 1979;17:233–266.

Dellamonica P. Cefuroxime axetil. *Int J Antimicrob Agents.* 1994;4:23–36.

Perry CM, Brogden RN. Cefuroxime axetil. A review of its antibacterial activity, pharmacokinetic properties and therapeutic efficacy. *Drugs.* 1996;52:125–158.

OTHER GROUP 3 CEPHALOSPORINS

CEFBUPERAZONE

A semisynthetic cephamycin antibiotic with properties similar to those of cefoxitin, but somewhat more active against *B. fragilis* and enterobacteria. It is not hydrolyzed by common β-lactamases and as a result its activity is not affected by inoculum size. Its activity against common pathogenic bacteria is shown in Table 13.3. It is not active against cefoxitin-resistant strains. It is available in Japan.

Further information

Del Bene VE, Carek PJ, Twitty JA, Burkey LI. In vitro activity of cefbuperazone compared with that of other new β-lactam agents against anaerobic Gram-negative bacilli and contribution of β-lactamase to resistance. *Antimicrob Agents Chemother.* 1985;27:817–820.

CEFMETAZOLE

A semisynthetic cephamycin antibiotic. Activity against common pathogenic bacteria is shown in Table 13.3. It is active against *Pr. mirabilis*, *Pr. vulgaris*, *Morganella morganii*, *Yersinia* spp.

and most anaerobes. *S. marcescens* is moderately susceptible, but *Ps. aeruginosa* and *E. faecalis* are resistant. It is active against *Mycobacterium fortuitum* and some strains of *M. chelonei*. It is resistant to a wide range of β-lactamases.

The serum concentration at the end of a 1 g intravenous infusion is around 77 mg/L. Plasma protein binding is 68%. It is principally excreted in the urine with a plasma half-life of *c.* 1.3 h; 70% is recovered over the first 6 h. In patients whose creatinine clearance is less than 10 mL/min, plasma levels are elevated and the plasma half-life is increased to around 15 h.

Side effects associated with the methylthiotetrazole group at position C-3 have been reported. Uses are similar to those of cefoxitin, but it is not widely available.

Further information

Cornick NA, Jacobus NV, Gorbach SL. Activity of cefmetazole against anaerobic bacteria. *Antimicrob Agents Chemother.* 1987;31:2010–2012.

Schentag JJ. Cefmetazole sodium: pharmacology, pharmacokinetics, and clinical trials. *Pharmacotherapy.* 1991;11:2–19.

CEFMINOX

A semisynthetic cephamycin. Activity is similar to that of cefoxitin and cefotetan, but the activity against enterobacteria and *B. fragilis* is somewhat better (Table 13.3). *C. difficile* is inhibited by 4–16 mg/L. It is stable to the common β-lactamases of enterobacteria and *Bacteroides* spp.

A 15-min intravenous infusion of 1 g achieves a serum concentration of 30 mg/L after 1 h. The plasma half-life is *c.* 2 h and around 68% is protein bound.

Its safety profile and uses are similar to those of other cephamycins. It is available in Japan.

Further information

Inouye S, Goi H, Watanabe T, et al. In vitro and in vivo antibacterial activities of a new semisynthetic cephalosporin compared with those of five cephalosporins. *Antimicrob Agents Chemother.* 1984;26:722–729.

Watanabe S, Omoto S. Pharmacology of cefminox, a new bactericidal cephamycin. *Drugs Exp Clin Res.* 1990;16:461–467.

CEFOTETAN

A semisynthetic cephamycin formulated as the disodium salt for intravenous administration. The activity is similar to that of cefoxitin, but cefotetan exhibits more potent activity against enterobacteria and more modest activity against *Staph. aureus* (Table 13.3).

A 1 g intravenous dose achieves a serum concentration of 140–180 mg/L. There is no evidence of accumulation on a dosage of 1 g every 12 h. Tissue fluid concentrations are about 30% of the simultaneous serum level. The plasma half-life is about 3 h and protein binding is around 88%.

About 85% of the drug is eliminated in the urine over 24 h. Accumulation in renal failure is inversely related to the creatinine clearance, the plasma half-life rising to 20 h in patients requiring hemodialysis. During hemodialysis the half-life falls to around 7.5 h and on peritoneal dialysis it falls to 15.5 h, 5–10% of the dose being recovered in the dialysate over 24 h.

Side effects are those typical of the group. Anaphylaxis has been described. Because of the methylthiotetrazole side chain there is some risk of hypoprothrombinemia, and disulfiram-like reactions can occur. Marked changes in the bowel flora, with appearance of *C. difficile*, have been reported. Uses are similar to those of other cephamycins, but it is not widely available.

 ### Further information

Ward A, Richards DM. Cefotetan. A review of its antibacterial activity, pharmacokinetic properties and therapeutic use. *Drugs*. 1985;30:382–426.

 ## CEFOTIAM

A semisynthetic cephalosporin formulated as the dihydrochloride for injection and as a prodrug ester, cefotiam hexetil, for oral administration. Activity is similar to that of cefuroxime, but it is somewhat more active against a range of enterobacteria (Table 13.3).

A 30-min intravenous infusion of the dihydrochloride produces a peak serum concentration of 35 mg/L; the corresponding concentration after a 1 g intramuscular dose is 17 mg/L. Oral absorption of the hexetil ester is around 65%. Food delays absorption of the ester. The plasma half-life is 0.6–1.1 h. Around 40% is bound to plasma protein.

Urinary excretion is almost complete 4 h after the end of intravenous infusion, but only 50–67% is recovered unchanged; there is substantial non-renal elimination and some evidence of saturation of renal tubular excretion at doses above 2 g. In anuria the plasma elimination half-life rises to 13 h and plasma and renal clearances parallel creatinine clearance. A small amount is excreted in bile. In patients with cholelithiasis given 0.5 or 1 g intravenously, mean concentrations in gallbladder bile and gallbladder wall 30 min after the dose were around 17 and 32 mg/L, respectively. In patients with normal liver function, hepatic bile concentrations can exceed 1 g/L.

It is generally well tolerated and has been used successfully to treat lower respiratory infections, skin and soft-tissue infection. It is not widely used, but is available in Japan and some other countries.

 ### Further information

Brogard JM, Jehl F, Willemin B, Lamalle AM, Blickle JF, Monteil H. Clinical pharmacokinetics of cefotiam. *Clin Pharmacokinet*. 1989;17:163–174.

Imada A, Hirai S. Cefotiam hexetil. *Int J Antimicrob Agents*. 1995;5:85–99.

GROUP 4 CEPHALOSPORINS

CEFOTAXIME

Molecular weight (sodium salt): 478.5.

A semisynthetic cephalosporin available as the sodium salt for parenteral administration.

 ## ANTIMICROBIAL ACTIVITY

The aminothiazoyl and methoximino groups at the 7-amino position confer, respectively, potent activity against many Gram-negative rods and cocci (Table 13.4) and stability to most β-lactamases. *Ps. aeruginosa*, *Sten. maltophilia* and other pseudomonads are often resistant. *Brucella melitensis* and some strains of *Nocardia asteroides* are susceptible. Activity against *L. monocytogenes* and *B. fragilis* is poor.

 ## ACQUIRED RESISTANCE

Many enterobacteria resistant to other β-lactam agents are susceptible, but selection of resistant strains with derepressed chromosomal molecular class C cephalosporinases (*see* p. 230) may occur. Gram-negative bacilli producing variants of the TEM enzymes (pp. 230–231) are resistant.

 ## PHARMACOKINETICS

C_{max} 500 mg intramuscular	10–15 mg/L after 0.5–1 h
1 g intravenous (15-min infusion)	90 mg/L end infusion
Plasma half-life	*c.* 1 h
Volume of distribution	32–37 L
Plasma protein binding	*c.* 40%

Distribution

It is widely distributed, achieving therapeutic concentrations in sputum, lung tissue, pleural fluid, peritoneal fluid, prostatic tissue and cortical bone. In patients receiving 2 g every 8 h, mean CSF concentrations in aseptic meningitis were

Table 13.4 Activity of group 4 cephalosporins against common pathogenic bacteria: MIC (mg/L)

	Cefmenoxime	Cefodizime	Cefotaxime	Ceftizoxime	Ceftriaxone	Latamoxef
Staphylococcus aureus	2–4	2–8	2–4	2–4	4	8–16
Streptococcus pyogenes	0.03	0.06–0.1	0.03–0.06	0.03	0.03	1
Str. pneumoniae[a]	0.06	0.03–0.25	0.1	0.1	0.25	1
Enterococcus faecalis	R	8–R	R	R	R	R
Neisseria gonorrhoeae	<0.01–0.03	0.008	<0.01–0.03	<0.01–0.03	<0.0 1–0.06	0.03–0.1
N. meningitidis	<0.01	0.008	0.01	<0.01	<0.01	<0.01
Haemophilus influenzae	0.03	0.008	<0.01–0.03	0.03	<0.01–0.03	0.1
Escherichia coli	0.06–0.1	0.1–1	0.03–0.1	0.03	0.06–0.1	0.1–0.25
Klebsiella pneumoniae	0.03	0.1–2	0.03–0.1	0.01	0.03–0.06	0.1–0.25
Pseudomonas aeruginosa	16–32	R	8–32	32–64	16–32	4–16
Bacteroides fragilis	8–64	8–R	2–32	8–64	16–64	0.5–4

[a] Penicillin-resistant strains are often less susceptible. R, resistant (MIC >64 mg/L).

0.8 mg/L. Levels of 2–15 mg/L can be found in the CSF in the presence of inflammation after doses of 50 mg/kg by intravenous infusion over 30 min. A single intraventricular dose of 40 mg/kg produced levels at 2, 4 and 6 h of 6.4, 5.7 and 4.5 mg/L, respectively.

Metabolism

About 15–25% of a dose is metabolized by hepatic esterases to the desacetyl form, which may have some clinical importance because of its concentration in bile and accumulation in renal failure. Desacetylcefotaxime has about 10% of the activity of the parent against enterobacteria, less against *Staph. aureus*. Its half-life in normal subjects is around 1.5 h.

Excretion

Elimination is predominantly by the renal route, more than half the dose being recovered in the urine over the first 24 h, about 25% as the desacetyl derivative. Excretion is depressed by probenecid and declines in renal failure with accumulation of the metabolite. In patients with creatinine clearances in the range 3–10 mL/min, the plasma half-life rose to 2.6 h while that of the metabolite rose to 10 h.

 ## TOXICITY AND SIDE EFFECTS

Minor hematological and dermatological side effects common to group 4 cephalosporins have been described. Superinfection with *Ps. aeruginosa* in the course of treatment has occurred. Occasional cases of pseudomembranous colitis have been reported.

 ## CLINICAL USES

Cefotaxime is widely used in neutropenic patients, respiratory infection, meningitis, intra-abdominal sepsis, osteomyelitis, typhoid fever, urinary tract infection, neonatal sepsis and gonorrhea.

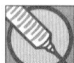 **Preparations and dosage**

Proprietary name: Claforan.

Preparation: Injection.

Dosage: Adults, i.m., i.v., 1–2 g every 8–12 h depending on severity of infection (maximum dose, 12 g per day). Neonates, <7 days, 25 mg/kg every 12 h; 7–21 days, 25 mg/kg every 8 h; 21–28 days, 25 mg/kg every 6–8 h; children >1 month, 50 mg/kg every 8–12 h (every 6 h in severe infections and meningitis; maximum 12 g daily).

Widely available.

 ## Further information

Anonymous. Cefotaxime (sodium). In: Dollery C, ed. *Therapeutic Drugs*. 2nd ed. Edinburgh: Churchill Livingstone; 1999:C100–C106.

Brogden RN, Spencer CM. Cefotaxime. A reappraisal of its antibacterial activity and pharmacokinetic properties, and a review of its therapeutic efficacy when administered twice daily for the treatment of mild to moderate infections. *Drugs*. 1997;53:483–510.

Prasad K, Kumar A, Singhal T, Gupta PK. Third generation cephalosporins versus conventional antibiotics for treating acute bacterial meningitis. *Cochrane Database Syst Rev*. 2007;(4) CD001832.

Todd PA, Brogden RN. Cefotaxime: an update of its pharmacology and therapeutic use. *Drugs*. 1990;40:608–651.

CEFTRIAXONE

Molecular weight (disodium salt) 600.6.

A semisynthetic cephalosporin supplied as the disodium salt.

ANTIMICROBIAL ACTIVITY

Activity is almost identical to that of cefotaxime (Table 13.4). Most β-lactamase-producing enterobacteria are highly susceptible, as are streptococci (but not enterococci) and fastidious Gram-negative bacilli, although brucellae are less sensitive (MIC 0.25–2 mg/L). Treatment failure has been reported in tularemia. *Ps. aeruginosa*, mycoplasmas, mycobacteria and *L. monocytogenes* are resistant.

ACQUIRED RESISTANCE

It is hydrolyzed by some chromosomal enzymes, including those of *Enterobacter* spp. and *B. fragilis*. Derepression of chromosomal β-lactamase production can cause resistance in some species of Gram-negative bacilli in vitro and has been observed in patients.

PHARMACOKINETICS

C$_{max}$ 500 mg/L intramuscular	c. 40 mg/L after 2 h
1 g intravenous (15–30-min infusion)	c. 120–150 mg/L end infusion
Plasma half-life	6–9 h
Volume of distribution	0.15 L/kg
Plasma protein binding	95%

Distribution

It penetrates well into normal body fluids and natural and experimental exudates. In children treated for meningitis with 50 or 75 mg/kg intravenously over 10–15 min, mean peak CSF concentrations ranged from 3.2 to 10.4 mg/L, with lower values later in the disease. In patients receiving 2 g before surgery, concentrations in cerebral tissue reached 0.3–12 mg/L. In patients with pleural effusions of variable etiology given a 1 g intravenous bolus, concentrations of 7–8.7 mg/L were found at 4–6 h. In patients with exacerbations of rheumatoid arthritis receiving the same dose, joint fluid contained concentrations close to those in the serum, but with wide individual variation. Tissue fluid:serum ratios have varied from around 0.05 in bone and muscle to 0.39 in cantharides blister fluid. The apparent volume of distribution is increased in patients with cirrhosis where the drug rapidly enters the ascitic fluid, but its elimination kinetics are unaffected.

It rapidly crosses the placenta, maternal doses of 2 g intravenously over 2–5 min producing mean concentrations in cord blood of 19.5 mg/L, a mean cord:maternal serum ratio of 0.18; and in amniotic fluid 3.8 mg/L, a fluid:maternal serum ratio of 0.04. The plasma elimination half-life appears to be somewhat shortened in pregnancy (5–6 h). Some appear in the breast milk, the milk:serum ratio being about 0.03–0.04, secretion persisting over a long period with a half-life of 12–17 h.

Metabolism and excretion

It is not metabolized. Biliary excretion is unusually high, 10–20% of the drug appearing in the bile in unchanged form, with concentrations up to 130 mg/g in biopsied liver tissue from patients receiving 1 g intravenously over 30 min. The insoluble calcium salt may precipitate in the bile leading to pseudolithiasis. About half the dose appears in the urine over the first 48 h, somewhat more (*c.* 70%) in neonates. Excretion is almost entirely by glomerular filtration, since there is only a small effect of probenecid on the excretion of the drug. The half-life is not linearly correlated with creatinine clearance in renal failure and, in keeping with the low free plasma fraction, it is not significantly removed by hemodialysis. The volume of distribution is not affected by renal failure.

TOXICITY AND SIDE EFFECTS

Reactions are those common to other cephalosporins. Mention has been made of thrombocytopenia, thrombocytosis, leukopenia, eosinophilia abdominal pain, phlebitis, rash, fever and increased values in liver function tests. Diarrhea is common and suppression of the aerobic and anaerobic fecal flora has been associated with the appearance of resistant bacteria·and yeasts.

Biliary pseudolithiasis due to concretions of insoluble calcium salt has been described in adults but principally in children. The precipitates can be detected in a high proportion of patients by ultrasonography and can occasionally cause pain, but resolve on cessation of treatment. The drug is better avoided in patients with pre-existing biliary disease, but the principal hazard appears to be misdiagnosis of gallbladder disease and unnecessary surgery.

CLINICAL USES

Uses are similar to those of cefotaxime, the long half-life offering the advantage of once-daily administration. It is used in the treatment of acute bacterial meningitis and as an alternative to rifampicin (rifampin) in the prophylaxis of meningococcal disease.

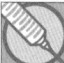

Preparations and dosage

Proprietary name: Rocephin.

Preparation: Injection.

Dosage: Adults, i.m., i.v., 1 g per day as a single dose, 2–4 g once or twice each day in severe infections. Neonates, i.v. infusion, 20–50 mg/kg once daily; children >1 month, 50 mg/kg once daily, increased up to 80 mg/kg in severe infections and meningitis; older children weighing >50 kg, 1 g daily, increased to 2–4 g daily in severe infections and meningitis. Widely available.

Further information

Anonymous. Ceftriaxone (sodium). In: Dollery C, ed. *Therapeutic Drugs*. 2nd ed. Edinburgh: Churchill Livingstone; 1999:C130–C135.

Brogden RN, Ward A. Ceftriaxone: a reappraisal of its antibacterial activity and pharmacokinetic properties, and an update on its therapeutic use with particular reference to once-daily administration. *Drugs*. 1988;35:604–645.

Gums JG, Boatwright DW, Camblin M, Halstead DC, Jones ME, Sanderson R. Differences between ceftriaxone and cefotaxime: microbiological inconsistencies. *Ann Pharmacother*. 2008;42:71–79.

Lopez AJ, O'Keefe P, Morrissey M, Pickleman J. Ceftriaxone-induced cholelithiasis. *Ann Intern Med*. 1991;115:712–714.

Monte SV, Prescott WA, Johnson KK, Kuhman L, Paladino JA. Safety of ceftriaxone at extremes of age. *Expert Opin Drug Saf*. 2008;7:515–523.

Yuk JH, Nightingale CH, Quintiliani R. Clinical pharmacokinetics of ceftriaxone. *Clin Pharmacokinet*. 1989;17:223–235.

OTHER GROUP 4 CEPHALOSPORINS

CEFMENOXIME

A semisynthetic cephalosporin supplied as the hydrochloride. Its activity is very similar to that of cefotaxime (Table 13.4). A 500 mg intramuscular injection achieves a plasma concentration of 15 mg/L after 40 min. A concentration of 200 mg/L is attained after intravenous administration of 1 g. The plasma half-life is *c*. 1 h. Around 77% is protein bound. Probenecid increases peak plasma levels and extends the plasma half-life to 1.8 h. Therapeutic concentrations are achieved in CSF. There is a degradation product with a long half-life (around 40 h), but 80–92% of the drug is recovered unchanged from the urine. In patients with renal insufficiency, no significant relation was found between creatinine clearance and peak serum concentrations but there was a linear relationship with plasma half-life and total body clearance. About 10% of the dose appears in the feces, mostly extensively degraded, possibly by the fecal flora.

Toxicity, side effects and clinical use are those common to group 4 cephalosporins.

Further information

Campoli-Richards DM, Todd PA. Cefmenoxime. A review of its antibacterial activity, pharmacokinetic properties and therapeutic use. *Drugs*. 1987;34:188–221.

CEFODIZIME

Activity is typical of the group (Table 13.4) but its overall activity is somewhat less than that of cefotaxime against enterobacteria. There has been some interest in its immunomodulating properties, which affect a number of functions.

A 1 g intramuscular dose achieves a plasma concentration of 55–60 mg/L after about 1.5 h. The plasma half-life is around 3.5 h. Protein binding is *c*. 88%. It penetrates into lung, sputum, serous fluids and prostate. Excretion is mainly renal with about 60% of the dose appearing in the urine over 12 h in adults and 80–90% in children. Elimination is inversely correlated with creatinine clearance.

It is well tolerated apart from some pain at the site of injection, mild gastrointestinal upset and rash in a few patients. It has been used mainly to treat respiratory and urinary tract infection.

Further information

Anonymous. Cefodizime (sodium). In: Dollery C, ed. *Therapeutic Drugs*. 2nd ed. Edinburgh: Churchill Livingstone; 1999:C96–C100.

Barradell LB, Brogden RN. Cefodizime: a review of its antibacterial activity, pharmacokinetic properties and therapeutic use. *Drugs*. 1992;44:800–834.

CEFTIZOXIME

A semisynthetic cephalosporin supplied as the sodium salt. The properties are very similar to those of cefotaxime, but it lacks the acetoxymethyl group at position C-4 and is therefore not subject to deacetylation. Activity against common pathogenic bacteria (Table 13.4) is very similar to that of cefotaxime.

A 500 mg intramuscular injection achieves a plasma concentration of around 14 mg/L. A concentration of 85–90 mg/L is produced 30 min at the end of a 30-min intravenous infusion. The plasma half-life is 1.3–1.9 h. Protein binding is 30%. It is well distributed. In children with meningitis receiving 200–250 mg/kg per day in four equally divided doses for 14–21 days, mean CSF concentrations 2 h after a dose were 6.4 mg/L on day 2 and 3.6 mg/L on day 14.

About 70–90% of the dose is recovered in the urine in the first 24 h, principally by glomerular filtration. Probenecid increases the plasma half-life by about 50%. In patients receiving 1 g intravenously over 30 min, the plasma elimination half-life rose to 35 h when the corrected creatinine clearance was <10 mL/min. It is partly removed by peritoneal and hemodialysis.

Adverse reactions and clinical use are similar to those of cefotaxime.

Further information

Anonymous. Ceftizoxime sodium. In: Dollery C, ed. *Therapeutic Drugs*. 2nd ed. Edinburgh: Churchill Livingstone; 1999:C125–C130.

Richards DM, Heel RC. Ceftizoxime. A review of its antibacterial activity, pharmacokinetic properties and therapeutic use. *Drugs*. 1985;29:281–329.

FLOMOXEF

An oxa-cephem which differs from latamoxef in the side chains carried at the 7-amino and C-3 positions, but which retains the 7-methoxy group that confers β-lactamase stability. The methyl group of the methylthiotetrazole side chain of latamoxef has been modified to hydroxymethyl in an attempt to avoid the undesirable side effects, while the side chain at the 7-amino position is F_2-CH-S-CH$_2$-.

Activity is similar to that of latamoxef, but activity against *Staph. aureus* is improved and it is claimed to be a poor inducer of penicillin-binding protein 2′, which is associated with resistance in methicillin-resistant strains.

Intravenous injection of 2 g achieves a peak plasma concentration of around 50 mg/L, falling to 2.6 mg/L after 6 h. The plasma half-life is about 50 min. It appears to be well distributed and penetrates moderately well into lung, mucosal tissue of the middle ear and bone.

Flomoxef does not seem to be prone to the effects on platelet function of latamoxef and it has a less marked effect on vitamin K metabolism. It does not cause a disulfiram-like reaction with alcohol.

It is available in Japan, where it appears safe and effective in a wide range of infections.

Further information

Ito M, Ishigami T. The meaning of the development of flomoxef and clinical experience in Japan. *Infection*. 1991;19(suppl 5):S253–S257.
Lee CH, Su LH, Tang YF, Liu JW. Treatment of ESBL-producing *Klebsiella pneumoniae* bacteraemia with carbapenems or flomoxef: a retrospective study and laboratory analysis of the isolates. *J Antimicrob Chemother*. 2006;58:1074–1077.
Shimada M, Takenaka K, Sugimachi K. A comprehensive multi-institutional study of empiric therapy with flomoxef in surgical infections of the digestive organs. The Kyushu Research Group for Surgical Infection. *J Chemother*. 1994;6:251–256.

LATAMOXEF

Moxalactam. A semisynthetic 7-methoxyoxacephem, supplied as the disodium salt. Activity against common pathogenic bacteria is shown in Table 13.4. It is generally slightly less active than cefotaxime, especially against *Staph. aureus*, but unlike other group 4 cephalosporins it exhibits fairly good activity against *B. fragilis*. Other *Bacteroides* spp. are generally less susceptible. The 7-methoxy substitution, also found in cephamycins such as cefoxitin, confers resistance to hydrolysis by a wide range of β-lactamases including those of *Staph. aureus*, various enterobacteria and *B. fragilis*. Resistance, predominantly in *Enterobacter* spp., *Ps. aeruginosa* and *Ser. marcescens* due to induction of chromosomal enzymes (p. 230), has been found in vitro and in some patients.

A 500 mg intramuscular injection achieves a serum concentration of 12–22 mg/L after 1.2 h. Infusion of 1 g over 30 min results in a concentration of 60 mg/L. The plasma half-life is *c.* 2 h and plasma protein binding 40–50%. There is

reasonably good penetration into serous fluids, the concentration in ascitic fluid reaching 75% and in pleural fluid 50% of the concentration simultaneously present in the serum. Levels of 5–35 mg/L have been obtained in inflamed meninges. Sputum levels are of the order of 2 mg/L following 1 g of the drug intravenously.

Renal elimination accounts for 90% of the clearance, but significant concentrations are found in the feces. Excretion is depressed in renal failure. Hemodialysis removes 48–51% of the drug in 4 h; peritoneal dialysis has little or no effect.

Increased bleeding and decreases in platelet function associated with the methylthiotetrazole side chain are sufficiently common to have been cited as reasons for restricting use of the agent. Use is contraindicated in patients on anticoagulant therapy. Uses are similar to those of group 4 cephalosporins. It is generally less successful in the treatment of infections due to Gram-positive organisms.

Further information

Anonymous. Moxalactam disodium. In: Dollery C, ed. *Therapeutic Drugs*, 2nd ed. Edinburgh: Churchill Livingstone; M232–M235.
Carmine AA, Brogden RN, Heel RC, Romankiewicz JA, Speight TM, Avery GS. Moxalactam (latamoxef). A review of its antibacterial activity, pharmacokinetic properties and therapeutic use. *Drugs*. 1983;26:279–333.

GROUP 5 CEPHALOSPORINS

CEFDITOREN

Molecular weight (pivoxil ester): 620.73

A semisynthetic cephalosporin formulated for oral use as the pivaloyloxymethyl ester, cefditoren pivoxil.

ANTIMICROBIAL ACTIVITY

Activity against common pathogens is shown in Table 13.5. It exhibits good activity against staphylococci, streptococci (but not enterococci), *H. influenzae* and *M. catarrhalis*, including β-lactamase-producing strains. Isolates of *Str. pneumoniae* exhibiting reduced susceptibility to penicillin are less susceptible (MIC 0.125–2 mg/L). Most enterobacteria, including many *Enterobacter*, *Citrobacter*, *Serratia* and *Proteus* spp., are susceptible. It is not active against *Ps. aeruginosa*, *Sten. maltophilia* or atypical respiratory pathogens such as *Chlamydophila pneumoniae* and *M. pneumoniae*. It is stable to staphylococcal and common enterobacterial β-lactamases.

Table 13.5   Activity of group 5 cephalosporins against common pathogenic bacteria: MIC (mg/L)

	Cefdinir	Cefditoren	Cefixime	Cefpodoxime	Ceftibuten
Staphylococcus aureus	0.002–1	1	4–16	0.5	32
Streptococcus pyogenes	<0.06–0.25	≤0.01	0.01–0.25	0.06	8–16
Str. pneumoniae	0.03–0.5	0.01	0.01–0.25	0.06	0.5–32
Enterococcus faecalis	2–R	R	R	R	R
Neisseria gonorrhoeae	0.002–0.06	≤0.025	0.01–0.1	<0.06	0.008–0.06
Haemophilus influenzae	0.25–1	0.01	0.06–0.25	0.06–0.12	0.01–1
Escherichia coli	0.008–1	0.25	0.25–8 0.25	0.25	0.01–16
Klebsiella pneumoniae	0.008–0.5	0.25–1	0.01–1	0.12	0.12
Pseudomonas aeruginosa	R	R	2–32	R	R
Bacteroides fragilis	R	4–32	R	R	R

R, resistant (MIC >64 mg/L).

 ## PHARMACOKINETICS

Oral absorption	*c.* 70%
C_{max} 200 mg oral	*c.* 1.8 mg/L after 1.5–3 h
Plasma half-life	0.8–1.3 h
Volume of distribution	9.3 L
Plasma protein binding	88%

After oral administration the pivaloyl ester is rapidly cleaved by esterases in the gut wall. Ingestion with food improves the bioavailability. Plasma concentrations are raised in elderly patients. There is no accumulation on repeated dosing.

It is excreted unchanged in the urine with a half-life of around 1.5 h, achieving a concentration of 150–200 mg/L within 4 h. Dosage adjustment is recommended in patients with deteriorating renal function.

 ## TOXICITY AND SIDE EFFECTS

In common with other pivoxil esters it may cause carnitine deficiency. Other side effects are those common to cephalosporins, mainly gastrointestinal disturbance.

 ## CLINICAL USE

It has been advocated for community-acquired upper and lower respiratory tract infections and skin infections.

 ### Preparations and dosage

Proprietary name: Spectracef.
Preparation: 200 mg tablets.
Dosage: 400 mg every 12 h for 10 days.
Available in USA and Japan; not available in the UK.

Further information

Balbisi A. Cefditoren: a new aminothiazolyl cephalosporin. *Pharmacotherapy.* 2002;22:1278–1293.
Darkes MJ, Plosker GL. Cefditoren pivoxyl. *Drugs.* 2002;62:319–336.
Wellington K, Curran MP. Spotlight on cefditoren pivoxil in bacterial infections. *Treat Respir Med.* 2005;4:149–152.

CEFIXIME

Molecular weight (anhydrous): 453.4; (trihydrate): 507.5.

An oral cephalosporin formulated as the anhydrous compound or the trihydrate.

ANTIMICROBIAL ACTIVITY

Activity against common pathogenic bacteria is shown in Table 13.5. It is active against *N. gonorrhoeae*, *M. catarrhalis*, *H. influenzae* and a wide range of enterobacteria, including most strains of *Citrobacter*, *Enterobacter* and *Serratia* spp. Its antistaphylococcal activity is poor. It is not active against *Acinetobacter* spp., *Ps. aeruginosa* or *B. fragilis*. It is resistant to hydrolysis by common β-lactamases.

 ## PHARMACOKINETICS

Oral absorption	c. 50%
C_{max} 400 mg oral	4–5.5 mg/L after 4 h
Plasma half-life	3–4 h
Volume of distribution	0.1 L/kg
Plasma protein binding	60–70%

Absorption and distribution

Oral absorption is slow and incomplete, but is unaffected by aluminum magnesium hydroxide. Penetration into cantharides blister fluid was very slow but exceeded the plasma level. CSF concentrations are poor even in the presence of meningeal inflammation, reaching an average of around 0.22 mg/L in children with meningitis.

Metabolism and excretion

It is not metabolized and is excreted unchanged in urine (mainly by glomerular filtration) and in bile, in which concentrations exceeding 100 mg/L have been found. Less than 20% of an oral dose is recovered from the urine over 24 h, falling to less than 5% in patients with severe renal impairment, with a corresponding increase in plasma concentration. It is not removed by peritoneal or hemodialysis.

 ## TOXICITY AND SIDE EFFECTS

It is well tolerated, but diarrhea is fairly common and pseudomembranous colitis has been reported. Other side effects common to cephalosporins are occasionally seen.

 ## CLINICAL USE

Cefixime has been used successfully in uncomplicated cystitis, upper and lower respiratory tract infections and various other infections. Its failure to provide adequate cover for staphylococci should be noted.

 ### Preparations and dosage

Proprietary name: Suprax.

Preparations: Tablets, suspension.

Dosage: Adults, oral, 200–400 mg per day as a single dose or in two divided doses. Children >6 months, 8 mg/kg per day (maximum 400 mg) as a single dose or in two divided doses.

Widely available.

 ### Further information

Anonymous. Cefixime. In: Dollery C, ed. *Therapeutic Drugs*. 2nd ed. Edinburgh: Churchill Livingstone; 1999:C93–C96.

Brogden RN, Campoli-Richards DM. Cefixime: a review of its antibacterial activity, pharmacokinetic properties and therapeutic potential. *Drugs*. 1989;38:524–550.

Markham A, Brogden RN. Cefixime. A review of its therapeutic efficacy in lower respiratory tract infections. *Drugs*. 1995;49:1007–1022.

Symposium. Clinical pharmacology and efficacy of cefixime. *Pediatr Infect Dis J*. 1987;6:949–1009.

Wu DHA. Review of the safety profile of cefixime. *Clin Ther*. 1993;15:1108–1119.

CEFPODOXIME

Molecular weight (proxetil ester): 557.6.

A semisynthetic cephalosporin supplied as the prodrug ester, cefpodoxime proxetil.

ANTIMICROBIAL ACTIVITY

The hydrolysis product is very similar to cefotaxime and it shares its potent, broad-spectrum activity (Table 13.5). It is stable to a wide range of plasmid-mediated β-lactamases. It induces the chromosomal β-lactamases of *Ps. aeruginosa*, *Enterobacter* spp., *S. marcescens* and *Citrobacter* spp., but is a less potent inducer than cefoxitin.

PHARMACOKINETICS

Oral absorption	c. 50%
C$_{max}$ 200 mg oral	2.1 mg/L after 3 h
Plasma half-life	c. 2.2 h
Volume of distribution	c. 35 L
Plasma protein binding	20–30%

Absorption and distribution

The ester is rapidly hydrolyzed to the parent compound in the small intestine. Bioavailability increases to 65% if taken with food, but antacids and H$_2$-receptor antagonists reduce absorption. Unabsorbed drug is hydrolyzed and excreted in the feces.

It is well distributed and penetrates well into tissues (including lung tissue) and inflammatory exudate to achieve concentrations inhibitory to common pathogens.

Metabolism and excretion

The hydrolyzed prodrug is not subject to further metabolism. About 80% of the absorbed compound (30–40% of the original dose) appears in the urine over 24 h. Excretion is by glomerular filtration and tubular secretion; probenecid delays secretion and increases the peak plasma concentration.

TOXICITY AND SIDE EFFECTS

The drug is well tolerated, but gastrointestinal disturbance with diarrhea is common. Pseudomembranous colitis has been reported occasionally. Other side effects are those common to cephalosporins.

CLINICAL USE

Cefpodoxime has been used principally for the treatment of upper and lower respiratory tract infections in children and adults.

Preparations and dosage

Proprietary name: Orelox, Vantin.

Preparations: Tablets, suspension.

Dosage: Adults, oral, 200–400 mg every 12 h depending on infection being treated. Children, 8 mg/kg per day in two divided doses.

Widely available.

Further information

Anonymous. Cefpodoxime proxetil. In: Dollery C, ed. *Therapeutic Drugs*. 2nd ed. Edinburgh: Churchill Livingstone; 1999:C113–C117.

Frampton JE, Brogden RN, Langtry HD, Buckley MM. Cefpodoxime proxetil: a review of its antibacterial activity, pharmacokinetic properties and therapeutic potential. *Drugs*. 1992;44:889–917.

Fulton B, Perry CM. Cefpodoxime proxetil: a review of its use in the management of bacterial infections in paediatric patients. *Paediatr Drugs*. 2001;3:137–158.

Moore EP, Speller DCE, White LO, Wilkinson PJ. Cefpodoxime proxetil: a third-generation oral cephalosporin. *J Antimicrob Chemother*. 1990;26(suppl E):1–100.

Todd WM. Cefpodoxime proxetil: a comprehensive review. *Int J Antimicrob Agents*. 1994;4:37–62.

OTHER GROUP 5 CEPHALOSPORINS

CEFCAPENE

A semisynthetic cephalosporin formulated for oral administration as the prodrug ester, cefcapene pivoxil. Activity and uses are similar to those of cefditoren.

Available in Japan.

CEFDINIR

An oral cephalosporin similar in structure to cefixime, but with a slightly modified side chain at the 7-amino position. Activity is similar to that of cefixime, but it is more active, especially against staphylococci (Table 13.5). It is not hydrolyzed by staphylococcal or the common plasmid-mediated enterobacterial β-lactamases. An enhancing effect on phagocytosis has been demonstrated in vitro.

Oral absorption is about 35%. A 200 mg oral dose achieves a plasma concentration of 1 mg/L after c. 3 h. Absorption is reduced after a fatty meal. Concentrations equal to or higher than corresponding plasma levels were present in blister fluid 6–12 h after administration of an oral dose. The plasma half-life is 1.5 h. Protein binding is 60–70%. A total of 12–20% of the dose was excreted in the urine within 12 h, the renal elimination declining with increasing dose. The elimination half-life and peak plasma concentration are increased in renal failure. About 60% of the drug is removed by hemodialysis.

Side effects and uses are those common to oral cephalosporins.

Further information

Guay DR. Cefdinir: an expanded-spectrum oral cephalosporin. *Ann Pharmacother*. 2000;34:1469–1477.

Perry CM, Scott LJ. Cefdinir: a review of its use in the management of mild-to-moderate bacterial infections. *Drugs*. 2004;64:1433–1464.

CEFETAMET

A semisynthetic cephalosporin formulated for oral use as the prodrug ester, cefetamet pivoxyl. It is less active than cefaclor and cefadroxil against *Staph. aureus*, but as active against streptococci and more active against enterobacteria, *H. influenzae* and *N. gonorrhoeae*, including β-lactamase-producing strains. *L. monocytogenes*, *C. difficile*, *Sten. maltophilia* and *Burk. cepacia* are all resistant. It is resistant to hydrolysis by common plasmid-mediated enzymes.

The absolute bioavailability is about 50%. The plasma peak is delayed by food. Binding to plasma protein is about 20%. The volume of distribution approximates to the extracellular water. It is excreted into urine with a half-life of 2–2.5 h, principally in the glomerular filtrate. Elimination is linearly related to creatinine clearance. Side effects and uses are similar to those of other group 5 cephalosporins.

Further information

Bryson HM, Brogden RN. Cefetamet pivoxil: a review of its antibacterial activity, pharmacokinetic properties and therapeutic use. *Drugs*. 1993;45:589–621.

CEFTERAM

A semisynthetic cephalosporin formulated for oral administration as the prodrug ester, cefteram pivoxil. Activity is similar to that of cefixime, but with slightly better activity against staphylococci and some Gram-negative rods.

Available in Japan.

CEFTIBUTEN

A semisynthetic cephalosporin formulated as the dihydrate for oral administration.

Activity against common pathogens is shown in Table 13.5. It exhibits good activity against many Gram-negative bacilli, but its activity against Gram-positive cocci is very poor. It is stable to hydrolysis by the common plasmid-mediated β-lactamases, but not derepressed chromosomal enzymes (*see* p. 230).

It is rapidly and almost completely absorbed by mouth and is excreted in the urine with a half-life of 1.5–3 h. An oral dose of 400 mg achieves a peak plasma concentration of around 15 mg/L. Binding to plasma proteins is 65–77%.

Side effects mostly consist of mild gastrointestinal symptoms and mild liver function test changes. Clinical trials have mainly been conducted in urinary tract and respiratory tract infections which, despite the poor in-vitro activity against *Str. pneumoniae*, have shown ceftibuten to be as efficacious as comparator agents.

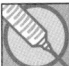

Preparations and dosage

Proprietary name: Cedax.

Preparations: Capsules, suspension.

Dosage: Adults and children >10 years (>45 kg), oral, 400 mg per day as a single dose. Children >6 months, 9 mg/kg per day as a single dose.

Available in USA and Japan; not available in the UK.

Further information

Guay DR. Ceftibuten: a new expanded-spectrum oral cephalosporin. *Ann Pharmacother*. 1997;31:1022–1033.

Owens RC, Nightingale CH, Nicolau DP. Ceftibuten: an overview. *Pharmacotherapy*. 1997;17:707–720.

Wiseman LR, Balfour JA. Ceftibuten. A review of its antibacterial activity, pharmacokinetic properties and clinical efficacy. *Drugs*. 1994;47:784–808.

GROUP 6 CEPHALOSPORINS

CEFEPIME

Molecular weight (dihydrochloride monohydrate): 571.5.

A semisynthetic parenteral cephalosporin formulated as the hydrochloride with arginine as a pH stabilizer.

ANTIMICROBIAL ACTIVITY

Its activity against common pathogens (Table 13.6) is comparable to that of group 4 cephalosporins, but it is somewhat more active against *Ps. aeruginosa*. Like cefpirome it has low affinity for the molecular class C cephalosporinases of many Gram-negative rods (p. 230) and is consequently active against most strains of *Citrobacter* spp., *Enterobacter* spp., *Serratia* spp. and *Ps. aeruginosa* that are resistant to cefotaxime and ceftazidime. It has poor activity against *L. monocytogenes* and against anaerobic organisms.

PHARMACOKINETICS

C$_{max}$ 2 g intravenous (30-min infusion)	*c.* 160 mg/L end infusion
Plasma half-life	*c.* 2 h
Volume of distribution	14–20 L
Plasma protein binding	10–19%

Table 13.6 Activity of group 6 cephalosporins against common pathogenic bacteria: MIC (mg/L)

	Cefoperazone	Cefpiramide	Cefsulodin	Ceftazidime	Cefepime	Cefpirome
Staphylococcus aureus	1–4	1	2–4	4–8	2–4	0.5–1
Streptococcus pyogenes	0.1	0.1	2	0.1–0.25	0.1	0.03
*Str. pneumoniae*ᵃ	0.1–0.25	0.1	4–8	0.25	<0.05	<0.05
Enterococcus faecalis	64–R	R	R	R	R	4–R
Neisseria gonorrhoeae	0.06		4–8	0.06–0.1	0.1	0.03
N. meningitidis	0.06		4–8	<0.01		
Haemophilus influenzae	0.1	0.5	32	0.1		0.1
Escherichia coli	0.1–2	0.5	64–R	0.1	0.1–0.5	0.1–0.5
Klebsiella pneumoniae	0.5–8	2	64–R	0.1	0.1–0.5	0.1–0.5
Pseudomonas aeruginosa	4–8	2	2	1–4	8–16	2–8
Bacteroides fragilis	16–32	R	R	16–64	R	R

ᵃPenicillin-resistant strains are often less susceptible. R, resistant (MIC >64 mg/L).

It is well distributed. Penetration into tissues, including lung, appears to be similar to that of other aminothiazoyl cephalosporins. Very low concentrations are achieved in CSF in the absence of meningeal inflammation. It is secreted in breast milk.

It is partially metabolized, but 85% of the dose is excreted unchanged in the urine, achieving a concentration approaching 1 g/L within 4 h of a 1 g intravenous dose. Dosage adjustment is required in patients with impaired renal function, but hepatic impairment does not affect the pharmacokinetic properties.

 ## TOXICITY AND SIDE EFFECTS

It is generally well tolerated, adverse events being those typical of the group.

 ## CLINICAL USE

It is used in the treatment of serious infections, particularly those in which resistant Gram-negative pathogens are known or suspected to be involved.

 ## Preparations and dosage

Proprietary name: Maxipime.
Preparation: Injection.
Dosage: Adult, i.m., i.v., 1–6 g per day in 2–3 divided doses.
Available in USA, most of Europe and Japan; not available in the UK.

 ## Further information

Barradell LB, Bryson HM. Cefepime: a review of its antibacterial activity, pharmacokinetic properties and therapeutic use. *Drugs.* 1994;47:471–505.
Brown EM, Finch RG, White LO. Cefepime: a β-lactamase-stable extended-spectrum cephalosporin. *J Antimicrob Chemother.* 1993;32(suppl B):1–214.
Wynd MA, Paladino JA. Cefepime: a fourth-generation parenteral cephalosporin. *Ann Pharmacother.* 1996;30:1414–1424.

CEFTAZIDIME

Molecular weight (anhydrous): 546.6; (pentahydrate): 636.7.

A semisynthetic parenteral cephalosporin formulated as the pentahydrate.

ANTIMICROBIAL ACTIVITY

Its activity against common pathogenic bacteria is shown in Table 13.6. Its activity is comparable to that of cefotaxime and ceftizoxime, but it is more active against *Ps. aeruginosa*, including almost all gentamicin-resistant strains, and *Burk. cepacia*. It is, however, less active against *Staph. aureus*. It is stable to a wide range of β-lactamases, but is hydrolyzed by some TEM variants (*see* pp. 230–231).

 PHARMACOKINETICS

C_{max} 500 mg intramuscular	18–20 mg/L
2 g intravenous (20-min infusion)	185 mg/L end infusion
Plasma half-life	1.5–2 h
Volume of distribution	16 L
Plasma protein binding	*c.* 10%

No accumulation was seen in subjects receiving 2 g every 12 h over 8 days. In premature infants given 25 mg/kg every 12 h, mean peak plasma concentrations were 77 mg/L after intravenous and 56 mg/L after intramuscular administration, with plasma elimination half-lives of 7.3 and 14.2 h, respectively. Postnatal age was the most important determinant of elimination rate, which was halved after 5 days. In newborn infants given 50 mg/kg intravenously over 20 min, mean peak plasma concentrations varied inversely with gestational age from 102 to 124 mg/L, with half-lives of 2.9–6.7 h.

Distribution

The concentration into serous fluids reaches 50% or more of the simultaneous serum level. In patients given 1 g intravenously during abdominal surgery, detectable concentrations appeared within a few minutes in the peritoneal fluid, reaching a peak around 67 mg/L with a half-life of 0.9 h. Following a similar intravenous dose, a mean peak of 9.4 mg/L was reached at 2 h in ascitic fluid. Concentrations in middle ear fluid after 1 g intravenously were broadly comparable to those of the plasma.

In patients with meningitis, CSF concentrations of 2–30 mg/L have been found 2–3 h after doses of 2 g intravenously over 30 min given every 8 h for four doses. Concentrations are substantially less in the absence of meningitis. Concentrations of 3–27 mg/g were found in patients with intracranial abscesses treated with 0.5–2 g every 8 h. Concentrations around 0.4 mg/g in skin, 0.6 mg/g in muscle and 0.2 mg/g in fatty tissue have been found in patients given 2 g intravenously over 5 min preoperatively. A similar dose has produced mean prostate tissue:serum ratios of around 0.14. Effective concentrations are achieved in bone: in patients given 1 g intravenously mean bone concentrations were 14.4 mg/kg 35–40 min after the dose. There is secretion in breast milk, peak concentrations being around 5 mg/L at about 1 h in patients receiving 2 g intravenously every 8 h.

Metabolism and excretion

No metabolites have been detected. Elimination is almost exclusively renal, predominantly via the glomerular filtrate, with 80–90% of the dose appearing in the urine in the first 24 h. Elimination half-life is inversely correlated with creatinine clearance: as the values fall to 2–12 mL/min, the mean plasma half-life rises to 16 h. In patients maintained on hemodialysis the half-life fell to 2.8 h on dialysis. No accumulation occurred over 10 days in severe renal impairment on a daily dose of 0.5–1 g.

Concentrations of 6.6–58 mg/L have been found in bile 25–160 min after the dose at times when the mean serum concentration was 77.4 mg/L. In T-tube bile there was considerable interpatient variation, with mean concentrations of 34 mg/L at 1–2 h after the dose. No accumulation occurs in patients with impaired hepatic function, but the presence of ascites, low plasma albumin and accumulation of protein-binding inhibitors may increase the volume of distribution.

 TOXICITY AND SIDE EFFECTS

It is generally well tolerated. Preparations containing arginine have replaced those with sodium carbonate, which causes pain on intramuscular injection. Reactions common to cephalosporins have been observed in some patients, including positive antiglobulin tests without hemolysis, raised liver function test values, eosinophilia, rashes, leukopenia, thrombocytopenia and diarrhea, occasionally associated with toxigenic *C. difficile.*

Failure of therapy has been associated with superinfection with resistant organisms, including *Staph. aureus*, enterococci and *Candida*. Resistance caused by induction of chromosomal β-lactamases may emerge in *Ps. aeruginosa*, *Ser. marcescens* or *Enterobacter* spp.

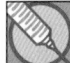 **CLINICAL USE**

It is used, often combined with an aminoglycoside, to treat a wide range of severe urinary, respiratory and wound infections, mostly due to enterobacteria or *Ps. aeruginosa*. Reference is made to its use in pneumonia, septicemia, meningitis (especially if caused by *Ps. aeruginosa*), peritonitis, osteomyelitis, neonatal sepsis, burns and melioidosis. Concern has been expressed at the relative frequency with which failure is associated with superinfection or the emergence of resistance.

Preparations and dosage

Proprietary names: Fortum, Kefadim, Ceptaz, Fortaz.

Preparation: Injection.

Dosage: Adults, i.m., i.v., 1–6 g per day in divided doses, depending on severity of infection. Neonates and children 25 mg/kg (neonates <7 days every 24 h; 7–21 days, every 12 h, older infants and children, every 8 h). The dose may be doubled in severe infection to a maximum of 6 g/day in children >1 month (9 g in cystic fibrosis).

Widely available.

Further information

Anonymous. Ceftazidime. In: Dollery C, ed. *Therapeutic Drugs*. 2nd ed. Edinburgh: Churchill Livingstone; 1999:C120–C125.

Boogaerts MA, Demuynck H, Mestdagh N, et al. Equivalent efficacies of meropenem and ceftazidime as empirical monotherapy of febrile neutropenic patients. *J Antimicrob Chemother*. 1995;36:185–200.

De Pauw BE, Deresinski SC, Feld R, Lane Allman EF, Donnelly JP, Elahi N. Ceftazidime compared with piperacillin and tobramycin for the empiric treatment of fever in neutropenic patients with cancer: a multicenter randomized trial. *Ann Intern Med*. 1994;120:834–844.

Fong IN, Tomkins KB. Review of *Pseudomonas aeruginosa* meningitis with special emphasis on treatment with ceftazidime. *Rev Infect Dis*. 1985;7:604–612.

Rains CP, Bryson HM, Peters DH. Ceftazidime: an update of its antibacterial activity, pharmacokinetic properties and therapeutic efficacy. *Drugs*. 1995;49:577–617.

OTHER GROUP 6 CEPHALOSPORINS

 ## CEFOPERAZONE

A semisynthetic parenteral cephalosporin. It is unstable, losing activity on storage even at –20°C. A formulation with sulbactam is available in some countries (*see* p. 241). Activity against common pathogenic bacteria is shown in Table 13.6. It exhibits moderate activity against carbenicillin-sensitive strains of *Ps. aeruginosa*. Activity against *Burk. cepacia* and *Sten. maltophilia* is unreliable. It is much less stable to enterobacterial β-lactamases than most other cephalosporins of groups 4–6 and consequently has unreliable activity against many species, including β-lactamase-producing strains of *H. influenzae* and *N. gonorrhoeae*. It is active against *Achromobacter*, *Flavobacterium*, *Aeromonas* and associated non-fermenters. *Past. multocida* is extremely susceptible (MIC <0.01–0.02 mg/L). It exhibits modest activity against most Gram-negative anaerobes, but not *B. fragilis*. Sulbactam increases activity against many, but not all, enterobacteria and non-fermenters, and almost all *B. fragilis*.

A 2 g intravenous infusion achieves a peak plasma concentration of 250 mg/L. The plasma half-life is 1.5–2 h. Over 85% is bound to plasma proteins. It achieves therapeutic concentrations in tissue and inflammatory exudates. Variable low levels are found in the sputum up to 1.5% of simultaneous serum levels. Penetration into CSF is unreliable even in the presence of meningeal inflammation.

The bile is a major route of excretion, accounting for almost 20% of the dose. About 20–30% is eliminated in urine, almost entirely by glomerular filtration. Clearance is effectively unchanged by renal failure or dialysis.

Side effects associated with the methylthiotetrazole side chain have been reported. Diarrhea has been notable in some studies. Marked suppression of fecal flora, with the appearance of *C. difficile*, has occasionally been found. There is a 5–10% incidence of mild transient increases in liver function tests.

Its potential toxicity and the availability of compounds with better β-lactamase stability and more reliable antipseudomonal activity have undermined its popularity.

 Further information

Brogden RN, Carmine A, Heel RC, Morley PA, Speight TM, Avery GS. Cefoperazone: a review of its in vitro antimicrobial activity, pharmacological properties and therapeutic efficacy. *Drugs*. 1981;22:423–460.

Symposium. Evaluation of cefoperazone. *Rev Infect Dis*. 1983;5(suppl 1):S108–S209.

 ## CEFOZOPRAN

An aminothiazole cephalosporin formulated as the hydrochloride. Activity is similar to that of ceftazidime, but it is more active against methicillin-susceptible staphylococci (MIC 1 mg/L). Representative MICs against Gram-negative species are: *Esch coli* 0.25 mg/L; *K. pneumoniae* 1 mg/L; *Ps. aeruginosa* 1–8 mg/L. Activity against *Acinetobacter* spp., *Sten. maltophilia* and *B. fragilis* group is poor.

A 20-min infusion of 1.5 g achieved a plasma concentration of around 125 mg/L at the end of infusion. Almost 90% of the dose was excreted in the urine over 24 h. The mean terminal half-life was around 2 h. Adverse reactions appear to be typical of those of other group 6 cephalosporins.

It is available in Japan.

 Further information

Iwahi T, Okonogi K, Yamazaki T, et al. In vitro and in vivo activities of SCE-2787, a new parenteral cephalosporin with a broad antibacterial spectrum. *Antimicrob Agents Chemother*. 1992;36:1358–1366.

Paulfeuerborn W, Muller HJ, Borner K, Koeppe P, Lode H. Comparative pharmacokinetics and serum bactericidal activities of SCE-2787 and ceftazidime. *Antimicrob Agents Chemother*. 1993;37:1835–1841.

 ## CEFPIMIZOLE

A semisynthetic parenteral cephalosporin. It exhibits modest activity compared to other antipseudomonal cephalosporins. Like cefoperazone, it is susceptible to many enterobacterial β-lactamases. In volunteers receiving 0.1–1 g intramuscularly, mean peak plasma concentrations reached 15–20 and 35–40 mg/L, respectively. There was no accumulation when the dose was repeated every 8 h for 7 days. No metabolites have been detected. The plasma elimination half-life is 1.8–2.1 h. The principal route of elimination is renal, 70–80% being recovered unchanged in the urine.

Significant pain at the site of infection has been a prominent adverse event. It is no longer widely available.

 ## CEFPIRAMIDE

A semisynthetic parenteral cephalosporin. It exhibits a broad range of activity, which includes *Ps. aeruginosa*, though the overall activity is rather modest (Table 13.6). It is moderately stable to most β-lactamases but less so than ceftazidime or cefpirome.

In volunteers given 0.5 or 1 g by intravenous bolus, the mean plasma concentration shortly after injection was around 150 or 300 mg/L, respectively. There was no accumulation when the same doses were repeated every 12 h for 11 doses. It is highly bound to plasma protein (c. 95%). The mean plasma half-life is around 5 h. Less than one-quarter of the dose appears in the urine over 24 h; the rest is excreted in bile and high concentrations are found in feces. Renal impairment has little effect on elimination in patients with normal liver function.

Diarrhea may be associated with marked suppression of gut flora resulting from biliary excretion of the drug. The molecule includes a C-3 methylthiotetrazole side chain and side effects associated with that substituent are to be expected.

It is available in Japan.

Further information

Conte JE. Pharmacokinetics of cefpiramide in volunteers with normal or impaired renal function. *Antimicrob Agents Chemother*. 1987;31:1585–1588.
Nakagawa K, Koyama M, Matsui H, et al. Pharmacokinetics of cefpiramide (SM-1652) in humans. *Antimicrob Agents Chemother*. 1984;25:221–225.

CEFPIROME

A semisynthetic aminothiazoyl cephalosporin formulated as the sulfate for parenteral administration. Activity against common pathogens (Table 13.6) is similar to that of cefotaxime and ceftriaxone, but it is more active against *Ps. aeruginosa*. Unlike other cephalosporins it exhibits activity against some strains of enterococci (MIC 4–16 mg/L), but this is of doubtful clinical benefit. It is generally very stable to β-lactamases. It is active against strains of *Enterobacter* spp., *Citrobacter* spp., *Hafnia* spp., *Providencia* spp., *Ser. marcescens* and *Pr. vulgaris* producing molecular class C cephalosporinases (*see* p. 230). *Sten. maltophilia* is resistant.

A 1 g intramuscular injection produces a plasma concentration of 25 mg/L after 1.6–2.3 h. A similar intravenous dose achieves a peak concentration of 97 mg/L. The plasma half-life is 1.4–2.3 h and protein binding is around 10%. It is well distributed, achieving therapeutic concentrations in tissues and exudates. It penetrates poorly into CSF in the absence of meningeal inflammation, but concentrations around 2–4 mg/L have been found in patients with purulent meningitis.

Little, if any, of the drug is metabolized and most is excreted unchanged in the urine within 12 h, mainly by glomerular filtration. Clearance declines in proportion to renal function. Around 60% of the drug is removed in 3 h by hemodialysis. Low concentrations are found in breast milk.

Side effects are those common to other cephalosporins. Diarrhea is common and occasional cases of pseudomembranous colitis have been reported.

It is mainly used in the treatment of serious sepsis, particularly nosocomial infections in which resistant Gram-negative pathogens are known or suspected to be involved. It is not widely available, but is marketed in Japan.

Further information

Anonymous. Cefpirome. In: Dollery C, ed. *Therapeutic Drugs*. 2nd ed. Edinburgh: Churchill Livingstone; 1999:C109–C113.
Wiseman LR, Lamb HM. Cefpirome. A review of its antibacterial activity, pharmacokinetic properties and clinical efficacy in the treatment of severe nosocomial infections and febrile neutropenia. *Drugs*. 1997;54:117–140.

CEFSULODIN

A semisynthetic parenteral cephalosporin supplied as the sodium salt. Activity against *Ps. aeruginosa* contrasts strikingly with poor activity against many other organisms (Table 13.6). Anaerobic Gram-negative rods, Gram-positive rods and cocci are all resistant. It is stable to many β-lactamases, including the *Ps. aeruginosa* chromosomal enzyme, and is a poor substrate for the enzymes of *Enterobacter* spp. and *Morg. morganii*. It is slowly hydrolyzed by TEM β-lactamases and more rapidly by the enzymes of some carbenicillin-resistant strains of *Ps. aeruginosa*, with which distinct inoculum effects may be seen.

A 500 mg intravenous bolus dose achieves a plasma concentration of c. 70 mg/L at the end of the injection; the corresponding intramuscular dose achieves a peak concentration of around 15 mg/L. The plasma half-life is 1.5 h. About 15–30% is protein bound.

There is some metabolism of the drug, but the main route of excretion is via the kidneys, most appearing in the urine in the first 6 h. The plasma half-life is linearly related to creatinine clearance, rising to a mean of 10–13 h in patients where clearance was <10 mL/min, falling to around 2 h on hemodialysis.

It is well tolerated, apart from nausea and vomiting in some subjects. It has been used in severe pseudomonas infections, usually in combination with an aminoglycoside, but treatment has been complicated on a number of occasions by the emergence of resistance or superinfection.

It is available in Japan.

Further information

Wright DB. Cefsulodin. *Drug Intell Clin Pharm*. 1986;20:845–849.
Young LS. *Pseudomonas aeruginosa* – biology, immunology and therapy: a cefsulodin symposium. *Rev Infect Dis*. 1984;6(suppl 3):S603–S776.

GROUP 7 CEPHALOSPORINS

CEFTOBIPROLE

Molecular weight: 534.57 (base); 712.64 (medocaril ester).

A semisynthetic cephalosporin formulated as the water-soluble medocaril prodrug for intravenous administration.

ANTIMICROBIAL ACTIVITY

The most important property distinguishing it from older cephalosporins is activity against methicillin-resistant staphylococci, a property conferred by a high affinity for penicillin-binding protein 2′ (2a). MICs for methicillin-resistant strains are nevertheless somewhat higher than those seen with fully susceptible strains. A similar situation exists with coagulase-negative staphylococci and with *Str. pneumoniae*, for which strains with reduced susceptibility to penicillin are less susceptible than fully resistant strains, while remaining within therapeutically achievable levels.

Otherwise activity approximates to that of cephalosporins of group 4 (Table 13.7). Activity against *Ps. aeruginosa* is modest and much reduced against ceftazidime-resistant strains.

ACQUIRED RESISTANCE

It is hydrolyzed by extended spectrum β-lactamases of enterobacteria (*see* p. 230), which are therefore resistant. The prospects for the emergence of resistance during extensive clinical use are presently unclear, though increased resistance in *Staph. aureus* appears to be difficult to induce under laboratory conditions.

PHARMACOKINETICS

C_{max} 500 mg (667 mg prodrug) intravenous (30-min infusion)	*c.* 35 mg/L end infusion
Plasma half-life	*c.* 3 h
Volume of distribution	18.4 L
Plasma protein binding	16%

The prodrug is rapidly hydrolyzed in plasma to release the active form together with diacetyl (2,3-butanediol) and CO_2. Distribution approximates to the extracellular fluid volume in adults. There is no accumulation on repeat dosing in subjects with normal renal function.

Table 13.7 Activity of group 7 cephalosporins against common pathogenic bacteria: MIC (mg/L)

	Ceftobiprole	Ceftaroline
Staphylococcus aureus (methicillin-sensitive)	0.25–0.5	0.25
Staph. aureus (methicillin-resistant)	1–2	0.5–1
Streptococcus pyogenes	0.06	0.008–0.03
Str. pneumoniae	0.015–0.25	0.008–0.12
Enterococcus faecalis	4	2–4
Neisseria gonorrhoeae	0.06	No data
Haemophilus influenzae	0.06	0.015–0.03
Escherichia coli	0.03–0.06	0.06–0.5
Klebsiella pneumoniae	0.03–0.12	0.06–0.25
Pseudomonas aeruginosa	2–8	0.5–R
Bacteroides fragilis	R	No data

R, resistant (MIC >64 mg/L).

It is chiefly excreted in urine by glomerular filtration. A urinary concentration exceeding 1 g/L is achieved within the first 2 h of a 500 mg (active drug equivalent) dose and 80–90% of active drug can be recovered within 24 h.

TOXICITY AND SIDE EFFECTS

Limited studies have so far revealed no unexpected side effects. Nausea, vomiting and altered taste sensation appear to be the most common.

CLINICAL USE

In countries in which approval has been granted, use is presently limited to complicated infections of skin and skin structures.

Preparations and dosage

Proprietary names: Zeftera, Zevtera.
Preparation: Infusion.
Dosage: i.v. infusion (1–2 h), 500 mg (667 mg medocaril prodrug) every 12 h. Limited availability. Available in Canada.

Further information

Anderson SD, Gums JG. Ceftobiprole: an extended-spectrum anti-methicillin-resistant *Staphylococcus aureus* cephalosporin. *Ann Pharmacother*. 2008;42:806–816.

Pillar CM, Aranza MK, Shah D, Sahm DF. *In vitro* activity profile of ceftobiprole, an anti-MRSA cephalosporin, against recent Gram-positive and Gram-negative isolates of European origin. *J Antimicrob Chemother*. 2008;61:595–602.

Schmitt-Hoffmann A, Nyman L, Roos B, et al. Multiple-dose pharmacokinetics and safety of a novel broad-spectrum cephalosporin (BAL5788) in healthy volunteers. *Antimicrob Agents Chemother*. 2004;48:2576–2580.

Schmitt-Hoffmann A, Roos B, Schleimer M, et al. Single-dose pharmacokinetics and safety of a novel broad-spectrum cephalosporin (BAL5788) in healthy volunteers. *Antimicrob Agents Chemother*. 2004;48:2570–2575.

Vidaillac C, Rybak MJ. Ceftobiprole: first cephalosporin with activity against methicillin-resistant *Staphylococcus aureus*. *Pharmacotherapy*. 2009;29:511–525.

OTHER GROUP 7 CEPHALOSPORINS

CEFTAROLINE

A semisynthetic cephalosporin formulated as the water-soluble fosamil acetate prodrug for intravenous administration.

Its properties are similar to those of ceftobiprole, with which it shares an enhanced affinity for penicillin-binding protein 2′ (2a) of methicillin-resistant *Staph. aureus*. Activity against common bacterial pathogens is shown in Table 13.7. It is hydrolyzed by extended-spectrum β-lactamases and is not active against Amp-C derepressed strains of Gram-negative bacilli (*see* p. 230).

C_{max} 600 mg intravenous (1-h infusion)	19 mg/L end infusion
Plasma half-life	2.6 h
Volume of distribution	0.37 L/kg
Plasma protein binding	<20%

Like ceftobiprole, ceftaroline fosamil is rapidly hydrolyzed in plasma after intravenous infusion and excreted principally in urine. In preliminary clinical studies it appears to be well tolerated.

Further information

Brown SD, Traczewski MM. In vitro antimicrobial activity of a new cephalosporin, ceftaroline and determination of quality control ranges for MIC testing. *Antimicrob Agents Chemother*. 2009;53:1271–1274.

Ge Y, Biek D, Talbot GH, Sahm DF. In vitro profiling of ceftaroline against a collection of recent bacterial clinical isolates from across the United States. *Antimicrob Agents Chemother*. 2008;52:3398–3407.

Zhanel GG, Sniezek G, Schweizer F, et al. Ceftaroline: a novel broad-spectrum cephalosporin with activity against methicillin-resistant *Staphylococcus aureus*. *Drugs*. 2009;69:809–831.

14 β-Lactam antibiotics: penicillins

Karen Bush

The penicillin class of antibiotics comprises a large group of bicyclic penam compounds (pp. 226–227) differing in the nature of the acyl side chain attached to the fused β-lactam–thiazolidine ring system. Most are semisynthetic derivatives of the penicillin nucleus, 6-aminopenicillanic acid (6-APA), prepared synthetically by the addition of acyl side chains at the 6-amino group.

Fleming reported the discovery of penicillin as the compound responsible for the antibacterial activity displayed by the mold *Penicillium notatum* in 1929, but it was not until 1940 that Florey and his collaborators at Oxford produced enough crude penicillin to start therapeutic tests in mice. Preliminary human trials followed in 1941. Later studies showed that the product derived from industrial fermentations of *Penicillium chrysogenum* was a family of closely related compounds differing only in the nature of the acyl side chain. These natural penicillins consisted of penicillins F (pentenylpenicillin), G (benzylpenicillin), K (heptylpenicillin) and X (*p*-hydroxybenzylpenicillin). From this family, benzylpenicillin (penicillin G) was selected as the penicillin most suitable for clinical development based on biological properties and ease of commercial production.

The limitations of benzylpenicillin as an antibacterial agent soon led to efforts to produce novel penicillins with superior properties. In early work acidic side-chain precursors that could be incorporated during biosynthesis were added during the fermentation. However, only a limited number of side chains could be introduced; the only penicillin produced by this process with any advantage over penicillin G was phenoxymethylpenicillin (penicillin V), the product of fermentations to which phenoxyacetic acid had been added as a precursor. This change conferred stability to gastric acid, allowing it to be administered orally.

The first semisynthetic penicillins, prepared by chemical substitution of the *p*-hydroxy group of the naturally occurring penicillin X (*p*-hydroxybenzylpenicillin) were, unfortunately, no better than penicillin G. A similar approach to modify the amino group of *p*-aminobenzylpenicillin was also unsuccessful, but research on this compound led to the important identification in 1957 of the penicillin nucleus, 6-aminopenicillanic acid (6-APA). It was later obtained more easily by removal of the benzylpenicillin side chain by microbial enzymes or by chemical modification, the process now used for commercial production.

The significance of the identification of 6-APA is that numerous semisynthetic penicillins can be prepared by adding acyl side-chain structures to the 6-amino group of the molecule. With the exceptions of penicillin G and penicillin V, the penicillins in clinical use are all derived from 6-APA, and display advantages over benzylpenicillin in antibacterial activity, stability to bacterial β-lactamases or pharmacokinetic properties. Attempts to further modify the penicillin nucleus have been disappointing. Only two clinically useful compounds resulted: mecillinam (amdinocillin), in which the side chain is joined in an amidino linkage; and temocillin, in which a 6-methoxy group has been incorporated in the β-lactam ring. After the late 1970s, research emphasis in the β-lactam field switched from penicillins to other β-lactam agents, notably the cephalosporins, cephamycins, carbapenems, penems, monobactams and penicillanic acid sulfones (Ch. 15), and the development of novel penams appears to have come to a halt.

CLASSIFICATION

Following the isolation of 6-APA, objectives in penicillin research were:

- synthesis of narrow-spectrum penicillins similar to benzylpenicillin in activity but with superior oral absorption
- preparation of penicillins stable to staphylococcal β-lactamase and active against benzylpenicillin-resistant staphylococci (excluding methicillin-resistant staphylococci)
- development of penicillins with broader spectra of antibacterial activity than benzylpenicillin and stability to plasmid-encoded class A β-lactamases (p. 230).

The first two objectives were achieved with some success but with the third there was less success, in that the extended-spectrum penicillins (with the exception of temocillin) are largely inactive against β-lactamase-producing bacteria, although some have achieved clinical success when combined with β-lactamase inhibitors (pp. 239–244).

The penicillins in clinical use may be divided into six major groups:

- *Group 1*: Benzylpenicillin and its long-acting parenteral forms.
- *Group 2*: Orally absorbed penicillins similar to benzylpenicillin.
- *Group 3*: Penicillins that are relatively stable to staphylococcal β-lactamase, but which have no useful activity against Gram-negative bacilli. Several are structurally related isoxazoylpenicillins.
- *Group 4*: Compounds with enhanced activity against certain Gram-negative bacilli, including many enterobacteria and *Haemophilus influenzae*, but which are inactivated by staphylococcal and many enterobacterial β-lactamases. They include several aminopenicillins, such as ampicillin and amoxicillin, and the amidinopenicillin mecillinam. Esters and condensates of ampicillin and a mecillinam ester, pivmecillinam, have been developed to improve oral absorption of the parent compounds.
- *Group 5*: Penicillins active against *Pseudomonas aeruginosa*. These include carboxypenicillins (and their orally absorbed esters) and acyl or acylureido derivatives of ampicillin.
- *Group 6*: Penicillins resistant to enterobacterial β-lactamase.

Group 1	Group 2	Group 3	Group 4	Group 5	Group 6
Benzylpenicillin	Azidocillin[a]	Cloxacillin[b]	Amoxicillin	Apalcillin[a]	Temocillin
Benzathine penicillin	Phenethicillin[a]	Dicloxacillin[b]	Ampicillin	Aspoxicillin	
Clemizole penicillin[a]	Phenoxymethyl penicillin	Flucloxacillin[b]	Ciclacillin	Azlocillin[a,c]	
Procaine penicillin	Propicillin[a]	Methicillin[a]	Epicillin[a]	Carbenicillin[a,d]	
		Nafcillin	Mecillinam	Mezlocillin[a,c]	
		Oxacillin[b]		Piperacillin[c]	
				Ticarcillin[d]	

[a]No longer available [b]isoxazolylpenicillins [c]acyureidopencillins [d]carboxypenicillins.

MODE OF ACTION

Penicillins and other β-lactam antibiotics prevent synthesis of the bacterial cell wall (pp. 12–13), a structure that is not found in mammalian cells – a feature responsible for the low toxicity and the consequent clinical popularity of this class of antibiotics.

ACQUIRED RESISTANCE

Bacteria may exhibit resistance to penicillins and other β-lactam antibiotics by several mechanisms (*see also* Ch. 3):

- Acquisition of penicillin-binding proteins (PBPs) with reduced affinity for penicillin. This is a frequent cause of resistance in Gram-positive bacteria such as staphylococci, pneumococci and enterococci. This mechanism may also be responsible for low-level penicillin resistance in *H. influenzae* and viridans streptococci.
- The production of a bacterial enzyme, β-lactamase, that opens the β-lactam ring, causing inactivation of the antibiotic.
- Modification of outer membrane proteins (porins) in Gram-negative bacteria, preventing passage of penicillins into the bacterial cell. Efflux mechanisms have been described in which bacteria pump out β-lactam antibiotics.

Bacteria frequently display more than one resistance mechanism – for example, methicillin-resistant staphylococci typically produce β-lactamase but demonstrate resistance primarily due to altered PBPs; Gram-negative bacteria may produce β-lactamases in organisms with efflux mechanisms or altered outer membrane proteins.

Methicillin-resistant strains of *Staphylococcus aureus* (MRSA) are considered to be resistant to all β-lactam antibiotics, with the exception of some newer cephalosporins, and are frequently multiresistant. The prevalence of MRSA is variable, with very low incidence in some countries of northern Europe, but high incidence in Japan and other countries. In the USA the frequency increased from 2.4% in 1975 to 64% in 2007. Although largely confined to hospitals, MRSA is increasingly seen in community settings.

When benzylpenicillin was introduced, all streptococci were sensitive to its action, and this situation remains largely unchanged. However, pneumococci exhibiting reduced susceptibility are now common, although the criteria for penicillin resistance differ in the USA and Europe (Table 14.1).

The interpretive criteria for non-meningitis isolates defined by the FDA in 2008 is based on clinical experience showing that high doses of penicillin provide efficacious drug concentrations, except in cerebrospinal fluid (CSF). The EUCAST or FDA pre-2008 definitions are generally used for epidemiological purposes.

Until the 1980s, clinical isolates of *Streptococcus pneumoniae* were uniformly susceptible to penicillin, except for a few reports from South Africa and elsewhere. By 1998, 24% of invasive pneumococci isolated in the USA displayed reduced susceptibility to penicillin and often to other classes of antibiotics. The frequency of isolation of penicillin-resistant pneumococci in Europe was 51% in Hungary (1990) and 9% in

Table 14.1 Interpretive criteria for susceptibility of *Str. pneumoniae* to penicillin

Organization	Source of isolate	MIC (mg/L)		
		Susceptible	Intermediate	Resistant
FDA (pre-2008)	Any	≤0.06	0.12–1	≥2
(post-2008)	Meningitis	≤0.06	Not defined	≥0.12
	Non-meningitis	≤2	4	>8
EUCAST	Any	≤0.06	0.12–2	≥4

FDA, United States Food and Drug Administration; EUCAST, European Committee on Antimicrobial Susceptibility Testing; MIC, minimum inhibitory concentration.

the UK (1998). Introduction of the heptavalent pneumococcal vaccine in 2000 caused a dramatic decrease in isolates of pneumococci insusceptible to penicillin, especially in the elderly and young children, in countries with effective vaccination programs.

As with pneumococci, enterococci were initially perceived always to be susceptible to ampicillin and benzylpenicillin, but resistant strains are now common. Resistance is less prevalent among the most common species, *Enterococcus faecalis*, in which β-lactamase has been reported at a low frequency. In *Enterococcus faecium*, the next most common enterococcal species, high-level penicillin resistance due to modified PBPs is usual.

IMPERMEABILITY RESISTANCE

β-Lactam antibiotics cross the outer membrane to reach PBPs in Gram-negative bacteria through porin proteins (p. 27; see also Figure 2.1, p.11). Alterations in porin production can lead to decreased permeability and concomitant β-lactam resistance. Porin deficiencies coupled with high β-lactamase production have been reported in clinical isolates of Enterobacteriaceae such as *Enterobacter cloacae* and *Serratia marcescens* that produce cephalosporinases. Resistance due to decreased permeability is also important among *Ps. aeruginosa* strains, which possess a less permeable membrane and contain efflux pump mechanisms for β-lactam antibiotics, coupled with production of chromosomally mediated β-lactamase activity. Because Gram-positive bacteria lack an outer membrane, this mechanism of resistance does not apply.

EFFLUX-MEDIATED RESISTANCE

Efflux mechanisms for β-lactam-containing antimicrobial agents were described in the 1990s. These multidrug, active efflux mechanisms have been best studied in *Ps. aeruginosa*, where an operon consisting of *mexA–mexB–oprM* is involved in an energy-dependent pumping out of diverse agents such as tetracyclines, fluoroquinolones and chloramphenicol, as well as penicillins. Related pumps have also been identified in the pseudomonads and Gram-negative bacteria.

TOXICITY AND SIDE EFFECTS

HYPERSENSITIVITY REACTIONS

Penicillins and other β-lactam agents are among the safest antibacterial agents used therapeutically. The most important untoward reactions are those resulting from hypersensitivity. Although serious or life-threatening reactions are rare, allergic reactions present a more serious problem with benzylpenicillin than with other antibiotics. There is cross-reaction among penicillins, and the agent to which the patient reacts is not necessarily the sensitizing agent.

The most dangerous form of drug allergy is acute anaphylactic shock, which may develop between a few minutes and 30 minutes after administration. It is characterized by profound circulatory collapse, nausea, vomiting, abdominal pain, severe bronchospasm and coma, and may be rapidly fatal. Anaphylaxis is said to occur in 0.005–0.05% of treated patients, with a mortality rate of approximately 10%.

The most common manifestations of hypersensitivity are various skin eruptions, usually maculopapular with itching but sometimes urticarial or mixed, and occasionally purpuric. Penicillins should not be applied to the skin as topical preparations are likely to lead to contact dermatitis or local swelling. Rashes occur in 1–7% of patient courses of penicillin. Although reactions can occur after any route of administration, the severe forms are much more common after injections than after oral administration. A serum sickness form of allergy can arise 7–10 days after treatment (earlier in previously sensitized patients).

Some patients develop allergic reactions only after repeated administration of penicillin but in others reactions develop after the initial treatment, often as a result of non-medicinal exposure to penicillin in the environment.

Anaphylaxis is much less common with penicillins other than benzylpenicillin. Ampicillin, however, is much more likely to produce rashes (9.5%), which may be severe, especially in patients with coexisting viral infections caused by cytomegalovirus or Epstein–Barr virus, notably infectious mononucleosis. It has been claimed that this propensity is not exhibited to the same degree by amoxicillin, ciclacillin or mecillinam.

ALLERGENS

The principal antigen responsible for these reactions is generated by opening the β-lactam ring, allowing the carbonyl group to react with the amino groups of proteins. This benzylpenicilloyl hapten, accounting for 95% of tissue-bound penicillin, is the major determinant for hypersensitivity. A number of other reactions within and between the molecules can occur, leading to the 'minor determinants' – minor components of the complex mixtures, but potentially important determinants of penicillin allergy. Penicillins with different side chains have different sensitizing capacities and may lead to different populations of antibodies in treated patients.

DETECTION AND CONTROL

Many patients without a history of penicillin allergy have circulating antibodies to the drug, and their presence is of no prognostic value. Skin testing for cutaneous reactivity to specific IgE is the most widely accepted test used to detect patients likely to suffer immediate hypersensitivity reactions to penicillins. Only about 10% of the patients who claim to have a history of penicillin hypersensitivity respond positively to the determinants used in skin testing. This testing, currently the most accepted and reliable testing method, uses all relevant antigens, including both major and minor determinants.

The use of benzylpenicillin itself for testing is generally regarded as hazardous because it may lead to a severe reaction in the highly susceptible patient and may sensitize the previously non-allergic individual. For this reason, agents such as penicilloyl–polylysine, in which the amino groups of an artificial peptide are virtually saturated with penicilloyl residues, are used. As there are other antigens involved, excellent predictive performance has been claimed for penicilloyl–polylysine plus a 'minor determinant' mixture. A positive penicillin skin test indicates that a patient is at risk for immediate hypersensitivity; a negative test cannot preclude a future hypersensitivity reaction upon subsequent therapy with penicillin. It is extremely rare, however, that life-threatening reactions occur in patients with a negative skin test.

The management of penicillin reactions relies on the use of antihistamines, corticosteroids and, in anaphylaxis or dangerous angioedema, adrenaline (epinephrine). It has sometimes been recommended that allergic patients may be successfully treated with the co-administration of corticosteroids or antihistamines, together with penicillin, where that is the most appropriate agent. However, this has major risks, as it is possible that any allergic reaction to the penicillin would be masked by the action of these agents.

CROSS-REACTIONS WITH CEPHALOSPORINS

About 3–9% of penicillin-allergic patients are cross-allergic to cephalosporins; specific allergy to cephalosporins in the absence of reactions to penicillin also occurs, albeit rarely. It is generally recommended that cephalosporins should be avoided in patients with a clear history of severe reaction to penicillin. Cross-reactivity between penicillins and carbapenems is even less frequent, while the monobactam aztreonam (p. 237) is only very weakly immunogenic and does not show cross-reactivity with penicillin.

OTHER REACTIONS

Leukopenia has occurred in patients receiving various penicillins, including methicillin and piperacillin. Neutropenia in patients treated with benzylpenicillin for bacterial endocarditis is related both to high dosage (18 g per day) and to low neutrophil counts before treatment. Prolonged bleeding times due to platelet abnormalities have been noted, particularly with carboxypenicillins and, to a lesser extent, with acylureidopenicillins. Various nephrotoxic manifestations have been described with carbenicillin, dicloxacillin and methicillin, and reversible abnormalities of liver function tests with carboxypenicillins and less frequently acylureidopenicillins.

Because penicillins are often administered in large doses as sodium salts, sodium overload and hypokalemia may develop. Large doses of penicillins, especially in patients with impaired renal function, may result in convulsions. Access to the central nervous system of neurotoxic concentrations is related to lipophilicity and protein binding of the compounds.

Further information

Brown DF, Hope R, Livermore DM, BSAC Working Parties on Resistance Surveillance, et al. Non-susceptibility trends among enterococci and non-pneumococcal streptococci from bacteraemias in the UK and Ireland, 2001–06. *J Antimicrob Chemother*. 2008;62(suppl 2):ii75–ii85.

Burton DC, Edwards JR, Horan TC, Jernigan JA, Fridkin SK. Methicillin-resistant *Staphylococcus aureus* central line-associated bloodstream infections in US intensive care units, 1997–2007. *J Am Med Assoc*. 2009;301:727–736.

Bush K. New β-lactamases in gram-negative bacteria: diversity and impact on the selection of antimicrobial therapy. *Clin Infect Dis*. 2001;32:1085–1089.

de Haan P, Bruynzeel P, van Ketel WG. Onset of penicillin rashes: relation between type of penicillin administered and type of immune reactivity. *Allergy*. 1986;41:75–78.

Garau J. Role of beta-lactam agents in the treatment of community-acquired pneumonia. *Eur J Clin Microbiol Infect Dis*. 2005;24:83–99.

Holgate ST. Penicillin allergy: how to diagnose and when to treat. *Br Med J*. 1988;296:1213–1214.

Kishiyama JL, Adelman DC. The cross-reactivity and immunology of β-lactam antibiotics. *Drug Safety*. 1994;10:318–327.

Lin RY. A perspective on penicillin allergy. *Arch Intern Med*. 1992;152:930–937.

Livermore DM. Mechanisms of resistance to β-lactam antibiotics. *Scand J Antibiot*. 1991;78(suppl):7–16.

Popovich KJ, Weinstein RA, Hota B. Are community-associated methicillin-resistant *Staphylococcus aureus* (MRSA) strains replacing traditional nosocomial MRSA strains? *Clin Infect Dis.* 2008;46:787–794.

Sogn DD, Evans R, Shepherd GM, et al. Results of the National Institute of Allergy and Infectious Diseases Collaborative Clinical Trial to test the predictive value of skin testing with major and minor penicillin derivatives in hospitalized patients. *Arch Intern Med.* 1992;152:1025–1032.

Srikumar R, Tsang E, Poole K. Contribution of the MexAB-OprM multidrug efflux system to the beta-lactam resistance of penicillin-binding protein and beta-lactamase-derepressed mutants of *Pseudomonas aeruginosa. J Antimicrob Chemother.* 1999;44:537–540.

Weiss ME, Adkinson NF. Immediate hypersensitivity reactions to penicillin and related antibiotics. *Clin Allergy.* 1988;18:515–540.

Whitney CG, Farley MM, Hadler J, et al. Active Bacterial Core Surveillance Program of the Emerging Infections Program Network. Increasing prevalence of multidrug-resistant *Streptococcus pneumoniae* in the United States. *N Engl J Med.* 2000;343:1917–1924.

Whitney CG, Farley MM, Hadler J, et al. Decline in invasive pneumococcal disease after the introduction of protein-polysaccharide conjugate vaccine. *N Engl J Med.* 2003;348:1737–1746.

GROUP 1: BENZYLPENICILLIN AND ITS LONG-ACTING PARENTERAL FORMS

Benzylpenicillin, the first naturally produced penicillin, is poorly absorbed orally and must be given by injection. Because the plasma half-life is short, insoluble salts of penicillin were prepared that act as intramuscular depots for the release of penicillin into the bloodstream. Repository penicillins that are in use include procaine penicillin and benzathine penicillin.

BENZYLPENICILLIN

Penicillin G. Molecular weight (free acid): 334.4.

Archetypal penicillin produced by *P. chrysogenum*; supplied as the highly soluble potassium or sodium salts for intramuscular or intravenous administration. Potency has traditionally been expressed in units (1 unit = 0.6 µg), but use of milligram or gram quantities is now preferred.

ANTIMICROBIAL ACTIVITY

Activity against common pathogenic bacteria is shown in Table 14.2. It has intrinsic activity against almost all Gram-positive pathogens, but is no longer effective against most staphylococci. Most species of streptococci are susceptible, including group B streptococci, an important cause of neonatal infections. Enterococci are more resistant than streptococci. Other susceptible Gram-positive organisms include non-β-lactamase-producing *Bacillus anthracis* and *Listeria*

Table 14.2 Activity of benzylpenicillin and phenoxymethylpenicillin against non-β-lactamase-producing strains of pathogenic bacteria; modal MIC (mg/L)

	Benzylpenicillin	Phenoxymethylpenicillin
Staphylococcus aureus (methicillin-susceptible)	0.03	0.06
Streptococcus pyogenes	0.02	0.02
Str. pneumoniae	0.02	0.02
Enterococcus faecalis	4	2
Neisseria gonorrhoeae	0.02	0.1
N. meningitidis	0.06	0.25
Haemophilus influenzae	0.25	2
Escherichia coli	64	R
Klebsiella pneumoniae	R	R
Pseudomonas aeruginosa	R	R
Bacteroides fragilis	32	ND

R, resistant (MIC >64 mg/L).

monocytogenes. The spirochetes *Borrelia burgdorferi* and *Treponema pallidum* are also susceptible.

The aerobic Gram-negative cocci *Neisseria gonorrhoeae* and *N. meningitidis* were initially highly susceptible to benzylpenicillin, but β-lactamase-producing strains of gonococci are now common. *H. influenzae* and *Moraxella catarrhalis* are usually resistant due to β-lactamase production. The Enterobacteriaceae and most other aerobic Gram-negative bacilli are resistant, as a result of β-lactamase production or the impermeability of the bacterial cell wall. Other resistant organisms include mycobacteria, mycoplasmas, *Nocardia* spp., rickettsiae and chlamydiae.

Anaerobic Gram-positive cocci are susceptible in the absence of β-lactamase production. Most clostridia strains are susceptible, but resistance can be observed. Anaerobic Gram-negative bacilli vary in their sensitivity: the *Bacteroides fragilis* group is resistant as the result of β-lactamase action, but many *Prevotella* and *Fusobacterium* spp. are susceptible.

Benzylpenicillin exhibits concentration-dependent bactericidal activity against growing organisms. Killing of highly susceptible Gram-positive cocci seldom proceeds to eradication, with measurable numbers of survivors ('persisters'), which are fully susceptible on retesting. Some strains of streptococci (including group B) and pneumococci show very large numbers of persisters, resulting in a large difference between the minimum inhibitory concentration (MIC) and the minimum bactericidal concentration (MBC), a phenomenon known as 'tolerance'.

Combination with aminoglycosides results in pronounced bactericidal synergy.

ACQUIRED RESISTANCE

Staph. aureus was originally highly susceptible to benzylpenicillin, but at least 85–90% of clinical isolates are now β-lactamase-producing strains. Most clinical isolates of coagulase-negative staphylococci are also resistant. β-Lactamase-producing strains of *E. faecalis* produce an enzyme identical to staphylococcal penicillinases, but these strains are increasingly uncommon. The emergence of penicillin-resistant staphylococci, enterococci and pneumococci, due to the acquisition of mosaic PBPs with decreased binding affinity for penicillin, has been described worldwide. Most strains of penicillin-resistant Gram-positive clinical isolates also demonstrate reduced susceptibility to other β-lactam agents but, in rare cases, cross-resistance is not seen for all cephalosporins.

Strains of *N. gonorrhoeae* for which the MIC of benzylpenicillin increased from 0.06 mg/L to >2 mg/L appeared in the 1970s, as the result of the production of modified PBPs with reduced affinity for β-lactam antibiotics; fully resistant strains producing TEM-1 β-lactamase also emerged. Currently penicillin resistance occurs in more than 60% of isolates in some parts of the world.

PHARMACOKINETICS

Oral absorption	2–25%
C_{max} 0.6 g intramuscular	12 mg/L
3 g intravenous (3–5 min)	400 mg/L
Plasma half-life	0.5 h
Volume of distribution	0.2–0.7 L/kg
Plasma protein binding	60%

Absorption

Benzylpenicillin is unstable in acid and destroyed in the stomach. As a result, plasma concentrations obtained after oral administration are variable, and are depressed by administration with food. It is absorbed from serous cavities, joints and the subarachnoid space. It is not absorbed following applications to the skin, which should be avoided because of the likelihood of sensitization.

Distribution

The drug is widely distributed in most tissues and body fluids. Highest levels are found in the kidney, with lower levels in the liver, skin and intestines. Low concentrations appear in saliva and in maternal milk. It does not enter uninflamed bone or the CSF. Its entry is limited by its low pK_a (2.6), which results in its almost complete ionization and very low lipid–water partition coefficient at pH 7.4. When the meninges are inflamed, the concentrations obtained in CSF are around 5% of the plasma level. In uremia, accumulated organic acids may enter the CSF and compete for transport of penicillin, causing the concentration to reach convulsive levels.

It diffuses into wound exudates and experimental transudates when the serum level is high, and enters glandular secretions and the fetal circulation, whence it is excreted in increased concentrations into the amniotic fluid.

Metabolism and excretion

About 40% is metabolized in the liver, mainly to penicilloic acid. After oral dosing, unabsorbed drug is largely degraded by colonic bacteria and little activity remains in the feces. Concentrations 2–4 times those of the plasma are found in bile, but 60–90% is excreted in the urine, largely in the first hour. Probenecid causes a doubling of the peak concentration and prolongation of the plasma half-life. Other drugs, including aspirin, sulfonamides and some non-steroidal anti-inflammatory drugs and diuretics, may prolong the half-life.

TOXICITY AND SIDE EFFECTS

Benzylpenicillin has low toxicity, except for the nervous system (into which it does not normally penetrate), where it is one of the most active convulsants among the β-lactam agents. Excessively high intravenous doses may induce convulsions and intrathecal doses should never exceed 12 mg (20 000 units) in adults or 3 mg (5000 units) in a child as a single daily dose. Inadvertent intravascular administration, especially direct injection into arteries, can cause serious neurotoxic damage, including hyperreflexia, myoclonic twitches, seizures and coma.

Massive intravenous doses of the sodium or potassium salts can lead to severe or fatal electrolyte disturbances. In patients treated with large doses of the potassium salt (60 g or more per day), hyponatremia, hyperkalemia and metabolic acidosis can develop.

Thrombocytopenia and platelet dysfunction resulting in coagulopathy and involving several different mechanisms have been described. Neutropenia associated with fever and allergic rash appears to be related to total dose, usually in excess of 90 g. Although it can be very severe, in most patients recovery occurs within a few days of withdrawal of treatment.

Large doses (24 g [40 megaunits] per day intravenously), or smaller doses given to patients with impaired renal function, may interfere with platelet function.

The most dramatic untoward response is anaphylactic shock due to allergy (p. 202). In addition to the generalized allergic reactions, particular organs may be damaged by a variety of immunological mechanisms. Hemolytic anemia occurs only in patients who have been treated previously with penicillin, and again receive a prolonged course of large doses (commonly 12 g per day). Reversible hemolysis is due to the action of anti-penicillin immunoglobulin G (IgG) on cells that have absorbed the antibiotic. Nephritis, resulting in dysuria, pyuria, proteinuria, azotemia and histological evidence of nephritis of allergic origin, is only rarely seen, usually in patients receiving large doses (12–36 g [20–60 mega-units] per day).

CLINICAL USE

Serious infections caused by streptococci (including *Str. pneumoniae*) other than meningitis caused by penicillin-resistant pneumococci

Serious infections caused by susceptible strains of staphylococci

Meningococcal septicemia and meningitis

Gonococcal infections caused by susceptible strains

Syphilis (including neurosyphilis) and other spirochetal infections

Anthrax

Actinomycosis

Clostridial infections

Diphtheria (adjunctive therapy to antitoxin and for prevention of carrier state)

Infections with other susceptible organisms, including *Listeria monocytogenes*, *Pasteurella multocida*, *Erysipelothrix insidiosa* and *Fusobacterium*

Preparations and dosage

Proprietary names: Crystapen, Pfizerpen and numerous generic forms.
Preparation: Injection.

Dosage: Adults, i.m., i.v., 600 mg to 1.2 g per day in 2–4 divided doses; adult meningitis, up to 14.4 g per day may be given in divided doses; bacterial endocarditis, 4.8 g per day or more in divided doses. Children, 1 month to 18 years, 25 mg/kg every 6 h (50 mg/kg every 4–6 h in severe infection); neonates preterm or <7 days, 25 mg/kg every 12 h (double in severe infection), 7–28 days, 25 mg/kg every 8 h (double in severe infection). Meningitis in neonates and children: neonates ≤7 days old, 75 mg/kg every 8 h; neonates >7 days old, 90–120 mg/kg per day in three divided doses; children 1 month to 12 years, 150–300 mg/kg per day in 4–6 divided doses (maximum 2.4 g/dose). Intrathecal, see manufacturer's literature.

Widely available.

Further information

Anonymous. Penicillin G (sodium or potassium). In: Dollery C, ed. *Therapeutic Drugs*. 2nd ed. Edinburgh: Churchill Livingstone; 1999:P32–P36.

Ducas J, Robson HG. Cerebrospinal fluid penicillin levels during therapy for latent syphilis. *J Am Med Assoc*. 1981;246:2583–2584.

Hovhannisyan G, von Schoen-Angerer T, Babayan K, Fenichiu O, Gaboulaud V. Antimicrobial susceptibility of *Neisseria gonorrhoeae* strains in three regions of Armenia. *Sex Transm Dis*. 2007;34:686–688.

Kim KS. Clinical perspectives on penicillin tolerance. *J Pediatr*. 1988;112:509–514.

Nicholls PJ. Neurotoxicity of penicillin. *J Antimicrob Chemother*. 1980;6:161–164.

Overbosch D, van Gulpen C, Hermans J, Mattie H. The effect of probenecid on the renal tubular excretion of benzylpenicillin. *Br J Clin Pharmacol*. 1988;25:51–58.

Schoth PE, Welters EC. Penicillin concentration in serum and CSF during high-dose intravenous treatment for neurosyphilis. *Neurology*. 1987;37:1214–1216.

Sullivan TJ. Cardiac disorders in penicillin-induced anaphylaxis. Association with intravenous epinephrine therapy. *J Am Med Assoc*. 1982;248:2116–2162.

COMPOUNDS LIBERATING BENZYLPENICILLIN

Antimicrobial activity and systemic effects of the long-acting forms are due to the liberation of benzylpenicillin. Intramuscular injection, particularly of benzathine penicillin, may produce local pain or tenderness, and accidental intravascular injection of procaine penicillin may produce acute agitation, hallucinations and collapse.

Long-acting forms have their principal use in the treatment of gonorrhea and syphilis, and in the follow-on treatment of patients requiring prolonged therapy after initial treatment with benzylpenicillin. They are also used in the prophylaxis of rheumatic fever.

BENZATHINE PENICILLIN

N, N′-dibenzolylethylene diamine dipenicillin salt of benzylpenicillin. It is poorly soluble (1:6000) in water. Available as an intramuscular preparation and in various mixtures with benzyl- and procaine penicillins. It has a local anesthetic effect comparable with that of procaine penicillin.

It is slowly absorbed after intramuscular injection, yielding very low plasma concentrations: a dose of 1.2 mega-units produces mean plasma concentrations of 0.1/0.02/0.002 mg/L 1, 2 and 4 weeks after injection.

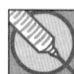

Preparations and dosage

Proprietary name: Permapen.
Preparation: Intramuscular injection.
Dosage: Varies according to infection being treated.

Limited availability; not available in the UK.

Further information

Kaplan EL, Berries X, Speth J, Siefferman T, Guzman B, Quesny F. Pharmacokinetics of benzathine penicillin G: serum levels during the 28 days after intramuscular injection of 1 200 000 units. *J Pediatr*. 1989;115:146–150.

Peter G, Dudley MN. Clinical pharmacology of benzathine penicillin G. *Pediatr Infect Dis*. 1985;4:586–591.

CLEMIZOLE PENICILLIN

A long-acting preparation of benzylpenicillin with the antihistamine, clemizole, given by deep intramuscular injection. It is of very limited availability.

PROCAINE PENICILLIN

The procaine salt of benzylpenicillin. Poorly soluble (1:200 in water). Administered intramuscularly as a suspension of crystals which slowly dissolve at the site of the injection.

It must not be given intravenously. Intramuscular administration produces a flat sustained plasma concentration of penicillin, which is much lower than that achieved by an equivalent dose of benzylpenicillin, with plasma levels still detectable 24 h later. An injection of 0.6 g yields a peak plasma concentration of 1–2 mg benzylpenicillin/L after 2–4 h. Free procaine is detectable in the plasma within 30 min.

Very severe and potentially fatal reactions resembling those of anaphylactic shock, but non-allergic in character, may occur, probably due to accidental entry into the vascular system at the site of injection and blockage of pulmonary and cerebral capillaries by crystals of the suspension. Reactions due to liberated procaine may include acute anxiety, hypertension, tachycardia, vomiting, audiovisual hallucinations and acute psychotic disturbance. The most severe reactions lead to convulsions and cardiac arrest. Other reactions are those to liberated benzylpenicillin.

Preparations and dosage

Proprietary names: Bicillin and numerous generic forms.

Preparation: Intramuscular injection.

Dosage: Adults, i.m., 300 mg (plus 60 mg benzylpenicillin) every 12–24 h. Widely available. No longer available in UK.

Further information

Shann F, Linnemann V, Gratten M. Serum concentration of penicillin after intramuscular administration of procaine, benzyl and benethamine penicillin in children with pneumonia. *J Pediatr*. 1987;110:299–302.

Silber TJ, D'Angelo L. Psychosis and seizures following the injection of penicillin G procaine. *Am J Dis Child*. 1985;139:335–337.

GROUP 2: ORALLY ABSORBED PENICILLINS RESEMBLING BENZYLPENICILLIN

The first natural penicillin to be identified as a useful oral agent was phenoxymethylpenicillin (penicillin V), produced by the addition of phenoxyacetic acid as a precursor in the fermentation. Penicillin V is more acid stable than benzylpenicillin and is absorbed after oral administration, producing therapeutically useful plasma penicillin concentrations. After the identification of the penicillin nucleus, 6-APA, a number of penicillin V analogs were developed, with claims for superior oral absorption characteristics. The most important of these semisynthetic penicillins were phenethicillin (the immediate homolog of penicillin V) and propicillin, which were both successful in the clinic, but are no longer readily available. Other orally active penicillins of this type include phenbenicillin (phenoxybenzylpenicillin) and azidocillin (D-azidobenzylpenicillin).

The phenoxypenicillins exhibit lower activity than benzylpenicillin against Gram-positive cocci and are distinctly less active against Gram-negative bacteria. All group 2 penicillins lack stability to β-lactamase.

In general, the absorption efficiency of these compounds increases in parallel with molecular weight. The peak plasma levels obtained from the phenoxypenicillins are well in excess of those required to inhibit the organisms for which benzylpenicillin is normally used.

Phenoxymethylpenicillin is the only member of this group to be considered here. Most of the related compounds are now obsolete.

PHENOXYMETHYLPENICILLIN

Penicillin V. Molecular weight (free acid): 350.4; (potassium salt): 388.5.

A naturally occurring penicillin produced by *P. chrysogenum* in media containing phenoxyacetic acid as a precursor. It is supplied as the potassium salt for oral administration.

ANTIMICROBIAL ACTIVITY

The antibacterial spectrum and level of activity are similar to that of benzylpenicillin (Table 14.2). Enteric Gram-negative bacilli are highly resistant.

PHARMACOKINETICS

Oral absorption	40–70%
C_{max} 250 mg oral	2 mg/L after 1 h
Plasma half-life	c. 0.5 h
Volume of distribution	0.2 L/kg
Plasma protein binding	80%

Absorption

Owing to acid stability, it is not destroyed in the stomach, but absorption is variable, about 30% remaining in the feces. Absorption is better after administration in the fasting state.

Metabolism and excretion

It is fairly extensively metabolized and degraded in the bowel. Some 60% of the dose is excreted in the urine, 25% in the unchanged form and the remainder as metabolites.

TOXICITY AND SIDE EFFECTS

Those common to penicillins (pp. 202–203). As with all penicillins, patients with a history of hypersensitivity to penicillins should be treated cautiously, as serious anaphylactic responses may occur.

CLINICAL USE

It may be prescribed for many indications for which benzylpenicillin is suitable, including streptococcal pharyngitis and skin sepsis, but is not recommended for initial therapy of serious infections. It is useful for continuation therapy after initial control of the disease by parenteral benzylpenicillin when prolonged treatment is required. It has been used prophylactically in recurrent pneumococcal meningitis after head injury and in rheumatic fever. It is not appropriate for infections caused by *H. influenzae* or Gram-negative bacteria, and is not recommended for the treatment of gonorrhea, syphilis or leptospirosis.

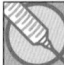

Preparations and dosage

Proprietary names: Numerous generic forms.

Preparations: Tablets, oral solution.

Dosage: Adults, oral, 250–500 mg every 6 h. Doses can be doubled. Children <1 year, 62.5 mg every 6 h; children 1–5 years, 125 mg every 6 h; children 6–12 years, 250 mg every 6 h.

Widely available.

Further information

Anonymous. Penicillin V (potassium). In: Dollery C, ed. *Therapeutic Drugs*. 2nd ed. Edinburgh: Churchill Livingstone; 1999:P36–P38.

Leung AK, Kellner JD. Group A beta-hemolytic streptococcal pharyngitis in children. *Adv Ther*. 2004;21:277–287.

Overbosch D, Mattie H, vanFurth R. Comparative pharmacodynamics and clinical pharmacokinetics of phenoxymethyl penicillin and pheneticillin. *Br J Clin Pharmacol*. 1985;19:657–668.

GROUP 3: ANTISTAPHYLOCOCCAL β-LACTAMASE-STABLE PENICILLINS

The members of this group include methicillin, nafcillin and four isoxazolylpenicillins: oxacillin, cloxacillin, dicloxacillin and flucloxacillin. All have less intrinsic microbiological activity than benzylpenicillin, but they are stable to staphylococcal β-lactamase and, as a result, display improved activity against penicillinase-producing strains of *Staph. aureus*. Oxacillin is rather less stable to hydrolysis by staphylococcal β-lactamase than the other compounds, with the order of stability: methicillin >nafcillin >cloxacillin, dicloxacillin and flucloxacillin >oxacillin.

Methicillin has been replaced in clinical practice because of low activity, poor oral absorption and a propensity to cause interstitial nephritis. Cloxacillin and flucloxacillin are used clinically in Europe and elsewhere, whereas nafcillin, oxacillin and dicloxacillin are preferred in North America.

ANTIMICROBIAL ACTIVITY

The compounds are active against staphylococci, streptococci, gonococci and meningococci but have no useful activity against enterococci, *H. influenzae* or enterobacteria (Table 14.3).

ACQUIRED RESISTANCE

The prevalence of strains of *Staph. aureus* resistant to methicillin (MRSA; pp. 35–36) has risen rapidly. Although MRSA and other methicillin-resistant staphylococci produce large amounts of β-lactamase, resistance is due primarily to the

Table 14.3 Activity of group 3 penicillins against susceptible strains of pathogenic bacteria: modal MIC (mg/L)

	Cloxacillin[a]	Methicillin	Nafcillin
Staphylococcus aureus (methicillin-susceptible)	0.25	1	0.1
Staph. epidermidis	0.25	1	0.1
Streptococcus pyogenes	0.06	0.25	0.06
Str. pneumoniae	0.12	0.25	0.1
Enterococcus faecalis	16	16–32	16
Neisseria gonorrhoeae	0.1	0.1–0.5	2
N. meningitidis	0.25	0.25	8
Haemophilus influenzae	8–16	2	4
Escherichia coli	R	R	R
Klebsiella pneumoniae	R	R	R
Pseudomonas aeruginosa	R	R	R
Bacteroides fragilis	R	R	R

[a]Activities of dicloxacillin, flucloxacillin and oxacillin are similar.
R, resistant (MIC >64 mg/L).

acquisition of the supplementary PBP 2a with low affinity for methicillin and almost all other β-lactam antibiotics. The bacterial population may be heterogeneous in its response to β-lactam compounds, and only a small minority of cells may appear to be resistant in conventional media. The population can be rendered homogeneously resistant by growth either at 30°C or in a medium containing an excess of electrolytes, such as 5% NaCl; or by lowering the pH. For these reasons, standard susceptibility testing may not detect MRSA and the use of large inocula plus media supplemented with NaCl and/ or incubation at 30°C is recommended. Oxacillin is the penicillin of choice for detection of these strains, although the use of the cephamycin cefoxitin (p. 181) may also increase testing sensitivity.

MRSA are resistant to almost all β-lactam agents, including imipenem and meropenem, and many isolates are also resistant to other antistaphylococcal antibiotics, with the exception of vancomycin and the related glycopeptide teicoplanin. Some newer agents, including quinupristin–dalfopristin (p. 334), linezolid (p. 301), daptomycin (p. 361) and tigecycline (p. 354) include MRSA in their spectrum of activity.

PHARMACOKINETICS

Methicillin is the most metabolically stable and least protein bound of the group 3 penicillins. Nafcillin is relatively acid labile and poorly and variably absorbed when dosed orally. Isoxazolylpenicillins are absorbed from the gut to varying degrees, although they are all absorbed considerably better than nafcillin. The mean peak plasma levels of cloxacillin are about twice those resulting from similar doses of oxacillin; those of dicloxacillin and flucloxacillin are about twice those of cloxacillin. Plasma levels are depressed when they are given with food.

Oxacillin is metabolized to a greater extent than dicloxacillin or flucloxacillin. All are highly protein bound. Levels obtained by intravenous bolus injection of isoxazolylpenicillins are higher than those produced by the extensively metabolized nafcillin, but this advantage is offset by their higher protein binding. Overall, dicloxacillin and flucloxacillin are superior to oxacillin and cloxacillin for oral administration. Flucloxacillin is better absorbed and provides more unbound drug than dicloxacillin.

They are widely distributed in the extracellular fluid and serous fluids, but as highly protein-bound agents their access to blister fluid is limited, though their persistence there is prolonged. They do not enter normal CSF, but their entry is somewhat erratically increased by inflammation, nafcillin penetrating better than others.

Little of these drugs appears in the bile, and they are excreted principally unchanged in the urine by both glomerular filtration and tubular secretion to produce very high urinary levels. Plasma half-lives are prolonged by probenecid and in the newborn and, with the exception of oxacillin, in renal failure. Patients with cystic fibrosis clear the drugs unusually rapidly.

TOXICITY AND SIDE EFFECTS

As with all penicillins, serious anaphylactic responses may occur, but acute anaphylaxis is much less common than with benzylpenicillin. Most side effects are similar to those observed for other penicillins. Pseudomembranous colitis has been reported. Renal damage (generally reversible) has been described, usually in patients receiving large doses.

CLINICAL USE

The only, but important, therapeutic use for these agents is in the treatment of proven staphylococcal infection or (usually in combination therapy) where staphylococcal infection is suspected, and the causative organism is susceptible to the agent. The oral drugs are valuable in the treatment of staphylococcal infections of soft tissues and as continuation therapy in infections of bone and joints. Empirical penicillin usage should be avoided in regions with high MRSA infection rates.

Further information

Abbanat D, Macielag M, Bush K. Novel antibacterial agents for the treatment of serious Gram-positive infections. *Expert Opin Investig Drugs*. 2003;12:379–399.

Rayner C, Munckhof WJ. Antibiotics currently used in the treatment of infections caused by *Staphylococcus aureus*. *Intern Med J*. 2005;35(suppl 2):S3–S16.

CLOXACILLIN

Molecular weight (free acid): 435.9.

A semisynthetic isoxazolylpenicillin supplied as the sodium salt for oral or parenteral administration.

ANTIMICROBIAL ACTIVITY

Cloxacillin is active against most Gram-positive cocci, but *E. faecalis* is relatively resistant (Table 14.3). It inhibits β-lactamase-producing strains of staphylococci (MIC 0.1–0.25 mg/L), but is not active against MRSA. Other susceptible bacteria include *N. gonorrhoeae*, *N. meningitidis* and Gram-positive anaerobes (MIC 0.1–0.25 mg/L). *H. influenzae*,

Enterobacteriaceae and *Ps. aeruginosa* are resistant, as are Gram-negative anaerobes. The compound is highly bound to serum protein and activity in vitro is substantially diminished in the presence of serum.

ACQUIRED RESISTANCE

Cloxacillin exhibits complete cross-resistance with other group 3 penicillins. Penicillin-tolerant strains are also tolerant to cloxacillin.

PHARMACOKINETICS

Oral absorption	40–60%
C_max 500 mg oral	8 mg/L (fasting) after 1 h
500 mg intramuscular	15 mg/L after 0.5–1 h
Plasma half-life	0.5 h
Plasma protein binding	93–95%

Absorption and distribution

Cloxacillin is moderately well absorbed by mouth but absorption is depressed by food. Being highly protein bound, it diffuses poorly into normal interstitial fluid, serous cavities and CSF, but enters pus and inflamed bones and joints. It crosses the placenta.

Metabolism and excretion

Some inactivation occurs in the liver and about 10% of the plasma content is in the form of metabolites.

About 10% of an oral dose is excreted in the bile, but the main route of excretion is renal. Around 30% of an oral dose and 40–60% of an intramuscular dose appears in the urine as active antibiotic, with 10–20% in the form of metabolites. Excretion is by both glomerular filtration and tubular secretion and is depressed by probenecid, which elevates and prolongs the plasma concentration. Excretion is impaired in renal failure and there is some accumulation of metabolites.

TOXICITY AND SIDE EFFECTS

In addition to hypersensitivity common to penicillins, nausea and diarrhea may occur on oral dosage, but are usually mild. Other effects are similar to those of benzylpenicillin.

CLINICAL USES

Clinical uses are those of group 3 penicillins (p. 209).

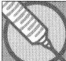

Preparations and dosage

Proprietary names: Orbenin (and other generic formulations).
Preparations: Capsules, injection, oral solution.
Dosage: Adults, oral, 250–500 mg every 6 h; i.m, i.v., 250–500 mg every 4–6 h, the dose may be doubled in severe infections. Children <2 years, all routes, quarter adult dose; children 2–12 years, all routes, half adult dose.
Widely available; not available in the UK.

Further information

Bergeron MG, Desaulnier SD, Lessard C, et al. Concentrations of fusidic acid, cloxacillin and cefamandole in sera and atrial appendages of patients undergoing cardiac surgery. *Antimicrob Agents Chemother.* 1985;27:928–932.
Spino M, Chai RP, Isles AF, et al. Cloxacillin absorption and disposition in cystic fibrosis. *J Pediatr.* 1984;105:829–835.

DICLOXACILLIN

Molecular weight (free acid): 470.4.

A semisynthetic isoxazolylpenicillin which differs from cloxacillin by an additional chlorine atom. It is supplied as the sodium monohydrate for oral administration.

ANTIMICROBIAL ACTIVITY

Its activities are generally similar to those of other isoxazolylpenicillins (Table 14.2). It is very highly bound to serum protein, and its activity in the presence of human serum in vitro is depressed to a greater extent than that of other isoxazolylpenicillins.

PHARMACOKINETICS

Oral absorption	c. 50%
C_max 250 mg oral	9 mg/L after 1 h
500 mg intramuscular	14–16 mg/L after 0.5–1 h
Plasma half-life	0.5 h
Plasma protein binding	95–97%

Absorption

Absorption in the very young is poor and unpredictable.

Metabolism and excretion

Dicloxacillin is partly metabolized in the liver and about 10% of the circulating drug is in the form of metabolites. Some 50–70% of a dose is excreted in the urine, about 20% as metabolites. It is eliminated both in the glomerular filtrate and by tubular secretion, and plasma concentrations are raised by probenecid. Parent drug and increased proportions of metabolites accumulate in renal failure. Elimination is increased through enhanced tubular secretion in patients with cystic fibrosis.

TOXICITY AND CLINICAL USE

Phlebitis is common after intravenous injection. Its toxicity is otherwise similar to that of other penicillins (pp. 202–203). Clinical uses are those of the group 3 penicillins (p. 209).

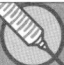

Preparations and dosage

Proprietary names: Diclocil.

Preparations: Capsules, oral suspension.

Dosage: Adults, oral, 125–250 mg every 6 h. Children, oral, 12.5–25 mg/kg per day in divided doses. Doses can be doubled in severe infections. Available in continental Europe and the USA.

Further information

Lofgren S, Bucht G, Hermansson B, Holm SE, Winblad B, Norrby SR. Single-dose pharmacokinetics of dicloxacillin in healthy subjects of young and old age. *Scand J Infect Dis*. 1986;18:365–369.

Pacifici GM, Viani A, Taddeuchi-Brunelli G, Rizzo G, Carrai M. Plasma protein binding of dicloxacillin: effects of age and disease. *Int J Clin Pharmacol Ther Toxicol*. 1987;25:622–626.

FLUCLOXACILLIN

Floxacillin. Molecular weight (free acid): 453.9; (sodium salt): 494.9.

A semisynthetic isoxazolylpenicillin that differs from dicloxacillin by the substitution of a fluorine atom for a chlorine atom. It is supplied as the sodium salt for oral or parenteral administration and as a suspension of the magnesium salt in a syrup formulation.

ANTIMICROBIAL ACTIVITY

Its antibacterial activity is almost identical to that of cloxacillin (Table 14.3). There is complete cross-resistance with other penicillinase-stable penicillins.

PHARMACOKINETICS

Oral absorption	c. 80%
C_{max} 250 mg (oral)	11 mg/L after 0.5–1 h
Plasma half-life	2 h
Plasma protein binding	95%

Absorption and distribution

It is well absorbed after oral administration and penetrates rapidly into extravascular exudates. Its high protein binding limits its diffusion, notably into the normal CSF.

Metabolism and excretion

Flucloxacillin is partly metabolized in the liver and about 10% of the plasma concentration is made up of metabolites. It is more slowly eliminated than cloxacillin. Some appears in the bile but about 50–80% of an oral dose is recovered from the urine, about 20% as metabolites.

TOXICITY AND SIDE EFFECTS

In patients treated by intravenous infusion, about 5% developed phlebitis by the first and 15% by the second day, after which the proportion rose dramatically. Side effects are otherwise those common to penicillins (pp. 202–203).

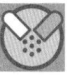

CLINICAL USE

Uses are those of group 3 penicillins (p. 209).

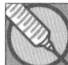

Preparations and dosage

Proprietary name: Floxapen.

Preparations: Capsules, oral solution, injection.

Dosage: Adults, oral, i.m., i.v., 500 mg to 1 g every 6 h, the dose may be doubled in severe infections. Endocarditis, 12 g per day in six divided doses. Children <2 years, any route, quarter adult dose; children 2–10 years, any route, half adult dose.

Widely available; not available in the USA.

Further information

Anonymous. Floxacillin (sodium). In: Dollery C, ed. *Therapeutic Drugs*. 2nd ed. Edinburgh: Churchill Livingstone; 1999:F57–F62.

Basker MJ, Edmondson RA, Sutherland R. Comparative stabilities of penicillins and cephalosporins to staphylococcal β-lactamase and activities against *Staph aureus*. *J Antimicrob Chemother*. 1980;6:333–341.

Bergan T, Engeset A, Olszewski W, Ostby N, Solberg R. Extravascular penetration of highly protein-bound flucloxacillin. *Antimicrob Agents Chemother*. 1986;30:729–732.

Bergdahl S, Eriksson M, Finkel Y. Plasma concentration following oral administration of di- and flucloxacillin in infants and children. *Pharmacol Toxicol*. 1987;60:233–234.

NAFCILLIN

Molecular weight (free acid): 414.4.

A semisynthetic penicillin supplied as the sodium salt for parenteral use.

 ANTIMICROBIAL ACTIVITY

The antibacterial spectrum is similar to that of the isoxazolylpenicillins but it is more active against streptococci and pneumococci (Table 14.3, p. 208). Activity in vitro is depressed in the presence of serum. It is more stable than the isoxazolylpenicillins to staphylococcal β-lactamase. There is complete cross-resistance with other group 3 penicillins.

 PHARMACOKINETICS

Oral absorption	c. 35%
C_max 1 g intramuscular	8 mg/L after 1 h
500 mg intravenous	30 mg/L after 5 min
Plasma half-life	0.5 h
Plasma protein binding	90%

Absorption and distribution

Nafcillin is poorly absorbed after oral administration, and absorption is further depressed if the drug is given with food. Most dosing is now intravenous. Penetration into tissues is similar to that of the isoxazolylpenicillins. Penetration into normal meninges is low, but is higher in inflamed meninges.

Metabolism and excretion

About 60–70% is inactivated in the liver. Following intramuscular administration, about 30% appears in the urine, producing concentrations up to 1000 mg/L. Administration of probenecid reduces the urinary excretion and raises and prolongs the plasma level. About 8% of the dose is excreted in the bile.

 TOXICITY AND SIDE EFFECTS

There is cross-allergenicity with other penicillins. Its side effects are similar to the penicillins. Pseudomembranous colitis has been reported.

 CLINICAL USE

Uses are those of group 3 penicillins (p. 209). Nafcillin has been particularly recommended for the treatment of staphylococcal bacteremia caused by susceptible strains.

Preparations and dosage

Proprietary name: Nallpen.

Preparation: Injection.

Dosage: Adults, i.m., i.v., 0.5–1.5 g every 4–6 h. Children, 25 mg/kg every 12 h; neonates, 10 mg/kg every 12 h.

Available in the USA.

 Further information

Banner W, Gooch WM, Burckart G, Korones SB. Pharmacokinetics of nafcillin in infants with low birth weights. *Antimicrob Agents Chemother*. 1980;17:691–694.

Paradisi F, Corti G, Messeri D. Antistaphylococcal (MSSA, MRSA, MSSE, MRSE) antibiotics. *Med Clin North Am*. 2001;85:1–17.

Stevens DL. The role of vancomycin in the treatment paradigm. *Clin Infect Dis*. 2006;42(suppl 1):S51–S57.

OXACILLIN

Molecular weight (free acid): 401.5.

A semisynthetic penicillin currently supplied primarily for intravenous administration. The first of the isoxazolyl series of β-lactamase-resistant penicillins.

ANTIMICROBIAL ACTIVITY

Its spectrum and activity are those of isoxazolylpenicillins (Table 14.3, p. 208). There is complete cross-resistance and tolerance with other group 3 penicillins. Oxacillin is frequently used to replace methicillin for standardized susceptibility testing to detect resistant staphylococci.

ACQUIRED RESISTANCE

In addition to methicillin-resistant strains producing the low affinity PBP 2a, rare methicillin-susceptible isolates of *Staph. aureus* display reduced susceptibility to oxacillin, due to incompletely defined chromosomal resistance mechanisms.

PHARMACOKINETICS

Oral absorption	30–35%
C$_{max}$ 500 mg intravenous	43 mg/L after 5 min
Plasma half-life	20–30 min
Plasma protein binding	92–96%

Absorption and distribution

It is the least well absorbed of the isoxazolylpenicillins when dosed orally. It is widely distributed at therapeutic levels into pleural, bile and amniotic fluid. Low concentrations penetrate the CSF.

Metabolism and excretion

Oxacillin is rapidly metabolized by opening of the β-lactam ring. Its main route of elimination is renal, about 25% of the dose being recovered from the urine as active material and another 25% as inactive metabolites. It is more rapidly eliminated in patients with cystic fibrosis.

TOXICITY AND SIDE EFFECTS

There is cross-allergy with other penicillins and reactions are generally typical of the group. Abnormalities of liver function, especially elevation of transaminase levels, may occur, sometimes accompanied by fever, nausea, vomiting and eosinophilia. As with benzylpenicillin, neurotoxicity may develop on high dosage in patients with renal failure. Pseudomembranous colitis has been reported

CLINICAL USE

Uses are those of group 3 penicillins (p. 209).

Preparations and dosage

Proprietary names: Bristopen and various other generic formulation.
Preparations: Injection.
Dosage: Adults, i.m., i.v., 250 mg to 1 g every 4–6 h. Children (<40 kg), 12.5–25 mg/kg every 4–6 h. Newborn and premature infants, 25 mg/kg per day in divided doses may be given, but used with caution.
Available widely in continental Europe, North America, South America and Japan. Not available in the UK.

Further information

Clinical and Laboratory Standards Institute. *Methods for dilution antimicrobial susceptibility tests for bacteria that grow aerobically. Approved standard – Eighth edition.* Vol. M07-A8. Wayne, PA: CLSI; 2009.

McDougal LK, Thornsberry C. The role of β-lactamase in staphylococcal resistance to penicillinase-resistant penicillins and cephalosporins. *J Clin Microbiol.* 1986;23:832–839.

Venglarcik JS, Blair LL, Dunkle LM. pH-dependent oxacillin tolerance of *Staphylococcus aureus. Antimicrob Agents Chemother.* 1983;23:232–235.

OTHER GROUP 3 PENICILLINS

METHICILLIN

2,6-Dimethoxyphenylpenicillin; methicillin (international non-proprietary name). The first β-lactamase-resistant semisynthetic penicillin. It was initially used widely but has been superseded by other group 3 members and is no longer commercially available.

It is less active than benzylpenicillin or other group 3 penicillins (Table 14.3, p. 208). It is very stable to staphylococcal β-lactamase and is active against β-lactamase-producing strains of *Staph. aureus* that do not produce a functional PBP 2a (p. 30). Resistance is common among staphylococci, with the incidence geographically diverse. Most methicillin-resistant staphylococcal isolates display multiresistance.

It is not acid resistant, and must therefore be administered parenterally. About 10% is metabolized, with 60–80% of the dose excreted in the urine. Toxicity is similar to that of other group 3 penicillins. Nephritis appears to be more common than with other penicillins.

Further information

Boucher HW, Corey GR. Epidemiology of methicillin-resistant *Staphylococcus aureus. Clin Infect Dis.* 2008;46(suppl 5):S344–S349.

Leclercq R. Epidemiological and resistance issues in multidrug-resistant staphylococci and enterococci. *Clin Microbiol Infect.* 2009;15:224–231.

Struelens MJ, Hawkey PM, French GL, Witte W, Tacconelli E. Laboratory tools and strategies for methicillin-resistant *Staphylococcus aureus* screening, surveillance and typing: state of the art and unmet needs. *Clin Microbiol Infect.* 2009;15:112–119.

GROUP 4: EXTENDED-SPECTRUM PENICILLINS

The introduction of an amino group in the α-position of the side chain of benzylpenicillin confers a high degree of acid stability together with enhanced activity against Gram-negative bacteria. Ampicillin, the first of the aminopenicillins to be developed, retains the activity of benzylpenicillin against Gram-positive cocci but exhibits increased activity against *H. influenzae* and certain non-β-lactamase-producing Gram-negative bacilli, notably *Escherichia coli*, *Salmonella enterica* serotypes, *Shigella* spp. and *Proteus mirabilis*. The aminopenicillins are readily inactivated by β-lactamases, but in combination with β-lactamase inhibitors (p. 239) they display enhanced activity against many β-lactamase-producing isolates.

The clinical success of ampicillin resulted in the development of a number of modified aminopenicillins with claims for superior properties. Compounds closely related structurally to ampicillin include amoxicillin and ciclacillin.

Amoxicillin differs from ampicillin in possessing a *p*-hydroxy group in the benzene ring of the side chain and has a spectrum of activity essentially identical to that of ampicillin, but is bactericidal to susceptible Gram-negative bacilli at rather lower concentrations. Amoxicillin with its superior absorption characteristics has largely displaced ampicillin for oral therapy, except against the enterococci.

The antibacterial activity of epicillin is virtually identical to that of ampicillin, while that of ciclacillin is substantially less. Neither of these agents is widely used.

Four esters of ampicillin (bacampicillin, lenampicillin, pivampicillin, talampicillin) were developed as prodrugs with oral absorption characteristics superior to those of the parent penicillin. The esters are lipophilic compounds that are devoid of antibacterial activity in their own right, but which are hydrolyzed by tissue esterases during absorption to liberate ampicillin. Two condensation products, hetacillin and metampicillin (formed by combination of ampicillin with acetone and formaldehyde, respectively), hydrolyze spontaneously to release ampicillin, but are no longer used clinically. The antibacterial activity of all these compounds is due solely to the ampicillin liberated.

Two other group 4 penicillins, mecillinam (amdinocillin) and its prodrug pivmecillinam, are structurally different from the aminopenicillins. Like other semisynthetic penicillins they are derived from 6-APA but differ in being 6-α-amidinopenicillanates rather than 6-α-acylaminopenicillanates. This is reflected in the antibacterial spectrum of mecillinam, which is atypical of the penicillins in displaying high activity against Gram-negative bacteria but poor activity against Gram-positive cocci. The mechanism of action of mecillinam differs from that of other penicillins in binding almost exclusively to PBP 2 (p. 13) in Gram-negative bacteria.

PHARMACOKINETICS

The aminopenicillins are acid stable and can be given orally. Ampicillin is the least well absorbed, about one-third of the dose appearing in the urine as active drug, and absorption is further reduced by food. The esters, ciclacillin and amoxicillin, are substantially better absorbed and not significantly affected by food, peak plasma levels generally being at least twice those achieved by equivalent doses of ampicillin. Plasma elimination half-lives are generally around 1 h and plasma protein binding is low (around 20%). Excretion is primarily renal, resulting in high concentrations of active antibiotic in urine; a proportion of an oral dose (10–20%) is metabolized in the liver and small amounts are found in the bile. The aminopenicillins may be administered by parenteral routes, but the esters are given only by mouth. Mecillinam is not absorbed by mouth but its pivaloyloxymethyl ester, pivmecillinam, is relatively well absorbed by the oral route.

TOXICITY AND SIDE EFFECTS

Patients with a history of hypersensitivity to penicillins should be treated cautiously, as serious anaphylactic responses may occur. Ampicillin appears to be less likely than benzylpenicillin to elicit true allergic reactions, but is much more likely to cause rashes that appear not to be of allergic origin, especially in patients with infectious mononucleosis or other lymphoid disorders. The prevalence of rashes in patients treated with amoxicillin is similar. Ampicillin esters naturally have the same potential to give rise to rashes.

Gastrointestinal side effects are relatively common in patients treated with oral ampicillin. Ampicillin esters, amoxicillin, ciclacillin and the ester of mecillinam are more likely to cause upper abdominal discomfort, nausea and vomiting, but are less likely, being better absorbed, to cause diarrhea. Upper abdominal symptoms are substantially ameliorated if the esters are taken with food. Liver function should be monitored in patients receiving prolonged courses, or in those in whom renal or hepatic function is impaired.

CLINICAL USE

Aminopenicillins are recommended for the wide range of infections that made ampicillin one of the most commonly prescribed agents, notably for urinary and respiratory infections, as well as for gastrointestinal infections caused by susceptible *Salmonella* spp. and *Shigella* spp. However, the increasing frequency of isolation of β-lactamase-producing pathogens has resulted in a reduction in the usefulness of aminopenicillins as monotherapy. This difficulty is overcome by combining ampicillin or amoxicillin with β-lactamase inhibitors (p. 239). Ampicillin and amoxicillin also have a role in the treatment of severe infections, including endocarditis, meningitis and septicemia, often in combination with other antibacterial agents, such as aminoglycosides. Mecillinam is suitable only for infections involving Gram-negative bacteria and should not be used where Gram-positive organisms may be implicated.

AMOXICILLIN

Amoxycillin. Molecular weight (free acid): 365.4; (trihydrate): 419.5.

Para-hydroxy ampicillin. Supplied as the trihydrate for oral administration and as the sodium salt for parenteral use. A formulation with clavulanic acid (co-amoxiclav) is also available (see p. 240).

 ## ANTIMICROBIAL ACTIVITY

The antibacterial spectrum is identical to that of ampicillin and there are few differences in antibacterial activity (Table 14.4). Like ampicillin, amoxicillin is unstable to most β-lactamases. It has useful activity against *Helicobacter pylori* (<1% resistance), and is included in most combination regimens for the treatment of *H. pylori* infections.

Table 14.4 Activity of group 4 penicillins against non-β-lactamase-producing strains of pathogenic bacteria; modal MIC (mg/L)

	Ampicillin	Amoxicillin	Mecillinam
Staphylococcus aureus (methicillin-susceptible)	1	0.1	128
Streptococcus pyogenes	0.03	0.01	2
Str. pneumoniae	0.02	0.02	2
Enterococcus faecalis	2	2	R
Neisseria gonorrhoeae	0.5	≤0.5	0.1
N. meningitidis	0.12–2	≤2	ND
Haemophilus influenzae	0.5	0.5	16
Escherichia coli	4	4	0.12
Klebsiella pneumoniae	R	R	0.25
Pseudomonas aeruginosa	R	R	R
Bacteroides fragilis	32	32	R

R, resistant (MIC >64 mg/L); ND, no data.

 ## ACQUIRED RESISTANCE

There is complete cross-resistance with ampicillin. Its action against many β-lactamase-producing strains can be restored by co-administration with β-lactamase inhibitors (p. 239).

 ## PHARMACOKINETICS

Oral absorption	75–90%
C_max 500 mg oral	5.5–7.6 mg/L after 1–2 h
500 mg intramuscular	c. 14 mg/L after 1–2 h
Plasma half-life	1 h
Volume of distribution	0.3 L/kg
Plasma protein binding	17–20%

Absorption and distribution

Oral absorption produces over twice the peak concentration achieved by comparable doses of ampicillin, allowing less frequent dosing intervals. Absorption is unaffected by food.

It is well-distributed in multiple body fluids, including pleural, peritoneal and middle ear fluid. It does not penetrate well into the CSF.

Metabolism and excretion

Some 10–25% is converted to the penicilloic acid. Between 50% and 70% of unchanged drug is recovered in the urine in the first 6 h after a dose of 250 mg. Plasma levels are elevated and prolonged by the administration of probenecid.

 ## TOXICITY AND SIDE EFFECTS

Amoxicillin is generally well tolerated, side effects being those common to penicillins, but including non-allergic rashes in patients with glandular fever. As the drug is well absorbed, diarrhea is generally infrequent and rarely sufficiently severe to require withdrawal of treatment.

CLINICAL USE

Isolates should be tested for susceptibility before use, especially for serious infections.

Ear, nose and throat infections other than pharyngitis, which may mask glandular fever

Tracheobronchitis, bronchitis, pneumonia

Genitourinary tract infections, including gonorrhea

Infections of skin and soft tissues due to streptococci and susceptible staphylococci

Helicobacter pylori infection (in combination with a proton pump inhibitor and at least one other antimicrobial agent such as clarithromycin)

Prophylaxis of endocarditis in patients undergoing dental treatment and other procedures

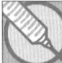

Preparations and dosage

Proprietary names: Amoxil (and many generic formulations).

Preparations: Capsules, suspension, injection, dispersible tablets, oral sachets.

Dosage: Adults, oral, 250–500 mg every 8 h high-dose therapy, 3 g every 12 h; short-course therapy, simple acute urinary tract infection, two 3 g doses with 10–12 h between doses, gonorrhea, single 3 g dose; i.m., i.v., 500 mg every 8 h, the dose may be increased to 1 g i.v. every 6 h in severe infections. Children up to 10 years, oral, 125–250 mg every 8 h. In severe otitis media, 750 mg every 12 h for 2 days may be used in children 3–10 years; i.m., i.v., 50–100 mg/kg per day in divided doses (increased to 180 mg/kg per day in severe infections). Widely available.

Further information

Anonymous. Amoxicillin. In: Dollery C, ed. *Therapeutic Drugs*. 2nd ed. Edinburgh: Churchill Livingstone; 1999:A162–A165.

Brogden RN, Speight TM, Avery GS. Amoxycillin: a review of its antibacterial and pharmacokinetic properties and therapeutic use. *Drugs*. 1975;9:88–140.

Egan BJ, Katicic M, O'Connor HJ, O'Morain CA. Treatment of *Helicobacter pylori*. *Helicobacter*. 2007;12(suppl 1):31–37.

Gordon C, Regamey C, Kirby WM. Comparative clinical pharmacology of amoxicillin and ampicillin administered orally. *Antimicrob Agents Chemother*. 1972;1:504–507.

Gould FK, Elliott TSJ, Foweraker J, et al. Guidelines for the prevention of endocarditis: report of the Working Party of the British Society for Antimicrobial Chemotherapy. *J Antimicrob Chemother*. 2006;57:1035–1042.

Mattie H, Van der Voet GB. The relative potency of amoxycillin and ampicillin in vitro and in vivo. *Scand J Infect Dis*. 1981;13:291–296.

AMPICILLIN

Molecular weight (free acid): 349.4; (sodium salt): 471.4.

A semisynthetic penicillin administered orally as the trihydrate and parenterally as the soluble sodium salt. Formulations with sulbactam are also available (see p. 242).

ANTIMICROBIAL ACTIVITY

Its activity against common pathogenic bacteria is shown in Table 14.4. Ampicillin is slightly less active than benzylpenicillin against most Gram-positive bacteria but is more active against *E. faecalis*. MRSA and strains of *Str. pneumoniae* with reduced susceptibility to benzylpenicillin are resistant. Most group D streptococci, anaerobic Gram-positive cocci and bacilli, including *L. monocytogenes*, *Actinomyces* spp. and *Arachnia* spp., are susceptible. Mycobacteria and nocardia are resistant.

Ampicillin has similar activity to benzylpenicillin against *N. gonorrhoeae*, *N. meningitidis* and *Mor. catarrhalis*. It is 2–8 times more active than benzylpenicillin against *H. influenzae* and many Enterobacteriaceae, but β-lactamase-producing strains are resistant. *Pseudomonas* spp. are resistant, but *Bordetella*, *Brucella*, *Legionella* and *Campylobacter* spp. are often susceptible. Certain Gram-negative anaerobes such as *Prevotella melaninogenica* and *Fusobacterium* spp. are susceptible, but *B. fragilis* is resistant, as are mycoplasmas and rickettsiae.

Activity against molecular class A β-lactamase-producing strains of staphylococci, gonococci, *H. influenzae*, *Mor. catarrhalis*, certain Enterobacteriaceae and *B. fragilis* is enhanced by the presence of β-lactamase inhibitors, specifically clavulanic acid.

Its bactericidal activity resembles that of benzylpenicillin. Bactericidal synergy occurs with aminoglycosides against *E. faecalis* and many enterobacteria, and with mecillinam against a number of ampicillin-resistant enterobacteria.

ACQUIRED RESISTANCE

β-Lactamase-producing pathogens, including most clinical isolates of *Staph. aureus*, are resistant. Strains of pneumococci, enterococci, gonococci and *H. influenzae* with altered PBPs have reduced susceptibility to ampicillin. Isolates of *N. gonorrhoeae* and *H. influenzae* with a TEM plasmid-mediated β-lactamase (which are more common) are fully resistant. Resistance among *H. influenzae* is often linked with resistance to chloramphenicol, erythromycin or tetracycline, due to plasmid-encoded resistance markers that are co-transferred with the gene for the TEM enzyme. However, at least 70% of current *H. influenzae* isolates remain susceptible to ampicillin worldwide.

The widespread use of ampicillin and other aminopenicillins has led to resistance becoming common in formerly susceptible species of enteric pathogens as a result of the widespread dissemination of plasmid-mediated β-lactamases. Surveillance data from North America and Europe indicate less than 50% susceptibility to ampicillin in *Esch. coli*. At least 90% of current isolates of *Mor. catarrhalis* are β-lactamase-producing strains. Ampicillin-resistant strains of salmonellae, notably *S. enterica* serotypes Typhi and Typhimurium (many of which are also resistant to chloramphenicol, sulfonamides and tetracyclines) present a serious problem in Africa, Asia and South America. Multiresistant strains of shigellae also predominate in many parts of the world.

PHARMACOKINETICS

Oral absorption	30–40%
C_{max} 500 mg oral	3.2 mg/L after c. 2 h
500 mg intramuscular	5–15 mg/L after 1 h
500 mg intravenous infusion	12–29 mg/L
Plasma half-life	1–1.5 h
Volume of distribution	0.38 L/kg
Plasma protein binding	20%

Absorption and distribution

Ampicillin is highly stable to acid: in 2 h at pH 2 and 37°C, only 5% of activity is lost. Absorption is impaired when it is given with meals.

It is distributed in the extracellular fluid. Adequate concentrations are obtained in serous effusions. Effective CSF levels are obtained only in the presence of inflammation, variable peak concentrations around 3 mg/L being found in the first 3 days of treatment in patients receiving 150 mg/kg per day. It accumulates and persists in the amniotic fluid.

Metabolism and excretion

A small proportion is converted to penicilloic acid. About 34% of an oral dose and 60–80% of parenteral doses are recoverable from the urine, where concentrations around 250–1000 mg/L appear. Excretion is partly in the glomerular filtrate and partly by tubular secretion, which can be blocked by probenecid. Impairment of renal function reduces the rate of excretion, the plasma half-life rising to 8–9 h in anuric patients.

Although excretion is mainly renal, up to 50 times the corresponding serum level may be attained in the bile. There is a degree of enterohepatic recirculation and significant quantities appear in the feces. Bioavailability may be affected in severe liver disease.

TOXICITY AND SIDE EFFECTS

Ampicillin is generally free from severe toxicity and, apart from gastrointestinal intolerance, the only significant side effects seen have been rashes. In common with other semisynthetic penicillins, it appears to be less likely than benzylpenicillin to elicit true allergic reactions. However, it is more likely to cause rashes, which are found in approximately 9% of treated patients and which occur more frequently in patients receiving large doses or in renal failure. Rashes occur in 95%

of patients with infectious mononucleosis or other lymphoid disorders. This unusual susceptibility disappears when the disease resolves. In keeping with a toxic rather than an allergic origin, skin tests to ampicillin and to mixed-allergen moieties of benzylpenicillin are negative. Since the typical maculopapular rash of ampicillin does not have an allergic origin, its development does not indicate penicillin allergy and is not a contraindication to the use of other penicillins.

Gastrointestinal side effects are relatively common (around 10%) in patients treated with oral ampicillin, and occur in 2–3% of patients given the drug parenterally, presumably as a result of drug entering the gut through the bile. The very young and the old are most likely to suffer. Diarrhea can be sufficiently severe to require withdrawal of treatment and pseudomembranous colitis may occur. Interference with the bowel flora, which is presumably implicated in diarrhea, can also affect enterohepatic recirculation of steroids, and the derangement can be sufficient to impair the absorption of oral contraceptives and affect the interpretation of estriol levels.

CLINICAL USE

Isolates should be tested for susceptibility before use, especially for serious infections. For oral therapy, amoxicillin is preferable to ampicillin.

Urinary tract infections
Bacterial meningitis
Respiratory tract infections
Gastrointestinal infections, including typhoid fever and bacillary dysentery
Enterococcal endocarditis and septicemia (in combination with an aminoglycoside)
Listeriosis (in combination with an aminoglycoside)

Preparations and dosage

Proprietary names: Penbritin, Omnipen and many generic preparations.
Preparations: Capsules, syrup, injection.
Dosage: Adults, oral, 250 mg to 1 g every 6 h; i.m., i.v., 500 mg every 4–6 h. Meningitis, i.v., 2 g every 4 h. Children <10 years, any route, half the adult dose. Meningitis, i.v., 150–200 mg/kg per day in divided doses.
Widely available.

Further information

Anonymous. Ampicillin. In: Dollery C, ed. *Therapeutic Drugs*. 2nd ed. Edinburgh: Churchill Livingstone; 1999:A172–A176.

Arias CA, Murray BE. Emergence and management of drug-resistant enterococcal infections. *Expert Rev Antiinfect Ther*. 2008;6:637–655.

Jacobs MR. Worldwide trends in antimicrobial resistance among common respiratory tract pathogens in children. *Pediatr Infect Dis J*. 2003;22(suppl 8):S109–S119.

Mazzulli T. Resistance trends in urinary tract pathogens and impact on management. *J Urol*. 2002;168(4 Part 2):1720–1722.

Mikhail IA, Sippel JF, Girgis NI, Yassin MW. Cerebrospinal fluid and serum ampicillin levels in bacterial meningitis patients after intravenous and intramuscular administration. *Scand J Infect Dis*. 1981;13:237–238.

Morrissey I, Maher K, Williams L, et al. Non-susceptibility trends among *Haemophilus influenzae* and *Moraxella catarrhalis* from community-acquired respiratory tract infections in the UK and Ireland, 1999–2007. *J Antimicrob Chemother*. 2008;62(suppl 2):ii97–ii103.

AMPICILLIN ESTERS

BACAMPICILLIN

The ethoxycarbonyloxyethyl ester of ampicillin. It is absorbed from the intestine more rapidly and more completely than ampicillin, with average peak plasma levels 2–3 times those produced by equivalent doses of ampicillin. Mean absorption differed considerably among hospital patients and was less than in healthy volunteers.

Preparations and dosage

Proprietary names: Various generic formulations.

Preparations: Tablets, oral suspension.

Dosage: Adults, oral, 400 mg, every 8–12 h; dose doubled in severe infections. Children >5 years, 200 mg every 8 h or 25–50 mg/kg per day in two divided doses.

Widely available; not available in the UK or the USA.

LENAMPICILLIN

The daloxate ester of ampicillin. In volunteers receiving 400 mg orally, peak concentrations were around 6.0 mg/L at about 1 h – about twice those seen with an equimolar dose (250 mg) of ampicillin. Peak plasma concentration is slightly lower and delayed by food.

PIVAMPICILLIN

The pivaloyloxymethyl ester of ampicillin. Its absorption is considerably better than that of the parent ampicillin and is less affected by food. Plasma levels rise more rapidly to 2–3 times those produced by corresponding doses of ampicillin.

TALAMPICILLIN

The phthalidyl thiazolidine carboxylic ester of ampicillin. It is well absorbed when administered orally, doses of 250 or 500 mg producing mean peak plasma levels of 4 or 11 mg/L, respectively, about 2 h after the dose. Administration with food delays and depresses the peak concentration. It is of limited commercial availability.

 Further information

Jones KH, Langley PF, Lees LJ. Bioavailability and metabolism of talampicillin. *Chemotherapy*. 1979;24:217–226.

Sjovall J. Tissue levels after administration of bacampicillin, a prodrug of ampicillin and comparisons with other aminopenicillins: a review. *J Antimicrob Chemother* 1981;8(suppl C):41–58.

Sum ZM, Sefton AM, Jepson AP, Williams JD. Comparative pharmacokinetic study between lenampicillin, bacampicillin and amoxycillin. *J Antimicrob Chemother*. 1989;23:861–868.

AMPICILLIN CONDENSATES

Hetacillin, a condensation product of ampicillin and acetone, and metampicillin, a condensation product of ampicillin and formaldehyde, hydrolyze rapidly in the body to liberate ampicillin, leaving little or none of the parent compound detectable in the plasma after oral dosing. For hetacillin, peak levels and excretion are reported to be lower than those for ampicillin. Their toxicity profiles are comparable to that of ampicillin. Both drugs are of very limited availability.

 Further information

Kahrimanis R, Pierpaoli P. Hetacillin vs ampicillin. *N Engl J Med*. 1971;285:236–237.

Sutherland R, Elson S, Croydon EA. Metampicillin: antibacterial activity and absorption and excretion in man. *Chemotherapy*. 1972;17:145–160.

MECILLINAM

Amdinocillin. Molecular weight (free acid): 325.4.

6-β-Amidinopenicillin. Supplied as the hydrochloride dihydrate for parenteral administration and as the hydrochloride salt of the pivaloyloxymethyl ester (pivmecillinam; amdinocillin pivoxil) for oral use.

ANTIMICROBIAL ACTIVITY

The antibacterial spectrum differs greatly from that of the aminopenicillins in that the compound displays high activity against many Gram-negative bacteria but limited activity against Gram-positive organisms (Table 14.4, p. 215). Mecillinam is active against many Enterobacteriaceae due to its selective binding to PBP 2, although the susceptibility of *Proteus* and *Providencia* spp. is variable. *H. influenzae* is less susceptible than enteric bacilli, and *Acinetobacter* spp., *B. fragilis* and *Ps. aeruginosa* are resistant.

It is readily inactivated by many β-lactamases, although it is more stable than ampicillin.

ACQUIRED RESISTANCE

Intrinsic resistance in susceptible species of enterobacteria is uncommon and many ampicillin-resistant strains are susceptible. Bacteria that are resistant to both ampicillin and mecillinam are usually those producing large amounts of β-lactamase, most commonly plasmid-mediated enzymes.

PHARMACOKINETICS

Oral absorption (pivmecillinam)	c. 75%
C_{max} 200 mg intravenous infusion	12 mg/L end infusion
200 mg intramuscular	c. 6 mg/L after 45 min
400 mg oral (pivmecillinam)	2–5 mg/L after c. 1 h
Plasma half-life	50 min
Volume of distribution	0.2–0.4 L/kg
Plasma protein binding	5–10%

Absorption

Oral absorption is very poor, with conventional doses producing plasma levels of <1 mg/L and recovery of only about 5% in the urine.

A 400 mg dose of the pivaloyl ester is equivalent to 273 mg mecillinam. It is relatively well absorbed and rapidly liberates the parent compound.

Metabolism and excretion

The amidino side chain undergoes spontaneous aqueous hydrolysis to the *N*-formyl derivative, which retains some antibacterial activity. Hydrolysis of the β-lactam ring also occurs.

Approximately 60% is excreted unchanged in the urine in the first 6 h, achieving concentrations exceeding 1 g/L. The concentration in bile can reach 40 or 50 mg/L in patients with normally functioning gallbladders treated with 800 mg intramuscularly.

TOXICITY AND SIDE EFFECTS

It is generally well tolerated, and serious anaphylactic responses are said to be rare. Nausea and vomiting, which may be persistent, occur with diarrhea in some patients treated with pivmecillinam.

CLINICAL USE

Urinary tract infection (pivmecillinam)
Other infections with susceptible Gram-negative bacilli (usually in combination with other agents)

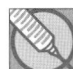

Preparations and dosage

Proprietary names: Selexid.

Preparations: Injection, suspension, tablets.

Dosage: Adults, mecillinam: 5–10 mg/kg every 6–8 h depending on the severity of the infection; pivmecillinam: 200–400 mg every 6–8 h.

Limited availability; pivmecillinam available in the UK.

Further information

Anonymous. Amdinocillin. In: Dollery C, ed. *Therapeutic Drugs.* 2nd ed.Edinburgh: Churchill Livingstone; 1999:A119–A122.
Patel IH, Bornemann LD, Brocks VM, Fang LST, Tolkoff-Rubin NE, Rubin RH. Pharmacokinetics of intravenous amdinocillin in healthy subjects and patients with renal insufficiency. *Antimicrob Agents Chemother.* 1985;28:46–50.
Symposium. An international review of amdinocillin: a new beta-lactam antibiotic. *Am J Med.* 1983;75(suppl):1–138.

OTHER GROUP 4 PENICILLINS

CICLACILLIN (CYCLACILLIN)

The structure differs from other aminopenicillins in that the benzene ring is completely saturated and the amino substituent is attached directly to it instead of being linked to an adjacent carbon atom. It is less active than ampicillin against staphylococci, streptococci and *H. influenzae*, but is better absorbed by mouth, peak plasma levels of 10–18 mg/L being reached after a 500 mg oral dose. Its pharmacokinetic properties, side effects and use resemble those of ampicillin. It has limited availability.

EPICILLIN

An analog of ampicillin in which the benzene ring is partially saturated. It closely resembles ampicillin in its antibacterial properties. It is moderately well absorbed, a 500 mg oral dose producing mean peak plasma levels of 2–3 mg/L. Its behavior on intramuscular injection, distribution, excretion, toxicity and uses resemble those of ampicillin. It is of very limited availability.

Further information

Gadebusch H, Miraglia G, Pansy F. Epicillin: experimental chemotherapy, pharmacodynamics and susceptibility testing. *Infect Immun.* 1971;4:50–53.
Gonzaga AJ, Antonio-Velmonte M, Tupasi TE. Cyclacillin: a clinical and in vitro profile. *J Infect Dis.* 1974;129:545–551.

GROUP 5: PENICILLINS ACTIVE AGAINST *PS. AERUGINOSA*

Certain derivatives of benzylpenicillin or ampicillin exhibit useful activity against *Ps. aeruginosa*. Three derivatives of benzylpenicillin possessing an acidic group in the acyl side chain were developed for clinical use: carbenicillin and ticarcillin are α-carboxypenicillins, and the third, sulbenicillin, possesses a sulfonic acid group in the side chain. Two oral prodrug forms of carbenicillin were formerly used: the phenyl ester, carfecillin, and the indanyl ester, carindacillin. The acyl derivatives of ampicillin active against *Ps. aeruginosa* include the acylureidopenicillins: azlocillin, mezlocillin and piperacillin. Apalcillin and aspoxicillin are also acylaminopenicillins, with properties generally similar to the ureidopenicillins, but lack the ureido group in the side chain. Only piperacillin and ticarcillin are now in widespread use.

 ## ANTIMICROBIAL ACTIVITY

The acylureidopenicillins and the carboxypenicillins display similar antibacterial spectra, but the ureidopenicillins are more active against streptococci and enterococci (Table 14.5). Both groups are as active as ampicillin against susceptible Gram-negative bacteria. However, strains producing elevated amounts of β-lactamase, such as those organisms with derepressed β-lactamase production, are resistant. Interest in these penicillins lies solely in their activity against *Ps. aeruginosa*. Apalcillin, azlocillin and piperacillin display greater activity in vitro than the carboxypenicillins. The superior activity of the ureidopenicillins against *Ps. aeruginosa* may be due to a combination of better penetration characteristics and greater affinity for PBPs. All these compounds exhibit reduced activity against *Bacteroides* spp.

 ## ACQUIRED RESISTANCE

Resistance in clinical isolates is due primarily to their hydrolysis by plasmid-encoded β-lactamases or by elevated levels of AmpC cephalosporinases found in many species of Enterobacteriaceae. Activity can often be restored by combinations with β-lactamase inhibitors; fixed combinations of ticarcillin with clavulanic acid (pp. 240–241) and piperacillin with tazobactam (p. 243) have been developed for clinical use.

 ## PHARMACOKINETICS

None of the compounds (other than the prodrugs of carbenicillin; *see above*) is orally absorbed.

The acylureidopenicillins produce peak plasma levels that are lower than those obtained with the carboxypenicillins. The half-lives and volumes of distribution of the ureidopenicillins are generally similar and increase with larger doses. Elimination from the body is largely by the renal route and most of the drug appears unchanged in the urine, but relatively high concentrations may appear in bile.

 ## CLINICAL USE

A major role of these compounds is the treatment of established pseudomonal infection, but they may also be active against some penicillin-resistant Gram-negative bacilli. They are also used in the treatment and prophylaxis of anaerobic and mixed infections, especially when combined with a β-lactamase inhibitor. A special role has been claimed, particularly for the acylureidopenicillins in providing broad prophylactic cover, notably in bowel surgery (*see* Ch. 39). An advantage claimed for acylureidopenicillins

Table 14.5   Activity of group 5 and 6 penicillins against non-β-lactamase-producing strains of pathogenic bacteria; modal MIC (mg/L)

	Azlocillin	Piperacillin	Ticarcillin	Temocillin
Staphylococcus aureus (methicillin-susceptible)	1	0.5	1	R
Streptococcus pyogenes	0.03	0.03	0.25	R
Str. pneumoniae	0.03	0.02	0.5	R
Enterococcus faecalis	2	1	32	R
Neisseria gonorrhoeae	<0.01	<0.01	0.06	0.01–1
N. meningitidis	ND	0.06	0.06	ND
Haemophilus influenzae	0.06	0.03	0.5	0.1–2
Escherichia coli	16	2	4	1–8
Klebsiella pneumoniae	64	16	R	1–16
Pseudomonas aeruginosa	4	4	16–32	R
Bacteroides fragilis	8	8	16	R

R, resistant (MIC >64 mg/L); ND, no data.

over carboxypenicillins is that they are mono- rather than di-sodium salts, thus presenting a substantially lower sodium load.

In neutropenic patients they should be combined with an aminoglycoside. However, it should be noted that penicillins and aminoglycosides should not be mixed in infusion fluids because of the possibility of mutual degradation (p. 149).

Combination therapy with an aminoglycoside is recommended in *Ps. aeruginosa* pneumonia. Soft-tissue and burn wound infections usually respond. Infections requiring treatment with these agents generally arise in patients with underlying disorders, and suppression rather than eradication of infection is often the best result obtainable. Good examples of such 'control' are provided by:

- cystic fibrosis (where accelerated elimination of the drugs requires high dosage)
- urinary tract infection in catheterized patients
- the grave necrotizing otitis externa of diabetes.

With all these agents, treatment failures are often due to the emergence of resistant variants.

 ## Further information

Tan JS, File Jr TM. Antipseudomonal penicillins. *Med Clin North Am.* 1995;79:679–693.

PIPERACILLIN

Molecular weight (free acid): 517.6; (sodium salt): 539.6.

A semisynthetic acylureidopenicillin supplied as the sodium salt for parenteral administration. A formulation with tazobactam is also available (p. 243).

 ## ANTIMICROBIAL ACTIVITY

The activity against common bacterial pathogens is shown in Table 14.5. It displays good activity against non-β-lactamase-producing strains of *N. gonorrhoeae*, ampicillin-susceptible *H. influenzae* and many Enterobacteriaceae. It is the most active of the antipseudomonal penicillins against *Ps. aeruginosa* and retains its activity in the absence of a β-lactamase inhibitor. Synergy with aminoglycosides has been demonstrated against many strains of Enterobacteriaceae and *Ps. aeruginosa*.

 ## ACQUIRED RESISTANCE

There is complete cross-resistance with other ureidopenicillins, but ticarcillin-resistant strains of *Ps. aeruginosa* may be susceptible. Piperacillin-resistant strains of *B. fragilis* and other *Bacteroides* spp. are common. Because piperacillin is hydrolyzed by most β-lactamases, many β-lactamase-producing isolates are resistant unless it is protected by β-lactamase inhibitors.

 ## PHARMACOKINETICS

Oral absorption	Negligible
C_{max} 2 g (2–3 min intravenous injection)	305 mg/L after 5 min
Plasma half-life	0.9 h
Volume of distribution	16–24 L/1.73 m^2
Plasma protein binding	16%

In patients with meningitis, mean CSF penetration of 30% has been found. The urine is the principal route of excretion, 50–70% of the dose appearing over 12 h, most in the first 4 h. Most is excreted via the tubules, 75–90% in active form. The half-life is prolonged in renal failure but much less than is the case with carboxypenicillins. There is substantial biliary excretion, levels in the common duct bile after a 1 g intravenous dose commonly reaching 500 mg/L or more. During hemodialysis the plasma half-life remains elevated and only 10–15% of the dose is removed.

 ## TOXICITY AND SIDE EFFECTS

Piperacillin is generally well tolerated, with mild to moderate pain on injection, thrombophlebitis and diarrhea in some patients. It otherwise exhibits side effects common to the group, including hypersensitivity, leukopenia and abnormalities of platelet aggregation without coagulation defect, except on prolonged treatment.

CLINICAL USES

Intra-abdominal infection
Urinary tract infections
Gynecological and gonococcal infections
Septicemia
Lower respiratory infections
Skin and skin structure infections
Bone and joint infections

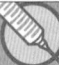

Preparations and dosage

Proprietary names: Pipril; Pipracil; Tazocin, Zosyn (with tazobactam).

Preparation: Injection.

Dosage: Piperacillin, adults, i.m., i.v., 100–150 mg/kg per day in divided doses, increased to 200–300 mg/kg per day in severe infections; in life-threatening infections a dose of not less than 16 g per day is recommended. Children 2 months to 12 years, 100–300 mg/kg per day in 3–4 divided doses; neonates and infants <2 months, 150–300 mg/kg per day in 2–3 divided doses. Piperacillin with tazobactam, adults and children >12 years, i.v., 2.25–4.5 g every 6–8 h.

Widely available.

Further information

Anonymous. Piperacillin (sodium). In: Dollery C, ed. *Therapeutic Drugs*. 2nd ed. Edinburgh: Churchill Livingstone; 1999:P133–P136.

Cunha BA. *Pseudomonas aeruginosa*: resistance and therapy. *Semin Respir Infect*. 2002;17:231–239.

Holmes B, Richards DM, Brogden RN, Heel RC. Piperacillin. A review of its antibacterial activity, pharmacokinetic properties and therapeutic use. *Drugs*. 1984;28:375–425.

Stefani S, Russo G, Nicolosi VM, Nicoletti G. Enterococci and aminoglycosides: evaluation of susceptibility and synergism of their combination with piperacillin. *Chemotherapia (Basel)*. 1987;6:12–16.

Tartaglione TA, Nye I, Vishniavsky N, Poynor W, Polk RE. Multiple dose pharmacokinetics of piperacillin and azlocillin in 12 healthy volunteers. *Clin Pharmacol*. 1986;5:941–946.

TICARCILLIN

Molecular weight (free acid): 384.4; (disodium salt): 428.4.

A semisynthetic carboxypenicillin supplied as the disodium salt for parenteral use. A formulation with clavulanic acid is also available (p. 240).

ANTIMICROBIAL ACTIVITY

The activity against common bacterial pathogens is shown in Table 14.5. Because it is hydrolyzed less rapidly than ampicillin, non-β-lactamase-producing strains of *N. gonorrhoeae*, ampicillin-susceptible *H. influenzae* and some Enterobacteriaceae are susceptible. Most aerobic and anaerobic Gram-positive bacteria are susceptible, with the exception of *E. faecalis* and β-lactamase-producing *Staph. aureus*. Anaerobic Gram-negative bacteria including *B. fragilis* are usually susceptible. Bactericidal synergy with aminoglycosides is demonstrable against *Ps. aeruginosa* and enterobacteria.

ACQUIRED RESISTANCE

Ticarcillin is generally cross-resistant with carbenicillin. It is somewhat stable to hydrolysis by AmpC-mediated β-lactamases of Gram-negative bacilli, but can be hydrolyzed by most other chromosomally and plasmid-mediated enzymes unless protected by a β-lactamase inhibitor.

PHARMACOKINETICS

Oral absorption	Negligible
C_{max} 1 g intramuscular	35 mg/L after 1 h
Plasma half-life	1.3 h
Volume of distribution	0.21 L/kg
Plasma protein binding	50–60%

Absorption and distribution

It is not orally absorbed. On parenteral co-administration with gentamicin, the plasma concentration of ticarcillin is unaffected, but the concentration of gentamicin is lowered. It enters the serous fluids, providing concentrations up to 60% of those of the plasma. It does not cross the normal meninges but levels of up to 50% of those of the plasma can be found in meningitis.

Metabolism and excretion

Up to 15% is excreted as penicilloic acid, a higher percentage than for carbenicillin (up to 5%). Some is excreted in the bile, producing levels 2–3 times those in the plasma, but the main route of excretion is through the kidneys (80%), principally as unchanged drug, appearing in the urine in the first 6 h. It is more rapidly eliminated in children with cystic fibrosis.

TOXICITY AND SIDE EFFECTS

As with all penicillins, hypersensitivity reactions may occur, but are less frequent and severe than those associated with benzylpenicillin. Rashes and eosinophilia occur; reversible abnormalities of liver function can develop. Since large doses of the drug have to be used, convulsions can occur, as with other penicillins, and being a disodium salt, electrolyte disturbances can result from the sodium load and from loss of potassium.

CLINICAL USE

Serious infection, including septicemia, respiratory tract infections, genitourinary tract infections and skin and soft-tissue infections caused by susceptible bacteria

Preparations and dosage

Proprietary names: Ticar, Timentin (with clavulanic acid).

Preparation: Injection.

Dosage: Ticarcillin, adults, i.v., 15–20 g per day in divided doses. Children, 200–300 mg/kg per day in divided doses. Ticarcillin with clavulanic acid, adults, i.v., 3.2 g every 6–8 h, increased to every 4 h in more severe infections. Children, 80 mg/kg every 6–8 h; neonates, 80 mg/kg every 6–8 h. Widely available.

Because of the increasing prevalence of bacteria possessing class A β-lactamases, it is now more commonly used in combination with clavulanic acid.

Further information

Anonymous. Ticarcillin (disodium). In: Dollery C, ed. *Therapeutic Drugs*. 2nd ed. Edinburgh: Churchill Livingstone; 1999:T106–T109.

Brogden RN, Heel RC, Speight TM, Avery GS. Ticarcillin: a review of its pharmacological properties and therapeutic efficacy. *Drugs*. 1980;20:325–352.

Symposium. *Ticarcillin (BRL 2288)*. International Congress Series No. 445. Oxford: Excerpta Medica; 1978:3–163.

OTHER GROUP 5 PENICILLINS

APALCILLIN

A semisynthetic acylaminopenicillin supplied as the sodium salt for parenteral administration. The antibacterial spectrum and toxicity profile are similar to those of the acylureidopenicillins. It is relatively labile to many β-lactamases, including the common TEM plasmid-mediated enzyme. It has very limited commercial availability.

ASPOXICILLIN

An acylaminopenicillin, synthesized from amoxicillin. It is more active than carbenicillin against *Ps. aeruginosa* and is less active than piperacillin against *Staph. aureus*, *H. influenzae*, the Enterobacteriaceae and *Ps. aeruginosa*. It is not absorbed when dosed orally; the plasma half-life is 87 min after intravenous infusion.

Aspoxicillin has been used in the treatment of respiratory, skin and soft tissue and urinary infections in adults and children, and, in combination with aminoglycosides, against gynecological infections and infections in patients with hematological disorders.

Further information

Geyer J, Hoffler D, Koeppe P. Pharmacokinetics of aspoxicillin in subjects with normal and impaired renal function. *Arzneimittelforschung*. 1988;11:1635–1639.

AZLOCILLIN

A semisynthetic acylureidopenicillin supplied as the sodium salt for parenteral administration. It is active against a wide range of other Gram-negative bacteria, but is distinguished mainly by its activity against *Ps. aeruginosa* (Table 14.5). *B. fragilis* and other anaerobes are moderately susceptible. Like other ureidopenicillins, azlocillin is active against Gram-positive cocci, *H. influenzae* and *N. gonorrhoeae*. Because it can be hydrolyzed by most β-lactamases, β-lactamase-producing isolates are resistant.

It attains peak concentrations of 250 mg/L after a 3 g intravenous infusion, with a plasma half-life of approximately 1 h. Protein binding is 20–30%. It distributes into multiple tissues and human body fluids at therapeutically useful concentrations. Up to 60% of the dose is recoverable from the urine, mostly unchanged, although some hydrolysis of the β-lactam ring takes place in the body.

Toxicity and side effects are similar to those associated with carboxypenicillins. Its clinical use is for serious infections with susceptible organisms, including lower respiratory tract, intra-abdominal, urinary tract and gynecological infections. Commercial availability is quite limited.

Further information

Anonymous. Azlocillin sodium. In: Dollery C, ed. *Therapeutic Drugs*. 2nd ed. Edinburgh: Churchill Livingstone; 1999:A265–A267.

CARBENICILLIN

α-Carboxybenzylpenicillin; the first antipseudomonal penicillin to be developed. A semisynthetic carboxypenicillin supplied as the disodium salt for parenteral administration. The two esterified prodrug formulations, carindacillin (carbenicillin indanyl sodium) and carfecillin (carbenicillin carboxyphenyl ester) are no longer available.

It is the least active of the group 5 agents, even against *Ps. aeruginosa* (MIC 64 mg/L) with notably reduced activity against Gram-positive cocci. It is labile to many plasmid-mediated β-lactamases, but is comparatively stable to class C chromosomal β-lactamases (pp. 228–230). Synergy is demonstrable with aminoglycosides against *Ps. aeruginosa* and other Gram-negative bacteria.

It is not orally absorbed, except in esterified form. A 1 g intramuscular injection achieves a plasma peak concentration of 20–30 mg/L after 0.5–1.5 h. The half-life is around 1 h. Plasma protein binding is 50–60%.

The drug is distributed in the extracellular fluid, providing concentrations up to 60% of those of the plasma. In patients with cystic fibrosis sputum concentrations may not reach inhibitory levels for *Ps. aeruginosa*. It does not cross the normal meninges but levels of up to 50% of those of the plasma can be found in patients with meningitis. Around 80% of the dose appears as unchanged drug in the urine, producing very high levels (2–4 g/L). It is more rapidly disposed of in patients with cystic fibrosis.

Hypersensitivity reactions may occur, but these are less frequent and severe than those associated with benzylpenicillin. High blood levels sometimes cause a coagulation defect that has occasionally progressed to life-threatening bleeding in patients with impaired excretion while receiving 500 mg/kg per day or more. Reversible abnormalities of liver function apparently occur more commonly than with other antipseudomonal penicillins. Since large doses of the drug have to be used, convulsions can occur (as with other penicillins; p. 203) and, being administered as the disodium salt, electrolyte disturbances can result. It was formerly used for treatment of serious infections, especially those involving *Ps. aeruginosa*. It has extremely limited availability.

Further information

Symposium. Symposium on carbenicillin: a clinical profile. *J Infect Dis.* 1970;122(suppl):S1–S116.

MEZLOCILLIN

A semisynthetic acylureidopenicillin supplied as the sodium salt for parenteral administration.

Ampicillin-susceptible strains of *H. influenzae* and *Neisseria* spp. are very susceptible, but β-lactamase-producing organisms are usually resistant. It is less active than azlocillin and piperacillin against *Ps. aeruginosa* and has variable activity against *B. fragilis*, independent of β-lactamase production. It exhibits typical β-lactam synergy with aminoglycosides against *Ps. aeruginosa* and enterobacteria.

It attains peak concentrations of 250 mg/L after a 2 g intravenous infusion, with a plasma half-life of 55 min. Protein binding is 20–30%. It distributes into multiple tissues and human body fluids at therapeutically useful concentrations. Up to 60% of the dose is recoverable unchanged from the urine, with up to 2.5% excreted in the bile.

Toxicity and side effects are similar to those associated with carboxypenicillins. Its clinical use is for serious infections with susceptible organisms, including lower respiratory tract, intra-abdominal, urinary tract and gynecological infections. Commercial availability is quite limited.

Further information

Anonymous. Mezlocillin. In: Dollery C, ed. *Therapeutic Drugs*. 2nd ed. Edinburgh: Churchill Livingstone; 1999:M158–M161.

SULBENICILLIN

α-Sulfobenzylpenicillin, a semisynthetic penicillin supplied as the disodium salt. Its antimicrobial spectrum and phar-

macokinetic behavior closely resemble those of carbenicillin. Following intravenous administration of 4 g, the mean plasma concentration at 1 h was approximately 160 mg/L, with a plasma elimination half-life of around 70 min. It is largely excreted in the urine, about 80% of the dose appearing in the first 24 h, less than 5% as the penicilloic acid. It has been noted that the penicilloic acid causes much stronger platelet aggregation than its parent. It is of very limited availability.

Further information

Hansen I, Jacobsen E, Weiss J. Pharmacokinetics of sulbenicillin, a new broad-spectrum semisynthetic penicillin. *Clin Pharmacol Ther.* 1975;17:339–347.

GROUP 6: β-LACTAMASE-RESISTANT PENICILLINS

The introduction of substituents into the 6-α-position of the penicillin nucleus generally results in loss of antibacterial activity, but the 6-α-methoxy derivative of ticarcillin, temocillin, possesses useful antibacterial and pharmacokinetic properties and has attained clinical status. Like the cephamycins (p. 170), which also contain an α-methoxy group on the β-lactam nucleus, it is highly resistant to most bacterial β-lactamases. As a result, it has attracted renewed attention for its potential utility to treat infections caused by class A and class C β-lactamase-producing Enterobacteriaceae (*see* pp. 228–230). It is not absorbed by the oral route, but it has a long serum half-life after parenteral administration. The *o*-methylphenyl ester produced substantial serum concentrations after oral dosing to human volunteers, but has not progressed to clinical trial.

TEMOCILLIN

Molecular weight (free acid): 414.4; (disodium salt): 458.4.

A semisynthetic 6-α-methoxylpenicillin supplied as the disodium salt for parenteral administration.

ANTIMICROBIAL ACTIVITY

Activity against common pathogenic bacteria is shown in Table 14.5 (p. 220). The introduction of the 6-α-methoxy group has resulted in loss of activity against Gram-positive cocci and anaerobic Gram-negative bacilli, but it is active against enterobacteria (MIC 1–8 mg/L), *H. influenzae* and *Mor. catarrhalis*, with somewhat elevated MICs against carbapenemase-producing isolates of *K. pneumoniae* (MIC

16–64 mg/L) and *Esch. coli* (modal MICs 8–16 mg/L). In most cases, β-lactamase-positive and negative strains are equally susceptible. In contrast to the structurally related ticarcillin, it is inactive against *Ps. aeruginosa*, but *Burkholderia cepacia*, *Ps. acidovorans* and *Aeromonas* spp. are susceptible (MIC 4 mg/L). Most *Acinetobacter* spp. are resistant, and *Ser. marcescens* exhibits variable susceptibility.

It is bactericidal at concentrations 2–4 times the MIC; filaments formed at lower concentrations slowly lyse at higher drug levels. Temocillin consists of diastereoisomers. The naturally predominant *R* epimer is more rapidly bactericidal than the *S* epimer. It is highly resistant to most bacterial β-lactamases, including those that confer resistance to extended-spectrum cephalosporins. It is hydrolyzed by β-lactamases produced by *Flavobacterium* spp. and by those of *Bacteroides* spp.

 ## PHARMACOKINETICS

Oral absorption	Negligible
C_{max} 1 g intramuscular injection	70 mg/L
1 g rapid intravenous infusion	172 mg/L after 5 min
Plasma half-life	4.3–5.4 h
Plasma protein binding	85%

Absorption and distribution

It is not absorbed when given orally and must be administered parenterally. Relatively high protein binding, together with its distribution in a volume less than the extracellular fluid, accounts for its relatively low renal clearance and subsequent high urinary concentrations that may be effective against some Enterobacteriaceae resistant to other β-lactam antibiotics. In artificial blister fluid and peritoneal fluid, concentrations reach 50% of the peak plasma level; in lymph, concentrations reach 25–60% of the simultaneous plasma level, with a similar half-life. The *R* epimer differs from the *S* epimer in lower protein binding, a 25% greater volume of distribution and a 60% shorter half-life.

Metabolism and excretion

Elimination is principally in the glomerular filtrate, with 80% of the dose appearing in the urine in the first 24 h. A small amount is disposed of in the bile and by degradation. Elimination declines in parallel with renal function, the half-life reaching 30 h in patients with creatinine clearance below 5%.

 ## TOXICITY AND SIDE EFFECTS

As with all penicillins, hypersensitivity reactions, including serious anaphylactic responses, may occur. It is generally well tolerated and administration of 4 g intravenously every 12 h produced no significant effect on template bleeding time, prothrombin time or ADP-induced platelet aggregation.

 ## CLINICAL USE

Severe infection with susceptible bacteria, including urinary and respiratory tract infections, peritonitis and septicemia.

 ### Preparations and dosage

Proprietary name: Negaban.
Preparation: Injection.
Dosage: Adults, i.m., i.v., 1–2 g every 12 h.
Available in UK and Belgium.

 ### Further information

Adams-Haduch JM, Potoski BA, Sidjabat HE, Paterson DL, Doi Y. Activity of temocillin against KPC-producing *Klebsiella pneumoniae* and *Escherichia coli*. Antimicrob Agents Chemother. 2009;53:2700–2701.

Brown RM, Wise R, Andrews JM. Temocillin, in-vitro activity and the pharmacokinetics and tissue penetration in healthy volunteers. *J Antimicrob Chemother*. 1982;10:295–302.

De Jongh R, Hens R, Basma V, Mouton JW, Tulkens PM, Carryn S. Continuous versus intermittent infusion of temocillin, a directed spectrum penicillin for intensive care patients with nosocomial pneumonia: stability, compatibility, population pharmacokinetic studies and breakpoint selection. *J Antimicrob Chemother*. 2008;61:382–388.

Glupczynski Y, Huang TD, Berhin C, et al. In vitro activity of temocillin against prevalent extended-spectrum beta-lactamases producing Enterobacteriaceae from Belgian intensive care units. *Eur J Clin Microbiol Infect Dis*. 2007;26:777–783.

Livermore DM, Tulkens PM. Temocillin revived. *J Antimicrob Chemother*. 2009;63:243–245.

Lode H, Verbist L, Williams JD, Richards DM. First international workshop on temocillin. *Drugs*. 1985;29(suppl 5):1–243.

15 Other β-lactam antibiotics

Karen Bush

In the penicillins and cephalosporins, the β-lactam ring is fused to a five- and six-membered ring, respectively, but monocyclic β-lactam compounds also exist. There are six chemical skeletons other than penicillins or cephalosporins which support β-lactam-containing agents that have current therapeutic use. Although many of these novel β-lactam structures are based on natural products, classes of agents such as the penems and the oxacephems are purely synthetic molecules that have relied on previous knowledge of β-lactam properties to design agents with broad-spectrum antibacterial activity. Characteristics of each of the various classes are listed below:

- **Penams (penicillins)** *N*-acylated derivatives of 6-β-aminopenicillanic acid. In these compounds the β-lactam ring is fused with a saturated five-membered thiazolidine ring containing sulfur.
- **Penicillanic acid sulfones** Penams that lack a 6-amino substituent and in which the sulfur is oxidized synthetically to a sulfone to yield β-lactamase inhibitors such as sulbactam or tazobactam.
- **Penems** These differ from penams by the presence of a double bond between C-2 and C-3.
- **Carbapenams and carbapenems** Compounds in which CH_2 replaces sulfur in the five-membered ring. Many natural and synthetic members of the group have been described, of which the most useful therapeutically are derivatives of the natural product thienamycin.
- **Cephems (cephalosporins)** *N*-acylated derivatives of 7-β-aminocephalosporanic acid. In these compounds, the β-lactam ring is fused with a six-membered dihydrothiazine ring containing sulfur and a double bond. Closely related are: cephamycins, which are substituted at the 7-position with an α-methoxy group; oxacephems, notably latamoxef, in which the sulfur of cephalosporins is replaced by oxygen; and carbacephems, including loracarbef, in which the sulfur is replaced by carbon.
- **Clavams** Compounds that differ from penams in the substitution of oxygen for sulfur. The only notable member of the clavam family at present is clavulanic acid, a compound that owes its therapeutic place to its ability to inhibit many class A (functional group 2) bacterial β-lactamases.

- **Monobactams** β-lactam compounds with no fused secondary ring. The monocyclic β-lactam antibiotics are represented therapeutically by aztreonam and carumonam, but the group also contains the nocardicins which have not been developed as antibacterial drugs.

The penicillins are considered in Chapter 14, and the cephalosporins and their close relatives, the cephamycins, oxacephems and carbacephems, in Chapter 13. This chapter deals with the remaining agents: carbapenems, penems and monobactams, which are notable for their antibacterial activity; and clavulanic acid and the penicillanic acid sulfones, which are primarily of interest as inhibitors of β-lactamases. The antibacterial activity of these inhibitors is associated with the synergistic activity seen with the accompanying penicillin in a β-lactamase inhibitor combination.

In-vitro activity of agents in each of these classes is highly dependent upon the chemical class to which it belongs. For example, carbapenems, penems and β-lactamase inhibitor combinations tend to have broad-spectrum activity covering Gram-positive and Gram-negative anaerobic and aerobic organisms, whereas the monobactams lack useful activity against Gram-positive bacteria and anaerobes.

Resistance to β-lactam agents is most frequently associated with production of enzymes that hydrolyze the β-lactam ring and since these novel compounds are all characterized by resistance to at least some β-lactamases, the classification of these enzymes is also dealt with in this chapter.

 Further information

Demain AL, Elander RP. The β-lactam antibiotics: past, present, and future. *Antonie Van Leeuwenhoek*. 1999;75:5–19.

Frere JM, Joris B, Varetto L, Crine M. Structure–activity relationships in the β-lactam family: an impossible dream. *Biochem Pharmacol*. 1988;37:125–132.

Rolinson GN. Forty years of β-lactam research. *J Antimicrob Chemother*. 1998;41:589–603.

Schofield CJ, Walter MW. β-lactam chemistry. *Amino Acids, Peptides, Proteins*. 1999;30:335–397.

Shah PM. Parenteral carbapenems. *Clin Microbiol Infect Dis*. 2008;14(suppl 1): 175–180.

Skeleton **Example**

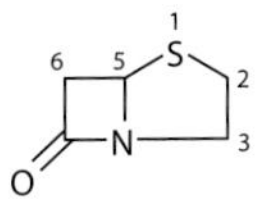

Penam — Sulbactam

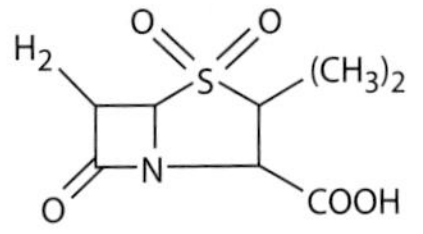

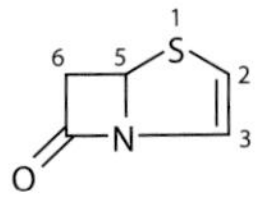

Penem — Faropenem

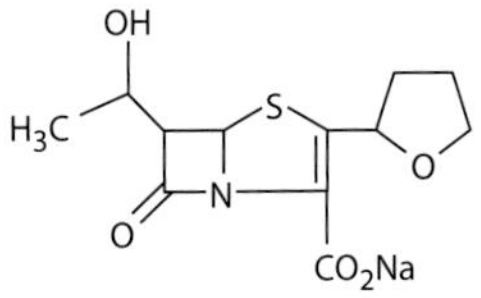

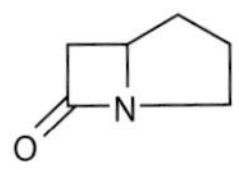

Carbapenam

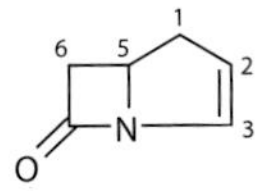

Carbapenem — Thienamycins

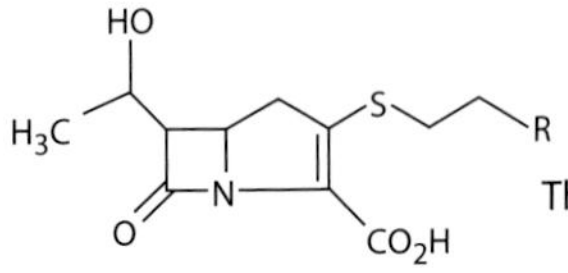

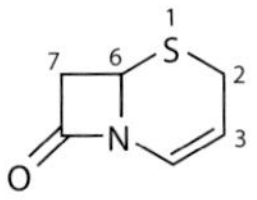

Cephem — Cephalosporins

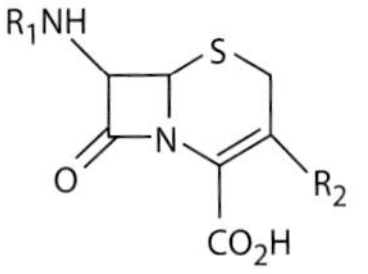

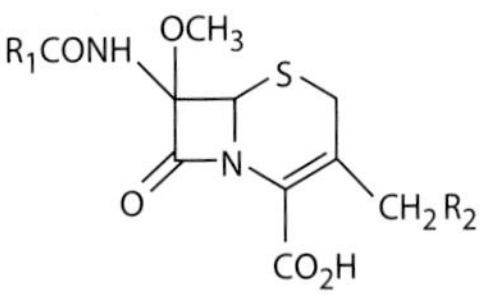

Cephamycins

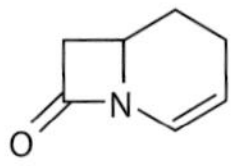

Carbacephem — Loracarbef

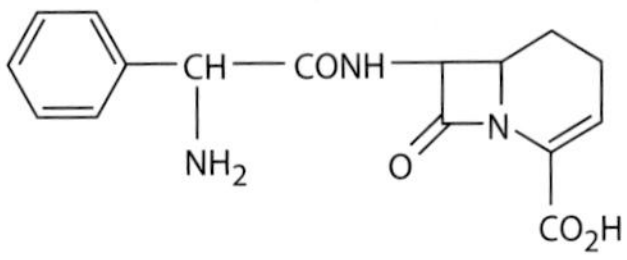

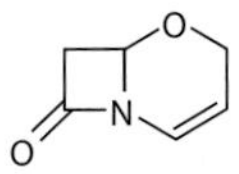

Oxacephem — Latamoxef

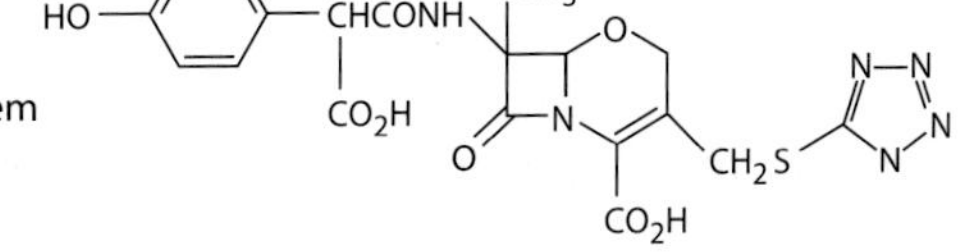

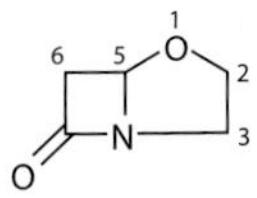

Oxapenam (clavam) — Clavulanic acid

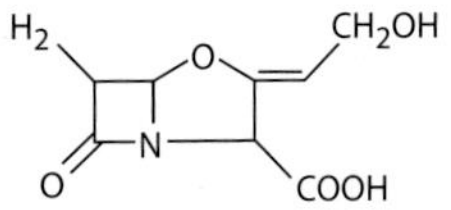

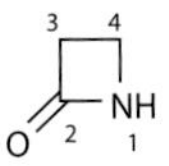

Azetidinone — Monobactams

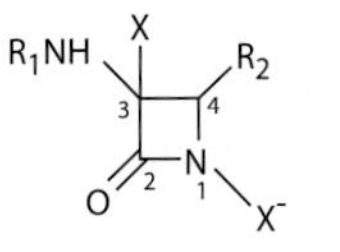

β-LACTAMASES

Even before penicillin was widely used clinically, bacteria such as *Escherichia coli* and *Staphylococcus aureus* were reported to have the capability of degrading this agent. The bacterial enzyme shown to hydrolyze the β-lactam ring was initially called 'penicillinase', and penicillinase-producing *Staph. aureus* became of great importance in outbreaks of hospital infection in the 1950s. Since that time, similar enzymes have become increasingly important as a cause of resistance in many pathogenic Gram-positive and Gram-negative bacteria, and even in legionellae, mycobacteria and nocardia. Because of their collective ability to destroy a wide range of β-lactam agents, the enzymes have been renamed β-lactamases. In the case of the penicillins the products are stable penicilloates, but in the case of cephalosporins the 'cephalosporoates' may rapidly undergo further degradation, liberating a variety of fragments depending on the C-3 substituent. Every β-lactam, including monobactams, β-lactamase inhibitors and carbapenems, can be inactivated by an appropriate β-lactamase.

β-Lactam antibiotics can be attacked at other chemical sites by microbial acylases and esterases, but these enzymes, which have important uses in semisynthetic processes, are of no significance as a cause of clinical resistance. The presence of esterases in mammalian tissues is exploited in the cleavage of oral prodrug esters of penicillins and cephalosporins with liberation of the active parent compound. Some penems and carbapenems can also be hydrolyzed by mammalian dehydropeptidases (see below).

GENERAL PROPERTIES

With the advent in the early 1960s of the broad-spectrum penicillins ampicillin and carbenicillin, resistance of Gram-negative bacilli to these agents was most often associated with β-lactamase production. Most aerobic and anaerobic Gram-negative bacilli produce chromosomally mediated β-lactamases characteristic of each species, which accounted for the intrinsic resistance to benzylpenicillin and ampicillin in organisms such as *Bacteroides fragilis*, *Klebsiella pneumoniae* and other enterobacteria. The discovery in 1965 that β-lactamases could be encoded by plasmids and readily transferred by conjugation among Gram-negative bacilli led to widespread dissemination of plasmid-mediated β-lactamase-producing Gram-negative bacilli that are currently a major and increasing clinical problem. In addition, β-lactamase-producing strains of *Haemophilus influenzae*, *Moraxella catarrhalis* and *Neisseria gonorrhoeae*, which were unknown before the mid-1970s, are now common causes of infection. The proliferation of β-lactamases and the identification of new β-lactamase entities have often followed the development and use of new β-lactam-containing agents that have served as the selecting agents for the next generation of enzymes.

Bacterial β-lactamases may be chromosomally encoded, with inducible or constitutive production; only rare reports of inducible plasmid-encoded enzymes have been documented. The β-lactamase genes may be translocated from or into the chromosome or into another plasmid by transposons (*see* Ch. 3), resulting in transfer within and between species or genera. For instance, the TEM β-lactamases are found in virtually every genus of Enterobacteriaceae. Plasmid-encoded cephalosporinases derived from common class C chromosomal cephalosporinases are being identified more frequently. Most seriously, plasmid-encoded carbapenemases capable of hydrolyzing almost all classes of β-lactam agent may also be refractory to inhibition by commercially available β-lactamase inhibitors.

Those β-lactamases found in Gram-positive organisms are often extracellular enzymes, but Gram-negative β-lactamases are almost invariably confined to the periplasmic space. Because the outer membrane of Gram-negative bacteria generally restricts transport of large molecules, little β-lactamase activity is detected extracellularly, unless cell lysis occurs. Quantitative measurement of β-lactamase activity in intact cells can be difficult, depending upon the permeability properties of the specific outer membrane of an organism, so that the enzymes are usually studied in extracts after disruption of the cell.

CLASSIFICATION

β-Lactamases are usually characterized on the basis of one of two properties: molecular characteristics, which routinely include a full nucleotide or amino acid sequence; or functional characteristics, including substrate and inhibition profiles (Table 15.1). Numerous classification schemes have been proposed. The two most cited schemes are that of Ambler, who proposed a classification based upon molecular structure, and that of Bush, Jacoby and Medeiros, who combined the functional properties with the known molecular sequences of β-lactamases from both Gram-positive and Gram-negative bacteria. The number of enzymes that have been classified using the latter scheme numbered at least 850 in 2009.

Hydrolytic activity is customarily defined by comparison with benzylpenicillin or cephaloridine, with rates of hydrolysis normalized to 100 for the reference compound. Inhibitory properties deemed to be significant include inhibition by clavulanic acid (an inactivator of many β-lactamases that contain an active site serine) and inhibition by the chelating agent ethylenediaminetetraacetic acid (EDTA), which is used to identify the zinc-containing metallo-β-lactamases. Characteristics of representative β-lactamases from each class are shown in Table 15.2.

Molecular classification of β-lactamases requires sequence determinations of either the gene encoding the enzyme or the amino acid sequence of the protein. Class A, C and D β-lactamases are all enzymes that require an active site serine to acylate the β-lactam substrate during the hydrolysis

Table 15.1 Classification of bacterial β-lactamases

| Functional group | Molecular class | Preferred substrates | Inhibited by | | Representative enzymes |
			CA	EDTA	
1	C	Ceph	–	–	AmpC, plasmid-encoded cephalosporinases (FOX-1, ACT-1 in Gram-negative bacteria), CMY-1
2a	A	Pen	+	–	Penicillinases from Gram-positive bacteria
2b	A	Pen, ceph	+	–	TEM-1, TEM-2, SHV-1
2be	A	Pen, ceph, extended-spectrum ceph, monobactam	+	–	TEM-3, TEM-26, TEM-168, SHV-2, SHV-120
2br	A	Pen	–	–	TEM-30 to TEM-39 (IRT 1 to IRT-26), SHV-10
2c	A	Pen, carbenicillin	+	–	PSE-1, PSE-3, PSE-4
2d	D	Pen, cloxacillin	+/–	–	OXA-1, OXA-10 = PSE-2
2de	D	Pen, oxacillin, extended spectrum cephs	–	–	OXA-11, OXA-15
2df	D	Pen, carbapenems	+/–	–	OXA-23, OXA-48
2e	A	Ceph	+	–	Inducible cephalosporinases from *Pr. vulgaris*, SFO-1
2f	A	Ceph, pen, carbapenems	+	–	IMI-1, KPC-2, SME-1
3	B	Carbapenems. Often, all ceph, pen. No monobactam	–	+	L1 from *Sten. maltophilia*, VIM-1, IMP-1, CfiA/CcrA from *B. fragilis*

CA, clavulanic acid; Ceph, cephalosporin; EDTA, ethylenediaminetetraacetic acid; Pen, penicillin.
Reproduced with permission from Greenwood D, Ogilvie MM, Antimicrobial Agents in: Greenwood D, Slack RCB, Peutherer JF, eds. 2002 Medical Microbiology 16th edn. Edinburgh: Churchill Livingstone, with permission of Elsevier.

Table 15.2 Characteristics of selected bacterial β-lactamases

| β-Lactamase | Functional group | Molecular class | Molecular mass (kDa) | Relative hydrolysis or relative k_{cat} for major substrates compared to benzylpenicillin as 100 | | | | | Clavulanic acid IC_{50} (μmol) |
				Amp	Lor	Ctx	Caz	Imp	
Enterobacter cloacae P99	1	C	40	0.3	6700	<7	<0.7	<0.7	>100
Staph. aureus PC1	2a	A	27	180	1.1	<0.1	No data	No data	0.03
TEM-1	2b	A	29	110	140	0.07	0.01	<0.01	0.09
TEM-3	2be	A	29	110	120	170	8.3	0.01	0.03
TEM-10	2be	A	29	130	77	1.6	68	<0.02	0.03
SHV-1	2b	A	29	150	48	0.18	0.02	<0.01	0.03
SHV-5	2be	A	29	240	140	130	49	<1	0.01
TEM-31 (IRT-1)	2br	A	29	250	13	<1	<1	<1	9.4
PSE-4 (Dalgleish)	2c	A	32	88	40	0.02	0.02	0.01	0.15
OXA-10 (PSE-2)	2d	A	28	270	32	1	0.12	0.05	0.81
Pr. vulgaris	2e	A	28	100	3000	13	0.17	No data	0.35
K. pneumoniae KPC-2	2f	A	29	410	1040	43	<0.2	29	1.5
B. fragilis CfiA/CcrA	3	B	26	98	22	51	68	100	>500[a]

[a]Inhibited by EDTA.
K_{cat}, catalytic constant (molecules of substrate hydrolyzed per molecule of enzyme per second); Amp, ampicillin; Lor, cephaloridine; Ctx, cefotaxime; Caz, ceftazidime; Imp, imipenem.
Data from Bush K, Jacoby GA, Medeiros AA 1995 *Antimicrobial Agents and Chemotherapy* 39: 1211–1233; Yigit H, Queenan AM, Rasheed JK, et al. 2003 *Antimicrobial Agents and Chemotherapy* 47: 3881–3889.

reaction. Class C β-lactamases tend to have higher molecular weights than the other classes. Class B β-lactamases contain at least one functional Zn^{2+} atom at the active site that participates in the hydrolytic process. A number of characteristic amino acid sequences have been identified to differentiate the various molecular classes.

Functional (Bush et al) groups are identified according to inhibitory properties based primarily upon clavulanic acid and EDTA. For many enzymes, the inhibitory activities of clavulanic acid and tazobactam are similar. Additional subgroups are identified according to substrate hydrolysis profiles.

Functional group 1 cephalosporinases include the chromosomal β-lactamases from Enterobacteriaceae that are not inhibited well by clavulanic acid. A second cephalosporinase class was segregated into group 2e due to high affinity for clavulanic acid, a good inhibitor of these enzymes. Sequencing data have shown that functional group 1 enzymes belong to molecular class C, whereas the functional group 2e enzymes are members of molecular class A, like most group 2 β-lactamases.

Other group 2 enzymes are generally inhibited by clavulanate, with the exception of the rare TEM-1 β-lactamase derivatives, the inhibitor-resistant TEM (IRT) enzymes, which have reduced affinity for the inhibitor, and many of the class D oxacillin-hydrolyzing enzymes. Group 2a enzymes are penicillinases; group 2b enzymes have a broader spectrum of activity, hydrolyzing penicillins and early cephalosporins almost equally well. Group 2be enzymes, the extended-spectrum β-lactamases (ESBLs), may be derived from group 2b enzymes, but exhibit enhanced hydrolytic properties that enable them to hydrolyze extended-spectrum cephalosporins and monobactams. Group 2c enzymes hydrolyze carbenicillin, and group 2d enzymes hydrolyze isoxazolyl penicillins such as cloxacillin or oxacillin. The 2d enzymes, the only β-lactamases that belong to molecular class D, may be further subdivided according to the ability to hydrolyze extended-spectrum cephalosporins (group 2de) or carbapenems (group 2df). Group 2f enzymes are carbapenem-hydrolyzing enzymes that are class A serine β-lactamases rather than metalloenzymes. The group 3 metallo-β-lactamases are readily distinguished from other β-lactamases because they can hydrolyze carbapenems and are not inhibited by clavulanic acid, but are inhibited by metal-ion chelators such as EDTA.

STAPHYLOCOCCUS AUREUS β-LACTAMASE

Today at least 90% of *Staph. aureus* causing infections in community and hospital practice are β-lactamase-producing strains. The enzyme produced occurs in four serologically distinct forms that are closely related on a molecular level. Production may be plasmid encoded or chromosomal. The chromosomal enzymes can be induced by penicillins such as methicillin or by the β-lactamase inhibitor sulbactam.

The enzymes are predominantly active against penicillins, but can be differentiated on the basis of hydrolysis of cephalosporins including cephaloridine, nitrocefin and cefazolin.

CHROMOSOMAL CEPHALOSPORINASES OF GRAM-NEGATIVE BACTERIA

Most Gram-negative bacteria elaborate chromosomally mediated enzymes, most of which fall into group 1. These hydrolyze cephalosporins up to 1000 times more rapidly than penicillins, some of which (e.g. cloxacillin) may inhibit them. Traditional β-lactamase-inhibitors work poorly against these enzymes, but monobactams such as aztreonam bind tightly and can act like potent inactivators.

In some species, including *Acinetobacter*, *Citrobacter*, *Enterobacter*, *Morganella*, *Pseudomonas* and *Serratia*, group 1 cephalosporinases are inducible and often species specific. Plasmid-encoded forms of these enzymes, such as those designated FOX-1, LAT-1, MIR-1 and MOX-1, have appeared, particularly in *K. pneumoniae* strains that have an additional β-lactamase. Sequence data indicate high homology with the AmpC cephalosporinases from *Pseudomonas aeruginosa*, *Serratia marcescens*, *Enterobacter cloacae* or *Citrobacter freundii*.

Induction is a clinically relevant phenomenon when the inducing molecule is a substrate that can be hydrolyzed by the enzyme, such as ampicillin or amoxicillin. Many good inducers, such as cefoxitin and imipenem, are not good substrates for these enzymes, and pose problems primarily when they are co-administered with a second β-lactam agent. Because induction is a transient event, the producing organisms revert to their original low basal production of β-lactamase on removal of the inducer. A more serious problem occurs if there is selection for a permanently altered organism with derepressed production of the chromosomal β-lactamase. Enterobacteriaceae that hyperproduce group 1 cephalosporinases are sometimes responsible for clinical failures of cephalosporins. Interestingly, β-lactam compounds that are good inducers rarely select for derepressed hyperproducing mutants.

PLASMID-ENCODED β-LACTAMASES

Plasmid-encoded enzymes account for perhaps the most important β-lactamase-related resistance mechanisms. The most common β-lactamase in Gram-negative organisms is the TEM-1 β-lactamase, responsible for transferable ampicillin resistance among Enterobacteriaceae worldwide. In *K. pneumoniae*, the broad-spectrum SHV-1 β-lactamase predominates, and appears as a chromosomal β-lactamase in most *K. pneumoniae* species. Other important families of plasmid-encoded β-lactamases include the OXA enzymes that hydrolyze oxacillin and the recently identified CTX-M family of extended spectrum β-lactamases (ESBLs).

In the mid-1980s, plasmid-encoded β-lactamases that conferred resistance to oxymino β-lactam agents, notably cefotaxime, and/or ceftazidime and aztreonam, began to appear in central Europe. The major families of ESBLs (functional group 2be) include numerous variants of TEM-1 and SHV-1 that are numbered through at least TEM-168 and SHV-120. It should be noted that the sequential numbers of each family include approximately 24 inhibitor-resistant TEM enzyme sequences, as well as sequences that have been withdrawn.

Organisms elaborating ESBLs may remain susceptible to cefoxitin and imipenem, or piperacillin–tazobactam, unless they produce multiple β-lactamases. The enzymes are readily inhibited by clavulanic acid or tazobactam. They differ from their parent TEM and SHV enzymes by selected point mutations; two or more amino acid substitutions often lead to high-level resistance (minimum inhibitory concentrations [MICs] of cephalosporins >32 mg/L). Such organisms have spread rapidly within localized metropolitan areas to cause hospital outbreaks and colonization in nursing homes. Infections caused by organisms producing TEM variants resistant to β-lactamase inhibitors do not respond to clavulanic acid or sulbactam–β-lactam combinations, but are often susceptible to early cephalosporins. Plasmid-encoded carbapenemases have become associated with one of the most serious multidrug resistance mechanisms in the Enterobacteriaceae, spreading throughout the world. Genes encoding enzymes such as the KPC β-lactamases can be transferred among species, together with resistance determinants for other antibiotic classes, resulting in pathogens that are susceptible to few antibiotics (e.g. only polymyxin B and tigecycline).

METALLO-β-LACTAMASES

Another formidable β-lactamase group includes the metallo-β-lactamases, which rapidly hydrolyze most β-lactam agents, especially the carbapenems, but not the monobactams, and are resistant to β-lactamase inhibitors. These enzymes were originally described as chromosomal enzymes in a few species, such as *Stenotrophomonas maltophilia*, *B. fragilis* and *Bacillus cereus*, but were then identified in Japan on plasmids found in *B. fragilis*, *S. marcescens*, *K. pneumoniae* and *Ps. aeruginosa*. Such strains have now been identified in most parts of the world, with the IMP and VIM families the predominant members. Because of the low catalytic efficiencies of these enzymes, they are almost always produced in combination with at least one other β-lactamase of a different class, thus expanding the hydrolytic repertoire for the organism.

 Further information

Bush K, Jacoby GA, Medeiros AA. A functional classification scheme for β-lactamases and its correlation with molecular structure. *Antimicrob Agents Chemother*. 1995;39:1211–1233.

Chaibi EB, Sirot D, Paul G, Labia R. Inhibitor-resistant TEM β-lactamases: phenotypic, genetic and biochemical characteristics. *J Antimicrob Chemother*. 1999;43:447–458.

Jacoby GA. AmpC beta-lactamases. *Clin Microbiol Rev*. 2009;22:161–182.

Jacoby GA, Bush K. β-Lactam resistance in the 21st century. In: White DG, Alekshun MN, McDermot PF, eds. *Frontiers in Antimicrobial Resistance: a Tribute to Stuart B. Levy*. Washington: ASM Press; 2005:53–65.

Medeiros AA. Evolution and dissemination of β-lactamases accelerated by generations of β-lactam antibiotics. *Clin Infect Dis*. 1997;24:S19–S45.

Philippon A, Dusart J, Joris B, Frère J-M. The diversity, structure, and regulation of β-lactamases. *Cell Mol Life Sci*. 1998;54:341–346.

Pitout JD, Laupland KB. Extended-spectrum beta-lactamase-producing Enterobacteriaceae: an emerging public-health concern. *Lancet Infect Dis*. 2008;8:159–166.

Queenan AM, Bush K. Carbapenemases: the versatile β-lactamases. *Clin Microbiol Rev*. 2007;20:440–458.

CARBAPENEMS AND PENEMS

Many novel molecules containing a β-lactam ring have been investigated, but few have survived the early stages of development. Prominent among those that have are the carbapenems, in which carbon replaces sulfur in the fused ring structure, and penems, which have a more conventional core structure (see above).

Only one penem, faropenem, has entered limited clinical use, but dozens of carbapenems have been isolated from fermentation products of various streptomycetes. Their nomenclature has been complicated by the use of multiple generic names to describe the same class of compounds, including thienamycins, olivanic acids, carpetimycins, asparenomycins and pluracidomycins. They demonstrate potent activity against a broad range of Gram-positive and Gram-negative bacteria and are resistant to hydrolysis by most β-lactamases. Some are also β-lactamase inhibitors. The most active of the natural compounds, thienamycin, is produced by *Streptomyces cattleya*, although concentration-related instability precludes its clinical use.

A search for more stable derivatives that retain potent antibacterial activity led to the development of *N*-formimidoyl-thienamycin, imipenem. This compound is stable to all bacterial β-lactamases other than the carbapenemases. It is rapidly degraded by the mammalian renal dipeptidase, dehydropeptidase I, which hydrolyzes carbapenems and penems, but not penicillins, cephalosporins or monobactams. Cilastatin is a dehydropeptidase inhibitor that is co-administered with imipenem for therapeutic use. Coincidentally, cilastatin also acts as a nephroprotectant when administered with imipenem.

Addition of a 1-β-methyl substituent on the carbapenem ring confers stability to hydrolysis by dehydropeptidase. As a result, semisynthetic carbapenems such as meropenem, ertapenem, biapenem and doripenem have been developed. These compounds retain broad-spectrum antimicrobial activity and β-lactamase stability, and do not need to be administered with a dehydropeptidase inhibitor.

DORIPENEM

Molecular weight (monohydrate): 438.52.

A 1-β-carbapenem, formulated as the monohydrate for parenteral administration. It is relatively stable to renal dehydropeptidase and can be administered as a single agent.

ANTIMICROBIAL ACTIVITY

Activity against aerobic and anaerobic Gram-negative pathogens is similar to that of other carbapenems (Table 15.3). MIC values against Gram-positive cocci are generally higher than for imipenem and those for Gram-negative bacilli are lower.

PHARMACOKINETICS

C_{max} 500 mg intravenous infusion (1 h)	c. 23 mg/L after 1 h
500 mg intravenous infusion (4 h)	c. 8 mg/L
Plasma half-life	1 h
Volume of distribution	16.8 L (steady state)
Plasma protein binding	8.1%

Absorption and distribution

Doripenem is not absorbed after oral administration. It penetrates well into most tissues and fluid, achieving concentrations matching or exceeding those required to inhibit most susceptible bacteria at the site of infection for the approved indications.

Metabolism and excretion

Metabolism of doripenem to the microbiologically inactive ring-opened metabolite occurs primarily by renal dehydropeptidase. Based on area under the concentration–time curve (AUC) values in plasma following a single 500 mg dose in healthy volunteers, 18% appears as metabolite and the rest as unchanged drug.

Excretion is primarily by the renal route. Within 24 h after dosing, 78.7% and 18.5% of the dose was recovered in urine as unchanged drug and the ring-opened metabolite, respectively. After administration of radiolabeled doripenem, 0.7% of the total radioactivity was recovered in feces after 1 week.

TOXICITY AND SIDE EFFECTS

Seizure and central nervous system (CNS) side effects are observed rarely (<1%), though headache is reported by 2.3% of patients. Other common drug-related adverse reactions are diarrhea (2.0%), nausea (1.9%), anemia (1.4%) and phlebitis (1.4%). Hypersensitivity reactions related to intravenous

Table 15.3 Activity of the carbapenems doripenem, ertapenem, imipenem and meropenem, the monobactam, aztreonam and the penem, faropenem against common bacterial pathogens: MIC (mg/L)[a]

Organism	Doripenem	Ertapenem	Imipenem	Meropenem	Aztreonam	Faropenem
Staphylococcus aureus (MSSA)	≤0.06	0.12	0.03	0.12	R	0.06
Staph. aureus (MRSA)	>2.0	2.0	0.5	2.0	R	2.0
Streptococcus pyogenes	≤0.02	≤0.03	≤0.01	≤0.01	8	0.015
Str. pneumoniae penicillin-susceptible	≤0.015	≤0.03	0.008	0.008	R	0.06
penicillin-resistant	1.0	1.0	0.03	0.12	No data	0.5
Enterococcus faecalis	2.0	16	1.0	4.0	R	1.0
Haemophilus influenzae	≤1.0	≤0.03	1.0	0.06	≤0.1	1.0
Neisseria spp.	No data	≤0.03	≤0.25	≤0.03	≤0.1	≤0.03
Escherichia coli	≤0.06	≤0.03	0.12	0.03	≤0.1	0.5
Klebsiella pneumoniae	≤0.12	≤0.03	≤0.25	0.03	≤0.1	0.5
Pseudomonas aeruginosa	4.0	4.0	4.0	4.0	8	R
Bacteroides fragilis	0.5	0.25	0.25	0.12	32	1.0
Chlamydia spp.	No data	No data	No data	No data	≤0.25	No data

[a]MIC against 50% of strains. R, resistant (MIC >32 mg/L). MSSA, methicillin-sensitive *Staph. aureus*; MRSA, methicillin-resistant *Staph. aureus*.

administration of the study drug and *Clostridium difficile* colitis occurred at a rate of less than 1%. However, patients with a history of hypersensitivity reactions to other β-lactam agents should be treated cautiously.

CLINICAL USE

Complicated intra-abdominal infections

Complicated urinary tract infections, including pyelonephritis

Nosocomial pneumonia, including ventilator-associated pneumonia (Europe)

Preparations and dosage

Proprietary names: Doribax, Finibax.

Preparation: Intravenous infusion.

Dosage: Adults, 500 mg by infusion over 1 h or 4 h every 8 h daily for 5–14 days depending on infection. Not recommended for use in children.

Available in the USA, Europe, Japan and Canada.

Further information

Cirillo I, Mannens G, Janssen C, et al. Disposition, metabolism, and excretion of [¹⁴C]doripenem after a single 500-milligram intravenous infusion in healthy men. *Antimicrob Agents Chemother.* 2008;52:3478–3483.

Keam SJ. Doripenem: a review of its use in the treatment of bacterial infections. *Drugs.* 2008;68:2021–2057.

Pillar CM, Torres MK, Brown NP, Shah D, Sahm DF. In vitro activity of doripenem, a carbapenem for the treatment of challenging infections caused by gram-negative bacteria, against recent clinical isolates from the United States. *Antimicrob Agents Chemother.* 2008;52:4388–4399.

ERTAPENEM

Molecular weight (monosodium salt): 497.5.

A 1-β-carbapenem, formulated as the sodium salt for parenteral administration. It is stable to renal dehydropeptidase and can be administered as a single agent.

ANTIMICROBIAL ACTIVITY

Activity against aerobic and anaerobic pathogens is comparable to that of imipenem (Table 15.3): MIC values for Gram-negative bacilli (with the exception of *Ps. aeruginosa*) are generally lower and those for Gram-positive cocci higher.

Ertapenem is stable to most serine β-lactamases, but is hydrolyzed by serine carbapenemases and metallo-β-lactamases.

PHARMACOKINETICS

C_{max} 1 g intramuscular	c. 67 mg/L after 2 h
1 g intravenous infusion (30 min)	c. 155 mg/L end infusion
Plasma half-life	c. 4 h
Volume of distribution	c. 0.12 L/kg (steady state)
Plasma protein binding	85–95%

Absorption after intramuscular injection is essentially complete with 90% bioavailability. The modestly extended plasma half-life allows once-daily dosing.

Excretion is predominantly by the renal route, about 80% being recovered in the urine within 24 h. About 40% is eliminated unchanged, the rest as a biologically inactive ring-opened metabolite. Dosage should be reduced in severe renal impairment.

TOXICITY AND SIDE EFFECTS

Ertapenem appears to be generally well tolerated. The most common drug-related adverse experiences are diarrhea (5.5%), infused vein complication (3.7%), nausea (3.1%), headache (2.2%), vaginitis (2.1%), phlebitis/thrombophlebitis (1.3%) and vomiting (1.1%). Seizures have occasionally been reported (0.5%) in patients with a history of disorders of the CNS.

CLINICAL USE

Complicated intra-abdominal infections

Complicated skin and skin structure infections, including diabetic foot infections without osteomyelitis

Community acquired pneumonia

Complicated urinary tract infections including pyelonephritis

Acute pelvic infections including postpartum endomyometritis, septic abortion and postsurgical gynecologic infections

Prophylaxis of surgical site infection following elective colorectal surgery

Preparations and dosage

Proprietary name: Invanz.

Preparation: Lyophilized powder for reconstitution for i.m. injection (with 1% lidocaine) or i.v. infusion over 30 min.

Dosage: Adults, 1 g i.m. or i.v. infusion per day for 3–14 days depending on infection type. Children >3 months, 15 mg/kg i.m. or i.v. infusion every 12 h for 3–14 days depending on infection type.

Available in the UK and the USA.

Further information

Fuchs PC, Barry AL, Brown SD. In-vitro antimicrobial activity of a carbapenem, MK-0826 (L-749,345) and provisional interpretive criteria for disc tests. *J Antimicrob Chemother.* 1999;43:703–706.

Gill CJ, Jackson JJ, Gerckens LS, et al. In vivo activity and pharmacokinetic evaluation of a novel long-acting carbapenem antibiotic, MK-826 (L-749,345). *Antimicrob Agents Chemother.* 1998;42:1996–2001.

Graham DR, Lucasti C, Malafaia O, et al. Ertapenem once daily versus piperacillin–tazobactam 4 times per day for treatment of complicated skin and skin-structure infections in adults: results of a prospective, randomized, double-blind multicenter study. *Clin Infect Dis.* 2002;34:1460–1468.

Livermore DM, Sefton AM, Scott GM. Properties and potential of ertapenem. *J Antimicrob Chemother.* 2003;52:331–344.

Teppler H, Gesser RM, Friedland IR, et al. Safety and tolerability of ertapenem. *J Antimicrob Chemother.* 2004;53:ii75–ii81.

IMPENEM

N-formimidoylthienamycin. Molecular weight (monohydrate): 317.37.

A semisynthetic carbapenem available as the monohydrate; formulated in a 1:1 ratio with the dehydropeptidase inhibitor, cilastatin sodium (molecular weight [monosodium salt] 380.43) for intramuscular and intravenous administration.

It is stable in the solid state for 6 months at 37°C. In aqueous solution at room temperature it decays at 10%/h.

 ## ANTIMICROBIAL ACTIVITY

Imipenem shows potent activity against a wide range of Gram-positive and Gram-negative aerobes and anaerobes, including many resistant to other agents. Its activity against common pathogenic organisms is shown in Table 15.3. Concentrations (mg/L) inhibiting 50% of strains of other organisms are: *Listeria monocytogenes*, 0.03; *Legionella pneumophila*, 0.03; *Enterococcus faecium*, 4; *Yersinia* spp., 0.06. *Mycobacterium fortuitum* is inhibited by 6.25 mg/L. Imipenem is active against many *Pseudomonas* species, but not *Sten. maltophilia*. It is active against most anaerobes, with the exception of *Cl. perfringens*, which is only moderately susceptible. It is bactericidal at 2–4 times the MIC for most species, but some strains of *Staph. aureus* exhibit 'tolerance' (see p. 204). Bactericidal synergy with aminoglycosides, glycopeptides, fosfomycin and rifampicin (rifampin) has been observed against many strains of *Staph. aureus* and enterococci.

Antibacterial activity is unaffected by the presence of cilastatin, which is itself devoid of antimicrobial activity.

Imipenem is stable to hydrolysis by most serine β-lactamases, with the exception of the group 2f carbapenem-hydrolyzing enzymes (*see above*). Strains of *B. fragilis*, *Aeromonas* spp. and *Sten. maltophilia* can produce metallo-β-lactamases that hydrolyze the drug rapidly. These strains, in addition to occasional strains of enterobacteria, *Acinetobacter baumannii* and *Ps. aeruginosa*, show variable resistance to imipenem depending upon the level of carbapenem-hydrolyzing enzymes and the presence or absence of imipenem-specific porins. Efflux pumps also exist that may extrude imipenem from Gram-negative bacteria.

 ## ACQUIRED RESISTANCE

Some strains of *Citrobacter*, *Enterobacter*, *Proteus vulgaris*, *Providencia*, *Ps. aeruginosa* and *Serratia* spp. may be resistant to imipenem and other β-lactam agents, often because of the selection of stably derepressed mutants expressing high levels of group 1 β-lactamases coupled with decreased intracellular drug levels due to porin mutations or increased efflux.

Induction of class 1 β-lactamases by imipenem in strains of *Aeromonas*, *Pseudomonas* and *Serratia* spp. is responsible for antagonism of β-lactamase-labile β-lactam agents in vitro. Imipenem resistance in *Ps. aeruginosa* can occur following selection of mutants that hyperproduce the group 1 cephalosporinase and which are also deficient in an outer membrane protein (OprD or D2) which specifically transports imipenem, but not cephalosporins or monobactams.

PHARMACOKINETICS

C$_{max}$ 500 mg intravenous (20-min infusion)	21–58 mg/L end infusion
Plasma half-life	1 h
Volume of distribution	c. 0.2 L/kg
Plasma protein binding	20%

Absorption and distribution

Imipenem is not absorbed by the oral route. No accumulation of imipenem is reported following multiple dosing with cilastatin. Imipenem and cilastatin are both widely distributed in multiple fluids and tissues. Although cerebrospinal fluid (CSF) concentrations of 1–2.6 mg/L have been reported, imipenem is not approved for use in meningitis.

Metabolism

In the absence of cilastatin, imipenem is slowly hydrolyzed, with a half-life of 0.7 h in serum in vitro. Most destruction occurs in the kidney and only 5–40% of the drug is recovered in the urine, where 80–90% is in the open-ring form. When imipenem is administered with cilastatin in a 1:1 ratio, urinary recovery of imipenem rises to c. 70%, with only 20% as the open-ring metabolite.

Excretion

In volunteers receiving 2 g of the mixture intravenously over 30 min, every 6 h for 40 doses, half-lives were 0.9 h after the first dose and 0.8 h after the last. Renal excretion was 55–60%. Probenecid has little effect on the plasma half-life, but markedly increases urinary recovery. Renal excretion of cilastatin closely follows that of imipenem, 75% being excreted unchanged in the urine over 6 h, with about 12% as the *N*-acetyl metabolite.

In patients with chronic renal failure, about 75% of the mixture was eliminated by 3 h hemofiltration. The half-lives of the two components differed markedly: around 3.4 h for imipenem and 16 h for cilastatin.

TOXICITY AND SIDE EFFECTS

CNS effects such as confusional states and seizures have been reported, especially when recommended doses were exceeded, and in patients with renal failure or creatinine clearances of ≤ 20 mL/min/1.73 m^2.

Other reactions include phlebitis/thrombophlebitis (3.1%), nausea (2.0%), diarrhea (1.8%) and vomiting (1.5%). Increased hepatic enzymes may be seen in adults and children. Superinfection with *Aspergillus*, *Candida* and resistant *Pseudomonas* spp. have been described and pseudomembranous colitis has been reported.

Patients with a history of hypersensitivity reactions to penicillins, cephalosporins or other β-lactam antibiotics should be treated cautiously with carbapenems.

CLINICAL USE

Lower respiratory tract infections
Urinary tract infections (complicated and uncomplicated)
Intra-abdominal infections
Gynecological infections
Bacterial septicemia
Bone and joint infections
Skin and skin structure infections
Endocarditis
Polymicrobial infections

Preparations and dosage

Proprietary name: Primaxin.

Preparations: Injection.

Dosage: Adults, deep i.m. injection, 500–750 mg every 12 h, depending on the severity of the infection; gonococcal urethritis or cervicitis, 500 mg as a single dose. (Not available in the USA.)

Adults, i.v., 1–2 g per day in 3–4 divided doses (maximum dose, 4 g per day); the dose is determined by the severity of the infection and the condition of the patient. Children 3 months (<40 kg body weight), 15 mg/kg every 6 h, with a maximum dose of 60 mg/kg per day (2 g per day), or 4 g per day if infections are caused by *Ps. aeruginosa*.

Widely available.

Further information

Clissold SP, Todd PA, Campoli-Richards DM. Imipenem/cilastatin: a review of its antibacterial activity, pharmacokinetic properties and therapeutic efficacy. *Drugs*. 1987;33:183–241.

Drusano GL. An overview of the pharmacology of imipenem/cilastatin. *J Antimicrob Chemother*. 1986;18(suppl E):79–92.

Livermore D. Interplay of impermeability and chromosomal β-lactamase activity in imipenem-resistant *Pseudomonas aeruginosa*. *Antimicrob Agents Chemother*. 1992;36:2046–2048.

Remington JS, ed. Carbapenems: a new class of antibiotics (Symposium on imipenem – cilastatin). *Am J Med*. 1985;78(suppl 6A):1–167.

Saxon A, Adelman DC, Patel A, Hajdu R, Calandra GB. Imipenem cross-reactivity with penicillin in humans. *J Allergy Clin Immunol*. 1988;82:213–217.

Trias J, Nikaido H. Outer membrane protein D2 catalyzes facilitated diffusion of carbapenems and penems through the outer membrane of *Pseudomonas aeruginosa*. *Antimicrob Agents Chemother*. 1990;34:52–57.

MEROPENEM

Molecular weight (trihydrate): 437.52.

A semisynthetic carbapenem formulated as the trihydrate for intravenous infusion. It is soluble in 5% monobasic potassium phosphate solution, sparingly soluble in water, and very slightly soluble in hydrated ethanol. The β-methyl group at C-1 confers increased stability to hydrolysis by most mammalian dehydropeptidase I enzymes (excluding rodents), thereby eliminating the need for a dehydropeptidase inhibitor in the dosing regimen.

ANTIMICROBIAL ACTIVITY

The unique side chain at C-2 is associated with increased activity against Gram-negative bacteria, including *H. influenzae*. It is slightly less active than imipenem against Gram-positive organisms (Table 15.3). It is active against anaerobes and more active against some strains that are less susceptible to imipenem. Its excellent activity against Gram-negative organisms is due to high affinity for multiple penicillin-binding proteins (PBPs; *see* p. 29). Activity is little affected by inoculum size or the presence of serum. It is bactericidal at concentrations close to the MIC.

Stability to β-lactamases is similar to that of other carbapenems: it is highly resistant to most serine β-lactamases, including extended-spectrum enzymes, but can be hydrolyzed by metallo-β-lactamases and by serine carbapenemases.

PHARMACOKINETICS

C_{max} 500 mg intravenous (30-min infusion)	23 mg/L end infusion
1 g intravenous (30-min infusion)	49 mg/L end infusion
Plasma half-life	1 h
Volume of distribution	c. 0.3 L/kg
Plasma protein binding	2%

Absorption and distribution

Meropenem is not absorbed after oral administration. It penetrates well into most body fluids and tissues, including CSF, achieving concentrations matching or exceeding those required to inhibit most susceptible bacteria. In pediatric patients (1 month to 15 years) with inflamed meninges it achieves CSF levels of 0.9–6.5 mg/L after a single intravenous infusion (40 mg/kg) over 30 min. After a single intravenous dose, the highest mean concentrations of meropenem were found in tissues and fluids at 1 h (0.5–1.5 h) after the start of infusion.

Metabolism and excretion

The mean recovery of unchanged meropenem is approximately 70%. The remainder consists of the microbiologically inactive open-ring form. Renal excretion is greater than 70% of unchanged drug over 12 h. Co-administration with probenecid prolongs the half-life 38%, but peak concentrations are not greatly affected. In patients with renal impairment the dose should be adjusted. Parent drug and metabolite are removed by hemodialysis.

TOXICITY AND SIDE EFFECTS

Seizures and other CNS adverse experiences have been reported in 0.7% of all adult patients, most commonly those with pre-existing CNS disorders. Pseudomembranous colitis has been reported. Other reactions include diarrhea (4.8%), nausea and vomiting (3.6%), inflammation at the site of injection (2.4%) and headache (2.3%). Moniliasis occurs in 1.9–3.1% of pediatric patients.

Patients with a history of hypersensitivity reactions to other β-lactam agents should be treated cautiously.

CLINICAL USE

Intra-abdominal infections
Bacterial meningitis (pediatric patients >3 months)
Complicated skin and skin structure infections

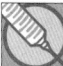

Preparations and dosage

Proprietary names: Merrem, Meronem.

Preparation: Injection.

Dosage: Adults, i.v., 0.5–2 g every 8 h. Children >3 months, 20 mg/kg every 8 h for intra-abdominal infections, or 40 mg/kg every 8 h for meningitis, or 10 mg/kg every 8 h for skin infections.

Widely available.

Further information

Craig WA. The pharmacology of meropenem, a new carbapenem antibiotic. *Clin Infect Dis.* 1997;24(suppl 2):S266–S275.

Dagan R, Velghe L, Rodda JL, Klugman KP. Penetration of meropenem into the cerebrospinal fluid of patients with inflamed meninges. *J Antimicrob Chemother.* 1994;34:175–179.

Lowe MN, Lamb HM. Meropenem: a review of its use in patients in intensive care. *Drugs.* 2000;59:653–680.

OTHER CARBAPENEMS AND PENEMS

BIAPENEM

A semisynthetic carbapenem with a 2-substituted triazolium moiety. It has broad-spectrum activity against most aerobic and anaerobic Gram-positive and Gram-negative organisms. It is equivalent to, or slightly more active than, imipenem against Gram-negative aerobic bacteria and slightly less active than imipenem against Gram-positive organisms. It is stable to hydrolysis by dehydropeptidase. It is not hydrolyzed by most serine β-lactamases, but like all carbapenems and penems is readily hydrolyzed by carbapenemases. It penetrates into bronchial epithelial lining fluid with peak concentrations of 2.4–4.4 mg/L. The plasma half-life is 1.5–1.9 h. The potential for neurotoxicity is less than that of imipenem.

Further information

Kikuchi E, Kikuchi J, Nasuhara Y, Oizumi S, Ishizaka A, Nishimura M. Comparison of the pharmacodynamics of biapenem in bronchial epithelial lining fluid in healthy volunteers given half-hour and three-hour intravenous infusions. *Antimicrob Agents Chemother.* 2009;53(7):2799–2803.

Petersen PJ, Jacobus NV, Weiss WJ, Testa RT. In vitro and in vivo activities of LJC10,627, a new carbapenem with stability to dehydropeptidase I. *Antimicrob Agents Chemother.* 1991;35:203–207.

Yang Y, Bhachech N, Bush K. Biochemical comparison of imipenem, meropenem and biapenem: permeability, binding to penicillin-binding proteins and stability to hydrolysis by β-lactamases. *J Antimicrob Chemother.* 1995;35:75–84.

FAROPENEM

An orally active penem with a broad spectrum of antibacterial activity, including activity against selected anaerobic pathogens (Table 15.3). Although it is active against most enterobacteria, it has reduced activity against *Ser. marcescens*, *Enterobacter* spp. and some *Providencia* spp. It generally retains activity against many Gram-positive organisms, but has no useful activity against *Ps. aeruginosa*. It has reduced activity against *E. faecium*, methicillin-resistant *Staph. aureus* (MRSA) and some strains of coagulase-negative staphylococci. It is stable to hydrolysis by extended spectrum β-lactamases, but is hydrolyzed by carbapenemases. Esterified prodrugs with increased bioavailability have been studied in clinical trials but have not received regulatory approval.

 Further information

Gettig JP, Crank CW, Philbrick AH. Faropenem medoxomil. *Ann Pharmacother.* 2008;42:80–90.
Woodcock JM, Andrews JM, Brenwald NP, Ashby JP, Wise R. The in vitro activity of faropenem, a novel oral penem. *J Antimicrob Chemother.* 1997;39:35–43.

 PANIPENEM

A 3-acetimidoylpyrrolidinyl-substituted carbapenem with no methyl group at the C-1 position. It has broad-spectrum antibacterial activity against Gram-positive and Gram-negative organisms very similar to that of other carbapenems. Activity against *Ps. aeruginosa* is similar to that of imipenem. It is co-administered in a ratio of 1:1 with betamipron (*N*-benzoyl-β-alanine), a renal anion transport inhibitor that decreases nephrotoxicity. Panipenem is slightly more stable to hydrolysis by dehydropeptidase than imipenem, but not as stable as meropenem or biapenem. It is hydrolyzed by carbapenemases.

Mean maximum blood concentrations following intravenous infusion of 0.5 g and 0.75 g of each component were 37 and 61 mg/L for panipenem and 24 and 39 mg/L for betamipron. Following intravenous infusion in children (10 mg or 20 mg of each component per kg), the half-life of panipenem was about 1.2 h; that of betamipron about 0.9 h. Drug levels in the CSF were at least eight-fold lower than serum concentrations.

Side effects are similar to those reported for other carbapenems (incidence <10%) and are generally mild. Patients with a history of previous hypersensitivity reactions to penicillins, cephalosporins or other β-lactam antibiotics should be treated cautiously.

Clinical use in serious infections is similar to that of other carbapenems.

 Further information

Shimada K. Panipenem/betamipron. *Jpn J Antibiot.* 1994;47:219–244.
Shimada J, Kawahara Y. Overview of a new carbapenem panipenem/betamipron. *Drugs Exp Clin Res.* 1994;20:241–245.

MONOBACTAMS

Study of the structural basis of activity of early β-lactam compounds led to the expectation that compounds in which the β-lactam ring was not strained by fusion to another ring would be inactive as antimicrobial agents. However, some natural monocyclic β-lactam antibiotics, including certain monobactams and nocardicins, are active in vitro against Gram-negative bacteria, including *Ps. aeruginosa*.

In contrast to penicillins and cephalosporins, which are commonly produced by fungi and actinomycetes, naturally occurring monobactams are produced by bacteria. Because of their simplicity of structure, they can be obtained easily by total synthesis. In some monobactams the β-lactam ring carries an α-methoxy group, similar to the β-lactamase-stable cephamycins, but the first monobactam used therapeutically, and the only one to achieve modest commercial acceptability, aztreonam, lacks this substituent.

Monobactams exhibit no useful activity against Gram-positive organisms or strict anaerobes because of poor binding to PBPs (p. 29). Activity against Gram-negative bacteria, including *Ps. aeruginosa*, is due to tight binding to PBP 3 (*Esch. coli* numbering). As a result, the organisms convert to filaments, which slowly lyse.

Monobactams are hydrolyzed poorly by many serine β-lactamases and all metallo-β-lactamases, but can be hydrolyzed by ESBLs and serine carbapenemases. Group 1 cephalosporinases have high affinities for non-methoxylated monobactams, whereas group 2 β-lactamases generally bind aztreonam poorly. They are generally not inducers of the group 1 chromosomal cephalosporinases of Gram-negative bacteria.

AZTREONAM

Molecular weight: 435.43.

A synthetic analog of a monobactam antibiotic from the bacterium *Chromobacterium violaceum*. Now obtained by chemical synthesis and available for intramuscular or intravenous administration.

ANTIMICROBIAL ACTIVITY

Its activity against common Gram-negative organisms is shown in Table 15.3 (p. 232). Concentrations (mg/L) inhibiting 50% of other organisms are: *Aeromonas* spp., 0.1;

Acinetobacter spp., 16; *Mor. catarrhalis*, 0.1; *Burkholderia cepacia*, 2; and *Yersinia* spp., 0.1. Synergy has been shown with gentamicin, tobramycin and amikacin against 52–89% of strains of *Ps. aeruginosa* and gentamicin-resistant Gram-negative bacteria.

PHARMACOKINETICS

C_max 1 g intravenous	90 mg/L end infusion
1 g intramuscular	46 mg/L after 1 h
Plasma half-life	1.7 h
Volume of distribution	0.18 L/kg
Plasma protein binding	56%

Absorption and distribution

Oral bioavailability is less than 1%. Peak concentrations above the median MIC for most Gram-negative pathogens are achieved in most tissues and body fluids after 1 g intramuscular or intravenous doses.

Metabolism and excretion

It is not extensively metabolized, the most prominent product, resulting from opening the β-lactam ring, being scarcely detectable in the serum and accounting for about 6% of the dose in the urine and 3% in the feces.

It is predominantly eliminated in the urine, where 58–72% appears within 8 h. Less than 12% is eliminated unchanged in the feces, suggesting low biliary excretion.

TOXICITY AND SIDE EFFECTS

Local reactions occasionally occur at the injection site. Systemic reactions include diarrhea, nausea and/or vomiting and rash (1–1.3%). Neutropenia was seen in 11.3% of the pediatric patients younger than 2 years. Pseudomembranous colitis has been reported.

There are no reactions in patients with immunoglobulin E (IgE) antibodies to benzylpenicillin or penicillin moieties. It is rarely cross-reactive with other β-lactam antibiotics and is weakly immunogenic.

CLINICAL USE

Urinary tract infections, including pyelonephritis and cystitis

Lower respiratory tract infections, including pneumonia and bronchitis caused by Gram-negative bacilli

Septicemia

Skin and skin structure infections, including postoperative wounds, ulcers and burns

Intra-abdominal infections, including peritonitis

Gynecological infections, including endometritis and pelvic cellulitis

Preparations and dosage

Proprietary name: Azactam.

Preparations: Injection, infusion.

Dosage: Adults, i.m., i.v., i.v. infusion, 1–8 g per day in 2–4 divided doses. Route, frequency and dose are determined by the severity of the infection and the condition of the patient. Children, 30 mg/kg every 6–8 h (up to 50 mg/kg every 6–8 h in severe infection and cystic fibrosis).

Widely available, including the USA and the UK.

Further information

Acar JF, Neu HC, eds. Gram-negative aerobic bacterial infections: a focus on directed therapy with special reference to aztreonam. *Rev Infect Dis.* 1985;7(suppl 4):S537–S843.

Brogden RN, Heel RC. Aztreonam: a review of its antibacterial activity, pharmacokinetic properties and therapeutic use. *Drugs.* 1986;31:96–130.

Swabb EA. Review of the clinical pharmacology of the monobactam antibiotic aztreonam. *Am J Med.* 1985;78(2A):11–18.

OTHER MONOBACTAMS

CARUMONAM

A synthetic monobactam with activity against common pathogenic organisms similar to that of aztreonam. It is resistant to hydrolysis by the common plasmid and chromosomal β-lactamases, but it can be hydrolyzed by ESBLs.

It is administered intravenously, achieving a concentration of *c.* 78 mg/L after a 20-min infusion of 1 g. The plasma half-life is 1.7 h and the plasma protein binding 18–28%.

Carumonam is almost entirely eliminated in the glomerular filtrate, probenecid having no effect on excretion; 96% of labeled compound is found in the urine, with 3% in the feces. Between 68% and 91% of the dose appears in the urine within 24 h.

Side effects and clinical use are similar to those of aztreonam.

Preparations and dosage

Preparation: Injection.

Dosage: Adult, i.m., i.v., 1–2 g per day in two divided doses.

Available in Japan. Not available in Europe or the USA.

Further information

Imada A, Kondo M, Okonogi K, Yukishige K, Kuno M. In vitro and in vivo antibacterial activities of carumonam (AMA-1080), a new *N*-sulfonated monocyclic β-lactam antibiotic. *Antimicrob Agents Chemother.* 1985;27:821–827.

Patel JH, Soni PP, Portmann R, Suter K, Banken L, Weidekamm E. Multiple intravenous dose pharmacokinetic study of carumonam in healthy subjects. *J Antimicrob Chemother.* 1989;23:107–111.

β-LACTAMASE INHIBITORS

Because β-lactamase production is the predominant cause of clinically important resistance to β-lactam antibiotics in most bacteria, an attractive therapeutic approach is to co-administer a β-lactamase inhibitor together with the labile antibiotic. Implicit in this approach, however, are some demanding requirements:

- The inhibitor must be active against a wide range of β-lactamases.
- The absorption, distribution and excretion characteristics of the inhibitor must match closely those of the β-lactam agent with which it is to be paired.
- Its use must not add materially to the toxicity.

The ability of certain β-lactam agents to inhibit selected β-lactamases has been known for a long time. A directed search for potent β-lactamase inhibitors resulted in the discovery of clavulanic acid as a natural product, and the subsequent synthesis of the sulfones, sulbactam and tazobactam. The β-lactamase inhibitors in therapeutic use have poor, or no, antimicrobial activity and act synergistically in combination with β-lactamase-labile penicillins or cephalosporins. None is effective against metallo-β-lactamases. In some organisms these inhibitors may act as inducers of β-lactamase activity.

Carbapenems and monobactams act like competitive inhibitors, or, more specifically, competitive substrates of some serine β-lactamases, with monobactams inhibiting group 1 cephalosporinases at nanomolar concentrations. Their action is reversible, leaving the enzyme intact, because they simply act as poor substrates that are bound tightly to the β-lactamase and are hydrolyzed slowly. The effective inhibitors that have been developed commercially are irreversible inactivators, or 'suicide' inhibitors. The enzyme and inhibitor interact competitively initially and then progressively form a complex in which the enzyme is inactivated over time, usually after a fixed amount of inhibitor has been hydrolyzed like a normal substrate. Clavulanic acid, sulbactam and tazobactam are all of this form, although the precise nature, rate and degree of inactivation differ considerably among the various combinations of agents and enzymes.

Inhibitory effects are dependent upon the amount of enzyme in the organism, so that increased β-lactamase production results in lower efficacy for inhibitor–β-lactam combinations. Resistance may arise through hyperproduction of a sensitive β-lactamase or the occurrence of relatively rare 'inhibitor-resistant' TEM or SHV variants with one or two amino acid changes in the parent enzymes.

 Further information

Buynak JD. Understanding the longevity of the beta-lactam antibiotics and of antibiotic/beta-lactamase inhibitor combinations. *Biochem Pharmacol.* 2006;71:930–940.

Canton R, Morosini MI, de la Maza OM, de la Pedrosa EG. IRT and CMT beta-lactamases and inhibitor resistance. *Clin Microbiol Infect.* 2008;14(suppl 1):53–62.

Payne DJ, Cramp R, Winstanley DJ, Knowles DJC. Comparative activities of clavulanic acid, sulbactam, and tazobactam against clinically important β-lactamases. *Antimicrob Agents Chemother.* 1994;38:767–772.

CLAVULANIC ACID

Molecular weight (potassium salt): 237.25.

An oxapenam (clavam) produced by *Streptomyces clavuligerus*. It is available as the potassium salt for oral and intravenous use in fixed-ratio combination with amoxicillin and for intravenous use in combination with ticarcillin. It is freely soluble in water.

ANTIMICROBIAL ACTIVITY

It exhibits broad-spectrum but low intrinsic activity, most MICs being in the range 16–128 mg/L. Enterobacteriaceae and *Staph. aureus* are among the more sensitive and *Ps. aeruginosa* the most resistant organisms. MICs of 8 mg/L against *H. influenzae* and 0.1–4 mg/L for penicillinase-producing *N. gonorrhoeae* are notable.

β-LACTAMASE INHIBITORY ACTIVITY

Clavulanic acid is a potent, progressive inhibitor of most group 2 β-lactamases, with the exception of some TEM and many OXA variants. It is very active against the *K. pneumoniae* K1 (group 2be) enzyme, the group 2e chromosomal enzymes produced by *Pr. vulgaris* and *B. fragilis*, both enzymes produced by *Mor. catarrhalis* and the group 2a penicillinases from *Staph. aureus*. It does not effectively inhibit the group 1 chromosomal cephalosporinases from Enterobacteriaceae or the group 3 metallo-β-lactamases.

In the presence of low concentrations of clavulanic acid (0.5–1 mg/L) the MICs of amoxicillin and ticarcillin for many β-lactamase-producing *Staph. aureus*, *Mor. catarrhalis*, *N. gonorrhoeae*, *H. influenzae*, enterobacteria and *B. fragilis* strains are reduced 8- to 64-fold. In *B. fragilis* strains resistant to penicillin, the addition of clavulanic acid renders most of the strains susceptible to amoxicillin or ticarcillin. Susceptibility of methicillin-resistant strains of *Staph. aureus* is unaffected by the presence of clavulanic acid.

Resistance that develops during therapy is generally due to overproduction of the sensitive β-lactamase, e.g. TEM-1 or SHV-1, which is no longer effectively inhibited by a limited quantity of clavulanic acid or to the production of occasional 'inhibitor-resistant' β-lactamases.

AMOXICILLIN–CLAVULANIC ACID

Co-amoxiclav. A mixture of potassium clavulanate and amoxicillin trihydrate (oral formulations) or amoxicillin sodium (parenteral formulations). The ratio of amoxicillin to clavulanic acid in the commercially available oral preparations is variable.

ANTIMICROBIAL ACTIVITY

Activity is that of amoxicillin (p. 215), the role of the inhibitor being to restore the activity against β-lactamase-producing strains that would otherwise hydrolyze the drug.

PHARMACOKINETICS

	Amoxicillin	Clavulanic acid
Oral absorption	c. 90%	c. 90%
C$_{max}$ 500 mg amoxicillin + 125 mg clavulanic acid oral	7.2 mg/L after 1 h	2.4 mg/L after 1 h
2000 g amoxicillin + 125 mg clavulanic acid (extended-release formulation)	17 mg/L after 1.5 h	2.05 mg/L after 1 h
400 mg amoxicillin + 57 mg clavulanic acid oral	6.9 mg/L	1.1 mg/L
Plasma half-life	1.3 h	1.0 h
Plasma protein binding	18%	25%

Absorption and distribution

There is little effect on the pharmacokinetics of each agent from the presence of the other, although clavulanic acid is marginally better absorbed in the presence of amoxicillin. There is wide individual variation in bioavailability (30–99%).

Effective levels are found in most body tissues and fluids. Total penetration into the CSF was 8% and 6% of the corresponding plasma values for clavulanate and amoxicillin, respectively. Clavulanate penetrates poorly into sputum after oral dosing.

Metabolism and excretion

Clavulanic acid appears to be metabolized extensively, with metabolites eliminated via the urine, bile, feces and lungs. Variation in bioavailability may be related to differences in first-pass effects through those organs.

Approximately 50–70% of the administered amoxicillin and 25–40% of clavulanic acid are recovered intact from the urine. Most renal excretion occurs in the first 6 h and is unaffected by probenecid, although probenecid prolongs the renal excretion of amoxicillin. In renal failure, the volume of distribution and systemic availability are unaffected after oral or intravenous administration, but clearance is progressively depressed with renal function.

TOXICITY AND SIDE EFFECTS

Cholestatic jaundice is more common with co-amoxiclav than with amoxicillin alone and the combination is contraindicated in patients with a history of hepatic dysfunction associated with the drug.

Other common side effects are diarrhea (9%), nausea (3%), skin rashes and urticaria (3%), vomiting (1%) and vaginitis (1%). The overall incidence of side effects, and in particular diarrhea, increases with the higher recommended dose. Pseudomembranous colitis has been reported.

For side effects attributable to amoxicillin, see page 215.

CLINICAL USE

Lower respiratory tract infections
Otitis media
Sinusitis
Skin and skin structure infections
Urinary tract infections

It is usually recommended for use against amoxicillin-resistant organisms if the susceptibility status is known.

Preparations and dosage

Proprietary name: Augmentin.

Preparations: Tablets, suspension, injection.

Dosage: Adults, oral, 250/125 mg every 8 h, or 500/125 mg every 12 h; 500/125 mg every 8 h, or 875/125 or 2000/125 mg every 12 h for more serious infections. Children, the dose varies according to age and severity of infection.

Adults, i.v., 1.2 g every 6–8 h depending on the severity of the infection. Infants <3 months, 30 mg/kg every 12 h; children 3 months to 12 years, 20–45 mg/kg every 8–12 h depending on the severity of the infection. (Not available in the USA.)

Widely available.

TICARCILLIN–CLAVULANIC ACID

A mixture of potassium clavulanate and ticarcillin disodium in a 1:15 or 1:30 ratio for parenteral administration.

ANTIMICROBIAL ACTIVITY

Activity is that of ticarcillin (p. 222), the role of the inhibitor being to restore the activity against β-lactamase-producing strains that would otherwise hydrolyze the drug.

PHARMACOKINETICS

	Ticarcillin	Clavulanic acid
C_{max} 3 g ticarcillin + 100 mg clavulanate intravenous infusion (30 min)	330 mg/L end infusion	8 mg/L end infusion
Plasma half-life	1.1 h	1.1 h
Plasma protein binding	45%	25%

The pharmacokinetics of the two agents are mutually unaffected by co-administration. Ticarcillin can be detected in tissues and interstitial fluid following parenteral administration. Penetration into bile, peritoneal fluid and pleural fluid has been demonstrated. Concentrations in blister fluid were significantly lower than those in serum.

Around 60–70% of ticarcillin and 35–45% of clavulanic acid are excreted unchanged in urine during the first 6 h after administration of a single dose of the mixture.

TOXICITY AND SIDE EFFECTS

Adverse reactions associated with ticarcillin occur (see p. 222). As with co-amoxiclav, there is a risk of cholestatic jaundice (see above). Pseudomembranous colitis has been reported.

CLINICAL USE

Septicemia, including bacteremia
Lower respiratory infections
Bone and joint infections
Skin and skin structure infections
Urinary tract infections (complicated and uncomplicated)
Gynecological infections, endometritis
Intra-abdominal infections, peritonitis

Its main use is in infections in which *Ps. aeruginosa* is suspected or proven.

Preparations and dosage

Proprietary name: Timentin.
Preparation: Infusion.
Dosage: Adults, i.v. infusion, 3.0/0.2 g every 4–6 h. Children <60 kg, 200–300 mg/kg per day in 4–6 divided doses; 60 kg, 3.0/0.2 g every 4–6 h depending on the severity of the infection.
Widely available.

Further information

Ferslew KE, Daigneault GA, Aten RM, Roseman RM. Pharmacokinetics and urinary excretion of clavulanic acid after oral administration of amoxicillin and potassium clavulanate. *J Clin Pharmacol.* 1984;24:452–456.
Geddes AM, Klugman KP, Rolinson GN. Introduction: historical perspective and development of amoxicillin/clavulanate. *Int J Antimicrob Agents.* 2007;30(suppl 2):S109–S112.
Leigh DA, Phillips I, Wise R. Timentin–ticarcillin plus clavulanic acid: a laboratory and clinical perspective. *J Antimicrob Chemother.* 1986;17(suppl C):1–240.
Sanders CC, Jaconis JP, Bodey GP, Samonis G. Resistance to ticarcillin–potassium clavulanate among clinical isolates of the family Enterobacteriaceae: the role of PSE-1 β-lactamase and high levels of TEM-1 and SHV-1 and problems with false susceptibility in disk diffusion tests. *Antimicrob Agents Chemother.* 1988;32:1365–1369.

SULBACTAM

Molecular weight (sodium salt): 255.22.

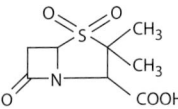

A penicillanic acid sulfone available as the sodium salt. Formulations combining ampicillin or cefoperazone with sulbactam in a 2:1 ratio are available for parenteral use. A methylene-linked double ester of penicillin and sulbactam, sultamicillin, is used for oral administration.

ANTIMICROBIAL ACTIVITY

Sulbactam has very weak antimicrobial activity against most bacteria. Its only notable activity is against *N. gonorrhoeae*, *N. meningitidis* and *Acinetobacter baumannii*.

β-LACTAMASE-INHIBITORY ACTIVITY

It inhibits a wide range of group 2 β-lactamases, including those from *Staph. aureus*, *K. pneumoniae* and *B. fragilis*. It is a good-to-moderate inhibitor of the TEM enzymes of groups 2b and 2be but has little effect on group 1, group 2br or group 3 β-lactamases. It does not induce the activity of cephalosporinases from Gram-negative bacteria but is a weak inducer of penicillinases from *Staph. aureus*.

A concentration of 4–8 mg/L restores the activity of ampicillin for many β-lactamase-producing strains of *Staph. aureus*, *H. influenzae*, *Mor. catarrhalis*, enterobacteria and *B. fragilis*, but there is a large inoculum effect.

AMPICILLIN–SULBACTAM

ANTIMICROBIAL ACTIVITY

Activity is that of ampicillin (p. 216), the role of the inhibitor being to restore the activity against β-lactamase-producing strains that would otherwise hydrolyze the drug.

PHARMACOKINETICS

	Ampicillin	Sulbactam
Oral absorption (sultamicillin)	>80%	>80%
C_{max}, ampicillin 2 g + sulbactam 1 g intravenous	109–150 mg/L end infusion	48–88 mg/L end infusion
750 mg oral (sultamicillin)	9.1 mg/L after 1 h	8.9 mg/L after 1 h
Plasma half-life	1 h	1 h
Plasma protein binding	28%	38%

Absorption and distribution

The sodium salt of sulbactam is poorly absorbed orally, but the linked prodrug sultamicillin is well absorbed; it undergoes first-pass hydrolysis to liberate equimolecular proportions of the components.

Ampicillin–sulbactam is completely bioavailable after intramuscular injection, doses of 1.0 and 0.5 g producing mean peak plasma levels of 8–37 and 6–24 mg/L, respectively. After intravenous administration both drugs penetrate peritoneal fluid, blister fluid (cantharides-induced), tissue fluid and intestinal mucosa to provide concentrations ≥7 mg/L. Penetration of both ampicillin and sulbactam into CSF in the presence of inflamed meninges has been demonstrated after intravenous infusion.

Metabolism and excretion

Sulbactam is not metabolized. Ampicillin metabolism is described on page 217. In normal volunteers 75–85% of both ampicillin and sulbactam are excreted unchanged in the urine during the first 8 h after administration.

TOXICITY AND SIDE EFFECTS

Local adverse reactions include pain at the injection site (intramuscular 16%, intravenous 3%) and thrombophlebitis (3%). Systemic adverse reactions include diarrhea (3%). Pseudomembranous colitis has been reported. For side effects attributable to ampicillin, see page 217.

CLINICAL USE

Skin and skin structure infections
Intra-abdominal infections
Gynecological infections

Preparations and dosage

Preparation: Injection.

Dosage: Adult, i.m., i.v., 1/0.5–2/1 g every 6 h; Children, 300 mg/kg per day in four divided doses.

Available in the USA, but not available in the UK.

Sulbactam–cefoperazone and sultamicillin are available in Japan.

Further information

Foulds G, McBride TJ, Knirsch AK, Rodriguez WJ, Khan WN. Penetration of sulbactam and ampicillin into cerebrospinal fluid of infants and young children with meningitis. *Antimicrob Agents Chemother*. 1987;31:1703–1705.

Frieder HA, Campoli-Richards DM, Goa KL. Sultamicillin. A review of its antibacterial activity, pharmacokinetic properties and therapeutic use. *Drugs*. 1989;37:491–522.

Karageorgopoulos DE, Falagas ME. Current control and treatment of multidrug-resistant *Acinetobacter baumannii* infections. *Lancet Infect Dis*. 2008;8:751–762.

Symposium. Enzyme-mediated resistance to β-lactam antibiotics. A symposium on sulbactam/ampicillin. *Rev Infect Dis*. 1986;8(suppl 5):S465–S650.

Rafailidis PI, Ioannidou EN, Falagas ME. Ampicillin/sulbactam: current status in severe bacterial infections. *Drugs*. 2007;67:1829–1849.

TAZOBACTAM

Molecular weight (sodium salt): 322.3.

A synthetic penicillanic acid sulfone available as the sodium salt. It is formulated with piperacillin in a piperacillin:tazobactam ratio of 8:1

ANTIMICROBIAL ACTIVITY

Tazobactam exhibits little useful antimicrobial activity, although weak activity against *Acinetobacter* spp. and *Borrelia burgdorferi* has been reported.

β-LACTAMASE INHIBITORY ACTIVITY

Tazobactam inhibits a wide range of β-lactamases, including the group 2 penicillinases from *Staph. aureus*, the TEM-1 and SHV-1 β-lactamases, many extended-spectrum enzymes, and the common group 2e cephalosporinases of *B. fragilis*. Against the group 1 cephalosporinases, activity is strongly influenced by the amount of enzyme produced. The inhibitor-resistant group 2br β-lactamases are poorly inhibited and group 3 metallo-β-lactamases are not inhibited at clinically useful levels. It is a poor inducer of β-lactamases of Gram-positive and Gram-negative organisms.

At a concentration of 4 mg/L it markedly reduces the MIC and enhances the bactericidal activity of piperacillin against many β-lactamase-producing organisms, but only moderately against those elaborating group 1 cephalosporinases. It enhances activity against β-lactamase-producing *Staph. aureus*, *H. influenzae*, *Mor. catarrhalis*, most of the *B. fragilis* group, *Acinetobacter* spp., many enterobacteria, especially *Pr. mirabilis* and *Morganella morganii*, and occasional *Enterobacter* spp. and *C. freundii*.

PIPERACILLIN–TAZOBACTAM

ANTIMICROBIAL ACTIVITY

Activity is that of piperacillin (p. 221), the role of the inhibitor being to restore the activity against β-lactamase-producing strains that would otherwise hydrolyze the drug. Although the activity of piperacillin against *Ps. aeruginosa* is not enhanced, it remains the most active inhibitor combination in vitro against *Ps. aeruginosa*.

PHARMACOKINETICS

	Piperacillin	Tazobactam
C_{max}, 3 g piperacillin + 375 mg tazobactam intravenous infusion	242 mg/L end infusion	24 mg/L end infusion
Plasma half-life	1 h	1.1 h
Plasma protein binding	30%	30%

Absorption and distribution

The components are not absorbed orally. The combination has good tissue distribution, with mean tissue concentrations 50–100% of those in plasma. Co-administration of tazobactam does not affect the pharmacokinetics of piperacillin. Co-administration of piperacillin and tazobactam with vancomycin resulted in no significant change in pharmacokinetic interactions.

Metabolism and excretion

A small amount of piperacillin is metabolized to a microbiologically active desethyl metabolite, and some undergoes cleavage of the β-lactam ring. Tazobactam is metabolized to a ring-opened compound that further degrades to a derivative devoid of pharmacological activity.

Renal clearance of both drugs occurs by glomerular filtration and tubular secretion. Urinary excretion of piperacillin is 68%, whereas tazobactam and its metabolite are eliminated primarily by renal excretion (80%). Biliary secretion of piperacillin, tazobactam and desethyl piperacillin are also observed.

TOXICITY AND SIDE EFFECTS

Most adverse events are mild to moderate, and transient. Most common drug-related events are rash and pruritus (1.3%) and gastrointestinal effects (0.9%). Pseudomembranous colitis has been reported.

For side effect attributable to piperacillin, see page 221.

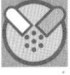

CLINICAL USE

Uncomplicated and complicated skin and skin structure infection
Postpartum endometritis or pelvic inflammatory disease
Community-acquired pneumonia (moderate severity)
Nosocomial pneumonia (moderate to severe)
Appendicitis and peritonitis

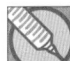

Preparations and dosage

Proprietary names: Tazocin, Zosyn.

Preparation: Injection.

Dosage: Adults and children over 12 years, by i.v. injection, 3.0/0.375 g every 6 h; may be dosed 4.0/0.5 g every 6 h plus amikacin or gentamicin for patients with nosocomial pneumonia caused by *Ps. aeruginosa*. Children >9 months, 100/12.5 mg/kg every 8 h. Children 2–9 months, 80 g/kg every 8 h.

Widely available.

Further information

Bush K, Macalintal C, Rasmussen BA, Lee VJ, Yang Y. Kinetic interactions of tazobactam with β-lactamases from all major structural classes. *Antimicrob Agents Chemother*. 1993;37:851–858.

Gin A, Dilay L, Karlowsky JA, Walkty A, Rubinstein E, Zhanel GG. Piperacillin–tazobactam: a beta-lactam/beta-lactamase inhibitor combination. *Expert Rev Anti Infect Ther*. 2007;5:365–383.

Greenwood D, Finch RG. Piperacillin/tazobactam: a new β-lactam/β-lactamase inhibitor combination. *J Antimicrob Chemother*. 1993;31(suppl A):1–124.

Kuck NA, Jacobus NV, Petersen PJ, Weiss WJ, Testa RT. Comparative in vitro and in vivo activities of piperacillin combined with the β-lactamase inhibitors tazobactam, clavulanic acid, and sulbactam. *Antimicrob Agents Chemother*. 1989;33:1964–1969.

Wise R, Logan M, Cooper M, Andrews JM. Pharmacokinetics and tissue penetration of tazobactam administered alone and with piperacillin *Antimicrob Agents Chemother*. 1991;35:1081–1084.

16 Chloramphenicol and thiamphenicol

Mark H. Wilcox

Chloramphenicol was the first broad-spectrum antibiotic to be discovered. It was isolated independently from streptomycetes from soil in Venezuela and a compost heap in Illinois. The commercial product is manufactured synthetically. There are four isomers, all of which have been synthesized, but none has greater activity than the natural compound. The major drawback is a rare, idiosyncratic, often fatal aplastic anemia, and numerous attempts have been made to manufacture related agents which retain the spectrum of activity and pharmacokinetics of the parent compound, but not the toxicity. The only derivative to come into commercial use in which this is believed to have been achieved is thiamphenicol, in which the nitro group of chloramphenicol is replaced by a sulfomethyl group. However, compounds in which the nitro group is replaced are all less active than the parent compound.

Substitution of the 3′-OH group or fluorine for chlorine has produced analogs of chloramphenicol and thiamphenicol that are active against strains of bacteria that owe their resistance to chloramphenicol acetylation, but not against organisms with reduced permeability. Fluorinated derivatives are not marketed for human use, but florfenicol is available in veterinary practice and aquaculture in some countries.

 Further information

Fuglesang J, Bergan T. Chloramphenicol and thiamphenicol. *Antibiot Chemother.* 1982;31:1–21.

Holt D, Harvey D, Hurley R. Chloramphenicol toxicity. *Adverse Drug React Toxicol Rev.* 1993;12:83–95.

Wareham DW, Wilson P. Chloramphenicol in the 21st century. *Hosp Med.* 2002;63:157–161.

CHLORAMPHENICOL

Molecular weight: 323.1.

$$O_2N - \bigcirc - \underset{\underset{OH}{|}}{\overset{\overset{H}{|}}{C}} - \underset{\underset{H}{|}}{\overset{\overset{NHCOCHCl_2}{|}}{C}} - CH_2OH$$

A fermentation product of *Streptomyces venezuelae*. Commercially manufactured synthetically. Formulated as the free compound (which is extremely bitter) or as the palmitate ester for oral administration; as the free compound for topical use; and as the sodium succinate for injection. Aqueous solutions are extremely stable, but some hydrolysis occurs on autoclaving.

ANTIMICROBIAL ACTIVITY

It is active against a very wide range of organisms. The susceptibility of common pathogenic bacteria is shown in Table 16.1. Minimum inhibitory concentrations (MICs) (mg/L) for other organisms are: *Staphylococcus epidermidis*, 1–8; *Corynebacterium diphtheriae*, 0.5–2; *Bacillus anthracis*, 1–4; *Clostridium perfringens*, 2–8; *Mycobacterium tuberculosis*, 8–32; *Legionella pneumophila*, 0.5–1; *Bordetella pertussis*, 0.25–4; *Brucella abortus*, 1–4; *Campylobacter fetus*, 2–4; *Pasteurella* spp., 0.25–4; *Serratia marcescens*, 2–8; *Burkholderia pseudomallei*, 4–8. Most Gram-negative bacilli are susceptible, but *Pseudomonas aeruginosa* is resistant. *Leptospira* spp., *Treponema pallidum*, chlamydiae, mycoplasmas and rickettsiae are all susceptible, but *Nocardia* spp. are resistant. It is widely active against anaerobes, including *Actinomyces israelii* (MIC 1–4 mg/L), *Peptostreptococcus* spp. (MIC 0.1–8 mg/L), and *Fusobacterium* spp. (MIC 0.5–2 mg/L), but *Bacteroides fragilis* is only moderately susceptible (MIC about 8 mg/L).

It is strictly bacteristatic against almost all bacterial species, but exerts a bactericidal effect at 2–4 times the MIC against some strains of Gram-positive cocci, *Haemophilus influenzae* and *Neisseria* spp. The minimum bactericidal concentrations (MBCs) for penicillin-resistant pneumococci are often significantly higher than those for penicillin-susceptible strains, although this cannot be detected by conventional disk susceptibility testing or MIC determination. Its bacteristatic effect may inhibit the action of penicillins and other β-lactam antibiotics against *Klebsiella pneumoniae* and other enterobacteria in vitro, but the clinical

Table 16.1 Activity of chloramphenicol and thiamphenicol: MIC (mg/L)

	Chloramphenicol	Thiamphenicol
Staphylococcus aureus	2–8	4–32
Streptococcus pyogenes	2–4	1–2
Str. pneumoniae	1–4	2–4
Enterococcus faecalis	4–16	8–32
Neisseria gonorrhoeae	0.5–2	0.5–2
N. meningitidis	0.5–2	0.5–2
Haemophilus influenzae	0.25–0.5	0.1–2
Escherichia coli	2–8	4–64
Klebsiella pneumoniae	0.5–32	4–32
Salmonella enterica	0.5–8	0.5–8
Shigella spp.	1–8	2–8
Pseudomonas aeruginosa	32–R	16–R
Bacteroides spp.	1–8	0.5–32

R, resistant (MIC >64 mg/L).

significance of this is doubtful. The presence of ampicillin does not affect the bactericidal effect of chloramphenicol on *H. influenzae*.

ACQUIRED RESISTANCE

The prevalence of resistant strains in many Gram-positive and Gram-negative organisms reflects usage of the antibiotic. Over-the-counter sales are believed to have compounded the problem in some countries. For example, it has long been the drug of choice for the treatment of typhoid and paratyphoid fevers, but widespread use led to a high prevalence of resistant *Salmonella enterica* serotype Typhi. Outbreaks of infection caused by chloramphenicol-resistant *S.* Typhi have been seen since the early 1970s. Use of co-trimoxazole and fluoroquinolones in typhoid has resulted in a decline in chloramphenicol resistance in some endemic areas. Many hospital outbreaks caused by multiresistant strains of enterobacteria, notably *Enterobacter*, *Klebsiella* and *Serratia* spp., have been described.

Plasmid-borne resistance was first noted in shigellae in Japan and subsequently spread widely in Central America, where it was responsible for a huge outbreak. Strains of *S.* Typhi resistant to many antibiotics including chloramphenicol are particularly common in the Indian subcontinent. Resistance in shigellae is also relatively common in some parts of the world.

Resistant strains of *H. influenzae* (some also resistant to ampicillin), *Staph. aureus* and *Streptococcus pyogenes* are also encountered. Most *N. meningitidis* strains remain susceptible,

but high-level resistance (MIC >64 mg/L) due to the production of chloramphenicol acetyltransferase (p. 27) has been described; the nucleotide sequence of the resistance gene was indistinguishable from that found on a transposon in *Cl. perfringens*. Resistant strains of *Enterococcus faecalis* are relatively common, and resistance to chloramphenicol is found in some multiresistant pneumococci.

Resistance in *Staph. aureus* is caused by an inducible acetyltransferase; additionally, the *cfr* (chloramphenicol–florfenicol resistance) gene encodes a 23S rRNA methyltransferase that also confers resistance to linezolid. In *Escherichia coli*, the capacity to acetylate chloramphenicol (at least three enzymes are involved) is carried by R factors. Replacement of the 3-OH group, which is the target of acetylation, accounts for the activity of fluorinated analogs against strains resistant to chloramphenicol and thiamphenicol. The resistance of *B. fragilis* and some strains of *H. influenzae* is also due to elaboration of a plasmid-encoded acetylating enzyme; in others it is due to reduced permeability resulting from loss of an outer membrane protein. Some resistant bacteria reduce the nitro group or hydrolyze the amide linkage. Resistance of *Ps. aeruginosa* is partly enzymic and partly due to impermeability.

PHARMACOKINETICS

Oral absorption	80–90%
C_{max} 500 mg oral	10–13 mg/L after 1–2 h
Plasma half-life	1.5–3.5 h
Volume of distribution	0.25–2 L/kg
Plasma protein binding	*c.* 25–60%

Absorption

The plasma concentration achieved is proportional to the dose administered. Suspensions for oral administration to children contain chloramphenicol palmitate, a tasteless and bacteriologically inert compound, which is hydrolyzed in the gut to liberate chloramphenicol. Following a dose of 25 mg/kg, peak plasma levels around 6–12 mg/L are obtained, but there is much individual variation.

Pancreatic lipase is deficient in neonates and, because of poor hydrolysis, the palmitate should be avoided. In very young infants, deficient ability to form glucuronides, and low glomerular and tubular excretion greatly prolong the plasma half-life.

For parenteral use, chloramphenicol sodium succinate, which is freely soluble and undergoes hydrolysis in the tissues with the liberation of chloramphenicol, can be injected intravenously or in small volumes intramuscularly. The plasma concentrations after administration by these routes are unpredictable, and approximate to only 30–70% of those obtained after the same dose by the oral route. Protein binding is reduced in cirrhotic patients and neonates, with correspondingly elevated concentrations of free drug.

Distribution

Free diffusion occurs into serous effusions. Penetration occurs into all parts of the eye, the therapeutic levels in the aqueous humor being obtained even after local application of 0.5% ophthalmic solution. Concentrations obtained in cerebrospinal fluid (CSF) in the absence of meningitis are 30–50% of those of the blood and greater in brain. It crosses the placenta into the fetal circulation and appears in breast milk.

Metabolism

It is largely inactivated in the liver by conjugation with glucuronic acid or by reduction to inactive arylamines; clearance of the drug in patients with impaired liver function is depressed in relation to the plasma bilirubin level. It has been suggested that genetically determined variance of hepatic glucuronyl transferase might determine the disposition and toxicity of the drug.

Excretion

It is excreted in the glomerular filtrate, and in the newborn elimination may be impaired by the concomitant administration of benzylpenicillin, which is handled early in life by the same route. Inactive derivatives are eliminated partly in the glomerular filtrate and partly by active tubular secretion. Over 24 h, 75–90% of the dose appears in the urine, 5–10% in biologically active forms and the rest as metabolites, chiefly as a glucuronide conjugate. Excretion diminishes linearly with renal function and at a creatinine clearance of <20 ml/min, maximum urinary concentrations are 10–20 mg/L rather than the 150–200 mg/L found in normal subjects. Because of metabolism, blood levels of active drug are only marginally elevated in renal failure, but microbiologically inactive metabolites accumulate. The plasma half-life of the products in the anuric patient is around 100 h, and little is removed by peritoneal or hemodialysis. Dosage modification is normally unnecessary in renal failure as the metabolites are less toxic than the parent compound. About 3% of the administered dose is excreted in the bile, but only 1% appears in the feces, and this mostly in inactive forms.

 INTERACTIONS

Induction of liver microsomal enzymes, for example by phenobarbital (phenobarbitone) or rifampicin (rifampin), diminishes blood levels of chloramphenicol; conversely, chloramphenicol, which inhibits hepatic microsomal oxidases, potentiates the activity of dicoumarol (dicumarol), phenytoin, tolbutamide and those barbiturates that are eliminated by metabolism. It also depresses the action of cyclophosphamide, which depends for its cytotoxicity on transformation into active metabolites. It is uncertain whether this interaction may lead to a clinically significant level of inhibition of the activity of cyclophosphamide. The half-life of chloramphenicol is considerably prolonged if paracetamol (acetaminophen) is given concurrently, and co-administration of these drugs should be avoided.

 TOXICITY AND SIDE EFFECTS

Glossitis, associated with overgrowth of *Candida albicans*, is fairly common if the course of treatment exceeds 1 week. Stomatitis, nausea, vomiting and diarrhea may occur, but are uncommon. Hypersensitivity reactions are very uncommon. Jarisch–Herxheimer-like reactions have been described in patients treated for brucellosis, enteric fever and syphilis.

Bone marrow effects

Chloramphenicol exerts a dose-related but reversible depressant effect on the marrow of all those treated, resulting in vacuolization of erythroid and myeloid cells, reticulocytopenia and ferrokinetic changes indicative of decreased erythropoiesis. Evidence of bone-marrow depression is regularly seen if the plasma concentration exceeds 25 mg/L, and leukopenia and thrombocytopenia may be severe. There is no evidence that this common marrow depression is the precursor of potentially fatal aplasia, which differs in that it is fortunately rare, late in onset, usually irreversible and may follow the smallest dose. Aplasia can follow systemic, oral and even ophthalmic administration and may be potentiated by cimetidine. Liver disease, uremia and pre-existing bone marrow dysfunction may increase the risk. It is unusual for manifestations to appear during treatment, and the interval between cessation of treatment and onset of dyscrasia can be months. A few patients survive with protracted aplasia, and myeloblastic leukemia then often supervenes.

It is thought that the toxic agent is not chloramphenicol itself but an as yet unidentified metabolite. Chloramphenicol is partially metabolized to produce oxidized, reduced and conjugated products. The toxic metabolite may be a short-lived product of reduction of the nitro group, which damages DNA by helix destabilization and strand breakage. Predisposition to aplasia may be explained by genetically determined differences in metabolism of the agent. Risk of fatal aplastic anemia has been estimated to increase 13-fold on average treatment with 4 g of chloramphenicol. Corresponding increases are 10-fold in patients treated with mepacrine (quinacrine) and 4-fold in patients treated with oxyphenbutazone.

Children

Infants given large doses may develop exceedingly high plasma levels of the drug because of their immature conjugation and excretion mechanisms. A life-threatening disorder called the 'gray baby' syndrome, characterized by vomiting, refusal to suck and abdominal distention followed by circulatory collapse, may appear when the plasma concentration exceeds 20 mg/L. If concentrations reach 200 mg/L, the disorder can develop in older children or even adults.

Optic neuritis has been described in children with cystic fibrosis receiving prolonged treatment for pulmonary infection. Most improve when the drug is discontinued, but central visual acuity can be permanently impaired. There is some experimental evidence that ear drops containing 5% chloramphenicol sodium succinate can damage hearing. One study identified an increased risk of acute leukemia following childhood administration of chloramphenicol, particularly for durations exceeding 10 days.

 ## CLINICAL USE

> Typhoid fever and other severe infections due to salmonellae
>
> Rickettsial infections
>
> Meningitis
>
> Invasive infection caused by *H. influenzae*
>
> Destructive lung lesions involving anaerobes
>
> Eye infections (topical)

Reference is made to its use in cholera, plague, tularemia and bartonellosis, melioidosis, Whipple's disease and relapsing fever. In enteric fever in adults, fluoroquinolones are associated with a lower clinical relapse rate. Treatment for other serious infections should be restricted to organisms that are resistant or much less susceptible to other antibiotics. A study in low resource countries found ampicillin plus gentamicin superior to injectable chloramphenicol for the treatment of very severe community-acquired pneumonia in children.

It has been used with varying success to treat infections caused by glycopeptide-resistant enterococci. Meningitis caused by penicillin-resistant pneumococci responds poorly, apparently due to failure to achieve bactericidal concentrations in CSF. It should never be given systemically for minor infections. Topical use in the treatment of eye infections is controversial given the unsubstantiated risk of bone marrow aplasia. A placebo-controlled study in children with infective conjunctivitis in the community found no clinical benefit in the use of chloramphenicol eye drops.

The daily dose should not normally exceed 2 g, and the duration of the course should be limited (e.g. 10 days). Although patients may show toxic manifestations after receiving very little drug, the danger is almost certainly increased by excessive or repeated dosage or by the treatment of patients with impaired hepatic or renal function, including those at the extremes of life. The wide pharmacokinetic variability of the antibiotic in neonates makes monitoring of serum concentrations advisable. Determination of full blood counts should be carried out twice weekly.

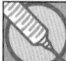 ## Preparations and dosage

Proprietary names: Chloromycetin, Kemicetine.

Preparations: Capsules, suspension, injection.

Dosage: Adults, oral, i.v., 50 mg/kg per day in four divided doses; the dose may be doubled for severe infections and reduced as soon as clinically indicated. Children, 50–100 mg/kg per day in divided doses; infants <2 weeks, 25 mg/kg per day in four divided doses; infants 2 weeks to 1 year, 50 mg/kg per day in four divided doses.

Widely available.

 ## Further information

Anonymous. Chloramphenicol. In: Dollery C, ed. *Therapeutic Drugs*. 2nd ed. Edinburgh: Churchill Livingstone; 1999:C168–C172.

Asghar R, Banajeh S, Egas J, et al. Chloramphenicol versus ampicillin plus gentamicin for community acquired very severe pneumonia among children aged 2–59 months in low resource settings: multicentre randomised controlled trial (SPEAR study). *Br Med J*. 2008;336:80–84.

Doona M, Walsh JB. Use of chloramphenicol as topical eye medication: time to cry halt? *Br Med J*. 1995;310:1217–1218.

Friedland IR, Shelton S, McCracken GH. Chloramphenicol in penicillin-resistant pneumococcal meningitis. *Lancet*. 1992;342:240–241.

Mirza SH, Beeching NJ, Hart CA. Multi-drug resistant typhoid: a global problem. *J Med Microbiol*. 1996;44:317–319.

Rose PW, Harnden A, Brueggemann AB, et al. Chloramphenicol treatment for acute infective conjunctivitis in children in primary care: a randomised double-blind placebo-controlled trial. *Lancet*. 2005;366:37–43.

Thaver D, Zaidi AK, Critchley J, Azmatullah A, Madni SA, Bhutta ZA. A comparison of fluoroquinolones versus other antibiotics for treating enteric fever: meta-analysis. *Br Med J*. 2009;338:b1865.

Wiholm BE, Kelly JP, Kaufman D, et al. Relation of aplastic anaemia to use of chloramphenicol eye drops in two international case-control studies. *Br Med J*. 1998;316:666.

THIAMPHENICOL

Molecular weight: 356.2.

A chloramphenicol analog in which a sulfomethyl group is substituted for the *p*-nitro group. Also available as the glycinate hydrochloride (1.26 g approximately equivalent to 1 g thiamphenicol). Aqueous solutions are very stable.

ANTIMICROBIAL ACTIVITY

It is generally less active than chloramphenicol (Table 16.1), but is equally active against *Str. pyogenes*, *Str. pneumoniae*, *H. influenzae* and *N. meningitidis*, including some strains resistant to chloramphenicol. It is more actively bactericidal against *Haemophilus* and *Neisseria* spp.

ACQUIRED RESISTANCE

There is complete cross-resistance with chloramphenicol in those bacteria which elaborate acetyltransferase, although the affinity of the enzyme for thiamphenicol is lower. Organisms that owe their resistance to other mechanisms may be susceptible.

PHARMACOKINETICS

An oral dose of 500 mg produces a peak plasma level of 3–6 mg/L after about 2 h. The plasma half-life is 2.6–3.5 h. It is said to reach the bronchial lumen in concentrations sufficient to exert a bactericidal effect on *H. influenzae*. Unlike chloramphenicol it is not a substrate for hepatic glucuronyl transferase; it is not eliminated by conjugation, and its half-life is not affected by phenobarbital induction.

About 50% of the dose can be recovered in an active form in the urine within 8 h and 70% over 24 h. The drug is correspondingly retained in the presence of renal failure, and in anuric patients the plasma half-life has been reported to be 9 h, a value not significantly affected by peritoneal dialysis. Biliary excretion is believed to account for removal of the antibiotic in anuric patients. The plasma concentration is elevated and half-life prolonged in patients with hepatitis or cirrhosis.

TOXICITY AND SIDE EFFECTS

There are no reports of irreversible bone-marrow toxicity. This has been related to the absence of the nitro group, and hence its reduction products, and differences in the biochemical effects of thiamphenicol and chloramphenicol on mammalian cells. It exerts a greater dose-dependent reversible depression of hemopoiesis and immunogenesis than chloramphenicol, and has been used for its immunosuppressive effect. Therapeutic doses (1–1.5 g) are likely to depress erythropoiesis in the elderly or others with impaired renal function.

CLINICAL USE

Similar to that of chloramphenicol.

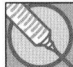

Preparations and dosage

Preparations: Oral, injection.

Dosage: Adults, i.m., oral, 1.5–3 g per day in divided doses depending on severity of infection. Children, 30–100 mg/kg per day in divided doses.

Limited availability in continental Europe and Japan. Not available in the UK or the USA.

Further information

Goris H, Loeffler M, Bungart B, Schmitz S, Nijhof W. Hemopoiesis during thiamphenicol treatment. *Exp Hematol*. 1989;17:957–961, 962–967.
Ravizzola G. In vitro antibacterial activity of thiamphenicol. *Chemioterapia*. 1984;3:163–166.

17 Diaminopyrimidines

Göte Swedberg and Lars Sundström

This group of agents comprises mainly 5-substituted 2,4-diaminopyrimidines, such as trimethoprim, cycloguanil and pyrimethamine, which have antibacterial or antiprotozoal activity. The diaminopyrimidine moiety can also be part of a pteridine or quinazoline ring system, as in the antineoplastic agents methotrexate and trimetrexate.

R$_2$: mostly H   X= C; N

They are potent inhibitors of the enzyme dihydrofolate reductase (*see* Ch. 2) and are generally termed antifolates.

Trimethoprim and pyrimethamine emerged from an antimetabolite program initiated in the 1940s by G.H. Hitchings and colleagues. Several trimethoprim analogs were subsequently synthesized, and derivatives with increased spectrum and activity against resistant strains remain under investigation. Activity against eukaryotic parasites is of special interest because of the relative lack of good alternatives. The determination of three-dimensional structures of the target enzyme is aiding further development of the field.

Clinical development of trimethoprim concentrated on a synergistic combination with sulfamethoxazole (co-trimoxazole), which exploits the sequential blockade of two steps in the biosynthesis of reduced folates. This double blockade results in greatly enhanced antibacterial activity, extends the antibacterial spectrum, slows down resistance development (at least under laboratory conditions) and increases the bactericidal potency. Co-trimoxazole became very successful, but the practice of applying a potent agent such as trimethoprim exclusively in combination with a sulfonamide was disputed on several grounds:

- Although the pharmacokinetic properties of trimethoprim and sulfamethoxazole match fairly well in the plasma, conditions far from those optimal for synergy prevail in different body compartments.

- Synergy is relevant only at sites in which concentrations fall below levels effective alone, whereas the combination is administered at doses that produce plasma levels of both components above the inhibitory concentration.
- Resistance to sulfonamides was already widespread at the time of launch of the combination, so that trimethoprim alone is the active component against such strains.
- The sulfonamide component, which is in five-fold excess over trimethoprim, is responsible for many of the undesirable side effects.
- The high concentrations of trimethoprim reached in urine are sufficient to treat uncomplicated cystitis and other infections of the urinary tract.

These considerations led to the clinical use of trimethoprim alone, especially in urinary tract infections. In other conditions it is often still used as a fixed combination with sulfonamides, usually sulfamethoxazole, although some licensing agencies recommend combined use solely for infections, such as the treatment and prophylaxis of *Pneumocystis jirovecii* (formerly *Pneumocystis carinii*) pneumonia, in which there are good grounds for preferring it over trimethoprim alone.

Further information

Baccanari DP, Kuyper LF. Basis of selectivity of antibacterial diaminopyrimidines. *J Chemother.* 1993;5:393–399.

Gangjee A, Kurup S, Namjoshi O. Dihydrofolate reductase as a target for chemotherapy in parasites. *Curr Pharm Des.* 2007;13:609–639.

Hawser S, Lucioro S, Islam K. Dihydrofolate reductase inhibitors as antibacterial agents. *Biochem Pharmacol.* 2006;71:941–948.

Liu J, Bolstad DB, Bolstad ES, Wright DL, Anderson AC. Towards new antifolates targeting eukaryotic opportunistic infections. *Eukaryot Cell.* 2009;8:483–486.

Then RL. Antimicrobial dihydrofolate reductase inhibitors – achievements and future options: review. *J Chemother.* 2004;16:3–12.

Wagenlehner FM, Weidner W, Naber KG. An update on uncomplicated urinary tract infections in women. *Curr Opin Urol.* 2009;19:368–374.

Yuthavong Y, Yuvaniyama J, Chitnumsub P, et al. Malarial (*Plasmodium falciparum*) dihydrofolate reductase-thymidylate synthase: structural basis for antifolate resistance and development of effective inhibitors. *Parasitology.* 2005;130:249–259.

PYRIMETHAMINE

2,4-Diamino-5-(p-chlorophenyl)-6-ethylpyrimidine.
Molecular weight: 248.717.

A synthetic diaminopyrimidine. Extremely insoluble. Available as a single agent (Daraprim) or in fixed combination with sulfadoxine (Fansidar), dapsone (Maloprim) or triple combination with mefloquine and sulfadoxine (Fansimef).

ANTIMICROBIAL ACTIVITY

Most notable activity is against *Plasmodium* spp., *Toxoplasma gondii* and *Pn. jirovecii*. It is about 1000 times more active against plasmodial dihydrofolate reductase than against the human enzyme. It has no useful antibacterial activity. Slow growing bradyzoite forms of *Tox. gondii* in tissue cysts are less sensitive than the intracellular tachyzoites. It is strongly recommended that it is used together with a sulfonamide for the treatment of malaria and toxoplasmosis, since the mixture lowers the ED_{50} and clinically curative dose approximately 10-fold.

ACQUIRED RESISTANCE

Plasmodium falciparum generally acquires resistance gradually by step-wise mutations in dihydrofolate reductase. The first mutation was a change from Ser to Asn in residue 108, with subsequent mutations at positions 51 (Asn to Ile), 59 (Cys to Arg) and 164 (Leu to Ile). Parasites with all four mutations have the highest level of resistance; they are still rare in Africa but much more prevalent in Asia. A further increase in resistance may be caused by an increased copy number of the gene coding for GTP cyclohydrolase, the first and rate-limiting enzyme in the folate biosynthetic pathway. Copy number mutations have so far been seen only in Asia. Resistance to pyrimethamine–sulfadoxine (Fansidar) is also affected by mutations in the gene coding for the dihydropteroate synthase target of sulfonamides, although the relation between such mutations and the level of resistance is less clear. The key mutation is a change at residue 437 (Ala to Gly), which in Africa is usually found in combination with a mutation at residue 540 (Lys to Glu), less commonly at residue 581 (Ala to Gly). Other mutations are found in Asia. Changes in membrane proteins like PfMRP1 have an effect on folate transport and may also influence antifolate action.

PHARMACOKINETICS

Oral absorption	Well absorbed
C_{max} (25 mg orally)	0.13–0.4 mg/L after 2–6 h
Plasma half-life	111 (54–148) h
Volume of distribution	0.68 L/kg
Plasma protein binding	87%

Absorption

Pyrimethamine is well absorbed orally. The plasma half-life is unaffected by partner drugs like dapsone and sulfadoxine. Absorption is markedly poorer in patients with HIV.

Distribution

Levels in cerebrospinal fluid (CSF) are around 10–25% of the simultaneous plasma level. A substantial part of the dose appears in maternal milk, the ratio of milk:serum area under the concentration–time curve (AUC) being 0.46–0.66, so that an infant might ingest almost half the maternal dose over 9 days. There is placental transfer of pyrimethamine, resulting in 50–100% of the maternal plasma concentrations in the neonate.

Metabolism and excretion

Plasma clearance is 0.3–0.4 mL/min/kg and elimination is mainly by hepatic metabolism. Few studies have been done on pyrimethamine metabolism, but some cytochrome P_{450} enzymes have been shown to be involved in the relatively slow metabolism.

TOXICITY AND SIDE EFFECTS

When administered with a sulfonamide or dapsone, all major side effects of these agents (including Stevens–Johnson syndrome) may occur, particularly hypersensitivity reactions. The principal toxic effect of pyrimethamine is on the bone marrow, producing megaloblastic anemia, leukocytopenia, thrombocytopenia or pancytopenia. This is particularly seen on prolonged administration and with the high doses used in toxoplasmosis. A relatively high incidence of side effects of pyrimethamine and other drugs was seen during treatment of ocular toxoplasmosis, with stomach problems as the main complaint. Very large doses in children have produced vomiting, convulsions, respiratory failure and death. Aggravation of subclinical folate deficiency may be alleviated by folinic acid. Pyrimethamine is teratogenic in animals and produces significant abnormalities. It should be used in pregnant women only after thoroughly weighing the risk–benefit for mother and child. However, the use of Fansidar in intermittent preventive treatment programs in Africa suggests that it is generally safe.

CLINICAL USE

Malaria (usually in combination with sulfadoxine, sulfalene [sulfametopyrazine] or dapsone)

Toxoplasmosis (usually in combination with sulfadiazine)

Pneumocystis pneumonia (usually in combination with dapsone)

Preparations and dosage

Proprietary names: Daraprim, Fansidar (with sulfadoxine), Maloprim (with dapsone).

Preparation: Tablets.

Dosage: Depends on indication. For acute malaria treatment 2–3 tablets (25 mg, plus sulfonamide) is the usual dose. Children 9–14 years, two tablets; 4–8 years, one tablet; under 4 years half a tablet. For prophylaxis (no longer recommended), adult dose one tablet per week, children 5–10 years half a tablet per week. For toxoplasmosis the starting dose is 50–75 mg of pyrimethamine daily, with 1–4 g of a sulfonamide.

Widely available as combination, limited availability of pyrimethamine alone.

Further information

Almond DS, Szwandt ISF, Edwards G, et al. Disposition of intravenous pyrimethamine in healthy volunteers. *Antimicrob Agents Chemother.* 2000;44:1691–1693.

Duombo OK, Kayentao K, Djimde A, et al. Rapid selection of *Plasmodium falciparum* dihydrofolate reductase mutants by pyrimethamine prophylaxis. *J Infect Dis.* 2000;182:993–996.

Gregson A, Plowe C. Mechanisms of resistance of malaria parasites to antifolates. *Pharmacol Rev.* 2005;57:117–145.

Iaccheri B, Fiore T, Papadaki T, et al. Adverse drug reactions to treatment for ocular toxoplasmosis: a retrospective chart review. *Clin Ther.* 2008;30:2069–2074.

Li XQ, Björkman A, Andersson TB, Gustafsson LL, Masimirembwa CM. Identification of human cytochrome P(450)s that metabolise anti-parasitic drugs and predictions of in vivo drug hepatic clearance from in vitro data. *Eur J Clin Pharmacol.* 2003;59:429–442.

Peters PJ, Thigpen MC, Parise ME, Newman RD. Safety and toxicity of sulfadoxine/pyrimethamine: implications for malaria prevention in pregnancy using intermittent preventive treatment. *Drug Safety.* 2007;30:481–501.

Sokhna C, Cissé B, Bâ el H. A trial of the efficacy, safety and impact on drug resistance of four drug regimens for seasonal intermittent preventive treatment for malaria in Senegalese children. *PLoS ONE.* 2008;23(3):e1471.

Winstanley P, Khoo S, Szwandt S, et al. Marked variation in pyrimethamine disposition in AIDS patients treated for cerebral toxoplasmosis. *J Antimicrob Chemother.* 1995;36:435–439.

TRIMETHOPRIM

2,4-Diamino-5-(3,4,5-trimethoxybenzyl)-pyrimidine. Molecular weight: 290.323.

The most frequently used synthetic diaminopyrimidine. It is poorly soluble in water and has a very bitter taste. It is available in oral formulations or, as trimethoprim lactate, as an injectable preparation.

ANTIMICROBIAL ACTIVITY

It has broad-spectrum activity (Table 17.1). It is active against Gram-positive bacilli and cocci, including *Staphylococcus aureus*, irrespective of β-lactamase production or methicillin resistance. *Enterococcus faecalis* is unusual in being able to utilize preformed folinic acid, thymine and thymidine. Folinic acid antagonizes the activity of trimethoprim and sulfamethoxazole in vitro and the efficacy in enterococcal infections is controversial.

Haemophilus spp., including β-lactamase-producing strains and *Haemophilus ducreyi* (minimum inhibitory concentration [MIC] 0.03–0.6 mg/L) are susceptible. Most enterobacteria are susceptible, as are *Bordetella*, *Legionella*, *Pasteurella* and *Vibrio* spp. Pseudomonads, with the exception of *Burkholderia cepacia* (MIC 1–2 mg/L) are resistant. Nocardiae, *Neisseria* spp. and *Brucella* spp. are relatively resistant, owing to their species-specific dihydrofolate reductase sensitivities, although they are susceptible to trimethoprim–sulfonamide combinations.

Most anaerobes are resistant, as are *Chlamydia*, *Coxiella*, *Leptospira*, *Mycoplasma*, *Rickettsia* and *Treponema* spp. *Mycobacterium tuberculosis* is resistant, but *M. marinum* (MIC 16 mg/L) and *M. smegmatis* (MIC 4 mg/L) are susceptible, as are *Listeria* spp.

Table 17.1 Representative minimum inhibitory concentrations of trimethoprim and co-trimoxazole for common pathogenic bacteria[a] (mg/L)

Organism	Trimethoprim	Co-trimoxazole[b]
Staphylococcus aureus	0.2–2	0.03–0.06
Streptococcus pneumoniae	0.5–2	0.06–2
Str. pyogenes	0.5–1	0.03–2
Enterococcus faecalis	0.15–0.5	0.015–0.4
Haemophilus influenzae	0.02–1	0.02–16
Neisseria gonorrhoeae	8–R	0.15–4
N. meningitidis	4–32	0.01–2
Escherichia coli	0.05–R	0.25–64
Klebsiella pneumoniae	0.5–8	0.5–4
Pseudomonas aeruginosa	R	R
Bacteroides fragilis	8–16	>4

[a]Data from various studies; a broad range indicates that resistant strains were included.
[b]Tested as a 1 + 19 fixed combination of trimethoprim with sulfamethoxazole. R, resistant (MIC >64 mg/L).

Among non-bacterial organisms, *Naegleria* spp., *Plasmodium* spp., *Pn. jirovecii*, and *Tox. gondii* exhibit some sensitivity to trimethoprim, which can often be potentiated by a sulfonamide.

ACQUIRED RESISTANCE

Resistance can be due to a variety of mechanisms. Chromosomal mutations in the structural gene for dihydrofolate reductase or in its promoter can result in modification or overproduction of the target enzyme. In addition, alterations in the metabolic pathway, or changes that affect the permeability of the cell or efflux pumps generally, confer moderate degrees of resistance. More than one mechanism can occur in the same cell, leading to higher resistance levels.

Plasmid-encoded resistance is widespread, especially in enteric Gram-negative bacilli including *Escherichia coli*, *Salmonella enterica* serotypes and *Acinetobacter* spp. It usually results in the synthesis of an additional, trimethoprim-resistant dihydrofolate reductase and confers high levels of resistance. Many distinct enzymes are known in Gram-negative bacteria and their prevalence varies with geographic region. Most frequently found are the enzyme types Ib, VIII, V and Ia.

Only a few of these enzymes have so far been described in Gram-positive bacteria, mainly in staphylococci but also in enterococci and *Listeria*. The most prevalent type in staphylococci is the S1 enzyme, which probably originated in *Staph. epidermidis*. Other resistance genes have been detected in *Staph. haemolyticus* and *E. faecalis*. Most cases of trimethoprim resistance in Gram-positive bacteria are due to alterations of chromosomally encoded enzymes. In *Streptococcus pneumoniae* a basic resistance-determining mutation has been identified at amino acid 100 (Ile to Leu). Other mutations may lead to higher levels of resistance. Corresponding mutations have been seen in the related commensal flora of streptococci.

Campylobacter jejuni owes its high level resistance to acquired *dfr1* and *dfr9* genes. In contrast, trimethoprim resistance in *H. influenzae* seems to be frequently caused by mutations in the *dfr* promoter region or the trimethoprim-binding domains of the structural gene. In *Pseudomonas aeruginosa* intrinsic resistance may be mediated by a multidrug efflux system.

Since thymidine can supply the metabolic requirement imposed by trimethoprim blockade, thymine-requiring bacteria are resistant. Such organisms are rarely implicated in infection, either because tissues generally fail to provide the necessary thymidine or because they escape detection owing to their slow growth on conventional media, which are low in thymine and thymidine. Infection with trimethoprim-resistant, thymine-requiring mutants has occasionally been observed in patients treated for prolonged periods with co-trimoxazole. Under certain pathological conditions these mutants seem to rescue enough thymidine from body fluid.

PHARMACOKINETICS

Oral absorption	95–100%
C_{max} (100 mg orally)	c. 1 mg/L after 1.5–3.5 h
Plasma half-life	8–11 h
Volume of distribution	69–133 L
Plasma protein binding	42–46%

Absorption and distribution

It is rapidly absorbed from the gut after oral administration. Plasma levels increase in a dose-proportional fashion. It is widely distributed in tissues and body fluids, including CSF, in which concentrations around half the simultaneous plasma level are achieved. It passes the placental barrier and is excreted in breast milk.

Metabolism and excretion

About 10–20% is metabolized, primarily in the liver. The remainder is excreted unchanged in the urine. Main metabolites are 1- and 3-oxide, and 3′- and 4′-hydroxy derivatives.

Elimination is mainly through glomerular filtration and tubular secretion. High concentrations are found in urine, reaching 30–160 mg/L within 4 h of a single 100 mg oral dose, and declining to 18–91 mg/L during the following 8–24 h. About 70% is excreted in the first 24 h, but detectable levels are present in the urine for 4–5 days, during which time about 90% of the dose can be recovered. The renal clearance of trimethoprim in normal subjects is 19–148 mL/min, the wide variation largely being accounted for by the influence of pH. Trimethoprim is a weak base, and urinary excretion rises sharply with falling pH as the drug ionizes and nonionic back diffusion in the tubules decreases. In patients with severely impaired renal function the half-life increases and a dose adjustment is needed.

TOXICITY AND SIDE EFFECTS

Rash, pruritus, nausea, vomiting and glossitis are the most common adverse effects. Hypersensitivity reactions (exfoliative dermatitis, erythema multiforme, Stevens–Johnson syndrome, Lyell's syndrome, anaphylaxis, aseptic meningitis) are rare, as are hematological side effects.

The induction of folate deficiency and consequent interference with hematopoiesis is rarely observed, even after high doses or prolonged administration. Trimethoprim should, however, be given with caution to pregnant women and to patients with possible folate deficiency. Reduced folates can be administered without interfering with the antibacterial activity.

Mutagenicity tests have been uniformly negative. Teratogenic effects have been observed in rats and rabbits only at doses far exceeding those used in humans.

Common clinical doses may inhibit the hepatic metabolism of phenytoin, increasing the half-life by 51% and lowering the metabolic clearance rate by 30%. Trimethoprim has some effect on the metabolism of antiretroviral drugs but these effects do not prevent the use of trimethoprim–sulfa drug combinations for prophylaxis during antiretroviral treatment.

 ## CLINICAL USE

> Urinary tract infections
> Enteric fever
> Prophylaxis and treatment of *Pn. jirovecii* infection

Topical preparations have been used in the treatment of burns and, combined with polymyxin, as eye drops to treat infective conjunctivitis.

 ### Preparations and dosage

Proprietary names: Ipral, Monotrim, Solotrim, Trimpex.

Preparations: Tablets, suspension, injection.

Dosage: Oral: Adults, acute infections, 100 mg every 12 h, 200 mg every 12 or 24 h. Children 6–12 years, 100 mg every 12 h; 6 months to 5 years, 50 mg every 12 h; 6 weeks to 5 years, 25 mg every 12 h (approx. 8 mg/kg day).

Long-term and prophylaxis: Adults, 100 mg at night. Children 6–12 years, 50 mg at night; 6 months to 5 years, 25 mg at night.

Intravenous injection: Adults, 150–250 mg every 12 h. Children <12 years, 6–9 mg/kg per day in 2–3 divided doses.

Widely available.

📖 Further information

Abou-Eisha A. Evaluation of cytogenic and DNA damage induced by the antibacterial drug, trimethoprim. *Toxicology in vitro.* 2006;20:601–607.

Brogden RN, Carmine AA, Heel RC, et al. Trimethoprim: a review of its antibacterial activity, pharmacokinetics and therapeutic use in urinary tract infections. *Drugs.* 1982;23:405–430.

Gibreel A, Skold O. High-level resistance to trimethoprim in clinical isolates of *Campylobacter jejuni* by acquisition of foreign genes (*dfr1* and *dfr9*) expressing drug-insensitive dihydrofolate reductases. *Antimicrob Agents Chemother.* 1998;42:3059–3064.

Huovinen P, Sundstrom L, Swedberg G, Skold O. Trimethoprim and sulfonamide resistance. *Antimicrob Agents Chemother.* 1995;39:279–289.

Maskell JP, Sefton AM, Hall LM. Multiple mutations modulate the function of dihydrofolate reductase in trimethoprim-resistant *Streptococcus pneumoniae*. *Antimicrob Agents Chemother.* 2001;45:1104–1108.

Then RL. Mechanisms of resistance to trimethoprim, the sulphonamides, and trimethoprim–sulphamethoxazole. *Rev Infect Dis.* 1982;4:261–269.

OTHER DIAMINOPYRIMIDINES AND RELATED STRUCTURES

 ### BRODIMOPRIM

A trimethoprim analog in which bromine replaces methoxy at position 4 of the phenyl substituent. It is used as a single agent for the oral treatment of bacterial infections of the respiratory tract, but has been withdrawn from most markets. Its antibacterial and toxicological properties are similar to those of trimethoprim, but its pharmacokinetic behavior is distinctly different. It has a long elimination half-life of 32–35 h, allowing once-daily dosing.

 ### CYCLOGUANIL

A 2,4-diaminotriazine inhibitor of plasmodial dihydrofolate reductase. It is the major human metabolite of proguanil (*see* p. 415).

 ### ICLAPRIM

A novel cyclopropyl dimethoxypyrimidine that shows increased hydrophobic interactions with the active site of dihydrofolate reductase including trimethoprim-resistant dihydrofolate reductase enzymes of *Staph. aureus*. It is active against *Staph. aureus* (including methicillin-resistant strains), β-hemolytic streptococci, penicillin-susceptible pneumococci and enterococci, as well as *Listeria*, *Legionella* and *Chlamydia* spp. Activity against *H. influenzae*, *Moraxella catarrhalis* and some Enterobacteriaceae is moderate. The action against Gram-positive pathogens, including methicillin-resistant *Staph. aureus* (MRSA), is rapidly bactericidal and unaffected by human plasma.

Oral bioavailability is approximately 40%. The plasma half-life is around 3 h. A standard dose maintains an inhibitory concentration against a range of pathogens for up to 7 h. It is metabolized by cytochromes and glucuronidation, with elimination of metabolites via the urine (about two-thirds) and feces (about one-third). The drug has a large volume of distribution and can accumulate intracellularly, suggesting that it could be used to treat infections caused by susceptible intracellular pathogens. It accumulates in epithelial lining fluid and alveolar macrophages but not bronchial mucosa. Protein binding is about 92–94%, but this does not impair the effective bactericidal effect.

At the time of writing it is not licensed for use.

📖 Further information

Andrews J, Honeybourne D, Ashby J, et al. Concentrations in plasma, epithelial lining fluid, alveolar macrophages and bronchial mucosa after a single intravenous dose of 1.6 mg/kg of iclaprim (AR-100) in healthy men. *J Antimicrob Chemother.* 2007;60:677–680.

Laue H, Valensise T, Seguin A, Lociuro S, Islam K, Hawser S. In vitro bactericidal activity of iclaprim in human plasma. *Antimicrob Agents Chemother.* 2009;53:4542–4544.

Oefner C, Bandera M, Haldimann A, et al. Increased hydrophobic interactions of iclaprim with *Staphylococcus aureus* dihydrofolate reductase are responsible for the increase in affinity and antibacterial activity. *J Antimicrob Chemother.* 2009;63:687–698.

Peppard WJ, Schuenke CD. Iclaprim, a diaminopyrimidine dihydrofolate reductase inhibitor for the potential treatment of antibiotic-resistant staphylococcal infections. *Curr Opin Investig Drugs.* 2008;9:210–225.

Sader H, Fritsche T, Jones R. Potency and bactericidal activity of iclaprim against recent clinical Gram-positive isolates. *Antimicrob Agents Chemother.* 2009;53:2171–2175.

TETROXOPRIM

A close analog of trimethoprim with a modified 3'-methoxy group. It was formerly used in some countries in combination with sulfadiazine, but has few, if any, advantages over co-trimoxazole.

TRIMETREXATE

A synthetic 2,4-diaminoquinazoline, structurally related to the anticancer drug methotrexate. Formulated as the glucuronate. It is a non-specific inhibitor of dihydrofolate reductase. It is more lipophilic than methotrexate and uses different routes for cellular uptake. It exhibits non-specific activity against dihydrofolate reductases, but is a much more potent inhibitor of the *Pn. jirovecii* and mammalian enzymes than trimethoprim.

After intravenous infusion of 30 mg/m² to adult patients with AIDS, concentrations of trimetrexate were around 2 μmol/L at 4 h. It is usually administered by intravenous infusion, but oral bioavailability is about 44% and concentrations comparable to those achieved by an intravenous infusion of 30 mg/m² were achieved 2 h after an oral dose of 60 mg/m². Elimination half-lives varied from 8.3 to 10 h for the early or late phase of a treatment course and terminal elimination half-lives were as long as 15–16 h. Protein binding is >95%. Excretion is largely by the renal route, with 10–20% of the dose being found in urine after 24–48 h; a substantial proportion of the dose is excreted as metabolites.

It is extremely toxic. The high affinity for the mammalian enzyme has to be circumvented by the concurrent administration of leucovorin (folinic acid), which *Pn. jirovecii* cannot take up. Important hematological side effects include neutropenia, thrombocytopenia, bone marrow suppression and anemia. Other adverse reactions are ulceration of the oral and gastric mucosa, and impairment of hepatic and renal function. Administration of leucovorin should be continued for 72 h after the last dose of trimetrexate in order to minimize these complications.

Trimetrexate glucuronate has been administered (together with leucovorin) in moderate to severe *Pn. jirovecii* pneumonia in patients who are intolerant of or refractory to co-trimoxazole, or those in whom co-trimoxazole is contraindicated. It is no longer available in the UK or the USA.

Further information

Fulton B, Wagstaff A, McTavish D. Trimetrexate: a review of its pharmacodynamic and pharmacokinetic properties and therapeutic potential in the treatment of *Pneumocystis carinii* pneumonia. *Drugs.* 1995;49:563–576.

Short CE, Gilleece YC, Fisher MJ, Churchill DR. Trimetrexate and folinic acid: a valuable salvage option for *Pneumocystis jirovecii* pneumonia. *AIDS.* 2009;23:1287–1290.

DIAMINOPYRIMIDINE–SULFONAMIDE COMBINATIONS

Several fixed-ratio combinations have been marketed over the years, but few have survived. By far the most widely used is co-trimoxazole, a 1:5 mixture of trimethoprim and sulfamethoxazole. Also used is co-trimazine, a 1:5 mixture of trimethoprim and sulfadiazine. Among other combinations the 4:5 mixture of trimethoprim and sulfamethoxypyridazine has higher activity than co-trimoxazole against *Pn. jirovecii* and may be better tolerated.

In addition to these preparations, the antiprotozoal agent pyrimethamine is used together with dapsone or sulfonamides (*see* Ch. 62). Proguanil, the metabolic precursor of cycloguanil, is used in combination with atovaquone (p. 417).

These combinations exhibit the activity of, and synergy between, the two components. They may also mutually cross-suppress the emergence of resistance. As well as lowering the concentration required to inhibit growth, the mixture is often bactericidal when the individual components are bacteristatic. Occasionally synergy may be so marked that organisms conventionally regarded as resistant to one or the other agent are rendered susceptible to the combination. The pharmacokinetic behavior of the different mixtures is that of the components, there being no significant interactions between them.

Synergy is most impressive against organisms that are only moderately susceptible to one of the components alone. In most cases maximum potentiation occurs when the drugs are present in the ratio of their MICs, but for some organisms, notably neisseriae and *Pn. jirovecii*, proportionally more trimethoprim is required as they are more susceptible to sulfonamide than trimethoprim. In some cases synergy is an in-vitro phenomenon with no clear clinical advantage, but with neisseriae, nocardiae, malaria parasites and *Pn. jirovecii* it clearly translates into clinical benefit.

Rifampicin (rifampin) and polymyxin also act synergistically with both sulfonamides and trimethoprim against Gram-negative bacilli. Formulations of trimethoprim with polymyxin B are widely available for topical use in eye drops and ointment. The triple mixture of sulfamethoxazole, trimethoprim and colistin may be more active than any pair of these agents against some organisms, including multiresistant *Serratia*.

CO-TRIMOXAZOLE

A fixed-ratio (1:5) combination of trimethoprim and sulfamethoxazole.

ANTIMICROBIAL ACTIVITY

The antimicrobial spectrum covers pathogens susceptible to the individual agents and is expanded by synergistic interaction. Some organisms that are refractory to many other antibiotics remain susceptible to co-trimoxazole. These include *Acinetobacter* spp., *Burk. cepacia*, *Stenotrophomonas maltophilia* and some fast-growing mycobacteria such as *M. marinum* and *M. kansasii*.

ACQUIRED RESISTANCE

There are large regional and local differences in rates of resistance. A study of MRSA isolates in 20 European hospitals found 71% to be susceptible to co-trimoxazole; higher rates have been reported in areas in which co-trimoxazole prophylaxis in HIV-positive patients is common. Large regional variations have been found for co-trimoxazole resistance in pneumococci, ranging from 8.6% in the Czech Republic in 1997 to 79.6% in Hong Kong. A large survey in Finland covering 1988–2004 found variance in resistance rates of 14.1–21.4% for *Str. pneumoniae*, 9.7–18.7% for *H. influenzae*, and 3.2–14.5% for *Mor. catarrhalis*, linked to regional variation in the use of co-trimoxazole. A similar study in the USA showed a resistance rate of 23.4%. Resistance is lowest in penicillin-susceptible pneumococci and highest in penicillin-resistant pneumococci. It has been suggested that the use of sulfadoxine–pyrimethamine in malaria and co-trimoxazole for pneumocystis prophylaxis may select for co-trimoxazole-resistant pneumococci. Accordingly, in parts of Africa, resistance rates close to 100% have been reported in pneumococci. The mechanism of resistance in Gram-positive cocci and in *Neisseria* spp. is generally mutational alteration of the chromosomally encoded target proteins.

Among Gram-negative organisms, a large study of bloodstream isolates from the USA, Canada and Latin America in 1998 reported susceptibility to co-trimoxazole in 47.5–77.9% of *Esch. coli* isolates, 81–87.7% of *Klebsiella* spp. and 69.8–83.1% of *Enterobacter* spp. The lower figure is for Latin America and the higher for the USA. A study from 2004 to 2006 found 18.1% resistance in patients with complicated urinary tract infection and 30.6% in patients with acute pyelonephritis. The resistance mechanism among Gram-negative bacilli is generally mediated by plasmid-encoded variants of the respective target genes.

Emergence of resistance in the course of treatment is not usually a problem.

PHARMACOKINETICS

	Trimethoprim	Sulfamethoxazole
Oral absorption	>95%	85%
C_{max} 160 mg trimethoprim + 800 mg sulfamethoxazole) orally	1–2 mg/L after 1 h	30–40 mg/L after 2 h
Plasma half-life	*c.* 7 h	*c.* 9 h
Volume of distribution	100–120 L	12–18 L
Plasma protein binding	*c.* 44%	*c.* 70%

Absorption

Trimethoprim is usually absorbed more rapidly than sulfamethoxazole when given as a single oral dose of the combination. After twice-daily administration of one tablet the steady state is reached in adults after 2–3 days; the steady state peak serum concentrations are approximately 50% greater than the peak levels after a single dose. Elderly patients behave as normal adults.

Distribution

Because of unequal distribution there is a wide range of concentration ratios of the two drugs in body tissues and fluids. The concentration of trimethoprim is equal to or greater than the simultaneous plasma level in saliva, intracellular fluid, breast milk, prostatic tissue, sputum, lung tissue, vaginal secretions, bile and urine. Concentrations of sulfamethoxazole in all these tissues and fluids, except urine, are lower than in plasma. Concentrations of trimethoprim in prostatic fluid are twice as high as in the plasma in elderly men. Trimethoprim and sulfamethoxazole both cross the human placenta and penetrate the CSF, where concentrations around half of the simultaneous plasma levels are usually reached.

Metabolism and excretion

Metabolism and excretion of the components of co-trimoxazole are described on pages 253 and 341. The excretion of trimethoprim increases in acid urine, while that of sulfonamide is unchanged; in alkaline urine the excretion of trimethoprim is depressed and that of sulfamethoxazole enhanced. As a result, the ratio of the urinary concentrations of active sulfonamide to trimethoprim is around 1 in acid urine and around 5 in alkaline urine. When the creatinine clearance falls below 30 mL/min the elimination half-lives of both drugs can increase up to 45–60 h and the quantity of the drug cleared by the kidney decreases.

 ## TOXICITY AND SIDE EFFECTS

Side effects are those described for the two components (*see* pp. 253–254 and 339); most adverse reactions are usually attributed to the sulfonamide. Serious toxicity is uncommon, but the increased risks of co-trimoxazole compared with trimethoprim alone, particularly in the elderly, have been sufficient to limit the licensed indications for the combination. Co-trimoxazole is less well tolerated in HIV-positive patients than in other patient groups. The production of a toxic hydroxylamine metabolite of sulfamethoxazole by the cytochrome P_{450} pathway is suspected to be the underlying reason for this.

Administration of co-trimoxazole (or trimethoprim alone) results in marked depression of fecal enterobacteria with little or no effect on fecal anaerobes. Corresponding clearance of enterobacteria from the perineal area is believed to be an important feature of the value of the drug in the control of recurrent urinary tract infection (*see* Ch. 54). While intrinsically resistant species, including *Ps. aeruginosa*, have naturally persisted, major overgrowth has not been a troublesome feature.

In the rat, doses greater than 200 mg/kg per day are teratogenic, but complete protection is afforded by folinic acid or dietary folate supplements. No abnormalities were produced in the rabbit or infants born to treated mothers, but use of the drug in pregnancy is not recommended. Although one extensive case control study in humans found an increased risk for congenital abnormalities during co-trimoxazole treatment, most reports state the risks as small.

Hyperkalemia is a well-described complication of therapy with high-dose trimethoprim (20 mg/kg per day) in patients with AIDS and may also develop in about 20% of patients under standard therapy with co-trimoxazole, and in up to 85% of patients with renal insufficiency. The reason is probably blocking of sodium channels, thus disturbing the sodium–potassium balance. The effect is reversible by supplementing sodium intake and restricting potassium.

 ## CLINICAL USE

Treatment and prophylaxis of *Pn. jirovecii* pneumonia
Toxoplasmosis
Urinary tract infections
Acute otitis media
Acne
Acute exacerbations of chronic bronchitis
Nocardiasis, listeriosis, brucellosis, melioidosis
Shigellosis and other enteric infections caused by pathogens susceptible to co-trimoxazole
Stenotrophomonas maltophilia infections
Chancroid, donovanosis (granuloma inguinale)
Whipple's disease, Wegener's granulomatosis

The only first-line indication in the UK is the treatment and prophylaxis of *Pn. jirovecii* pneumonitis. It can also be used in other conditions in which there is microbiological evidence of sensitivity to the combination and good reason (including resistance to other front-line drugs) to prefer the combination to trimethoprim alone. Leucovorin is sometimes used to reduce the incidence of neutropenia; this may, however, interfere with the efficacy of co-trimoxazole against *Pn. jirovecii*. Co-trimoxazole has activity against some protozoa and is used for treatment of human *Isospora belli* and *Cyclospora cayetanensis* infections.

 ### Preparations and dosage

Proprietary names: Bactrim, Septrin, Cotrim and others.

Preparations: Tablets (400 mg sulfamethoxazole plus 80 mg trimethoprim, or double-strength tablet: 800 mg sulfamethoxazole plus 160 mg trimethoprim), injections, pediatric suspension.

Dosage: Adults, oral, 960 mg every 12 h, increased to 1.44 g every 12 h in severe infections. Children >12 years, as for adults; 6 weeks to 5 months, 120 mg every 12 h; 6 months to 5 years, 240 mg every 12 h; 6–12 years, 480 mg every 12 h.

High dose therapy for *Pn. jirovecii* infections: 120 mg/kg per day, in 2–4 divided doses, for 14 days.

Pn. jirovecii prophylaxis: Many recommended regimens; consult local formularies.

Widely available.

Further information

Czeizel AE, Rockenbauer M, Sørensen HT, Olsen J. The teratogenic risk of trimethoprim–sulfonamides: a population based case-control study. *Reprod Toxicol*. 2001;15:637–646.

Diekema DJ, Pfaller MA, Jones RN, et al. Trends in antimicrobial susceptibility of bacterial pathogens isolated from patients with blood stream infections in the USA, Canada and Latin America. *Int J Antimicrob Agents*. 2000;13:257–271.

Dibbern DA, Montanaro A. Allergies to sulfonamide antibiotics and sulfur-containing drugs. *Ann Allergy Asthma Immunol*. 2008;100:91–100.

Feikin DR, Dowell SF, Nwanyanwu OC, et al. Increased carriage of trimethoprim/sulfamethoxazole resistant *Streptococcus pneumoniae* in Malawian children after treatment for malaria with sulfadoxine/pyrimethamine. *J Infect Dis*. 2000;181:1501–1505.

Forna F, McConnell M, Kitabire FN, et al. Systematic review of the safety of trimethoprim–sulfamethoxazole for prophylaxis in HIV-infected pregnant women: implications for resource-limited settings. *AIDS Rev*. 2006;8:24–36.

Jick H, Derby LE. Is co-trimoxazole safe? *Lancet*. 1995;345:1118–1119.

Jones RN, Croco MAT, Kugler KC, et al. Respiratory tract pathogens isolated from patients hospitalized with suspected pneumonia: frequency of occurrence and antimicrobial susceptibility patterns from the SENTRY antimicrobial surveillance program (United States and Canada, 1997). *Diagn Microbiol Infect Dis*. 2000;37:115–125.

Kärpänoja P, Nyberg ST, Bergman M, et al. Connection between trimethoprim–sulfamethoxazole use and resistance in *Streptococcus pneumoniae*, *Haemophilus influenzae*, and *Moraxella catarrhalis*. *Antimicrob Agents Chemother*. 2008;52:2480–2485.

Lee BL. Adverse reactions to trimethoprim–sulfamethoxazole. *Clin Rev Allergy Immunol*. 1996;14:451–455.

Masters PA, O'Bryan TA, Zurlo J, et al. Trimethoprim–sulfamethoxazole revisited. *Arch Intern Med*. 2003;163:402–410.

Mori H, Kuroda Y, Imamura S. Hyponatremia and/or hyperkalemia in patients treated with the standard dose of trimethoprim–sulfamethoxazole. *Inter Med*. 2003;42:665–669.

Schmitz FJ, Krey A, Geisel R, et al. Susceptibility of 302 methicillin-resistant *Staphylococcus aureus* isolates from 20 European university hospitals to vancomycin and alternative antistaphylococcal compounds. *Eur J Clin Microbiol Infect Dis*. 1999;18:528–530.

Wilén M, Buwembo W, Sendagire H, Kironde F, Swedberg G. Co-trimoxazole resistance of *Streptococcus pneumoniae* and commensal streptococci from Kampala, Uganda. *Scand J Infect Dis*. 2009;41:113–121.

OTHER DIAMINOPYRIMIDINE–SULFONAMIDE COMBINATIONS

 ## CO-TRIMAZINE

A fixed-ratio (1:5) combination of trimethoprim and sulfadiazine. Its antimicrobial activity is that of its components and synergistic interaction between them. Following a dose of 1 g, mean peak serum concentrations of sulfadiazine are around 25 mg/L, with a plasma elimination half-life of 9.3 h. Untoward effects resemble those of co-trimoxazole and its clinical uses are similar. It is no longer much used except in veterinary medicine.

 Further information

Bergan T, Ortengan B, Westerlund D. Clinical pharmacokinetics of co-trimazine. *Clin Pharmacokinet*. 1986;11:372–386.

18 Fosfomycin and fosmidomycin

David Greenwood

Fosfomycin (originally called phosphonomycin) was discovered in Spain in 1969 and jointly developed in Spain and the USA. Fosmidomycin was synthesized in Japan a decade later. They are phosphonic acid derivatives, with unique structures that set them apart from other antimicrobial agents and, probably, from each other.

Uptake of these compounds in many Gram-negative bacteria, notably *Escherichia coli*, is induced by glucose 6-phosphate and this substance greatly potentiates the activity in vitro. Glucose 6-phosphate is present in places where glycolysis takes place, but the tissue content generally is low and located intracellularly. It is not present in the serum or cerebrospinal fluid (CSF) and is probably suboptimal at sites of infection, since the efficacy of the agents in experimental infection is increased by co-administration of glucose 6-phosphate. Nonetheless, the correlation between their in-vivo and in-vitro activity is better when tested in the presence of the inducer.

Synergy with aminoglycosides and with other cell-wall active agents, notably β-lactam antibiotics, has been demonstrated against some organisms.

Resistant mutants, typically exhibiting loss of the hexose phosphate transport system induced by glucose 6-phosphate, arise in vitro with relatively high frequency (10^{-4}–10^{-5}). Resistance that emerges in vivo is generally associated with deletion of the α-glycerophosphate transport mechanism. Plasmid-encoded resistance to fosfomycin also occurs in some species and such strains may remain susceptible to fosmidomycin.

FOSFOMYCIN

cis-1,2-Epoxypropylphosphonic acid. Molecular weight: 138.

A fermentation product of *Streptomyces fradiae*, *Streptomyces viridochromogenes* and *Streptomyces wedmorensis*. Commercially produced synthetically. It is stable for several years in powder form and for 48 h in aqueous solution. Fosfomycin tromethamine (*syn*: trometamol; tris(hydroxymethyl)aminomethane) and the much less soluble calcium salt are used in oral preparations; the very soluble sodium and disodium salts are used for parenteral administration.

ANTIMICROBIAL ACTIVITY

Fosfomycin is moderately active against a wide range of pathogens, but its activity in vitro is reduced at an alkaline pH and in the presence of glucose, phosphates or sodium chloride. Consequently, different results may be obtained depending on the medium used: inhibitory concentrations observed in simple nutrient broth or agar are usually lower than those in Mueller–Hinton medium. Addition of glucose 6-phosphate (25 mg/L) to the medium enhances the activity of the drug against most enterobacteria. Its activity against common pathogens (in the presence of glucose-6-phosphate) is shown in Table 18.1. It is, in general, more active against Gram-negative bacilli than Gram-positive cocci, although most strains of *Staphylococcus aureus* (including methicillin-resistant strains) are susceptible and *Pseudomonas aeruginosa* is usually resistant. Synergy with a variety of β-lactam antibiotics, aminoglycosides and other agents has been exhibited against some enterococci, methicillin-resistant *Staph. aureus* and enterobacteria. The tromethamine salt exhibits half the activity of other derivatives in tests in vitro since the tromethamine component has a molecular weight similar to that of fosfomycin itself.

It has been suggested that fosfomycin has immunomodulatory activity that may be of value in respiratory syncytial virus infection by suppressing cytokines involved in the pathogenesis of the disease.

ACQUIRED RESISTANCE

Bacterial populations contain variants that are resistant to the drug, but these are not highly prevalent even in those countries in which it has been widely used. There is no cross-resistance

Table 18.1 Activity of fosfomycin and fosmidomycin, in the presence of glucose 6-phosphate against common pathogenic bacteria: MIC (mg/L)

	Fosfomycin	Fosmidomycin
Staphylococcus aureus	2–32	R
Streptococcus pyogenes	8–64	R
Str. pneumoniae	8–64	R
Enterococcus faecalis	64	R
Haemophilus influenzae	4	0.5–R
Neisseria spp.	32–64	R
Escherichia coli	1–4	1
Klebsiella pneumoniae	2–64	0.5
Enterobacter spp.	2–R	0.1
Pseudomonas aeruginosa	4–R	2–R
Bacteroides fragilis	R	R

R, resistant (MIC >64 mg/L).

with other antibiotics, and it is active against many strains resistant to other agents. A type of enzyme-mediated resistance in which the epoxide ring is opened in the presence of glutathione is transferred by plasmids and may be associated with multidrug resistance.

 ## PHARMACOKINETICS

Oral absorption	
calcium salt	*c.* 30–40%
tromethamine salt	*c.* 60%
C_{max}, calcium salt 1 g oral	7 mg/L after 4 h
tromethamine salt 50 mg/kg oral	32 mg/L after 2 h
sodium salt 1 g intramuscular	28 mg/L after 1 h
sodium salt 20 mg/kg intravenous	130 mg/L end infusion
Plasma half-life	2–5 h
Volume of distribution	20–22 L
Plasma protein binding	<3%

Absorption

Absorption of the tromethamine salt is dose dependent, the fraction recovered from the urine falling from about one-half after 2 g to one-fifth after 5 g. The effect of food is variable, but generally depresses absorption. The sodium salt causes gastric irritation and is used only for parenteral administration. There is some accumulation after repeated doses given every 6 h. Constant intravenous infusion of 500 mg/h produced a steady-state blood level of about 60 mg/L.

Distribution

Fosfomycin diffuses freely into interstitial fluid and tissues. Diffusion into CSF is modest, but improves with meningeal inflammation. In patients with acute meningitis, CSF levels were 10.9 mg/L when the serum level was 65.2 mg/L. In patients with pleural effusions given 30 mg/kg as an intravenous bolus, average peak concentrations in pleural fluid around 43 mg/L were found at 3.7 h; clearance was slower than from plasma. Relatively high concentrations have been found in fetal blood (17.6 mg/L) and amniotic fluid (45 mg/L). Concentrations in breast milk are about 10% of the mother's plasma levels.

Metabolism and excretion

Fosfomycin is not metabolized in human beings. The drug is excreted into urine by glomerular filtration. About 80% of an intravenous dose is recoverable in urine in the first 24 h, achieving a peak concentration in excess of 1000 mg/L. Less than 20% of an oral dose of the calcium salt finds its way into urine, but a single 50 mg/kg dose of the tromethamine salt provides a urinary concentration that remains above 1000 mg/L for 12 h. Renal impairment increases the half-life proportional to the fall in creatinine clearance, reaching around 50 h as the creatinine clearance level falls below 10 mL/min. Most of the drug is removed by hemodialysis. Fosfomycin is excreted into bile, but is returned to the circulation by enterohepatic recycling.

 ## TOXICITY AND SIDE EFFECTS

Adverse reactions have been observed in about 10–17% of patients, mostly slight gastrointestinal disorders. There may be a transient rise in transaminase levels.

Sodium salt

Respiratory, gastrointestinal, generalized and genitourinary infections

Tromethamine salt

Single-dose treatment of cystitis
Prophylaxis in transurethral surgery

 ### Preparations and dosage

Fosfomycin trometamol

Proprietary names: Monuril, Monurol.

Preparations: Granules in 3 g sachets.

Dosage: Urinary tract infection: Adults, oral, 3 g as a single dose.
Surgical prophylaxis: 3 g preoperatively; 3 g after 24 h.

Widely available. Not available in the UK.

Fosfomycin sodium

Limited availability; not available in the UK or the USA.

Further information

Falagas ME, Kastoris AC, Karageorgopoulos DE, Rafailidis PI. Fosfomycin for the treatment of infections caused by multidrug-resistant non-fermenting Gram-negative bacilli: a systematic review of microbiological, animal and clinical studies. *Int J Antimicrob Agents*. 2009;34(2):111–120.

Okabayashi T, Yokota SI, Yoto Y, Tsutsumi H, Fujii N. Fosfomycin suppresses chemokine induction in airway epithelial cells infected with the respiratory syncytial virus. *Clin Vaccine Immunol*. 2009;16(6):859–865.

Patel SS, Balfour JA, Bryson HM. Fosfomycin tromethamine. A review of its antibacterial activity, pharmacokinetic properties and therapeutic efficacy as a single-dose oral treatment for uncomplicated lower urinary tract infections. *Drugs*. 1997;53:637–656.

Rudenko N, Dorofeyev A. Prevention of lower urinary tract infections by long-term administration of fosfomycin trometamol. Double blind, randomized, parallel group, placebo controlled study. *Arzneimittelforschung*. 2005;55:420–427.

Stein GE. Comparison of single-dose fosfomycin and a 7-day course of nitrofurantoin in female patients with uncomplicated urinary tract infection. *Clin Ther*. 1999;21:1864–1872.

FOSMIDOMYCIN

Sodium hydrogen-3 (*N*-hydroxyformamido) propyl phosphate. Molecular weight (sodium salt): 191.

$$HCNCH_2CH_2CH_2 \overset{\overset{\displaystyle O}{\|}}{\underset{\underset{\displaystyle ONa}{|}}{P}} OH$$

 ANTIMICROBIAL ACTIVITY

Fosmidomycin is active against a broad range of enterobacteria, but not against Gram-positive organisms or anaerobes (Table 18.1). Activity is affected by medium composition and enhanced by glucose 6-phosphate. It is slowly bactericidal at concentrations close to the minimum inhibitory concentration and shows synergy with aminoglycosides and β-lactam antibiotics. Bacteria resistant to fosfomycin are usually, but not always, cross-resistant to fosmidomycin.

Interest in fosmidomycin has been revived by demonstration of activity against malaria parasites.

 PHARMACOKINETICS

Oral absorption	*c.* 25%
C_{max} 500 mg oral 7.5 mg/kg intramuscular 30 mg/kg intravenous	2.3 mg/L after 2.4 h 11 mg/L after 1 h 160 mg/L end infusion
Plasma half-life	1.6–1.8 h
Plasma protein binding	<5%

It is not metabolized and there is no evidence of accumulation after multiple dosing. Elimination is almost entirely renal: mean urinary recoveries in the first 24 h after oral, intramuscular and intravenous administration are around 25%, 65% and 85%, respectively.

 TOXICITY, SIDE EFFECTS AND CLINICAL USE

Fosmidomycin appears to be well tolerated. Uses are similar to those of fosfomycin against Gram-negative organisms. Fosmidomycin is being investigated as a potential antimalarial agent in combination with clindamycin, with which it appears to interact synergically, or artemisinin.

 Further information

Missinou MA, Borrmann S, Schindler A, et al. Fosmidomycin for malaria. *Lancet*. 2002;360:1941–1942.

Neu HC, Kamimura T. In vitro and in vivo antibacterial activity of FR-31564, a phosphonic acid antimicrobial agent. *Antimicrob Agents Chemother*. 1981;19:1013–1023.

Ruangweerayut R, Looareesuwan S, Hutchinson D, Chauemung A, Banmairuroi V, Na-Bangchang K. Assessment of the pharmacokinetics and dynamics of two combination regimens of fosmidomycin–clindamycin in patients with uncomplicated falciparum malaria. *Malar J*. 2008;7:225.

CHAPTER

19   Fusidanes

David Greenwood

The fusidanes are antibiotics with a steroid-like structure, but the stereochemistry differs from that of metabolically active steroids and they do not exert any hormonal or anti-inflammatory activity. The group includes helvolic acid, cephalosporin P₁ and fusidic acid. Helvolic acid, a product of *Aspergillus fumigatus*, attracted some early attention because of its weak antimycobacterial activity; cephalosporin P₁ was a component of the antibiotic complex of the mold that also yielded the first true cephalosporin.

Fusidic acid is much the most active member of the group and is the only one commercially available. It was discovered in Denmark in 1960 as a product of *Fusidium coccineum*, a fungus originally isolated in Japan from monkey dung. The principal interest of fusidic acid lies in its antistaphylococcal activity.

FUSIDIC ACID

Molecular weight (sodium salt): 538.7.

Supplied as the sodium salt, which is readily soluble in water, or suspension of the acid. Intravenous preparations (sodium or diethanolamine salt) are dissolved in phosphate–citrate buffer. Several formulations are available for topical application. The dry powder is stable for 3 years.

ANTIMICROBIAL ACTIVITY

Fusidic acid is active against most Gram-positive bacteria, but all aerobic Gram-negative bacilli are resistant (Table 19.1). Streptococci and pneumococci are much less susceptible than staphylococci. *Bacteroides fragilis*, *Nocardia asteroides* (minimum inhibitory concentration [MIC] 0.5–4 mg/L), *Corynebacterium diphtheriae* (MIC <0.01 mg/L) and *Clostridium* spp. (MIC 0.01–0.5 mg/L) are susceptible. It is moderately active against many mycobacteria, including *Mycobacterium tuberculosis*, *M. bovis*, *M. malmoense* and *M. leprae*, but other species are resistant. Fusidic acid shows some activity against certain protozoa, including *Giardia lamblia* and *Plasmodium falciparum*.

In 50% serum, the MIC may double and it is slightly more effective at pH 6–7 than at pH 8. It is bactericidal in concentrations close to the MIC.

ACQUIRED RESISTANCE

Large inocula of *Staphylococcus aureus* contain a small number of chromosomal mutants, designated *fusA*, which emerge rapidly in vitro and sometimes during therapy. Other bacterial properties, such as growth rate and coagulase production remain unimpaired. Plasmid-mediated resistance caused by acquisition of *fusB*, *fusC* and *fusD* determinants also occur in *Staph. aureus* and other staphylococci and may, indeed, be more common in clinical isolates. The end result in all cases seems to be the prevention of binding of the drug at the target site, the EFG–ribosome complex (*see* p. 16). Genes for β-lactamase production and fusidic acid resistance are commonly carried on the same plasmid.

Despite the ease of emergence of resistance in vitro, resistance remained uncommon in clinical isolates (1–2%) for many years, but has risen significantly. Topical applications are liable to facilitate the emergence of resistant mutants and

Table 19.1 Activity of sodium fusidate against some common pathogenic bacteria

Species	MIC (mg/L)
Staphylococcus aureus	0.03–0.1
Streptococcus pyogenes	4–16
Str. pneumoniae	2–16
Enterococcus faecalis	1–4
Neisseria spp.	0.03–1
Escherichia coli	R
Klebsiella pneumoniae	R
Pseudomonas aeruginosa	R
Bacteroides fragilis	2
Mycobacterium tuberculosis	8–32

R, resistant (MIC >64 mg/L).

there is evidence that increased use has contributed to the pool of resistant strains in circulation.

PHARMACOKINETICS

Oral absorption: sodium salt	>90%
suspension	70%
C_{max} 500 mg oral	30 mg/L after 2–3 h
500 mg i.v. infusion	50 mg/L end infusion
Plasma half-life	c. 9 h
Volume of distribution	c. 12 L
Plasma protein binding	97%

Absorption

The suspension is less well absorbed than the sodium salt of the tablet formulation. In children absorption is more rapid than in adults. Milk appears to delay absorption, peak concentrations not being reached for 4–8 h. Because of slow elimination, accumulation of the drug occurs on repeated administration of both oral and intravenous formulations.

Distribution

It is well distributed in the tissues and most organs of the body. It does not reach the cerebrospinal fluid, but penetrates into cerebral abscesses. Inhibitory levels are obtained in muscle, kidney, lungs and pleural exudate. Bone concentrations in samples taken at operation from patients with chronic osteomyelitis treated for at least 5 days were 1.7–14.9 mg/g in patients receiving 1.5 g per day and 3.4–14.8 mg/g in patients receiving 3 g per day.

Levels in excess of 7 mg/L have been found in aspirated synovial fluid from patients with osteo- or rheumatoid arthritis after 3–7 days' treatment with 0.75 g or 1.5 g per day. The drug has been detected in brain, milk and placenta, which it crosses to reach the fetus. In patients treated with 1.5 g per day, levels of 0.08–0.84 mg/L were found in the aqueous humor after 1 day and 1.2–2.0 mg/L after 3 days' treatment. In the post-distribution phase, about half of the drug is in the peripheral compartment, in keeping with the known ability of the drug to penetrate into tissues including bone.

Metabolism and excretion

It is extensively metabolized in the liver and is excreted in the bile in the form of glucuronides and various other metabolites. Only about 2% of the administered dose can be recovered in active form in the feces. Less than 1% of active drug is excreted in the urine. Very little is removed by dialysis.

TOXICITY AND SIDE EFFECTS

Mild gastrointestinal disturbance and occasional rashes have been reported. Some patients develop abnormalities in liver function tests and jaundice which resolve on withdrawal of therapy. Jaundice is less common with oral than with parenteral therapy. The drug is not recommended in hepatic insufficiency. Rapid infusion of diethanolamine fusidate may lead to venospasm or thrombosis, and occasionally to hypocalcemia, possibly as an effect of the buffer.

CLINICAL USE

Systemic formulations

Severe staphylococcal infections, particularly bone and joint infections (in combination with other antistaphylococcal agents)

Prosthetic valve endocarditis due to 'diphtheroids' (in combination with erythromycin)

Topical formulations

Skin infections, principally those involving staphylococci, but including erythrasma

Acute staphylococcal conjunctivitis

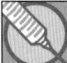

Preparations and dosage

Proprietary name: Fucidin.

Preparations: Tablets, suspension, injection, topical preparations.

Dosage: Adults, oral (as sodium fusidate): 500 mg every 8 h, doubled for severe infections. Children (as fusidic acid) ≤1 year, 50 mg/kg per day in three divided doses; 1–5 years, 250 mg every 8 h; 5–12 years, 500 mg every 8 h.

Intravenous infusion (as sodium fusidate): adults >50 kg, 500 mg every 8 h; adults <50 kg and children, 6–7 mg/kg every 8 h.

Widely available; not available in the USA.

Further information

Dobie D, Gray J. Fusidic acid resistance in *Staphylococcus aureus*. *Arch Dis Child*. 2004;89:74–77.

Howden BP, Grayson ML. Dumb and dumber – the potential waste of a useful antistaphylococcal agent: emerging fusidic acid resistance in *Staphylococcus aureus*. *Clin Infect Dis*. 2006;42:394–400.

Mason BW, Howard AJ, Magee JT. Fusidic acid resistance in community isolates of methicillin-susceptible *Staphylococcus aureus* and fusidic acid prescribing. *J Antimicrob Chemother*. 2003;51:1033–1036.

McLaws F, Chopra I, O'Neill AJ. High prevalence of resistance to fusidic acid in clinical isolates of *Staphylococcus epidermidis*. *J Antimicrob Chemother*. 2008;61:1040–1043.

O'Neill AJ, McLaws F, Kahlmeter G, Henriksen AS, Chopra I. Genetic basis of resistance to fusidic acid in staphylococci. *Antimicrob Agents Chemother*. 2007;51:1737–1740.

Reeves DS. The pharmacokinetics of fusidic acid. *J Antimicrob Chemother*. 1987;20:467–476.

Various authors. Fusidic acid. *Int J Antimicrob Agents*. 1999;12(suppl 2):S1–S93.

CHAPTER 20

Glycopeptides

Neil Woodford

The natural glycopeptides are a group of chemically complex antibacterial compounds obtained originally from various species of soil actinomycetes. They all contain a core heptapeptide to which are attached sugar moieties, some of which are unique. Vancomycin and teicoplanin, the only representatives presently in clinical use, are used for the treatment of serious infections caused by Gram-positive bacteria, particularly *Staphylococcus aureus*. Three semisynthetic glycopeptides – dalbavancin, oritavancin and telavancin – are presently undergoing clinical trial (*see* p. 271).

Among other glycopeptides, avoparcin and actaplanin have been used as animal feed additives, while actinoidin and ristocetin have been used as investigational aids in the diagnosis of von Willebrand's disease and platelet aggregation dysfunction.

A naturally occurring lipoglycodepsipeptide, ramoplanin, shares many of the microbiological properties of vancomycin and teicoplanin. It is, however, chemically distinct and has a different mode of action. It is too toxic for systemic use, but remains under investigation as a topical agent, as a component of oral gut decontamination regimens, and for the oral therapy of antibiotic-associated colitis.

ANTIMICROBIAL ACTIVITY

The activity of glycopeptides is essentially restricted to Gram-positive organisms, notably staphylococci and streptococci of all kinds. However, *Lactobacillus, Leuconostoc, Pediococcus* and *Erysipelothrix* spp. are inherently resistant. Their large molecular size prevents them from penetrating the Gram-negative outer membrane and, with rare exceptions (e.g. some *Prevotella* and *Porphyromonas* spp.), they are inactive against Gram-negative bacteria.

ACQUIRED RESISTANCE

 ## ENTEROCOCCI

Seven distinct resistance genotypes are recognized, of which the first two are most prevalent, especially in *Enterococcus faecium* (*see also* p. 30).

- VanA resistance is associated with the substitution of D-alanyl-D-alanine by D-alanyl-D-lactate at the carboxy terminus of the pentapeptide side chain of N-acetylmuramic acid (*see* p. 11; Figure 2.2), with a consequent loss of binding affinity for both vancomycin and teicoplanin. The modification is brought about by the functioning of an inducible cluster of genes that are on a transposable element and may be present on a transferable plasmid.
- VanB resistance also results from a D-lac substitution that is inducible by vancomycin but not by teicoplanin, to which susceptibility is retained. It is usually chromosomally mediated and transferability has been shown in some cases.
- VanC resistance is an intrinsic characteristic of *Ent. gallinarum* and *Ent. casseliflavus*, which are infrequently encountered as pathogens. It is non-transferable, chromosomally mediated, expressed constitutively and is conferred by substitution of D-alanyl-D-alanine by D-alanyl-D-serine. It is characterized by low-level resistance to vancomycin alone.
- VanD resistance has been found in a few strains of *E. faecium*. It results from a D-lac substitution, is usually expressed constitutively, and confers non-transferable resistance to vancomycin and reduced susceptibility to teicoplanin.
- VanE resistance has been described in a few strains of *E. faecalis* that display reduced susceptibility to vancomycin alone and harbor a D-ser substitution. Resistance may be expressed inducibly or constitutively.
- VanG and VanL resistance have also been found in a few strains of *E. faecalis*. Isolates have low-level resistance to vancomycin, but not to teicoplanin, owing to a D-ser substitution. The inducible resistance genes are located on the chromosome, but may be transferable from some strains.

None of the newer glycopeptides has increased binding to peptidoglycan precursors with D-lac or D-ser substitutions.

STAPHYLOCOCCI

Low-level resistance is described in clinical isolates and laboratory mutants of staphylococci, usually in *Staph. epidermidis* and *Staph. haemolyticus*, less often in *Staph. aureus*. Most glycopeptide-non-susceptible staphylococci show resistance to teicoplanin, but retain susceptibility to vancomycin, at least in vitro. This phenotype has not been reported in enterococci. Isolates of *Staph. aureus* with intermediate vancomycin resistance and reduced teicoplanin susceptibility are reported; in some such strains a raised minimum inhibitory concentration (MIC) is displayed by only a small subpopulation of cells.

The various resistance phenotypes each result from chromosomal mutation(s), rather than horizontal acquisition of resistance genes, and have been variously attributed to alterations in cell wall structure, overproduction of the cell-wall peptidoglycan and binding to cell-wall sites other than the primary target. However, the genetic basis has not yet been precisely defined and it seems probable that there are several genetic paths to low-level glycopeptide resistance.

There are several substantiated reports from the USA of high-level resistance to glycopeptides in *Staph. aureus* mediated by horizontal transfer of the enterococcal *vanA* gene cluster, but these isolates remain rare and the resistance often unstable.

DETECTION OF GLYCOPEPTIDE RESISTANCE

The routine detection of glycopeptide resistance may present problems, especially with strains exhibiting low-level resistance, such as glycopeptide-intermediate *Staph. aureus*. Disk tests are notoriously unreliable for this purpose and problems may occur with automated systems. In general, quantitative methods are recommended for accurate determination of MICs whenever possible. Population analysis may aid confirmation of strains showing intermediate resistance.

Further information

Cetinkaya Y, Falk P, Mayhall CG. Vancomycin-resistant enterococci. *Clin Microbiol Rev.* 2000;13:686–707.

Courvalin P. Vancomycin resistance in gram-positive cocci. *Clin Infect Dis.* 2006;42(suppl 1):S25–S34.

Hiramatsu K. Vancomycin-resistant *Staphylococcus aureus*: a new model of antibiotic resistance. *Lancet Infect Dis.* 2001;1:147–155.

Tenover FC, Biddle JW, Lancaster MV. Increasing resistance to vancomycin and other glycopeptides in *Staphylococcus aureus*. *Emerg Infect Dis.* 2001;7:327–332.

Werner G, Strommenger B, Witte W. Acquired vancomycin resistance in clinically relevant pathogens. *Future Microbiology.* 2008;3:547–562.

TEICOPLANIN

Molecular weight: (A_2-1): 1877.7; (A_2-2 and A_2-3): 1879.7; (A_2-4 and A_2-5): 1893.7.

A complex of several molecules of similar antibiotic potency produced by *Actinoplanes teichomyceticus*. It is formulated as the sodium salt for intramuscular or intravenous administration.

ANTIMICROBIAL ACTIVITY

In general, teicoplanin is 2–4 times more active than vancomycin against susceptible strains (Table 20.1). However, against some coagulase-negative staphylococci, especially *Staph. haemolyticus*, it may be less active (MIC 16–64 mg/L compared with ≤4 mg vancomycin/L). For these strains, the MIC of teicoplanin, but not vancomycin, is greatly affected by the composition of the medium, including the presence of lysed horse blood, and the bacterial inoculum density. Isolates inhibited by ≤4 mg/L are usually considered susceptible.

ACQUIRED RESISTANCE

Vancomycin-resistant enterococci of the VanA type are resistant, as are *Staph. aureus* strains with intermediate or full resistance to vancomycin. Strains of other resistance genotypes are usually susceptible, although resistance may develop in VanB enterococci by mutations that cause the resistance genes to be expressed constitutively. Coagulase-negative

Table 20.1 Comparative in vitro activity of glycopeptides against some common pathogenic bacteria: MIC range (mg/L)

Species	Vancomycin	Teicoplanin	Dalbavancin	Oritavancin	Telavancin
Staphylococcus aureus	1–2	0.12–1	≤0.008–2	≤0.008–4	≤0.015–2
Streptococcus pyogenes	0.12–0.25	0.03–0.12	≤0.008–0.06	0.015–0.5	0.03–0.12
Str. pneumoniae	0.12–0.25	0.03–0.12	≤0.008–0.25	≤0.008–0.5	≤0.008–0.06
Enterococcus faecalis and *E. faecium*	1–4	0.12–0.5	≤0.015–4	≤0.008–0.5	≤0.015–4
Haemophilus influenzae	16–R	R	R	R	R
Neisseria spp.	8–32	No data	No data	No data	No data
Escherichia coli	R	R	R	R	R
Klebsiella pneumoniae	R	R	R	R	R
Pseudomonas aeruginosa	R	R	R	R	R
Clostridium difficile	0.06–1	0.03–0.25	0.125–0.5	0.06–1	0.125–0.5
Bacteroides fragilis	R	R	R	R	R

R, resistant (MIC >32 mg/L).

staphylococci exhibiting low-level glycopeptide resistance are usually more resistant to teicoplanin than vancomycin even when they emerge during vancomycin therapy.

 # PHARMACOKINETICS

Oral absorption	Very low
C_{max} 400 mg intravenous bolus	25–40 mg/L after 1 h
6 mg/kg intramuscular	c. 10 mg/L after 2 h
Plasma half-life (terminal)	90 h (mean)
Volume of distribution (steady state)	0.9–1.6 L/kg
Plasma protein binding	>90%

Absorption

It is very poorly absorbed from the gastrointestinal tract. Bioavailability after intramuscular administration is about 90%. The area under the concentration–time curve (AUC) is similar after intravenous or intramuscular administration. In children, a dose of 6 mg/kg per day produced a mean trough concentration of 4.6 mg/L and a peak concentration of 19.1 mg/L. After a dose of 10 mg/kg the corresponding concentrations were 15.8 and 36.9 mg/L, respectively.

Distribution

Teicoplanin is widely distributed and penetrates readily into tissues, peritoneal fluid, synovial fluid and bone. It crosses the placenta, but not the blood–brain barrier.

Metabolism and excretion

No metabolic products have been identified. The drug is removed from the body almost entirely by glomerular filtration. The terminal half-life ranges from 33 to 190 h or longer, depending upon the pharmacokinetic model used for analysis and the last sampling time. The half-life may be shorter in children and is substantially altered in patients with renal failure (and the elderly), so that adjustment of dosage may be necessary. It is not removed during hemodialysis or hemofiltration and clearance by peritoneal dialysis is less than 20% of total body clearance. In all three procedures, management of plasma concentration is best achieved by giving a loading dose followed by monitoring at appropriate intervals.

 # TOXICITY AND SIDE EFFECTS

Unlike vancomycin, teicoplanin does not cause significant histamine release and the 'red-man' syndrome is very seldom seen. Nephrotoxicity is uncommon and, when it does occur, is not related to dose, plasma concentration or concomitant therapy with an aminoglycoside. Ototoxicity has been reported rarely and is not dose related.

Other, reversible, adverse effects include allergy, local intolerance, fever and altered liver function. Thrombocytopenia has been seen in patients with raised trough levels (about 60 mg/L). None of these effects occurs with a frequency greater than 3%. Teicoplanin should be used with caution in patients with a history of hypersensitivity to vancomycin.

Safety in pregnancy has not been established. Accidental overdosing in two children, in whom plasma levels in excess of 300 mg/L were found, was not associated with symptoms or laboratory abnormalities.

CLINICAL USE

Infections caused by *Staph. aureus* and other Gram-positive pathogens (especially those caused by methicillin-resistant staphylococci and in patients hypersensitive to β-lactam antibiotics)

Treatment of infections caused by vancomycin-resistant enterococci (other than VanA strains)

Treatment and prophylaxis of endocarditis caused by Gram-positive species (often in combination with an aminoglycoside)

Peritonitis associated with continuous ambulatory peritoneal dialysis (intraperitoneal)

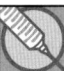

Preparations and dosage

Proprietary name: Targocid.

Preparation: Injection.

Dosage: Adults, i.v., 400 mg initial loading dose on day 1 then 200 mg per day; severe infections, 400 mg loading dose every 12 h for the first three doses, then 400 mg per day. Children ≥2 months, 10 mg/kg every 12 h for three doses then 6 mg/kg per day; severe infections, 10 mg/kg every 12 h for three doses, then 10 mg/kg per day. Neonates, 16 mg/kg initial loading dose on day 1, subsequently 8 mg/kg per day.

Widely available; not available in the USA.

Further information

Anonymous. Teicoplanin. In: Dollery C, ed. *Therapeutic Drugs.* 2nd ed. Edinburgh: Churchill Livingstone; 1999:T20–T24.

Brogden RN, Peters DH. Teicoplanin. A reappraisal of its antimicrobial activity, pharmacokinetic properties and therapeutic efficacy. *Drugs.* 1994;47:823–854.

Parenti F, Schito GC, Courvalin P. Teicoplanin chemistry and microbiology. *J Chemother.* 2000;12:5–14.

Wilson APR. Clinical pharmacokinetics of teicoplanin. *Clin Pharmacokinet.* 2000;39:167–183.

Wood MJ. Comparative safety of teicoplanin and vancomycin. *J Chemother.* 2000;12:21–25.

VANCOMYCIN

Molecular weight (free base): 1449; (hydrochloride): 1485.7.

A tricyclic glycopeptide isolated from the fermentation products of the actinomycete, *Amycolatopsis orientalis* (formerly *Streptomyces orientalis*). It is formulated as the water-soluble hydrochloride for intravenous infusion or oral administration.

ANTIMICROBIAL ACTIVITY

The antibacterial activity is essentially restricted to Gram-positive species (Table 20.1), including methicillin-resistant strains of staphylococci; viridans streptococci, *Listeria monocytogenes*, *Propionibacterium acnes* and corynebacteria are all susceptible (MIC 0.25–2 mg/L), as are Gram-positive anaerobes, including *Clostridium difficile* (MIC 0.06–1 mg/L) and *C. perfringens* (MIC 0.12–0.5 mg/L). Mycobacteria are resistant.

Vancomycin is slowly bactericidal for most susceptible bacteria. However, against isolates of *Enterococcus* spp., some viridans streptococci and *Staph. haemolyticus* it is effectively bacteristatic. Gentamicin enhances the bactericidal effect, provided the isolate is susceptible (staphylococci) or lacks high-level resistance (enterococci and streptococci). There is growing evidence that vancomycin is less effective against methicillin-resistant *Staph. aureus* (MRSA) infections caused by strains with MICs at the high end of the susceptible range.

ACQUIRED RESISTANCE

Resistance is uncommon, except in enterococci. In this genus, acquired resistance is far more common in *E. faecium* than in *E. faecalis* or other species, and has emerged in response to widespread use of vancomycin in hospitals. The use of avoparcin (a related glycopeptide) as a growth promoter in animal husbandry may also have played a part in encouraging resistance in enterococci.

Low-level resistance (MIC 8–32 mg/L) has been described in coagulase-negative staphylococci, usually *Staph. epidermidis* or *Staph. haemolyticus*, sometimes emerging during protracted treatment. Strains of *Staph. aureus* exhibiting intermediate vancomycin susceptibility (MIC 8–16 mg/L) have been found, but the prevalence of these strains, many of which exhibit hetero-resistance, appears to be very low, though they may be under-reported owing to the difficulties in detecting them in vitro. Rare strains of *Staph. aureus* highly resistant to glycopeptides (MIC: 32–128 mg vancomycin/L; 8–32 mg teicoplanin/L) have been reported from the USA, India and Iran.

PHARMACOKINETICS

Oral absorption	Very low
C_{max} 500 mg slow intravenous infusion (>1 h)	10–25 mg/L 1 h after end infusion
1 g slow intravenous infusion (>1 h)	20–50 mg/L 1 h after end infusion
Plasma half-life	5–11 h
Volume of distribution	0.6 L/kg
Plasma protein binding	c. 55%

Rapid infusion (<1 h) or bolus administration is dangerous. The intramuscular route of administration causes pain and necrosis and is not used. Slow intravenous infusion over at least 100 min is recommended. Dosage should be adjusted to give a peak concentration of 25–40 mg/L and a trough of 5–10 mg/L. In some centers, continuous infusion is used and may be pharmacodynamically optimal.

Absorption

It is very poorly absorbed from the gastrointestinal tract and large concentrations of unaltered drug are found in the feces after oral administration.

Distribution

After slow intravenous infusion vancomycin is distributed widely, reaching therapeutic concentrations in most body compartments. It does not penetrate appreciably into the cerebrospinal fluid of subjects with normal meninges, but levels may approach therapeutic concentrations in patients with meningitis; however, intrathecal administration may be necessary to achieve adequate levels.

Metabolism and excretion

Vancomycin is not metabolized and 90% of an intravenous dose is eliminated in the urine, almost exclusively by glomerular filtration. The elimination half-life in patients with normal renal function is usually 6–8 h, but is altered substantially in patients with impaired renal function, necessitating dosage modification. This can be predicted to some extent by creatinine clearance values but adequately optimized only by monitoring plasma concentrations.

Renal clearance may be more rapid in intravenous drug abusers and children (with the exception of neonates in whom the half-life may be prolonged) and plasma monitoring is indicated in such patients, particularly those receiving therapy for endocarditis or other life-threatening sepsis. A prolonged half-life has been observed in some patients with hepatic failure. Plasma monitoring is also indicated in these patients.

It is not removed efficiently by hemodialysis or hemofiltration. Patients undergoing these procedures should be given an appropriate loading dose and the frequency and size of further doses determined by monitoring plasma concentrations. Vancomycin crosses the peritoneal membrane in both directions with a transfer half-life of about 3 h, resulting in about 75% equilibration over a 6 h dialysis period. Because of the large dilution effect, many exchanges may be required before the plasma concentration reaches that of the dialysate, and to achieve rapid equilibration a loading dose of about three times the maintenance dose has been suggested. Thus, in patients on continuous ambulatory peritoneal dialysis, incorporation of 50 mg vancomycin/L of dialysate eventually produces plasma concentrations of 5–20 mg/L.

Alternatively, a loading dose of 0.5 g vancomycin, administered by intravenous infusion, followed by 7.5 mg/L dialysate with exchange every 4–6 h, produces plasma concentrations of 6.5–37 mg/L.

 ## INTERACTIONS

Gentamicin, also furosemide (frusemide) or other loop diuretics, may increase the potential for nephrotoxicity and ototoxicity. Owing to the acidic nature of solutions, vancomycin is incompatible in vitro with various agents, including β-lactam antibiotics, aminophylline and heparin.

 ## TOXICITY AND SIDE EFFECTS

Rapid administration (<60 min) may result in release of histamine from basophils and mast cells, leading to the so-called 'red-man' or 'red-neck' syndrome, characterized by one or more of pruritus, erythema, flushing of the upper torso, anaphylactoid reaction, angioedema and, rarely, cardiovascular depression and collapse.

Vancomycin is potentially nephrotoxic and ototoxic, although the highly purified drug preparations in current use are safer than early preparations. Increased risk of nephrotoxicity has been associated with treatment for longer than 3 weeks, trough plasma concentrations continually in excess of 10 mg/L, and concurrent therapy with an aminoglycoside or a loop diuretic. Ototoxicity, often irreversible, used to be seen particularly in elderly patients and in patients receiving excessive dosage, but is unusual with the more highly purified preparations. The risk of ototoxicity is minimized if the peak serum level is kept below 50 mg/L and is very unusual if the level is less than 30 mg/L, unless the patient has prior auditory nerve damage or is receiving another potentially ototoxic drug. Reversible neutropenia and/or thrombocytopenia, which can be profound, may occur, notably in patients with renal impairment.

 ## CLINICAL USE

Infections caused by *Staph. aureus* and other Gram-positive pathogens (especially those caused by methicillin-resistant staphylococci and in patients hypersensitive to β-lactam antibiotics)

Empirical therapy of febrile and profoundly neutropenic patients (in combination with agents active against Gram-negative bacteria)

Treatment and prophylaxis of endocarditis caused by Gram-positive species (often in combination with an aminoglycoside)

Peritonitis associated with continuous ambulatory peritoneal dialysis (intraperitoneal)

Oral formulation: Antibiotic-associated colitis

Oral formulation: Suppression of bowel flora in neutropenic patients (in combination with other agents)

Preparations and dosage

Proprietary name: Vancocin.

Preparations: Injection, capsules.

Dosage: Adults, oral, 125 mg every 6 h for 7–10 days, up to 2 g per day in severe infections; i.v., 500 mg every 6 h or 1 g every 12 h. Children, oral, 5–10 mg/kg every 6 h; >5 years, half the adult dose. Children, i.v., >1 month, 15 mg/kg every 8 h; infants 1–4 weeks, 15 mg/kg initially then 10 mg/kg every 8 h; neonates up to 1 week, 15 mg/kg initially then 10 mg/kg every 12 h.

Widely available.

Further information

Anonymous. Vancomycin (hydrochloride). In: Dollery C, ed. *Therapeutic Drugs*. 2nd ed. Edinburgh: Churchill Livingstone; 1999:V6–V10.

Gold HS. Vancomycin-resistant enterococci: mechanisms and clinical observations. *Clin Infect Dis*. 2001;33:210–219.

Perichon B, Courvalin P. Heterologous expression of the enterococcal *vanA* operon in methicillin-resistant *Staphylococcus aureus*. *Antimicrob Agents Chemother*. 2004;48:4281–4285.

Rybak MJ, Albrecht LM, Boike SC, Chandreesekar PH. Nephrotoxicity of vancomycin, alone and with an aminoglycoside. *J Antimicrob Chemother*. 1990;25:679–687.

Sakoulas G, Moise-Broder PA, Schentag J, Forrest A, Moellering RC, Eliopoulos GM. Relationship of MIC and bactericidal activity to efficacy of vancomycin for treatment of methicillin-resistant *Staphylococcus aureus* bacteremia. *J Clin Microbiol*. 2004;42:2398–2402.

Sievert DM, Rudrik JT, Patel JB, McDonald LC, Wilkins MJ, Hageman JC. Vancomycin-resistant *Staphylococcus aureus* in the United States, 2002–2006. *Clin Infect Dis*. 2008;46:668–674.

Soriano A, Marco F, Martinez JA, et al. Influence of vancomycin minimum inhibitory concentration on the treatment of methicillin-resistant *Staphylococcus aureus* bacteremia. *Clin Infect Dis*. 2008;46:193–200.

INVESTIGATIONAL GLYCOPEPTIDES

DALBAVANCIN

A teicoplanin-like lipoglycopeptide derived from a product of the actinomycete *Nonomura* spp.

It displays excellent activity in vitro, especially against staphylococci (Table 20.1) and including many strains with mutational resistance to teicoplanin. Activity against glycopeptide-resistant enterococci is similar to that of teicoplanin (Table 20.1). Activity against strains of enterococci and *Staph. aureus* with VanA resistance is much reduced. Susceptibility testing is complicated since dalbavancin binds to surfaces of labware, which may result in artificially high MICs. This can be overcome by the addition of 0.002% polysorbate-80 to liquid media.

The serum half-life of 6–11 days allows once weekly dosing, which may facilitate outpatient intravenous therapy.

Further information

Billeter M, Zervos MJ, Chen AY, Dalovisio JR, Kurukularatne C. Dalbavancin: a novel once-weekly lipoglycopeptide antibiotic. *Clin Infect Dis*. 2008;46:577–583.

Jones RN, Biedenbach DJ, Johnson DM, Pfaller MA. *In vitro* evaluation of BI 397, a novel glycopeptide antimicrobial agent. *J Chemother*. 2001;13:244–254.

Mushtaq S, Warner M, Johnson AP, Livermore DM. Activity of dalbavancin against staphylococci and streptococci, assessed by BSAC and NCCLS agar dilution methods. *J Antimicrob Chemother*. 2004;54:617–620.

Zhanel GG, Trapp S, Gin AS, et al. Dalbavancin and telavancin: novel lipoglycopeptides for the treatment of Gram-positive infections. *Expert Rev Anti Infect Ther*. 2008;6:67–81.

ORITAVANCIN

A semisynthetic vancomycin-like derivative of chloroeremomycin, which has an alkyl side chain that promotes strong dimerization and membrane anchoring, both of which enhance its complex antibacterial activity.

It is highly active against a wide range of Gram-positive organisms in vitro (Table 20.1). It remains active against many strains with reduced susceptibility or resistance to vancomycin or teicoplanin, although strains with VanA resistance are usually less susceptible. Like dalbavancin, it binds rapidly to labware; susceptibility testing media (broth) should be supplemented with 0.002% polysorbate-80.

It is in development as a once-daily injectable agent.

 Further information

Anderson DL. Oritavancin for skin infections. *Drugs Today*. 2008;44:563–575.

Crandon J, Nicolau DP. Oritavancin: a potential weapon in the battle against serious Gram-positive pathogens. *Future Microbiology*. 2008;3:251–263.

Jones RN, Barrett MS, Erwin ME. In vitro activity and spectrum of LY333328, a novel glycopeptide derivative. *Antimicrob Agents Chemother*. 1997;41:488–493.

Poulakou G, Giamarellou H. Oritavancin: a new promising agent in the treatment of infections due to Gram-positive pathogens. *Expert Opin Investig Drugs*. 2008;17:225–243.

 ## TELAVANCIN

A bactericidal, vancomycin-like lipoglycopeptide currently under clinical trial for injectable treatment of infections caused by Gram-positive pathogens, including hospital-acquired pneumonia and complicated skin and skin structure infections.

It exhibits excellent activity in vitro against enterococci and staphylococci (Table 20.1), though it has reduced activity against many glycopeptide-resistant strains, especially VanA strains. The half-life is 7–9 h, which allows once-daily dosing. Telavancin was approved by the US Food and Drug Administration (FDA) in September 2009 for the treatment of adult patients with complicated skin and skin structure infections (cSSSI) caused by susceptible Gram-positive bacteria, including *Staph. aureus*, both methicillin-resistant (MRSA) and methicillin-susceptible (MSSA) strains.

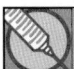 ## Preparations and dosage

Proprietary Name: Vibativ.

Preparation: Injection

Dosage: Adults, i.v., 10 mg/kg infused over 60 minutes, once every 24 hours for 7 to 14 days. Adjustment is needed for patients with reduced renal function. No adjustment is needed for those with reduced hepatic function.

Animal data suggest that telavancin may cause adverse developmental outcomes in the fetus if given to pregnant women. A pregnancy test should be performed in all women of childbearing age and use should be avoided in pregnant women unless the benefits for the mother outweigh the risks to the fetus.

Available in US.

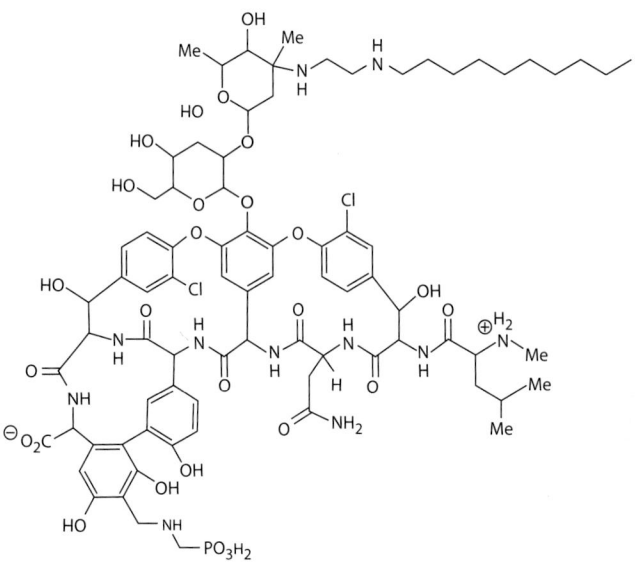

 Further information

Jansen WTM, Verel A, Verhoef J, Milatovic D. In vitro activity of telavancin against Gram-positive clinical isolates recently obtained in Europe. *Antimicrob Agents Chemother*. 2007;51:3420–3424.

Nannini EC, Stryjewski ME. A new lipoglycopeptide: telavancin. *Expert Opin Pharmacother*. 2008;9:2197–2207.

Saravolatz LD, Pawlak J, Johnson LB. Comparative activity of telavancin against isolates of community-associated methicillin-resistant *Staphylococcus aureus*. *J Antimicrob Chemother*. 2007;60:406–409.

Zhanel GG, Trapp S, Gin AS, et al. Dalbavancin and telavancin: novel lipoglycopeptides for the treatment of Gram-positive infections. *Expert Review in Anti-infective Therapy*. 2008;6:67–81.

21 Lincosamides

David Greenwood

The lincosamides are a small group of agents with a novel structure unlike that of any other antibiotic. The naturally occurring members of the group are lincomycin and the much less active celesticetin. Attempts to prepare semisynthetic derivatives with improved properties have been largely unsuccessful, with the exception of the chlorinated derivative, clindamycin, and pirlimycin, which is used in bovine mastitis.

Lincosamides are widely active against Gram-positive bacteria and most anaerobes, but not Gram-negative aerobes. They are also active against some mycoplasmas and protozoa. Their principal therapeutic indications are staphylococcal infections, particularly of bones and joints, and anaerobic infections, including mixed infections for which they must be combined with an agent active against aerobic Gram-negative bacilli. They are moderately well absorbed when administered by mouth and distributed widely to tissues, including penetration into cells and bone. They are generally well tolerated, except for the relative frequency with which they have been associated with severe diarrhea, including *Clostridium difficile*-associated pseudomembranous colitis.

 Further information

Spízek J, Novotná J, Rezanka T. Lincosamides: chemical structure, biosynthesis, mechanism of action, resistance and applications. *Adv Appl Microbiol.* 2004;56:121–154.

CLINDAMYCIN

7-Chloro-7-deoxylincomycin. Molecular weight (anhydrous free base): 425.

A semisynthetic derivative of lincomycin. Aqueous suspensions are stable for up to 2 weeks at room temperature. Capsules contain clindamycin hydrochloride, which has a very bitter taste, detectable in concentrations as low as 8 mg/L; the syrup contains a suspension of the ester, clindamycin palmitate, which is palatable for children. Clindamycin phosphate, which is more soluble at neutral pH and less irritating than the hydrochloride, is used parenterally. The palmitate and phosphate salts are inactive in vitro and must be hydrolyzed to liberate clindamycin.

ANTIMICROBIAL ACTIVITY

The spectrum includes most Gram-positive organisms, notably staphylococci (including many methicillin-resistant strains) and streptococci, but not enterococci (Table 21.1). Aerobic Gram-negative rods are uniformly resistant, but most anaerobic bacteria are highly susceptible. Typical minimum inhibitory concentrations (MICs) are: *Prevotella* and *Porphyromonas* spp., 0.1–2 mg/L; *Fusobacterium* spp., <0.5 mg/L; *Peptostreptococcus* spp., 0.1–0.5 mg/L. Clostridia, with the notable exception of *Clostridium perfringens* (MIC <0.1–8 mg/L) are less susceptible. Corynebacteria, *Bacillus anthracis* and *Nocardia asteroides* are all susceptible, but mycobacteria are resistant. The MIC for *Chlamydia trachomatis* is 16 mg/L, that for *Mobiluncus* spp. is 0.5 mg/L, and that for *Gardnerella vaginalis* is 0.03 mg/L. *Mycoplasma hominis* is susceptible (MIC <1 mg/L), *M. pneumoniae* somewhat less so (MIC 1–4 mg/L). Ureaplasmas are resistant. Clindamycin exhibits useful activity against some protozoa, including *Toxoplasma gondii*, *Plasmodium falciparum* and *Babesia* spp. and against the fungus *Pneumocystis jirovecii*.

ACQUIRED RESISTANCE

Resistant strains of staphylococci, streptococci (including pneumococci) and *Bacteroides* spp. are found with variable frequency and are commonly also resistant to erythromycin. Resistance may be caused by changes in a ribosomal protein

Table 21.1 Susceptibility of common pathogenic bacteria: MIC (mg/L)

	Clindamycin	Lincomycin
Staphylococcus aureus	0.1–1	0.5–2
Streptococcus pyogenes	0.01–0.25	0.05–1
Str. pneumoniae	0.05	0.1–1
Enterococcus faecalis	4–R	2–R
Haemophilus influenzae	0.5–16	4–16
Neisseria spp.	0.5–4	8–64
Escherichia coli	R	R
Klebsiella pneumoniae	R	R
Pseudomonas aeruginosa	R	R
Bacteroides fragilis	0.02–2	2–4

R, resistant (MIC >64 mg/L).

or, less commonly, by enzymic inactivation. There is complete cross-resistance to lincomycin. A form of resistance that embraces macrolides, lincosamides and type B streptogramins is associated with methylation of adenine residues at a common binding site. The methylase is inducible by macrolides, but not lincosamides (or streptogramins), which consequently remain active in the absence of macrolides.

 PHARMACOKINETICS

Oral absorption	80–90%
C_{max}: hydrochloride 300 mg oral	3.6 mg/L after 1–2 h
palmitate 300 mg oral	1.4–4.2 mg/L after 1 h
phosphate 300 mg intramuscular	4–5 mg/L after 2 h
phosphate 300 mg intravenous	5–6 mg/L end infusion
Plasma half-life	c. 2–3 h
Volume of distribution	43–74 L/m²
Plasma protein binding	94%

Absorption

Oral absorption is not depressed or delayed by food. The palmitate is rapidly and completely hydrolyzed in the gut. In contrast, clindamycin phosphate is absorbed intact after intramuscular injection and relatively slowly hydrolyzed by alkaline phosphatases. A substantial amount of unhydrolyzed clindamycin phosphate (1–2 mg/L) is detectable in the serum at 30–60 min and up to 10% of the dose may still be present as phosphate after 8 h. The bioavailability in relation to dose is linear, but not proportional.

Plasma levels in pregnant women following a single 450 mg oral dose were similar to those in non-pregnant women. After intravaginal administration of 5 mL of 2% clindamycin phosphate cream (100 mg) to healthy women and women suffering from bacterial vaginosis, less than 5% of the dose was subsequently found in the plasma.

Distribution

After hydrolysis in the serum, clindamycin phosphate is rapidly and widely distributed, but cerebrospinal fluid (CSF) concentrations are low (0.14–0.46 mg/L after a single 150 mg dose) and levels in brain are low or absent.

The drug is excreted in breast milk and crosses the placenta. In patients undergoing cesarean section, mean peak fetal plasma concentrations (c. 3 mg/L) were 46% of the maternal level after a 600 mg intravenous dose of the phosphate.

Therapeutic concentrations are achieved in cancellous and cortical bone. The tissue:serum concentration ratio has been found to be 1.0 in bone marrow, 0.5–0.75 in spongy bone and 0–0.15 in compact bone. Hydroxyapatite binds clindamycin and probably also the ester.

Uptake of clindamycin phosphate into neutrophils is rapid, temperature dependent, saturable and depressed by acid pH. Clindamycin is accumulated by lysosomes to active concentrations around 40 times those of the extracellular fluid. After an initially high rate of hydrolysis by intracellular alkaline phosphatase, enzyme activity declines; after 4 h around half of the drug is still unhydrolyzed. Similar product inhibition may prevent the complete hydrolysis of the phosphate in pus where alkaline phosphatase is liberated from neutrophils.

Metabolism

It is extensively metabolized in the liver to clindamycose, desmethyl clindamycin, and sulfoxide derivatives. Desmethyl clindamycin and clindamycin sulfoxide retain antibacterial activity, but clindamycose and desmethyl clindamycin sulfoxide are much less active than the base.

Excretion

About 13% of an oral dose is excreted unchanged in urine, somewhat less after a parenteral dose of the phosphate. Bioactivity persists in the urine for up to 4 days, suggesting slow release of the drug or its active metabolites from tissues or body fluids. In patients with severe renal disease, plasma levels may be 3–4 times normal and persist for over 24 h. Urinary recovery of the drug can fall below 1% in severe renal failure. Clindamycin is not removed by hemodialysis or peritoneal dialysis.

The liver plays a significant part in the metabolism and elimination of the drug. Concentrations 2–3 times those in serum have been found in the bile gallbladder wall and liver of patients with patent common ducts undergoing biliary tract surgery, most of the activity being due to the desmethyl metabolite. Where the common duct was obstructed, none could be detected in bile and the level was lower in gallbladder wall, but the concentration in liver was slightly higher than in those without obstruction. Patients with proven hepatic cirrhosis show significant impairment of clindamycin elimination. Clindamycin phosphate may be slowly converted to the base in patients with hepatic impairment. Less than 5% of an oral dose can be recovered from the feces, but excretion of bioactive drug persists for several days and may continue to affect the normal gut flora.

The plasma half-life in premature infants (8.7 h) is significantly longer than in term infants (3.6 h).

TOXICITY AND SIDE EFFECTS

Up to 30% of patients experience diarrhea, especially when taking the drug orally. This is often due to *C. difficile* toxins and in a small proportion of cases leads to pseudomembranous colitis. Diarrhea is more common in women and in patients over 60 years of age. Diarrhea may abate if treatment is continued; however, because of the risk of pseudomembranous colitis, administration of the drug should be stopped.

Parenteral administration can cause elevation of transaminases and serum alkaline phosphatase, but these are generally reversible. Intravenous administration may be complicated by thrombophlebitis.

Rashes occur in about 10% of patients, but severe eruptions are rare. Isolated episodes of toxic epidermal necrolysis, blood dyscrasias and erythema multiforme have been reported and there is a single report of prolonged neuromuscular blockade after an accidental intravenous overdose.

CLINICAL USE

Staphylococcal soft tissue, bone and joint infection

Streptococcal infection (as a penicillin substitute in allergic patients, including prophylaxis of endocarditis in special risk patients undergoing dental procedures)

Prophylaxis and treatment of anaerobic infections (with appropriate agents where infection is likely to include aerobic Gram-negative rods)

Bacterial vaginosis

Acne

Toxoplasmosis

Babesiosis (in combination with quinine)

Pneumocystis jirovecii pneumonia (in combination with primaquine)

Preparations and dosage

Proprietary names: Dalacin C, Dalacin T.

Preparations: Capsules, suspension, injection.

Dosage: Adults, oral, 150–300 mg every 6 h, increased to 450 mg every 6 h for severe infections. Children, oral, 3–6 mg/kg every 6 h. Adults, i.m., i.v., 600 mg to 1.2 g per day in 2–4 equal doses; more severe infections, 1.2–2.7 g per day in 2–4 equal doses; life-threatening infections, up to 4.8 g per day. Children >1 month, i.m., i.v., 15–25 mg/kg per day in 3–4 divided doses; severe infections, 25–40 mg/kg per day in 3–4 divided doses; in severe infections it is recommended that children are given no less than 300 mg per day, regardless of body weight. Neonates have been given 15–20 mg/kg per day in 3–4 divided doses.

Widely available.

Further information

Anonymous. Clindamycin (hydrochloride). In: Dollery C, ed. *Therapeutic Drugs*. 2nd ed. Edinburgh: Churchill Livingstone; 1999:C257–C261.

Bartlett JG. Historical perspectives on studies of *Clostridium difficile* and *C. difficile* infection. *Clin Infect Dis*. 2008;46(suppl 1):S4–S11.

Guay D. Update on clindamycin in the management of bacterial, fungal and protozoal infections. *Expert Opin Pharmacother*. 2007;8:2401–2444.

Guay DR. Topical clindamycin in the management of acne vulgaris. *Expert Opin Pharmacother*. 2007;8:2625–2664.

McDonald HM, Brocklehurst P, Gordon A. Antibiotics for treating bacterial vaginosis in pregnancy. *Cochrane Database Syst Rev*. 2007;(1) CD000262.

Wilson W, Taubert KA, Gewitz M, et al. Prevention of infective endocarditis: guidelines from the American Heart Association. *Circulation*. 2007;116:1736–1754.

LINCOMYCIN

Molecular weight (hydrochloride monohydrate): 461.

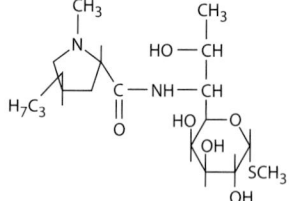

A fermentation product of *Streptomyces lincolnensis* var. *lincolnensis* supplied as the hydrochloride. The dry crystalline hydrochloride is very soluble in water and very stable.

ANTIMICROBIAL ACTIVITY

The spectrum closely resembles that of clindamycin, but it is generally less potent (Table 21.1).

ACQUIRED RESISTANCE

There is complete cross-resistance between clindamycin and lincomycin. Clinical isolates of streptococci and enterococci are commonly cross-resistant to erythromycin. A transposon carrying a lincomycin resistance gene similar to that found in *Staphylococcus aureus* has been reported in *Bacteroides* strains.

PHARMACOKINETICS

Oral absorption (fasting)	20–35%
C_{max} 500 mg oral	2–3 mg/L after 2–4 h
600 mg intramuscular	8–18 mg/L after 1–2 h
600 mg intravenous	18–20 mg/L end infusion
Plasma half-life	4–6 h
Plasma protein binding	72%

Absorption

It is less well absorbed than clindamycin. Food significantly delays and decreases absorption, the mean peak plasma level from a dose given immediately after a meal being only about half the fasting levels.

Distribution

It is widely distributed in a volume approximating to the total body water. Levels in normal CSF are low, but in the presence of inflammation, CSF:serum concentration ratios around 0.4 have been found. Penetration occurs into cerebral abscesses. Concentrations in saliva and sputum approximate to the simultaneous serum level. Concentrations of 1.5–6.9 mg/L have been found in cord serum or amniotic fluid after the mother received 600 mg intramuscularly, and 0.5–2.4 mg/L in human milk after the second of two maternal 500 mg doses.

In patients undergoing total hip replacement given 600 mg intramuscularly 6 h preoperatively, and again by intravenous infusion perioperatively, mean concentrations achieved were: capsule 9.4 mg/kg; synovial fluid 5.4 mg/L; cancellous bone 7.2 mg/kg; cortical bone 5.4 mg/kg.

Peak concentrations of 30–135 mg/L have been found in aqueous humor 1–2 h after subconjunctival injection of 75 mg; plasma levels were around 2–3 mg/L within 10 min.

Metabolism and excretion

Like clindamycin, it is metabolized in the liver and excreted in the bile. About 40% of an oral dose can be recovered from the feces. Less than 5% of an oral dose appears in the urine over 24 h, but up to 60% after intravenous administration, mostly in the first 4 h. In patients with severe hepatic dysfunction the plasma half-life is approximately doubled and the proportion of the dose appearing in the urine increases. It is not removed by dialysis.

 ## TOXICITY AND SIDE EFFECTS

Nausea, vomiting and abdominal cramps may occur. Diarrhea affects at least 10% of patients, usually within a few days of oral or parenteral administration. It is more common in older patients and uncommon in children. Symptoms range from watery diarrhea without fever or leukocytosis to severe, often bloody, diarrhea, with abdominal pain progressing to profound shock and dehydration with high mortality.

Hypersensitivity reactions are rare. Transient changes occur in liver function tests, probably due to interference with the tests, since abnormalities in specific enzyme tests and clinical evidence of hepatic dysfunction are rare.

In some patients receiving large doses by rapid intravenous injection, the blood pressure falls precipitately with nausea, vomiting, arrhythmias and, exceptionally, cardiac arrest. It can transiently depress neuromuscular transmission and might weakly depress respiration after anesthesia.

There is no evidence of risk in pregnancy.

 ## CLINICAL USE

Uses are similar to those of clindamycin, by which it has been generally superseded.

Preparations and dosage

Proprietary name: Lincocin.

Preparations: Capsules, syrup, injection.

Dosage: Adults, oral, 500 mg, every 6–8 h; i.m., 600 mg, every 12–24 h; i.v. infusion, 600 mg to 1 g, every 8–12 h, up to 8 g per day in severe infections. Children >1 month, oral, 30–60 mg/kg per day in divided doses; i.m., i.v., 10–20 mg/kg per day in divided doses.

Limited availability; available in the USA, but not available in the UK.

 ## Further information

Rosato A, Vicarini H, Leclerc R. Inducible or constitutive expression of resistance in clinical isolates of streptococci and enterococci cross-resistant to erythromycin and lincomycin. *J Antimicrob Chemother.* 1999;43:559–562.

Spízek J, Rezanka T. Lincomycin, clindamycin and their applications. *Appl Microbiol Biotechnol.* 2004;64:455–464.

22 Macrolides

André Bryskier

The macrolides form a large group of closely related antibiotics produced mostly by *Streptomyces* and related species. They are characterized by a macrolactone ring (to which they owe their generic name), to which typically two sugars, one an amino sugar, are attached. The original macrolide complex, erythromycin A, was isolated in 1952 as a natural product of *Saccharopolyspora erythraea* (formerly *Streptomyces erythreus*). Other natural products followed. The search for analogs has focused on compounds with an extended antibacterial spectrum (notably against fastidious Gram-negative pathogens), improved pharmacokinetic properties (e.g. increased acid stability) and reduced gastrointestinal intolerance.

The most important therapeutic macrolides are characterized by a 14-, 15- or 16-membered lactone ring. Macrolides with a 12-membered ring are also known, but only as research compounds. In the group that includes erythromycin A, the lactone ring contains 14 atoms and one or two sugar groups attached by α- or β-glycosidic linkages to the aglycone. In the 16-membered-ring macrolides, two sugars are linked together and attached to the lactone ring through the amino sugar.

Insertion of a nitrogen atom into the erythronolide A ring of erythromycin A yielded a chemical subclass with a 15-membered ring, known as azalides, one of which, azithromycin, is used clinically. It shares the properties of other macrolide antibiotics, but exhibits increased potency against fastidious Gram-negative bacteria and some Enterobacteriaceae, and has a longer elimination half-life.

A further development came with the ketolides, semisynthetic derivatives of erythromycin A in which α-L cladinose at position 3 of the erythronolide A ring is replaced with a ketone function and a cyclic carbamate residue is present at C11–C12. Ketolides are highly stable, even at pH 1.0, and remain active against many erythromycin-resistant Gram-positive cocci. They do not induce resistance to macrolides, lincosamides and streptogramins caused by methylation of the ribosomal binding site (*see below*). One such compound, telithromycin, is clinically available.

More than 100 other ketolide derivatives have been reported. Three – cethromycin, modithromycin and CEM 101 – are in clinical development at the time of writing. Modithromycin has a bicyclic bridge between positions 6 and 11 of the lactone ring, and because of this structure the name 'bicyclolide' has been proposed for this type of ketolide.

Several macrolides, including tylosin, mycinamycin, tilmicosin (a derivative of tylosin), tulathromycin and gamithromycin are used only in veterinary medicine and are not discussed further here.

ANTIBACTERIAL ACTIVITY

The 14-, 15- and 16-membered-ring macrolides share the same antibacterial spectrum, including most Gram-positive organisms, *Neisseria* spp., *Haemophilus* spp., *Bordetella pertussis*, *Moraxella catarrhalis* and both Gram-positive and Gram-negative anaerobes. Activity against common pathogenic bacteria is shown in Table 22.1. They are inactive or poorly active against Enterobacteriaceae and non-fermentative Gram-negative bacteria such as *Pseudomonas aeruginosa*.

Group 1 14-membered ring compounds	Group 2 16-membered ring compounds	Group 3 Azalides (15-membered ring)	Group 4 Ketolides (14-membered ring)
Clarithromycin[a]	Josamycin	Azithromycin[a]	Cethromycin[a]
Dirithromycin[a]	Kitasamycin (leucomycin)		Modithromycin[a]
Erythromycin A	Midecamycin		Telithromycin[a]
Flurithromycin[a]	Miokamycin[a]		CEM 101[a]
Oleandomycin	Rokitamycin[a]		
Roxithromycin[a]	Spiramycin		

[a]Semisynthetic compounds

The semisynthetic macrolides do not provide a significant advantage over erythromycin A against staphylococci and streptococci, and are poorly active against enterococci. They are active against *Mor. catarrhalis, B. pertussis, Neisseria gonorrhoeae, Campylobacter jejuni, Rhodococcus equi, Haemophilus ducreyi, Gardnerella vaginalis, Mobiluncus* spp., *Propionibacterium acnes, Borrelia burgdorferi* and *Treponema pallidum.* The minimum inhibitory concentrations (MICs) against *H. influenzae* range from 0.25 to 8 mg/L, the azalide azithromycin being the most active. Variable susceptibilities are reported for *B. bronchiseptica, Listeria monocytogenes, Corynebacterium jeikeium, Eikenella corrodens, Pasteurella multocida, Bacteroides fragilis, Prevotella melaninogenica, Fusobacterium* spp. and *Clostridium perfringens.*

In-vitro activity against common respiratory pathogens is shown in Table 22.2. The ketolide, telithromycin, is the most active compound and retains activity against erythromycin-resistant strains.

The semisynthetic macrolides exert important activity against intracellular pathogens, including *Chlamydia trachomatis* (MIC$_{50}$ clarithromycin 0.007 mg/L; azithromycin 0.125 mg/L; roxithromycin 0.06 mg/L), *Chlamydophila* (formerly *Chlamydia*) *pneumoniae, Legionella pneumophila* and other *Legionella* spp., the *Mycobacterium avium* complex (MIC: clarithromycin 0.25–4.0 mg/L; azithromycin and roxithromycin 4–32 mg/L), *M. leprae* and *Rickettsia* spp. (MIC 1–2 mg/L). Azithromycin appears to be the most active of the compounds against *Brucella melitensis* and atypical pathogens such as *Ureaplasma urealyticum* and *Mycoplasma* spp. They are inactive against *M. tuberculosis.*

ACQUIRED RESISTANCE

Widespread use of erythromycin and semisynthetic analogs has led to the emergence of resistance in *Staphylococcus aureus, Streptococcus pneumoniae* and Lancefield group A streptococci (*Str. pyogenes*). Chromosomal or plasmid-mediated resistance to erythromycin may be inducible or constitutive. Intrinsic resistance of Gram-negative bacilli is probably due to the relative impermeability of the outer membrane to the hydrophobic compounds and/or to an efflux mechanism of resistance.

Table 22.1 Susceptibility (MIC range: mg/L) of some common pathogenic bacteria to macrolides

	Azithromycin	Erythromycin A	Josamycin	Midecamycin	Oleandomycin	Roxithromycin	Spiramycin	Telithromycin
Staphylococcus aureus	0.25–1	0.1–1	0.25–4	0.5–2	0.25–4	0.1–2	0.25–1	0.12–0.25
Streptococcus pyogenes	0.03–0.1	0.01–0.25	0.06–0.5	0.1–2	0.1–1	0.06–0.25	0.1–2	0.01–0.06
Str. pneumoniae	0.03–0.25	0.01–0.25	0.03–0.5	–	0.1–0.25	0.01–4	–	0.004–0.06
Enterococcus faecalis	0.5–R	0.5–4	0.5–4	1–4	2–4	0.5–8	2–4	–
Neisseria gonorrhoeae	0.03–2	0.03–0.5	0.5–2	–	2–4	0.03–2	2–4	–
N. meningitidis	0.01–0.06	0.03–1	0.06–2	–	2–4	0.03–2	–	0.03–0.25
Haemophilus influenzae	0.25–2	0.5–8	2–16	1–4	0.1–2	0.5–16	2–8	0.5–4
Escherichia coli	0.5–2	8–32	R	R	R	R	32	–
Pseudomonas aeruginosa	R	R	R	R	R	R	R	R
Bacteroides fragilis	0.5–16	0.1–16	0.06–1	2–32	–	0.25–64	–	–

Table 22.2 In vitro activity of selected macrolides against respiratory pathogens: MIC$_{50}$ (mg/L)

	Erythromycin A	Azithromycin	Clarithromycin	Dirithromycin	Roxithromycin	Telithromycin	Cethromycin
Streptococcus pneumoniae	0.06	0.06	0.015	0.06	0.06	0.008	0.015
Str. pyogenes	0.06	0.06	0.015	0.12	0.12	0.01	0.015
Haemophilus influenzae	4	1	4	8	8	1	2
Moraxella catarrhalis	0.12	0.03	0.06	0.12	0.25	0.06	0.03
Mycobacterium pneumoniae	0.01	0.004	0.004	0.03	0.03	0.001	<0.001
Chlamydophila pneumoniae	0.03	0.06	0.03	1	0.06	0.01	0.015
Legionella pneumophila	0.25	0.12	0.03	1	0.12	0.03	0.015

Acquired resistance to macrolides involves three mechanisms: modification of the target, active efflux or inactivation. In the first type, a single alteration in 23S ribosomal RNA in the 50S ribosomal subunit confers cross-resistance to macrolides, azalides, lincosamides and streptogramin-B-type antibiotics (the so-called MLS$_B$ phenotype); the other types confer resistance to structurally related antibiotics only.

Modification of the 50S ribosomal targets is a complex mechanism. Several types have been described:

- Monomethylation of adenine 2058, located in the 23S rRNA, results in blockade of the N^6 amino group of adenine and inhibition of binding of erythromycin A or its derivatives. It can be induced by 14-membered-ring macrolides and azalides, but not by 16-membered-ring macrolides or ketolides. Monomethylation or bimethylation of adenine 2058 or 2059 may be constitutive and affects all available macrolides. Monomethylation does not affect telithromycin.
- Mutation of adenine 2058 to guanine has been described in many bacterial species, such as staphylococci, streptococci (including *Str. pneumoniae* and *Str. pyogenes*), *Helicobacter pylori*, the *M. avium* complex and *T. pallidum*. Other point mutations on the peptidyltransferase site, such as adenine 2611 to guanine, lead to resistance to 14- and 15-membered-ring macrolides.
- Mutations at ribosomal proteins L4 and L22, which are close to the exit channel, have been reported in clinical isolates of *Str. pneumoniae*, *Str. oralis* and *Str. pyogenes*.

An efflux pump, Mef, encoded by a *mef* gene, accounts for resistance in over 50% of *Str. pneumoniae* or *Str. pyogenes* isolates in certain geographic areas. It has been described in all streptococci, including the viridans group. Other pumps involved in macrolide resistance include Msr A/B in staphylococci, Acr-like in *H. influenzae*, Mre A in *Str. agalactiae* and Mtr (which also removes penicillin G) in *N. gonorrhoeae*.

Macrolide-inactivating esterases that hydrolyze the lactone ring are found mainly in *Escherichia coli*. Enzymes that fix either a glucose or a phosphate at the 2′ OH group of D-desosamine have been reported in *Nocardia* spp., which are resistant to all macrolides having a D-desosamine substituent. Inactivation mechanisms have also been reported in 16-membered-ring macrolides.

PHARMACOKINETICS

Erythromycin is characterized by poor water solubility and rapid inactivation by stomach acidity, resulting in widely varying bioavailability after oral administration. Derivatives of erythromycin A have improved pharmacological properties, including bioavailability, gastrointestinal tolerance, higher peak plasma levels, longer apparent elimination plasma half-lives and improved tissue concentrations.

Oral absorption is rapid, with plasma peaks varying between 0.4 mg/L (azithromycin) and 11 mg/L (roxithromycin). Maximum concentrations are reached between 0.5 h (rokitamycin) and 3 h (clarithromycin) and are dose dependent.

The apparent elimination half-life varies from 1 h (miokamycin) to 44 h (dirithromycin); the absolute bioavailability varies between 10% (dirithromycin) and 55–60% (roxithromycin, clarithromycin). The main elimination route is via the bile and feces; a proportion of clarithromycin is excreted via the intestinal mucosa. A substantial part of the administered dose of clarithromycin is eliminated in urine. The long apparent elimination half-lives of roxithromycin, azithromycin and dirithromycin allow them to be administered as single daily oral doses.

INTRACELLULAR CONCENTRATION

Rates of uptake into cells and efflux vary for each compound (Table 22.3). Azithromycin, dirithromycin and telithromycin concentrate progressively, with a high concentration after 3 h. Macrolides usually concentrate in the granule zone of polymorphonuclear neutrophils. They are concentrated in the bronchial mucosa and tonsils (Table 22.4).

INTERACTIONS

Erythromycin A and oleandomycin induce hepatic microsomal enzymes and interfere via the cytochrome P$_{450}$ system with clearance of other drugs such as theophylline, antipyrine and carbamazepine, increasing their plasma levels. The induced isoenzymes of cytochrome P$_{450}$ rapidly demethylate and oxidize macrolides to nitrosoalkanes, which combine with the iron of the enzymes, thereby inactivating them. The 16-membered-ring macrolides such as josamycin and

Table 22.3 Uptake of macrolides into polymorphonuclear neutrophils

Macrolide	Uptake^a	Efflux^b	Percentage in granule
Azithromycin	>300	≤20	60
Clarithromycin	9–100	80	30
Dirithromycin	60–80	52	73
Erythromycin A	4–18	80	35
Erythromycylamine	25	63	45
Flurithromycin	>10	–	–
Josamycin	21	>20	13
Rokitamycin	30	>70	–
Roxithromycin	40–100	80	49
Telithromycin	348	45	56–75

^{a}Ratio of intracellular: extracellular concentration; ^{b}over 60 min.

Table 22.4 Concentration of macrolides in respiratory tissue

Macrolide	Dose (mg)	Plasma (mg/L)	Bronchial mucosa (mg/kg)	Tonsils (mg/kg)
Azithromycin	500 (S)	–	3.9	–
Clarithromycin	500 (R)	2.5	–	1.9
Dirithromycin	500 (R)	0.22	1.9	3.5
Erythromycin	500 (R)	3.08	7.2	2.9
Josamycin	1000 (R)	0.39	–	21.4
Oleandomycin	2000 (S)	–	–	4.1
Miokamycin	600 (R)	2.3	–	3.2
Roxithromycin	150 (R)	6.3	–	2.9
Spiramycin	2000 (R)	2.4	13–36	21.5–40
Telithromycin	800 (S)	1.9–2.7	0.7–3.9	0.7–3.95

S, single dose; R, repeated dose.

spiramycin have no such effect. Erythromycin base, estolate and stearate, and a metabolite of triacetyloleandomycin all form stable complexes with cytochrome P_{450}. Josamycin base forms an unstable complex. Josamycin propionate and spiramycin (base and adipate) do not bind.

TOXICITY AND SIDE EFFECTS

Macrolides are generally safe and serious adverse events are rare. A notable exception is erythromycin estolate, which is hepatotoxic and may cause severe hepatitis, probably as a result of the mixture of lauryl sulfate and the 2′-propionyl ester. Gastrointestinal complaints (nausea, vomiting, abdominal pain or, less frequently, diarrhea) are most common; they present a problem mainly with erythromycin doses higher than those recommended and are partly due to a hemiketal degradation product that acts on motilin, an intestinal endopeptide.

The semisynthetic 14- and 15-membered-ring macrolides are more acid stable than erythromycin A and are better tolerated.

CLINICAL USE

The macrolides retain the classic clinical applications of erythromycin, including activity against Gram-positive cocci and intracellular pathogens such as *Legionella*, *Chlamydia* and *Rickettsia* spp. The improved pharmacokinetic properties and tissue distribution of some semisynthetic compounds may prove useful in more unusual settings such as infections due to mycobacteria (*M. avium* complex) and protozoa (e.g.

Toxoplasma gondii, *Entamoeba histolytica*, *Plasmodium falciparum*). Other target infections are chronic gastritis (*H. pylori*) and borreliosis.

 Further information

Abu-Gharbieh E, Vasina V, Poluzzi E, De Ponti F. Antibacterial macrolides: a drug class with a complex pharmacological profile. *Pharmacol Res.* 2004;50:211–222.

Bryskier A. Novelties in the field of macrolides. *Expert Opin Investig Drugs.* 1997;6:1697–1709.

Bryskier A. *Antibiotiques et agents antibactériens et antifongiques.* Paris: Ellipses; 1999.

Bryskier A, Labro MT. Macrolides – nouvelles perspectives thérapeutiques. *Presse Méd.* 1994;23:1762–1766.

Bryskier A, Butzler JP, Neu HC, Tulkens PM, eds. *Macrolides: chemistry, pharmacology and clinical uses* Paris: Blackwell-Arnette; 1993:698.

Bryskier A, Agouridas C, Chantot JF. New insights into the structure-activity relationship of macrolides and azalides. In: Zinner SH, Young LS, Acar JF, Neu HC, eds. *New macrolides, azalides and streptogramins in clinical practice.* New York: Marcel Dekker; 1995:3–30.

Bryskier A, Agouridas C, Chantot JF. Ketolides: new semisynthetic 14-membered ring macrolides. In: Zinner SH, Young LS, Acar JF, Neu HC, eds. *Expanding indications for the new macrolides, azalides, and streptogramins.* New York: Marcel Dekker; 1997:39–50.

Drusano GL. Infection site concentrations: their therapeutic importance and the macrolide and macrolide-like class of antibiotics. *Pharmacotherapy.* 2005;25:150S–158S.

Hoban DJ, Zhanel GG. Clinical implications of macrolide resistance in community-acquired respiratory tract infections. *Expert Rev Anti Infect Ther.* 2006;4:973–980.

Zhu ZJ, Krasnykh O, Pan D, et al. Structure–activity relationships of macrolides against *Mycobacterium tuberculosis*. *Tuberculosis (Edinburgh).* 2008;88(suppl 1):S49–S63.

Zuckerman JM. Macrolides and ketolides: azithromycin, clarithromycin, telithromycin. *Infect Dis Clin North Am.* 2004;18:621–649.

GROUP 1: 14-MEMBERED RING MACROLIDES

CLARITHROMYCIN

Molecular weight: 748.

A semisynthetic erythromycin A derivative (6-*O*-methylerythromycin A) formulated for oral and intravenous use.

ANTIBACTERIAL ACTIVITY

Activity against susceptible common pathogens is two to four times greater than that of erythromycin A (Table 22.1). Most respiratory pathogens, with the exception of *H. influenzae*, are inhibited at a concentration of ≤0.25 mg/L. It inhibits *Mycoplasma pneumoniae* at 0.004 mg/L and *Mor. catarrhalis* at 0.06 mg/L. It is eight times more active than erythromycin A against *Legionella* spp., *C. trachomatis* and *Ch. pneumoniae*. Against anaerobic species, activity is similar to that of erythromycin A. Against *H. influenzae* the 14-hydroxy metabolite is twice as active as the parent compound.

PHARMACOKINETICS

Oral absorption	55%
C_{max} 250 mg oral	0.75 mg/L after 1.7 h
500 mg oral	1.65 mg/L after 2 h
Terminal half-life	2.7–3.5 h
Volume of distribution	250 L
Plasma protein binding	80%

Absorption and distribution

It is more stable to gastric acid than erythromycin, but internal ketalization between the 9-keto group and the C-12 hydroxyl group has been described resulting in an inactive product: pseudo clarithromycin. It is rapidly absorbed orally and absorption is not affected by food.

Concentrations in tonsil and lung tissues exceed the simultaneous plasma level by a factor of two and four, respectively.

Metabolism and excretion

The primary metabolic pathway is *N*-demethylation of the D-desosamine and stereospecific hydroxylation at the 14-position of the erythronolide A ring. Metabolism to the 14-hydroxy derivative is saturable above 800 mg.

Around 20–40% of the administered dose is eliminated in urine. The apparent elimination half-life of the 14-hydroxy metabolite is around 7 h. The parent compound and its principal metabolite are retained in renal impairment, resulting in long apparent elimination half-lives, exceeding 30 and 45 h, respectively, in patients whose creatinine clearance is less than 30 mL/min.

TOXICITY AND SIDE EFFECTS

Clarithromycin is well tolerated, producing little gastrointestinal disturbance and only transient changes in some liver function tests.

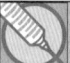

Upper and lower respiratory tract infections, including streptococcal pharyngitis, acute bacterial maxillary sinusitis, bacterial exacerbations of chronic bronchitis and community-acquired pneumonia

Skin and soft-tissue infections

H. pylori infection (in combination with other agents)

Preparations and dosage

Proprietary names: Klaricid, Biahin.

Preparations: Tablets, suspension, granules, injection.

Dosage: Adults, oral, 250–500 mg every 12 h for 7–14 days, depending on severity of infection. Children, oral, <8 kg, 7.5 mg/kg every 12 h; 8–11 kg, 62.5 mg every 12 h; 12–19 kg, 125 mg every 12 h; 20–29 kg, 187.5 mg every 12 h; 30–40 kg, 250 mg every 12 h. Adults, i.v. infusion, 500 mg every 12 h. Widely available.

Further information

Anonymous. Clarithromycin. In: Dollery C, ed. *Therapeutic Drugs*. 2nd ed. Edinburgh: Churchill Livingstone; 1999:C248–C253.

Finch RG, Speller DCE, Daly PJ. Clarithromycin: new approaches to the treatment of respiratory tract infections. *J Antimicrob Chemother*. 1991;27(suppl A).

ERYTHROMYCIN

Molecular weight (erythromycin A base): 733.9; (ethyl succinate): 862.1; (stearate): 1018.4; (estolate): 1056.4.

A natural antibiotic produced as a complex of six components (A–F) by *Saccharopolyspora erythraea*. Only erythromycin A has been developed for clinical use. It is available in a large number of forms for oral administration: the base compound (enteric- or film-coated to prevent destruction by gastric acidity); 2′-propionate and 2′-ethylsuccinate esters; a stearate salt; estolate and acistrate salts of 2′-esters. The 2′-esters and their salts have improved pharmacokinetic and pharmaceutical properties and are less bitter than erythromycin. It is also formulated as the lactobionate and gluceptate for parenteral use.

ANTIBACTERIAL ACTIVITY

Activity against common bacterial pathogens is shown in Table 22.1 (p. 277). Gram-positive rods, including *Clostridium* spp. (MIC$_{50}$ 0.1–1 mg/L), *C. diphtheriae* (MIC$_{50}$ 0.1–1 mg/L), *L. monocytogenes* (MIC$_{50}$ 0.1–0.3 mg/L) and *Bacillus anthracis* (MIC$_{50}$ 0.5–1.0 mg/L), are generally susceptible. Most strains of *M. scrofulaceum* and *M. kansasii* are susceptible (MIC$_{50}$ 0.5–2 mg/L), but *M. intracellulare* is often and *M. fortuitum* regularly resistant. *Nocardia* isolates are resistant. *H. ducreyi*, *B. pertussis* (MIC$_{50}$ 0.03–0.25 mg/L), some *Brucella*, *Flavobacterium*, *Legionella* (MIC$_{50}$ 0.1–0.5 mg/L) and *Pasteurella* spp. are susceptible. *H. pylori* (MIC 0.06–0.25 mg/L) and *C. jejuni* are usually susceptible, but *C. coli* may be resistant. Most anaerobic bacteria, including *Actinomyces* and *Arachnia* spp., are susceptible or moderately so, but *B. fragilis* and *Fusobacterium* spp. are resistant. *T. pallidum* and *Borrelia* spp. are susceptible, as are *Chlamydia* spp. (MIC ≤0.25 mg/L), *M. pneumoniae* and *Rickettsia* spp. *M. hominis* and *Ureaplasma* spp. are resistant. Enterobacteriaceae are usually resistant.

Activity rises with increasing pH up to 8.5. Incubation in 5–6% CO_2 raises the MIC for *H. influenzae* from 0.5–8 to 4–32 mg/L; MICs for *Str. pneumoniae* and *Str. pyogenes* also rise steeply. Activity is predominantly bacteristatic.

ACQUIRED RESISTANCE

In Europe, the USA and other countries the incidence of resistance in *Str. pneumoniae* ranges from 5% to over 60%. In *Str. pneumoniae* strains resistant or intermediately susceptible to penicillin G, resistance rates above 80% have been reported. Increasing rates of resistance in clinical isolates of *Str. pyogenes* have also been reported, threatening its use as an alternative to penicillin G in allergic patients.

Lower rates of resistance have been reported in other bacterial species, including methicillin-resistant *Staph. aureus*, coagulase-negative staphylococci, *Str. agalactiae*, Lancefield group C and G streptococci, viridans group streptococci, *H. pylori*, *T. pallidum*, *C. diphtheriae* and *N. gonorrhoeae*.

PHARMACOKINETICS

Oral absorption	Variable
C$_{max}$	
base 250 mg oral	1.3 mg/L after 3–4 h
500 mg oral	2 mg/L after 2–4 h
1000 mg oral	1.3–1.5 mg/L after 4 h
stearate 250 mg oral (fasting)	0.88 mg/L after 2.2 h
500 mg oral (fasting)	2.4 mg/L after 2–4 h
500 mg oral (after food)	0.1–0.4 mg/L after 2–4 h
2′-propionate 500 mg oral (fasting)	0.4–1.9 mg/L after 2–4 h
500 mg oral (after food)	0.3–0.5 mg/L after 4 h
2′-estolate 250 mg oral (fasting)	0.36–3 mg/L after 2–4 h
500 mg oral (fasting)	1.4–5 mg/L after 1–2 h
250 mg oral (after food)	1.1–2.9 mg/L after 2–4 h
500 mg oral (after food)	1.8–5.2 mg/L after 2–4 h
lactobionate 500 mg intravenous	11.5–30 mg/L end infusion
gluceptate 250 mg intravenous	3.5–10.7 mg/L end infusion
Plasma half-life:	
base	1.6–2 h
stearate	1.6–4 h
2′-propionate	3–5 h
2′-estolate	2–4 h
lactobionate/gluceptate	1–2 h
Volume of distribution	0.75 L/kg
Plasma protein binding:	
base	70%
propionate	93%

Absorption and metabolism

The acid lability of erythromycin base necessitates administration in a form giving protection from gastric acid. In acid media it is rapidly degraded (10% loss of activity at pH 2 in less than 4 s) by intramolecular dehydrogenation to a hemiketal and hence to anhydroerythromycin A, neither of which exerts antibacterial activity. Delayed and incomplete absorption is obtained from coated tablets and there is important inter- and intra-individual variation, adequate levels not being attained at all in a few subjects. Food delays absorption of erythromycin base. After 500 mg of the 2′-ethylsuccinyl ester, mean peak plasma levels at 1–2 h were 1.5 mg/L. In subjects given 1 g of the 2′-ethylsuccinate every 12 h for seven doses, the mean plasma concentration 1 h after the last dose was around 1.4 mg/L. Intra- and inter-subject variation and delayed and erratic absorption in the presence of food have not yet been eliminated by new formulations. Improved 500 mg preparations of erythromycin stearate are claimed to produce peak plasma levels of 0.9–2.4 mg/L that are little affected by the presence of food. 2′-Esters of erythromycin are partially hydrolyzed to erythromycin; 2′-acetyl erythromycin is hydrolyzed more rapidly than the 2′-propionyl ester, but more slowly than the 2′-ethylsuccinate.

The stoichiometric mixture with stearate does not adequately protect erythromycin from acid degradation. After an oral dose of erythromycin stearate, equivalent concentrations of erythromycin and its main degradation product, anhydroerythromycin, could be detected.

Doses of 10 mg/kg produced mean peak plasma concentrations around 1.8 mg/L in infants weighing 1.5–2 kg and 1.2 mg/L in those weighing 2–2.5 kg. In infants less than 4 months old, doses of 10 mg/kg of the 2′-ethylsuccinate every 6 h produced steady state plasma levels of around 1.3 mg/L. The apparent elimination half-life was 2.5 h. In children given 12.5 mg/kg of erythromycin 2′-ethylsuccinate every 6 h, the concentration in the plasma 2 h after the fourth dose was around 0.5–2.5 mg/L.

Distribution

Very low levels are obtained in cerebrospinal fluid (CSF), even in the presence of meningeal inflammation, and after parenteral administration. Levels of 0.1 mg/L in aqueous humor were found when the serum level was 0.36 mg/L, but there was no penetration into the vitreous. In children with otitis media given 12.5 mg/kg of erythromycin 2′-ethylsuccinate every 6 h, concentrations in middle ear exudate were 0.25–1 mg/L. In patients with chronic serous otitis media given 12.5 mg/kg up to a maximum of the equivalent of 500 mg, none was detected in middle ear fluid, but on continued treatment levels up to 1.2 mg/L have been described.

Penetration also occurs into peritoneal and pleural exudates. Mean concentrations of 2.6 mg/L have been found in sputum in patients receiving 1 g of erythromycin lactobionate intravenously every 12 h and 0.2–2 mg/L in those receiving an oral stearate formulation. Levels in prostatic fluid are about 40% of those in the plasma. Salivary levels of around 4 mg/L were found in subjects receiving doses of 0.5 g every 8 h at 5 h after a dose, when the plasma concentration was around 5.5 mg/L. Intracellular:extracellular ratios of 4–18 have been found in polymorphonuclear neutrophils.

Fetal tissue levels are considerably higher after multiple doses; when the mean peak maternal serum level was 4.94 (0.66–8) mg/L, the mean fetal blood concentration was 0.06 (0–0.12) mg/L. Concentrations were more than 0.3 mg/L in amniotic fluid and most other fetal tissues, but the concentrations were variable and unmeasurable in some. Erythromycin appears to be concentrated by fetal liver.

Excretion

Erythromycin is excreted both in urine and in the bile but only a fraction of the dose can be accounted for in this way. Only about 2.5% of an oral dose or 15% of an intravenous dose is recovered unchanged in the urine. It is not removed to any significant extent by peritoneal dialysis or hemodialysis. Reported changes in apparent elimination half-life in renal impairment may be related to the saturable nature of protein binding. Fairly high concentrations (50–250 mg/L) are found in the bile. In cirrhotic patients receiving 500 mg of the base, peak plasma levels were higher and earlier than in healthy volunteers (2.0 and 1.5 mg/L at 4.6 and 6.3 h, respectively). The apparent elimination half-life was 6.6 h. It is possible that the smaller excretion of the 2′-propionyl ester in the bile in comparison to the base accounts in part for its better-maintained serum levels. There is some enterohepatic recycling, but some of the administered dose is lost in the feces, producing concentrations of around 0.5 mg/g.

 ## INTERACTIONS

Interaction with the hepatic metabolism of other drugs can result in clinically significant potentiation of the action of carbamazepine, ciclosporin (cyclosporine), methylprednisolone, theophylline, midazolam, terfenadine and warfarin, and in adverse responses to digoxin and ergot alkaloids.

 ## TOXICITY AND SIDE EFFECTS

Oral administration, especially of large doses, commonly causes epigastric distress, nausea and vomiting, which may be severe. Solutions are very irritant: intravenous infusions almost invariably produce thrombophlebitis. Cholestatic hepatitis occurs rarely. Transient auditory disturbances have been described after intravenous administration of the lactobionate salt, and occasionally in patients with renal and hepatic impairment in whom oral dosage has produced high plasma levels. Sensorineural hearing impairment can occur and, although this is usually a reversible effect which occurs at high dosage, can be permanent. Prolongation of the apparent elimination half-life of carbamazepine, due to inhibition of its conversion to the epoxide, usually results in central nervous system (CNS) disturbances. Nightmares are troublesome in some patients. Allergic effects occur in about 0.5% of patients.

The estolate is particularly prone to give rise to liver abnormalities, consisting of upper abdominal pain, fever, hepatic enlargement, a raised serum bilirubin, pale stools and dark urine and eosinophilia. The condition is rare and usually seen 10–20 days after the initiation of treatment, with complete recovery on stopping the drug. Recurrence of symptoms can be induced by giving the estolate but not the base or stearate. There is evidence that erythromycin estolate is more toxic to isolated liver cells than is the 2′-propionate or the base, and it is suggested that the essential molecular feature responsible for toxicity is the propionyl–ester linkage. The relative frequency of the reaction, its rapidity of onset (within hours) after second courses of the drug, evidence of hypersensitivity and the histological appearance suggest a mixture of hepatic cholestasis, liver cell necrosis and hypersensitivity. Abnormal liver function tests in patients receiving the estolate must be interpreted with caution, since increased levels of transaminases is often the only abnormality and some metabolites of the estolate can interfere with the measurement commonly used. Elevated levels of transaminases return to normal after cessation of treatment. Serum bilirubin is generally unchanged in these patients, but γ-glutamyl transpeptidase may also be affected.

Lower and upper respiratory tract infections (including those caused by atypical and intracellular pathogens)

Legionellosis (alone or in combination with rifampicin [rifampin])

Skin and soft-tissue infections

Campylobacter infection

Syphilis (penicillin-allergic patients)

Whooping cough

Diphtheria (including treatment of carriers)

Concentrations found in middle ear exudate are unlikely to be sufficient to inhibit *H. influenzae* isolates, which is a common cause of otitis media in children.

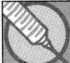

Preparations and dosage

Proprietary names: Erythrocin, Ilosone and many generic forms.

Preparations: Film-coated tablets (as ethyl succinate and stearate), suspension (as ethyl succinate), capsules, injection (as lactobionate).

Dosage: Adults and children >8 years, oral, 250–500 mg every 6 h or 0.5–1 g every 12 h, up to 4 g per day for severe infections. Children up to 2 years, oral, 125 mg every 6 h; 2–8 years, 250 mg every 6 h; doses doubled for severe infection. Adults, children, i.v., 50 mg/kg per day by continuous i.v. infusion or in divided doses every 6 h for severe infections; 25 mg/kg per day for mild infections when oral treatment is not possible.
Widely available.

Further information

Anonymous. Erythromycin. In: Dollery C, ed. *Therapeutic Drugs*. 2nd ed. Edinburgh: Churchill Livingstone; 1999:E50–E54.

Barre J, Mallat A, Rosembaum J, et al. Pharmacokinetics of erythromycin in patients with severe cirrhosis. Respective influence of decreased serum binding and impaired liver metabolic capacity. *Br J Clin Pharmacol.* 1987;23:753–757.

Carter BL, Woodhead JC, Cole KJ, Milavetz G. Gastrointestinal side effects with erythromycin preparations. *Drug Intell Clin Pharm.* 1987;21:734–738.

Eady EA, Ross JJ, Cove JH. Multiple mechanisms of erythromycin resistance. *J Antimicrob Chemother.* 1990;26:461–465.

Inman WAW, Rawson NSB. Erythromycin estolate and jaundice. *Br Med J.* 1983;286(1):1954–1957.

Kanfer A, Stamatakis G, Torlotin JC, Fredt G, Kenouch S, Mery JP. Changes in erythromycin pharmacokinetics induced by renal failure. *Clin Nephrol.* 1987;27:147–150.

ROXITHROMYCIN

Molecular weight: 837.04.

A semisynthetic derivative of erythromycin A formulated for oral use.

ANTIBACTERIAL ACTIVITY

Activity against common pathogens (Table 22.1, p. 277) is comparable to that of erythromycin. It is active against *L. monocytogenes, C. jejuni, H. ducreyi, G. vaginalis, Bord. pertussis, C. diphtheriae, B. burgdorferi, H. pylori,* the *M. avium* complex, *Chlamydia* spp., and *U. urealyticum*. Activity against respiratory pathogens is shown in Table 22.2 (p. 277).

PHARMACOKINETICS

Oral absorption	50–55%
C_{max} 150 mg oral	7.9 mg/L after 1.9 h
300 mg oral	10.8 mg/L after 1.5 h
Plasma half-life	10.5–11.9 h
Plasma protein binding	*c.* 90%

Absorption

Absorption is not affected by food. Oral administration with antacids or H_2-receptor antagonists does not significantly affect bioavailability. In a direct comparison, the area under the time–concentration curve (AUC) produced by a 150 mg dose was 16 times greater than that produced by 250 mg erythromycin A. Behavior in children is broadly similar to that in adults, repeated doses of 2.5 mg/kg producing age-independent mean peak plasma concentrations around 10 mg/L at 1–2 h, but the apparent elimination half-life was longer (approximately 20 h).

It is saturably bound to α-acid glycoprotein in plasma. The plasma clearance appears to be dose dependent or plasma concentration dependent.

Distribution

It is widely distributed, but does not reach the CSF. Concentrations close to the simultaneous serum level have been found in tonsillar, lung, prostatic and other tissues. It achieves high levels in skin.

Metabolism and excretion

Less than 5% of the administered dose is eliminated as degradation products. Rather more than half the dose appears in the feces and only 7–10% (including metabolites) in the urine; up to 15% is eliminated via the lungs. Renal clearance increased in volunteers as the dose was raised from 150 to 450 mg, and is decreased in elderly subjects. In patients in whom the creatinine clearance was <10 mL/min, the apparent elimination half-life rose to around 15.5 h and total body clearance was significantly reduced. The apparent elimination half-life was somewhat increased in patients with hepatic cirrhosis.

INTERACTIONS

The half-life of simultaneously administered theophylline is increased by about 10%, but there is no effect on that of carbamazepine and no interaction with warfarin or ciclosporin.

TOXICITY AND SIDE EFFECTS

It is generally well tolerated, adverse effects being described in 3–4% of patients, mostly gastrointestinal disturbance (abdominal pain, nausea and diarrhea). Headache, weakness, dizziness, rash and reversible changes in liver function tests and increased eosinophils and platelets have also been described.

Upper and lower respiratory tract infections
Skin and soft-tissue infections
Urogenital infections
Orodental infections

Preparations and dosage

Proprietary names: Rulid, Surlid.

Preparations: Tablets, oral suspension.

Dosage: Adults, oral, 150 mg every 12 h or 300 mg per day. Children, oral, 2.5–5 mg/kg every 12 h.

Widely available. Not available in the UK or the USA.

Further information

Bryskier A. Roxithromycin: review of its antimicrobial activity. *J Antimicrob Chemother.* 1998;41:1–21.

Phillips I, Péchère J-C, Speller D. Roxithromycin: a new macrolide. *J Antimicrob Chemother.* 1987;21(suppl B).

OTHER GROUP 1 MACROLIDES

DIRITHROMYCIN

A prodrug of erythromycylamine, a semisynthetic erythromycin A derivative, formulated for oral administration. Activity against respiratory pathogens (Table 22.2, p. 277) is generally poorer than that of erythromycin A.

The long apparent elimination half-life (30–44 h) allows once-daily administration. Around 60–90% of a dose is converted to erythromycylamine within 35 min after intravenous administration. After oral administration of single doses of 500–1000 mg to healthy volunteers, the peak plasma concentrations ranged from 0.29 to 0.64 mg/L after 4–5 h. The absolute bioavailability after oral administration is about 10%. It achieves a higher concentration than erythromycin in some tissues. After a 500 mg single oral dose, the mean peak biliary concentration was 139 mg/L. Renal and non-renal clearance was lower in patients with biliary disease than in other patients or healthy volunteers.

About 60–80% of an oral dose and over 80% of an intravenous dose are eliminated in the feces, predominantly as erythromycylamine. Dosage adjustments do not appear necessary in patients with mild or moderate hepatic, biliary or renal impairment. Negligible amounts of the drug are removed during hemodialysis.

Adverse events are similar to those found with other macrolides. Gastrointestinal events are most common; around 5% of patients experience abdominal pain, diarrhea or nausea.

It has been used in community-acquired infections of the respiratory tract and skin and soft-tissue infections. It is no longer widely available.

Further information

Brogden RN, Peters DH. Dirithromycin – a review of its antimicrobial activity, pharmacokinetic properties and therapeutic efficacy. *Drugs.* 1994;48:599–616.

FLURITHROMYCIN

A semisynthetic derivative of erythromycin A, supplied for oral administration. It is stable at acid pH due to the presence of the fluorine atom at C-8 of the erythronolide A ring.

It is active against most streptococci (including *Str. pneumoniae* and *Str. agalactiae*; MIC_{50} 0.03 mg/L), *Mor. catarrhalis*, *N. gonorrhoeae* (MIC_{50} 0.04 mg/L), *C. trachomatis* (MIC 0.06–0.125 mg/L), *M. genitalium* (MIC_{50} 0.007 mg/L) and *U. urealyticum* (MIC_{50} 0.03 mg/L). It has little or no activity against *H. influenzae* and *M. hominis*. Activity against anaerobes is similar to that of erythromycin A. It displays cross-resistance with erythromycin A.

A single 500 mg oral dose achieved a mean peak plasma concentration of 1.2–2 mg/L after 1–2 h. The apparent elimination half-life was 8 h and the volume of distribution 5.5 L/kg. With repeated doses (500 mg orally every 8 h for 10 doses), plasma concentrations were 0.72 mg/L immediately before and 0.67 mg/L at 4 h after the last dose. Absorption is not significantly affected by food. After administration of a single 375 mg tablet of flurithromycin ethylsuccinate, the mean serum levels at 0.5 h were 0.43 ± 0.35 mg/L. The mean peak serum concentration (1.41 ± 0.49 mg/L) was achieved at 1 h. At 8 and 12 h, the serum levels were 0.14 (± 0.05) and 0.04 (± 0.04) mg/L, respectively. The apparent elimination half-life is 3.94 (± 1.42) h. The apparent half-life in artificial gastric juice was about 40 min.

It is generally well tolerated and has been used successfully for the treatment of lower respiratory tract infections. Availability is limited.

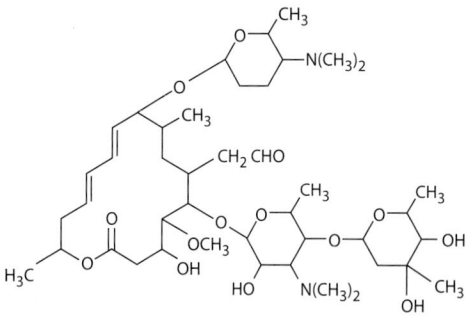

 Further information

Benonl G, Cuzzolin L, Leone R, et al. Pharmacokinetics and human tissue distribution of flurithromycin. *Antimicrob Agents Chemother.* 1988;32:1875–1878.

Cocuza CE, Mattina R, Lanzafame A, Romoli L, Lepore AM. Serum levels of flurithromycin ethylsuccinate in healthy volunteers. *Chemotherapy.* 1994;40:157–160.

Nord CE, Lindmark A, Persson I. Comparative antimicrobial activity of the new macrolide flurithromycin against respiratory pathogens. *Eur J Clin Microbiol Infect Dis.* 1988;7:71–73.

 # OLEANDOMYCIN

A natural 14-membered-ring macrolide produced by *Streptomyces antibioticus*. It is stable in acid conditions. It is less active than erythromycin A in vitro, but four times more active than spiramycin (Table 22.1, p. 277). Several attempts have been made to improve its potency by chemical modification while retaining its relative acid stability.

It is incompletely absorbed, but an ester, triacetyloleandomycin, gives improved plasma levels. Following doses of 0.5 g, mean peak serum levels around 0.8 mg/L were reached by the base and 2 mg/L by the triacetyl ester. A single oral dose of 1 g of the ester produced a mean plasma oleandomycin concentration of 4 mg/L at 1 h after dosing, with an AUC of 14 mg.h/L. The apparent elimination half-life was 4.2 h. Significant quantities of mostly inactivated compound are eliminated in the bile. About 10% of the dose appears in the urine after administration of the base and about 20% after the ester.

Nausea, vomiting and diarrhea are common. Like erythromycin estolate, triacetyloleandomycin can cause liver damage. Abnormal liver function tests were found in about one-third of patients treated for 2 weeks. Hepatic dysfunction resolved when treatment was discontinued. The action of drugs eliminated via the cytochrome P_{450} system may be potentiated.

Its uses are similar to those of erythromycin. It is of restricted availability.

 Further information

Koch R, Asay LD. Oleandomycin, a laboratory and clinical evaluation. *J Pediatr.* 1958;53:676–682.

Ticktin HE, Zimmerman HJ. Hepatic dysfunction and jaundice in patients receiving triacetyloleandomycin. *N Engl J Med.* 1962;267:964–968.

GROUP 2: 16-MEMBERED-RING MACROLIDES

SPIRAMYCIN

Molecular weight (spiramycin 1): 843.

A fermentation product of *Streptomyces ambofaciens*, composed of several closely related compounds. Spiramycin 1 is the major component (*c.* 63%); spiramycins 2 and 3 are the acetate and monopropionate esters, respectively. It is available for oral administration and as spiramycin adipate for intravenous infusion. Spiramycins are relatively stable in acid conditions. A derivative, acetylspiramycin, is available in Japan.

 ## ANTIBACTERIAL ACTIVITY

Activity against common pathogens is shown in Table 22.1 (p. 277). *L. pneumophila* is inhibited by 1–4 mg/L and *Campylobacter* spp. by 0.5–16 mg/L. Enterobacteriaceae are resistant. Spiramycin is also active against anaerobic species: *Actinomyces israelii* (MIC 2–4 mg/L), *Cl. perfringens* (MIC 2–8 mg/L) and *Bacteroides* spp. (MIC 4–14 mg/L). It is also active against *Tox. gondii*.

 ## PHARMACOKINETICS

Oral absorption	Variable
C_{max} 1 g oral	2.8 mg/L after 2 h
Plasma half-life	4–8 h
Volume of distribution	383 L
Plasma protein binding	15%

In healthy volunteers given 2 g orally followed by 1 g every 6 h, peak plasma levels were 1.0–6.7 mg/L. After 1 g orally the AUC was 10.8 mg.h/L, with an apparent elimination half-life of 2.8 h. It is widely distributed in the tissues. It does not reach the CSF. Levels 12 h after a dose of 1 g were 0.25 mg/L in serum, 5.3 mg/L in bone and 6.9 mg/L in pus. Levels of 10.6 mg/L have been found 4 h after dosing in saliva, and concentrations at least equal to those in the serum are seen in bronchial secretions. A concentration of 27 mg/g was found in prostate tissues after repeated dosage. Only 5–15% is recovered from the urine. Most is metabolized, but significant quantities are eliminated via the bile, in which concentrations up to 40 times those in the serum may be found.

TOXICITY AND SIDE EFFECTS

Spiramycin is generally well tolerated, the most common adverse reactions being gastrointestinal disturbances, notably abdominal pain, nausea and vomiting, rashes and sensitization following contact.

> Respiratory tract infections
> Toxoplasmosis (especially in pregnancy)

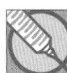

Preparations and dosage

Proprietary name: Rovamycine.

Preparations: Tablets, capsules, intravenous formulation (spiramycin adipate).

Dosage: Adults, oral, 2–4 g per day in two divided doses; i.v., 0.5–1 g every 8 h. Children, oral, 50–100 mg/kg per day in divided doses.

Limited availability.

Further information

Anonymous. Spiramycin. In: Dollery C, ed. *Therapeutic Drugs*. 2nd ed. Edinburgh: Churchill Livingstone; 1999:S85–S88.

Davey P, Speller D, Daly PJ. eds. Spiramycin reassessed. *J Antimicrob Chemother*. 1988;22(suppl B).

OTHER GROUP 2 MACROLIDES

JOSAMYCIN

A naturally occurring antibiotic produced by *Streptomyces narbonensis* var. *josamyceticus* and belonging to the leucomycin group of macrolides. It is formulated for oral administration.

Activity is comparable to that of erythromycin A (Table 22.1, p. 277), susceptible organisms being inhibited by ≤2 mg/L. Many Gram-positive and Gram-negative anaerobes are susceptible, including *Peptostreptococcus* spp., *Propionibacterium* spp., *Eubacterium* spp. and *Bacteroides* spp.

After a single 1 g oral dose, a peak serum concentration of 2.74 mg/L was achieved 0.75 h after dosing. The AUC was 4.2 mg.h/L, and the apparent elimination half-life 1.5 h. Several inactive metabolites could be detected. It penetrates into saliva, tears and sweat, and achieves high levels in bile and lungs. It is mostly metabolized and excreted in the bile in an inactive form. Less than 20% of the dose appears in the urine, producing levels of around 50 mg/L.

The drug is generally well tolerated, producing only mild gastrointestinal disturbance. Its uses are similar to those of erythromycin. It is of limited availability.

Further information

Chabbert YA, Modai J. Perspectives josamycine – Symposium International du 16–18 mai 1985, Lisbones. *Médicine et Maladies Infectieuses*. 1985;(suppl).

KITASAMYCIN (LEUCOMYCIN)

A naturally occurring product of *Streptomyces kitasatoensis*, available in Japan for parenteral and oral use, and as acetylkitasamycin for topical application. Elsewhere it is chiefly used in veterinary medicine.

MIDECAMYCIN

A naturally occurring metabolite of *Streptomyces mycarofaciens*, supplied as the native compound and as midecamycin acetate for oral administration.

The antibacterial spectrum is comparable to that of erythromycin A, but it is less active (Table 22.1, p. 277). It is rapidly and extensively metabolized and is said to exhibit less toxicity than earlier macrolides. It is of limited availability.

Further information

Neu HC. In vitro activity of midecamycin, a new macrolide antibiotic. *Antimicrob Agents Chemother*. 1983;24:443–444.

MIOKAMYCIN

A semisynthetic diacetyl derivative of midecamycin A_1. It is generally less active than erythromycin and some strains of *H. influenzae* and *E. faecalis* are resistant. It is rapidly and extensively metabolized, though some metabolites retain antibacterial activity.

Absorption of the dry formulation is unaffected by food, whereas that of the oral suspension is delayed. In various studies the peak plasma concentration was 1.65, 1.31–3 and 1.3–2.7 mg/L after doses of 400, 600 and 800 mg, respectively.

It is said to exhibit less toxicity than earlier macrolides. Attention has been paid to its interaction with theophylline, which resembles that of other macrolides. It is of limited availability.

ROKITAMYCIN

3 -Propionyl leucomycin A_5. A semisynthetic macrolide. Unstable in acid media.

The antibacterial spectrum is identical to that of erythromycin, but it is less active against Gram-positive cocci. It is poorly active against *H. influenzae* (MIC_{50} 8 mg/L) and *Mor. catarrhalis* (MIC_{50} 4 mg/L). It displays good activity against *Campylobacter* spp. (MIC_{50} 0.1 mg/L), *L. pneumophila* (MIC_{50} 0.1 mg/L) and *M. pneumoniae* (MIC_{50} 0.003 mg/L). It is active against anaerobes, including some *Bacteroides* spp. (MIC_{50} <0.05 mg/L).

After a single oral dose of 600 mg, the peak plasma concentration was 1.9 mg/L after 0.6 h. Oral doses of 5, 10 and 15 mg/kg of a syrup formulation given to children achieved plasma concentrations of 0.26, 0.55 and 0.79 mg/L, respectively, after about 40 min. The half-life is around 2 h.

It is mainly eliminated in the bile; only about 2% appears in the urine. Its major metabolites are leucomycin A_7, 10″-OH-rokitamycin (which show some antibacterial activity) and leucomycin V. In healthy adult volunteers, the proportions of rokitamycin and its metabolites in serum 30 min after a single oral dose of 1200 mg were 18% (leucomycin A_7), 33% (10″-OH-rokitamycin) and 9% (leucomycin V). The pharmacokinetic behavior is not altered in patients with liver cirrhosis. It is available in Italy and Japan.

GROUP 3: AZALIDES

AZITHROMYCIN

Molecular weight (dihydrate): 785.

A semisynthetic derivative of erythromycin A, supplied as the dihydrate for oral administration.

ANTIBACTERIAL ACTIVITY

Activity in vitro against common bacterial pathogens is shown in Table 22.1 (p. 277). It is less potent than erythromycin A against Gram-positive isolates, but is more active against Gram-negative bacteria. It is four times more potent than erythromycin A against *H. influenzae*, *N. gonorrhoeae* and *Campylobacter* spp., and twice as active against *Mor. catarrhalis*. It also exhibits superior potency against Enterobacteriaceae, notably *Esch. coli*, *Salmonella enterica* serotypes, and *Shigella* spp. It is active against *Mycobacteria*, notably the *M. avium* complex and against intracellular micro-organisms such as *Legionella* and *Chlamydia* spp.

PHARMACOKINETICS

Oral absorption	37%
C_{max} 250 mg oral	0.17 mg/L after 2.2 h
500 mg oral	0.4 mg/L after 2 h
Plasma half-life (terminal)	11–40 h
Volume of distribution	31 L/kg
Plasma protein binding	7–50%

Chemical modification at the 9 position of the erythronolide A ring of erythromycin A blocks the internal ketalization and markedly improves acid stability. At pH 2, loss of 10% activity occurred in less than 4 s with erythromycin A, but took 20 min with azithromycin. The AUC at 0–24 h is 4.5 mg.h/L. The level is only slightly increased on repeated dosing.

Binding to plasma protein varies with the concentration, from around 50% at 0.05 mg/L to 7.1% at 1 mg/L. The apparent elimination half-life is dependent upon sampling interval: between 8 and 24 h it ranged from 11 to 14 h; between 24 and 72 h it was 35–40 h.

It rapidly penetrates the tissues, reaching levels that approach or, in some cases, exceed the simultaneous plasma levels and persist for 2–3 days. Only about 6% of the dose is found in urine in the first 24 h.

TOXICITY AND SIDE EFFECTS

Azithromycin is well tolerated with little gastrointestinal disturbance.

Lower and upper respiratory tract infections
Skin and soft-tissue infections
Uncomplicated urethritis/cervicitis associated with *N. gonorrhoeae, C. trachomatis* or *U. urealyticum*
Trachoma

Preparations and dosage

Proprietary name: Zithromax.

Preparations: Capsules, tablets, suspension.

Dosage: Adults, oral, 500 mg per day for 3 days. Children >6 months, 10 mg/kg per day for 3 days; 15–25 kg, 200 mg per day for 3 days; 26–35 kg, 300 mg per day for 3 days; 36–45 kg, 400 mg per day for 3 days. Widely available.

Further information

Anonymous. Azithromycin. In: Dollery C, ed. *Therapeutic Drugs.* 2nd ed. Edinburgh: Churchill Livingstone; 1999:A261–A265.

Leigh DA, Ridgway GL, Leeming JP, Speller DCE. Azithromycin (CP 62,993): the first azalide antimicrobial agent. *J Antimicrob Chemother.* 1990;25(suppl A).

GROUP 4: KETOLIDES

TELITHROMYCIN

Molecular weight: 812.

A 14-membered-ring ketolide, obtained by semisynthesis from erythromycin A. Formulated for oral administration.

ANTIBACTERIAL ACTIVITY

Activity against common bacterial pathogens is shown in Table 22.1 (p. 277). The spectrum covers Gram-positive and Gram-negative cocci, Gram-positive bacilli, fastidious Gram-negative bacilli, atypical mycobacteria, *M. leprae*, *H. pylori*, anaerobes, *T. pallidum*, intracellular pathogens and atypical organisms.

It exhibits bactericidal activity in vitro against isolates of *Str. pneumoniae* regardless of the underlying resistance to penicillin G, erythromycin A and other agents. It is 2–4 times more active than clarithromycin against erythromycin A-susceptible isolates of *Str. pneumoniae* and other streptococci. Against *H. influenzae* the MIC range is 1–4 mg/L. It also exhibits good in-vitro activity against *Coxiella burnetii* (MIC 1 mg/L) and various Gram-positive species, including viridans streptococci (MIC ≤0.015–0.25 mg/L), *C. diphtheriae* (MIC 0.004–0.008 mg/L) and *Listeria* spp. (MIC 0.03–0.25 mg/L).

ACQUIRED RESISTANCE

It retains activity against isolates resistant to erythromycin A. *Str. pneumoniae* and *Str. pyogenes* isolates for which the MIC of telithromycin is above the resistance breakpoint of 2 mg/L are presently rare. It is not active against *Staph. aureus* isolates that owe their resistance to erythromycin to constitutive methylation of adenine 2058 on domain V of the peptidyl transferase loop.

PHARMACOKINETICS

Oral absorption	90%
C_{max} 800 mg oral	1.9–2.27 mg/L (steady state after 2–3 days)
Plasma half-life	10–12 h
Volume of distribution	210 L
Plasma protein binding	60–70%

After oral administration the absolute bioavailability is 57% in both young and elderly subjects. The rate and extent of absorption are not influenced by food. In a study of ascending doses administered to healthy volunteers, peak plasma concentration ranged from 0.8 mg/L (400 mg dose) to 6 mg/L (2400 mg dose). The peak plasma concentration was reached after 1–2 h. The apparent elimination half-lives ranged from 10 to 14 h, with an AUC of 2.6 mg.h/L (400 mg dose) to 43.3 mg.h/L (2400 mg dose). After repeated oral doses the ratios between day 1 and day 10 ranged from 1.3 to 1.5. After once-daily oral dosing with 800 mg, the AUC is 8.25 mg.h/L. Concentrations in alveolar macrophages, epithelial lining fluid and bronchial tissue are shown in Table 22.5.

TOXICITY AND SIDE EFFECTS

It is generally well tolerated. The main adverse event is diarrhea.

> Lower and upper respiratory tract infections in adult patients (community-acquired pneumonia, acute exacerbations of chronic bronchitis, acute bacterial maxillary sinusitis and pharyngitis)

Preparations and dosage

Proprietary name: Ketek.
Preparation: Tablet (400 mg).
Dosage: Adults, oral, 800 mg per day.
Widely available.

Further information

Brown SD. Benefit–risk assessment of telithromycin in the treatment of community-acquired pneumonia. *Drug Safety.* 2008;31:561–575.
Bryskier A. Telithromycin – an innovative ketolide antimicrobial. *Jpn J Antibiot.* 2001;54(suppl A):64–69.
Carbon C, van Rensburg D, Hagberg L, et al. Clinical and bacteriologic efficacy of telithromycin in patients with community-acquired pneumonia. *Respir Med.* 2006;100:577–585.
Wellington K, Noble S. Telithromycin. *Drugs.* 2004;64:1683–1694.

Table 22.5 Telithromycin concentration in respiratory tissue (800 mg oral daily dose)

	Mean concentrations (mg/L)			
	2–3 h	6–8 h	12 h	24 h
Epithelial lining fluid	5.4–14.9	4.2	3.3	0.8–1.2
Alveolar macrophages	65–69	100	3.8	41–162
Bronchial tissues	0.68–3.9	2.2	1.4	0.7
Tonsils	3.95	–	0.9	0.7

OTHER KETOLIDES

CETHROMYCIN (ABT 773)

A semisynthetic derivative of erythromycin A. It is a C11–C12 carbamate ketolide and has an unsaturated chain with a quinoline ring at the C-6 position. It has the same antibacterial spectrum as telithromycin and exhibits comparable activity against respiratory tract pathogens (Table 22.2, p. 277). Erythromycin-susceptible *Staph. aureus* strains are inhibited by 0.015–0.06 mg/L irrespective of susceptibility to methicillin.

The apparent elimination half-life ranges from 3.6 to 6.7 h. In an escalating oral dose study, the peak plasma concentration ranged from 0.14 mg/L (100 mg dose) to 1.2 mg/L (1200 mg dose) after 0.5–5.1 h. The AUC ranged from 0.63 mg.h/L (100 mg dose) to 11.0 mg.h/L (1200 mg dose) with a total clearance of 183–254 L/h.

Clinical efficacy in respiratory tract infections is under investigation.

Further information

Barry AL, Fuchs PC, Brown SD. In vitro activity of ABT 773. *Antimicrob Agents Chemother.* 2001;45:2922–2924.

Brueggemann AB, Doern GV, Huynh HK, Wingert EM, Rhomberg PR. In vitro activity of ABT 773, a new ketolide, against recent clinical isolates of *Streptococcus pneumoniae, Haemophilus influenzae* and *Moraxella catarrhalis. Antimicrob Agents Chemother.* 2000;44:447–449.

Hammerschlag MR, Sharma R. Use of cethromycin, a new ketolide, for treatment of community-acquired respiratory infections. *Expert Opin Investig Drugs.* 2008;17:387–400.

Strigl S, Roblin PM, Reznik T, Hammerschlag MR. In vitro activity of ABT 773, a new ketolide antibiotic, against *Chlamydia pneumoniae. Antimicrob Agents Chemother.* 2000;44:1112–1113.

Waites KB, Crabb DM, Duffy LB. In vitro activities of ABT-773 and other antimicrobials against human mycoplasmas. *Antimicrob Agents Chemother.* 2003;47:39–42.

MODITHROMYCIN (EDP 420)

A bicyclolide ketolide with a 9-substituted oxime group and a bicyclic substituted (pyridine and imidazole rings) bridge between position 6 and position 11 of the lactone ring. It exhibits good antipneumococcal activity (MIC 0.008–0.25 mg/L). Typical MICs for *Staph. aureus* are 0.125–32 mg/L and for

H. influenzae 1–64 mg/L. In-vitro activity against intracellular pathogens (*Legionella, Chlamydophila* spp.) and atypical pathogens such as *M. pneumoniae* is good. Gram-positive cocci resistant to erythromycin A by an efflux mechanism remain susceptible; those resistant by methylation (*erm* gene) exhibit variable susceptibility.

After a single oral ascending dose to healthy volunteers, the peak plasma concentrations were *c.* 0.2 mg/L (100 mg dose) and 1 mg/L (1200 mg dose) after 1.75–5 h (average 3 h). The lag time between administration and first detection in plasma was about 0.25 h. The apparent elimination half-life is around 15 h. Approximately 6–12% of the administered dose is eliminated in urine.

Further information

Jiang LJ, Wang M, Or YS. Pharmacokinetics of EDP 420 after ascending doses in healthy adult volunteers. *Antimicrob Agents Chemother.* 2009;57:1786–1792.

Wang Q, Niu D, Qiu Y-L, et al. Synthesis of novel 6, 11-O-bridged bicyclic ketolides via a palladium-catalyzed bis-alkylation. *Org Lett.* 2004;6:4455–4458.

CEM 101

A 2-fluoroketolide. The side chain substituting the C11–C12 carbamate is composed of a substituted triazolyl (aminophenyl) ring. It displays good in-vitro and in-vivo activity against *Streptococcus* spp., including *Str. pneumoniae* (MIC 0.0015–0.25 mg/L), *Str. pyogenes* (MIC ≤0.008–0.015 mg/L) and viridians group streptococci (MIC ≤0.008–0.06 mg/L). Activity against *H. influenzae* is close to that of azithromycin (MIC 1.0–2.0 mg/L). Vancomycin-susceptible strains of *E. faecalis* are inhibited by 0.003–2.0 mg/L and *E. faecium* by 0.25–2.0 mg/L. It exhibits good activity against *Ch. pneumoniae* (MIC 0.25–1.0 mg/L), *C. trachomatis* (MIC 0.123–0.5 mg/L) and *Mycoplasma* spp. (MIC ≤0.0008 mg/L). In vitro *H. pylori* is susceptible (MIC 0.006–0.25 mg/L), but *C. jejuni* less so (MIC 1–4 mg/L). It is extremely active in vitro against *B. anthracis* (MIC <0.008–0.015 mg/L) and other agents of bioterrorism such as *Francisella tularensis* (MIC <0.08–4.0 mg/L), *Yersinia pestis* and *Burkholderia mallei* (MIC 0.25–2.0 mg/L). It exhibits a good activity against the *M. avium* complex.

In healthy adult volunteers the proposed therapeutic dose of 400 mg achieved a peak plasma concentration of 0.78 mg/L after 4 h. The apparent elimination half-life was 5.1 h.

23 Mupirocin

Adam P. Fraise

Mupirocin is an antimicrobial substance originally derived from *Pseudomonas fluorescens*. It is a mixture of pseudomonic acids with more than 90% of the commercial product being pseudomonic acid A:

It has activity predominantly against Gram-positive bacteria and its main use is as a topical agent for the eradication of carriage of methicillin-resistant *Staphylococcus aureus* (MRSA). It is also used as a topical treatment for superficial skin infections caused by Gram-positive organisms such as impetigo.

ANTIMICROBIAL ACTIVITY

Activity against common pathogens is shown in Table 23.1. It is active against staphylococci and streptococci, but also *Neisseria* and *Haemophilus* spp. *Enterococcus faecalis* tends to be sensitive whereas *E. faecium* is usually resistant. Activity against *Staph. aureus* is affected by inoculum such that a 10-fold increase in the inoculum causes doubling of the minimum inhibitory concentration (MIC) in vitro. Activity also decreases as pH increases above the normal skin pH of 5.5.

ACQUIRED RESISTANCE

Before the introduction of mupirocin, resistance in *Staph. aureus* was uncommon, with a natural mutation frequency of 1 in 10^9. However, shortly after the agent was introduced, mupirocin-resistant strains began to emerge. They are of two types: low level (MIC 8–256 mg/mL) and high level (MIC >256 mg/mL).

Table 23.1 Activity of mupirocin against some common pathogenic bacteria: MIC (mg/L)

Species	MIC
Staphylococcus aureus (including MRSA)	0.01–0.25
Coagulase-negative staphylococci	0.01–4.0
Streptococcus pyogenes	0.06–0.5
Str. pneumoniae	0.06–0.5
Enterococcus faecalis	16–R
E. faecium	1.0–4.0
Neisseria gonorrhoeae	0.03–0.25
N. meningitidis	0.03–0.25
Haemophilus influenzae	0.003–0.25
Enterobacter spp.	R
Pseudomonas aeruginosa	R
Bacteroides fragilis	R

R, resistant (MIC >64 mg/L).

Low-level resistance appears to be due to mutations in the target enzyme, isoleucyl-tRNA synthetase (*see* p. 16); it is probably not transmissible and seems of little clinical significance as these strains respond to standard treatment.

High-level resistance, in contrast, is linked to the acquisition of a transmissible resistance gene *MupA* that may co-transfer with other antimicrobial resistance genes. Strains that express *MupA* are not clinically susceptible to mupirocin.

Several studies suggest that widespread use of prophylactic mupirocin may result in increased levels of resistance. In Canada increasing use of mupirocin across the country led to high-level mupirocin resistance, rising from 1.6% to 7% over a 9-year period.

PHARMACOKINETICS

Following parenteral administration, mupirocin is rapidly destroyed by non-specific esterases (possibly in renal or liver tissues since it is reasonably stable in blood) to inactive monic acid and its conjugates. It is strongly protein bound. About 0.25% is absorbed from intact skin. The skin ointment, but not the cream, contains polyethylene glycol, which may be absorbed significantly when applied to open wounds or damaged skin, including burns.

TOXICITY AND SIDE EFFECTS

Topical applications are well tolerated. Conjunctival application is contraindicated as it may cause irritation. Minor side effects such as irritation and unpleasant or abnormal taste have been recorded for very few patients following nasal application.

Polyethylene glycol from the ointment base may, if absorbed from application to open wounds or damaged skin, cause renal toxicity.

CLINICAL USE

Mupirocin is mainly used as a nasal cream as part of the regimen to decolonize patients who have been found to carry methicillin-resistant *Staph. aureus*. It can also be applied to tracheostomy, gastrostomy and other sites that are frequently colonized with MRSA.

The use of mupirocin as a means of controlling outbreaks of infection due to MRSA appears to be of only marginal benefit in an endemic situation.

A Cochrane Review of nine randomized controlled trials of use of mupirocin to prevent subsequent *Staph. aureus* infections in nasal carriers of the organism found a statistically significant reduction in such infections at any site.

A small study of local therapy to reduce the risk of peritonitis in patients on continuous ambulatory peritoneal dialysis (CAPD) found that mupirocin applied three times weekly to the dialysis catheter exit site resulted in a 92% reduction in the rate of peritonitis

Preparations and dosage

Proprietary name: Bactroban.

Preparations: 2% mupirocin as ointment, cream or nasal ointment.

Dosage: Topical application, up to three times daily for a maximum of 10 days. Nasal application, up to three times daily for 3–5 days.

Widely available.

Further information

Casewell MW, Hill RLR. In vitro activity of mupirocin (pseudomonic acid) against clinical isolates of *Staphylococcus aureus. J Antimicrob Chemother.* 1985;15:523–531.

Coia JE, Duckworth GJ, Edwards DI, et al. Guidelines for the control and prevention of meticillin-resistant *Staphylococcus aureus* (MRSA) in healthcare facilities. *J Hosp Infect.* 2006;63(suppl 1):S1–S44.

Hill RLR, Duckworth GD, Casewell MW. Elimination of nasal carriage of methicillin-resistant *Staphylococcus aureus* with mupirocin during a hospital outbreak. *J Antimicrob Chemother.* 1988;22:377–384.

Simor AE, Stuart TL, Louie L, et al. Mupirocin-resistant, methicillin-resistant *Staphylococcus aureus* strains in Canadian hospitals. *Antimicrob Agents Chemother.* 2007;51:3880–3886.

Van Rijen M, Bonten M, Wenzel R, Kluytmans J. Mupirocin ointment for preventing *Staphylococcus aureus* infection in nasal carriers. *Cochrane Database Syst Rev.* 2008;(4): CD006216. DOI: 10.1002/14651858.CD006216.pub2.

24 Nitroimidazoles

Peter J. Jenks

An imidazole ring is an important feature of many natural compounds with a wide range of biological activities. Nitroimidazoles with antimicrobial activity emerged from a search for a drug that would provide an effective treatment for infections caused by protozoa of the *Trichomonas* genus, including the human pathogen, *Trichomonas vaginalis*. The first active compound was an antibiotic, azomycin (2-nitroimidazole) produced by a streptomycete. It was soon abandoned, but led to the synthesis of several hundred related compounds, one of which, the 5-nitroimidazole metronidazole, combined activity against the parasites with acceptable animal toxicity. The compound was marketed in 1960 and 2 years later was fortuitously found also to possess potent activity against anaerobic bacteria.

Numerous 5-nitroimidazoles were subsequently developed. Metronidazole and tinidazole are in widespread clinical use; others include nimorazole, ornidazole and secnidazole. The 2-nitroimidazole, benznidazole, is uniquely used in the treatment of South American trypanosomiasis (Chagas disease); fexinidazole is under investigation in African trypanosomiasis (sleeping sickness). Carnidazole, dimetridazole, ipronidazole and ronidazole are used in veterinary medicine and are not discussed further here.

Other imidazole derivatives are used as antifungal agents (Chapter 32) and anthelmintics (Chapter 34). Some, chiefly 2-nitroimidazoles, have been examined as possible radiosensitizers for the treatment of hypoxic tumors.

ANTIMICROBIAL ACTIVITY

BACTERIA

The 5-nitroimidazoles exhibit excellent potency against anaerobic bacteria (Table 24.1), including *Bacteroides* spp., *Clostridium* spp., *Prevotella* spp. and *Fusobacterium* spp. Most isolates of *Mobiluncus curtisii* are resistant to metronidazole and its hydroxy metabolite, while *Mobiluncus mulieris* is often sensitive. Other susceptible bacteria include *Capnocytophaga* spp. and *Campylobacter fetus*. Most *Actinomyces* and

Propionibacterium spp. are resistant. Among facultative anaerobes, *Actinobacillus actinomycetemcomitans* and *Eikenella corrodens* are usually resistant, while *Gardnerella vaginalis* is frequently sensitive, more so to the hydroxy metabolite of metronidazole.

PROTOZOA

Susceptible protozoa include *T. vaginalis*, *Giardia lamblia*, *Entamoeba histolytica*, *Balantidium coli* and *Blastocystis hominis*. The spectrum of benznidazole is restricted to *Trypanosoma cruzi*.

FACTORS AFFECTING ACTIVITY IN VITRO

All nitroimidazoles exert their antimicrobial activity via reduction of the nitro group, which only occurs at low redox potentials. The major factor affecting in-vitro activity is therefore the failure to achieve anaerobic conditions, which can lead to reporting of false resistance. The presence of traces of oxygen may inhibit or reverse reduction of the drug through 'futile cycling'. It is essential, therefore, to ensure that fully anaerobic conditions are maintained during susceptibility testing.

All nitroimidazoles are capable of being photodegraded and should be protected from light.

ACQUIRED RESISTANCE

PROTOZOA

While resistant strains of *E. histolytica* and *T. vaginalis* are rarely encountered, up to 20% of *G. lamblia* isolates may be resistant in general clinical practice. Although resistance rates of *T. vaginalis* are low, millions of cases of infection occur each

Table 24.1 Activity of nitroimidazoles against anaerobic bacteria: MIC (mg/L)

	Metronidazole	Ornidazole	Tinidazole
Bacteroides fragilis	0.5–4	<0.1–4	0.1–4
B. melaninogenicus	<0.1	<0.1	<0.1
Fusobacterium spp.	<0.1–1	<0.1–1	0.1–2
Clostridium perfringens	0.25–2	0.25–2	0.25–2
Peptococcus and *Peptostreptococcus* spp.	<0.1–4	<0.1–2	<0.1–2
Veillonella spp.	1–2	0.5–1	0.5–2
Eubacterium spp.	0.5–2	0.5–1	0.5–2
Propionibacterium spp.	R	R	R

R, resistant (MIC >16 mg/L).

year and the number of treatment failures due to resistance is significant. The minimum inhibitory concentration (MIC) of metronidazole for strains of *T. vaginalis* from refractory vaginitis is frequently 3–8 times the value for susceptible strains.

The development of high-level resistance is frequently multifactorial and many protozoa develop nitroimidazole resistance either by reducing or by abolishing activity of elements of the electron transport reactions, particularly ferredoxin oxidoreductase (FOR) and ferredoxin, with appropriate compensatory modifications of the normal fermentative pathway. Reduced or abolished FOR activity and decreased transcription of the ferredoxin gene resulting in decreased levels of a functional pyruvate:ferredoxin oxidoreductase (PFOR) system have been reported in both *Trichomonas* and *Giardia* spp. The consequences are that pyruvate oxidation is diverted to alternative pathways which favor the formation of lactate (in *T. vaginalis*) or ethanol (in *T. fetus*). Decreased levels of the PFOR system with compensatory changes in the electron transport chain are also associated with resistance in *Giardia* spp.

Increased expression of superoxide dismutase without a reduction of PFOR activity has been reported in metronidazole-resistant ameba and appears to contribute to the resistant phenotype, rather than being the result of a general stress response.

BACTEROIDES AND *CLOSTRIDIUM* SPP

Reduced susceptibility to metronidazole and other nitroimidazoles has been described in *B. fragilis*, *B. distasonis* and *B. bivius*. Mechanisms such as reduced uptake of nitroimidazoles, reduced nitroreductase activity or decreased PFOR activity have been proposed. Reduction in PFOR activity is compensated by increased pyruvate dehydrogenase activity, and results in reduced activation and hence uptake of

nitroimidazoles. Resistance in *Bacteroides* spp. may also be associated with specific nitroimidazole (nim) resistance genes that can be either plasmid or chromosomally encoded. These are thought to encode a nitroimidazole reductase which converts nitroimidazole to aminoimidazole, preventing formation of bactericidal nitroso residues.

Metronidazole-resistant strains of clostridia have not been reported clinically, but a laboratory strain of *Clostridium perfringens* made resistant by mutation possessed decreased levels of PFOR.

HELICOBACTER SPP

Most nitroimidazole-resistant strains of *H. pylori* contain mutations within the gene encoding the oxygen-insensitive NADPH nitroreductase, RdxA. This usually arises by de-novo mutation of the *rdxA* gene, but resistance transfer may occur in patients infected with two strains of *H. pylori*.

Inactivation of other reductase-encoding genes, including *frxA* (which encodes NADPH flavin oxidoreductase) and *fdxB* (which encodes a ferredoxin-like protein), are also occasionally associated with resistance to metronidazole. Mutations in these genes often result in transition to high-level resistance once inactivation of the *rdxA* gene has occurred, but resistance may also arise as a result of inactivation of *frxA* alone.

Other mechanisms of metronidazole resistance may remain to be discovered in *H. pylori*. These are most likely to involve inactivation of other nitroreductase enzyme-encoding genes, but mutations affecting membrane transport and DNA repair may also contribute to the resistant phenotype. Combinations of these factors are likely to account for wide interstrain differences in susceptibility of *H. pylori*.

PHARMACOKINETICS

Nitroimidazoles are generally well absorbed following oral administration. Following rectal or vaginal administration, bioavailability is approximately 60% and 20%, respectively, with considerable variation between individuals. Binding to proteins is low. Peak plasma levels are achieved 3–5 h after an oral dose. The decay from the peak is exponential, with the rate depending on the half-life of the drug. Dose-proportional kinetics are observed for clinically relevant doses. The concentrations after normal oral doses are well above the MICs for anaerobes but are borderline for *G. vaginalis*. The nitroimidazoles are well distributed to peripheral compartments, including brain tissue and cerebrospinal fluid, but concentrations in subcutaneous fat are 15% or less of concurrent serum levels.

Nitroimidazoles are metabolized mainly by the liver and excreted in the urine. Derivatives with a 2-methyl group (except nimorazole) are metabolized to the corresponding methoxy derivative and those with an alcohol side chain are metabolized to the corresponding acid metabolite. All can form glucuronide conjugates and, occasionally, the ethereal sulfate conjugate.

TOXICITY AND SIDE EFFECTS

The most common side effects are gastrointestinal (including nausea and diarrhea) and a metallic taste, especially when high doses are used. A reversible peripheral neuropathy may occur in patients receiving high doses for prolonged periods, particularly in the treatment of hypoxic tumors. Central neurotoxicity has also been reported and the drug should be discontinued if any abnormal neurological symptoms are reported. If combined with alcohol, metronidazole may cause a disulfiram-like reaction, with nausea, vomiting, flushing of the skin, tachycardia, hypotension and palpitations.

Although nitroimidazoles have been found to be mutagenic and carcinogenic in animal studies, there is no evidence that they are carcinogenic to humans. Nevertheless, they should only be used in pregnancy when the benefits outweigh the risks, and should be avoided altogether in the first trimester. Because the concentrations in breast milk are similar to those in serum, a risk assessment should be performed before use in lactating mothers.

CLINICAL USE

Nitroimidazoles are the most active antibiotics for the treatment and prevention of infections involving anaerobic bacteria. They are therefore important in the treatment of intra-abdominal and gynecological sepsis, abscesses and specific clinical syndromes such as tetanus. They are also an important component of prophylactic regimens for surgical procedures where contamination with anaerobic flora is likely. They are used to treat bacterial vaginosis (frequently associated with *G. vaginalis*) and dental infections, including acute necrotizing ulcerative gingivitis (Vincent's angina). Metronidazole is the treatment of choice for antibiotic-associated diarrhea caused by *C. difficile* for all but those with recurrent, complicated or fulminant disease, for whom oral vancomycin is recommended. Metronidazole and tinidazole are also used as part of eradication regimens for *H. pylori*, although resistance may affect 10–50% of strains isolated in developed countries and virtually all strains from developing countries.

The nitroimidazoles provide the first-line treatment for giardiasis, amebiasis and trichomonal vaginitis, and may also be used to treat balantidiasis. Benznidazole is used for the treatment of *Trypanosoma cruzi* infections (Chagas disease).

These drugs have also been used as hypoxic cell sensitizers in the radiotherapy of tumors, in the treatment of bacterial overgrowth syndromes and in the prevention of recurrence of Crohn's disease.

 Further information

Carlier JP, Sellier N, Rager M-N, Reysset G. Metabolism of a 5-nitroimidazole in susceptible and resistant isogenic strains of *Bacteroides fragilis*. *Antimicrob Agents Chemother*. 1997;41:1495–1499.

Dans L, Martinez E. Amoebic dysentery. *Clin Evid*. 2006;15:1007–1013.
Edwards DI. Nitroimidazole drugs – action and resistance mechanisms. I. Mechanisms of action. *J Antimicrob Chemother*. 1993;31:9–20.
Edwards DI. Nitroimidazole drugs – action and resistance mechanisms. II. Mechanisms of resistance. *J Antimicrob Chemother*. 1993;31:201–210.
Gardner TB, Hill DR. Treatment of giardiasis. *Clin Microbiol Rev*. 2001;14:114–128.
Jenks PJ, Ferrero RL, Labigne A. The role of the *rdxA* gene in the evolution of metronidazole resistance in *Helicobacter pylori*. *J Antimicrob Chemother*. 1999;43:753–758.
Lamp KC, Freeman SD, Klutman NE, Lacy MK. Pharmacokinetics and pharmacodynamics of the nitroimidazole antimicrobials. *Clin Pharmacokinet*. 1999;36:353–373.
Raether W, Hänel H. Nitroheterocyclic drugs with broad spectrum activity. *Parasitol Res*. 2003;90(suppl 1):S19–S39.
Upcroft P, Upcroft JA. Drug targets and mechanisms of resistance in the anaerobic protozoa. *Clin Microbiol Rev*. 2001;14:150–164.
Van Der Wouden E-J, Thijs JC, Kusters JG, van Zwet AA, Kleibeuker JH. Mechanism and clinical significance of metronidazole resistance in *Helicobacter pylori*. *Scand J Gastroenterol*. 2001;36:10–14.

BENZNIDAZOLE

Molecular weight: 260.26.

A synthetic 2-nitroimidazole, formulated for oral administration. Solubility in water 400 mg/L.

ANTIMICROBIAL ACTIVITY

It exhibits antiprotozoal activity, particularly against *Trypanosoma cruzi*.

PHARMACOKINETICS

Oral bioavailability	High
C$_{max}$ 100 mg oral	2.2–2.8 mg/L after 3–4 h
Plasma half-life	10.5–13.6 h
Volume of distribution	c. 0.56 L/kg
Plasma protein binding	c. 44%

The 2-nitro group undergoes reduction to the amine and hydrolysis to the hydroxy derivative.

TOXICITY AND SIDE EFFECTS

Adverse effects are more common in the elderly and include nausea, vomiting, abdominal pain, peripheral neuropathy and severe skin reactions.

CLINICAL USE

Benznidazole is used in treatment of South American trypanosomiasis (Chagas disease).

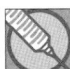

Preparations and dosage

Preparation: Tablets.

Dosage: Adults, 5–10 mg/kg per day for 30–60 days. Children, 5–10 mg/kg per day for 30–60 days.

Available in South America.

Further information

de Andrade AL, Zicker F, de Oliveira RM, et al. Randomised trial of efficacy of benznidazole in treatment of early *Trypanosoma cruzi* infection. *Lancet.* 1996;348:1407–1413.

Mady C, Ianni BM, de Souza JL. Benznidazole and Chagas disease: can an old drug be the answer to an old problem? *Expert Opin Investig Drugs.* 2008;17:1427–1433.

Reyes PA, Vallejo M. Trypanocidal drugs for late stage, symptomatic Chagas disease (*Trypanosoma cruzi* infection). *Cochrane Database Syst Rev.* 2005;(4): CD004102.

Viotti R, Vigliano C, Lococo B, et al. Side effects of benznidazole as treatment in chronic Chagas disease: fears and realities. *Expert Rev Anti Infect Ther.* 2009;7:157–163.

METRONIDAZOLE

Molecular weight (free compound): 171.16; (hydrochloride): 207.6; (benzoate): 275.3.

A 5-nitroimidazole available for oral administration or as a suppository; also formulated as the hydrochloride for intravenous use, and as the benzoate in an oral suspension and a dental gel. Aqueous solubility: 10 g/L at 20°C. Soluble in dilute acids. It is photolabile and preparations should be protected from light. Metronidazole hydrochloride has a low pH (0.5–2.0) when reconstituted, and reacts with aluminum in equipment, including needles, to produce a reddish-brown discoloration. It is incompatible with several agents and other drugs should not be added to intravenous solutions.

ANTIMICROBIAL ACTIVITY

It is a potent inhibitor of obligate anaerobic bacteria (Table 24.1, p. 293) and protozoa, but not of any organism that is aerobic or incapable of anaerobic metabolism. Susceptible protozoa include *T. vaginalis*, *G. lamblia*, *E. histolytica*, *Balantidium coli* and *Blastocystis hominis*, which are inhibited by concentrations of 0.2–0.25 mg/L. *Clostridium* spp. (including *C. difficile*) are inhibited at concentrations of 0.5–8 mg/L. It is also active against the microaerophilic *H. pylori* (MIC for susceptible strains <8 mg/L). The 2-methoxy metabolite of metronidazole is more active (MIC about 0.3 mg/L), but the acid metabolite shows less activity than the parent drug (MIC about 3 mg/L). *G. vaginalis* shows similar susceptibility (MIC 1–8 mg/L); the methoxy metabolite is more active (MIC 0.02–2 mg/L).

ACQUIRED RESISTANCE

Although resistance in *Bacteroides* spp. and *T. vaginalis* is well documented, it is uncommon. Resistance occurs more frequently in *H. pylori* and failure of treatment with triple drug regimens may be associated with resistance to the metronidazole component.

PHARMACOKINETICS

Oral absorption	>90%
C_{max} 400 mg oral	c. 10 mg/L after 3–5 h
Plasma half-life	6–11 h
Volume of distribution	0.6–1.1 L/kg
Plasma protein binding	<20%

Absorption

Peak plasma concentrations after oral administration are proportional to the dose. Plasma levels are usually lower in men because of weight differences. In patients treated intravenously with a loading dose of 15 mg/kg followed by 7.5 mg/kg every 6 h, peak steady state plasma concentrations averaged 25 mg/L with minimum trough concentrations averaging 18 mg/L.

The bioavailability of metronidazole in rectal suppositories is around 60%. Effective blood concentrations occur 5–12 h after the first suppository and are maintained by an 8 h regimen.

There are conflicting data on the effects of age on absorption. One study, which did not distinguish between metronidazole and its metabolites, indicated that the area under the curve (AUC) for plasma was almost doubled in the elderly. However, the general consensus is that there is no requirement for a decreased dosage for the elderly, unless there is significant renal impairment.

Distribution

It is widely distributed in body tissues after oral or intravenous administration. It appears about 90 min after an oral dose in brain tissue, cerebrospinal fluid (CSF), saliva and breast milk in concentrations similar to those found in plasma; and in vaginal secretions, pleural and prostatic fluid at levels about 40% of those of the plasma. In patients receiving 500 mg every 12 h or 1 g every 6 h, CSF levels of up to 2 and 8 mg/L, respectively, have been found. Bactericidal concentrations of metronidazole are achieved in pus from hepatic abscesses. Concentrations in placenta and fetal tissue are related to the corresponding maternal plasma levels: concentrations of 3.5 mg/kg (placenta) and 9 mg/kg (fetus) when the plasma concentration was 13.5 mg/L.

Metabolism

It is metabolized in the liver to a glucuronide conjugate and to acid and hydroxy derivatives. The acid metabolite, produced by oxidation of the N-1 ethanol side-chain, is microbiologically inactive and appears in the urine because of its high water solubility. The hydroxy derivative, which is as active as the parent drug against *G. vaginalis*, is formed by oxidation of the methyl group on C-2 of the imidazole ring, first to the hydroxymethyl derivative and subsequently to the carboxylic acid. Hydroxymetronidazole has a half-life of 10–13 h. Both metronidazole itself and the hydroxymethyl metabolite can form sulfate or glucuronide conjugates; the acid metabolite may be excreted as the glycine conjugate. Traces of metabolites derived from reduction of the nitro group are found in urine and are assumed to be formed by the intestinal flora.

Excretion

About 60–80% of the dose appears in the urine and 6–15% in the feces. The hydroxy and acid metabolites are also excreted in the urine. Glucuronide conjugates account for approximately 20% of the total. Renal clearance is approximately 10 mL/min per 1.73 m². Decreased renal function does not alter the single-dose kinetics and dose adjustment is not normally required in patients with renal impairment. However, the hydroxy metabolite may accumulate in patients with end-stage disease and dose reduction may be necessary. Elimination is prolonged in patients with impaired liver function necessitating dose reduction. Hemodialysis increases the clearance of metronidazole, shortening the half-life to 2–3 h.

Newborn infants possess a decreased capacity to eliminate metronidazole. In one study, the elimination half-life measured during the first 3 days of life was inversely related to gestational age. In premature newborns and infants whose gestational ages were between 28 and 40 weeks, the corresponding half-life elimination rates ranged from 10.9 to 22.5 h.

 ## TOXICITY AND SIDE EFFECTS

Precautions

Alcohol should not be taken during and for 48 h after therapy because of a possible disulfiram-like reaction, nor should it be combined with formulations containing alcohol. It should not be given in cases of known hypersensitivity to nitroimidazoles.

It enhances the anticoagulant effect of warfarin and may impair the clearance of phenytoin and lithium. Phenytoin may increase the metabolism of metronidazole. Plasma concentrations are decreased by the concomitant administration of phenobarbital (phenobarbitone). The drug may also mask the immunological response of untreated early syphilis cases because of its antitreponemal activity.

It should be used with care in patients with blood dyscrasias or with any central nervous system (CNS) disease.

The drug should be avoided in pregnancy, especially during the first trimester and particularly if high doses are being administered. Use during the second and third trimesters may be acceptable if alternative therapies for trichomoniasis have failed, but single-dose (2 g oral) therapy should be avoided. The drug may cause the breast milk to taste bitter. Breast feeding should be discontinued until 24 h after the last dose to allow excretion of the drug. It appears safe when given to nursing mothers at doses of up to 400 mg every 8 h.

Adverse effects

An unpleasant sharp, metallic taste is not unusual. Furry tongue, glossitis and stomatitis have occurred; stomatitis may be associated with overgrowth of *Candida* spp. during treatment. Gastrointestinal disturbances include nausea, vomiting, abdominal discomfort and diarrhea, and occur with intravenous and oral preparations. Pseudomembranous colitis has also been reported.

Nervous system effects associated with intravenous and oral preparations include convulsive seizures, peripheral neuropathy, dizziness, vertigo, incoordination, ataxia, confusion, irritability, depression, weakness and insomnia. Peripheral neuropathy was found in 11 of 13 patients aged 12–22 years treated for Crohn's disease. The symptoms disappeared when the dose was discontinued or markedly reduced. Peripheral neuropathy or CNS toxicity is more likely in patients treated for 10 days or more and treatment should be discontinued. The co-administration of cimetidine increases plasma levels of metronidazole and may increase the risk of neurological side effects.

Reversible neutropenia has been reported after administration of both intravenous and oral preparations. Bone marrow aplasia and thrombocytopenia are rare. Hemolytic uremic syndrome was reported in six children who had been given metronidazole for non-specific diarrhea or for prophylaxis after bowel surgery.

Erythematous rash and pruritus have been reported after use of the intravenous preparation. The risk of thrombophlebitis can be minimized by avoiding prolonged indwelling catheters for intravenous infusion.

Rarely, flattening of the T wave may be seen in electrocardiographic tracings. A number of cases of deafness have been reported. Myopia related to 11 days' oral treatment for trichomoniasis disappeared 4 days after treatment was stopped, but returned when treatment was resumed. There have been isolated reports of pancreatitis and gynecomastia.

Mutagenicity and carcinogenicity

Metronidazole and some of its metabolites are weakly mutagenic by the Ames test, but only under anaerobic or microaerophilic conditions that lead to reduction of the nitro group, an essential prerequisite for its bactericidal action. Other mutagenicity and genotoxicity studies in experimental animals and in-vitro tests of human cells have proved negative.

Several large studies have found no increase in the incidence of cancer.

 ## CLINICAL USE

Trichomonal vaginitis, giardiasis and amebiasis
Treatment and prophylaxis of anaerobic infections
Acute necrotizing ulcerative gingivitis (Vincent's stomatitis)
Bacterial vaginosis
C. difficile-associated disease
Gastric colonization with *H. pylori* (in combination with other agents)
Surgical prophylaxis (abdominal and gynecological)

It is also used in acne rosacea, balantidiasis and Guinea worm infection. *T. vaginalis* infections resistant to the usual dosage require special treatment (p. 836).

 ## Preparations and dosage

Proprietary names: Flagyl and numerous generic preparations.
Preparations: Tablets, suppositories, topical gel and cream, i.v. infusion, oral suspension.
Dosage:

Trichomonal vaginitis: Adults, 2 g as a single oral dose or a 7-day course of 400 mg every 12 h. All sexual partners should be treated concomitantly. Children aged 1–3 years, 50 mg every 8 h for 7 days; aged 3–7 years, 100 mg every 12 h for 7 days; aged 7–10 years, 100 mg every 8 h for 7 days; aged 10–18 years, 200 mg every 8 h for 7 days or 2 g as a single dose. *In the USA:* 250–500 mg every 8 h for 7 days or 2 g as a single dose.

Anaerobic bacterial infections: Adults, an initial dose of 800 mg orally followed by 400 mg every 8 h, for 7–10 days; i.v. administration is 500 mg every 8 h. Children: 7.5 mg/kg every 8 h orally or i.v. By rectal suppository: child 1 month–1 year, 125 mg every 8 h for 3 days, then every 12 h thereafter; child 1–5 years, 250 mg every 8 h for 3 days, then every 12 h thereafter; child 5–12 years, 500 mg every 8 h for 3 days, then every 12 h thereafter; child 12–18 years, 1 g every 8 h for 3 days, then every 12 h thereafter. *In the USA:* Adults 500 mg every 6–12 h orally or 15 mg/kg by i.v. infusion over 1 h, followed by 7.5 mg/kg every 6 h. No more than 4 g in 24 h.

Surgical prophylaxis. Adults, 400 mg orally or 500 mg i.v. as a single dose, repeated every 3 h for prolonged procedures. Children, 7.5 mg/kg administered as above. Alternatively, rectal suppositories of 500 mg may be used for children 5–10 years and 1 g for children 10–18 years. *In the USA:* Adults 15 mg/kg by i.v. infusion over 30–60 min and completed about 1 h before surgery, followed by two further i.v. doses of 7.5 mg/kg infused at 6 and 12 h after the initial dose.

C. difficile-associated disease: 800 mg orally then 400 mg every 8 h for 10–14 days. *In the USA:* 250 mg every 6 h or 500 mg every 8 h.

Intestinal amebiasis: Adults, 800 mg orally every 8 h for 5–10 days. Children aged 1–3 years, 200 mg every 8 h for 5 days; aged 3–7 years, 200 mg every 6 h; aged 7–10 years, 400 mg every 8 h for 5 days; aged 10–18 years, 800 mg every 8 h for 5 days. *In the USA:* 500–750 mg every 8 h for 10 days.

Extraintestinal amebiasis: Adults, 800 mg orally every 8 h for 10 days. Children aged 1–3 years, 100–200 mg every 8 h for 5–10 days; aged 3–7 years, 100–200 mg every 6 h for 5–10 days; aged 7–10 years, 200–400 mg every 8 h for 5–10 days; aged 10–18 years, 400–800 mg every 8 h for 5–10 days. *In the USA:* 500–750 mg every 8 h for 10 days.

Symptomless cyst passers: Adults, 400–800 mg orally every 8 h for 5–10 days. Children aged 1–3 years, 100–200 mg every 8 h for 5–10 days; aged 3–7 years, 100–200 mg every 6 h for 5–10 days; aged 7–10 years, 200–400 mg every 8 h for 5–10 days. Similar doses to those given for amebiasis may be used for balantidiasis and *Blastocystis hominis* infections.

Giardiasis: Adults, 2 g metronidazole orally per day as a single dose for 3 days; alternatively, 400 mg every 8 h for 5–7 days. Children aged 1–3 years, 500 mg once per day for 3 days; aged 3–7 years, 600–800 mg once per day for 3 days; aged 7–10 years, 1 g once per day for 3 days; aged 10–18 years, 2 g once per day for 3 days or 400 mg every 8 h for 5 days. *In the USA:* 250 mg every 8–12 h.

Acute ulcerative gingivitis: Adults, 200 mg orally every 8 h for 3 days. Children aged 1–3 years, 50 mg every 8 h for 3 days; aged 3–7 years, 100 mg every 12 h for 3 days; aged 7–10 years, 100 mg every 8 h for 3 days; aged 10–18 years, 200 mg every 8 h for 3 days.

Bacterial vaginosis: 400 mg orally every 12 h for 5–7 days or 2 g as a single dose. *In the USA:* 500 mg every 12 h.

Gastroduodenal ulcers (H. pylori): 400 mg every 8 h for 7–14 days (in combination with other agents). *In the USA:* 250 mg every 6 h.

Widely available.

 ## Further information

Bendesky A, Ménendez D, Ostrosky-Wegman P. Is metronidazole carcinogenic? *Mutat Res.* 2002;511:133–144.

Burtin P, Taddio A, Aruburno O, Einarson TR, Koren G. Safety of metronidazole in pregnancy: a meta-analysis. *Am J Obstet Gynecol.* 1995;172:525–529.

Caro-Paton T, Carvajal A, Martin de Diego I, et al. Is metronidazole teratogenic? A meta-analysis. *Br J Clin Pharmacol.* 1997;44:179–182.

Gerding DN, Muto CA, Owens RC. Treatment of *Clostridium difficile* infection. *Clin Infect Dis.* 2008;46(suppl 1):S32–S42.

Jenks PJR, Ferrero L, Labigne A. The role of the *rdxA* gene in the evolution of metronidazole resistance in *Helicobacter pylori. J Antimicrob Chemother.* 1999;43:753–758.

Lau AH, Lam NP, Piscitelli SC, Wilkes L, Danziger LH. Clinical pharmacokinetics of metronidazole and other nitroimidazole anti-infectives. *Clin Pharmacokinet.* 1992;23:328–364.

Lossick JG. Treatment of sexually transmitted vaginosis/vaginitis. *Rev Infect Dis.* 1990;12(suppl 6):S665–S681.

Snydman DR, Jacobus NV, McDermott LA, et al. Multicenter study of in vitro susceptibility of *Bacteroides fragilis* group, 1995 to 1996 with comparison of resistance trends from 1990 to 1996. *Antimicrob Agents Chemother.* 1999;43:2417–2422.

TINIDAZOLE

Molecular weight: 247.3.

A 5-nitroimidazole available for oral administration and, in some countries, for intravenous infusion.

ANTIMICROBIAL ACTIVITY

Its antibacterial and antiprotozoal activity is similar to that of metronidazole. Activity against the common anaerobic bacterial pathogens is shown in Table 24.1 (p. 293). The MIC against *G. vaginalis* is 0.2–2 mg/L; the hydroxy metabolite is significantly more active than that of metronidazole. *H. pylori* is inhibited by 0.5 mg/L. *T. vaginalis* and *T. fetus* at 2.5 mg/L and *E. histolytica* is inhibited by about 0.3–2.5 mg/L.

PHARMACOKINETICS

Oral absorption	>95%
C_{max} 2 g oral	40 mg/L after 2 h
800 mg (30-min infusion)	12 mg/L 6 min after end infusion
Plasma half-life	12–14 h
Volume of distribution	0.64 L/kg
Plasma protein binding	12%

Absorption and distribution

After a 2 g oral dose, concentrations remain at *c.* 10 mg/L at 24 h and 2.5 mg/L at 48 h. Daily doses of 1 g maintain plasma levels in excess of 8 mg/L, irrespective of whether the dose is oral or intravenous.

It is well distributed, with concentrations in bile, CSF, breast milk and saliva similar to those reached in plasma. The drug readily crosses the placenta. In women undergoing first trimester abortion, concentrations of 4.9 mg/kg (placenta) and 7.6 mg/kg (fetus) were found when the plasma concentration was 13.2 mg/L.

Metabolism and excretion

Metabolites include the 2-hydroxymethyl derivative, its glucuronide and two unidentified minor derivatives. In urine about half the drug remains unmetabolized.

The parent drug and its metabolites are excreted primarily in the urine and to a minor extent in the feces. The clearance rate is about 0.73 mL/min per kg and the urinary excretion is about 21% of the dose. Total clearance of the drug is 51 mL/min, renal clearance 10 mL/min. In healthy volunteers given an intravenous infusion of 800 mg [^{14}C]tinidazole over 30 min, a mean of 44% of the dose was excreted in the urine during the first 24 h, increasing to 63% over 5 days; only 12% of the dose appeared in the feces. Unchanged tinidazole comprised 32% of urinary ^{14}C in 0–12 h urine. The 2-hydroxymethyl metabolite accounted for about 9% of the urinary ^{14}C and was also present in plasma.

In renal failure the pharmacokinetics are not significantly different from those in healthy individuals. It is rapidly removed by hemodialysis and a normal dose should be given after each dialysis; if treatment precedes dialysis a half dose should be infused after the end of the procedure.

TOXICITY AND SIDE EFFECTS

Tinidazole is generally well tolerated. Infrequent and transient effects include nausea, vomiting, diarrhea and a metallic taste. Disulfiram-like reactions may occur and rare neurological disturbances and transient leukopenia have been described. Rash, which may be severe, urticaria and angioneurotic edema can occur.

CLINICAL USE

Anaerobic bacterial infections (prophylaxis and treatment)
Trichomoniasis
Giardiasis (single dose)
Amebiasis (including amebic liver abscess)
Bacterial vaginosis
Gastric colonization with *H. pylori* (in combination with other agents)

Preparations and dosage

Proprietary names: Fasigin, Fasigyn, Fasigyne Simplotan, Sorquetan, Tricolam, Tindamax.

Preparations: Tablets, intravenous infusion.

Dosage: In general, tinidazole in tablet form is taken with or after food.

Trichomoniasis, giardiasis, bacterial vaginosis and acute necrotizing gingivitis: Adults, 2 g as a single oral dose. In trichomoniasis all sexual partners should be treated. Children, 50–75 mg/kg, repeating the dose once if necessary.

Anaerobic bacterial infection: 2 g orally, then 1 g per day as a single dose or two divided doses for 5–6 days; i.v. infusion: 800 mg as 400 mL of a 2 mg/mL solution at 10 mL/min, followed by 800 mg per day or 400 mg every 12 h until oral therapy can be substituted.

Surgical prophylaxis: 2 g orally about 12 h before surgery; alternatively, 1.6 g as a single i.v. infusion before surgery, or in two divided doses, one just before surgery, the other during or not longer than 12 h after surgery.

Intestinal amebiasis: Adults, 2 g per day as a single dose for 2–3 days. Children, 50–60 mg/kg per day as a single dose for 3 days.

Liver amebiasis: Adults, 1.5–2 g per day as a single dose for 3–6 days. Children, 50–60 mg/kg per day as a single dose for 5 days.

Gastroduodenal ulcers (H. pylori): 500 mg every 12 h for 7 days in combination with other drugs.

Widely available as tablets; restricted availability as infusion.

Further information

Bercu TE, Petri WA, Behm JW. Amebic colitis: new insights into pathogenesis and treatment. *Curr Gastroenterol Rep.* 2007;9:429–433.

Evaldson GR, Lindgren S, Nord CE, Rane AT. Tinidazole milk excretion and pharmacokinetics in lactating women. *Br J Clin Pharmacol.* 1985;13:503–507.

Fung HB, Doan TL. Tinidazole: a nitroimidazole antiprotozoal agent. *Clin Ther.* 2005;27:1859–1884.

Manes G, Balzano A. Tinidazole: from protozoa to *Helicobacter pylori* – the past, present and future of a nitroimidazole with peculiarities. *Expert Rev Anti Infect Ther.* 2004;2:695–705.

Nailor MD, Sobel JD. Tinidazole for the treatment of vaginal infections. *Expert Opin Investig Drugs.* 2007;16:743–751.

Wood SG, John BA, Chasseaud LF, et al. Pharmacokinetics and metabolism of ¹⁴C-tinidazole in humans. *J Antimicrob Chemother.* 1986;17:801–809.

OTHER NITROIMIDAZOLES

NIMORAZOLE (NITRIMIDAZINE)

An orally administered 5-nitroimidazole. It is slightly soluble in water at room temperature, soluble in alcohols, acetone and chloroform. The spectrum includes *T. vaginalis*, *G. lamblia*, *E. histolytica*, anaerobic bacteria and *G. vaginalis*. Activity against *B. fragilis* and *Fusobacterium* spp. is similar to or slightly less than that of metronidazole (mean MIC 0.25–1 mg/L).

A peak blood concentration of about 32 mg/L occurs within 2 h of a 500 mg oral dose. High concentrations are achieved in saliva and vaginal secretions. Excretion is principally via the urine where the drug appears as metabolites which display antimicrobial and antiprotozoal activity less than that of the parent drug.

It is generally well tolerated even at the high doses required in conjunction with radiotherapy for the treatment of head and neck tumors. Adverse effects are the same as those of metronidazole. Disulfiram-like reactions appear to be rare.

Clinical uses are similar to those of metronidazole. It is also used as a hypoxic radiosensitizer in the radiotherapy of head and neck tumors.

Preparations and dosage

Proprietary names: Esclama, Naxogin, Naxogyn.

Preparation: Tablets.

Dosage:

Trichomoniasis: 2 g as a single dose with a main meal; can be repeated after 1 month. Sexual partners should be treated concomitantly.

Giardiasis or amebiasis: Adults, 500 mg to 1 g every 12 h for 5–10 days. Children >10 kg body weight, 500 mg per day for 5 days; <10 kg body weight, 250 mg per day for 5 days.

Ulcerative gingivitis: 500 mg every 12 h for 2 days.

Available in continental Europe and South Africa.

Further information

Bache M, Kappler M, Said HM, Staab A, Vordermark D. Detection and specific targeting of hypoxic regions within solid tumors: current preclinical and clinical strategies. *Curr Med Chem.* 2008;15:322–338.

Pamba HO. Comparative study of aminosidine, etophamide and nimorazole alone or in combination in the treatment of intestinal amebiasis in Kenya. *Eur J Clin Pharmacol.* 1990;39:353–357.

Raether W, Hänel H. Nitroheterocyclic drugs with broad spectrum activity. *Parasitol Res.* 2003;90(supp 1):S19–S39.

ORNIDAZOLE

A 5-nitroimidazole available for oral administration, intravenous infusion and as a vaginal pessary. Its activity closely parallels that of metronidazole and tinidazole (Table 24.1, p. 293).

Peak plasma levels after a single 750 mg or 1.5 g oral dose reach 11 mg/L and 30 mg/L, respectively, within about 2 h. The half-life is 12–14 h. It is well absorbed from the vagina, with peak plasma concentrations of 5 mg/L being reached 12 h after the insertion of a 500 mg vaginal pessary. After a single 1 g intravenous infusion for colorectal surgery, serum levels reached about 24 mg/L after 15 min and about 6 mg/L after 24 h. It has wide tissue distribution, including CSF. Plasma protein binding is 10–15%.

It is metabolized in the liver, mainly to hydroxymethyl derivatives. The plasma clearance rate decreases in hepatic failure because of reduced liver metabolism and decreased biliary elimination. About 60% of an oral dose is recovered in the urine and 20% in the feces. The dosing interval should be doubled in patients with severe hepatic impairment, but it is unnecessary to reduce the dose in patients with impaired renal function. It is removed by hemodialysis.

Toxicity and side effects are similar to those of metronidazole and tinidazole and it has similar clinical uses. It has been shown to be effective for the prevention of recurrence of Crohn's disease after ileocolonic resection.

Preparations and dosage

Preparations: Tablets, vaginal pessary, i.v. infusion.

Dosage:

Amebiasis: Adults, oral, 500 mg every 12 h for 5–10 days; 1.5 g as a single dose for 3 days for amebic dysentery. Children, 25 mg/kg per day as a single dose for 5–10 days; 40 mg/kg per day in amebic dysentery. In severe cases of amebic dysentery or severe amebic liver abscess, 0.5–1 g i.v. over 15–30 min, followed by 500 mg every 12 h for 3–6 days. Children, 20–30 mg/kg per day.

Giardiasis: Adults, oral, 1–1.5 g per day as a single dose for 1–2 days. Children, 30–40 mg/kg per day.

Trichomonal vaginitis: Adults, oral, a single 1.5 g tablet, or 1 g orally together with 500 mg vaginally; alternatively, 500 mg every 12 h for 5 days with or without a 500 mg vaginal pessary. Children, 25 mg/kg per day.

Anaerobic bacterial infections: Adults, an initial dose of 0.5–1.0 g i.v., followed by 500 mg every 12 h for 5–10 days. Oral therapy with 500 mg every 12 h should be substituted as soon as possible. Children, 10 mg/kg every 12 h.

Surgical prophylaxis: 1 g i.v. about 30 min before surgery.

Restricted availability. Not available in the UK or the USA.

Further information

Rutgeerts P, Van Assche G, Vermeire S, et al. Ornidazole for prophylaxis of post-operative Crohn's disease recurrence: a randomized, double-blind, placebo-controlled trial. *Gastroenterology.* 2005;128:856–861.

Turcant A, Granry JC, Allain P, Cavellat M. Pharmacokinetics of ornidazole in neonates and infants after a single intravenous infusion. *Eur J Clin Pharmacol.* 1987;32:111–113.

SECNIDAZOLE

A 5-nitroimidazole with properties similar to those of metronidazole. It is rapidly absorbed after oral administration and is distinguished by having the longest plasma half-life (18 h) of clinically used nitroimidazole drugs. It is used in the treatment of intestinal amebiasis, giardiasis, trichomoniasis and bacterial vaginosis.

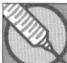

Preparations and dosage

Proprietary name: Flagentyl.

Preparation: Tablets.

Dosage: Adults, oral, 2 g as a single dose. Children, 30 mg/kg as a single dose. In invasive amebiasis, 15 g per day for 5 days. Children, 30 mg/kg per day for 5 days.

Available in France.

Further information

Gillis JC, Wiseman LR. Secnidazole: a review of its antimicrobial activity, pharmacokinetic properties and therapeutic use in the management of protozoal infections and bacterial vaginosis. *Drugs.* 1996;51:621–638.

Toppare MF, Kitapçi F, Senses DA, Yalcinkaya F, Kaya IS, Dilmen U. Ornidazole and secnidazole in the treatment of symptomatic intestinal amoebiasis in childhood. *Trop Doct.* 1994;24:183–184.

Oxazolidinones

Una Ni Riain and Alasdair P. MacGowan

The oxazolidinones are a novel class of synthetic antimicrobial agents unrelated to any other antibacterial drug class. They were originally developed as monoamine oxidase inhibitors for treatment of depression, with subsequent recognition of their antimicrobial properties. The first members of the group to emerge exhibited potent activity against Gram-positive organisms, but were not developed for human use owing to toxicity in animal models. In the 1990s two less toxic oxazolidinones were developed: eperezolid, a piperazine derivative, and linezolid, a morpholine derivative. Linezolid exhibited the more favorable pharmacokinetic profile and was subsequently licensed for human use.

Numerous chemical analogs have been screened in a search for compounds with enhanced potency, a broader spectrum of activity or a more favorable side effect profile. Several promising candidates have been described, but linezolid remains the only oxazolidinone currently available.

These drugs are characterized by activity against Gram-positive organisms including methicillin-resistant *Staphylococcus aureus*, penicillin-resistant pneumococci and vancomycin-resistant enterococci. They are inactive against most Gram-negative species, although some investigational compounds are active against fastidious Gram-negative bacteria including *Haemophilus influenzae*. They have potentially useful activity against mycobacteria, including multiresistant isolates of *Mycobacterium tuberculosis*. Resistance among Gram-positive organisms remains very uncommon (<0.5%) among clinical isolates.

 Further information

Diekema DJ, Jones RN. Oxazolidinones. *Drugs*. 2000;59:7–16.

Dresser LD, Rybak MD. The pharmacologic and bacteriologic properties of oxazolidinones, a new class of synthetic antimicrobials. *Pharmacotherapy*. 1998;18:456–462.

Ford C, Hamel JC, Stapert D, et al. Oxazolidinones: new antibacterial agents. *Trends Microbiol*. 1997;5:196–200.

LINEZOLID

Molecular weight: 337.35.

A synthetic oxazolidinone available for oral or intravenous administration. Soluble in water at a pH range of 5–9. Aqueous solutions (2 g/L) are stable at 25°C, 4°C and −20°C for at least 3 months.

ANTIMICROBIAL ACTIVITY

The in-vitro activity against common pathogenic bacteria is shown in Table 25.1. It exhibits potent activity against a wide range of Gram-positive organisms, including those that are resistant to other antimicrobial agents. Methicillin-resistant *Staph. aureus* and coagulase-negative staphylococci are susceptible, as are enterococci, including vancomycin-resistant *Enterococcus faecalis* and *Ent. faecium*. Penicillin-sensitive and resistant isolates of *Streptococcus pneumoniae* are equally susceptible. Less common Gram-positive pathogens are also susceptible; the minimum inhibitory concentrations (MICs) for *Bacillus* spp., *Corynebacterium* spp., *Listeria monocytogenes*, *Aerococcus* spp., *Micrococcus* spp. and *Rhodococcus equi* are all ≤2 mg/L. *M. tuberculosis* is susceptible, with typical MICs ≤1 mg/L for sensitive and multidrug-resistant strains.

All enterobacteria, *Pseudomonas* spp. and other non-fermentative aerobic Gram-negative bacilli, including *Acinetobacter* spp., are resistant. *Moraxella catarrhalis*, *Legionella* spp.,

Table 25.1 Activity of linezolid against common pathogenic bacteria: MIC (mg/L)

		MIC
Staphylococcus aureus	(methicillin susceptible)	0.06–4
	(methicillin resistant)	0.12–4
Coagulase-negative staphylococci		0.5–2
Streptococcus pyogenes		0.5–2
Str. pneumoniae	(penicillin susceptible)	0.12–2
	(penicillin resistant)	0.5–2
Enterococcus faecalis	(vancomycin susceptible)	0.5–4
	(vancomycin resistant)	1–4
E. faecium	(vancomycin susceptible)	1–4
	(vancomycin resistant)	0.5–4
Haemophilus influenzae		8–16
Neisseria gonorrhoeae		4–>16
Escherichia coli		R
Klebsiella pneumoniae		R
Pseudomonas aeruginosa		R
Bacteriodes fragilis		1–8

R, resistant (MIC >32 mg/L).

Mycoplasma spp. and *Chlamydia* spp. are inhibited by 4–8 mg/L. Activity against *Haemophilus influenzae* is modest.

Among anaerobes, *Clostridium perfringens* and *Peptostreptococcus* spp. are inhibited by <2 mg/L. Typical MICs (mg/L) for Gram-negative anaerobes include: *Bacteroides* spp., 4–8; *Prevotella* spp., 1–4; *Fusobacterium* spp., 0.125–1.

Activity is bacteristatic against most susceptible species, but modest bactericidal activity has been demonstrated against some strains of *Str. pneumoniae*, *C. perfringens* and *Bacteroides fragilis*. Inhibition of toxin production by staphylococci and streptococci in the presence of sub-MIC concentrations has been described.

Linezolid may antagonize the bactericidal action of some antibiotics (e.g. gentamicin). No evidence of synergy has been found in various experimental systems with gentamicin against vancomycin-resistant *Enterococcus* spp. or with vancomycin, gentamicin, ciprofloxacin, fusidic acid or rifampicin (rifampin) against methicillin-resistant *Staph. aureus*.

ACQUIRED RESISTANCE

Isolates of *Staph. aureus* and *E. faecalis* for which the MIC of linezolid is raised have been obtained following serial exposure to gradients of the drug. However, induction of resistance requires many passages over several weeks. Resistance in these laboratory mutants is associated with modifications of the 23S rRNA gene.

Overall, resistance rates in clinical isolates are very low at <0.5%. Resistance is reported primarily in coagulase-negative staphylococci (1.77%) and enterococci (1.13%; mostly *E. faecium*), with exceptionally low resistance rates in *Staph. aureus* (0.06%). Risk factors for emergence of resistance include prolonged use of the drug, the presence of irremovable indwelling devices, sequestered sites of infection and low-dose therapy for infections caused by vancomycin-resistant enterococci or methicillin-resistant *Staph. aureus*. Resistance in clinical isolates is most often associated with gene mutations in which guanosine is replaced by uracil in the 23S rRNA. Nosocomial clonal spread of such mutants has been described in coagulase-negative staphylococci and enterococci. Resistance conferred by a novel mobile element, *cfr*, has been described in two isolates of staphylococci.

PHARMACOKINETICS

Oral absorption	>95%
C_{max} 400 mg oral	11–12 mg/L after 1–2 h
600 mg oral	18–21 mg/L after 1–2 h
600 mg intravenous	>15 mg/L after 1 h
Plasma half-life	c. 5.5 h
Volume of distribution	45–50 L
Plasma protein binding	31%

Absorption

Bioavailability after oral administration is almost complete. Plasma trough concentrations following oral doses of 400 mg and 600 mg every 12 h are >3.0 and >4.0 mg/L, respectively. With the higher dose, administered orally or intravenously, plasma concentrations remain above the MIC for most susceptible species throughout a 12 h dosage interval. After administration with high fat content food the maximum serum concentration achieved is lower and the peak delayed, but the area under the concentration–time curve (AUC) is unaltered.

Distribution

Linezolid is distributed widely in tissues and fluids. In human volunteers, maximum concentrations in inflammatory blister fluid averaged over 16 mg/L, with a mean penetrance of 104%. In patients undergoing hip arthroplasty, linezolid rapidly penetrates into bone, fat and muscle, achieving levels in excess of the MICs for susceptible organisms, with therapeutic concentrations maintained in the perioperative site hematoma fluid for more than 16 h. Mean penetration of linezolid into inflamed diabetic foot infection tissue is 101%, producing a concentration of 9.6 µg/g. Studies with human volunteers have also indicated good concentrations in pulmonary alveolar fluid with a mean fluid to plasma ratio of 3.2:1. When the meninges are not inflamed, the concentration in cerebrospinal fluid (CSF) is lower than that of plasma, with a CSF:plasma ratio of approximately 0.7:1. The concentration in sweat is about half that of plasma.

Other sites at which local concentrations exceed corresponding plasma concentrations, based on animal studies, include kidney, adrenal, liver and gastrointestinal tract. In a rat model of endocarditis, heart valve tissue and plasma concentrations were approximately equivalent.

Pharmacokinetic properties are unaltered in elderly patients and dose adjustment is unnecessary. Single-dose pharmacokinetic studies indicate that plasma clearance and volume of distribution are greater in children than in adults, while peak and trough serum concentrations are lower. Shorter dosing intervals (every 8 h) are therefore recommended for most therapeutic indications in children.

Metabolism

Linezolid undergoes non-renal as well as renal metabolism. Non-renal metabolism is by slow chemical oxidation in a process that does not discernibly interact with the hepatic cytochrome P_{450} system. The oxidants contributing to metabolism of the drug have not yet been fully elucidated, but in-vivo studies suggest the process is mediated by reactive oxygen species produced throughout the body. The metabolites produced following non-renal metabolism are an aminoethoxyacetic acid and a hydroxyethylglycine metabolite, neither of which has any significant antimicrobial activity. Non-renal clearance rates are 120 mL/min and account for almost 65% of total body clearance. Since it does not appear to act as an inducer or inhibitor of cytochrome P_{450} enzymes, interactions with drugs metabolized by these enzymes are unlikely to occur.

Excretion

Renal clearance accounts for approximately 50 mL/min of the total body clearance of 170 mL/min. Under steady-state conditions, approximately 30% of the dose is excreted unchanged in the urine.

In populations with varying degrees of renal function (creatinine clearance range of 10–>80 mL/min) there is no evidence of alteration in total body clearance, and adjustment of dose in patients with renal insufficiency is not recommended. However, accumulation of metabolites, up to 10-fold, occurs in patients with severe renal impairment (creatinine clearance <30 mL/min). The clinical significance of this is unknown, but linezolid should be used with caution in patients with severe renal impairment. Approximately one-third of the dose is removed by hemodialysis and since total apparent clearance is increased during dialysis, one of the 12-hourly doses should be administered after the procedure. Accumulation of metabolites also occurs in patients on dialysis, with unknown clinical significance, and caution in use in hemodialysis is advised. There are no available data on pharmacokinetics in patients undergoing peritoneal dialysis or hemofiltration.

In patients with mild to moderate hepatic impairment there is no significant change to the pharmacokinetic profile. Accordingly, dosage adjustment is not recommended in patients with mild to moderate liver disease. The pharmacokinetics of linezolid in severe hepatic failure have not been studied, but as its metabolism is predominantly non-enzymatic, the pharmacokinetics would not be expected to alter significantly.

PHARMACODYNAMICS

Human and animal studies indicate that the parameters that best correlate with efficacy are AUC divided by MIC and the period for which the drug concentration remains above the MIC. In 288 patients with significant infection caused by Gram-positive organisms, optimal efficacy was observed when plasma concentrations remained above the MIC for >85% of the dosage interval, and when the AUC:MIC ratio was 80–20.

A post-antibiotic effect, which was more prolonged at 4 × MIC than at 1 × MIC, has been demonstrated for staphylococci and enterococci in vitro. A modest post-antibiotic effect of 3–4 h has been described in a mouse thigh model of infection with *Staph. aureus*.

TOXICITY AND SIDE EFFECTS

Most reported adverse events are mild or moderate, with reactions severe enough to lead to withdrawal of therapy occurring in less than 3% of patients. The most common adverse events are shown in Table 25.2. The most frequent side effects are gastrointestinal disturbances (diarrhea, nausea, vomiting and taste alteration) and headache. The reported incidence of *Clostridium difficile* complications is 0.2%.

Mild and transient abnormalities of liver function tests (elevation of transaminases and/or alkaline phosphatase) occur in more than 1% of patients. Skin reactions, including rashes, dermatitis, pruritus and diaphoresis, are uncommon.

Serious but infrequent adverse drug effects include myelosuppression, peripheral neuropathy, optic neuropathy and lactic acidosis. These adverse events, which probably result from inhibition of mitochondrial protein synthesis, occur primarily in patients treated for >28 days. Myelosuppression

Table 25.2 Common adverse drug reactions to linezolid

Adverse event	Frequency (%)
Diarrhea	4.3
Nausea	3.4
Headache	2.2
Vaginal candidiasis	1
Taste alteration (metallic taste)	0.9
Vomiting	1.2
Abnormal liver function tests	1.3

generally occurs only after more than 2 weeks of treatment and increases with longer durations. It occurs more frequently in patients with severe renal insufficiency and is reversible on discontinuation of therapy.

Reversal of cytopenias by concomitant administration of vitamin B_6 has been described. Weekly monitoring of full blood count is recommended for all patients, with more frequent monitoring of those in the following categories: pre-existing anemia or thrombocytopenia; receiving concomitant drugs that may cause anemia or thrombocytopenia; severe renal insufficiency; treatment for more than 10–14 days.

Peripheral and optic neuropathy are serious but infrequent. Most cases are associated with treatment for more than 28 days (median 5 months), but neuropathies have occurred with shorter courses. In most cases optic neuropathy improved or resolved on cessation of therapy but peripheral neuropathy did not.

Lactic acidosis can occur within a week of commencing therapy but is most often seen in patients receiving prolonged treatment (median 6 weeks).

Linezolid is a weak, reversible monoamine oxidase inhibitor (MAOI) with potential interaction with adrenergic and serotonergic drugs. Co-administration of sympathomimetics, vasopressors or dopaminergic agents may lead to an enhanced pressor response. It should be co-administered with these drugs only under conditions where close observation and monitoring of blood pressure is available, and their initial doses should be reduced and then titrated to achieve the desired pressor effect. Similarly, concomitant administration of linezolid with agents that increase central nervous system serotonin concentrations can lead to serotonin toxicity (serotonin syndrome). This most commonly follows concurrent administration of selective serotonin receptor inhibitors, but can occur with tricyclic antidepressants or any MAOI. Since MAOIs and their active metabolites have long elimination half-lives, linezolid is contraindicated in patients who are taking these drugs or have taken them in the previous 2 weeks.

 ## CLINICAL USE

Community-acquired pneumonia

Nosocomial pneumonia

Skin and soft-tissue infections

Vancomycin-resistant *E. faecium* infections, including cases with concurrent bacteremia

Linezolid is primarily used for the treatment of infections caused, or likely to be caused, by methicillin-resistant *Staph. aureus*, vancomycin-resistant enterococci and penicillin-resistant *Str. pneumoniae*. Combination therapy with an antimicrobial active against Gram-negative bacteria is indicated if concomitant infection with a Gram-negative pathogen is suspected or confirmed.

Outside of licensed indications, it has been used in the treatment of bone and joint infections, endocarditis, central nervous system infections, infections in neutropenic patients and drug-resistant tuberculosis.

 ## Preparations and dosage

Proprietary name: Zyvox.

Preparations: Tablets, suspension, injection.

Dosage: Adults, oral or i.v. infusion over 30–120 min, 600 mg every 12 h. Children (unlicensed in the UK), oral or i.v. infusion over 30–120 min, neonate <7 days, 10 mg/kg every 8–12 h; neonate >7 days, 10 mg/kg every 8 h; 1 month–12 years, 10 mg/kg (max. 600 mg) every 8 h; 12–18 years, 600 mg every 12 h.

Widely available.

Further information

Alcala L, Ruiz-Serrano MJ, Perez-Fernandez Turegano C, et al. In vitro activities of linezolid against clinical isolates of *Mycobacterium tuberculosis* that are susceptible or resistant to first-line antituberculous drugs. *Antimicrob Agents Chemother.* 2003;47:416–417.

Beekman SE, Gilbert DN, Polgreen PM. Toxicity of extended courses of linezolid: results of an Infectious Diseases Society of America Emerging Infections Network survey. *Diagn Microbiol Infect Dis.* 2008;62:407–410.

Brier M, Stalker D, Aronoff G, et al. Pharmacokinetics of linezolid in subjects with renal dysfunction. *Antimicrob Agents Chemother.* 2003;47:2775–2780.

Clemett D, Markham A. Linezolid. *Drugs.* 2000;59:815–827.

Dobbs TE, Patel M, Waites KB, et al. Nosocomial spread of *Enterococcus faecium* resistant to vancomycin and linezolid in a tertiary care medical centre. *J Clin Microbiol.* 2006;44:3368–3370.

Gee T, Ellis R, Marshall G, et al. Pharmacokinetics and tissue penetration of linezolid following multiple oral doses. *Antimicrob Agents Chemother.* 2001;45:1843–1846.

Gemmell CG. Susceptibility of a variety of clinical isolates to linezolid: a European inter-country comparison. *J Antimicrob Chemother.* 2001;48:47–52.

Jones RN, Ross JE, Castanheira M, et al. United States resistance surveillance results for linezolid (LEADER Program for 2007). *Diagn Microbiol Infect Dis.* 2008;62:416–426.

Jones RN, Stilwell MG, Hogan PA, et al. Activity of linezolid against 3, 251 strains of uncommonly isolated Gram-positive organisms: report from the SENTRY antimicrobial surveillance program. *Antimicrob Agents Chemother.* 2007;51:1491–1493.

Kearns GL, Abdel-Rahman SM, Blumer JL, et al. Single dose pharmacokinetics of linezolid in infants and children. *Pediatr Infect Dis J.* 2000;19:1178–1184.

Prammananan T, Chaiprasert A, Leechawengwongs M. In vitro activity of linezolid against multidrug-resistant tuberculosis (MDR-TB) and extensively drug-resistant (XDR)-TB isolates. *Int J Antimicrob Agents.* 2009;33:183–192.

Richter E, Rusch-Gerdes S, Hillemann D. First linezolid-resistant clinical isolates of *Mycobacterium tuberculosis. Antimicrob Agents Chemother.* 2007;51:1534–1536.

Rubinstein E, Isturiz R, Standiford H, et al. Worldwide assessment of linezolid's clinical safety and tolerability: comparator-controlled phase III studies. *Antimicrob Agents Chemother.* 2003;47:1824–1831.

Stalker D, Jungbluth G, Hopkins N, et al. Pharmacokinetics and tolerance of single- and multiple-dose oral or intravenous linezolid, an oxazolidinone antibiotic, in healthy volunteers. *J Antimicrob Chemother.* 2003;51:1239–1246.

INVESTIGATIONAL OXAZOLIDINONES

Numerous chemical analogs have been described. Among the most promising candidates are:

- RWJ-416457, a pyrrolopyrazolyl-substituted oxazolidinone, with greater potency than that of linezolid against staphylococci and enterococci in vitro
- Radezolid (RX-1741), one of a family of biaryloxazolidinones that demonstrate improved potency against Gram-positive bacteria including methicillin-resistant *Staph. aureus* and vancomycin-resistant enterococci, and which are also active against *H. influenzae* and *Mor. catarrhalis*
- PF-00422602, an oxazolidinone with a novel C-5 side chain, which has antibacterial activities similar to those of linezolid but reduced in-vivo myelotoxicity in animal models.

 Further information

Lawrence L, Danese P, DeVito J, et al. In vitro activities of the Rx-01 oxazolidinones against hospital and community pathogens. *Antimicrob Agents Chemother.* 2008;52:1653–1662.

Livermore DM, Warner M, Mushtaq S, et al. In vitro activity of the oxazolidinone RWJ-416457 against linezolid-resistant and -susceptible staphylococci and enterococci. *Antimicrob Agents Chemother.* 2007;51:1112–1114.

Vara Prasad JVN. New oxazolidinones. *Curr Opin Microbiol.* 2007;10:454–460.

26 Quinolones

Peter C. Appelbaum and André Bryskier

The pyridone-β-carboxylic acid derivatives or quinolones comprise a large and expanding number of synthetic compounds. Since the first analog, nalidixic acid, was synthesized in 1962, many types have been reported based on a few common structures: most are 1,8 naphthyridone or quinoline derivatives:

1,8 naphthyridone derivatives   Quinoline derivatives

Changes to various parts of the molecules confer different properties and this is the basis of the variation in activity of various members of the group. The main structure–activity relationships are shown in the accompanying figure:

The first 4-quinolone, nalidixic acid, is a 1,8-naphthyridinone with a narrow spectrum of activity, chiefly against Enterobacteriaceae. Several compounds with improved antibacterial activity were subsequently synthesized. These included pipemidic acid, which expanded the spectrum to include weak activity against *Pseudomonas aeruginosa*, and piromidic acid, which exhibited useful activity against *Staphylococcus aureus*. Further development led to the discovery in the late 1970s of fluorine-substituted derivatives with much enhanced intrinsic activity against both organisms, a group now known as the fluoroquinolones. Numerous fluoroquinolones with altered

pharmacokinetic properties and additional improvements in spectrum, including in some cases useful activity against *Mycobacterium tuberculosis* and *M. leprae*, became available in the next 30 years. Current research efforts are directed to overcome problems of resistance, which is increasingly encountered in both Gram-positive and Gram-negative bacteria.

CLASSIFICATION

The varied properties of the quinolones make them difficult to classify accurately. According to their antibacterial activity and spectrum, four broad groups are recognized:

Group 1:	Compounds with a narrow antibacterial spectrum directed mainly against Enterobacteriaceae.
Group 2:	Fluoroquinolones, which exhibit potent activity against Gram-negative bacilli including *Ps. aeruginosa* and many Gram-positive bacteria excluding *Streptococcus pneumoniae*. These compounds are characterized by a 6-fluorine atom and often by a 7-piperazinyl group.
Group 3:	Compounds with improved activity against *Str. pneumoniae* and *Staph. aureus*. Some derivatives do not contain a fluorine atom.
Group 4:	Compounds with properties similar to those of groups 2 and 3 and additional activity against anaerobes.

Group 1	Group 2	Group 3	Group 4
Cinoxacin	Ciprofloxacin	Garenoxacin	Gemifloxacin
Flumequine	Enoxacin	Gatifloxacin	Delafloxacin[b]
Nalidixic acid	Norfloxacin	Levofloxacin	Moxifloxacin
Oxolinic acid	Ofloxacin	Sparfloxacin[a]	Nemonoxacin[b]
Pipemidic acid	Pazufloxacin	Tosufloxacin	Sitafloxacin[b]
Piromidic acid	Pefloxacin		Trovafloxacin[a]
Rosoxacin	Prulifloxacin		WCK 771[b]
	Rufloxacin		Zabofloxacin[b]

[a]Compounds withdrawn from use in the USA and Europe.
[b]Compounds under development.

Two additional quinolones, besifloxacin and nadifloxacin, are marketed solely for topical use. Other derivatives, including danofloxacin, difloxacin, enrofloxacin, ibafloxacin, marbofloxacin, orbifloxacin and sarafloxacin, are used in veterinary medicine and are not dealt with here.

ANTIBACTERIAL ACTIVITY

Group 1 quinolones exhibit moderate activity against a wide range of Enterobacteriaceae as well non-fastidious Gram-negative bacilli such as *Haemophilus influenzae* and *Neisseria* spp. They have weak (pipemidic acid) or no activity against *Ps. aeruginosa*, anaerobes and Gram-positive bacteria (Table 26.1).

Introduction of a fluorine atom and a nitrogen-containing heterocycle on the quinoline or a naphthyridone core resulted in compounds with greater potency and a broader antibacterial spectrum (Table 26.2). Minimum inhibitory concentrations (MICs) of the group 2 fluoroquinolones are up to 100-fold lower than those of group 1 compounds for Enterobacteriaceae, *Aeromonas* spp., *Campylobacter* spp. and *Yersinia* spp., as well as against fastidious Gram-negative bacilli such as *H. influenzae*, *Neisseria* spp. and *Moraxella catarrhalis*. Some of these compounds (such as ciprofloxacin) also exhibit significant antibacterial activity against *Ps. aeruginosa*; some compounds presently under investigation are active against non-fermentative Gram-negative bacilli such as *Acinetobacter* spp. and *Stenotrophomonas maltophilia*. Fluoroquinolones display variable in-vitro activity against *Staph. aureus* and coagulase-negative staphylococci. Methicillin-resistant strains are often quinolone resistant.

Compounds of groups 3 and 4, including levofloxacin, moxifloxacin and gemifloxacin, are very potent against *Str. pneumoniae* but exhibit poor activity against *Enterococcus* spp.

Table 26.1 Activity of selected group 1 quinolones against common pathogenic bacteria: MIC (mg/L)

Species	Cinoxacin	Nalidixic acid	Pipemidic acid
Staphylococcus aureus	64–R	R	R
Streptococcus pyogenes	R	R	R
Str. pneumoniae	R	R	R
Enterococcus faecalis	R	R	R
Neisseria gonorrhoeae	1–8	1	2
Haemophilus influenzae	1	1	2
Escherichia coli	1–4	4–8	2
Klebsiella pneumoniae	2–32	8–16	2
Pseudomonas aeruginosa	R	R	8–32
Acinetobacter spp.	R	R	R
Bacteroides fragilis	R	R	32–R

R, resistant (MIC >64 mg/L).

and *Listeria monocytogenes*. Among group 4 compounds, some, such as moxifloxacin, claim to exert improved activity against anaerobes.

Most fluoroquinolones exhibit antibacterial activity against atypical bacteria (mycoplasmas, ureaplasmas) and intracellular pathogens including *Legionella* spp., *Chlamydophila* (formerly *Chlamydia*) *pneumoniae*, *Chlamydia trachomatis*, *Coxiella burnetii* and *Rickettsia* spp. Fluoroquinolones, particularly those with a quinoline core, exhibit variable activity against *Mycobacterium tuberculosis* and *M. leprae*, the most active being pefloxacin, ofloxacin, levofloxacin, gatifloxacin, sparfloxacin and moxifloxacin. Other mycobacteria, including organisms of the *M. avium* complex, are less susceptible.

Table 26.2 Activity of group 2 fluoroquinolones against common pathogenic bacteria: MIC (mg/L)

	Ciprofloxacin	Enoxacin	Fleroxacin	Lomefloxacin	Norfloxacin	Ofloxacin	Pefloxacin	Rufloxacin
Staphylococcus aureus	0.25–1	2	1–2	1–2	1	0.12–1	0.5–1	2
Streptococcus pyogenes	0.5–2	8–16	4–16	4–8	4	2	4–8	16
Str. pneumoniae	1–4	8–16	4–16	2–8	8	1–4	8	32
Enterococcus faecalis	0.5–2	≥8	4–16	8–16	8	2–4	4	32
Neisseria spp.	≥0.06	0.12	<0.06–0.5	<0.06–0.12	≥0.06	≥0.06	≥0.06	0.12
Haemophilus influenzae	≥0.06	0.12	<0.06–0.25	≥0.06–0.25	≥0.06	≥0.06	≥0.06	0.5
Escherichia coli	≥0.06	0.25	0.12–0.5	0.25	0.25	0.06–0.25	0.25	2
Klebsiella pneumoniae	0.06–0.25	0.25	0.12–2	0.25	0.5	0.25	0.5	32
Pseudomonas aeruginosa	0.25–2	2–8	1–8	0.25–4	1–2	2–4	2–4	8
Bcteroides fragilis	4–16	≥32	8–64	8–64	8–32	8	16	32
Chlamydia trachomatis	0.5–2	0.5–2	4–8	0.5–2	4–16	0.5–2	2–8	4–8
Mycobacterium tuberculosis	0.25–4	0.3–>4	>4	>4	2–8	0.3–1.2	0.3–2	No data

Quinolones are rapidly bactericidal to most susceptible bacterial species at concentrations exceeding the MIC by no more than four-fold. However, there is usually an optimal bactericidal concentration above which the lethal action is diminished. This paradoxical effect is probably caused by dose-dependent inhibition of RNA synthesis.

Fluoroquinolones rapidly accumulate in polymorphonuclear neutrophils, monocytes, macrophages and other cells, achieving bactericidal concentrations. The ratio of cellular to extracellular concentrations is compound dependent and ranges from 2:1 to 10:1.

INTERACTIONS

Combinations of quinolones with carbapenems, aminoglycosides and polymyxin may interact synergistically in vitro, particularly against *Ps. aeruginosa* and *Acinetobacter* spp. Against *Sten. maltophilia*, marked synergy has been observed when quinolones are combined with cephalosporins such as ceftazidime, ceftriaxone and cefoperazone. Testing for synergy in vitro has not been standardized and there is no solid evidence of correlation between in vitro and clinical results.

ACQUIRED RESISTANCE

MECHANISMS

Four mechanisms of resistance within the quinolone family have been described:

- Mutations at the level of the gene targets (*gyrA*, *parC*, *gyrB* and *parcE*).
- Decreased cellular uptake and/or active expulsion (efflux).
- Protection of DNA gyrase by plasmid-encoded pentapeptides.
- Inactivation of quinolones (rare).

The frequency with which bacteria develop resistance to the quinolones is much lower for the fluoroquinolones (10^{-12}) than for nalidixic acid (10^{-8}). Moreover, Gram-positive bacteria mutate to resistance at higher frequencies than do Gram-negative organisms. Single-step mutations generally lead to two- to eight-fold increases in MICs. There is cross-resistance within available quinolones. The species that are most likely to become resistant to group 2 fluoroquinolones in a single mutational step are those of borderline susceptibility (e.g. *Ps. aeruginosa*, *Serratia* spp., *Acinetobacter* spp., *Staphylococcus* spp.).

Gram-positive cocci (*Staph. aureus*, *Str. pneumoniae*) express fluoroquinolone efflux systems that utilize the energy of the proton motive force and generally provide modest resistance. In Gram-negative bacilli, efflux systems recognize fluoroquinolones and other antibacterial agents. An efflux pump, QepA in *Escherichia coli*, may decrease susceptibility of hydrophilic fluoroquinolones such as ciprofloxacin and norfloxacin by a factor of 8–32.

Plasmid-mediated resistance conferred by pentapeptides that protect DNA gyrase has become a worrying problem among Enterobacteriaceae and mycobacteria. It may be associated with other resistance genes. Inactivation of ciprofloxacin and norfloxacin by *N*-acetylation of the free N4′ of the piperazinyl ring has also been described.

EPIDEMIOLOGY

Epidemiological surveys of fluoroquinolone resistance in *Str. pneumoniae* found a prevalence rate below 1% in Europe and North America, but a higher rate in Hong Kong (≥3%). However, clinically significant resistance has been detected among bacterial species such as *Ps. aeruginosa*, *Staph. aureus* (particularly methicillin-resistant strains, for which resistance rates of up to 80% have been reported), coagulase-negative staphylococci and *Acinetobacter* spp. and *Esch. coli* (up to 20% in some countries and hospitals). Clinical isolates of *N. gonorrhoeae* with reduced susceptibility or resistance to fluoroquinolones are commonly isolated in many parts of the world.

PHARMACOKINETICS

ABSORPTION

Most quinolones are rapidly absorbed when given orally, although there is considerable variation among different compounds. Absorption is inhibited by co-administration with antacids containing divalent metals, such as magnesium, calcium and iron, with which they form insoluble chelates. When the oral bioavailability is absolute, fluoroquinolones may be administered by this route instead of intravenously in many diseases.

DISTRIBUTION

Protein binding of fluoroquinolones varies. They have large volumes of distribution; concentrations approximating those in the plasma are found in tissue fluid and they are highly distributed into bone and prostate. Concentrations in the bronchial mucosa, lung epithelial lining fluid and alveolar macrophages are usually higher than in plasma. Concentrations in cerebrospinal fluid (CSF) are about one-third to one-half the corresponding plasma level; the presence of inflammation does not appear to enhance penetration significantly.

ELIMINATION

Most available fluoroquinolones are eliminated by the renal route but many are metabolized, to a greater or lesser extent, in the liver. Liver metabolism of <5% occurs with ofloxacin and levofloxacin. Some metabolites exhibit antibacterial activity (pefloxacin metabolized to norfloxacin; prulifloxacin metabolized to ulifloxacin).

If the dominant elimination route is the kidney, adjustment of doses or times of administration may be needed depending upon the degree of renal impairment. In elderly subjects, changes in pharmacokinetics are drug dependent and usually low; dosage modification may sometimes be indicated.

TOXICITY AND ADVERSE EVENTS

Several quinolones (temafloxacin, sparfloxacin, grepafloxacin, trovafloxacin) have been withdrawn or their use severely limited soon after their clinical introduction owing to severe and sometimes life-threatening adverse events.

The frequency of mild adverse events in patients receiving ciprofloxacin, levofloxacin, moxifloxacin and gemifloxacin (particularly short courses) is comparable to that seen with other commonly used antibacterial agents. Rates of 6–10% have been described, with less than 1% being regarded as serious. Fluoroquinolones are not recommended during pregnancy, for lactating women or for children unless there are overriding reasons for their use.

The most common serious adverse events are:

- phototoxicity (lomefloxacin, sitafloxacin, pefloxacin); bone and joint arthropathies (occurring mainly in elderly patients when a steroid is co-administered)
- central nervous system abnormalities when administered with anti-inflammatory drugs such as ibuprofen; drug interactions (co-administration with theophylline)
- hypotension (garenoxacin)
- cardiotoxicity (QTc prolongation and/or torsade de pointes) resulted in withdrawal of grepafloxacin and restriction on the use of sparfloxacin; it may occur rarely with other fluoroquinolones
- hypoglycemia or interference with diabetic drugs (gatifloxacin)
- tendon rupture (especially of the Achilles tendon) rarely occurs with ciprofloxacin and levofloxacin.

CLINICAL USE

GROUP 1 QUINOLONES

The narrow Gram-negative spectrum of group 1 quinolones makes them suitable for treatment of urinary tract infection. Nalidixic acid is prescribed for enteric infection due to *Shigella* in some part of the world.

FLUOROQUINOLONES (GROUPS 2–4)

Many fluoroquinolones are available in both oral and parenteral formulations but because they are well absorbed when given by mouth, many infectious diseases can be treated successfully with oral therapy. The following comprise common indications:

- Lower respiratory tract infections (i.e. acute bacterial exacerbations of chronic bronchitis, community-acquired pneumonia)
- Sinusitis
- Uncomplicated and some complicated urinary tract infections
- Bacterial prostatitis
- Community-acquired skin and soft-tissue infections
- Bone and joint infections
- Gastrointestinal tract infections, particularly infectious diarrhea caused by toxigenic *Esch. coli*, *Salmonella enterica* (including typhoid and paratyphoid fevers, and the chronic salmonella carrier state), *Shigella*, *Campylobacter*, *Aeromonas* and *Vibrio* species (including *Vibrio cholerae*), as well as *Plesiomonas shigelloides*
- Sexually transmitted diseases (including pelvic infections) other than syphilis, which does not respond to quinolones
- Tuberculosis, leprosy, plague.

Specific pharmaceutical formulations (eye drops and creams) are available for topical application.

Further information

Andriole VT, ed. *The Quinolones*. 3rd ed.San Diego, CA: Academic Press; 2000.

Bryskier A, ed. Fluoroquinolones. In: *Antibacterial and Antifungal Agents*. 2nd ed. Washington DC: ASM Press; 2005.

Bryskier A, Chantot JF. Classification and structure–activity relationships of fluoroquinolones. *Drugs*. 1995;49(suppl 2):16–28.

Bryskier A, Lowther J. Fluoroquinolones and tuberculosis. *Expert Opin Investig Drugs*. 2002;11:233–255.

Cattoir V, Nordmann P. Plasmid-mediated quinolone resistance in Gram-negative bacterial species: an update. *Curr Med Chem*. 2009;16:1028–1046.

Dembry LM, Farrington JM, Andriole VT. Fluoroquinolone antibiotics: adverse effects and safety profiles. *Infect Dis Clin Pract*. 1999;8:9–16.

Hooper DC. Mechanisms of action of antimicrobials: focus on fluoroquinolones. *Clin Infect Dis*. 2001;32(suppl 1):S9–S15.

Mitscher LA. Bacterial topoisomerase inhibitors: quinolone and pyridone antibacterial agents. *Chem Rev*. 2005;105:559–592.

Zhanel GG, Fontaine S, Adam H, et al. A review of new fluoroquinolones. Focus on their use in respiratory tract infections. *Treat Respir Med*. 2006;5:437–465.

GROUP 1 QUINOLONES

NALIDIXIC ACID

Molecular weight: 232.2.

A 1,8 naphthyridone derivative available for oral administration.

ANTIBACTERIAL ACTIVITY

It displays good activity in vitro against a wide range of Enterobacteriaceae. *Ps. aeruginosa*, Gram-positive bacteria and anaerobes are resistant (Table 26.1, p. 307).

PHARMACOKINETICS

Oral absorption	>90%
C_{max} 1 g oral	c. 25 mg/L
Plasma half-life	c. 1.5 h
Volume of distribution	0.4 L/kg
Plasma protein binding	93%

The plasma concentrations achieved after oral administration vary widely. In infants with acute shigellosis, absorption is much impaired by diarrhea. Administration with an alkaline compound leads to higher plasma concentrations, partly as the result of enhanced solubility (nalidixic acid is much more soluble at higher pH) and absorption and partly because of reduced tubular reabsorption.

It is rapidly metabolized, principally to the hydroxy acid, which is bacteriologically active, and glucuronide conjugates, which are not. The entire administered dose appears in the urine over a 24 h period. Elimination is reduced by probenecid. In the presence of renal impairment there is little accumulation of the active compound because it continues to be metabolized. However, elimination of metabolites is progressively delayed as renal function declines. About 4% of a dose appears in the feces.

TOXICITY AND SIDE EFFECTS

Adverse reactions are generally those common to all quinolones: gastrointestinal tract and CNS disturbances and skin rashes, including eruptions related to photosensitivity. About half of the reported CNS reactions involve visual disturbances, hallucinations or disordered sensory perception. Severe excitatory states, including acute psychoses and convulsions, are usually observed in patients receiving high dosages. The drug should be avoided in patients with psychiatric disorders or epilepsy.

Acute intracranial hypertension has been observed in children, some of whom have also manifested cranial nerve palsies. Hemorrhage has occurred in patients who were also receiving warfarin, presumably due to displacement of the anticoagulant from its protein binding sites by the nalidixic acid. Hemolytic anemia has been described several times in infants with or without glucose-6-phosphate dehydrogenase deficiency; in adults, death has occurred from autoimmune hemolytic anemia. Arthralgia and severe metabolic acidosis have rarely been reported.

CLINICAL USE

Urinary tract infection

Prophylaxis in patients undergoing transurethral surgery

Treatment of acute shigellosis

Preparations and dosage

Proprietary names: Mictral, Negram, Uriben.

Preparations: Tablets, suspension.

Dosage: Adults, oral, 900 mg–1 g every 6 h for 7 days; for chronic infections, 500–600 mg every 6 h. Children >3 months, oral, 50 mg/kg per day in four divided doses; reduced in prolonged therapy to 30 mg/kg per day.

Widely available.

Further information

Anonymous Nalidixic acid. In: Dollery C, ed. *Therapeutic Drugs*. 2nd ed. Edinburgh: Churchill Livingstone; 1999:N17–N20.

Barbeau G, Belanger P-M. Pharmacokinetics of nalidixic acid in old and young volunteers. *J Clin Pharmacol.* 1982;22:490–496.

Schaad UB, Wedgwood-Krucko J. Nalidixic acid in children: retrospective matched controlled study for cartilage toxicity. *Infection.* 1987;15:165–168.

OTHER GROUP 1 QUINOLONES

ROSOXACIN (ACROSOXACIN)

The antibacterial spectrum and potency are similar to those of other members of this group, but it is particularly active against *N. gonorrhoeae* (MIC 0.06–0.1 mg/L).

A single oral dose of 300 mg produces a mean peak plasma concentration of 4–5 mg/L at about 2–4 h, with an apparent elimination half-life of about 6 h. Elimination in the urine is partly as the *N*-oxide metabolite and the glucuronide of this metabolite.

Side effects are those common to quinolones, notably gastrointestinal tract and CNS disturbances. About 50% of patients treated with single oral doses of 100–400 mg developed dizziness, drowsiness, altered visual perception and other CNS effects.

It is effective as single-dose treatment of patients with urethral and anorectal gonorrhea, but coexistent *C. trachomatis* infection is not eliminated from most patients and postgonococcal urethritis develops in up to 30%.

Preparations and dosage

Proprietary name: Eradacil.

Preparation: Capsules.

Dosage: Adult, oral, 300 mg as a single dose.

Limited availability.

Further information

Park GB, Saneski J, Weng T, Edelson J. Pharmacokinetics of rosoxacin in human volunteers. *J Pharm Sci.* 1982;71:461–462.

Romanowski B, Austin TW, Pattison FLM, et al. Rosoxacin in the therapy of uncomplicated gonorrhea. *Antimicrob Agents Chemother.* 1984;25:445–457.

 ## CINOXACIN

A cinnoline derivative formulated for oral administration. It is active against most Enterobacteriaceae, but *Ps. aeruginosa*, Gram-positive bacteria and anaerobes are resistant (Table 26.1, p. 307).

It is well-absorbed when given orally. Administration with food reduces the peak concentration by about one-third, but the area under the concentration–time curve (AUC) remains unchanged. Concentrations in prostatic and bladder tissues reach 60% and 80%, respectively, of the simultaneous serum concentrations.

It is almost entirely eliminated in the urine, about 40–60% as unchanged drug and the rest as metabolites, most of which have no antibacterial activity. Urinary concentrations of active drug in the first 2 h after administration of a dose is 100–500 mg/L. Elimination is reduced by probenecid and by renal impairment, the half-life rising to about 12 h in end-stage renal failure.

Adverse reactions that are common to the group are reported in 4–5% of patients; these are primarily gastrointestinal tract disturbances, but rashes occur in up to 3% and CNS disturbances in less than 1%. Use is restricted to uncomplicated urinary tract infection.

Preparations and dosage

Proprietary name: Cinobac.

Preparation: Capsules.

Dosage: 500 mg every 12 h or 250 mg every 6 h; prophylaxis 250–500 mg per day for 7–14 days.

No longer widely available.

 Further information

Anonymous. Cinoxacin. In: Dollery C, ed. *Therapeutic Drugs.* 2nd ed. Edinburgh: Churchill Livingstone; 1999:C224–C226.

Sisca TS, Heel RC, Romakiewicz JA. Cinoxacin. A review of its pharmacological properties and therapeutic efficacy in the treatment of urinary tract infections. *Drugs.* 1983;25:544–569.

 ## PIPEMIDIC ACID

An orally administered pyridopyrimidine derivative with a 7-piperazinyl moiety. The piperazinyl moiety at C-7 increases in-vitro activity against *Ps. aeruginosa*. Pipemidic acid is inactive against Gram-positive bacteria or anaerobes (Table 26.1, p. 307).

It is well absorbed orally. The drug is rapidly metabolized, primarily to acetyl, formyl and oxo derivatives, which exhibit much reduced antibacterial activity. It is eliminated in the urine, 50–85% of a dose appearing over the first 24 h, less than 2% as inactive metabolites. Non-renal clearance accounts for 10–40% of a dose in the young, rising to 40–70% in elderly subjects, thereby compensating for possible renal insufficiency. No dosage adjustment is necessary in patients with mild renal insufficiency. Some of the drug is eliminated in the bile and a significant portion appears in the feces.

Nausea and vomiting are common; dizziness, weakness and grand mal seizures have been observed, principally in the elderly. A number of reactions have been sufficiently severe to require discontinuation of therapy. Clinical use is restricted to urinary tract infections.

Preparations and dosage

Proprietary name: Pipram.

Preparation: Tablets.

Dosage: Adults, oral, 400 mg every 12 h.

Available in Europe (not UK) and Japan.

 Further information

Klinge E, Mannisto PT, Mantyla R, Mattila J, Hanninen U. Single- and multiple-dose pharmacokinetics of pipemidic acid in normal human volunteers. *Antimicrob Agents Chemother.* 1984;26:69–73.

Mannisto P, Solkinen A, Mantyla R, et al. Pharmacokinetics of pipemidic acid in healthy middle-aged volunteers and elderly patients with renal insufficiency. *Xenobiotica.* 1984;14:339–347.

 ## FLUMEQUINE

A tricyclic fluorinated 4-quinolone, with activity similar to that of nalidixic acid in vitro, although it is somewhat more active against some Enterobacteriaceae.

Following escalating oral doses of 400, 800 or 1200 mg, mean peak plasma levels reached at 2 h are 13.5, 23.8 and 31.9 mg/L, respectively. The apparent elimination half-life is about 7 h. The main metabolite, hydroxyflumequine, is much more rapidly eliminated. About 60% of a dose appears in the urine, mostly in the form of conjugates. Urinary concentrations following an 800 mg dose are 10–35 mg/L, with a peak of 105 mg/L. It has no effect on the pharmacokinetics of theophylline.

Flumequine is generally well tolerated, side effects being mainly mild gastrointestinal tract disturbances, rashes, dizziness and confusion.

It is principally used in uncomplicated urinary tract infections.

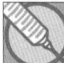

Preparations and dosage

Proprietary name: Apurone.

Preparation: Tablets.

Dosage: Adult, oral, 400 mg every 8–12 h.

Limited availability in Europe.

Further information

Schuppan D, Harrison LI, Rohlfing SR, et al. Plasma and urine levels of flumequine and 7-hydroxyflumequine following single and multiple oral dosing. *J Antimicrob Chemother*. 1985;15:337–343.

OXOLINIC ACID

An oral 4-quinolone with a tricyclic structure. Its antibacterial spectrum is very similar to that of nalidixic acid, but it is more active against Enterobacteriaceae (MIC 0.25–2 mg/L). Gram-positive bacteria, *Ps. aeruginosa* and anaerobes are resistant.

After repeated doses of 750 mg twice daily, mean plasma concentrations are initially very low, but steady state is reached at the third day and C_{max} is around 3.5 mg/L. Administration with food delays absorption. Binding to plasma protein is about 80%. It undergoes complex biotransformation, and an enterohepatic cycle may account for the increase in the apparent elimination half-life from 4 to 15 h over 7 days of treatment as well as for the 20% of dose which can be recovered from the feces. About 50% of the dose appears in the urine in the first 24 h, partly in the form of metabolites, some of which display antibacterial activity.

Side effects common to the quinolones occur frequently. About one-quarter of patients treated with 750 mg every 12 h suffer nausea and vomiting or restlessness and insomnia. Its only use is in the treatment of lower urinary tract infections.

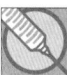

Preparations and dosage

Proprietary name: Urotrate.

Preparation: Tablets.

Dosage: Adults, oral, 750 mg every 12 h. Children, 50–600 mg every 12 h (age dependent).

Available in some European countries.

Further information

Gleckman R, Alvarez S, Joubert DW, Matthews SJ. Drug therapy reviews: oxolinic acid. *Am J Hosp Pharm*. 1979;36:1077–11010.

PIROMIDIC ACID

A pyrimidopyrimidine derivative with a C7-pyrrolidinyl ring, allowing a slight increase in activities against Gram-positive cocci. Its main antibacterial activity is close to that of nalidixic acid and there have been reports of renal toxicity. It is available in only a few countries.

GROUP 2 QUINOLONES

CIPROFLOXACIN

Molecular weight (free base): 331.4.

A 6-fluoro, 7-piperazinyl quinolone formulated as the hydrochloride for oral administration and as the lactate for intravenous use.

ANTIBACTERIAL ACTIVITY

Activity against common bacterial pathogens is shown in Table 26.2 (p. 307). It exhibits potent activity against most Enterobacteriaceae, as well as against *Acinetobacter* spp. (MIC 0.25–1 mg/L), fastidious Gram-negative bacilli such as *Mor. catarrhalis* (MIC 0.06–0.25 mg/L) and *Campylobacter jejuni* (MIC 0.12 mg/L). In common with other quinolones, it is active against *Bacillus anthracis*. Ciprofloxacin is the most active quinolone against *Ps. aeruginosa* and exhibits good activity in vitro against other non-fermenting Gram-negative bacilli. In-vitro activity against *Staph. aureus* coagulase-negative staphylococci, *Str. pyogenes*, *Str. pneumoniae* and *Enterococcus* spp. (MIC c. 0.5–2 mg/L) is moderate. Most methicillin-resistant strains of staphylococci are resistant. It has poor activity against anaerobes, but is active against *M. tuberculosis*, *Mycoplasma* spp. and intracellular pathogens such as *Chlamydia*, *Chlamydophila* and *Legionella*.

PHARMACOKINETICS

Oral absorption	50–80%
C_{max} 500 mg oral	1.5–2 mg/L after 1–2 h
200 mg intravenous (15-min infusion)	3.5 mg/L end infusion
Plasma half-life	3–4 h
Volume of distribution	3–4 L/kg
Plasma protein binding	20–40%

Absorption

After escalating oral doses, mean peak plasma levels increase proportionately with dose. However, accumulation occurs after repeated doses of 500 mg orally or 200 mg intravenously every 12 h; the apparent elimination half-life has been reported to rise to about 6 h after a regimen of 250 mg every 12 h for 6 days. Absorption is delayed, but seems unaffected by food and, in common with other quinolones, is reduced by certain antacids. Co-administration of sucralfate reduces the peak plasma concentrations to undetectable levels in many subjects (mean value from 2 to 0.2 mg/L) and the AUC is reduced to 12% of the value obtained when ciprofloxacin is administered alone. Ferrous sulfate and multivitamin preparations containing zinc significantly reduce absorption, which is also impaired in patients receiving cytotoxic chemotherapy for hematological malignancies. Calculated total bioavailability is 60–70%.

Distribution

It is widely distributed in body fluids, concentrations in most tissues and in phagocytic cells approximating those in plasma. Concentrations in the CSF, even in the presence of meningitis, are about half the simultaneous plasma levels.

Metabolism and excretion

It is partly metabolized to four metabolites, all but one of which (desethylciprofloxacin) display antibacterial activity. About 95% of a dose can be recovered from feces and urine. Around 40% of an oral and 75% of an intravenous dose appear in the urine over 24 h. Elimination is by both glomerular filtration and tubular secretion (60–70%) and is reduced by concurrently administered probenecid and by renal insufficiency. It is poorly removed by hemodialysis. Part of the administered drug is eliminated in the bile. An enterohepatic cycle results in prolongation of the half-life. The four metabolites are eliminated in the urine and feces at low concentration in comparison to the parent compound.

 ## TOXICITY AND SIDE EFFECTS

Untoward reactions are uncommon, those encountered being typical of the group (p. 309). Reactions severe enough to require withdrawal of treatment have occurred in <2% of patients. The most common reactions, gastrointestinal tract disturbances, have been seen in 5% of patients and rashes in about 1%. CNS disturbances typical of quinolones have been reported in 1–2% of patients. Tendinitis and tendon rupture (especially of the Achilles tendon) may occur in a small number of patients and ciprofloxacin should be avoided in patients at risk for these conditions. Potentiation of the action of theophylline and other drugs metabolized by microsomal enzymes may occur. Crystalluria and transient arthralgia have been reported.

In volunteers, dosages of up to 750 mg produced no change in the numbers of fecal streptococci and anaerobes, but did produce a $2.5 \times \log_{10}$ decline in the numbers of enterobacteria, which lasted 1 week. There was no change in the susceptibility of the affected organisms and no overgrowth by resistant strains. As with other quinolones, ciprofloxacin is not recommended for use in children or in pregnant or lactating women.

Urinary tract infections (especially pathogens resistant to standard agents)

Prostatitis

Uncomplicated urogenital and rectal gonorrhea (single dose)

Purulent bronchitis, bronchopneumonia, acute exacerbations of chronic obstructive airways disease, pneumonia (other than pneumococcal pneumonia) and bronchiectasis; pulmonary exacerbations in cystic fibrosis; legionellosis; atypical pneumonia (*Mycoplasma*, *Chlamydophila*)

Osteomyelitis caused by Gram-negative bacteria

Enteric fever (including chronic carriage), severe bacterial gastroenteritis, cholera

Mycobacterial infections caused by multidrug-resistant *M. tuberculosis*

Eradication of nasopharyngeal carriage of *N. meningitidis*

Anthrax (skin and inhalation)

The drug should be avoided in suspected or confirmed infections caused by *Str. pneumoniae*. It is inferior to conventional agents and some other fluoroquinolones in the treatment of genital tract infections caused by *C. trachomatis*.

Ciprofloxacin has also been shown to be effective in the treatment of patients with malignant otitis externa, cat-scratch disease, prevention of infection in patients undergoing biliary tract surgery, and treatment of biliary tract infections. A topical preparation for use in the treatment of ocular infections is available, but is neither more effective nor safer than established topical agents; it may be indicated for superficial eye infections caused by pathogens resistant to conventional drugs or in patients unable to tolerate standard therapeutic agents.

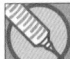 ### Preparations and dosage

Proprietary names: Ciproxin, Ciflox, Cipro, Ciloxan (ophthalmic)

Preparations: Tablets (including extended-release tablets), oral suspension, infusion, ophthalmic solution.

Dosage: Adults, oral, 250–750 mg every 12 h; i.v. infusion, 100–400 mg every 12 h. Children, where the benefits outweigh the risks, oral, 7.5–15 mg/kg per day in two divided doses; i.v., 5–10 mg/kg per day in two divided doses. Higher doses (400 mg every 12 h) needed in pseudomonal lower respiratory tract infection in cystic fibrosis.

Widely available.

Further information

Akali AU, Niranjan NS. Management of bilateral Achilles tendon rupture associated with ciprofloxacin: a review and case presentation. *J Plastic Reconstr Aesthet Surg.* 2008;61:830–834.

Anonymous. Ciprofloxacin (hydrochloride). In: Dollery C, ed. *Therapeutic Drugs.* 2nd ed. Edinburgh: Churchill Livingstone; 1999:C230–C235.

Garretts JC, Godley PJ, Peterie JD, Gerlach EH, Yakshe CC. Sucralfate significantly reduces ciprofloxacin concentrations in serum. *Antimicrob Agents Chemother.* 1990;34:931–933.

Hirata CAI, Guay DRP, Awni WM, Stein DJ, Peterson PK. Steady-state pharmacokinetics of intravenous and oral ciprofloxacin in elderly patients. *Antimicrob Agents Chemother.* 1989;33:1927–1931.

Jacobs F, Marchal M, de Francquen P, Kains J-P, Ganji D, Thys J-P. Penetration of ciprofloxacin into human pleural fluid. *Antimicrob Agents Chemother.* 1990;34:934–936.

Lettieri JT, Rogge MC, Kaiser K, Echols RM, Meller AN. Pharmacokinetic profile of ciprofloxacin after single intravenous and oral doses. *Antimicrob Agents Chemother.* 1992;36:993–996.

Nau R, Prange HW, Martell J, Sharifi S, Kolenda H, Bircher J. Penetration of ciprofloxacin into the cerebrospinal fluid of patients with uninflamed meninges. *J Antimicrob Chemother.* 1990;25:956–973.

Piddock LJV. Clinically relevant chromosomally encoded multidrug resistance efflux pumps in bacteria. *Clin Microbiol Rev.* 2005;19:382–402.

NORFLOXACIN

Molecular weight: 319.3.

A 6-fluoro, 7-piperazinyl quinoline available for oral administration and as an ophthalmic ointment.

ANTIBACTERIAL ACTIVITY

Activity against common bacterial pathogens is shown in Table 26.2 (p. 307). It is active against a wide range of Gram-negative bacteria, including Enterobacteriaceae and *Campylobacter* spp. *Ps. aeruginosa*, *Acinetobacter*, *Serratia* and *Providencia* spp. are weakly susceptible (and often resistant). It has no useful activity against anaerobes, *Chlamydia*, *Mycoplasma* and *Mycobacterium* spp.

PHARMACOKINETICS

Oral absorption	50–70%
C_{max} 400 mg oral	1.5 mg/L after 1–1.5 h
Plasma half-life	3–4 h
Volume of distribution	2.5–3.1 L/kg
Plasma protein binding	15%

Absorption and distribution

Norfloxacin displays linear kinetics. There is no significant accumulation with the recommended dosage of 400 mg every 12 h. Food slightly delays but does not otherwise impair absorption. Antacids reduce absorption. It is widely distributed, but concentrations in tissues other than those of the urinary tract are low; levels in the prostate are around 2.5 mg/g.

Metabolism and excretion

Six or more inactive metabolites are produced. Around 30% of a dose appears as unchanged drug in the urine and <10% as metabolites, producing peak concentrations of microbiologically active drug of around 100–400 mg/L. Urinary recovery is halved by probenecid, with little effect on the plasma concentration. The apparent plasma elimination half-life increases with renal impairment, rising to around 8 h in the anuric patient. Some of the drug appears in the bile where concentrations three- to seven-fold greater than the simultaneous plasma levels are achieved, but this is not a significant route of elimination and hepatic impairment is without effect. Very variable quantities, averaging 30% of a dose, appear in the feces, producing concentrations of active agent of around 200–2000 mg/kg.

TOXICITY AND SIDE EFFECTS

Untoward reactions are those common to the fluoroquinolones (p. 309). Gastrointestinal tract disturbances, which are generally mild, have been reported in 2–4% of patients. CNS disturbances have largely been limited to headache, drowsiness and dizziness. Co-administration with theophylline results in increased plasma theophylline levels.

CLINICAL USE

Complicated and uncomplicated urinary tract infections (including prophylaxis in recurrent infections), prostatitis

Uncomplicated gonorrhea

Gastroenteritis caused by *Salmonella*, *Shigella* and *Campylobacter* spp., *Vibrio cholerae*

Conjunctivitis (ophthalmic preparation)

Preparations and dosage

Proprietary names: Utinor, Noroxin, Chibroxin (ophthalmic).

Preparations: Tablets, ophthalmic solution.

Dosage: Adults, oral, 400 mg every 12 h for 7–10 days; uncomplicated lower urinary tract infections, 400 mg every 12 h for 3 days; chronic relapsing urinary tract infections, 400 mg every 12 h for 12 weeks, reduced to 400 mg per day if adequate suppression within the first 4 weeks.

Widely available.

Further information

Anonymous. Norfloxacin. In: Dollery C, ed. *Therapeutic Drugs*. 2nd ed. Edinburgh: Churchill Livingstone; 1999:N137–N141.

Holmes B, Brogden RN, Richards DM. Norfloxacin. A review of its antibacterial activity, pharmacokinetic properties and therapeutic use. *Drugs*. 1985;30:482–513.

Symposium. Norfloxacin: a fluoroquinolone carboxylic acid antimicrobial agent. *Am J Med*. 1987;82(suppl 6B):1–92.

OFLOXACIN

Molecular weight: 361.38.

A tricyclic 6-fluoro, 7-piperazinyl quinoline with a methyl substituted oxazine ring substituted. It is a racemic mixture of L- (levofloxacin, *see* p. 319) and D-isomers.

 ## ANTIBACTERIAL ACTIVITY

Activity against common bacterial pathogens is shown in Table 26.2 (p. 307). It exhibits good activity against a wide range of enterobacteria, including strains resistant to nalidixic acid, as well as against *Aeromonas*, *Campylobacter*, *Vibrio* and *Moraxella* spp. Activity against methicillin-sensitive *Staph. aureus* is good, but streptococci, including *Str. pneumoniae* and enterococci, are less susceptible. Most anaerobes are moderately or completely resistant. It is active against *L. pneumophila*, *Ch. pneumoniae*, *C. trachomatis*, mycoplasmas, ureaplasmas and *M. tuberculosis*. Other mycobacteria such as *M. fortuitum*, *M. kansasii*, *M. chelonei* and the *M. avium* complex are moderately susceptible.

PHARMACOKINETICS

Oral absorption	*c.* 95%
C$_{max}$ 400 mg oral	3–5 mg/L after 1–1.5 h
200 mg intravenous (30-min infusion)	1.8 mg/L 1 h after end infusion
Plasma half-life	5–7 h
Volume of distribution	1–2.5 L/kg
Plasma protein binding	*c.* 25%

Absorption and distribution

There is no significant interference with absorption by magnesium–aluminum hydroxide or calcium carbonate compounds,

providing administration is separated by at least 2 h. In patients receiving repeated 200 mg doses, the mean peak plasma concentration rose from 2.7 mg/L after the first dose to 3.4 mg/L after the seventh.

It is widely distributed, achieving levels ≥50% of simultaneous plasma concentrations in many tissues, including lung and bronchial secretions. In cantharides and suction blisters, peak concentrations exceed those in plasma, while the elimination half-life is similar. In patients with non-inflamed meninges, 200 mg administered orally or by intravenous infusion over 30 min produced CSF concentrations of around 0.4–1 mg/L at 2–4 h while the plasma concentration was 1.7–4 mg/L; a 400 mg intravenous infusion yielded a CSF concentration of 2 mg/L, which is adequate for some Gram-negative bacteria, but not for Gram-positive bacteria or *Ps. aeruginosa*.

Metabolism and excretion

It is poorly metabolized into desmethyl and *N*-oxide derivatives (<5% of the administered dose), only about 20% of a dose being eliminated by non-renal routes. There is a very slight effect on cytochrome P$_{450}$-related isoenzymes and no significant effect on the metabolism of theophylline in dosages of up to 800 mg.

About 60% of a dose appears in the urine over 12 h and 80–90% over 48 h. The apparent elimination half-life is prolonged in renal failure, reaching 30–50 h in anuria, necessitating a dosage reduction. The desmethyl metabolite accumulates in all patients and the *N*-oxide in 50%. Absorption and distribution are not affected by renal failure. Significant amounts of the drug appear in the feces, producing very variable concentrations up to 100 mg/kg.

 ## TOXICITY AND SIDE EFFECTS

Untoward reactions have been described in 2.5–7.5% of patients, and are those common to the group: gastrointestinal tract disturbances, rashes, tendon rupture and insomnia. CNS effects rarely occur.

 ## CLINICAL USE

Complicated and uncomplicated infections of the urinary tract, chronic prostatitis
Uncomplicated urogenital and anorectal gonorrhea (single-dose), chancroid (3-day course), genital chlamydial infections (7-day course)
Lower respiratory tract infections, including bronchopneumonia, community-acquired pneumonia (except pneumococcal pneumonia), acute bacterial exacerbations of chronic bronchitis (unless pneumococci are involved) and bronchiectasis
Enteric fever, including the chronic carrier state; gastroenteritis caused by enterotoxigenic *Escherichia coli*, *Salmonella*, *Shigella* and *Campylobacter* spp.
Ocular infections (ophthalmic preparation)

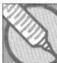

Preparations and dosage

Proprietary names: Floxin, Oflocet, Tarivid, Exocin (ophthalmic).

Preparations: Tablets, injection, ophthalmic.

Dosage: Adults, oral, 200–400 mg per day, increased to 400 mg every 12 h in severe infections; i.v., 200–400 mg every 12 or 24 h depending on severity of infection.

Widely available.

Further information

Flors S, Guay DRP, Opsahl JA, Tack K, Matzke GR. Effects of magnesium–aluminium hydroxide and calcium carbonate antacids on bioavailability of ofloxacin. *Antimicrob Agents Chemother.* 1990;34:2436–2438.

Guay DRP, Opsahl JA, McMahon FG, Vargas R, Matzke GR, Flor S. Safety and pharmacokinetics of multiple doses of intravenous ofloxacin in healthy volunteers. *Antimicrob Agents Chemother.* 1992;36:308–312.

Navarro AS, Lanao JM, Recio MMS, et al. Effect of renal impairment on distribution of ofloxacin. *Antimicrob Agents Chemother.* 1990;34:455–459.

Symposium. Ofloxacin – developments in therapy. *J Antimicrob Chemother.* 1990;26(suppl D):1–142.

OTHER GROUP 2 QUINOLONES

BALOFLOXACIN

A 6-fluoro-8-methoxy quinolone derivative. It has good antistaphylococcal activity (MIC 0.4–4 mg/L), but is inactive against methicillin-resistant *Staph. aureus* (MRSA) and quinolone-resistant *Staph. aureus*; *Str. pneumoniae* is inhibited by 0.4 mg/L. It has good activity against Enterobacteriaceae, but is inactive against *Ps. aeruginosa* (MIC 8–16 mg/L). After a 200 mg oral dose a peak level of 1.7 mg/L is reached in 1 h. The apparent elimination half-life is about 8 h, rising to 13 h in elderly subjects. Plasma protein binding is about 16%. It was withdrawn from the market in Japan because of adverse events, but is available in China.

ENOXACIN

A 1,8 naphthyridone derivative available as an oral drug. It exhibits good activity in vitro against many species of Enterobacteriaceae. It is inactive against *Ps. aeruginosa*, *Serratia*, *Citrobacter*, *Acinetobacter* and *Mycobacterium* spp., as well as anaerobes, chlamydiae and ureaplasmas.

It is well absorbed and widely distributed when given orally. Absorption is not significantly affected by food, but ranitidine, sucralfate and some antacids or mineral supplements may interfere with absorption. After repeated doses of 400 mg every 12 h for 14 days, mean peak plasma levels reach 3.5–4.5 mg/L, a steady state being achieved in 3–4 days.

About 40–60% of the administered dose is eliminated unchanged in the urine with <10% as the 3-oxo metabolite, which is 10–20 times less active than the parent compound. In renal failure, the apparent elimination half-life rises to >20 h, with marked reduction in the elimination of the oxo metabolite. Hemodialysis removes insignificant amounts of both compounds. Part is eliminated in bile, where concentrations of 4.5–25 mg/L have been noted when the corresponding serum levels were 0.5–2 mg/L.

About 6% of patients experience mild and transient effects typical of the quinolones: gastrointestinal tract disturbances, rashes, headaches and dizziness. Epileptiform and asthmatic attacks have occurred, but serious effects have been rare. Enoxacin interferes with theophylline metabolism.

It is no longer widely used, but is available in some countries for the treatment of urinary tract infection.

Preparations and dosage

Proprietary name: Enoxor.

Preparation: Tablets.

Dosage: Adults, oral, 200–400 mg every 12 h.

Available in Japan and parts of Europe.

Further information

Henwood JM, Monk JP. Enoxacin. A review of its antibacterial activity, pharmacokinetic properties and therapeutic use. *Drugs.* 1988;36:32–66.

FLEROXACIN

A trifluorinated quinolone formulated as the hydrochloride for oral use. The antibacterial spectrum and activity are similar to those of norfloxacin and ofloxacin (p. 307).

It is well absorbed, achieving a mean plasma concentration of 6 mg/L 1–2 h after a 400 mg dose. The apparent elimination half-life is 9–12 h. Absorption is unaffected by food. Bioavailability is absolute and binding to plasma protein is around 30%. It is widely distributed with tissue or fluid: plasma ratios of 0.6 in saliva, 0.3–2 in prostate and 1.7 in seminal fluid. About 50% of a dose appears in the urine as unchanged drug, giving urinary concentrations of the active compound of around 150–300 mg/L. The dosage interval (normally 24 h) should be increased in patients with renal failure.

Fleroxacin has been withdrawn from clinical use in many countries and is no longer recommended for the systemic treatment of infections.

Further information

Balfour JA, Todd PA, Peters DH. Fleroxacin. A review of its pharmacology and therapeutic efficacy in various infections. *Drugs.* 1995;49:794–850.

LOMEFLOXACIN

A difluoropiperazinyl quinolone formulated as the hydrochloride salt for oral administration. The in-vitro activity is very similar to that of norfloxacin (p. 307). It is active against Enterobacteriaceae and fastidious Gram-negative bacilli, including *L. pneumophila*. Activity against *Campylobacter* spp., *Ps. aeruginosa*, *Acinetobacter* and *Chlamydia* spp. is poor. It has reduced activity against staphylococci and poor activity against streptococci, *L. monocytogenes*, anaerobes and *Mycobacterium* spp.

A 400 mg oral dose achieves a concentration of 3–5 mg/L after 1–1.5 h. In escalating oral doses of 100, 400 and 800 mg to volunteers, the AUC was essentially proportional to the dosage, the mean plasma concentrations following 100, 400 and 800 mg doses being approximately 1.1, 4.7 and 7.5 mg/L, respectively.

Several metabolites have been described, accounting for <5% of the oral dose. Elimination occurs principally via the kidneys and 50–70% of a dose appears in the urine over 24 h. In patients with impaired renal function given 400 mg orally, the apparent elimination half-life ranged from 8 to 44 h, depending on the degree of renal failure. Non-renal clearance was also impaired, but there was no significant change in other pharmacokinetic parameters. The daily dosage (400 mg) should be reduced to 280 mg when the creatinine clearance falls below 30 mL/min. Hemodialysis has no effect on the plasma concentration. The effect of lomefloxacin on the plasma concentration of theophylline is clinically insignificant and no dosage adjustment is required.

The main adverse event is phototoxicity; other adverse events (mainly diarrhea, abdominal pain, skin reactions, dizziness, headache and insomnia) occur in about 10% of patients.

It is chiefly used in urinary tract infection, but is no longer widely available.

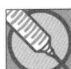

Preparations and dosage

Proprietary names: Maxaquin, Okacin.
Preparations: Tablets, ophthalmic.
Dosage: Adults, oral, 400 mg once daily.
Available in Japan, Russia and some European countries.

Further information

Anonymous. Lomefloxacin (hydrochloride). In: Dollery C, ed. *Therapeutic Drugs*. 2nd ed. Edinburgh: Churchill Livingstone; 1999:L80–L86.
Blum RA, Schultz RW, Schentag JJ. Pharmacokinetics of lomefloxacin in renally compromised patients. *Antimicrob Agents Chemother*. 1990;34:2364–2368.
Freeman CD, Nicolan DP, Belliveau PP, Nightingale CH. Lomefloxacin clinical pharmacokinetics. *Clin Pharmacokinet*. 1993;25:6–19.

PAZUFLOXACIN

A tricyclic fluoroquinolone, formulated as mesylate and hydrochloride salts for oral or parenteral use or as a methane sulfonate (eye ointment).

It displays good activity in vitro against methicillin-susceptible *Staph. aureus* (MIC 0.2 mg/L), but is inactive against *Str. pyogenes*, *Str. pneumoniae* (MIC ≥4 mg/L) and enterococci. *L. pneumophila* is inhibited by 0.03 mg/L. Activity against Enterobacteriaceae, fastidious Gram-negative bacilli, *Ps. aeruginosa* and *Acinetobacter* spp. is similar to that of ofloxacin. It is weakly active against *Sten. maltophilia* and *Burkholderia cepacia* (MIC *c.* 2 mg/L). Against *M. tuberculosis*, MICs range from 0.8 to 4 mg/L. It is inactive against anaerobes.

After oral doses of 100 or 400 mg, peak plasma concentrations range from 0.94 mg/L (100 mg) to 4.5 mg/L (400 mg) after <1 h. The apparent elimination half-life is around 2 h. Most of the administered dose is eliminated in urine, about 70% within 24 h. Four metabolites have been reported. In elderly patients, according to the renal function, the peak plasma concentration may be elevated (up to 5.6 mg/L) and significantly delayed (2–6 h). The plasma protein binding ranges from 17% to 28%.

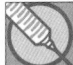

Preparations and dosage

Proprietary names: Pasil, Pazucross.
Preparations: Tablets, injection, eye ointment.
Dosage: 600 mg per day.
Available in China and Japan.

Further information

Fukuoka Y, Ikeda Y, Yamashiro Y, Takahata M, Todo Y, Narita H. in vitro and in vivo antibacterial activities of T-3761, a new fluoroquinolone. *Antimicrob Agents Chemother*. 1993;37:384–392.
Yamaki K-I, Hasegawa T, Matsuda I, Nadai M, Aoki H, Takagi K. Pharmacokinetic characteristics of a new fluoroquinolone, pazufloxacin in elderly patients. *J Infect Chemother*. 1997;3:97–102.

PEFLOXACIN

A 6-fluoro, 7-piperazinyl quinoline available for oral and intravenous administration. The in-vitro activity is very similar to that of norfloxacin (p. 307). It is active against *H. ducreyi*, *V. cholerae* and *Legionella* spp., but *Campylobacter* and *Acinetobacter* spp. and pseudomonads are not susceptible. It has poor activity against pneumococci, chlamydiae, mycoplasmas and ureaplasmas. *L. monocytogenes*, *Nocardia* spp. and anaerobes are resistant.

A plasma concentration of *c.* 5 mg/L is achieved 1–1.5 h after a 400 mg oral dose. The plasma elimination half-life is 8.5–15 h. It is widely distributed, concentrations in bone, brain, blister fluid, CSF, saliva, sputum and prostate all approximating, and in some cases exceeding, the simultaneous plasma concentration. It is extensively metabolized to the desmethyl (= norfloxacin) and *N*-oxide derivatives. Some 60–70% of a dose, only about 10% of which is unchanged, appears in the urine; 25% of a dose appears in the feces, a small part contributed by elimination in the bile.

The half-life increases with hepatic impairment, but is virtually unaffected by renal failure. In patients on continuous ambulatory peritoneal dialysis (CAPD) given 800 mg followed by 400 mg every 12 h for 10–12 days, there was no significant accumulation of pefloxacin or its metabolite, norfloxacin, but concentrations of pefloxacin *N*-oxide rose continuously in plasma and dialysate; all concentrations fell rapidly when treatment was discontinued.

Adverse reactions are those common to the group (p. 309). Most common are gastrointestinal tract disturbances, although some typical CNS reactions have been encountered. Skin eruptions (some photosensitive) occur and rashes appeared in about one-third of a group of patients who were given long-term therapy. Clinical uses are similar to those of ofloxacin.

Preparations and dosage

Proprietary name: Peflacine.
Preparations: Tablets, injection.
Dosage: Adults, oral, i.v., 400 mg every 12 h.
Available in Europe, Africa and Asia.

Further information

Gonzalez JP, Henwood JM. Pefloxacin: a review of its antibacterial activity, pharmacokinetic properties and therapeutic use. *Drugs.* 1989;37:628–668.
Symposium. Pefloxacin in clinical practice. *J Antimicrob Chemother.* 1990;26(suppl B):1–229.

PRULIFLOXACIN

A lipophilic prodrug which is very rapidly metabolized by esterase into ulifloxacin, a 6-fluoro, 7-piperazinyl thiazetoquinoline.

Ulifloxacin is moderately active against *Staph. aureus* (MIC 0.4–0.8 mg/L) and inactive against *Str. pneumoniae* (MIC 2–8 mg/L) as well as against *Enterococcus* spp. Against Enterobacteriaceae (MIC 0.05–0.8 mg/L) and *Ps. aeruginosa* (MIC 0.2–0.8 mg/L) activity is similar to that of ciprofloxacin. It is active against fastidious Gram-negative bacilli, but not against anaerobes and non-fermentative Gram-negative bacilli. Activity against *Acinetobacter* spp. is modest.

Prulifloxacin is rapidly converted into ulifloxacin and after 3 h is no longer detected in blood. In volunteers receiving a single oral dose, peak plasma concentrations of 0.68 mg/L (300 mg dose) to 1.88 mg/L (for 400 mg dose) were attained between 0.67 and 1.25 h. The mean apparent elimination half-life was 8 h and the mean cumulative elimination rate in urine within 48 h was 31–46%. Other inactive metabolites account for 7% of the dose. Half the administered dose is eliminated in feces within 72 h as ulifloxacin and 4% as prulifloxacin. Protein binding is 45%.

Preparations and dosage

Proprietary names: Glimbax, Keraflox, Primax, Pruquin, Unidrox.
Preparations: Tablets.
Dosage: Adults, oral, 600 mg per day.
Available in Italy and in Asia; under development in North America for treatment of traveler's diarrhea.

Further information

Nakashima M, Uematsu T, Kosuge K, et al. Pharmacokinetic and safety of NM 441, a new quinolone, in healthy volunteers. *J Clin Pharmacokinet.* 1994;34: 930–937.
Prats G, Rossi V, Salvatori E, Mirelis B. Prulifloxacin: a new antibacterial fluoroquinolone. *Expert Rev Anti Infect Ther.* 2006;4:27–41.
Yagi Y, Shibutani S, Hodoshima N, et al. Involvement of multiple transport systems in the disposition of an active metabolite of a pro-drug-type new quinolone antibiotic: prulifloxacin. *Drug Metab Pharmacokinet.* 2003;18:381–389.
Yoshida T, Mitshuashi S. Antibacterial activity of NM-394, the active form of prodrug NM 441, a new quinolone. *Antimicrob Agents Chemother.* 1993;37:793–800.

RUFLOXACIN

A tricyclic fluoroquinolone formulated as the hydrochloride salt. It is inactive against Gram-positive cocci with MICs >2 mg/L. It displays weak activity in vitro against Enterobacteriaceae with the MIC for most species >1 mg/L. Activity against *Ps. aeruginosa* is poor (MIC 16–32 mg/L). After loading doses of 400 and 600 mg followed with 9 days of either 200 or 300 mg, mean peak plasma levels were around 4.5–7 mg/L, respectively. The mean apparent elimination half-life was 44 h. Approximately 50% is eliminated in the urine.

It has been used in urinary tract infection and chronic prostatitis, but clinical experience is limited.

Preparations and dosage

Proprietary name: Monos, Qari, Ruflox, Tebraxin, Uroclar, Uroflox.
Preparation: Tablets.
Dosage: Adults, oral, 400 mg on day 1, followed by 200 mg per day.
Available in some countries such as Italy, Mexico and Thailand.

Further information

Boerema JBJ, Bischoff W, Focht J, Naber KG. An open multicentre study on the efficacy and safety of rufloxacin in patients with chronic bacterial prostatitis. *J Antimicrob Chemother.* 1991;28:587–597.

Kisicki JC, Griess RS, Ott CI, et al. Multiple dose pharmacokinetics and safety of rufloxacin in normal volunteers. *Antimicrob Agents Chemother.* 1992;36:1296–1301.

Mattina R, Bonfiglio G, Cocuzza CE, Gulisano G, Cesana M, Imbimbo BP. Pharmacokinetics of rufloxacin in healthy volunteers after repeated oral doses. *Chemotherapy.* 1991;37:389–397.

GROUP 3 QUINOLONES

LEVOFLOXACIN

For molecular weight and structure, see ofloxacin (p. 315). Levofloxacin is the L-isomer of ofloxacin.

ANTIBACTERIAL ACTIVITY

Levofloxacin is the active component of ofloxacin; D-ofloxacin is without significant antibacterial activity. The activity against common bacterial pathogens is shown in Table 26.3. It exhibits good activity in vitro against Gram-positive cocci (including *Str. pneumoniae*), Enterobacteriaceae, some fastidious Gram-negative bacilli and *Ps. aeruginosa* as well as chlamydiae, *Mycoplasma pneumoniae*, *L. pneumophila* and *M. tuberculosis*. MICs for *Acinetobacter* spp. and *Sten. maltophilia* are 0.06–0.25 and 0.5–2.0 mg/L, respectively. Activity against anaerobes is moderate to low.

PHARMACOKINETICS

Oral absorption	>95%
C$_{max}$ 500 mg oral	*c.* 5 mg/L after 1.5–2 h
750 mg oral	*c.* 8 mg/L after 1.5–2 h
500 mg intravenous (90-min infusion)	*c.* 6 mg/L end infusion
750 mg intravenous (90-min infusion)	*c.* 12 mg/L end infusion
Plasma half-life	6–8 h
Volume of distribution	0.6–0.8 L/kg
Plasma protein binding	<25%

Co-administration with antacids, calcium, sucralfate and heavy metals decreases bioavailability and AUC. No interactions with warfarin or theophylline have been observed. Co-administration of a non-steroidal anti-inflammatory drug may increase the risk of convulsions. It undergoes limited metabolism and is primarily eliminated unchanged in urine by both glomerular filtration and tubular secretion. The free AUC:MIC ratio for *Str. pneumoniae* increases from about 55 to 70 when the daily dosage is raised from 500 mg to 750 mg.

It is stable in plasma and does not revert to D-ofloxacin. It undergoes limited metabolism and is primarily eliminated

Table 26.3 Activity of group 3 and group 4 fluoroquinolones against common pathogenic bacteria: MIC (mg/L)

	Garenoxacin	Gatifloxacin	Gemifloxacin	Levofloxacin	Moxifloxacin	Sparfloxacin	Tosufloxacin	Trovafloxacin
Staphylococcus aureus	0.06	0.125	0.06	0.25	0.06	0.12–4	0.12	0.03–2
Streptococcus pyogenes	0.25	0.5	0.016	0.5	0.5	0.5	0.25	0.12
Str. pneumoniae	0.012	1	0.03	2	0.25	0.5	0.5	0.12
Enterococcus faecalis	2	2	2	2	0.5	1	1	0.5
Neisseria spp.	0.008	0.016	0.004	<0.06	0.016	0.004	0.06	0.015
Haemophilus influenzae	0.008	0.016	0.004	<0.06	0.06	0.025	0.06	0.03
Escherichia coli	0.016	0.06	0.008	0.25	0.06	0.05	0.5	0.12
Klebsiella pneumoniae	0.016	1	0.06	0.5	0.5	0.12	0.5	0.5
Pseudomonas aeruginosa	2	32	2	1	8	8	8	8
Bactoides fragilis	1	1	2	1	2	8	2	4
Chlamydophilia pneumoniae	0.008	0.25	0.25	0.05	0.03–0.06	0.03–0.25	0.25	0.5
Legionella pneumophilia	0.008	0.03	0.03	0.03	0.06	0.016–0.03	0.008–0.03	≤0.004
Mycoplasma pneumoniae	0.06	0.06–0.25	0.012	0.06–1	0.125–0.25	0.125	0.125–0.5	0.125–0.25
Clostridium trachomatis	0.016	0.25	No data	0.5	0.03–0.06	0.06	0.25	1
Mycobacterium tuberculosis	2	0.12	>8	0.125–1	0.25–1.0	0.5	>8	>8

unchanged in the urine. Renal clearance in excess of the glomerular filtration rate suggests that tubular secretion also occurs. Concomitant administration of either cimetidine or probenecid reduces renal clearance by approximately one-third. Clearance is reduced and half-life is prolonged in patients with impaired renal function (creatinine clearance <50 mL/min) requiring dosage adjustment in such patients.

 ## TOXICITY AND SIDE EFFECTS

Side effects have been reported in 6–7% of patients and include fever, rash and other events common to the group. Elderly patients are at increased risk of developing severe tendon disorders including rupture, a risk increased by concomitant corticosteroid therapy.

 ## CLINICAL USE

Acute bacterial sinusitis

Acute bacterial exacerbations of chronic bronchitis, community-acquired pneumonia

Uncomplicated and complicated skin and skin structure infections

Uncomplicated and complicated urinary infections including acute pyelonephritis

Chronic bacterial prostatitis

 ### Preparations and dosage

Proprietary names: Cravit, Levaquin, Oftaquix, Quixin, Tavanic.

Preparations: Tablets, injection, ophthalmic solution.

Dosage: Adults, oral, 250–750 mg per day; i.v., 250–750 mg per day. Community-acquired pneumonia, acute bacterial sinusitis, 750 mg once daily. Ophthalmic solution 0.5% (Oftaquix, Quixin).

Widely available.

 ### Further information

American Thoracic Society. Guidelines for the management of adults with community-acquired pneumonia. Diagnosis, assessment of severity, antimicrobial therapy, and prevention. *Am J Respir Crit Care Med.* 2001;163:1730–1754.

Chien S-C, Wong FA, Fowler CL, et al. Double-blind evaluation of the safety and pharmacokinetics of multiple oral once-daily 750-milligram and 1-gram doses of levofloxacin in healthy volunteers. *Antimicrob Agents Chemother.* 1998;42:885–888.

Dunbar LM, Wunderink RG, Habib MP, et al. High-dose short-course levofloxacin for community-acquired pneumonia: a new treatment paradigm. *Clin Infect Dis.* 2003;37:752–760.

Sprandel KA, Schreiver CA, Pendland SL, et al. Pharmacokinetics and pharmacodynamics of intravenous levofloxacin at 750 milligrams and various doses of metronidazole in healthy adult subjects. *Antimicrob Agents Chemother.* 2004;48:4597–4605.

 ## GATIFLOXACIN

Activity against common bacterial pathogens is shown in Table 26.3 (p. 319). The spectrum includes *Acinetobacter* spp. and *Aeromonas* spp. but it is not very active against *Ps. aeruginosa* and other non-fermentative Gram-negative rods. It is more active against methicillin-susceptible strains of staphylococci than methicillin-resistant strains. It is also active against *Chlamydia*, *Mycoplasma* and *Legionella* spp. and has some activity against anaerobes.

It is almost completely absorbed when given orally and is widely distributed throughout the body into many body tissues and fluids. The plasma half-life is 6–8 h. More than 70% of the drug is excreted unchanged in the urine. Renal clearance is reduced by 57% in moderate renal insufficiency and by 77% in severe renal insufficiency.

Prolongation of the QTc interval in some patients and interference with diabetes mellitus have resulted in withdrawal of the drug in most countries for systemic usage. Gatifloxacin remains in use in North America only as an ophthalmic solution.

 ### Further information

Dembry LM, Farrington JM, Andriole VT. Fluoroquinolone antibiotics: adverse effects and safety profiles. *Infect Dis Clin Pract.* 1999;8:9–16.

Hosaka M, Kinoshita S, Royama A, Otsuki M, Nishino T. Antibacterial properties of AM-1155, a new methoxy quinolone. *J Antimicrob Chemother.* 1995;36:293–301.

Park-Wyllien LY, Juurlink DN, Kopp A, et al. Outpatient gatifloxacin therapy and dysglycemia in older patients. *N Engl J Med.* 2006;354:1352–1361.

 ## SPARFLOXACIN

Activity against common bacterial pathogens is shown in Table 26.3 (p. 319). It is highly active against most aerobic Gram-positive cocci and Gram-negative bacilli, including fastidious Gram-negative bacilli, *Acinetobacter* spp., *Campylobacter* spp. and *Legionella* spp. *Ps. aeruginosa* is weakly susceptible. Activity also extends to the genital mycoplasmas, *M. tuberculosis* and *M. avium* complex isolates. It is moderately active against some anaerobes (including the *B. fragilis* group); *L. monocytogenes* is resistant.

It is well absorbed, achieving a plasma concentration of 1–1.5 mg/L 4.5 h after a 400 mg oral dose. Absorption is decreased in the presence of antacids owing to the formation of chelates with metallic ions. Concentrations in many tissues, including lung, exceed those in plasma. The plasma half-life is 15–20 h. CSF penetration is limited. Around 5–10% of a dose is eliminated unchanged in the urine, with about 30% appearing as the glucuronide. Total clearance is 10–15 L/h. The plasma half-life increases only modestly in renal failure to 30–40 h. About 50–60% of the dose appears as unchanged drug in the feces, mainly as the glucuronide, accounting for 10–20% of the administered dose.

Adverse events are those common to fluoroquinolones (p. 309), in particular gastrointestinal tract disturbances, CNS effects (mainly headache and insomnia) and rashes. Photosensitivity reactions have been observed in 2–11% of patients. It can prolong the QTc interval and cases of torsade de pointes have been reported. It does not potentiate the toxicity of theophylline.

It has been used for respiratory and other infections caused by susceptible bacteria, but use has been restricted in the USA and Europe because of phototoxicity and cardiotoxicity.

Preparations and dosage

Proprietary name: Zagam.

Preparation: Tablets.

Dosage: Adult, oral, loading dose of 400 mg on day 1; maintenance doses of 200 mg per day thereafter.

Restricted use in the USA and the European Union but available in Asia.

Further information

Andriole VT, ed. *The Quinolones.* 3rd ed. San Diego: Academic Press; 2000.

Canton N, Peman J, Jimenez MT, Ramon MS, Gobemado M. In vitro activity of sparfloxacin compared with those of five other quinolones. *Antimicrob Agents Chemother.* 1992;36:558–565.

Shimada J, Nogita T, Ishibashi Y. Clinical pharmacokinetics of sparfloxacin. *Clin Pharmacokinet.* 1993;25:358–369.

TOSUFLOXACIN

Activity against common bacterial pathogens is shown in Table 26.3 (p. 319). It is active against a wide range of Gram-positive and Gram-negative bacteria, including *Acinetobacter* spp., *L. pneumophila* and *Campylobacter* spp. Unlike many quinolones it is moderately active against *L. monocytogenes. C. trachomatis* is also moderately susceptible. It is active against some anaerobes, including the *B. fragilis* group. Activity against *Mycobacterium* spp. is limited. It is well absorbed by the oral route, achieving a plasma concentration of *c.* 1 mg/L 4 h after a 300 mg dose. Around 30–35% of the dose is eliminated in the urine, with an apparent elimination half-life of 6–7 h.

Clinical experience is limited, but high clinical and bacteriological cure rates have been obtained in patients with skin and soft-tissue infections.

Preparations and dosage

Proprietary names: Ozex, Tosuxacin.

Preparation: Tablets.

Dosage: Adult, oral, 150 mg every 8 h.

Available in Japan; not available in the USA or the European Union.

Further information

Barry AL, Fuchs PC. In vitro activities of sparfloxacin, tosufloxacin, ciprofloxacin and fleroxacin. *Antimicrob Agents Chemother.* 1991;35:955–960.

GROUP 4 QUINOLONES

GEMIFLOXACIN

Molecular weight: 389.4.

A fluoronaphthyridone derivative with a dual substituted pyrrolidine moiety at the C-7 position. It is formulated as the mesylate.

ANTIBACTERIAL ACTIVITY

Activity against common bacterial pathogens is shown in Table 26.3 (p. 319). The broad antibacterial spectrum embraces most Gram-positive cocci (including high potency against *Str. pneumoniae*) and Gram-negative bacilli. It possesses a high affinity for pneumococcal topoisomerase IV. Activity against Gram-negative respiratory tract pathogens such as *H. influenzae, Mor. catarrhalis, Ch. pneumoniae, L. pneumophila* and *Mycoplasma pneumonia* is good. It is relatively inactive against *Ps. aeruginosa* and *Enterococcus* spp. Activity against Enterobacteriaceae is similar to that of moxifloxacin but it is less potent against anaerobes. Gemifloxacin is inactive against *M. tuberculosis.* Activity against *Nocardia asteroides* (MIC 0.5–1 mg/L) is better than that of other quinolones other than the investigational compound nemonoxacin (*see below*).

Multistep resistance studies suggest that it is less likely than other quinolones to select for quinolone-resistant *Str. pneumoniae* strains. Because it inhibits both DNA gyrase and DNA topoisomerase IV enzyme systems at therapeutically relevant drug levels in *Str. pneumoniae*, single mutations in *parC* or *gyrA* result in only a small increase in the MIC. In *Str. pneumoniae gyrA* mutations arise at a lower rate (1.6×10^{-11}) than mutations in *parC*. It seems to be unaffected clinically by quinolone efflux mechanisms in *Str. pneumoniae*. Low rates of resistance selection have also been reported in *H. influenzae*.

PHARMACOKINETICS

Oral absorption	71%
C_{max} 320 mg oral	1.6 mg/L after 0.5–2 h
Plasma half-life	c. 7 h
Volume of distribution	4.97 L/kg
Plasma protein binding	60–70%

Absorption and distribution

In oral escalating dose studies (single doses of 20–800 mg), C_{max} ranged from 0.12 to 4.33 mg/L after an average of 1 h.

Antacids significantly reduce the systemic availability and protein binding is relatively high. Excellent concentrations are achieved in serum as well as various tissues such as bronchial mucosa, epithelial lining fluid and alveolar macrophages. Absolute bioavailability of the 320 mg oral tablet is around 71%. Pharmacokinetics are not significantly altered when administered with a high fat meal.

Metabolism and excretion

The apparent elimination half-life ranges from 6 to 9 h, and 26–40% of administered doses are eliminated in urine. It is metabolized to a limited extent in the liver. Cytochrome P_{450} enzymes do not play an important role in metabolism, and the metabolic activity of these enzymes is unaffected. Around 65% of the parent compound and its metabolites are eliminated in the feces and the remainder in the urine. The mean renal clearance after repeated doses of 320 mg is about 11.6 L/h, indicating active renal secretion. The mean apparent elimination half-life at steady state following administration of 320 mg to healthy subjects was approximately 7 h. No dosage adjustment is recommended in patients with mild, moderate or severe hepatic impairment. Clearance is reduced and plasma elimination is prolonged in patients with renal insufficiency, leading to an average increase in AUC values of c. 70%. Hemodialysis removes approximately 20–30% of an oral dose from plasma.

 ## TOXICITY AND SIDE EFFECTS

The most commonly reported side effects are diarrhea (3.6%), rash (2.8%) and nausea (2.7%). No evidence has emerged of a clinically significant prolongation in QTc interval. The phototoxicity potential is low and similar to that seen with ciprofloxacin. The overall incidence of drug-related rash is 2.8%. The rash is most commonly mild, macropapular (occasionally urticarial), predominantly self-limiting, and mainly occurs in women under 40 years and in postmenopausal women on hormone replacement therapy after ≥10 days.

 ## CLINICAL USE

Community-acquired pneumonia in adults

Acute exacerbations of chronic bronchitis in adults

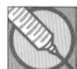 ### Preparations and dosage

Proprietary name: Factive.

Preparation: Tablets.

Dosage: Adults, 320 mg once daily for 5–7 days.

Available in the USA; not available in Europe.

 ### Further information

Allen A, Bygate E, Oliver S, et al. Pharmacokinetics and tolerability of gemifloxacin (SB-265805) after administration of single oral doses to healthy volunteers. *Antimicrob Agents Chemother.* 2000;44:1604–1608.

Appelbaum PC, Gillespie SH, Burley CJ, Tillotson GS. Antimicrobial selection for community-acquired lower respiratory tract infections in the 21st century: a review of gemifloxacin. *Int J Antimicrob Agents.* 2004;23:533–546.

MOXIFLOXACIN

Molecular weight: 401.4.

A fluoroquinolone substituted with an 8-methoxy group and a 7-diazabicyclononyl moiety, formulated as the hydrochloride for oral or intravenous use.

 ## ANTIBACTERIAL ACTIVITY

Activity against common bacterial pathogens is shown in Table 26.3 (p. 319). It displays good activity in vitro against Enterobacteriaceae and fastidious Gram-negative bacilli such as *H. influenzae* and *Mor. catarrhalis*, as well as against Gram-positive cocci including *Str. pneumoniae*, but is poorly active against *Enterococcus* spp. Activity against non-fermentative Gram-negative bacilli is species dependent: *Acinetobacter* spp. (MIC 0.006–2.0 mg/L) and *Sten. maltophilia* (MIC 0.5–2.0 mg/L) are partially susceptible in vitro, but it has poor activity against *Ps. aeruginosa* and other non-fermenting Gram-negative rods. It displays good in-vitro activity against *Ch. pneumoniae*, *C. trachomatis*, mycoplasmas (including *M. pneumoniae*), *L. pneumophila* and *B. fragilis*. Although highly active against *M. tuberculosis*, it is less active against the *M. avium* complex, *M. intracellulare*, *M. chelonei* and *M. fortuitum*.

PHARMACOKINETICS

Oral absorption	86%
C$_{max}$ 400 mg oral	1.62–3.8 mg/L after 1–2 h
400 mg i.v. infusion (1 h, single dose)	3.6 mg/L end infusion
Plasma half-life	12–15 h
Volume of distribution	11.6 L/kg
Plasma protein binding	40%

Absorption and distribution

By the oral route, drug uptake is rapid, with moderate variability. As with all quinolones iron and antacids significantly reduce the bioavailability. No significant drug interactions with theophylline, itraconazole, probenecid or oral contraceptives have been found. In escalating dose studies (50–80 mg doses), C$_{max}$ and AUC values increased proportionally to the dose.

It is widely distributed throughout the body and into many tissues in concentrations exceeding those in plasma. Around 50–80% of plasma concentrations penetrate into CSF if the meninges are inflamed. The apparent plasma half-life is 15.6 h.

Metabolism and excretion

Biliary elimination and metabolism are the main elimination pathways. About 19.3% of the administered dose is eliminated in the urine, with a bioavailability of 86.2%. Urinary excretion is via glomerular filtration and tubular reabsorption. Two main metabolites are recovered: M1 (a sulfocompound) and M2 (a glucuronide). M1 is mainly eliminated in feces (34.4%) and only 2.5% in urine; M2 is eliminated in urine (13.8%).

TOXICITY AND SIDE EFFECTS

Adverse events are similar to those for other fluoroquinolones. Phototoxicity rates are not significantly above placebo levels. Gastrointestinal side effects are the most common, particularly nausea, diarrhea, abdominal pain and vomiting. Dizziness and headache may occur as well as allergic reactions. Attention has been drawn to a potential to cause life-threatening hepatotoxicity. Moxifloxacin has the potential to prolong the QTc interval in some patients but the clinical significance of this phenomenon is unclear.

CLINICAL USE

> Acute bacterial exacerbations of chronic bronchitis and community-acquired pneumonia
>
> Acute bacterial sinusitis
>
> Treatment of complicated skin and soft-tissue infections caused by methicillin-susceptible *Staph. aureus* and Gram-negative rods (i.v. formulation)
>
> Treatment of complicated intra-abdominal infections (i.v. formulation)

Preparations and dosage

Proprietary name: Avelox.

Preparations: Tablets, ophthalmic drops, i.v. infusion.

Dosage: Adults, oral, 400 mg tablets once daily; i.v. infusion 400 mg per day for 5–14 days.

Widely available.

Further information

Ackerman G, Schaumann R, Pless B, et al. Comparative activity of moxifloxacin in vitro against obligately anaerobic bacteria. *Eur J Clin. Microbiol Infect Dis.* 2000;19:229–232.

Church D, Haverstock D, Andriole VT. Moxifloxacin: a review of its safety profile based on worldwide clinical trials. *Today's Therapeutic Trends.* 2000;18:205–223.

Stass H, Dahloff A, Kubitza D, Schühly U. Pharmacokinetics, safety and tolerability of ascending single doses of moxifloxacin, a new 8-methoxy quinolone, administered in healthy subjects. *Antimicrob Agents Chemother.* 1998;42:2060–2065.

Stass H, Kubitza D. Pharmacokinetics and elimination of moxifloxacin after oral and intravenous administration in man. *J Antimicrob Chemother.* 1999;43(suppl B):83–90.

OTHER GROUP 4 QUINOLONES

GARENOXACIN

An oral and parenteral des-fluoro(6) quinolone formulated as the mesylate. Activity against common bacterial pathogens is shown in Table 26.3 (p. 319). Activity in vitro against Enterobacteriaceae is similar to that of moxifloxacin. It is extremely active against *L. pneumophila* and is one of the most active quinolones against *Ch. pneumoniae* and *C. trachomatis*, as well as *M. pneumoniae* and *Ureaplasma urealyticum* (MIC 0.12–0.25 mg/L). It is poorly active or inactive against non-fermentative Gram-negative bacilli including *Ps. aeruginosa* but exhibits very good activity against Gram-positive cocci including methicillin-susceptible *Staph. aureus* and *Str. pneumoniae*. It is one of the most active quinolones against Gram-positive and Gram-negative anaerobes: 93% of isolates are inhibited by a concentration of 2 mg/L. Activity in vitro against *M. tuberculosis* is weak and it has no useful activity against *M. leprae* in mouse footpad tests.

After a single dose peak plasma levels vary between 1.2 mg/L (100 mg dose) and 16.3 mg/L (1200 mg dose). The apparent terminal half-life is around 11 h and protein binding is *c.* 80%. Main metabolites found in plasma, urine and feces include sulfate conjugates and glucuronides. Urinary elimination rates of approximately 31% and 43% at 24 h and 72 h, respectively, are found. Maximum plasma concentrations decrease by 20–52% in patients with severely impaired renal function and activity is slightly reduced in patients with moderately or severely impaired hepatic function. About 1.5–11% is removed by CAPD and hemodialysis.

Drugs containing aluminum, magnesium, calcium, iron and zinc decrease the activity. The incidence of hypotension tends to increase when it is co-administered parenterally with nitroglycerine or isosorbide nitrate. It is hardly metabolized by cytochrome P_{450}.

Clinically significant adverse effects include: shock or anaphylactoid reactions; hypotension; Stevens–Johnson syndrome; bradycardia; sinus arrest or atrioventricular block; hepatic function disorder with raised liver enzymes; hypoglycemia; pseudomembranous colitis; agranulocytosis; and rhabdomyolysis.

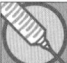

Preparations and dosage

Proprietary name: Geninax.
Preparation: Tablets.
Dosage: 400 mg once daily.
Available in Japan.

Further information

Fung-Tomc JC, Minassian B, Kolek B, et al. Antibacterial spectrum of a novel desfluoro(6) quinolone, BMS-284756. *Antimicrob Agents Chemother.* 2000;44:3351–3356.
Liebetrau A, Rodloff AC, Behra-Miellet J, Dubreuil L. In vitro activities of a new desfluoro(6) quinolone, garenoxacin, against clinical anaerobic bacteria. *Antimicrob Agents Chemother.* 2003;47:3667–3671.

SITAFLOXACIN

A group 4 quinolone formulated for oral or intravenous use. In-vitro activity is similar to or better than that of moxifloxacin. The antibacterial spectrum covers Gram-positive and Gram-negative bacteria including anaerobes. It has a chlorine atom at the C-8 position, and therefore has potential for phototoxicity. Early interest in this compound has not been maintained, but it is available in Japan.

Preparations and dosage

Proprietary name: Gracevit.
Preparations: Tablets, i.v. infusion.
Dosage: 400 mg once daily.
Available in Japan.

TROVAFLOXACIN

A trifluoroquinolone, formulated as the mesylate for oral administration and as a prodrug formulation (alatrofloxacin mesylate) for parenteral use. Activity against common bacterial pathogens is shown in Table 26.3 (p. 319). It is active against a wide range of Gram-positive and Gram-negative micro-organisms, including *L. pneumophila* and *L. monocytogenes*. It is inactive against *Ps. aeruginosa* and against non-fermentative Gram-negative bacilli such as *Sten. maltophilia* and *Burkholderia cepacia*. Most anaerobes other than *Clostridium difficile* are susceptible.

The mesylate is very well absorbed, achieving a plasma concentration of *c.* 2.5 mg/L 1 h after an oral dose. The apparent plasma half-life is 11 h.

Hepatotoxicity, sometimes with clinical jaundice and life-threatening acute liver failure, has been reported, resulting in withdrawal of the oral and intravenous formulations of the drug. It is no longer recommended for clinical use except as noted below.

Preparations and dosage

Proprietary name: Trovan.
Dosage: Adult, 200–300 mg i.v. infusion once daily. Oral, 100–200 mg once daily.
Available in the USA only as a compliance pack with azithromycin (see p. 287) for single-dose treatment of gonococcal and non-gonococcal urethritis. Limited availability elsewhere.

Further information

Garey KW, Amsden GW. Trovafloxacin: an overview. *Pharmacotherapy.* 1999;19:21–34.
Haria M, Lamb HM. Trovafloxacin. *Drugs.* 1997;54:435–445.

QUINOLONES USED SOLELY FOR TOPICAL INFECTIONS

BESIFLOXACIN

An amino-azepinyl quinolone formulated as a suspension for ophthalmic usage. It exhibits good antistaphylococcal activity, as well as activity against *Str. pneumoniae*, Enterobacteriaceae, *H. influenzae* and *Mor. catarrhalis*. It is weakly active against *Corynebacterium* spp. and has no useful activity against *Ps. aeruginosa*. After instillation into the eye, less than 0.1% of the drug reaches the plasma. It is used for bacterial conjunctivitis.

Preparations and dosage

Proprietary name: Besivance.

Preparation: 0.6% suspension.

Available in the USA.

Further information

Tepedino ME, Heller WH, Usner DW, et al. Phase II efficacy and safety study of besifloxacin ophthalmic suspension 0.6% in the treatment of bacterial conjunctivitis. *Curr Med Res Opin*. 2009;25:1159–1169.

NADIFLOXACIN

A lipophilic tricyclic fluorobenzoquinoline with a 4-hydroxylpiperinyl moiety at the C-8 position, formulated as a cream for topical use. It is active against many Gram-positive bacteria involved in skin infections, including *Propionibacterium acnes* (MIC 0.25–2.0 mg/L), and *Staph. aureus* (MIC 0.015–2 mg/L). It appears to inhibit the generation of reactive oxygen species by neutrophils. The sodium salt is used as a 1% cream for use in acne vulgaris and cutaneous staphylococcal infections.

Preparations and dosage

Proprietary name: Acuatim, Nadiflox, Nadixa, Nadoxin.

Preparation: 1% cream.

Available in Japan and some European countries (e.g. Spain, Germany, Russia).

INVESTIGATIONAL QUINOLONES

Current research is mainly focused on derivatives able to overcome quinolone resistance or with activity against mycobacteria. Compounds in development at the time of writing include the following:

- **Delafloxacin** (WQ 3034, ABT 492). It exhibits a broad antibacterial spectrum with expanded activity against Gram-positive organisms, including *Enterococcus* spp., and quinolone-resistant *Str. pneumoniae* and *Staph. aureus* that owe their resistance to efflux. Activity against *Ps. aeruginosa* is similar to that of ciprofloxacin (MIC 0.06–0.25 mg/L), but it is not active against ciprofloxacin-resistant Enterobacteriaceae. It has good in-vitro activity against *Helicobacter pylori*, *M. tuberculosis* and anaerobes. It is active against *Ch. pneumoniae* (MIC 0.125 mg/L) and *M. pneumoniae* (MIC 0.25–8 mg/L). In oral dosing studies peak plasma concentrations of 1.4 mg/L (100 mg dose) to 11.5 mg/L (1200 mg dose) were reached in around 1 h. The apparent elimination half-life is about 4 h.

- **Levonadifloxacin** (WCK 771). A derivative of nadifloxacin formulated for parenteral use; an oral prodrug (WCK 2349) has also been synthesized. The *S* (−) isomer is 64–256 times more active than the *R* (+) isomer and twice as active as the racemate (nadifloxacin). It is more active than levofloxacin against *Str. pneumoniae* (MIC 0.5 mg/L) and displays potent antistaphylococcal activity (MIC 0.03 mg/L); strains resistant to methicillin and quinolones are inhibited by 0.5–1 mg/L. It has good overall activity in vitro against Gram-positive and Gram-negative anaerobic bacteria. At the end of a 1 h infusion, plasma concentrations ranged from 2 mg/L (50 mg dose) to 28 mg/L (800 mg dose). The apparent elimination half-life was around 5–6 h. Less than 5% of the parent compound is eliminated in urine, and 20% as glucuronate and sulfate metabolites.

- **Nemonoxacin**. A 6(des)-fluoro quinolone. It displays good activity in vitro against *Staph. aureus* (MIC 0.03–0.06 mg/L) including strains resistant to other quinolones (MIC 1–2 mg/L) and is highly active against *Str. pneumoniae* (MIC ≤0.03–0.06 mg/L). It is inactive against *M. tuberculosis*. Absorption after oral administration is rapid; the peak plasma concentration ranges from 0.37 mg/L (50 mg dose) to 12.1 mg/L (1500 mg dose) with a long apparent elimination half-life (*c*. 10–13 h). It is mainly eliminated in urine (around 50%). The protein binding is 16%. Food affects the pharmacokinetics by delaying absorption. After repeated doses, the half-life increases significantly and steady state is reached after 3–5 days.

- **Zabofloxacin** (DW 224a). An analog of gemifloxacin anticipated to have better tolerability. It exhibits good in-vitro activity against Gram-positive cocci including *Str. pneumoniae* and *Staph. aureus*. It displays a bimodal distribution of activity against *Ps. aeruginosa* and *Sten. maltophilia*. Activity against Enterobacteriaceae is similar to that of ofloxacin. It is inactive against *Enterococcus* spp. but is very active against *H. influenzae*. After single oral ascending doses, peak plasma concentrations ranged from 0.7 mg/L (200 mg dose) to 3.6 mg/L (800 mg dose) after an average of 2 h. The mean apparent elimination half-life was 6 h. Protein binding was 77%.

Further information

De Souza NJ, Gupte SV, Deshpande PK, et al. A chiral benzoquilizine-2-carboxylic acid arginine salt active against vancomycin-resistant *Staphylococcus aureus*. *J Med Chem*. 2005;48:5232–5242.

Jacobs MR, Appelbaum PC. Nadifloxacin: a quinolone for topical treatment of skin infections and potential for systemic use of its active isomer, WCK 771. *Expert Opin Pharmacother*. 2006;7:1957–1966.

Kwon AR, Min YH, Ryu JM, Choi DR, Shim MJ, Choi CC. In vitro and in vivo activities of DW-224a, a novel fluoroquinolone antibiotic agent. *J Antimicrob Chemother*. 2006;58:684–688.

Nilius AM, Shen LL, Hensey-Rudloff D, et al. In vitro antibacterial potency and spectrum of ABT-492, a new fluoroquinolone. *Antimicrob Agents Chemother*. 2003;47:3260–3269.

Patel M, de Souza NJ, Gupta SV, et al. Antistaphylococcal activity of WCK 771, a tricyclic fluoroquinolone, in an animal infection model. *Antimicrob Agents Chemother*. 2004;48:4754–4761.

CHAPTER

27 Rifamycins

Francesco Parenti and Giancarlo Lancini

The rifamycins are a family of antibiotics produced by an actinomycete now classified as *Amycolatopsis mediterranei*. All the therapeutically useful rifamycins are semisynthetic derivatives of rifamycin B, a fermentation product that is poorly active, but easily produced and readily converted chemically into rifamycin S, from which most active derivatives are prepared. They all share the general structure:

Natural products like rifamycins, which are characterized by an aromatic ring spanned by an aliphatic bridge (ansa) are called 'ansamycins'. To this class belong the streptovaricins and the tolypomycins (chemically and biologically similar to rifamycins) and geldanamycin and the maytansines, which have quite different, antiblastic, biological activities. Among the vast number of rifamycin derivatives investigated, rifampicin (rifampin) is by far the most important and most widely used. Various others, notably rifabutin, rifapentine and rifaximin, are also in use in various parts of the world. Rifamycin SV and rifamide are much less widely available.

Interest in these antibiotics centers on their potent activity against pathogenic Gram-positive cocci and mycobacteria. Knowledge of the general properties of the group is largely based on extensive study and use of rifampicin but, insofar as they have been investigated, the main features are exhibited also by the other congeners:

- Bactericidal action through inactivation of bacterial DNA-dependent RNA polymerase
- Mechanism of resistance consisting of mutation of specific amino acids in the β-chain of RNA polymerase

- Relatively high frequency of resistant mutants; resistance is not horizontally transferable
- Significant biliary excretion and stimulation of hepatic metabolism.

The structure of RNA polymerase is highly conserved among bacteria and when tested in cell-free systems all rifamycins present similar intrinsic activity. Differences in the minimum inhibitory concentration (MIC) values among the various congeners are caused by different abilities to penetrate into cells. Rifamycins also inhibit the RNA polymerase of eukaryotic organelles, such as mitochondria, since these are of a prokaryotic type. Some rifamycins carrying a large lipophilic chain inhibit eukaryotic RNA and DNA polymerases and viral reverse transcriptases. These effects have no clinical significance.

The different congeners differ substantially in their pharmacokinetic behavior and in their therapeutic efficacy. The principal use of rifampicin and rifapentine is in the treatment of tuberculosis and leprosy. Rifabutin is approved for the prevention of mycobacterial infections in AIDS patients. Rifampicin proved so important in the treatment of tuberculosis that in many countries its use was restricted to that indication for fear that more widespread use would encourage the emergence of resistant *Mycobacterium tuberculosis* strains. Those fears have proven to be exaggerated and interest has been increasingly refocused on what was originally anticipated to be an important use: treatment of severe Gram-positive infections. To prevent emergence of resistance, co-administration of another effective agent is required.

Rifaximin does not encourage emergence of resistance in mycobacteria and is used in the treatment of gastrointestinal infections. Rifamycin SV and rifamide were originally released for the treatment of infections with susceptible Gram-positive organisms and infections of the biliary tract.

Further information

Pelizza G, Lancini GC, Allievi GC, Gallo GG. The influence of lipophilicity on the antibacterial activity of rifamycins. *Farmaco (Società Chimica Italiana)*. 1973;28:298–315.

Riva S, Silvestri G. Rifamycins: a general view. *Annu Rev Microbiol*. 1972;26:199–224.

Sensi P, Lancini GC. Inhibitors of transcribing enzymes: rifamycins and related agents. In: Hansch C, Sammes PG, Taylor JB, eds. *Comprehensive medicinal chemistry*. Vol. 2. Oxford: Pergamon; 1990:793–811.

RIFABUTIN

Rifabutine; ansamycin. Molecular weight: 847.02.

A semisynthetic spiropiperidyl derivative of rifamycin S, available for oral administration. It is slightly soluble in water and soluble in organic solvents.

ANTIMICROBIAL ACTIVITY

The activity is similar to that of rifampicin, but it is more active against the *Mycobacterium avium* complex (MIC 0.01–2 mg/L) (Table 27.1) and several other atypical mycobacteria.

It inhibits the replication of human immunodeficiency virus 1 (HIV-1) in concentrations (10 mg/L) that are not toxic to lymphoid cells, but no efficacy on HIV infections has been demonstrated.

ACQUIRED RESISTANCE

The frequency of spontaneously resistant mutants in several bacterial species, including *M. tuberculosis*, *M. leprae*, *Staphylococcus aureus* and *Chlamydia trachomatis*, is somewhat lower than with rifampicin.

Table 27.1 Activity of rifabutin and rifampicin on clinical isolates of *M. avium* complex strains (MIC for 90% of strains)

Organism	Rifampicin	Rifabutin
Mycobacterium avium	4	0.4
M. intracellulare	2	0.5
M. avium complex (AIDS patients)	2	1
(non-AIDS patients)	4	2

PHARMACOKINETICS

Oral absorption	12–20%
C_{max} 300 mg oral	0.38 mg/L after 3.3 h
Plasma half-life	16 h
Volume of distribution	9.3 L/kg
Plasma protein binding	85%

Absorption and distribution

Oral absorption is rapid but incomplete, with considerable interpatient variation. It is well distributed, concentrations in many organs being higher than that in plasma. The average concentration in lungs is 6.5 times the simultaneous plasma concentration.

Metabolism and excretion

Rifabutin is mainly metabolized to the active desacetyl derivative, although several other oxidation products have been detected in urine, where some 10% of the dose is eliminated. About 30–50% of the dose can be recovered from the feces. Elimination from plasma is biphasic, with a terminal half-life of 45 h. The drug is a weak inducer of hepatic enzymes. The rate of metabolism increases, and the plasma area under the concentration–time curve (AUC) declines as the treatment continues.

INTERACTIONS

Clarithromycin and ritonavir both inhibit cytochrome P_{450}, resulting in decreased metabolism and increased plasma levels of rifabutin when the drugs are used together. Association with delavirdine should be avoided.

TOXICITY AND SIDE EFFECTS

Rash (4% of patients), gastrointestinal intolerance (3%) and neutropenia (2%) are fairly common and may require discontinuation of treatment. Uveitis and general arthralgia are rare with a 300 mg dosage, but frequent with higher dosages, especially with concomitant use of fluconazole or macrolide antibiotics.

CLINICAL USE

Prevention of infections with *M. avium* complex in AIDS patients

Treatment of non-tuberculous mycobacterial disease (in combination with other agents)

Rifabutin in combination with other agents has been proposed as a rescue therapy after *Helicobacter pylori* treatment failures.

Although some efficacy has been observed in the treatment of tuberculosis, its use for this condition is not recommended.

Preparations and dosage

Proprietary name: Mycobutin.

Preparation: Capsules.

Dosage: Adults, oral, prophylaxis of *M. avium* complex infections in immunocompromised patients with low CD4 count, 300 mg per day as a single dose. Treatment of non-tuberculous mycobacterial disease, in combination with other drugs, 450–600 mg per day as a single dose for up to 6 months after cultures become negative. Treatment of pulmonary tuberculosis, in combination with other drugs, 150–450 mg per day as a single dose for at least 6 months.

Widely available, including the UK and the USA.

Further information

Brogden RN, Fitton A. Rifabutin – a review of its antimicrobial activity, pharmacokinetic properties and therapeutic efficacy. *Drugs.* 1994;47:983–1009.

Gisbert JP, Gisbert JL, Marcos S, Jimenez-Alonso I, Moreno-Otero R, Pajares JM. Empirical rescue therapy after *Helicobacter pylori* treatment failure: a 10 year single-centre study of 500 patients. *Aliment Pharmacol Ther.* 2008;27:346–354.

Griffith DE, Brown BA, Girard WM, Wallace RJ. Adverse events associated with high dose rifabutin in macrolide containing regimens for the treatment of *Mycobacterium avium* complex lung disease. *Clin Infect Dis.* 1995;21:594–598.

Kuper JJ, D'Aprile M. Drug–drug interactions of clinical significance in the treatment of patients with *Mycobacterium avium* disease. *Clin Pharmacokinet.* 2000;39:203–214.

Skinner MH, Hsieh M, Torseth J, et al. Pharmacokinetics of rifabutin. *Antimicrob Agents Chemother.* 1989;33:1237–1241.

RIFAMPICIN

Rifampin (USAN). Molecular weight: 822.95.

A semisynthetic derivative of rifamycin SV, available for oral administration or intravenous infusion and in several combined formulations with other antimycobacterial drugs. It is poorly soluble in water, but soluble in organic solvents.

ANTIMICROBIAL ACTIVITY

The activity against common bacterial pathogens is shown in Table 27.2. It exhibits potent activity in vitro against Gram-positive cocci, including methicillin-resistant staphylococci (MIC <0.025–0.5 mg/L) and penicillin-resistant pneumococci. Enterococci are less susceptible. Gram-positive bacilli, including *Bacillus* spp., *Clostridium difficile*, *Corynebacterium* spp. and *Listeria monocytogenes*, are highly susceptible (MIC 0.025–0.5 mg/L). The pathogenic *Neisseria* and *Moraxella* spp. are also highly susceptible.

Enteric Gram-negative bacteria are generally less sensitive (MIC 1–32 mg/L), but *Bacteroides fragilis* is highly susceptible. Among other Gram-negative bacilli, *Haemophilus influenzae*, *H. ducreyi*, *Flavobacterium meningosepticum* and *Legionella* spp. are highly susceptible (MIC <0.025–2 mg/L). *Chlamydia trachomatis* and *Chlamydophila psittaci* are inhibited by low concentrations (0.025–0.5 mg/L).

Most strains of *M. tuberculosis*, *M. kansasii* and *M. marinum* are inhibited by <0.01–0.1 mg/L, but *M. fortuitum* and members of the *M. avium* complex are resistant. *M. leprae* is highly sensitive.

Rifampicin is active against some eukaryotic parasites through inhibition of the prokaryote-like polymerase of kinetoplasts or mitochondria. Maturation of *Plasmodium falciparum* is inhibited by 2–10 mg/L; at higher concentrations *Leishmania* spp. are also inhibited.

High concentrations inhibit growth of a variety of poxviruses by interference with viral particle maturation; viral reverse transcriptase is unaffected.

Table 27.2 Activity of rifampicin against common pathogenic bacteria

Organism	MIC (mg/L)
Staphylococcus aureus	0.008–0.06
Streptococcus pyogenes	0.03–0.1
Str. pneumoniae	0.06–4
Enterococcus faecalis	1–4
Mycobacterium tuberculosis	0.1–1
Neisseria gonorrhoeae	0.06–0.5
N. meningitidis	0.01–0.5
Haemophilus influenzae	0.5–1
Escherichia coli	8–16
Klebsiella pneumoniae	16–32
Pseudomonas aeruginosa	32–64

ANTIMICROBIAL INTERACTIONS

Because of the relative ease with which resistant mutants emerge, rifampicin is normally used in combination with unrelated antibiotics. Combination with β-lactam agents or glycopeptides (vancomycin and teicoplanin) in vitro usually results in antagonism or indifference, but synergy with penicillins is found in some strains of *Staph. aureus* and the combination has proved effective in some cases in vivo. Rifampicin antagonizes the bactericidal effect of ciprofloxacin against *Staph. aureus*. Synergy with aminoglycosides occurs in vitro against *Escherichia coli* and with polymyxin B against multiresistant *Serratia marcescens*. Synergy with trimethoprim against enterobacteria, streptococci and staphylococci has been reported, but others have found indifference, or sometimes antagonism, and there appears to be substantial individual strain variation. Synergy with erythromycin, clindamycin and other antistaphylococcal agents has been demonstrated against some strains of *Staph. aureus*.

In-vitro activity against *M. tuberculosis* is increased in the presence of streptomycin and isoniazid, but not ethambutol. Synergy with amphotericin B against *Candida albicans* and against the mycelial phase of *Coccidioides immitis* is seen in vitro. However, this is not a clinically useful interaction.

 ## ACQUIRED RESISTANCE

Most large bacterial populations contain resistant mutants, which readily emerge in the presence of the drug and can emerge during treatment. The mutation rate to resistance in *Staph. aureus*, *Str. pyogenes*, *Str. pneumoniae*, *Esch. coli* and *Proteus mirabilis* is about 10^{-7} and that to *M. tuberculosis* and *M. marinum* 10^{-9}–10^{-10}. Primary resistance in *M. tuberculosis* remained low for many years, but is increasing.

Resistance is of the one-step type, and several classes of mutants exhibiting different degrees of resistance can be selected by exposing a large population to a relatively low concentration of the drug. Some of these mutants may be susceptible to other rifamycin derivatives.

Resistance is due to a change in a single amino acid of the β subunit of DNA-dependent RNA polymerase, which no longer forms a stable complex with rifampicin. It is not transferable and there is no cross-resistance with any other antibiotic class. The susceptible strains of the gastrointestinal flora become rapidly resistant during rifampicin treatment without alteration in the flora composition, and revert to susceptibility within a few weeks of cessation of treatment.

 ## PHARMACOKINETICS

Oral absorption	>90%
C_{max} 300 mg oral	4 mg/L after 2 h
600 mg oral	10 mg/L after 2 h
Plasma half-life	2.5 h
Volume of distribution	1.5 L/kg
Plasma protein binding	80%

Absorption

Rifampicin is virtually completely absorbed when administered orally, but substantial differences in blood levels have been reported in comparisons of capsules or tablets from different manufacturers. Peak plasma levels differ noticeably between individuals. Food affects absorption, the peak plasma levels being delayed and about 2 mg/L lower after a meal. Although the AUC and the length of time for which effective antibacterial levels are maintained are little affected, it is preferable that patients take the drug before meals.

Intravenous administration produces AUCs and elimination half-lives similar to those obtained after oral doses.

Distribution

The lipid solubility of the drug facilitates its distribution. It is widely distributed in the internal organs, bones and fluids, including tears, saliva, ascitic fluid and abscesses. It penetrates into cells and is active against intracellular bacteria. Low concentrations are found in the cerebrospinal fluid (CSF), but these are substantially higher when the meninges are inflamed. Concentrations around 60% of the simultaneous plasma value were found in the heart valves of patients receiving a 600 mg dose before surgery.

Metabolism

Rifampicin is metabolized principally to its desacetyl derivative, which is also antimicrobially active, and this process is accelerated by its stimulatory effect on hepatic microsomal enzymes. As a consequence, hepatic clearance increases on continuous administration and, especially with high doses, the serum half-life becomes shorter after a few days of treatment.

Excretion

The main route of elimination is secretion into the bile, a process that is dose dependent, being efficient at low dosage but limited at high dosage. As a result, the dose determines the proportion excreted via the bile or passing the liver to be excreted in the urine. Because there is a limit to the rate at which the liver can deliver the drug to the bile, the elimination half-life after a 600 mg dose rises to 3 h and may be as long as 5 h with a 900 mg dose.

The desacetyl compound is mainly found in the bile, where the parent compound accounts for only 15% of the total. Plasma levels are increased by hepatic insufficiency and biliary obstruction, and by probenecid, which depresses hepatic uptake. The drug escaping biliary excretion appears in the urine, to which it imparts an orange–red color, the parent compound and the desacetyl metabolites being present in about equal proportions. The plasma concentration and half-life are not significantly affected by renal failure. The drug is not removed by hemodialysis.

DRUG INTERACTIONS

The antibiotic is a potent inducer of hepatic cytochrome P_{450} microsomal enzymes, which leads not only to more rapid self-elimination but also to enhanced metabolism of other agents handled by the same process. The effect is selective and it is not possible to predict which drugs may be affected. The most important are warfarin, the anticoagulant effect of which is thereby diminished, and oral contraceptives, with possible breakthrough bleeding and unwanted pregnancy. Addisonian crises have been described, and adjustments to steroid dosage in patients with Addison's disease may be necessary. Plasma concentrations of a number of other drugs may be affected, including digoxin, quinidine, methadone, hypoglycemic agents and barbiturates, with corresponding pharmacological effects.

Among antiretroviral drugs, use in combination with indinavir and its congeners is not recommended, but it can be used with ritonavir or nevirapine.

TOXICITY AND SIDE EFFECTS

Rifampicin is relatively non-toxic, even when administered for a long period (as in the treatment of tuberculosis). However, several unwanted effects, including pink staining of soft contact lenses, are associated with its use. Other reactions can be divided into those associated with daily or intermittent administration, and those found only with intermittent therapy.

Adverse events associated with daily or intermittent therapy

Most common are skin reactions (mostly flushing with or without rash, and often transient even when therapy is continued), gastrointestinal disturbances (usually mild and most common in the early weeks of treatment) and disturbance of hepatic function. Transient abnormalities of liver function, especially a rise in serum transaminases (and, less often, a raised bilirubin level), are common, and clinical hepatitis, usually of mild degree, also occurs. Hepatitis was commonly recorded in some early studies, but the incidence in short-course regimens appears to be low. Early suggestions that hepatic damage was more common in rapid acetylators when given in combination with isoniazid have not been confirmed.

Thrombocytopenia, associated with complement-fixing serum antibodies, is uncommon. The platelet count falls within a few hours, returning to normal within a day or two. Rifampicin administration should be discontinued at once. Thrombocytopenia is more common with intermittent schemes, but is also encountered in patients receiving daily treatment.

Adverse events confined to patients receiving intermittent therapy

The most important is the 'flu' syndrome, with fever, chills and malaise usually developing after 3–6 months of treatment. Its incidence is less with frequent than infrequent dosage; less with lower than higher doses; and less when intermittent therapy is preceded by an initial phase of daily treatment. It was not, however, prevented by a daily supplement of 25 mg in an intermittent regimen. Circulating immunoglobulin M (IgM) antibodies to rifampicin are found in serum, and the 'flu' syndrome may be caused by resulting complement activation.

Other rare syndromes associated with intermittent administration are acute renal failure, sometimes associated with acute hemolysis. Shortness of breath, wheezing and fall of blood pressure have occasionally been recorded. Immunosuppressive properties are demonstrable in a number of experimental systems, but no resultant adverse effect has been described in humans.

CLINICAL USE

Tuberculosis (in combination with other antituberculosis agents; *see* Ch. 58)

Leprosy (in combination with other antileprotic agents; *see* Ch. 57)

Serious infection with multiresistant staphylococci and pneumococci (in combination with a glycopeptide)

Elimination of nasopharyngeal carriage of *Neisseria meningitidis* and *H. influenzae*.

Reference is made to its use in legionellosis (Ch. 45), meningitis (Ch. 50) and brucellosis (Ch. 61).

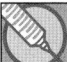

Preparations and dosage

Proprietary names: Rifadin, Rimactane. In combination with isoniazid: Rifinah, Rimactazid. In combination with isoniazid and with pyrazinamide: Rifater.

Preparations: Capsules, syrup, i.v. infusion.

Dosage: Adults, oral, 450–600 mg per day as a single dose, based on approx. 10 mg/kg per day. Children, up to 20 mg/kg per day as a single dose (maximum dose, 600 mg per day). Premature and newborn infants, 5–10 mg/kg once daily; treat only in cases of emergency and with extreme caution because their liver enzyme system may not be fully developed. Adults, i.v. infusion, 450–600 mg per day as a single dose, based on approx. 10 mg/kg per day. Lower doses are recommended for small or frail patients. Children, 20 mg/kg per day (maximum dose, 600 mg per day). Premature and newborn infants, 10 mg/kg per day with caution, as for oral dose. Chemoprophylaxis of meningococcal meningitis: adults, oral, 600 mg every 12 h for 2 days; children 1–12 years, 10 mg/kg every 12 h for 2 days; infants up to 1 year, 5 mg/kg every 12 h for 2 days.

Widely available.

Further information

Acocella G. Clinical pharmacokinetics of rifampicin. *Clin Pharmacokinet.* 1978;3:108–127.

Bemer-Melchior P, Bryskier A, Drugeon HB. Comparison of in vitro activities of rifapentine and rifampicin against *Mycobacterium tuberculosis* complex. *J Antimicrob Chemother.* 2000;46:571–576.

Ellard GA, Fourie PB. Rifampicin bioavailability: a review of its pharmacology and the chemotherapeutic necessity for ensuring optimal absorption. *Int J Tuberc Lung Dis.* 1999;3(suppl 3):301S–308S.

Havlir DV, Barnes PF. Tuberculosis in patients with human immunodeficiency virus infection. *N Engl J Med.* 1999;340:367–373.

Loeffler AM. Uses of rifampin for infections other than tuberculosis. *Pediatr Infect Dis.* 1999;18:631–632.

Martinez E, Collazos J, Mayo J. Hypersensitivity reactions to rifampin. Pathogenic mechanisms, clinical manifestations, management strategies, and review of anaphylactic-like reactions. *Medicine (Baltimore).* 1999;78:361–369.

Venkatesan K. Pharmacokinetic drug interactions with rifampicin. *Clin Pharmacokinet.* 1992;22:47–65.

RIFAPENTINE

Molecular weight: 877.04.

An analog of rifampicin in which a cyclopentyl group is substituted for a methyl group on the piperazine ring. It is available for oral administration.

ANTIMICROBIAL ACTIVITY

Activity is similar to that of rifampicin, but it is more active against atypical mycobacteria, especially the *M. avium* complex (MIC <0.06–0.5 mg/L). It has good activity on staphylococci and streptococci (MIC 0.01–0.5 mg/L), *L. monocytogenes* and *Brucella* spp.; less against *Enterococcus faecalis* (MIC 1–4 mg/L). *Bacteroides* spp. are inhibited by 0.5–2 mg/L. Gram-negative cocci are susceptible and, although some Gram-negative bacilli are inhibited by 4–32 mg/L, most are resistant.

PHARMACOKINETICS

Oral absorption	c. 70%
C_{max} 600 mg oral	12 mg/L after 5 h
Plasma half-life	13 h
Volume of distribution	1.5 L/kg
Plasma protein binding	97%

Absorption

The absolute oral bioavailability of rifapentine has not been determined. The relative bioavailability of capsules (with an oral solution as reference) is 70%. Food increases absorption: a 600 mg dose taken after a meal gives C_{max} and AUC values 44% higher than under fasting conditions. The extended half-life provides therapeutic concentrations for at least 72 h after administration, allowing less frequent dosing.

Distribution

Animal data suggest that it is well distributed in the body, with tissue concentrations exceeding the plasma concentration, except in bone, testes and brain. The ratio of intracellular:extracellular concentration in macrophages was estimated as 24:1.

Metabolism

The main metabolite is an antimicrobially active 25-desacetyl derivative. Although it induces liver cytochromes it is not an inducer of its own metabolism, which is mediated by an esterase. The peak concentration of 25-desacetyl rifapentine is about one-third of that of the unchanged drug, and is attained after about 11 h.

Excretion

The main route of elimination is through the bile. In healthy volunteers about 70% of a 600 mg dose of ^{14}C rifapentine was recovered in the feces, and less than 17% in the urine. There is evidence of enterohepatic recycling in humans.

DRUG INTERACTIONS

The metabolism of several drugs concurrently administered can be substantially accelerated and adjustment of their dosage may be necessary. In particular, treatment of AIDS patients with rifapentine resulted in a 70% reduction in the AUC of indinavir. It should be used with extreme caution, if at all, in patients who are also taking protease inhibitors.

TOXICITY AND SIDE EFFECTS

Signs of teratogenic effects and fetal toxicity have been observed when administered during pregnancy to rats and rabbits. Rifapentine should be used during pregnancy only if the potential benefit justifies the potential risk to the fetus.

The most common adverse effect observed in combinations with other antimycobacterial agents was hyperuricemia, most probably due to pyrazinamide. Effects likely to be due to rifapentine were neutropenia (3.7% of patients) and hepatitis (increased transaminases in 1.6% of patients).

CLINICAL USE

Tuberculosis (in combination with other antituberculosis drugs)

Preparations and dosage

Proprietary name: Priftin.

Preparation: 150 mg tablets.

Dosage: Adults, oral, 600 mg (4 tablets) twice a week during the 2-month intensive phase treatment; 600 mg once a week in the 4-month continuation phase.

Available in the USA.

Further information

Burman WJ, Gallicano K, Peloquin C. Comparative pharmacokinetics and pharmacodynamics of the rifamycin antibacterials. *Clin Pharmacokinet.* 2001;40:327–341.

Jarvis B, Lamb MM. Rifapentine. *Drugs.* 1998;56:607–616.

Klemens SP, Grossi MA, Cynamon MH. Comparative in vivo activities of rifabutin and rifapentine against *Mycobacterium avium* complex. *Antimicrob Agents Chemother.* 1994;38:234–237.

Mor N, Simon B, Mezo N, Heifets LB. Comparison of activities of rifapentine and rifampin against *Mycobacterium tuberculosis* residing in human macrophages. *Antimicrob Agents Chemother.* 1995;39:2073–2077.

Temple ME, Nahata MC. Rifapentine: its role in treatment of tuberculosis. *Ann Pharmacother.* 1999;33:1203–1210.

RIFAXIMIN

Molecular weight: 785.879.

A semisynthetic derivative of rifamycin S formulated for oral administration. It is poorly absorbed from the gastrointestinal tract, where its high concentrations are effective against a variety of gastrointestinal pathogens.

ANTIMICROBIAL ACTIVITY

The in-vitro activity is slightly inferior to that of rifampicin. The MIC_{90} for Gram-positive cocci is well below 1 mg/L, with the exception of enterococci (MIC 2–8 mg/L). Among intestinal pathogens *C. difficile* is sensitive (MIC_{90} 0.8 mg/L), *Esch. coli*, *Salmonella* spp. and *Shigella* spp. are inhibited by 4–8 mg/L. *Campylobacter jejuni* is mostly insensitive.

PHARMACOKINETICS

Oral absorption is very low. However, a fraction of the dose may be absorbed and rapidly eliminated through the bile. A 400 mg oral dose produces a maximum plasma concentration of 3.8 μg/L after 1.2 h. The plasma half-life is 5.8 h. Up to 90% of the administered dose is concentrated in the gut, less than 0.2% in the liver and kidney, and less than 0.01% in other tissues.

TOXICITY AND SIDE EFFECTS

Oral doses up to 100 mg/kg for 6 months produced no significant signs of toxicity to rats. Teratogenic effects in rats and rabbits have been reported (pregnancy category C).

Very few adverse effects were reported during human treatment, mostly gastrointestinal discomfort. Prolonged therapy was associated with infrequent urticarial skin reactions.

CLINICAL USE

It is used for a variety of gastrointestinal diseases, including the treatment of traveler's diarrhea. Preliminary results suggest clinical efficacy in the therapy of hepatic encephalopathy and of *C. difficile* infections.

Preparations and dosage

Proprietary names: Normix, Rifacol, Xifaxan, Rifaximina, Rifaximine and others.
Preparations: Tablets, granules, topical.
Dosage: Adults, oral, 10–15 mg/kg per day. Children, oral, 20–30 mg/kg per day.
Widely available.

Further information

Garey KW, Salazar M, Shah H, Rodrigue R, DuPont HL. Rifamycin antibiotics for the treatment of *Clostridium difficile*-associated diarrhea. *Ann Pharmacother.* 2008;42:827–835.
Gerard L, Garey KW, DuPont HL. Rifaximin: a non-absorbable rifamycin antibiotic for use in nonsystemic gastrointestinal infections. *Expert Rev Anti Infect Ther.* 2005;3:201–211.
Gillis JC, Brogden RN. Rifaximin: a review of its antibacterial activity, pharmacokinetic properties and therapeutic potential in conditions mediated by gastrointestinal bacteria. *Drugs.* 1995;49:467–484.
Lawrence KR, Klee JA. Rifaximin for the treatment of hepatic encephalopathy. *Pharmacotherapy.* 2008;28:1019–1032.
Scarpignato C, Pelosini I. Rifaximin, a poorly absorbed antibiotic: pharmacology and clinical potential. *Chemotherapy.* 2005;51(suppl 1):36–66.

OTHER RIFAMYCINS

RIFAMIDE

The diethyl amide of rifamycin B, formulated as the sodium salt for parenteral administration. It exhibits high activity against Gram-positive organisms and *M. tuberculosis* typical of the group. MICs for Gram-negative bacilli are of the order of 20–50 mg/L.

It is absorbed orally and is rapidly eliminated through the bile, achieving concentrations sufficient to inhibit Gram-negative bacilli. In contrast to rifampicin, it can be administered as the sodium salt by intramuscular injection. A dose of 150 mg produces mean plasma levels of about 1 mg/L. The plasma half-life is about 2 h. The same dosage produces concentrations over 1 g/L in bile and *c.* 40 mg/L in the gallbladder wall.

Toxicity and side effects are similar to those of other rifamycins. It has been used in staphylococcal infections and infections of the biliary tract. It is unsuitable for the treatment of tuberculosis because of insufficient distribution to the tissues.

Preparations and dosage

Preparations: Parenteral injection, i.m., i.v., topical.
Dosage: i.m., 250 mg every 8 h; i.v. infusion (slow), up to 750 mg every 12 h. Limited availability.

Further information

Acocella G, Lamarina F, Tenconi LT, Nicolis FB. Study of the secretion in bile and concentration in gall bladder wall of rifamide. *Gut.* 1966;7:380–386.
Pallanza R, Furesz S, Timbal MT, Carniti G. In vitro bacteriological studies on rifamycin B diethylamide (rifamide). *Arzneimittelforschung.* 1965;15:800–802.

RIFAMYCIN SV

The simplest rifamycin in clinical use, obtained by elimination of a glycolic moiety from rifamycin B. Formulated as sodium salt for parenteral administration. Also available for topical use. Its activity, general properties and pharmacokinetics are very similar to those of rifamide. It is orally absorbed and excreted mainly in the bile. Intramuscular doses of 250 mg produce mean plasma levels of about 2 mg/L. The plasma half-life is around 2 h.

In addition to uses similar to those of rifamide, it is administered topically in surgery and has been proposed for the treatment of synovitis by intra-articular injections. A topical preparation is used for application to wounds and bedsores. Cases of anaphylactic reactions have been reported after local administration of the drug.

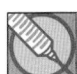

Preparations and dosage

Proprietary names: Chibro-Rifamycin, Otofa, Rifocine.
Preparations: Parenteral injection, i.m, i.v., topical.
Dosage: i.m., 250 mg every 8 h; i.v. infusion (slow), up to 750 mg every 12 h. Available in Italy, Switzerland and Germany.

Further information

Bergamini G, Fowst G, Rifamycin SV. A review. *Arzneimittelforschung.* 1965;15:951–1002.
Cardot E, Tillie-Leblond I, Jeannin P, et al. Anaphylactic reaction to local administration of rifamycin SV. *J Allergy Clin Immunol.* 1995;95:1–7.
Radossi P, Baggio R, Petris U, et al. Intra-articular rifamycin in haemophilic arthropathy. *Haemophilia.* 2003;9:60–63.

Streptogramins

Francisco Soriano

Streptogramins are natural mixtures of cyclic peptides produced by *Streptomyces* spp., which display a synergistic inhibitory effect on some bacteria. They are macrocyclic lactone peptolides, having two basic chemical structures classified as either group A or group B. Compounds of group A are polyunsaturated cyclic peptolides, the best known being virginiamycin M_1, pristinamycin II_A, pristinamycin II_B and dalfopristin (a pristinamycin II_B derivative). Compounds of group B are cyclic hexa-depsipeptides, with virginiamycin S and pristinamycins I_A, I_B, and I_C as the principal compounds. Quinupristin is a pristinamycin I_A derivative.

Streptogramins behave as bacteriostatic drugs, but a mixture of group A and group B antibiotics causes a 10–100-fold greater inhibition of bacterial growth than the individual components. Useful activity is mainly restricted to Gram-positive organisms (Table 28.1). Naturally occurring group A and group B components are both highly water insoluble and have to be administered by mouth. Quinupristin and dalfopristin are water soluble and can be administered parenterally in a fixed 30:70 ratio marketed as Synercid.

Further information

Bonfiglio G, Furneri PM. Novel streptogramin antibiotics. *Expert Opin Investig Drugs*. 2001;10:185–198.

QUINUPRISTIN–DALFOPRISTIN

Molecular weight quinupristin: 1022; dalfopristin: 690

Quinupristin

Table 28.1   In-vitro activity of three streptogramins against Gram-positive organisms: MIC (mg/L)

	Quinupristin–dalfopristin	Pristinamycin	NXL 103
Staphylococcus aureus			
methicillin-susceptible	0.12–0.5	≤0.06–1	0.06–0.25
methicillin-resistant	0.12–1	0.25–2	0.06–0.5
Staphy. epidermidis	≤0.06–0.5	≤0.06–2	0.06–1
Streptococcus pneumoniae	0.12–1	0.12–1	0.06–1
Str. pyogenes	0.25–1	≤0.06–0.12	≤0.06
Str. agalactiae	0.5–2	0.12–0.25	≤0.03–0.06
Viridans group streptococci	0.12–4	0.25–1	0.06–0.25
Enterococcus faecium	0.5–2	0.12–2	≤0.06–1
E. faecalis	1–32	0.5–16	0.12–2

Dalfopristin

PHARMACOKINETICS

	Quinupristin and metabolites	Dalfopristin and metabolites
C_{max} 7.5 mg/kg i.v. infusion (1 h)	2.5–3.2 mg/L	6.5–7.96 mg/L
Plasma half-life	1 h	0.75 h
Volume of distribution	c. 1.0 L/kg	c. 1.0 L/kg
Plasma protein binding	55–78%	11–26%

A fixed combination of two purified water-soluble compounds derived from natural pristinamycin I_A and II_B, respectively. Both compounds are formulated as the mesylate for intravenous infusion. It is the only streptogramin combination presently available for parenteral use.

ANTIMICROBIAL ACTIVITY

Quinupristin–dalfopristin is mainly active against Gram-positive organisms, with modest activity against selected Gram-negative and anaerobic pathogens. It inhibits vancomycin-sensitive and -resistant *Enterococcus faecium*, including multidrug-resistant strains with a minimum inhibitory concentration required to inhibit the growth of 90% of organisms (MIC_{90}) of ≤4 mg/L, but has little activity against *E. faecalis* (MIC_{90} 16 mg/L). It is active against *Staphylococcus aureus*, including methicillin-resistant *Staph. aureus* (MRSA), coagulase-negative staphylococci, *Streptococcus pneumoniae* and *Str. pyogenes*. The drug is also active against *Moraxella catarrhalis*, *Chlamydophila* (formerly *Chlamydia*) *pneumoniae*, *Legionella pneumophila*, *Mycoplasma hominis* and *Ureaplasma urealyticum*. The use of this drug should be governed by susceptibility testing.

Quinupristin–dalfopristin exhibits a significant post-antibiotic effect estimated at 5–7.5 h for staphylococci and 4 h for enterococci.

ACQUIRED RESISTANCE

Resistance can be chromosomal or plasmid mediated and is mainly due to methylation of the drug target, resulting in resistance to all macrolides, lincosamides and group B streptogramins, but not to group A streptogramins. Resistance can also occur by drug-modifying enzymes or active efflux. Other mechanisms of resistance to macrolides and lincosamides, including those of target modification and active efflux, do not affect streptogramins.

Quinupristin–dalfopristin is usually administered by 1 h intravenous infusion at a dose of 7.5 mg/kg in 5% glucose–dextrose every 8–12 h. Reported values for protein binding vary considerably. The compound does not cross the non-inflamed blood–brain barrier or placenta to any significant degree and is rapidly converted in the liver to several active metabolites. In experimental endocarditis quinupristin is homogeneously distributed in cardiac vegetations whereas dalfopristin shows a gradient concentration. Biliary excretion into feces is the main route of elimination for both compounds and their metabolites with only 15–19% eliminated in the urine. Dosage adjustments may be needed in patients with hepatic dysfunction but it seems unnecessary in patients with renal impairment, those undergoing peritoneal dialysis, the obese or the elderly.

INTERACTIONS

The metabolism is not affected by the cytochrome P_{450} 3A4 system but may alter the metabolism of other drugs metabolized by this pathway, such as ciclosporin (cyclosporine). Quinupristin–dalfopristin can also interfere with the metabolism of drugs associated with QTc prolongation and co-administration of these compounds should be avoided.

TOXICITY AND SIDE EFFECTS

The drug has significant toxicity problems, including arthralgia–myalgia syndrome (7.3–9.5%), venous intolerance experienced as pain at the infusion site (14.8%) and inflammation (6.2–11.1%). Hyperbilirubinemia and liver toxicity can also occur.

CLINICAL USE

Serious, refractory infections caused by multiresistant Gram-positive organisms, including *Staph. aureus* and *E. faecium*

If mixed infection is documented or suspected, the drug should be used in combination with an agent active against Gram-negative organisms.

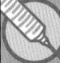

Preparations and dosage

Proprietary name: Synercid.

Preparation: Intravenous infusion. Vials of 500 and 600 mg containing quinupristin–dalfopristin in a 30:70 ratio (mesylate salts).

Dosage: Adults, i.v., 7.5 mg/kg every 8 h.

Widely available.

Further information

Allington DR, Rivey MP. Quinupristin/dalfopristin: a therapeutic review. *Clin Ther.* 2001;23:24–44.

Drew RH, Perfect JR, Srinath L, et al. Treatment of methicillin-resistant *Staphylococcus aureus* infections with quinupristin–dalfopristin in patients intolerant of or failing prior therapy. For the Synercid Emergency-Use Study Group. *J Antimicrob Chemother.* 2000;46:775–784.

Fantin B, Leclercq R, Merlé Y, et al. Critical influence of resistance to streptogramin B-type antibiotics on activity of RP 59500 (quinupristin–dalfopristin) in experimental endocarditis due to Staphylococcus aureus. *Antimicrob Agents Chemother.* 1995;39:400–405.

Metzger R, Bonatti H, Sawyer R. Future trends in the treatment of serious Gram-positive infections. *Drugs of Today.* 2009;45:33–45.

Moellering RC, Linden PK, Reinhardt J, et al. The efficacy and safety of quinupristin/dalfopristin for the treatment of infections caused by vancomycin-resistant *Enterococcus faecium.* Synercid Emergency-Use Study Group. *J Antimicrob Chemother.* 1999;44:251–261.

Nichols RL, Graham DR, Barriere SL, et al. Treatment of hospitalized patients with complicated gram-positive skin and skin structure infections: two randomized, multicentre studies of quinupristin/dalfopristin versus cefazolin, oxacillin or vancomycin. Synercid Skin and Skin Structure Infection Group. *J Antimicrob Chemother.* 1999;44:263–273.

Rubinstein E, Bompart F. Activity of quinupristin/dalfopristin against gram-positive bacteria: clinical applications and therapeutic potential. *J Antimicrob Chemother.* 1997;39(suppl A):139–143.

Wang JL, Hsueh PR. Therapeutic options for infections due to vancomycin-resistant enterococci. *Expert Opin Pharmacother.* 2009;10:785–796.

OTHER STREPTOGRAMINS

PRISTINAMYCIN

The two major components are pristinamycin I_A and pristinamycin I_B. It is available in some countries for the oral treatment of upper respiratory, bronchopulmonary, dental, skin, genital and bone infections caused by susceptible organisms. In-vitro activity is summarized in Table 28.1. The drug is usually well tolerated, although minor gastrointestinal disturbances and rash may occur.

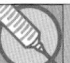

Preparations and dosage

Proprietary name: Pyostacine.

Preparation: Tablets (250 and 500 mg).

Dosage: Adults, oral, 2–4 g per day, in three equal doses, with meals. Children, 50–100 mg/kg per day in three equal doses, with meals.

Available in Belgium and France.

VIRGINIAMYCIN

A natural product of *Streptomyces virginiae* with antimicrobial activity similar to that of other streptogramins. It has chiefly been used as an animal feed additive, but is available in some countries for oral administration and in topical preparations.

NXL103

NXL103 (formerly XRP 2868) is one of several new oral streptogramins under development. It is a 30:70 mixture of streptogramins B and A (RPR 202868 and RPR 132552) and is in clinical trial as a treatment for mild to moderate community-acquired pneumonia. It is somewhat more active than quinupristin–dalfopristin in vitro (Table 28.1). Clinical efficacy and safety appear to be good, with the most frequent adverse events related to gastrointestinal intolerance. Available information suggests that the relationship between its pharmacokinetics and efficacy is similar to that of quinupristin–dalfopristin.

Further information

Andes D, Craig WA. Pharmacodynamics of a new streptogramin, XRP 2868, in murine thigh and lung infection models. *Antimicrob Agents Chemother.* 2006;50:243–249.

Eliopoulos GM, Ferraro MJ, Wennersten CB, et al. In vitro activity of an oral streptogramin antimicrobial, XRP2868, against Gram-positive bacteria. *Antimicrob Agents Chemother.* 2005;49:3034–3039.

29 Sulfonamides

David Greenwood

The original sulphonamide, sulphanilamide, is the active principle of Prontosil, which holds a special place in medicine as the first agent to exhibit broad-spectrum activity against systemic bacterial disease (*see* Ch. 1). Within a few years of the introduction of Prontosil, numerous sulfonamide derivatives were synthesized. Advances included increased antibacterial potency, decreased toxicity, and the introduction of compounds with special properties such as high or low solubility and prolonged duration of action. Most have since been discarded, as safer and more active antibacterial agents have overtaken them, but a few are still in use for particular purposes, often in combination with diaminopyrimidines (*see* Ch. 17). Some survive in topical preparations, often in multi-ingredient formulations. Discussion here is limited to the most important sulfonamides that are still widely available; a short description is included of some of the many other compounds that are of more restricted availability.

ANTIBACTERIAL ACTIVITY

Sulfonamides exhibit broad-spectrum activity against common Gram-positive and Gram-negative pathogens, although the potency against many bacteria within the spectrum is modest by present standards. Meningococci are generally much more susceptible than gonococci. Other organisms commonly susceptible include *Bordetella pertussis*, *Yersinia pestis*, *Actinomyces* spp., *Nocardia* spp., *Bacillus anthracis*, *Corynebacterium diphtheriae*, *Legionella pneumophila*, *Brucella* spp. and several important causes of sexually transmitted diseases (*Chlamydia trachomatis*, *Haemophilus ducreyi* and *Calymmatobacterium granulomatis*). Activity against anaerobes is generally poor. *Pseudomonas aeruginosa* is usually resistant, as are *Leptospira*, *Treponema* and *Borrelia* spp., rickettsiae, *Coxiella burnetii* and mycoplasmas. Mycobacteria are resistant, although the related sulfone, dapsone, exhibits good activity against *M. leprae* (*see* p. 387) and *para*-aminosalicylic acid, which is structurally similar, was formerly widely used in tuberculosis (p. 392). Sulfonamides act synergistically with certain diaminopyrimidines against many bacteria and some protozoa, including plasmodia and *Toxoplasma gondii* (*see* Ch. 17).

In-vitro tests are markedly influenced by the composition of the culture medium and the size of the inoculum. The different derivatives vary somewhat in antibacterial activity (Table 29.1). Among those that are still fairly widely available as antibacterial agents, sulfadimidine shows comparatively low activity, whereas sulfadiazine, sulfisoxazole (sulphafurazole) and sulfamethoxazole, the sulfonamide commonly combined with trimethoprim (p. 256), are relatively more active.

ACQUIRED BACTERIAL RESISTANCE

Resistance is now widespread and there is complete cross-resistance among sulfonamides. Plasmid-mediated resistance in all enterobacteria is common. Resistance is found in 25–40% of strains of *Escherichia coli* and other enterobacteria infecting the urinary tract. Many strains of meningococci and *H. ducreyi* are now resistant.

PHARMACOKINETICS

Most sulfonamides are well absorbed after oral administration, reaching a peak concentration in the blood of 50–100 mg/L 2–4 h after a dose of 2 g. After absorption, the behavior of the individual compounds varies widely, depending on the extent of protein-binding and metabolization. The main metabolic pathway is conjugation by acetylation in the liver, although glucuronidation and oxidation also occur. Sulfonamide acetylation shows a bimodal distribution in the population, rapid and slow inactivators corresponding with rapid and slow inactivators of isoniazid (p. 390). The conjugates are inactive antibacterially and the low solubility of the acetyl conjugates of some of the earlier compounds may give rise to renal toxicity.

A proportion, varying considerably with different compounds, is contained in the red cells, some is free in the plasma and some is bound to plasma albumin. Protein binding varies widely, the highest levels being seen with long-acting

Table 29.1 Activity of selected sulfonamides against common pathogenic bacteria: MIC (mg/L)

	Sulfadiazine	Sulfadimidine	Sulfamethoxazole	Sulfisoxazole
Staphylococcus aureus	16–32	32–R	4–32	4–16
Streptococcus pyogenes	0.5–64	1–64	0.25–16	0.25–4
Str. pneumoniae	8–64	4–64	4–64	2–16
Enterococcus faecalis	R	R	R	R
Haemophilus influenzae	2–4	8–16	2–4	0.5–2
Neisseria gonorrhoeae	1–32	16–R	1–32	1–64
N. meningitidis	0.12–1	0.5–8	0.12–1	0.12–0.5
Escherichia coli	4–16	16–64	4–8	8–16
Klebsiella pneumoniae	8–16	64–R	4–16	8–16
Pseudomonas aeruginosa	64	R	R	R

R, resistant (MIC >64 mg/L).

sulfonamides such as sulfadoxine. Sulfonamides can be displaced from their protein binding sites by a variety of compounds, the most important clinically being oral anticoagulant drugs. Administration of these compounds with sulfonamides potentiates the anticoagulant effect and produces higher concentrations of diffusible sulfonamide. Competition for plasma albumin binding sites causes sulfonamides to displace albumin-bound bilirubin.

Sulfonamides are distributed throughout the body tissues. Access to the cerebrospinal fluid (CSF) is normally limited to the unbound drug, but with increasing capillary permeability and the passage of protein into the CSF in inflammation, protein-bound sulfonamide enters and the total concentration of drug in the CSF rises. The concentration of short-acting sulfonamides in CSF varies between 30% and 80% of the corresponding plasma concentration. Sulfonamides also enter other body fluids, including the eye. They pass readily through the placenta into the fetal circulation and also reach the infant via the breast milk.

Sulfonamides are excreted mainly in the urine, the free drug and its conjugates being frequently excreted at different rates and by different mechanisms. Excretion is partly by glomerular filtration and partly by tubular secretion, during which some of the drug is reabsorbed. Substances with high clearances (e.g. sulfisoxazole) are rapidly eliminated from the plasma and achieve high concentrations in the urine. Substances with low clearances are slowly excreted, plasma levels are maintained for long periods, and low concentrations appear in the urine. If renal function is impaired, excretion may be delayed still further and therapeutic levels may persist for considerably longer; if the drugs are given repeatedly, high and possibly toxic levels may develop. Less than 1% of the dose of most sulfonamides is excreted in the bile, but the proportion is 2.4–6.3% for the long-acting compounds.

TOXICITY AND SIDE EFFECTS

With proper attention to dosage, side effects are relatively uncommon, but some are serious. Crystals of less soluble compounds, such as sulfadiazine, or of less soluble conjugates may deposit in the urine and block the renal tubules or the upper orifice of the ureter. Hematuria is a common early sign. However, renal damage during sulfonamide therapy is often due to a hypersensitivity reaction, rather than to tubular blockage, with changes of tubular necrosis or vasculitis. Renal failure has been recorded in several patients after treatment with sulfamethoxazole, as a component of co-trimoxazole.

Hypersensitivity reactions usually occur as moderate fever with a rash on about the ninth day of a course of treatment. Repetition after an interval elicits the reaction immediately. Rashes are commonly erythematous, maculopapular or urticarial, and recur if the drug is given again. Well documented, but uncommon, is a severe serum-sickness-like reaction with fever, urticarial rash, polyarthropathy and eosinophilia. Eosinophilia may occur without other allergic manifestations.

Stevens–Johnson syndrome is a rare but potentially fatal complication (one estimate puts the risk at 1–2 cases per 10 million doses). The relative risks of different sulfonamides are not known accurately, but there are many reports of this complication following the use of long-acting sulfonamides. The time of onset varies from 2 to 24 days, and sometimes as long as 6 weeks after discontinuing the drug. Toxic epidermal necrolysis (Lyell's syndrome) has also been recorded after administration of long-acting sulfonamides.

Drug fever without other features may occur. A special problem of hypersensitivity to the sulfonamide component of co-trimoxazole is its frequency in the treatment of AIDS.

Sulfonamides are among the compounds reported to provoke systemic lupus erythematosus. An intractable type of sensitization may result from local applications.

In patients with inherited glucose-6-phosphate dehydrogenase deficiency, intravascular hemolysis and hemoglobinuria may occur. Hemolysis may also occur as part of a generalized sensitivity reaction. Agranulocytosis, aplastic anemia and thrombocytopenia have been occasionally reported, especially with earlier sulfonamides. Liver injury is rare.

Interference with bilirubin transport in the fetus by sulfonamide administered to the mother may increase the free plasma bilirubin level and result in kernicterus. Many other interactions arise as a result of competition for plasma albumin binding sites. Those of greatest potential clinical importance are increases in the actions of oral anticoagulants and sulfonylureas (but not biguanides) and increased toxicity of methotrexate.

CLINICAL USE

Sulfonamides were formerly much used, alone or in combination with trimethoprim, for the treatment of urinary tract infection, but are no longer recommended because of potential adverse reactions. Use in the treatment of respiratory infections is now confined to a few special problems, notably nocardiasis (and also for cerebral nocardiasis) and, in combination with trimethoprim, in the prevention and treatment of *Pneumocystis jirovecii* pneumonia. The value of sulfonamides in the prophylaxis and treatment of meningococcal infection is now greatly reduced by bacterial resistance. Sulfonamides are sometimes used for chlamydial infections and chancroid but are unreliable. Some formulations are used topically in eye infections and bacterial vaginosis. Combined preparations with pyrimethamine are used in the treatment of drug-resistant malaria and for toxoplasmosis (*see* Chs 62 and 63).

 Further information

Dibbern DA, Montanaro A. Allergies to sulfonamide antibiotics and sulfur-containing compounds. *Ann Allergy Asthma Immunol.* 2008;100:91–100.
Smith CL, Powell KR. Review of the sulfonamides and trimethoprim. *Pediatr Rev.* 2000;21:368–371.

SULFADIAZINE

2-Sulfanilamidopyrimidine. Molecular weight: 250.3.

Sulfadiazine is almost insoluble in water and unstable on exposure to light. It is administered orally or, as the sodium salt, by intravenous injection. It is a component of several multi-ingredient preparations. Its low solubility in urine led to its general replacement by other compounds. The intravenous solution is highly alkaline and should not be given by any other route.

ANTIMICROBIAL ACTIVITY

Sulfadiazine is somewhat more active than other sulphonamides (Table 29.1).

PHARMACOKINETICS

Oral absorption	Very good
C_{max} 3 g oral	*c.* 50 mg/L after 3–4 h
Plasma half-life	7–12 h
Volume of distribution	0.36 L/kg
Plasma protein binding	*c.* 40%

Absorption and distribution

Adequate blood concentrations are easily achieved and maintained after oral administration. It is well distributed and penetrates in therapeutic concentrations into the CSF, but because of resistance it is no longer the drug of choice in meningitis. It crosses the placenta and enters breast milk to achieve concentrations around 20% of plasma levels.

Metabolism and excretion

Sulfadiazine is subject to acetylation in the liver. The acetyl derivative lacks antibacterial activity and is excreted more slowly (half-life 8–18 h). Parent compound and metabolite are both excreted mainly by glomerular filtration.

TOXICITY AND SIDE EFFECTS

In addition to side effects common to the group, sulfadiazine inhibits the metabolism of phenytoin. The risk of crystalluria can be reduced by high fluid intake and alkalization of the urine.

CLINICAL USE

Urinary tract infection
Nocardiasis
Chancroid
Toxoplasmosis (in combination with pyrimethamine)
Meningococcal infections
Prophylaxis of rheumatic fever

See also silver sulfadiazine (p. 343).

Preparations and dosage

Preparations: 4 mL ampoules, each containing 1 g for i.v. injection; tablets.

Dosage: Adult, i.v., 1–1.5 g every 4 h for 2 days, then oral.

Available in the UK, the USA, Canada, Belgium and Australia. Widely available in multi-ingredient preparations.

Further information

Anonymous. Sulfadiazine. In: Dollery C, ed. *Therapeutic Drugs*. 2nd ed. Edinburgh: Churchill Livingstone; 1999:S126–S129.

Dusseault BN, Croce KJ, Pais VM. Radiographic characteristics of sulfadiazine urolithiasis. *Urology*. 2009;73:928.

SULFADOXINE

4-Sulfanilamido-5,6-dimethoxypyrimidine. Molecular weight: 310.3.

An ultra-long-acting sulfonamide. It is no longer prescribed alone, but is used in combination with pyrimethamine as the antimalarial agent Fansidar (*see* Ch. 62). It is poorly soluble in water.

ANTIMICROBIAL ACTIVITY

Its antibacterial activity is relatively poor. Used alone it has a slow and uncertain effect against malaria parasites. Resistance of malaria parasites to the combination with pyrimethamine is common in many endemic areas.

PHARMACOKINETICS

Oral absorption	Extensive
C_{max} 500 mg oral	c. 60 mg/L after 3–4 h
Plasma half-life	c. 6 days
Volume of distribution	0.13 L/kg
Plasma protein binding	94%

The extremely long half-life allows administration at weekly intervals. The acetyl metabolite has a similarly long half-life, but sulfadoxine is less extensively metabolized than many other sulfonamides.

TOXICITY AND SIDE EFFECTS

Side effects are those common to the group. There have been many reports of Stevens–Johnson syndrome following its use and the combination with pyrimethamine is no longer recommended for the prophylaxis of malaria.

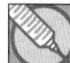

CLINICAL USE

Sulfadoxine is used only in combination with pyrimethamine.

Preparations and dosage

Proprietary names: Fansidar, Fanasil, in combination with pyrimethamine.

Preparation: Tablets containing 500 mg sulfadoxine and 25 mg pyrimethamine.

Dosage: Adults, oral, three tablets as a single dose. Children 10–14 years, two tablets; 7–9 years, 1½ tablets; 4–6 years, one tablet; under 4 years, half a tablet.

Limited availability. No longer available in UK and Europe.

Further information

Anonymous. Sulfadoxine. In: Dollery C, ed. *Therapeutic Drugs*. 2nd ed. Edinburgh: Churchill Livingstone; 1999:S132–S135.

Barnes KI, Little F, Smith PJ, Evans A, Watkins WM, White NJ. Sulfadoxine–pyrimethamine pharmacokinetics in malaria: pediatric dosing implications. *Clin Pharmacol Ther*. 2006;80:582–596.

SULFAMETHOXAZOLE

5-Methyl-3-sulfanilamidoisoxazole. Molecular weight: 253.2.

This is the sulfonamide component of co-trimoxazole (p. 256). It is slightly soluble in water.

ANTIMICROBIAL ACTIVITY

The intrinsic activity is similar to that of sulfadiazine (Table 29.1).

PHARMACOKINETICS

Oral absorption	85%
C_{max} 800 mg oral	c. 50 mg/L after 3–6 h
Plasma half-life	6–20 h
Volume of distribution	12–18 L
Plasma protein binding	65%

Penetration of extravascular sites, including the CSF, is good. It crosses the placenta and achieves levels in breast milk of about 10% of the simultaneous plasma concentration. It is extensively metabolized, but about 30% of the dose is excreted unchanged in urine so that high concentrations are achieved.

TOXICITY AND SIDE EFFECTS

Unwanted effects are those common to sulfonamides. In addition, benign intracranial hypertension has been reported in children. Most side effects of co-trimoxazole are thought to be attributable to the sulfonamide component.

CLINICAL USE

Sulfamethoxazole is used only in combination with the diaminopyrimidine trimethoprim (*see* p. 256).

 Preparations

Very limited availability as a single agent.

 Further information

Anonymous. Sulfamethoxazole and trimethoprim combination. In: Dollery C, ed. *Therapeutic Drugs.* 2nd ed. Edinburgh: Churchill Livingstone; 1999:S136–S140.

OTHER SULFONAMIDES

SULFACETAMIDE

N-acetylsulfanilamide. It is very soluble in water and was formerly used in urinary tract infection. It is available in some countries in ophthalmic preparations and as a component (with sulfathiazole and sulfabenzamide) of a triple sulfonamide cream for the topical treatment of bacterial vaginosis.

Sulfacetamide is one of the least active sulfonamides. It is well absorbed when given orally and is excreted in the urine with a half-life of around 9 h. About 70% is excreted unchanged, the remainder being present as the acetyl metabolite. Adverse reactions are those common to the group. Stevens–Johnson syndrome has been reported several times after topical use in conjunctivitis.

SULFADIMETHOXINE

2,4-Dimethoxy-6-sulfanilamido-1,3-diazine. A rapidly absorbed compound with a long half-life (38–40 h) and a high degree of protein binding (98%). Renal clearance is very slow, and daily dosage maintains adequate plasma levels.

SULFADIMIDINE

2-Sulfanilamido-4,6-methylpyrimidine (*syn:* sulphamethazine, sulfamezathine). A water-soluble compound, unstable on exposure to light. It is usually administered by mouth and is a component of some triple sulfonamide combinations.

The spectrum is typical of the group, but sulfadimidine exhibits relatively low potency (Table 29.1). It is well absorbed after oral administration. It is extensively metabolized, predominantly by acetylation. The mean plasma half-life (1.5–5 h) varies with acetylator status.

In addition to side effects common to the group, a serious interaction between ciclosporin (cyclosporin A) and sulfadimidine, leading to reduced ciclosporin levels, has been reported.

SULFAFURAZOLE (SULFISOXAZOLE)

3,4-Dimethyl-5-sulfanilamidoisoxazole. It is highly soluble, even in acid urine. The spectrum and potency are typical of the group. It is well absorbed, achieving a concentration of around 20 mg/L 3–4 h after a 2 g oral dose.

Side effects are those common to other sulfonamides. It is less prone than some other members of the group to cause renal problems. Its principal use is in urinary tract infection, and is present in some ophthalmic preparations.

SULFAGUANIDINE

1-Sulfanilylguanidine. A poorly absorbed compound, less potent than succinylsulfathiazole but with similar uses. Blood concentrations of 15–40 mg/L have been found after single doses of 1–7 g. Excretion in the urine is rapid.

SULFALENE (SULFAMETOPYRAZINE)

2-Sulfanilamido-3-methoxypyrazine. A very long-acting compound (plasma half-life 60 h). Adequate blood levels can be maintained by giving a dose of 2 g once weekly. The protein binding is *c.* 70%. It has been successfully used in the single-dose treatment of urinary tract infection. As with other long-acting compounds, sulfametopyrazine has been associated with an increased incidence of erythema multiforme.

SULFALOXATE

A poorly absorbed compound formulated as the calcium salt. About 5% is absorbed from the gastrointestinal tract. Formerly used to treat intestinal infections.

SULFAMERAZINE

2-Sulfonamido-4-methylpyrimidine. A component of some triple sulfa combinations. Plasma half-life is *c.* 24 h and protein binding *c.* 75%. It is less active than sulfadiazine.

SULFAMETHIZOLE

2-Sulfanilamido-5-methyl-1,3,4-thiodiazole. A short-acting sulfonamide (plasma half-life 2.5 h). Protein binding is *c.* 85%. About 60% is excreted in the urine within 5 h. It was formerly widely used in the treatment of urinary tract infection.

SULFAMETHOXYDIAZINE

2-Sulfanilamido-5-methoxypyrimidine. A long-acting compound with activity similar to that of sulfadiazine. Binding to plasma proteins is about 75%.

SULFAMETHOXYPYRIDAZINE

3-Sulfanilamido-6-methoxypyridazine. Properties are similar to those of sulfadimethoxine. A rapidly absorbed, long-acting compound (half-life 38 h) with a high degree of protein binding (96%). A 1 g oral dose achieves a peak plasma concentration of around 100 mg/L after 5 h. Its use has been largely discontinued because of frequent adverse effects, but there are reports of benefit in dermatitis herpetiformis. It has been used in combination with trimethoprim.

SULFATHIAZOLE

2-Sulfanilamidothiazole. A short-acting compound (half-life *c.* 4 h) with relatively high activity. Protein binding is *c.* 75%. Its use has declined because of a high incidence of side effects. It is one of the constituents of triple sulfonamide mixtures, of which local preparations are still available.

Two compounds, phthalylsulfathiazole (sulfathalidine) and succinylsulfathiazole (sulfasuxidine) owe their activity to the slow liberation of sulfathiazole in the bowel. They are poorly soluble and very little is absorbed after oral administration. They were formerly used in the treatment of intestinal infections and in bowel preparation before surgery. They are available in multi-ingredient preparations in some countries.

SULFISOMIDINE

6-Sulfanilamido-2,4-dimethylpyrimidine (*syn:* sulphasomidine). A highly soluble sulfonamide with a plasma half-life of 6–8 h. Protein binding is about 90%. Activity is similar to that of sulfadiazine. It is less extensively metabolized than most other sulfonamides and is largely excreted unchanged in the urine.

SULFONAMIDES FOR SPECIAL PURPOSES

MAFENIDE

p-Aminomethylbenzene sulfonamide; Sulfamylon.

A topical agent formerly used extensively in burns, especially for its action in suppressing *Ps. aeruginosa*. It is rapidly absorbed through burned skin and is unusual in that it is not neutralized by *p*-aminobenzoic acid or by tissue exudates. Disadvantages of its use are local pain and burning, a variety of allergic reactions including erythema multiforme and its capacity to inhibit carbonic anhydrase, necessitating careful observation to detect the development of metabolic acidosis. Its metabolite, *p*-carboxybenzene sulfonamide, also inhibits carbonic anhydrase but has no antibacterial activity. Mafenide propionate was formerly used in ophthalmic preparations.

SILVER SULFADIAZINE

Silver sulfadiazine is extremely insoluble. In addition to the usual activity of sulfonamides it exhibits activity – almost certainly attributable to the silver component – against *Ps. aeruginosa* and some fungi.

It is variably absorbed after topical application depending on the integrity of the skin. Toxic concentrations may be achieved in patients with extensive burns. It is used topically, mainly for burns, pressure sores and leg ulcers. Central venous catheters impregnated with chlorhexidine and silver sulfadiazine have been developed to reduce bacterial colonization. Other suggested uses include the prevention of infection in skin graft donor sites and cord care in newborn infants.

Preparations

Proprietary name: Flamazine.

Preparation: Topical cream containing 1% w/w silver sulfadiazine.
Widely available.

Further information

Anonymous. Silver sulfadiazine. In: Dollery C, ed. *Therapeutic Drugs*. 2nd ed. Edinburgh: Churchill Livingstone; 1999:S32–S35.
Atiyeh BS, Costagliola M, Hayek SN, Dibo SA. Effect of silver on burn wound infection control and healing: review of the literature. *Burns*. 2007;33:139–148.
Fuller FW. The side effects of silver sulfadiazine. *J Burn Care Res*. 2009;30:464–470.

SULFASALAZINE

One of the earliest and most successful sulfonamides to be developed was sulfapyridine, which fell into disuse because of unwanted effects such as crystalluria. Later, a number of salicylazosulfonamides, developed because of their increased water solubility, showed anti-inflammatory properties; one of them, sulfasalazine (salicylazosulfapyridine), has come into general use for ulcerative colitis.

After oral administration, some intact compound is absorbed from the upper gastrointestinal tract, appearing in the blood in 1–2 h, but most is cleaved by colonic bacteria to yield sulfapyridine and 5-aminosalicylic acid (mesalamine, mesalazine). Controlled trials have confirmed the efficacy of 5-aminosalicylic acid alone in ulcerative colitis, the sulfonamide component merely acting as a carrier. Thus, in remarkable extension of the good fortune that attended the discovery of sulfanilamide as the unexpected active principle of Prontosil (*see* Ch. 1), a cleavage product appears to be responsible for the beneficial effect of sulfasalazine. Since most of the side effects associated with sulfasalazine are attributable to sulfapyridine, there seems little reason, other than cost, to use it in preference to mesalamine.

Sulfasalazine is also of benefit in Crohn's disease and rheumatoid arthritis, but the role, if any, of sulfapyridine in the overall effect is unclear.

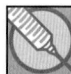

Preparations

Proprietary name: Salazopyrin.

Preparations: Tablets, enema, suppositories, suspension.
Widely available.

Further information

Anonymous. Sulfasalazine. In: Dollery C, ed. *Therapeutic Drugs*. 2nd ed. Edinburgh: Churchill Livingstone; 1999:S140–S144.
Anonymous. Mesalamine. In: Dollery C, ed. *Therapeutic Drugs*. 2nd ed. Edinburgh: Churchill Livingstone; 1999:M61–M65.
Plosker GL, Croom KF. Sulfasalazine: a review of its use in the management of rheumatoid arthritis. *Drugs*. 2005;65:1825–1849.

Ian Chopra

A group of natural products derived from *Streptomyces* spp. and their semisynthetic derivatives. The minimum pharmacophore is a linear fused tetracyclic molecule, 6-deoxy-6-demethyltetracycline:

The various members of the class contain a variety of functional groups attached to the rings designated A, B, C and D. Natural products include chlortetracycline, oxytetracycline, tetracycline and demeclocycline (demethychlortetracycline). Semisynthetic derivatives include doxycycline, minocycline, methacycline, lymecycline, rolitetracycline and tigecycline, a glycylcycline that has been specifically developed to overcome problems of bacterial resistance to earlier tetracyclines.

ANTIMICROBIAL SPECTRUM

Tetracyclines are broad-spectrum, essentially bacteristatic agents. They share a similar spectrum of activity, though that of tigecycline is somewhat different from that of earlier tetracyclines.

In general, tetracyclines are active against many Gram-positive and Gram-negative bacteria, chlamydiae, mycoplasmas, rickettsiae, coxiellae, spirochetes and some mycobacteria. Most streptococci are sensitive, except *Streptococcus agalactiae*, and enterococci. Susceptible Gram-positive bacilli include *Actinomyces israelii*, *Arachnia propionica*, *Listeria monocytogenes*, most clostridia and *Bacillus anthracis*. *Nocardia* spp. are much less susceptible, minocycline demonstrating the greatest activity against them.

Among Gram-negative bacteria most enterobacteria and most strains of *Moraxella catarrhalis*, *Neisseria meningitidis* and *Haemophilus influenzae* are sensitive. Legionellae, brucellae, *Francisella tularensis*, *Vibrio cholerae*, *Campylobacter* spp., *Helicobacter pylori*, *Plesiomonas shigelloides* and *Aeromonas hydrophila* are all susceptible. Many anaerobic bacteria are susceptible, doxycycline and minocycline being the most active. Rickettsiae are generally sensitive, especially to doxycycline, minocycline and tetracycline. None is active against *Pseudomonas aeruginosa*, *Proteus* spp. or *Providencia* spp., but *Burkholderia pseudomallei* and *Stenotrophomonas maltophilia* are usually susceptible.

ACQUIRED RESISTANCE

Resistance to tetracyclines has emerged in an ever-increasing number of bacterial species and is geographically widespread. Resistance arises primarily from acquisition of genes that either encode transporters of the major facilitator superfamily (MFS), which remove the antibiotics from the cell (e.g. TetB, TetK), or encode proteins that protect the ribosome from inhibition (e.g. TetM, TetO). Tigecycline is not affected by these resistance mechanisms and consequently is active against many species resistant to earlier tetracyclines. In some Gram-negative bacteria resistance can also be due to the activity of innate (endogenous) bacterial efflux proteins such as the chromosomally encoded resistance–nodulation–cell division efflux pumps that confer resistance to several structurally unrelated biocides and antibiotics, as well as all classes of tetracyclines. The presence of these pumps explains the inherent resistance of most *Ps. aeruginosa* and *Proteus* spp. to all tetracyclines.

PHARMACOKINETICS

ABSORPTION

Tetracyclines are usually administered by mouth. However, tigecycline is available only for intravenous infusion.

Absorption of oral tetracyclines occurs largely in the proximal small bowel, but may be diminished by the simultaneous presence of food, milk or cations, which form nonabsorbable tetracycline chelates. Cimetidine and presumably other H_2-receptor antagonists also impair absorption of tetracyclines by interfering with their dissolution, which is pH dependent.

The absorption problems of earlier compounds have been essentially overcome in the later tetracyclines. Improved absorption is claimed for lymecycline, demeclocycline and methacycline, but is best established for doxycycline and minocycline, which may be administered with food and for which the proportion of administered dose absorbed is more than 90%.

DISTRIBUTION

For orally administered tetracyclines, peak serum concentrations follow 1–4 h after ingestion. Serum levels achieved after normal dosage of orally bioavailable tetracyclines are of the order of 1.5–4.0 mg/L. Most tetracyclines must be given four times daily to maintain therapeutic concentrations in the blood, but demeclocycline and minocycline can be administered twice daily and doxycycline once daily.

Tetracyclines penetrate moderately well into body fluids and tissues, reflected in relatively large volumes of distribution. Concentrations of most tetracyclines in the cerebrospinal fluid (CSF) are usually about 10–25% of those in the blood, although penetration of tigecycline into the CSF is poor. A unique feature of tetracyclines is deposition and persistence in areas where bone is being laid down. Radioactive tracer studies in animals suggest that tigecycline also concentrates in the bone but concentration at this site in humans remains unproven owing to technical difficulties with assay methods.

Older tetracyclines are known to penetrate into the sebum and are excreted in perspiration, properties which contribute to their usefulness in the management of acne. The older tetracyclines are also known to be concentrated in the eye.

EXCRETION

Excretory routes are the kidney and feces. Fecal excretion occurs even after parenteral administration as a result of passage of the drug into the bile. The concentrations obtained in bile are 5–25 times those in the blood, doxycycline attaining especially high levels. These concentrations are lowered in the presence of biliary obstruction. The proportion of administered dose found in the urine is, for most tetracyclines, in the range 20–60%, but is less for chlortetracycline and doxycycline and least for minocycline and tigecycline.

TOXICITY AND SIDE EFFECTS

Known adverse effects are primarily based on studies with older tetracyclines and it is not yet clear whether they also apply to tigecycline. However, it might be expected that tigecycline will share at least some of the unwanted side effects associated with all members of the class.

The most important adverse effect is gastrointestinal intolerance, reported for all tetracyclines including tigecycline. Photosensitivity is a class phenomenon; it is most marked for demeclocycline but is not yet reported for tigecycline. Deposition in developing bones and teeth precludes the use of older tetracyclines in young children and during late pregnancy; tigecycline may also exhibit these properties and is contraindicated in these situations. Most compounds accumulate in renal failure, with the exception of doxycycline and tigecycline. Nausea and vomiting are presumed to be due to a direct irritant effect of the drug on the gastric mucosa, but diarrhea is probably the result of disturbance of the normal flora. The frequency and nature of superinfection with resistant organisms depends much on local ecology. Pseudomembranous colitis has been associated with the use of older tetracyclines, but they do not appear to be a common precursor of that complication. Other organisms that often become dominant in the fecal flora after administration of tetracyclines are *Candida*, *Proteus* or *Pseudomonas* spp. *Staph. aureus* enterocolitis, which was described in hospital patients when tetracyclines were widely prescribed, now seems to be rare.

Glossitis and pruritus ani, vulvitis and vaginitis are well-recognized side effects associated with the use of older tetracyclines; less common side effects include esophageal ulceration and acute pancreatitis. Changes occur in the surface lipids of the skin, notably a decrease in fatty acids and reciprocal increase in triglycerides that probably results from inhibition of extracellular bacterial lipase production by *Propionibacterium acnes*.

Deaths have been reported in pregnant women given large intravenous doses (>1 g per day), usually for the treatment of pyelonephritis. The main lesion found at autopsy was diffuse fatty degeneration of the liver, which may also involve the pancreas, kidneys and brain. Mild derangements of liver enzyme function are not uncommon.

A number of infants have developed bulging of the anterior fontanelle; benign intracranial hypertension has also been described in older children and even in adults, with headache, photophobia and papilledema. Symptoms disappear quickly after the drug is withdrawn, but papilledema may persist in some patients for many months or reappear when tetracyclines are given again. The mechanism is unknown.

Hypersensitivity rashes, including exfoliation, occasionally occur, but skin reactions are more often manifestations of photosensitivity. A reaction may occur after administration of any tetracycline, but is especially associated with demeclocycline and may be less common with doxycycline and minocycline. Fixed drug eruptions, onycholysis and nail and

Table 30.1 Current applications of tetracyclines (excluding tigecycline)

Type of infection	First choice	Acceptable alternative to other agents
Respiratory	Atypical pneumonia due to *Mycoplasma pneumoniae, Chlamydophila* (formerly *Chlamydia*) *pneumoniae, Ch. psittaci*	Community-acquired pneumonia[a] Infective exacerbations of chronic bronchitis[a] Legionellosis (doxycycline)
Bowel	Cholera Prophylaxis of traveler's diarrhea	
Genital	Non-gonococcal urethritis; cervicitis Lymphogranuloma venereum Pelvic inflammatory disease Granuloma inguinale	Syphilis Epididymitis Prostatitis
Other infections	Rocky Mountain spotted fever Endemic and epidemic typhus Trachoma (topical or oral) Q fever Brucellosis[b] Lyme disease Relapsing fever Periodontal infection (topical tetracycline or minocycline) Acne vulgaris (topical and systemic treatment)	Plague Tularemia Bartonellosis Leptospirosis Whipple's disease Cutaneous *Mycobacterium marinum* infections *Helicobacter pylori* infections[b] Prophylaxis of drug-resistant *Plasmodium falciparum* malaria

[a]Except in situations where there is a high rate of resistance among pneumococci and/or *H. influenzae.*
[b]In combination with other agents.

thyroid pigmentation have also been reported. Angiodema and anaphylaxis are rare. Hypersensitivity reactions to one tetracycline generally infer cross-hypersensitivity to the other agents. Reported inhibitory effects on several human polymorphonuclear leukocyte and lymphocyte functions in vitro have yet to be shown to have any therapeutic significance.

Drug interactions include complexes with divalent and trivalent cations together with chelation by iron-containing preparations. The anticonvulsants carbamazepine, phenytoin and barbiturates decrease the half-life of doxycycline through enzyme induction. The anesthetic methoxyflurane has been reported to cause nephrotoxicity when co-administered with older tetracyclines. Tigecycline is reported to affect the pharmacokinetic profile of warfarin such that anticoagulation tests should be performed if it is administered with warfarin. The efficiency of oral contraceptives is reduced by tetracyclines, as with many other broad-spectrum antibiotics.

CLINICAL USE

The use of tetracyclines has significantly declined in most countries as the incidence of bacterial resistance has increased and more active and better tolerated antimicrobial agents have been introduced. However, some new applications have emerged, such as their use as part of multidrug regimens for the management of gastritis and peptic ulcer disease associated with *H. pylori*. Their activity against malaria has become important for prophylaxis following the rapid increase of chloroquine- and mefloquine-resistant *Plasmodium falciparum*.

Current applications of the older tetracyclines are summarized in Table 30.1. Tigecycline is currently approved only for use in complicated skin and skin structure infections (including those caused by methicillin-resistant *Staph. aureus*), complicated intra-abdominal infections and community-acquired bacterial pneumonia, but use for other indications, including those listed in Table 30.1, may emerge if there is suitable clinical evidence.

 Further information

Bryskier A. Tetracyclines. In: Bryskier A, ed. *Antimicrobial agents: antibacterials and antifungals.* Washington, D.C.: American Society for Microbiology; 2005:642–651.

Chopra I. Glycylcyclines: third-generation tetracycline antibiotics. *Curr Opin Pharmacol.* 2001;1:464–469.

Chopra I, Roberts M. Tetracycline antibiotics: mode of action, applications, molecular biology and epidemiology of bacterial resistance. *Microbiology and Molecular Microbiology Reviews.* 2001;65:232–260.

Dean CR, Visalli MA, Projan SJ, et al. Efflux-mediated resistance to tigecycline (GAR-936) in *Pseudomonas aeruginosa* PAO1. *Antimicrob Agents Chemother.* 2003;47:972–978.

Maurin M, Raoult D. Q fever. *Clin Microbiol Rev.* 1999;12:518–553.

Pankey GA. Tigecycline. *J Antimicrob Chemother.* 2005;56:470–480.

Petersen PJ, Jacobus NV, Weiss WJ, Sum PE, Testa RT. In vitro and in vivo antibacterial activities of a novel glycylcycline, the 9-t-butylglycylamido derivative of minocycline (GAR-936). *Antimicrob Agents Chemother.* 1999;43:738–744.

Roberts MC. Tetracycline therapy: update. *Clin Infect Dis.* 2003;36:462–467.

Van Steenberghe D, Rosling B, Soder PO, et al. A 15-month evaluation of the effects of repeated subgingival minocycline in chronic adult periodontitis. *J Periodontol.* 1999;70:657–667.

Zhanel GC, Homenuik K, Nichol K, et al. The glycylcyclines: a comparative review with the tetracyclines. *Drugs.* 2004;64:63–88.

CHLORTETRACYCLINE

Molecular weight (free base): 478.9; (hydrochloride): 515.3.

7-Chlortetracycline. A fermentation product of certain strains of *Streptomyces aureofaciens*. Formulated as the hydrochloride or the free base for oral or topical application.

ANTIMICROBIAL ACTIVITY

The activity against a range of pathogenic bacteria is shown in Table 30.2. It is slightly less active than tetracycline against many bacteria, with the exception of Gram-positive organisms.

PHARMACOKINETICS

Oral absorption	30–60%
C$_{max}$ 500 mg oral	2.5–7 mg/L
Plasma half-life	5–6 h
Volume of distribution	*c.* 2 L/kg
Plasma protein binding	47–65%

Absorption is relatively poor compared with other tetracyclines. It undergoes rapid metabolism and is largely eliminated by biliary excretion, with only a small proportion eliminated via the kidney. Despite this, chlortetracycline is not recommended for patients in renal failure, since accumulation occurs as a consequence of the half-life increase to approximately 7–11 h.

TOXICITY AND SIDE EFFECTS

Side effects are typical of the group (p. 345). Contact hypersensitivity has been reported with topical application to abraded skin and varicose ulcers.

CLINICAL USE

Its uses are those common to the group (Table 30.1, p. 346). It has also been used topically in the management of recurrent aphthous ulcers of the mouth, but experience is limited and the mechanism of action is unknown.

Preparations and dosage

Proprietary name: Aureomycin.
Preparations: Topical, ophthalmic, capsules.
Dosage: Adults, oral, 250–500 mg, every 6 h.
Widely available; oral preparation not available in the UK.

Table 30.2 Activity of the most important tetracyclines against common pathogenic bacteria: MIC (mg/L). Data compiled from a variety of sources

Organism	Chlortetracycline	Demeclocycline	Doxycycline	Minocycline	Oxytetracycline	Tetracycline	Tigecycline
Staphylococcus aureus	0.5–R	1–R	0.5–16	0.5–16	2–R	2–R	0.25–2
Streptococcus pyogenes	0.1–32	0.25–32	0.1–16	0.1–16	0.25–32	0.25–32	0.06–0.25
Str. pneumoniae	No data	No data	0.06–32	0.06–16	No data	0.12–R	0.03–0.25
Enterococcus faecalis	4–R	2–R	2–R	2–R	8–R	8–R	0.12–1
Neisseria gonorrhoeae	0.25–>8	0.5–>8	0.1–>8	0.25–8	1–>8	0.5–>8	0.008–0.12
N. meningitidis	No data	No data	No data	0.06–0.12	No data	0.06–0.25	0.015–0.12
Haemophilus influenzae	1–>8	2–>8	1–2	0.12–2	4–16	0.25–>8	1–4
Escherichia coli	8–16	4–16	2–16	4–8	2–16	2–16	0.12–0.25
Klebsiella pneumoniae	8–R	8–R	8–R	4–32	16–R	4–R	0.5–4
Proteus mirabilis	R	32–R	R	R	R	32–R	2–R
Seratia marcescens	R	R	R	32	R	4–16	1–8
Pseudomonas aeruginosa	R	32–R	32–R	R	R	32–R	0.5–32
Bacteroides fragilis	No data	No data	No data	0.25–R	0.5–R	No data	0.5–8

R, resistant (MIC >32 mg/L).

Further information

Anonymous. Chlortetracycline (hydrochloride). In: Dollery C, ed. *Therapeutic Drugs*. 2nd ed. Edinburgh: Churchill Livingstone; 1999:C199–C201.

DEMECLOCYCLINE

Molecular weight (free base): 464.9; (hydrochloride): 501.3.

6-Demethyl-7-chlortetracycline. A fermentation product of a mutant strain of *Streptomyces aureofaciens* formulated as the hydrochloride for oral administration.

 ANTIMICROBIAL ACTIVITY

Activity against a range of pathogenic bacteria is shown in Table 30.2. Occasional strains of viridans streptococci, *N. gonorrhoeae* and *H. influenzae* are more susceptible than to tetracycline. It is the most active tetracycline against *Brucella* spp.

 PHARMACOKINETICS

Oral absorption	60–70%
C_{max} 300 mg oral	2 mg/L after 3–6 h
Plasma half-life	c. 12 h
Volume of distribution	c. 1.7 L/kg
Plasma protein binding	90%

Absorption

It is promptly yet incompletely absorbed by mouth, giving mean peak plasma levels after a single dose that are slightly higher than those produced by oxytetracycline and chlortetracycline, but lower than those achieved by tetracycline. However, with repeat dosing, steady-state concentrations exceed those for tetracycline. Simultaneous administration of antacids markedly depresses blood levels.

Distribution and excretion

It is widely distributed, achieving concentrations in pleural exudates similar to those of blood. CSF penetration is poor, especially in the absence of inflammation. Biliary concentrations are 20–30 times higher than those of plasma,

and 40–50% of the drug can be recovered from feces. The other route of elimination is via glomerular filtration without reabsorption and accumulation occurs in renal failure.

 TOXICITY AND SIDE EFFECTS

Untoward reactions, notably gastrointestinal intolerance, are generally those typical of the group (p. 345). Occasional patients develop transient steatorrhea.

Of particular note is the occurrence of nephrogenic diabetes insipidus with development of vasopressin-resistant polyuria. The effect is dose dependent and occurs with daily doses in excess of 1.2 g. The drug inhibits activation of adenylate cyclase and protein kinase, which are both important in the interaction of antidiuretic hormone (ADH) with receptors within the renal tubule, thus decreasing the effect of ADH on the kidney. As a result, it has found a place in the treatment of inappropriate ADH secretion.

Renal failure may occur, particularly if prescribed for those with advanced liver cirrhosis. The mechanism is uncertain but may in part be related to the antianabolic effect of the tetracyclines as well as a direct toxic effect.

Photosensitivity may be severe and accompanied by vesiculation, edema and onycholysis. It is largely restricted to exposed skin; patients should avoid prolonged exposure to sunlight.

 CLINICAL USE

Its uses are those common to the group (Table 30.1, p. 346). It has been extensively used in the management of the syndrome of inappropriate ADH secretion in a dose of at least 1.2 g per day; therapeutic response may take several days, but is superior to that of lithium. It has also found occasional use in patients with water retention as a result of congestive cardiac failure and in those with alcoholic cirrhosis and water and electrolyte retention.

Preparations and dosage

Proprietary names: Declomycin, Ledermycin.
Preparations: Capsules, tablets.
Dosage: Adults, oral, 150 mg every 6 h, or 300 mg every 12 h.
Widely available.

 Further information

Anonymous. Demeclocycline (hydrochloride). In: Dollery C, ed. *Therapeutic Drugs*. 2nd ed. Edinburgh: Churchill Livingstone; 1999:D29–D31.
Geheb M, Cox M. Renal effects of demeclocycline. *J Am Med Assoc*. 1980;243:2519–2520.
Miller PD, Linas SL, Schrier RW. Plasma demeclocycline levels and nephrotoxicity. Correlation in hyponatremic cirrhotic patients. *J Am Med Assoc*. 1980;243:2513–2515.

DOXYCYCLINE

Molecular weight (free base): 444.5; (hyclate): 512.9.

6-Deoxy-5 β-hydroxytetracycline. A semisynthetic product supplied as the hyclate, calcium salt or the hydrochloride for oral and intravenous administration.

ANTIMICROBIAL ACTIVITY

Its activity and spectrum are typical of the group (Table 30.2). It is active against some tetracycline-resistant *Staph. aureus* and is more active than other tetracyclines against *Str. pyogenes*, enterococci and *Nocardia* spp. *Mor. catarrhalis* (MIC 0.5 mg/L), *Legionella pneumophila* and most strains of *Ureaplasma urealyticum* (MIC 0.5 mg/L) are susceptible.

PHARMACOKINETICS

Oral absorption	90%
C_{max} 100–200 mg oral	1.7–5.7 mg/L after 2–3.5 h
100 mg intravenous infusion (1 h)	2.5 mg/L end infusion
Plasma half-life	18 h
Volume of distribution	0.9–1.8 L/kg
Plasma protein binding	90%

Absorption

Doxycycline is rapidly absorbed from the upper gastrointestinal tract and absorption appears to be linearly related to the administered dose. Food, especially dairy products, reduces peak serum concentrations by 20%. Alcohol also delays absorption. As with other tetracyclines, divalent and trivalent cations, as in antacids and ferrous sulfate, form chelates which reduce absorption.

Distribution

The greater lipophilicity of doxycycline is responsible for its widespread tissue distribution. Concentrations in liver, biliary system, kidneys and the digestive tract are approximately twice those in plasma. Within the respiratory tract, it achieves concentrations of 2.3–6.7 mg/kg in tonsils and 2.3–7.5 mg/kg in maxillary sinus mucosa. In bronchial secretions concentrations are about 20% of plasma levels, increasing to 25–35% in the presence of pleurisy. Gallbladder concentrations are approximately 75% those of plasma, and prostate concentrations are 60–100%. It penetrates well into the aqueous humor. CSF concentrations range from 11% to 56% of plasma levels and are not affected by inflammation. In the elderly, tissue concentrations are 50–100% higher than in young adults. The half-life remains unaltered and one explanation is reduced fecal elimination.

Metabolism and excretion

Doxycycline is largely excreted unchanged. Around 35% is eliminated through the kidneys and the remainder through the digestive tract. Renal clearance ranges from 1.8 to 2.1 L/h, and is largely via glomerular filtration, with approximately 70% tubular reabsorption. Alkalinization enhances renal clearance. Fecal elimination partly reflects biliary excretion but also includes diffusion across the intestinal wall. Provided the drug is not chelated, reabsorption occurs with enterohepatic recycling. The elimination half-life is long (15–25 h).

The half-life and the area under the concentration–time curve (AUC) are little altered in renal insufficiency, with no evidence of accumulation after repeat dosing, even in anuric patients, evidently as a result of increased clearance through the liver or gastrointestinal tract, since biliary and fecal concentrations increase in renal failure. Although the plasma elimination half-life is unchanged, the drug appears to accumulate in tissues with increasing renal failure, and it has been suggested that less drug is bound to plasma protein and red cells through competition with other metabolites, which in turn increases hepatic elimination. Pharmacokinetics are unaltered by hemodialysis or peritoneal dialysis. Clearance is decreased by about half in patients with type IIa and type IV hyperlipidemia.

The plasma elimination half-life is shortened by various antiepileptic agents including phenytoin, barbiturates and carbamazepine, presumably as a result of liver enzyme induction, although there is also evidence for some interference with the protein binding of doxycycline.

TOXICITY AND SIDE EFFECTS

Untoward reactions are generally those typical of the group but gastrointestinal side effects are less common than with other tetracyclines due to the lower total dosage and the ability to administer the drug with meals. Esophageal ulceration as a result of capsule impaction has been reported. Dental and bone deposition appear to be less common than with other tetracycline derivatives. Other adverse phenomena include occasional vestibular toxicity.

Hypersensitivity reactions include photosensitivity and eosinophilia, but rarely anaphylaxis. In common with demeclocycline and chlortetracycline it may be a more powerful sensitizer than other tetracyclines. It is contraindicated in patients with acute porphyria because it has been demonstrated to be porphyrinogenic in animals.

CLINICAL USE

Uses are those common to the group (Table 30.1, p. 346). Its once-daily administration and safety in renal insufficiency make it one of the most widely used tetracyclines. It is used in the prophylaxis and treatment of malaria in areas in which resistance to conventional antimalarial agents is common.

Preparations and dosage

Proprietary name: Vibramycin.

Preparations: Capsules, tablets, suspension.

Dosage: Adults, oral, 200 mg on day 1 then 100 mg per day; severe infections, 200 mg per day; acne, 50 mg per day for 6 weeks or longer. Widely available.

Further information

Anonymous. Doxycycline hyclate. In: Dollery C, ed. *Therapeutic Drugs*. 2nd ed. Edinburgh: Churchill Livingstone; 1999:D229–D232.
Cunha BA. Doxycycline re-visited. *Arch Intern Med.* 1999;159:1006–1007.

MINOCYCLINE

7-Dimethylamino-6-demethyl-6-deoxy-tetracycline. Molecular weight (free base): 457.5; (hydrochloride): 493.9.

A semisynthetic tetracycline derivative supplied as the hydrochloride for oral administration.

ANTIMICROBIAL ACTIVITY

Activity against common bacterial pathogens is shown in Table 30.2 (p. 347). It exhibits the broad-spectrum activity typical of the group, but retains activity against some strains of *Staph. aureus* resistant to older tetracyclines. It is active against β-hemolytic streptococci and some tetracycline-resistant pneumococci. It is also active against some enterobacteria resistant to other tetracyclines, probably because some Gram-negative efflux pumps remove minocycline less effectively than other tetracyclines. Some strains of *H. influenzae* resistant to other tetracyclines are susceptible. *Sten. maltophilia* is susceptible, as are most strains of *Acinetobacter* spp. and *L. pneumophila*.

It is notable for its activity against *Bacteroides* and *Fusobacterium* spp., and is more active than other tetracyclines against *C. trachomatis*, brucellae and nocardiae. It inhibits *Mycobacterium tuberculosis*, *M. bovis*, *M. kansasii* and *M. intracellulare* at 5–6 mg/L. *Candida albicans* and *C. tropicalis* are also slightly susceptible.

PHARMACOKINETICS

Oral absorption	95–100%
C_{max} 150 mg oral	2 mg/L after 2 h
300 mg oral	4 mg/L after 2h
Plasma half-life	12–24 h
Volume of distribution	80–115 L
Plasma protein binding	76%

Absorption

Food does not significantly affect absorption, which is depressed by co-administration with milk. It is chelated by metals and suffers the effects of antacids and ferrous sulfate common to tetracyclines. On a regimen of 100 mg every 12 h, steady-state concentrations ranged between 2.3 and 3.5 mg/L.

Distribution

The high lipophilicity of minocycline provides wide distribution and tissue concentrations that often exceed those of the plasma. The tissue:plasma ratio in maxillary sinus and tonsillar tissue is 1.6; that in lung is 3–4. Sputum concentrations may reach 37–60% of simultaneous plasma levels. In bile, liver and gallbladder the ratios are 38, 12 and 6.5, respectively.

Prostatic and seminal fluid concentrations range from 40% to 100% of those of serum. CSF penetration is poor, especially in the non-inflamed state. Concentrations in tears and saliva are high, and may explain its beneficial effect in the treatment of meningococcal carriage.

Metabolism

Biotransformation to three microbiologically inactive metabolites occurs in the liver; the most abundant is 9-hydroxyminocycline.

Excretion

Only 4–9% of administered drug is excreted in the urine, and in renal failure elimination is little affected. Neither hemodialysis nor peritoneal dialysis affects drug elimination. Fecal excretion is relatively low and evidence for enterohepatic recirculation remains uncertain. Despite high hepatic excretion, dose accumulation does not occur in liver disease, such as cirrhosis. Type IIa and type IV hyperlipidemic patients show a decreased minocycline clearance of 50%, suggesting that dose modification may be necessary.

 ## TOXICITY AND SIDE EFFECTS

Minocycline shares the untoward reactions common to the group with gastrointestinal side effects being most common, and more prevalent in women. Diarrhea is relatively uncommon, presumably as a result of its lower fecal concentrations. Hypersensitivity reactions, including rashes, interstitial nephritis and pulmonary eosinophilia, are occasionally seen.

Staining of the permanent dentition occurs with all tetracyclines; a side effect that appears to be unique to minocycline is that of tissue discoloration and skin pigmentation. Tissues that may become pigmented include the skin, skull and other bones and the thyroid gland, which at autopsy appears blackened. The pigmentation tends to resolve slowly with discontinuation of the drug and is related to the length of therapy. Three types of pigmentation have been identified:

- A brown macular discoloration ('muddy skin syndrome'), which occurs in sun-exposed parts and is histologically associated with melanin deposition.
- Blue–black macular pigmentation occurring within inflamed areas and scars associated with hemosiderin deposition.
- Circumscribed macular blue–gray pigmented areas occurring in sun-exposed and unexposed skin, which appears to be linked to a breakdown product of minocycline.

CNS toxicity has been prominent, notably benign intracranial hypertension, which resolves on discontinuation of the drug, and, more commonly, dizziness, ataxia, vertigo, tinnitus, nausea and vomiting, which appear to be more frequent in women. These primarily vestibular side effects have ranged in frequency from 4.5% to 86%. They partly coincide with plasma concentration peaks, but their exact pathogenesis has yet to be determined.

 ## CLINICAL USE

There appear to be few situations in which it has a unique therapeutic advantage over other tetracyclines. Its use has been tempered by the high incidence of vestibular side effects.

Although used in the long-term management of acne, the potential for skin pigmentation must be considered. Because of its high tissue concentrations, it may occasionally provide a useful alternative to other agents for the treatment of chronic prostatitis. It has a role in the treatment of sexually transmitted chlamydial infections.

 ### Further information

Anonymous. Minocycline (hydrochloride). In: Dollery C, ed. *Therapeutic Drugs.* 2nd ed. Edinburgh: Churchill Livingstone; 1999:M187–M190.
Dykhuizen RS, Zaidi AM, Godden DJ, Jegarajah S, Legge JS. Minocycline and pulmonary eosinophilia. *Br Med J.* 1995;310:1520–1521.
Freeman CD, Nightingale CH, Quintiliani R. Minocycline: old and new therapeutic uses. *Int J Antimicrob Agents.* 1994;4:325–335.
Okada N, Moriya K, Nishida K, et al. Skin pigmentation associated with minocycline therapy. *Br J Dermatol.* 1989;121:247–257.
Saivin S, Houin G. Clinical pharmacokinetics of doxycycline and minocycline. *Clin Pharmacokinet.* 1988;15:355–366.

OXYTETRACYCLINE

5-Hydroxytetracycline. Molecular weight (free base): 460.4; (dihydrate): 496.5.

A fermentation product of certain strains of *Streptomyces rimosus*, supplied as the dihydrate or hydrochloride for oral or parenteral administration.

 ## ANTIMICROBIAL ACTIVITY

Its spectrum and activity are typical of the group (Table 30.2, p. 347). It is slightly less active than other tetracyclines against most common pathogenic bacteria.

PHARMACOKINETICS

Oral absorption	c. 60%
C_{max} 500 mg oral	3–4 mg/L after 2–4 h
Plasma half-life	c. 9 h
Volume of distribution	c. 1.8 L/kg
Plasma protein binding	20–35%

Oxytetracycline is moderately well absorbed from the upper gastrointestinal tract. Food decreases plasma levels by approximately 50%. Although widely distributed in the tissues, it achieves lower concentrations than related agents such as mino-cycline. Sputum concentrations of 1 mg/L have been recorded on a daily dosage of 2 g. Approximately 60% is excreted in the urine and the half-life is prolonged in renal insufficiency.

 ## TOXICITY AND SIDE EFFECTS

Gastrointestinal intolerance is responsible for most side effects, and tends to be more severe than with other tetra-cyclines. Esophageal irritation may result from the local effects of the swallowed drug. Potentially serious adverse reactions have included neuromuscular paralysis follow-ing intravenous administration to patients with myasthenia gravis. Thrombocytopenic purpura and lupus erythematosus syndrome have been reported, although a direct role for the drug in the latter remains uncertain. Apart from the effect on nitrogen balance common to many tetracyclines, a metabolic effect on glucose homeostasis has been noted in type 1 dia-betes mellitus. Allergic contact sensitivity reactions have also been reported.

 ## CLINICAL USE

Its uses are those common to the group (Table 30.1, p. 346). It offers no unique therapeutic advantages, although it is one of the cheaper preparations.

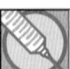 ### Preparations and dosage

Proprietary name: Terramycin.

Preparations: Tablets, capsules.

Dosage: Adults, oral, 250–500 mg every 6 h; acne, 250 mg–1 g per day as a single dose or two divided doses.

Widely available.

 ### Further information

Anonymous. Oxytetracycline (dihydrate). In: Dollery C, ed. *Therapeutic Drugs*. 2nd ed. Edinburgh: Churchill Livingstone; 1999:O55–O58.

TETRACYCLINE

Molecular weight (free base): 444.4; (hydrochloride): 480.9.

 ## ANTIMICROBIAL ACTIVITY

Its activity against common pathogenic bacteria is shown in Table 30.2 (p. 347). It is also active against *V. cholerae*, chla-mydiae, rickettsiae and spirochetes.

 ## PHARMACOKINETICS

Oral absorption	c. 75%
C_{max} 500 mg oral	2–4 g/L
Plasma half-life	8.5 h
Volume of distribution	c. 1.3 L/kg
Plasma protein binding	c. 50–60%

Absorption

When taken with food, absorption is reduced by approxi-mately 50%. Steady-state plasma concentrations of 4–5 mg/L occur after oral doses of 500 mg every 6 h. Women appear to produce higher concentrations than men. Divalent and trivalent cations such as calcium and aluminum pres-ent in antacids and milk interfere with absorption through chelation, as does ferrous sulfate. H_2-receptor antagonists, by raising gastric pH, also interfere with absorption through impaired drug dissolution. Despite the effect of gastric pH, oral absorption is not affected in elderly patients with achlorhydria.

Distribution

Tetracycline is widely distributed in the body tissues. In particular, it penetrates well into the prostate, uterus, ovary and bladder, and also appears to be preferentially taken up by the gastrointestinal tract. It is also detectable within reticuloendothelial cells of the liver, spleen and bone marrow.

Protein binding is reduced in states of malnutrition. It is also bound to bone, dentine and tooth enamel of unerupted teeth. Sputum concentrations of 0.4–2.6 mg/L have been detected after 250 mg oral dosage every 8 h. Maxillary sinus secretions and bronchial mucosal tissue have concentrations comparable to those of serum.

CSF penetration is poor, but increases with meningeal inflammation. It crosses the placenta readily to enter the fetal circulation, where it achieves 25–75% of the maternal plasma concentration. It is also present in breast milk.

A fermentation product of *Streptomyces aureofaciens*, also pro-duced from chlortetracycline. Available as the hydrochloride for oral and topical use.

Metabolism

A small amount is metabolized to 4-epitetracycline.

Excretion

Tetracycline is largely eliminated unchanged by glomerular filtration, with more than 50% excreted within 24 h after oral administration. This rises to approximately 70% following parenteral administration. Urinary concentrations of 300 mg/L occur within the first 2 h and persist for up to 12 h. Urinary excretion is enhanced in alkaline urine. Renal clearance is reduced in severe protein calorie malnutrition, possibly through reduced glomerular filtration. It accumulates in the presence of renal failure and is only slowly removed by hemodialysis and minimally by peritoneal dialysis.

The bile is an important route of excretion, accounting for about one-third of the dose. Biliary concentrations may be 10–25 times those found in serum. Impaired hepatic function or biliary obstruction leads to an increase in blood levels.

TOXICITY AND SIDE EFFECTS

The gastrointestinal side effects common to the group are the most frequent cause of intolerance. Metallic taste and glossitis are less burdensome than diarrhea. Antibiotic-associated enterocolitis caused by *Clostridium difficile* toxin and staphylococcal enterocolitis have been reported. Steatorrhea and acute pancreatitis has also been described. Irritation and ulceration of the esophagus has occurred with local impaction of the drug. *C. albicans* overgrowth is common and may result in symptomatic oral or vaginal candidiasis and occasionally candida diarrhea.

Hypersensitivity reactions include contact dermatitis, urticaria, facial edema and asthma. Anaphylaxis is rare. A lupus syndrome has been reported, but its cause is uncertain. Photosensitivity can be severe and cause vesiculation, desquamation and onycholysis. The Jarisch–Herxheimer reaction has been observed in the treatment of syphilis, louse-borne relapsing fever, leptospirosis, brucellosis and tularemia. Deposition in deciduous teeth and bone (where it may temporarily inhibit growth) is of continuing concern. Between 3% and 44% of administered tetracycline is incorporated in the inorganic phase of bone, which may become visibly discolored and fluoresce. Concentrations as high as 290 mg/g have been recorded in bone in those on long-term tetracycline treatment for acne.

Existing renal insufficiency may be aggravated and is probably related to the antianabolic effect of this class of drugs; interference with protein synthesis places an additional burden on the kidney from amino acid metabolism. Acute renal failure may occur and can be aggravated by drug-induced diarrhea. Dehydration and salt loss from diuretic therapy may aggravate nephrotoxicity. Methoxyflurane and tetracycline in combination may be synergistically nephrotoxic.

An uncommon but serious adverse reaction is acute fatty liver, which may be complicated by renal insufficiency and electrolyte abnormalities. This is most likely to occur with high-dose intravenous administration, especially during pregnancy.

Hematological toxicity is uncommon. Leukopenia, thrombocytopenia and hemolytic anemia have been reported. Altered coagulation may also occur with high intravenous dosage. Phagocyte function may be impaired as a result of the increased excretion of vitamin C.

Neurological toxicity is uncommon but includes benign intracranial hypertension (p. 345). A transient myopathy has complicated long-term oral use for the treatment of acne, while intravenous administration has caused increased muscle weakness in those with myasthenia gravis and has also potentiated curare-induced neuromuscular blockade.

Metabolic effects include: precipitation of lactic acidosis in diabetic patients receiving phenformin; a reduction in vitamins B_{12}, B_6 and pantothenic acid with long-term therapy; interference with laboratory tests of urinary catecholamines and urinary tests for glucose (Clinitest and Benedict's); and elevation of serum lithium concentrations. In addition, warfarin is potentiated and failure of oral contraception occurs.

CLINICAL USE

Uses are those listed in Table 30.1 (p. 346). Along with doxycycline it is one of the most commonly used tetracyclines.

Preparations and dosage

Proprietary names: Achromycin, Sustamycin, Tetrabid-Organon, Tetrachel, Decteclo (in combination with chlortetracycline and demeclocycline), Mysteclin (in combination with nystatin).
Preparations: Tablets, capsules.
Dosage: Adults, oral, 250–500 mg every 6–8 h, depending on severity of infection; acne, 500 mg–1 g per day as a single dose or two divided doses.
Widely available as oral formulation.

Further information

Anonymous. Tetracycline (hydrochloride). In: Dollery C, ed. *Therapeutic Drugs*. 2nd ed. Edinburgh: Churchill Livingstone; 1999:T66–T69.

Boer de WA, Driessen WM, Potters VP, Tytgat GN. Randomized study comparing 1 with 2 weeks of quadruple therapy for eradicating Helicobacter pylori. *Am J Gastroenterol*. 1994;89:1993–1997.

Feurle GE, Marth T. An evaluation of antimicrobial treatment for Whipple's disease. Tetracycline versus trimethoprim–sulfamethoxazole. *Dig Dis Sci*. 1994;39:1642–1648.

Labenz J, Ruhl GH, Bertrams J, Borsch G. Effective treatment after failure of omeprazole plus amoxycillin to eradicate *Helicobacter pylori* infection in peptic ulcer disease. *Alimen Pharmacol Ther*. 1994;8:323–327.

Looareesuwan S, Vanijanota S, Viravan C, et al. Randomised trial of mefloquine–tetracycline and quinine–tetracycline for acute uncomplicated falciparum malaria. *Acta Trop*. 1994;57:47–53.

Murphy AA, Zacur HA, Charache P, Burkman RT. The effect of tetracycline on levels of oral contraceptives. *Am J Obstet Gynecol.* 1991;164:28–33.

Nicolau DP, Mengedoht DE, Kline JJ. Tetracycline-induced pancreatitis. *Am J Gastroenterol.* 1991;86:1669–1671.

TIGECYCLINE

Molecular weight: 585.6

9-T-butylglycylamido-minocycline. A compound of the glycyl-cycline class available as a powder for intravenous infusion.

ANTIMICROBIAL ACTIVITY

Activity against common bacterial pathogens is shown in Table 30.2 (p. 347). It is as potent as, or more potent than, earlier tetracyclines and activity is retained against strains expressing acquired tetracycline resistance determinants. It displays better activity than tetracycline, doxycycline or minocycline against *Streptococcus* spp. and against *Enterococcus faecalis* and *E. faecium*. Among Gram-negative organisms it displays improved activity against *Citrobacter freundii*, *Escherichia coli*, *Enterobacter cloacae*, *Klebsiella pneumoniae*, *Salmonella* spp., *Serratia marcescens* and *Shigella* spp. The spectrum includes rapidly growing mycobacteria. *Ps. aeruginosa*, *Pr. mirabilis*, other *Proteus* spp. and some strains of *Corynebacterium jeikeium* are resistant. Activity against strains expressing acquired resistance to earlier tetracyclines is attributed to failure of the MFS efflux pumps to recognize tigecycline, and to a novel mechanism of ribosome binding that permits tigecycline to overcome ribosomal protection mechanisms.

Comparative susceptibility data for some atypical pathogens are not available. However, in common with earlier tetracyclines, it is active against *Chlamydophila* and *Mycoplasma* spp. and rapidly growing *Mycobacteria* spp. It is less active than minocycline or tetracycline against *U. urealyticum*.

PHARMACOKINETICS

C_{max} 100 mg intravenous infusion (1 h)	0.85–1 mg/L
Plasma half-life	37–67 h
Volume of distribution	7–10 L/kg
Plasma protein binding	68%

Distribution and excretion

It is widely distributed and is concentrated in the gallbladder, colon and lung. The volume of distribution is dose related and variable, but is generally greater than that of older tetracyclines. CSF penetration is poor. Tigecycline is excreted in the feces and urine predominantly as the unchanged molecule. The elimination half-life is long (37–67 h). Tigecycline clearance is decreased by 20% in patients with renal failure. No dosage adjustments are apparently necessary for tigecycline in patients with renal impairment.

TOXICITY AND SIDE EFFECTS

Side effects typical of the group, including nausea, vomiting, diarrhea and headache, occur. Occasional cases of pancreatitis, hypoproteinemia, antibiotic-associated colitis and thrombocytopenia have also been reported.

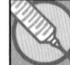

CLINICAL USE

Complicated skin and skin structure infections
Complicated intra-abdominal infections
Community-acquired bacterial pneumonia

Recommended principally for the treatment of infections with multiresistant organisms.

Preparations and dosage

Proprietary name: Tygacil.

Preparation: Powder.

Dosage: Adults, i.v. infusion of 100 mg followed by 50 mg every 12 h for 5–14 days.

Available in the USA, Europe and Japan.

Further information

Muralidharan G, Micalizzi M, Speth J, et al. Pharmacokinetics of tigecycline after single and multiple doses in healthy subjects. *Antimicrob Agents Chemother.* 2005;49:220–229.

Olson MW, Ruzin A, Feyfant E, et al. Functional, biophysical and structural bases for antibacterial activity of tigecycline. *Antimicrob Agents Chemother.* 2006;50:2156–2166.

Rodvold KA, Gotfried MH, Cwik M, et al. Serum, tissue and body fluid concentrations of tigecycline after a single 100 mg dose. *J Antimicrob Chemother.* 2006;58:1221–1229.

Various authors. Tigecycline, a therapeutic option from a new antibiotic class (the glycylcyclines) in an era of increasing resistance. *J Antimicrob Chemother.* 2008;62(supp 1):i1–i40.

OTHER TETRACYCLINES

LYMECYCLINE

2-*N*-lysinomethyl-tetracycline. A water-soluble prodrug of tetracycline available for oral administration.

Its antimicrobial activity is due to the tetracycline content. It is lipophilic, rapidly absorbed from the gastrointestinal tract and widely distributed. Concentrations around 1 mg/kg have been found in maxillary sinus tissue some 3 h after administration of a conventional dose. The half-life is 7–14 h. Approximately 30% of an orally administered dose is excreted as active drug in the urine, where it achieves concentrations of 300 mg/L.

Its untoward effects and clinical uses are those of tetracycline, although it is claimed to be better tolerated.

 Preparations and dosage

Proprietary name: Tetralysal 300.
Preparation: Capsules.
Dosage: Adults, oral, 408 mg every 12 h.
Available in the UK and continental Europe.

METHACYCLINE

6-Methylene-5-hydroxy-tetracycline. A semisynthetic derivative supplied as the hydrochloride for oral administration.

Mean peak plasma concentrations of 2–6 mg/L are found about 4 h after a 300 mg oral dose. Both food and milk reduce uptake by half. Protein binding is 80–90%. The plasma elimination half-life varies between 7 and 15 h and increases to 44 h in severe renal impairment. It is widely distributed, producing lung concentrations similar to, or greater than, the simultaneous plasma concentration. About one-third is excreted in the urine.

Gastrointestinal intolerance is reported to be less frequent than with other tetracyclines, largely because of the lower dosages used. There are no unique adverse drug reactions, although skin and conjunctival pigmentation have been reported.

 Preparations and dosage

Proprietary name: Rondomycin.
Preparation: Capsules.
Dosage: Adults, oral, 600 mg per day in two or four divided doses.
Widely available in continental Europe.

ROLITETRACYCLINE

2-*N*-pyrrolidinomethyl-tetracycline. A semisynthetic derivative of tetracycline supplied as the nitrate sesquihydrate for parenteral use.

It is not absorbed from the gastrointestinal tract. It is highly soluble and therefore can be administered parenterally. Peak plasma concentrations of 4–6 mg/L occur at 0.5–1 h after 350 mg intravenously. The plasma elimination half-life is 5–8 h. About 50% of the dose is excreted in the urine, producing high concentrations.

Intravenous administration is occasionally accompanied by abnormal taste, shivering and rigors, hot flushes, facial reddening, dizziness and, rarely, circulatory collapse. Symptoms of myasthenia gravis have occasionally been exacerbated.

 Preparations and dosage

Proprietary name: Reverin.
Preparation: Injection.
Dosage: Adults, i.m., 350 mg per day; i.v., 275 mg per day.
Limited availability in continental Europe.

Miscellaneous antibacterial agents

David Greenwood

This chapter is concerned with various antimicrobial compounds that are structurally different from the major antimicrobial drug families and from each other. Most are of limited use in human medicine, except in specific diseases or as topical agents.

NITROFURANS

Antimicrobial nitrofurans are based on the 5-nitro-2-furaldehyde molecule:

Antimicrobial activity requires the 5-nitro group. Substitutions on the aldehyde at the 2 position produce compounds with varying activities and pharmacokinetic properties. They are yellow or orange compounds and are relatively easy to synthesize. They are poorly soluble in water, but often dissolve well in solvents such as dimethyl sulfoxide or dimethylformamide.

Many nitrofurans have been developed since their antibacterial activity was discovered in the early 1940s, but few have survived into medical and veterinary practice. Nitrofurantoin is the most important, but furazolidone is also widely used in some countries for non-specific treatment of gastrointestinal infections.

Nitrofurans are active in vitro against a wide range of bacteria, including staphylococci, streptococci, enterococci, corynebacteria, clostridia and many species of enterobacteria (Table 31.1). *Serratia marcescens*, *Pseudomonas aeruginosa* and members of the Proteae tribe are resistant. They are less active under alkaline conditions.

They are active against strains of *Helicobacter pylori* that have acquired resistance to metronidazole, but it is not clear whether this reflects therapeutic efficacy. Nifurtimox is one of the few antimicrobial agents with activity against trypanosomes.

Many nitrofurans are mutagenic, and some are said to be co-carcinogenic. However, therapeutic use of nitrofurans over many years has shown no evidence of long-term harmful effects. Nitrofurans share a class side effect of causing nausea. They may also bring about hemolysis in patients with a deficiency of glucose-6-phosphate dehydrogenase.

Further information

Buzás GM, Józan J. Nitrofuran-based regimens for the eradication of *Helicobacter pylori* infection. *J Gastroenterol Hepatol.* 2007;22:1571–1581.
Raether W, Hänel H. Nitroheterocyclic drugs with broad spectrum activity. *Parasitological Research.* 2003;90(supp 1):S19–S39.

FURAZOLIDONE

Molecular weight: 225.2.

A non-ionic synthetic compound, available for oral use only. It is poorly soluble in water (40 mg/L) and ethanol (90 mg/L), but dissolves well in dimethylformamide (10 g/L). It decomposes in the presence of alkali.

ANTIMICROBIAL ACTIVITY

Activity against common bacterial pathogens is shown in Table 31.1. It is active against a wide range of enteric pathogens, including *Salmonella enterica*, *Shigella* spp., enterotoxigenic *Escherichia coli*, *Campylobacter jejuni*, *Aeromonas hydrophila*, *Plesiomonas shigelloides*, *Vibrio cholerae* and *V. parahaemolyticus*. *Yersinia enterocolitica* is intrinsically resistant. Furazolidone is also active against the protozoa *Giardia lamblia* and *Trichomonas vaginalis*.

Table 31.1   Activity of nitrofurans against common pathogenic bacteria: MIC (mg/L)

	Furazolidone	Nitrofurantoin	Nitrofurazone
Staphylococcus aureus	2–8	4–32	8–16
Streptococcus pyogenes	4–8	4–16	8–64
Enterococcus faecalis	8–32	4–128	32–128
Neisseria gonorrhoeae	No data	0.25–2	0.1–8
Escherichia coli	<0.5–4	0.5–16	4–16
Proteus spp.	32–128	8–R	8–128
Klebsiella pneumoniae	2–8	32–R	8–128
Salmonella enterica	0.25–2	4–128	4–16
Shigella spp.	0.25–4	4–128	4–32
Pseudomonas aeruginosa	R	R	R
Bacteroides fragilis	8–16	8–16	4–32
Helicobacter pylori	0.06–0.25	8–32	No data

R, resistant (MIC >128 mg/L).

ACQUIRED RESISTANCE

Acquired resistance has been observed in *V. cholerae* O1 and O139, *S. enterica* serotypes Typhi and Enteritidis, *A. hydrophila* and *Shigella* spp. Such resistance may be transferable, and there is cross-resistance with nitrofurantoin. Many of these reports come from the Indian subcontinent, where furazolidone is used widely for treating diarrheal diseases.

PHARMACOKINETICS

There is substantial absorption (65–70%) after oral administration, but the drug is heavily metabolized, so that only about 5% of the material excreted is microbiologically active. A dose of 5 mg/kg achieves a maximum plasma concentration of around 1 mg/L. Protein binding is about 30%. Intact drug can be found in various body fluids in concentrations approximating to the minimum inhibitory concentration (MIC) for various intestinal pathogens. Less than 1% of the drug is excreted into urine.

TOXICITY AND SIDE EFFECTS

Most reported side effects are mild and only rarely cause discontinuation of treatment. Nausea and vomiting are experienced by around 8% of patients. Other adverse events include neurological reactions (mainly headache; 1.3% of patients), 'systemic' reactions such as fever and malaise (0.6%) and skin rashes (0.54%). Administration of furazolidone may give rise to inhibition of monoamine oxidase, and disulfiram-like reactions have been reported.

CLINICAL USE

Furazolidone is used in gastrointestinal infections and vaginitis. It is mainly used in developing countries to treat diarrheal diseases of varying etiology, but it is not the drug of choice if a specific pathogen has been identified. Use as a second-line agent in giardiasis and as part of multidrug regimens in *Helicobacter* infection has been advocated.

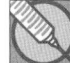

Preparations and dosage

Preparations: Tablets, suspension.

Dosage: Adults, oral, 100 mg, every 6 h for 7–10 days. Children, 1.25 mg/kg every 6 h (suspension available).

Limited availability in the USA and continental Europe.

Further information

Gardner TB, Hill DR. Treatment of giardiasis. *Clin Microbiol Rev.* 2001;14:114–128.

Graham DY, Qureshi WA. Antibiotic-resistant *H. pylori* and its treatment. *Curr Pharm Des.* 2000;6:1537–1544.

Samal SK, Khuntia HK, Nanda PK, et al. Incidence of bacterial enteropathogens among hospitalized diarrhea patients from Orissa, India. *Jpn J Infect Dis.* 2008;61:350–355.

NITROFURANTOIN

Molecular weight: 238.2.

A synthetic compound available only for oral administration. There are three formulations, differing in their crystalline nature: microcrystalline, macrocrystalline, and a delayed-release preparation containing a combination of the two. The macrocrystalline form is said to be less liable to give rise to the most common adverse event, nausea. However, pharmacokinetic and clinical trial evidence for this assertion is not very strong.

It is slightly soluble in water (*c.* 200 mg/L) but more so in dilute alkali. Solubility in ethanol is modest (500 mg/L), but the compound dissolves very well in dimethylformamide (80 g/L). If packaged in light-resistant containers and kept at room temperature, it is stable for more than 5 years. The yellow solution should be kept in the dark.

 ## ANTIMICROBIAL ACTIVITY

Activity against common bacterial pathogens is shown in Table 31.1. It is active against almost all the common urinary pathogens, except *Proteus mirabilis*. It is bactericidal.

It antagonizes the activity of nalidixic acid and other quinolones in vitro, but this combination is unlikely to be used clinically.

 ## ACQUIRED RESISTANCE

Surprisingly for an agent that has been used for so long, resistance remains uncommon. R-factor-mediated resistance has been reported, but this appears to be very unusual. The mechanism of resistance seems to be a decreased nitroreductase activity in the target organism.

There is cross-resistance within the nitrofuran group, but none with antibiotics of other chemical classes.

 ## PHARMACOKINETICS

Oral absorption	>95%
C_{max} 100 mg oral	<2 mg/L after 1–4 h
Plasma half-life	0.5–1 h
Volume of distribution	0.6 L/kg
Plasma protein binding	60–70%

Absorption

It is absorbed mainly from the proximal small intestine and the plasma peak concentration may not be achieved for as long as 4 h. The recommendation to take the drug with food may be motivated by reducing the incidence of nausea rather than increasing bioavailability.

Bioavailability varies widely between different brands and this may not be apparent from results of standard in-vitro pharmaceutical tests. Therefore, different brands should not be substituted unless therapeutic equivalence has been formally established.

Distribution

Serum levels are low, owing to extensive metabolism and the short plasma half-life. Tissue concentrations are too low for adequate treatment of systemic infection, including pyelonephritis. Negligible concentrations are found in breast milk and only a small amount crosses the placenta.

Metabolism and excretion

About 20% of the dose is excreted in microbiologically active form in the urine, sufficient to give inhibitory concentrations against urinary pathogens for up to 6 h. With reduced renal function (creatinine clearance <60 mL/min), urinary excretion falls, and virtually ceases when creatinine clearance is below 20 mL/min. This gives rise to the risk of accumulation in the blood and inadequate urine levels. With this proviso, it can be given to elderly patients. Infants over the age of 3 months may also be treated, but in the absence of a suitable suspension, and at the recommended dosage, a 6-month baby would need to be given one-tenth of a standard 50 mg tablet.

 ## TOXICITY AND SIDE EFFECTS

Nausea, which may be combined with anorexia or vomiting, or both, occurs in about 30% of patients taking the microcrystalline form, causing about 10% to stop treatment. The frequency of nausea is approximately halved with the macrocrystalline formulation. Nausea is due to a direct effect on the vomiting center; it occurs early in the course, and its incidence may be reduced by taking the medication with food or milk.

Pulmonary, hepatic, neurological and hematological side effects have been reported, but are very uncommon. There are two kinds of pulmonary reaction. Acute reactions are the more common, starting within 5–10 days of the first dose, or within a few hours on re-challenge. Symptoms may resemble those found in asthma, tracheobronchitis or pneumonia, and usually resolve permanently within 2 days. There may be an eosinophilia. Subacute or chronic reactions, often referred to as pneumonitis, are of more gradual onset, and resolve only slowly when the drug is stopped. Prolonged dyspnea and cough may be accompanied by fibrosis.

Hepatic reactions follow prolonged drug usage and usually manifest as chronic active hepatitis, sometimes with cirrhosis. The prognosis is good, but recovery may take months.

Peripheral neuropathy has been reported mainly in patients with pre-existing impaired renal function. The prognosis depends upon the severity of the symptoms. Unlike hepatic and pulmonary effects, for which immunological phenomena seem to be responsible, neurological events have been attributed to a direct toxic effect of the drug, one of its metabolites or the superoxide generated in vivo.

In common with other nitrofurans, nitrofurantoin may cause hemolysis in patients who lack glucose-6-phosphate dehydrogenase.

CLINICAL USE

Acute dysuria and frequency
Bacteriuria in pregnancy
Prophylaxis of recurrent cystitis (reduced dosage)

Preparations and dosage

Proprietary names: Furadantin (microcrystalline), Macrodantin (macrocrystalline), Macrobid (mixture).

Preparations: Tablets, capsules, suspension.

Dosage: Adults, oral, 50 or 100 mg every 6 h for 5 or 7 days for acute infection; 50–100 mg at night for prophylaxis. Children >3 months, 3 mg/kg per day in four divided doses; 1 mg/kg at night for prophylaxis.

Widely available.

A nitrofurantoin analog, furagin (furazidin), with similar properties and use is available in eastern Europe.

Further information

Anonymous. Nitrofurantoin. In: Dollery C, ed. *Therapeutic Drugs*. 2nd ed. Edinburgh: Churchill Livingstone; 1999:N114–N117.

Arya SC, Agarwal N. Nitrofurantoin: the return of an old friend in the wake of growing resistance. *BJU Int*. 2009;103:994–995.

Dybowski B, Jabłoska O, Radziszewski P, Gromadzka-Ostrowska J, Borkowski A. Ciprofloxacin and furagin in acute cystitis: comparison of early immune and microbiological results. *Int J Antimicrob Agents*. 2008;31:130–134.

Guay DR. Contemporary management of uncomplicated urinary tract infections. *Drugs*. 2008;68:1169–1205.

Gupta K, Hooton TM, Roberts PL, Stamm WE. Short-course nitrofurantoin for the treatment of acute uncomplicated cystitis in women. *Arch Intern Med*. 2007;167:2207–2212.

Lumbiganon P, Villar J, Laopaiboon M, et al. (World Health Organization Asymptomatic Bacteriuria Trial Group). One-day compared with 7-day nitrofurantoin for asymptomatic bacteriuria in pregnancy: a randomized controlled trial. *Obstet Gynecol*. 2009;113(2 Part 1):339–345.

NIFURATEL

A synthetic compound available as tablets and vaginal preparations. It is poorly soluble in water, but readily soluble in dimethylformamide.

The activity is similar to that of nitrofurantoin but it is more active, especially against Gram-negative anaerobes. It also has modest, but clinically useful, activity against *Candida albicans*. Little is known about the pharmacokinetics. It structurally resembles furazolidone, and may undergo a similar degree of metabolism. It does not achieve therapeutic concentrations in the bloodstream after oral administration and it seems likely that the antibacterial activity in urine is due to active metabolites. There is little or no systemic absorption when vaginal suppositories are used.

As with other members of the group, side effects are mostly associated with the upper gastrointestinal tract. It is used to treat urinary infections and vaginal candidiasis.

Preparations and dosage

Preparations: Tablets and vaginal pessaries.

Dosage: Adults, oral, 200–400 mg every 8 h. A 250 mg vaginal pessary may be used concurrently once a day for 10 days.

Available in some countries in continental Europe.

Further information

Mendling W, Mailland F. Microbiological and pharmaco-toxicological profile of nifuratel and its favourable risk/benefit ratio for the treatment of vulvo-vaginal infections: a review. *Arzneimittelforschung*. 2002;52:8–13.

Mendling W, Poli A, Magnani P. Clinical effects of nifuratel in vulvovaginal infections. A meta-analysis of metronidazole-controlled trials. *Arzneimittelforschung*. 2002;52:725–730.

NIFURTIMOX

A water-soluble synthetic compound available for oral use. It exhibits antibacterial activity typical of the group, but its most notable property is its activity against trypanosomes, especially *Trypanosoma cruzi*.

A plasma concentration of 0.5–1 mg/L is achieved *c.* 2 h after an oral dose of 15 mg/kg. The plasma half-life is 2–4 h. In common with other nitrofurans, it is rapidly and extensively metabolized, so that less than 1% of a dose is excreted intact in the urine. In renal failure, clearance is somewhat reduced but the half-life is unchanged.

Adverse events are common. Many patients experience anorexia, which may be combined with vomiting and abdominal pain. There may also be neurological reactions such as restlessness, insomnia, headache and disorientation.

It is used in the treatment of Chagas disease (South American trypanosomiasis). It has also found some use in the treatment of African sleeping sickness in combination with eflornithine (p. 419).

Preparations and dosage

Preparation: Oral.

Dosage: Adults, oral, 8–10 mg/kg per day in divided doses. Children: 1–10 years, 15–20 mg/kg per day in divided doses; 11–16 years, 12.5–15 mg/kg per day in divided doses. Treatment should last 60–120 days.

Available in South America.

Further information

Anonymous. Nifurtimox. In: Dollery C, ed. *Therapeutic Drugs*. 2nd ed. Edinburgh: Churchill Livingstone; 1999:N91–N95.

Castro JA, de Mecca MM, Bartel LC. Toxic side effects of drugs used to treat Chagas' disease (American trypanosomiasis). *Hum Exp Toxicol*. 2006;25:471–479.

Jannin J, Villa L. An overview of Chagas disease treatment. *Memórias do Instituto Oswaldo Cruz*. 2007;102(supp 1):95–97.

Kennedy PG. The continuing problem of human African trypanosomiasis (sleeping sickness). *Ann Neurol*. 2008;64:116–126.

NIFURTOINOL

The hydroxymethyl derivative of nitrofurantoin, formulated for oral administration. The activity is similar to that of nitrofurantoin. Little is known about the pharmacokinetic behavior. It is said to be more rapidly absorbed than nitrofurantoin and excreted into the urine to a greater extent. Available in some countries in continental Europe.

NITROFURAZONE (NITROFURAL)

A synthetic compound used in the topical treatment of wounds and burns and as an instillation for bladder washout. A nitrofurazone-impregnated urinary catheter is said to reduce infection in catheterized patients. Activity against the common bacterial pathogens is sufficient to cover most pathogens that cause infections of burns and wounds, with the important exception of *Ps. aeruginosa*. Attention has been drawn to its activity against methicillin-resistant *Staphylococcus aureus*, and its use in clearing carriage has been suggested. Slight absorption occurs from intact skin (*c.* 1%) and burned skin (5%). It is neither a primary irritant nor a sensitizer, but some preparations contain polyethylene glycol as a vehicle, and absorption can cause problems in patients with reduced renal function. Of limited availability.

Further information

Schumm K, Lam TB. Types of urethral catheters for management of short-term voiding problems in hospitalized adults: a short version Cochrane review. *Neurourol Urodyn*. 2008;27:738–746.

Stensballe J, Tvede M, Looms D, et al. Infection risk with nitrofurazone-impregnated urinary catheters in trauma patients: a randomized trial. *Ann Intern Med*. 2007;147:285–293.

PEPTIDE ANTIBIOTICS

Peptides of various kinds were among the earliest antibiotics isolated from natural sources. The recovery of tyrothricin from *Bacillus brevis* was reported in 1939 and its separation into gramicidin (a linear peptide) and tyrocidine (a cyclic peptide) in 1940. Gramicidin S (Soviet), which is also produced by a strain of *B. brevis*, is a cyclic peptide similar to tyrocidine. It was developed in the former Soviet Union and is not generally available.

Another cyclic peptide, bacitracin, was isolated from *Bacillus licheniformis* in 1945 and named after Margaret Tracy, the young girl from whom the organism was isolated. Polymyxin B, which was discovered almost simultaneously in the USA as a product of *Bacillus polymyxa* and in the UK as a product of *Bacillus aerosporus* followed in 1947.

The disruptive activity of these peptides on cell membranes, to which they owe their mammalian toxicity, has limited their therapeutic use largely to topical application, but the polymyxins, notably as colistimethate sodium (colistin sulfomethate), are still occasionally used systemically against otherwise resistant organisms. Daptomycin, a lipopeptide originally developed and discarded in the 1980s, has been revived for the treatment of infections with resistant Gram-positive cocci.

Antibacterial oligopeptides are virtually ubiquitous throughout the natural world and are thought to play a part in native defences against infection. Such peptides include, among many others: cecropins (originally described in insects); magainins (from the skin of the toad *Xenopus laevis*); lantibiotics (lanthionine-containing peptides, like nisin, from bacteria); and defensins (from mammalian phagocytes). Many of these compounds interfere with membrane integrity and exhibit differential activity against various species. Some of them, and related synthetic oligopeptides, continue to be investigated, but none has yet emerged as a possible therapeutic agent.

DAPTOMYCIN

A semisynthetic lipopeptide derived from a fermentation product of *Streptomyces roseosporus*.

Daptomycin is a cyclic peptide with a lipophilic tail and thus resembles the polymyxins structurally. Its useful activity is restricted to Gram-positive cocci, notably *Staph. aureus* and its chief attraction is that it retains activity against multiresistant strains. Its activity in vitro is greatly potentiated by the presence of calcium (but not magnesium) ions and in these conditions it is more potently bactericidal than the glycopeptides.

PHARMACOKINETICS

Oral absorption	Poor
C_{max} 4 mg/kg intravenous infusion	55 mg/L end infusion
Plasma half-life	8–9 h
Volume of distribution	c. 0.1 L/kg
Plasma protein binding	92–95%

Oral absorption is poor and it is administered intravenously. It is eliminated predominantly by the kidneys, about half the dose being excreted unchanged within 24 h. The plasma half-life increases in patients with impaired renal function so that the dosage interval should be extended. Around 10% of an administered dose is removed by peritoneal and hemodialysis.

TOXICITY AND SIDE EFFECTS

It is generally well-tolerated, but gastrointestinal side effects, headache and various other adverse reactions occur with varying frequency. Less commonly, but more seriously, myalgia, muscle weakness and myositis may occur requiring regular monitoring of creatine kinase during treatment. Rhabdomyolysis has been reported, but is very rare.

Further information

Hair PI, Keam SJ. Daptomycin: a review of its use in the management of complicated skin and soft tissue infections and *Staphylococcus aureus* bacteraemia. *Drugs*. 2007;67:1483–1512.

Hawkey PM. Pre-clinical experience with daptomycin. *J Antimicrob Chemother*. 2008;62(supp 3):iii7–iii14.

Sauermann R, Rothenburger M, Graninger W, Joukhadar C. Daptomycin: a review 4 years after first approval. *Pharmacology*. 2008;81:79–91.

Tally FP, DeBruin MF. Development of daptomycin for gram-positive infections. *J Antimicrob Chemother*. 2000;46:523–526.

POLYMYXINS

Polymyxin B and colistin (polymyxin E); mixtures of sulfates of polypeptides produced by strains of *B. polymyxa* and *B. polymyxa* var. *colistinus*. Colistimethate sodium (colistin sulfomethate sodium). Molecular weights: polymyxin B_1 1203; polymyxin B_2 1189; colistimethate sodium 1748.

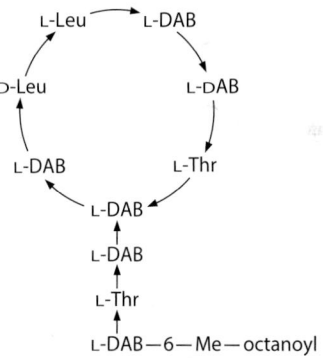

DAB= diaminobutyric acid

A group of basic polypeptide antibiotics with a side chain terminated by characteristic fatty acids. Five polymyxins (A–E) were originally characterized and others have since been added. Polymyxin B and colistin (polymyxin E) sulfates have been commercially developed.

By treatment with formalin and sodium bisulfite, five of the six diaminobutyric acid groups of the polymyxins can be modified by sulfomethyl groups to form undefined mixtures of the mono-, di-, tri-, tetra- and penta-substituted derivatives. Sulfomethyl polymyxins differ considerably in their properties from the parent antibiotics: they are less active antibacterially, less painful on injection, more rapidly excreted by the kidney and less toxic. Only colistimethate sodium is now commercially available for systemic use, but polymyxin B and colistin sulfates are found as ingredients of several topical formulations.

 ## ANTIMICROBIAL ACTIVITY

All the polymyxins have a similar antibacterial spectrum, although there are slight quantitative differences in their activity in vitro. They are inactive against Gram-positive organisms, but nearly all enterobacteria, except *Proteus* spp., *Burkholderia cepacia* and *Ser. marcescens*, are highly susceptible. The MIC of polymyxin B or colistin sulfate for *Esch. coli* and *Klebsiella* spp. is 0.01–1 mg/L; the corresponding concentration for *Ps. aeruginosa* is 0.03–4 mg/L. *Bacteroides fragilis* is resistant, but other *Bacteroides* spp. and fusobacteria are susceptible. Resistance of *V. cholerae* eltor to polymyxin B distinguishes it from the classic vibrio.

The sulfomethyl derivatives are generally 4–8 times less active than the sulfates, but their activity is difficult to measure precisely since on incubation they spontaneously decay to the parent compound, with a corresponding progressive increase in antibacterial activity.

Binding of polymyxins to the bacterial cell membrane can increase permeability to hydrophilic compounds, including sulfonamides and trimethoprim, producing significant synergy. Synergy with ciprofloxacin is also described. Calcium ions exert a strong pH-dependent competition for membrane binding sites, and the presence of calcium and magnesium ions in certain culture media adversely affects the bactericidal activity, notably against *Ps. aeruginosa*.

 ## ACQUIRED RESISTANCE

There is complete cross-resistance between the polymyxins, but stable acquired resistance in normally susceptible species is very rare. Adaptive resistance, probably due to changes in cell-wall permeability, is readily achieved by passage of a variety of enterobacteria in the presence of the agents in vitro.

 ## PHARMACOKINETICS

Oral absorption	Negligible
C$_{max}$ (colistimethate sodium) 2 mega-units (c. 16 mg colistin base) i.m.	6–7 mg/L after 2–3 h
Plasma half-life (colistimethate sodium)	c. 4–6 h
Plasma protein binding	Very low

Absorption

Polymyxins are not absorbed from the alimentary tract or mucosal surfaces, but can be absorbed from denuded areas or large burns.

Distribution

After parenteral administration of the sulfates, blood levels are usually low (1–4 mg/L 2 h after a 500 000 unit intramuscular dose). Substantially higher plasma levels are obtained from intramuscular injections of sulfomethyl polymyxins. There is some accumulation in patients receiving 120 mg every 8 h. In patients treated intravenously with a priming dose of 1.5–2.5 mg/kg followed by continuous infusion of 4.8–6.0 mg/h for 20–30 h, steady state levels were around 5–10 mg/L.

The volume of distribution is unknown, but polymyxins diffuse poorly into tissue fluids and penetration to cerebrospinal fluid is poor. As a result of binding to mammalian cell membranes (sulfomethates less so), they persist in the tissues, where they accumulate on repeated dosage, although they disappear from the serum. Polymyxin crosses the placenta, but the levels achieved are low. A small amount appears in the breast milk.

Metabolism and excretion

The sulfates are excreted almost entirely by the kidney, but after a considerable lag, with very little of the dose appearing in the first 12 h. The sulfomethyl derivatives are much more rapidly excreted, accounting for their shorter half-lives. Around 80% of a parenteral dose of colistimethate sodium is eventually found in the urine, with concentrations reaching around 100–300 mg/L at 2 h. The fate of the remainder is unknown, but no metabolic products have been described and none is excreted in the bile. Polymyxins accumulate in renal failure and are not removed by peritoneal dialysis.

 ## TOXICITY AND SIDE EFFECTS

Pain and tissue injury can occur at the site of injection of the sulfates, but this is less of a problem with the sulfomethyl derivatives. Neurological symptoms such as paresthesia with typical numbness and tingling around the mouth, dizziness and weakness are relatively common, and neuromuscular blockade, sometimes severe enough to impede respiration, occurs. Evidence of nephrotoxicity is observed in about 20% of patients, leading to acute tubular necrosis in about 2%. Damage is more likely in patients with pre-existing renal disease. The appearance of any evidence of deterioration of renal function or of neuromuscular blockade calls for immediate cessation of treatment. All the toxic manifestations appear to be reversible, but complete recovery may be slow.

Although less toxic than the sulfate, untoward effects have been observed in up to one-quarter of those treated with colistimethate sodium. Nephrotoxicity is common, with an increase in urea and creatinine over the first few days of treatment. Acute tubular necrosis is heralded by the appearance of proteinuria, hematuria and casts, sometimes without prior evidence of functional impairment. Renal damage usually continues to progress for up to 2 weeks after withdrawal of therapy. Renal damage is likely to increase with the dose and with the simultaneous administration of other potentially nephrotoxic agents.

Manifestations of central and peripheral neurotoxicity occur particularly in patients with impaired renal function. Neuromuscular blockade is seen principally in patients also receiving anesthetics or other agents that impair neuromuscular transmission. Complete flaccid paralysis with respiratory arrest and subsequent complete recovery has been seen in a patient with myasthenia gravis. Allergy is occasionally seen, and nebulized colistin has caused bronchial hyperreactivity with tightness in the chest in adults with cystic fibrosis. Application of colistin or polymyxin B ear drops can lead to ototoxicity.

CLINICAL USE

Colistimethate sodium

Infections due to *Ps. aeruginosa* and other Gram-negative rods resistant to less toxic agents

Cystic fibrosis (inhalation therapy for pseudomonas infection)

Polymyxin B and colistin sulfate

Component of preparations for local application

Superficial infections with *Ps. aeruginosa* and to prevent the colonization of burns

Selective decontamination of the gut (p. 531) and as a paste for control of upper respiratory tract colonization in patients on prolonged mechanical ventilation (in combination with other agents)

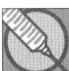

Preparations and dosage

Proprietary name: Aerosporin.

Preparations: Injection, ear and eye drops and ointment. Also in multi-ingredient topical preparations.

Dosage: Adults, i.v., 1.5–2.5 mg/kg per day.

Topical preparations widely available.

Proprietary name: Colomycin.

Preparations: Injection, tablets, syrup, multi-ingredient topical applications.

Dosage: Adults, oral, 1.5–3 million units every 8 h. Children, oral, 15–30 kg, 750 000 units–1.5 million units every 8 h; <15 kg, 250 000–500 000 units every 8 h. Adults i.m., i.v., 2 million units every 8 h. Children, i.m., i.v., <60 kg, 50 000 units/kg per day in three divided doses; inhalation of nebulized solution, patients >40 kg, 1 million units every 12 h, <40 kg, 500 000 units every 12 h.

Widely available.

Further information

Anonymous. Colistin (sulfate) and colistimethate (sodium). In: Dollery C, ed. *Therapeutic Drugs*. 2nd ed. Edinburgh: Churchill Livingstone; 1999:C326–C329.

Anonymous. Polymyxin B (sulfate). In: Dollery C, ed. *Therapeutic Drugs*. 2nd ed. Edinburgh: Churchill Livingstone; 1999:P162–P164.

Evans ME, Feola DJ, Rapp RP. Polymyxin B sulfate and colistin: old antibiotics for emerging gram-negative bacteria. *Ann Pharmacother*. 1999;33:960–967.

Landman D, Georgescu C, Martin DA, Quale J. Polymyxins revisited. *Clin Microbiol Rev*. 2008;21:449–465.

Li J, Nation RL, Turnidge JD, et al. Colistin: the re-emerging antibiotic for multidrug-resistant Gram-negative bacterial infections. *Lancet Infect Dis*. 2006;6:589–601.

Littlewood JM, Koch C, Lambert PA, et al. A ten year review of colomycin. *Respir Med*. 2000;94:632–640.

Nation RL, Li J. Optimizing use of colistin and polymyxin B in the critically ill. *Semin Respir Crit Care Med*. 2007;28:604–614.

OTHER PEPTIDE ANTIBIOTICS

BACITRACIN

A mixture of peptides produced by *Bacillus licheniformis*. Bacitracin A is the major constituent of commercial preparations. The more stable zinc salt is used in topical formulations. It has been widely used as a growth promoter in animals, but has been banned for that purpose in the European Union.

It is highly active against many Gram-positive bacteria and is mainly used as a component of topical preparations. Although strains of *Staph. aureus* are usually susceptible, they are rather less so than most other Gram-positive bacteria. *Streptococcus pyogenes* is so much more susceptible than other hemolytic streptococci that bacitracin susceptibility is used as a screening test for identification. *Clostridium difficile* and *Actinomyces* spp. are susceptible, but enterobacteria and *Pseudomonas* spp. are resistant. *Entamoeba histolytica* is inhibited by 0.6–10 mg/L.

Resistance is uncommon, but has been detected in *Staph. aureus* following topical treatment.

It is nephrotoxic and unsuitable for parenteral use. Systemic toxicity from application to skin or ulcerated areas is rare, but it may cause allergic reactions and occasional anaphylaxis has been described. It is found in many ointments and ophthalmic preparations, usually together with other components, including polymyxins, neomycin and corticosteroids.

Bacitracin is not absorbed by mouth but oral preparations have been used for suppression of gut flora, including *C. difficile*.

Further information

Andrews BJ, Bjorvatn B. Chemotherapy of *Entamoeba histolytica*: studies in vitro with bacitracin and its zinc salt. *Trans R Soc Trop Med Hyg*. 1994;88:98–100.

Jacob SE, James WD. From road rash to top allergen in a flash: bacitracin. *Dermatol Surg*. 2004;30:521–524.

Nelson R, 2007; Antibiotic treatment for *Clostridium difficile*-associated diarrhoea in adults. *Cochrane Database Syst Rev*. (3):CD004610.

GRAMICIDIN

Gramicidin as used in topical formulations is a mixture of several closely related compounds, of which about 80% is in the form of gramicidin A. It is part of the tyrothricin complex originally isolated from *B. brevis*.

It is active against most species of Gram-positive bacteria, including mycobacteria. Gram-negative bacilli are completely insensitive.

It is highly toxic to erythrocytes, liver and kidney, and is used only in topical formulations, usually as one of several components.

PLEUROMUTILINS

A group of compounds with a structure and mechanism of activity that distinguishes them from other agents, hence offering the attraction of lack of cross-resistance to existing drugs. The original pleuromutilin is a naturally occurring diterpene product of *Clitopilus scyphoides* (formerly *Pleurotus mutilis*). Two of these compounds, tiamulin and valnemulin, are used in veterinary medicine. Interest now centers on other semisynthetic derivatives, of which one, retapamulin, has been marketed for human use as a topical agent.

RETAPAMULIN

A semisynthetic pleuromutilin formulated as a 1% ointment for topical use. It is active against staphylococci (MIC 0.12 mg/L), including methicillin-resistant strains, and against streptococci (MIC 0.03–0.25 mg/L), including *Str. pyogenes* and *Str. pneumoniae*. Most enterococci and Gram-negative bacilli are resistant. Propionibacteria are susceptible, suggesting that it might be useful in acne. Early indications suggest that resistance does not emerge readily, but experience with veterinary pleuromutilins indicates that chromosomal resistance may develop with extended use.

It is metabolized in the liver and rapidly excreted, precluding use in systemic infection. Systemic exposure is said to be low following topical application and it appears safe, but there are few data on absorption through broken and unbroken skin. Principal side effects noted include local irritation and occasional allergic reactions. Licensed use is presently restricted to the treatment of impetigo and uncomplicated skin infections. Possible value in methicillin-resistant *Staph. aureus* (MRSA) infection or carriage has not yet been established.

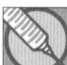

Preparations and dosage

Proprietary names: Altabax, Altargo.

Preparations: 1% ointment

Dosage: Adults and children >9 months, apply twice daily for 5 days.
Widely available.

Further information

Pankuch GA, Lin G, Hoellman DB, Good CE, Jacobs MR, Appelbaum PC. Activity of retapamulin against *Streptococcus pyogenes* and *Staphylococcus aureus* evaluated by agar dilution, microdilution, E-test and disk diffusion methodologies. *Antimicrob Agents Chemother.* 2006;50:1727–1730.

Traczewski MM, Brown SD. Proposed MIC and disk diffusion microbiological cutoffs and spectrum of activity of retapamulin, a novel topical antimicrobial agent. *Antimicrob Agents Chemother.* 2008;52:3863–3867.

Yang LP, Keam SJ. Retapamulin: a review of its use in the management of impetigo and other uncomplicated superficial skin infections. *Drugs.* 2008;68:855–873.

COUMARINS

A group of naturally occurring antibiotics chemically related to the coumarin group of anticoagulants. The best known is novobiocin, but a few naturally occurring coumarins and some semisynthetic derivatives have been studied. They share a narrow range of antimicrobial activity largely directed against aerobic Gram-positive organisms. Novobiocin inhibits susceptible strains of *Staph. aureus* (including β-lactamase-producing and methicillin-resistant strains), *Str. pyogenes* and *Str. pneumonia* at a concentration of 0.1–2 mg/L and it has been considered for the treatment of infection with multiresistant *Staph. aureus* and other Gram-positive cocci. However, since resistance arises readily and side effects are common, the general consensus is that it no longer has a place in antibacterial therapy.

There has been some revived interest in coumarins as potentiating agents of antineoplastic drugs.

Further information

Anderle C, Stieger M, Burrell M, et al. Biological activities of novel gyrase inhibitors of the aminocoumarin class. *Antimicrob Agents Chemother.* 2008;52:1982–1990.

Donnelly A, Blagg BS. Novobiocin and additional inhibitors of the Hsp90 C-terminal nucleotide-binding pocket. *Curr Med Chem.* 2008;15:2702–2717.

OTHER ANTIBACTERIAL AGENTS

FIDAXOMICIN

Formerly known as difimicin. An 18-membered macrocyclic compound related to the tiacumicin group of antibiotics rather than conventional macrolides. It is active against staphylococci (MIC 0.5–2 mg/L) and most anaerobic Gram-positive bacilli and cocci, but Gram-negative bacilli, including Gram-negative anaerobes, are resistant. It is very poorly absorbed when given orally and most interest surrounds its activity against *C. difficile* (MIC 0.12–0.25 mg/L). Such data as are presently available from clinical trials suggest that it is as safe and effective in the treatment of *C. difficile*-associated diarrhea as vancomycin.

Further information

Finegold SM, Molitoris D, Vaisanen M-L, Song Y, Liu C, Bolaños M. In vitro activities of OPT-80 and comparator drugs against intestinal bacteria. *Antimicrob Agents Chemother.* 2004;48:4898–4902.

Gerber M, Ackermann G. OPT-80, a macrocyclic antimicrobial agent for the treatment of *Clostridium difficile* infections: a review. *Expert Opin Investig Drugs.* 2008;17:547–553.

Shue YK, Sears PS, Shangle S, et al. Safety, tolerance, and pharmacokinetic studies of OPT-80 in healthy volunteers following single and multiple oral doses. *Antimicrob Agents Chemother.* 2008;52:1391–1395.

METHENAMINE

Methenamine (hexamine, hexamethylenetetraamine), under the name Urotropin, was successfully used in cystitis by the German physician Nicolaier in 1895. It has no intrinsic antibacterial activity and owes its effect to decomposition in acid conditions to formaldehyde, which is non-specifically microbicidal, and ammonia. It is often used in the form of organic acid salts, methenamine hippurate and methenamine mandelate, which have been claimed (unconvincingly) to keep the urinary pH low. Mandelic acid has some antibacterial activity in its own right and is sometimes given alone as a urinary antiseptic, usually as the calcium or ammonium salt. Infection with urea-splitting organisms such as *Proteus* spp. causes the urine to become alkaline and methenamine is unsuitable for these infections.

Methenamine is absorbed from the gut and mainly excreted unchanged in the urine, achieving concentrations of around 2–60 mg/L, sufficient to inhibit most bacteria and yeasts. Higher concentrations are achieved by the hippurate salt.

It is given in enteric-coated tablets to prevent the liberation of formaldehyde by gastric acid. There is little breakdown in the blood and no systemic effect or toxicity.

Some patients complain of gastrointestinal upset or frequent and burning micturition. Attempts to control these side effects with alkali will abolish the antibacterial effect of the drug. Contact dermatitis and anterior uveitis have occasionally been encountered. Prolonged administration or high dosage may produce proteinuria, hematuria and bladder changes. Methenamine should not be given to patients with acidosis, gout or hepatic insufficiency. There have been fears about the potential carcinogenicity of formaldehyde.

Methenamine and its salts are unsuitable for the treatment of acute urinary tract infection. Their main use, now largely supplanted by other agents, has been in the long-term prophylaxis of recurrent cystitis.

Preparations and dosage

Preparation: Tablets.

Dosage: Adults, oral, 1 g every 8–12 h. Children, oral, 6–12 years, 500 mg every 12 h (maximum dose, 2 g per day).

Widely available.

Further information

Lee BB, Simpson JM, Craig JC, Bhuta T. Methenamine hippurate for preventing urinary tract infections. *Cochrane Database Syst Rev.* 2007;(4):CD003265.

32 Antifungal agents

David W. Warnock

Effective drugs are available for a wide range of fungal infections, covering most of the major systemic pathogens and providing a choice for many conditions. In the more common superficial infections it is possible to cure many patients with topical treatment, and the details of administration are often more important than the choice of agent. There are now few conditions for which there is no effective treatment.

There are four main families of antifungal agents: the allylamines, the azoles, the echinocandins and the polyenes. In addition, there is a miscellaneous group of drugs that includes flucytosine, griseofulvin and various agents that are used for topical treatment. Resistance, although not a major problem, has been recorded with some azole antifungals and with the echinocandins, usually in situations where the drugs have been given for long periods of time in the face of persistent infection.

 Further information

Barker KS, Rogers PD. Recent insight into the mechanisms of antifungal resistance. *Curr Infect Dis Rep*. 2006;8:449–456.

Dodds Ashley ES, Lewis R, Lewis JS, et al. Pharmacology of systemic antifungal agents. *Clin Infect Dis*. 2006;43(suppl 1):S28–S39.

Goodwin ML, Drew RH. Antifungal serum concentration monitoring: an update. *J Antimicrob Chemother*. 2008;61:17–25.

Gubbins PO, Amsden JR. Drug–drug interactions of antifungal agents and implications for patient care. *Expert Opin Pharmacother*. 2005;6:2231–2243.

Rex JH, Pfaller MA, Walsh TJ, et al. Antifungal susceptibility testing: practical aspects and current challenges. *Clin Microbiol Rev*. 2001;14:643–658.

Sanglard D, Odds FC. Resistance of *Candida* species to antifungal agents: molecular mechanisms and clinical consequences. *Lancet Infect Dis*. 2002;2:73–85.

Spanakis EK, Aperis G, Mylonakis E. New agents for treatment of fungal infections: clinical efficacy and gaps in coverage. *Clin Infect Dis*. 2006;43:1060–1068.

ALLYLAMINES

A group of synthetic compounds effective in the topical and oral treatment of dermatophytoses and superficial forms of candidosis. Two drugs, naftifine and terbinafine, are in clinical use.

NAFTIFINE

A topical antifungal used as a 1% cream for the treatment of dermatophytoses, including tinea pedis, tinea corporis and tinea cruris.

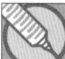 **Preparation and dosage**

Proprietary name: Naftin, Exoderil.

Preparation: Topical.

Dosage: For fungal skin infections dosage and duration of treatment varies according to condition.

Available in a number of countries, including the USA; not available in the UK..

 Further information

Gupta AK, Ryder JE, Cooper EA. Naftifine: a review. *J Cutan Med Surg*. 2008;12:51–58.

TERBINAFINE

Molecular weight (free base): 291.4; (hydrochloride): 327.9.

A synthetic allylamine available as the hydrochloride for oral and topical administration.

ANTIFUNGAL ACTIVITY

Terbinafine is active against a wide range of pathogenic fungi, including dermatophytes (*Epidermophyton*, *Microsporum* and *Trichophyton* spp.), various *Candida* spp., *Aspergillus* spp., some dimorphic fungi (*Blastomyces dermatitidis*, *Histoplasma capsulatum* and *Sporothrix schenckii*) and many dematiaceous fungi.

 ## ACQUIRED RESISTANCE

Resistance has not been reported.

 ## PHARMACOKINETICS

Oral absorption	70–80%
C_{max} 250 mg oral	c. 1 mg/L after 2 h
Plasma half-life	c. 17 h
Volume of distribution	1000 L
Plasma protein binding	>99%

Blood concentrations increase in proportion to dosage. It is lipophilic and is rapidly and extensively distributed to body tissues. It reaches the stratum corneum by diffusion through the dermis and epidermis, and secretion in sebum. Diffusion from the nail bed is the major factor in its rapid penetration of nails. It is metabolized by the liver and the inactive metabolites are mostly excreted in the urine. The elimination half-life is prolonged in patients with hepatic or renal impairment.

 ## INTERACTIONS

It is a potent competitive inhibitor of the human hepatic cytochrome P_{450} CYP-2D6 enzyme system, and concomitant administration with drugs predominantly metabolized by this system (e.g. tricyclic antidepressants, neuroleptics, antihypertensives, opioids and antiarrhythmics) should be carefully monitored. Blood concentrations are reduced following concomitant administration with drugs such as rifampicin (rifampin) that induce the hepatic cytochrome P_{450} enzyme system. Conversely, levels are increased if it is given with drugs such as cimetidine that inhibit hepatic metabolism.

 ## TOXICITY AND SIDE EFFECTS

These include abdominal discomfort, loss of appetite, nausea, diarrhea, headache, impairment of taste, rash and urticaria. Serious skin reactions, including Stevens–Johnson syndrome, and rare hepatotoxic reactions, including jaundice, cholestasis and hepatitis, are occasionally encountered.

 ## CLINICAL USE

Tinea pedis, tinea corporis, tinea cruris, tinea capitis
Onychomycosis caused by dermatophytes

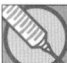 ### Preparations and dosage

Proprietary name: Lamisil.

Preparations: Tablets, cream, oral granules.

Dosage: Adults, oral, 250 mg per day for 2–6 weeks in tinea pedis, 2–4 weeks in tinea cruris, 2–4 weeks in tinea corporis, at least 4 weeks in tinea capitis, 6–12 weeks or longer in nail infections. Children, oral granules, 250 mg per day if >35 kg, 187.5 mg per day if 25–35 kg, 125 mg per day if <25 kg for 6 weeks in tinea capitis.

Widely available.

 ## Further information

Darkes MJ, Scott LJ, Goa KL. Terbinafine: a review of its use in onychomycosis in adults. *Am J Clin Dermatol*. 2003;4:39–65.

Elewski BE, Caceres HW, DeLeon L, et al. Terbinafine hydrochloride oral granules versus oral griseofulvin suspension in children with tinea capitis: results of two randomized, investigator-blinded, multicenter, international controlled trials. *J Am Acad Dermatol*. 2008;59:41–54.

McClellan KJ, Wiseman LR, Markham A. Terbinafine: an update of its use in superficial mycoses. *Drugs*. 1999;58:179–202.

Revankar SG, Nailor MD, Sobel JD. Use of terbinafine in rare and refractory mycoses. *Future Microbiol*. 2008;3:9–17.

AZOLES

A large group of synthetic agents, which includes drugs used in bacterial and parasitic infections (5-nitroimidazoles, Ch. 24; benzimidazoles, Ch. 34). Antifungal azoles have in common an imidazole or triazole ring with *N*-carbon substitution. The activity is essentially fungistatic, but some of the newer triazoles exert fungicidal effects at therapeutic concentrations. They are effective in the topical treatment of dermatophytoses and superficial forms of candidosis; several are suitable for systemic administration.

Several molecular mechanisms of resistance have been elucidated. These include overexpression of efflux pump genes, point mutations in the gene that encodes the target enzyme, lanosterol demethylase, and overexpression of this gene. Changes in other enzymes involved in ergosterol biosynthesis, such as sterol desaturase, may also contribute to azole resistance.

INTERACTIONS

Azoles are metabolized by the human hepatic cytochrome P_{450} enzyme system, and are potent inhibitors of CYP-3A4; some also inhibit CYP-2C9 and CYP-2C19. Administration with drugs that are metabolized by these enzymes can result in increased concentrations of the azole, the interacting drug, or both. Administration with drugs that are potent inducers of the human cytochrome P_{450} enzyme system, such as rifampicin, results in a marked reduction in blood levels, especially with itraconazole and ketoconazole.

Among systemically administered azoles, fluconazole and voriconazole weakly inhibit CYP-3A4, whereas itraconazole, ketoconazole and posaconazole are potent inhibitors of the enzyme.

 ## Further information

Aperis G, Mylonakis E. Newer triazole antifungal agents: pharmacology, spectrum, clinical efficacy and limitations. *Expert Opin Investig Drugs*. 2006;15:579–602.

Gubbins PO. Mould-active azoles: pharmacokinetics, drug interactions in neutropenic patients. *Curr Opin Infect Dis*. 2007;20:579–586.

Hope WW, Billaud EM, Lestner J, Denning DW. Therapeutic drug monitoring for triazoles. *Curr Opin Infect Dis*. 2008;21:580–586.

FLUCONAZOLE

Molecular weight 306.3.

A synthetic bis(triazole) available for oral or parenteral administration. A prodrug formulation, fosfluconazole, is available for intravenous use in Japan.

 ## ANTIFUNGAL ACTIVITY

The spectrum is limited, but includes most *Candida* spp., *Cryptococcus* spp., dermatophytes and dimorphic fungi (*Blast. dermatitidis*, *Coccidioides* spp., *Hist. capsulatum* and *Paracoccidioides brasiliensis*). Strains of *C. krusei* appear to be insensitive.

 ## ACQUIRED RESISTANCE

Resistant strains of *C. albicans* have been isolated from AIDS patients given long-term treatment for oral or esophageal candidosis. Strains of *C. glabrata* frequently become resistant during short courses of treatment. There are a few reports of fluconazole-resistant strains of *Cryp. neoformans* recovered from AIDS patients with relapsed meningitis. Most, but not all, *C. albicans* and *C. glabrata* strains resistant to fluconazole are cross-resistant to other azoles.

 ## PHARMACOKINETICS

Oral absorption	>93%
C_{max} 50 mg oral	c. 1 mg/L after 2 h
Plasma half-life	25–30 h
Volume of distribution	0.6–0.8 L/kg
Plasma protein binding	<10%

Absorption

Oral absorption is rapid (1–3 h) and is not affected by food or intragastric pH. Blood concentrations increase in proportion to dosage. Maximum serum concentrations increase to about 2–3 mg/L after repeated dosing with 50 mg.

Distribution

It is widely distributed, achieving therapeutic concentrations in most tissues and body fluids. Concentrations in cerebrospinal fluid (CSF) are 50–60% of the simultaneous serum concentration in normal individuals and even higher in patients with meningitis.

Metabolism and excretion

More than 90% of an oral dose is eliminated in the urine: about 80% as unchanged drug and 10% as inactive metabolites. The drug is cleared by glomerular filtration, but there is significant tubular reabsorption. The plasma half-life is prolonged in renal failure, necessitating adjustment of the dosage. Fluconazole is removed during hemodialysis and, to a lesser extent, during peritoneal dialysis. In children the volume of distribution and plasma clearance are increased, and the half-life is considerably shorter (15–25 h).

 ## INTERACTIONS

It is a potent inhibitor of CYP-2C9 and CYP-2C19, and administration with other drugs metabolized by these P_{450} enzymes should be avoided.

 ## TOXICITY AND SIDE EFFECTS

These are rare, but untoward reactions include nausea, abdominal discomfort, diarrhea and headache. Transient abnormalities of liver enzymes and rare serious skin reactions, including Stevens–Johnson syndrome, have been reported.

CLINICAL USE

Mucosal, cutaneous and systemic candidosis
Coccidioidomycosis
Cryptococcosis
Dermatophytosis
Pityriasis versicolor

Preparation and dosage

Proprietary names: Diflucan, Prodif (Japan).

Preparations: Capsules, oral suspension, i.v. infusion.

Dosage: Adults, oral, vaginal candidosis or balanitis, 150 mg as a single dose; oropharyngeal candidosis, 200 mg on the first day, followed by 100 mg once daily for at least 14 days; esophageal candidosis, 200 mg on the first day, followed by 100 mg once daily for at least 3 weeks. Tinea pedis, corporis, cruris, pityriasis versicolor, 50 mg per day for 2–4 weeks. Systemic candidosis, cryptococcal meningitis and other forms of cryptococcosis, oral or i.v. infusion, 200–400 mg on the first day, then 100–400 mg per day; treatment is continued according to response. For the prevention of relapse of cryptococcal meningitis in AIDS patients, 200 mg per day, indefinitely. Prevention of fungal infections in neutropenic patients, 400 mg per day.

Children >1 year, oral, i.v. infusion, superficial candidosis, 3 mg/kg per day; systemic candidosis and cryptococcosis, 6–12 mg/kg per day (maximum dose, 400 mg per day).

Widely available.

Further information

Charlier C, Hart E, Lefort A, et al. Fluconazole for the management of invasive candidiasis: where do we stand after 15 years? *J Antimicrob Chemother.* 2006;57:384–410.

Debruyne D. Clinical pharmacokinetics of fluconazole in superficial and systemic mycoses. *Clin Pharmacokinet.* 1997;33:52–77.

Pfaller MA, Diekema DJ. Twelve years of fluconazole in clinical practice: global trends in species distribution and fluconazole susceptibility of bloodstream isolates of *Candida. Clin Microbiol Infect.* 2004;10(suppl 1):11–23.

ITRACONAZOLE

Molecular weight: 705.6.

A synthetic dioxolane triazole available for oral or parenteral administration.

ANTIFUNGAL ACTIVITY

The spectrum includes dermatophytes, dimorphic fungi (*Blast. dermatitidis, Coccidioides* spp., *Hist. capsulatum, Paracocc.* brasiliensis, *Penicillium marneffei* and *Spor. schenckii*), molds (including *Aspergillus* spp.), dematiaceous fungi and yeasts (*Candida* spp. and *Cryptococcus* spp.).

ACQUIRED RESISTANCE

This is uncommon, but fluconazole-resistant *C. albicans* and *C. glabrata* are often cross-resistant to itraconazole. There are reports of itraconazole-resistant strains of *A. fumigatus.*

PHARMACOKINETICS

Oral absorption	30% (capsules); 55% (solution)
C_{max} 100 mg oral	0.1–0.2 mg/L after 2–4 h
Plasma half-life	20–30 h
Volume of distribution	11 L/kg
Plasma protein binding	>99%

Absorption

Absorption is improved if the drug is given with food or an acidic beverage. In contrast, absorption is reduced if it is given together with compounds that reduce gastric acid secretion. Higher concentrations are obtained with repeated dosing, but there is much individual variation. Incorporation into a solution of hydroxypropyl-β-cyclodextrin enhances bioavailability and leads to much higher blood levels in neutropenic individuals and persons with AIDS. This formulation is better absorbed if given without food. Increases in dosage produce disproportionate changes in blood concentrations.

Distribution

Levels in the CSF are low, but concentrations in lung, liver and bone are 2–3 times higher than in serum, and concentrations in the genital tract are 3–10 times higher. High concentrations are also found in the stratum corneum, as a result of drug secretion in sebum. The drug persists in the skin and nails for weeks to months after treatment is discontinued.

Metabolism and excretion

It is degraded by the liver into a large number of (mostly inactive) metabolites which are excreted with the bile and urine. Itraconazole is unusual because the major metabolite, hydroxyitraconazole, is bioactive and has a similar spectrum of activity as the parent compound. In the steady state, this metabolite is found at serum concentrations about two-fold higher than those of the parent drug. About 80–90% of the intravenous carrier, hydroxypropyl-β-cyclodextrin, is excreted unchanged in the urine. No adjustment of dosage is required in hepatic or renal failure, or during hemodialysis or peritoneal dialysis.

INTERACTIONS

Itraconazole and its metabolites potently inhibit CYP-3A4, and it should not be given with drugs metabolized by this enzyme. Concomitant administration with drugs that induce the cytochrome P$_{450}$ system, such as phenytoin, phenobarbital (phenobarbitone), carbamazepine, rifamycins and nevirapine, results in a marked reduction in blood levels of the azole.

TOXICITY AND SIDE EFFECTS

Unwanted effects are more common with oral solution than with capsules, and are more severe. They include nausea, abdominal discomfort, dyspepsia, diarrhea, headache, pruritus and skin rash. Rare side effects include Stevens–Johnson syndrome, transient abnormalities of liver enzymes, reversible idiosyncratic hepatitis and hypokalemia.

Intravenous itraconazole has been associated with congestive heart failure. Neither intravenous nor oral itraconazole should be used to treat infections in patients with evidence of ventricular dysfunction unless the expected benefit clearly exceeds the risk. Patients with risk factors for congestive heart failure should be treated with caution and their condition monitored.

CLINICAL USE

Aspergillosis

Systemic mycoses with dimorphic fungi (blastomycosis, coccidioidomycosis, histoplasmosis, paracoccidioidomycosis, penicilliosis)

Subcutaneous mycoses (chromoblastomycosis, sporotrichosis)

Mucosal and cutaneous candidosis.

Dermatophytosis

Phaeohyphomycosis

Pityriasis versicolor

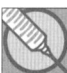

Preparations and dosage

Proprietary name: Sporanox.

Preparations: Capsules, oral solution, i.v. infusion.

Dosage: Adults, oral, oropharyngeal candidosis, 100 mg per day (200–400 mg per day in AIDS or neutropenia) for 15 days. Vaginal candidosis, 200 mg every 12 h for 1 day. Pityriasis versicolor, 200 mg per day for 7 days; tinea corporis, tinea cruris, 100 mg per day for 15 days; tinea pedis, tinea manuum, 100 mg per day for 30 days or 200 mg every 12 h for 7 days. Onychomycosis, 200 mg once daily for 3 months or 200 mg every 12 h for 7 days, repeated once after 21 days for fingernails and repeated twice at 21-day intervals for toenails. Aspergillosis and other systemic or subcutaneous fungal infections, oral or i.v. infusion, 200 mg every 12 or 24 h; treatment is continued according to response. For the prevention of relapse of histoplasmosis or penicilliosis in AIDS patients, 200 mg per day, indefinitely. Prevention of fungal infections in neutropenic patients, 200–400 mg per day.

Widely available.

Further information

Caputo R. Itraconazole (Sporanox) in superficial and systemic fungal infections. *Expert Rev Anti Infect Ther.* 2003;1:531–542.

De Beule K, Van Gestel J. Pharmacology of itraconazole. *Drugs.* 2001;61 (suppl 1):27–37.

Maertens J, Boogaerts M. The place for itraconazole in treatment. *J Antimicrob Chemother.* 2005;56(suppl 1):i33–i38.

KETOCONAZOLE

Molecular weight: 531.4.

A synthetic dioxolane imidazole available for oral and topical use.

ANTIFUNGAL ACTIVITY

The spectrum includes dermatophytes, some dimorphic fungi and *Candida* spp.

ACQUIRED RESISTANCE

Resistance has been documented in patients treated for chronic mucocutaneous candidosis and AIDS patients with oropharyngeal or esophageal candidosis. Some fluconazole-resistant *C. albicans* and *C. glabrata* are cross-resistant to ketoconazole.

PHARMACOKINETICS

Oral absorption	Variable
C$_{max}$ 400 mg oral	c. 5–6 mg/L after 2 h
Plasma half-life	6–10 h
Volume of distribution	0.36 L/kg
Plasma protein binding	>95%

It is erratically absorbed after oral administration. Absorption is favored by an acid pH. Food delays absorption, but does not significantly reduce the peak serum concentration. Absorption is reduced if it is given with compounds that reduce gastric acid secretion. Penetration into CSF is generally poor and unreliable, although effective concentrations have been recorded with high doses in some cases of active meningitis. It is extensively metabolized by the liver, and the metabolites are excreted in the bile. Less than 1% of an oral dose is excreted unchanged in the urine.

INTERACTIONS

It is a potent inhibitor of CYP-3A4 and administration with other drugs metabolized by this enzyme can lead to potentially dangerous levels of the azole, the interacting drug, or both. Concomitant administration with rifampicin results in a marked reduction in blood levels of the azole.

TOXICITY AND SIDE EFFECTS

Unwanted effects include nausea, vomiting, abdominal pain, headache, rashes, urticaria and pruritus. Transient abnormalities of liver enzymes, interference with testosterone synthesis (leading to gynecomastia, alopecia and oligospermia) and rare fatal hepatic damage have been reported.

CLINICAL USE

Mucosal candidosis

Pityriasis versicolor

Seborrheic dermatitis

Non-life-threatening forms of blastomycosis, coccidioidomycosis, histoplasmosis and paracoccidioidomycosis

Preparations and dosage

Proprietary name: Nizoral.

Preparations: Tablets, suspension, topical cream, shampoo.

Dosage: Adult, oral, 200–400 mg per day for 14 days. Children, oral, 3 mg/kg per day.

Widely available.

Further information

Daneshmend TK, Warnock DW. Clinical pharmacokinetics of ketoconazole. *Clin Pharmacokinet*. 1988;14:13–34.

Lake-Bakkar G, Scheuer PJ, Sherlock S. Hepatic reactions associated with ketoconazole in the United Kingdom. *Br Med J*. 1987;294:419–422.

Sugar AM, Alsip SG, Galgiani JN, et al. Pharmacology and toxicity of high-dose ketoconazole. *Antimicrob Agents Chemother*. 1987;31:1874–1878.

POSACONAZOLE

Molecular weight: 700.8.

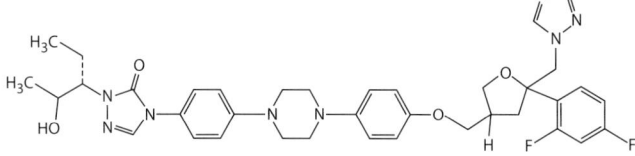

A synthetic triazole available for oral administration.

ANTIFUNGAL ACTIVITY

The spectrum includes dimorphic fungi (*Blast. dermatitidis*, *Coccidioides* spp., *Hist. capsulatum*, *Pen. marneffei*, and *Spor. schenckii*), molds (*Aspergillus* spp., *Mucor* spp., *Rhizomucor* spp. and *Rhizopus* spp.), some dematiaceous fungi and yeasts (*Candida* spp. and *Cryptococcus* spp.).

ACQUIRED RESISTANCE

This has not yet been described.

PHARMACOKINETICS

C_{max} 200 mg oral	0.5 mg/L after 4 h
Plasma half-life	35 h
Volume of distribution	1774 L
Plasma protein binding	>98%

Absorption

Oral absorption is slow. Absorption from the gastrointestinal tract is improved if the drug is given with a high-fat meal. Blood concentrations increase in proportion to dosage up to 800 mg.

Distribution

It is extensively distributed into body tissues.

Metabolism and excretion

It is not as extensively metabolized by the hepatic cytochrome P_{450} system as other triazole antifungals. More than 70% of an administered dose is eliminated in the feces, predominantly as unchanged drug. The remainder is excreted as glucuronidated derivatives in the urine. Posaconazole is a substrate for intestinal P-glycoprotein, an adenosine triphosphate-dependent plasma membrane transporter responsible for drug efflux from cells. Multiple peaks in blood concentrations have been observed, suggesting that effluxed drug is reabsorbed into the systemic circulation.

 ## INTERACTIONS

Because it is primarily metabolized through glucuronidation and is a substrate for P-glycoprotein efflux, drugs that inhibit or induce these clearance pathways may increase or decrease blood concentrations of posaconazole. It inhibits the CYP-3A4 system, and co-administration may lead to increased serum concentrations of drugs metabolized by this enzyme. When posaconazole is discontinued, dosage of the other drugs may need to be decreased.

 ## TOXICITY AND SIDE EFFECTS

It is generally well tolerated even for long periods. Unwanted effects include gastrointestinal discomfort and mild to moderate, transient abnormalities of liver enzymes. Rare side effects include cholestasis and hepatic failure.

 ## CLINICAL USE

Invasive aspergillosis
Fusarium infection
Chromoblastomycosis and mycetoma
Coccidioidomycosis
Oropharyngeal candidosis
Prophylaxis of invasive fungal infections in patients at serious risk

With the exception of oropharyngeal candidosis and prophylaxis, use is presently restricted to patients with disease that is refractory to other antifungal drugs, or who are intolerant to them.

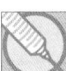 ### Preparation and dosage

Proprietary name: Noxafil.

Preparation: Oral suspension.

Dosage: Adults, oral, oropharyngeal candidosis, 200 mg (5 mL) once a day on the first day, then 100 mg (2.5 mL) once daily for 13 days with food. Invasive fungal infections, 400 mg (10 mL) every 12 h with food. Prevention of invasive fungal infections, 200 mg (5 mL) every 8 h with food. Not recommended for children under 18 years.

Widely available.

 ## Further information

Kwon DS, Mylonakis E. Posaconazole: a new broad-spectrum antifungal agent. *Expert Opin Pharmacother.* 2007;8:1167–1178.

Raad II, Graybill JR, Bustamante AB, et al. Safety of long-term oral posaconazole use in the treatment of refractory invasive fungal infections. *Clin Infect Dis.* 2006;42:1726–1734.
Rachwalski EJ, Wieczorkiewicz JT, Scheetz MH. Posaconazole: an oral triazole with an extended spectrum of activity. *Ann Pharmacother.* 2008;42:1429–1438.

VORICONAZOLE

Molecular weight: 349.3.

A synthetic triazole formulated for oral and parenteral use.

 ## ANTIFUNGAL ACTIVITY

The spectrum includes most fungi that cause human disease: dimorphic fungi (*Blast. dermatitidis*, *Coccidioides* spp., *Hist. capsulatum*, *Paracocc. brasiliensis*, *Pen. marneffei* and *Spor. schenckii*), molds (*Aspergillus* spp., *Fusarium* spp. and *Scedosporium* spp.), dematiaceous fungi and yeasts (*Candida* spp., *Cryptococcus* spp. and *Trichosporon* spp.).

 ## ACQUIRED RESISTANCE

Some fluconazole- and itraconazole-resistant strains of *Candida* and *Aspergillus* spp. show reduced susceptibility to voriconazole.

PHARMACOKINETICS

Oral absorption	96%
C_{max} 400 mg oral	*c.* 2 mg/L after 2 h
Plasma half-life	*c.* 6 h
Volume of distribution	4.6 L/kg
Plasma protein binding	58%

Absorption

Oral absorption is rapid and almost complete, and is unaffected by intragastric pH. In adults, there is a disproportionate increase in blood concentrations with increasing oral and parenteral dosage, due to partial saturation of first-pass metabolism. In children given low dosages of the drug, proportional changes in drug levels are seen.

Distribution

It is widely distributed into body tissues and fluids, including brain and CSF.

Metabolism and excretion

It is extensively metabolized by the liver. More than 80% of a dose appears in the urine, but less than 2% is excreted in unchanged form. It is metabolized by several different hepatic cytochrome P_{450} enzymes. Some people with point mutations in the genes encoding these enzymes are poor metabolizers while others are extensive metabolizers. Drug levels are as much as four-fold lower in individuals who metabolize the drug more extensively.

 ## INTERACTIONS

Like fluconazole, voriconazole inhibits several cytochrome P_{450} enzymes, and there is considerable potential for the drug and its metabolites to increase the serum concentrations of other drugs metabolized by this system. Blood levels of voriconazole are significantly reduced by administration with drugs that induce hepatic cytochrome P_{450} enzyme activity.

 ## TOXICITY AND SIDE EFFECTS

Unwanted effects include mild to moderate visual disturbance, rashes, and transient abnormalities of liver enzymes. Rare side effects include life-threatening hepatitis.

Clinical use

Acute and chronic invasive aspergillosis
Serious invasive *Candida* infections
Serious infections caused by *Scedosporium* and *Fusarium* spp.

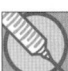 ### Preparations and dosage

Proprietary name: Vfend.

Preparations: Film-coated tablets (50 mg and 200 mg); lyophilized power (200 mg) for reconstitution for infusion.

Dosage: Adult, oral, 200–400 mg every 12 h for 24 h, then 100–300 mg every 12 h; i.v. 6 mg/kg every 12 h for 24 h, then 4 mg/kg every 12 h. Not recommended for children under 2 years.

Widely available.

 ### Further information

Maschmeyer G, Haas A. Voriconazole: a broad spectrum triazole for the treatment of serious and invasive fungal infections. *Future Microbiol.* 2006;1:365–385.

Pascual A, Calandra T, Bolay S, et al. Voriconazole: therapeutic drug monitoring in patients with invasive mycoses improves efficacy and safety outcomes. *Clin Infect Dis.* 2008;46:201–211.

Scott LJ, Simpson D. Voriconazole: a review of its use in the management of invasive fungal infections. *Drugs.* 2007;67:269–298.

Theuretzbacher U, Ihle F, Derendorf H. Pharmacokinetic/pharmacodynamic profile of voriconazole. *Clin Pharmacokinet.* 2006;45:649–663.

OTHER AZOLES

In addition to the systemic agents, numerous imidazoles are presently available for topical use. They include:

- **Bifonazole.** Used for the topical treatment of dermatophytoses and pityriasis versicolor.
- **Butoconazole.** Used for the topical treatment of vaginal candidosis.
- **Clotrimazole.** Used for the topical treatment of dermatophytoses, and oral, cutaneous and genital candidosis.
- **Econazole nitrate.** Used for the topical treatment of dermatophytoses, and oral, cutaneous and genital candidosis. It has also been used to treat corneal infection.
- **Fenticonazole nitrate.** Used for the topical treatment of vaginal candidosis.
- **Isoconazole nitrate.** Used for the topical treatment of dermatophytoses, and cutaneous and vaginal candidosis.
- **Miconazole nitrate.** Used for the topical treatment of dermatophytoses, pityriasis versicolor, and oral, cutaneous and genital candidosis. (Formerly also available for intravenous use.)
- **Oxiconazole.** Used for the topical treatment of dermatophytoses and cutaneous candidosis.
- **Sertaconazole nitrate.** Used for the topical treatment of dermatophytoses and vaginal candidosis.
- **Sulconazole nitrate.** Used for the topical treatment of dermatophytoses and cutaneous candidosis.
- **Terconazole.** Used for the topical treatment of dermatophytoses, and cutaneous and vaginal candidosis.
- **Tioconazole.** Used for the topical treatment of dermatophytoses (including nail infections), and cutaneous and vaginal candidosis.

 ### Preparations and dosages

Bifonazole

Proprietary names: Amycor, Mycospor.

Preparation: Topical.

Dosage: For fungal skin infections dosage and duration of treatment varies according to condition.

Widely available.

Butoconazole

Proprietary name: Femstat.

Preparations: Pessaries, vaginal cream.

Dosage: Adults, pessaries, 100 mg per day for 3–6 consecutive days.

Widely available.

Preparations and dosages—cont'd

Clotrimazole

Proprietary names: Canesten, Gyne-Lotrimin, Lotrimin, Mycelex.

Preparations: Pessaries, vaginal cream, oral troche, topical.

Dosage: Adults, pessaries, 500 mg as a single dose, or 200 mg per day for 3 consecutive days, or 100 mg per day for 6 days. Oral troches, 10 mg five times daily for 2 weeks or longer. For fungal skin infections dosage and duration of treatment varies according to condition.

Widely available.

Econazole nitrate

Proprietary names: Ecostatin, Gyno-Pevaryl, Pevaryl, Spectazole.

Preparations: Pessaries, topical.

Dosage: Adults, pessaries, 150 mg per day for 3 consecutive days. For fungal skin infections dosage and duration of treatment varies according to condition.

Widely available.

Fenticonazole nitrate

Proprietary name: Lomexin.

Preparation: Pessaries.

Dosage: Adult, pessaries, 600 mg as a single dose or 200 mg per day for 3 consecutive days.

Widely available.

Isoconazole

Proprietary names: Fazol, Travogen, Travogyn.

Preparations: Pessaries, topical.

Dosage: Adult, pessaries, 600 mg as a single dose or 300 mg per day for 3 days. For fungal skin infections dosage and duration of treatment varies according to condition.

Widely available.

Miconazole nitrate

Proprietary names: Daktarin, Femeron, Gyno-Daktarin, Micatin, Micozole, Monistat.

Preparations: Pessaries, vaginal cream, oral gel, topical.

Dosage: Adults, pessaries, 200 mg per day for 7 consecutive days, or 100 mg per day for 14 days; oral gel, 125 mg every 6 h. Children 2–6 years, 125 mg every 12 h; infants <2 years, 62.5 mg every 12 h. For fungal skin infections dosage and duration of treatment varies according to condition.

Widely available.

Oxiconazole

Proprietary names: Oxistat, Oxizole.

Preparation: Topical.

Dosage: For fungal skin infections dosage and duration of treatment varies according to the condition being treated.

Widely available.

Sertaconazole nitrate

Proprietary name: Ertaczo

Preparation: Topical.

Dosage: For fungal skin infections dosage and duration of treatment varies according to condition.

Widely available.

Sulconazole nitrate

Proprietary name: Exelderm.

Preparation: Topical.

Dosage: For fungal skin infections dosage and duration of treatment varies according to the condition being treated.

Widely available.

Terconazole

Proprietary name: Terazol.

Preparations: Pessaries, vaginal cream.

Dosage: Adults, pessaries, 80 mg per day for 3 consecutive days.

Widely available.

Tioconazole

Proprietary names: Trosyd, Trosyl, Vagistat.

Preparations: Pessaries, nail solution, cream.

Dosage: Adults, pessaries, 300 mg as a single dose. For fungal skin and nail infections dosage and duration of treatment varies according to the condition being treated.

Widely available.

Further information

Sheehan DJ, Hitchcock CA, Sibley CM. Current and emerging azole antifungal agents. *Clin Microbiol Rev.* 1999;12:40–79.

ECHINOCANDINS

Semisynthetic cyclic lipopeptides that interfere with the synthesis of the cell wall of susceptible fungi (p. 19). They are active against *Candida* spp. resistant to azoles and amphotericin B. Three agents of this type – anidulafungin, caspofungin and micafungin – have been licensed for use in systemic fungal infections.

Echinocandins do not interact with the human hepatic cytochrome P_{450} enzyme system, and their use has been associated with very few significant drug interactions.

Further information

Cappelletty D, Eiselstein-McKitrick K. The echinocandins. *Pharmacotherapy.* 2007;27:369–388.

Perlin D. Resistance to echinocandin-class antifungal drugs. *Drug Resist Updat.* 2007;10:121–130.

Wagner C, Graninger W, Presteri E, et al. The echinocandins: comparison of their pharmacokinetics, pharmacodynamics and clinical applications. *Pharmacology.* 2006;78:161–177.

ANIDULAFUNGIN

Molecular weight: 1140.3.

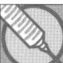

A semisynthetic lipopeptide derived from a fermentation product of *Aspergillus nidulans*. Formulated for intravenous infusion.

ANTIFUNGAL ACTIVITY

It is active against *Aspergillus* spp., *Candida* spp. and the cyst stage of *Pneumocystis jirovecii*. Resistance has not yet been reported.

PHARMACOKINETICS

C_{max} 100 mg 1-h infusion	c. 9 mg/L end infusion
Plasma half-life	18–27 h
Volume of distribution	0.6 L/kg
Plasma protein binding	84%

Blood concentrations increase in proportion to dosage. The steady state is achieved on the first day after a loading dose (twice the daily maintenance dose).

Distribution

Levels in the CSF are negligible.

Metabolism and excretion

Unlike caspofungin and micafungin, anidulafungin is not metabolized by the liver, but undergoes slow non-enzymatic degradation in the blood to a peptide breakdown product which is enzymatically degraded and excreted in the feces and bile. About 30% of a dose is eliminated in the feces, of which less than 10% is unchanged drug. Less than 1% of a dose is excreted in the urine. No dosage adjustment is required in patients with hepatic or renal impairment. Anidulafungin is not cleared by hemodialysis.

Toxicity and side effects

Occasional histamine-mediated infusion-related reactions, injection site reactions and transient abnormalities of liver enzymes have been reported.

Interactions

No clinically significant interactions have yet been reported.

Clinical use

Candidemia and certain invasive forms of candidosis
Esophageal candidosis

Preparations and dosage

Proprietary names: Eraxis, Ecalta.

Preparation: i.v. infusion.

Dosage: Adult, candidemia and invasive candidosis, 200 mg on the first day, then 100 mg per day; treatment is continued according to response. Esophageal candidosis, 100 mg on the first day, then 50 mg per day for at least 2 weeks. The rate of infusion should not exceed 1.1 mg/min.

Widely available.

Further information

Joseph JM, Kim R, Reboli AC. Anidulafungin: a drug evaluation of a new echinocandin. *Expert Opin Pharmacother.* 2008;9:2339–2348.

Vazquez JA, Sobel JD. Anidulafungin: a novel echinocandin. *Clin Infect Dis.* 2006;43:215–222.

CASPOFUNGIN

Molecular weight: 1213.42.

A semisynthetic lipopeptide derived from a fermentation product of *Glarea lozoyensis*. Formulated as the diacetate for intravenous infusion.

ANTIFUNGAL ACTIVITY

It is active against *Aspergillus* spp., *Candida* spp. and the cyst form of *Pn. jirovecii*.

 ## ACQUIRED RESISTANCE

This is rare, but resistant strains of *C. albicans*, *C. glabrata* and *C. parapsilosis* have been recovered from patients failing caspofungin treatment. These strains are typically cross-resistant to other echinocandins.

 ## PHARMACOKINETICS

C_{max} 70 mg 1-h infusion	*c.* 10 mg/L 1 h post infusion
Plasma half-life	9–11 h
Volume of distribution	0.15 L/kg
Plasma protein binding	97%

Blood concentrations increase in proportion to dosage.

Distribution

The drug is widely distributed, the highest concentrations being found in the liver. Levels in the CSF are negligible.

Metabolism and excretion

It is slowly metabolized by the liver through non-enzymatic peptide hydrolysis and *N*-acetylation, and the two inactive metabolites are excreted in the feces and bile. No dosage adjustment is required in patients with renal impairment; however, a dose reduction to 35 mg following the 70 mg loading dose is recommended for patients with moderate hepatic impairment. Caspofungin is not cleared by hemodialysis.

 ## INTERACTIONS

It has few documented interactions. In some patients, administration with ciclosporin (cyclosporin) results in transaminase elevations two to three times the upper limit of normal, resolving when both drugs are discontinued. Co-administration of these drugs is not recommended unless the expected benefit outweighs the risk. Caspofungin interacts with tacrolimus, reducing its serum concentrations. Tacrolimus concentrations should be monitored and the dosage adjusted if required. Caspofungin concentrations are reduced when it is given with rifampicin.

 ## TOXICITY AND SIDE EFFECTS

Occasional histamine-mediated infusion-related reactions, injection site reactions and transient abnormalities of liver enzymes have been reported. Rare cases of significant hepatic dysfunction, hepatitis or worsening liver failure have also been described.

 ## CLINICAL USE

Candidemia and certain invasive forms of candidosis

Esophageal candidosis

Invasive aspergillosis unresponsive to other antifungal drugs

Empirical treatment of presumed fungal infections in febrile neutropenic patients

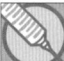 ### Preparations and dosage

Proprietary name: Cancidas.

Preparation: i.v. infusion.

Dosage: Adult, i.v., 70 mg on the first day, then 50 mg per day; treatment is continued according to response.

Widely available.

 ### Further information

Hope WW, Shoham S, Walsh TJ. The pharmacology and clinical use of caspofungin. *Expert Opin Drug Metab Toxicol.* 2007;3:263–274.

Kartsonis NA, Nielsen J, Douglas CM. Caspofungin: the first in a new class of antifungal agents. *Drug Resist Updat.* 2003;6:197–218.

McCormack PL, Perry CM. Caspofungin: a review of its use in the treatment of fungal infections. *Drugs.* 2005;65:2049–2068.

MICAFUNGIN

Molecular weight: 1292.26.

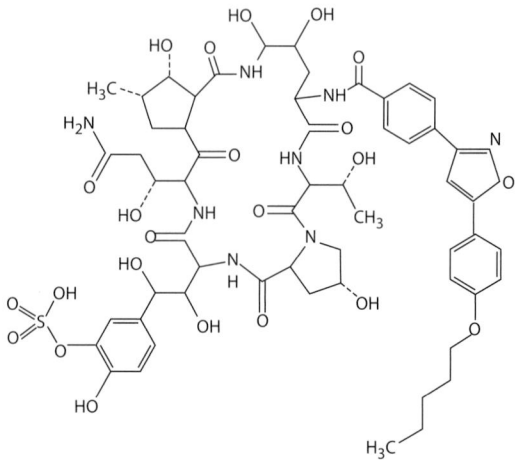

A semisynthetic lipopeptide derived from a fermentation product of *Coleophoma empetri*. Formulated as the monosodium salt for intravenous infusion.

ANTIFUNGAL ACTIVITY

It is active against *Aspergillus* spp., *Candida* spp. and the cyst form of *Pn. jirovecii*. Resistance has rarely been reported.

PHARMACOKINETICS

C_{max} 50 mg 1-h infusion	*c.* 5 mg/L 1 h post infusion
Plasma half-life	11–15 h
Volume of distribution	0.4 L/kg
Plasma protein binding	99%

Blood concentrations increase in proportion to dosage. Unlike anidulafungin and caspofungin, a loading dose is not required.

Distribution

The drug is widely distributed, the highest concentrations being found in the liver. Levels in the CSF and urine are negligible.

Metabolism and excretion

It is metabolized by the liver and the three inactive metabolites are excreted in the feces (70%). Less than 1% of a dose is eliminated as unchanged drug in the urine. No dosage adjustment is required in patients with severe renal impairment or mild to moderate hepatic impairment. The effect of severe hepatic impairment on micafungin pharmacokinetics has not been studied. Micafungin is not cleared by hemodialysis.

INTERACTIONS

Micafungin inhibits the cytochrome P_{450} CYP-3A4 metabolism of sirolimus and nifedipine, and may increase blood concentrations of these drugs. Patients receiving concurrent treatment with these drugs should be monitored for signs of toxicity, and the dosage of sirolimus or nifedipine should be reduced if necessary.

TOXICITY AND SIDE EFFECTS

Occasional histamine-mediated infusion-related reactions, injection site reactions and transient abnormalities of liver enzymes have been reported. Isolated cases of significant hepatic or renal dysfunction, hepatitis, or liver or renal failure have also been described.

CLINICAL USE

Candidemia and certain invasive forms of candidosis

Esophageal candidosis

Prophylaxis of *Candida* infections in hematopoietic stem cell transplant (HSCT) recipients

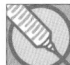

Preparations and dosage

Proprietary name: Mycamine.

Preparation: i.v. infusion.

Dosage: Adult, i.v., invasive candidosis, 100 mg per day; treatment is continued according to response. Esophageal candidosis, 150 mg per day. Prevention of *Candida* infections in HSCT recipients, 50 mg per day. Widely available.

Further information

Cross SA, Scott LJ. Micafungin: a review of its use in adults for the treatment of invasive and oesophageal candidiasis, and as prophylaxis against *Candida* infections. *Drugs*. 2008;68:2225–2255.

Joseph JM, Jain R, Danziger LH. Micafungin: a new echinocandin antifungal. *Pharmacotherapy*. 2007;27:53–67.

Wiederhold NP, Lewis JS. The echinocandin micafungin: a review of the pharmacology, spectrum of activity, clinical efficacy and safety. *Expert Opin Pharmacother*. 2007;8:1155–1166.

POLYENES

Around 100 polyene antibiotics have been described, but few have been developed for clinical use. They are large amphipathic molecules: closed macrolide rings with a variable number of hydroxyl groups along the hydrophilic side, and along the hydrophobic side a variable number of conjugated double bonds to which they owe the name 'polyene'; e.g. tetraene (four double bonds), heptaene (seven double bonds). They bind to sterols in the membranes of susceptible fungal cells (p. 19), causing impairment of membrane function and cell death. Polyenes can also damage fungal cells through a cascade of oxidative reactions linked to lipoperoxidation of the cell membrane. Non-selective binding of polyenes to cholesterol in mammalian cell membranes may account for some of the toxic side effects.

The most important member of the group is amphotericin B, a heptaene that is administered parenterally for the treatment of systemic fungal infections.

Further information

Sugar AM. The polyene macrolide antifungal drugs. In: Peterson PK, Verhoef J, eds. The Antimicrobial Agents Annual. Vol. 1. Amsterdam: Elsevier; 1986:229–244.

AMPHOTERICIN B

Molecular weight: 924.1.

A fermentation product of *Streptomyces nodosus* available for intravenous infusion or oral administration. The traditional micellar suspension formulation is often associated with serious toxic effects, in particular renal damage, and this has stimulated efforts to develop chemical modifications and new formulations. Three lipid-associated formulations have been licensed for use (Table 32.1):

- Liposomal amphotericin B, in which the drug is encapsulated in phospholipid-containing liposomes.
- Amphotericin B colloidal dispersion, in which the drug is packaged into small lipid disks containing cholesterol sulfate.
- Amphotericin B lipid complex, in which the drug is complexed with phospholipids to produce ribbon-like structures.

These formulations are less toxic than the micellar suspension because of their altered pharmacological distribution, allowing higher doses to be given.

 ANTIFUNGAL ACTIVITY

The spectrum includes most fungi that cause human disease: *A. fumigatus*, *Blast. dermatitidis*, *Candida* spp., *Coccidioides* spp., *Cryptococcus* spp., *Hist. capsulatum*, *Paracocc. brasiliensis* and *Spor. schenckii*. Dermatophytes, *Fusarium* spp. and some other *Aspergillus* spp., including *A. terreus* and *A. flavus*, may be less susceptible, while *Scedosporium* spp., *Trichosporon asahii* (formerly *T. beigelii*) and some fungi that cause mucormycosis are resistant.

It also exhibits useful activity against *Prototheca* spp., some protozoa, including *Leishmania* spp., and the genera *Naegleria* and *Hartmanella*.

 ACQUIRED RESISTANCE

Resistant strains of *C. tropicalis*, *C. lusitaniae*, *C. krusei* and *C. guilliermondii*, with alterations in the cell membrane, including reduced amounts of ergosterol, have occasionally been isolated after prolonged treatment, particularly of infections in partially protected sites, such as the vegetations of endocarditis. Significant resistance in yeasts, including *C. albicans* and *C. glabrata*, has been reported in isolates from cancer patients with prolonged neutropenia. In some cases resistant strains have caused disseminated infection. There are a few reports of amphotericin-resistant strains of *Cryp. neoformans* recovered from AIDS patients with relapsed meningitis.

PHARMACOKINETICS

Less than 10% of a parenteral dose of the conventional micellar suspension of amphotericin B remains in the blood 12 h after administration. The remainder is thought to bind to tissue cell membranes, the highest concentrations being found in the liver (up to 40% of the dose). Levels in the CSF are less than 5% of the simultaneous blood concentration. The conventional formulation has a terminal half-life of about 2 weeks. About 75% of a given dose is excreted unchanged in the urine and feces. No metabolites have been identified.

The pharmacokinetics of lipid-based formulations are quite diverse (Table 32.1). Maximal serum concentrations of the liposomal formulation are much higher than those of the conventional micellar formulation, while levels of colloidal dispersion and lipid complex formulations are lower due to more rapid distribution of the drug to tissue. Administration of lipid-associated formulations of amphotericin B results in much higher drug concentrations in the liver and spleen than are achieved with the conventional formulation. Renal concentrations of the drug are much lower and its nephrotoxic side effects are greatly reduced.

Table 32.1 Pharmacokinetics of amphotericin B formulations

	Amphotericin B	Amphotericin B lipid complex	Amphotericin B colloidal dispersion	Liposomal amphotericin B
Dose	0.5 mg/kg	5 mg/kg for 1 week	5 mg/kg for 1 week	5 mg/kg for 1 week
C_{max}	1.2 mg/L	1.7 mg/L	3.1 mg/L	83 mg/L
Plasma half-life	91 h	173 h	28.5 h	6.8 h
Volume of distribution	3–5 L/kg	131 L/kg	4.3 L/kg	0.1 L/kg
Plasma protein binding	>95%	>95%	>95%	>95%

Blood concentrations are unchanged in hepatic or renal failure. Hemodialysis does not influence serum concentrations unless the patient is hyperlipidemic, in which case there is some drug loss due to adherence to the dialysis membrane.

INTERACTIONS

Amphotericin B can augment the nephrotoxic effects of other drugs, such as aminoglycoside antibiotics, ciclosporin, interleukin-2 and certain antineoplastic agents. It can also augment corticosteroid-induced potassium loss. Reducing the risk of amphotericin B-induced nephrotoxicity is central to avoiding toxicity due to delayed clearance of other agents.

TOXICITY AND SIDE EFFECTS

Common side effects of conventional amphotericin B include hypotension, fever, rigors, chills, headache, backache, nausea, vomiting, anorexia, anemia, disturbances in renal function (including hypokalemia and hypomagnesemia), renal toxicity, abnormal liver function (discontinue treatment), rash and anaphylactoid reactions. Risk factors for nephrotoxicity include average daily dose, concomitant treatment with other nephrotoxic drugs and elevated baseline serum creatinine.

The lipid-associated formulations all lower the risk of amphotericin B-induced renal failure. However, infusion-related side effects, such as fever, rigors and hypotension, develop in up to 40% of patients treated with the colloidal dispersion, and hypoxic events also occur; as a result this formulation is not widely used. In contrast, infusion-related reactions are uncommon with liposomal amphotericin B or the lipid complex. Patients who have developed renal impairment while receiving the conventional formulation of amphotericin B have improved or stabilized when lipid-associated amphotericin B was substituted, even when the dose was increased. Renal function should be measured at regular intervals, particularly in patients receiving other nephrotoxic drugs.

CLINICAL USE

Aspergillosis

Systemic mycoses with dimorphic fungi (blastomycosis, coccidioidomycosis, histoplasmosis, paracoccidioidomycosis, penicilliosis)

Candidosis

Cryptococcosis

Hyalohyphomycosis, mucormycosis, phaeohyphomycosis

Visceral leishmaniasis

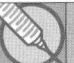

Preparations and dosage

Proprietary names: Abelcet (lipid complex), AmBisome (liposomal), Amphocil (colloidal dispersion), Amphocin, Amphotec (colloidal dispersion), Fungilin, Fungizone.

Preparations: Tablets, lozenges, oral suspension, i.v. infusion.

Dosage: Adults, oral, 100–200 mg every 6 h. Lozenges, 1–2, every 6h. Infants and children, 1 mL of suspension every 6 h. Intravenous infusion, adults and children, 0.25 mg/kg per day, gradually increasing to 1 mg/kg per day. In severely ill patients the dose can be increased to 1.5 mg/kg per day. Lipid formulations, adults and children, i.v. infusion, 1–5 mg/kg per day.

Widely available.

Further information

Barrett JP, Vardulaki KA, Conlon C, et al. A systematic review of the antifungal effectiveness and tolerability of amphotericin B formulations. *Clin Ther.* 2003;25:1295–1320.

Gallis HA, Drew RH, Packard WW. Amphotericin B: 30 years of clinical experience. *Rev Infect Dis.* 1990;12:308–329.

Moen MD, Lyseng-Williamson KA, Scott LJ. Liposomal amphotericin B: a review of its use as empirical therapy in febrile neutropenia and in the treatment of invasive fungal infections. *Drugs.* 2009;69:361–392.

Ostrosky-Zeichner L, Marr KA, Rex JH, et al. Amphotericin B: time for a new 'gold standard'. *Clin Infect Dis.* 2003;37:415–425.

Sterling TR, Merz WG. Resistance to amphotericin B: emerging clinical and microbiological patterns. *Drug Resist Updat.* 1998;1:161–165.

Ullmann AJ, Sanz MA, Tramarin A, et al. Prospective study of amphotericin B formulations in immunocompromised patients in 4 European countries. *Clin Infect Dis.* 2006;43:e29–e38.

Wong-Beringer A, Jacobs RA, Guglielmo BJ. Lipid formulations of amphotericin B: clinical efficacy and toxicities. *Clin Infect Dis.* 1998;27:603–618.

OTHER POLYENES

Other clinically useful polyenes, which in general resemble amphotericin B in antifungal action and spectrum of activity, are mostly used only topically.

- **Mepartricin**; methyl partricin (heptaene).
  A product of *Str. aureofaciens* used for intravenous treatment of deep candidosis and for the topical treatment of vaginal candidosis. It offers no conspicuous advantages over amphotericin B as a systemic antifungal.
- **Natamycin**; pimaricin (tetraene). A product of *Str. chatanoogensis* or *Str. natalensis* used for the topical treatment of ophthalmic and bronchopulmonary infections and vaginal candidosis.
- **Nystatin** (tetraene). A product of *Str. albulus* or *Str. noursei* used for the topical treatment of oral, esophageal, gastrointestinal and genital candidosis, and gastrointestinal prophylaxis.

Preparations and dosages

Mepartricin

Preparations: Tablets, vaginal preparations, topical cream, oral suspension.

Available in continental Europe; not available in the UK.

Natamycin

Preparations: Oral suspension, ophthalmic suspension, cream, vaginal preparations, lozenges.

Dosage: Adults, oral, tablets: oral candidiasis 10 mg every 4–6 h; intestinal candidiasis 100 mg every 4–6 h.

Available in continental Europe; not available in the UK.

Nystatin

Proprietary names: Mycostatin, Nystan.

Preparations: Tablets, pastilles, oral suspension, vaginal and topical preparations.

Dosage: Adults, oral: oral candidiasis 100 000 units every 6 h; intestinal candidiasis 500 000 units every 6 h. Prophylaxis: adults, 1 million units per day; children, 100 000 units every 6 h; neonates, 100 000 units per day as a single dose. Vaginal pessaries, 1–2 at night for at least 14 nights.

Widely available.

OTHER SYSTEMIC AGENTS

FLUCYTOSINE

5-Fluorocytosine. Molecular weight: 129.1.

A synthetic fluorinated pyrimidine available for intravenous infusion or oral administration.

ANTIFUNGAL ACTIVITY

The spectrum of activity is restricted to *Candida* spp., *Cryptococcus* spp. and some fungi causing chromoblastomycosis.

ACQUIRED RESISTANCE

About 2–3 of *Candida* spp. isolates (more in some centers) are resistant before treatment starts, and resistance may develop during treatment. The most common cause of resistance appears to be loss of the enzyme uridine monophosphate pyrophosphorylase.

PHARMACOKINETICS

Oral absorption	Complete
C_{max} 25 mg/kg 6-hourly oral	70–80 mg/L after 1–2 h
Plasma half-life	3–6 h
Volume of distribution	0.7–1 L/kg
Plasma protein binding	c. 12%

Absorption is slower in persons with impaired renal function, but peak concentrations are higher. Levels in the CSF are around 75% of the simultaneous serum concentration. More than 90% of a dose of flucytosine is excreted in the urine in unchanged form. The serum half-life is much longer in renal failure, necessitating modification of the dosage regimen: for patients with a creatinine clearance below 40 mL/min the dosage interval should be doubled to 12 h; in severe renal failure the dosage interval should be further increased to once daily or less, based on frequent serum drug concentration measurements.

INTERACTIONS

Cytosine arabinoside has been reported to inactivate flucytosine. Drugs that are known to be myelosuppressive, such as zidovudine and ganciclovir, should be used with caution in individuals receiving flucytosine.

TOXICITY AND SIDE EFFECTS

Nausea, vomiting, abdominal pain and diarrhea are common. Serious side effects include myelosuppression and hepatic toxicity; they occur more frequently when serum concentrations exceed 100 mg/L.

The nephrotoxic effects of amphotericin B can result in elevated blood concentrations of flucytosine, and levels of the latter drug should be monitored when these compounds are administered together.

CLINICAL USE

Candidosis (in combination with amphotericin B or fluconazole)
Cryptococcosis (in combination with amphotericin B or fluconazole)

Monitoring of flucytosine concentrations is desirable in all patients, and mandatory in those with renal impairment.

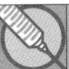
Preparations and dosage

Proprietary names: Alcobon, Ancobon, Ancotil.
Preparations: Tablets, capsules, i.v. infusion.
Dosage: Adults, oral, i.v., 200 mg/kg per day in four divided doses. For extremely sensitive organisms, 50–150 mg/kg per day in four divided doses may be sufficient.
Widely available.

Further information

Francis P, Walsh TJ. Evolving role of flucytosine in immunocompromised patients: new insights into safety, pharmacokinetics, and antifungal therapy. *Clin Infect Dis.* 1992;15:1003–1018.
Vermes A, Guchelaar HJ, Dankert J. Flucytosine: a review of its pharmacology, clinical indications, pharmacokinetics, toxicity and drug interactions. *J Antimicrob Chemother.* 2000;46:171–179.

GRISEOFULVIN

Molecular weight: 352.8.

A fermentation product of various species of *Penicillium*, including *Pen. griseofulvum*. Available as fine-particle or ultra-fine-particle formulations for oral use.

ANTIFUNGAL ACTIVITY

The spectrum of useful activity is restricted to dermatophytes causing skin, nail and hair infections (*Epidermophyton*, *Microsporum* and *Trichophyton* spp.). Resistance has seldom been reported.

PHARMACOKINETICS

Absorption from the gastrointestinal tract is dependent on drug formulation. Administration with a high-fat meal will increase the rate and extent of absorption, but individuals tend to achieve consistently high or low blood concentrations. It appears in the stratum corneum within 4–8 h as a result of secretion in perspiration. However, levels begin to fall soon after the drug is discontinued, and within 48–72 h it can no longer be detected. It is metabolized in the liver, the metabolites being excreted in the urine. The elimination half-life is 9–21 h.

INTERACTIONS

Griseofulvin can diminish the anticoagulant effect of warfarin. Its absorption is reduced in persons receiving concomitant treatment with phenobarbital.

TOXICITY AND SIDE EFFECTS

Adverse reactions occur in about 15% of patients and include headache, nausea, vomiting, rashes and photosensitivity.

CLINICAL USE

Dermatophyte infections of hair, skin and nail

Preparations and dosage

Proprietary names: Fulcin, Fulvicin, Grifulvin V, Grisactin, Grisovin, Grisol.
Preparations: Tablets, capsules, oral suspension.
Dosage: Adults, oral, 500 mg per day as a single or divided dose. In severe infections the dose may be doubled, reducing when response occurs. Children, 10 mg/kg per day in divided doses, or as a single dose.
Widely available.

Further information

Bennett ML, Fleischer AB, Loveless JW, et al. Oral griseofulvin remains the treatment of choice for tinea capitis in children. *Pediatr Dermatol.* 2000;17:304–309.

OTHER TOPICAL AGENTS

There is a large and miscellaneous group of topical antifungal agents, all of which are effective treatments for superficial mycoses. They include the following:

- **Amorolfine hydrochloride.** A synthetic morpholine derivative that inhibits ergosterol biosynthesis. It is used for the treatment of tinea corporis, tinea cruris, tinea pedis and onychomycosis.
- **Butenafine hydrochloride.** A synthetic benzylamine derivative which acts as an ergosterol biosynthesis inhibitor. It is used for the treatment of tinea corporis, tinea cruris and tinea pedis.
- **Ciclopirox.** A synthetic pyridinone used in onychomycosis and as the olamine salt in tinea corporis, tinea cruris, tinea pedis, cutaneous candidosis and pityriasis versicolor.
- **Haloprogin.** A halogenated phenolic which is effective in tinea corporis, tinea cruris, tinea pedis and pityriasis versicolor.
- **Tolnaftate.** A thiocarbamate used in tinea cruris and tinea pedis.

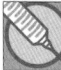 **Preparations and dosages**

Amorolfine hydrochloride

Proprietary name: Loceryl.

Preparations: Nail solution, cream.

Dosage: For fungal skin infections, apply once daily for at least 2–3 weeks (up to 6 weeks for tinea pedis). For nail infections, apply solution 1–2 times weekly; treat fingernails for 6 months, toenails for 9–12 months.

Widely available.

Butenafine hydrochloride

Proprietary name: Mentax.

Preparation: Topical.

Dosage: For fungal skin infections dosage and duration of treatment varies according to condition.

Widely available.

Ciclopirox

Proprietary names: Loprox, Penlac.

Preparations: Nail solution, cream, powder.

Dosage: For fungal skin infections, apply twice daily for at least 2–4 weeks. For nail infections, apply solution once daily for at least 6 months.

Widely available.

Haloprogin

Proprietary name: Halotex.

Preparation: Topical.

Dosage: For fungal skin infections dosage and duration of treatment varies according to condition.

Widely available.

Tolnaftate

Proprietary names: Aftate, Mycil, Tinactin.

Preparation: Topical.

Dosage: For fungal skin infections dosage and duration of treatment varies according to condition.

Widely available.

 Further information

Haria M, Bryson HM. Amorolfine, a review of its pharmacological properties and therapeutic potential in the treatment of onychomycosis and other superficial fungal infections. *Drugs*. 1995;49:103–120.

McNeely W, Spencer CM. Butenafine. Drugs. 1998;55:405–412.

The use of product names in this chapter does not imply their endorsement by the U.S. Department of Health and Human Services. The findings and conclusions in this chapter are those of the author and do not necessarily represent the views of the Centers for Disease Control and Prevention.

33 Antimycobacterial agents

John M. Grange

The mycobacteria causing human disease, and therefore requiring treatment by antibacterial agents, are divisible into three groups: the tuberculosis complex (principally *Mycobacterium tuberculosis*, *M. bovis* and *M. africanum* in humans); the leprosy bacillus (*M. leprae*); and various environmental saprophytes that occasionally cause human disease. Patients with AIDS are particularly likely to develop disease due to the latter species, notably the *Mycobacterium avium* complex (MAC), although the incidence of such infection has declined in regions where antiretroviral therapy is widely available.

Antimycobacterial agents include natural and semisynthetic antibiotics and synthetic agents. Some, such as rifampicin (rifampin; Ch. 27) and streptomycin (Ch. 12), are active against a wide range of bacteria, although their use is mostly restricted to the treatment of mycobacterial disease, and some are synthetic agents, mostly with activity only against mycobacteria. The four first-line drugs used in modern short-course antituberculosis regimens (Ch. 58) are rifampicin, isoniazid, pyrazinamide and ethambutol, with the latter three being synthetic agents.

Resistance to one or more of these agents requires the use of second-line drugs of which there are six classes – aminoglycosides (streptomycin, kanamycin, amikacin), cyclic peptides (capreomycin and, rarely, viomycin), thioamines (ethionamide, prothionamide), fluoroquinolones (Ch. 26), cycloserine and *p*-aminosalicylic acid.

As a result of the increasing prevalence of tuberculosis resistant to many or most of the currently available antituberculosis agents, there is a pressing need for new drugs but there was little financial incentive for the pharmaceutical industry to meet this need. This serious deficit has been addressed by the establishment of the Global Alliance for TB Drug Development by various agencies, especially the World Health Organization (WHO), and private foundations. This Alliance has facilitated the development and clinical evaluation of several new agents, the progress of which is shown on the Alliance website, http://www.tballiance.org. As at April 2010 PA-824, a nitroimidazole (Ch. 24), moxifloxacin, a fluoroquinolone (Ch. 26), and TMC 207, a diarylquinolone, were in clinical trial, and several other agents were undergoing preclinical evaluation. In addition, the sequencing of the entire genome of *M. tuberculosis* and innovations in computer modeling have paved the way to the development of 'designer' agents based on unique mycobacterial structures and metabolic pathways. There is also growing interest in the use of adjunct immunotherapy to improve the treatment outcome in tuberculosis, particularly in drug-resistant cases.

The principal drugs for the treatment of leprosy (Ch. 57) are dapsone, rifampicin and clofazimine, with prothionamide for patients who will not take clofazimine. An alternative and increasingly used regimen is based on rifampicin, ofloxacin and minocycline.

Treatment of opportunist disease due to environmental mycobacteria poses serious problems as many patients have underlying complicating conditions, notably various causes of immunosuppression. Drugs and regimens (see below) that are active in vitro are often ineffective clinically against these mycobacteria and novel approaches to treatment are required.

ANTIMICROBIAL ACTIVITY

The action of antimycobacterial agents in vivo depends on the population dynamics of the mycobacteria within the lesions. In the case of tuberculosis, some bacilli replicate freely in the walls of well-oxygenated cavities, some replicate more slowly in acidic and anoxic tissue and within macrophages and a few are in a near-dormant 'persister' state. Isoniazid exerts a powerful and rapid bactericidal activity against the freely replicating bacilli and kills the great majority of such bacilli, with a substantial reduction of infectiousness, within a few days of commencing treatment. It has little or no effect against the near-dormant bacilli, which are killed by rifampicin. The slowly replicating bacilli in acidic, often anoxic, environments are killed by pyrazinamide, which is active only at low pH. Thus a distinction may be drawn between agents that are bactericidal in vitro and those that actually 'sterilize' lesions in vivo. Accordingly, the most widely used short-course antituberculosis regimen is based on a 2-month intensive phase of treatment with isoniazid, rifampicin, pyrazinamide and ethambutol, during which all except a few persisters are killed, and a 4-month continuation phase of rifampicin (which kills persisters during shorter bursts of metabolic activity) and isoniazid to kill any rifampicin-resistant mutants that might commence replication (Ch. 58). In both tuberculosis and leprosy, the great majority of bacilli are killed during the first few weeks of therapy; prolonged therapy, with its associated problems of cost, compliance and the need for supervision, is required to kill a few remaining metabolically inactive persisters and thus prevent relapse.

In the absence of acquired drug resistance, strains of *M. tuberculosis* and related members of the tuberculosis complex are very similar in their susceptibility to the antituberculosis drugs, although strains of *M. bovis* and some strains of *M. africanum* are naturally resistant to pyrazinamide. Environmental mycobacteria show very variable resistance to antituberculosis drugs and other antimicrobial agents, and in vitro susceptibility tests do not accurately reflect clinical responses.

DRUG RESISTANCE

Mutation to drug resistance occurs at a low but constant rate in all mycobacterial populations and such mutants (Table 33.1) are readily selected if the patient is treated with a single drug. Successful therapy thus requires the use of at least two drugs to which the strain is susceptible. An exception is the use of a single drug, usually isoniazid, to prevent the emergence of active tuberculosis in infected but healthy persons who are assumed to have very small numbers of bacilli in their tissues. Emergence of drug resistance is uncommon in patients receiving a fully supervised course of modern short-course chemotherapy based on drugs of known quality.

Unfortunately, poor prescribing habits, unavailability of drugs, inadvertent use of time-expired or even counterfeit drugs, poor supervision of therapy and unregulated 'over-the-counter' sales of drugs have led to the emergence of drug-resistant tubercle bacilli in many countries. Even fixed dose combination formulations occasionally lead to the development of single- or multiple-drug resistance if taken irregularly.

Tuberculosis resistant to rifampicin and isoniazid, with or without additional resistances, is termed multidrug-resistant (MDR) tuberculosis. Extensive drug resistance (XDR) has arisen in many countries and is variously defined as MDR with additional resistance to three or more of the six classes of second-line drugs, or to fluoroquinolones and at least one injectable drug (aminoglycosides and cyclic peptides). The exact definition is an academic one as, despite the establishment of regional and supraregional reference laboratories, few countries have adequate facilities for conducting drug susceptibility tests.

Drug resistance may develop in an inadequately treated patient (acquired or secondary resistance) or a person may become infected with a resistant strain (initial or primary resistance). Likewise, primary and acquired drug resistance is encountered in leprosy and the WHO has advised that all cases of leprosy should be treated by combination therapy.

The WHO recommends that periodic surveys of primary drug resistance should be undertaken as these give a good measure of the efficiency of control programs. The extent to which such surveys are carried out varies considerably from country to country: whereas in developed nations drug susceptibility tests are carried out on most or all clinical isolates of *M. tuberculosis*, such testing is often carried out only sporadically, and perhaps on unrepresentative isolates, in many developing countries.

Table 33.1 Targets of antimycobacterial agents and genes determining resistance[a]

Agent	Target	Gene(s) encoding target(s) or in which mutations conferring resistance occur
p-Aminosalicylic acid	Folic acid metabolism	Unknown
Clofazimine	Uncertain	Unknown
Cyclic peptides (capreomycin and viomycin)	50S or 30S ribosomal subunit	*vicA* (50S) or *vicB* (30S)
Cycloserine	Peptidoglycan synthesis	*alrA*
Dapsone	Folic acid synthesis	*folP1*
Ethambutol	Cell wall arabinogalactan synthesis	*embA*, *embB* and *embC*
Isoniazid	Mycolic acid synthesis	*katG*, *inhA* gene or its promoter region, intergenic region of the *oxyR–ahpC* locus
Pyrazinamide	? Bacterial membrane energetics and transport	*pncA*
Thioacetazone (amithiozone)	Synthesis of cyclopropane rings in mycolic acid	Genes coding for cyclopropane mycolic acid synthetase enzymes
Thioamines (ethionamide and prothionamide)	Mycolic acid synthesis	*inhA*

[a]For details on aminoglycosides and rifampicin, see Chapters 12 and 27, respectively.

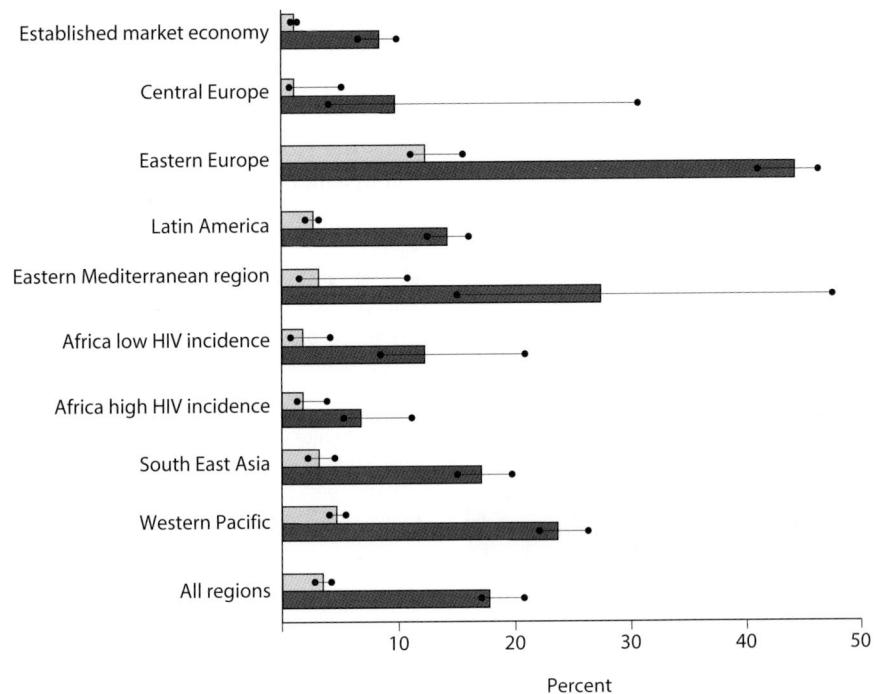

Fig. 33.1 Estimates, as a percentage, of multidrug-resistant tuberculosis among new (upper bar) and previously treated (lower bar) cases by World Health Organization epidemiological regions. Black bars show the 95% confidence ranges.

In four global surveys of resistance undertaken between 1994 and 2007, the global prevalence of various patterns of drug resistance varied enormously from region to region, with particularly high levels in certain regions. In 2008 the reported prevalence of MDR TB was over 5% in 14 regions: Armenia, Azerbaijan, the Baltic States (Estonia, Latvia, Lithuania), two provinces of China, Georgia, Moldova, three districts (Oblasts) of Russia, Ukraine and Uzbekistan. The incidence of MDR TB in new and previously treated cases in the WHO epidemiological regions is shown in Figure 33.1. The precise incidence of XDR tuberculosis is unknown as resistance to the full range of antituberculosis agents is determined in a minority of laboratories worldwide, but in June 2008 cases had been reported in 49 countries. In 2008, there were an estimated 490 000 cases of MDR TB and 40 000 cases of XDR TB.

PHARMACOKINETICS

With the exception of streptomycin, other aminoglycosides and the cyclic peptides, all the antimycobacterial agents currently in use are absorbed adequately when given orally. They are distributed to all tissues and organs and adequate amounts of the first-line antituberculosis agents cross the blood–brain barrier. Thus, in principle, standard regimens and doses are suitable for treatment of all forms of tuberculosis, although many clinicians prescribe more prolonged courses of therapy for extrapulmonary tuberculosis, particularly tuberculous meningitis, and for cases of HIV-related tuberculosis. Rifampicin,

isoniazid, pyrazinamide, ethionamide and protionamide are either eliminated in the bile or metabolized, and may therefore be given in standard doses to patients with impaired renal function. Ethambutol and aminoglycosides, which are eliminated predominantly or entirely by the kidney, should be avoided, if possible, in patients with impaired renal function.

Only small amounts of isoniazid and even smaller amounts of the other antituberculosis drugs enter the milk, so breast feeding is not contraindicated.

TOXICITY AND SIDE EFFECTS

Unwanted side effects occur with all antituberculosis agents, but those caused by the first-line drugs (rifampicin, isoniazid, pyrazinamide, ethambutol) are less frequent and severe than those due to the older agents (streptomycin, *p*-aminosalicylic acid, thioacetazone). Side effects are particularly likely to occur in HIV-positive patients, who should never be given thioacetazone as fatal exfoliative dermatitis may occur (specific toxicities are discussed under the individual drugs). A transient and clinically insignificant rise in serum hepatic enzyme levels commonly occurs during the first few weeks of therapy and, unless the patient is known to have liver disease, routine assay of these enzymes is generally regarded as unnecessary. Clinically evident hepatitis occurs in about 1% of patients and the incidence increases with age, although it usually resolves rapidly when therapy ends; usually therapy with the same drugs can be continued. More generalized reactions, with rashes, influenza-like symptoms and sometimes lymphadenopathy and hepatic enlargement, with or without jaundice, may occur in the first 2 months of therapy. Therapy must be stopped, the responsible drug identified by giving small challenge doses sequentially, and treatment resumed without that drug.

Interactions between the antimycobacterial drugs themselves have been described: pyrazinamide and ethionamide may increase serum concentrations of isoniazid while pyrazinamide may decrease that of rifampicin, but these effects are of no known clinical significance. More significant interactions occur between the antimycobacterial agents and drugs used for other purposes, particularly antiretroviral drugs (Chs. 36 and 43). Most recorded drug interactions involve rifampicin and quinolones but some interactions with isoniazid have been described, especially in slow acetylators (p. 390).

CLINICAL USE

Definite recommendations for the treatment of tuberculosis and leprosy have been made by the WHO (Chs 57 and 58). These regimens are also used for treating human tuberculosis due to *M. bovis* and for the rare cases of disseminated disease due to the vaccine strain bacille Calmette-Guérin (BCG), although both are naturally resistant to pyrazinamide.

Isoniazid preventive therapy has a controversial history, but the HIV pandemic, leading to a greatly enhanced risk of tuberculosis, has led to re-evaluation of its protective role. It can be safely used in HIV-infected persons as long as they do not have active tuberculosis and it prevents the risk of the latter by 33–67% for up to 4 years. It is recommended for HIV-infected persons living in regions with a prevalence of latent tuberculosis of over 30% and for all those with known latent disease or exposure to a case of infectious tuberculosis. Where available, a combination of isoniazid and antiretroviral therapy provides even greater protection.

Treatment of opportunist mycobacterial disease continues to pose problems, with a high failure rate, often due to coexistent HIV infection or other forms of immunosuppression. Disease caused by slowly growing mycobacteria, principally the *Mycobacterium avium* complex, *M. kansasii*, *M. xenopi* and *M. malmoense*, is usually treated with rifampicin (or rifabutin) and ethambutol, together with clarithromycin or a fluoroquinolone.

In the absence of clinical trials, therapy of disease due to the rapidly growing mycobacteria, principally *M. abscessus*, *M. chelonae* and *M. fortuitum*, is empirical. Limited infections such as post-injection abscesses respond to co-trimoxazole together with erythromycin. More serious infections have responded to cefoxitin with amikacin. The outcome of therapy is, however, unpredictable. In-vitro drug susceptibility tests do not give an accurate indication of clinical response.

 ## FORMULATIONS

Compliance with antituberculosis therapy is aided by use of fixed drug combination preparations and calendar blister-packs. Several preparations containing rifampicin + isoniazid, rifampicin + isoniazid + pyrazinamide or all four of the first-line drugs are commercially available but only those approved by the WHO should be used as in some combinations the bioavailability of the component drugs, especially rifampicin, is inadequate.

 ## Further information

Blomberg B, Spinaci S, Fourie B, Laing R. The rationale for recommending fixed-dose combination tablets for treatment of tuberculosis. *Bull World Health Org.* 2001;79:61–68.

Colombo RE, Olivier KN. Diagnosis and treatment of infections caused by rapidly growing mycobacteria. *Semin Respir Crit Care Med.* 2008;29:577–588.

Crofton J, Chaulet P, Maher D. *Guidelines for the management of drug-resistant tuberculosis.* Geneva: WHO; 1997.

Dorman SE, Chaisson RE. From magic bullets back to the magic mountain: the rise of extensively drug-resistant tuberculosis. *Nat Med.* 2007;13:295–298.

Gillespie SH. Evolution of drug resistance in *Mycobacterium tuberculosis*: clinical and molecular perspective. *Antimicrob Agents Chemother.* 2002;46:267–274.

Ginsberg AM. Emerging drugs for active tuberculosis. *Semin Respir Crit Care Med.* 2008;29:552–559.

Grange JM, Winstanley PA, Davies PDO. Clinically significant drug interactions with antituberculosis agents. *Drug Safety.* 1994;11:242–251.

Jenkins PA, Campbell IA, Banks J, Gelder CM, Prescott RJ, Smith AP. Clarithromycin vs ciprofloxacin as adjuncts to rifampicin and ethambutol in treating opportunist mycobacterial lung diseases and an assessment of *Mycobacterium vaccae* immunotherapy. *Thorax.* 2008;63:627–634.

Mitchison DA. How drug resistance emerges as a result of poor compliance during short course chemotherapy of tuberculosis. *Int J Tuberc Lung Dis.* 1998;2:10–15.

Mitchison DA. Role of individual drugs in the chemotherapy of tuberculosis. *Int J Tuberc Lung Dis.* 2000;4:796–806.

Mitnick CD, Shin SS, Seung KJ, et al. Comprehensive treatment of extensively drug-resistant tuberculosis. *N Engl J Med.* 2008;359:563–574.

Onyebujoh P, Zumla A, Ribiero I, et al. Treatment of tuberculosis: present status and future prospects. *Bull World Health Org.* 2005;83:857–865.

Peloquin CA. Clinical pharmacology of antituberculosis drugs. In: Davies PDO, Barnes PF, Gordon SB, eds. *Clinical tuberculosis.* 4th ed. London: Hodder Arnold; 2008:205–224.

Raviglione MC, Smith IM. XDR tuberculosis – implications for global public health. *N Engl J Med.* 2007;356:656–659.

World Health Organization/International Union Against Tuberculosis and Lung Disease. *Global project on anti-tuberculosis drug resistance surveillance 2008. Anti-tuberculosis drug resistance in the world.* Report no. 4. Geneva: WHO; 2008.

World Health Organization 2003 (revision). *Treatment of tuberculosis.* 3rd ed. Guidelines for national programmes. Geneva: WHO; 2005.

World Health Organization. *Report of the expert consultation on immunotherapeutic interventions for tuberculosis.* Geneva: WHO; 2007.

World Health Organization. *Guidelines for the programmatic management of drug-resistant tuberculosis.* Emergency update. Geneva: WHO; 2008.

World Health Organization. HIV/AIDS Department. *WHO Three I's Meeting. Intensified case finding (ICF), isoniazid preventive therapy (IPT) and TB infection control (IC) for people living with HIV.* WHO: Geneva; 2008.

Zhang Y, Vilchèze C, Jacobs WR. Mechanisms of drug resistance in *Mycobacterium tuberculosis*. In: Cole ST, Eisenach K, McMurray D, Jacobs WR, eds. *Tuberculosis and the Tubercle Bacillus.* 2nd ed. Washington, DC: American Society for Microbiology; 2005:115–140.

CLOFAZIMINE

Molecular weight: 473.4.

One of a number of substituted iminophenazine dyes originally synthesized as potential antituberculosis agents. It is almost insoluble in water. It stimulates various phagocyte functions including release of free oxygen radicals, but it is not clear whether this contributes to its antimicrobial activity. It also has anti-inflammatory properties, attributed to its ability to inhibit certain patterns of intracellular T-cell receptor-mediated signaling, making it a useful drug for treating leprosy reactions and possibly other autoimmune processes.

ANTIMICROBIAL ACTIVITY

The mode of action is not fully understood. It has bacteriostatic and weak bactericidal activity against several species of mycobacteria and some species of *Actinomyces* and *Nocardia*. In-vitro minimum inhibitory concentrations (MICs) are: *M. tuberculosis* 0.5 mg/L and *M. leprae* (assayed in a mouse model) 0.1–1 mg/L, but these MICs have limited clinical relevance as clofazimine shows marked differences in accumulation in various tissues. Activity against *M. leprae* is demonstrable in humans only after 50 days of therapy. Clofazimine resistance, although reported, appears to be rare.

PHARMACOKINETICS

Clofazimine is well absorbed by the intestine and is taken up by adipose tissue and cells of the macrophage/monocyte series, including those in the intestinal wall. It has a very long half-life (variously estimated as 10–70 days) and is eliminated, mostly unchanged, in the urine and feces.

TOXICITY AND SIDE EFFECTS

Clofazimine is usually well tolerated, but some patients develop nausea, abdominal pain and diarrhea, relieved to some extent by taking the drug with a meal or glass of milk. Dose-related, reversible, skin discoloration is very common and is unacceptable to some patients. Discoloration of the hair, cornea, urine, sweat and tears also occurs. Infants born to mothers receiving clofazimine are reversibly pigmented at birth. Edema of the wall of the small intestine leading to subacute obstruction is

a rare but serious complication of prolonged high-dose therapy for leprosy reactions. Deposition of clofazimine in lymph nodes may interfere with lymphatic drainage, occasionally manifesting as edema of the feet.

CLINICAL USE

Multibacillary leprosy (in combination with other anti-leprosy drugs)
Erythema nodosum leprosum (anti-inflammatory activity)

Clofazimine has been suggested as a drug for treatment of MDR tuberculosis, although its efficacy is unproven. It has been used to treat *M. ulcerans* infection (Buruli ulcer) but with limited responses. Use in disease caused by mycobacteria of the *M. avium* complex is no longer recommended as more effective and less toxic alternative agents are available.

Preparations and dosage

Proprietary name: Lamprene.
Preparation: Capsules.
Dosage: Multibacillary forms of leprosy: adults, oral, 300 mg once a month, supervised, and 50 mg per day or 100 mg on alternate days self-administered. Erythema nodosum leprosum: 300 mg once a day for no longer than 3 months.

Further information

Grange JM. Detection of drug resistance in *Mycobacterium leprae* and the design of treatment regimens for leprosy. In: Heifets L, ed. *Drug susceptibility in the chemotherapy of mycobacterial infections.* Boca Raton, FL: CRC Press; 1991:161–177.
Jamet P, Traore I, Husser JA, Ji B. Short-term trial of clofazimine in previously untreated lepromatous leprosy. *Int J Lepr.* 1992;60:542–548.
Oommen ST, Natu MV, Mahajan MK, Kadyan RS. Lymphangiographic evaluation of patients with clinical lepromatous leprosy on clofazimine. *Int J Lepr.* 1994;62:32–36.
Reddy VM, O'Sullivan JF, Gangadharam PR. Antimycobacterial activities of riminophenazines. *J Antimicrob Chemother.* 1999;43:615–623.
Schaad-Lanyi Z, Dieterle W, Dubois JP, Theobold W, Vischer W. Pharmacokinetics of clofazimine in healthy volunteers. *Int J Lepr.* 1987;55:9–15.
Steel HC, Matlola NM, Anderson R. Inhibition of potassium transport and growth of mycobacteria exposed to clofazimine and B669 is associated with a calcium-independent increase in microbial phospholipase A2 activity. *J Antimicrob Chemother.* 1999;44:209–216.

DAPSONE

Diaminodiphenyl sulphone (DDS). Molecular weight: 248.3.

The most effective of a number of sulfonamide derivatives to be tested against leprosy. The dry powder is very stable. It is only slightly soluble in water.

ANTIMICROBIAL ACTIVITY

Dapsone is active against many bacteria and some protozoa. Fully susceptible strains of *M. leprae* are inhibited by a little as 0.003 mg/L. It is predominantly bacteristatic. Resistance is associated with mutations in the *folP1* gene involved in the synthesis of *para*-aminobenzoic acid.

ACQUIRED RESISTANCE

Resistance to high levels is acquired by several sequential mutations. As a result of prolonged use of dapsone monotherapy, acquired resistance emerged in patients with multibacillary leprosy in many countries. Initial resistance also occurs in patients with both paucibacillary and multibacillary leprosy. Thus, leprosy should always be treated with multidrug regimens. Resistance of *M. leprae* to dapsone (and other anti-leprosy drugs) may now be determined by use of DNA microarrays.

PHARMACOKINETICS

Oral absorption	>90%
C_{max} 100 mg oral	c. 2 mg/L after 3–6 h
Plasma half-life	10–50 h
Plasma protein binding	c. 50%

It is slowly but almost completely absorbed from the intestine and widely distributed in the tissues, but selectively retained in skin, muscle, kidneys and liver. It is metabolized by *N*-oxidation and also by acetylation, which is subject to the same genetic polymorphism as isoniazid (p. 390). The elimination half-life is consequently very variable, but on standard therapy the trough levels are always well in excess of inhibitory concentrations. It is mostly excreted in the urine: in the unchanged form (20%), as *N*-oxidation products (30%) and as a range of other metabolites.

TOXICITY AND SIDE EFFECTS

Although usually well tolerated at standard doses, gastrointestinal upsets, anorexia, headaches, dizziness and insomnia may occur. Less frequent reactions include skin rashes, exfoliative dermatitis, photosensitivity, peripheral neuropathy (usually in non-leprosy patients), tinnitus, blurred vision, psychoses, hepatitis, nephrotic syndrome, systemic lupus erythematosus and generalized lymphadenopathy.

The term 'dapsone syndrome' is applied to a skin rash and fever occurring 2–8 weeks after starting therapy and sometimes accompanied by lymphadenopathy, hepatomegaly, jaundice and/or mononucleosis.

Blood disorders include anemia, methemoglobinemia, sulfhemoglobinemia, hemolysis (notably in patients with glucose-6-phosphate dehydrogenase deficiency), mononucleosis, leukopenia and, rarely, agranulocytosis. Severe anemia should be treated before patients receive dapsone.

The incidence of adverse reactions declined in the 1960s but reappeared around 1982 when multidrug therapy was introduced, and may represent an unexplained interaction with rifampicin.

CLINICAL USE

Leprosy (multidrug regimens)
Prophylaxis of malaria, treatment of chloroquine-resistant malaria (in combination with pyrimethamine)
Prophylaxis of toxoplasmosis (in combination with pyrimethamine)
Prophylaxis (monotherapy) and treatment (in combination with trimethoprim) of *Pneumocystis jirovecii* pneumonia
Dermatitis herpetiformis and related skin disorders

Preparations and dosage

Preparation: Tablets.

Dosage: For all forms of leprosy (in combination with other anti-leprosy drugs): Adults, 100 mg per day, children 1–2 mg/kg (maximum dose, 100 mg per day). Duration of treatment depends on type of leprosy and the other agents used.

Further information

Ahrens EM, Meckler RJ, Callen JP. Dapsone-induced peripheral neuropathy. *Int J Dermatol*. 1986;25:314–316.

Byrd SR, Gelber RH. Effect of dapsone on haemoglobin concentration in patients with leprosy. *Lepr Rev*. 1991;62:171–178.

Matsuoka M, Aye KS, Kyaw K, et al. A novel method for simple detection of mutations conferring drug resistance in *Mycobacterium leprae*, based on a DNA microarray, and its applicability in developing countries. *J Med Microbiol*. 2008;57:1213–1219.

Rai PP, Aschhoff M, Lilly L, Balakrishnan S. Influence of acetylator phenotype of the leprosy patient on the emergence of dapsone resistant leprosy. *Indian J Lepr*. 1988;60:400–406.

Richardus JH, Smith TC. Increased incidence in leprosy of hypersensitivity reactions to dapsone after introduction of multidrug therapy. *Lepr Rev*. 1989;60:267–273.

Williams DL, Spring L, Harris E, Roche P, Gillis TP. Dihydropteroate synthase of *Mycobacterium leprae* and dapsone resistance. *Antimicrob Agents Chemother*. 2000;44:1530–1537.

Zuidema J, Hilbers-Modderman ES, Merkus FW. Clinical pharmacokinetics of dapsone. *Clin Pharmacokinet*. 1986;11:299–315.

ETHAMBUTOL

Hydroxymethylpropylethylene diamine. Molecular weight (dihydrochloride): 277.2.

$$HC \underset{\underset{C_2H_5}{|}}{\overset{\overset{CH_2OH}{|}}{-}} NH - CH_2 - CH_2 - NH - \underset{\underset{CH_2OH}{|}}{\overset{\overset{C_2H_5}{|}}{CH}}$$

A synthetic ethylenediamine derivative formulated as the dihydrochloride for oral administration. The dry powder is very soluble and stable.

ANTIMICROBIAL ACTIVITY

Ethambutol is active against several species of mycobacteria and nocardiae. MICs on solid media are: *M. tuberculosis* 0.5–2 mg/L; *M. kansasii* 1–4 mg/L; other slowly growing mycobacteria 2–8 mg/L; rapidly growing pathogens 2–16 mg/L; *Nocardia* spp. 8–32 mg/L.

Resistance is uncommon and is a multistep process due to mutations in the *embA*, *embB* and *embC* gene cluster. A mutation in codon 306 of the *embB* gene predisposes to the development of resistance to a range of antituberculosis agents, possibly by affecting cell-wall permeability.

PHARMACOKINETICS

Oral absorption	*c.* 80%, but some patients absorb it poorly
C_{max} 25 mg/kg oral	2–6 mg/L after 2–3 h
Plasma half-life	10–15 h
Volume of distribution	>3 L/kg
Plasma protein binding	20–30%

Absorption is impeded by aluminum hydroxide and alcohol. It is concentrated in the phagolysosomes of alveolar macrophages. It does not enter the cerebrospinal fluid (CSF) in health but CSF levels of 25–40% of the plasma concentration, with considerable variation between patients, are achieved in cases of tuberculous meningitis.

Various metabolites are produced, including dialdehyde, dicarboxylic acid and glucuronide derivatives. Around 50% is excreted unchanged in the urine, with an additional 10–15% as metabolites, and 20% is excreted unchanged in feces.

TOXICITY AND SIDE EFFECTS

The most important side effect is optic neuritis, which may be irreversible if treatment is not discontinued. This complication is rare if the higher dose (25 mg/kg) is given for no more than 2 months. National codes of practice for prevention of ocular toxicity should be adhered to; in particular, patients should be advised to stop therapy and seek medical advice if they notice any change in visual acuity, peripheral vision or color perception, and the drug should not be given to young children and others unable to comply with this advice.

Other side effects include gastrointestinal upsets, peripheral neuritis, arthralgia, nephritis, myocarditis, hyperuricemia, dermal hypersensitivity and, rarely, thrombocytopenia and hepatotoxicity.

CLINICAL USE

Tuberculosis (initial intensive phase of short-course therapy)
Other mycobacterioses (*M. kansasii*, *M. xenopi*, *M. malmoense* and the *M. avium* complex) (with appropriate additional drugs)

Preparations and dosage

Proprietary name: Myambutol.

Preparations: Tablets (and syrup on special request).

Dosage: Adults and children, oral, 15–25 mg/kg per day for 2 months or 25–30 mg/kg three times a week or 45–50 mg/kg twice a week. If more prolonged therapy is indicated, the daily dose should not exceed 15 mg/kg; retreatment 25 mg/kg per day for the first 60 days.

Widely available.

Further information

Citron KM. Ocular toxicity from ethambutol. *Thorax.* 1986;41:737–739.
Donald PR, Maher D, Maritz JS, Qazi S. Ethambutol dosage for the treatment of children: literature review and recommendations. *Int J Tuberc Lung Dis.* 2006;10:1318–1330.
Safi H, Sayers B, Hazbón MH, Alland D. Transfer of embB codon 306 mutations into clinical *Mycobacterium tuberculosis* strains alters susceptibility to ethambutol, isoniazid, and rifampin. *Antimicrob Agents Chemother.* 2008;52:2027–2034.
McIlleron H, Wash P, Burger A, Norman J, Folb PI, Smith P. Determinants of rifampin, isoniazid, pyrazinamide, and ethambutol pharmacokinetics in a cohort of tuberculosis patients. *Antimicrob Agents Chemother.* 2006;50:1170–1177.

ISONIAZID

Isonicotinic acid hydrazide (INH). Molecular weight: 137.1.

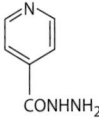

One of a number of nicotinamide analogs found to have antituberculosis activity, following the observation that nicotinamide inhibited the replication of *M. tuberculosis*. It is soluble in water. The dry powder is stable if protected from light. It is a prodrug requiring oxidative activation by KatG, a mycobacterial catalase–peroxidase enzyme.

ANTIMICROBIAL ACTIVITY

Susceptibility to isoniazid is virtually restricted to the *M. tuberculosis* complex (MIC 0.01–0.2 mg/L). It is highly bactericidal against actively replicating *M. tuberculosis*. Other mycobacteria are resistant, except for some strains of *M. xenopi* (MIC 0.2 mg/L) and a few strains of *M. kansasii* (MIC 1 mg/L).

 ## ACQUIRED RESISTANCE

Mutations in the *katG* gene, the *inhA* gene or its promoter region, and in the intergenic region of the *oxyR–ahpC* locus confer resistance to isoniazid (Table 33.1, p. 384). The relative proportions of such mutations vary geographically and are related to the distribution of the various lineages or superfamilies of *M. tuberculosis*.

Isoniazid resistance is the commonest form of drug resistance worldwide and the great majority of strains resistant to another agent are also resistant to isoniazid (see pp. 384–385).

 ## PHARMACOKINETICS

Oral absorption	>95%
C_{max} 300 mg oral	3–5 mg/L after 1–2 h
Plasma half-life	0.5–1.5 h (rapid acetylators)
	2–4 h (slow acetylators)
Volume of distribution	0.6–0.8 L/kg
Plasma protein binding	Very low

Absorption and distribution

Isoniazid is almost completely absorbed from the gut and is well distributed. Absorption is impaired by aluminum hydroxide. Therapeutic concentrations are achieved in sputum and CSF. It crosses the placenta and is found in breast milk.

Metabolism

Isoniazid is extensively metabolized to a variety of pharmacologically inactive derivatives, predominantly by acetylation. As a result of genetic polymorphism, patients are divisible into rapid and slow acetylators. About 50% of Caucasians and Blacks, but 80–90% of Chinese and Japanese, are rapid acetylators. Acetylation status does not affect the efficacy of daily administered therapy. The rate of acetylation is reduced in chronic renal failure.

Excretion

Nearly all the dose is excreted in the urine within 24 h, as unchanged drug and metabolic products.

 ## TOXICITY AND SIDE EFFECTS

Toxic effects are unusual on recommended doses and are more frequent in slow acetylators. Many side effects are neurological, including restlessness, insomnia, muscle twitching and difficulty in starting micturition. More serious but less common neurological side effects include peripheral neuropathy, optic neuritis, encephalopathy and a range of psychiatric disorders, including anxiety, depression and paranoia.

Neurotoxicity is usually preventable by giving pyridoxine (vitamin B_6) 10 mg per day. Pyridoxine should be given to patients with liver disease, pregnant women, alcoholics, renal dialysis patients, HIV-positive patients, the malnourished and the elderly. Encephalopathy, which has been reported in patients on renal dialysis, may not be prevented by, or respond to, pyridoxine, but usually resolves on withdrawal of isoniazid.

Isoniazid-related hepatitis occurs in about 1% of patients receiving standard short-course chemotherapy. The incidence is unaffected by acetylator status. It is more common in those aged over 35 years and preventive isoniazid monotherapy should be used with care in older people.

Less common side effects include arthralgia, a 'flu'-like syndrome, hypersensitivity reactions with fever, rashes and, rarely, eosinophilia, sideroblastic anemia, pellagra (which responds to treatment with nicotinic acid) and hemolysis in patients with glucose-6-phosphate dehydrogenase deficiency. It exacerbates acute porphyria and induces antinuclear antibodies, but overt systemic lupus erythematosus is rare.

 ## DRUG INTERACTIONS

Isoniazid increases the plasma concentrations of phenytoin and carbamazepine, sometimes enough to cause toxicity; antiepileptic therapy requires monitoring and adjustment of dosage as necessary. It enhances defluorination of the anesthetic enflurane. Drug interactions may be more pronounced in slow acetylators. Prednisolone reduces isoniazid levels in both slow and rapid acetylators, but the mechanism is unclear.

 ## CLINICAL USE

Tuberculosis (intensive and continuation phases)
Prevention of primary tuberculosis in close contacts and reactivation disease in infected but healthy persons (monotherapy)

 ### Preparations and dosage

Preparations: Tablets, elixir and injectable form.

Dosage: Adults, oral, 300 mg per day; children, 5–10 mg/kg per day (maximum dose, 300 mg per day). Neonates, 3–5 mg/kg per day (maximum dose, 10 mg/kg per day).

Widely available.

Further information

Baker LV, Brown TJ, Maxwell O, et al. Molecular analysis of isoniazid-resistant *Mycobacterium tuberculosis* isolates from England and Wales reveals the phylogenetic significance of the ahpC–46A polymorphism. *Antimicrob Agents Chemother.* 2005;49:1455–1464.

Banerjee A, Dubnau E, Quemard A, et al. InhA, a gene encoding a target for isoniazid and ethionamide in *Mycobacterium tuberculosis. Science.* 1994;263:227–230.

Cheung WC, Lo CY, Lo WK, Ip M, Cheng IKP. Isoniazid induced encephalopathy in dialysis patients. *Tuber Lung Dis.* 1993;74:136–139.

Ellard GA. The potential clinical significance of the isoniazid acetylator phenotype in the treatment of pulmonary tuberculosis. *Tubercle.* 1984;65:211–217.

Gagneux S, Burgos MV, DeRiemer K, et al. Impact of bacterial genetics on the transmission of isoniazid-resistant *Mycobacterium tuberculosis. PLoS Pathog.* 2006;2:e61.

Guo H, Seet Q, Denkin S, Parsons L, Zhang Y. Molecular characterization of isoniazid-resistant clinical isolates of *Mycobacterium tuberculosis* from the USA. *J Med Microbiol.* 2006;55:1527–1531.

International Union Against Tuberculosis and Lung Disease/World Health Organization. Tuberculosis preventive therapy in HIV-infected individuals. *Tuber Lung Dis.* 1994;75:96–98.

Israel HL, Gottleib JE, Maddrey WC. Perspective: preventive isoniazid therapy and the liver. *Chest.* 1992;101:1298–1301.

Lee H, Cho SN, Bang HE, et al. Exclusive mutations related to isoniazid and ethionamide resistance among *Mycobacterium tuberculosis* isolates from Korea. *Int J Tuberc Lung Dis.* 2000;4:441–447.

Snider DE, Tabas GJ. Isoniazid associated hepatitis deaths: a review of available information. *Am Rev Respir Dis.* 1992;145:494–497.

PYRAZINAMIDE

Pyrazinoic acid amide. Molecular weight: 123.1.

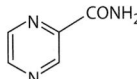

Like isoniazid, pyrazinamide is a synthetic nicotinamide analog, although its mode of action is quite distinct.

ANTIMICROBIAL ACTIVITY

It is principally active against actively metabolizing intracellular bacilli and those in acidic, anoxic inflammatory lesions. Activity against *M. tuberculosis* is highly pH dependent: at pH 5.6 the MIC is 8–16 mg/L, but it is almost inactive at neutral pH. Other mycobacterial species, including *M. bovis*, are resistant. Activity requires conversion to pyrazinoic acid by the mycobacterial enzyme pyrazinamidase, encoded for by the *pncA* gene, which is present in *M. tuberculosis* but not *M. bovis*. A few resistant strains lack mutations in *pncA*, indicating alternative mechanisms for resistance, including defects in transportation of the agent into the bacterial cell.

ACQUIRED RESISTANCE

Drug resistance is uncommon and cross-resistance to other antituberculosis agents does not occur. Susceptibility testing is technically demanding as it requires very careful control of the pH of the medium, but molecular methods for detection of resistance-conferring mutations are available.

PHARMACOKINETICS

Oral absorption	>90%
C_{max} 20–22 mg/kg oral	10–50 mg/L after 2 h
Plasma half-life	*c.* 9 h
Plasma protein binding	*c.* 50%

It readily crosses the blood–brain barrier, achieving CSF concentrations similar to plasma levels. It is metabolized to pyrazinoic acid in the liver and oxidized to inactive metabolites, which are excreted in the urine, although about 70% of an oral dose is excreted unchanged.

TOXICITY AND SIDE EFFECTS

It is usually well tolerated. Moderate elevations of serum transaminases occur early in treatment. Severe hepatotoxicity is uncommon with standard dosage, except in patients with pre-existing liver disease.

Its principal metabolite, pyrazinoic acid, inhibits renal excretion of uric acid, but gout is extremely rare. An unrelated arthralgia, notably of the shoulders and responsive to analgesics, also occurs.

Other side effects include anorexia, nausea, mild flushing of the skin and photosensitization.

CLINICAL USE

Tuberculosis (a component of the early, intensive phase of short-course therapy)

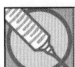

Preparations and dosage

Proprietary names: Tebrazid, Zinamide.

Preparation: Tablets.

Dosage: Adult, oral, 2 g per day (>50 kg), 1.5 g per day (<50 kg); children, 25–35 mg/kg per day in 3–4 divided doses. Alternatively, adults and children, oral, 50 mg/kg three times a week or up to 75 mg/kg twice a week. Widely available.

Further information

Denkin S, Volokhov D, Chizhikov V, Zhang Y. Microarray-based PncA genotyping of pyrazinamide-resistant strains of *Mycobacterium tuberculosis. J Med Microbiol.* 2005;54:1127–1131.

Lacroix C, Hoang TP, Nouveau J, et al. Pharmacokinetics of pyrazinamide and its metabolites in healthy subjects. *Eur J Clin Pharmacol.* 1989;36:395–400.

Raynaud C, Laneelle MA, Senaratne RH, et al. Mechanisms of pyrazinamide resistance in mycobacteria: importance of lack of uptake in addition to lack of pyrazinamidase activity. *Microbiology.* 1999;145:1359–1367.

Scorpio A, Zhang Y. Mutations in *pncA*, a gene encoding pyrazinamidase/nicotinamidase, cause resistance to the antituberculous drug pyrazinamide in tubercle bacillus. *Nat Med.* 1996;2:662–667.

Stamatakis G, Montes C, Trouvin JH, et al. Pyrazinamide and pyrazinoic acid pharmacokinetics in patients with chronic renal failure. *Clin Nephrol.* 1988;30:230–234.

Zhang Y, Mitchison D. The curious characteristics of pyrazinamide: a review. *Int J Tuberc Lung Dis.* 2003;7:6–21.

OTHER ANTIMYCOBACTERIAL AGENTS

PARA-AMINOSALICYLIC ACID

A salicylic acid derivative formulated as the dihydrate or sodium salt for oral administration. The activity is bacteriostatic and against extracellular bacteria. Inhibitory concentrations for *M. tuberculosis* are 0.5–10 mg/L, depending on the medium used and the inoculum size. It appears to act by interfering with folic acid metabolism. Resistance is very uncommon as the drug is rarely used.

It is well absorbed, achieving a plasma concentration of 70–80 mg/L 1–2 h after a 4 g oral dose. High tissue concentrations are achieved. The drug is rapidly acetylated in the liver and about 80% is excreted in the urine within 7 h, mostly in the acetylated form.

Adverse effects, leading to problems of compliance, occur in 10–30% of patients. Gastrointestinal effects, including abdominal pain, nausea, vomiting and diarrhea, are very common. It interferes with iodine metabolism in the thyroid, and prolonged therapy may lead to goiter, and less frequently to myxedema, which respond to thyroxine therapy. Allergic skin reactions are common. Less common side effects include blood dyscrasias, crystalluria, eosinophilic pneumonia, malabsorption, encephalopathy and optic neuritis. It is used only in MDR tuberculosis.

Preparations and dosage

Preparations: Tablets, oral granules.

Dosage: Adults 200–300 mg/kg per day in 3 divided doses (maximum dose, 12 g per day). Children 150 mg/kg in 2–3 divided doses (maximum dose, 12 g per day).

Limited availability.

Further information

Peloquin CA. *Para*-aminosalicylic acid. In: Yu VL, Edwards G, McKinnon PS, Peloquin CA, Morse GD, eds. *Antimicrobial Chemotherapy and Vaccines.* 2nd ed. Vol. 2. Pittsburgh, PA: Esun Technologies; 2005:551–558.

Peloquin CA, Berning SE, Huitt GA, Childs JM, Singleton MD, Jones GT. Once-daily and twice daily doses of *p*-aminosalicylic acid granules. *Am J Respir Crit Care Med.* 1999;159:932–934.

Rengarajan J, Sassetti CM, Naroditskaya V, Sloutsky A, Bloom BR, Rubin EJ. The folate pathway is a target for resistance to the drug *para*-aminosalicylic acid (PAS) in mycobacteria. *Mol Microbiol.* 2004;53:275–282.

CAPREOMYCIN AND VIOMYCIN

These are naturally occurring cyclic peptide antibiotics synthesized by several *Streptomyces* species. Both are supplied as water-soluble sulfates. There is evidence that capreomycin is active against non-replicating cells of *M. tuberculosis*. They inhibit *M. tuberculosis*, including strains resistant to most other antituberculosis agents, at a concentration of 1.25–2.5 mg/L in liquid media. MICs are higher (8–16 mg/L) on egg media owing to protein binding. There is complete cross-resistance between capreomycin and viomycin and part cross-resistance of both to aminoglycosides.

They are not absorbed from the intestine and do not readily enter cells or the CSF. Intramuscular injection of 1 g gives peak serum concentrations of 20–50 mg/L. They are mostly excreted unchanged in the urine. No metabolites have been described.

Pain, induration and excessive bleeding may occur at the injection site. Cyclic peptides are ototoxic, affecting both cochlear and vestibular functions, and nephrotoxic, causing loss of K$^+$, Ca^{2+} and Mg^{2+}, leading to neuromuscular blockade. Anorexia, thirst and polyuria occasionally occur. These toxic effects are uncommon if the drugs are given two or three times weekly. Auditory and vestibular functions and serum potassium levels should be monitored before and regularly during therapy. Capreomycin is used for MDR tuberculosis (with other antituberculosis drugs). Viomycin is rarely, if ever, used (for the same purpose) and is of very limited availability. A derivative, enviomycin, is available in Japan and is said to be less ototoxic.

Preparations and dosage (capreomycin)

Proprietary name: Capastat.

Preparation: Injection.

Dosage: Adults, deep i.m. injection, 1 g per day (maximum dose, 20 mg/kg per day) for 2–4 months, then 1 g 2–3 times a week for the remainder of therapy. Children, 20 mg/kg per day (maximum dose, 1 g per day).

Further information

Black HR, Griffith RS, Peabody AM. Absorption, excretion and metabolism of capreomycin in normal and diseased states. *Ann N Y Acad Sci.* 1966;135:974–982.

Heifets L, Simon J, Pham V. Capreomycin is active against non-replicating *M. tuberculosis. Ann Clin Microbiol Antimicrob.* 2005;4:6.

Lehmann CR, Garrett LE, Winn RE, et al. Capreomycin kinetics in renal impairment and clearance by hemodialysis. *Am Rev Respir Dis.* 1988;138:1312–1313.

Maus CE, Plikaytis BB, Shinnick TM. Molecular analysis of cross-resistance to capreomycin, kanamycin, amikacin, and viomycin in *Mycobacterium tuberculosis. Antimicrob Agents Chemother.* 2005;49:3192–3197.

CYCLOSERINE

A fermentation product of *Strep. orchidaceus* and other related organisms now produced synthetically. Aqueous solutions are stable at pH 7.8 but the agent is rapidly destroyed in acid conditions. It is active against a wide range of Gram-negative and Gram-positive bacteria, including *Staphylococcus aureus*, streptococci, including *Enterococcus faecalis*, various enterobacteria, *Nocardia* and *Chlamydia* spp. *M. tuberculosis* is inhibited by 8–16 mg/L. Some environmental mycobacteria, including *M. avium*, are also susceptible. Its action is specifically antagonized by D-alanine, from which media for in-vitro tests should be free. Its use is limited by neurological and psychiatric side effects. Primary resistance in *M. tuberculosis* is rare and develops only slowly in patients treated with cycloserine alone. Its inclusion in combinations deters the development of resistance to other drugs. There is no cross-resistance with other therapeutic antibiotics.

It is well absorbed when given orally, achieving a concentration of *c.* 10 mg/L 3–4 h after a 250 mg dose. Doubling the dose approximately doubles the plasma level. Some accumulation occurs over the first 3 or 4 days of treatment. In children receiving 20 mg/kg orally, plasma levels of 20–35 mg/L have been found. It is widely distributed throughout the body fluids, including the CSF. About 50% is excreted unchanged in the glomerular filtrate over 24 h and 65–70% over the subsequent 2 days. The remainder is metabolized. There is no tubular secretion and no effect of probenecid. Cycloserine accumulates in renal failure, reaching toxic levels if dosage is uncontrolled. It can be removed by hemodialysis.

Evidence of central nervous system toxicity, including headache, somnolence, vertigo, visual disturbances, confusion, depression, acute psychotic reactions and tremors, may develop over the first 2 weeks of treatment. The effects may be exacerbated by alcohol and can be reduced, to some extent, by administering pyridoxine. Treatment should be stopped promptly if any mental or neurological signs develop. Convulsions are said to occur in about 50% of patients when the plasma concentration exceeds 20–25 mg/L, but the relationship to dose is not particularly close. No permanent damage appears to be caused. Cycloserine inhibits mammalian transaminases and this and the convulsant effects of the drug have been attributed to a metabolite, amino-oxyalanine. Use of the drug should be avoided in patients with previous fits or other neurological or psychiatric abnormalities. Rare side effects include rashes, cardiac arrhythmia and deficiency in folate and vitamin B_{12} leading to peripheral neuritis.

It is occasionally used in MDR tuberculosis (with other antituberculosis drugs) and other mycobacterioses (with appropriate additional drugs).

Preparations and dosage

Proprietary names: Cycloserine, Seromycin.

Preparation: Capsules.

Dosage: Adults, oral, 250 mg every 12 h (maximum dose, 500 mg every 12 h) for 2 weeks. Children, initially 10 mg/kg per day, adjusted according to blood levels and response.

Further information

Wolinsky E. Statement of the Tuberculosis Committee of the Infectious Diseases Society of America. *Clin Infect Dis.* 1993;16:627–628.

ETHIONAMIDE AND PROTIONAMIDE (PROTHIONAMIDE)

These are closely related thioamides structurally similar to isoniazid. They are almost insoluble in water and are unstable on exposure to light. Their antibacterial activity and pharmacokinetics are almost identical, but protionamide is said to be better tolerated. Ethionamide is a second-line agent for treatment of MDR tuberculosis. Protionamide is seldom used in tuberculosis but is used in place of clofazimine for the treatment of leprosy in patients who find skin pigmentation caused by that drug unacceptable. It is more effective than an equivalent dose of ethionamide for killing *M. leprae*, but not as effective as some other agents (fluoroquinolones, minocycline and newer macrolides) currently used in leprosy. If given simultaneously with isoniazid, the blood levels of thioamides may be raised, resulting in more side effects unless the dosage is adjusted.

The MIC for *M. tuberculosis* on solid egg media is 0.8–1.6 mg/L; MICs for the *M. avium* complex, *M. kansasii* and *M. malmoense* are similar. There is complete cross-resistance between ethionamide and protionamide but complete cross-resistance to isoniazid does not occur and partial cross-resistance is uncommon.

They are almost completely absorbed, achieving a plasma concentration of *c.* 1.8 mg/L 2–3 h after a 250 mg oral dose given as an enteric-coated formulation. The uncoated drugs are less well tolerated, but produce serum levels double those of enteric-coated tablets. The plasma half-life is about 2 h. CSF concentrations approach the unbound plasma levels. Thioamides are degraded in the liver to several metabolites, including a biologically active sulfoxide and various inert compounds including nicotinic acid. Less than 1% is excreted unchanged in the urine.

The principal side effect is gastric irritation, which is more common in adults and in women. This effect is reduced by commencing with a low dose and gradually increasing to the full dose, by the use of antacids and by taking the drug at bedtime. As gastric irritation often leads to non-compliance, supervised therapy is recommended. Hypersensitivity reactions and hepatitis also occur. Rare side effects include hypothyroidism, menstrual irregularities, alopecia, convulsions, deafness, diplopia, peripheral neuropathy, mental disturbances (including depression) and, in male patients, impotence and gynecomastia.

Ethionamide is used with other antituberculosis drugs in MDR tuberculosis. Protionamide is used with other anti-leprosy drugs in non-responsive multibacillary leprosy.

Preparations and dosage

Proprietary names: Trecator (ethionamide), Peteha (protionamide).
Preparation: Tablets.

Dosage: Adult, oral, 15–20 mg/kg per day in divided doses with meals. Children, 12–15 mg/kg per day to a maximum of 750 mg in divided doses, with meals.

Further information

Donald PR, Seifart HL. Cerebrospinal fluid concentrations of ethionamide in children with tuberculous meningitis. *J. Pediatr.* 1989;115:483–486.
Fajardo TT, Guinto RS, Cellona RV, Abalos RM, Dela Cruz EC, Gelber RH. A clinical trial of ethionamide and prothionamide for treatment of lepromatous leprosy. *Am J Trop Med Hyg.* 2006;74:457–461.
Jenner PJ, Ellard GA, Gruer PJK, Aber VR. Plasma levels and urinary excretion of ethionamide and prothionamide in man. *J Antimicrob Chemother.* 1984;13:267–277.

THIOACETAZONE (AMITHIOZONE)

Thioacetazone (USAN amithiozone) is a synthetic compound discovered during initial work on the sulfonamides, to which it is structurally related. It is only slightly soluble in water. It is a weak bacteristatic drug, with frequent serious side effects, particularly in HIV-positive persons to whom it must never knowingly be given. On the advice of the WHO it no longer has a place in the treatment of tuberculosis, except as a last resort in cases of extreme drug resistance.

In-vitro MICs vary considerably according to the medium used and bear little relation to in-vivo efficacy. Many strains of *M. tuberculosis* isolated in East Africa, India and Hong Kong are naturally more resistant than strains from Europe. Acquired resistance, as a result of monotherapy, is prevalent in the developing countries.

Thioacetazone is well absorbed, achieving a plasma concentration of 1–4 mg/L 2–4 h after a 100 mg oral dose.

The plasma half-life is 8–12 h. Little is known about the distribution of the drug. Several metabolites are described. About 20% is eliminated in the urine; the fate of the remainder is unknown. Rashes are common, occurring in 2–4% of patients in Africa but much more frequently in those of Chinese ethnic origin. More severe skin reactions, exfoliative dermatitis and Stevens–Johnson syndrome occur in less than 0.5% of HIV-negative patients, but there is a 10-fold increase of these reactions in HIV-positive patients, proving fatal in up to 3% of such patients. Other common side effects include gastrointestinal reactions, vertigo and conjunctivitis. Less common reactions include hepatitis, erythema multiforme, hemolytic anemia and, rarely, agranulocytosis. Prolonged therapy may rarely lead to hypertrichosis, gynecomastia and osteoporosis. It is very rarely used, but may occasionally be considered (with other antituberculosis drugs) in extremely drug resistant tuberculosis.

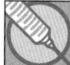

Preparations and dosage

Preparation: Tablets.

Dosage: Adults, oral, 150 mg per day. Children, 2.5 mg/kg (maximum dose, 150 mg per day).

Limited availability and very rarely used.

Further information

Alahari A, Trivelli X, Guérardel Y, et al. Thiacetazone, an antitubercular drug that inhibits cyclopropanation of cell wall mycolic acids in mycobacteria. *PLoS ONE.* 2007;2:e1343.
Heifets LB, Lindholm-Levy PJ, Flory M. Thiacetazone in vitro activity against *Mycobacterium avium* and *M. tuberculosis. Tubercle.* 1990;71:287–292.
Lawn SD, Griffin GE. Further consequences of thiacetazone-induced cutaneous reactions. *Int J Tuberc Lung Dis.* 2000;4:92–93.

34 Anthelmintics

George A. Conder

The helminths, or parasitic worms, comprise the nematodes (roundworms), trematodes (flukes), cestodes (tapeworms) and acanthocephalans (thorny-headed worms). Most anthelmintics were discovered and developed for use in the veterinary field, where helminths significantly impact health and productivity. Few companies are searching for new compounds for use in human medicine, but commercial competition has produced a steady supply of new products for the veterinarian. Three new classes of anthelmintic (cyclic octadepsipeptides, amino-acetonitrile derivatives and paraherquamides) have entered or will soon enter the veterinary market and these have potential for human medicine. In addition, some members of established classes have exhibited promising results in preliminary investigations (moxidectin for filariasis; artemisinins for schistosomiasis).

Despite the lack of new anthelmintics for human treatment, satisfactory results can be achieved with current products for nearly all helminth infections. In some cases such as for filariasis, combinations of available drugs are being used to enhance treatment. Side effects usually include gastrointestinal upsets, but these are as likely to be related to the worm burden as to the drug. As helminths are often large and/or present in large numbers, their death and disintegration after chemotherapy can result in an obstruction or an allergic–anaphylactic type reaction.

The biggest problems still remaining to be solved are treatment of infections with larval cestodes, especially *Echinococcus* spp. There is no satisfactory drug against these parasites; although benzimidazole carbamates have useful activity, they are poorly absorbed from the gut when administered orally and painful injection-site reactions preclude parenteral use. Praziquantel also may be useful in some cases for larval cestodes. Another problem is the treatment of disseminated strongyloidiasis, which occurs when patients with a latent infection are immunosuppressed (*see* pp. 844–845). No satisfactory chemotherapy is available for the macrofilarial stages in filarial infections, or to treat Guinea worm (*Dracunculus medinensis*) infection, although an eradication program has greatly reduced its incidence.

Although drug resistance is common in the veterinary field it is not yet a problem in human medicine, except with regard to schistosomiasis where resistance is known for hycanthone and praziquantel. This discrepancy is because anthelmintics are very widely and frequently used in the veterinary world but much less so in human medicine, in part due to the poverty of most of the people who are infected. With increasing wealth in tropical countries where these infections are common, anthelmintics are being used much more widely and there is concern that drug resistance will develop.

Further information

Cioli D, Pica-Mattoccia L, Archer S. Antischistosomal drugs: past, present... and future? *Pharmacol Ther*. 1995;68:35–85.

Conder GA. Chemical control of animal-parasitic nematodes. In: Lee D, ed. *The biology of nematodes*. London: Taylor & Francis; 2001:521–529.

Johnson SS, Coscarelli EM, Davis JP, et al. Interrelationships among physicochemical properties, absorption and anthelmintic activities of 2-desoxoparaherquamide and selected analogs. *J Vet Pharmacol Ther*. 2004;27:169–181.

Kaminsky R, Ducray P, Jung M, et al. A new class of anthelmintics effective against drug-resistant nematodes. *Nature*. 2008;452:176–180.

Vercruysse J, Rew RS. *Macrocyclic Lactones in Antiparasitic Therapy*. New York: CABI Publishing; 2002.

Welz C, Harder A, Schnieder T, et al. Putative G protein-coupled receptors in parasitic nematodes – potential targets for the new anthelmintic class cyclooctadepsipeptides? *Parasitol Res*. 2005;97(suppl 1):S22–S32.

World Health Organization. *WHO model prescribing information. Drugs used in parasitic diseases*. 2nd ed. Geneva: WHO; 1995.

BENZIMIDAZOLES

These synthetic compounds exhibit useful activity against cestodes, trematodes and nematodes. They are widely used in veterinary medicine. The first compound of this class to be marketed for human use, tiabendazole (thiabendazole), has been largely superseded by the benzimidazole carbamates, especially albendazole and mebendazole.

ACQUIRED RESISTANCE

There are no published records of any human nematode developing resistance to benzimidazole derivatives.

Since mebendazole is now available without prescription in some countries, there is a risk that resistance may develop in patients who do not complete the full course of treatment and such resistance may extend to related benzimidazoles. Experience in the veterinary world shows that if resistance to one benzimidazole occurs the parasite very rapidly becomes resistant to all members of the class.

Further information

Various authors. Benzimidazole anthelmintics. *Parasitol Today.* 1990;6:106–136.

ALBENDAZOLE

Molecular weight: 265.33.

A benzimidazole carbamic acid methyl ester available for oral administration. Insoluble in water, soluble in dimethyl sulfoxide. Stable at room temperature.

ANTHELMINTIC ACTIVITY

Activity against the common intestinal nematodes is shown in Table 34.1. Albendazole is active against trichostrongyles and exhibits useful activity against tissue-dwelling larvae of *Trichinella spiralis*, larvae of animal hookworms (causing cutaneous larva migrans) and microfilariae of various filarial species. It also exhibits some activity against cysticercosis and hydatid stages of *Echinococcus granulosus* and *Echinococcus multilocularis*. It has been successfully used in infections with the protozoon *Giardia lamblia* and for microsporidiosis.

PHARMACOKINETICS

Albendazole is better absorbed after oral absorption than other benzimidazole carbamates. It is extensively metabolized to the anthelmintically active albendazole sulfoxide, producing plasma concentrations of the metabolite of about 1.3 mg/L 2–5 h after a 400 mg oral dose. The half-life is about 8 h and the major route of excretion is via the bile. Plasma protein binding of the sulfoxide is around 70%.

TOXICITY AND SIDE EFFECTS

Various mild intestinal and other upsets usually resolve without treatment. With extended use, as for larval tapeworm infections, hepatic abnormalities or leukopenia may require discontinuation of treatment. In rare cases granulocytopenia, pancytopenia, agranulocytosis or thrombocytopenia may occur. It should not be given during pregnancy since it may cause fetal harm; women should be cautioned against becoming pregnant within a month of completing treatment.

CLINICAL USE

Intestinal worm infections
Trichinosis (including chronic stage)
Cutaneous larva migrans
Hydatid disease (as an adjunct, or alternative, to surgery)
Neurocysticercosis
Lymphatic filariasis (alone or in combination with ivermectin)
Giardiasis
Microsporidiosis

Table 34.1 Activity of currently used anthelmintics against common intestinal nematodes

Agent	Enterobius vermicularis	Ascaris lumbricoides	Ancylostoma duodenale	Necator americanus	Strongyloides stercoralis	Trichuris trichiura
Piperazine	++	+++	–	–	–	–
Levamisole	–	+++	+++	+++	–	–
Pyrantel	+++	+++	+++	++	–	–
Mebendazole	+++	+++	+++	+++	++	++
Albendazole	+++	+++	+++	+++	++	++
Ivermectin	+	+++	+	+	+++	+

+++, Highly effective; ++, moderately effective; +, poorly effective; –, no useful activity.

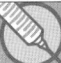
Preparations and dosage

Proprietary names: Albenza, Eskazole, Zentel, etc.

Preparation: Tablets, 200 or 400 mg.

Dosage

Ascariasis, pinworm, hookworms, trichostrongyliasis: 400 mg as a single oral dose; for pinworm, a second dose may be needed after 2–3 weeks.

Strongyloidiasis, whipworm: 400 mg orally on three consecutive days.

Echinococcosis: therapy, presurgery or postsurgery, ≥60 kg, 400 mg orally every 12 h with meals for 28 days followed by 14 tablet-free days; up to three cycles of treatment may be given; <60 kg, 15 mg/kg per day orally every 12 h with meals (maximum dose, 800 mg per day).

Neurocysticercosis: ≥60 kg, 400 mg orally every 12 h with meals for 8–30 days; <60 kg, 15 mg/kg per day orally every 12 h with meals (maximum dose, 800 mg per day).

Widely available.

Further information

Anonymous. Albendazole. In: Dollery C, ed. *Therapeutic Drugs*. 2nd ed. Edinburgh: Churchill Livingstone; 1999:A51–A56.

Horton J. Albendazole: a review of anthelmintic efficacy and safety in humans. *Parasitology*. 2000;121:5113–5132.

Ottesen E. Lymphatic filariasis: treatment, control and elimination. *Adv Parasitol*. 2006;61:395–441.

MEBENDAZOLE

Molecular weight: 295.29.

A benzimidazole carbamic acid methyl ester available for oral administration. It is insoluble in water and stable at room temperature.

ANTHELMINTIC ACTIVITY

Activity against common intestinal nematodes is shown in Table 34.1.

PHARMACOKINETICS

Oral absorption is poor. Plasma concentrations achieved after oral administration of 100 mg every 12 h for three consecutive days do not exceed 0.03 mg/L. All metabolites are inactive. Most of the dose, as unchanged drug or a primary metabolite, is retained in the intestinal tract and passed in the feces, with the remainder, approximately 2% of the dose, excreted in the urine.

TOXICITY AND SIDE EFFECTS

Diarrhea and gastrointestinal discomfort may occur, but adverse reactions are generally mild. Woman of childbearing age should be informed of a potential risk to the fetus if treated during pregnancy, particularly during the first trimester.

CLINICAL USE

Intestinal nematode infections
Trichinosis (larval stage)

Preparations and dosage

Proprietary name: Vermox (many others).

Preparations: Tablets, 100 mg; suspension 100 mg/5 mL.

Dosage: Adults and children >2 years, not recommended for children <2 years of age.

Pinworm: 100 mg as a single dose; if reinfection occurs, a second dose may be needed after 2–3 weeks.

Ascariasis, hookworms and whipworm: 100 mg every 12 h on three consecutive days.

Widely available.

Further information

Anonymous. Mebendazole. In: Dollery C, ed. *Therapeutic Drugs*. 2nd ed. Edinburgh: Churchill Livingstone; 1999:M12–M15.

OTHER BENZIMIDAZOLES

FLUBENDAZOLE

A benzimidazole carbamate used in some countries in place of mebendazole for the treatment of ascariasis. It is even less well absorbed after oral administration than mebendazole.

Preparations and dosage

Dosage: Adults and children, oral, enterobiasis, 100 mg as a single dose, repeated if necessary after 2–3 weeks. Ascariasis, trichuriasis and hookworm, 100 mg every 12 h on three consecutive days.

Limited availability.

TIABENDAZOLE

Thiabendazole; a thiazolyl benzimidazole available for oral administration. It is active against most common intestinal nematodes. As a result of its larvicidal and ovicidal activity, it is effective in strongyloidiasis, trichinosis, visceral larva migrans and cutaneous larva migrans.

It is well absorbed from the small intestine. Peak plasma levels are reached about 1–2 h after a single oral dose of the suspension. It is extensively metabolized in the liver to the 5-hydroxy derivative, which is inactive. Most of the drug is excreted within 24 h. About 90% is excreted in the urine, chiefly as glucuronide or sulfate conjugates; the remainder is passed in the feces.

A wide range of unpleasant side effects occur, including nausea and other gastrointestinal upsets, fever and neurological effects. It has been largely replaced by the less toxic benzimidazole carbamates. Although active against *Ascaris lumbricoides*, *E. vermicularis* and hookworms, it should not be used as primary therapy for these infections.

Preparations and dosage

Proprietary names: Mintezol, Triasox.

Preparations: Tablets, 500 mg; oral suspension 500 mg/5 mL.

Dosage: Oral, based on patient's weight.

Strongyloidiasis: Two doses a day on two successive days or 50 mg/kg as a single dose.

Trichinosis: Two doses a day on 2–4 successive days, depending on response.

Cutaneous larva migrans: Two doses a day on two successive days; repeat if active lesions are still present 2 days after completion of therapy.

Visceral larva migrans: Two doses a day on 5–7 successive days.

Widely available.

 Further information

Anonymous. Thiabendazole. In: Dollery C, ed. *Therapeutic Drugs*. 2nd ed. Edinburgh: Churchill Livingstone; 1999:T81–T83.

MISCELLANEOUS ANTHELMINTIC AGENTS

DIETHYLCARBAMAZINE

Molecular weight (free base): 199.29; (citrate): 391.42.

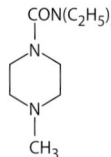

A carbamyl derivative of piperazine formulated as the citrate. It is readily soluble in water and slightly hygroscopic.

 ANTHELMINTIC ACTIVITY

Useful activity is restricted to filarial worms. It is adulticidal and microfilaricidal against *Loa loa*. Against *Wuchereria bancrofti* and *Brugia malayi* it is predominantly microfilaricidal, but slowly kills adult worms. It kills microfilariae, but not adults, of *Onchocerca volvulus*.

 PHARMACOKINETICS

Oral absorption	>90%
C_{max} 200 mg	1.5–2 mg/L after 2 h
Plasma half-life	c. 6–12 h
Volume of distribution	107–371 L
Plasma protein binding	Very low

Like piperazine (to which it is related), diethylcarbamazine is rapidly and completely absorbed. About half the dose is excreted unchanged in the urine; the rest is metabolized and eliminated by renal and extrarenal routes.

 TOXICITY AND SIDE EFFECTS

In uninfected people, diethylcarbamazine has virtually no side effects, but in those with various forms of filariasis it has unpleasant effects primarily due to the death of blood- or skin-dwelling microfilariae. Severe reactions ('Mazzotti reactions'), most frequently of the skin, occur in patients with onchocerciasis and may also be systemic with fever, headache, prostration, nausea, joint and muscle pain, vertigo, tachycardia, cough and respiratory distress, hypotension and ocular signs. In patients with *L. loa* who harbor very large numbers of microfilariae in their blood, neurological problems may be very severe. Cardiological damage has also been reported. In patients with *W. bancrofti* and *B. malayi* high fever occurs in the first few days after treatment. Reversible proteinuria may occur.

 CLINICAL USE

Filariasis

It has also been used for visceral larva migrans, but experience is limited and there is little evidence of its efficacy.

Preparations and dosage

Proprietary names: Banocide, Hetrazan, etc.

Preparation: Tablets, 50 or 100 mg.

Dosage:

Loiasis: Adults, oral, 1 mg/kg as a single dose, doubled on two successive days, and then adjusted to 2–3 mg/kg every 8 h for a further 18 days.

Wuchereria bancrofti: Adults and children >10 years of age, oral, 6 mg/kg per day for 12 days, preferably in divided doses after meals.

Brugia spp.: Adults and children >10 years of age, oral, 3–6 mg/kg per day for 6–12 days, preferably as divided doses after meals.

Limited availability.

Further information

Anonymous. Diethylcarbamazine (citrate). In: Dollery C, ed. *Therapeutic Drugs.* 2nd ed. Edinburgh: Churchill Livingstone; 1999:D103–D106.

Mackenzie CD, Kron MA. Diethylcarbamazine: a review of its action in onchocerciasis, lymphatic filariasis and inflammation. *Trop Dis Bull.* 1985;82:R1–R37.

Maizels RM, Denham DA. Diethylcarbamazine (DEC): immunopharmacological interactions of an anti-filarial drug. *Parasitology.* 1993;105:S49–S60.

IVERMECTIN

Molecular weight: (dihydroavermectin B_{1a}): 875.1; (dihydroavermectin B_{1b}): 861.07.

R	
secbutyl (80%)	
isopropyl (20%)	

A mixture of two closely related semisynthetic derivatives of avermectins, a complex of macrocyclic lactone antibiotics produced by *Streptomyces avermitilis*. In commercial preparations the ratio of the two components, dihydroavermectin B_{1a} and dihydroavermectin B_{1b}, are present within the limits 80–90% and 10–20%, respectively.

ANTHELMINTIC ACTIVITY

Activity against intestinal nematodes is shown in Table 34.1 (p. 396). It is also active against *O. volvulus* and other filarial worms, but the effect is chiefly directed against the larval forms (microfilariae). Uniquely among anthelmintic agents it exhibits activity against some ectoparasites, including *Sarcoptes scabiei*.

PHARMACOKINETICS

Oral absorption	c. 60%
C_{max} 12 mg oral	c. 30–47 ng/mL after 4 h
Plasma half-life	c. 12 h
Volume of distribution	46.9 L
Plasma protein binding	93%

It is rapidly metabolized in the liver and the metabolites are excreted in the feces over about 12 days with minimal (<1%) urinary excretion. Highest concentrations occur in the liver and fat. Extremely small amounts are found in the brain.

TOXICITY AND SIDE EFFECTS

In the treatment of onchocerciasis mild Mazzotti-type reactions occur, with occasional neurological problems. Although it is highly effective against *L. loa*, care must be taken to avoid treating patients with high microfilarial counts: there is one report of a patient with a concomitant *L. loa* infection who died when treated for onchocerciasis. Mild gastrointestinal and nervous system signs may occur following treatment for strongyloidiasis.

CLINICAL USE

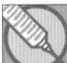

Onchocerciasis
Non-disseminated strongyloidiasis
Lymphatic filariasis (in combination with albendazole)
Scabies

If the patient is harboring *Asc. lumbricoides*, the worms will be passed in the feces. Head lice will also be killed, which is very much welcomed by the treated patients. Ivermectin has been widely used in the veterinary field, where use is also made of its effect on ectoparasites.

Preparations and dosage

Proprietary names: Mectizan, Stromectol.

Preparation: Tablets, 3 or 6 mg.

Dosage:

Onchocerciasis: ≥15 kg, oral, 150 µg/kg as a single dose. Re-treat at 6–12-month intervals.

Strongyloidiasis: ≥15 kg, oral, 200 µg/kg as a single dose on two consecutive days.

Ivermectin should not be used during pregnancy or in nursing mothers. Limited availability.

Further information

Anonymous. Ivermectin. In: Dollery C, ed. *Therapeutic Drugs*. 2nd ed. Edinburgh: Churchill Livingstone; 1999:I127–I130.

Brown KR, Ricci FM, Ottesen EA. Ivermectin: effectiveness in lymphatic filariasis. *Parasitology*. 2000;121:S133–S146.

Campbell WC. Ivermectin as an antiparasitic agent for use in humans. *Annu Rev Microbiol*. 1991;45:445–474.

Goa KL, McTavish D, Clissold SP. Ivermectin: a review of its antifilarial activity, pharmacokinetic properties and clinical efficacy in onchocerciasis. *Drugs*. 1991;42:640–658.

Ottesen EA, Campbell WC. Ivermectin in human medicine. *J Antimicrob Chemother*. 1994;32:195–203.

LEVAMISOLE

Molecular weight (free base): 204.29; (hydrochloride): 240.75.

The L-isomer of tetramisole, available as the monohydrochloride. The D-isomer has no anthelmintic activity. It is very soluble in water and is stable in the dry state.

ANTHELMINTIC ACTIVITY

Its principal activity is against *Asc. lumbricoides* and hookworms (Table 34.1, p. 396). Worms are paralyzed and passed out in the feces within a few hours.

PHARMACOKINETICS

Oral absorption	c. 90%
C_{max} 150 mg oral	0.5 mg/L after c. 2 h
Plasma half-life	c. 4 h
Volume of distribution	100–120 L

Levamisole is rapidly absorbed from the gut and extensively metabolized in the liver. It is excreted chiefly in the urine.

TOXICITY AND SIDE EFFECTS

Nausea, gastrointestinal upsets and very mild neurological problems have been reported.

CLINICAL USE

Ascariasis
Hookworm infection

Levamisole has been used in rheumatoid arthritis and some other conditions that are said to respond to its immunomodulatory activity.

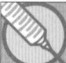

Preparations and dosage

Proprietary names: Ergamisol, Ketrax, Solaskil.

Preparation: Tablets, 40 or 50 mg.

Dosage:

Ascariasis: Adults, oral, 120–150 mg as a single dose; children, 3 mg/kg as a single dose.

Hookworm: Oral, 2.5–5 mg/kg as a single dose; in severe cases, a second dose may be given 7 days after the first.

Limited availability.

Further information

Anonymous. Levamisole (hydrochloride). In: Dollery C, ed. *Therapeutic Drugs*. 2nd ed. Edinburgh: Churchill Livingstone; 1999:L26–L29.

METRIFONATE

Trichlorfon (USAN). Molecular weight: 257.44.

$$Cl_3CCH \overset{OH}{\underset{}{|}} \overset{O}{\underset{}{||}} P(OCH_3)_2$$

An organophosphorus compound. It is soluble in water and stable at room temperature. At higher temperatures it decomposes to the insecticide dichlorvos.

ANTHELMINTIC ACTIVITY

Useful activity is restricted to *Schistosoma haematobium*. It has little activity against other schistosomes (Table 34.2). Although it exhibits activity against several other helminths, it is not used for their treatment.

PHARMACOKINETICS

Metrifonate is rapidly absorbed after oral administration, achieving a peak concentration in plasma within 1–2 h. It undergoes chemical transformation to dichlorvos, which is the active molecule. Dichlorvos is rapidly and extensively metabolized and excreted mainly in the urine.

TOXICITY AND SIDE EFFECTS

Various side effects such as abdominal pain, gastrointestinal upsets and vertigo occur in many patients. As the worms

Table 34.2 Activity of commonly used antischistosome agents

Agent	Schistosoma mansoni	Schistosoma haematobium	Schistosoma japonicum	Schistosoma intercalatum	Schistosoma mekongi
Praziquantel	+++	+++	+++	+++	+++
Metrifonate	–	+++	–	–	–
Oxamniquine	+++	–	–	–	–

+++, Highly effective; –, no useful activity.

release their hold of the veins in the bladder they pass through the blood system to the lungs, where they disintegrate; this may cause some of the side effects. Cholinesterase levels in the blood and on erythrocytes are depressed, but the significance of this is unknown.

CLINICAL USE

Urinary schistosomiasis (especially mass chemotherapy control programs)

Preparations and dosage

Proprietary name: Bilarcil.

Preparation: Tablets, 100 mg.

Dosage: Adults and children, oral. *S. haematobium*: three doses of 75–10 mg/kg may be given at intervals of 14 days.
Limited availability.

Further information

Anonymous. Trichlorfon. In: Dollery C, ed. *Therapeutic Drugs*. 2nd ed. Edinburgh: Churchill Livingstone; 1999:T174–T179.

NICLOSAMIDE

Molecular weight: 327.12.

A synthetic chlorinated nitrosalicylanilide available for oral administration.

ANTHELMINTIC ACTIVITY

Useful activity is restricted to intestinal tapeworms, including *Taeniarhynchus saginatus* (syn. *Taenia saginata*), *Taenia solium*,

Diphyllobothrium latum and *Hymenolepis nana*. It is not effective against larval stages of tapeworms.

PHARMACOKINETICS

Conflicting data exist relative to the level of absorption of niclosamide from the gut. The metabolized drug is passed in the feces and urine, staining them yellow.

TOXICITY AND SIDE EFFECTS

Very few side effects have been reported, but these include mild nausea, abdominal cramps and dizziness.

CLINICAL USE

Intestinal tapeworm infections

Preparations and dosage

Proprietary names: Niclocide, Tredemine, Yomesan.

Preparation: Tablets, 500 mg.

Dosage:

T. saginatus, T. solium (intestinal stage) and *D. latum*: Adults, oral, 2 g as a single dose; children 10–35 kg, 1 g as a single dose; infants <10 kg, 0.5 g as a single dose. Chronically constipated patients should receive a purgative on the evening preceding treatment.

H. nana: A 7-day treatment is recommended; adults, 2 g on the first day and 1 g on each of the next 6 days; children 10–35 kg, 1 g on the first day and 0.5 g on each of the next 6 days; infants <10 kg, a total of 2 g should be given over 7 days.
Widely available.

OXAMNIQUINE

Molecular weight: 279.33.

A synthetic quinolinemethanol, available for oral administration.

ANTHELMINTIC ACTIVITY

Activity is restricted to *Schistosoma mansoni* (Table 34.2). Some strains, particularly those in Egypt and Southern Africa, require higher doses for efficacy owing to innate tolerance.

PHARMACOKINETICS

It is rapidly absorbed after oral administration, achieving a peak concentration of 0.3–2.5 mg/L 1–3 h after an oral dose of 15 mg/kg body weight. Peak levels following intramuscular treatment at 7.5 mg/kg generally do not exceed 0.15 mg/L. It is extensively metabolized to biologically inactive 6-carboxylic and 2-carboxylic acid derivatives, which are excreted in the urine, mostly within 12 h.

TOXICITY AND SIDE EFFECTS

Dizziness, sleepiness, nausea and headache occur frequently. Other side effects are probably due to the death and disintegration of the worms in the liver. Following treatment, urine may become red.

CLINICAL USE

Infection with *S. mansoni*

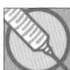

Preparations and dosage

Proprietary name: Vansil.
Preparations: Capsule, 250 mg; syrup, 50 mg/mL.
Dosage:
West Africa, South America, Caribbean Islands: Adults, 15 mg/kg as a single oral dose; children <30 kg, 10 mg/kg orally every 12 h for 1 day.
East and Central Africa and Arabian Peninsula: Adults and children, 15 mg/kg orally every 12 h for 1 day.
Egypt, Southern Africa and Zimbabwe: Adults and children, 60 mg/kg orally over 2–3 days with no single dose to exceed 20 mg/kg.
Limited availability.

Further information

Anonymous. Oxamniquine. In: Dollery C, ed. *Therapeutic Drugs*. 2nd ed. Edinburgh: Churchill Livingstone; 1999:O35–O37.

PIPERAZINE

Molecular weight: piperazine: 86.14; (edetate calcium): 416.44; (anhydrous citrate): 642.65.

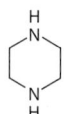

A synthetic chemical, most commonly formulated as the citrate, but also available as the adipate, edetate calcium and tartrate salts.

ANTHELMINTIC ACTIVITY

Activity against common intestinal nematodes is shown in Table 34.1 (p. 396). It has no other useful anthelmintic activity.

PHARMACOKINETICS

Activity against intestinal worms requires that a substantial amount remains in the gut. However, after oral administration a variable amount is rapidly absorbed from the small intestine and subsequently excreted in the urine. Its half-life is extremely variable.

TOXICITY AND SIDE EFFECTS

Some people develop hypersensitivity, requiring cessation of treatment. Transient, mild gastrointestinal or neurological symptoms may occur.

CLINICAL USE

Ascariasis
Pinworm

Preparations and dosage

Proprietary names: Many (e.g. Antepar, Pripsen).

Preparations: Various oral presentations.

Dosage:

The dosage of piperazine is generally expressed relative to piperazine hexahydrate.

Ascariasis: Adults and children >12 years, the equivalent of 75 mg/kg to a maximum of 35 g of piperazine hexahydrate as a single oral dose or divided over two consecutive days; children 2–12 years, as for adults but to a maximum of 25 g; children <2 years, the equivalent of 50 mg/kg of piperazine hexahydrate administered under medical supervision. Alternative regimens exist.

Pinworm: Adults and children, the equivalent of 50 mg/kg of piperazine hexahydrate given orally on seven consecutive days. Treatment should be repeated at an interval of 2 weeks and all family members should be treated. Alternative regimens exist.

Widely available without prescription in many countries under numerous trade names.

Further information

Anonymous. Piperazine. In: Dollery C, ed. *Therapeutic Drugs*. 2nd ed. Edinburgh: Churchill Livingstone; 1999:P137–P139.

PRAZIQUANTEL

Molecular weight: 312.41.

A synthetic pyrazinoquinoline formulated for oral administration. It is stable in the dry state, but hygroscopic.

ANTHELMINTIC ACTIVITY

All species of human schistosomes are susceptible (Table 34.2, p. 401), but there is a relative lack of efficacy against immature stages. It is also effective against adult and tissue-dwelling larval tapeworms; against the intestinal flukes *Fasciolopsis buski*, *Metagonimus yokogawi*, *Heterophyes heterophyes* and *Nanophyetus salmincola*; against *Clonorchis* and *Opisthorchis* spp. in the bile ducts; and against *Paragonimus* spp. in the lungs. It has variable activity against zoonotic *Fasciola hepatica* infections.

ACQUIRED RESISTANCE

There is evidence that resistance to praziquantel is emerging in schistosomes, although there is debate as to whether treatment failures are due to resistance or innate tolerance.

PHARMACOKINETICS

Oral absorption	>80%
C_{max} 50 mg/kg oral	1 mg/L after 1–2 h
Plasma half-life: parent drug	1–1.5 h
metabolites	4–6h
Plasma protein binding	80%

Praziquantel is rapidly absorbed when given orally, but it undergoes extensive first-pass biotransformation and the concentration of unchanged drug in plasma is low. The major metabolite, a 4-hydroxy derivative, retains little to no antiparasitic activity. About 80% of the oral dose, as parent drug and its metabolites, is excreted in the urine by the fourth day post-treatment, 90% of this in 24 h. A higher peak plasma concentration is achieved in infected people, but other pharmacokinetic values are unchanged.

TOXICITY AND SIDE EFFECTS

Very few side effects have been reported. In the treatment of cerebral cysticercosis the death of cysts in the brain may cause local inflammation and edema, but this usually subsides quickly. Ocular cysticercosis should not be treated with this drug, because parasite destruction in the eye can lead to irreparable lesions. Adverse events seen in the treatment of schistosomiasis, including abdominal pain, nausea, anorexia, diarrhea and mild neurological effects, are almost certainly due to the death and disintegration of the large adult worms.

CLINICAL USE

Schistosomiasis
Other trematode infections (except *F. hepatica*)
Tapeworm infection, including cerebral cysticercosis

Treatment may need to be prolonged in cerebral cysticercosis.

Preparations and dosage

Proprietary names: Biltricide, Distocide.

Preparation: Tablets, 600 mg.

Dosage:

Adults and children >4 years.

Schistosomiasis: 20 mg/kg orally three times a day at 4–6 h intervals on 1 day or 40 mg/kg as a single dose.

Liver and lung flukes: 25 mg/kg orally three times a day at 4–6 h intervals on one day or two consecutive days.

Intestinal flukes: 25 mg/kg as a single oral dose.

Intestinal taeniasis: 5–10 mg/kg as a single oral dose.

Intestinal diphyllobothriasis: 5–10 mg/kg as a single oral dose.

Intestinal hymenolepiasis: 15–25 mg/kg as a single oral dose.

Cysticercosis: A total of 50 mg/kg per day in three divided doses on 14 consecutive days. A corticosteroid should be administered for 2–3 days before and throughout treatment.

Limited availability.

Further information

Anonymous. Praziquantel. In: Dollery C, ed. *Therapeutic Drugs.* 2nd ed. Edinburgh: Churchill Livingstone; 1999:P184–P189.

Botros SS, Bennett J. Praziquantel resistance. *Expert Opin Drug Discov.* 2007;2: (suppl 1):S35–S40.

Groll E. Praziquantel. *Adv Pharmacol Chemother.* 1984;20:219–238.

Kumar V, Gryseels B. Use of praziquantel against schistosomiasis: a review of current status. *Int J Antimicrob Agents.* 1994;4:313–320.

Pica-Mattoccia L, Ciola D. Sex- and stage-related sensitivity of *Schistosoma mansoni* to *in vivo* and *in vitro* praziquantel treatments. *Int J Parasitol.* 2004;34:527–533.

PYRANTEL

Molecular weight: (free base): 206.3; (pamoate): 594.68.

A tetrahydropyrimidine, formulated as the pamoate (embonate) in a 1:1 ratio and available as a suspension for oral administration. It is practically insoluble in water, but soluble in dimethyl sulfoxide. It is stable at room temperature.

ANTHELMINTIC ACTIVITY

Activity against the common intestinal nematodes is shown in Table 34.1 (p. 396). Pyrantel is less active against *Necator americanus* than against *Ancylostoma duodenale*.

PHARMACOKINETICS

By synthetic design most of the dose is passed unchanged in the feces. The portion that is absorbed (<5%) is metabolized and excreted in the urine.

TOXICITY AND SIDE EFFECTS

Pyrantel should not be used at the same time as piperazine as their modes of action are antagonistic. Gastrointestinal upsets and, rarely, very mild neurological symptoms occur.

CLINICAL USE

Ascariasis
Pinworm
Hookworm (especially *A. duodenale*)
Trichostrongyliasis

Higher and more prolonged doses may be necessary in hookworm infection caused by *N. americanus*. Pyrantel has been used in combination with an analog (oxantel) where concurrent whipworm infection was likely.

Preparations and dosage

Proprietary names: Antiminth, Combantrin.

Preparations: Tablets, 250 mg; oral suspension, 50 mg/mL.

Dosage: Adults and children >6 months, 10 mg/kg as a single oral dose; treatment for pinworm should be repeated after 2 weeks; more severe infections of *N. americanus* require 20 mg/kg as a single dose on two consecutive days, or 10 mg/kg as a single dose on 3–4 consecutive days. Widely available.

Further information

Anonymous. Pyrantel (pamoate). In: Dollery C, ed. *Therapeutic Drugs.* 2nd ed. Edinburgh: Churchill Livingstone; 1999:P284–P286.

SURAMIN

A complex symmetrical molecule originally developed in Germany in the early 1920s for the treatment of African trypanosomiasis. Its useful anthelmintic activity is restricted to *O. volvulus* and it has been used to achieve a radical cure of onchocerciasis by killing the adult worms. However, it is an extremely toxic drug and its use has become increasingly uncommon since ivermectin became available. Its properties are described in Chapter 35 (pp.424–425).

OTHER ANTHELMINTIC AGENTS

Potassium antimony tartrate (tartar emetic), sodium antimony tartrate, the thioxanthone, hycanthone, and the 5-nitrothiazole, niridazole, were formerly used in the treatment of schistosomiasis, but have been largely superseded by less toxic compounds. Niridazole has also been used in Guinea worm infection, but no drug interrupts transmission, and metronidazole or benzimidazole carbamates are much safer and as useful in providing symptomatic relief.

The chlorinated hydrocarbon tetrachloroethylene has been used since the 1920s in the treatment of hookworm infection. It is more effective in eliminating *N. americanus* than *Ancyl. duodenale* and has no useful effect against other intestinal worms. Bephenium, a quaternary ammonium compound formulated as the hydroxynaphthoate, is effective against several nematodes, including *Asc. lumbricoides* and *Ancyl.duodenale*, but not *N. americanus*. Pyrvinium, a cyanine dye formulated as the almost insoluble pamoate, was formerly used to treat pinworm infections. It is not absorbed from the gut, is very bright red in color, and stains the feces red. All of these drugs have been replaced by safer and more effective agents.

35 Antiprotozoal agents

Simon L. Croft and Karin Seifert

Protozoa are unicellular, eukaryotic cells with an enormous diversity of biological characteristics. This is reflected in the requirements for different drugs and limited overlap in sensitivity. Several antiprotozoal agents developed in the 1920s and 1930s (e.g. suramin, mepacrine, chloroquine and sodium stibogluconate) are still widely used. Standard drugs for the treatment of the most neglected diseases – human African trypanosomiasis (sleeping sickness), leishmaniasis and South American trypanosomiasis (Chagas disease) – remain inadequate, although the introduction of miltefosine for leishmaniasis has seen a significant improvement in potential for treatment of this condition. There is still a need to identify more effective drugs for diseases such as cryptosporidiosis and toxoplasmosis, which have emerged as important opportunistic pathogens in immunocompromised patients.

Awareness of the impact of protozoal diseases such as malaria on the development of many countries, and the spread of drug resistance (Ch. 62), has led to initiatives to discover and develop new drugs. Large screening programs are now in place through philanthropic and public funding and the development of public–private partnerships.

 Further information

Croft SL, Barrett MP, Urbina JA. Chemotherapy of trypanosomiasis and leishmaniasis. *Trends Parasitol.* 2005;28:508–512.

Olliaro P, Wells TNC. The global portfolio of new antimalarial medicines under development. *Clin Pharmacol Ther.* 2009;85:584–599.

Renslo AR, McKerrow JH. Drug discovery and development for neglected diseases. *Nat Chem Biol.* 2006;2:701–710.

Stuart K, Brun R, Croft S, et al. Kinetoplastids: related protozoan pathogens, different diseases. *J Clin Invest.* 2008;118:1301–1310.

Witkowski B, Berry A, Benoit-Vical F. Resistance to antimalarial compounds: methods and applications. *Drug Resistance Updates.* 2009;12:42–50.

ORGANOMETALS

Arsenical and antimonial compounds such as atoxyl and tartar emetic have been used for the treatment of African sleeping sickness and leishmaniasis for over a century. The compounds presently used (sodium stibogluconate, melarsoprol, meglumine antimonate) were developed in the 1940s and are considerably less toxic than their predecessors.

MELARSOPROL

Molecular weight: 398.34.

Mel B. A derivative of trivalent melarsen oxide and dimercaprol (BAL), possessing a melaminyl moiety. Formulated in 3.6% propylene glycol for intravenous administration. It is almost insoluble in water.

ANTIMICROBIAL ACTIVITY

It is highly and rapidly active against *Trypanosoma brucei gambiense* and *T. brucei rhodesiense* in vitro at submicromolar concentrations. It is much less active against the trypanosomes that infect domestic animals, *T. congolense* and *T. vivax*. Co-administration with eflornithine is effective against central nervous system (CNS) infection with *T. brucei* in rodent models, but clinical studies have found the combination less effective than nifurtimox–eflornithine.

ACQUIRED RESISTANCE

Up to 25% of cases of *T. brucei gambiense* in Central Africa relapse. Patients infected with *T. brucei rhodesiense* normally respond to a second course of the drug, but those with *T. brucei gambiense* do not. In laboratory-generated resistant strains, decreased sensitivity results from reduced uptake of the drug by bloodstream trypomastigotes that either lack an adenine/adenosine transporter (TbAT1) or contain a transporter gene with point mutations. There is conflicting evidence about the role of this mechanism of resistance in isolates from patients unresponsive to treatment.

PHARMACOKINETICS

Serum levels of 2–4 mg/L were achieved 24 h after administration of 3.6 mg/kg, falling to 0.1 mg/L at 120 h after the fourth daily injection. Elimination was biphasic with a half-life of 35 h. The volume of distribution was 100 L. It is rapidly metabolized by microsomal enzymes to melarsen oxide, reaching maximum plasma concentration by 15 min and eliminated with a half-life of 3.9 h. This metabolite can cross the blood–brain barrier and effect a CNS cure in mice. Levels of melarsoprol in the cerebrospinal fluid (CSF) reached around 300 μg/L, about 50 times lower than serum levels.

TOXICITY AND SIDE EFFECTS

The propylene glycol formulation can cause tissue trauma and long-term damage to veins. Drug-induced reactions include fever on first administration, abdominal colic pain, dermatitis and arthralgia. Polyneuropathy has been reported in about 10% of patients. Reactive arsenical encephalopathy is a serious side effect that occurs in around 10% of those treated, with death in 1–3% of cases. The frequency of encephalopathy increases with a rise in the white cell count or the presence of trypanosomes in the CSF. The causes of the immunological responses involved in the encephalopathy and the possible existence of two forms (reactive and hemorrhagic) are not completely resolved. Studies to identify anti-inflammatory approaches to reduce reactive encephalopathy in late-stage *T. brucei gambiense* infection have produced limited results.

CLINICAL USE

Late-stage sleeping sickness caused by *T. brucei gambiense* and *T. brucei rhodesiense*

It is not recommended for early-stage disease, in which alternatives with less serious side effects are available.

Preparations and dosage

Proprietary name: Arsobal.

Preparation: Injection.

Dosage: Adults, i.v., 3.6 mg/kg per day for 3–4 days and repeat 2–3 times with an interval of at least 7 days between courses. An alternative regimen of 10 daily doses of 2.2 mg/kg, with no interval, did not improve safety but reduced time in hospital.

Limited availability.

Further information

Balasegaram M, Young H, Chappuis F, et al. Effectiveness of melarsoprol and eflornithine as first-line regimes for sleeping sickness in nine Médicines sans Frontières programmes. *Trans R Soc Trop Med Hyg.* 2009;103:280–290.

Barrett MP, Boykin DW, Brun R, Tidwell RR. Human African trypanosomiasis: pharmacological re-engagement with a neglected disease. *Br J Pharmacol.* 2007;152:1155–1171.

Bernhard SC, Nerima B, Mäser P, Brun R. Melarsoprol- and pentamidine-resistant *Trypanosoma brucei rhodesiense* populations and their cross-resistance. *Int J Parasitol.* 2007;37:1443–1448.

Keiser J, Ericsson O, Burri C. Investigations of the metabolites of the trypanocidal drug melarsoprol. *Clin Pharmacol Ther.* 2000;67:478–488.

SODIUM STIBOGLUCONATE

Pentavalent sodium antimony gluconate.

A pentavalent antimonial of uncertain chemical composition; probably a complex mixture of polymeric forms. There is batch-to-batch variation and solutions may contain 32–34% pentavalent antimony (Sb^V). The structural formula is conjectural as studies have identified a mixture of non-complexed Sb^V and large polymeric gluconate complexes. Chemical composition also depends on concentration and time. It is freely soluble in water.

ANTIMICROBIAL ACTIVITY

It has low activity against the extracellular promastigote stage of *Leishmania* spp. in vitro, but is active against amastigotes in macrophages. The trivalent form is considered to be the toxophore, with metabolism of Sb^V to toxic Sb^{III} in the host cell macrophage and the parasite; the level of metabolism is higher in amastigotes than promastigotes. Variation in the sensitivity of different *Leishmania* species may contribute to differences in clinical response. It is more active against visceral than cutaneous leishmaniasis in animal models. Sodium stibogluconate cures CNS infections with *T. brucei* in rodents.

ACQUIRED RESISTANCE

Unresponsiveness and relapse of *L. donovani* infections in Bihar State, India (over 60% of cases), is due to increasing acquired resistance. In laboratory-generated and clinical isolates, resistant *Leishmania* promastigotes show increased levels of intracellular thiols, for example trypanothione, to which Sb^{III} is conjugated and extruded by efflux pumps.

Lack of response is also reported in patients with mucosal leishmaniasis caused by *L. braziliensis*. Relapse is common in patients with visceral leishmaniasis who are immunosuppressed, for example by HIV infection, but this is due to pathogen interaction and the immune dependence of drug activity and not acquired resistance. High mortality has been reported in treatment of these co-infection cases.

PHARMACOKINETICS

Peak concentrations of about 12–15 mg antimony/L are achieved in serum 1 h after a dose of 10 mg/kg. There is a slow accumulation in the central compartment, and tissue concentrations reach a maximum after several days. In contrast to trivalent derivatives, pentavalent antimonials are not accumulated by erythrocytes, but there is evidence of protein binding. Antimony is detected in the skin for at least 5 days after treatment. Some of the dose of Sb^V is converted to Sb^{III}, possibly by the liver or by macrophages. It is rapidly excreted into urine with a half-life of about 2 h; 60–80% of the dose appears in the urine within 6 h of parenteral administration. In a study on structurally related meglumine antimonate (*see below*) the pharmacokinetics of Sb^V and Sb^{III} were similar as measured by serum and urine levels.

TOXICITY AND SIDE EFFECTS

The toxic effects are limited by the rapid excretion, but cumulative toxicity increases in proportion to dose. Myalgia, arthralgia, anorexia and electrocardiographic changes have been reported with high-dose regimens. In particular, development of ventricular tachyarrhythmias associated with prolongation of the QT interval has been recorded. Hepatocellular damage, hepatic and renal functional impairment and pancreatitis have also been reported. The changes are reversible on discontinuation of treatment.

CLINICAL USE

Visceral, cutaneous and mucocutaneous leishmaniasis

The combination with paromomycin has been used in unresponsive cases and in relapses of visceral and cutaneous leishmaniasis.

Preparations and dosage

Proprietary name: Pentostam.

Preparation: Injection.

Dosage: Adults, i.m., i.v., 10–20 mg/kg per day with a maximum of 850 mg for at least 20 days; the dose varies with different geographical regions.

Limited availability; not available in the USA.

Further information

Croft SL, Sundar S, Fairlamb AH. Drug resistance in leishmaniasis. *Clin Microbiol Rev.* 2006;19:116–126.

Frézard F, Martins PS, Barbosa MC, et al. New insights into the chemical structure and composition of the pentavalent antimonial drugs, meglumine antimonate and sodium stibogluconate. *J Inorg Biochem.* 2008;102:656–665.

Mittal MK, Rai S, Ashutosh R, et al. Characterisation of natural antimony resistance in *Leishmania donovani* isolates. *Am J Trop Med Hyg.* 2007;76:681–688.

Olliaro PL, Guerin PJ, Gerstl S, Haaskjold AA, Rottingen JA, Sundar S. Treatment options for visceral leishmaniasis: a systematic review of clinical studies done in India, 1980–2004. *Lancet Infect Dis.* 2005;5:763–774.

Ritmeijer K, Dejenie A, Assefa Y, et al. A comparison of miltefosine and sodium stibogluconate for treatment of visceral leishmaniasis in an Ethiopian population with high prevalence of HIV infection. *Clin Infect Dis.* 2006;43:357–364.

MEGLUMINE ANTIMONATE

N-Methylglucamine antimonate; methylaminoglucitol antimonate. The Sb^V content varies around 28% between batches. The major moieties are Sb^V–ligand complexes which are zwitterionic in solution.

The activity, pharmacology and toxicology are similar to those of sodium stibogluconate, with which it is essentially interchangeable.

CLINICAL USE

Treatment of visceral and cutaneous leishmaniasis

Studies in Central and South America have indicated that the combination with interferon-γ is effective in the treatment of visceral and cutaneous leishmaniasis cases unresponsive to antimony alone.

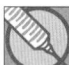

Preparations and dosage

Proprietary name: Glucantime.

Preparation: Injection.

Dosage: Adults, i.m., i.v., 20 mg/kg per day for 20–28 days. The course can be repeated.

Limited availability, not available in the UK.

QUINOLINES

Quinine and related alkaloids have been the mainstay of antimalarial chemotherapy since the 17th century, originally in the form of *Cinchona* bark. Synthetic quinolines were developed in the 1920s and 1930s. The most important of these, the 4-aminoquinoline chloroquine, has succumbed to global resistance in *Plasmodium falciparum*. Quinine is still used for the therapy of severe malaria. The search for new derivatives led to the discovery of mefloquine. Amodiaquine, another 4-aminoquinoline, is active against chloroquine-resistant strains of *P. falciparum*, but is not recommended for prophylaxis. Identification of the structure–function relationships for activity and resistance has enabled the development of quinolines active against chloroquine-resistant *P. falciparum*; two bis(quinolines), piperaquine and hydroxypiperaquine, have been used in the treatment of drug-resistant malaria in China and are in development in co-formulations with artemisinin derivatives. The 8-aminoquinoline primaquine is used for the radical cure of benign tertian malaria. Others of this class are in clinical trial: tafenoquine for malaria and sitamaquine for visceral leishmaniasis.

Further information

Egan TJ. Haemazoin formation. *Mol Biochem Parasitol*. 2008;157:127–136.
O'Neill PM, Ward SA, Berry NG, et al. A medicinal chemistry perspective on 4-aminoquinoline antimalarial drugs. *Curr Top Med Chem*. 2006;6:479–507.
Tekwani BL, Walker LA. 8-Aminoquinolines: future role as antiprotozoal drugs. *Curr Opin Infect Dis*. 2006;19:623–631.

CHLOROQUINE

Molecular weight: 319.9.

A synthetic 4-aminoquinoline, formulated as the phosphate or sulfate for oral administration and as the hydrochloride or sulfate for parenteral use. The salts are soluble in water.

ANTIMICROBIAL ACTIVITY

Chloroquine accumulates 300-fold in infected erythrocytes and acts against the early erythrocytic stages of all four species of *Plasmodium* that cause human malaria. It is also active against the gametocytes of *P. vivax*, *P. ovale* and *P. malariae*, but not against the hepatic stages or mature erythrocytic schizonts and merozoites.

ACQUIRED RESISTANCE

Resistance of *P. falciparum* is widespread and has become a major problem. The mechanism appears to be either decreased uptake or increased efflux of the drug by the parasite, or both. Changes in genes encoding a P-glycoprotein homolog, *Pfmdr1*,

and another putative transporter, *Pfcrt*, are associated with resistance. Reversal of resistance with, for example, verapamil or probenecid has been demonstrated in experimental models, but human trials have been disappointing. Chloroquine-resistant *P. vivax* has been reported in South America and South East Asia.

PHARMACOKINETICS

Oral absorption	80–90%
C_{max} 300 mg oral	0.25 mg/L after 1–6 h
Plasma half-life	*c*. 9 days (mean)
Volume of distribution	200 L/kg
Plasma protein binding	50–70%

There is extensive tissue binding and a high affinity for melanin-containing tissues. Chloroquine is extensively metabolized to a biologically active monodesethyl derivative that forms about 20% of the plasma level of the drug. The mean elimination half-life results from an initial phase (3–6 days), a slow phase (12–14 days) and a terminal phase (40 days). Renal clearance is about 50% of the dose.

TOXICITY AND SIDE EFFECTS

Minor side effects such as dizziness, headache, rashes, nausea and diarrhea are common. Pruritus occurs in up to 20% of Africans taking chloroquine. Long-term treatment can induce CNS effects and cumulative dosing over many years may cause retinopathy. Rarely, photosensitization, tinnitus and deafness have occurred.

CLINICAL USE

| Prophylaxis and treatment of all types of malaria |
| Hepatic amebiasis (in sequential combination with dehydroemetine) |

A combination with azithromycin has been suggested for intermittent preventive treatment.

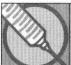

Preparations and dosage

Proprietary names: Avloclor, Nivaquine.

Preparations: Tablets, syrup, injection.

Dosage: Treatment of benign malarias: adult, oral, 600 mg chloroquine base as initial dose then a single dose of 300 mg after 6–8 h, then a single dose of 300 mg per day for 2 days. Children, oral, initial dose of 10 mg/kg of chloroquine base then a single dose of 5 mg/kg after 6–8 h, then a single dose of 5 mg/kg per day for 2 days. Malaria prophylaxis: consult specialist guidelines.

Widely available.

Further information

Chico RM, Pittrof R, Greenwood B, et al. Azithromycin–chloroquine and the intermittent preventive treatment of malaria in pregnancy. *Malar J.* 2008;7:255.
Fidock DA, Eastman RT, Ward SA, et al. Recent highlights in antimalarial drug resistance and chemotherapy research. *Trends in Parasitolology.* 2008;24:537–544.
Jensen M, Melhorn H. Seventy-five years of Resochin in the fight against malaria. *Parasitol Res.* 2009;105:609–622.

AMODIAQUINE

Molecular weight: 355.86.

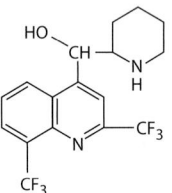

A mono-Mannich-base 4-aminoquinoline, formulated as the dihydrochloride dihydrate or free base for oral administration.

It is active against *P. falciparum* and *P. vivax* and is more active than chloroquine for the treatment of uncomplicated *P. falciparum* malaria. Chloroquine-resistant strains may remain susceptible, but resistance to amodiaquine is also spreading in some regions of Africa. The pharmacological properties are similar to those of chloroquine. The terminal elimination half-life is 1–3 weeks. It is rapidly and extensively metabolized to the desethyl derivative which has reduced antiplasmodial activity.

Prophylactic use has been abandoned because of agranulocytosis and hepatotoxicity due to formation of a quinone-imine metabolite.

A fixed dose combination with artesunate and derivatives (for example, isoquine) with altered metabolism and reduced toxicity is in development.

 ## CLINICAL USE

Treatment of falciparum malaria

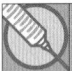 ## Preparations and dosage

Preparation: Tablets. Also co-formulation artesunate–amodiaquine tablets.
Dosage: Amodiaquine recommended at 30 mg/kg (range 25–35 mg/kg) given over 3 days (e.g. 10 mg/kg/day). Artesunate: amodiaquine fixed dose combination at 4 mg/kg (range 2–10 mg/kg) artesunate and 10 mg/kg (range 7.5–15 mg/kg) amodiaquine once daily for 3 days.
Limited availability.

 ## Further information

Olliaro P, Mussano P. Amodiaquine for treating malaria. *Cochrane Database Syst Rev.* 2003;(2) CD000016.
O'Neill PM, Park BK, Shone AE, et al. Candidate selection and preclinical evaluation of *N*-tert-butyl isoquine (GSK369796), an affordable and effective 4-aminoquinoline antimalarial for the 21st century. *J Med Chem.* 2009;52(5):1408–1415.
Sasi P, Abdulrahaman A, Mwai L, et al. In vivo and in vitro efficacy of amodiaquine against *Plasmodium falciparum* in an area of continued use of 4-aminoquinolines in East Africa. *J Infec Dis.* 2009;199:1575–1582.

MEFLOQUINE

Molecular weight (free base): 378.3; (hydrochloride): 414.8.

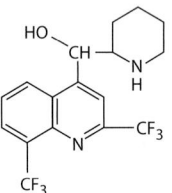

A synthetic 4-quinolinemethanol, formulated as the hydrochloride for oral administration. It is slightly soluble in water.

 ## ANTIMICROBIAL ACTIVITY

Mefloquine is a lipophilic drug with a high affinity to membranes. A concentration of 10–40 nM has rapid dose-related activity against erythrocytic stages of *Plasmodium* spp., including strains resistant to chloroquine, sulfonamides and pyrimethamine. The C-11 (hydroxy) enantiomers have equal antimalarial activity. It also exhibits activity against bacteria (including methicillin-resistant *Staphylococcus aureus*), and some fungi and helminths.

 ## ACQUIRED RESISTANCE

Resistance in *P. falciparum* is widespread in South East Asia where high-grade resistance was found in 15% of patients and low-grade resistance in about 50%. There is cross-resistance with quinine and halofantrine, and an inverse relationship with chloroquine resistance has been reported. The molecular basis of resistance remains unclear but polymorphisms of the *pfmdr1* gene, associated with chloroquine resistance, led to increased sensitivity to mefloquine. Resistant strains of *P. falciparum* appeared in Africa before the drug was used in that continent, perhaps because of quinine abuse or intrinsic resistance. In South East Asia, declining response rates to combination therapy with mefloquine and artesunate are reported.

PHARMACOKINETICS

Oral absorption	70–80%
C_{max} 1 g oral	1 mg/L after 2–12 h
Plasma half-life	20 days
Volume of distribution	16–25 L/kg
Plasma protein binding	98%

Mefloquine is concentrated two- to five-fold in erythrocytes. The major metabolites do not have antimalarial activity. Pregnant women require larger doses than non-pregnant women to achieve comparable blood levels. It is predominantly excreted in the bile. Less than 10% is excreted in urine.

TOXICITY AND SIDE EFFECTS

At prophylactic doses risks of serious toxicity are about 1 in 10 000, similar to chloroquine. Doses used in therapy are more commonly associated with nausea, dizziness, fatigue, mental confusion and sleep loss. Psychosis, encephalopathy and convulsions are seen in about 1 in 1200–1700 patients. Mefloquine(+), the enantiomer with potential lower toxicity, is currently in development.

CLINICAL USE

Antimalarial prophylaxis in areas of chloroquine resistance
Treatment of uncomplicated multidrug-resistant malaria

A mefloquine–artesunate co-formulation is available. Mefloquine has been used for the treatment of cutaneous leishmaniasis in South America.

Preparations and dosage

Proprietary names: Lariam, Mephaquine.
Preparation: Tablets. Co-formulation mefloquine–artesunate tablets.
Dosage: Malaria treatment, oral, 20–25 mg/kg as a single dose or in 2–3 divided doses 6–8 h apart. A lower dose of 15 mg/kg may suffice for partially immune individuals. Malaria prophylaxis, see specialist guidelines. Widely available.

Further information

Carrara VI, Zwang J, Ashley EA, et al. Changes in the treatment responses to artesunate–mefloquine on the northwestern border of Thailand during 13 years of continuous deployment. *PLoS ONE*. 2009;4:e4551.
Gutman J, Green M, Durand S, et al. Mefloquine pharmacokinetics and mefloquine–artesunate effectiveness in Peruvian patients with uncomplicated *Plasmodium falciparum* malaria. *Malar J*. 2009;8:58.

Sidhu AB, Uhlemann AC, Valderramos SG, et al. Decreasing *pfmdr1* copy number in *Plasmodium falciparum* malaria heightens susceptibility to mefloquine, lumefantrine, halofantrine, quinine and artemisinin. *J Infect Dis*. 2006;194:528–535.
Simpson JA, Watkins ER, Price RN, et al. Mefloquine pharmacokinetic–pharmacodynamic models: implications for dosing and resistance. *Antimicrob Agents Chemother*. 2000;44:3414–3424.

PRIMAQUINE

Molecular weight (free compound): 259.3; (diphosphate): 455.3.

A synthetic 8-aminoquinoline, formulated as the diphosphate for oral administration.

ANTIMICROBIAL ACTIVITY

Primaquine is highly active against the hepatic stages of the malaria life cycle, including the latent hypnozoite stage of *P. vivax*. It has poor activity against erythrocytic stages of malaria parasites, other than gametocytes. The isomers have similar antiplasmodial activity but differ in toxicity. It exhibits activity against *Pneumocystis jirovecii* and, in experimental models, against *Babesia* spp. and the intracellular stages of *Leishmania* spp. and *Trypanosoma cruzi*.

ACQUIRED RESISTANCE

Failure rates of up to 35% have been reported in South East Asia in patients treated with a standard course for *P. vivax* infections.

PHARMACOKINETICS

Oral absorption	>75%
C_{max} 45 mg oral	0.2 mg/L after 2–3 h
Plasma half-life	4–10 h
Volume of distribution	2 L/kg
Plasma protein binding	Extensive

Bioavailability is variable after oral administration. There is extensive tissue distribution. About 60% of the dose is metabolized to carboxyprimaquine, which can reach levels 50 times that of the parent drug; this metabolite has a half-life of 16 h, a low tissue distribution and is detectable at 120 h. Methoxy and hydroxy metabolites are also detectable. Less than 4% of the original dose is excreted unchanged in urine.

TOXICITY AND SIDE EFFECTS

At standard doses side effects are mild: abdominal cramps, anemia, leukocytosis and methemoglobinemia. However, primaquine is often associated with serious adverse effects due to the toxic metabolites 5-hydroxyprimaquine or 6-methoxy-8-aminoquinoline which are considered to be directly responsible for complications such as hemolytic anemia. Toxicity is worse in people deficient of glucose-6-phosphate dehydrogenase (G6PD) or glutathione synthetase. Adverse effects can be further increased by the repeated administration of high doses, due to its limited oral bioavailability.

CLINICAL USE

Radical cure of malaria caused by *P. vivax* or *P. ovale*

Mild or moderately severe infections with *Pn. jirovecii* (in combination with clindamycin).

Because of its gametocytocidal properties, primaquine has been used rarely in a single dose to prevent the spread of chloroquine-resistant *P. falciparum*.

Preparations and dosage

Dosage: Malaria treatment, adults, oral, 15 mg per day for 14–21 days (after chloroquine). Children, oral, 250 µg/kg per day as per adult. Malaria prophylaxis, see specialist guidelines.

Limited availability in the UK.

Further information

Bolchoz U, Budinsky RA, McMillan DC, Jollow DJ. Primaquine-induced hemolytic anemia: formation and hemotoxicity of the arylhydroxylamine metabolite 6-methoxy-8-hydroxyaminoquinoline. *J Pharmacol Exp Ther.* 2001;297:509–515.

Vale N, Moreira R, Gomes P. Primaquine revisited six decades after its discovery. *Eur J Med Chem.* 2009;44:937–953.

QUININE

Molecular weight (free base): 324.4.

A quinolinemethanol from the bark of the *Cinchona* tree; the laevorotatory stereoisomer of quinidine. Formulated as the sulfate, bisulfate or ethylcarbonate for oral use and as the dihydrochloride for parenteral administration. The salts are highly soluble in water.

ANTIMICROBIAL ACTIVITY

Quinine inhibits the erythrocytic stages of human malaria parasites at <1 mg/L, but not the liver stages. It is active against the gametocytes of *P. vivax*, *P. ovale* and *P. malariae*, but not *P. falciparum*. The dextrorotatory stereoisomer, quinidine, is more active than quinine, but epiquinine (cinchonine) and epiquinidine (cinchonidine) have much lower antimalarial activities.

ACQUIRED RESISTANCE

Resistance is now widespread in South East Asia, where some strains are also resistant to chloroquine, sulfadoxine–pyrimethamine and mefloquine. Cross-resistance with mefloquine has been demonstrated in *P. falciparum*, but genetic polymorphisms associated with chloroquine resistance are not associated with quinine resistance.

PHARMACOKINETICS

Oral absorption	80–90%
C_{max} 600 mg oral	5 mg/L after 1–3 h
Plasma half-life	8.7 h
Volume of distribution	1.8 L/kg
Plasma protein binding	*c.* 70%

Quinine is well absorbed by the oral route. Intramuscular administration gives more predictable data than intravenous administration and may be more useful in children. Plasma protein binding rises to 90% in uncomplicated malaria and 92% in cerebral malaria due to high levels of acute-phase proteins. Similarly, the elimination half-life rises to 18.2 h in severe malaria. There is extensive hepatic metabolism to hydroxylated derivatives. Urinary clearance is <20% of total clearance.

TOXICITY AND SIDE EFFECTS

Up to 25% of patients experience cardiac dysrhythmia, hypoglycemia, cinchonism (tinnitus, vomiting, diarrhea, headache). Severe effects, including hypotension and hypoglycemia, are of particular importance in children, pregnant women and the severely ill. Rarely, it can induce hemolytic anemia ('blackwater fever'). Quinine inhibits tryptophan uptake into cells.

CLINICAL USE

Falciparum malaria (alone or in combination with tetracycline, doxycycline, clindamycin or pyrimethamine–sulfadoxine)

Babesiosis (in combination with clindamycin)

It is particularly used in cerebral malaria if chloroquine resistance is suspected (Ch. 62). It is not recommended for treatment of uncomplicated falciparum malaria.

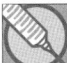

Preparations and dosage

Preparations: Tablets, injection.

Dosage: Treatment of falciparum malaria: Adults, oral, 600 mg of quinine salt every 8 h for 7 days; i.v., initial loading dose of 20 mg/kg quinine salt (maximum dose, 1.4 g) infused over 4 h, then after 8–12 h a maintenance dose of 10 mg/kg (maximum dose, 700 mg) infused over 4 h, every 8–12 h until oral therapy can be taken to complete the 7-day course. Children, oral, 10 mg/kg of quinine salt every 8 h for 7 days. Malaria prophylaxis: see specialist guidelines.

Widely available.

Further information

Khozoie C, Pleass RJ, Avery SV. The antimalarial drug quinine disrupts Tat2p-mediated tryptophan transport and causes tryptophan starvation. *J Biol Chem*. 2009;284:17968–17974.

Krishna S, Nagaraja NV, Planche T, et al. Population pharmacokinetics of intramuscular quinine in children with severe malaria. *Antimicrob Agents Chemother*. 2001;45:1803–1809.

Yeka A, Achan J, D'Alessandro U, Talisuna AO. Quinine monotherapy for treating uncomplicated malaria in the era of artemisinin-based combination therapy: an appropriate public health policy? *Lancet Infect Dis*. 2009;9:448–452.

OTHER QUINOLINES

DIIODOHYDROXYQUINOLINE

Iodoquinol (USAN). Molecular weight: 396.98. An 8-hydroxyquinoline derivative formulated for oral use.

It has weak activity against *Entamoeba histolytica* and *Dientamoeba fragilis* in vitro and in vivo. It is slowly and incompletely absorbed, with less than 10% of an oral dose reaching the circulation. Absorbed drug is metabolized to sulfate or glucuronide conjugates and excreted.

Side effects include nausea, diarrhea, rashes and cramps. Other halogenated hydroxyquinolines have been shown to cause subacute myelo-optic neuropathy from prolonged dosage and are banned in some countries. It is used in asymptomatic or mild intestinal amebiasis, but is not widely available.

PIPERAQUINE

A bisquinoline used to treat malaria in China since 1978. It is structurally related to chloroquine, but active against chloroquine-resistant *P. falciparum*. A combination with dihdyroartemisinin has shown excellent tolerability and high cure rates for multidrug-resistant falciparum malaria.

It is highly lipid-soluble and orally well absorbed. The elimination half-life is 20–30 days and there is extensive metabolism. Adverse effects are similar to chloroquine, but pruritus is uncommon.

Further information

Davis TM, Hung TY, Sim IK, et al. Piperaquine: a resurgent antimalarial drug. *Drugs*. 2005;65:75–87.

Karunajeewa HA, Ilett KF, Mueller I, et al. Pharmacokinetics and efficacy of piperaquine and chloroquine in Melanesian children with uncomplicated malaria. *Antimicrob Agents Chemother*. 2008;52:237–243.

Myint HY, Ashley EA, Day NPJ, et al. Efficacy and safety of dihydroartemisinin–piperaquine. *Trans R Soc Trop Med Hyg*. 2007;101:858–866.

TAFENOQUINE

Etaquine. A synthetic 8-aminoquinoline, formulated as the succinate for oral administration. Tafenoquine is an effective schizonticide against *P. falciparum* and *P. vivax*. It is also active against the pre-erythrocytic stages of these species and the hypnozoites of *P. vivax*. A dosage of 100 mg base corresponds to 125 mg salt. Oral absorption is slow with a maximum plasma concentration reached after 12 h. The half-life is 2 weeks, significantly longer than that of primaquine. It is not eliminated via the kidneys. Toxicity and side effects are similar to those of primaquine. Development of methemoglobinemia is common. Patients with G6PD deficiency may develop severe hemolysis.

It is in clinical development for the treatment and prophylaxis of *P. vivax* malaria and for the treatment of *P. falciparum* infection.

Further information

Charles BG, Miller AK, Nasveld PE, Reid MG, Harris IE, Edstein MD. Population pharmacokinetics of tafenoquine during malaria prophylaxis in healthy subjects. *Antimicrob Agents Chemother*. 2007;51:2709–2715.

Kitchener S, Nasveld P, Edstein MD. Tafenoquine for the treatment of recurrent *Plasmodium vivax* malaria. *Am J Trop Med Hyg*. 2007;76:494–496.

DIAMIDINES

Stilbamidine, propamidine, pentamidine and diminazene were initially developed for the treatment of African trypanosomiasis. Pentamidine has been used extensively for early stage infections with *T. brucei gambiense*, but has also been used in the prophylaxis and treatment of *Pn. jirovecii* infections. Diminazene aceturate (Berenil) is used for cattle trypanosomiasis, but is not registered for human use.

Propamidine and hexamidine have been used for the topical treatment of amebic keratitis, often in combination, caused by *Acanthamoeba* spp.; therapeutic activity is also reported for the structurally related polyhexamethylene biguanide.

Further information

Schuster FL, Visvesvara GS. Opportunistic amoeba: challenges in prophylaxis and treatment. *Drug Resist Updat.* 2004;7:41–51.

Werbowetz K. Diamidines as antitrypanosomal, antileishmanial and antimalarial agents. *Curr Opin Investig Drugs.* 2006;7:147–157.

Wilson WD, Tanious FA, Mathis A, Tevis D, Hall JE, Boykin DW. Antiparasitic compounds that target DNA. *Biochimie.* 2008;90:999–1014.

PENTAMIDINE

Molecular weight (isethionate): 592.7.

A synthetic diamidine, available as the isethionate (2-hydroxymethane sulfonate) salt for parenteral use. It is also administered by instillation of a nebulized solution directly into the lungs.

ANTIMICROBIAL ACTIVITY

Pentamidine has broad activity in experimental models against *P. falciparum*, *Toxoplasma gondii*, *Leishmania* spp., *Trypanosoma* spp. and *Babesia* spp. It also has activity against *Pn. jirovecii*.

ACQUIRED RESISTANCE

Relapse rates of 7–16% have been reported in the treatment of human African trypanosomiasis in West Africa. Patients usually respond to a subsequent course of treatment with melarsoprol. A membrane transporter is involved in cross-resistance of arsenic-resistant *T. brucei* to diamidines, affecting diminazene and stilbamidine more than pentamidine.

PHARMACOKINETICS

Oral absorption	Negligible
C_{max} 4 mg/kg intramuscular	c. 0.5 mg/L after 1 h
Plasma half-life	c. 6.5 h
Volume of distribution	3 L/kg
Plasma protein binding	c. 70%

Pentamidine is rapidly and extensively metabolized by rat liver, and high concentrations are retained in renal and hepatic tissue for up to 6 months after administration. In humans distribution is mainly in the liver, kidney, adrenal glands and spleen, with lower accumulation in the lung. This tissue retention is

the basis for its prophylactic use. Although transport across the blood–brain barrier has been demonstrated in experimental models, it is probably unable to cross the blood–brain barrier in sufficient quantity to be trypanocidal: <1% of the plasma concentration has been measured in the CSF of sleeping sickness patients. About 15–20% of the dose is excreted in the urine but because of retention in tissues there is an extremely long terminal half-life (>12 days).

TOXICITY AND SIDE EFFECTS

Side effects range from local irritation and sterile abscess at the site of injection to transient effects (vomiting, abdominal discomfort) and serious systemic effects (hypotension, effects on the heart, hypoglycemia and hyperglycemia, leukopenia, thrombocytopenia). In a study of the treatment of South American cutaneous leishmaniasis, 17% of patients prematurely terminated treatment due to toxicity and another 30% reported side effects.

CLINICAL USE

Human African trypanosomiasis (early stages before CNS involvement)

Prophylaxis and therapy of *Pn. jirovecii* pneumonia

Visceral leishmaniasis unresponsive to pentavalent antimonials and cutaneous leishmaniasis caused by *L. guyanensis*

There is limited evidence for its use in the treatment of babesiosis.

Preparations and dosage

Proprietary name: Pentacarinat.

Preparations: Injection, nebulizer solution.

Dosage:

Visceral leishmaniasis: Adults, i.m., 3–4 mg/kg once or twice weekly until the condition resolves; i.v., 3–4 mg/kg on alternate days to a maximum of 10 injections.

Trypanosomiasis: Adults, i.m., 4 mg/kg per day or on alternate days to a total of 7–10 injections.

Pn. jirovecii pneumonia: i.v., 4 mg/kg per day for at least 14 days.

Widely available.

Further information

de Koning HP. Ever-increasing complexities of diamidine and arsenical cross resistance in African trypanosomes. *Trends Parasitol.* 2008;24:345–349.

Dorlo TP, Kager PA. Pentamidine dosage: a base/salt confusion. *PLoS Neglected Tropical Diseases.* 2008;2:e225.

Sanderson L, Dogruel M, Rodgers J, De Koning HP, Thomas SA. Pentamidine movement across the murine blood–brain and blood–cerebrospinal fluid barriers: effect of trypanosome infection, combination therapy, P-glycoprotein, and multidrug resistance-associated protein. *J. Pharmacol Exp Ther.* 2009;329:967–977.

van der Meide WF, Sabajo LO, Jensema AJ, et al. Evaluation of treatment with pentamidine for cutaneous leishmaniasis in Suriname. *Int J Dermatol.* 2009;48:52–58.

PROPAMIDINE

A synthetic diamidine formulated as the isethionate or as dibromopropamidine isethionate for topical administration to the eye. Resistant clinical isolates of *Acanthamoeba* have been identified. It is available over the counter in eye drops.

Its activity against bacterial pathogens is poor, but it exhibits specific activity against *Acanthamoeba* spp. Reduction in sensitivity of *Acanthamoeba* during encystation might reflect changes in drug uptake. It is still recommended for aggressive treatment of amebic keratitis (in combination with neomycin or other agents), but is not well tolerated.

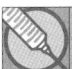

Preparations and dosage

Proprietary name: Brolene.

Preparations: Ophthalmic ointment and eye drops.

Widely available.

Further information

Schuster FL, Visvesvara GS. Opportunistic amoeba: challenges in prophylaxis and treatment. *Drug Resist Updat.* 2004;7:41–51.

Turner NA, Russell AD, Furr JR, Lloyd D. Emergence of resistance to biocides during differentiation of *Acanthamoeba castellanii. J Antimicrob Chemother.* 2000;46:27–34.

BIGUANIDES

The biguanides proguanil and chlorproguanil are pro-drugs, metabolized in vivo to the triazines cycloguanil and chlorcycloguanil, which have much enhanced activity in malaria treatment. Along with the diaminopyrimidines (Ch. 17), they are often referred to as antifolates due to their mechanism of action (p. 17). Proguanil is also used in combination with atovaquone, but the interaction has a different basis; antifolates do not enhance the effect of atovaquone.

PROGUANIL

Chlorguanide. Molecular weight (free base): 253.8; (hydro-chloride): 290.2.

Proguanil → Cycloguanil

A synthetic arylbiguanide, formulated as the hydrochloride for oral use. It is slightly soluble in water.

ANTIMICROBIAL ACTIVITY

Proguanil has low antiplasmodial action, but useful activity is attributable to the metabolite cycloguanil, which inhibits the early erythrocytic stages of all four *Plasmodium* spp. that cause human malaria and the primary hepatic stage of *P. falciparum*. Proguanil acts synergistically with atovaquone and probably enhances its effect on mitochondrial membrane charge.

ACQUIRED RESISTANCE

Resistance of *P. falciparum* associated with point mutations of dihydrofolate reductase has been reported worldwide. Resistance in *P. vivax* and *P. malariae* has been reported in South East Asia. Cross-resistance with pyrimethamine is not absolute, because differential resistance can arise from different point mutations on the dihydrofolate reductase gene.

PHARMACOKINETICS

Oral absorption	>90%
C_{max} 100 mg oral	0.4 mg/L after 2–4 h
Plasma half-life	10 h
Plasma protein binding	75%

Oral absorption is slow. It is 75% protein bound and is concentrated 10- to 15-fold by erythrocytes. About 20% of the drug is metabolized to dihydrotriazene derivatives, most importantly cycloguanil, by hepatic cytochrome P_{450} processes. Cycloguanil is detectable 2 h after administration of proguanil. High proportions of 'non-metabolizers' have been identified in Japan and Kenya, indicating another source of resistance. About 60% of the dose is excreted in the urine.

TOXICITY AND SIDE EFFECTS

It is well tolerated at recommended doses. Gastrointestinal and renal effects have been reported at doses exceeding 600 mg per day.

CLINICAL USE

Antimalarial prophylaxis (usually in combination with chloroquine)

Treatment and prophylaxis for drug-resistant falciparum malaria (in combination with atovaquone)

Preparations and dosage

Proprietary names: Paludrine, Malarone (combination with atovaquone).

Preparation: Tablets.

For malaria prophylaxis, see specialist guidelines.

Widely available.

Further information

Boggild AK, Parise ME, Lewis LS, Kain KC. Atovaquone–proguanil: report from the CDC expert meeting on malaria chemoprophylaxis (II). *Am J Trop Med Hyg.* 2007;76:208–223.

Khositnithikul R, Tan-Ariya P, Mungthin M. In vitro atovaquone/proguanil susceptibility and characterization of the cytochrome b gene of *Plasmodium falciparum* from different endemic regions of Thailand. *Malar J.* 2008;7:23.

Painter HJ, Morrisey JM, Mather MW, Vaidya AB. Specific role of mitochondrial electron transport in blood-stage *Plasmodium falciparum. Nature.* 2007;446:88–91.

Srivastava IK, Vaidya AB. A mechanism for the synergistic antimalarial action of atovaquone and proguanil. *Antimicrob Agents Chemother.* 1999;43:1334–1339.

SESQUITERPENE LACTONES

Artemisinin (qinghaosu), a compound derived from a plant used in traditional Chinese medicine, *Artemisia annua*, has been used extensively in East Asia and Africa for the treatment of malaria. This drug, and derivatives that have higher intrinsic antimalarial activity (artesunate, artemether and arteether), have replaced quinine as a treatment of falciparum malaria in many countries, normally in combination with other antimalarials. A semisynthetic derivative, artemisone, which has higher efficacy than artesunate and lower toxicity potential, is in development. Artemisinin and its derivatives also show broad antiprotozoal, anthelmintic and antiviral activities.

The novel structure, containing an endoperoxide bridge, has stimulated the development of semisynthetic and synthetic dioxane, trioxane and tetroxane compounds with activity against *Plasmodium* spp. and *Schistosoma* spp. Some of these synthetic trioxalanes are now in clinical development with Medicines for Malaria Venture and other organizations.

Further information

Efferth T, Romero MR, Wolf DG, Stamminger T, Marin JJ, Marschall M. The antiviral activities of artemisinin and artesunate. *Clin Infect Dis.* 2008;47:804–811.

Keiser J, Utzinger J. Artemisinins and synthetic trioxolanes in the treatment of helminth infections. *Curr Opin Infect Dis.* 2007;20:605–612.

Krishna S, Bustamante L, Haynes RK, Staines HM. Artemisinins: their growing importance in medicine. *Trends Pharmacol Sci.* 2008;29:520–527.

Vennerstrom JL, Arbe-Barnes S, Brun R, et al. Identification of an antimalarial synthetic trioxolane drug development candidate. *Nature.* 2004;430:900–904.

White NJ. Qinghaosu (artemisinin): the price of success. *Science.* 2008;320:330–334.

ARTEMISININ

Qinghaosu. Molecular weight (native compound): 282.3; (artemether): 298.4; (sodium artesunate): 407.4: (dihydroartemisinin): 284.3

A sesquiterpene peroxide derived from *A. annua*, chiefly used in the form of artemether, the methyl ester synthesized from dihydroartemisinin, or artesunate, the water-soluble hemisuccinate. Formulated for administration by the oral, intramuscular or intrarectal routes; artesunate can also be given intravenously.

ANTIMICROBIAL ACTIVITY

Artemisinins are active against the erythrocytic and gametocyte stages of chloroquine-sensitive and chloroquine-resistant strains of *P. falciparum* and other malaria parasites. Two anomers of artemether are produced on synthesis, α-artemether and β-artemether, of which the latter has higher antimalarial activity. Activity against the protozoa *Tox. gondii* and *Leishmania major* and the helminth *Schistosoma mansoni* has been demonstrated in experimental models.

ACQUIRED RESISTANCE

Resistance caused, for example, by changes in the plasmodial endoplasmic reticulum ATPase has been shown in experimental models. There have been clinical reports of reduced susceptibility to treatment with artesunate in Cambodia.

PHARMACOKINETICS

Oral absorption	Incomplete
C_{max} 500 mg oral	0.4 mg/L after 1.8 h
Plasma half-life (dihydroartemisinin)	40–60 min
Volume of distribution	c. 0.25 L/kg
Plasma protein binding (artemether)	77%

Artemisinins are concentrated by erythrocytes and are rapidly hydrolyzed to dihydroartemisinin. They are hydroxylated by cytochromes 2B6, 2C19 and 3A4; the derivatives induce this metabolism. After injection, peak plasma concentrations are reached within 1–3 h, when levels of dihydroartemisinin are included. The elimination half-life of intravenous artesunate is <30 min; artemether appears to have a much longer half-life (4–11 h).

TOXICITY AND SIDE EFFECTS

A few toxic effects in addition to drug-induced fever and a reversible decrease in reticulocyte counts have been reported. High-dose studies in animal models show neurotoxicity and reproducible dose-related neuropathic lesions; dihydroartemisinin is a toxic metabolite but the precise causes of neurotoxicity are not clear. Embryotoxicity of artemisinin and derivatives has been reported in rodent and primate models, probably due to depletion of erythroblasts.

CLINICAL USE

Malaria (including cerebral malaria), in combination with other antimalarials

Preparations and dosage

Preparations: Tablets, injection, suppositories.

Available in artesunate–amodiaquine, artesunate–mefloquine and artemether–lumefantrine co-formulations

Dosage: Adults, oral, 25 mg/kg on the first day, then 12.5 mg/kg on days two and three (plus mefloquine on day two to effect a radical cure). Other derivatives can also be given.

Limited availability.

Further information

Dondorp AM, Nosten F, Yi P, et al. Artemisinin resistance in *Plasmodium falciparum* malaria. *New Eng J Med.* 2009;361:455–467.

Giao PT, de Vries PJ. Pharmacokinetic interactions of antimalarial drugs. *Clin Pharmacokinet.* 2001;40:343–373.

Hartwig CL, Rosenthal AS, D'Angelo J, Griffin CE, Posner GH, Cooper RA. Accumulation of artemisinin trioxane derivatives within neutral lipids of *Plasmodium falciparum* malaria parasites is endoperoxide-dependent. *Biochem Pharmacol.* 2009;77:322–336.

Nagelschmitz J, Voith B, Wensing G, et al. First assessment in humans of the safety, tolerability, pharmacokinetics, and ex vivo pharmacodynamic antimalarial activity of the new artemisinin derivative artemisone. *Antimicrob Agents Chemother.* 2008;52:3085–3091.

Smith SL, Sadler CJ, Dodd CC, et al. The role of glutathione in the neurotoxicity of artemisinin derivatives in vitro. *Biochem Pharmacol.* 2001;61:409–416.

Sinclair D, Zani B, Donegan S, Olliaro P, Garner P. Artemisinin-based combination therapy for uncomplicated malaria. *Cochrane Database Syst Rev.* 2009;(3) CD007483.

MISCELLANEOUS ANTIPROTOZOAL AGENTS

ATOVAQUONE

Molecular weight: 366.8.

A hydroxynaphthoquinone. Available as the *trans* isomer (which is more active than the *cis* form) for oral use. It is insoluble in water.

ANTIMICROBIAL ACTIVITY

It is active against erythrocytic, liver and sexual stages of malaria parasites. It shows synergy with proguanil and tetracyclines in vitro. It is also active against *Babesia* spp. and both tachyzoites and cysts of *Tox. gondii*. *Pn. jirovecii* is sensitive in vitro at 0.1–3.0 mg/L and high doses are effective in the rat.

ACQUIRED RESISTANCE

Point mutations on parasite cytochrome b, in particular at codon 268, cause resistance and readily occur when the drug is used alone. The rapid selection of resistance led to the development of the synergistic combination with proguanil. Failure of *Pn. jirovecii* prophylaxis has also been associated with cytochrome b mutations.

PHARMACOKINETICS

Oral absorption	Poor
C_{max} 750 mg oral	27 mg/L (steady state)
Plasma half-life	70 h
Plasma protein binding	>99%

It is highly lipophilic and is poorly absorbed from the gastrointestinal tract following oral administration. Bioavailability is improved when administered with meals, particularly those with a high fat content. Steady-state plasma concentrations are up to 50% lower in AIDS patients than in asymptomatic HIV-positive cases and the elimination half-life is lower (55 h) in patients with AIDS. The concentration in CSF is <1% of the plasma level. Unlike some other naphthoquinones it is not metabolized by human liver microsomes. Combinations with co-trimoxazole (in HIV patients) and with proguanil plus artesunate in healthy adults did not produce any changes in atovaquone pharmacokinetics.

TOXICITY AND SIDE EFFECTS

Most clinical trials of atovaquone alone have involved patients with AIDS in whom adverse effects are often difficult to detect; however, more than 20% reported fever, nausea, diarrhea and rashes. There were limited changes in hepatocellular function. In malaria, in combination with proguanil, there are few reported side effects.

CLINICAL USE

> *Pn. jirovecii* pneumonia; alternative therapy for mild to moderate illness (prophylaxis and treatment)
>
> Prophylaxis and treatment of malaria in combination with proguanil

It has also been used in cerebral toxoplasmosis in AIDS patients and in a few cases of human babesiosis.

Preparations and dosage

Proprietary names: Malarone (atovaquone–proguanil), Mepron (atovaquone suspension), Wellvone.

Preparations: Tablets, oral suspension.

Dosage:

Pn. jirovecii pneumonia treatment: adults, oral, 750 mg every 12 h (suspension) or every 8 h (tablets) for 21 days.

Malaria treatment: adults, oral, 1 g per day (plus proguanil 400 mg per day) for 3 days.

Malaria prophylaxis: see specialist guidelines.

Widely available.

Further information

Baggish AL, Hill DR. Antiparasitic agent atovaquone. *Antimicrob Agents Chemother.* 2002;46:1163–1173.

Mather MW, Henry KW, Vaidya AB. Mitochondrial drug targets in apicomplexan parasites. *Curr Drug Targets.* 2007;8:49–60.

Painter HJ, Morrisey JM, Mather MW, Vaidya AB. Specific role of mitochondrial electron transport in blood-stage *Plasmodium falciparum*. *Nature.* 2007;446:88–91.

Rosenberg DM, McCarthy W, Slavinsky J, et al. Atovaquone suspension for treatment of *Pneumocystis carinii* pneumonia in HIV-infected patients. *AIDS.* 2001;15:211–214.

DEHYDROEMETINE

The synthetic racemic derivative of the plant alkaloid emetine. Formulated as the hydrochloride for intramuscular administration. Like the parent compound, emetine, it inhibits *E. histolytica* at concentrations of 1–10 mg/L in vitro, but it is more active than the parent in animal models. Drug-resistance in *E. histolytica* is rare.

No human pharmacokinetic data are available. A half-life of 2 days, compared with 5 days for emetine, has been reported. There is selective tissue binding and accumulation in the liver, lung, spleen and kidney.

It is considerably less toxic than emetine, possibly because it is more rapidly eliminated. Nevertheless, nausea, vomiting, diarrhea and abdominal cramps frequently occur. Neuromuscular effects have also been reported. More serious cardiotoxic effects can lead to electrocardiogram (EGG) changes, tachycardia and a drop in blood pressure.

It was formerly used as a second-line treatment in severe intestinal or hepatic amebiasis, but is no longer recommended for use.

DILOXANIDE

Molecular weight (furoate): 328.1.

Dichloro(hydroxyphenyl)methylacetamide. Available as an insoluble ester, the furoate, for oral administration.

ANTIMICROBIAL ACTIVITY

Diloxanide inhibits *E. histolytica* with unusually high specificity at concentrations of 0.01–0.1 mg/L.

ACQUIRED RESISTANCE

No resistance has been reported. Patients with dysentery have lower cure rates than cyst excreters.

PHARMACOKINETICS

Human pharmacokinetic data are limited. Animal data show that diloxanide furoate is rapidly absorbed from the intestine. The furoate is hydrolyzed in the gut, leaving high intraluminal concentrations of free diloxanide. About 75% is excreted via the kidney within 48 h, mostly as a glucuronide.

TOXICITY AND SIDE EFFECTS

It is well tolerated, but flatulence is common, and nausea and vomiting may occur.

CLINICAL USE

Asymptomatic intestinal infection with *E. histolytica*

It is also used in invasive amebiasis in conjunction with nitroimidazoles in order to eradicate luminal cysts.

Preparations and dosage

Proprietary names: Entamizole, Furamide.

Preparation: Tablets.

Dosage: Adults, oral, 500 mg every 8 h for 10 days. Children >25 kg, oral, 20 mg/kg per day in three divided doses for 10 days.

Limited availability. Available in the UK and the USA.

Further information

Blessmann J, Tannich E. Treatment of asymptomatic intestinal *Entamoeba histolytica* infection. *N Engl J Med.* 2002;347:1384.

Pritt BS, Clark CG. Amebiasis. *Mayo Clin Proc.* 2008;83:1154–1160.

EFLORNITHINE

α-Difluoromethylornithine. Molecular weight (free base): 182.2; (hydrochloride monohydrate): 236.6.

$$H_2N\,(CH_2)_3 - \underset{\underset{CHF_2}{|}}{\overset{\overset{NH_2}{|}}{C}} - COOH$$

An analog of ornithine, formulated as the hydrochloride for intravenous infusion. It is freely soluble in water.

ANTIMICROBIAL ACTIVITY

Cultured bloodstream trypomastigotes of *T. brucei* are relatively insensitive, but high doses are effective against bloodstream and CNS infections of *T. brucei brucei* and *T. brucei gambiense* in rodents, provided a strong antibody response is also present. Eflornithine entry into the CNS can be enhanced with suramin (*see* p. 424-425). *T. brucei rhodesiense* infections do not respond. Synergy with some arsenicals has been demonstrated.

Eflornithine is active against *P. falciparum* in experimental models and against *Leishmania* promastigotes and *Giardia lamblia* in culture.

ACQUIRED RESISTANCE

Acquired resistance in *T. brucei gambiense* in West Africa has not been reported. East African *T. brucei rhodesiense* strains are innately less sensitive. Reported treatment failures are thought to be associated with severity of disease.

PHARMACOKINETICS

Oral absorption	55%
C_{max} 10 mg/kg oral	c. 7 mg/L after 4 h
200 mg/kg intravenously	15.9 mg/L (87.5 nmol/mL) (mean)
Plasma half-life	3.3 h
Volume of distribution	0.34 L/kg
Plasma protein binding	Very low

Renal clearance is 83%, with most eliminated unchanged. In a study in Zaire the mean serum concentration in children under 12 years old was half that of adults, probably due to more rapid renal clearance. CNS penetration is good in adult patients, with a CSF:plasma ratio of 0.91 at the end of administration for 14 days. However, the CSF:plasma ratio in children under 12 years old was 0.58. Relapses have been recorded in patients in whom CSF levels dropped below 9 mg/L (50 nmol/mL) at the end of treatment.

TOXICITY AND SIDE EFFECTS

Osmotic diarrhea and bone marrow suppression are common, and up to 50% of sleeping sickness patients develop leukopenia. Reversible anemia and thrombocytopenia have been observed. Convulsions and seizures, different from those observed in melarsoprol-induced encephalopathy, have been reported in 4–18% of treated sleeping sickness patients but not in patients treated for *Pn. jirovecii* pneumonia. This difference might be due to the CNS inflammation associated with sleeping sickness.

CLINICAL USE

Late-stage *T. brucei gambiense* infections (including arsenic-resistant cases)

It has been used speculatively for treatment of *Pn. jirovecii* infections in AIDS patients. Co-administration with oral nifurtimox has been added to the World Health Organization (WHO) List of Essential Medicines for second-stage sleeping sickness caused by *T. brucei gambiense*.

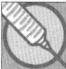

Preparations and dosage

Proprietary name: Ornidyl.

Preparation: Injection.

Dosage: Trypanosomiasis: adults, i.v., 400 mg/kg per day in divided doses for at least 14 days.

Limited availability.

Further information

Barrett MP, Boykin DW, Brun R, Tidwell RR. Human African trypanosomiasis: pharmacological re-engagement with a neglected disease. *Br J Pharmacol.* 2007;152:1155–1171.

Pepin J, Khonde N, Maiso F, et al. Short-course eflornithine in Gambian trypanosomiasis: a multicentre randomized controlled trial. *Bull World Health Org.* 2000;78:1284–1295.

Priotto G, Kasparian S, Mutombo W, et al. Nifurtimox–eflornithine combination therapy for second-stage African *Trypanosoma brucei gambiense* trypanosomiasis: a multicentre, randomised, phase III, non-inferiority trial. *Lancet.* 2009;374:56–64.

Sanderson L, Dogruel M, Rodgers J, Bradley B, Thomas SA. The blood–brain barrier significantly limits eflornithine entry into *Trypanosoma brucei brucei* infected mouse brain. *J Neurochem.* 2008;107:1136–1146.

HALOFANTRINE

Molecular weight (free base): 500.4; (hydrochloride): 536.9.

A phenanthrene methanol, formulated as the hydrochloride for oral administration. Parenteral formulations are not available. The enantiomers have equivalent activity in vitro. Aqueous solubility is extremely low.

ANTIMICROBIAL ACTIVITY

It inhibits erythrocytic stages of chloroquine-sensitive and chloroquine-resistant *P. falciparum* and other *Plasmodium* spp. in vitro at concentrations of 0.4–4.0 mg/L. It is more active than mefloquine and the combination of proguanil and atovaquone against *P. falciparum*, but less effective than mefloquine or chloroquine against *P. vivax*.

ACQUIRED RESISTANCE

Resistance in *P. falciparum* has been reported in Central and West Africa, where it has been used widely. Cross-resistance with mefloquine has been reported in Thailand, where it has not been used.

PHARMACOKINETICS

Absorption shows high intra- and inter-subject variability and depends on co-administration with fats. Bioavailability is increased more than six-fold after a fatty meal or by lipid-based formulations. Bioavailability is significantly lower in patients with malaria than in healthy individuals. Peak plasma levels are variable and occur 3–6 h after administration. Unlike many other antimalarials, halofantrine is not concentrated by infected or uninfected erythrocytes. Distribution to lipoproteins is stereo-selective. About 20–30% of the dose is metabolized to an *N*-desbutyl derivative by cytochrome P_{450} (CYP) 3A4 and 3A5. The elimination half-life of the parent drug is generally 1–2 days and that of the metabolite 3 days. Little unchanged drug is excreted in urine.

TOXICITY AND SIDE EFFECTS

Abdominal pain, diarrhea and pruritus are the most frequent. High doses (24 mg/kg) induce prolongation of the PR and QTc intervals; this is not stereo-selective. There are individual reports of fatal cardiac arrest and torsade de pointes. To reduce the risk of cardiac toxicity it should be taken on an empty stomach. It should not be administered with other antimalarials that have the potency to induce cardiac arrhythmias (mefloquine, chloroquine, quinine). Halofantrine has also been associated with intravascular hemolysis.

CLINICAL USE

Treatment of multidrug-resistant falciparum malaria

Its use has been questioned due to the existence of safer alternatives.

Preparations and dosage

Proprietary name: Halfan.

Preparation: Tablets.

Dosage: Treatment of falciparum malaria: Adults, oral, 1.5 g divided into three doses of 500 mg given at intervals of 6 h on an empty stomach; repeat the course after an interval of 1 week. Children, oral, 24 mg/kg divided into three doses as adult.

Widely available.

Further information

Abernethy DR, Wesche DL, Barbey JT, et al. Stereoselective halofantrine disposition and effect: concentration-related QTc prolongation. *Br J Clin Pharmacol.* 2001;51:231–237.

Baune B, Flinois JP, Furlan V, et al. Halofantrine metabolism in microsomes in man: major role of CYP 3A4 and CYP 3A5. *J Pharm Pharmacol.* 1999;51:419–426.

Bouchaud O, Monlun E, Muanza K, et al. Atovaquone plus proguanil versus halofantrine in the treatment of imported acute uncomplicated *Plasmodium falciparum* malaria in non-immune adults: a randomized comparative trial. *Am J Trop Med Hyg.* 2000;63:274–279.

White NJ. Cardiotoxicity of antimalarial drugs. *Lancet Infect Dis.* 2007;7:549–558.

LUMEFANTRINE

Benflumetol. Molecular weight: 528.9

A dichlorobenzylidene derivative given orally in combination with artemether.

ANTIMICROBIAL ACTIVITY

Lumefantrine has marked blood schizonticidal activity against a wide range of plasmodia, including chloroquine-resistant *P. falciparum*. The 50% and 90% effective concentrations (EC_{50} and EC_{90}) in vitro are similar: <10 and 40 nmol/L, respectively. The racemate and the two enantiomers exhibit similar activities. Blood schizonticidal activity of desbutylbenflumetol is four to five times greater than benflumetol in vitro.

ACQUIRED RESISTANCE

Treatment with artemether–lumefantrine can select for polymorphisms in the *P. falciparum pfmdr1* gene. Resistance has been selected experimentally in murine malaria.

PHARMACOKINETICS

Bioavailability after oral administration is variable; absorption is substantially increased by co-administration with food, particularly with a high fat content. Peak plasma concentrations occur after 6–8 h. The elimination half-life is 4–6 days. It is almost completely protein bound and metabolized mainly in the liver by CYP3A4.

 ## TOXICITY AND SIDE EFFECTS

The most common adverse effects in combination with artemether include headache, dizziness and gastrointestinal disturbances.

 ## CLINICAL USE

Treatment of *P. falciparum* infections (including mixed infections) in a fixed-dose combination treatment with artemether.

> ### Preparations and dosage
>
> **Proprietary name:** Coartem, Riamet (contains 20 mg artemether and 120 mg lumefantrine).
>
> **Dosage:** see specialist guidelines.

 Further information

Dokomajilar C, Nsobya SL, Greenhouse B, Rosenthal PJ, Dorsey G. Selection of *Plasmodium falciparum pfmdr1* alleles following therapy with artemether–lumefantrine in an area of Uganda where malaria is highly endemic. *Antimicrob Agents Chemother.* 2006;50:1893–1895.

Kiboi DM, Irungu BN, Langat B, et al. *Plasmodium berghei* ANKA: selection of resistance to piperaquine and lumefantrine in a mouse model. *Exp Parasitol.* 2009;122:196–202.

Noedl H, Allmendinger T, Prajakwong S, Wernsdorfer G, Wernsdorfer WH. Desbutyl-benflumetol, a novel antimalarial compound: *in vitro* activity in fresh isolates of *Plasmodium falciparum* from Thailand. *Antimicrob Agents Chemother.* 2001;45:2106–2109.

Sidhu AB, Uhlemann AC, Valderramos SG, Valderramos JC, Krishna S, Fidock DA. Decreasing *pfmdr1* copy number in *Plasmodium falciparum* malaria heightens susceptibility to mefloquine, lumefantrine, halofantrine, quinine, and artemisinin. *J Infect Dis.* 2006;194:528–535.

Wernsdorfer WH, Landgraf B, Kilimali VA, Wernsdorfer G. Activity of benflumetol and its enantiomers in fresh isolates of *Plasmodium falciparum* from East Africa. *Acta Trop.* 1998;70:9–15.

MEPACRINE

Quinacrine (USAN). Molecular weight (dihydrochloride): 508.9.

A synthetic acridine derivative, formulated as the hydrochloride for oral use.

ANTIMICROBIAL ACTIVITY

Mepacrine is active against the asexual erythrocytic stage of all four *Plasmodium* spp. that infect humans and the gametocytes of *P. vivax* and *P. malariae*. The enantiomers have equal antimalarial activity. It exhibits broad activity in experimental models against *T. cruzi*, *Leishmania* spp., *E. histolytica*, *Trichomonas vaginalis*, *G. lamblia* and *Blastocystis hominis*. It is also active against tapeworms.

ACQUIRED RESISTANCE

The structural resemblance to chloroquine suggests the likelihood of cross-resistance with that drug, but evidence for this is equivocal.

PHARMACOKINETICS

Oral absorption	Good
C_{max} 100 mg oral	50 µg/L after 1–3 h
Plasma half-life	5 days
Plasma protein binding	85%

There is extensive tissue binding and a six-fold concentration into leukocytes from plasma. About 10% of the daily dose is excreted in the urine. It is widely distributed throughout the body.

TOXICITY AND SIDE EFFECTS

Dizziness, headache and gastric problems are common. Toxic psychoses, bone marrow depression, yellow skin and exfoliative dermatitis are described. Poor toleration is noted, especially in children. It should not be used in combination with 8-aminoquinolines.

CLINICAL USE

Giardiasis
Prophylaxis of malaria
Tapeworm infections

Preparations and dosage

Preparation: Tablets.

Dosage: Adults, oral, 100 mg every 8 h for 5–7 days. A second course of treatment after 2 weeks is sometimes required. Children, oral, 2 mg/kg every 8 h.

Limited availability.

It has been superseded by other drugs, but is useful in giardiasis if treatment with nitroimidazoles fails. Intralesional injections have been tried in cutaneous leishmaniasis.

Further information

Gardner TB, Hill DR. Treatment of giardiasis. *Clin Microbiol Rev.* 2001;14: 114–128.
Vdovanko AA, Williams JE. *Blastocystis hominis:* neutral red supravital staining and its application to in vitro drug sensitivity testing. *Parasitol Res.* 2000;86:573–581.

MILTEFOSINE

Hexadecylphosphocholine. Molecular weight: 407.58.

$$H_3C\,(CH_2)_{14}—CH_2—O—P(=O)(O^-)—O—CH_2\,CH_2N^+\,(CH_3)_3$$

An alkylphospholipid, originally investigated as an anticancer compound, formulated for oral administration.

ANTIMICROBIAL ACTIVITY

Concentrations of 1–5 µM inhibit the promastigotes and amastigotes of *Leishmania* spp. and the epimastigotes and amastigotes of *T. cruzi*. Inhibitory concentrations against *T. brucei* spp. and *E. histolytica* are closer to 50 µM. *Acanthamoeba* spp. are variably susceptible, depending on the experimental conditions.

ACQUIRED RESISTANCE

There are no reports of clinical resistance in *Leishmania* so far. Experimental resistance has been induced in vitro against the promastigote stage of *Leishmania* and two plasma membrane proteins, LdMT and Ld Ros3, are necessary for miltefosine uptake. There is evidence that reduced sensitivity of promastigotes is passed on to intracellular amastigotes.

PHARMACOKINETICS

In rodent models the drug is almost completely absorbed after oral administration. About 90% is bound to plasma proteins. It is widely distributed in the body; studies in rats showed highest uptake in kidney, liver and spleen. In rats and dogs bioavailability was 82% and 94%, with maximum values reached after 4–48 h.

In adult human trials repeated oral dosing with 100 mg per day achieved a peak plasma concentration of 70 mg/L after 8–24 h (day 23). The half-life is 6–8 days.

TOXICITY AND SIDE EFFECTS

Mild to moderate gastrointestinal side effects are reported in 40–60% of patients. Moderate to severe nephrotoxicity was seen in 2% and 1% of patients, respectively; increases in creatinine levels were reversible. Miltefosine is contraindicated in pregnancy, based on findings of teratogenicity in rats. It causes hemolysis and cannot be given intravenously.

CLINICAL USE

Visceral leishmaniasis
Cutaneous leishmaniasis

Preparations and dosage

Proprietary name: Impavido, Miltex.

Preparation: Capsules (10 and 50 mg miltefosine).

Dosage: 2.5 mg/kg per day orally for 28 days (usually 100–150 mg per day) (maximum dose, 150 mg per day).

Available through private and public sources in India.

Studies to investigate short-course combination treatments with miltefosine are in progress.

Further information

Bhattacharya SK, Sinha PK, Sundar S, et al. Phase 4 trial of miltefosine for the treatment of Indian visceral leishmaniasis. *J Infect Dis.* 2007;196:591–598.

Croft SL, Seifert K, Duchene M. Antiprotozoal activities of phospholipid drugs. *Mol Biochem Parasitol.* 2003;126:165–172.

Perez-Victoria FJ, Sanchez-Canete MP, et al. Mechanisms of experimental resistance of *Leishmania* to miltefosine: implications for clinical use. *Drug Resist Updat.* 2006;9:26–39.

Pérez-Victoria FJ, Sánchez-Cañete MP, Castanys S, Gamarro F. Phospholipid translocation and miltefosine potency require both *L. donovani* miltefosine transporter and the new protein LdRos3 in *Leishmania* parasites. *J Biol Chem.* 2006;281:23766–23775.

NITAZOXANIDE

Molecular weight: 307.3

A synthetic broad-spectrum antiparasitic nitroheterocycle (2-acetyloxy-*N*-(5-nitro-2-thiazolyl) benzamide), formulated for oral use.

ANTIMICROBIAL ACTIVITY

In vitro *Cryptosporidium parvum* sporocytes and oocysts are inhibited by <33 μM, and *Giardia lamblia* (*intestinalis*) trophozoites by <10 μM. The metabolite tizoxanide is more active than the parent compound against some isolates. *E. histolytica* is inhibited by 6–23 μM (parent compound) and 5.6–28 μM (metabolite), and *T. vaginalis* by 0.5–15.5 μM (parent compound) and 0.3–12.2 μM (metabolite). Activity against other microorganisms, including some helminths, bacteria (*Clostridium difficile*) and viruses (hepatitis C) has also been demonstrated.

ACQUIRED RESISTANCE

Resistance caused by altered expression of genes involved in stress response has been demonstrated in experimental studies with *G. lamblia*.

PHARMACOKINETICS

After oral administration the major circulating metabolites are tizoxanide (desacetyl nitazoxanide) and its glucuronide. Minor metabolites include salicyluric acid and tizoxanide sulfate. Maximum concentrations of the active metabolites tizoxanide and tizoxanide glucuronide are observed within 1–4 h. Following a single oral dose of 500 mg given with food, the C_{max} of both metabolites was around 10 mg/L. Tizoxanide has a half-life of around 1–2 h and is >99.9% bound to plasma proteins.

TOXICITY AND SIDE EFFECTS

Nitazoxanide appears well tolerated. Side effects may include abdominal pain diarrhea, headache and nausea.

CLINICAL USE

It is indicated for the treatment of diarrhea caused by *G. lamblia* or *C. parvum*.

Preparations and dosage

Proprietary name: Alinia.

Preparations: Oral suspension, tablets.

Dosage: 1–3 years of age, 5 mL (100 mg nitazoxanide) oral suspension every 12 h with food for 3 days; 4–11 years: 10 mL (200 mg nitazoxanide) oral suspension every 12 h with food for 3 days; ≥12 years: 1 tablet (500 mg nitazoxanide) every 12 h with food for 3 days or 25 mL oral suspension (500 mg nitazoxanide) every 12 h with food for 3 days.

Available in USA.

Further information

Adagu IS, Nolder D, Warhurst DC, Rossignol JF. *In vitro* activity of nitazoxanide and related compounds against isolates of *Giardia intestinalis, Entamoeba histolytica* and *Trichomonas vaginalis. J Antimicrob Chemother.* 2002;49:103–111.

Muller J, Ley S, Felger I, Hemphill A, Muller N. Identification of differentially expressed genes in a *Giardia lamblia* WB C6 clone resistant to nitazoxanide and metronidazole. *J Antimicrob Chemother.* 2008;62:72–82.

Rossignol JF, Ayoub A, Ayers MS. Treatment of diarrhea caused by *Cryptosporidium parvum*: a prospective double-blind, placebo-controlled study of nitazoxanide. *J Infect Dis.* 2001;184:103–106.

Rossignol JF, Kabil SM, El-Gohary Y, Younis AM. Nitazoxanide in the treatment of amebiasis. *Trans R Soc Trop Med Hyg.* 2007;101:1025–1031.

Rossignol JF. *Cryptosporidium* and *Giardia*: Treatment options and prospects for new drugs. *Exp Parasitol.* 2010;124: 45–53.

PYRONARIDINE

Molecular weight: 518.06.

An aza-aminoacridine formulated for oral use. A Mannich-base derivative of mepacrine (*see* p. 421).

ANTIMICROBIAL ACTIVITY

Pyronaridine is active against the asexual erythrocytic stage of *P. falciparum* with little or no activity against gametocytes or the hepatic stage. In-vitro blood schizonticide activities are in the range of 0.001–0.03 mg/L, showing a moderate correlation to chloroquine resistance. However, this correlation varies between studies and does not seem to be clinically significant. It is also active against *P. vivax, P. ovale* and *P. malariae*. Antagonistic interactions with artemisinins were reported in vitro, but synergy with artesunate has been observed in rodent models.

ACQUIRED RESISTANCE

Decreasing in-vitro sensitivity has been observed in China.

PHARMACOKINETICS

Peak plasma concentrations are reached after 3–14 h depending upon the formulation; there is also considerable interindividual variation. Elimination half-lives of 63–190 h have been reported, again dependent upon the formulation.

TOXICITY AND SIDE EFFECTS

It is well tolerated and no outstanding toxic effects have been reported.

CLINICAL USE

Treatment of uncomplicated *P. falciparum* and *P. vivax* malaria

A fixed-dose combination with artesunate (Pyramax) is being developed for uncomplicated *P. falciparum* and *P. vivax* malaria.

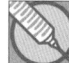

Preparations and dosage

Not widely available. Oral formulations have been used in China and in clinical trials in Thailand and Africa.

Further information

Auparakkitanon S, Chapoomram S, Kuaha K, Chirachariyavej T, Wilairat P. Targeting of hematin by the antimalarial pyronaridine. *Antimicrob Agents Chemother.* 2006;50:2197–2200.

Kurth F, Pongratz P, Bélard S, Mordmüller B, Kremsner PG, Ramharter M. *In vitro* activity of pyronaridine against *Plasmodium falciparum* and comparative evaluation of anti-malarial drug susceptibility assays. *Malar J.* 2009;8:79.

Vivas L, Rattray L, Stewart L, et al. Anti-malarial efficacy of pyronaridine and artesunate in combination *in vitro* and *in vivo. Acta Trop.* 2008;105:222–228.

SURAMIN

Molecular weight (hexasodium salt): 1429.21.

A sulfated naphthylamine formulated for intravenous administration. It is freely soluble in water. The dry powder is stable, but it is hygroscopic and unstable in solution.

ANTIMICROBIAL ACTIVITY

Suramin has no significant trypanocidal activity in vitro, but is effective in animals infected with *T. brucei*. Trypanosomes take up suramin bound to plasma protein by a combination of fluid phase and receptor-mediated endocytosis. It acts synergistically with nitroimidazoles and eflornithine in the elimination of trypanosomes from CSF of infected mice.

ACQUIRED RESISTANCE

Relapse rates of 30–50% have been recorded in Kenya and Tanzania but there is no evidence of resistant parasites. Stable resistance has been described in the related camel parasite *Trypanosoma evansi*.

PHARMACOKINETICS

Oral absorption	Poor
C_{max} 1 g intravenous doses (6 doses at weekly intervals)	100 mg/L
Plasma half-life	44–54 days
Volume of distribution	20–80 L
Plasma protein binding	>99%

It is normally administered by slow intravenous infusion. It can be detected in blood for 3 months; plasma levels >100 mg/L were observed for several weeks after a 6-week course of treatment. No metabolism was observed and 80% was removed by renal clearance. Distribution to mononuclear phagocytes, especially liver macrophages, the adrenal glands and the kidney is high. It does not enter erythrocytes and penetrates the blood–brain barrier poorly.

TOXICITY AND SIDE EFFECTS

Suramin is toxic, especially in malnourished patients. A test dose of 200 mg has been recommended. Immediate febrile reactions (nausea, vomiting, loss of consciousness) can be avoided by slow intravenous administration. Intramuscular or subcutaneous injections are painful and irritating, and can be followed by fever and urticaria. Anaphylactic shock occurs in fewer than 1 in 2000 patients. Delayed reactions include renal damage, exfoliative dermatitis, anemia, leukopenia, agranulocytosis, jaundice and diarrhea.

CLINICAL USE

African sleeping sickness (early stage before CNS involvement) Onchocerciasis

Preparations and dosage

Preparation: Injection.
Dosage: The dose schedule varies depending on the stage of the disease. Limited availability.

Further information

Amin DN, Masocha W, Ngan'dwe K, Rottenberg M, Kristensson K. Suramin and minocycline treatment of experimental African trypanosomiasis at an early stage of parasite brain invasion. *Acta Trop.* 2008;106:72–74.

Barrett MP, Boykin DW, Brun R, Tidwell RR. Human African trypanosomiasis: pharmacological re-engagement with a neglected disease. *Br J Pharmacol.* 2007;152:1155–1171.

Kaminsky R, Maser P. Drug resistance in African trypanosomes. *Curr Opin Anti Infect Investig Drugs.* 2000;2:76–82.

ANTIBACTERIAL AND OTHER ANTIMICROBIAL AGENTS USED FOR PROTOZOAL DISEASES

Properties of the diaminopyrimidines (Ch. 17), sulfonamides (Ch. 29) nitroimidazoles (Ch. 24) and nitrofurans (Ch. 31) that are used as antiprotozoal agents are described in the appropriate chapters. Among antibiotics, tetracyclines (Ch. 30), clindamycin (Ch. 21) and certain macrolides (Ch. 22) have a place in the treatment of some protozoal diseases, including malaria and toxoplasmosis. The aminoglycoside paromomycin (Ch. 12) is sometimes used in amebiasis, leishmaniasis and in intractable cryptosporidiosis.

Antifungal polyene and azole derivatives (Ch. 32) are increasingly used in diseases caused by protozoa. Both extracellular and intracellular forms of *Leishmania* spp. and *T. cruzi* are highly sensitive to amphotericin B in vitro at concentrations below 1 mg/L. Lipid formulations, in particular liposomal amphotericin B (p. 378), are highly effective in visceral leishmaniasis. Amphotericin B is also used for the treatment of primarily amebic meningoencephalitis caused by *Naegleria fowleri*.

The imidazoles miconazole and ketoconazole (p. 370) and the triazole itraconazole (p. 369) are active against *Leishmania* spp. and *T. cruzi* in experimental models, but results have been equivocal in clinical trials. The triazoles posaconazole (p. 371) and ravuconazole are effective against *T. cruzi* in experimental models and may be useful in the treatment of Chagas disease. The anthelmintic benzimidazole albendazole (p. 396) is effective in infections caused by *G. lamblia*.

Further information

Bern C, Adler-Moore J, Berenguer J, et al. Liposomal amphotericin B for the treatment of visceral leishmaniasis. *Clin Infect Dis*. 2006;43:917–924.

Dahl EL, Rosenthal PJ. Multiple antibiotics exert delayed effects against the *Plasmodium falciparum* apicoplast. *Antimicrob Agents Chemother*. 2007;51:3485–3490.

Davidson RN, den Boer M, Ritmeijer K. Paromomycin. *Trans R Soc Trop Med Hyg*. 2009;103:653–660.

Pukrittayakamee S, Clemens R, Chantra A, et al. Therapeutic responses to antibacterial drugs in vivax malaria. *Trans R Soc Trop Med Hyg*. 2001;95:524–528.

Sosa-Estani S, Segura EL. Etiological treatment in patients infected by *Trypanosoma cruzi*: experiences in Chagas' disease. *Curr Opin Infect Dis*. 2006;19:583–587.

Sundar S, Jha TK, Thakur CP, et al. Injectable paromomycin for visceral leishmaniasis in India. *N Engl J Med*. 2007;356:2571–2581.

Urbina JA. Ergosterol synthesis and drug development for Chagas' disease. *Memorias Instituto Oswaldo Cruz*. 2009;104:311–318.

CHAPTER

36 Antiretroviral agents

Mark Boyd and David A. Cooper

Recognition of the serious threat that the human immunodeficiency virus (HIV) presents to global health and security has stimulated an enormous investment in the development of anti-HIV therapies. This has occurred in parallel with advances in the understanding of HIV replication; in particular, the identification of steps in the replicative cycle that are unique to the virus and thus potential targets for chemotherapy (Figure 36.1).

The human immunodeficiency virus is a member of the lentivirus subfamily of human retroviruses with a double-stranded RNA genome encoding at least nine functional or regulatory proteins. There are several potential points at which the process of virus replication could be blocked:

- Entry into host-cell membranes
- Reverse-transcription of the virus genome
- Integration of virus into the host genome
- Virus assembly and maturation.

The use of combination antiretroviral therapy has resulted in significant and sustained reductions in morbidity and mortality in people with HIV infection, but no currently available therapy is curative. Once initiated, treatment is a lifelong commitment. Adverse effects and toxicities arise during long-term exposure but the causal relationship between individual drugs and specific adverse effects, and the degree to which HIV infection or immunodeficiency itself contributes to pathogenesis, continues to be difficult to define. Many other challenges remain, arising from drug interactions, problems of long-term adherence to therapy and drug resistance.

Because antiretroviral drugs act intracellularly, where relative concentrations are virtually impossible to predict or measure, little reliable information is available that relates plasma concentrations to in-vivo effectiveness. Clinical studies continue to attempt to determine the extent to which plasma drug level monitoring may be of clinical use in the treatment of HIV disease. Of all the available ART classes the

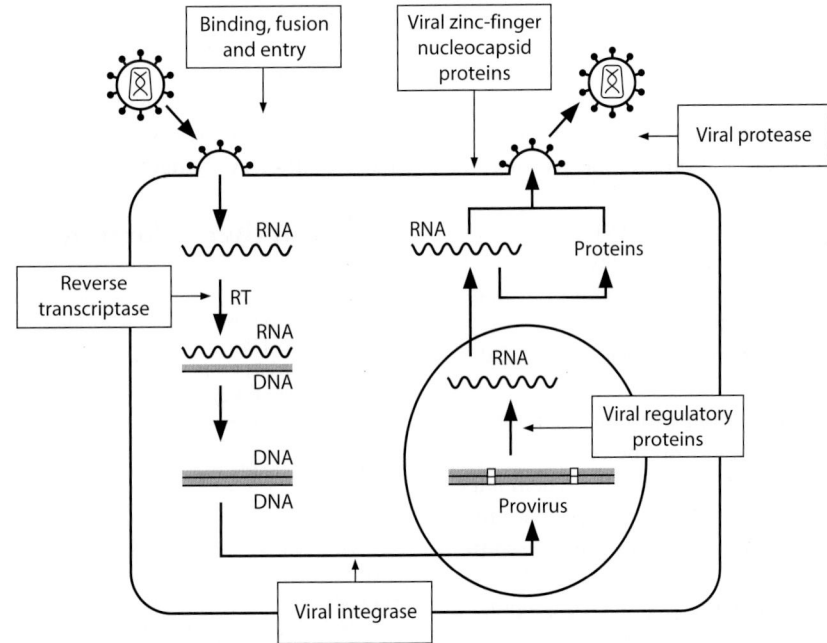

Fig. 36.1 Schematic representation of the HIV replicative cycle. Points at which antiretroviral therapies can inhibit virus replication are shown in boxed arrows.

most evidence exists for a possible role of therapeutic drug monitoring (TDM) in the management of HIV Protease Inhibitors (PIs) and Non-Nucleoside Reverse Transcriptase Inhibitors (NNRTIs). In the pharmacokinetic tables that accompany each drug in this chapter Cmin values for the PIs and NNRTIs have therefore been included.

Data on the human use of antiretroviral agents are mostly derived from developed countries in which HIV subtype B is most common. With the availability of cheap generic versions of antiretrovirals in low- and middle-income countries, data are emerging which suggest that other subtypes may be associated with different resistance pathways. Thus it seems that HIV subtype C is more likely to select for resistance to thymidine analogs through the K65R mutation. This bias in the database should be borne in mind when reading this chapter.

 Further information

Brown KC, Paul S, Kashuba AD. Drug interactions with new and investigational antiretrovirals. *Clin Pharmacokinet*. 2009;48:211–241.

Calmy A, Hirschel B, Cooper DA, Carr A. A new era of antiretroviral drug toxicity. *Antivir Ther*. 2009;14:165–179.

Letendre S, Marquie-Beck J, Capparelli E, et al. Validation of the CNS penetration–effectiveness rank for quantifying antiretroviral penetration into the central nervous system. *Arch Neurol*. 2008;65:65–70.

Martin AM, Nolan D, Gaudieri S, Phillips E, Mallal S. Pharmacogenetics of antiretroviral therapy: genetic variation of response and toxicity. *Pharmacogenomics*. 2004;5:643–655.

Orrell C, Walensky RP, Losina E, Pitt J, Freedberg KA, Wood R. HIV type-1 clade C resistance genotypes in treatment-naive patients and after first virological failure in a large community antiretroviral therapy programme. *Antivir Ther*. 2009;14:523–531.

http://www.hivpharmacology.com/
http://www.hiv-druginteractions.org/

CLASSIFICATION

Drugs that interfere with HIV replication are categorized into five types based on where in the HIV replicative cycle they exert inhibitory effects:

- Nucleoside reverse transcriptase inhibitors (NRTIs) and nucleotide reverse transcriptase inhibitors (N(t)RTIs) are analogs of naturally occurring deoxynucleotides and compete with them for incorporation into the growing viral DNA chain.
- Non-nucleoside reverse transcriptase inhibitors (NNRTIs) bind to a site distant to the catalytic site of reverse transcriptase, inhibiting the movement of protein domains required for DNA synthesis.
- HIV protease inhibitors block enzymic cleavage of HIV *gag–pol* proteins.
- HIV entry inhibitors prevent virion entry into cells in two ways: by preventing fusion with the cellular membrane; or as antagonists of one of the two chemokine co-receptors (CCR5 and CXCR4) that HIV attaches to in combination with the CD4 molecule to gain entry into the human cell.
- HIV integrase inhibitors block the enzyme responsible for incorporation of viral DNA into the host chromosome.

INTERACTIONS

HIV protease inhibitors, NNRTIs or CCR5 antagonists should not be co-administered with certain other drugs because of the potential for serious interactions or loss of efficacy. These interactions are described in detail at the US Department of Health and Human Services website (http://aidsinfo.nih.gov/contentfiles/AdultandAdolescentGL.pdf), which is updated regularly. Readers are also referred to the website of the Liverpool HIV Pharmacology Group at the University of Liverpool (http://www.hiv-druginteractions.org), another useful and frequently updated tool, and to Chapter 6 in this book.

NUCLEOSIDE REVERSE TRANSCRIPTASE INHIBITORS

NRTIs are dideoxynucleosides that undergo intracellular phosphorylation to yield triphosphates, which inhibit HIV-1 and HIV-2 replication.

In addition to sharing a common mode of action, these drugs have a number of overlapping toxicities that may arise through a common pathway. They inhibit some mammalian DNA polymerases, in particular those found exclusively within mitochondria. Interference with mitochondrial replication and function is likely to be a mechanism through which several significant toxicities, including fatal and non-fatal cases of lactic acidosis with hepatomegaly, are mediated. Laboratory investigations indicate that the potency of this class of drugs for inhibition of cellular DNA polymerases is: zalcitabine ≥didanosine ≥stavudine >zidovudine >abacavir =tenofovir =lamivudine =emtricitabine.

Resistance is well described, often associated with failure of combination therapy to control viral replication. Resistant isolates may show varying degrees of cross-resistance to other drugs within the class, and a switch to an apparently active alternative drug(s) within the class can be accompanied by selection of highly resistant variants at the cost of only minimal evolutionary changes to the virus.

 Further information

Brinkmann K, ter Hofstede HJM, Burger DM, et al. Adverse effects of reverse transcriptase inhibitors: mitochondrial toxicity as a common pathway. *AIDS*. 1998;12:1735–1744.

Brinkmann K, Smeitink JA, Romjin JA, Reiss P. Mitochondrial toxicity induced by nucleoside analogue reverse transcriptase inhibitors is a key factor in the pathogenesis of antiretroviral therapy related lipodystrophy. *Lancet*. 1999;354:1112–1115.

Clavel F, Hance AJ. HIV drug resistance. *N Engl J Med*. 2004;350:1023–1035.

Johnson VA, Brun-Vézinet F, Clotet B, et al. Update of the drug resistance mutations in HIV-1: December 2008. *Top HIV Med*. 2008;16:138–145.

Lewis W, Dalakas MC. Mitochondrial toxicity of antiviral drugs. *Nat Med*. 1995;1:417–421.

Moyle GJ, Datta D, Mandalia S, Morlese J, Asboe D, Gazzard BG. Hyperlactataemia and lactic acidosis during antiretroviral therapy: relevance, reproducibility and possible risk factors. *AIDS*. 2002;16:1341–1349 Erratum in: AIDS 2002; 16: 1708.

ABACAVIR

Molecular weight: 670.76.

A synthetic analog of guanine formulated for oral use.

ANTIVIRAL ACTIVITY

Abacavir has activity against HIV-1, HIV-2 and human T-cell lymphotrophic virus type-1 (HTLV-1).

ACQUIRED RESISTANCE

Resistance is associated with specific changes in codons 184 with 65, 74 or 115 in the HIV reverse transcriptase codon region.

PHARMACOKINETICS

Oral absorption	83%
C_{max} 300 mg oral twice daily	3.0 ± 0.89 mg/L
600 mg once daily	4.26 mg/L
Plasma half-life	1.5 h
Volume of distribution	0.8 L/kg
Plasma protein binding	c. 49%

Absorption

After oral administration abacavir sulfate undergoes rapid and extensive absorption unaffected by food.

Distribution

It penetrates well into the cerebrospinal fluid (CSF) and is an NRTI of choice if this characteristic is thought desirable. Good penetration into the male genital tract has been observed. The drug is secreted into human breast milk.

Metabolism

It is primarily metabolized in the liver, mainly by alcohol dehydrogenase and glucuronidation.

Excretion

Around 83% of the dose is eliminated in the urine, <2% as unchanged drug; the remainder is excreted in the feces.

Dose adjustment is unnecessary in renal impairment. It can be used in moderate hepatic impairment, but is contraindicated if dysfunction is severe.

TOXICITY AND SIDE EFFECTS

Life-threatening hypersensitivity reactions occur in 5–8% of all individuals, necessitating discontinuation of the drug. Typically patients present within the first 6 weeks of starting treatment with fever, rash or other symptoms that worsen in severity with continued drug exposure. Hypersensitivity is associated with carriage of the major histocompatibility complex class I allele HLA-B57*01 and screening for this allele can significantly reduce the incidence of this effect.

Current or recent (within the preceding 6 months) use of abacavir has been associated with a risk of myocardial infarction, but studies have yielded conflicting data.

CLINICAL USE

Treatment of HIV infection in adults and children (in combination with other antiretroviral drugs)

Preparations and dosage

Proprietary name: Ziagen.

Preparations: Tablets (300 and 600 mg), oral solution (20 mg/mL). The oral solution contains sorbitol, which is metabolized to fructose and is unsuitable for patients with hereditary fructose intolerance.

Dosage: Adults, oral, 300 mg every 12 h or 600 mg once daily. Children target dosing range: 8–10 mg/kg per dose every 12 h (maximum dose, 300 mg every 12 h).

Available alone, in combination with lamivudine, and in combination with zidovudine and lamivudine.

Further information

D:A:D Study Group. Use of nucleoside reverse transcriptase inhibitors and risk of myocardial infarction in HIV-infected patients enrolled in the D:A:D study: a multi-cohort collaboration. *Lancet.* 2008;371:1417–1426. Erratum in: *Lancet* 372: 292.

Mallal S, Phillips E, Carosi G, et al. HLA-B*5701 screening for hypersensitivity to abacavir. *N Engl J Med.* 2008;358:568–579.

DIDANOSINE

Molecular weight: 236.2.

An analog of deoxyadenosine, formulated for oral administration.

ANTIVIRAL ACTIVITY

Didanosine is active against HIV-1, HIV-2 and HTLV-1.

ACQUIRED RESISTANCE

Codon changes at positions 65 or 74 in HIV reverse transcriptase are associated with reduced susceptibility.

PHARMACOKINETICS

Oral absorption	c. 40%
Cmax 400 mg once daily	0.93 mg/L
Plasma half-life	c. 1.4 h
Volume of distribution	c. 1 L/kg
Plasma protein binding	<5%

Absorption

Bioavailability is reduced by about half when taken with food and the drug should be given at least 30 min before a meal. The peak plasma concentration achieved by enteric-coated tablets is less than half that of buffered tablets.

Distribution

Central nervous system (CNS) penetration is relatively poor. Median concentrations in semen (455 ng/mL; range <50–2190 ng/mL) are greater than those in blood (<50 ng/mL; range <50–860 ng/mL). It is secreted in breast milk.

Metabolism

Based upon animal studies it is presumed that metabolism occurs by the pathways responsible for the elimination of endogenous purines by xanthine oxidase. Metabolism may be altered in patients with severe hepatic impairment; however, no specific dose adjustment is recommended.

Excretion

Renal clearance by glomerular filtration and active tubular secretion accounts for 50% of total body clearance. Urinary recovery accounts for about 20% of the oral dose in adults. The half-life increases three-fold in patients requiring dialysis. Patients with a creatinine clearance <60 mL/min may be at greater risk of toxicity.

TOXICITY AND SIDE EFFECTS

Most serious are pancreatitis (fatal and non-fatal), lactic acidosis and severe hepatomegaly with steatosis (fatal and non-fatal), retinopathy, optic neuritis and dose-related peripheral neuropathy. Patients with low body weight may require dose modification. A strong association with non-cirrhotic portal hypertension has been described.

The combination with stavudine should be avoided in pregnant women as fatal cases of lactic acidosis have been reported. Caution should also be exercised in patients with known risk factors for liver disease. Therapy should be stopped in patients who develop clinical or laboratory evidence of lactic acidosis or hepatotoxicity. Monitoring lactate levels prospectively is not recommended as mild hyperlactatemia occurs in asymptomatic patients and has a poor positive predictive value for the development of lactic acidosis.

Caution should be exercised in co-administering other drugs with known neurotoxicity and in patients with a history of neuropathy. Treatment should stop if symptoms and signs of neuropathy are observed, but the condition is usually reversible and patients with resolved neuropathy may be retreated at a reduced dosage. Retinal depigmentation has been observed in children and twice-yearly dilated retinal examination is recommended.

CLINICAL USE

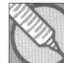

Treatment of HIV infection (in combination with other antiretroviral drugs)

Preparations and dosage

Proprietary name: Videx.

Preparations: Enteric-coated capsules (125, 200, 250 and 400 mg). Also available as tablets (25, 50, 100, 150 and 200 mg) and as a powder for reconstitution.

Dosage: Adults, oral, 400 mg once daily (weight ≥60 kg) or 250 mg once daily (weight <60 kg). Children <3 months, 50 mg/m² per dose every 12 h; children >3 months, 120 mg/m² per dose every 12 h. Children 20–<25 kg, 200 mg once daily; 25–<60 kg, 250 mg once daily; ≥60 kg, 400 mg once daily. For patients <20 kg the recommended dose is based on age and body surface area: children aged 2 weeks–8 months should receive 100 mg/m² every 12 h; those older than 8 months should receive 120 mg/m² every 12 h.

Widely available.

Further information

Carr A, Amin J. Efficacy and tolerability of initial antiretroviral therapy: a systematic review. *AIDS*. 2009;23:343–353.

Kovari H, Ledergerber B, Peter U, et al. Association of noncirrhotic portal hypertension in HIV-infected persons and antiretroviral therapy with didanosine: a nested case-control study. *Clin Infect Dis*. 2009;49:626–635.

Lactic Acidosis International Study Group. Risk factors for lactic acidosis and severe hyperlactataemia in HIV-1-infected adults exposed to antiretroviral therapy. *AIDS*. 2007;21:2455–2464.

Moreno S, Hernández B, Dronda F. Didanosine enteric-coated capsule: current role in patients with HIV-1 infection. *Drugs*. 2007;67:1441–1462.

EMTRICITABINE

Molecular weight: 247.2.

A synthetic nucleoside analog of cytosine, formulated for oral use.

 ANTIVIRAL ACTIVITY

Emtricitabine is active against HIV-1, HIV-2 and hepatitis B virus (HBV).

 ACQUIRED RESISTANCE

Resistance is associated with a substitution in the HIV-1 reverse transcriptase gene at codon 184 (M184V/I). Emtricitabine-resistant isolates are cross-resistant to lamivudine. HIV-1 isolates with the K65R substitution in the reverse transcriptase coding region have reduced susceptibility.

 PHARMACOKINETICS

Oral absorption: capsules	93%
C_{max} 200 mg oral once daily	1.8 ± 0.7 mg/L
Plasma half-life	c. 10 h
Volume of distribution	1.4 ± 0.3 L/kg
Plasma protein binding	<4%

Absorption and distribution

It is rapidly and extensively absorbed. There is moderate CNS penetration. The estimated semen:plasma ratio is approximately 4. There are presently no data on levels in breast milk.

Metabolism and excretion

It does not inhibit human cytochrome P_{450} enzymes. About 80% is excreted in the urine, the rest in feces. Renal clearance is greater than the estimated creatinine clearance, suggesting elimination by both glomerular filtration and active tubular secretion. There may be competition for elimination with other compounds that are renally excreted. Exposure is significantly increased in renal insufficiency, but dose reductions are not generally recommended. It is unlikely that a dose adjustment would be required in the presence of hepatic impairment.

 TOXICITY AND SIDE EFFECTS

At least 10% of patients suffer headache, diarrhea, nausea, fatigue, dizziness, depression, insomnia, abnormal dreams, rash, abdominal pain, asthenia, increased cough and rhinitis. Skin hyperpigmentation is common (≥10%) in pediatric patients. Emtricitabine competes with lamivudine for the enzymes involved in intracellular phosphorylation; their co-administration is contraindicated.

 CLINICAL USE

Treatment of HIV infection (in combination with other antiretroviral drugs)

 Preparations and dosages

Proprietary name: Emtriva.

Preparations: Capsules (200 mg), oral solution (240 mg/24 mL).

Dosage: Adults: one 200 mg capsule or 24 mL solution orally once daily. Children, 0–3 months, 3 mg/kg oral solution once daily; 3 months–17 years, 6 mg/kg up to a maximum of 240 mg (24 mL); children weighing >33 kg who can swallow an intact capsule, 4.8–6 mg/kg once daily or one 200 mg capsule once daily.

Available alone, in combination with tenofovir, and in combination with tenofovir and efavirenz.

 Further information

Anderson PL. Recent developments in the clinical pharmacology of anti-HIV nucleoside analogs. *Curr Opin HIV AIDS*. 2008;3:258–265.

Saag MS. Emtricitabine, a new antiretroviral agent with activity against HIV and hepatitis B virus. *Clin Infect Dis*. 2006;42:126–131.

LAMIVUDINE

Molecular weight: 229.3.

An analog of cytidine available for oral administration.

ANTIVIRAL ACTIVITY

Lamivudine is active against HIV-1, HIV-2, HBV and HTLV-1.

ACQUIRED RESISTANCE

A single codon change at position 184 in the HIV reverse transcriptase gene confers high-level resistance. The K65R mutation is also associated with resistance. In-vitro data indicate that lamivudine resistance may restore HIV sensitivity to zidovudine- and tenofovir-resistant virus.

PHARMACOKINETICS

Oral absorption	80–85%
C_{max}, 300 mg once daily	2.0 mg/L
Plasma half-life	5–7 h
Volume of distribution	1.3 L/kg
Plasma protein binding	<36%

Absorption

It is rapidly absorbed and there is no significant difference in bioavailability when taken with food.

Distribution

It penetrates moderately well into the CNS. The semen:plasma ratio is about 9.1 (2.3–16.1). It is secreted into breast milk.

Metabolism and excretion

Less than 10% of the administered dose undergoes hepatic metabolism. Over 70% of the dose is subject to renal clearance via active tubular secretion. Dosage adjustments are not routinely recommended in the presence of renal or hepatic impairment.

TOXICITY AND SIDE EFFECTS

Lamivudine is relatively safe and non-toxic. Animal studies of very high doses did not result in any organ toxicity. In patients co-infected with HIV and HBV, cessation of lamivudine therapy may result in clinical and/or laboratory evidence of recurrent hepatic disease that may be more severe in patients with hepatic decompensation. Tests of liver function and inflammation and markers of HBV replication should be periodically monitored.

Lamivudine competes with emtricitabine for the enzymes involved in intracellular phosphorylation and co-administration is contraindicated.

> Treatment of HIV infection (in combination with other antiretroviral drugs)
> Treatment of hepatitis B infection

Preparations and dosage

Proprietary name: Epivir.

Preparations: Tablets (150 and 300 mg). Also available as an oral solution (10 mg/mL) and as granules (25 and 50 mg).

Dosage: Adults, oral, 150 mg every 12 h or 300 mg once daily.
Children target dosing range: 4 mg/kg every 12 h (maximum dose, 300 mg per day).

Available alone, in combination with zidovudine, and in combination with zidovudine and abacavir. Various combinations with other antiretrovirals are available in generic formulations.

Lower doses are used in hepatitis B therapy.

Further information

Carr A, Amin J. Efficacy and tolerability of initial antiretroviral therapy: a systematic review. *AIDS*. 2009;23:343–353.

Perry CM, Faulds D. Lamivudine: a review of its antiviral activity, pharmacokinetic properties and therapeutic efficacy in the management of HIV infection. *Drugs*. 1997;54:657–680.

STAVUDINE

Molecular weight: 224.2.

An analog of thymidine formulated for oral administration.

ANTIVIRAL ACTIVITY

Stavudine is active against HIV-1, HIV-2 and HTLV-1.

ACQUIRED RESISTANCE

Resistance to stavudine is identical to that seen for zidovudine. Mutations at positions 41, 67 and 70, and positions 210, 215 and 219 (the 'thymidine analog mutations') of the reverse transcriptase genes are associated with diminished antiretroviral efficacy.

PHARMACOKINETICS

Oral absorption	86%
C_{max} 40 mg twice daily	0.54 mg/L
Plasma half-life	1.4 h
Volume of distribution	0.66 L/kg
Plasma protein binding	<5%

Absorption and distribution

It is rapidly absorbed with or without food. CNS penetration is moderate. The estimated semen:plasma ratio is >1. It is secreted into breast milk.

Metabolism and excretion

The metabolic fate in humans has not been elucidated. Renal elimination accounts for approximately 40% of overall clearance at a rate almost twice that of endogenous creatinine, indicating glomerular filtration and active tubular secretion.

Clearance decreases as creatinine clearance decreases and the dosage should be adjusted in patients with reduced renal function. Pharmacokinetics are not significantly altered in patients with hepatic impairment.

TOXICITY AND ADVERSE EFFECTS

Toxicity includes peripheral neuropathy, lactic acidosis, hepatomegaly with steatosis and liver failure, lipoatrophy and pancreatitis. Combination therapy with didanosine results in higher frequency of these toxicities, and fatalities have been reported in pregnant women. The use of the two drugs in combination is no longer recommended. It competes with zidovudine for the same intracellular phosphorylating enzymes and co-administration is contraindicated.

CLINICAL USE

Treatment of HIV infection in adults and children

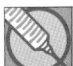

Preparations and dosage

Proprietary name: Zerit.

Preparations: Capsules (15, 20, 30 and 40 mg). Also available as a powder (1 mg/mL) for reconstitution and in granules (5 and 10 mg).

Dosage: Adults weighing at least 60 kg, oral, 40 mg every 12 h. Adults weighing <60 kg, 30 mg every 12 h. The World Health Organization (WHO) recommends the use of 30 mg every 12 h in adults and adolescents regardless of body weight. Children target dosing range: 1 mg/kg per dose every 12 h.

Available in various dual or triple combinations from generic manufacturers.

Further information

Anonymous. Stavudine. In: Dollery C, ed. *Therapeutic Drugs*. 2nd ed. Edinburgh: Churchill Livingstone; 1999:S94–S98.

Hill A, Ruxrungtham K, Hanvanich M, et al. Systematic review of clinical trials evaluating low doses of stavudine as part of antiretroviral treatment. *Expert Opin Pharmacother*. 2007;8:679–688.

Lea AP, Faulds D. Stavudine: a review of its pharmacodynamic and pharmacokinetic properties and clinical potential in HIV infection. *Drugs*. 1996;51:846–864.

ZIDOVUDINE

Molecular weight: 267.2.

An analog of thymidine formulated for oral or intravenous use.

ANTIVIRAL ACTIVITY

Zidovudine is active against HIV-1, HIV-2 and HTLV-1.

ACQUIRED RESISTANCE

As with stavudine, mutations at position 41, 67 and 70, and positions 210, 215 and 219 (the 'thymidine analog mutations') of the reverse transcriptase genes are associated with diminished antiretroviral efficacy.

PHARMACOKINETICS

Oral absorption	65%
C_{max} 300 mg twice daily	2.3 mg/L
Plasma half-life	1.1 h
Volume of distribution	1.6 L/kg
Plasma protein binding	34–38%

Absorption and distribution

It is absorbed rapidly and almost completely following oral administration. Absorption is not significantly affected by food. It appears to undergo widespread body distribution. CNS penetration is fairly good. The semen:plasma ratio varies from 0.95 to 13.5 (mean 5.9). It is secreted into breast milk.

Metabolism and excretion

Following hepatic metabolism (glucuronidation), elimination is primarily renal. After oral administration, urinary recovery of zidovudine and its glucuronide metabolite accounted for 14% and 74% respectively of the dose, with a total urinary recovery of 90%.

In severe renal impairment, clearance was about half that reported in subjects with normal renal function Accumulation may occur in patients with hepatic impairment due to decreased glucuronidation.

TOXICITY AND ADVERSE EFFECTS

In common with other drugs in this class, use has been associated with episodes of fatal and non-fatal lactic acidosis and hepatomegaly with steatosis. Careful clinical evaluation is needed in patients with evidence of hepatic abnormality. Myelosuppression may occur within the first 4–6 weeks of therapy. Hematological parameters should be monitored during this period, with prompt dose modification or switch if abnormalities are observed. Treatment with reduced doses may be attempted in some patients once bone marrow recovery has been observed. Myopathy is rarely seen with the use of the current dosing regimens.

Co-administration with drugs known to cause nephrotoxicity, cytotoxicity or which interfere with red or white blood cell number and function may increase the risk of toxicity.

Probenecid and trimethoprim may reduce renal clearance of zidovudine, and other drugs that are metabolized by glucuronidation may interfere with its metabolism.

CLINICAL USE

Treatment of HIV infection in adults and children (in combination with other antiretroviral drugs)

Reduction of maternal transmission of HIV to the fetus

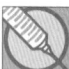

Preparations and dosage

Proprietary name: Retrovir.

Preparations: Capsules (100 and 250 mg), tablets (300 mg), syrup (10 mg/mL), granules (25 and 50 mg), injection.

Dosage: Adults, oral, 500–600 mg per day in two divided doses. The optimal dose in children has not been established, although a dose of 180–240 mg/m²/dose every 12 h has been advocated by some investigators.

Available alone, in combination with lamivudine, and in combination with lamivudine and abacavir. Various combinations with other antiretrovirals are available in generic formulations.

Further information

Anonymous. Zidovudine. In: Dollery C, ed. *Therapeutic Drugs*. 2nd ed. Edinburgh: Churchill Livingstone; 1999:Z12–Z18.

Volmink J, Siegfried NL, van der Merwe L, Brocklehurst P. Antiretrovirals for reducing the risk of mother-to-child transmission of HIV infection. *Cochrane Database Syst Rev*. 2007;(1): CD003510.

NUCLEOTIDE ANALOGS

Nucleotides are monophosphorylated derivatives of nucleosides. Phosphorylation of nucleosides normally occurs within the cytoplasm of cells entering mitotic division and represents the rate-limiting step in the synthesis of bases for addition to growing nucleic acid chains. Nucleotides are actively taken up by most cells irrespective of the stage in the cell cycle. Several such drugs have been synthesized and some have activity against HIV reverse transcriptase. They also inhibit mitochondrial DNA polymerases.

TENOFOVIR

Molecular weight (disoproxil fumarate salt): 635.5.

An acyclic nucleoside phosphonate, formulated as the disoproxil fumarate salt for oral administration.

ANTIVIRAL ACTIVITY

Tenofovir is effective against simian immunodeficiency virus (SIV), HIV-1, HIV-2, HBV and HTLV-1.

ACQUIRED RESISTANCE

HIV variants with the K65R mutation and the K70E mutation in the reverse transcriptase demonstrate reduced susceptibility to tenofovir.

PHARMACOKINETICS

Oral absorption	c. 25%
C_{max} 300 mg once daily	0.3 mg/L
Plasma half-life	17 h
Volume of distribution	1.3 ± 0.6 L/kg at 3.0 mg/kg intravenous dose
Plasma protein binding	<0.7% (in vitro)

Absorption and distribution

Oral bioavailability is poor, but is enhanced by administration as the disoproxil prodrug. It may be taken with or without food. CSF penetration is likely to be minimal due to the anionic charge of the molecule at physiological pH. It accumulates in semen at higher concentrations than in plasma. It is not known if it is distributed into breast milk.

Metabolism and excretion

Tenofovir is not metabolized and is principally eliminated by the kidneys by a combination of glomerular filtration and active tubular secretion. In patients with renal dysfunction the dose should be adjusted accordingly.

Compounds such as cidofovir, aciclovir (acyclovir), valaciclovir, ganciclovir, valganciclovir and probenecid may compete for renal excretion. Tenofovir levels are increased when prescribed with some HIV protease inhibitors. The co-administration of tenofovir with didanosine leads to didanosine accumulation which is thought to occur through inhibition of purine nucleoside phosphorylase. This has been associated with impaired immune recovery and several cases of lactic acidosis and pancreatitis. If tenofovir is combined with didanosine the dose of didanosine should be reduced to 200 mg (<60 kg) or 250 mg (≥60 kg) per day and the patient monitored for symptoms of didanosine toxicity.

TOXICITY AND SIDE EFFECTS

In clinical trials of antiretroviral treatment-naive participants, the most commonly reported adverse events were mild to moderate gastrointestinal upset (nausea 8%, diarrhea 11%), headache (14%) and depression (11%). Tenofovir has the potential to result in nephrotoxicity, particularly through proximal tubular damage, but the risk of clinically significant renal dysfunction appears relatively low and seems to occur mainly in subjects with other identifiable risks for renal impairment. Minor elevations in serum creatinine and reductions in creatinine clearance occur, but rarely require drug discontinuation.

A few (<0.1%) cases of osteomalacia and decreased bone density have been reported.

CLINICAL USE

Treatment of HIV infection in adults and children (in combination with other antiretroviral drugs)

Preparations and dosages

Proprietary name: Viread.

Preparation: Tablets (300 mg).

Dosage: Adults, oral, 300 mg per day in a single daily dose.

Available alone, in combination with emtricitabine, and in combination with emtricitabine and efavirenz.

Further information

Carr A, Amin J. Efficacy and tolerability of initial antiretroviral therapy: a systematic review. *AIDS*. 2009;23:343–353.

Matthews G. Tenofovir disoproxil fumarate. In: Kucers' *The Use of Antibiotics*. A clinical review of antibacterial, antifungal and antiviral drugs. Grayson ML, Kucers A, Crowe SM, et al. eds. 6th ed. London: Hodder Arnold; 2010.

Pozniak A. Tenofovir: what have over 1 million years of patient experience taught us? *Int J Clin Pract*. 2008;62:1285–1293.

NON-NUCLEOSIDE REVERSE TRANSCRIPTASE INHIBITORS

This group of structurally unrelated compounds selectively inhibits HIV-1 reverse transcriptase through allosteric inhibition following binding to the enzyme at regions remote from the active site. The unique mechanism of action results in a pattern of resistance distinct from other antiretroviral drug classes.

These drugs can inhibit or induce cytochrome P_{450} isozymes. As a consequence, use with several medications is contraindicated or cautioned. Importantly, nevirapine and efavirenz can reduce methadone concentrations by up to half, resulting in clinical features of opiate withdrawal that require careful management.

Further information

Brown KC, Paul S, Kashuba DM. Drug interactions with new and investigational antiretrovirals. *Clin Pharmacokinet.* 2009;48:211–241.

Waters L, John L, Nelson M. Non-nucleoside reverse transcriptase inhibitors: a review. *Int J Clin Pract.* 2007;1:105–118.

DELAVIRDINE

Molecular weight: 552.68.

A complex piperazine derivative, formulated for oral administration.

ANTIVIRAL ACTIVITY

Delavirdine is active against HIV-1 but not HIV-2.

ACQUIRED RESISTANCE

The predominant amino acid substitution associated with resistance is at position 236 of the HIV reverse transcriptase.

PHARMACOKINETICS

Oral absorption	Not known/available
C_{max} 400 mg oral thrice daily	c. 19.3 mg/L
C_{min} 400 mg oral thrice daily	c. 8.3 mg/L
Plasma half-life	c. 6 h
Volume of distribution	c. 0.7 L/kg
Plasma protein binding	c. 98%

Absorption and distribution

It is rapidly absorbed following oral administration. Food has no significant effect on absorption. It is distributed predominantly into blood plasma and CNS penetration is poor.

The semen:plasma ratio is about 0.02. It is not known if it is distributed into breast milk.

Metabolism and excretion

Several metabolites are formed by the CYP3A4 isoform of cytochrome P_{450} and it is a potent inhibitor of this enzyme system. Around 44% of the drug is recovered in feces and 51% in urine, about 5% as unchanged drug. Given the predominant hepatic metabolism, caution should be exercised in patients with impaired hepatic function.

TOXICITY AND SIDE EFFECTS

Around 18% of patients experience a diffuse, maculopapular, erythematous and often pruritic rash. Dose titration does not appear to reduce the incidence of this side effect. The rash usually first appears within 1 month of commencing therapy and resolves within 2 weeks without dose modification. In about 4% of cases it is severe enough to warrant discontinuation of treatment.

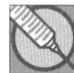

CLINICAL USE

Treatment of HIV disease in adults and children over 12 years of age (in combination with other antiretroviral agents)

Delavirdine has fallen out of favor with the increasing preference for antiretrovirals than can be dosed twice or once daily.

Preparations and dosage

Proprietary name: Rescriptor.

Preparation: Tablets (100 and 200 mg).

Dosage: Adults, oral, 400 mg every 8 h.

Widely available.

Further information

Scott LJ, Perry CM. Delavirdine: a review of its use in HIV infection. *Drugs.* 2000;60:1411–1444.

EFAVIRENZ

Molecular weight: 315.68.

A synthetic heterocyclic compound formulated for oral administration.

ANTIVIRAL ACTIVITY

Efavirenz is active against HIV-1 but not HIV-2.

ACQUIRED RESISTANCE

One or more single-codon substitutions in the HIV reverse transcriptase genome at positions 100, 103, 106, 108, 181, 188, 190 and 225 confer reduced susceptibility. Many, but not all, of these point mutations confer reduced susceptibility to other non-nucleoside reverse transcriptase inhibitors.

PHARMACOKINETICS

Oral absorption	Not known/available
C_{max} 600 mg oral once daily	c. 4.07 mg/L
C_{min} 600 mg oral once daily	c. 1.77 mg/L
Plasma half-life	c. 45 h
Volume of distribution	c. 2.4 L/kg
Plasma protein binding	>99%

Absorption and distribution

Bioavailability following a standard high-fat meal was increased by an average of 50%, but was unaffected by a standard meal. Distribution into body tissues and fluids has not been fully characterized. It penetrates moderately well into the CNS. The semen:plasma ratio is 0.09 (0.03–0.43). The mean concentration in breast milk is 3.51 mg/L; significant linear correlations have been found between maternal plasma and breast milk.

Metabolism and excretion

It is metabolized by cytochrome P_{450} systems to hydroxylated intermediates and excreted after subsequent glucuronidation. Metabolites are not active against HIV.

It is excreted principally in the feces, both as metabolites and unchanged drug. Up to 34% is recovered in the urine, <1% as unchanged drug. Given this, the impact of renal impairment on efavirenz is likely to be minimal. Caution is recommended in patients with mild–moderate liver disease; it is contraindicated in patients with severe hepatic impairment.

Dose adjustment is unnecessary when it is co-administered with HIV protease inhibitors or rifampicin (rifampin).

TOXICITY AND SIDE EFFECTS

The most common (>5%, moderate–severe) adverse effects associated with efavirenz therapy are rash, dizziness, nausea, headache, fatigue, insomnia and vomiting. Rash occurs in up to 26% of patients, mostly in the first 2 weeks of therapy. It usually resolves within 1 month, but is sufficiently severe to limit treatment in a few cases.

Dizziness, insomnia, somnolence, impaired concentration, abnormal dreaming and other CNS disturbances have been reported in around 52% of clinical trial participants, with events of moderate to severe intensity occurring in about 3% of patients. Rare (0.2% of patients) episodes of severe delusional or inappropriate behavior and severe acute depression have also been reported. The symptoms commonly begin in the first 2 weeks of treatment but often resolve or substantially improve within a month.

Elevations in serum hepatic transaminase to levels more than five times the upper limit of normal are observed in about 3% of patients and 8% of those co-infected with viral hepatitis B or C.

CLINICAL USE

Treatment of HIV-1 infection in adults and children (in combination with other antiretroviral drugs)

Preparations and dosage

Proprietary names: Stocrin, Sustiva.

Preparations: Capsules (50, 100, 200 and 600 mg), oral solution (30 mg/mL).

Dosage: Adults, oral, 600 mg once a day. Children target dosing range: 15–18.75 mg/kg solid form or 19.5 mg/kg syrup given once daily. Dosage has not been established for children <3 years. In order to alleviate some of the CNS side effects it is recommended the daily dose be taken at bedtime.

Available alone or in combination with tenofovir and emtricitabine, zidovudine and lamivudine, and stavudine and lamivudine.

Further information

Riddler SA, Haubrich R, DiRienzo AG, et al. Class-sparing regimens for initial treatment of HIV-1 infection. *N Engl J Med.* 2008;358:2095–2106.

van Leth F, Phanuphak P, Ruxrungtham K, et al. Comparison of first-line antiretroviral therapy with regimens including nevirapine, efavirenz, or both drugs, plus stavudine and lamivudine: a randomised open-label trial, the 2NN Study. *Lancet.* 2004;363:1253–1263.

Vrouenraets SM, Wit FW, van Tongeren J, Lange JM. Efavirenz: a review. *Expert Opin Pharmacother.* 2007;8:851–871.

ETRAVIRINE

Molecular weight: 435.31.

A comprehensive analysis of baseline resistance data from the DUET-1 and DUET-2 studies has identified a list of 17 etravirine resistance associated mutations: V901, A98G, L100L, K101E/H/I, V1061, E138A, V179D/F/T, Y181C/L/V, G190A/S, and M230L. A single K103N mutation is not associated with resistance to etravirine.

ANTIVIRAL ACTIVITY

Etravirine is active only against HIV-1.

ACQUIRED RESISTANCE

Various mutations are associated with a decreased virological response. Single codon substitutions at positions 100, 101 and 181 are considered major mutations. A single K103N mutation is not associated with resistance.

PHARMACOKINETICS

Oral absorption	Not known/available
C_{max} 200 mg oral twice daily	c. 959 ng/mL
C_{min} 200 mg oral twice daily	c. 469 ng/mL
Plasma half-life	c. 36 h
Volume of distribution	Not known/available
Plasma protein binding	>99%

Administration with food improves the bioavailability and reduces interpatient variability. It undergoes oxidative metabolism by cytochrome P_{450} systems. Around 93.7% and 1.2% of an administered dose can be retrieved in the feces and urine, respectively, mostly as unchanged drug.

Details of distribution into CSF, semen and breast milk and recommendations for dose adjustment in patients with hepatic impairment are not yet available.

TOXICITY AND SIDE EFFECTS

In the phase III studies around 15% of patients experienced erythematous or maculopapular rashes of mild or moderate severity; most resolved with continued dosing, but treatment was discontinued in 2% of patients. Rare cases of Stevens–Johnson syndrome have been reported.

Other common adverse events are diarrhea, nausea, headache and fatigue. Dyslipidemia and raised pancreatic amylase occur in some patients.

CLINICAL USE

Treatment of HIV-1 infection in adults (in combination with other antiretroviral drugs)

Preparations and dosage

Proprietary name: Intelence.
Preparation: Tablets (100 mg).
Dosage: Adults, oral, 200 mg every 12 h.
Widely available.

Safety and efficacy in children and adolescents are not yet established.

Further information

Deeks ED, Keating GM. Etravirine. *Drugs*. 2008;68:2357–2372.
Lazzarin A, Campbell T, Clotet B, et al. Efficacy and safety of TMC125 (etravirine) in treatment-experienced HIV-1-infected patients in DUET-2: 24-week results from a randomised, double-blind, placebo-controlled trial. *Lancet*. 2007;370:39–48.
Madruga JV, Cahn P, Grinsztejn B, et al. Efficacy and safety of TMC125 (etravirine) in treatment-experienced HIV-1-infected patients in DUET-1: 24-week results from a randomised, double-blind, placebo-controlled trial. *Lancet*. 2007;370:29–38.

NEVIRAPINE

Molecular weight (anhydrous): 266.3.

A synthetic heterocyclic compound formulated for oral use as anhydrous compound or as the hemihydrate in a liquid oral suspension.

ANTIVIRAL ACTIVITY

Nevirapine is active only against HIV-1.

ACQUIRED RESISTANCE

One or more changes within the HIV reverse transcriptase at amino acid positions 100, 103, 106, 108, 181, 188 and 190 are associated with resistance. These point mutations have also been implicated, either alone or in combination, in HIV resistance to other non-nucleoside reverse transcriptase inhibitors.

PHARMACOKINETICS

Oral absorption	*c.* 93%
C_{max} 200 mg twice daily	*c.* 5.74 mg/L
C_{min} 200 mg twice daily	*c.* 2.88 mg/L
Plasma half-life	*c.* 36 h
Volume of distribution	*c.* 1.21 L/kg
Plasma protein binding	*c.* 60%

Absorption and distribution

Nevirapine is orally very well absorbed and widely distributed. CNS penetration is good and the semen:plasma ratio is in the range of 0.6–1. It is distributed into breast milk.

Metabolism and excretion

It is extensively metabolized by cytochrome P_{450} enzymes into a number of hydroxylated intermediates that are subsequently conjugated with glucuronide.

Around 81% of the dose is excreted in urine (<5% as unchanged compound) and 10% in feces. There is no significant change in the pharmacokinetics in renal impairment. It is contraindicated in patients with severe hepatic impairment; caution should be exercised in patients with moderate hepatic dysfunction.

INTERACTIONS

Administration with boosted protease inhibitors does not require dose adjustment. Adjustment of methadone dose in patients experiencing narcotic withdrawal symptoms may be needed. Studies of the effect of rifampicin have yielded conflicting results. In general, efavirenz is preferred to nevirapine if possible.

TOXICITY AND SIDE EFFECTS

Life-threatening hepatic events, including fulminant hepatitis, have been observed in treatment-naive patients, generally within the first few weeks of treatment, but sometimes later. Approximately half the patients also develop skin rash, with or without fever or constitutional symptoms. Women with elevated CD4 counts (>250 cells/mm³) appear to be at highest risk. Men with pretreatment CD4 counts >400 cells/mm³ are also at increased risk. These risks exist in the absence of underlying hepatic abnormalities and, in some cases, hepatic injury continues to progress despite discontinuation of treatment. Treatment should stop, and not be restarted, in patients with clinical evidence of hepatitis. A starting dose of 200 mg per day, with escalation to full dose if no adverse reaction occurs, reduces the frequency of reaction. Single doses given to mothers or infants for prevention of perinatal HIV infection appear safe.

CLINICAL USE

Treatment of HIV-1 infection in adults and children over 2 months old (in combination with other antiretroviral therapies)
Reduction of maternal transmission of HIV to the fetus (recommended only for use in HIV-infected treatment-naive women in labor who have had no prior HIV therapy)

Preparations and dosage

Proprietary name: Viramune.

Preparations: Tablets (200 mg), oral suspension (10 mg/mL), granules (25 and 50 mg).

Dosage: Adults, oral, 200 mg once daily for the first 14 days, followed by 200 mg every 12 h or 400 mg once daily, in combination with other antiretroviral therapies. Children target dosing range: 150–200 mg/m² per dose every 12 h, with a reduced dose for the first 2 weeks.

Available alone or in combination in generic formulations with stavudine and lamivudine, and zidovudine and lamivudine.

Further information

Kesselring AM, Wit FW, Sabin CA, et al. Risk factors for treatment-limiting toxicities in patients starting nevirapine-containing antiretroviral therapy. *AIDS.* 2009;23:1689–1699.

Sheran M. The nonnucleoside reverse transcriptase inhibitors efavirenz and nevirapine in the treatment of HIV. *HIV Clin Trials.* 2005;6:158–168.

Volmink J, Siegfried NL, van der Merwe L, Brocklehurst P. Antiretrovirals for reducing the risk of mother-to-child transmission of HIV infection. *Cochrane Database Syst Rev.* 2007;(1):CD003510.

HIV PROTEASE INHIBITORS

Protease inhibitors are active against HIV-1 and HIV-2. As they have significant metabolic interactions, co-administration with many other drugs is either contraindicated or cautioned. Most also possess specific toxicities, some of which are treatment limiting. The extent to which protease inhibitors contribute to the lipodystrophy syndrome is debated, but they are associated with dyslipidemia, particularly when combined with low doses of ritonavir. Some early protease inhibitors (notably indinavir) have been associated with glucose intolerance, insulin resistance and diabetes mellitus, but evidence suggests that later protease inhibitors are not. Since the description of the use of ritonavir as an agent to potently inhibit the cytochrome P_{450}-mediated metabolism of other HIV protease inhibitors, 'ritonavir boosting' has become a routine aspect of the prescription of protease inhibitor-containing antiretroviral regimens and clinical trials. An important limitation of this drug class in patients experiencing treatment-limiting side effects is the lack of recommended reductions in unit dose. For such patients treatment regimens that may include an alternative protease inhibitor must be prescribed. Efforts have been made to determine whether the use of lower unit doses of a protease inhibitor, particularly when administered in combination with ritonavir-boosting for pharmacokinetic enhancement, may offer equal potency and improved tolerability for use in specific populations. However, to date no adequately powered comparative studies have been conducted to help guide recommendations and policy.

While virus isolates from patients who are no longer responding to treatment with single protease inhibitors usually possess resistance mutations within the protease amino acid sequence, regimens containing ritonavir-boosted protease inhibitors usually do not, at least in settings in which routine virological monitoring is performed frequently (i.e. 3–4 times per year). When resistance mutations are selected, mutations to one protease inhibitor may confer high-level resistance to others. Increasing levels of viral resistance appear usually to be conferred by increasing numbers of primary mutations.

 ## Further information

Flexner C. HIV protease inhibitors. *N Engl J Med*. 1998;338:1281–1292.

Friis-Møller N, Sabin CA, Weber R, et al. Combination antiretroviral therapy and the risk of myocardial infarction. *N Engl J Med*. 2003;349:1993–2003. Erratum in *N Engl J Med* 2004; 350: 955.

Kempf DJ, Marsh KC, Kumar G, et al. Pharmacokinetic enhancement of inhibitors of the human immunodeficiency virus protease by coadministration with ritonavir. *Antimicrob Agents Chemother*. 1997;41:654–660.

van der Lugt J, Colbers A, Burger D. Clinical pharmacology of HIV protease inhibitors in pregnancy. *Curr Opin HIV AIDS*. 2008;3:620–626.

AMPRENAVIR

Molecular weight: 505.6; (fosamprenavir): 625.7.

A synthetic compound formulated as the calcium salt of the oral prodrug fosamprenavir.

 ## ANTIVIRAL ACTIVITY

Amprenavir is active against HIV-1 and, to a lesser extent, HIV-2.

 ## ACQUIRED RESISTANCE

Mutations at position 50, 76 and 84 of the protease enzyme gene are associated with significantly reduced susceptibility.

 ## PHARMACOKINETICS

Oral absorption	Not known/available
C_{max} 700 mg + ritonavir 100 mg twice daily	c. 6.08 mg/L
C_{min} 700 mg + ritonavir 100 mg twice daily	c. 2.12 mg/L
Plasma half-life	c. 7.7 h
Volume of distribution	c. 430 L
Plasma protein binding	c. 90%

Absorption

Fosamprenavir is rapidly and almost completely hydrolyzed to amprenavir and inorganic phosphate by cellular phosphatases in the gut epithelium as it is absorbed. Absolute bioavailability has not been established. It can be taken without regard to food.

Distribution

It penetrates moderately well into the CNS. The semen:plasma ratio is negligible. It is not known if it is distributed into breast milk.

Metabolism and excretion

It is extensively metabolized by the cytochrome P_{450} (CYP) 3A4 enzyme system. Two major metabolites have been identified that appear to result from the oxidation of the tetrahydrofuran and aniline moieties.

Around 14% of a dose is eliminated in the urine and 75% in feces, <3% as unchanged drug. Metabolites account for >90% of administered drug found in fecal samples. It should be used with caution and at reduced doses in adults with mild or moderate hepatic impairment; it is contraindicated in patients with severe hepatic impairment.

 ## TOXICITY AND SIDE EFFECTS

The most common adverse events in patients receiving boosted fosamprenavir were diarrhea, nausea, headache, fatigue, vomiting and rash. Ritonavir-boosted fosamprenavir is associated with a dyslipidemia profile characteristic of those treated with other protease inhibitors boosted with 200 mg of ritonavir.

CLINICAL USE

Treatment of HIV infection (in combination with other antiretroviral drugs)

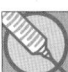

Preparations and dosage

Proprietary names: Lexiva, Telzir.

Preparations: Capsules (700 mg), oral solution (50 mg/mL).

Dosage (fosamprenavir): Adults, oral, 700 mg + ritonavir 100 mg every 12 h or 1400 mg + ritonavir 100 mg once daily. Children 6–12 years, 20 mg/kg every 12 h or 15 mg/kg every 8 h (maximum dose, 2400 mg per day in each instance). Children <6 years, no previous antiretroviral treatment: 30 mg/kg every 12 h (maximum dose, 1400 mg every 12 h) or 18 mg/kg + ritonavir 3 mg/kg every 12 h; previous antiretroviral treatment: 18 mg/kg + ritonavir 3 mg/kg every 12 h.

Limited availability.

Further information

Arvieux C, Tribut O. Amprenavir or fosamprenavir plus ritonavir in HIV infection: pharmacology, efficacy and tolerability profile. *Drugs*. 2005;65:633–659.

Chapman TM, Plosker GL, Perry CM. Fosamprenavir: a review of its use in the management of antiretroviral therapy-naive patients with HIV infection. *Drugs*. 2004;64:2101–2124.

Eron Jr J, Yeni P, Gathe Jr J, et al. The KLEAN study of fosamprenavir–ritonavir versus lopinavir–ritonavir, each in combination with abacavir–lamivudine, for initial treatment of HIV infection over 48 weeks: a randomised non-inferiority trial. *Lancet*. 2006;368:476–482. Erratum in: *Lancet* 2006; 368: 1238.

ATAZANAVIR

Molecular weight (free base): 704.9; (sulfate) 802.9.

An azapeptide formulated as the sulfate for oral use.

ANTIVIRAL ACTIVITY

Atazanavir is active against HIV-1 group M clades A–D, AE, AG, F, G and J. Information on activity against HIV-1 groups N and O and on HIV-2 is lacking.

ACQUIRED RESISTANCE

Mutations at positions 50 (I50L), 84 (I84V) and 88 (N88S) of the protease gene are associated with resistance.

PHARMACOKINETICS

Oral absorption	*c.* 68%
C_{max} 400 mg once daily	*c.* 3.15 µg/L
300 mg + ritonavir 100 mg once daily	*c.* 4.47 µg/L
C_{min} 400 mg once daily	*c.* 0.27 µg/L
300 mg + ritonavir 100 mg once daily	*c.* 0.65 µg/L
Plasma half-life	*c.* 8.6 h (300 mg+ ritonavir 100 mg)
Volume of distribution	*c.* Not known/available
Plasma protein binding	*c.* 86%

Absorption

Administration with food enhances bioavailability and reduces pharmacokinetic variability. Absorption is dependent on gastric pH. It should be given separately from proton-pump inhibitors or H_2-receptor antagonists. Buffered or enteric-coated formulations should be given (with food) 2 h before or 1 h after co-administration of didanosine.

Distribution

It penetrates moderately well into the CNS. The semen:plasma ratio is 0.11–4.42. It is distributed into breast milk.

Metabolism

It is extensively metabolized by CYP3A4. Administration with ritonavir prevents metabolization and enhances the pharmacokinetic profile.

Excretion

Following a single 400 mg dose, 79% and 13% of the dose was recovered in the feces and urine, respectively. It should be used with caution in the presence of mild hepatic impairment and should not be used in patients with more severe hepatic impairment.

TOXICITY AND SIDE EFFECTS

The most common adverse reactions (≥2%) are nausea, jaundice/scleral icterus, rash, headache, abdominal pain, vomiting, insomnia, peripheral neurological symptoms, dizziness, myalgia, diarrhea, depression and fever.

CLINICAL USE

Treatment of HIV infection (in combination with other antiretroviral drugs)

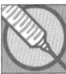

Preparations and dosage

Proprietary name: Reyataz.

Preparation: Capsules (100, 150, 200 and 300 mg).

Dosage: Treatment-naive patients, 400 mg (or 300 mg + ritonavir 100 mg) once daily with food. Not recommended for children under 6 years. Children 6–18 years, adjust dose according to weight.

Widely available.

Further information

Croom KF, Dhillon S, Keam SJ. Atazanavir: a review of its use in the management of HIV-1 infection. *Drugs*. 2009;69:1107–1140.

Goldsmith DR, Perry CM. Atazanavir. *Drugs*. 2003;63:1679–1693.

Molina JM, Andrade-Villanueva J, Echevarria J, et al. Once-daily atazanavir/ritonavir versus twice-daily lopinavir/ritonavir, each in combination with tenofovir and emtricitabine, for management of antiretroviral-naive HIV-1-infected patients: 48 week efficacy and safety results of the CASTLE study. *Lancet*. 2008;372:646–655.

Pett SL, Emery S. Atazanavir. In: Kucers', *The Use of Antibiotics*. A clinical review of antibacterial, antifungal and antiviral drugs. Grayson ML, Kucers A, Crowe SM, et al. eds. 6th ed. London: Hodder Arnold; 2010.

DARUNAVIR

Molecular weight: 547.7.

A synthetic compound formulated as the ethanolate for oral use in combination with ritonavir.

ANTIVIRAL ACTIVITY

It is active against HIV-1 and HIV-2.

ACQUIRED RESISTANCE

Darunavir is less affected than other protease inhibitors by mutations to resistance, but subgroups with more than 10 cumulative mutations show a >10-fold (median value) decrease in susceptibility. The major resistance mutations occur at positions 50 (I50V), 54 (I50M/L), 76 (L76V) and 84 (I84V) of the protease gene.

PHARMACOKINETICS (IN COMBINATION WITH RITONAVIR 100 mg)

Oral absorption	c. 82%
C_{max} 600 mg once daily + ritonavir 100 mg twice daily	c. 6500 µg/L
C_{min} 600 mg oral + ritonavir 100 mg twice daily	c. 3578 µg/L
Plasma half-life	c. 15 h
Volume of distribution	c. 131 L
Plasma protein binding	c. 95%

A single 600 mg dose given orally in combination with ritonavir 100 mg every 12 h increased the systemic exposure of darunavir approximately 14-fold. The relative bioavailability is 30% lower when administered with food in the presence of low-dose ritonavir. Distribution into human CSF, semen or breast milk has not yet been determined.

At least three oxidative metabolites, mediated predominantly through CYP3A4, have been identified in humans; all are at least 10-fold less active than the parent compound against HIV. Around 80% and 14% of the dose is found in the feces and urine, respectively. It should be used with caution in mild–moderate hepatic impairment and avoided in patients with more severe impairment.

TOXICITY AND SIDE EFFECTS

In phase III studies the most common adverse events were diarrhea, nausea, headache and nasopharyngitis. Patients co-infected with hepatitis B or C did not have a higher incidence of adverse events.

CLINICAL USE

Treatment of HIV infection (in combination with other antiretroviral drugs)

Preparations and dosage

Proprietary name: Prezista.

Preparation: Tablets (200, 300 and 600 mg).

Dosage: Adults, oral, 600 mg in combination with ritonavir 100 mg every 12 h in treatment-experienced patients; 800 mg in combination with ritonavir 100 mg once daily in treatment-naive patients. Children, 6–18 years (according to weight): 20–30 kg, 375 mg + 50 mg ritonavir every 12 h; >30–40 kg, 450 mg + 100 mg ritonavir every 12 h.

Widely available.

Further information

Back D, Sekar V, Hoetelmans RM. Darunavir: pharmacokinetics and drug interactions. *Antivir Ther.* 2008;13:1–13.

Madruga JV, Berger D, McMurchie M, et al. Efficacy and safety of darunavir–ritonavir compared with that of lopinavir–ritonavir at 48 weeks in treatment-experienced, HIV-infected patients in TITAN: a randomised controlled phase III trial. *Lancet.* 2007;370:49–58.

McKeage K, Perry CM, Keam SJ. Darunavir: a review of its use in the management of HIV infection in adults. *Drugs.* 2009;69:477–503.

Ortiz R, Dejesus E, Khanlou H, et al. Efficacy and safety of once-daily darunavir/ritonavir versus lopinavir/ritonavir in treatment-naive HIV-1-infected patients at week 48. *AIDS.* 2008;22:1389–1397.

INDINAVIR

Molecular weight (free base): 613.8; (sulfate): 711.88.

A synthetic compound formulated as the sulfate for oral administration.

ANTIVIRAL ACTIVITY

Indinavir is active against HIV-1 and HIV-2.

ACQUIRED RESISTANCE

The major mutations in the protease enzyme associated with loss of the antiretroviral activity occur at positions 46, 82 and 84. Generally, the level of resistance rises with the number of point mutations.

PHARMACOKINETICS

Oral absorption	c. 65%
C_{max} 800 mg thrice daily	c. 8.97 mg/L
C_{min} 800 mg thrice daily	c. 0.15 mg/L
Plasma half-life	c. 2 h
Volume of distribution	c. 0.4–1.74 L/kg
Plasma protein binding	c. 60%

Absorption and distribution

It is rapidly absorbed and not significantly affected by intake with food. Distribution in the body has not been fully characterized. It penetrates well into the CNS. The semen:plasma ratio is 1.9. It is distributed into breast milk.

Metabolism and excretion

Seven major metabolites have been described, including a glucuronide conjugate and six oxidative metabolites. Around 83% of the dose is recovered in feces and 18% in urine, 10% as unchanged drug. The effect of renal impairment has not been studied. It should be used with caution in the presence of hepatic impairment, particularly if severe.

TOXICITY AND SIDE EFFECTS

The principal side effect is nephrolithiasis, including flank pain with or without hematuria. There is good evidence that indinavir directly causes nephrolithiasis as a result of crystallization in the urinary tract. Indirect hyperbilirubinemia occurs in about 10% of patients associated with inhibition of bilirubin-conjugating activity occurring as a result of competitive inhibition of uridine diphosphate (UDP)-glucuronosyltransferase.

Ritonavir-boosted indinavir is associated with a dyslipidemia profile characteristic of those treated with other protease inhibitors boosted with a 200 mg dose of ritonavir per day. Insulin resistance and hyperglycemia have also been associated with ritonavir-boosted indinavir.

CLINICAL USE

Treatment of adult HIV infection (in combination with other antiretroviral drugs)

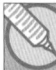

Preparations and dosage

Proprietary name: Crixivan.

Preparation: Capsules (100, 200, 333.33 and 400 mg).

Dosage: Adults, oral, 800 mg + ritonavir 100 mg every 12 h Children, 50 mg/kg every 8 h taken away from food; when boosted with ritonavir can be given without food restrictions.

Widely available, including generic versions.

Further information

Boyd MA, Crowe S. Indinavir. In: Kucers' *The Use of Antibiotics. A clinical review of antibacterial, antifungal and antiviral drugs*. Grayson ML, Kucers A, Crowe SM, et al, eds. 6th ed. London: Hodder Arnold; 2010.

Burger D, Boyd MA, Duncombe C, et al. Pharmacokinetics and pharmacodynamics of indinavir with or without low-dose ritonavir. *J Antimicrob Chemother*. 2003;51:1231–1238.

Cressey TR, Plipat N, Fregonese F, Chokephaibulkit K. Indinavir/ritonavir remains an important component of HAART for the treatment of HIV/AIDS, particularly in resource-limited settings. *Expert Opin Drug Metab Toxicol*. 2007; 3:347–361.

LOPINAVIR

Molecular weight: 628.80.

A synthetic compound, co-formulated with ritonavir for oral administration. In this formulation, ritonavir functions to inhibit the metabolic clearance of lopinavir, and does not contribute to the antiretroviral activity.

ANTIVIRAL ACTIVITY

Lopinavir is active against HIV-1 and HIV-2.

ACQUIRED RESISTANCE

Significant resistance to the antiretroviral efficacy of ritonavir-booted lopinavir occurs as a result of amino acid substitutions at positions 32, 47 and 82 in the protease region. Protease inhibitor resistance is uncommon in patients identified with early failure of combination therapy with ritonavir boosted-lopinavir and nucleotide reverse transcriptase inhibitors.

PHARMACOKINETICS

Oral absorption	Not known/available
C_{max} 400 mg + ritonavir 100 mg twice daily	c. 9.6 mg/L
C_{min} 400 mg + ritonavir 100 mg twice daily	c. 5.5 mg/L
Plasma half-life	c. 5–6 h
Volume of distribution	Not known/available
Plasma protein binding	c. 98–99%

Absorption and distribution

The absorption of lopinavir–ritonavir in capsule or liquid form is favorably affected by the presence of food, particularly if high in fat. The CNS penetration is good. It has a semen:plasma ratio of 0.07. It is distributed into breast milk.

Metabolism

Lopinavir is extensively metabolized by the CYP3A4 system, but this is inhibited by ritonavir.

Excretion

Over an 8-day period after single dosing with the combined formulation, around 10% and 83% of the administered dose is recovered in urine and feces, respectively. Less than 3% of the dose is recovered as unchanged drug in urine and 20% in feces. In mild to moderate hepatic impairment, an increase in exposure of approximately 30% is observed, but is probably not clinically relevant. It should be avoided in severe hepatic impairment.

TOXICITY AND SIDE EFFECTS

The most common adverse events seen in trials of complex antiretroviral regimens were diarrhea, nausea, headache, fatigue, vomiting and rash. Ritonavir-boosted lopinavir is associated with a dyslipidemia profile characteristic of those treated with other protease inhibitors boosted with 200 mg of ritonavir.

CLINICAL USE

Treatment of HIV infection (in combination with ritonavir and other antiretroviral agents)

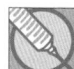

Preparations and dosages

Proprietary names: Aluvia, Kaletra.

Preparations: Tablets (lopinavir–ritonavir 200 + 50 mg and 100 + 25 mg), capsules (lopinavir–ritonavir 133.3 + 33.3 mg); oral solution (lopinavir–ritonavir 80 + 20 mg/mL).

Dosage: Adults, oral, lopinavir–ritonavir 400 + 100 mg every 12 h or 800 + 200 mg once daily. Children, 7–15 kg, lopinavir 12 mg/kg + ritonavir 3 mg/kg every 12 h; ≥15–40 kg, lopinavir 10 mg/kg + ritonavir 2.5 mg/kg every 12 h. Widely available, including generic versions.

Further information

Barragan P, Podzamczer D. Lopinavir/ritonavir: a protease inhibitor for HIV-1 treatment. *Expert Opin Pharmacother.* 2008;9:2363–2375.

Gathe J, da Silva BA, Cohen DE, et al. A once-daily lopinavir/ritonavir-based regimen is noninferior to twice-daily dosing and results in similar safety and tolerability in antiretroviral-naive subjects through 48 weeks. *J Acquir Immune Defic Syndr.* 2009;50:474–481.

Klein CE, Chiu YL, Awni W, et al. The tablet formulation of lopinavir/ritonavir provides similar bioavailability to the soft-gelatin capsule formulation with less pharmacokinetic variability and diminished food effect. *J Acquir Immune Defic Syndr.* 2007;44:401–410.

Riddler SA, Haubrich R, DiRienzo AG, et al. Class-sparing regimens for initial treatment of HIV-1 infection. *N Engl J Med.* 2008;358:2095–2106.

NELFINAVIR

Molecular weight: 663.9.

A synthetic chemical formulated as the mesylate for oral administration.

 ## ANTIVIRAL ACTIVITY

Nelfinavir inhibits HIV-1 and HIV-2 proteases. Bioavailability is affected to only a limited degree by combination with low-dose ritonavir.

 ## ACQUIRED RESISTANCE

Resistance is most frequently selected through a D30N mutation in the HIV protease. An L90M mutation also confers resistance.

PHARMACOKINETICS

Oral absorption	c. 70–80% (with food)
C_{max} 750 mg thrice daily	c. 3–4 mg/L
1250 mg twice daily	c. 4 mg/L
C_{min} 750 mg thrice daily	c. 1–3 mg/L
1250 mg twice daily	c. 0.7–2.2 mg/L
Plasma half-life	c. 3.5 h
Volume of distribution	c. 2–7 L/kg
Plasma protein binding	>98%

Absorption and distribution

Food improves the bioavailability and the drug should be administered with a light meal. The semen:plasma ratio is 0.07. It is distributed into breast milk.

Metabolism and excretion

One major and several minor oxidative metabolites are found in plasma. Most of an oral dose is recovered in feces as unchanged drug (22%) and metabolites (78%). The remainder is recovered in urine, mainly unchanged.

An increase in the area under the time–concentration curve (AUC) has been observed in patients with hepatic impairment, but specific dose recommendations have not been made.

 ## TOXICITY AND SIDE EFFECTS

The most common adverse effect is diarrhea of mild to moderate severity. Other side effects include nausea, fatigue, vomiting and headache. It is associated with less dyslipidemia in comparison with ritonavir-boosted protease inhibitors.

 ## CLINICAL USE

Treatment of HIV infection (in combination with other antiretroviral drugs)

 ### Preparations and dosage

Proprietary name: Viracept.

Preparations: Tablets (250 and 625 mg), oral powder containing nelfinavir free base 50 mg per 1 g powder.

Dosage: Five 250 mg tablets or two 625 mg tablets every 12 h, or three 250 mg tablets every 8 h. Children ≥2 years, 45–55 mg/kg every 12 h, or 25–35 mg/kg every 8 h.

Widely available.

 Further information

Olmo M, Podzamczer D. A review of nelfinavir for the treatment of HIV infection. *Expert Opin Drug Metab Toxicol.* 2006;2:285–300.

Walmsley S, Bernstein B, King M, et al. Lopinavir–ritonavir versus nelfinavir for the initial treatment of HIV infection. *N Engl J Med.* 2002;346:2039–2046.

RITONAVIR

Molecular weight: 720.95.

A synthetic chemical available for oral use as soft capsules and a liquid formulation. It is now almost exclusively used as a pharmacokinetic enhancer to 'boost' the pharmacokinetic properties of HIV protease inhibitors in the treatment of HIV-1 infection in patients over 1 month in age.

ANTIVIRAL ACTIVITY

Ritonavir is active against HIV-1 and, to a lesser extent, HIV-2.

ACQUIRED RESISTANCE

At antiretroviral doses resistance is associated with the presence of specific amino acid substitutions in the HIV protease at positions 82 and 84. Concern about the risk for selection of ritonavir resistance when used at a subtherapeutic 'booster' dose has so far not been borne out by clinical experience.

PHARMACOKINETICS

Oral absorption	Not known/available
C_{max} 600 mg twice daily	c. 11.2 mg/L
C_{min} 600 mg twice daily	c. 3.7 mg/L
Plasma half-life	c. 3–5 h
Volume of distribution	c. 0.3–0.6 L/kg
Plasma protein binding	c. 97%

Absorption and distribution

Fasting and high-fat meals had no appreciable effect on oral absorption. It penetrates poorly into the CNS. The semen:plasma ratio is <0.04. It is distributed into breast milk.

Metabolism and excretion

Four oxidized metabolites have been identified, the major of which retains antiretroviral activity. Around 11% of the dose is excreted in urine, 4% as unchanged drug. The remainder is found in feces. Metabolites are eliminated primarily via the feces.

No dose adjustment is recommended in mild to moderate hepatic impairment. It should not be given to patients with severe hepatic impairment, nor should it be given as a pharmacokinetic enhancer to patients with decompensated liver disease.

TOXICITY AND SIDE EFFECTS

Full (antiretroviral) doses are associated with nausea, vomiting, diarrhea and fatigue in >20% of subjects. The degree to which ritonavir at low dose is associated with specific adverse events is uncertain. In HIV-negative healthy volunteers given 'booster' doses of 100 mg every 12 h, the concentration of total cholesterol, low-density cholesterol and triglycerides all increased, and the concentration of high-density cholesterol concentration fell.

CLINICAL USE

Treatment of HIV infection in adults and children >1 month old (in combination with other antiretroviral agents)

Preparations and dosage

Proprietary name: Norvir.

Preparations: Soft capsules (100 mg), oral solution (80 mg/mL).

Dosage: Adults, starting dose no less than 300 mg every 12 h, increased by 100 mg at 2–3 day intervals to 600 mg every 12 h. Children, starting dose 250 mg/m², increased by 50 mg/m² at 2–3 day intervals to 350–400 mg/m² every 12 h (maximum dose, 600 mg every 12 h). For use as a pharmacokinetic enhancer, please refer to the prescribing information for the specific protease inhibitor in this chapter.

Widely available.

Further information

Hurst M, Faulds D. Ritonavir. *Drugs*. 2000;60:1371–1379.

Kempf DJ, Marsh KC, Kumar G, et al. Pharmacokinetic enhancement of inhibitors of the human immunodeficiency virus protease by coadministration with ritonavir. *Antimicrob Agents Chemother*. 1997;41:654–660.

SAQUINAVIR

Molecular weight: 766.95.

A peptidomimetic protease inhibitor formulated as the mesylate for oral use.

ANTIVIRAL ACTIVITY

Saquinavir is active against HIV-1 and HIV-2.

ACQUIRED RESISTANCE

Resistance is associated with an amino acid substitution at position 48 in the HIV protease (G48V). An L90M mutation also confers resistance, as it does for most protease inhibitors. Saquinavir-resistant isolates from patients on long-term therapy often show cross-resistance to other protease inhibitors.

PHARMACOKINETICS

Oral absorption	c. 4%
C_{max} 1200 mg thrice daily	c. 1–2.2 mg/L
C_{min} 1200 mg thrice daily	c. 0.1–0.22 mg/L
Plasma half-life	c. 7–12 h
Volume of distribution	c. 700 L
Plasma protein binding	c. 98%

Absorption and distribution

It is poorly absorbed and penetrates poorly into the CNS. The semen:plasma ratio is 0.04. It is not known if it is distributed into human breast milk.

Metabolism and excretion

It is metabolized via CYP3A4, principally to mono- and dihydroxylated derivatives. Around 88% of the dose is excreted in feces and 1% in urine. Caution should be exercised in severe renal impairment and moderate hepatic impairment; use in decompensated hepatic impairment is contraindicated.

TOXICITY AND SIDE EFFECTS

The most frequently reported adverse effects include abdominal discomfort, diarrhea and nausea. Ritonavir-boosted saquinavir is associated with a dyslipidemic profile characteristic of those

treated with a boosted protease inhibitor requiring 200 mg of the ritonavir 'booster'.

CLINICAL USE

Treatment of HIV infection (in combination with other antiretroviral drugs)

Preparations and dosage

Proprietary name: Invirase.
Preparations: Tablets (500 mg), hard gelatin capsules (200 mg).
Dosage: Two 500 mg tablets or five 200 mg capsules co-administered with 100 mg ritonavir every 12 h.
Widely available.

Further information

Plosker GL, Scott LJ. Saquinavir: a review of its use in boosted regimens for treating HIV infection. *Drugs*. 2003;63:1299–1324.
Walmsley S, Avihingsanon A, Slim J, et al. Gemini: a noninferiority study of saquinavir/ritonavir versus lopinavir/ritonavir as initial HIV-1 therapy in adults. *J Acquir Immune Defic Syndr*. 2009;50:367–374.

TIPRANAVIR

Molecular weight: 602.7.

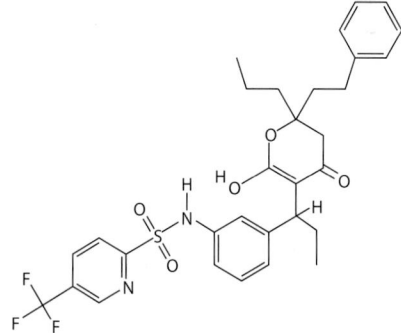

A non-peptidic protease inhibitor formulated as capsules or solution for oral use.

ANTIVIRAL ACTIVITY

Tipranavir is active against HIV-1 and HIV-2.

ACQUIRED RESISTANCE

In a study of 105 viruses resistant to other protease inhibitors, 90% exhibited a more than four-fold decrease in susceptibility and 2% high-level resistance (>10-fold decrease). The predominant emerging mutations in use with ritonavir are L33F/I/V, V82T/L and I84V. Combination of all three of these mutations is usually required for reduced susceptibility. Mutations at positions 47, 58 and 74 are also associated with resistance.

 ## PHARMACOKINETICS

Oral absorption	Not known/available
C_{max} 500 mg + 200 mg ritonavir twice daily	c. 57.2 mg/L (female); 46.8 mg/L (male)
C_{min} 500 mg + 200 mg ritonavir twice daily	c. 25.1 mg/L (female); 21.5 mg/L (male)
Plasma half-life	c. 5.5 h (female); 6 h (male)
Volume of distribution	Not known/available
Plasma protein binding	>99.9%

Absorption and distribution

The combination with ritonavir may be taken with or without food. No studies have been conducted to determine the distribution into human CSF, semen or breast milk.

Metabolism and excretion

Metabolism in the presence of 200 mg ritonavir is minimal. Around 82% is excreted in the feces and 4% in the urine. In mild hepatic impairment it should be used with caution; it should not be used in moderate or severe hepatic impairment.

 ## TOXICITY AND SIDE EFFECTS

Adverse effects include nausea, vomiting, diarrhea, fatigue and headache. In studies of ritonavir-boosted regimens higher rates of hepatotoxicity have been observed with tipranavir than with other protease inhibitors. In addition, 14 reports of intracranial bleeding (eight fatal cases) associated with tipranavir have been reported. It has been associated with dyslipidemia to a greater extent than other protease inhibitors.

 ## CLINICAL USE

Treatment (in combination with other antiretroviral drugs) of HIV-1 infection in patients unresponsive to more than one other protease inhibitor

 ### Preparations and dosage

Proprietary name: Aptivus.
Preparations: Capsules (250 mg), oral solution (100 mg/mL).
Dosage: Adults, oral, 500 mg + 200 mg ritonavir every 12 h, with or without food. Children, 2–18 years: dose based on body weight or body surface area, not to exceed adult dose.
Widely available.

 ## Further information

King J, Acosta E. Tipranavir: a novel nonpeptidic protease inhibitor of HIV. *Clin Pharmacokinet.* 2006;45:665–682.

ENTRY INHIBITORS

These drugs inhibit fusion of the virion with the CD4 and CCR5 co-receptor complex on the outer surface of the human cellular membrane. The fusion inhibitor enfuvirtide prevents the formation of the pore through which HIV gains entry to the cell. Maraviroc is a specific antagonist of the CCR5 co-receptor that interacts with the gp120 envelope glycoprotein, thereby inhibiting the entrance of HIV into the cell. It is the first agent to inhibit HIV replication by targeting a host cell protein rather than a viral enzyme.

 ## Further information

Kuritzkes DR. HIV-1 entry inhibitors: an overview. *Curr Opin HIV AIDS.* 2009;4:82–87.

ENFUVIRTIDE

Molecular weight: 4492.

A linear 36-amino acid synthetic peptide with an acetylated N-terminus and a carboxamide C-terminus. It is formulated as a lyophilized powder to be reconstituted for subcutaneous injection.

 ## ANTIVIRAL ACTIVITY

Enfuvirtide selectively inhibits HIV-1, but has no activity against HIV-2.

 ## ACQUIRED RESISTANCE

Resistance is mediated by amino acid substitutions within the first heptad repeat region of gp41 at amino acids 36–45. Resistance emerges fairly rapidly in patients experiencing virological failure with an enfuvirtide-containing antiretroviral regimen, and is associated with the return of the plasma HIV load toward baseline within a few weeks.

 ## PHARMACOKINETICS

Subcutaneous absorption	c. 84.3%
C_{max} 90 mg s/c twice daily	c. 4.59 mg/L
Plasma half-life	c. 3.8 h
Volume of distribution	5.5 L
Plasma protein binding	c. 92%

Absorption and distribution

Absorption of the 90 mg dose is comparable when injected into the subcutaneous tissue of the abdomen, thigh or arm. It does not penetrate the CSF or semen. Distribution into breast milk has not been described.

Metabolism and excretion

It probably undergoes catabolism to its constituent amino acids, with subsequent recycling of the amino acids in the body pool.

TOXICITY AND SIDE EFFECTS

It does not seem to have any long-term toxicities (including the HIV lipodystrophy syndrome) associated with other commonly used antiretrovirals. Reaction at the injection site, variously characterized by local pain, erythema, pruritus, induration, ecchymosis, nodules or cysts, is experienced by more than 90% of patients and may lead to treatment fatigue.

CLINICAL USE

Treatment of HIV infection (in combination with other antiretroviral drugs) in adults and children older than 6 years who show evidence of HIV-1 replication despite ongoing antiretroviral therapy

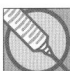

Preparations and dosage

Proprietary name: Fuzeon.

Preparation: Vial containing 108 mg lyophilized powder for reconstitution in 1.1 mL sterile water (end volume 1.2 mL).

Dosage: 90 mg (1 mL of solution) by subcutaneous injection twice daily. Widely available.

Further information

Makinson A, Reynes J. The fusion inhibitor enfuvirtide in recent antiretroviral strategies. *Curr Opin HIV AIDS.* 2009;4:150–158.

Matthews T, Salgo M, Greenberg M, Chung J, DeMasi R, Bolognesi D. Enfuvirtide: the first therapy to inhibit the entry of HIV-1 into host CD4 lymphocytes. *Nat Rev Drug Discov.* 2004;3:215–225.

Nelson M, Arastéh K, Clotet B, et al. Durable efficacy of enfuvirtide over 48 weeks in heavily treatment-experienced HIV-1-infected patients in the T-20 versus optimized background regimen only 1 and 2 clinical trials. *J Acquir Immune Defic Syndr.* 2005;40:404–412.

MARAVIROC

Molecular weight: 513.67.

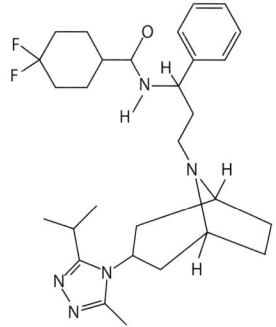

A spirodiketopiperazine formulated as tablets for oral use.

ANTIVIRAL ACTIVITY

Maraviroc is active against HIV-1. Activity against HIV-2 has not been evaluated.

ACQUIRED RESISTANCE

In most patients (*c.* 60%) failure of response is associated with the selection of virus that can use CXCR4 as its entry co-receptor. Evidence for the selection of virus that continues to use CCR5 has also been described.

PHARMACOKINETICS

Oral absorption	c. 33% (300 mg dose)
C_{max} 150 mg twice daily	c. 332 µg/L*
C_{min} 150 mg twice daily	c. 101 µg/L*
Plasma half-life	c. 13.2 h (30 mg iv administration)
Volume of distribution	c. 194 L
Plasma protein binding	c. 76%

*Treatment experienced patients receiving a CYP3A inhibitor.

Absorption

The absolute bioavailability of a 100 mg dose is 23% and is predicted to be 33% after a 300 mg dose. Co-administration of a 300 mg tablet and a high-fat meal has resulted in reduced C_{max} and AUC by 33% in healthy volunteers. However, because no food restrictions were enacted during clinical trials, maraviroc may be taken with or without food.

Distribution

Animal experiments suggest low CSF concentrations around 10% of free plasma concentrations. It is not known whether it passes into breast milk. A study of genital tract secretions and vaginal tissue in healthy HIV-uninfected female volunteers suggest a concentration in cervicovaginal fluid more than four-fold higher than that in plasma.

Metabolism

It is a substrate for CYP3A4 and P-glycoprotein, but does not appear to inhibit or induce CYP3A4.

Excretion

Seventy-six and 19% of a radiolabeled maraviroc dose were recovered in the feces and urine, respectively.

 ## TOXICITY AND SIDE EFFECTS

There has been some concern that CCR5 blockade may result in decreased immune surveillance and a subsequent increased risk of development of malignancies (e.g. lymphomas). Genetic deficiency of the CCR5 co-receptor is also known to be a risk factor for the development of symptomatic West Nile virus infection. No evidence for an increase in either of these potential risks has so far emerged.

The toxicity profile appears relatively benign. The most common adverse events described so far include diarrhea, fatigue, headache and nausea. In placebo-controlled studies the only differences to emerge were fever (6% versus 4% in the placebo group) and headache (2% versus 6% with placebo). Discontinuation because of adverse events was uncommon and the same in both groups.

 ## CLINICAL USE

Treatment of HIV infection (in combination with other antiretroviral drugs) in treatment-experienced patients

On November 20, 2009, the US Food and Drug Administration approved a supplemental new drug application to expand the indication for maraviroc to include combination antiretroviral treatment of treatment-naive adults infected with CCR5-tropic HIV virus

 ### Preparations and dosage

Proprietary name: Celsentri.

Preparation: Tablets (150 and 300 mg).

Dosage: 300 mg every 12 h. Dosage adjustments are recommended in the presence of CYP3A4 inducers and inhibitors.

Widely available.

 ### Further information

Fätkenheuer G, Nelson M, Lazzarin A, et al. Subgroup analyses of maraviroc in previously treated R5 HIV-1 infection. *N Engl J Med*. 2008;359:1442–1455.
Gulick RM, Lalezari J, Goodrich J, et al. Maraviroc for previously treated patients with R5 HIV-1 infection. *N Engl J Med*. 2008;359:1429–1441.

MacArthur RD, Novak RM. Reviews of anti-infective agents: maraviroc: the first of a new class of antiretroviral agents. *Clin Infect Dis*. 2008;47:236–241.

HIV INTEGRASE INHIBITORS

The HIV integrase enzyme incorporates viral DNA into the host chromosome through a three-step process: formation of the preintegration viral DNA complex; 3′ processing; and strand transfer. Raltegravir inhibits the final step by preventing formation of covalent bonds between the preintegration complex and the host DNA.

 ### Further information

Correll T, Klibanov OM. Integrase inhibitors: a new treatment option for patients with human immunodeficiency virus infection. *Pharmacotherapy*. 2008;28:90–101.

RALTEGRAVIR

Molecular weight: 482.51.

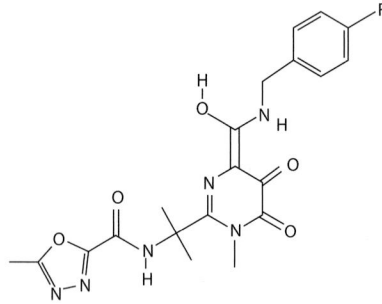

Formulated as the potassium salt for oral administration.

 ## ANTIVIRAL ACTIVITY

Raltegravir is active against HIV-1 and HIV-2.

 ## ACQUIRED RESISTANCE

Several characteristic mutations leading to typical amino acid exchanges have been characterized in cell culture studies and confirmed in clinical trial participants with virological failure while receiving raltegravir in combination with other antiretrovirals. Virological failure has generally been associated with mutations at one of three residues – Y143, Q148 or N155 – usually in combination with at least one other mutation.

PHARMACOKINETICS

Oral absorption	Not known/available
C_{max} 400 mg twice daily	c. 2.17 mg/L
Plasma half-life	c. 9 h
Volume of distribution	Not known/available
Plasma protein binding	c. 83%

Absorption and distribution

It may be administered without regard to food. There are few data regarding its capacity to penetrate into genital secretions or breast milk. A study of 25 HIV-infected individuals receiving raltegravir as a component of combination antiretroviral therapy found that 24 had detectable levels and that 50% of these reached a level exceeding the 95% inhibitory concentration reported to inhibit HIV-1 strains fully susceptible to integrase inhibition.

Metabolism and excretion

It is not a substrate, and does not appear to inhibit or induce the cytochrome P_{450} enzyme complex. It is primarily metabolized through hepatic glucuronidation mediated by the UGT-1A1 enzyme. It is excreted in the feces (51%) and the urine (32%) as unaltered compound and its glucuronide.

There are no recommended dose adjustments for weight, sex and race, or for hepatic or renal insufficiency. The pharmacokinetic handling in children has not been determined.

TOXICITY AND SIDE EFFECTS

Its toxicity profile to date is remarkably benign. Clinical trial participants experienced similar types and frequencies of adverse events as those receiving placebo. The most frequently reported adverse events were nausea, diarrhea and headache and were mostly mild to moderate in intensity. Myopathy, rhabdomyolysis and elevations of creatinine phosphokinase have been noted in a few trial participants and it should be used cautiously in combination with drugs associated with muscle toxicity.

CLINICAL USE

Treatment of HIV infection (in combination with other antiretroviral drugs)

Preparations and dosage

Proprietary name: Isentress.

Preparation: Film-coated tablets (434.4 mg, equivalent to 400 mg active drug).

Dosage: Adults 400 mg every 12 h.

Widely available.

Further information

Cooper DA, Steigbigel RT, Gatell JM, et al. Subgroup and resistance analyses of raltegravir for resistant HIV-1 infection. *N Engl J Med.* 2008;359:355–365.

Croxtall JD, Keam SJ. Raltegravir: a review of its use in the management of HIV infection in treatment-experienced patients. *Drugs.* 2009;69:1059–1075.

Lennox JL, DeJesus E, Lazzarin A, et al. Safety and efficacy of raltegravir-based versus efavirenz-based combination therapy in treatment-naive patients with HIV-1 infection: a multicentre, double-blind randomized controlled trial. *Lancet.* 2009;374:796–806.

Steigbigel RT, Cooper DA, Kumar PN, et al. Raltegravir with optimized background therapy for resistant HIV-1 infection. *N Engl J Med.* 2008;359:339–354.

37 Other antiviral agents

Richard J. Whitley

The impact of chronic viral infections such as hepatitis B and C and HIV, together with the achievements of molecular virologists in defining the life cycle of many viral pathogens and the availability of rapid viral diagnostic procedures, have stimulated the development of effective antiviral therapy. Various ways of inhibiting viral replication have been exploited:

- Direct inactivation of the virus prior to cell attachment and entry
- Blocking attachment of virus to host-cell membrane receptors and penetration
- Prevention of viral uncoating
- Impeding transcription or translation into viral messenger RNA and proteins
- Interfering with glycosylation steps
- Alteration of viral assembly and prevention of release
- Inhibition of host pathways that impede these events.

This chapter addresses compounds other than antiretroviral agents that are licensed for clinical use.

ADAMANTANES

 ### AMANTADINE

1-Aminoadamantane hydrochloride. Molecular weight (hydrochloride): 187.7.

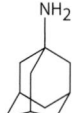

A symmetrical synthetic C-10 tricyclic amine with an unusual cage-like structure, supplied as the hydrochloride for oral administration.

 ### ANTIVIRAL ACTIVITY

It inhibits influenza A virus replication at concentrations of 0.2–0.6 mg/L, but has little or no activity against influenza B or C.

 ### ACQUIRED RESISTANCE

Resistance is the consequence of mutations in amino acid positions 27, 30 and 31 in the M2 transmembrane sequence. Cross-resistance between amantadine and rimantadine is universal. Influenza H3N2 strains worldwide are now resistant, but seasonal H1N1 strains remain susceptible. Postexposure family prophylaxis results in the prompt emergence of drug resistance after onset of treatment.

 ### PHARMACOKINETICS

Oral absorption	>90%
C_{max} 200 mg oral per day	0.4–0.9 mg/L after c. 4–6 h
Plasma half-life	9.7–14.5 h
Volume of distribution	10.4 L/kg
Plasma protein binding	65%

Absorption and distribution

Absorption after oral administration is almost complete. Levels in secretions approach plasma concentrations.

Metabolism and excretion

About 56% of a single oral dose is excreted unchanged within 24 h by the kidney. Altogether 90% of an oral dose is excreted in the urine with a mean elimination half-life of 11.8 h in subjects with normal renal function. In elderly men, the half-life is 28.9 h and in patients with renal insufficiency half-lives of 18.5 h to 33.8 days have been observed. The renal clearance is around 398 mL/min (range 112–772 mL/min), indicating active secretion as well as glomerular filtration. Less than 5% of a dose is removed during hemodialysis and average half-lives of 8.3 and 13 days have been reported in patients on chronic hemodialysis. Extreme care must be taken to ensure that drug does not accumulate to toxic levels.

INTERACTIONS

Central nervous system (CNS), gastrointestinal or other side effects provoked by anticholinergic drugs or L-dopa may be aggravated. Patients have developed visual hallucinations while concurrently taking amantadine and trihexyphenidyl (benzhexol); these respond to a reduction of the dose of trihexyphenidyl. Hemodialysis is not helpful because of the large volume of distribution.

 ## TOXICITY AND SIDE EFFECTS

Embryotoxicity and teratogenicity have been observed in rats receiving 50 mg/kg per day, about 15 times the usual human dose. Neurological side effects include drowsiness, insomnia, light-headedness, difficulty in concentration, nervousness, dizziness and headache in up to 20% of individuals. Other side effects include anorexia, nausea, vomiting, dry mouth, constipation and urinary retention. All develop during the first 3–4 days of therapy and are reversible by discontinuing the drug. An exception to rapid onset of adverse reactions is livedo reticularis. Convulsions, hallucinations and confusion are dose related, usually occurring at levels in excess of 1.5 mg/L; convulsions may occur at a lower threshold in patients with a history of epilepsy and the drug is best avoided in such patients.

 ## CLINICAL USE

Prevention and treatment of influenza A H1N1 infections

 ### Preparations and dosage

Proprietary name: Symmetrel.
Preparations: Capsules, syrup.
Dosage: Treatment or prophylaxis. Adults, oral, 100 mg once or twice daily for 5–7 days. Children, 1–9 years, 4–8 mg/kg per day; 10–15 years, 100 mg per day.
Widely available.

 ## Further information

Anonymous. Update: drug susceptibility of swine-origin influenza A (H1N1) viruses, April 2009. *Morb Mortal Wkly Rep.* 2009;58:433–435.

Deyde VM, Xu X, Bright RA, et al. Surveillance of resistance to adamantanes among influenza A(H3N2) and A(H1N1) viruses isolated worldwide. *J Infect Dis.* 2007;196:249–257.

Higgins RR, Eshaghi A, Burton L, Mazzulli T, Drews SJ. Differential patterns of amantadine-resistance in influenza A (H3N2) and (H1N1) isolates in Toronto, Canada. *J Clin Virol.* 2009;44:91–93.

Monto AS. Antivirals and influenza: frequency of resistance. *Pediatr Infect Dis J.* 2008;27:S110–S112.

RIMANTADINE

Molecular weight (hydrochloride): 215.7.

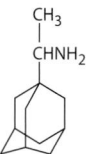

An analog of amantadine, supplied as the hydrochloride for oral administration.

 ## ANTIVIRAL ACTIVITY

In cell culture and animal models rimantadine is more effective than amantadine on a weight-for-weight basis. There is complete cross-resistance with amantadine.

 ## PHARMACOKINETICS

Oral absorption	>90%
C_{max} 100 mg oral (every 12 h)	0.4–0.5 mg/L after 2–6 h
Plasma half-life	c. 35 h
Volume of distribution	Very large
Plasma protein binding	c. 40%

Absorption and distribution

Single- and multiple-dose pharmacokinetic studies in elderly patients and young adults are remarkably similar. The steady-state concentration in nasal mucus develops by day 5 at a concentration approximately 1.5-fold higher than plasma.

Metabolism

In contrast to amantadine, rimantadine is extensively metabolized in the liver by hydroxylation and glucuronidation.

Excretion

Less than 20% is excreted unchanged in the urine and most of the breakdown products are excreted by this route. Thus, the plasma half-life is much less affected by renal dysfunction than that of amantadine.

 ## TOXICITY AND SIDE EFFECTS

Rimantadine has significantly fewer side effects than amantadine at equivalent doses, perhaps because of differences in pharmacokinetics, since with equal doses the blood levels are considerably lower. CNS side effects are not significantly higher than placebo.

CLINICAL USE

| Prophylaxis and treatment of influenza A H1N1 infections |

Since prolonged administration is well tolerated by elderly patients, the drug is preferable to amantadine.

Preparations and dosage

Proprietary name: Flumadine.

Preparations: Tablets, syrup.

Dosage: Adults, oral, 200 mg per day in single or divided doses, if >40 kg. Children, 5 mg/kg per day in 1–2 divided doses (maximum dose, 150 mg per day).

Available in continental Europe and the USA.

Further information

Alves Galvão MG, Rocha Crispino Santos MA, Alves da Cunha AJ. Amantadine and rimantadine for influenza A in children and the elderly. *Cochrane Database Syst Rev.* 2008;(1) CD002745.

Drinka PJ, Haupt T. Emergence of rimantadine-resistant virus within 6 days of starting rimantadine prophylaxis with oseltamivir treatment of symptomatic cases. *J Am Geriatr Soc.* 2007;55:923–926.

Jefferson T, Demicheli V, Di Pietrantonj C, Rivetti D. Amantadine and rimantadine for influenza A in adults. *Cochrane Database Syst Rev.* 2006:2: CD001169.

INTERFERONS

Interferons are low molecular weight proteins produced by mammalian cells in vitro and in vivo in response to viral infection and certain other stimuli. There are three classes:

- Interferon-α, produced by lymphocytes
- Interferon-β, produced by fibroblasts
- Interferon-γ, produced by lymphoid cells in response to mitogens.

Interferons are generally species specific and are now produced by recombinant genetic techniques. Only interferon-α is used in the context of viral disease, where its effectiveness may be due as much to immunomodulatory as antiviral properties.

INTERFERON-α

Molecular weight: approximately 19 kDa.

A human protein produced by recombinant DNA technology in *Escherichia coli*, formulated for administration by intramuscular, subcutaneous or intralesional injection. A pegylated form, peginterferon, developed by attaching a 40 kDa branched-chain polyethylene glycol moiety to interferon-α-2a, has a prolonged half-life and is better tolerated. Potency is expressed as international units (IU), defined as the amount needed to prevent lysis of 50% of cells by vesicular stomatitis virus in tissue culture assay.

ANTIVIRAL ACTIVITY

Interferon-α renders cells resistant to infection by a wide range of viruses and mediates immunoregulation, inflammation, inhibition of cell multiplication, interaction with mixed histocompatibility genes, and differentiation. It has no effect on extracellular virus and does not prevent virus from penetrating cells. It reversibly binds to specific cellular receptors, thereby activating cytoplasmic enzymes affecting messenger RNA translation and protein synthesis; the antiviral state takes several hours to develop but persists for days. Peginterferon has the same spectrum of activity as interferon-α.

PHARMACOKINETICS

Oral absorption	Poor
C_{max} 3 × 10⁶ IU intramuscularly	20 IU/mL after 2–4 h
9 × 10⁶ IU intramuscularly	50–100 IU/mL after 2–4h
Plasma half-life	3–8 h
Peginterferon	36 h
Plasma protein binding	Not known

Cerebrospinal fluid (CSF) penetration is poor. It is not cleared by hemodialysis. Little or none is excreted in the urine, and its fate after release from the cell receptor is largely unknown. The extent of excretion in breast milk is unknown.

INTERACTIONS

Human hepatic cytochrome P_{450} systems and oxidative drug metabolism are inhibited, causing a modest prolongation in the half-life of drugs such as theophylline.

TOXICITY AND SIDE EFFECTS

Toxicity has become increasingly apparent with the advent of purer preparations. 'Flu'-like symptoms (fever, arthralgia, myalgia, headache, malaise, chills) occur, which can usually be ameliorated by acetaminophen (paracetamol) administration. Lymphocytopenia is common, generally arising 2–4 h after administration of several million units. Liver function test values are frequently elevated at doses above 10^7 IU/day. These effects are rapidly reversible and tolerance may develop after several doses. Other toxic effects include gastrointestinal disturbances (anorexia, nausea, diarrhea, vomiting), weight loss, local pain, severe fatigue, alopecia, paresthesias, confusion, dizziness, drowsiness, nervousness and bone marrow suppression. Neutropenia and thrombocytopenia are dose dependent (threshold around 3×10^6 IU/day) and reversible. Hypotension may develop during, or up to 2 days after, treatment, and arrhythmias and cardiac failure have been observed.

Administration of excessive doses to pregnant rhesus monkeys in the early to mid-trimester caused abortions. Its effect on human pregnancy is unknown. Neutralizing antibodies have been reported in about 25% of treated patients but no clinical sequelae to their presence have been documented. Intralesional administration in the treatment of condylomata acuminata is generally well tolerated.

Peginterferon is also associated with fatigue, headache, myalgia and fever; most other side effects occur less frequently.

 ## CLINICAL USE

Chronic hepatitis B
Chronic hepatitis C (in combination with ribavirin)
Condyloma acuminata (intralesional)

It may also be of benefit in hairy cell and chronic myelogenous leukemias and Kaposi's sarcoma.

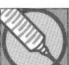 ### Preparations and dosage

Proprietary names: Interferon-α, Intron A, Roferon A, Wellferon, Viraferon, Interferon-γ1b, Imukin, Pegasys (peginterferon).
Preparation: Injection.
Dosage: Dose varies according to the condition being treated.
Widely available.

 ### Further information

de Almeida PR, de Mattos AA, Amaral KM, et al. Treatment of hepatitis C with peginterferon and ribavirin in a public health program. *Hepatogastroenterology*. 2009;56:223–226.

Gonzalez SA, Keeffe EB. Management of chronic hepatitis C treatment failures: role of consensus interferon. *Biologics*. 2009;3:141–150.

McHutchison JG, Lawitz EJ, Shiffman ML, et al. Peginterferon alfa-2b or alfa-2a with ribavirin for treatment of hepatitis C infection. *N Engl J Med*. 2009;361:580–593.

Witthoft T. Review of consensus interferon in the treatment of chronic hepatitis C. *Biologics*. 2008;2:635–643.

NEURAMINIDASE INHIBITORS

NEURAMINIDASE INHIBITORS

OSELTAMIVIR

Molecular weight (ethyl ester): 312.

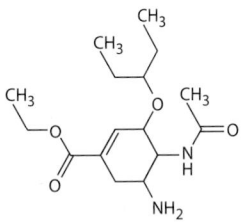

A selective neuraminidase inhibitor, formulated as the phosphate salt of the ethyl ester for oral administration.

 ## ANTIVIRAL ACTIVITY

Oseltamivir is active against influenza A and B, but no other virus.

 ## ACQUIRED RESISTANCE

Mutations in the neuraminidase (H274Y) have been detected in treated patients with seasonal H1N1 infection. Cross-resistance with zanamivir has been described in vitro.

 ## PHARMACOKINETICS

Oral absorption	c. 75%
C_{max} 75 mg oral	0.35–0.55 mg/L after 4 h
Plasma half-life	7–9 h
Plasma protein binding	Not known

The ethyl ester prodrug is hydrolyzed by hepatic esterases to release the active compound, oseltamivir carboxylate. Drug is excreted in the urine as the carboxylate derivative.

 ## TOXICITY AND SIDE EFFECTS

Adverse events relate to the gastrointestinal tract; the most common is nausea with or without vomiting in 10% of patients. Food alleviates side effects.

CLINICAL USE

Treatment and prevention of susceptible influenza A (H3N2) and B infections in adults and young children

Preparations and dosage

Proprietary name: Tamiflu.

Preparations: 75 mg tablets, capsules.

Dosage: Adults, oral, 75–150 mg per day in 1–2 divided doses. Children: 0–9 months, 3.0 mg/kg twice daily; 9 months–2 years, 3.5 mg/kg twice daily; >2 years old, 30–75 mg once or twice daily. Treatment twice daily for 5 days; prophylaxis once daily.

Widely available.

Further information

Lennon S, Barrett J, Kirkpatrick C, Rayner C. Oseltamivir oral suspension and capsules are bioequivalent for the active metabolite in healthy adult volunteers. *Int J Clin Pharmacol Ther.* 2009;47:539–548.

Mossong J, Opp M, Gerloff N, et al. Emergence of oseltamivir-resistant influenza A H1N1 virus during the 2007–2008 winter season in Luxembourg: clinical characteristics and epidemiology. *Antiviral Res.* 2009;84:91–94.

Whitley RJ. The role of oseltamivir in the treatment and prevention of influenza in children. *Expert Opin Drug Metab Toxicol.* 2007;3:755–767.

Yu K, Luo C, Qin G, et al. Why are oseltamivir and zanamivir effective against the newly emerged influenza A virus (A/H1N1)? *Cell Res.* 2009;19:1221–1224.

ZANAMIVIR

Molecular weight: 332.

A synthetic neuraminidase inhibitor formulated for administration by inhalation.

ANTIVIRAL ACTIVITY

Zanamivir is active against influenza A and influenza B.

ACQUIRED RESISTANCE

Resistance is presently uncommon, including strains resistant to oseltamivir. In clinical trials the frequency was no more than 1% of exposed patients.

PHARMACOKINETICS

Oral bioavailability is poor. After inhalation local respiratory mucosal concentrations greatly exceed those that are inhibitory for influenza A and B replication. The median concentrations in the sputum exceed 1 mg/L 6 h after inhalation and remain detectable for 24 h.

TOXICITY AND SIDE EFFECTS

Most adverse effects are related to the respiratory tree. These include rhinorrhea and, rarely, bronchospasm. Nausea and vomiting have been reported at low incidence.

CLINICAL USE

Treatment of influenza A and B infections in patients over 7 years of age, and prophylaxis of patients ≥5 years of age

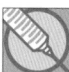

Preparation and dosage

Proprietary name: Relenza.

Preparation: Powder for inhalation.

Dosage: Adults and children >5 years, by inhalation, 10 mg every 12 h for 5 days. Prophylaxis, 10 mg once daily.

Widely available.

An intravenous preparation is under development

Further information

Eiland LS, Eiland EH. Zanamivir for the prevention of influenza in adults and children age 5 years and older. *Thera Clin Risk Manag.* 2007;3:461–465.

Hurt AC, Holien JK, Parker M, Kelso A, Barr IG. Zanamivir-resistant influenza viruses with a novel neuraminidase mutation. *J Virol.* 2009;83:10366–10373.

Wen WH, Lin M, Su CY, et al. Synergistic effect of zanamivir–porphyrin conjugates on inhibition of neuraminidase and inactivation of influenza virus. *J Med Chem.* 2009;52:4903–4910.

OTHER NEURAMINIDASE INHIBITORS

PERAMIVIR

An intravenously administered neuraminidase inhibitor currently under investigation for the treatment of influenza infections in normal and high-risk patient populations. No drug interactions of note have yet been identified.

Further information

Hayden F. Developing new antiviral agents for influenza treatment: what does the future hold?. *Clin Infect Dis.* 2009;48: (suppl 1):S3–S13.

Li Y, Zhang X, Wang X, Li S, Ruan J, Zhang Z. Quantification of peramivir (a novel anti-influenza drug) in human plasma by hydrophilic interaction chromatography/tandem mass spectrometry. *J Chromatogr.* 2009;877:933–938.

Yun NE, Linde NS, Zacks MA, et al. Injectable peramivir mitigates disease and promotes survival in ferrets and mice infected with the highly virulent influenza virus, A/Vietnam/1203/04 (H5N1). *Virology.* 2008;374:198–209.

NUCLEOSIDE ANALOGS

ACICLOVIR

Acyclovir (USAN); valacyclovir (USAN). Molecular weight (aciclovir): 225; (valaciclovir): 324.

| (A) Aciclovir | (B) Valaciclovir |

A synthetic acyclic purine nucleoside analog of the natural nucleoside 2′ deoxyguanosine, formulated for oral and topical use, and as the sodium salt for intravenous infusion. Valaciclovir (the L-valyl ester) is a prodrug formulation supplied as the hydrochloride for oral use.

ANTIVIRAL ACTIVITY

Activity is restricted to viruses of the herpes group. Herpes simplex virus (HSV) types 1 and 2, simian herpes virus B and varicella zoster viruses (VZV) are susceptible to concentrations readily attainable in human plasma. The 50% inhibitory concentration (ID_{50}) is 0.1 µmol for HSV-1 and HSV-2 and 3 µmol for VZV, concentrations much below those toxic to cells. Valaciclovir is metabolized to aciclovir, and has the same antiviral profile.

Thymidine-kinase-negative HSV mutants and cytomegalovirus (CMV) do not code for thymidine kinase and are generally resistant. Although Epstein–Barr virus (EBV) may have reduced thymidine kinase activity, its DNA polymerase is susceptible to aciclovir triphosphate and shows intermediate susceptibility. Human herpes viruses 6 and 7 are less susceptible than EBV.

ACQUIRED RESISTANCE

Mutations in HSV that involve deficient thymidine kinase or an altered substrate are most common; alterations in the DNA polymerase gene also result in resistance. Resistant mutants may be found in wild virus populations; mutants lacking thymidine kinase activity may be readily induced by passage of HSV in the presence of the drug. Resistant strains have mostly been reported in immunocompromised patients, are generally thymidine-kinase negative, and have decreased virulence. Resistant mutants that retain thymidine kinase activity appear to retain virulence. Emergence of resistant HSV strains is less frequent in immunocompetent patients, occurring in about 2% of those receiving prolonged treatment.

PHARMACOKINETICS

Oral absorption, aciclovir	*c.* 20%
valaciclovir	*c.* 60%
C_{max} 200 mg oral 4-hourly	1.4–4 µmol after 1.5–1.75 h
5 mg/kg 8-hourly intravenous infusion	43.2 µmol steady state
10 mg/kg 8-hourly intravenous infusion	88.9 µmol steady state
Plasma half-life	3–3.3 h
Plasma protein binding	15%

Absorption

Therapeutic drug levels are readily attained after oral or intravenous administration, although concentrations achieved by an oral dose are over 90% lower than those after intravenous therapy. Accumulation of the drug is unlikely in patients without renal dysfunction.

Valaciclovir is readily absorbed and is converted rapidly and almost completely to aciclovir; absorption is unaffected by food. Peak plasma concentrations of 22 µmol are found in subjects after an oral dose of 1000 mg every 8 h; systemic exposure is comparable to that of intravenous aciclovir 5 mg/kg every 8 h. The peak plasma concentration and area under the concentration–time curve (AUC) do not increase proportionally with increasing doses, presumably due to reduced absorption. The time to peak aciclovir concentration is also dose dependent, ranging from 0.9 to 1.8 h after single oral doses of 100–1000 mg.

Distribution

Aciclovir is widely distributed in various tissues and body fluids. Delivery of the drug to the basal epidermis after topical administration is about 30–50% of that obtained by oral dosing. Aciclovir ointment penetrates the corneal epithelium. CSF concentrations are about 50% of simultaneous plasma concentrations. Vesicular fluid concentrations approximate those in plasma. The drug is actively secreted into breast milk at a concentration several times that of plasma. Placental cord blood contains levels of 69–99% of maternal plasma and the drug is 3–6 times more concentrated in amniotic fluid.

Metabolism

About 15% of an intravenous dose is metabolized in persons with normal renal function. The only significant urinary metabolite is 9-carboxymethoxymethylguanine, which has no antiviral activity. Less than 0.2% of the dose is recovered as the 8-hydroxylation product.

Excretion

Around 45–79% of a dose is recovered unchanged in urine, the percentage declining with decreasing creatinine clearance. In patients with renal failure, mean peak plasma concentrations nearly doubled and the elimination half-life increased to 19.5 h. Dosage reductions are advised for various stages of renal impairment. During hemodialysis the half-life is 5.7 h and after dialysis the plasma concentration is about 60% less than the predialysis concentration. Half-lives of 12–17 h have been reported for patients undergoing continuous peritoneal dialysis, with only 13% or less of administered drug being recovered in the 24-h dialysate. The half-life in patients undergoing arteriovenous hemofiltration/dialysis is about 20 h.

Less than 1% of a dose of valaciclovir is recovered as unchanged drug in the urine. In multidose studies the amount of aciclovir recovered across dose levels ranged from about 40% to 50%. Between 7% and 12% of the dose is found as the 9-carboxymethoxymethylguanine metabolite. Overall, aciclovir accounts for 80–85% of total urinary recovery.

 ## TOXICITY AND SIDE EFFECTS

Few adverse reactions to topical, ocular, oral or intravenous formulations have been reported. Allergic contact dermatitis occasionally occurs with aciclovir cream. Superficial punctate keratopathy occurs in 10% of patients receiving the ophthalmic preparation; stinging or burning on application occurs in 4%. Less common complications include conjunctivitis, blepharitis and pain.

Transient increases in blood urea nitrogen and creatinine occur in 10% of patients given bolus injections. It can be largely avoided by reducing the rate of infusion, adequate hydration and dosage adjustment in renal failure. Nausea, vomiting, diarrhea and abdominal pain occasionally occur, particularly in association with a raised creatinine concentration. Acute reversible renal failure has been reported. Reconstituted aciclovir has a pH of about 11; severe inflammation and ulceration have been reported after extravasation at the infusion site. Encephalopathy, tremors, confusion, hallucinations, convulsions, psychiatric disorders, bone marrow depression and abnormal liver function have occasionally arisen. Skin rashes have been reported in a few patients but resolve on discontinuation of the drug.

Headache and nausea have been reported as side effects of valaciclovir, but occurred with similar frequency in subjects taking placebo.

Results of mutagenicity tests in vitro and in vivo indicate that aciclovir is unlikely to pose a genetic risk to humans, and the drug was not found to be carcinogenic in long-term studies in mice and rats. No detectable drug-related effects have been detected in pregnancy.

 ## CLINICAL USE

Aciclovir

Herpes simplex keratitis
Chickenpox and herpes zoster
Herpes simplex encephalitis and neonatal herpes
Prophylaxis of HSV infections in the severely immunocompromised

Valaciclovir

Herpes zoster and genital HSV infections

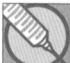 ## Preparations and dosage

Proprietary names: Zovirax (aciclovir), Valtrex (valaciclovir).

Preparations: Tablets, suspension, i.v. infusion, cream, eye ointment (aciclovir), tablets (valaciclovir).

Dosage: Adults, children, oral, dose varies according to the condition being treated. I.v. infusion, adults, HSV or VZV, 5 mg/kg every 8 h, doubled in primary and VZV in the immunocompromised and in herpes simplex encephalitis. Children, 1–3 months, 10 mg/kg every 8 h; 3 months–12 years, 250 mg/m² every 8 h; dose doubled in the immunocompromised and HSV encephalitis; for neonatal HSV, 20 mg every 8 h for 21 days.

Valaciclovir: herpes zoster, 1000 mg every 8 h for 7 days. Episodic therapy of genital herpes, 500 mg every 8 h for 3–5 days. Suppressive treatment, 500 or 1000 mg per day in two divided doses.

Widely available.

 ## Further information

Fife KH, Warren TJ, Justus SE, Heitman CK. An international, randomized, double-blind, placebo-controlled, study of valacyclovir for the suppression of herpes simplex virus type 2 genital herpes in newly diagnosed patients. *Sex Transm Dis*. 2008;35:668–673.

Paz-Bailey G, Sternberg M, Puren AJ, et al. Improvement in healing and reduction in HIV shedding with episodic acyclovir therapy as part of syndromic management among men: a randomized, controlled trial. *J Infect Dis*. 2009;200:1039–1049.

Rha B, Kimberlin DW, Whitley RJ. Laboratory diagnosis of viral infections. In: Jerome K, ed. *Antiviral Therapy*. London: Informa Healthcare; 2010 In press.

ENTECAVIR

Molecular weight (monohydrate): 295.3.

An analog of guanosine formulated as tablets and suspension for oral use.

ANTIVIRAL ACTIVITY

Entecavir is active only against hepatitis B virus. The 50% effective dose (ED_{50}) is approximately 0.004 μM.

RESISTANCE

Development of resistance after 96 weeks of therapy was uncommon (<1%).

PHARMACOKINETICS

Oral absorption	100%
C_{max} 0.5 mg/kg oral	4.2 ng/mL
Intracellular half-life	c. 16 h
Volume of distribution	In excess of body water
Plasma protein binding	13%

Entecavir is rapidly absorbed after administration on an empty stomach, achieving peak plasma concentrations in 1–1.5 h. Plasma steady state is achieved in 6–10 days.

It is renally eliminated. Dosage adjustment is required with impaired creatinine clearance. The drug is not metabolized by cytochrome P_{450}. No drug interactions have been identified.

TOXICITY AND SIDE EFFECTS

Severity of adverse reactions was comparable to that of lamivudine, with headache, fatigue, upper respiratory infections and abdominal pain being most common. Lactic acidosis and hepatic steatosis were rarely observed.

CLINICAL USE

Treatment of chronic hepatitis B virus infection in patients >16 years of age

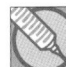

Preparations and dosage

Proprietary name: Baraclude.

Preparations: Tablets (0.5 and 1.0 mg), oral suspension (0.05 mg/mL).

Dosage: 0.5 mg per day; for known lamivudine or telbivudine resistance, 1 mg per day.

Available in Europe and the USA.

Further information

Cho SW, Koh KH, Cheong JY, et al. Low efficacy of entecavir therapy in adefovir-refractory hepatitis B patients with prior lamivudine resistance. *J Viral Hepat.* 2009; 17:171–177.

Kobashi H, Fujioka S, Kawaguchi M, et al. Two cases of development of entecavir resistance during entecavir treatment for nucleoside-naive chronic hepatitis B. *Hepatol Int.* 2009;3:403–410.

Lai CL, Yuen MF. The saga of entecavir. *Hepatol Int.* 2009;3:421–424.

Tse KC, Yap DY, Tang CS, Yung S, Chan TM. Response to adefovir or entecavir in renal allograft recipients with hepatic flare due to lamivudine-resistant hepatitis B. *Clin Transplant.* 2010; 24:207–212.

Uchiyama M, Tamai Y, Ikeda T. Entecavir as prophylaxis against hepatitis B virus reactivation following chemotherapy for lymphoma. *Int J Infect Dis.* 2010;14:e265–266.

GANCICLOVIR

Molecular weight (free acid): 255; (sodium salt): 277; (valganciclovir): 354.

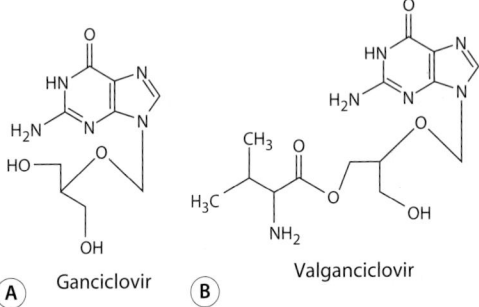

(A) Ganciclovir (B) Valganciclovir

A synthetic 2'-deoxyguanosine nucleoside analog, supplied as the L-valine ester, valganciclovir, for oral administration and as the sodium salt for parenteral use. A slow-release ocular implant device is also available.

ANTIVIRAL ACTIVITY

Ganciclovir is phosphorylated to the monophosphate by a cellular deoxyguanosine kinase more rapidly in infected than uninfected cells. HSV and VZV thymidine kinases monophosphorylate ganciclovir, after which it is further metabolized to the active triphosphate by cellular enzymes. The UL97 open reading frame of CMV encodes a phosphonotransferase, which can regulate phosphorylation. In CMV-infected cells the concentration of the triphosphate is approximately 10-fold higher than in uninfected cells.

HSV-1 and HSV-2 are inhibited by 0.2–8.0 μmol (0.05–2.0 mg/L). Its activity is similar to that of aciclovir against HSV-1 in vitro, but is slightly superior against HSV-2. The ID_{50} for CMV ranges from 0.5 to 11 μmol (0.125–2.75 mg/L). EBV is inhibited by 1–4 μmol and VZV by 4–40 μmol.

ACQUIRED RESISTANCE

Prolonged, repeated courses lead to the selection of resistant strains, occurring in 8% of patients receiving the drug for >3 months. Studies of laboratory-derived resistant strains indicate that drug resistance can result from alterations in the phosphonotransferase encoded by the gene region UL 27, the viral DNA polymerase (gene region UL 54), or both.

PHARMACOKINETICS

Oral absorption, ganciclovir	c. 5.4–7.1%
valganciclovir	80%
C_{max} 5 mg/kg 1-h infusion	33.2 μmol end infusion
Plasma half-life (intravenous infusion)	2.9 h
Volume of distribution	c. 1.17 L/kg
Plasma protein binding	1–2%

Absorption

After an intravenous infusion of 5 mg/kg, the plasma level after 11 h was 2.2 μmol. After repeated 5 mg/kg doses every 8 h, the mean peak serum levels were 25 μmol and mean trough levels 3.6 μmol, levels in excess of, or in the same range as, the ID_{50} for CMV. In patients treated for 8–22 days with 1 or 2.5 mg/kg every 8 h, the mean steady-state plasma concentrations after a 1 h infusion of 1 mg/kg ranged from 7.2 μmol immediately after infusion to 0.8 μmol after 8 h. Corresponding values after a dose of 2.5 mg/kg were 19.6 and 3.2 μmol, respectively.

Multiple dosing with oral ganciclovir 1 g every 8 h resulted in peak levels of 1.1 mg/L (4.3 μmol) and a trough of 0.52 mg/L (2.1 μmol). Valganciclovir is rapidly converted to ganciclovir, doses of 900 mg producing plasma levels similar to those achieved with 5 mg/kg ganciclovir every 12 h.

Distribution

Data on distribution are limited. The levels of the drug in CSF are estimated to be 24–67% of those in plasma. Mean intravitreal levels of 14 μmol were reported for samples taken a mean of 12 h after therapy with a mean dose of 6 mg/kg per day. However, no significant correlations are noted between time after the last dose and intravitreal concentration. The observed mean value in the eye is below the concentration required to achieve 50% or 90% inhibition of CMV plaque

formation by clinical isolates, which may explain the difficulty in controlling CMV retinitis.

Metabolism and excretion

About 80% of the drug is eliminated unchanged in the urine within 24 h. Probenecid and other drugs that impact renal tubular secretion or absorption may reduce renal clearance. In severe renal impairment, the mean plasma half-life is 28.3 h. Dosage must be reduced in patients with impaired renal function. Plasma levels of the drug can be reduced by approximately 50–90% with hemodialysis. The half-life on dialysis is about 4 h. Patients undergoing dialysis should be given 1.25 mg/kg per day; therapy should also be administered after dialysis.

No significant pharmacokinetic interaction occurs when ganciclovir and foscarnet are given as concomitant or daily alternate therapy.

TOXICITY AND SIDE EFFECTS

The 50% inhibitory concentration (IC_{50}) for human bone marrow colony-forming cells is 39 (± 73) μmol; for other cell lines it ranges from 110 to 2900 μmol. Toxicity frequently limits therapy. Marrow suppression may develop on as little as 5 mg/kg on alternate days and is exacerbated when the drug is given with zidovudine. Neutropenia of <1000/mm³ occurs in nearly 40% of recipients and <500/mm³ in upwards of 30% for those given induction therapy of 10 mg/kg per day for 14 days, followed by 5 mg/kg per day. Neutropenia is reversible and develops during the early treatment or maintenance phase, but may occur later. Thrombocytopenia of <20 000/mm³ and <50 000/mm³ develops in about 10% and 19% of patients, respectively. Frequent monitoring of the full blood count is recommended.

Adverse effects on the CNS, including confusion, convulsions, psychosis, hallucinations, tremor, ataxia, coma, dizziness, headaches and somnolence, occur in around 5% of patients. Liver function abnormalities, fever and rash occur in about 2%. Intraocular injection of ganciclovir is associated with intense pain, and occasionally amaurosis lasting for 1–10 min.

Animal studies indicate that inhibition of spermatogenesis and suppression of female fertility occurs. Ganciclovir is also potentially embryolethal, mutagenic and teratogenic, and is contraindicated during pregnancy or lactation. It can cause local tissue damage and should not be administered intramuscularly or subcutaneously; patients should be adequately hydrated during treatment.

CLINICAL USE

Life- or sight-threatening CMV infections in immunocompromised individuals
Prevention and treatment of CMV disease in patients receiving immunosuppressive therapy for organ transplantation

An ocular implant has been developed for the treatment of CMV retinitis.

Use in congenital CMV infections has not yet gained regulatory approval.

Preparations and dosage

Proprietary names: Cytovene, Cymevene, Vitrasert (ocular implant), Valcyte (valganciclovir).

Preparations: Capsules, i.v. infusion, ophthalmic solution (ganciclovir); tablets (valganciclovir).

Dosage: Adults, i.v., treatment, 5 mg/kg every 12 h for 14–21 days. Maintenance dose, i.v., 6 mg/kg per day on 5 days per week or 5 mg/kg once every day. Oral, 1 g every 8 h or 500 mg every 4 h, following at least 3 weeks i.v. therapy.

Valganciclovir: 900 mg every 12 h.

Widely available.

Further information

Acosta EP, Brundage RC, King JR, et al. Ganciclovir population pharmacokinetics in neonates following intravenous administration of ganciclovir and oral administration of a liquid valganciclovir formulation. *Clin Pharmacol Ther.* 2007;81:867–872.

Brady RL, Green K, Frei C, Maxwell P. Oral ganciclovir versus valganciclovir for cytomegalovirus prophylaxis in high-risk liver transplant recipients. *Transpl Infect Dis.* 2009;11:106–111.

Kimberlin DW, Acosta EP, Sanchez PJ, et al. Pharmacokinetic and pharmacodynamic assessment of oral valganciclovir in the treatment of symptomatic congenital cytomegalovirus disease. *J Infect Dis.* 2008;197:836–845.

LAMIVUDINE

An antiretroviral agent that also exhibits activity against hepatitis B virus and duck hepatitis B virus. Its properties are described in Ch. 36 (p. 432). Use is limited by the development of resistance within 1 year in up to 25% of treated patients. It is likely to be used with other drugs in the future.

CLINICAL USE

Therapy of chronic hepatitis B

Preparations and dosage

Proprietary name: Epivir.

Preparations: 100 mg tablets, oral solution.

Dosage: Adults, oral, 150 mg every 12 h. Children, 3 months–12 years, 4 mg/kg every 12 h (maximum dose, 300 mg per day).

Widely available.

Further information

Huang H, Cai Q, Lin T, et al. Lamivudine for the prevention of hepatitis B virus reactivation after high-dose chemotherapy and autologous hematopoietic stem cell transplantation for patients with advanced or relapsed non-Hodgkin's lymphoma single institution experience. *Expert Opin Pharmacother.* 2009;10:2399–2406.

Hoa PT, Huy NT, Thu LT, et al. A randomized-controlled study investigating viral suppression and serological response following PreS1/PreS2/S vaccine therapy combined with lamivudine in HBeAg-positive chronic hepatitis B patients. *Antimicrob Agents Chemother.* 2009;53(12):5134–5140.

PENCICLOVIR

Molecular weight (penciclovir): 253.3; (famciclovir): 321.3.

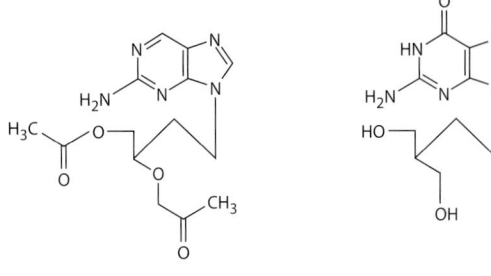

Famciclovir   Penciclovir

A synthetic acyclic purine nucleoside analog, usually administered orally as the diacetyl ester, famciclovir, which acts as a prodrug undergoing rapid first-pass metabolism to release the active compound in vivo. The parent compound has virtually no oral bioavailability, but is supplied as a topical formulation.

ANTIVIRAL ACTIVITY

It is active against members of the herpes virus family, with greatest activity against HSV-1 (ID_{50} 1.6 μmol), somewhat lower activity against HSV-2 (ID_{50} 6.0 μmol), and less activity against VZV (ID_{50} 12 μmol). The ID_{50} values for aciclovir in the same cells were 0.9, 2.7 and 17 μmol, respectively. CMV is relatively resistant and EBV has intermediate susceptibility. The activity of hepatitis B virus is inhibited in vitro.

In cells infected with HSV-1, HSV-2 and VZV monophosphorylation is more efficient than that of aciclovir. It has less affinity for viral DNA polymerases than aciclovir triphosphate and does not act as a DNA chain terminator; however, it has a much longer half-life.

ACQUIRED RESISTANCE

Penciclovir is inactive against thymidine kinase-deficient strains of HSV.

PHARMACOKINETICS

Oral absorption, penciclovir	5%
famciclovir	77%
Cmax famciclovir 250 mg oral	1.6 mg/L after 0.5–1.5 h
famciclovir 500 mg oral	3.3 mg/L after 0.5–1.5 h
famciclovir 750 mg oral	5.1 mg/L after 0.5–1.5 h
Plasma half-life	2.1–2.7 h
Volume of distribution	c. 1.5 L/kg
Plasma protein binding	<20%

Following absorption famciclovir is converted rapidly by enzyme-mediated deacetylation and oxidation to penciclovir. Food does not lead to any significant change in the availability or elimination.

The pharmacokinetics in elderly subjects are similar to those seen in younger subjects, although small increases in AUC and plasma half-lives were seen, consistent with slightly decreased renal clearance.

Renal excretion is the major route of elimination, 50–60% of an oral dose being recovered in the urine. After intravenous infusion, about 70% is excreted unchanged in the urine. After oral administration of famciclovir, penciclovir accounts for 82% of urinary drug-related material. The remainder includes metabolites, of which the largest is the 6-deoxy precursor of penciclovir. Renal clearance exceeds glomerular filtration, indicating renal tubular secretion.

TOXICITY AND SIDE EFFECTS

In clinical trials the incidence of adverse events after famciclovir, aciclovir and placebo were similar, the most common adverse events being headache and nausea.

CLINICAL USE

| Herpes zoster and genital herpes |
| Orolabial herpes (topical) |

Preparations and dosage

Proprietary names: Denavir, Famvir, Vectavir.

Preparations: Tablets and topical cream.

Dosage: Adults, oral, 125–500 mg every 6–8 h for 7 days for HSV and VZV infections. Alternative 1-day treatment regimens include 1000 mg every 12 h for 1 day in the treatment of genital and labial herpes. Topical, every 6 h.

Widely available.

Further information

Bartlett BL, Tyring SK, Fife K, et al. Famciclovir treatment options for patients with frequent outbreaks of recurrent genital herpes: the RELIEF trial. *J Clin Virol.* 2008;43:190–195.

Bodsworth N, Bloch M, McNulty A, et al. 2-Day versus 5-day famciclovir as treatment of recurrences of genital herpes: results of the FaST study. *Sex Health.* 2008;5:219–225.

Bodsworth N, Fife K, Koltun W, et al. Single-day famciclovir for the treatment of genital herpes: follow-up results of time to next recurrence and assessment of antiviral resistance. *Curr Med Res Opin.* 2009;25:483–487.

RIBAVIRIN

Molecular weight: 244.2.

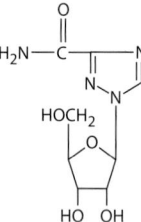

A synthetic nucleoside. It is neither a classic pyrimidine nor a purine, but stereochemical studies indicate that it is a guanosine analog. It is usually formulated for administration by inhalation, but oral and intravenous preparations are also used.

ANTIVIRAL ACTIVITY

Laboratory tests indicate that herpes viruses are the most sensitive. Of the RNA viruses, activity has been noted with influenza types A and B; parainfluenza virus types 1, 2 and 3; mumps, measles and respiratory syncytial virus (RSV); Lassa fever and Machupo viruses; Rift Valley fever, sandfly fever, Hantaan and yellow fever viruses. RSV plaques are reduced 85–98% by 16 mg/L.

Ribavirin is phosphorylated in cells and inhibits inosine monophosphate dehydrogenase, which is involved in the synthesis of guanosine triphosphate. Decrease in intracellular thymidine triphosphate has also been noted. In most cell lines the antiviral activity is much lower than the cytostatic dose, which ranges from 200 to 1000 mg/L.

Ribavirin and interferon-α, particularly the pegylated forms, act synergistically in the treatment of chronic hepatitis C virus (HCV) infection, resulting in sustained reduction in alanine aminotransferase levels and loss of HCV RNA in 40% of patients who failed to respond to interferon previously.

ACQUIRED RESISTANCE

Development of resistant virus strains has not been demonstrated.

PHARMACOKINETICS

Oral absorption	36–46%
C_{max} 3 mg/kg oral	4.1–8.2 µmol/L after 1–1.5 h
600 mg intravenous	43.6 µmol/L end infusion
Plasma half-life	c. 24 h
Volume of distribution	647 L
Plasma protein binding	<10%

Absorption

It is rapidly absorbed after oral administration. Mean peak concentrations after 1 week of oral doses of 200, 400 and 800 mg every 8 h were 5.0, 11.1 and 20.9 µmol/L, respectively. Trough levels 9–12 h after the end of 2 weeks' therapy were 5.1, 13.2 and 18.4 µmol/L, respectively, indicating continued accumulation of the drug. Drug was still detectable 4 weeks later. Mean peak plasma concentrations after intravenous doses of 600, 1200 and 2400 mg were 43.6, 72.3 and 160.8 µmol/L, respectively; at 8 h the mean plasma concentrations were 2.1, 5.6 and 10.2 µmol/L.

Aerosolized doses (6 g in 300 mL distilled water) are generally administered at a rate of 12–15 mL/h using a Collison jet nebulizer, the estimated dosage being 1.8 mg/kg per h for infants and 0.9 mg/kg per h for adults. When administered by small particle aerosol for 2.5–8 h, plasma concentrations ranged from 0.44 to 8.7 µmol/L.

Metabolism and excretion

It is rapidly degraded by deribosylation or amide hydrolysis, and together with its metabolites is slowly eliminated by the kidney. About 50% of the drug or its metabolites appear in the urine within 72 h and 15% is excreted in the stools. The remainder seems to be retained in body tissues, principally in red blood cells, which concentrate the drug or metabolites to a peak at 4 days, with a half-life of around 40 days. After intravenous administration 19.4% of the dose was eliminated during the first 24 h (compared with 7.3% after an oral dose), the difference reflecting the bioavailability.

TOXICITY AND SIDE EFFECTS

It is generally well tolerated, though adverse reactions appear to be related to dose and duration of therapy. Minor adverse reactions include metallic taste, dry mouth sensation and increased thirst, flatulence, fatigue and CNS complaints, including headache, irritability and insomnia. Daily doses of 1 g may cause unconjugated bilirubin levels to double and the reticulocyte count to increase. Hemoglobin concentrations may decrease with treatment or higher dosages; with doses of 3.9–12.6 g per day, a drop in hemoglobin was noted by days 7–13 of treatment, which was generally 'rapidly'

reversible on withdrawal of the drug, but in some instances necessitated blood transfusion.

Aerosol administration of about 2 g in 36 or 39 h during 3 days is well tolerated, does not affect results of pulmonary function tests, and seems non-toxic.

It is both teratogenic and embryotoxic in laboratory animals, so precautions must be observed in women of child bearing age.

CLINICAL USE

RSV infections in infants (by nebulizer) in emergency situations (i.e. transplant recipients)
Lassa fever
Hepatitis C (in combination with interferon-α)

Use in RSV pneumonia in infants is no longer routine. It reduces mortality from Hantaan virus, the agent responsible for hemorrhagic fever with renal syndrome.

Preparations and dosage

Proprietary names: Virazole (for inhalation); Rebotal, Copegus (oral).

Preparations: Inhalation, tablets, capsules, oral solution.

Dosage: By aerosol inhalation or nebulization (via small-particle aerosol generator) of solution containing 20 mg/mL for 12–18 h per day for at least 3 days and a maximum of 7 days. Adults, oral, <65 kg, 400 mg every 12 h; 65–85 kg, 400 mg in the morning and 600 mg at night; >85 kg, 600 mg every 12 h. Oral dosage recommendation vary according to formulations: see manufacturer's literature.

Widely available.

Further information

Boeckh M, Englund J, Li Y, et al. Randomized controlled multicenter trial of aerosolized ribavirin for respiratory syncytial virus upper respiratory tract infection in hematopoietic cell transplant recipients. *Clin Infect Dis.* 2007;44:245–249.

Richards GA, Sewlall NH, Duse A. Availability of drugs for formidable communicable diseases. *Lancet.* 2009;373:545–546.

Zeuzem S, Buti M, Ferenci P, et al. Efficacy of 24 weeks treatment with peginterferon alfa-2b plus ribavirin in patients with chronic hepatitis C infected with genotype 1 and low pretreatment viremia. *J Hepatol.* 2006;44:97–103.

TELBIVUDINE

Molecular weight: 242.2.

A synthetic thymidine nucleoside analog formulated for oral use in the treatment of chronic hepatitis B infection.

ANTIVIRAL ACTIVITY

Telbivudine is active at therapeutic concentrations only against hepatitis B. After phosphorylation it competitively inhibits HBV DNA polymerase. It inhibits HBV first strand (EC_{50} 1.3 ± 1.6 μM) and second strand synthesis (EC_{50} 0.2 ± 0.2 μM). Concentrations of telbivudine 5′-triphosphate ≤100 μM did not inhibit human cellular DNA polymerases. No appreciable mitochondrial toxicity was observed in HepG2 cells at concentrations up to 10 μM.

ACQUIRED RESISTANCE

After 1 year resistance occurred in 7–20% of patients on telbivudine depending upon past exposure to other drugs used in the treatment of hepatitis B and the type of infection. Development of resistance was less frequent in those receiving telbivudine than in those receiving lamivudine.

PHARMACOKINETICS

Oral absorption	100%
C_{max} 600 mg/kg oral	3.7 μg/mL
Volume of distribution	In excess of body water
Plasma protein binding	3.3%

It is eliminated renally, necessitating dose adjustment in patients with renal insufficiency.

It should not be administered with pegylated interferon because of an increased risk of neuropathy.

TOXICITY AND SIDE EFFECTS

Adverse effects are similar to those of lamivudine and include upper respiratory tract infection, headache, fatigue and gastrointestinal upset. Myopathy and peripheral neuropathy are rare but have been observed in some patients several weeks into the course with associated rise in serum creatine kinase levels. Acute exacerbations of hepatitis have been observed on discontinuation of therapy. Lactic acidosis may occur, necessitating drug discontinuation.

CLINICAL USE

Treatment of chronic hepatitis B in patients >16 years of age

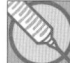

Preparations and dosage

Proprietary name: Tzeka, Sebire.

Preparations: Tablets (600 mg), oral suspension (100 mg/5 mL).

Dosage: 600 mg once daily.

Available in Europe and the USA.

Further information

Buti M. Is telbivudine superior to lamivudine for the treatment of patients with chronic hepatitis B? *Nat Clin Pract Gastroenterol and Hepatol.* 2008;5:494–495.

Hou J, Yin YK, Xu D, et al. Telbivudine versus lamivudine in Chinese patients with chronic hepatitis B: results at 1 year of a randomized, double-blind trial. *Hepatology.* 2008;47:447–454.

Lai CL, Gane E, Liaw YF, et al. Telbivudine versus lamivudine in patients with chronic hepatitis B. *N Engl J Med.* 2007;357:2576–2588.

Zhou XJ, Lim SG, Lloyd DM, Chao GC, Brown NA, Lai CL. Pharmacokinetics of telbivudine following oral administration of escalating single and multiple doses in patients with chronic hepatitis B virus infection: pharmacodynamic implications. *Antimicrob Agents Chemother.* 2006;50:874–879.

OTHER NUCLEOSIDE ANALOGS

IDOXURIDINE

A halogenated pyrimidine analog originally synthesized as an anticancer agent. Formulated in dimethylsulfoxide for topical application and as a solution for ophthalmic use.

Activity is largely limited to DNA viruses, primarily HSV-1, HSV-2 and VZV. HSV-1 plaque formation in BHK 21 cells is sensitive to 6.25–25 mg/L; type 2 microplaques required 62.5–125 mg/L. RNA viruses are not affected, with the exception of oncogenic RNA viruses such as Rous sarcoma virus. Drug resistance is easily generated in vitro, and may be an obstacle to treatment. However, there is little or no cross-resistance with newer nucleoside analogs.

It is poorly soluble in water, and aqueous solutions are ineffective against infections other than those localized to the eye. In animals, therapeutic levels are achieved in the cornea within 30 min of ophthalmic application and persist for 4 h. Penetration is otherwise poor, with only the biologically inactive dehalogenated metabolite uracil entering the eye.

The drug is too toxic for systemic administration. Contact dermatitis, punctate epithelial keratopathy, follicular conjunctivitis, ptosis, stenosis and occlusion of the puncta and keratinization of the lid margins occur in up to 14% of those receiving ophthalmic preparations.

It is used in herpes keratitis, but has largely been superseded by trifluridine or aciclovir.

TRIFLURIDINE

Trifluorothymidine. A synthetic halogenated pyrimidine nucleoside, first synthesized as an antitumor agent. It inhibits enzymes of the DNA pathway and is incorporated into both cellular and progeny viral DNA, causing faulty transcription of late messenger RNA and the production of incompetent virion protein. It does not require a viral thymidine kinase for monophosphorylation and is far less selective and more toxic than other analogs. It is active against HSV-1 and HSV-2, vaccinia virus, CMV and possibly adenovirus. When applied as a 1% ophthalmic solution, it rapidly enters the aqueous humor of HSV-infected rabbits' eyes but is cleared within 60–90 min.

It causes sister chromatid exchange – an indicator of mutagenicity – at 0.5 mg/L in human lymphocytes and fibroblasts. It is teratogenic to chick embryos when injected directly into the yolk sac. Its principal adverse effects in humans following systemic administration include leukopenia, anemia, fever and hypocalcemia. Accordingly, it is restricted to topical ophthalmic use in HSV ocular infections. The ophthalmic 1% aqueous solution produces occasional punctate lesions; other side effects are similar to those of idoxuridine but arise less frequently.

NUCLEOTIDE ANALOGS

ADEFOVIR

Molecular weight (base): 273.2; (dipivoxil): 501.5.

A nucleotide analog of adenosine monophosphate, administered orally as its prodrug, adefovir dipivoxil.

ANTIVIRAL ACTIVITY

It is phosphorylated by cellular kinases to adefovir diphosphate, which competitively inhibits HBV reverse transcriptase and terminates DNA synthesis upon incorporation into the growing chain. The inhibition constant (K_i) for adefovir diphosphate for HBV DNA polymerase was 0.1 μM. The diphosphate is a weak inhibitor of human DNA polymerases α and γ, with K_i values of 1.18 μM and 0.97 μM, respectively. It inhibits HIV in vitro, but an effective dose with a margin of safety could not be achieved in human studies.

ACQUIRED RESISTANCE

It has a lower propensity to induce drug resistance than lamivudine. Clinical trials of patients receiving 48 weeks of therapy did not identify any cases of resistance. Longer courses

yield resistant strains of HBV with mutations in the DNA polymerase gene; other rare variants of resistant strains have been identified. Lamivudine-resistant strains of HBV retain susceptibility to adefovir.

PHARMACOKINETICS

Oral absorption	c. 60%
C_{max} 10 mg/kg oral	18.4 ng/mL
Plasma half-life	c. 7.5 h.
Volume of distribution	392 mL/kg
Plasma protein binding	Not known

The prodrug is metabolized to adefovir, which is excreted by the kidneys and therefore requires dose adjustment in patients with impaired renal function. It does not induce cytochrome P_{450} at standard doses and does not influence the metabolism or plasma concentrations of the other licensed medications used in the treatment of hepatitis B.

TOXICITY AND SIDE EFFECTS

It is generally well tolerated, with headache, pharyngitis, abdominal pain and peripheral neuropathy being the most common side effects. Nephrotoxicity has been observed in some patients, with those receiving higher doses and longer courses of therapy at greater risk. Exacerbation of hepatitis has been reported in patients immediately following discontinuation of treatment. Most exacerbations occur within 12 weeks of stopping therapy, and elevations of alanine aminotransferase (ALT) up to 10 times the upper limit of normal can be observed in over 25% of patients. Lactic acidosis has been reported in a few patients and is an indication for immediate discontinuation.

CLINICAL USE

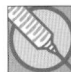

Treatment of chronic hepatitis B virus infection in patients >12 years of age

Preparations and dosage

Proprietary name: Hepsera.

Preparation: 10 mg tablet.

Dosage: 10 mg tablet.

Widely available in Europe and the USA.

Further information

Hadziyannis SJ, Tassopoulos NC, Heathcote EJ, et al. Long-term therapy with adefovir dipivoxil for HBeAg-negative chronic hepatitis B. *N Engl J Med.* 2005;352:2673–2681.

Marcellin P, Chang TT, Lim SG, et al. Long-term efficacy and safety of adefovir dipivoxil for the treatment of hepatitis B e antigen-positive chronic hepatitis B. *Hepatology.* 2008;48:750–758.

Schildgen O, Sirma H, Funk A, et al. Variant of hepatitis B virus with primary resistance to adefovir. *N Engl J Med.* 2006;354:1807–1812. Comment and author reply: Chang TT, Lai CL. 2006 Hepatitis B virus with primary resistance to adefovir. *N Engl J Med.* 355:322–323.

CIDOFOVIR

Molecular weight: 279.

An acyclic cytosine analog administered by intravenous infusion.

ANTIVIRAL ACTIVITY

The phosphonate group enables it to mimic a nucleotide and bypass virus-dependent phosphorylation. Cellular enzymes convert it to the triphosphate, which has in-vitro and in-vivo activity against CMV and other herpesviruses, including aciclovir-resistant HSV. Oral hairy leukoplakia resolved on therapy, suggesting that it has activity against EBV. Activity against adenovirus and papillomaviruses is also reported.

RESISTANCE

Resistance can be generated in the laboratory but has not yet been encountered during treatment of patients.

PHARMACOKINETICS

Oral absorption	<5%
C_{max} 3 mg/kg intravenous infusion	7.7 mg/L end infusion
10 mg/kg intravenous infusion	23 mg/L end infusion
Plasma half-life	c. 3–4 h
Volume of distribution	c. 0.6 L/kg
Plasma protein binding	<6%

The intracellular half-life of the diphosphate is 17–65 h. It is excreted unchanged by the kidney by glomerular filtration and tubular secretion.

TOXICITY AND SIDE EFFECTS

Nephrotoxicity, heralded by proteinuria, occurred at weekly doses of ≤3 mg/kg in two of five patients after 6 and 14 consecutive weeks of therapy. Two of five patients given 10 mg/kg developed nephrotoxicity, manifested as a Fanconi-like syndrome, after only two doses. Biopsy revealed proximal tubular effects. Prehydration and extended dosing intervals seem to be nephroprotective.

CLINICAL USE

Treatment of CMV retinitis

Because of nephrotoxicity it is a drug of last resort. It has been used experimentally in the treatment of adenovirus pneumonia and BK virus in transplant patients and juvenile laryngeal papillomatosis.

Preparations and dosage

Proprietary name: Vistide.

Preparation: Injection.

Dosage: Induction: adults, i.v., 5 mg/kg with hydration and probenecid once weekly for 2 weeks, then every other week.

Available in the USA and Europe, including the UK.

Further information

Coremans G, Snoeck R. Cidofovir: clinical experience and future perspectives on an acyclic nucleoside phosphonate analog of cytosine in the treatment of refractory and premalignant HPV-associated anal lesions. *Expert Opin Pharmacother.* 2009;10:1343–1352.

Cesaro S, Hirsch HH, Faraci M, et al. Cidofovir for BK virus-associated hemorrhagic cystitis: a retrospective study. *Clin Infect Dis.* 2009;49:233–240.

Dvorak CC, Cowan MJ, Horn B, Weintrub PS. Development of herpes simplex virus stomatitis during receipt of cidofovir therapy. *Clin Infect Dis.* 2009;49:e92–e95.

Jesus DM, Costa LT, Goncalves DL, et al. Cidofovir inhibits genome encapsidation and affects morphogenesis during the replication of vaccinia virus. *J Virol.* 2009;83:11477–11490.

TENOFOVIR

A nucleotide analog structurally similar to adefovir. It is also used as an antiretroviral agent and its properties are described in Chapter 36 (pp. 434–435).

EC_{50} values for HBV, assessed in the HepG2 2.2.15 cell line, ranged from 0.14 to 1.5 μM; the cytotoxic concentration exceeded 100 μM. A decline in HBV DNA levels below 10^5 copies/mL at 48 weeks of therapy in 100% of patients receiving tenofovir compared with 44% on adefovir therapy has been reported. There are also case reports of patients with primary resistance to adefovir responding to tenofovir.

It is generally well tolerated in patients with chronic HBV; the most common side effects include nausea and gastrointestinal upset, headache, dizziness, fatigue and rash.

 ## CLINICAL USE

Chronic hepatitis B infection

 ## Preparations and dosage

Proprietary name: Viread.

Preparation: 300 mg tablets.

Dosage: 300 mg once daily.

Widely available.

 ## Further information

Peters MG, Andersen J, Lynch P, et al. Randomized controlled study of tenofovir and adefovir in chronic hepatitis B virus and HIV infection: ACTG A5127. *Hepatology*. 2006;44:1110–1116.

van Bommel F, Zollner B, Sarrazin C, et al. Tenofovir for patients with lamivudine-resistant hepatitis B virus (HBV) infection and high HBV DNA level during adefovir therapy. *Hepatology*. 2006;44:318–325.

OLIGONUCLEOTIDES

FOMIVIRSEN

Molecular weight: 6682.

An antisense oligonucleotide, 21 bases in length, representing the mirror image of a region of mRNA coding for a regulatory protein of CMV. It is administered as the sodium salt by intraocular injection. Experiments in monkeys suggest that it has a very long elimination half-life (*c.* 3 days). Because of its unique mode of action fomivirsen retains activity against strains of CMV resistant to other antiviral agents.

Side effects commonly include ocular inflammation, which is responsive to topical steroids, and raised intraocular pressure.

 ## CLINICAL USE

CMV retinitis in AIDS patients intolerant of, or unresponsive to, other treatments

 ## Preparations and dosage

Proprietary name: Vitravene.

Preparation: Injection.

Dosage: 0.33 mg intravitreal injection every 2 weeks for two doses, then every 4 weeks (half this dose for previously untreated patients). Limited availability.

 ## Further information

Andrei G, De Clercq E, Snoeck R. Drug targets in cytomegalovirus infection. *Infect Disord Drug Targets*. 2009;9:201–222.

De Clercq E. Antiviral drugs in current clinical use. *J Clin Virol*. 2004;30:115–133.

Schreiber A, Harter G, Schubert A, Bunjes D, Mertens T, Michel D. Antiviral treatment of cytomegalovirus infection and resistant strains. *Expert Opin Pharmacother*. 2009;10:191–209.

PHOSPHONIC ACIDS

FOSCARNET

Phosphonoformic acid; trisodium phosphonoformate. Molecular weight (anhydrous): 126; (trisodium salt): 300.1.

A synthetic non-nucleoside pyrophosphate analog formulated as the trisodium hexahydrate for intravenous use. The solubility in water at pH 7 is only about 5% (w/w).

 ## ANTIVIRAL ACTIVITY

The RNA polymerase of influenza A virus, the DNA polymerases of HSV-1 and HSV-2, CMV, EBV, VZV and HBV are inhibited more efficiently than host-cell DNA polymerases. Concentrations of 6–55 μmol inhibit CMV plaque formation by 50%, but clinical isolates are generally 1.5–8 times less sensitive. In-vitro inhibition of CMV replication is reversed by withdrawal of the drug. Most strains of HSV that are resistant to aciclovir respond, but when treatment is discontinued, relapse is frequent. Foscarnet acts as a non-competitive inhibitor for substrates and templates of HIV reverse transcriptase in concentrations of 0.1–5.0 μmol, but 680 μmol was required to block replication of the virus in H9 cell cultures.

ACQUIRED RESISTANCE

Resistance can be generated in vitro, and CMV strains resistant to both ganciclovir and foscarnet have occasionally been recovered from humans.

PHARMACOKINETICS

Oral absorption	c. 17%
C_{max} 60 mg/kg intravenous 8-hourly	557 μmol/L
Plasma half-life	3.3–6.8 h
Volume of distribution	0.52–0.74 L/kg
Plasma protein binding	14–17%

Absorption and distribution

Oral bioavailability is poor. A wide range of plasma concentrations was noted (75–500 μmol/L) during 3–21 days of continuous intravenous infusion of 0.14–0.19 mg/kg per min. During continuous intravenous therapy the concentrations reached a plateau on day 3. Considerable differences in steady-state plasma concentrations exist between individuals. Drug penetrates the CSF; the mean concentration is about 40–60% of the mean plasma concentration, depending upon dose.

Metabolism and excretion

Elimination appears to be triphasic, with two initially short half-lives of 0.5–1.4 h and 3.3–6.8 h, followed by a long terminal phase of 88 h. About 88% of the cumulative intravenous dose is recovered unchanged in the urine within a week of stopping an infusion, indicating that the drug is not significantly metabolized. Non-renal clearance accounts for 14–18% of total clearance and may relate to uptake into bone. Plasma clearance decreases markedly with decreased renal function and the elimination half-life may be increased by up to 10-fold. Conventional dialysis eliminates about 25% of a dose while high-flux dialysis can remove nearly 60%.

INTERACTIONS

There is no significant pharmacokinetic interaction with zidovudine, or with ganciclovir given as concomitant or daily alternating therapy.

In view of its nephrotoxicity, co-administration with potentially nephrotoxic drugs – for example, aminoglycosides, amphotericin B, pentamidine and ciclosporin (cyclosporin) – should be avoided.

TOXICITY AND SIDE EFFECTS

Treatment is more frequently limited by toxicity than with ganciclovir. Renal toxicity is most common. A two- to three-fold increase in serum creatinine levels occurs in 20–60% (mean 45%) of patients given 130–230 mg/kg per day as a continuous intravenous infusion. Renal impairment usually develops within the first few weeks of treatment and is generally reversible within several weeks of discontinuing therapy. Foscarnet chelates metal ions, and serum electrolyte abnormalities – predominantly hypocalcemia, hypomagnesemia, hypokalemia and hypophosphatemia – occur in about 30, 15, 16 and 8% of patients, respectively. Convulsions occur in 10–15%. Other side effects include anemia (25–50%), penile or vulval ulceration (3–9%), nausea and vomiting (20–30%), local irritation and thrombophlebitis at the infusion site, abdominal pain and occasional pancreatitis, headache (c. 25%), dizziness, involuntary muscle contractions, tremor, hypoesthesia, ataxia, neuropathy, anxiety, nervousness, depression and confusion, and skin rash. Nephrogenic diabetes insipidus has been reported.

Foscarnet is contraindicated in pregnancy. Topical application does not result in dermal toxicity similar to that produced by phosphonacetic acid.

CLINICAL USE

Treatment of CMV retinitis in patients for whom ganciclovir is contraindicated, inappropriate or ineffective

It is also potentially of value in the treatment of aciclovir-resistant HSV infection.

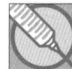

Preparations and dosage

Proprietary name: Foscavir.

Preparation: Injection.

Dosage: Adults, i.v., 60 mg/kg every 8 h for 2–3 weeks, then 60 mg/kg per day, increasing to 90–120 mg/kg per day if tolerated.

Widely available.

Further information

Claro C, Ruiz R, Cordero E, et al. Determination and pharmacokinetic profile of liposomal foscarnet in rabbit ocular tissues after intravitreal administration. *Exp Eye Res*. 2009;88:528–534.

Nigro G, Sali E, Anceschi MM, et al. Foscarnet therapy for congenital cytomegalovirus liver fibrosis following prenatal ascites. *J Matern Fetal Neonatal Med*. 2004;15:325–329.

OTHER ANTIVIRAL COMPOUNDS

DOCOSANOL

A 22-carbon straight chain alcohol licensed for over-the-counter sales for the topical treatment of herpes labialis. It is thought to act by blocking viral fusion with the host cell, although definitive studies are lacking. The clinical relevance of the antiviral activity has been debated and the place of this medication as a treatment of herpes labialis remains to be established.

 IMIQUIMOD

An imidazoquinoline used for the treatment of genital and perianal warts. While the mechanism of action is not precisely known, it is thought to induce interferon. It has no direct antiviral activity. The 5% cream applied three times a week for up to 16 weeks resulted in total wart clearance in 50% of patients, with a better response in women than in men. Local reactions are common and include erythema, erosion, excoriation and edema.

 PLECONARIL

An oxadiazole active against most enteroviruses and rhinoviruses. It binds to the hydrophobic pocket of the virus capsid protein VP1, inducing conformational changes that lead to altered receptor binding and viral uncoating. Concerns over safety and efficacy have constrained development of the drug.

38 Sepsis

Anna Norrby-Teglund and Carl Johan Treutiger

In the second half of the 20th century, the use of antibiotics resulted in a sharp decline in morbidity and mortality from bacterial infectious disease. However, mortality has remained high when acute infection induces sepsis with shock, metabolic acidosis, oliguria or hypoxemia. In the USA alone, there are at least 500 000 episodes of sepsis annually; mortality rates range from 30% to 50%, despite intensive medical care, including antibiotics, intravenous fluids, nutrition, mechanical ventilation for respiratory failure and surgical eradication of the source of the infection.[1,2] However, our understanding of sepsis and sepsis syndrome has increased markedly over the last decade. It is now well established that sepsis is an overwhelming, systemic host response to infection, resulting from complex interactions between the infecting pathogen and the host inflammatory, coagulation and fibrinolytic systems. The processes that lead to the sepsis syndrome are the result of microbial products that profoundly dysregulate mediator release and the homeostasis of several important pathways.[3,4] One of the major advances has been the identification of mediators, both host and pathogen derived, which contribute to these pathophysiological changes and hence represent potential targets for intervention.[4,5] Attempts to treat sepsis by blocking individual mediators or some of the common pathways have largely failed to reduce the overall mortality. This is probably due partly to the fact that where multiple cellular activation processes are involved and many humoral cascades triggered, merely blocking a single component may be insufficient to arrest the inflammatory process. However, the dysregulation that characterizes sepsis may be amenable to blockade of the bacterial components or to the intracellular pathways triggered by these products. Alternatively, intervention with pleiotropic and late-acting inflammatory mediators such as caspases, C5a, migration inhibitory factor or high mobility group box 1 may be possible.[5]

EPIDEMIOLOGY

Mortality and morbidity data from the US National Center for Health Statistics reported a 58% increase in death rates due to infectious diseases between 1980 to 1992[6] and a rate of admission to hospital for infectious diseases that declined less steeply than for all admissions.[7] Among the 15 leading reported causes of death in the USA since 1950, the greatest increase in mortality has been due to septicemia. Recent data suggest that the incidence of sepsis continues to increase, but that the survival rates have gradually improved over the last 25 years.[8]

BACTEREMIA

Clinically significant bacteremia occurs with a frequency of 5–10 per 1000 hospital admissions, a figure that has been rising slowly over the last 10 years, largely due to an increasing number of nosocomial infections. Mylotte et al[9] compared the epidemiology and outcome of community-acquired bacteremia in a teaching hospital and a non-teaching hospital and found incidences of community-acquired bacteremia to be 12.6 and 11.9 episodes per 1000 admissions, respectively. A number of sites are possible sources of bacteremia (Table 38.1). The type of pathogen and resistance pattern can vary according to the site of infection, the type of hospital and the location within the hospital in which the patient is being treated (Table 38.2). Such information may be of assistance in deciding on the most likely pathogen and most appropriate antimicrobial therapy. Mylotte et al[9] found the proportion of episodes due to methicillin-sensitive *Staphylococcus aureus* significantly higher at the teaching hospital, in contrast to the proportion of episodes due to *Escherichia coli*, which was significantly higher at the non-teaching hospital (Table 38.2). Except for these differences, the proportion of episodes due to other organisms was similar. Community-acquired bacteremia caused by Gram-positive organisms (staphylococci, streptococci and enterococci) occurred significantly more often at the teaching hospital; conversely, community-acquired bacteremia caused by Gram-negative bacilli from a urinary tract source occurred more often at the non-teaching hospital.

The intensive care unit (ICU) is a common focus for nosocomial infections. In a 1-day point-prevalence infection surveillance performed in 1417 European ICUs, 45% of 10 038 patients were infected and 21% had ICU-acquired infections.[10] Richards et al[11] reported on the epidemiology of nosocomial infections in adults in 112 medical ICUs in 97 hospitals in the

Table 38.1 Sources of micro-organisms isolated from blood of patients with community-acquired bacteremia[9]

Source	Site of acquisition (%)	
	Teaching hospital	Non-teaching hospital
Intravenous catheter	8	0
Respiratory tract	31	21
Urinary tract	29	40
Skin/soft tissue	9	3
Intra-abdominal	4	12
Other	6	5
Unknown	12	19

From Mylotte JM, Kahler L, McCann C. Community-acquired bacteremia at a teaching versus a nonteaching hospital: impact of acute severity of illness on 30-day mortality. **Am J Infect Control.** 2001;29:13–19.

Table 38.2 Micro-organisms isolated from the blood of patients with community-acquired bacteremia by study hospital[9]

Organism	Number of episodes (%)	
	Teaching hospital	Non-teaching hospital
Staphylococcus aureus		
Methicillin-sensitive	25	9
Methicillin-resistant	5	<1
Coagulase-negative staphylococci	Not included in study	
Streptococcus pneumoniae	10	15
Enterococci	10	5
Escherichia coli	14	41
Klebsiella pneumoniae	4	9
Pseudomonas aeruginosa	5	4
Proteus mirabilis	6	4
Others	21	11
% Gram-positives	59	38
% Gram-negatives	41	62

From Mylotte JM, Kahler L, McCann C. Community-acquired bacteremia at a teaching versus a nonteaching hospital: impact of acute severity of illness on 30-day mortality. **Am J Infect Control.** 2001;29:13–19.

USA that were part of the National Nosocomial Infections Surveillance (NNIS) system of the Centers for Disease Control and Prevention between January 1992 and July 1997. The most commonly reported pathogens were coagulase-negative staphylococci (36%), enterococci (16%), *Staph. aureus* (13%) and Gram-negative aerobes (17%). The most frequent Gram-negatives were *Klebsiella pneumoniae* and *Pseudomonas aeruginosa*. *Candida* species were found to be associated with urinary catheters, coagulase-negative staphylococci with central lines, and *Ps. aeruginosa* and *Acinetobacter* species with ventilators.

In other reports from the NNIS, trends of increasing proportions of Gram-positive infections and decreasing proportions of Gram-negative infections during the last 15 years have become apparent.

Shorr et al[12] reported on the epidemiology of 6697 patients with bloodstream infections during 2002–2003. In this study, healthcare-associated bloodstream infections accounted for 53% of all bloodstream infections, and were associated with a higher morbidity and mortality compared to community-acquired bloodstream infection. The most prevalent community-acquired pathogen was *Esch. coli* (25.2%) and *Staph. aureus* the most common hospital-acquired or healthcare-associated pathogen (25.7% and 29.7%, respectively). Of all bacterial bloodstream infections, methicillin-resistant *Staph. aureus* (MRSA) was associated with the highest mortality rate (22.5%) and the longest hospital stay.

Community-associated MRSA has recently received considerable attention due to its association with highly aggressive infections in otherwise healthy individuals outside the healthcare system.[13,14] These infections include severe skin and soft-tissue infections, necrotizing fasciitis and necrotizing pneumonia, all associated with substantial morbidity and mortality. Several studies have highlighted the importance of *Staph. aureus* bloodstream infections, and the emergence of MRSA, as an increasing health problem.[12,15]

SEPTICEMIA

There have been major increases in the rates of admission to hospital due to septicemia: between 1980 and 1994, the annual change in the number of admissions due to septicemia was 10.5%, second only to that for HIV AIDS infection.[7] Simonsen et al[7] found septicemia to be the fourth leading cause of hospital admission due to infectious diseases in the USA in 1994 (a total of 301 800, or 116 admissions per 100 000 persons). The age-adjusted death rate due to septicemia increased from 0.3 per 100 000 in 1950 to 4.2 per 100 000 in 1997, a 14-fold increase, which makes septicemia the thirteenth leading cause of death in 1997.[16] The unadjusted rate in 1997 was 8 per 100 000. Among elderly people, the mortality rate was 23 per 100 000 for persons 65–74 years old, 60 per 100 000 for those 75–84 years old, and 178 per 100 000 for people of 85 years or more. Recently, Melamed and Sorvillo[17] concluded that the rapid rise in sepsis mortality seen in previous decades has slowed, but population aging continues to drive the growth of sepsis-associated mortality in the USA. The age-adjusted rate of sepsis-associated mortality was 50.37 deaths per 100 000 between 1999 and 2005.

McBean and Rajamani[18] examined the rates of hospital admission of elderly people due to septicemia in the period 1986–1997. The sex- and race-adjusted annual rates in 1997 were more than double the rates in 1986. For people between 65 and 74 years old, the rate in 1997 was 2.2 times the rate in 1986; for those 75–84 years it was double and 2.3 times greater for patients ≥85 years in whom rates of admission for septicemia were significantly higher (*p* <0.001).

The overall 30-day mortality rate for persons admitted for the treatment of septicemia in 1997 was 246.5 per 1000 patients admitted and was 6.9% greater among Black Americans (262 per 1000) than among White Americans (245 per 1000). The 30-day mortality rates for patients for whom the presumed source of infection was decubitus ulcer was 372 per 1000 admissions; for pneumonia it was 336 per 1000, for urinary tract infections and cystitis 193 per 1000, for cellulitis 177 per 1000 and 66 per 1000 for kidney infections. Reasons for the increase in septicemia over the 12-year study period included an increased prevalence (due to both increased incidence and increased duration) of chronic diseases such as diabetes, cancer and end-stage renal disease in the elderly, putting them at higher risk for infectious diseases. Medical devices, either temporary or permanent, may also increase the risk of septicemia.

Drombovskiy et al[19] reported on 8 402 766 patients hospitalized with sepsis in the USA from 1993 to 2003. The rate of severe sepsis hospitalization almost doubled during this 11-year period from 66.8 to 132 per 100 000 population. Age-adjusted, population-based mortality rates from severe sepsis also increased significantly from 30.3% to 49.7%.

PATHOPHYSIOLOGY

Severe sepsis is a consequence of microbial antigenemia inducing a generalized activation of numerous host defense systems, including the adaptive and the innate immune responses of which the complement, coagulation, contact-phase and fibrinolytic systems are prominent contributors.[20,21] Activation of these proinflammatory and procoagulatory cascades results in release of proinflammatory cytokines, nitric oxide, endothelins, tissue-damaging proteinases, lipid mediators and hypotensive molecules such as kinins (see Figure 38.1). These mediators regulate cellular and humoral immune responses and are essential to an adequate and efficient host defense against infecting micro-organisms. However, excessive and dysregulated release of these mediators is the key event leading to the clinical features of sepsis and shock, namely circulatory collapse, organ failure, tissue necrosis and death. In addition to this systemic inflammatory response (SIRS), sepsis is also associated with an exacerbated release of anti-inflammatory mediators such as interleukin-10 (IL-10), IL-1 receptor antagonist (IL-1ra) and transforming growth factor-β (TGF-β). Consequently, in 1997 Bone et al coined the term 'compensatory anti-inflammatory response syndrome' (CARS) to illustrate this immunosuppressive response of SIRS patients.[22] CARS is considered an adapted response to dampen the overzealous inflammatory response.[23] Multiple mechanisms, including release of anti-inflammatory cytokines, downregulation and shedding of cytokine receptors, induction of T-regulatory cells and myeloid-derived suppressor cells, as well as cell death, contribute to the immunosuppressive state in sepsis. Increased apoptosis has been observed in lymphocytes and dendritic cells in septic patients,

whereas monocytes remain unchanged and neutrophils display decreased apoptosis.[24] The immunosuppressive state has been suggested to contribute to the susceptibility to secondary infections and/or reactivation of otherwise dormant viruses such as cytomegalovirus.[25,26]

Gram-positive and Gram-negative bacteria produce numerous factors capable of activating the host systems involved in sepsis. Lipopolysaccharide (LPS), a major constituent of the outer membrane of Gram-negative bacteria, has long been recognized as the principal mediator of sepsis.[27] The cell wall of Gram-positive bacteria also contains potent proinflammatory components, including peptidoglycan and lipoteichoic acid.[28] LPS, lipoteichoic acid and peptidoglycan are all examples of microbial molecules that display pathogen-associated molecular patterns (PAMPs), which are detected by pattern recognition receptors (PRRs), primarily toll-like receptors (TLRs) and nucleotide-oligomerization domain leucin-rich repeat (NOD-LRR) proteins, expressed on immune cells.[29,30] This results in activation of the innate immune response and regulation of the adaptive immune response to infection. The PRRs are also important sensors of endogenous alarmins, i.e. intracellular proteins or mediators that are released from damaged cell and tissues. Together, endogenous alarmins and exogenous PAMPs are called damage-associated molecular patterns (DAMPs).[29] During sepsis, the microbial infection and damaged tissues result in high levels of DAMPs and consequently an overstimulation of immune cells resulting in the pathological cytokine storm seen in septic patients.

Streptococcus pyogenes and *Staph. aureus* express and secrete exotoxins with superantigenic activity that induce very powerful immune responses.[31] Superantigens interact, without prior cellular processing, with the Vβ region of the T-cell receptor and the major histocompatibility complex (MHC) class II molecules on antigen-presenting cells. Cross-linking of T cells and antigen-presenting cells by superantigens results in potent activation of these cells and the excessive production of proinflammatory cytokines.[32] Other virulence factors expressed by pathogenic bacteria include pili, M protein, hemolysins and proteases, which have all been shown to be important contributors to pathogenesis.[28,33,34] In addition, synergistic or additive effects have been shown for many of these virulence factors and it is increasingly evident that the pathogenesis of sepsis involves a complex interplay between multiple microbial factors, host cells and mediators.

One of the initial events in sepsis is the induction of proinflammatory cytokines; these trigger the cytokine cascade, complement and coagulation systems, resulting in injury to endothelium and vessels, and the release of proteases, arachidonic acid metabolites and nitric oxide (Figure 38.1). The leading proinflammatory mediators are IL-1, IL-6, IL-8 and IL-12, tumor necrosis factor (TNF)-α, interferon (IFN)-γ, macrophage migration inhibitory factor (MIF) and high mobility group box 1 (HMGB1).[35,36] IL-1 and TNF-α are commonly referred to as 'early cytokines' in the sepsis cascade. They induce potent pyrogenic and hypotensive responses, and the experimental administration of either cytokine reproduces

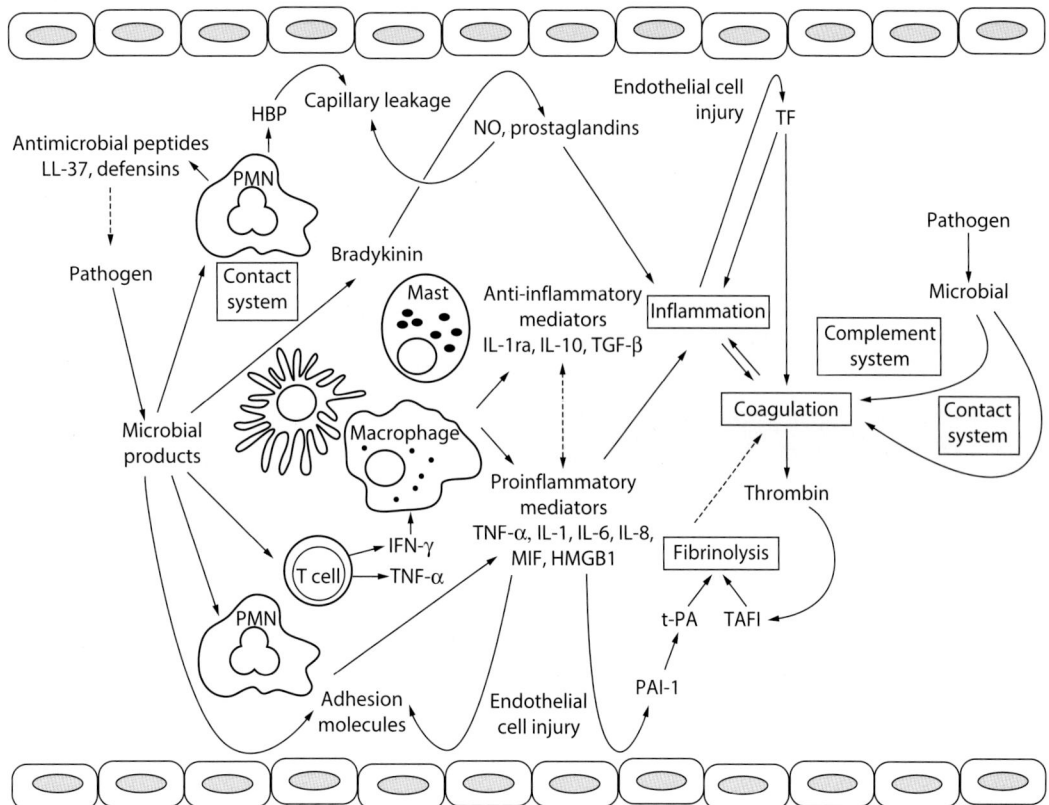

Fig. 38.1 Schematic illustration of some of the host–microbe interactions that contribute to the pathophysiology of sepsis. Microbial factors interact with specific receptors on immune cells, including macrophages, T cells, neutrophils (PMN), dendritic cells (DC) and mast cells. This results in activation of the cells and release of proinflammatory cytokines, which activate the coagulation system through induction of tissue factor (TF). TF results in production of thrombin and subsequent formation of fibrin deposition. Tissue-plasminogen activator (t-PA) triggers conversion of plasminogen to plasmin, the main effector molecule of fibrinolysis. Proinflammatory cytokines and thrombin stimulate release of plasminogen activator inhibitor-1 (PAI-1) from platelets and the endothelium. Thrombin activates thrombin-activatable fibrinolysis inhibitor (TAFI). TAFI and PAI-1 are key inhibitors of t-PA, consequently fibrinolysis is effectively suppressed during sepsis. Solid and dashed arrows indicate activation and inhibition, respectively. HBP, heparin binding protein; HMBG1, high mobility group box 1; IFN, interferon; IL, interleukin; MIF, migration inhibitory factor; NO, nitric oxide; TGF, transforming growth factor; TNF, tumor necrosis factor.

the clinical symptoms of sepsis.[37–40] Similarly MIF, a pituitary- and macrophage-derived factor, behaves as a proinflammatory cytokine and has been shown to be a critical mediator of septic shock.[41] However, in contrast to other known cytokines, MIF production is induced rather than suppressed by glucocorticoids, and MIF has been found to override the immunosuppressive effects of glucocorticoids.[42] HMGB1 increases LPS-induced IL-1 and TNF-α, and is a late mediator of septic shock in mice.[43] Elevated levels of HMGB1 could be demonstrated in patient plasma up to a week after the diagnosis of severe sepsis or septic shock.[44] Although described as a proinflammatory cytokine,[45] recent studies have shown HMGB1 to enhance inflammatory responses by acting as a carrier of LPS,[46] CpG DNA[47] and proinflammatory cytokines such as IL-1β.[48] HGMB1 acts via interaction with TLR2, TLR4 and the receptor for advanced glycation end-products (RAGE), and is considered an endogenous alarmin.

A positive correlation between the development of shock in sepsis and activation of the coagulation response was reported some 30 years ago.[21] Microbial factors can activate the coagulation cascade either directly or indirectly via induction of proinflammatory cytokines and subsequent expression of tissue factor on endothelial cells and monocytes, which is the main pathway for coagulation activation in sepsis (see Figure 38.1). A drastic reduction in the levels of important endogenous coagulation inhibitors, such as antithrombin III and activated protein C (APC), due to consumption, expression deficiency or proteolytic inactivation, further contributes to the procoagulatory state in sepsis. Sepsis and disseminated intravascular coagulation are associated with decreased antithrombin III and protein C, and a disruption of the balance between coagulation and fibrinolysis.[21] Furthermore, there is a correlation between deficiency in these inhibitors and increased morbidity and mortality in sepsis.[21] Dysregulated expression of antithrombin III and activated protein C also affects the inflammatory processes due to increased thrombin production which promotes upregulation of adhesion molecule expression and microvascular thrombosis, which further increases the inflammatory response through tissue ischemia and neutrophil/endothelium activation.

Activation of the complement and contact systems has also been linked to the sepsis process, mainly by the release of hypotensive mediators, anaphylatoxins such as C5a, and the consumption of coagulatory factors.[49,50] Herwald et al[51] demonstrated that the fibrous surface components of Gram-positive and Gram-negative bacteria bind to and trigger assembly of the components of the contact system, resulting in the release of hypotensive kinins, hypocoagulatory state, and dysregulated fibrin and clot formation. Other virulence factors, such as the streptococcal M protein and the streptococcal proteinase, also interact with components of the contact system.[51]

DIAGNOSTIC ISSUES

Sepsis is not a single disease. It is a syndrome that can result from diverse causes, with a spectrum of severity that ranges from fever associated with transitory hypotension through to profound shock and high mortality. The same clinical picture is seen in some non-infective conditions, which has given rise to some confusion.

Identifying and naming subgroups is worthwhile only if doing so aids design of better treatment or more accurate prediction of outcome. In 1991 the American College of Chest Physicians (ACCP) and the Society of Critical Care Medicine (SCCM)[52] published consensus definitions of sepsis. Sepsis was defined as the presence of systemic inflammatory response syndrome (SIRS; Box 38.1) with a confirmed infectious process. Sepsis associated with organ dysfunction, hypoperfusion abnormality or sepsis-induced hypotension was named severe sepsis, and septic shock was defined as severe sepsis with sepsis-induced hypotension persisting despite adequate fluid resuscitation.

The critical difference between SIRS and sepsis is the requirement for clinical or laboratory evidence of infection. The relationships between SIRS, sepsis, shock and death is well illustrated by a prospective study of nearly 4000 patients admitted to ICUs in the USA.[53] The incidence of SIRS on surgical ICUs was 857 episodes per 1000 patient-days, and the mortality of these patients was just 7%, emphasizing that SIRS is a very sensitive definition. However, in the small proportion (4%) that developed septic shock, mortality was 46%.

With further advances in the understanding of the pathophysiology of sepsis and identification of new biomarkers, a new consensus sepsis definition conference was held in 2001 by SCCM, the European Society of Intensive Care Medicine (ESICM), the ACCP, the American Thoracic Society (ATS) and the Surgical Infection Societies (SIS).[54]

The previous definitions of sepsis, severe sepsis and septic shock, as defined in 1991, remain useful, but the diagnostic criteria for SIRS were too sensitive and non-specific. An expanded list of signs and symptoms of sepsis was proposed to better reflect the clinical response to infection (Box 38.2). The list of signs and markers should be considered as a guide to diagnosis. Not all patients with sepsis will have all the markers included on the list, and many patients without sepsis may have several. The unexplained presence of several of the listed signs in a patient, however, should be used to raise suspicion of sepsis.

There are two major reasons why an infectious etiology is not identified in a patient presenting with sepsis:

- Antibiotics are often used empirically in the outpatient and home care setting and the hospital before testing.
- Bacteremia may be intermittent, except in the patient with endovascular infection.

However, in patients with sepsis, it is more important to promptly initiate appropriate antimicrobial therapy in order to ensure optimal outcome than to wait for further blood culture sets.[55,56] Although 75–80% of neutropenic fevers are thought to be caused by infections, a causal organism can be confirmed in only 30–50% of episodes. In a prospective study of sepsis and septic shock, at least 15% of patients had no documented infection. Even among patients with presumed infection, less than half had bacteremia.[57] Ideally two or three blood cultures should be obtained several hours apart to increase the likelihood for detection.[58] The total volume of blood cultured is one of the most important factors in the

Box 38.1 Systemic inflammatory response syndrome (SIRS)

SIRS is defined as the presence of two or more of the following criteria:
- Temperature >38°C or <36°C
- Heart rate >90 beats/min
- Respiratory rate >20 breaths/min or $Paco_2$ <32 mmHg
- White blood cell count >12 × 10^9/L or <4 × 10^9/L.

Box 38.2 Clinical signs of sepsis[110]

General signs and symptoms

Rigor – fever (sometimes hypothermia)
Tachypnea/respiratory alkalosis
Positive fluid balance – edema

General inflammatory reaction

Altered white blood cell count
Increased C-reactive protein, interleukin-6, procalcitonin concentrations

Hemodynamic alterations

Arterial hypotension
Tachycardia
Increased cardiac output/low systemic vascular resistance/high Svo_2
Altered skin perfusion
Decreased urine output
Hyperlactatemia – increased base deficit

Signs of organ dysfunction

Hypoxemia
Coagulation abnormalities
Altered mental status
Hyperglycemia
Thrombocytopenia, disseminated intravascular coagulation
Altered liver function (hyperbilirubinemia)
Intolerance to feeding (altered gastrointestinal motility)

From Levy MM, Fink MP, Marshall JC, et al. SCCM/ESICM/ACCP/ATS/SIS 2001 SCCM/ESICM/ACCP/ATS/SIS International Sepsis Definitions Conference. **Crit Care Med.** 2003;31:1250–1256.

recovery of bacterial pathogens: in one study, increasing the volume over a 24-h period from 40 to 60 mL increased recovery by 10%.[59]

TREATMENT

Studies have demonstrated that the first 6 h of management of sepsis are especially important, and that measures taken during this period have a significant impact on outcome.[60,61]

The need for evidence-based recommendations regarding the acute management of sepsis and septic shock led to a consensus meeting in 2004. Following that, an international group of experts in the diagnosis and management of infection and sepsis, representing 11 organizations, published the first internationally accepted clinical guidelines for the practicing clinician to improve outcomes in severe sepsis and septic shock.[62,63] A new consensus meeting held in 2008 has updated the original Surviving Sepsis Campaign recommendations.[64]

TRADITIONAL THERAPEUTIC STRATEGIES

ANTIMICROBIAL THERAPY

Antimicrobial therapy remains fundamental to the treatment of sepsis; many studies have demonstrated that inadequate initial antimicrobial and/or delayed therapy is associated with marked increases in all-cause and infection-related mortality in patients admitted to the ICU with life-threatening infection.[55,65–68] Duration of hypotension before initiation of effective antimicrobial therapy is the critical determinant of survival in human septic shock.[55] Such findings support the empirical use of broad-spectrum therapy before the results of laboratory culture are known.

The number of effective antimicrobial agents available is becoming increasingly limited because of the emergence of multidrug resistance in both Gram-negative and Gram-positive pathogens.[69] One of the consequences of drug-resistant infections is the increased likelihood of inappropriate initial therapy. Leroy et al[70] found that ineffective initial antimicrobial therapy was the best predictor for poor prognosis in community-acquired pneumonia.

Which antimicrobial or antimicrobial combination to use empirically depends on the source of the infection, whether it is community or nosocomially acquired, whether or not the patient has an underlying illness that alters the predictability of the offending pathogen, and the local antimicrobial resistance rates. A broad-spectrum empirical antibiotic should be started as soon as possible for suspected severe infections, especially in the presence of hypotension. Every effort should be made to obtain proper site-specific cultures. However, such efforts should not delay antimicrobial therapy. There are studies suggesting that, in certain circumstances, outcomes may

improve if two or more effective agents are used;[71,72] however, whether possible pathogens should be covered by multiple antibiotics or not is still under debate. So far there are no prospective controlled studies that compare multiple versus single drug therapy in severe sepsis or septic shock. Importantly, empirical antimicrobial therapy should be adjusted and narrowed within 48–72 h if a pathogen is identified or if there is a resolution of septic shock.

VOLUME REPLACEMENT

The first goal of management of severe sepsis is to adequately monitor vital signs so that any hemodynamic changes can be promptly detected and treated. Insertion of a central venous pressure monitoring device, arterial catheter and Swan-Ganz catheters to determine the left atrial end-diastolic pressure allows for optimal monitoring and fluid replacement.

To expand intravascular fluid volume and colloid oncotic pressure, a number of solutions may be used, including normal and hypertonic saline, fresh-frozen plasma, albumin and various dextran preparations. There is general agreement that volume therapy is an essential component of early resuscitation and that the goal is to optimize systemic oxygen delivery (cardiac preload, afterload, arterial oxygen content, contractility, or stroke volume) and ultimately to balance tissue oxygen demand.[73]

Crystalloid solutions are the first choice to correct fluid and electrolyte deficits in non-hemorrhagic shock. In the case of major hypovolemia, particularly in situations of increased capillary permeability, colloid solutions are favored to achieve sufficient tissue perfusion. However, different colloids have different molecular weights and therefore vary in the length of time they remain in the circulation. Because of this and their other characteristics, colloids may differ in their safety and efficacy. Bunn et al[74] reviewed randomized and quasi-randomized trials comparing colloid solutions in critically ill and surgical patients thought to need volume replacement. They found no evidence that one colloid solution was more effective or safer than another.

The use of colloids for the treatment of septic shock has been challenged: they are more expensive than crystalloids, some colloid solutions may be associated with adverse outcomes, and some clinical trials have found them to be no better than crystalloids. Schierhout and Roberts[75] carried out a systematic review of randomized controlled trials of resuscitation with colloids or crystalloids for volume replacement of critically ill patients. The overview concluded that the use of colloids for volume resuscitation in critically ill patients is not supported by the literature. Concern has also been raised about the use of albumin, often the colloid of choice for replacement therapy.[76] The Cochrane Group carried out a review of randomized controlled trials comparing administration of albumin or plasma protein fraction with no administration, or with administration of crystalloid solution, in critically ill patients with hypovolemia, burns or hypoalbuminemia. They concluded that use of human albumin in critically ill patients should be urgently reviewed and that it should not be used outside the context of rigorously conducted, randomized controlled trials. However, a saline versus albumin study compared fluid resuscitation with albumin or saline on mortality in critically ill patients and found no difference between them.[77]

VASOPRESSOR AGENTS

If fluid therapy alone fails to restore adequate arterial pressure and organ perfusion, vasopressor agents should be used. The goal of mean arterial pressure should be at least 65 mmHg.[78] For many years, noradrenaline (norepinephrine) and adrenaline (epinephrine) were the principal agents available. However, because of their intense peripheral vasoconstricting activity and increase in myocardial irritability, they have been replaced with isoproterenol, dopamine and dobutamine. These agents have an inotropic effect on myocardial function but because of β-adrenergic activity are capable of enhancing peripheral tissue perfusion. The recent Surviving Sepsis Campaign recommendations were published with six evidence-graded statements for vasopressor use, concluding that there is no high-quality primary evidence to recommend one catecholamine over another; consequently, neither noradrenaline (norepinephrine) nor dopamine can be recommended over the other. Furthermore, adrenaline (epinephrine) should be limited for use in patients unresponsive to other agents.[73]

NOVEL THERAPEUTIC STRATEGIES

During the last two decades, significant advances have been made in the field of sepsis that have allowed the development of novel therapeutic strategies, ranging from interventions with defined microbial factors to the various host systems (Table 38.3).

NEUTRALIZATION OF MICROBIAL FACTORS

Anti-endotoxin therapies, including polyclonal and monoclonal antibodies and various lipid analogs, have been extensively tested in clinical trials, but have so far failed to have a significant effect on mortality.[27] Other anti-endotoxin approaches under investigation include:

- Eritoran, a synthetic lipid A antagonist, now in phase III[79]
- bactericidal-permeability-increasing protein[80]

Table 38.3 Some novel therapeutic strategies in septic shock

Strategies[a]	Type of agent	References
Neutralization of microbial factors		
Anti-endotoxin	Polyclonal antiserum (J5, anti-Lipid A, IVIG)	27, 111
	Polymyxin B immobilized hemofiltration columns	83
	Monoclonal antibodies (HA-1A, E5, T88)	27, 111
	Lipid A analogs (lipid X, monophosphoryl lipid A, etc.)	28, 112
	Recombinant bactericidal/permeability-increasing protein	80, 112, 113
Anti-superantigen	IVIG	90, 114
Modulation of proinflammatory mediators		
Anti-cytokines	Corticosteroids	64
Anti-tumor necrosis factor	Monoclonal antibodies, receptor fusion proteins, cytofab	111, 115, 116
Anti-interleukin-1	Interleukin-1 receptor antagonist	111, 115
Anti-PAF	PAF antagonist	115
Anti-bradykinin	Bradykinin antagonist	115
Anti-prostaglandin	Ibuprofen (cyclo-oxygenase inhibitor)	111
Statins	3-Hydroxymethyl-3methylglutaryl coenzyme A	117, 118
Modulation of coagulation		
Antithrombin III	Inhibitor of coagulation	103–105
Activated protein C	Inhibitor of coagulation	102, 108, 109
Recombinant tissue factor pathway inhibitor	Inhibitor of coagulation	119

IVIG, intravenous polyclonal immunoglobulin; PAF, platelet-activating factor.
[a]Includes therapeutic agents that have been tested in controlled human sepsis trials.

- recombinant human lactoferrin[81]
- TAK-242, a small molecule blocking the MyD-88 pathway[82]
- polymyxin B immobilized hemofiltration columns[83]
- anti-endotoxin vaccines.[84]

Neutralization of Gram-positive microbial factors has mainly been achieved by intravenous polyspecific immunoglobulin G (IVIG), which contains a broad spectrum of neutralizing antibodies against streptococcal and staphylococcal superantigens, as well as opsonic antibodies against a variety of micro-organisms.[85] In addition to its direct toxin-neutralizing and opsonic activities, IVIG has a general immunomodulatory effect due to its interaction with Fc receptors, complement, immune cell functions, cytokines and cytokine antagonists.[85] Recent meta-analyses have reported an overall reduction in mortality with the use of IVIG as adjunctive therapy in critically ill patients with sepsis.[86–89] However, due to heterogeneity of the trials and small patient cohorts, the power is insufficient to allow solid conclusion.[86,87]

Certain subgroups of patients may benefit more than others from IVIG-treatment, such as those with superantigen-mediated toxic shock.[90] Two studies have reported that adjunctive therapy with IVIG reduces the mortality associated with streptococcal toxic shock syndrome.[91,92] The first is an observational cohort study, which showed significant improvement in survival among IVIG-treated cases.[92] However, confounding factors that could have affected the outcome of the trial included the fact that the majority of the controls were historical and IVIG-treated cases were more likely to have received clindamycin therapy than the controls.

Further support for the use of IVIG in streptococcal toxic shock syndrome is provided by a multicenter placebo-controlled trial.[91] Due to a low incidence of invasive streptococcal infections during the study period, the trial was prematurely terminated after enrolment of 21 patients. The results revealed a trend towards a reduced mortality rate in IVIG-treated cases as compared to those receiving placebo (10% versus 36%). Importantly, this trend in reduced mortality was supported by significantly better improvement of organ dysfunction following treatment in the IVIG group, whereas no such change could be noted in the placebo group.

INHIBITION OF PROINFLAMMATORY MEDIATORS

As principal mediators of sepsis and shock, TNF-α and IL-1 were obvious therapeutic targets. However, none of these agents succeeded in lowering the mortality of sepsis in large phase III clinical trials (Table 38.3). There are several potential reasons why these therapies failed:

- Blockage of one mediator may not suffice to arrest the whole process.
- Agents directed against early mediators have a narrow therapeutic window.
- Peak cytokine production may have passed by the time treatment started, and downstream cascades may already be triggered.

Corticosteroids have been extensively studied in sepsis, with results ranging from beneficial to harmful. Recommendations have included the use of low-dose corticosteroids in the management of septic shock.[62,93,94] A recent European trial of corticosteroid therapy in septic shock (CORTICUS)[95] has confirmed early shock reversal, although by day 28 the overall number of patients with shock reversed was not significantly greater in the treated versus the placebo group. The updated Surviving Sepsis Campaign guidelines advise hydrocortisone only in adults with septic shock in whom there is a poor response of low blood pressure to fluid replacement and vasopressor therapy.[73]

Another approach directed at attenuating the pathogenic proinflammatory response involves the parasympathetic anti-inflammatory pathway by which the brain modulates systemic inflammatory responses.[96] Vagus nerve stimulation inhibits proinflammatory cytokines via the alpha7 nicotinic acetylcholine receptor subunit.[97] Lethal endotoxic shock in rats can be prevented by direct electric stimulation of the peripheral vagus nerve, which decreases in-vivo levels of TNF.[98]

Other potential targets for intervention include the danger protein HMGB1 and the receptor for advanced glycation end-products (RAGE). HMGB1 have been shown to be a persistent mediator of severe sepsis and its neutralization results in protection against experimental septic shock.[43] In contrast to the early cytokines TNF-α and IL-1, HMGB1 is a late mediator of sepsis and is produced over an extended period of time,[44] which would provide a wider therapeutic window.[5,43,99] The RAGE recognizes several ligands, among others HMGB1. Inhibition of RAGE in experimental sepsis increases survival.[100,101]

MODULATORS OF COAGULATION

Patients with severe sepsis are deficient in important coagulation inhibitors, suggesting that modulation of coagulation might be a potential therapeutic strategy.[72] Several anticoagulant strategies have been proposed, among which the most promising are the natural coagulation inhibitors antithrombin III and activated protein C.[102,103] However, the KyberSept study published in 2001[104] showed no significant benefit overall with high-dose antithrombin III, but rather an excess risk of bleeding in patients receiving antithrombin. However, in a prespecified subgroup of patients (i.e. patients with severe sepsis and with a predicted high risk of death) there was a modest improvement in survival.[105]

The Recombinant Human Protein C Worldwide Evaluation in Severe Sepsis (Prowess) study was a phase III, double-blind, randomized, placebo-controlled, multicenter trial which showed a significant treatment effect on 28-day mortality rate.[102] There are several reasons as to why activated protein C might be effective in patients with sepsis:

- Most patients with severe sepsis have diminished levels of activated protein C because of the reduction in the components of the coagulation system necessary for the conversion of inactive protein C to activated protein C.[106]

- Activated protein C inhibits activated factors V and VIII, thereby decreasing the formation of thrombin and stimulating fibrinolysis by reducing the concentration of plasminogen-activator inhibitor type 1.
- In addition to its central regulatory role in coagulation, protein C has been shown to have a strong anti-inflammatory effect, some of which may be mediated by its inhibition of the proinflammatory cytokines MIF and TNF-α.[107]

Bernard et al[102] conducted a randomized, double-blind, placebo-controlled, multicenter trial, assigning patients with systemic inflammation and organ failure due to acute infection to receive an intravenous infusion of either placebo or activated protein C (APC). Patients receiving APC demonstrated a dose-dependent reduction in the plasma levels of D-dimer and serum IL-6, markers of coagulopathy and inflammation, respectively. The absolute reduction in the 28-day mortality rate was 6.1% (in the placebo group it was 30.8%, compared with 24.7% in the APC group), and the relative risk of death was reduced by nearly 20% in the treated group. The exact role of APC has been questioned. A study in which APC was given to patients defined to have mild to moderate sepsis was terminated prematurely due to lack of efficacy after a second interim analysis.[108] A recent Cochrane systematic review suggested that the use of APC should be suspended pending results from additional trials as they found no evidence suggesting that APC should be used for treating patients with severe sepsis or septic shock, and, additionally, APC seems to be associated with a higher risk of bleeding.[109]

CONCLUSION

As the number of patients with chronic underlying disease and temporary or permanent implanted medical devices has increased, so has the number of episodes of sepsis. The microbial etiology of these episodes reflects the patient population and the geographical location of the healthcare facility in which they are treated. Patients with severe underlying illness or chronic disease will always be at increased risk of endotoxin-mediated Gram-negative sepsis, whereas those with intravascular catheters or prosthetic devices are at greater risk for Gram-positive infections. Complicating the management of these infections has been the emergence of multidrug resistance in such pathogens, both in the hospital and the community. In some countries and regions, multidrug-resistant strains are endemic and account for the majority of infections. This often means that first- and second-line antimicrobials are ineffective, leaving few and often less acceptable alternatives. Infections caused by multiresistant organisms are associated with increased morbidity and mortality.

However, despite the advancements in medical treatment, the outcome of patients with sepsis syndrome and septic shock has not improved greatly. This is because we treat only the cause and not the consequences of such infections. We now recognize that these conditions reflect a generalized activation of numerous host defense systems, resulting in excessive and dysregulated release of inflammatory and coagulatory mediators.

Blockade or antagonism of the actions of individual intermediary messenger molecules has proved unsuccessful. The most promising therapies today seem to be agents that target several different microbial factors and/or host systems involved in sepsis. Furthermore, several clinical trials have shown clinical efficacy in subgroups of patients, but not in the whole study population. This indicates that by targeting more defined patient populations based on specific clinical, immunological and/or microbiological parameters, a more favorable outcome may be seen in future trials of treatment for these syndromes.

 References

1. Angus DC, Linde-Zwirble WT, Lidicker J, Clermont G, Carcillo J, Pinsky MR. Epidemiology of severe sepsis in the United States: analysis of incidence, outcome, and associated costs of care. *Crit Care Med*. 2001;29:1303–1310.
2. Martin GS, Mannino DM, Eaton S, Moss M. The epidemiology of sepsis in the United States from 1979 through 2000. *N Engl J Med*. 2003;348:1546–1554.
3. Cinel I, Opal SM. Molecular biology of inflammation and sepsis: a primer. *Crit Care Med*. 2009;37:291–304.
4. Hotchkiss RS, Karl IE. The pathophysiology and treatment of sepsis. *N Engl J Med*. 2003;348:138–150.
5. Parrish WR, Gallowitsch-Puerta M, Czura CJ, Tracey KJ. Experimental therapeutic strategies for severe sepsis: mediators and mechanisms. *Ann N Y Acad Sci*. 2008;1144:210–236.
6. Pinner RW, Teutsch SM, Simonsen L, et al. Trends in infectious diseases mortality in the United States. *J Am Med Assoc*. 1996;275:189–193.
7. Simonsen L, Conn LA, Pinner RW, Teutsch S. Trends in infectious disease hospitalizations in the United States, 1980–1994. *Arch Intern Med*. 1998;158:1923–1928.
8. Christaki E, Opal SM. Is the mortality rate for septic shock really decreasing? *Curr Opin Crit Care*. 2008;14:580–586.
9. Mylotte JM, Kahler L, McCann C. Community-acquired bacteremia at a teaching versus a nonteaching hospital: impact of acute severity of illness on 30-day mortality. *Am J Infect Control*. 2001;29:13–19.
10. Vincent JL, Bihari DJ, Suter PM, et al. The prevalence of nosocomial infection in intensive care units in Europe. Results of the European Prevalence of Infection in Intensive Care (EPIC) Study. EPIC International Advisory Committee. *J Am Med Assoc*. 1995;274:639–644.
11. Richards MJ, Edwards JR, Culver DH, Gaynes RP. Nosocomial infections in medical intensive care units in the United States. National Nosocomial Infections Surveillance System. *Crit Care Med*. 1999;27:887–892.
12. Shorr AF, Tabak YP, Killian AD, Gupta V, Liu LZ, Kollef MH. Healthcare-associated bloodstream infection: a distinct entity? Insights from a large U.S. database. *Crit Care Med*. 2006;34:2588–2595.
13. Hidron AI, Low CE, Honig EG, Blumberg HM. Emergence of community-acquired meticillin-resistant *Staphylococcus aureus* strain USA300 as a cause of necrotising community-onset pneumonia. *Lancet Infect Dis*. 2009;9:384–392.
14. Zetola N, Francis JS, Nuermberger EL, Bishai WR. Community-acquired meticillin-resistant *Staphylococcus aureus*: an emerging threat. *Lancet Infect Dis*. 2005;5:275–286.
15. Naber CK. *Staphylococcus aureus* bacteremia: epidemiology, pathophysiology, management strategies. *Clin Infect Dis*. 2009;48:231–237.
16. Hoyert DL, Kochanek KD, Murphy SL. Deaths: final data for 1997. *Natl Vital Stat Rep*. 1999;47:1–104.
17. Melamed A, Sorvillo FJ. The burden of sepsis-associated mortality in the United States from 1999 to 2005: an analysis of multiple-cause-of-death data. *Critical Care*. 2009;13:R28.
18. McBean M, Rajamani S. Increasing rates of hospitalization due to septicemia in the US elderly population, 1986–1997. *J Infect Dis*. 2001;183:596–603.

19. Dombrovskiy VY, Martin AA, Sunderram J, Paz HL. Rapid increase in hospitalization and mortality rates for severe sepsis in the United States: a trend analysis from 1993 to 2003. *Crit Care Med*. 2007;35:1244–1250.

20. Rittirsch D, Flierl MA, Ward PA. Harmful molecular mechanisms in sepsis. *Nat Rev Immunol*. 2008;8:776–787.

21. Schouten M, Wiersinga WJ, Levi M, van der Poll T. Inflammation, endothelium and coagulation in sepsis. *J Leukoc Biol*. 2008;83:536–545.

22. Bone RC, Grodzin CJ, Balk RA. Sepsis: a new hypothesis for pathogenesis of the disease process. *Chest*. 1997;112:235–243.

23. Adib-Conquy M, Cavaillon J-M. Compensatory anti-inflammatory response syndrome. *Thromb Haemost*. 2009;101:36–47.

24. Hotchkiss RS, Nicholson DW. Apoptosis and caspases regulate death and inflammation in sepsis. *Nat Rev Immunol*. 2006;6:813–822.

25. Hotchkiss RS, Coopersmith CM, McDunn JE, Ferguson TA. The sepsis seesaw. Tilting towards immunosuppression. *Nat Med*. 2009;15:496–497.

26. Limaye AP, Kirby KA, Rubenfeld GD, et al. Cytomegalovirus reactivation in critically ill immunocompetent patients. *J Am Med Assoc*. 2008;300:413–422.

27. Lynn WA. Anti-endotoxin therapeutic options for the treatment of sepsis. *J Antimicrob Chemother*. 1998;41(Suppl):71–80.

28. Sriskandan S, Cohen J. Gram-positive sepsis. Mechanisms and differences from gram-negative sepsis. *Infect Dis Clin North Am*. 1999;13:397–412.

29. Bianchi ME. DAMPs, PAMPs and alarmins: all we need to know about danger. *J Leukoc Biol*. 2007;81:1–5.

30. Janeway CA, Medzhitov R. Innate immune recognition. *Annual Reviews of Immunology*. 2002;20:197–216.

31. Kotb M. Superantigens of gram-positive bacteria: structure–function analyses and their implications for biological activity. *Curr Opin Microbiol*. 1998;1:56–65.

32. Kotb M. Bacterial pyrogenic exotoxins as superantigens. *Clin Microbiol Rev*. 1995;8:411–426.

33. Herwald H, Cramer H, Mörgelin M, et al. M protein, a classical bacterial virulence determinant, forms complexes with fibrinogen that induce vascular leakage. *Cell*. 2004;116:367–379.

34. Uhlén P, Laestadius Å, Jahnukainen T, et al. α-Haemolysin of uropathogenic *E. coli* induces Ca^{2+} oscillations in renal epithelial cells. *Nature*. 2000;405:694–697.

35. Calandra T, Roger T. Macrophage migration inhibitory factor: a regulator of innate immunity. *Nat Rev Immunol*. 2003;3:791–800.

36. Cavaillon JM, Adib-Conquy M, Fitting C, Adrie C, Payen D. Cytokine cascades in sepsis. *Scand J Infect Dis*. 2003;35:535–544.

37. Fischer E, Marano MA, Barber AE, et al. Comparison between effects of interleukin-1 alpha administration and sublethal endotoxemia in primates. *Am J Physiol*. 1991;261:R442–R452.

38. Okusawa S, Gelfand JA, Ikejima T, Connolly RJ, Dinarello CA. Interleukin 1 induces a shock-like state in rabbits. Synergism with tumor necrosis factor and the effect of cyclooxygenase inhibition. *J Clin Invest*. 1988;81:1162–1172.

39. Tracey KJ, Beutler B, Lowry SF, et al. Shock and tissue injury induced by recombinant human cachectin. *Science*. 1986;234:470–474.

40. Tracey KJ, Lowry SF, Fahey 3rd TJ, et al. Cachectin/tumor necrosis factor induces lethal shock and stress hormone responses in the dog. *Surgery, Gynecology and Obstetrics*. 1987;164:415–422.

41. Calandra T, Echtenacher B, Roy DL, et al. Protection from septic shock by neutralization of macrophage migration inhibitory factor. *Nat Med*. 2000;6:164–170.

42. Bernhagen J, Calandra T, Bucala R. Regulation of the immune response by macrophage migration inhibitory factor: biological and structural features. *J Mol Med*. 1998;76:151–161.

43. Wang H, Bloom O, Zhang M, et al. HMG-1 as a late mediator of endotoxin lethality in mice. *Science*. 1999;285:248–251.

44. Sundén-Cullberg J, Norrby-Teglund A, Rouhiainen A, et al. Persistent elevation of high mobility group box-1 protein (HMGB1) in patients with severe sepsis or septic shock. *Crit Care Med*. 2005;33:564–573.

45. Andersson U, Erlandsson-Harris H, Yang H, Tracey KJ. HMGB1 as a DNA-binding cytokine. *J Leukoc Biol*. 2002;72:1084–1091.

46. Youn JH, Oh YJ, Kim ES, Choi JE, Shin JS. High mobility group box 1 protein binding to lipopolysaccharide facilitates transfer of lipopolysaccharide to CD14 and enhances lipopolysaccharide-mediated TNF-alpha production in human monocytes. *J Immunol*. 2008;180:5067–5074.

47. Tian J, Avalos AM, Mao SY, et al. Toll-like receptor 9-dependent activation by DNA-containing immune complexes is mediated by HMGB1 and RAGE. *Nat Immunol*. 2007;8:487–496.

48. Sha Y, Zmijewski J, Xu Z, Abraham E. HMGB1 develops enhanced proinflammatory activity by binding to cytokines. *J Immunol*. 2008;180:2531–2537.

49. Colman RW, Schmaier AH. Contact system: a vascular biology modulator with anti-coagulant, profibrinolytic, antiadhesive, proinflammatory attributes. *Blood*. 1997;90:3819–3843.

50. Ward PA. The dark side of C5a in sepsis. *Nat Rev Immunol*. 2004;4:133–142.

51. Herwald H, Mörgelin M, Olsén A, et al. Activation of the contact-phase system on bacterial surfaces – a clue to serious complications in infectious diseases. *Nat Med*. 1998;4:298–302.

52. American College of Chest Physicians/Society of Critical Care Medicine Consensus Conference. Definitions for sepsis and organ failure and guidelines for the use of innovative therapies in sepsis. *Crit Care Med*. 1992;20:864–874.

53. Rangel-Frausto MS, Pittet D, Costigan M, Hwang T, Davis CS, Wenzel RP. The natural history of the systemic inflammatory response syndrome (SIRS). A prospective study. *J Am Med Assoc*. 1995;273:117–123.

54. Levy MM, Fink MP, Marshall JC, et al. SCCM/ESICM/ACCP/ATS/SIS 2001SCCM/ESICM/ACCP/ATS/SIS International Sepsis Definitions Conference. *Crit Care Med*. 2003;31:1250–1256.

55. Kumar A, Roberts D, Wood KE, et al. Duration of hypotension before initiation of effective antimicrobial therapy is the critical determinant of survival in human septic shock. *Crit Care Med*. 2006;34:1589–1596.

56. Meehan TP, Fine MJ, Krumholz HM, et al. Quality of care, process, outcomes in elderly patients with pneumonia. *J Am Med Assoc*. 1997;278:2080–2084.

57. Bone RC. Toward an epidemiology and natural history of SIRS (systemic inflammatory response syndrome). *J Am Med Assoc*. 1992;268:3452–3455.

58. Weinstein MP, Murphy JR, Reller LB, Lichtenstein KA. The clinical significance of positive blood cultures: a comprehensive analysis of 500 episodes of bacteremia and fungemia in adults. II. Clinical observations, with special reference to factors influencing prognosis. *Rev Infect Dis*. 1983;5:54–70.

59. Li J, Plorde JJ, Carlson LG. Effects of volume and periodicity on blood cultures. *J Clin Microbiol*. 1994;32:2829–2831.

60. Rivers E, Nguyen B, Havstad S, Early Goal-Directed Therapy Collaborative Group, et al. Early goal-directed therapy in the treatment of severe sepsis and septic shock. *N Engl J Med*. 2001;345:1368–1377.

61. Rivers EP, Coba V, Visbal A, Whitmill M, Amponsah D. Management of sepsis: early resuscitation. *Clin Chest Med*. 2008;29:689–704.

62. Dellinger RP, Carlet JM, Masur H, et al. Surviving Sepsis Campaign guidelines for management of severe sepsis and septic shock. *Intensive Care Med*. 2004;30:535–555.

63. Dellinger RP, Carlet JM, Masur H, et al. Surviving Sepsis Campaign Management Guidelines Committee. Surviving Sepsis Campaign guidelines for management of severe sepsis and septic shock. *Crit Care Med*. 2004;32:858–873.

64. Dellinger RP. Steroid therapy of septic shock: the decision is in the eye of the beholder. *Crit Care Med*. 2008;36:1987–1989.

65. Ibrahim EH, Sherman G, Ward S, Fraser VJ, Kollef MH. The influence of inadequate antimicrobial treatment of bloodstream infections on patient outcomes in the ICU setting. *Chest*. 2001;118:146–155.

66. Kollef MH, Sherman G, Ward S, Fraser VJ. Inadequate antimicrobial treatment of infections: a risk factor for hospital mortality among critically ill patients. *Chest*. 1999;115:462–474.

67. Ibrahim EH, Sherman G, Ward S, Fraser VJ, Kollef MH. The influence of inadequate antimicrobial treatment of bloodstream infections on patient outcomes in the ICU setting. *Chest*. 2000;118:146–155.

68. Kreger BE, Craven DE, McCabe WR. Gram-negative bacteremia. IV. Re-evaluation of clinical features and treatment in 612 patients. *Am J Med*. 1980;68:344–355.

69. Neu HC. The crisis in antibiotic resistance. *Science*. 1992;257:1064–1073.

70. Leroy O, Georges H, Beuscart C, et al. Severe community-acquired pneumonia in ICUs: prospective validation of a prognostic score. *Intensive Care Med*. 1996;22:1307–1314.

71. Baddour LM, Yu VL, Klugman KP, et al. International Pneumococcal Study Group. Combination antibiotic therapy lowers mortality among severely ill patients with pneumococcal bacteremia. *American Journal of Respiratory Critical Care Medicine*. 2004;170:440–444.

72. Rodríguez A, Rello J. Mono versus combination antibiotic therapy: who is right? *Crit Care Med*. 2007;35:668.

73. Dellinger RP, Levy MM, Carlet JM, et al. International Surviving Sepsis Campaign Guidelines Committee, American Association of Critical-Care Nurses, American College of Chest Physicians, American College of Emergency Physicians, Canadian Critical Care Society, European Society of Clinical Microbiology and Infectious Diseases, European Society of Intensive Care Medicine, European Respiratory Society, International Sepsis Forum, Japanese Association for Acute Medicine, Japanese Society of Intensive Care Medicine, Society of Critical Care Medicine, Society of

Hospital Medicine, Surgical Infection Society, World Federation of Societies of Intensive and Critical Care Medicine. Surviving Sepsis Campaign: international guidelines for management of severe sepsis and septic shock: 2008. *Crit Care Med*. 2008;36:296–327.

74. Bunn F, Alderson P, Hawkins V. Colloid solutions for fluid resuscitation. *Cochrane Database Syst Rev*. 2000;2: CD001319.

75. Schierhout G, Roberts I. Fluid resuscitation with colloid or crystalloid solutions in critically ill patients: a systematic review of randomised trials. *Br Med J*. 1998;316:961–964.

76. Cochrane Injuries Group Albumin Reviewers. Human albumin administration in critically ill patients: systematic review of randomised controlled trials. *Br Med J*. 1998;317:235–240.

77. Finfer S, Bellomo R, Boyce N, et al. A comparison of albumin and saline for fluid resuscitation in the intensive care unit. *N Engl J Med*. 2004;350:2247–2256.

78. LeDoux D, Astiz ME, Carpati CM, Rackow EC. Effects of perfusion pressure on tissue perfusion in septic shock. *Crit Care Med*. 2000;28:2729–2732.

79. Bennett-Guerrero E, Grocott HP, Levy JH, et al. A phase II, double-blind, placebo-controlled, ascending-dose study of Eritoran (E5564), a lipid A antagonist, in patients undergoing cardiac surgery with cardiopulmonary bypass. *Anesth Analg*. 2007;104:378–383.

80. Levin M, Quint PA, Goldstein B, et al. Recombinant bactericidal/permeability-increasing protein (rBPI21) as adjunctive treatment for children with severe meningococcal sepsis: a randomised trial. rBPI21 Meningococcal Sepsis Study Group. *Lancet*. 2000;356:961–967.

81. Zimecki M, Artym J, Chodaczek G, Kocieba M, Kruzel ML. Protective effects of lactoferrin in *Escherichia coli*-induced bacteremia in mice: relationship to reduced serum TNF alpha level and increased turnover of neutrophils. *Inflamm Res*. 2004;53:292–296.

82. Land W. Innate immunity-mediated allograft rejection and strategies to prevent it. *Transplant Proc*. 2007;39:667–672.

83. Ronco C. The place of early haemoperfusion with polymyxin B fibre column in the treatment of sepsis. *Critical Care*. 2005;9:631–633.

84. Opal SM, Palardy JE, Chen WH, Parejo NA, Bhattacharjee AK, Cross AS. Active immunization with a detoxified endotoxin vaccine protects against lethal polymicrobial sepsis: its use with CpG adjuvant and potential mechanisms. *J Infect Dis*. 2005;192:2074–2080.

85. Norrby-Teglund A, Low DE, Kotb M. Intravenous immunoglobulin adjunctive therapy in patients with streptococcal toxic shock syndrome and necrotizing fasciitis. In: Kotb M, Calandra T, eds. *Cytokines and chemokines in infectious diseases handbook*. New Jersey: Humana Press; 2003:409–423.

86. Alejandria MM, Lansang MA, Dans LF, Mantaring JBV. Intravenous immunoglobulin for treating sepsis and septic shock. *Cochrane Database Syst Rev*. 2002;1: CD14001090.

87. Laupland KB, Kirkpatrick AW, Delaney A. Polyclonal intravenous immunoglobulin for the treatment of severe sepsis and septic shock in critically ill adults: a systematic review and meta-analysis. *Crit Care Med*. 2007;35:2686–2692.

88. Norrby-Teglund A, Haque KN, Hammarström L. Intravenous polyclonal IgM-enriched immunoglobulin therapy in sepsis: a review of clinical efficacy in relation to microbiological aetiology and severity of sepsis. *J Intern Med*. 2006;260:509–516.

89. Turgeon AF, Hutton B, Fergusson DA, et al. Meta-analysis: intravenous immunoglobulin in critically ill adult patients with sepsis. *Ann Intern Med*. 2007;146:193–203.

90. Norrby-Teglund A, Ihendyane N, Darenberg J. Intravenous immunoglobulin adjunctive therapy in sepsis with special emphasis on severe invasive group A streptococcal infections. *Scand J Infect Dis*. 2003;35:683–689.

91. Darenberg J, Ihendyane N, Sjölin J, et al. the Streptlg Study Group. Intravenous immunoglobulin G therapy in streptococcal toxic shock syndrome – a European randomized double-blind placebo-controlled trial. *Clin Infect Dis*. 2003;37:333–340.

92. Kaul R, McGeer A, Norrby-Teglund A, et al The Canadian Streptococcal Study Group. Intravenous immunoglobulin therapy for streptococcal toxic shock syndrome – a comparative observational study. *Clin Infect Dis*. 1999;28:800–807.

93. Annane D, Bellissant E, Bollaert PE, Briegel J, Keh D, Kupfer Y. Corticosteroids for severe sepsis and septic shock: a systematic review and meta-analysis. *Br Med J*. 2004;329:480.

94. Minneci PC, Deans KJ, Banks SM, Eichacker PQ, Natanson C. Corticosteroids for septic shock. *Ann Intern Med*. 2004;141:742–743.

95. Sprung CL, Annane D, Keh D, CORTICUS Study Group, et al. Hydrocortisone therapy for patients with septic shock. *N Engl J Med*. 2008;358:111–124.

96. Tracey KJ. Physiology and immunology of the cholinergic anti-inflammatory pathway. *Journal of Clinical Investigations*. 2007;117:289–296.

97. Wang H, Yu M, Ochani M, et al. Nicotinic acetylcholine receptor alpha7 subunit is an essential regulator of inflammation. *Nature*. 2003;421:384–388.

98. Borovikova LV, Ivanova S, Zhang M, et al. Vagus nerve stimulation attenuates the systemic inflammatory response to endotoxin. *Nature*. 2000;405:458–462.

99. Andersson U, Wang H, Palmblad K, et al. High mobility group 1 protein (HMG-1) stimulates proinflammatory cytokine synthesis in human monocytes. *J Exp Med*. 2000;192:565–570.

100. Bopp C, Bierhaus A, Hofer S, et al. Bench-to-bedside review: the inflammation-perpetuating pattern-recognition receptor RAGE as a therapeutic target in sepsis. *Critical Care*. 2008;12:210.

101. Liliensiek B, Weigand MA, Bierhaus A, et al. Receptor for advanced glycation end products (RAGE) regulates sepsis but not the adaptive immune response. *J Clin Invest*. 2004;113:1641–1650.

102. Bernard GR, Vincent JL, Laterre PF, et al. Efficacy and safety of recombinant human activated protein C for severe sepsis. *N Engl J Med*. 2001;344:699–709.

103. Thijs LG. Coagulation inhibitor replacement in sepsis is a potentially useful clinical approach. *Crit Care Med*. 2000;28(suppl):S68–S73.

104. Warren BL, Eid A, Singer P, KyberSept Trial Study Group, Caring for the Critically Ill Patient, et al. High-dose antithrombin III in severe sepsis: a randomized controlled trial. *J Am Med Assoc*. 2001;286:1869–1878.

105. Wiedermann CJ, Hoffmann JN, Juers M, KyberSept Investigators, et al. High-dose antithrombin III in the treatment of severe sepsis in patients with a high risk of death: efficacy and safety. *Crit Care Med*. 2006;34:285–292.

106. Esmon CT. Regulation of blood coagulation. *Biochim Biophys Acta*. 2000;1477:349–360.

107. Schmidt-Supprian M, Murphy C, While B, et al. Activated protein C inhibits tumor necrosis factor and macrophage migration inhibitory factor production in monocytes. *Eur Cytokine Netw*. 2000;11:407–413.

108. Abraham E, Laterre PF, Garg R, et al. Administration of Drotrecogin Alfa (Activated) in Early Stage Severe Sepsis (ADDRESS) Study Group. Drotrecogin alfa (activated) for adults with severe sepsis and a low risk of death. *N Engl J Med*. 2005;353:1332–1341.

109. Martí-Carvajal A, Salanti G, Cardona AF. Human recombinant activated protein C for severe sepsis. *Cochrane Database Syst Rev*. 2008;1: CD004388.

110. Levy MM, Fink MP, Marshall JC, et al. SCCM/ESICM/ACCP/ATS/SIS 2001 SCCM/ESICM/ACCP/ATS/SIS International Sepsis Definitions Conference. *Crit Care Med*. 2003;31:1250–1256.

111. Cohen J. Adjunctive therapy in sepsis: a critical analysis of the clinical trial programme. *Br Med Bull*. 1999;55:212–215.

112. LaRosa SP, Opal SM. Sepsis strategies in development. *Clin Chest Med*. 2009;29:735–747.

113. Giroir BP, Scannon PJ, Levin M. Bactericidal/permeability-increasing protein – lessons learned from the phase III, randomized, clinical trial of rBPI21 for adjunctive treatment of children with severe meningococcemia. *Crit Care Med*. 2001;29:S130–S2135.

114. Werdan K, Pilz G. Supplemental immune globulins in sepsis: a critical appraisal. *Clinical Experimental Immunology*. 1996;104(suppl):83–90.

115. Abraham E. Why immunomodulatory therapies have not worked in sepsis. *Intensive Care Med*. 1999;25:556–566.

116. Rice TW, Wheeler AP, Morris PE, et al. Safety and efficacy of affinity-purified, anti-tumor necrosis factor-alpha, ovine fab for injection (CytoFab) in severe sepsis. *Crit Care Med*. 2006;34:2271–2281.

117. Chua D, Tsang RS, Kuo IF. The role of statin therapy in sepsis. *Ann Pharmacother*. 2007;41:647–652.

118. Kopterides P, Falagas ME. Statins for sepsis: a critical and updated review. *Clin Microbiol Infect*. 2009;15:325–334.

119. Laterre PF, Opal SM, Abraham E, et al. A clinical evaluation committee assessment of recombinant human tissue factor pathway inhibitor (tifacogin) in patients with severe community-acquired pneumonia. *Critical Care*. 2009;13:R36.

39 Abdominal and other surgical infections

Eimear Brannigan, Peng Wong and David Leaper

Surgical site infection (SSI) represents 20% of healthcare-associated infections (HCAIs) in the UK.[1,2] Superficial SSIs are the most common but the more serious and complex deep and organ/space remainder lead to abscesses, bacteremia, sepsis and death, with an associated strain on healthcare resources because of prolonged hospital, high dependency unit (HDU) and intensive care unit (ITU) stays.[4–6] These infections mostly involve the patient's own organisms (endogenous) but others materialize later, probably relating to poor infection control practices (exogenous).

The surgically presenting community-acquired complicated skin and soft tissue, orthopedic, urological and gynecological infections are covered elsewhere (see Chs 49, 52, 54–56). Peritonitis and abdominal infections are addressed in this chapter.

ETIOLOGY OF COMMUNITY-ACQUIRED AND POSTOPERATIVE ABDOMINAL INFECTIONS

Community-acquired abdominal infections are polymicrobial and potential pathogens act in synergy. Treatment must be directed against colonic organisms that have breached the bowel lumen to cause peritonitis. These potential pathogens are typically endogenous flora, mostly anaerobes, predominantly the *Bacteroides fragilis* group, clostridial species and peptostreptococci, and aerobic Gram-negative organisms.[7–9] Peritonitis may be generalized or focal, or be divided into primary, secondary and tertiary forms (*see below*).

Postoperative abdominal infections also involve enterococci, *Candida* spp. and drug-resistant organisms in addition to the enteric pathogens seen in community-acquired infection. Complex surgical procedures, undertaken on patients with increasing co-morbidity, longer hospital stays and prolonged exposure to antimicrobials and hospital flora, lead to infections with resistant organisms. This has driven the search for new antimicrobial agents with activity against organisms with these new defenses, including extended spectrum β-lactamases (ESBL) and AmpC, which render third-generation cephalosporins inactive. These include the carbapenems and drugs such as tigecycline, although resistance to these agents has also emerged, notably among *Klebsiella* spp.[10] This requires unorthodox antimicrobial combination strategies, with the guidance of infection expertise[11] and excellence in antimicrobial stewardship.[12]

Superficial SSIs are predominantly caused by organisms carried on the skin or anterior nares of patients or healthcare staff. These are *Staphylococcus aureus* and coagulase-negative staphylococci (CNS), but *Enterococcus* spp. and *Escherichia coli* may also be implicated. Increasing numbers are drug resistant, reflecting increased broad-spectrum use in more severely ill, debilitated surgical patients.

Deep SSIs are caused by similar organisms, and can be lessened by good surgical technique and limitation of tissue damage at operation, with prevention of hematomas and seromas. Transient bacteremia with seeding of a hematoma or devitalized tissue, and translocation of gut organisms are alternative mechanisms leading to SSIs. Superficial or deep SSIs originate from intraoperative wound contamination. Tissue invasion leads to local infection, as cellulitis or an abscess, or dissemination to cause systemic inflammatory response syndrome, sepsis, septic shock syndrome and multiorgan failure. Influential factors include the load of contamination, the extent of tissue damage at operation, and host defense.

BACTERIAL CONTAMINATION

In the pathogenesis of SSI, contamination of the site precedes tissue invasion. When there are more contaminating organisms present at the end of an operation, infection is more likely. This has been demonstrated in quantitative studies; the increased risk of infection matches the four hypothetical categories of clean, clean-contaminated, contaminated and dirty surgery.[13] However, the source of contamination attributable to organisms of either exogenous (surgical team or instruments) or endogenous (patient skin, nasal carriage, gut flora) origins may not be identifiable in an individual case of SSI.

Bacterial contamination of an operative site is inevitable, and organisms survive on the skin despite optimal aseptic technique and sterilization procedures. Operating room ventilation, attention to preoperative preparation of the patient's general health, and the appropriate use of antimicrobial prophylaxis are additionally directed at achieving the lowest possible contaminating bacterial load, thereby minimizing infection. Despite the ultra-clean environment of the orthopedic theatre – with laminar flow, high efficiency particle air (HEPA) filtration and intensive focus on aseptic technique – organisms can still be found on surfaces[14] and in wounds at the close of clean elective surgical cases.[15] Air sampling shows that these are mainly Gram-positive organisms.[16] As more procedures are performed involving prosthetic material, on patients who are more debilitated, and with an increased incidence of antimicrobial-resistant organisms, it is not surprising that SSIs still occur.

A combination of strategies to minimize bacterial contamination is optimal, although there may not always be robust supportive evidence. Many operating theater practices, skin preparation and draping, theatre staff apparel and the surgical team's handwashing are largely directed against exogenous sources of infection. However, there is little scientific evidence to show that the use of caps, masks, gloves or overshoes alters the infection rate after most non-implant operations. Novel strategies such as antiseptic impregnated drapes and microbial sealants for wounds have been studied, with variable outcomes.[15] Incise drapes, adhesive polyethylene sheets designed to 'isolate' the incision site, increase the risk of SSI, but when impregnated with povidone–iodine the risk is lessened. Antimicrobial sealants[17,18] and antiseptic-coated sutures[19,20] also show promise in early evaluation.[21] Prevention of infection from endogenous sources includes decolonization of nasal *Staph. aureus* or bowel preparation for colonic surgery. In the former case, application of mupirocin reduces nasal carriage and as most *Staph. aureus* infections result from autoinfection, SSIs should also fall, although this has not been proven.[22]

Bowel preparation of patients undergoing elective colorectal surgery reduces colonic fecal content and microbial load. Dietary restriction, cathartic agents and whole gut lavage are used, and many surgeons additionally use oral and parenteral antimicrobials.[23] A number of studies suggest that this common practice may need re-evaluation as the proof they reduce infection is lacking.[24]

TISSUE DAMAGE

The proliferation of endogenous bacteria also depends on intraoperative tissue damage, which varies between wounds, operations and surgeons. Virulence factors and pathogenicity of micro-organisms, as well as their numbers in the wound at closure, are also influential. Gram-negative bacterial cell walls, rich in lipopolysaccharide, initiate a chain of responses via toll-like receptor 4 (TLR4) mediated activation of immune defenses. These trigger stimulation of adaptive immune defenses and the systemic inflammatory response and, if inappropriate or excessive, may lead to sepsis. Gram-positive

organisms such as *Staph. aureus* can produce a similar end result.[25] Optimal operative technique is essential in limiting such damage. Delicate handling of tissues, together with hemostatic control to prevent seromas or hematomas, removal of devitalized tissues, avoidance of inadvertent entry into hollow viscera and use of electrocautery all positively influence the risk of infection.[26] Choice of suture and prosthetic material contributes to optimal wound healing and minimization of postoperative infection. In many operations prosthetic, non-absorbable materials are used which reduce the number of organisms necessary to cause infection.

Suction or open drains also increase the risk of infection by providing a portal of entry for bacteria and acting as foreign bodies.[27] Placement of drains distant from the operative incision, with early drain removal, is optimal, as sterile drains soon become colonized with potential pathogens.[28] Meta-analyses of the use of surgical drains do not encourage their use.[29–31]

HOST RESISTANCE

Tobacco smoking, diabetes, malignancy, and renal and liver disease are recognized influences on health outcomes, but also specifically on infection after surgery. Host resistance to infection is adversely affected by malnutrition (including obesity) and perioperative hyperglycemia. These factors impair a patient's ability to overcome bacterial contamination at operation and the incidence of postoperative infection.

In obesity, for example, there is evidence that immune and inflammatory responses are diminished. This has implications for the increasing numbers of obese patients embarking upon bariatric surgery.[32] Immunosuppressive drugs influence the risk of infection and include corticosteroids, cytotoxic chemotherapeutic agents and immune-targeted biologically active agents such as etanercept and monoclonal antibody therapies such as natalizumab. Although they have specific intentional immunological consequences, they may additionally result in vulnerability to infection.

Genetically influenced variations in immune defense mechanisms predict postoperative infection, and coordination of innate immune responses to, for example, secondary peritonitis is central in determining clinical outcome depending on whether responses are contained or become more generalized and systemic.[33] Individuals with TLR4 polymorphisms have aberrant responses to some Gram-negative infections with increased susceptibility and severity of infection.[25]

INCIDENCE AND SURVEILLANCE OF SURGICAL SITE INFECTION

The intensity of post discharge surveillance (PDS) of SSI, and other surgical infections, may lead to different figures of incidence and prevalence. Audit surveillance is less accurate than research surveillance, relating as it does to the definitions used, and the rigor and extent of follow-up. Defining SSI is central to measuring incidence, but is difficult. Although no generally accepted guidelines exist, the most widely used and accepted clinical definitions used in surveillance and research are the Centers for Disease Control (CDC) definition[3] and the ASEPSIS score.[34]

The CDC definition of SSI requires identification of a number of features within 30 days of surgery, or up to 1 year after prosthetic surgery, although the majority are usually apparent between the fifth and tenth postoperative day. These diagnostic features are:

- a purulent discharge or abscess
- organisms isolated from the wound
- at least one Celsian sign
- wound separation or need for drainage
- the attending surgeon records the presence of an SSI.

In addition there are three categories of SSI: superficial incisional which affect the skin and superficial tissues, usually with the classical Celsian signs of calor, rubor, dolor and tumor (and functio laesa); deep incisional which affect the fascial and muscle layers; and organ/space infection involving anatomical sites other than the incision, for example joint or peritoneum.

The ASEPSIS score acronym (see below) is an excellent tool for research and allows collection of continuous or interval scale data as opposed to the categorical data of other systems:

- **A**dditional treatment
- **S**erous discharge
- **E**rythema
- **P**urulent exudates
- **S**eparation of deep tissues
- **I**solation of bacteria
- hospital **S**tay for longer than 14 days.

The ASEPSIS score allows distinction of life-threatening SSIs (needing readmission or prolonged inpatient stay) from less serious infections (such as discharge of pus that interferes minimally with postoperative recovery).

Many surgeons believe that their SSI rate after clean wound surgery is low. The often quoted Cruse and Foord data on SSI after clean surgery, using questionnaire by telephone, does indicate rates of <2%;[35] however, more intensive methods, employing an independent, blinded, trained and validated observer, produce higher figures. The cost and management of SSIs are transferred to primary care where instead of appropriately opening a wound to release pus, empirical antibiotics with an inappropriate spectrum of activity may be given (adding to the risk of resistance).

Audit of all surgical wounds with extensive PDS is expensive. However, an early study in this field (Study on the Efficacy of Nosocomial Infection Control, SENIC) showed that surveillance, which included collection, analysis and feedback of data to surgeons, significantly reduced SSI rates.[36] Many surveillance systems have been established since then and are mandatory for orthopedic SSIs in the UK.[37,38] A drawback of these systems is that they tend to be recorded only during the increasingly short, postoperative, inpatient hospital stays.[39,40]

Up to 75% of elective clean surgery is now undertaken on a day-case basis so that the high incidence of SSI is often not recognized by the operating team in secondary care. To allow feedback to surgeons or for the evaluation of related research, data relating to rates and incidence of SSI must be valid. It may be possible to undertake an intensive audit of SSI in rotation between hospital-based specialties but accurate recognition after every type of surgery requires significant resources. These data cannot be easily collected by a surveillance coordinator or infection control team, with standardization and validation of definitions and approach, unless they are adequately funded.

PATIENT FACTORS WHICH INFLUENCE POSTOPERATIVE INFECTIONS (particularly SSIs)

The logic of having a risk score or recognized risk factors to predict infection in surgical patients is attractive. Healthcare resources could thereby be directed at pre-empting or avoiding risk, or at anticipating and managing infection earlier. The risk of SSI has been identified by the National Nosocomial Infections Surveillance System (NNISS) in North America to relate to the parameters of the American Society of Anesthesiologists (ASA) score, length of operation and wound class.[41]

Longer operations reflect severe underlying illness and greater blood loss; conversely, endoscopic surgical approaches have reduced the risk of SSI, even though they often have a longer operative time.[42] Statistical analysis to identify independent variables is clearly important.

Concern that the NNIS system would not necessarily work for all surgical operations, particularly in predicting the more clinically significant deep and organ/space infections,[43,44] led Haridas and Malangoni[45] to hypothesize that additional risk factors could be identified. A previous operation and hypoalbuminemia were significant risks for deep or organ/space infections. Many other patient risk factors have been suggested, including age, a history of cardiac failure, diabetes and hyperglycemia in non-diabetic patients, immunological insufficiency, high body mass index (BMI), low hemoglobin and blood transfusion, remote infection, excessive alcohol use and smoking. This is well summarized in the National Institute for Health and Clinical Excellence (NICE) guideline on prevention and treatment of SSI in which few systematic assessments of patient risk factors were found.[46] However, in the first of the American College of Surgeons Best Practices Initiative, many of these factors were addressed.[47]

PRINCIPLES OF ANTIBIOTIC AND OTHER PROPHYLACTIC MEASURES IN SURGERY

ANTIBIOTIC PROPHYLAXIS

The choice of antibiotic prophylaxis prior to surgery depends on the type of surgery. There is now level I evidence that intravenous prophylactic antibiotics should be given at induction of anesthesia for optimal tissue levels during the operation (above the minimum inhibitory concentration $(MIC)_{90}$ of anticipated bacteria), and repeated *only* if there is excess blood loss, a long operation time or the placement of a prosthesis, as in hip replacement. Even then, three-dose prophylaxis should not be exceeded; extension beyond this is therapy with all the risks of resistance and emergence. Excessive, unanticipated fecal spillage during an elective colorectal operation serves as an example where prophylaxis should be extended to 5 days of antibiotic therapy.

Use of antibiotic prophylaxis to prevent SSI is based on the work of John Burke.[48] After staphylococci were injected into rabbit skin, a 4-hour delay in the host response was described (the 'decisive period'). Administering an antibiotic before this period prevented abscess development. In surgical patients, this decisive period immediately follows surgery when host defenses are being mounted and the wound is most at risk of contamination and subsequent SSI; antibiotic prophylaxis is protective during this period of vulnerability. Level I evidence in Cochrane systematic reviews recommends antibiotic prophylaxis in colorectal surgery and in prosthetic hip surgery to prevent SSIs.[49,50]

Four categories of operative wound contamination have been defined.[51] Prior to antibiotic prophylaxis the corresponding SSI rates were:[52]

- clean (5%+)
- clean-contaminated (<10%)
- contaminated (15–20%)
- dirty (>40%).

Rates of SSIs have been significantly reduced since the introduction of antibiotic prophylaxis.[53] The choice of a prophylactic regimen depends on availability and cost, and local guidelines which consider local resistance patterns, and microbiological and pharmaceutical advice. Guidelines adapted from the previous edition of *Antibiotics and Chemotherapy* are listed in Table 39.1.

Paradoxically, the reported rates of SSI after clean, non-prosthetic surgery are variable, and use of prophylactic antibiotics for non-prosthetic operations is controversial. The National Research Council definition[51] of clean wound surgery is that no other inflammation is encountered, the respiratory, alimentary and gastrointestinal tracts are not opened, and there is no breach in aseptic technique. Cruse and Foord,[35] in a clean wound audit, estimated that the superficial SSI rate was 1.4%. While this figure is widely quoted, other papers report much higher rates of SSIs ranging from 4.5% to 18%.[54–59] This variation in rate can be accounted for in part by the different audit techniques used. Higher rates are found in studies that incorporate surveillance by a trained unbiased observer than in studies employing telephone or postal enquiry.[60,61] Keeling and Morgan[57] reported that the observed infection rate increased 10-fold if surgical patients were followed up after discharge.

Should perioperative antibiotic prophylaxis be given for clean wound surgery? Platt et al[62] reported a reduced infection rate following hernia or breast surgery in patients given antibiotic prophylaxis versus placebo. However, the analysis included chest and urinary tract infections; if these are excluded the SSI rates do not differ significantly. Taylor and colleagues[58] reported no effect of co-amoxiclav in patients undergoing open groin hernia repair (9%). High rates of SSI following breast surgery (17–19%) have been reported,[59] whether patients were given co-amoxiclav prophylaxis or placebo. A Cochrane meta-analysis of antibiotic prophylaxis in hernia repair, involving eight randomized controlled trials (RCTs) and 2907 patients, found no significant difference in infection rates after prophylaxis (2.9%) compared to placebo (4.3%). It was concluded that antibiotic prophylaxis could neither be firmly recommended nor discarded.[63] Thus, SSI after clean surgery is probably underestimated, the value of antibiotic prophylaxis is uncertain and the cost of infection can be high. A better picture will only develop from studies that employ a rigorous definition of SSI, accurate audit, an independent trained observer and a scoring system, such as ASEPSIS.

There is compelling evidence supporting antibiotic prophylaxis in clean-contaminated and contaminated wounds but the value in non-prosthetic clean wound surgery is less clear. There is also controversy over the true incidence of infection, and even whether these wound complications are superficial SSIs or represent a 'failure to heal'. Adjuvant approaches which may also be effective are discussed next.

MAINTENANCE OF PERIOPERATIVE NORMOTHERMIA

Patient warming, systemic or local, is logical in preventing SSIs because of the known link between warming and tissue viability; low tissue perfusion increases the risk of infection[64,65] and warming increases tissue oxygenation.[65] Operating theatres are designed for operating personnel comfort, not that of patients (21°C, 55% relative humidity); gases and intravenous fluids need to be warmed for patients losing heat following exposure and the vasodilatation caused by anesthesia. The pathophysiological consequences are an increased basal metabolic rate, with shivering; increased oxygen demand, acidosis, shift in the oxygen dissociation curve; relative organ ischemia and cardiac dysfunction; and prolonged drug actions. The result is an increased risk of infection and poor healing.

Warming patients systemically during elective colorectal surgery significantly reduces SSIs[66] and the value of prewarming before anesthesia and surgery has been shown.[67] A meta-analysis by Mahoney and Odom[68] combined 18 studies involving 1575 patients and identified significant reductions in the use of blood products, length of hospital stay, length of time in the intensive care unit (ICU), reduced infection and mortality by the avoidance of hypothermia, with considerable cost savings.

Local warming of patients prior to clean wound surgery at the intended surgical incision site has also been shown to reduce SSI rates.[69] Infection rates were 13.7% for standard

Table 39.1 Antibiotic prophylaxis in surgery

Type of operation	Principal pathogens	Antibiotic regimens and recommended doses[a]	
Clean operations			
In hospitals without endemic MRSA			
Implanted prosthesis Other clean operations for which prophylaxis is indicated	*Staphylococcus* spp. including MRSA	Amoxicillin–clavulanic acid Flucloxacillin + gentamicin Cefuroxime	1.2 g i.v. 2 g i.v. 2 mg/kg i.v. 1.5 g i.v.
In hospitals with endemic MRSA		Vancomycin Teicoplanin or linezolid	1 g i.v. infusion over 60 min 600 mg i.v.
For penicillin-allergic patients		(Clindamycin) (Clarithromycin + gentamicin)	(500 mg i.v.) (2 mg/kg i.v.)
Clean-contaminated operations			
Head and neck			
(if sinus, nasal, oral or pharyngeal mucosa breached)	Staphylococci Streptococci Oral anaerobes	Amoxicillin–clavulanic acid Cefuroxime + metronidazole (Clindamycin)	1.2 g i.v. 1.5 g i.v. 500 mg i.v. (600 mg i.v.)
Thoracic			
Bronchial	Staphylococci	Amoxicillin–clavulanic acid	1.2 g i.v.
Esophageal	Streptococci GNAB Oral anaerobes	Cefuroxime + metronidazole (Cefuroxime + metronidazole)	1.5 g i.v. 500 mg i.v. (1.5 g i.v.) + (500 mg i.v.)
Upper gastrointestinal			
Gastric	GNAB	Amoxicillin–clavulanic acid Gentamicin + metronidazole Clarithromycin Cefuroxime	1.2 g i.v. 5 mg/kg i.v. 500 mg i.v. 500 mg i.v. 1.5 g i.v.
Biliary	GNAB	Amoxicillin–clavulanic acid	1.2 g i.v.
ERCP	Enterococci	Piperacillin + gentamicin Cefuroxime (Vancomycin)	2 g i.v. 2 mg/kg i.v. 1.5 g i.v. (1 g i.v. infusion over 1 h)
Urology			
TURP	GNAB Enterococci	Amoxicillin–clavulanic acid Gentamicin (Ciprofloxacin)	1.2 g i.v. 2 mg/kg i.v. (500 mg orally with premed)
Obstetrics and gynecology			
Hysterectomy	GNAB *Bacteroides* spp.	Amoxicillin–clavulanic acid Gentamicin + metronidazole Cefotetan (Clindamycin)	1 g i.v. 2 mg/kg i.v. 500 mg/kg i.v. 1 g i.v. (600 mg i.v.)
Cesarean section	β-Hemolytic streptococci *Bacteroides* spp Enterococci *Staph. aureus* *Chlamydia*[b]	Options as above	As above
Amputation	*Clostridium* spp.	Benzylpenicillin + gentamicin + metronidazole (Clarithromycin + metronidazole) (Clindamycin)	1.2 g i.v. 2 mg/kg i.v. 500 mg i.v. (500 mg i.v.) + (500 mg i.v.) 600 mg i.v.

(Continued)

Table 39.1 Antibiotic prophylaxis in surgery—cont'd

Type of operation	Principal pathogens	Antibiotic regimens and recommended doses[a]	
Contaminated operations			
Colorectal			
Elective operations	GNAB	Amoxicillin–clavulanic acid	1.2 g i.v.
	Bacteroides fragilis	Amoxicillin	1 g i.v.
		+ gentamicin	2 mg/kg i.v.
		+ metronidazole	500 mg i.v.
		Cefotetan	1 g i.v.
		(Cefuroxime + metronidazole)	(1.5 g i.v. + 500 mg i.v.)
Intestinal obstruction	*Bacteroides* spp.	Options as above	As above
	GNAB		
Compound trauma (within 4 h)	Other anaerobes	Penicillin	1.2–2.4 g
	Staph. aureus	+ gentamicin	5 mg/kg i.v.
	GNAB	+ metronidazole	500 mg i.v.
	Bacillus spp.	(Clarithromycin + metronidazole)	(500 mg i.v. + 500 mg i.v.)

[a]The evidence indicates that single-dose prophylaxis is adequate, although some surgeons administer antibiotic prophylaxis for 24 h.
[b]Is not an acute surgical infection risk, although it may be spread by surgery. If prophylaxis is considered appropriate, azithromycin 1 g is recommended.
ERCP, endoscopic retrograde cholangiopancreatogram; GNAB, Gram-negative aerobic bacilli; MRSA, methicillin-resistant *Staphylococcus aureus*; TURP, transurethral prostatectomy.
Antibiotics shown in brackets are replacements for β-lactam antibiotics in the above regimen for patients allergic to penicillin.

treatment, 3.6% for local warming ($p = 0.003$) and 5.8% for systemic warming ($p = 0.028$). Other surgical complications were also reduced in the warmed patients and significantly fewer antibiotics were prescribed for wound complications on return to primary care.

Prudent antibiotic prescribing and warming have not been widely or consistently adopted, despite directives and 'checklists' from the Department of Health[70] and from the World Health Organization.[71,72]

PERIOPERATIVE SUPPLEMENTAL OXYGENATION

Another intervention that has been shown to reduce the incidence of SSIs is the use of supplemental perioperative oxygen.[73,74] Although taken up widely in the USA, together with other factors such as tight perioperative blood glucose control,[75] this intervention has not been adopted in the UK. A fall in SSI rates from 2.3% to 1.7% was reported in the 44-hospital US collaborative. In the UK it is normal recovery-room practice to ensure that oxygenation is optimal (95% hemoglobin saturation) and that patients are routinely given an $F\text{io}_2$ of >60%, which, after extubation, is not likely to offer any further benefit.[46] The results of further studies are anticipated.

SELECTIVE DECONTAMINATION OF THE DIGESTIVE TRACT

Selective decontamination of the digestive tract (SDD) was developed to reduce the incidence of morbidity and mortality resulting from nosocomial acquisition of infection by Gram-negative aerobic bacilli (GNAB) in patients treated in the ICU. The intention is to remove GNAB and yeasts from the oropharynx and upper and lower gastrointestinal tract using non-absorbable antibiotics, thereby reducing the risk of ventilator-associated pneumonia (VAP) and mortality (this topic, and the use of probiotic bacteria, is discussed in more detail in Ch. 41). The challenge is related to the time it takes to eradicate GNAB from the gastrointestinal tract: in very sick patients it can take 5–10 days, by which time the organisms have already caused infection. There appears to be little to choose between SDD and selective oropharyngeal decontamination (SOD) alone.[76]

Meta-analyses of trials of SDD[77,78] have shown significant reduction in mortality in critically ill patients. Webb[79] has expressed concern about the impact on antibiotic resistance of such use. He notes that other methods of preventing VAP carry no such risks and have yet to be evaluated in comparison with SDD. Ebner and colleagues[80] share Webb's concern. Certainly outbreaks of infection, resulting from GNAB containing plasmid-mediated ESBL genes, have been reported. This may be related to the use of third-generation cephalosporins during SDD in the ICU, and laboratory identification of multiple drug-resistant GNAB ought to guide the use of SDD.[81] Nevertheless, the proponents of SDD report no clear increase in resistance in a review of RCTs.[82] The practice has not been taken up widely in the UK and there is also controversy as to whether SDD should be part of the surviving sepsis campaign bundles.[83]

The organisms responsible for the development of postoperative sepsis, multiple organ dysfunction syndrome (MODS) and multiple organ failure (MOF) are mainly derived from the colon, described as the 'motor' of sepsis, MODS and MOF.[84] Although aerobic and anaerobic colonic flora act synergistically, preoperative eradication of anaerobes from the colon may not be possible because of their large numbers, and not desirable because of their influence on colonization and resistance.[85] The aerobes in the colon can be suppressed by SDD and it has been shown that SDD mainly targets GNAB with little increase in Gram-positive infections.[86]

In health the small bowel remains relatively sterile but in disease it is colonized rapidly by GNAB which adds to the risk of bacterial translocation and sepsis. The value of SDD has been favorably assessed to prevent these infective complications after cardiopulmonary bypass,[87] esophageal surgery,[88] liver transplantation,[89] small-bowel transplantation[90] and colorectal surgery.[91]

SPECIFIC ANTIBIOTIC THERAPY IN ABDOMINAL AND OTHER SURGICAL AREAS

HEAD AND NECK SURGERY

Endogenous oropharyngeal organisms are the most common cause of infection. Antimicrobial prophylaxis is not required for clean surgery for benign disease, but should be considered for malignant disease. Prophylaxis for clean-contaminated or contaminated procedures is recommended, but for a maximum of 24 h. For procedures such as complex septorhinoplasty or grommet insertion, a single dose or short duration (<24 h) antimicrobial prophylaxis is recommended. The agents should have activity against both aerobic and anaerobic organisms.

Following tonsillectomy or adenoidectomy, bacteremia occurs with a frequency dependent upon the indication for the procedure. Children operated on for recurrent acute otitis media or otitis media with effusion had higher rates of bacteremia than children whose surgery was for other indications.[92]

After tracheostomy, it is common to culture organisms from tracheal aspirates, but this most often represents bacterial colonization of the tube surface. As the length of time the tracheostomy tube is in place is extended, colonization is more likely, with *Pseudomonas* spp. or resistant GNAB. Optimal management includes attention to limiting antimicrobial exposure, and chest physiotherapy to expectorate secretions and prevent mucous stasis.

Deep space neck infections are the most severe, but have decreased since the introduction of penicillin and the appropriate use of antimicrobial prophylaxis in head and neck procedures. Community-acquired pharyngitis and tonsillitis were primarily responsible for precipitating deep neck infections, but this has decreased and has been overtaken by those related to odontogenic infection. The complex anatomy of the fascial planes and potential spaces within the neck has been reviewed by Vieira et al[93] and this should direct clinical examination and appropriate imaging during evaluation of a patient with such an infection.

Poor oral hygiene increases odontogenic infection, including Ludwig's angina, while altered states of immunity such as malignancy, diabetes and HIV infection result in atypical presentations of deep neck infections. Predominant organisms are viridans streptococci, staphylococci and anaerobes such as *Prevotella* and peptostreptococci.

The priority in managing a patient presenting with fever, pain and swelling in the neck, up to the parotid and mastoid, and down to the supraclavicular fossae, is airway protection. This is followed closely by antibiotics, with a spectrum of activity sufficiently broad to treat the anticipated organisms, and surgical decompression of any collection. Surgical management, particularly of deeper space infections, requires extensive debridement, antimicrobial-impregnated dressings to permit frequent review and tracheostomy. Complications include mediastinitis, osteomyelitis, bacteremia and empyema.[93]

THORACIC SURGERY

For non-cardiac thoracic surgery antimicrobial prophylaxis is standard, although in health the lower respiratory tract is usually sterile. In complex or recalcitrant infection requiring surgical intervention, prophylaxis is warranted. A single dose of an agent active against aerobic and anaerobic organisms common to the oropharyngeal and upper respiratory tract is adequate for esophageal surgery or resection of lung tissue. When a complex loculated infection or abscess is present, treatment should be directed by microbiological analysis of drained pus or culture of resected tissue and often needs to be prolonged for several weeks. *Staph. aureus*, *Streptococcus pneumoniae*, CNS and GNAB are the usual organisms encountered.

Complicated parapneumonic effusions or empyemas may require open surgical management if tube drainage or aspiration procedures have failed. Later indications for surgery include thoracotomy and restoration of normal chest mechanics by decortication of adherent thickened pleura. Thoracostomy allows irrigation and gradual closure over months in more complicated cases. Decortication is a procedure with significant morbidity and mortality;[94] however, in severely ill patients, the best outcomes are achievable by this approach.[95] The esophagus is normally colonized by oropharyngeal and upper respiratory tract organisms. Esophageal operations are frequently combined with gastric surgery for malignancy; in these operations, and where there is an esophageal stricture, overgrowth of both aerobic and anaerobic organisms with Enterobacteriaceae, enterococci and streptococci may occur. Single-dose prophylaxis with cefuroxime, cefotaxime or piperacillin (possibly with the addition of metronidazole) or amoxicillin–clavulanate is recommended.

STERNOTOMY WOUND INFECTIONS AND MEDIASTINITIS

The reported rate for deep sternal wound infections (DSWIs) is 1–2%.[96] Established patient risk factors include increased BMI, chronic airways disease, renal impairment, diabetes, steroid use, concurrent infection and immunosuppression. Operative factors also influence risk and include perioperative glycemic control, surgical technique including off-midline incisions, and prolonged cardiopulmonary bypass time. Preventive strategies include primary sternal plating and materials such as titanium in sternal plates, which limits mobility during chest wall movement, such as coughing, thereby decreasing the opportunity for infection.[97] The diagnosis of deep infection is largely clinical, supported by microbiological data, but neither CT nor MRI adequately differentiates usual benign postoperative findings from abscesses and deep space infections.

DSWIs include mediastinitis, osteomyelitis, pericarditis, sepsis and wound dehiscence. Infection of prosthetic valves and of coronary grafts may occur and be fatal. The predominant pathogens are *Staph. aureus* and CNS, and hematoma formation, bone debris and suture wires in the sternotomy site are ideal substrates on which to form biofilm in which these organisms thrive.

Superficial infections should be drained, material sent for microbiological analysis and treatment initiated with an anti-staphylococcal agent, often a combination of a β-lactam and vancomycin until culture and sensitivity data are available.

Deeper infections can be catastrophic and require aggressive surgical debridement and high-dose, long-term antibiotic therapy directed by bacterial cultures from the deep tissues and local sensitivity patterns. The precise pathophysiology of mediastinitis is unclear but is related to imperfect asepsis, perioperative bleeding, sternal instability and operative time, as well as patient-related factors. Microbiological analysis of deep tissue samples directs appropriate therapy as infection often needs prolonged courses with parenteral agents. Where methicillin-resistant *Staph. aureus* (MRSA) is isolated, treatment with a glycopeptide is required, although novel agents such as linezolid, daptomycin and tigecycline may have a role.

Mediastinitis may complicate cardiac or esophageal surgery, penetrating trauma and spontaneous or instrumental perforation. Surgical management depends upon the underlying cause and may need thoracotomy with drainage of the mediastinum. The use of broad-spectrum antibiotics covering both aerobic and anaerobic organisms (e.g. cefotaxime and metronidazole, imipenem or amoxicillin–clavulanate) is required, and evidence of MRSA infection should be sought. Once the patient has stabilized and the operative management of the infection is completed, long-term antimicrobials can be chosen and managed in an outpatient antimicrobial therapy (OPAT) program.

Reoperation and rewiring may be required. Chest wall reconstruction has evolved, including omental interpositioning and the use of muscle flaps from the abdominal wall. Vacuum-assisted closure (negative pressure) devices are increasingly widely used with improved outcomes after DSWI.[98] Hyperbaric oxygen therapy over prolonged courses has been used with some success. The theory is attractive, with delivery of increased 'antimicrobial' oxygenation to tissues, but the supporting evidence is limited. A review of the available evidence specifically for sternal infections[99] found only a handful of papers encompassing the experience from four centers which had used hyperbaric oxygen in approximately 150 patients, and concluded that the evidence base was very weak and in need of RCT data.

With regard to SSIs at the saphenous vein harvest site, the usual pathogens are staphylococci and streptococci, but can include enterococci and *Esch. coli*. The presentation ranges from cellulitis to wound dehiscence and necrosis requiring debridement. Low rates of infection relate to the technique of vein harvesting and the introduction of endoscopic methods. Therapy should be directed against skin organisms, and where MRSA is endemic, glycopeptides should be included.

CARDIAC SURGERY

Before the advent of antibiotics, infective endocarditis had a mortality of 100%. A more recent study of endocarditis in London reported an 18% mortality at discharge, with a 6-month mortality of 27%.[100]

The common organisms identified in endocarditis are streptococci, *Staph. aureus*, CNS and occasionally yeasts. Appropriate antimicrobial therapy should always accompany surgery on an infected valve. Other foci of infection such as dental disease should be identified and controlled.

Surgical technique is central in preventing early postoperative infection of prosthetic valves, although accompanying interventions are also portals of entry (central venous access devices, pacing wires, intra-aortic balloon pumps and urinary catheters). Management should now follow the care bundle concept to reduce infection risk. Postoperative infection after valve surgery is usually caused by CNS, *Staph. aureus*, streptococci and occasionally GNAB. Late infection of prosthetic valves may follow subsequent bacteremia, particularly after dental procedures. MRSA has become prevalent in many cardiac units and in ICUs where these patients are managed postoperatively.

CARDIAC PACEMAKERS

Patients undergoing cardiac pacemaker insertion or open heart surgery should receive antimicrobial prophylaxis not exceeding 24 h. Typically postoperative infections are caused by CNS and *Staph. aureus* from the patient's skin and this, together with the catastrophic consequences of such infections, has led to the use of prophylaxis, although cardiac surgery is in the clean surgery category. After coronary artery bypass grafting (CABG), the sternotomy wound and the saphenous vein harvest site wound are vulnerable to infection. Screening for MRSA and decolonization of nasal carriage in advance of elective CABG or valvular cardiac surgery can reduce infections, but CNS also play a significant role. The most dreaded complication is mediastinitis.

Over 3 million people worldwide have a permanent pacing device.[101] Following insertion of a cardiac pacemaker or implantable cardioverter defibrillator (ICD), infection may occur in the pocket created to contain the device, on the subcutaneous electrodes or in tissues surrounding the leads. Infection originates in the external elements such as the pocket, and advances into the deeper regions along the electrodes or wires. The incidence of infection is higher for temporary external pacemakers (1–5%) than for permanent pacemakers (1%). ICD infection rates are around 1%[101] and skin organisms predominate as pathogens, mainly *Staph. aureus* and CNS. Local evidence of infection – such as pain and erythema, swelling, discharge of pus or exteriorization of the lead or generator – indicates a pocket abscess but deeper or invasive infection including bacteremia and endocarditis can be predicted.[102] Extraction of hardware is needed and blood cultures underestimate deep infection. Optimal management requires removal of the pacemaker and leads, a significant procedure with an associated mortality risk and which may need open heart surgery with cardiopulmonary bypass.

Antibiotics are widely used prophylactically at the time of pacemaker implantation, as infection probably arises from peri-implantation contamination. However, evidence for the efficacy of this approach is lacking as the infection rate is low (around 1%) and valid trials are virtually impossible. Nevertheless, as the consequences of infection can be life-threatening, it is pragmatic to continue administration of single-dose prophylaxis with activity against the commonly implicated organisms (flucloxacillin, oxacillin or amoxicillin–clavulanate, or a glycopeptide where MRSA is endemic).

PERIPHERAL VASCULAR SURGERY

Vascular graft infection, in particular prosthetic graft infection, is uncommon (1–5%)[103] but carries a high amputation risk (10–25%) and mortality (20%).[104] Most graft infections originate from direct contamination at surgery or by hematogenous seeding from intravascular line, urinary tract or respiratory tract infection. Grafts to or below the groin are the most vulnerable, particularly when there is distal tissue necrosis or infection.

Prosthetic graft infection can present as local abscesses, sinuses, graft exposure, thrombosis or anastomotic hemorrhage. Infected aortic grafts can erode the fourth part of the duodenum or bowel, forming an aortoenteric fistula, and present with catastrophic gastrointestinal bleeding.

Most graft infections are due to skin organisms and the vast majority are due to *Staph. epidermidis*, *Staph. aureus* and *Esch. coli*. CNS and other organisms, when present within a biofilm bound to the prosthesis, are protected from antibiotics. MRSA infection is associated with a high morbidity and mortality. Fungal infections are rare and tend to occur in immunocompromised patients.

Prompt treatment is required to prevent catastrophic hemorrhage or graft thrombosis. Conservative measures are rarely curative. Treatment often involves explantation of the graft and revascularization via an extra-anatomical, uninfected route. The use of the sartorius muscle flap has been shown to be effective in facilitating complicated groin wound healing, while maintaining vascular graft salvage and patency. There is no evidence to guide the optimal duration of antibiotic therapy.[105] As *Staph. aureus* is the organism most likely to be isolated in early infection,[106] and as MRSA is increasingly common, empirical treatment of early-onset infection should include a glycopeptide.[107] The serious consequences of graft infection have led to almost universal prescribing of perioperative antibiotic prophylaxis. Antibiotics active against *Staph. aureus* and *Staph. epidermidis*, and if the operation extends to or below the groin, activity against Enterobacteriaceae are recommended. Where MRSA is endemic, a glycopeptide may be needed. There is little evidence to indicate that prophylaxis for more than 24 h is necessary.[108]

GASTROINTESTINAL SURGERY

PERITONITIS

Bacterial peritonitis following an ischemic, inflammatory or perforated pathology in an abdominal viscus is one of the major infective challenges in surgery. Despite advances in diagnosis, surgical and anesthetic techniques, antimicrobial agents and supportive care, mortality remains high (20–60%).

Peritonitis can be subclassified into primary, secondary or tertiary according to the underlying etiology. Primary peritonitis occurs in the absence of any loss of integrity of the gastrointestinal tract. The most characteristic syndrome of primary peritonitis is spontaneous bacterial peritonitis, in which the peritoneum is infected via the bloodstream. In contrast, secondary peritonitis is an acute infection of the peritoneal cavity, usually arising from a perforation, anastomotic disruption or transmural necrosis. Tertiary peritonitis has been described as a diffuse and persistent form of peritonitis with impaired host defenses following overwhelming infection of the peritoneal cavity, the result of which is often fatal. Understanding the classification of peritonitis is important in guiding management as the pathogenesis and the microbial nature of the different causes vary.

 ## PRIMARY PERITONITIS

Primary peritonitis usually occurs in the presence of ascites. Primary or spontaneous bacterial peritonitis (SBP) develops in up to 25% of patients with alcoholic cirrhosis.[109] It is accepted that colonization of the ascitic fluid from an episode of bacteremia initiates peritoneal infection, made possible by the constant fluid exchange between the circulatory and ascitic compartments.

The diagnosis of SBP is based on the polymorphonuclear (PMN) cell count in ascitic fluid. A PMN count of more than $250/mm^3$ is highly suspicious of SBP and is an indication to start empirical antibiotic treatment. A bedside leukocyte esterase reagent strip with spectrophotometric analysis is available to rapidly exclude SBP.[110] *Esch. coli* is the commonest pathogen responsible for SBP, followed by *Klebsiella pneumoniae*, *Str. pneumoniae* and other streptococcal species, including enterococci.[109] Anaerobes are rare; the presence of aerobes and anaerobes suggests secondary peritonitis.

Third-generation cephalosporins are the antibiotics of choice because of their safer profile, despite the lack of evidence found in a systematic review.[111] Antibiotic prophylaxis has been advocated for cirrhotic patients with ascites[112,113] using oral fluoroquinolones.[114]

 ## SECONDARY PERITONITIS

The microbial flora of the gastrointestinal tract increase in numbers and diversity from proximal to distal end. Gram-positive organisms predominate in the oral cavity, while the stomach and small bowel are relatively sterile. Increased numbers of Gram-negative organisms occur in the distal small bowel and anaerobes appear in large numbers in the colon.[115] Patients with secondary peritonitis are most frequently encountered on surgical wards.

These abdominal infections are accompanied by a significant systemic inflammatory response and endotoxin production, which often leads to multiple organ failure.

The organisms isolated in secondary peritonitis vary depending on the site of the pathology. The stomach in the fasting state contains few, relatively acid-resistant species (e.g. lactobacilli or *Candida* spp.). Gastric perforation is therefore associated initially with a sterile chemical peritonitis. In contrast, perforation of the colon results in a peritoneal influx of an enormous number of organisms that constitute the normal colonic flora. *B. fragilis* is the most frequently isolated anaerobe and *Esch. coli* is the most frequently isolated facultative anaerobe.[109] They act in synergy.

Treatment of secondary peritonitis involves judicious fluid and oxygen resuscitation, correction of physiological derangements, administration of empirical antibiotics and source control by surgical closure, resection or excision of the diseased segment. Source control should be followed by extensive peritoneal lavage to remove fibrin (which traps bacteria), blood, bacteria, toxin and debris. If the source of infection cannot be controlled, continuous postoperative lavage, staged relaparotomy or treatment by an open abdomen (laparostomy) could be considered to prevent secondary or recurrent infection. The use of the APACHE (Acute Physiology and Chronic Health Evaluation) II scoring system of stratification provides objective discrimination between low-risk and high-risk patients with intra-abdominal infection.[116]

Antimicrobial therapy should include narrow-spectrum agents to treat community-acquired infections, and broader-spectrum agents for hospital-acquired infections,[117] as this latter group of patients often harbors resistant pathogens. The Surgical Infection Society of North America[118] has made recommendations for antimicrobial therapy for intra-abdominal infections (Boxes 39.1 and 39.2). Furthermore, a Cochrane review of antibiotic regimens in secondary peritonitis has shown equivocal efficacy of several regimens.[120] The choice of antibiotics must be influenced by toxicity, local nosocomial patterns of microbiological sensitivity and cost. The optimal duration of antibiotic therapy must be individualized and

Box 39.1 Surgical Infection Society recommended antimicrobial regimens for patients with intra-abdominal infections

Single agents
Ampicillin–sulbactam
Cefotetan
Cefoxitin
Ertapenem
Imipenem–cilastatin
Meropenem
Piperacillin–tazobactam
Ticarcillin–clavulanic acid

Combination therapy
Aminoglycoside (amikacin, gentamicin, netilmicin, tobramycin) plus an anti-anaerobe
Aztreonam plus clindamycin
Cefuroxime plus metronidazole
Ciprofloxacin plus metronidazole
Third/fourth generation cephalosporin (cefepime, cefotaxime, ceftazidime, ceftizoxime, ceftriaxone) plus an anti-anaerobe

With kind permission from Springer Science+Business Media: Varela JE, Wilson SE, Nguyen NT. Laparoscopic surgery significantly reduces surgical-site infections compared with open surgery. Surgical Endoscopy, Jan 2009.

Box 39.2 Surgical Infection Society recommended antimicrobial regimens for higher-risk patients with intra-abdominal infections

Single agents
Imipenem–cilastatin
Meropenem
Piperacillin–tazobactam

Combination therapy
Aminoglycoside (amikacin, gentamicin, netilmicin, tobramycin) plus an anti-anaerobe (clindamycin or metronidazole)
Aztreonam plus clindamycin
Ciprofloxacin plus metronidazole
Third/fourth generation cephalosporin (cefepime, cefotaxime, ceftazidime, ceftizoxime, ceftriaxone) plus an anti-anaerobe

With kind permission from Springer Science+Business Media: Varela JE, Wilson SE, Nguyen NT. Laparoscopic surgery significantly reduces surgical-site infections compared with open surgery. Surgical Endoscopy, Jan 2009.

depends on the underlying pathology, severity of infection, speed and effectiveness of source control, and the patient response to therapy.

A recent randomized controlled trial has shown that procalcitonin levels effectively differentiate patients with sepsis from those with the systemic inflammatory response syndrome, thereby reducing the duration of antimicrobial use.[121]

 ## TERTIARY PERITONITIS

Tertiary peritonitis is a sepsis-like syndrome not induced by endotoxin and seen in patients who, despite being 'adequately treated', have persistent signs of sepsis. These patients exhibit impaired host defenses and multiple organ dysfunction, and are unable to compartmentalize and clear the initial infection, or subsequently develop a superinfection of the entire peritoneal cavity. As a result of impaired host defense, low virulence pathogens (usually enterococci and fungi) can overgrow. The microbial nature of tertiary peritonitis is therefore difficult to predict when compared with primary and secondary peritonitis. *Staph. epidermidis*, *Pseudomonas* and *Candida* spp. are the predominant micro-organisms, with *Esch. coli* and *B. fragilis* only being occasionally found. The main source of these micro-organisms is thought to be the patient's own gastrointestinal tract, intestinal hypoperfusion, intestinal starvation or elimination of normal gut flora by antimicrobial agents. Adequate perfusion and enteral feeding aid preservation and restoration of the gastrointestinal tract and maintenance of barrier function.

Management of tertiary peritonitis entails correction of physiological derangements, administration of antimicrobial therapy, and surgical or other means of source control. The antibiotics commonly used are those listed in Box 39.1.[118] Yeasts and other fungi can be major pathogens in tertiary peritonitis, particularly in patients who have received prolonged antimicrobial therapy or immunosuppression. It is critical that all patients with tertiary peritonitis have cultures of blood and infected peritoneal fluid.

GASTRODUODENAL SURGERY

The stomach is essentially sterile as a result of its high acidity and swift peristalsis. It contains mainly acid-tolerant lactobacilli and streptococci. The acidity of the stomach can be reduced or neutralized by drug therapy, proton-pump inhibitors, gastroduodenal bleeding or in the presence of obstruction. Combined failure of intestinal clearance and the gastric acid barrier results in more severe colonization with increased numbers of GNAB. Antibiotic prophylaxis in gastroduodenal surgery has been advocated and the commonly used antibiotic regimens include cephalosporins (commonly cefuroxime) plus metronidazole, and amoxicillin–clavulanate; third- or fourth-generation cephalosporins are reserved for high-risk patients.[122] Empirical *Helicobacter pylori* eradication treatment has been proposed for perforated peptic ulcers to prevent recurrence of ulcers.[123]

LIVER SURGERY

Patients undergoing liver surgery, specifically hepatectomy, are at increased risk of SSI and liver failure due to impaired glucose tolerance, long operation time, large blood loss and bile spillage. *Staphylococcus* and *Enterococcus* spp., *K. pneumoniae*, *Enterobacter* spp., *Esch. coli* and *B. fragilis* are the commonly encountered micro-organisms.[124,125]

Cefazolin[125,126] and flomoxef[127] have both proven efficacious in clinical trials as prophylactic agents in hepatectomy. *B. fragilis* is, however, resistant to cefazolin and the addition of metronidazole can improve cover. (In view of the latter, and as cefazolin is no longer available in many countries, we would advocate the use of cefuroxime as an appropriate substitute.) Only two randomized trials have examined the effects of antibiotic prophylaxis after hepatectomy and are conflicting.[126,127] Antibiotic prophylaxis is recommended by the Scottish Intercollegiate Guidelines Network (SIGN) based on evidence inferred from biliary surgery.[128] There is no consensus with regard to the duration of antibiotic prophylaxis, but current evidence suggests that there is no benefit in extending beyond 24 h[127] in patients undergoing hepatectomy.

LIVER ABSCESS

Liver abscesses can be classified according to their etiology:
- Pyogenic abscess, usually polymicrobial, accounts for 80% of hepatic abscesses
- Amebic abscess due to *Entamoeba histolytica* accounts for 10%
- Fungal abscess, most often due to *Candida* spp., accounts for less than 10%.

Liver abscess can be solitary or multiple and commonly affects the right lobe. Biliary tract infection is the main cause of pyogenic abscess and accounts for 21–30%. Biliary obstruction encourages bacterial proliferation and can cause multiple liver abscesses.

Infections within organs drained by the portal vein (portal pyemia) can result in localized septic thrombophlebitis, leading to liver abscess. Diverticulitis, pancreatitis and diffuse peritonitis are now some of the more frequently reported causes. Septic emboli are released into the portal circulation and are trapped by the hepatic sinusoids, each becoming the nidus for micro-abscess formation. These micro-abscesses usually coalesce into a solitary lesion. Micro-abscess formation can also follow hematogenous dissemination in association with systemic bacteremia, endocarditis, pyelonephritis, pneumonia, osteomyelitis or following intravenous drug abuse. Cases are also reported in immunocompromised children affected by diseases such as chronic granulomatous disease and leukemia. Hematogenous spread from non-gastrointestinal sources accounts for 10–20% of liver abscesses. In 15–35% of patients, the etiology of hepatic abscess remains obscure (cryptogenic abscess). The incidence of cryptogenic abscess is increased in patients with diabetes and metastatic cancer. Unusual pathogens such as *Mycobacterium avium* complex are seen in patients with AIDS and *Yersinia enterocolitica* in patients with cirrhosis, diabetes mellitus, alcoholism or malnutrition. Mortality from liver abscess has decreased steadily and ranges from 2.5% to 10.9%.[129,130]

Most liver abscesses are polymicrobial and are commonly due to *Esch. coli*, *K. pneumonia*, *Bacteroides* and *Streptococcus* spp. and microaerophilic streptococci. The incidence of *K. pneumonia* is rising[129] in the western world, and streptococci of the *anginosus* group (formerly *Str. milleri*), which are microaerophilic commensals of the gastrointestinal tract, have emerged as important causes of hepatic abscess.

The clinical presentation of liver abscess is insidious; many patients have symptoms for weeks prior to presentation, which may include fever, malaise, anorexia, weight loss and right upper quadrant pain. Ultrasonography or CT scan are usually diagnostic.

Antibiotic therapy as a sole treatment modality is not routinely advocated. Regimens using β-lactam/β-lactamase inhibitor combinations, carbapenems or second-generation cephalosporins with anaerobic coverage are excellent empirical choices for the coverage of enteric bacilli and anaerobes. Fluoroquinolones are an acceptable alternative in patients who are allergic to penicillin. Metronidazole or clindamycin should be added for anaerobic coverage. The optimal duration of parenteral therapy, as well as of subsequent oral therapy, remains unclear.[129] Amebic abscesses are cured by metronidazole in 90% of cases, which should be initiated before serological test results are available. This should be followed by an agent with luminal activity such as diloxanide furoate or paromomycin. Systemic antifungal agents should be initiated if a fungal abscess is suspected and after the abscess has been drained percutaneously or surgically. Initial therapy for fungal abscess is currently amphotericin. All patients should have serial radiological investigations to assess efficacy of medical treatment.

Percutaneous drainage and aspiration have become the standard of care and are advocated for abscesses larger than 5 cm.[131] Laparoscopic drainage has been shown to be a safe alternative.[132] Liver resection may be indicated in management of complicated liver abscesses.

BILIARY TRACT SURGERY

Laparoscopic cholecystectomy is the 'gold standard' in managing gallstone disease. It has an extremely low rate of postoperative infection (0.4–1.1%)[133] in comparison to open cholecystectomy, consisting mostly of superficial SSIs around the trocar site. Two meta-analyses have revealed no beneficial effects of antibiotic prophylaxis in low-risk patients (those without cholecystitis, choledocholithiasis and cholangitis) undergoing elective laparoscopic cholecystectomy in reducing postoperative infection rates.[133,134] SIGN guidance[128] reflects this, and advocates that antibiotics are not required. However, antibiotic prophylaxis remains appropriate in complicated patients and patients requiring open cholecystectomy.

Bacterial colonization of bile occurs as a result of either obstruction of the biliary tree or biliary stasis. In the former, it is commonly due to gallstones but can be as a result of benign or malignant obstruction to the common bile duct. Biliary stasis is seen in critically ill patients as a consequence of increased bile viscosity due to fever and dehydration. Patients on long-term total parenteral nutrition (TPN), prolonged fasting, gallbladder dysmotility and occasionally diabetes are at increased risk of biliary stasis, which can lead to acalculous cholecystitis. Bacterial infection is thought to be a consequence, not a cause, of cholecystitis. In early acute cholecystitis, bile is sterile.

Bacteria can enter bile by ascending the common bile duct from the duodenum (across an incompetent sphincter of Oddi or following instrumentation); entering directly from the small bowel after choledochoenterostomy; or by translocation from the gut into the portal vein, resulting in cholangitis. Some 20–75% of bile cultures are positive, with the most common organisms being *Esch. coli*, *Klebsiella* spp., enterococci, *Enterobacter* and *Ps. aeruginosa*. Anaerobes are rare. Recurrent pyogenic cholangitis (oriental cholangiohepatitis) is common in South East Asia and is characterized by recurrent attacks of primary bacterial cholangitis. The cause is unknown, although *Clonorchis sinensis*, ascariasis and nutritional insufficiency have been suggested.

Antimicrobial treatment of biliary tract infections usually requires single-agent therapy, or combination treatment with broad-spectrum cover for more serious infections. High biliary concentration of antimicrobials is vital, but the range of antimicrobial activity is a more important factor. When there is biliary obstruction, it is doubtful whether any antibiotic is excreted effectively into the bile. Cephalosporins have the required spectrum of activity and suitable pharmacokinetics, while quinolones achieve high concentrations in the biliary tract and are active against biliary pathogens. Suitable single-agent regimens include the following:

- Mild to moderate cholecystitis: ampicillin–sulbactam, ticarcillin–clavulanate, ertapenem, quinolones, cefuroxime, ceftriaxone or cefoxitin
- Severe cholecystitis, nosocomially acquired or prior antibiotic exposure: piperacillin–tazobactam, imipenem or meropenem.

Combination regimens include penicillin (including piperacillin, ampicillin, or penicillin) and metronidazole; penicillin with an aminoglycoside (gentamicin or tobramycin); or an aminoglycoside and third-generation cephalosporin. In cholangitis or biliary obstruction, biliary secretion of antibiotics may be impaired. Treatment may therefore require decompression and drainage of the biliary system depending on the cause of the infection and the severity of illness. This could be performed via endoscopic retrograde cholangiopancreatography (ERCP) or percutaneous transhepatic biliary (PTC) drainage. The incidence of infective complications after ERCP for acute cholangitis and cholecystitis is less than 2%.[135] *Ps. aeruginosa* cholangitis has been reported in post-ERCP patients as a result of inadequate endoscope disinfection.[136]

Early laparoscopic cholecystectomy for acute cholecystitis is controversial as there is a higher complication rate with conversion to open surgery. However, a meta-analysis[137] has shown that early laparoscopic cholecystectomy is safe and shortens hospital stay.

PANCREATITIS

Acute pancreatitis is a common emergency hospital admission and carries a mortality rate of 5–10%. The diagnosis is supported by a raised total serum amylase (at least three times the upper limit of normal). Pancreatic duct obstruction (e.g. by gallstones) induces activation of proenzymes within the acinar cell by intracellular lysosomal enzymes, resulting in a cascade of enzymatic reactions. The mechanism of alcohol-induced acute pancreatitis (second commonest cause of pancreatitis) is less clear. These reactions cause release of mediators of inflammation resulting in increased pancreatic vascular permeability, leading to hemorrhage, edema and eventually pancreatic necrosis. The initial management of acute pancreatitis involves aggressive fluid resuscitation, pain control and correction of underlying physiological derangements. Uncontrolled local and systemic inflammatory responses from the initial insult can lead, apart from pancreatic necrosis, to multiorgan failure and death.

Acute necrotizing pancreatitis develops in 15% of patients with pancreatitis and is associated with mortality rates of 12–35%.[138] Pancreatic necrosis results in three potential outcomes: resolution, pseudocyst or abscess formation. Infections complicating necrotizing pancreatitis are often polymicrobial. Causative organisms most commonly originate from the gastrointestinal tract and include *Esch. coli*, *Ps. aeruginosa*, *Klebsiella*, *Enterobacter*, *Proteus*, *Bacteroides* and *Clostridium* spp. and enterococci. Why, and by what route, the necrotic pancreas becomes infected is not clear. It is most probable that passage of bacteria from the bowel lumen or from the bile into the pancreatic duct is the route of infection, although bacterial translocation from the colon into lymphatics and retroperitoneal inflammatory edema is possible.

Antibiotics are used to treat both infected pancreatic necrosis and extrapancreatic infections, and to prevent infection in patients with pancreatic necrosis. Guidelines suggest that a carbapenem should be used prophylactically and continued for 14 days, and infected necrosis should be assessed using fine-needle aspiration and culture.[139] For extrapancreatic infections, the most commonly used antibiotics are cephalosporins whereas carbapenems, glycopeptides and antifungals are used in the treatment of proven infected pancreatic necrosis.[140] Prophylactic antibiotic use in acute pancreatitis is controversial. A systematic review concluded that antibiotics in severe acute pancreatitis do not reduce mortality or protect against infected necrosis or the frequency of surgical intervention,[141] contrasting with two other meta-analyses.[142,143] There was a benefit for non-pancreatic infections. Only five of the studies reviewed were considered to be of high quality and used various antibiotic regimens.

The choice of antibiotics in preventing infection during necrotizing pancreatitis should be based on their antimicrobial activity, penetration rate, persistence and therapeutic concentrations. This is achieved by pefloxacin and metronidazole, imipenem and mezlocillin. In the absence of strong evidence, an expert group has recommended that prophylactic antibiotic therapy should be considered only for patients with CT evidence of more than 30% necrosis of the pancreas.[144]

All patients with persistent symptoms and greater than 30% pancreatic necrosis, and those with smaller areas of necrosis and clinical suspicion of sepsis, should undergo image-guided fine-needle aspiration to obtain material for culture 7–14 days after the onset of pancreatitis. Patients with infected necrosis require drainage of infected pseudocysts or abscess, with debridement.

COLORECTAL SURGERY

Surgery in the colon is associated with a high incidence of postoperative infection and mortality. Complication rates of 10–20% have been reported. A systematic review[145] found a statistically significant benefit in favor of antibiotic prophylaxis with a variety of antibiotics. The overall SSI rate was reduced from 39% to 10%. There is no advantage in extending the duration of antibiotic prophylaxis beyond the single preoperative antibiotic dose unless there is gross spillage. Additional dosing increases the risk of resistant organisms and *Clostridium difficile* infection.

Antimicrobial prophylaxis for colorectal operations can involve oral antimicrobial bowel preparation, a preoperative parenteral antimicrobial, or the combination of both. A combination of oral and parenteral prophylaxis is common practice in the USA.[146] The regimen should cover Gram-positive and -negative, aerobic and anaerobic enteric bacteria, particularly *Bacteroides* spp. Although a number of anaerobically active drugs such as clindamycin, cefoxitin and tinidazole have been used, metronidazole (intravenous, oral or rectal) has been the mainstay of therapy and prophylaxis.

Recommended oral prophylaxis consists of neomycin plus erythromycin or neomycin plus metronidazole, started no more than 18–24 h preoperatively. Mechanical bowel preparation is controversial, being phased out in the enhanced recovery program, as it has not been shown to confer any benefits in terms of anastomotic leak and SSI rates.[24] Furthermore, there is no trial examining the effects of oral antibiotic prophylaxis in uncleansed colon. Oral, non-absorbable antibiotics in bowel preparation in a retrospective case-controlled study may have an associated higher rate of *Clostridium difficile* infection.[147] Cefotetan or cefoxitin are recommended for parenteral prophylaxis and the combination of parenteral cefuroxime and metronidazole is recommended as a cost-effective alternative. In patients with confirmed allergy to β-lactams, one of the following regimens is recommended: clindamycin plus gentamicin, aztreonam or ciprofloxacin; or metronidazole plus gentamicin or ciprofloxacin. A single 750 mg dose of levofloxacin can be substituted for ciprofloxacin.[148]

Two significant advances in colorectal surgery within the last decade are the enhanced recovery program and laparoscopic-assisted colorectal surgery. The enhanced recovery after surgery (ERAS) program does not recommend mechanical bowel preparation, uses carbohydrate loading preoperatively, and advocates early introduction of enteral feeding and patient mobilization. Patients so treated are less likely to develop postoperative complications.[149] A meta-analysis of RCTs of patients having laparoscopic colorectal surgery had a statistically significant reduction in SSI rates.[150]

APPENDICECTOMY

Appendicitis is a common acute surgical presentation. Obstruction of the appendiceal lumen leads to ineffective lymphatic and venous drainage and bacterial invasion which progresses to perforation and peritoneal contamination.

Open or laparoscopic appendicectomy is the treatment of choice. Interval appendicectomy is occasionally performed as part of treatment of appendiceal abscess/mass following resolution. A large retrospective study has shown a statistically significant reduction in SSIs rate from 1.9% in open, to 0.7% in laparoscopic appendicectomy.[119] The contributing factors are believed to be a shorter surgical incision, decreased tissue trauma and contamination, and elimination of mechanical retraction of the abdominal wall.

Wound infection is more common in patients with a perforated or gangrenous appendix, and antibiotic therapy, rather than prophylaxis, is indicated.

The predominant microbial flora associated with acute appendicitis include *Esch. coli*, *Klebsiella* and *Proteus* spp. Other anaerobic organisms, particularly *Bacteroides*, are common in wound infections after appendicectomy, leading to the widespread use of metronidazole. Postoperative complication rates parallel those found from a perforated viscus of any cause and rates of as high as 40% have been reported.[151] The most common complications are intra-abdominal abscesses and superficial SSI. In a meta-analysis[152] it was shown that antibiotic administration pre-, peri- or postoperatively significantly reduces SSI or intra-abdominal abscess following appendicectomy. The most common antibiotics used were cephalosporin and imidazole derivatives, followed by aminoglycosides and clindamycin. Use of piperacillin–tazobactam, tigecycline, ertapenem or doripenem is more appropriate for severe cases of intra-abdominal infection or patients with recent antibiotic exposure.

Duration of antibiotic dosing logically depends on the severity of the peritoneal contamination. In an RCT in nonperforated appendicitis,[153] single dose, three doses and 5-day doses of cefuroxime and metronidazole were compared. Postoperative infective complication rates were the same (6.5%, 6.4% and 3.6%, respectively). A single-dose prophylactic antibiotic is therefore probably adequate for uncomplicated appendicitis. The duration of therapy required for high-risk patients with perforated or gangrenous appendicitis is unclear. If source control is optimal, it is likely that 24–48 h therapy will be effective, although 5-day treatment is usually administered. Controversially, Hansson et al[154] reported efficacy rates of 90.8% and 89.2% for antibiotic therapy only and surgery, respectively. However, this study was flawed as a result of its methodology.

SPLENECTOMY

Overwhelming postoperative splenectomy infection (OPSI) is an uncommon condition but has a mortality rate up to 50%. This follows the loss of splenic macrophages which filter and phagocytose bacteria and other pathogens. OPSI is usually caused by the encapsulated bacteria *Str. pneumoniae*, *Haemophilus influenzae* and *Neisseria meningitidis*. Other pathogens may include *Esch. coli*, *Ps. aeruginosa*, *Capnocytophaga canimorsus*, group B streptococci, *Enterococcus* and *Ehrlichia* spp., and protozoa such as *Plasmodium* and *Babesia* spp. It is most common during the first 2 years following splenectomy but can also occur decades later.

The main risk factors are the age of the patient (young children are more prone, particularly those with sickle-cell disease), timing of the procedure (emergency splenectomy carries a higher incidence of OPSI), splenectomy for hematological malignancies and the time interval from surgery.[155] Most postoperative infections can be avoided by preoperative immunization, at least 2 weeks prior to elective splenectomy, or within 2 weeks after emergency splenectomy.[156] Vaccines should include conjugated pneumococcal and meningococcal C vaccine, in addition to the conjugated Hib vaccine. Pneumococcal and meningococcal vaccination boosters should be given every 5–10 years. Patients should also be offered influenza immunization yearly.

The role and efficacy of antibiotic prophylaxis are controversial, further compounded by problems with patient compliance. Young children should be given oral phenoxymethyl penicillin or erythromycin to at least age 5 years or for 5 years, and adults for 2 years following splenectomy.[156]

Patients with OPSI require urgent blood culture and parenteral penicillin, ceftriaxone or similar antibiotics. A combination of antibiotics should be given to cover the wide spectrum of bacteria implicated. Where moderately or highly penicillin-resistant pneumococci are prevalent, ceftriaxone plus vancomycin or teicoplanin (plus rifampicin [rifampin] for highly resistant pneumococci) provide suitable initial cover.

TRAUMA SURGERY

Early deaths after major trauma follow brain, spinal, cardiac or vascular injury. Hypothermia, acidosis and coagulopathy which follow blood loss conspire against the patient, but 'damage control' surgery can improve survival.[157,158] Deaths continue over subsequent weeks, resulting from trauma-related infection or indirectly related to critical care: endotracheal intubation, blood transfusion, catheterization or nasogastric suction (see Selective decontamination of the digestive tract, above). Infection after abdominal trauma is related to the mechanism of injury and organs involved. The interval between injury and treatment, and the occurrence of hypovolemic shock, are also important, particularly after vascular injury. Catastrophic injuries in the military arena have led to great advances in surgical and infection management, including early and aggressive debridement, pedicle flaps for repair of tissue defects and ABC resuscitation. Recognition of nosocomial infection, with infection control practices enforced through the leadership and command, have had an impact on wound outcome. Resistant organisms have appeared in infections of injured extremities, particularly multidrug-resistant GNAB such as *Acinetobacter* and *Klebsiella* spp.[159]

Traumatic injury leads to conditions favorable for infection: tissue damage, impairment of vascular supply, breach of skin defenses and exposure to contaminated environmental materials and micro-organisms. Military wounds are compounded by high-velocity injuries where the kinetic energy ($1/2\ mv^2$) of a bullet or shrapnel can cause massive tissue damage with cavitation that causes suction of clothing and other foreign bodies, including soil, into the wound.

The greatest risk of infection follows trauma involving colonic injury and peritoneal contamination.[160] The options of stoma versus primary anastomosis must be considered in this context. Nutritional support, particularly parenteral nutrition, also influences infection after visceral injury. Empirical antimicrobial choice should anticipate polymicrobial exposure, and cover GNAB, Gram-positive cocci and anaerobes. Antimicrobials can be limited to 24 h after early surgery, but extension to 48–72 h is required if colonic contents have contaminated the peritoneum. Local microbiological data and guidelines should guide choice.[120] Broad-spectrum regimens can be narrowed according to clinical response and microbiological culture data.

In orthopedic trauma with open fractures, anticipated organisms are *Staph. aureus*, coagulase-negative staphylococci and Gram-negative rods, and perioperative antimicrobials targeting these organisms are recommended. In penetrating abdominal trauma, anaerobes are also implicated. In chest trauma, parenteral antibiotics after chest tube insertion in prevention of empyema and pneumonia are recommended when there is an associated hemopneumothorax.

Weigelt[8] found a higher incidence of infection after shotgun injuries (20–25%) than after gunshot wounds (3.6–16%) or stab injuries (4–4.7%), and particularly after four or more intra-abdominal organs were injured. Together with thermal injury, there is widespread soft-tissue injury, which favors infection of devitalized tissues. Extensive irrigation and debridement with removal of foreign material and dead tissue is recommended with 48–72 h of intravenous antibiotics. Activity against clostridia and β-hemolytic streptococci is essential, and cephalosporins are widely used because of penicillin-resistant streptococci, with an aminoglycoside for significant soft-tissue defect. Intra-articular injuries require 24 h antimicrobial prophylaxis, with extension for significantly contaminated wounds.[161]

Factors that predicted infection in patients with intra-abdominal vascular injuries who survived beyond 48 h of hospitalization have been examined: 40% of survivors developed intra-abdominal infection when blood pressure was initially unrecordable, but was 11% in those with a blood pressure over 90 mmHg on admission. Resuscitation to restore blood pressure to a level of >70 mmHg, with early control of bleeding, resulted in a serious infection risk of 20% but failure of resuscitation resulted in a 77% risk.[162]

Bacterial translocation may occur more commonly in patients with hypovolemic shock but does occur after traumatic injury. Its clinical significance in humans continues to be debated.[163] Nutrition is as important after trauma as in other patients requiring major surgery. Concepts linked to bacterial translocation have underpinned the practice of preferring enteral nutrition to parenteral nutrition. However, it is only in trauma patients that there is firm evidence that morbidity from sepsis is improved in enterally nourished patients.[163] Early introduction of nutrition (i.e. within 36 h of surgery) benefits severely injured patients who have undergone damage control surgery with open abdomens.[164] Specifically, the rate of pneumonia was significantly lower in patients fed early (43%) than those for whom feeding was delayed (72%).

The abdominal trauma index and the presence of a colostomy were found to be independent risk factors associated with intra-abdominal abscesses in an analysis of patients sustaining penetrating injuries of the colon.[165] In patients with bullet injuries of the colon, primary repair of the colon led to less abdominal sepsis.[166] In the civilian context, the majority of colon injuries can be managed by repair or resection with primary anastomosis;[167] however, in the military context, with the adversity of conditions and complexity of assessment and access to care, there may still be a role for the use of temporary stomas.[168]

Infection following abdominal trauma involves aerobic and anaerobic bacteria. Enterobacteriaceae are the main pathogens in early peritonitis, whereas anaerobes, particularly *B. fragilis*, are predominantly responsible for the later abscess stage. Therefore, antibiotics chosen must have activity against aerobic and anaerobic organisms.

The pharmacokinetics of antibiotics in trauma patients may be important, following changes in volume of distribution and total body clearance of drugs.[169] Significant expansion in the apparent volume of distribution for amikacin, which correlated with fluid resuscitation, has been shown.[170] Similar variability in other aminoglycoside pharmacokinetics has also been shown,[171] suggesting that higher doses of antibiotic are more effective than longer courses, provided there is adequate source control. The Surgical Infection Society of North America has endorsed this approach in patients who have traumatic enteric perforations and operated on within 12 h of injury.[118]

 References

1. National Institute for Health and Clinical Excellence. *Surgical site infection. Prevention and treatment of surgical site infection.* Clinical Guideline CG74. London: NICE; 2008.

2. Smyth ET, McIlvenny G, Enstone JE, et al. Hospital Infection Society Prevalence Survey Steering Group. Four country healthcare associated infection prevalence survey 2006: overview of the results. *J Hosp Infect.* 2008;69:230–248.

3. Horan TC, Gaynes RP, Martone WJ, Jarvis WR, Emori TG. CDC definitions of nosocomial surgical site infections, 1992: a modification of CDC definitions of surgical wound infections. *Infect Control Hosp Epidemiol.* 1992;13:606–608.

4. Mangram AJ, Horan TC, Pearson ML, Silver LC, Jarvis WR. Guideline for prevention of surgical site infection, 1999. Centers for Disease Control and Prevention (CDC) Hospital Infection Control Practices Advisory Committee. *Am J Infect Control*. 1999;27:97–132.

5. Leaper DJ, van Goor H, Reilly J, et al. Surgical site infection – a European perspective of incidence and economic burden. *Int Wound J*. 2004;1:247–273.

6. Coello R, Charlett A, Wilson J, Ward V, Pearson A, Borriello P. Adverse impact of surgical site infections in English hospitals. *J Hosp Infect*. 2005;60:93–103.

7. Laterre PF. Progress in medical management of intra-abdominal infection. *Curr Opin Infect Dis*. 2008;21:393–398.

8. Weigelt JA. Empiric treatment options in the management of complicated intra-abdominal infections. *Cleve Clin J Med*. 2007;74(suppl 4):S29–S37.

9. Brook I. Microbiology and management of abdominal infections. *Dig Dis Sci*. 2008;53:2585–2591.

10. Centers for Disease Control and Prevention (CDC). Guidance for control of infections with carbapenem-resistant or carbapenemase-producing Enterobacteriaceae in acute care facilities. *MMWR Morb Mortal Wkly Rep*. 2009;58:256–260.

11. Livermore DM, Hope R, Mushtaq S, Warner M. Orthodox and unorthodox clavulanate combinations against extended-spectrum beta-lactamase producers. *Clin Microbiol Infect*. 2008;14(suppl 1):189–193.

12. Paterson D. Resistance in gram-negative bacteria: Enterobacteriaceae. *Am J Infect Control*. 2006;34(suppl 1):S20–S28.

13. Raahave D. Wound contamination and post-operative infection. In: Taylor EW, ed. *Infection in Surgical Practice*. Oxford: Oxford Medical Publications; 1992.

14. Davis N, Curry A, Gambhir AK, et al. Intraoperative bacterial contamination in operations for joint replacement. *J Bone Joint Surg*. 1999;81:886–889.

15. Towfigh S, Cheadle WG, Lowry SF, Malangoni MA, Wilson SE. Significant reduction in incidence of wound contamination by skin flora through use of microbial sealant. *Arch Surg*. 2008;143:885–891.

16. Edmiston Jr CE, Seabrook GR, Cambria RA, et al. Molecular epidemiology of microbial contamination in the operating room environment: is there a risk for infection? *Surgery*. 2005;138:573–579.

17. Bady S, Wongworawat MD. Effectiveness of antimicrobial incise drapes versus cyanoacrylate barrier preparations for surgical sites. *Clin Orthop Relat Res*. 2009;467:1674–1677.

18. Dohmen PM. Antibiotic resistance in common pathogens reinforces the need to minimise surgical site infections. *J Hosp Infect*. 2008;70(suppl 2):15–20.

19. Edmiston CE, Seabrook GR, Goheen MP, et al. Bacterial adherence to surgical sutures: can antibacterial-coated sutures reduce the risk of microbial contamination? *J Am Coll Surg*. 2006;203:481–489.

20. Fleck T, Moidl R, Blacky A, et al. Triclosan-coated sutures for the reduction of sternal wound infections: economic considerations. *Ann Thorac Surg*. 2007;84:232–236.

21. Deliaert AE, Van den Kerckhove E, Tuinder S, et al. The effect of triclosan-coated sutures in wound healing. A double blind randomised prospective pilot study. *J Plast Reconstr Aesthet Surg*. 2009;62:771–773.

22. Coates T, Bax R, Coates A. Nasal decolonization of *Staphylococcus aureus* with mupirocin: strengths, weaknesses and future prospects. *J Antimicrob Chemother*. 2009;64:9–15.

23. Nichols RL. Preventing surgical site infections: a surgeon's perspective. *Emerg Infect Dis*. 2001;7:220–224.

24. Guenaga K.K.F.G., Matos D, Wille-Jørgensen P. Mechanical bowel preparation for elective colorectal surgery. *Cochrane Database Syst Rev*. 2009;(1) CD001544.

25. Arcaroli J, Fessler MB, Abraham E. Genetic polymorphisms and sepsis. *Shock*. 2005;24:300–312.

26. Gårdlund B. Postoperative surgical site infections in cardiac surgery – an overview of preventive measures. *APMIS*. 2007;115:989–995.

27. Simchen E, Rozin R, Wax Y. The Israeli study of surgical infection of drains and the risk of wound infection in operations for hernia. *Surg Gynecol Obstet*. 1990;170:331–337.

28. Kawai M, Tani M, Terasaw H, et al. Early removal of prophylactic drains reduces the risk of intra-abdominal infections in patients with pancreatic head resection: prospective study for 104 consecutive patients. *Ann Surg*. 2006;244:1–7.

29. Karthikesalingam A, Walsh SR, Sadat U, Tang TY, Koraen L, Varty K. Efficacy of closed suction drainage in lower limb arterial surgery: a meta-analysis of published clinical trials. *Vasc Endovascular Surg*. 2008;42:243–248.

30. Gurusamy KS, Samraj K, Mullerat P, Davidson BR. Routine abdominal drainage for uncomplicated laparoscopic cholecystectomy. *Cochrane Database Syst Rev*. 2007;(4):CD006004.

31. Parker MJ, Livingstone V, Clifton R, McKee A. Closed suction surgical wound drainage after orthopaedic surgery. *Cochrane Database Syst Rev*. 2007;(3): CD001825.

32. Cottam DR, Mattar SG, Barinas-Mitchell E, et al. The chronic inflammatory hypothesis for the morbidity associated with morbid obesity: implications and effects of weight loss. *Obes Surg*. 2004;14:589–600.

33. Van Till OJW, Van Veen SQ, Van Ruler O, Lamme B, Gouma DJ, Boermeester MA. The innate immune response to secondary peritonitis. *Shock*. 2007;28:504–517.

34. Wilson APR, Treasure T, Sturridge MF, Gruneberg RN. A scoring method (ASEPSIS) for postoperative wound infections for use in clinical trials of antibiotic prophylaxis. *Lancet*. 1986;327:311–312.

35. Cruse PJ, Foord R. The epidemiology of wound infection. A 10-year prospective study of 62,939 wounds. *Surg Clin North Am*. 1980;60:27–40.

36. Haley RW, Culver DH, White JW, et al. The efficacy of infection surveillance and control programs in preventing nosocomial infections in US hospitals. *Am J Epidemiol*. 1985;121:182–205.

37. Health Protection Agency. *Surveillance of surgical site infection in England: October 1997–September 2005*. London: Health Protection Agency; 2006.

38. Wilson J, Ramboer I, Suetens C; HELICS-SSI Working Group. Hospitals in Europe Link for Infection Control through Surveillance (HELICS). Inter-country comparison of rates of surgical site infection – opportunities and limitations. *J Hosp Infect*. 2007;65(suppl 2):165–170.

39. Whitby M, McLaws ML, Collopy B, et al. Post discharge surveillance: can patients reliably diagnose surgical wound infections? *J Hosp Infect*. 2002;52:155–160.

40. Mannien J, Wille JC, Snoeren RL, van hen Hof S. Impact of postdischarge surveillance on surgical site infection rates for several surgical procedures; results from the nosocomial surveillance network in the Netherlands. *Infect Control Hosp Epidemiol*. 2006;27:809–816.

41. Gaynes RP, Culver DH, Horan TC, Edwards JR, Richards C, Tolson JS. Surgical site infection (SSI) rates in the United States, 1992–1998: the National Nosocomial Infections Surveillance System basic SSI risk index. *Clin Infect Dis*. 2001;33(suppl 2):S69–S77.

42. De Oliveira AC, Ciosak SI, Ferraz EM, Grinbaum RS. Surgical site infection in patients submitted to digestive surgery: risk prediction and NNIS risk index. *Am J Infect Control*. 2006;34:201–207.

43. Konishi T, Watanabe T, Kishimoto J, Nagawa H. Elective colon and rectal surgery differ in risk factors for wound infection: results of prospective surveillance. *Ann Surg*. 2006;244:758–763.

44. Leong G, Wilson J, Charlett A. Duration of operation as a risk factor for surgical site infection: comparison of English and US data. *J Hosp Infect*. 2006;63:255–262.

45. Haridas M, Malangoni MA. Predictive factors for surgical site infection in general surgery. *Surgery*. 2008;144:496–503.

46. National Institute for Health and Clinical Excellence. *Surgical site infection. Prevention and treatment of surgical site infection*. Clinical Guideline CG74. London: NICE; 2008.

47. Campbell DA, Henderson WG, Englesbe MJ, et al. Surgical site infection: the importance of operative duration and blood transfusion – results of the first American College of Surgeons–National Surgical Quality Improvement Program Best Practices Initiative. *J Am Coll Surg*. 2008;207:810–820.

48. Burke JF. The effective period of preventive antibiotic action in experimental incisions and dermal lesions. *Surgery*. 1961;50:161–168.

49. Glenny AM, Song F. Antimicrobial prophylaxis in colorectal surgery. *Quality Health Care*. 1999;8:132–136.

50. Glenny AM, Song F. Antimicrobial prophylaxis in total hip replacement: a systematic review. *Health Technol Assess*. 1999;3:1–57.

51. National Research Council Ad Hoc Committee on Trauma. Postoperative wound infections: factors influencing the incidence of wound infections. *Ann Surg*. 1964;160(suppl 2):33–75.

52. Keighley MRB, Burdon DW, eds. *Antimicrobial prophylaxis in surgery*. Tunbridge Wells, England: Pitman Medical; 1979.

53. Williams NA, Leaper DJ. Infection. In: Leaper DJ, Harding KG, eds. *Wounds: biology and management*. Oxford: Oxford Medical Publications; 1998.

54. Zoutman D, Pearce P, McKenzie M, Taylor G. Surgical wound infections occurring in day surgery patients. *Am J Infect Control*. 1990;18:277–282.

55. Bailey IS, Karran SE, Toyn K, Brough P, Ranaboldo C, Karran SJ. Community surveillance of complications after hernia repair. *Br Med J*. 1992;304:469–471.

56. Byrne DJ, Lynch W, Napier A, Davey P, Malek M, Cuschieri A. Wound infection rates: the importance of definition and post-discharge wound surveillance. *J Hosp Infect.* 1994;26:37–43.

57. Keeling NJ, Morgan MWE. Inpatient and post-discharge wound infections in general surgery. *Ann R Coll Surg Engl.* 1995;77:245–247.

58. Taylor EW, Byrne DJ, Leaper DJ, Karran SJ, Browne MK, Mitchell KJ. Antibiotic prophylaxis and open groin hernia repair. *World J Surg.* 1997;21:811–815.

59. Gupta R, Sinnett D, Carpenter R, Preece PE, Royle GT. Antibiotic prophylaxis for post-operative wound infection in clean elective breast surgery. *Eur J Surg Oncol.* 2000;26:363–366.

60. Holmes J, Readman R. A study of wound infections following inguinal hernia repair. *J Hosp Infect.* 1994;28:153–156.

61. Horwitz JR, Chwals WJ, Doski JJ, Suescun EA, Cheu HW, Lally KP. Pediatric wound infections: a prospective multicenter study. *Ann Surg.* 1998;227:553–558.

62. Platt R, Zalenik DF, Hopkins CC, et al. Perioperative antibiotic prophylaxis for herniorrhaphy and breast surgery. *N Engl J Med.* 1990;322:153–160.

63. Sanchez-Manuel FJ, Seco-Gil JL. Antibiotic prophylaxis for hernia repair. *Cochrane Database Syst Rev.* 2004;(4):CD00343769. Updated: Sanchez-Manuel FJ, Lozano-García J, Seco-Gil JL. Antibiotic prophylaxis for hernia repair. *Cochrane Database of Syst Rev* 2007;(3):CD003769.

64. Hopf HW, Hunt TK, West JM, et al. Wound tissue oxygen tension predicts the risk of wound infection in surgical patients. *Arch Surg.* 1997;132:997–1004.

65. Ikeda T, Tayafeh F, Sessler DI, et al. Local radiant heat increases subcutaneous oxygen tension. *Am J Surg.* 1998;175:33–37.

66. Kurz A, Sessler DI, Lenhardt R. Perioperative normothermia to reduce the incidence of surgical wound infection and shorten hospitalization. *N Engl J Med.* 1996;334:1209–1215.

67. Wong PF, Kumar S, Bohra A, Whetter D, Leaper DJ. Randomised clinical trial of perioperative systemic warming in major elective abdominal surgery. *Br J Surg.* 2007;94:421–426.

68. Mahoney CB, Odom J. Maintaining intraoperative normothermia: a meta-analysis of outcomes with costs. *J Am Assoc Nurse Anesth.* 1999;67:155–164.

69. Melling AC, Ali B, Scott EM, Leaper DJ. Effects of preoperative warming on the incidence of wound infection after clean surgery: a randomised controlled trial. *Lancet.* 2001;358:876–880.

70. National Audit Office. *Reducing healthcare associated infections in England.* London: The Stationery Office; 2009.

71. World Health Organization. *Safe surgery saves Lives. WHO surgical safety checklist.* Geneva: WHO; 2009.

72. Haynes AB, Weiser TG, Berry WR, et al. Safe Surgery Saves Lives Group. A surgical safety checklist to reduce morbidity and mortality in a global population. *N Engl J Med.* 2009;360:491–499.

73. Greif R, Akca O, Horn EP, Kurz A, Sessler DI. Supplemental perioperative oxygen to reduce the incidence of surgical wound infection. *N Engl J Med.* 2000;342:161–167.

74. Belda FJ, Aguilera L, Garcia de la Asuncion J, et al. Spanish Reduccion de la Tasa de Infeccion Quirurgica Group. Supplemental perioperative oxygen and the risk of surgical wound infection: a randomized controlled trial. *J Am Med Assoc.* 2005;294:2035–2042.

75. Dellinger EP, Hausmann SM, Bratzler DW, et al. Hospitals collaborate to decrease surgical site infections. *Am J Surg.* 2005;190:9–15.

76. de Smet AM, Kluytmans JA, Cooper BS, et al. Decontamination of the digestive tract and oropharynx in ICU patients. *N Engl J Med.* 2009;360:20–31.

77. Silvestri L, Mannucci F, van Saene HK. Selective decontamination of the digestive tract: a life saver. *J Hosp Infect.* 2000;45:185–190.

78. Silvestri L, van Saene HK, Weir J, Gullo A. Survival benefit of the full selective digestive decontamination regimen. *J Crit Care.* 2009;24(3):474.e7–474. e14.

79. Webb CH. Selective decontamination of the digestive tract: a commentary. *J Hosp Infect.* 2000;46:106–109.

80. Ebner W, Kropec-Hubner A, Daschner FD. Bacterial resistance and overgrowth due to selective decontamination of the digestive tract. *Eur J Clin Microbiol Infect Dis.* 2000;19:243–247.

81. Al Naiemi N, Heddema ER, Bart A, et al. Emergence of multi-drug resistant Gram negative bacteria during selective decontamination of the digestive tract on an intensive care unit. *J Antimicrob Chemother.* 2006;58:853–856.

82. Silvestri L, van Saene HK. Selective decontamination of the digestive tract does not increase resistance in critically ill patients: evidence from randomised controlled trials. *Crit Care Med.* 2006;34:2027–2029.

83. Machado FR, Freitas FG. Controversies of surviving sepsis campaign bundles: should we use them? *Shock.* 2008;30(suppl 1):34–40.

84. Carrico CJ, Meakins JL, Marshall JC, Fry D, Maier RV. Multiple-organ-failure syndrome. *Arch Surg.* 1986;121:196–208.

85. Tetteroo GWM, Wagenvoort JHT, Bruining HA. Bacteriology of selective decontamination: efficacy and rebound colonization. *J Antimicrob Chemother.* 1994;34:139–148.

86. Silvestri L, van Saene HK, Casarin A, Berlot G, Gullo A. Impact of selective decontamination of the digestive tract on carriage and infection due to Gram negative and Gram positive bacteria: a systematic review of randomised trials. *Anaesth Intensive Care.* 2008;36:324–338.

87. Martinez-Pellus AE, Merino P, Bru M, et al. Endogenous endotoxemia of intestinal origin during cardiopulmonary bypass. Role of type of flow and protective effect of selective digestive decontamination. *Intensive Care Med.* 1997;23:1251–1257.

88. Tetteroo GWM, Wagenvoort JHT, Castelein A, Tilanus HW, Ince C, Bruining HA. Selective decontamination to reduce Gram-negative colonization and infections after oesophageal resection. *Lancet.* 1990;335:704–707.

89. Emre S, Sebastian A, Chodoff L, et al. Selective decontamination of the digestive tract helps prevent bacterial infections in the early postoperative period after liver transplant. *Mt Sinai J Med.* 1999;66:310–313.

90. Beath SV, Kelly DA, Booth IW, Freeman J, Buckels JAC, Mayer AD. Postoperative care of children undergoing small bowel and liver transplantation. *British Journal of Intensive Care.* 1994;4:302–308.

91. Taylor EW, Lindsay G. West of Scotland Surgical Infection Study Group. Selective decontamination of the colon before elective colorectal operations. *World J Surg.* 1994;18:926–931.

92. Esposito S, Marchisio P, Capaccio P, et al. Risk factors for bacteremia during and after adenoidectomy and/or adenotonsillectomy. *J Infect.* 2009;58:113–118.

93. Vieira F, Allen SM, Stocks RMS, Thompson JW. Deep neck infection. *Otolaryngol Clin North Am.* 2008;41:459–483.

94. Koegelenberg CFN, Diacon AH, Bolliger CT. Parapneumonic pleural effusion and empyema. *Respiration.* 2008;75:241–250.

95. Renner H, Gabor S, Pinter H, Maier A, Friehs G, Smolle-Juettner F-M. Is aggressive surgery in pleural empyema justified? *Eur J Cardiothorac Surg.* 1998;14:117–122.

96. Mauermann WJ, Sampathkumar P, Thompson RL. Sternal wound infections. *Best Pract Res Clin Anaesthesiol.* 2008;22:423–436.

97. Song DH, Lohman RF, Renucci JD, Jeevanandam V, Raman J. Primary sternal plating in high-risk patients prevents mediastinitis. *Eur J Cardiothorac Surg.* 2004;26:367–372.

98. Tocco MP, Costantino A, Ballardini M, et al. Improved results of the vacuum assisted closure and Nitinol clips sternal closure after postoperative deep sternal wound infection. *Eur J Cardiothorac Surg.* 2009;35:833–838.

99. Mills C, Bryson P. The role of hyperbaric oxygen therapy in the treatment of sternal wound infection. *Eur J Cardiothorac Surg.* 2006;30:153–159.

100. Wallace SM, Walton BI, Kharbanda RK, Hardy R, Wilson APR, Swanton RH. Mortality from infective endocarditis: clinical predictors of outcome. *Heart.* 2002;88:53–60.

101. Uslan DZ, Baddour LM. Cardiac device infections: getting to the heart of the matter. *Curr Opin Infect Dis.* 2006;19:345–348.

102. Klug D, Lacroix D, Savoye C, et al. Systemic infection related to endocarditis on pacemaker leads: clinical presentation and management. *Circulation.* 1997;95:2098–2107.

103. Seeger JM. Management of patients with prosthetic vascular graft infection. *American Surgery.* 2000;66:166–177.

104. Yeager RA, Porter JM. Arterial and prosthetic graft infection. *Ann Vasc Surg.* 1992;5:485–491.

105. FitzGerald SF, Kelly C, Humphreys H. Diagnosis and treatment of prosthetic aortic graft infections: confusion and inconsistency in the absence of evidence or consensus. *J Antimicrob Chemother.* 2005;56:996–999.

106. Darouiche RO. Treatment of infections associated with surgical implants. *N Engl J Med.* 2004;350:1422–1429.

107. Gemmell CG, Edwards DI, Fraise AP, Gould FK, Ridgway GL, Warren RE, on behalf of the Joint Working Party of the British Society for Antimicrobial Chemotherapy, Hospital Infection Society and Infection Control Nurses Association. Guidelines for the prophylaxis and treatment of methicillin-resistant *Staphylococcus aureus* (MRSA) infections in the UK. *J Antimicrob Chemother.* 2006;57:589–608.

108. Stewart AH, Eyers PS, Earnshaw JJ. Prevention of infection in peripheral arterial reconstruction: a systematic review and meta-analysis. *J Vasc Surg.* 2007;46:148–155.

109. Johnson CC, Baldesarre J, Levison ME. Peritonitis: update on pathophysiology, clinical manifestations, and management. *Clin Infect Dis.* 1997;24:1035–1047.

110. Gaya DR, David B, Lyon T, et al. Bedside leucocyte esterase reagent strips with spectrophotometric analysis to rapidly exclude spontaneous bacterial peritonitis: a pilot study. *Eur J Gastroenterol Hepatol.* 2007;19:289–295.

111. Chavez-Tapia NC, Soares-Weiser K, Brezis M, Leibovici L. Antibiotics for spontaneous bacterial peritonitis in cirrhotic patients. *Cochrane Database Syst Rev.* 2009;1: CD002232.

112. Cohen MJ, Sahar T, Benenson S, Elinav E, Brezis M, Soares-Weiser K. Antibiotic prophylaxis for spontaneous bacterial peritonitis in cirrhotic patients with ascites, without gastro-intestinal bleeding. *Cochrane Database Syst Rev.* 2009;2: CD004791.

113. Koulaouzidis A, Bhat S, Saeed AA. Spontaneous bacterial peritonitis. *World J Gastroenterol.* 2009;15:1042–1049.

114. Loomba R, Wesley R, Bain A, Csako G, Pucino F. Role of fluoroquinolones in the primary prophylaxis of spontaneous bacterial peritonitis: meta-analysis. *Clin Gastroenterol Hepatol.* 2009;7:487–493.

115. Marshall J. The microbial ecology of the gastrointestinal flora. In: Tellado J, Christou N, eds. *Intra-abdominal infections.* Madrid: Harcourt International; 2000:13–30.

116. Bosscha K, Reijnders K, Hulstaert P, Algra A, Van der Werken C. Prognostic scoring systems to predict outcome in peritonitis and intra-abdominal sepsis. *Br J Surg.* 1997;84:1532–1534.

117. Mazuski JE, Solomkin JS. Intra-abdominal infections. *Surg Clin North Am.* 2009;89:421–437, ix.

118. Mazuski J, Sawyer RG, Nathens AB, et al. The Surgical Infection Society guidelines on antimicrobial therapy for intra-abdominal infections: evidence for the recommendations. *Surg Infect (Larchmt).* 2002;3:175–234.

119. Varela JE, Wilson SE, Nguyen NT. Laparoscopic surgery significantly reduces surgical-site infections compared with open surgery. *Surg Endosc.* 2009;. [Epub ahead of print] Online. Available at http://www.springerlink.com/content/dq72p57th7257087/fulltext.pdf.

120. Wong P, Gilliam AD, Kumar S, Shenfine J, O'Dair GN, Leaper DJ. Antibiotic regimens for secondary peritonitis of gastrointestinal origin in adults. *Cochrane Database Syst Rev.* 2005;2: CD004539.

121. Hochreiter M, Köhler T, Schweiger AM, et al. Procalcitonin to guide duration of antibiotic therapy in intensive care patients: a randomized prospective controlled trial. *Critical Care.* 2009;13:R83.

122. Solomkin JS, Mazuski JE, Baron EJ, et al. Infectious Diseases Society of America. Guidelines for the selection of anti-infective agents for complicated intra-abdominal infections. *Clin Infect Dis.* 2003;37:997–1005.

123. Gisbert JP, Pajares JM. *Helicobacter pylori* infection and perforated peptic ulcer prevalence of the infection and role of antimicrobial treatment. *Helicobacter.* 2003;8:159–167.

124. Shigeta H, Nagino M, Kamiya J, et al. Bacteremia after hepatectomy: an analysis of a single-center, 10-year experience with 407 patients. *Langenbecks Arch Surg.* 2002;387:117–124.

125. Kobayashi S, Gotohda N, Nakagohri T, Takahashi S, Konishi M, Kinoshita T. Risk factors of SSI after hepatectomy for liver cancers. *World J Surg.* 2009;33:312–317.

126. Wu CC, Yeh DC, Lin MC, Liu TJ, Peng FK. Prospective randomized trial of systemic antibiotics in patients undergoing liver resection. *Br J Surg.* 1998;85:489–493.

127. Togo S, Tanaka K, Matsuo K, et al. Duration of antimicrobial prophylaxis in patients undergoing hepatectomy: a prospective randomized controlled trial using flomoxef. *J Antimicrob Chemother.* 2007;59:964–970.

128. Scottish Intercollegiate Guidelines Network. *Antibiotic prophylaxis in surgery: a national clinical guideline.* Edinburgh: SIGN; 2008. Online. Available at http://www.sign.ac.uk/pdf/sign104.pdf.

129. Rahimian J, Wilson T, Oram V. Pyogenic liver abscess: recent trends in etiology and mortality. *Clin Infect Dis.* 2004;39:1654–1659.

130. Tsai FC, Huang YT, Chang LY, Wang JT. Pyogenic liver abscess as endemic disease, Taiwan. *Emerg Infect Dis.* 2008;14:1592–1600.

131. Chung YF, Tan YM, Lui HF, et al. Management of pyogenic liver abscesses – percutaneous or open drainage? *Singapore Med J.* 2007;48:1158–1165.

132. Wang W, Lee WJ, Wei PL, Chen TC, Huang MT. Laparoscopic drainage of pyogenic liver abscesses. *Surg Today.* 2004;34:323–325.

133. Choudhary A, Bechtold ML, Puli SR, Othman MO, Roy PK. Role of prophylactic antibiotics in laparoscopic cholecystectomy: a meta-analysis. *J Gastrointest Surg.* 2008;12:1847–1853; discussion 1853.

134. Zhou H, Zhang J, Wang Q, Hu Z. Meta-analysis: antibiotic prophylaxis in elective laparoscopic cholecystectomy. *Aliment Pharmacol Ther.* 2009;29:1086–1095.

135. Kimura Y, Takada T, Kawarada Y, et al. Definitions, pathophysiology, and epidemiology of acute cholangitis and cholecystitis: Tokyo Guidelines. *J Hepatobiliary Pancreat Surg.* 2007;14:15–26.

136. Fraser TG, Reiner S, Malczynski M, Yarnold PR, Warren J, Noskin GA. Multidrug- resistant *Pseudomonas aeruginosa* cholangitis after endoscopic retrograde cholangiopancreatography: failure of routine endoscope cultures to prevent an outbreak. *Infect Control Hosp Epidemiol.* 2004;25:856–859.

137. Gurusamy KS, Samraj K. Early versus delayed laparoscopic cholecystectomy for acute cholecystitis. *Cochrane Database Syst Rev.* 2006;18: CD005440.

138. Dellinger EP, Tellado JM, Soto NE, et al. Early antibiotic treatment for severe acute necrotizing pancreatitis: a randomized, double-blind, placebo-controlled study. *Ann Surg.* 2007;245:674–683.

139. Pezzilli R, Uomo G, Zerbi A, et al. Italian Association for the Study of the Pancreas Study Group. Diagnosis and treatment of acute pancreatitis: the position statement of the Italian Association for the Study of the Pancreas. *Dig Liver Dis.* 2008;40:803–808.

140. Pezzilli R, Uomo G, Gabbrielli A, et al. ProInf-AISP Study Group. A prospective multicentre survey on the treatment of acute pancreatitis in Italy. *Dig Liver Dis.* 2007;39:838–846.

141. Jafri NS, Mahid SS, Idstein SR, Hornung CA, Galandiuk S. Antibiotic prophylaxis is not protective in severe acute pancreatitis: a systematic review and meta-analysis. *Am J Surg.* 2009;197:806–813.

142. Villatoro E, Bassi C, Larvin M. Antibiotic therapy for prophylaxis against infection of pancreatic necrosis in acute pancreatitis. *Cochrane Database Syst Rev.* 2006;(4):CD002941.

143. Mazaki T, Ishii Y, Takayama T. Meta-analysis of prophylactic antibiotic use in acute necrotizing pancreatitis. *Br J Surg.* 2006;93:674–684.

144. Working Party of the British Society of Gastroenterology; Association of Surgeons of Great Britain and Ireland; Pancreatic Society of Great Britain and Ireland; Association of Upper GI Surgeons of Great Britain and Ireland. UK guidelines for the management of acute pancreatitis. *Gut.* 2005;54(suppl III):iii1–iii9.

145. Nelson RL, Glenny AM, Song F. Antimicrobial prophylaxis for colorectal surgery. *Cochrane Database Syst Rev.* 2009;(1): CD001181.

146. Bratzler DW, Houck PM, Surgical Infection Prevention Guidelines Writers Workgroup; American Academy of Orthopedic Surgeons; American Association of Critical Care Nurses; American Association of Nurse Anesthetists; American College of Surgeons; American College of Osteopathic Surgeons; American Geriatrics Society; American Society of Anesthesiologists; American Society of Colon and Rectal Surgeons; American Society of Health-System Pharmacists; American Society of Peri-Anesthesia Nurses; Ascension Health; Association of Perioperative Registered Nurses; Association for Professionals in Infection Control and Epidemiology; Infectious Diseases Society of America; Medical Letter; Premier; Society for Healthcare Epidemiology of America; Society of Thoracic Surgeons; Surgical Infection Society. Antimicrobial prophylaxis for surgery: an advisory statement from the National Surgical Infection Prevention Project. *Clin Infect Dis.* 2004;38:1706–1715.

147. Nichols RL, Smith JW, Garcia RY, Waterman RS, Holmes JW. Current practices of preoperative bowel preparation among North American colorectal surgeons. *Clin Infect Dis.* 1997;24:609–619.

148. Wren SM, Ahmed N, Jamal A, Safadi BY. Preoperative oral antibiotics in colorectal surgery increase the rate of *Clostridium difficile* colitis. *Arch Surg.* 2005;140:752–756.

149. Eskicioglu C, Forbes SS, Aarts MA, Okrainec A, McLeod RS. Enhanced Recovery after Surgery (ERAS) programs for patients having colorectal surgery: a meta-analysis of randomized trials. *J Gastrointest Surg.* 2009;13:2321–2329.

150. Yamamoto S, Fujita S, Ishiguro S, Akasu T, Moriya Y. Wound infection after laparoscopic resection for colorectal cancer. *Surg Today.* 2008;38:618–622.

151. Almqvist P, Leandoer L, Törnqvist A. Timing of antibiotic treatment in non-perforated gangrenous appendicitis. *Eur J Surg.* 1995;161:431–433.

152. Andersen BR, Kallehave FL, Andersen HK. Antibiotics versus placebo for prevention of postoperative infection after appendicectomy. *Cochrane Database Syst Rev.* 2005; CD001439.

153. Mui LM, Ng CS, Wong SK, et al. Optimum duration of prophylactic antibiotics in acute non-perforated appendicitis. *Aust N Z J Surg.* 2005;75:425–428.

154. Hansson J, Körner U, Khorram-Manesh A, Solberg A, Lundholm K. Randomized clinical trial of antibiotic therapy versus appendicectomy as primary treatment of acute appendicitis in unselected patients. *Br J Surg*. 2009;96:473–481.

155. Kyaw MH, Holmes EM, Toolis F, et al. Evaluation of severe infection and survival after splenectomy. *Am J Med*. 2006;119:276.e1–276.e7.

156. Davies JM, Barnes R, Milligan D. Update of guidelines for the prevention and treatment of infection in patients with an absent or dysfunctional spleen. *Clin Med*. 2002;2:440–443.

157. Sagraves SG, Toschlog EA, Rotondo MF. Damage control surgery – the intensivist's role. *J Intensive Care Med*. 2006;21:5.

158. Lee JC, Peitzman AB. Damage-control laparotomy. *Curr Opin Crit Care*. 2006;12:346–350.

159. Murray CK. Infectious disease complications of combat-related injuries. *Crit Care Med*. 2008;36(suppl 7):S358–S364.

160. Zheng YX, Chen L, Tao SF, Song P, Xu SM. Diagnosis and management of colonic injuries following blunt trauma. *World J Gastroenterol*. 2007;13:633–636.

161. Simpson BM, Wilson RH, Grant RE. Antibiotic therapy in gunshot wound injuries. *Clin Orthop Relat Res*. 2003;408:82–85.

162. Wilson RF, Wiencek RG, Balog M. Predicting and preventing infection after abdominal vascular injuries. *J Trauma*. 1989;29:1371–1375.

163. MacFie J. Current status of bacterial translocation as a cause of surgical sepsis. *Br Med Bull*. 2004;71:1–11.

164. Dissanaike S, Pham T, Shalhub S, et al. Effect of immediate enteral feeding on trauma patients with an open abdomen: protection from nosocomial infections. *J Am Coll Surg*. 2008;207:690–697.

165. Ivatury RR, Gaudino J, Nallathambi MN, Simon RJ, Kazigo ZJ, Stahl WM. Definitive treatment of colon injuries: a prospective study. *Am J Surg*. 1993;591:43–49.

166. Demetriades D, Pantanowitz D, Charalambides D. Gunshot wounds of the colon: role of a primary repair. *Ann R Coll Surg Engl*. 1992;74:381–384.

167. Woo K, Wilson MT, Killeen K, Margulies DR. Adapting to the changing paradigm of management of colon injuries. *Am J Surg*. 2007;194:746–749.

168. Duncan JE, Corwin CH, Sweeney WB, et al. Management of colorectal injuries during operation Iraqi freedom: patterns of stoma usage. *J Trauma*. 2008;64:1043–1047.

169. Mimoz O, Schaeffer V, Incagnoli P, et al. Co-amoxiclav pharmacokinetics during posttraumatic hemorrhagic shock. *Crit Care Med*. 2001;29:1350–1355.

170. Reed 2nd RL, Ericsson CD, Wu A, Miller-Crotchett P, Fischer RP. The pharmacokinetics of prophylactic antibiotics in trauma. *J Trauma*. 1992;32:21–27.

171. Barletta JF, Johnson SB, Nix DE, Nix LC, Erstad BL. Population pharmacokinetics of aminoglycosides in critically ill trauma patients on once-daily regimens. *J Trauma*. 2000;49:869–872.

40 Infections associated with neutropenia and transplantation

Emmanuel Wey and Chris C. Kibbler

Neutropenic patients and transplant recipients are at risk of a number of life-threatening opportunistic infections. Neither patient group suffers from a single specific immunological deficit, there being a subtle blend of physical and immunological defects which evolve with time. Judgments about management need to be based upon knowledge of the balance of these defects and the timing of the infection.

The majority of hemato-oncology centers and transplant units base patient management (including that of infection) upon agreed protocols and the evidence base for these has become more robust in recent years. In addition there are now more national and international guidelines on which to base these. It is important that protocols are regularly updated and take account of local variations in risk, organisms and antimicrobial sensitivities.

INFECTIONS IN NEUTROPENIC PATIENTS

The inverse relationship between the numbers of circulating neutrophils and the risk of infection was established more than four decades ago.[1] This effect becomes apparent when the absolute neutrophil count is less than 1.0×10^9/L. The risk increases considerably as the count falls below 0.5×10^9/L and all patients with a count of less than 0.1×10^9/L for more than 3 weeks have been found to develop an infective episode.[1] Criteria for enrollment in a febrile neutropenia trial usually include a neutrophil count less than 0.5×10^9/L.

CAUSES OF NEUTROPENIA

Most of these patients are neutropenic following chemotherapy for leukemia while some leukemic patients will present with neutropenia before chemotherapy. In addition, the neutrophils of patients with myelodysplastic syndrome (MDS) or leukemia, particularly those with acute myeloid leukemia (AML), may have impaired microbicidal activity.[2,3]

Patients receiving chemotherapy for high-risk or relapsed leukemia may be neutropenic for 2–3 weeks, and longer if receiving regimens containing fludarabine. Those undergoing standard chemotherapy for lymphoma or for solid tumors may also suffer a reduction in circulating neutrophils, but this is rarely less than 0.1×10^9/L and is often not below 0.5×10^9/L with the duration of neutropenia often less than 7 days. In patients with aplastic anemia, or bone marrow transplant (BMT) recipients who fail to engraft, neutropenia is often profound and prolonged. Normal engraftment in allogeneic BMT recipients takes place between 2 and 3 weeks after transplantation.

There has been a steady increase in the numbers of peripheral blood stem cell transplants (PBSCT) performed in Europe and autologous PBSCT has virtually replaced autologous bone marrow transplantation. Autologous PBSCT recipients have a shorter duration of neutropenia.

Patients undergoing allogeneic bone marrow transplantation behave essentially like neutropenic patients during the early post-transplant phase, but remain immunosuppressed for up to 2 years, even without complications such as graft-versus-host disease (GVHD).

Other causes of neutropenia are shown in Box 40.1.

Box 40.1 Non-malignant causes of neutropenia

Congenital
- Cyclical neutropenia
- Chronic benign neutropenia
- Severe congenital neutropenia

Acquired
- Drug-induced
  - Cytotoxic chemotherapy (the most common cause of neutropenia)
  - Antimicrobial associated: chloramphenicol; β-lactams; sulfonamides; trimethoprim; nitrofurantoin; flucytosine; ganciclovir; zidovudine
  - Other drugs (e.g. phenothiazines, tolbutamide)
- Alcohol
- Radiation
- Megaloblastic anemia
- Autoimmune neutropenia

FACTORS PREDISPOSING TO INFECTION

The pathogenesis of infection in these patients is multifactorial and is often the consequence of a breach in the skin or oral mucosa plus defects in cellular or humoral immunity.

Some defects are associated with specific infections (Table 40.1). Lymphopenia, as a consequence of lymphoid malignancy or treatment, is associated with reactivation of intracellular organisms such as mycobacteria, the herpes viruses, *Toxoplasma gondii* and *Pneumocystis jirovecii* (formerly *Pneumocystis carinii*). Patients with chronic lymphoid malignancies and those receiving immunosuppressive chemotherapy, such as BMT recipients, have impaired antibody production which predisposes to infection with encapsulated organisms such as *Streptococcus pneumoniae*. The use of indwelling central venous catheters and mucosal damage caused by chemotherapy and herpes simplex virus (HSV) infection[4] allows penetration by commensal flora. In recent years changes in cytotoxic chemotherapy have rendered the oropharynx a major portal of entry for α-hemolytic streptococci. Likewise, splenectomy undertaken as treatment or for diagnosis renders the patient susceptible to infection with encapsulated organisms such as *Str. pneumoniae*. Others have pre-existing sites of chronic infection such as middle-ear disease or bronchiectasis, which may act as reservoirs of infection with organisms such as *Pseudomonas aeruginosa*. Ethnic origin and foreign travel may increase exposure to infections such as tuberculosis, malaria or strongyloidiasis.

CAUSATIVE ORGANISMS

Between 30% and 50% of febrile episodes in neutropenic patients can be confirmed microbiologically, and of these, most are due to bacteremia. Infections with Gram-positive bacteria, especially the coagulase-negative staphylococci and α-hemolytic streptococci, have increased in frequency over the past two decades. In the EORTC (European Organisation for Research and Treatment of Cancer) participatory centers the incidence of bacteremia due to Gram-positive organisms increased from 29%[5] to 67% during the 1970s and 1980s.[6] This increase correlates with the escalating use of central venous catheters, the development of alternative high-dose chemotherapy with attendant mucositis, and better prevention of Gram-negative infections. However, subsequent trials have shown a fall again, possibly associated with the decline in quinolone prophylaxis usage associated with emerging resistance. Of recent interest is the finding that cell-wall deficient (mostly Gram-positive) bacteria may be responsible for up to 25% of episodes of neutropenic fever in BMT recipients.[7]

Gram-negative bacteria continue to cause some of the most serious episodes of sepsis. Infections caused by the Enterobacteriaceae and *Ps. aeruginosa* carry a mortality of 40–60%.[8,9] Oropharyngeal candidosis is extremely common in patients not receiving prophylaxis, while invasive candidosis and aspergillosis account for 20–30% of fatal infections when treating acute leukemia.[10,11] Invasive aspergillosis is the most important infective cause of death in childhood acute myeloid leukemia[12] and in adult allogeneic bone marrow transplant/hematopoietic stem cell transplant patients. Other important infectious agents are listed in Box 40.2.

CHEMOPROPHYLAXIS

Allogeneic hematopoietic stem cell transplant (HSCT) recipients are at risk of a wide range of infections based upon extent of exposure and degree of immunosuppression. Autologous HSCT recipients are also at risk of infection although to a lesser degree due to shorter periods of neutropenia and time to engraftment. However, patients receiving CD34-enriched autografts appear to be at a similar level of risk as allogeneic HSCT recipients for cytomegalovirus (CMV) and other opportunistic infections.[13] These risks are summarized in Box 40.3.

Prevention of these serious infections has been the goal of clinicians for many years. Strategies for preventing acquisition of organisms, such as the provision of a low microbial diet, or the use of high-efficiency particulate air (HEPA) filtration, appear important in some profoundly neutropenic patients at risk from aspergillosis and have been increasingly emphasized in recent years.[14]

Table 40.1 Factors predisposing to infection in the neutropenic patient

Immune defect/risk factor	Example of opportunistic organisms
Neutropenia	*Streptococcus oralis* *Pseudomonas aeruginosa* *Candida* spp. *Aspergillus* spp.
Lymphoid cell defect	*Mycobacterium* spp. *Toxoplasma gondii* Herpes viruses *Pneumocystis jirovecii*
Humoral	*Str. pneumoniae*
Mucosal barrier (e.g. HSV/chemo-therapy-induced mucositis)	*Str. oralis* Enterobacteriaceae Fungi
Vascular access	Coagulase-negative staphylococci Fungi Non-tuberculous and environmental mycobacteria
Foreign travel/ethnic origin	*Mycobacterium* spp. *Strongyloides stercoralis* *Blastomyces dermatitidis* *Coccidioides immitis* *Histoplasma capsulatum*
Anatomical defect/reservoir (e.g. chronic sinusitis)	*Pseudomonas* spp.
Splenectomy	*Str. pneumoniae* Other encapsulated bacteria

Box 40.2   Important infectious agents in neutropenic and hematopoietic stem cell transplant patients

Bacteria	Viruses
Staphylococci	Herpes simplex virus
Streptococci	Varicella zoster virus
Enterobacteriaceae	Cytomegalovirus
Pseudomonads	Epstein–Barr virus
Mycobacterium spp.	Hepatitis A, B, C viruses
Legionella spp.	Parvovirus
Clostridium septicum	Adenovirus
Clostridium difficile	Polyomavirus
Rothia spp.	Measles virus
	Human herpesvirus-6
Fungi	
Candida spp.	**Protozoa/helminths**
Aspergillus spp.	*Toxoplasma gondii*
Zygomycetes	*Strongyloides stercoralis*
Cryptococcus neoformans	
Pneumocystis jirovecii	

Box 40.3   Summary of overall infection risk

Overall infection risk	Disease/chemotherapy regimen/ duration of neutropenia
Low	Standard solid tumor chemotherapy regimens
	Duration of neutropenia <7 days
Intermediate	Autologous HSCT
	Lymphoma
	Multiple myeloma
	Chronic lymphocytic leukemia
	Purine analog therapy (fludarabine, 2-CdA)
	Duration of neutropenia 7–10 days
High	Allogenic HSCT
	Acute leukemia, induction and consolidation phases
	Campath (alemtuzumab) therapy
	Graft-versus-host disease treated with high-dose steroids
	Duration of neutropenia >10 days

HSCT, hematopoietic stem cell transplant.

The infections to which these HSCT recipients are most vulnerable can be temporally categorized into three periods following transplantation:

- Pre-engraftment – less than 3 weeks
- Immediate postengraftment – 3 weeks to 3 months
- Late postengraftment – more than 3 months.

These periods, pathogens, immune defects and associated host factors in HSCT recipients are illustrated in Figure 40.1.

 BACTERIAL CHEMOPROPHYLAXIS

Various trials have examined the efficacy of oral non-absorbable antibiotics. Although a number of these were flawed, several controlled trials showed a benefit only when they were combined with a protective environment.[15–23]

Although trimethoprim–sulfamethoxazole was first used in patients with acute leukemia to prevent *Pn. jirovecii* pneumonitis, it also reduced the incidence of bacterial infection.[24] Further studies demonstrated the greatest benefit in patients with prolonged neutropenia, where a reduction in Gram-negative bacterial infections was seen.[25–28] However, the incidence of side effects (including bone marrow suppression) and the selection of multiresistant organisms led to a decline in its use for this indication.

Oral quinolones are currently the most commonly used prophylactic antibacterial agents in adult patients with chemotherapy-induced neutropenia. Initially oral quinolones (ciprofloxacin, ofloxacin and norfloxacin) were compared in a number of studies with placebo, trimethoprim–sulfamethoxazole and non-absorbable antibiotics. In the majority of these the 4-quinolone treated patients had significantly fewer Gram-negative bacterial infections, a delayed onset of fever and a reduction in the number of days of fever. Importantly, a reduction in mortality was not demonstrated.[29] There has been concern that quinolone resistance is increasing in some units[30] and this has led to the discontinuation of quinolone prophylaxis. However, initial meta-analysis did not show this to be a significant problem, and recent EORTC and Health Protection Agency (HPA) data further support these findings. A sequential study has shown that combining ciprofloxacin with colistin was associated with no significant change in quinolone resistance over a 12-year period.[31]

However, a more recent meta-analysis[32] that evaluated 95 randomized trials in afebrile neutropenic patients (the majority of whom had hematological malignancies) comparing antibiotic prophylaxis with placebo, no intervention or with another antibiotic class has shown a significant reduction in the risk for death when compared with placebo or no treatment (relative risk [RR], 0.67). The survival benefit was more substantial when the analysis was limited to fluoroquinolones. Fluoroquinolone prophylaxis reduced the risk for all-cause mortality (RR 0.52, 95% CI, 0.35–0.77), as well as infection-related mortality, fever, clinically documented infections and microbiologically documented infections. Although there was no significant increase in resistant bacteria with fluoroquinolone prophylaxis, the length of observation may have been insufficient to detect the emergence of resistant bacteria. All prophylactic antibiotics were associated with an increased risk for adverse events.

Following on from this meta-analysis, two randomized, double-blind, placebo-controlled trials of levofloxacin prophylaxis in neutropenic patients undergoing chemotherapy were performed.[33,34] Levofloxacin has similar activity against Gram-negative bacteria in comparison with ciprofloxacin, with the exception of pseudomonads; however, it has improved activity against certain Gram-positive pathogens, including streptococci. The first trial evaluated levofloxacin prophylaxis from the initiation of chemotherapy until neutrophil recovery, in higher-risk, mainly inpatient adult leukaemic or stem cell transplant patients in whom chemotherapy-induced neutropenia was expected to last for more than 7 days. The second

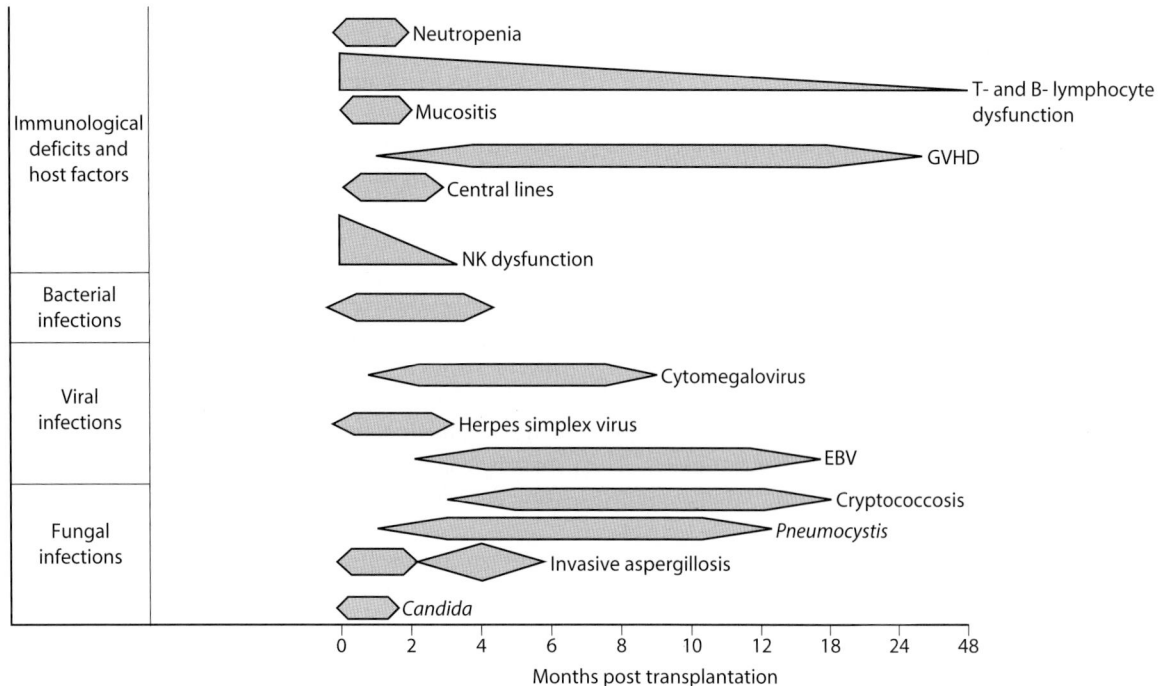

Fig. 40.1 The time course of infections after HSCT. EBV, Epstein–Barr virus; GVHD, graft-versus-host disease; LRTI, lower respiratory tract infection; NK, natural killer [cell]; UTI, urinary tract infection.

trial was in the outpatient setting and evaluated levofloxacin prophylaxis after chemotherapy for solid tumors and lymphomas for patients anticipated to have periods of neutropenia of 7 days or less. The effects of prophylaxis were similar between both patient groups in the two trials, as were mortality and tolerability. Both trials failed to demonstrate a significant survival benefit with prophylaxis. The results reflected previous meta-analyses and a review of both trials demonstrated that the numbers needed to treat to prevent one death by any cause was 24 in all patients and 43 in patients with an expected duration of neutropenia of >7 days.

The decision whether to use antibiotic prophylaxis and the selection of agent is a fine balance between calculated risk and expected benefit. Risks to consider include associations between fluoroquinolone use and severe *Clostridium difficile* and methicillin-resistant *Staphylococcus aureus* (MRSA), adverse drug reactions, antibiotic resistance, and whether prophylaxis will preclude the use of quinolones in empirical therapy of neutropenic fever in those patients stratified as low risk. The benefit of prophylactic antibiotics in other patient subsets with chemotherapy-induced neutropenia remains controversial.

With regard to timing and length of prophylaxis, guidelines from the European Conference on Infections in Leukemia (ECIL) suggest it should start with chemotherapy and continue until resolution of neutropenia or initiation of empirical antibacterial therapy for febrile neutropenia.

The problem of Gram-positive infections, particularly those due to α-hemolytic streptococci, has been addressed by a number of studies using different agents, including oral penicillins,[35] macrolides[36,37] and rifampicin (rifampin).[38] However, these have given mixed results and have been associated with the emergence of resistance. It is difficult, therefore, to make recommendations for prophylaxis of Gram-positive pathogens other than to use levofloxacin which has been shown to be of benefit. Some centers advocate prophylaxis against pneumococcal infection in allogeneic HSCT recipients, functionally asplenic patients and in patients receiving immunosuppressive therapy for GVHD. Where pneumococcal isolates have intermediate to high-level resistance rates to penicillin approaching 35%, alternative agents should be considered based on local susceptibility patterns. Trimethoprim–sulfamethoxazole prophylaxis for *Pn. jirovecii* is likely to be protective against pneumococcal disease.

 FUNGAL CHEMOPROPHYLAXIS

Attempts at antifungal prophylaxis have met with variable success. Initial studies examined oral polyenes. Nystatin, in doses up to 12×10^6 units per day, had little effect on the incidence of invasive candidosis in neutropenic patients,[11] whereas amphotericin B was superior to placebo in preventing the disease.[39]

While most invasive candidal infections are thought to gain entry via the gut,[39] non-absorbable antifungal agents do not protect against fungal infections at other sites, namely the skin, intravenous catheter sites and the respiratory tract. The oral, systemically active azoles have the potential to control colonization as well as prevent dissemination.

Ketoconazole reduces yeast carriage and the incidence of both local and systemic candidosis compared with placebo or non-absorbable agents.[39] Absorption is impaired in neutropenic patients, particularly in BMT recipients,[40] and breakthrough infections have occurred.[41] Ketoconazole also causes elevated ciclosporin A levels as a result of activity on hepatic P_{450} enzymes and serious idiosyncratic hepatotoxicity.

Fluconazole reduces colonization, mucosal thrush and the number of disseminated yeast infections.[42,43] Two placebo-controlled studies in HSCT recipients showed a significant reduction in invasive fungal infections (IFI).[44,45] Fluconazole was associated with a reduced mortality,[45] and fluconazole prophylaxis reduced the incidence of IFI, overall mortality and empirical antifungal therapy in allogeneic HSCT recipients but not autologous HSCT recipients. Unfortunately, its use in some centers has been associated with an increase in colonization and infection with *Candida krusei*, which is intrinsically resistant to fluconazole.[46] Fluconazole is also inactive against the important invasive molds that affect this population, especially *Aspergillus* spp. and the zygomycetes.

In contrast, itraconazole has activity against the molds, particularly *Aspergillus* spp. (*see* Ch. 32). However, in its original capsule formulation it was poorly absorbed in HSCT patients. This has been overcome by the introduction of an itraconazole–cyclodextrin complex in solution. Meta-analysis has shown this formulation to be associated with a lower overall incidence of fungal infection, lower mortality from fungal infection and a reduction in the use of intravenous amphotericin for suspected invasive fungal infection than fluconazole, oral amphotericin and placebo.[47–49] There was also a reduction in the incidence of invasive aspergillosis.

In a randomized trial involving neutropenic patients with AML or MDS, prophylaxis with posaconazole led to a decrease in IFI due to aspergillosis and reduced overall mortality compared with the comparator group receiving fluconazole or itraconazole prophylaxis.[50] A similar effect was shown in allogeneic HSCT patients with GVHD.[51] However, posaconazole prophylaxis has not been evaluated to date in allogeneic HSCT recipients in the neutropenic period post conditioning. Voriconazole has been used in prophylaxis, although large trial data of its use in this setting are still awaited. Extended-spectrum triazole prophylaxis should be avoided in patients receiving vinca alkaloid-based chemotherapy regimens such as vincristine in acute lymphoblastic leukemia. In these cases amphotericin regimens or an echinocandin could be considered.

Micafungin, an echinocandin, is approved for prophylaxis of candidal infections in patients undergoing HSCT. In a randomized, double-blind trial of neutropenic autologous and allogeneic HSCT recipients, comparing 50 mg per day of micafungin with 400 mg per day of fluconazole for antifungal prophylaxis, micafungin was superior to fluconazole based on the absence of breakthrough fungal infection.[52]

In the absence of trial data it would be appropriate to recommend that prophylaxis continue until absolute neutrophil counts are above 0.5×10^9/L in chemotherapy patients. In allogeneic HSCT there is an argument for continuing prophylaxis until at least day +75 or until the end of immunosuppression (in the case of supervening GVHD).

Amphotericin administered as a nasal spray has produced conflicting results in preventing invasive aspergillosis,[53,54] although some studies have shown greater benefit when it is aerosolized.[55,56] One study showed no significant difference in proven, probable or possible invasive aspergillosis between aerosolized amphotericin and no inhalation (4% vs 7%).[57]

Prophylaxis against *Pn. jirovecii* infection has proved remarkably effective in those undergoing treatment for acute lymphoblastic leukaemia[24] and for the first 6 months post-BMT. Trimethoprim–sulfamethoxazole three times weekly has been most studied, although some units are now using a 2-day regimen. Nebulized pentamidine is often used during marrow engraftment to avoid the myelosuppressive effects of trimethoprim–sulfamethoxazole, although data suggest that it may be inferior when used prophylactically in allogeneic transplant recipients. Other alternatives include dapsone and atovaquone.

 ## VIRAL CHEMOPROPHYLAXIS

Most virus infections in the neutropenic patient are due to reactivation of the human herpes viruses. Up to 80% of adult patients with leukemia are herpes simplex virus (HSV) seropositive and the incidence of HSV infection among HSV-seropositive HSCT recipients is about 80%. HSV infection in patients with leukemia is subsequent to reactivation of latent virus in most cases.

Aciclovir (acyclovir), 200 mg every 8 h to 800 mg every 12 h, is effective as prophylaxis against HSV infection in HSV-seropositive patients with leukemia undergoing chemotherapy or in BMT recipients.[58,59] An alternative regimen is valaciclovir 500 mg every 12 h.

Chemoprophylaxis against CMV infection, defined as the use of antiviral agents to prevent a primary CMV infection or a CMV reactivation, has been investigated in detail only in HSCT recipients, although CMV disease also occurs in patients with acute leukemia receiving chemotherapy. Allogeneic HSCT recipients comprise the group at highest risk of CMV reactivation and disease.

High-dose aciclovir has been shown to be partially effective in preventing CMV infection and disease post-BMT. A multicenter randomized trial compared 500 mg/m² intravenously every 8 h for 1 month followed by 800 mg every 6 h by mouth for 6 months with 200 or 400 mg every 6 h orally for 1 month followed by placebo.[60] The incidence of CMV infection reduced and survival increased by day 210 post-BMT, although the rates of CMV pneumonia were similar in the two groups. Valaciclovir is also being used in this setting.

The use of ganciclovir as prophylaxis against CMV infection has shown some benefit in reducing the incidence of CMV disease but has no effect on survival during the first 4 months post-BMT.[42,61]

Pre-emptive therapy, defined as the use of antiviral agents in an asymptomatic patient with CMV detected by a screening assay, includes ganciclovir, valganciclovir and foscarnet. The choice depends on the risk of toxicity and which antiviral drugs have been used previously. Weekly monitoring in allogeneic HSCT recipients using a CMV antigenemia assay or a technique for detection of either CMV DNA or RNA is of use for the pre-emptive management of CMV infection.[62,63] Centers vary with regard to the cut-off value used after which therapy is commenced and studies are in progress to better define this. When ganciclovir has been used as pre-emptive therapy following detection of CMV infection, survival was improved at 100 and 180 days post-transplant.[64] Foscarnet may be considered for second-line pre-emptive therapy, or in combination. Cidofovir can be considered for second-line pre-emptive therapy (3–5 mg/kg) but careful monitoring of renal function is required. Other therapeutic options in patients with multiresistant CMV disease are leflunomide and artesunate; however, experience with these agents is very limited.

To date there is no evidence to support the use of prophylaxis for other human herpesvirus (HHV) infections such as HHV-6 following HSCT.

A summary of prophylactic regimens is shown in Table 40.2.

EMPIRICAL THERAPY

The use of empirical antibiotic therapy in febrile neutropenic patients is almost universally practiced, because to await microbiological diagnosis is associated with a high mortality, particularly in patients with Gram-negative bacteremia. The trigger for this is usually a single oral temperature of 38.3°C or two separate temperatures of 38.0°C at least 1 h apart.

The regimen chosen should be active against the common organisms likely to result in overwhelming sepsis or death, and influenced by local antibiotic sensitivity patterns, the incidence of particular infections, the specific needs of the patient and the prophylactic regimen used. Traditionally the significant organisms have been the Enterobacteriaceae and *Ps. aeruginosa*, which carry a mortality of 40–60%.[8,9] Earlier regimens included an aminoglycoside in combination with a β-lactam antibiotic in an attempt to achieve broad-spectrum and synergistic activity against organisms such as *Ps. aeruginosa*. Aminoglycoside use carries the inherent risk of renal and ototoxicity, and data for its combination with β-lactams in empirical therapy have been conflicting. National Comprehensive Cancer Network (NCCN) guidelines recommend aminoglycosides in patients at high risk of pseudomonal infections (history of previous pseudomonal infections or the presence of ecthyma gangrenosum) whereas Infectious Diseases Society of America (IDSA) guidelines suggest they may be added in cases of progressive infection or documented resistant Gram-negative infection. A Cochrane review of 68 randomized controlled trials[65] concluded that for the primary outcome measure of all-cause mortality, there was no significant difference between monotherapy and combination (RR = 0.85). For the second outcome measure of treatment failure there was an advantage to monotherapy in 37 trials comparing different β-lactams (this was for patients with documented infection or hematological malignancy) (RR = 0.86). There was no difference between the two comparator arms in the number of superinfections but significantly more adverse events in the combination group for nephrotoxicity. Another meta-analysis also concluded that monotherapy is as

Table 40.2 Current antimicrobial prophylactic regimens for patients with prolonged neutropenia

Prophylaxis	Agent	Dosage	Duration
Antibacterial	Ciprofloxacin Levofloxacin	500 mg 12-hourly 500 mg daily	During period of neutropenia During period of neutropenia
Antifungal (high-risk patients)	Itraconazole suspension Posaconazole Voriconazole	See Chapter 60 for recommended regimens	During period of neutropenia 6 months post-BMT
Anti-*Pn. jirovecii*	Trimethoprim–sulfamethoxazole (Nebulized pentamidine in adults)	960 mg 12-hourly (150 mg fortnightly)	1 week pre- and 6 months post-BMT 3 times/week throughout treatment in acute lymphoblastic leukemia During period of neutropenia
Antituberculosis[a]	Isoniazid	5 mg/kg daily	During period of neutropenia 6 months post-BMT
Herpes simplex virus[b]	Aciclovir	400–800 mg 4–5 times per day	During period of neutropenia
Cytomegalovirus[c]	Seronegative blood products Aciclovir Ganciclovir	High dose	Not yet established Not yet established

[a]At-risk patients only.
[b]Seropositive patients only.
[c]HSCT recipients only.

effective as aminoglycoside–β-lactam combinations.[66] Data from patients in non-neutropenic studies have shown that once-daily dosing aminoglycoside regimens are as efficacious as multiple-dose regimens.

The first studies of double β-lactam therapy gave results inferior to aminoglycoside-containing regimens,[5,67,68] but later studies using ceftazidime, latamoxef and cefoperazone in combination with a ureidopenicillin[69–71] concluded that such combinations were of equal efficacy and less nephrotoxic than aminoglycoside-containing regimens. However, it was unclear whether they were any better than β-lactam monotherapy. A number of antibiotic regimens have subsequently been evaluated for empirical therapy in febrile neutropenic patients[70–77] and are listed in Box 40.4.

There have been reports that *Stenotrophomonas maltophilia* is selected out by the carbapenems, to which it is intrinsically resistant.[78] In addition, there have been concerns over central nervous system (CNS) toxicity with high-dose imipenem[71] or in patients receiving ciprofloxacin prophylaxis.[79]

One advantage of the carbapenems is their activity against the α-hemolytic streptococci,[80] allowing them to be used alone without the need for early glycopeptide therapy. Similar streptococcal activity can be provided by piperacillin–tazobactam.[81]

A recent meta-analysis of randomized trials examining the choice of β-lactam agent as empirical therapy for the treatment of febrile neutropenia reported that cefepime was associated with an increase in all-cause mortality but not with an increase in infection-related mortality.[82] The authors have concluded that ceftazidime, imipenem, meropenem and piperacillin–tazobactam are suitable monotherapy agents.

The high incidence of Gram-positive infections suggests that empirical therapy should contain a broad-spectrum anti-Gram-positive agent. Clinical trials of glycopeptides have provided conflicting evidence as to whether and when to add such an agent.

Early studies in centers in which there were significant numbers of Gram-positive infections showed that initial vancomycin or teicoplanin increased response rates and reduced morbidity,[83,84] although no study showed a reduction in mortality. In addition, vancomycin is associated with increased toxicity.[84,85] A large joint study conducted by the EORTC and the National Cancer Institute of Canada showed that including vancomycin in the initial therapy conferred no additional benefit,[86] and this has been reinforced by a meta-analysis showing no benefit of empirical Gram-positive therapy either initially or for persistent fever.[87]

The increasing isolation of vancomycin-resistant enterococci (VRE)[88,89] prompted the Centers for Disease Control and Prevention (CDC) to issue guidelines on the use of vancomycin that specifically excluded its use as empirical therapy in the neutropenic patient. This seemed prudent, although the IDSA suggests that vancomycin may be used in initial regimens in institutions where fulminant Gram-positive infections are common, particularly where MRSA may be a problem, and discontinued 3–4 days later if such an infection is not identified.[90]

Box 40.4 Representative antibiotic regimens that have been evaluated for empirical therapy in febrile neutropenic patients[73]

Penicillin and aminoglycoside combinations

Carbenicillin and gentamicin/amikacin/sisomicin
Ticarcillin and gentamicin/tobramycin/amikacin/netilmicin
Mezlocillin and tobramycin
Piperacillin and gentamicin/amikacin/netilmicin/tobramycin
Azlocillin and amikacin/netilmicin
Piperacillin–tazobactam and amikacin

Penicillin/β-lactam allergy

Vancomycin–teicoplanin + ciprofloxacin + gentamicin/amikacin

Cephalosporin and aminoglycoside combinations

Cefalotin and gentamicin
Latamoxef and gentamicin/amikacin
Cefotaxime and amikacin
Ceftazidime and tobramycin/amikacin
Cefoperazone and amikacin
Ceftriaxone and amikacin/netilmicin

Double β-lactam combinations

Carbenicillin and cefalotin
Carbenicillin and cefamandole
Ceftazidime and flucloxacillin
Ticarcillin and latamoxef
Piperacillin and latamoxef
Ceftazidime and azlocillin
Ceftazidime and piperacillin

Triple agent combinations

Carbenicillin, cefalotin and gentamicin
Carbenicillin, cefazolin and amikacin
Cefotaxime, piperacillin and netilmicin

Monotherapy regimens

Latamoxef
Ceftazidime
Cefoperazone
Ceftriaxone
Imipenem
Meropenem
Ciprofloxacin
Cefpirome
Cefepime
Piperacillin–tazobactam

Outpatient empirical regimens

Co-amoxiclav and ciprofloxacin p.o. (clindamycin and ciprofloxacin in penicillin allergy)
Ceftriaxone ± aminoglycoside

Other agents and combinations

Aztreonam and vancomycin
Imipenem and vancomycin
Trimethoprim–sulfamethoxazole and amikacin
Ticarcillin–clavulanate

From Liang R, Yung R, Chiu E, et al. Ceftazidime versus imipenem–cilastatin as initial monotherapy for febrile neutropenic patients. **Antimicrob Agents Chemother.** 1990;34:1336–1341.

Table 40.3 Options for initial empirical therapy

Regimen	Advantages	Disadvantages
Aminoglycoside + β-lactam	Broad spectrum Proven efficacy Synergy vs Gram-negative bacteria and streptococci	Poor activity vs coagulase-negative staphylococci Nephrotoxic and ototoxic Serum assays required
Double β-lactam therapy	Broad spectrum Avoids aminoglycoside toxicity No monitoring required	No more effective than single-agent therapy Possible prolongation of neutropenia Electrolyte imbalance Possible antagonism
Monotherapy	Broad spectrum Avoids aminoglycoside toxicity Avoids antagonism No monitoring required Cheaper	Lack of synergy (? less effective vs *Ps. aeruginosa*) Less active versus Gram-positive bacteria (with ceftazidime) Risk of resistance Potential central nervous system toxicity (with imipenem)
Single agent + glycopeptide	Broad spectrum including coagulase-negative staphylococci and α-hemolytic streptococci No monitoring required (with teicoplanin)	Expensive Unnecessary in some units Nephro- and ototoxicity (with vancomycin) Monitoring required (with vancomycin) Risk of glycopeptide resistance

There is also evidence that the choice of broad-spectrum agent for empirical therapy can influence the emergence of glycopeptide-resistant enterococci (GRE).[91] At present glycopeptide-intermediate *Staph. aureus* (GISA) infections are not a significant problem in the UK, but provide another reason for selective use of glycopeptides in institutions where they do occur.

The oxazolidinone linezolid, the streptogramin quinupristin–dalfopristin and daptomycin are alternatives in patients intolerant of vancomycin and teicoplanin and for treatment of GRE and GISA infections. A multicenter, randomized study of febrile neutropenic patients comparing the safety of linezolid and vancomycin showed that clinical success rates 7 days after completion of therapy were equivalent, as was mortality at 16 days after completion of therapy. Drug adverse events were more frequent in the vancomycin arm and time to defervescence was shorter in the linezolid arm in patients with documented Gram-positive infections. Slower times to neutrophil recovery seen in the linezolid arm may have been secondary to the myelosuppressive effects of linezolid but were not statistically significant.

The duration of treatment has not been studied independently, but since the first EORTC trial the evidence has suggested that prolonged treatment is associated with more superinfections, often fungal, but no improvement in outcome. Current EORTC trials are conducted on the basis of discontinuing antibiotics after 7 days minimum treatment and four consecutive afebrile days, and this is similar to the IDSA and NCCN guidelines where 5–7 days without fever is recommended.[90] Options are summarized in Table 40.3.

With health services moving towards earlier discharge of all groups of patients, attempts have been made to achieve this in the neutropenic population. Talcott and colleagues derived a risk assessment model in which patients were divided into four groups.[92] The fourth group was found to be at low risk and was studied in subsequent trials, which showed that amoxicillin–clavulanate plus ciprofloxacin was as effective as intravenous ceftazidime or ceftriaxone plus amikacin in treating these patients.[93,94]

Examples of outpatient oral/intravenous regimens are included in Box 40.4.

MANAGEMENT OF THE PATIENT WITH PERSISTENT PYREXIA

Approximately 20–30% of febrile patients who remain persistently neutropenic fail to respond to apparently appropriate antibiotic therapy. Some remain febrile until recovery of their neutrophil counts, irrespective of the antimicrobial therapy administered. Many patients with persistent fever will have an occult fungal infection. Patients with acute leukemia and allogeneic HSCT recipients are at highest risk due to prolonged neutropenia and immunosuppression for GVHD. Autopsy studies have shown that up to 25% of those neutropenic patients who die have an undiagnosed fungal infection.[10]

In view of the difficulties in diagnosis, the use of empirical antifungal therapy has been advocated. Recent ECIL 2009 guidelines are consistent with this viewpoint and current British Committee for Standards in Haematology (BCSH) guidelines advocate empirical antifungal therapy where IFI is suspected in conjunction with high-resolution computed tomography (HRCT) scanning and mycological tests (*see* Ch. 60). The main randomized study on which empirical antifungal therapy is based compared the effect of amphotericin (0.6 mg/kg per day or equivalent) with no treatment in patients remaining febrile 4 days after empirical therapy.[95] Although more responded in the amphotericin-treated group, the effect was only significant in patients not given antifungal prophylaxis (78% vs 45%; *p* = 0.04). Following this a number of other agents have been shown to be at least as effective as conventional amphotericin. Liposomal amphotericin B (AmBisome) is less nephrotoxic than conventional amphotericin, at least as effective in rendering patients afebrile and is associated with significantly fewer breakthrough fungal infections.[96,97] Subsequently, caspofungin has been shown to be at least as effective as AmBisome in this setting.[97]

Patients who deteriorate during the first 48 h of empirical therapy pose a particularly difficult therapeutic challenge. It is important that there are no gaps in the spectrum of the selected regimen. Deterioration may be due to Gram-negative or Gram-positive organisms, such as α-hemolytic streptococci, which may cause features similar to those of sepsis syndrome (including acute respiratory distress syndrome and septic shock), or enterococci. Gram-negative activity (including antipseudomonal activity) is essential. Consequently, the addition of an aminoglycoside to initial β-lactam monotherapy is recommended, and this is also supported by the ECIL guidelines for patients with septic shock. A glycopeptide should also be considered. The above approach is summarized in Figure 40.2.

ASPECTS OF THERAPY FOR SPECIFIC ORGANISMS AND INFECTIONS

INTRAVENOUS CATHETER-ASSOCIATED INFECTIONS

Most neutropenic patients undergoing chemotherapy have an indwelling central line, which commonly becomes infected. The predominant pathogens are coagulase-negative staphylococci and *Staph. aureus*.[98] Others include *Candida* spp., coryneforms, *Acinetobacter*, *Stenotrophomonas* and *Pseudomonas* spp.[99] Ideally, infected catheters should be removed, but coagulase-negative staphylococcal infections may be effectively suppressed or eliminated by administering antibiotics via the catheter until neutropenia has resolved.[98] A high percentage of coagulase-negative staphylococci isolated on hematology units are resistant to methicillin and other β-lactams.

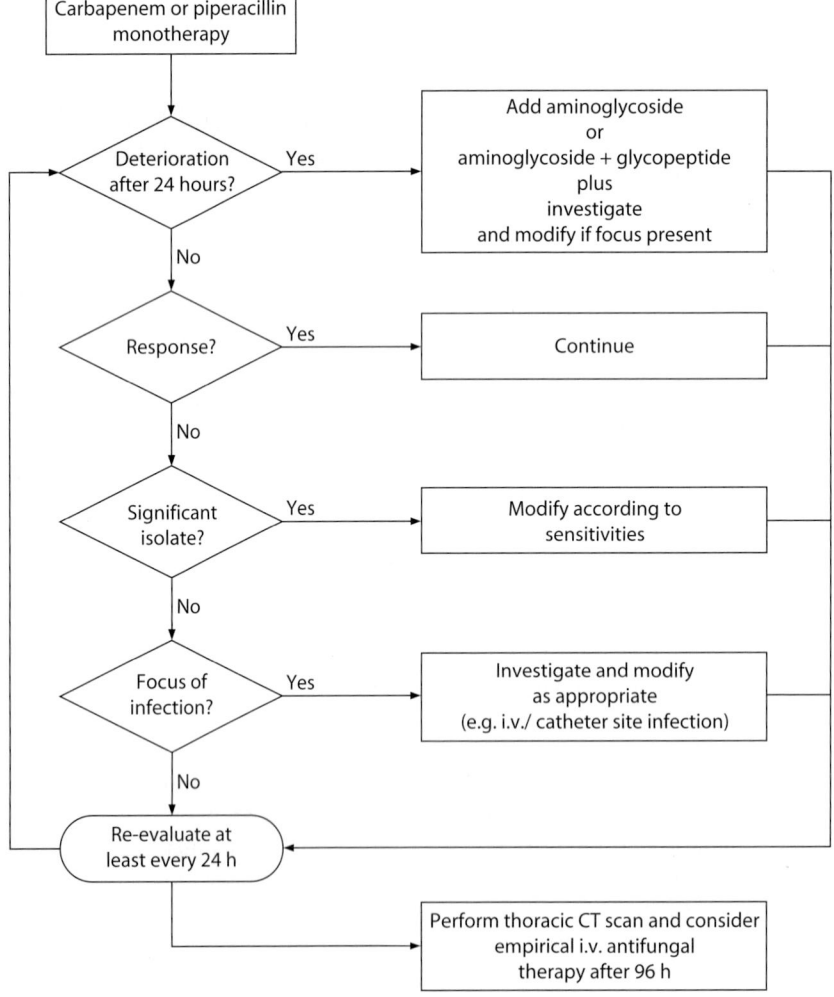

Fig. 40.2 An algorithm for the initial management of febrile neutropenic patients receiving prophylaxis.

A glycopeptide (most frequently vancomycin) is given for these, with the chance of successful resolution of bacteremia and fever being more than 50%. Similar response rates can be obtained with coryneform infections but those due to *Candida* spp., Enterobacteriaceae, *Staph. aureus*, *Ps. aeruginosa*, *Acinetobacter*, *Sten. maltophilia*, non-tuberculous mycobacteria, and any form of tunnel infection, require the catheter to be removed and appropriate antimicrobial therapy administered.[100] The presence of port infection or septic phlebitis in association with long-term indwelling catheters are also indications for catheter removal and antimicrobial therapy.

PULMONARY INFECTIONS OF UNKNOWN CAUSE

Pulmonary infiltrates commonly occur in the febrile neutropenic patient and have a number of causes, especially in the BMT recipient. These include non-infective conditions such as pulmonary edema, alveolar hemorrhage, adverse drug reactions, radiation injury and the idiopathic pneumonitis syndrome. Focal lesions are more indicative of fungal infection, and HRCT or MRI scanning may reveal characteristic features of these.[101] If clinical status permits, the causative organism(s) may be obtained by bronchoalveolar lavage. However, in many cases treatment has to be given empirically.

Initial therapy should certainly include agents effective against common respiratory pathogens such as *Str. pneumoniae* and *Haemophilus influenzae*, as well as Gram-negative organisms including *Ps. aeruginosa*, and hence a carbapenem, piperacillin–tazobactam or ceftazidime, with or without an aminoglycoside, is recommended.

Atypical pneumonias are extremely uncommon in this population and, unless there are particular clinical or epidemiological reasons to suggest Legionnaires' disease, erythromycin can be omitted from the initial therapy unless the infection appears to be community related. Mycobacterial infections may occasionally complicate hematological malignancies. Patients with lymphoid malignancy and BMT recipients who have not been receiving trimethoprim–sulfamethoxazole prophylaxis are at risk of *Pn. jirovecii* pneumonitis; empirical high-dose trimethoprim–sulfamethoxazole therapy (120 mg/kg per day in divided doses) is warranted in such patients. BMT recipients are particularly at risk of CMV pneumonitis post-transplant. However, CMV or *Pn. jirovecii* pneumonitis usually presents a month or so post-transplant, when the patient is no longer neutropenic, and the timing of the presentation should be taken into account when decisions are being made regarding empirical therapy. CMV pneumonitis is treated with intravenous ganciclovir (5 mg/kg every 12 h) plus intravenous immunoglobulin (200–400 mg/kg on alternate days for 14–21 days).[102–104] Despite this, mortality from CMV pneumonitis is still in excess of 50% in BMT recipients. Furthermore, the myelosuppressive effect of ganciclovir can present a particular problem in these patients.

Patients discharged into the community are at risk of respiratory viral infections with agents such as respiratory syncytial virus, influenza and paramyxoviruses, which occasionally cause outbreaks on hematology units.[105]

INVASIVE FUNGAL INFECTIONS

Despite recent advances in the diagnosis and treatment of invasive fungal infections (IFI), failure rates approach 50% in invasive aspergillosis. Case fatality rates of 87% for HSCT and 50% for leukemia patients are quoted,[106] with 30-day mortality rates of 45% for candidemia in hematological malignancy.[107] Current BCSH guidelines advocate the use of caspofungin and liposomal amphotericin for empirical therapy of suspected IFI as they have the lowest rates of toxicity and are of equal efficacy. This is also in keeping with the current ECIL guidelines. Other options include voriconazole and posaconazole. The therapy of fungal infection is considered in detail in Chapter 60.

INVASIVE CANDIDAL INFECTIONS

A trend towards non-*albicans* species such as *C. glabrata* and *C. krusei* displaying a decreased susceptibility or resistance to azoles has been documented in both Europe and North America. These species are responsible for more than 60% of invasive candidal infections in patients with hematological malignancy.[108]

Recent trials of the three licensed echinocandins – caspofungin, micafungin and anidulafungin – have demonstrated response rates in excess of 70% and these are now considered to be among the first-line agents for invasive candidal infections, especially where the species is not known, where the patient has received azole prophylaxis or in severe sepsis. This is supported by the ECIL-2 guideline update and IDSA candida guidelines, together with the use of AmBisome and other lipid formulations of amphotericin. Voriconazole is an alternative agent but should be used with care in patients where previous azole prophylaxis has been used. Recommendations for duration of therapy consist of 14 days following the last positive blood culture, together with extensive investigation for dissemination of infection. Further trials regarding the use of efungumab (Mycograb), a human recombinant antibody consisting of an Fv fragment that binds to the domain structure HSP90 of *Candida* spp., are needed before recommendations regarding its use in combination with antifungals can be made, and it is currently not licensed.

INVASIVE ASPERGILLOSIS

Mortality due to invasive aspergillosis remains high in neutropenic patients; the infection is now the most important cause of death in childhood AML and adult BMT recipients. In BMT recipients case fatality rates are as high as 87%.[106] Successful outcome is dependent upon early treatment and, to a considerable extent, on bone marrow recovery. Agents active against *Aspergillus* spp. include amphotericin deoxycholate and its lipid-associated preparations, the extended-spectrum triazoles and echinocandins. High-dose conventional amphotericin is also associated with a high incidence of nephrotoxicity. Lipid-associated formulations of the drug have been licensed for use in patients failing treatment or experiencing unacceptable toxicity with conventional amphotericin. Liposomal amphotericin (AmBisome) has been studied in a randomized prospective trial comparing two doses (1 mg/kg per day and 4 mg/kg per day) for the treatment of invasive aspergillosis in neutropenic patients:[109] 6-month mortality was approximately 60% with attributable mortality of around 20% in the two arms. A double-blind comparison of AmBisome 3 mg/kg and AmBisome 10 mg/kg in primary therapy by Cornely and colleagues demonstrated no additional benefit of 10 mg/kg dosing over 3 mg/kg dosing of liposomal amphotericin B.[110]

Voriconazole has been assessed by Denning and colleagues in two open-labeled studies in which response rates of 44% and 48% were reported, respectively.[111,112] Superiority of voriconazole over amphotericin deoxycholate in terms of efficacy, safety and survival has been demonstrated by Herbrecht and colleagues in a randomized trial.[112] Superiority was irrespective of the host group, site of lesion or neutropenic status. Voriconazole has been given the highest graded recommendation in the recent ECIL-2 guideline update, followed by AmBisome. In North America the NCCN currently recommends voriconazole as the agent of choice for first-line therapy of invasive pulmonary aspergillosis. There are insufficient data to recommend the use of caspofungin, itraconazole and posaconazole as agents in first-line therapy of invasive aspergillosis, but these have all been used in salvage therapy with similar efficacy. There are also currently insufficient data to recommend combination therapy in first-line therapy. One retrospective study[113] comparing the combination of voriconazole and caspofungin given as salvage therapy after failure of amphotericin formulations in allogeneic HSCT recipients with voriconazole monotherapy in a historical control group demonstrated substantially improved 3-month survival.

The development of mycotic lung sequestra (which have been mistakenly termed mycetomas) may require additional therapy. These lesions appear once the bone marrow is regenerating. Patients are at risk of life-threatening hemoptysis.[114] In addition, patients who require further chemotherapy or bone marrow transplantation are at considerable risk of relapse of the original infection. Resection of these lesions has been shown to be effective, preventing relapse following bone marrow transplantation, and is associated with a lower mortality than antifungal therapy alone in some studies,[115] although there are no large randomized studies in this setting.

ADDITIONAL THERAPIES

 ### GROWTH FACTORS

Hematopoietic growth factors have been extensively used to treat neutropenic patients. Studies have consistently shown that granulocyte–colony-stimulating factor (G-CSF) reduces the duration of neutropenia. However, the reduction in infectious complications has been modest and most trials have been unable to demonstrate a reduction in infectious morbidity and mortality.[116–118] This is probably because the major effect of G-CSF is to accelerate the recovery of neutrophils, whereas it has no impact on the critical lag period of profound neutropenia.[119] The American Society of Oncology and the NCCN have published guidelines for the use of these agents in the setting of anti-cancer chemotherapy.

Granulocyte–macrophage colony-stimulating factor (GM-CSF) and macrophage colony-stimulating factor (M-CSF) may be beneficial in the treatment of invasive fungal infections,[120] although large-scale trials demonstrating this are regrettably still lacking.

 ## GRANULOCYTE TRANSFUSIONS

Renewed interest is now being shown in this modality, coupled with improved methods of harvesting and increased yield following the use of growth factors.[121,122]

 ## IMMUNOGLOBULIN THERAPY

Routine prophylactic use of intravenous immunoglobulin does not reduce viral infections; however, the addition of intravenous immunoglobulin to ganciclovir may improve survival in CMV pneumonitis and post-exposure immunoglobulin is indicated for the prevention of hepatitis A, measles and varicella-zoster infection.

INFECTIONS IN TRANSPLANT RECIPIENTS

IMMUNOSUPPRESSIVE THERAPY

Since the first successful human cadaveric kidney transplant in 1954, solid organ transplantation has proceeded to become a viable option in the management of end-organ failure worldwide. Current 1- and 5-year graft survival for cadaveric (non-extended criteria donor) renal transplants in the USA is 95% and 82%, respectively.[123] The results are similar for Europe. Developments in surgery and better control of rejection and infective complications have allowed a steady improvement in the survival of other organ grafts.

Most transplant units use a triple regimen of azathioprine or mycophenolate, a calcineurin inhibitor such as ciclosporin A, and corticosteroids for immunosuppression. Azathioprine is a purine analog which inhibits both B- and T-cell proliferation; as a consequence, both cell-mediated immunity (CMI) and humoral immunity are inhibited. The drug may take weeks or months to exert its full effect. Ciclosporin, a calcineurin inhibitor, arrests the lymphocyte cell cycle in the resting phase, having most effect on CD4-positive T cells and a minimal effect on B cells. This results in effective suppression of CMI, has little effect on humoral immunity and no effect on phagocytosis. The inflammatory response is preserved.

Corticosteroids in high dose have a very broad immunosuppressive action, producing a reduction in antigen-stimulated lymphocyte proliferation and a blunting of the primary antibody response. They also inhibit neutrophil chemotaxis and monocyte phagocytosis, dramatically reducing inflammatory responses at high dosage and disguising the presence of infection.

The aim of these regimens is to achieve a balance between graft rejection and risk of infection. Episodes of subsequent acute rejection require considerable immunosuppression and are accompanied by an increased risk of opportunistic infections. The phase of acute rejection varies in length for different transplants. Most episodes occur in the first 3 months of liver transplantation, whereas the phase of acute rejection lasts for 6 months for renal transplants.[124] Rejection episodes are usually treated with high-dose methylprednisolone or various antibody preparations such as polyclonal antithymocyte globulin (ATG), antilymphocyte globulin (ALG) or the pan-T-cell monoclonal antibody OKT3. Patients requiring a second or third graft are usually even more immunosuppressed and at increased risk of opportunistic infection.

Tacrolimus (FK506), another calcineurin antagonist, has been substituted for ciclosporin for certain indications; several studies have demonstrated it to have fewer infective complications,[125–128] which may be a consequence of the need for less episodic antirejection therapy. Mycophenolate mofetil, an inhibitor of inosine monophosphate dehydrogenase which inhibits purine synthesis, has been used as a substitute for calcineurin inhibitors. Although it has no associated renal toxicity (and allows improvement in renal function), some studies have shown it to result in increased risk of rejection.[124] A recent review comparing the use of azathioprine with mycophenolate in liver transplantation concluded that, to date, little if any clinical benefit could be observed of mycophenolate mofetil over azathioprine.[129] There is still considerable scope for refining immunosuppression with these and other new agents, hopefully enabling a further reduction in infective complications.

THE SEQUENCE OF INFECTIONS FOLLOWING TRANSPLANTATION

The risk of infection in the organ transplant patient is influenced by previous epidemiological exposures and the degree of immunosuppression. Epidemiological exposures can be divided into donor-derived infections, recipient-derived infections, nosocomial infections and community infections. The extent of immunosuppression is determined by the type of immunosuppressive therapy, its dose and duration (*see* Box 40.5), underlying diseases and co-morbid conditions, the presence of devitalized tissues or fluid collections in the transplanted organ, and the presence of invasive devices. Other important factors include concomitant infection with immunomodulating

viruses such as CMV and other human herpes viruses, HIV-1, and hepatitis B and C viruses. Infectious complications follow a relatively predictable chronological order after any transplantation procedure. Knowledge of this is helpful in guiding the use and duration of prophylaxis, establishing a diagnosis through appropriate investigations and administering empirical treatment if necessary. This is summarized in Figure 40.3.

In the first month after transplant, infections are largely associated with the transplant surgical procedure, particularly those complicating the anastomoses associated with the specific procedure. Some infections are transmitted with the allograft or are present in the recipient before transplantation. An important component of the pretransplant evaluation is to recognize and treat such infections. Nosocomial infections such as those due to VRE or MRSA, and *Clostridium difficile* colitis are also important at this time.

Between the first and the sixth month following transplantation the most important infections are caused by the herpes group viruses (especially CMV), *Nocardia* species, *Listeria monocytogenes*, *Toxoplasma gondii*, *Pn. jirovecii* and other fungi. In addition, latent infections such as tuberculosis or histoplasmosis may reactivate at this time. The risk of infection correlates with the severity of immunosuppression required to treat rejection episodes.

Subsequent infections are usually the result of community-acquired organisms. A few patients will suffer chronic viral infections affecting the graft, while others who have been intensively immunosuppressed remain at risk of opportunistic infections. Other rare infections in the late post-transplant period have been described, including chronic infection with hepatitis E virus causing cirrhosis as a late complication.[130]

 ## BACTERIAL INFECTIONS

Bacterial infections occur in approximately 50% of renal transplant recipients and in up to 70% of liver transplant patients. In some series patients have suffered at least one bacterial infection in the post-transplant period.[131] The common infections are intra-abdominal abscess, cholangitis, bacteremia, wound infection, lower respiratory tract infection and urinary tract infection, with intra-abdominal infection responsible for approximately 30% in liver transplantation.[131–134] The overall mortality is less than 5%, but varies according to site and organ.

Subsequently resistant organisms have become established as endemic pathogens in many transplant units. MRSA was found to be the leading cause of bacteremia in liver transplant recipients in one center, responsible for 37% of all episodes.[135] VRE and extended-spectrum β-lactamase-producing Gram-negative organisms are also increasingly causing infections in these patients.

Representative organisms isolated from infected patients in the postoperative period are shown in Box 40.6. Bacteria isolated from the graft perfusion fluid differ in their propensity to cause post-transplantation infection. Positive

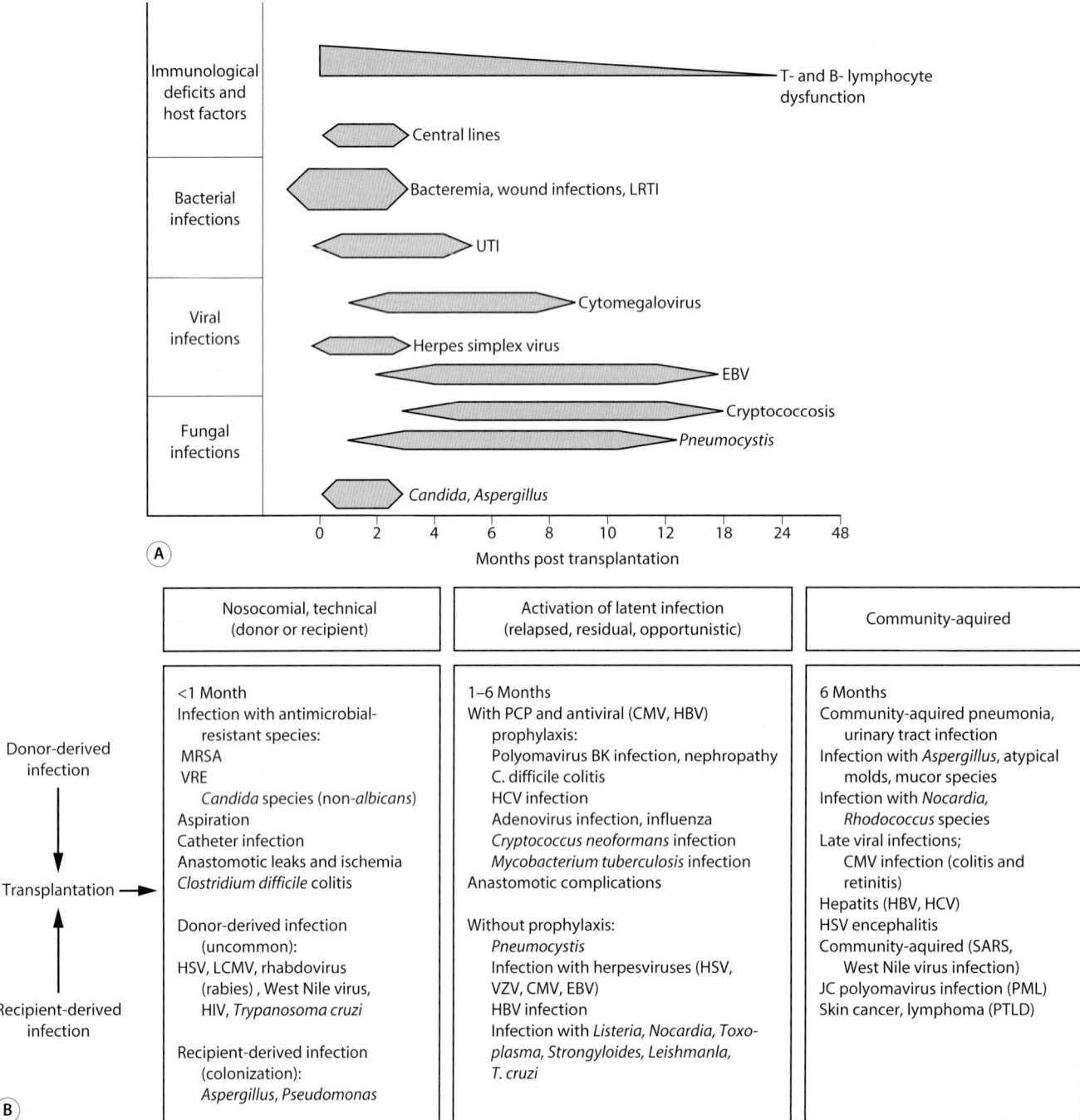

Fig. 40.3 (A) The time course of infections after solid organ transplantation. (B) Changing timeline of infection after transplantation. Infections occur in a generally predictable pattern. The development of infection is delayed by prophylaxis and accelerated by intensified immunosuppression, drug toxic effects that may cause leukopenia, or immunomodulatory viral infections such as infection with cytomegalovirus (CMV), hepatitis C virus (HCV) or Epstein–Barr virus (EBV). At the time of transplantation, a patient's short-term and long-term risk of infection can be stratified according to donor and recipient screening, the technical outcome of surgery, and the intensity of immunosuppression required to prevent graft rejection. Subsequently, an ongoing assessment of the risk of infection is used to adjust both prophylaxis and immunosuppressive therapy. HBV, hepatitis B virus; HIV, human immunodeficiency virus; HSV, herpes simplex virus; LCMV, lymphocytic choriomeningitis virus; MRSA, methicillin-resistant *Staphylococcus aureus*; PCP, *Pneumocystis jirovecii* pneumonia; PML, progressive multifocal leukoencephalopathy; PTLD, post-transplantation lymphoproliferative disorder; SARS, severe acute respiratory syndrome; VRE, vancomycin-resistant *Enterococcus* spp.; VZV, varicella-zoster virus. (Adapted from Fishman, JA. Infection in solid organ transplant recipients. *New England Journal of Medicine* 2007; 357:2601. Copyright ©2007 Massachusetts Medical Society.)

- *Antilymphocyte globulins*: T-cell depleting antibodies mimic the alloimmune response with activation of latent (herpes) virus, fever, cytokine release
- *Corticosteroids*: Bacteria, *Pneumocystis* pneumonia, activation of hepatitis C and hepatitis B
- *Azathioprine*: Neutropenia, uncertain role in human papillomavirus infection
- *Mycophenolate mofetil*: Early bacterial infection, B-cell depression, late cytomegalovirus infection
- *Ciclosporin/tacrolimus*: Increased viral replication, B-cell depression, gingival infection, intracellular pathogens
- *Rapamycin*: Excess infections in combination with current agents (requires monitoring), idiosyncratic pulmonary syndrome, often with other respiratory pathogens
- *Plasmapheresis*: Encapsulated bacteria
- *Co-stimulatory blockade*: Unknown so far
- *Rituximab*: B-cell depletion, bacterial and viral infections
- *Alemtuzumab*: Cytomegalovirus infection, viral infection, fungal infections

Box 40.6 Organisms causing post-transplant infections

Gram-positive bacteria	*Pneumocystis jirovecii*
Coagulase-negative staphylococci	*Cryptococcus neoformans*
Staphylococcus aureus	*Blastomyces dermatitidis*
Enterococci	*Coccidioides immitis*
Streptococci	*Histoplasma capsulatum*
Listeria monocytogenes	
Nocardia spp.	**Viruses**
	Herpes simplex virus
Gram-negative bacteria	Cytomegalovirus
Enterobacteriaceae	Hepatitis B virus
Pseudomonas spp.	Hepatitis C virus
Stenotrophomonas maltophilia	Varicella zoster virus
Legionella spp.	Polyoma viruses
	Adenovirus
Anaerobic bacteria	Human herpesvirus-6
Bacteroides spp.	Human herpesvirus-8
Clostridium spp.	
	Others
Fungi	*Mycobacterium* spp.
Candida spp.	*Toxoplasma gondii*
Aspergillus spp.	

cultures have been found in up to 40% of cases in renal transplantation, but most of these have been due to Gram-positive skin bacteria and do not seem to have serious consequences. However, the isolation of the Enterobacteriaceae and *Ps. aeruginosa* correlate with vascular infection and postoperative sepsis,[136–138] and warrant systemic antibiotic therapy following transplantation.

Infections due to *Nocardia* spp. are important late complications following transplantation, usually occurring after the first month, and which correlate with the degree of immunosuppression. Outbreaks in renal transplant units have been described[139] and the incidence is up to 4% in this group.

Tuberculosis tends to occur several months after transplantation. The onset is significantly later in renal transplants than

in other groups of organ transplant recipients.[140] Approximately one-third have disseminated infection and the overall mortality is 29%. The overall incidence of mycobacterial infection in the transplant population is 1%, more than 50-fold greater than the incidence in the general population.[141]

Transplant recipients are at increased risk of Legionnaires' disease by virtue of their immunosuppression. In addition, a UK study demonstrated that *Legionella* spp. could be isolated from the water in approximately 50% of transplant units[142] and *Legionella* control is now an important component of water and air conditioning management in hospitals.

 ## FUNGAL INFECTIONS

Colonization with yeasts is common in this population, although the incidence varies according to the number and frequency of sites sampled and the use of antifungal prophylaxis. Infection rates vary, with the lowest in renal transplant recipients (approximately 5%).[143] The incidence of fungal infections is falling, possibly as a consequence of reduced immunosuppression and improvement in surgical technique.[144] Most infections are caused by *Candida* spp. (approximately 80%), with *Aspergillus* spp. accounting for the majority of invasive mold infections.[143,145] *Pn. jirovecii* pneumonitis occurred in 4–10% of kidney, 10–11% of liver, 5–41% of heart, and 16–43% of heart–lung and lung transplant recipients before routine prophylaxis was implemented.[146] It is closely linked with CMV disease.

Candidal infections are associated with death in more than 50% and invasive aspergillosis is almost universally fatal in this group.[143] The site of infection is transplant dependent. Thus urinary tract candidosis is mostly confined to the renal transplant group and lung transplant recipients have a much increased risk of pulmonary infections. Although occurring very infrequently, focal brain infection in solid organ transplant patients is almost exclusively due to fungi, usually *Aspergillus* spp.;[147–149] *Cryptococcus neoformans* is the most frequent cause of meningitis.

Most fungal infections occur in the first 2 months after transplant,[143] although *Pn. jirovecii* infection tends to be delayed and cryptococcosis usually affects patients in the late transplant period. Infections due to the endemic fungi, including *Coccidioides immitis* (most often following exposure in the southwestern United States), *Histoplasma capsulatum* (most often following exposure in the Ohio River Valley, but also elsewhere in the world) and *Blastomyces dermatitidis*, may also be seen in the late post-transplant period. In one series, the median time to symptoms from histoplasmosis was 11 months after transplantation.[150] The management of these infections is discussed further in Chapter 60.

 ## VIRAL INFECTIONS

Since the earliest days of transplantation, virus infections have caused problems in transplant recipients. Members of the Herpesviridae are the most commonly implicated.

Cytomegalovirus is responsible for the greatest number of all types of infection in these patients. The incidence varies from 45% to 100%,[151] reflecting the incidence of seropositivity among the recipient population and the numbers of seropositive to seronegative transplantations. However, the incidence of disease is transplant dependent, being lowest in renal transplant recipients, in whom it is symptomatic in less than 10%.[152]

Overall, 25–30% of infected patients develop disease,[151–153] although of those at highest risk (seropositive to seronegative transplants) 50–60% will develop clinical disease.[141] The site of disease is transplant dependent, being focused on the graft. About 3% of all transplant recipients affected will develop CMV pneumonitis.[153]

Post-transplant hepatitis occurs in more than 10% of solid organ transplant recipients overall. The most common cause is hepatitis C virus (HCV). In liver transplant patients most of these infections occur as a result of reinfection in patients who have been transplanted for HCV-related cirrhosis. Polymerase chain reaction (PCR) techniques have shown that virtually all infected patients suffer reinfection post-transplant. Before universal screening of blood donors and awareness of donor status, primary HCV infections occurred in more than 35%;[154] the incidence is now much lower. In one study, 95% of patients with pretransplant infection developed post-transplant hepatitis, mostly due to HCV.

Reinfection with hepatitis B virus (HBV) following liver transplantation is almost inevitable unless long-term prophylaxis is used. The highest recurrence is seen in those who are HBV-DNA positive before transplant.[155]

Epstein–Barr virus (EBV) infection following transplant is probably underdiagnosed. Most clinical disease is due to reactivation, although primary infection does occur, usually after the patient is discharged, and is responsible for more severe disease. The most important complication of EBV infection is post-transplant lymphoproliferative disorder (PTLD). The overall incidence of this condition is approximately 1%.[156] In a large series of various solid organ graft recipients, viremia was found in 3.9%, and 75% of those with primary viremia developed PTLD compared with 11% of secondary viremia cases.[156] The risk of this disease is also increased by the use of antirejection therapy such as OKT3 anti-T-cell antibodies.

Before the advent of aciclovir, HSV infections (almost exclusively the consequence of reactivation) were responsible for clinical disease in approximately 50% of seropositive patients.[141] HSV infections are now much less clinically significant than other herpes group infections.

Human herpesvirus-6 (HHV-6) may be responsible for central nervous system disease post transplantation. CNS symptoms occurred in 25% of liver transplant recipients with HHV-6 viremia compared with 12% of those without.[157] Infection with HHV-6 may also have an immunomodulatory role, being associated with an increased risk of CMV infection and fungal infection.[158]

Human herpesvirus-8 (HHV-8) is transmitted from donor to recipient, resulting in Kaposi's sarcoma in up to 8% of cases who seroconvert.[159]

Polyomavirus causes latent infection in the kidney in the immunocompetent subject, and in renal transplant recipients may be responsible for tubulointerstitial nephritis and graft dysfunction.[160]

 ## INFECTIONS DUE TO OTHER ORGANISMS

The incidence of toxoplasmosis varies according to the type of transplant and is most common in heart transplant recipients, of whom more than 50% of seronegative patients receiving a heart from a seropositive donor will seroconvert.[161] In addition, toxoplasmosis is governed by the seroprevalence of the infection (20% in the UK and higher in other countries such as France) and the serological status of donor and recipient: the highest rate and most severe infections occur when transplanting a seropositive donor to a seronegative recipient. In renal transplant recipients less than 1% develop primary toxoplasmosis. Most such cases occur within 2 months of transplant and are characterized by encephalitis, brain abscess, retinitis, pneumonitis, cardiac involvement and hepatitis.[162–164]

CHEMOPROPHYLAXIS

Antimicrobial prophylaxis, along with vaccination and preemptive therapy, form the mainstay of preventive strategies against infection. Until recently, most prophylactic regimens used in transplant recipients have been based on the risk of infection and likely organisms. Regimens shown to be effective in the neutropenic patient or in surgical prophylaxis have been adopted, yet few have been subject to randomized comparative trials. A short course of prophylactic antibiotics is probably appropriate to prevent wound infection related to the procedure itself. Selective decontamination of the digestive tract may be of benefit in some transplant groups, although there is conflicting evidence. Gram-negative infections are reduced in liver transplant recipients[165] but an increase in Gram-positive infections, including MRSA and VRE, has been seen in several heart transplant centers.[166]

A number of studies have demonstrated the benefit of long-term prophylaxis for urinary tract infections in renal transplant recipients. Both trimethoprim–sulfamethoxazole (960 mg nightly) and ciprofloxacin have been effective, although the former has the additional benefit of preventing *Pn. jirovecii* infection.[167,168]

The issue of mycobacterial prophylaxis remains controversial and policies vary internationally. As there is a significant risk of isoniazid hepatic toxicity, this drug should be used selectively. However, this risk varies according to the transplant, from 2.5% in renal transplant recipients to 41% in liver transplant recipients.[140] Patients in whom such prophylaxis is justified are those of Asian or other high-risk ethnic origin, those with a history of tuberculosis and those with radiographic changes suggesting past chest infection.

The high risk of fungal infection in liver transplant recipients has led to the administration of antifungal agents in the post-transplant period. Non-absorbable agents such as amphotericin or nystatin, sometimes in combination with oral antibiotics such as gentamicin and polymyxin B, have been widely used. Fluconazole and itraconazole have been studied in randomized comparative trials in liver transplantation and both are better than placebo in preventing superficial and invasive candidosis.[169,170]

Prophylaxis against *Pn. jirovecii* pneumonia with trimethoprim–sulfamethoxazole is probably only necessary during the first year post-transplant, except in lung transplant recipients when there is a significant persisting risk of the disease.[171]

The current American Society of Transplantation guidelines recommend antiviral prophylaxis in all CMV donor-positive, recipient-negative solid organ transplant recipients.[172] Several randomized comparative studies have demonstrated that early (first 14 days or until discharge) post-transplant ganciclovir, with[173] or without[174] gammaglobulin, is more effective than aciclovir (various doses) in preventing CMV symptomatic infection in liver transplants. Symptomatic infection was reduced to 5–9%.

Pre-emptive prophylaxis targets patients at highest risk of disease and limits duration of drug administration, reducing toxicity and cost. Hence, kidney–pancreas transplant patients receiving OKT3 pan-T-cell monoclonal antibody therapy and CMV-shedding liver transplant recipients both appear to benefit from pre-emptive prophylaxis with ganciclovir or foscarnet.[175,176] CMV antigenemia or PCR-guided pre-emptive therapy based on attainment of a pre-defined viral load is as effective as, but less expensive than, universal oral ganciclovir prophylaxis for 90 days or intravenous ganciclovir for 14 days.[177] The duration of this pre-emptive therapy is not fixed and is determined by viral load and varies in length between centers.

Trials of prophylaxis with lamivudine to prevent recurrence of HBV following liver transplantation have shown that, although HBV-DNA levels become undetectable in virtually all patients, this effect is not sustained because of the emergence of resistant mutants.[178] As a consequence, alternative strategies involving a combination of adefovir, lamivudine and hepatitis B immune globulin are being employed.

TREATMENT

Although transplant recipients are severely immunocompromised, they do not have the same paucity of signs as neutropenic patients in the face of serious sepsis and, in the immediate postoperative period, behave more like non-transplant patients with surgical sepsis.[179] Consequently, the concept of early empirical therapy in response to fever alone has not been applied to these patients.

All attempts should be made to identify a focus of sepsis or the non-infective cause for fever in a transplant patient. Antimicrobial therapy may reasonably be withheld if the patient is otherwise well and there is no identifiable infective cause, but this should be kept under review. If empirical treatment is considered necessary, the choice of antimicrobials should be governed by the timing of the infection (and hence the probable organisms), the type of transplant, the site of sepsis, knowledge of colonization with resistant organisms (such as MRSA and VRE), and local antimicrobial resistance patterns, as discussed previously.

ASPECTS OF THERAPY FOR SPECIFIC INFECTIONS

 ### FUNGAL INFECTIONS

Fungal infections should be managed using the same agents as used in the neutropenic patient. No antifungal is contraindicated but care is required in their use because of toxicity (especially in renal and liver transplant recipients) and drug interaction (especially flucytosine with antimetabolites and triazoles with ciclosporin and tacrolimus – *see below*).

It is probably appropriate to reduce immunosuppression in the face of a progressive life-threatening fungal infection such as invasive aspergillosis, especially in the setting of a non-essential organ graft such as a kidney transplant, although the evidence for benefit is anecdotal. Other attempts at immunomodulation have included the use of colony-stimulating factors. G–CSF antagonizes the effect of triazoles in an immunocompromised mouse model of invasive aspergillosis.[180] GM-CSF has been used with some success in the neutropenic patient and might prove of more use than G-CSF in the transplant setting.

 ### PULMONARY INFECTIONS OF UNKNOWN CAUSE

Patients presenting with pulmonary infiltrates and fever 1 month or more post-transplant are most likely to have CMV or *Pn. jirovecii* infection (unless they are receiving trimethoprim–sulfamethoxazole prophylaxis). These infections should be managed as in the HSCT recipient. The possibility of other community-acquired respiratory tract infections, including those due to influenza and respiratory syncytial viruses, should always be borne in mind.

 ### POST-TRANSPLANT LYMPHOPROLIFERATIVE DISORDER

The incidence of this occurring in renal transplant recipients is 1–2%,[181,182] is related to the degree of immunosuppression (it is seen particularly in patients receiving OKT3) and is more likely in primary EBV infection.[183] At present, the mainstay of therapy is the reduction of immunosuppression together with intravenous aciclovir (10 mg/kg every 8 h). However, many patients will require local resection or radiotherapy of affected tissue and/or antilymphoma chemotherapy. Developments in this field include the possibility of immunotherapy by means of donor leukocyte infusions.[184] Most recently the efficacy of rituximab, an anti-CD20 monoclonal antibody in the treatment of EBV-driven PTLD, has been described.[185]

DRUG INTERACTIONS DURING TREATMENT OF INFECTION

Ciclosporin and tacrolimus are metabolized by the cytochrome P_{450} enzyme system and therefore interact with a number of important antimicrobial agents likely to be prescribed in transplant recipients (Table 40.4). Levels of these drugs may be altered by the induction or inhibition of this system and it is essential that these are measured to prevent toxicity, as well as to avoid inadequate or excessive immunosuppression with the consequences of rejection or infection. Rifampicin is a potent inducer of these cytochrome isoenzymes and causes increased metabolism of ciclosporin and tacrolimus, as well as reducing the bioavailability of corticosteroids. Erythromycin, some of the newer macrolides (particularly clarithromycin), and the azole antifungal agents, especially ketoconazole, itraconazole and voriconazole (and fluconazole at high doses), competitively inhibit this pathway, thus increasing levels of ciclosporin and tacrolimus.

Renal function is often impaired in the transplantation setting and there may be a complex interaction between ciclosporin (itself potentially nephrotoxic, particularly during initial therapy) and nephrotoxic antimicrobial agents such as the aminoglycosides, high-dose trimethoprim–sulfamethoxazole, vancomycin and amphotericin. Therapeutic drug monitoring is mandatory (with the exception of amphotericin) to prevent additional toxicity and alternative agents should be chosen whenever possible (Table 40.4).

CONCLUSION

Prevention should always be the goal in the management of infective complications in neutropenia and organ transplantation. This has become increasingly important over the past decade with the advent of MRSA, VRE and other resistant organisms. Despite the development of antimicrobials with good activity against the infecting agents, the mortality from many of these infections remains high. The spectrum of immunocompromised patients is changing with the evolution of chemotherapy, stem-cell transplantation, immunosuppression regimens, and tissue and organ transplantation techniques – thus we can expect to see the pattern of opportunistic infections shift as well.

Table 40.4 Potential drug interactions during management of infections in organ transplant recipients

Antimicrobial agent	Immunosuppressive agent	Effect
Aminoglycosides	Ciclosporin	Exacerbation of nephrotoxicity
Amphotericin	Ciclosporin	Exacerbation of nephrotoxicity
Trimethoprim–sulfamethoxazole	Ciclosporin	Possible exacerbation of nephrotoxicity Reduced levels of ciclosporin
Doxycycline	Ciclosporin	Increased ciclosporin levels
Erythromycin[a]	Ciclosporin	Increased ciclosporin levels
Fluconazole	Ciclosporin	Increased ciclosporin levels
Flucytosine	Azathioprine	Possible exacerbation of myelosuppression
Ganciclovir	Azathioprine	Possible exacerbation of myelosuppression
Itraconazole	Ciclosporin Vincristine	Increased ciclosporin levels Increased neurotoxicity
Ketoconazole	Ciclosporin	Increased ciclosporin levels
Pentamidine (i.v.)	Ciclosporin	Possible exacerbation of nephrotoxicity
Rifampicin (rifampin)	Ciclosporin Prednisone	Reduced levels of ciclosporin Reduced levels of prednisone
Sulfonamides	Azathioprine	Possible exacerbation of myelosuppression
Trimethoprim	Azathioprine	Possible exacerbation of myelosuppression
Vancomycin	Ciclosporin	Exacerbation of nephrotoxicity

[a]And other macrolides.

References

1. Bodey GP, Buckley M, Sathe YS, Freireich EJ. Quantitative relationships between circulating leucocytes and infection in patients with acute leukaemia. *Ann Intern Med.* 1966;64:328–340.

2. Cline MJ. A new white cell test which measures individual phagocyte function in a mixed leukocyte population. I. A neutrophil defect in acute myelocytic leukemia. *J Lab Clin Med.* 1973;81:311–316.

3. Cline MJ. Defective mononuclear phagocytic function in patients with myelomonocytic leukemia and in some patients with lymphomas. *J Clin Invest.* 1973;52:2815–12190.

4. Hann I, Prentice HG, Blacklock HA, et al. Acyclovir prophylaxis against herpes virus infections in severely immunocompromised patients: randomised double blind trial. *Br Med J.* 1983;287:384–388.

5. The EORTC International Antimicrobial Therapy Project Group. Three antibiotic regimens in the treatment of infection in febrile granulocytopenic patients with cancer. *J Infect Dis.* 1978;137:14–29.

6. Cometta A, Zinner S, De Bock R, et al. Piperacillin–tazobactam plus amikacin as empiric therapy for fever in granulocytopenic patients with cancer. *Antimicrob Agents Chemother.* 1995;39:445–452.

7. Woo PCY, Wong SSY, Lum PNL, Hui W-T, Yuen K-Y. Cell-wall-deficient bacteria and culture-negative febrile episodes in bone-marrow-transplant recipients. *Lancet.* 2001;357:675–679.

8. Schimpff SC, Greene WH, Young VW, Wiernik PH. Significance of *Pseudomonas aeruginosa* in the patient with leukemia or lymphoma. *J Infect Dis.* 1974;130:S24–S31.

9. Bodey GP, Jadeja J, Elting L. Pseudomonas bacteremia. Retrospective analysis of 410 episodes. *Arch Intern Med.* 1985;145:1621–1629.

10. Bodey GP, Bueltmann B, Duguid W, et al. Fungal infections in cancer patients – an international autopsy survey. *Eur J Clin Microbiol.* 1992;11:99–109.

11. DeGregorio MW, Lee WMF, Linker CA, et al. Fungal infections in patients with acute leukemia. *Am J Med.* 1982;73:543–548.

12. Riley LC, Hann IM, Wheatley K, Stevens RF. Treatment-related deaths during induction and first remission of acute myeloid leukaemia in children treated on the Tenth Medical Research Council Acute Myeloid Leukaemia Trial (MRC AML 10). *Br J Haematol.* 1999;106:436–444.

13. Crippa F, Holmberg L, Carter RA, et al. Infectious complications after autologous CD34-selected peripheral blood stem cell transplantation. *Biol Blood Marrow Transplant.* 2002;8:281–289.

14. Manuel RJ, Kibbler CC. The epidemiology and prevention of invasive aspergillosis. *J Hosp Infect.* 1998;39:95–109.

15. Jameson B, Gamble DR, Lynch J, Kay HEM. Five-year analysis of protective isolation. *Lancet.* 1971;i:1034–1040.

16. Levine AS, Siegal SE, Schreiber AD, et al. Protected environments and prophylactic antibiotics. A prospective controlled study of their utility in the therapy of acute leukemia. *N Engl J Med.* 1973;288:477–483.

17. Yates JW, Holland JF. A controlled study of isolation and endogenous microbial suppression in acute myelocytic leukemia patients. *Cancer.* 1973;32:1490–1498.

18. Schimpff SC, Greene WH, Young VW, et al. Infection prevention in acute nonlymphocytic leukemia. Laminar air flow room reverse isolation with oral nonabsorbable antibiotic prophylaxis. *Ann Intern Med.* 1975;82:351–358.

19. Dietrich M, Gaus W, Vossen J, et al. Protective isolation and antimicrobial decontamination in patients with high susceptibility to infection. A prospective co-operative study of gnotobiotic care in acute leukemia patients. I. Clinical results. *Infections.* 1977;5:107–114.

20. Storring RA, Jameson B, McElwain TJ, Wiltshire E. Oral nonabsorbed antibiotics prevent infection in acute non-lymphoblastic leukaemia. *Lancet.* 1977;ii:837–840.

21. Rodriguez V, Bodey GP, Freireich EJ, et al. Randomized trial of protected environment prophylactic antibiotics in 145 adults with acute leukemia. *Medicine.* 1978;57:253–266.

22. Buckner CD, Clift RA, Sanders JE, et al. Protective environment for marrow transplant recipients. *Ann Intern Med.* 1978;89:893–901.

23. Bodey GP. Treatment of acute leukemia in protected environment units. *Cancer.* 1979;44:431–436.

24. Hughes WT, Price RA, Kim HK, et al. *Pneumocystis carinii* pneumonia in children with malignancies. *J Pediatr.* 1973;82:404–415.

25. Gurwith MJ, Brunton JL, Lank BL, et al. A prospective controlled investigation of prophylactic trimethoprim–sulfamethoxazole in hospitalized granulocytopenic patients. *Am J Med.* 1979;66:248–256.

26. Dekker AW, Rozenberg-Arska M, Sixma JJ, et al. Prevention of infection by trimethoprim–sulfamethoxazole plus amphotericin B in patients with acute nonlymphocytic leukemia. *Ann Intern Med.* 1981;95:555–559.

27. Wade JC, Schimpff SC, Hargadon MT, et al. A comparison of trimethoprim–sulfamethoxazole plus nystatin with gentamicin plus nystatin in the prevention of infections in acute leukemia. *N Engl J Med.* 1981;304:1057–1062.

28. EORTC International Antimicrobial Therapy Project Group. Trimethoprim–sulfamethoxazole in the prevention of infection in neutropenic patients. *J Infect Dis.* 1984;150:372–379.

29. Cruciani M, Rampazzo R, Malena M, et al. Prophylaxis with fluoroquinolones for bacterial infections in neutropenic patients: a meta-analysis. *Clin Infect Dis.* 1996;23:795–805.

30. Krcmery Jr V, Spanik S, Krupova I, Trupl J, Kunova A, Smid MPE. Bacteremia due to multiresistant gram-negative bacilli in neutropenic cancer patients: a case controlled study. *J Chemother.* 1998;10:320–325.

31. Prentice HG, Kibbler CC, Prentice AG. Towards a targeted, risk-based, antifungal strategy in neutropenic patients. *Br J Haematol.* 2000;110:273–284.

32. Gafter-Gvili A, Fraser A, Paul M, Leibovici L. Meta-analysis: antibiotic prophylaxis reduces mortality in neutropenic patients. *Ann Intern Med.* 2005;142:979–995.

33. Bucaneve G, Micozzi A, Menichetti F, et al. Levofloxacin to prevent bacterial infection in patients with cancer and neutropenia. *N Engl J Med.* 2005;353:977.

34. Cullen M, Steven N, Billingham L, et al. Antibacterial prophylaxis after chemotherapy for solid tumors and lymphomas. *N Engl J Med.* 2005;353:988.

35. Fanci R, Leoni F, Bosi A, et al. Chemoprophylaxis of bacterial infections in granulocytopenic patients with ciprofloxacin vs ciprofloxacin plus amoxicillin. *J Chemother.* 1993;5:119–123.

36. Kern WV, Hay B, Kern P, Marre R, Arnold R. A randomized trial of roxithromycin in patients with acute leukemia and bone marrow transplant recipients receiving fluoroquinolone prophylaxis. *Antimicrob Agents Chemother.* 1994;38:465–472.

37. Wimperis JZ, Baglin TP, Marcus RE, Warren RE. An assessment of the efficacy of antimicrobial prophylaxis in bone marrow autografts. *Bone Marrow Transplant.* 1991;8:363–367.

38. Bow EJ, Mandell LA, Louie TJ, et al. Quinolone-based antibacterial chemoprophylaxis in neutropenic patients: effect of augmented gram-positive activity on infectious morbidity. National Cancer Institute of Canada Clinical Trials Group. *Ann Intern Med.* 1996;125:183–190.

39. Odds FC. *Candida and candidosis.* 2nd ed. London: Baillière Tindall; 1988.

40. Hann IM, Corringham R, Keaney M, et al. Ketoconazole versus nystatin plus amphotericin B for fungal prophylaxis in severely immunocompromised patients. *Lancet.* 1982;i:826–829.

41. Hansen RM, Reinerio N, Sohnle PG, et al. Ketoconazole in the prevention of candidiasis in patients with cancer. A prospective, randomized, controlled, double-blind study. *Arch Intern Med.* 1987;147:710–712.

42. Winston DJ, Ho WG, Bartoni K, et al. Ganciclovir prophylaxis of cytomegalovirus infection and disease in allogeneic bone marrow transplant recipients. Results of a placebo-controlled, double-blind trial. *Ann Intern Med.* 1993;118:179–184.

43. Philpott-Howard JN, Wade JJ, Mufti GJ, Brammer KW, Ehninger G. Randomized comparison of oral fluconazole versus oral polyenes for the prevention of fungal infection in patients at risk of neutropenia. Multicentre Study Group. *J Antimicrob Chemother.* 1993;31:973–984.

44. Goodman JL, Winston DJ, Greenfield RA, et al. A controlled trial of fluconazole to prevent fungal infections in patients undergoing bone marrow transplantation. *N Engl J Med.* 1992;326:845–851.

45. Slavin MA, Osborne B, Adams R, et al. Efficacy and safety of fluconazole prophylaxis for fungal infections after marrow transplantation – a prospective, randomised, double-blind study. *J Infect Dis.* 1995;171:1545–1552.

46. Wingard JR, Merz WG, Rinaldi MG, et al. Increase in *Candida krusei* infection among patients with bone marrow transplantation and neutropenia treated prophylactically with fluconazole. *N Engl J Med.* 1991;325:1274–1277.

47. Morgenstern GR, Prentice AG, Prentice HG, Ropner JE, Schey SA, Warnock DW. A randomized controlled trial of itraconazole versus fluconazole for the prevention of fungal infections in patients with haematological malignancies. *Br J Haematol.* 1999;105:901–911.

48. Harousseau JL, Dekker A, Stamatoullas A, Bassaris H, Linkesch W, Fassas A. Prophylaxis of fungal infections in haematological malignancies: a double blind trial comparing itraconazole oral solution to amphotericin B capsules. *Antimicrob Agents Chemother*. 2000;44:1887–1893.

49. Menichetti F, Del Favero A, Martino P, et al. Itraconazole oral solution as prophylaxis for fungal infections in neutropenic patients with hematologic malignancies: a randomised, placebo-controlled, double blind, multicentre trial. GIMEMA infection programme. Groupo Italiano Malattie Ematologiche del Adulto. *Clin Infect Dis*. 1999;28:250–255.

50. Cornely O, Maertens J, Winston D, et al. Posaconazole vs. fluconazole or itraconazole prophylaxis in patients with neutropenia. *N Engl J Med*. 2007;356(4):348–359.

51. Ullmann A, Lipton J, Vesole D, et al. Posaconazole or fluconazole for prophylaxis in severe graft-versus-host disease. *N Engl J Med*. 2007;356:335–347.

52. van Burik JA, Ratnatharathorn V, Stepan DE, et al. Micafungin versus fluconazole for prophylaxis against invasive fungal infections during neutropenia in patients undergoing hematopoietic stem cell transplantation. *Clin Infect Dis*. 2004;39:1407–1416.

53. Meunier F. Prevention of mycoses in immunocompromised patients. *Rev Infect Dis*. 1987;9:408–416.

54. Jorgensen CJ, Dreyfus F, Vaixeler J, et al. Failure of amphotericin B spray to prevent aspergillosis in granulocytopenic patients. *Nouv Rev Fr Hématol*. 1989;31:327–328.

55. Conneally E, Cafferkey MT, Daly PA, et al. Nebulized amphotericin B as prophylaxis against invasive aspergillosis in granulocytopenic patients. *Bone Marrow Transplant*. 1990;5:403–406.

56. Myers SE, Devine SM, Topper RL, et al. A pilot study of prophylactic aerosolized amphotericin B in patients at risk for prolonged neutropenia. *Leuk Lymphoma*. 1992;8:229–233.

57. Schwartz S, Behre G, Heinemann V, et al. Aerosolized amphotericin B inhalations as a prophylaxis of invasive aspergillus infections during prolonged neutropenia: results of a prospective randomized multicenter trial. *Blood*. 1999;93:3654–3661.

58. Zaia JA. Viral infections associated with bone marrow transplantation. *Hematol Oncol Clin North Am*. 1990;4:603–623.

59. Wade JC. Management of infection in patients with acute leukemia. *Hematol Oncol Clin North Am*. 1993;1:293–315.

60. Prentice HG, Gluckman E, Powles RL, et al. Impact of long-term acyclovir on cytomegalovirus infection and survival after allogeneic bone marrow transplantation. European Acyclovir for CMV Prophylaxis Study Group. *Lancet*. 1994;343:749–753.

61. Goodrich JM, Bowden RA, Fisher L, et al. Ganciclovir prophylaxis to prevent cytomegalovirus disease after allogeneic marrow transplant. *Ann Intern Med*. 1993;118:173–178.

62. Einsele H, Steidle M, Vallbracht A, et al. Early occurrence of human cytomegalovirus infection after bone marrow transplantation as demonstrated by polymerase chain reaction technique. *Blood*. 1991;77:1104–1110.

63. Kidd M, Fox JC, Pillay D, et al. Provision of prognostic information in immunocompromised patients by routine application of the polymerase chain reaction for cytomegalovirus. *Transplantation*. 1993;56:867–871.

64. Goodrich JM, Mori M, Gleaves CA, et al. Prevention of cytomegalovirus disease after allogeneic marrow transplantation by early treatment with ganciclovir. *N Engl J Med*. 1991;325:1601–1607.

65. Paul M, Soares-Weiser K, Grozinsky S, Leibovici L. Beta-lactam versus beta-lactam aminoglycoside combination therapy in cancer patients with neutropaenia. *Cochrane Database Syst Rev*. 2003;3: CD003038.

66. Furno P, Bucaneve G, Del Favero A. Monotherapy or aminoglycoside containing combinations for empirical treatment of febrile neutropenic patients: a meta-analysi. *Lancet Infect Dis*. 2002;2(4):231–242.

67. Bodey GP, Buckley Valdivieso M, Feld R, Rodriguez V, McCredie K. Carbenicillin plus cephalothin or cefazolin as therapy for infections in neutropenic patients. *Am J Med Sci*. 1977;273:309–318.

68. Gurwith M, Brunton JL, Lank B, et al. Granulocytopenia in hospitalised patients. II. A prospective comparison of two antibiotic regimens in the empiric therapy of febrile patients. *Am J Med*. 1978;64:127–132.

69. Winston DJ, Barnes RC, Ho WG, et al. Moxalactam plus piperacillin versus moxalactam plus amikacin in febrile granulocytopenic patients. *Am J Med*. 1984;77:442–450.

70. Winston DJ, Ho WG, Bruckner DA, Gale RP, Champlin RE. Controlled trials of double beta-lactam therapy with cefoperazone plus piperacillin in febrile granulocytopenic patients. *Am J Med*. 1988;85(suppl IA):21–30.

71. Kibbler CC, Prentice HG, Sage RJ, et al. Do double beta-lactam combinations prolong neutropenia in patients undergoing chemotherapy or bone marrow transplantation for haematological disease? *Antimicrob Agents Chemother*. 1989;33(4):503–507.

72. Sanders JW, Powe NR, Moore RD. Ceftazidime monotherapy for empiric treatment of febrile neutropenic patients: a meta-analysis. *J Infect Dis*. 1991;164:907–916.

73. Liang R, Yung R, Chiu E, et al. Ceftazidime versus imipenem–cilastin as initial monotherapy for febrile neutropenic patients. *Antimicrob Agents Chemother*. 1990;34:1336–1341.

74. Rikonen P. Impenem compared with ceftazidime plus vancomycin as initial therapy for fever in neutropenic children with cancer. *Pediatr Infect Dis J*. 1991;10:918–923.

75. Cornelissen JJ, DeGraeff A, Verdonck LF, et al. Imipenem versus gentamicin combined with either cefuroxime or cephalothin as initial therapy for febrile neutropenic patients. *Antimicrob Agents Chemother*. 1992;36:801–807.

76. Rolston KV, Berkey P, Bodey GP, et al. A comparison of imipenem ceftazidime with or without amikacin as empiric therapy in febrile neutropenic patients. *Arch Intern Med*. 1992;152:283–291.

77. Cometta A, Calandra T, Gaya H, et al. Monotherapy with meropenem versus combination therapy with ceftazidime plus amikacin as empiric therapy for fever in granulocytopenic patients with cancer. *Antimicrob Agents Chemother*. 1996;40:1108–1115.

78. Kerr KG, Hawkey PM, Child JA, Norfolk DR, Anderson AW. *Pseudomonas maltophilia* infections in neutropenic patients and the use of imipenem. *Postgrad Med J*. 1990;66:1090.

79. McWhinney PHM, Kibbler CC, Prentice HG, et al. A prospective trial of imipenem versus ceftazidime/vancomycin as empirical therapy for fever in neutropenic patients. In: *Proceedings of the 17th International Congress of Chemotherapy, Berlin*. 1991 abstract 1276.

80. McWhinney PH, Patel S, Whiley RA, et al. Activities of potential therapeutic and prophylactic antibiotics against blood culture isolates of viridans group streptococci from neutropenic patients receiving ciprofloxacin. *Antimicrob Agents Chemother*. 1993;37:2493–2495.

81. Klastersky J. Science and pragmatism in the treatment and prevention of neutropenic infection. *J Antimicrob Chemother*. 1998;41(suppl D):13–24.

82. Yahav D, Paul M, Fraser A, et al. Efficacy and safety of cefepime: a systematic review and meta-analysis. *Lancet Infect Dis*. 2007;7(5):338–348.

83. Karp JE, Merz WG, Dick JD, Saral R. Strategies to prevent or control infections after bone marrow transplants. *Bone Marrow Transplant*. 1991;8:1–6.

84. Chow AW, Jewesson PJ, Kureishi A, Phillips GL. Teicoplanin versus vancomycin in the empirical treatment of febrile neutropenic patients. *Eur J Haematol*. 1993;51:18–24.

85. Ramphal R, Bolger M, Oblon DJ, et al. Vancomycin is not an essential component of the initial empiric treatment regimen for febrile neutropenic patients receiving ceftazidime: a prospective randomized study. *Antimicrob Agents Chemother*. 1992;36:1062–1067.

86. EORTC International Antimicrobial Therapy Cooperative Group and the National Cancer Institute of Canada – Clinical Trials Group. Vancomycin added to empirical combination antibiotic therapy for fever in granulocytopenic cancer patients. *J Infect Dis*. 1991;163:951–958.

87. Paul M, Borok S, Fraser A, Vidal L, Leibovici L. Empirical antibiotics against Gram-positive infections for febrile neutropenia: systematic review and meta-analysis of randomized controlled trials. *J Antimicrob Chemother*. 2005;55:436–444.

88. Shlaes DM, Binczewski B, Rice LB. Emerging antibiotic resistance and the immunocompromised host. *Clin Infect Dis*. 1993;17(suppl 2):S527–S536.

89. Handwerger S, Rancher B, Alterac D, et al. Outbreak due to *Enterococcus faecium* highly resistant to vancomycin, penicillin, and gentamicin. *Clin Infect Dis*. 1993;16:750–755.

90. Hughes WT, Armstrong D, Bodey GP, et al. guidelines for the use of antimicrobial agents in neutropenic patients with unexplained fever. *Clin Infect Dis*. 1997;25:551–573.

91. Bradley SJ, Wilson ALT, Allen MC, Sher HA, Goldstone AH, Scott GM. The control of hyperendemic glycopeptide-resistant *Enterococcus* spp. on a haematology unit by changing antibiotic usage. *J Antimicrob Chemother*. 1999;43:261–266.

92. Talcott JA, Siegel RD, Finberg R, Goldman L. Risk assessment in cancer patients with fever and neutropenia: a prospective, two-center validation of a prediction rule. *J Clin Oncol*. 1992;10:316–322.

93. Freifeld A, Marchigiani D, Walsh T, et al. A double-blind comparison of empirical oral and intravenous antibiotic therapy for low-risk febrile patients with neutropenia during cancer chemotherapy. *N Engl J Med.* 1999;341:305–311.

94. Kern WV, Cometta A, De Bock R, et al. for the International Antimicrobial Therapy Cooperative Group of the European Organization for Research and Treatment of Cancer. Oral versus intravenous empirical therapy for fever in patients with granulocytopenia who are receiving cancer chemotherapy. *N Engl J Med.* 1999;341:312–318.

95. Anonymous. Empiric antifungal therapy in febrile granulocytopenic patients. EORTC International Antimicrobial Therapy Cooperative Group. *Am J Med.* 1989;86:668–672.

96. Prentice HG, Hann IM, Herbrecht R, et al. A randomized comparison of liposomal versus conventional amphotericin B for the treatment of pyrexia of unknown origin in neutropenic patients. *Br J Haematol.* 1997;98:711–718.

97. Walsh TJ, Finberg RW, Arndt C, et al. Liposomal amphotericin B for empirical therapy in patients with persistent fever and neutropenia. *N Engl J Med.* 1999;340:764–771.

98. Winston DJ, Dudnick DV, Chapin M, et al. Coagulase-negative staphylococcal bacteremia in patients receiving immunosuppressive therapy. *Arch Intern Med.* 1983;143:32–36.

99. Bodey GP. Infection in cancer patients. A continuing association. *Am J Med.* 1986;81(suppl 1A):11–26.

100. Smith JG, Summerfield GP, Adam A, et al. BCSH guidelines on the insertion and management of central venous lines. *Br J Haematol.* 1997;98:1041–1047.

101. Berger LA. Imaging in the diagnosis of infections in immunocompromised patients. *Curr Opin in Infect Dis.* 1998;11:431–436.

102. Emanuel D, Cunningham I, Jules-Elysee K, et al. Cytomegalovirus pneumonia after bone marrow transplantation successfully treated with the combination of ganciclovir and high-dose intravenous immune globulin. *Ann Intern Med.* 1988;109:777–782.

103. Reed EC, Bowden RA, Dandliker PS, Lilleby KE, Meyers JD. Treatment of cytomegalovirus pneumonia with ganciclovir and intravenous cytomegalovirus immunoglobulin in patients with bone marrow transplants. *Ann Intern Med.* 1988;109:783–788.

104. Ljungman P, Engelhard D, Link H, et al. Treatment of interstitial pneumonitis due to cytomegalovirus with ganciclovir and intravenous immune globulin: experience of European Bone Marrow Transplant Group. *Clin Infect Dis.* 1992;14(4):831–835.

105. Harrington RD, Hooton TM, Hackman RC, et al. An outbreak of respiratory syncytial virus in a bone marrow transplant center. *J Infect Dis.* 1992;165:987–993.

106. Lin S-J, Schranz J, Teutsch SM. Aspergillus case-fatality rate: systematic review of the literature. *Clin Infect Dis.* 2001;32:358–366.

107. Tortorano AM, Peman J, Bernhardt H, et al. ECMM Working Group on Candidaemia. Epidemiology of candidaemia in Europe: results of 28-month European Confederation of Medical Mycology (ECMM) hospital-based surveillance study. *Eur J Clin Microbiol Infect Dis.* 2004;23(4):317–322.

108. Kibbler CC, Seaton S, Barnes RA, et al. Management and outcome of bloodstream infections due to *Candida* species in England and Wales. *J Hosp Infect.* 2003;54:18–24.

109. Ellis M, Spence D, De Pauw B, et al. An EORTC international multicenter randomized trial (EORTC number 1992) comparing two dosages of liposomal amphotericin B for treatment of invasive aspergillosis. *Clin Infect Dis.* 1998;27:1406–1412.

110. Cornely OA, Maertens J, Bresnik M, et al. AmBiLoad Trial Study Group. Liposomal amphotericin B as initial therapy for invasive mold infection: a randomized trial comparing a high-loading dose regimen with standard dosing (AmBiLoad trial). *Clin Infect Dis.* 2007;44:1289–1297.

111. Denning D, Ribaud P, Milpied N, et al. Efficacy and safety of voriconazole in the treatment of acute invasive aspergillosis. *Clin Infect Dis.* 2002;34:563–571.

112. Herbrecht R, Denning DW, Patterson TF, et al. Voriconazole versus amphotericin B for primary therapy of invasive aspergillosis. *N Engl J Med.* 2002;347:408–415.

113. Marr KA, Boeckh M, Carter RA, Kim HW, Corey L. Combination antifungal therapy for invasive aspergillosis. *Clin Infect Dis.* 2004;39:797–802.

114. Kibbler CC, Milkins SR, Bhamra A, et al. Apparent pulmonary mycetoma following invasive aspergillosis in neutropenic patients. *Thorax.* 1988;43:108–112.

115. Yeghen T, Kibbler CC, Prentice HG, et al. Management of invasive pulmonary aspergillosis in hematology patients: a review of 87 consecutive cases at a single institution. *Clin Infect Dis.* 2000;31:859–868.

116. Demetri GD, Antman KHS. Granulocyte–macrophage colony-stimulating factor (GMCSF): preclinical and clinical investigations. *Semin Oncol.* 1992;19:362–385.

117. Glaspy JA, Golde DW. Granulocyte colony-stimulating factor (GCSF): preclinical and clinical investigations. *Semin Oncol.* 1992;19:386–394.

118. Pettengell R, Gurney H, Radford JA, et al. Granulocyte colony-stimulating factor to prevent dose-limited neutropenia in non-Hodgkin's lymphoma: a randomized controlled trial. *Blood.* 1992;80:1430–1436.

119. Singer JW. Role of colony-stimulating factors in bone marrow transplantation. *Semin Oncol.* 1992;19:27–31.

120. Bodey GP, Anaissie E, Gutterman J, Vadhan-Raj S. Role of granulocyte–macrophage colony-stimulating factor as adjuvant therapy for fungal infection in patients with cancer. *Clin Infect Dis.* 1993;17:705–707.

121. Hubel K, Dale DC, Engbert A, Liles WC. Current status of granulocyte (neutrophil) transfusion therapy for infectious diseases. *J Infect Dis.* 2001;183(2):321–328.

122. Price TH, Bowden RA, Boeckh M, et al. Phase I/II trial of neutrophil transfusions from donors stimulated with G-CSF and dexamethasone for treatment of patients with infections in hematopoietic stem cell transplantation. *Blood.* 2000;95(11):3302–3309.

123. *OPTN/SRTR annual report.* Online Available at http://www.ustransplant.org; 2008.

124. Ascher NL. Immunosuppressant substitutes in liver transplantation. *Lancet.* 2001;357:571–572.

125. Torre-Cisneros J, Manez R, Kusne S, Alessiani M, Martin M, Starzl TE. The spectrum of aspergillosis in liver transplant patients: comparison of FK506 and cyclosporin immunosuppression. *Transplant Proc.* 1991;23:3040–3041.

126. Sakr M, Hassanein T, Gaveler J, et al. Cytomegalovirus infection of the upper gastrointestinal tract following liver transplantation: incidence, location and severity in cyclosporin and FK506 treated patients. *Transplantation.* 1992;53:786–791.

127. Kusne S, Fung J, Alessiani M, et al. Infections during a randomized trial comparing cyclosporine to FK506 immunosuppression in liver transplantation. *Transplant Proc.* 1992;24:429–430.

128. European FK506 Multicentre Liver Study Group. Randomised trial comparing tacrolimus (FK506) and cyclosporin in prevention of liver allograft rejection. *Lancet.* 1994;344:423–428.

129. Germani G, Pleguezuelo M, Villamil F, et al. Azathioprine in liver transplantation: a reevaluation of its use and a comparison with mycophenolate mofetil. *Am J Transplant.* 2009;9(8):1725–1731.

130. Gerolami R, Moal V, Colson P, Chronic hepatitis E. with cirrhosis in a kidney-transplant recipient. *N Engl J Med.* 2008;358:859–860.

131. George DL, Arnow PM, Fox AS, et al. Bacterial infection as a complication of liver transplantation: epidemiology and risk factors. *Rev Infect Dis.* 1991;13:387–396.

132. Kusne S, Dummer JS, Singh N, et al. Infections after liver transplantation. An analysis of 101 consecutive cases. *Medicine (Baltimore).* 1988;67:132–143.

133. Colonna JO, Winston DJ, Brill JE, et al. Infectious complications in liver transplantation. *Arch Surg.* 1988;123:360–364.

134. Paya CV, Hermans PE, Washington JA, et al. Incidence, distribution and outcome of episodes of infection in 100 orthotopic liver transplantations. *Mayo Clin Proc.* 1989;64:555–564.

135. Chang FY, Singh N, Gayowski T, Drenning SD, Wagener MM, Marino R. *Staphylococcus aureus* nasal colonisation and association with infections in liver transplant recipients. *Transplantation.* 1998;65:1169–1172.

136. Fernando ON, Higgins AF, Moorhead JF. Secondary haemorrhage after renal transplantation. *Lancet.* 1976;ii:368.

137. Weber TR, Freier DT, Turcotte JF. Transplantation of infected kidneys. *Transplantation.* 1979;27:63–65.

138. Nelson PW, Delmonicao FL, Tolkoff-Rubin NE, et al. Unsuspected donor Pseudomonas infection causing arterial disruption after renal transplantation. *Transplantation.* 1984;37:313–314.

139. Leaker B, Hellyar A, Neild GH, et al. Nocardia infection in a renal transplant unit. *Transplant Proc.* 1989;21:2103–2104.

140. Singh N, Paterson DL. *M. tuberculosis* infection in solid organ transplant recipients: impact and implications for management. *Clin Infect Dis.* 1998;27:1266–1277.

141. Rubin RH. Infection in the organ transplant recipient. In: Rubin RH, Young LS, eds. *Clinical approach to infection in the compromised host.* 3rd ed. New York: Plenum; 1994:629–705.

142. Patterson WJ, Hay J, Seal DV, McLuckie JC. Colonization of transplant unit water supplies with *Legionella* and protozoa: precautions required to reduce the risk of legionellosis. *J Hosp Infect.* 1997;37:7–17.

143. Paya CV. Fungal infections in solid organ transplantation. *Clin Infect Dis.* 1993;16:677–688.

144. Singh N. Infectious diseases in the liver transplant patient. *Semin Gastrointest Dis.* 1998;9:136–146.

145. Wajszczuk CP, Dummer JS, Ho M, et al. Fungal infections in liver transplant recipients. *Transplantation.* 1985;40:347–353.

146. Sepkowitz KA, Brown AE, Armstrong D. *Pneumocystis carinii* pneumonia without acquired immunodeficiency syndrome: more patients, same risk. *Arch Intern Med.* 1995;155:1125–1128.

147. Martinez AJ, Ahdab-Barmada M. The neuropathology of liver transplantation: comparison of main complications in children and adults. *Mod Pathol.* 1993;6:25–32.

148. Singh N, Yu VL, Gayowski T. Central nervous system lesions in adult liver transplant recipients – clinical review with implications for management. *Medicine.* 1994;73:110–118.

149. Bonham CA, Dominguez EA, Fukui MB, Paterson DL, Pankey GA, Wagener MM. Central nervous system lesions in liver transplant recipients: prospective assessment of indications for biopsy and implications for management. *Transplantation.* 1998;66:1596–1604.

150. Freifeld AG, Iwen PC, Lesiak BL, Gilroy RK, Stevens RB, Kalil AC. Histoplasmosis in solid organ transplant recipients at a large Midwestern university transplant center. *Transpl Infect Dis.* 2005;7(3–4):109–115.

151. Umana JP, Mutimer DJ, Shaw JC, et al. Cytomegalovirus surveillance following liver transplantation: does it allow presymptomatic diagnosis of CMV disease? *Transplant Proc.* 1992;24:2643–2645.

152. Ho M. Advances in understanding cytomegalovirus infection after transplantation. *Transplant Proc.* 1994;26:7–11.

153. Mustafa MM. Cytomegalovirus infection and disease in the immunocompromised host. *Pediatr Infect Dis J.* 1994;13:249–259.

154. Wright TL, Donegan E, Hsu HH, et al. Recurrent and acquired hepatitis C viral infection in liver transplant recipients. *Gastroenterology.* 1992;103:317–322.

155. Samuel D, Muller R, Alexander G. Liver transplantation in European patients with the hepatitis B surface antigen. *N Engl J Med.* 1993;329:1842–1847.

156. Rostaing L, Icart J, Durand D, et al. Clinical outcome of Epstein–Barr viraemia in transplant patients. *Transplant Proc.* 1993;25:2286–2287.

157. Rogers J, Singh N, Carrigan DR, et al. Clinical relevance of human herpesvirus-6 infection in liver transplant recipients: role in pathogenesis of fungal infections, neurologic complications and impact on outcome. In: *Program and abstracts of the 39th Interscience Conference on Antimicrobial Agents and Chemotherapy, San Francisco, USA.* 1999:457–472.

158. Dockrell DH, Mendez JC, Jones M, et al. Human herpesvirus 6 seronegativity before transplantation predicts the occurrence of fungal infection in liver transplant recipients. *Transplantation.* 1999;67:399–403.

159. Ragamey N, Tamm M, Wernli M, et al. Transmission of human herpesvirus 8 infection from renal-transplant donors to recipients. *N Engl J Med.* 1998;339:1358–1363.

160. Nickeleit V, Hirsch HH, Binet IF, et al. Polyomavirus infection of renal allograft recipients: from latent infection to manifest disease. *J Am Soc Nephrol.* 1999;10:1080–1089.

161. Gallino A, Maggioroni M, Kiowski W. Toxoplasmosis in heart transplant recipients. *Eur J of Clin Microbiol Infect Dis.* 1996;15:389–393.

162. Speirs GE, Hakim M, Wreghitt TG. Relative risk of donor transmitted *Toxoplasma gondii* infection in heart, liver and kidney transplant recipients. *Clin Transpl.* 1998;2:257–269.

163. Michaels MG, Wald ER, Fricker FJ, del Nido PJ, Armitage J. Toxoplasmosis in pediatric recipients of heart transplant. *Clin Infect Dis.* 1992;14:847–851.

164. Singer MA, Hagler WS, Grossniklaus HE. *Toxoplasma gondii* retinochoroiditis after liver transplantation. *Retina.* 1993;13:40–45.

165. Smith SD, Jackson RJ, Hannaken CJ, Wadowsky RM, Tzakis AG, Rowe ML. Selective decontamination in paediatric liver transplantation. A randomised prospective study. *Transplantation.* 1993;55:1306–1309.

166. Murphy OM, Gould FK. Prevention of nosocomial infection in solid organ transplantation. *J Hosp Infect.* 1999;42:177–183.

167. Tolkoff-Rubin NE, Cosimi AB, Russell PS, et al. A controlled study of trimethoprim–sulfamethoxazole prophylaxis of urinary tract infections in renal transplant recipients. *Rev Infect Dis.* 1982;4:614–618.

168. Fox BC, Sollinger HW, Belzer FO, et al. A prospective, randomized, double-blind study of trimethoprim–sulfamethoxazole for prophylaxis of infections in renal transplantation: clinical efficacy, absorption of trimethoprim–sulfamethoxazole, effects on the microflora, and the cost–benefit of prophylaxis. *Am J Med.* 1990;89:255–274.

169. Winston DJ, Pakrasi A, Busuttil RW. Prophylactic fluconazole in liver transplant recipients. A randomised, double-blind, placebo-controlled trial. *Ann Intern Med.* 1999;131:729–737.

170. Colby WD, Sharpe MD, Ghent CN, et al. Efficacy of itraconazole prophylaxis against systemic fungal infection in liver transplant recipients. In: *Program and abstracts of the 39th Interscience Conference on Antimicrobial Agents and Chemotherapy, San Francisco, USA;* 1999, Abstract 1650.

171. Gordon SM, LaRossa SP, Kalmadi S, et al. Should prophylaxis for *Pneumocystis carinii* pneumonia in solid organ transplant recipients ever be discontinued? *Clin Infect Dis.* 1999;28:240–246.

172. Anonymous. Cytomegalovirus. *Am J Transplant.* 2004;4(suppl 10):51–58.

173. Kakazato PZ, Burns W, Moore P, Garcia-Kennedy R, Cox K, Esquivel C. Viral prophylaxis in hepatic transplantation: preliminary report of a randomized trial of acyclovir and ganciclovir. *Transplant Proc.* 1993;25:1935–1937.

174. Martin M. Antiviral prophylaxis for CMV infection in liver transplantation. *Transplant Proc.* 1993;25(suppl 4):10–14.

175. Hopt UT, Pfeffer F, Schareck W, Busing M, Ming C. Ganciclovir for prophylaxis of CMV disease after pancreas/kidney transplantation. *Transplant Proc.* 1994;26:434–435.

176. Singh N, Yu VL, Mieles L, et al. High-dose acyclovir compared with short-course preemptive ganciclovir therapy to prevent cytomegalovirus disease in liver transplant recipients: a randomized trial. *Ann Intern Med.* 1994;120:375–381.

177. Kusne S, Grossi P, Irish W, et al. Cytomegalovirus PP65 antigenaemia monitoring as a guide for preemptive therapy: a cost effective strategy for prevention of cytomegalovirus disease in adult liver transplant recipients. *Transplantation.* 1999;68:1125–1131.

178. Dodson SF, Balart LA, Shakil O, et al. Lack of efficacy of lamivudine for HBV infection after liver transplantation. *Hepatology.* 1998;28:262A.

179. Sawyer RG, Crabtree TD, Gleason TD, et al. Impact of solid organ transplantation and immunosuppression on fever, leukocytosis and physiologic response during bacterial and fungal infections. *Clin Transpl.* 1999;13:260–265.

180. Graybill J, Loebenberg R, Bocanegra R, Najvar L. Granulocyte colony stimulating factor (G-CSF) and azole antifungal therapy in murine aspergillosis: surprises. In: *Program and abstracts of the 38th International Conference on Antimicrobial Agents and Chemotherapy, San Diego, USA;* 1998.

181. Cockfield SM, Preiksatis JK, Jewell LD, Parfrey NA. Post-transplant lymphoproliferative disorder in renal allograft recipients. *Transplantation.* 1993;56:88–96.

182. Strauss SE, Cohen JI, Tosato G, et al. Epstein–Barr virus infection: biology, pathogenesis, and management. *Ann Intern Med.* 1993;118:45–58.

183. Nalesnik MA, Starzl TE. Epstein–Barr virus, infectious mononucleosis, and posttransplant lymphoproliferative disorders. *Transplant Sci.* 1994;4:61–79.

184. Papadopoulos EB, Ladanyi M, Emanuel D, et al. Infusions of donor leukocytes to treat Epstein–Barr virus-associated lymphoproliferative disorders after allogeneic bone marrow transplantation. *N Engl J Med.* 1994;330:1185–1191.

185. Frey NV, Tsai DE. The management of posttransplant lymphoproliferative disorder. *Med Oncol.* 2007;24:125–136.

 Further information

American Society of Clinical Oncology. http://www.asco.org.

Apperley J, Carreras E, Gluckman E, Gratwohl A, Masszi T. *Haematopoietic stem cell transplantation. The EBMT Handbook.* 5th ed. Paris: European Society of Hypertension; 2008.

Brammer KW. Management of fungal infection in neutropenic patients with fluconazole. *Hamatol Bluttransfus.* 1990;33:546–550.

British Committee for Standards in Haematology (BCSH). *Guidelines on the management of invasive fungal infection during therapy for haematological malignancy.* London: BCSH; 2008. Online Available at http://www.bcshguidelines.com/pdf/IFI_therapy.pdf.

British Transplantation Society. *Standards for solid organ transplantation in the United Kingdom.* 2nd ed. Macclesfield, Cheshire: BTS; 2003.

Calandra T, Zinner SH, Viscoli C, et al. Efficacy and toxicity of single daily doses of amikacin and ceftriaxone versus multiple daily doses of amikacin and ceftazidime for infection in patients with cancer and granulocytopenia. *Ann Intern Med.* 1993;119:584–593.

Castaldo P, Stratta RJ, Wood RP, et al. Clinical spectrum of fungal infections after orthotopic liver transplantation. *Arch Surg.* 1991;126:149–156.

Castaldo P, Stratta RJ, Wood RP, et al. Fungal infections in liver allograft recipients. *Transplant Proc.* 1991;23:1967.

De Pauw BE, Deresinski SC, Feld R, et al. Ceftazidime compared with piperacillin and tobramycin for the empiric treatment of fever in neutropenic patients with cancer – a multicenter randomized trial. *Ann Intern Med.* 1994;120:834–844.

Donnelly JP, Maschmeyer G, Daenen S. Selective oral antimicrobial prophylaxis for the prevention of infection in acute leukaemia – ciprofloxacin versus co-trimoxazole plus colistin. *Eur J Cancer.* 1992;28A:873–878.

ECIL-3 (3rd European Conference on Infections in Leukemia) update of the ECIL-1 guidelines for antifungal therapy in leukemia patients. September 25–26, 2009. Juan-les-Pins, France: 2009.

Eickhoff TC, Olin DB, Anderson RJ, et al. Current problems and approaches to diagnosis of infection in renal transplant recipients. *Transplant Proc.* 1972;4:693–697.

EORTC International Antimicrobial Therapy Group. Ceftazidime combined with a short or long course of amikacin for empirical therapy of Gram-negative bacteremia in cancer patients with granulocytopenia. *N Engl J Med.* 1987;317:1692–1698.

Fisher BD, Armstrong D, Yu B, Gold JW. Invasive aspergillosis: progress in early diagnosis and treatment. *Am J Med.* 1981;71:571–577.

Fishman, JA. Infection in solid organ transplant recipients. *N Engl J Med.* 2007;357:2601.

GIMENA Infection Program. Prevention of bacterial infection in neutropenic patients with hematologic malignancies. A randomized multicenter trial comparing norfloxacin with ciprofloxacin. *Ann Intern Med.* 1991;115:7–12.

Green H, Paul M, Vidal L, Leibovici L. Prophylaxis for Pneumocystis pneumonia (PCP) in non-HIV immunocompromised patients. *Cochrane Database Syst Rev.* 2007;(3) CD005590.

Hawkins C, Armstrong D. Fungal infections in the immunocompromised host. *Clin Haematol.* 1984;13:599–630.

Hughes WT, Rivera GK, Schell MJ, Thornton D, Lott L. Successful intermittent chemoprophylaxis for *Pneumocystis carinii* pneumonitis. *N Engl J Med.* 1987;316(26):1627–1632.

Infectious Diseases Society of America (IDSA). Guidelines for preventing opportunistic infections among hematopoietic stem cell transplant recipients. *Morb Mortal Wkly Rep.* 2000;49(RR-10).

Kern WV. Epidemiology of fluoroquinolone-resistant *Escherichia coli* among neutropenic patients. *Clin Infect Dis.* 1998;27:235–237.

Kibbler CC, Prentice HG, Sage RJ, et al. A comparison of double beta-lactam combinations with netilmicin/ureidopenicillin regimens in the empirical therapy of febrile neutropenic patients. *J Antimicrob Chemother.* 1989;23:759–771.

Kirby RM, McMaster P, Clements D, et al. Orthotopic liver transplantation: postoperative complications and their management. *Br J Surg.* 1987;74:3–11.

Klastersky J, Glauser MP, Schimpff SC, Gaya H. Antimicrobial Therapy Project Group for Research on Treatment of Cancer. Prospective randomised comparison of three antibiotic regimens for empirical therapy of suspected bacteremic infection in febrile granulocytopenic patients. *Antimicrob Agents Chemother.* 1986;29:263–270.

Majeski JA, Alexander JW, First MR, et al. Transplantation of microbially contaminated cadaver kidneys. *Arch Surg.* 1982;117:221–224.

McCoy GC, Loening S, Braun WE, et al. The fate of cadaver renal allografts contaminated before transplantation. *Transplantation.* 1975;20:467–472.

McWhinney PH, Kibbler CC, Hamon MD, et al. Progress in the diagnosis and management of aspergillosis in bone marrow transplantation: 13 years' experience. *Clin Infect Dis.* 1993;17:397–404.

Mills W, Chopra R, Linch DC, Goldstone AH. Liposomal amphotericin B in the treatment of fungal infections in neutropenic patients: a single-centre experience of 133 episodes in 116 patients. *Br J Haematol.* 1994;86:754–760.

Montgomery JR, Barrett FF, Williams Jr TW. Infectious complications in cardiac transplant patients. *Transplant Proc.* 1973;5:1239–1243.

National Comprehensive Cancer Network (NCCN). Clinical practice guidelines in oncology Online Available at http://www.nccn.org.

Pizzo PA, Commers J, Cotton D, et al. Approaching the controversies in the antibacterial management of cancer patients. *Am J Med.* 1984;76:436–449.

Pizzo PA, Hathorn JW, Hiemenz J, et al. A randomised trial comparing ceftazidime alone with combination antibiotic therapy in cancer patients with fever and neutropenia. *N Engl J Med.* 1986;315:552–558.

Pizzo PA, Rubin M, Freifeld A, Walsh TJ. The child with cancer and infection. I. Empiric therapy for fever and neutropenia, and preventive strategies. *J Pediatr.* 1991;119:679–694.

Schroter GPJ, Hoelscher M, Putnam CW, Porter KA, Starzl TE. Fungus infections after liver transplantation. *Ann Surg.* 1977;186:115–122.

Shenep JL, Hughes WT, Roberson PK, et al. Vancomycin, ticarcillin, and amikacin compared with ticarcillin–clavulanate and amikacin in the empirical treatment of febrile, neutropenic children with cancer. *N Engl J Med.* 1988;319:1053–1058.

The International Antimicrobial Therapy Project Cooperative Group of the European Organization for Research and Treatment of Cancer. Efficacy and toxicity of single daily doses of amikacin and ceftriaxone versus multiple daily doses of amikacin and ceftazidime for infection in patients with cancer and granulocytopenia. *Ann Intern Med.* 1993;119:584–593.

Viviani MA, Tortorano AM, Malaspina C, et al. Surveillance and treatment of liver transplant recipients for candidiasis and aspergillosis. *Eur J Epidemiol.* 1992;8:433–436.

Winston DJ, Chandrasekar PH, Lazarus HM, et al. Fluconazole prophylaxis of fungal infections in patients with acute leukemia. Results of a randomized placebo-controlled, double-blind, multicenter trial. *Ann Intern Med.* 1993;118:495–503.

Working Party of the British Society for Antimicrobial Chemotherapy. Chemoprophylaxis for candidosis and aspergillosis in neutropenia and transplantation: a review and recommendation. *J Antimicrob Chemother.* 1993;32:5–21.

Yale SH, Limper AH. *Pneumocystis carinii* pneumonia in patients without acquired immunodeficiency syndrome: associated illness and prior corticosteroid therapy. *Mayo Clin Proc.* 1996;71(1):5–13.

41 Infections in intensive care patients

Mark G. Thomas and Stephen J. Streat

Infection is a common reason for admission to an intensive care unit (ICU) and a common complication of stay in such units. Approximately one in three patients in the ICU will have an infection. Approximately half of these are acquired before admission to the ICU, usually before admission to hospital.[1,2] Community-acquired infection is common in pediatric and adult medical and surgical ICUs but infrequent in neonatal and cardiac surgical ICUs.[1] Between 2000 and 2008, 1131 patients with sepsis were admitted to the adult ICU in our hospital in Auckland, New Zealand. These patients comprised 14.8% of the 7640 ICU admissions but used 22.8% of ICU hours and accounted for 19.3% of the 866 ICU deaths over the 9-year period. Most received ventilatory (61%) or inotropic (84%) support; only 10% received neither form of support. Renal replacement therapy was given to 8.7%. Their overall mortality within the ICU was 14.8%. Table 41.1 shows the number of ICU admissions for all septic sites or sources together with the mean age, length of ICU stay and ICU survival for each site. The most common sites of infection were intraperitoneal from a gastrointestinal source (35.5% of admissions), respiratory tract (22%), urinary tract (13.9%), soft-tissue infections (8.1%), bacteremia with an unknown source (6.1%) and meninges (4.6%). ICU survival varied by septic site, being excellent for brain abscess (100%), meningitis (96%), genital tract infection (96%) and endovascular infection (94%), and good for urinary tract infection (90%), soft-tissue infection (90%), gastrointestinal-source infection (89%) and infections in joints and bone (86%). Survival was poorer for respiratory infection (75%), bacteremia (74%) and for infections in other less common sites (73%). ICU admissions for sepsis continue to rise while their survival is improving very slowly (at 1% per year). The reasons for the improvement in ICU mortality for sepsis are not clear and are likely to be multifactorial – including perhaps earlier attention to shock resuscitation,[3] surgical source control[4] and appropriate empirical antibiotic therapy. Currently, the total cost per ICU survivor of treating all patients with sepsis is approximately NZ$21 333 (£8750).

Approximately half the infections present in patients in an ICU are acquired following admission to the unit. Richards et al[5] found six nosocomial infections per 100 patients in medical–surgical ICUs in the USA, while 21% of patients in European ICUs had nosocomial infections. The most important sites of nosocomial infection in these patients are the respiratory tract, the urinary tract and the bloodstream (Table 41.2). The spectrum of organisms responsible for infections acquired in the ICU differs from that causing community-acquired infections: *Neisseria meningitidis* and *Streptococcus pneumoniae* are important causes of community-acquired infection in adults[6] but are unusual causes of ICU-acquired infection; enteric Gram-negative

Table 41.1 Admissions with infection to the Department of Critical Care Medicine, Auckland City Hospital, during the period 2000–2008

Septic site/ source	Number of admissions	Mean age (years)	Mean length of stay (days)	ICU survival (%)
Gastrointestinal	402	61	4.5	89
Respiratory	249	53	4.7	75
Urinary tract	157	58	2.9	90
Soft tissues	92	51	4.6	90
Bacteremia (unknown source)	69	47	3.4	74
Meninges	52	38	2.5	96
Joints/bone	29	65	4.3	86
Genital	24	43	1.5	96
Endovascular and endocarditis	16	52	2.3	94
Epidural abscess	16	54	8.1	75
Brain (abscess, ventriculitis)	11	45	2.7	100
Vascular line-related	9	50	1.3	78
Mediastinum	3	56	1	67
CAPD peritonitis	2	75	2.6	50
Total	**1131**	**56**	**4.1**	**85**

CAPD, continuous ambulatory peritoneal dialysis.

Table 41.2 Site of nosocomial infection in intensive care units[a]

	Study	
	Vincent et al[2]	Richards et al[5]
Total no. of infections	2485	29041
Site of infection (%)		
Respiratory tract	54	37
Genitourinary tract	15	23
Wound	6	8
Gastrointestinal	4	4
Bacteremia	10	14
Skin	4	3
Other	8	11

[a]Infection at each site as a proportion of total infection rate.

bacilli, *Staphylococcus aureus* and *Staphylococcus epidermidis* are responsible for most nosocomial ICU infections.[2,7]

The presence of infection in patients in the ICU is an important risk factor for increased mortality and morbidity.[8] Infection on admission to the ICU and nosocomial intra-abdominal infection have been shown to be independently predictive of fatality, after allowing for other variables such as acute physiology (APACHE score) or the use of steroids or chemotherapy.[9] Commonly death is due to inadequate treatment of a nosocomial infection (often caused by an unusually resistant organism) following successful treatment of a community-acquired infection.[10]

In recent decades the incidence of infection due to multidrug resistant organisms (MROs) has begun to outstrip the pharmaceutical industry's ability to develop effective new antimicrobial agents. This has led to increased interest in practices that can limit the spread of infection within the ICU. Routine screening, on admission and then weekly, to detect colonization with MROs such as methicillin-resistant *Staph. aureus* (MRSA), extended spectrum β-lactamase (ESBL)-positive Enterobacteriaceae, *Acinetobacter* spp. and vancomycin-resistant enterococci (VRE), linked to enhanced infection control precautions, can reduce the incidence of infection due to these MROs within the ICU. The dramatic reduction in central venous-line-associated infection that follows consistent application of infection control procedures is an excellent illustration of the opportunities to reduce nosocomial infection within the ICU. Prescribing practices within the ICU inevitably contribute to the selection of resistant organisms in ICU patients and provide an influential exemplar for the rest of the hospital. ICU prescribing guidelines should contribute to a hospital-wide policy of prudent antimicrobial stewardship.

PNEUMONIA

Pneumonia (Ch. 45) is a common reason for admission to the ICU and among the most common nosocomial infections in patients in these units. Both community-acquired and nosocomial pneumonia have a high mortality and management is complicated by the need to cover a wide range of pathogens.

COMMUNITY-ACQUIRED PNEUMONIA

The presence of clinical features such as tachypnea (>30/min), hypotension (systolic BP <90 and/or diastolic BP <60 mmHg), confusion, multilobar involvement, hypoxemia (Pao_2/Fio_2 <250) and renal impairment (serum creatinine >180 µmol/L) can help identify patients with severe community-acquired pneumonia.[11,12] *Str. pneumoniae, Staph. aureus, Haemophilus influenzae*, enteric Gram-negative bacilli and *Legionella pneumophila* are the most commonly identified bacterial causes of community-acquired pneumonia in patients admitted to the ICU (Table 41.3). It seems likely that *Str. pneumoniae* is the etiological agent for many patients in whom no microbial cause can be proven. Enteric Gram-negative bacilli, particularly *Pseudomonas aeruginosa* and *Klebsiella pneumoniae*, are uncommon causes of community-acquired pneumonia in patients admitted to the ICU, but are associated with a mortality of 50–75%, in contrast to an overall mortality of 20–50%.[17,18]

The clinical presentation is usually an unreliable guide to the etiology of community-acquired pneumonia,[18–20] and initial treatment will often need to cover the most common pathogens. Occasionally the clinical features on admission may provide useful clues to the etiology. For example, a history of chronic respiratory disease, alcoholism, immunosuppression or bronchiectasis should alert the doctor to the possibility that the pneumonia is due to an enteric Gram-negative bacillus. Other clues to a specific diagnosis include admission during an epidemic due to mycoplasma or influenza. During an influenza epidemic, secondary infection with *Staph. aureus* should be suspected. The admission radiographic findings in patients admitted with pneumonia usually do not allow a reliable discrimination between the various possible etiologies. Sputum Gram stain suggests the etiology in approximately 10% of patients, while sputum culture and blood culture are diagnostic in 12–44% and 10–35%, respectively.[13,17,19] Urinary antigen tests for *Str. pneumoniae* and *L. pneumophila* serogroup 1 should be performed on all patients with community-acquired pneumonia admitted to the ICU. Although a variety of methods (including fiberoptic

Table 41.3 Etiology of community-acquired pneumonia in intensive care units

	BTS[13]	Moine et al[14]	Leroy et al[15]	Oleacha et al[16]
Total no. of patients	185	132	299	262
Organism (%)				
Streptococcus pneumoniae	22	33	27	11
Staphylococcus aureus	9	4	19	4
Haemophilus influenzae	4	11	8	4
Enteric Gram-negative bacilli	2	11	18	3
Legionella pneumophila	18	3	0	8
Unknown	32	28	34	41

bronchoscopy with protected brush sampling or bronchoalveolar lavage; percutaneous lung aspiration with ultra-thin needles) have been proposed to increase the rate of microbiological diagnosis, none has entered routine clinical practice. Bronchoscopy with bronchoalveolar lavage should at present be reserved for selected patients, such as those in whom infection with *Mycobacterium tuberculosis*, *Pneumocystis jirovecii* (formerly *Pneumocystis carinii*) or cytomegalovirus is thought likely.

TREATMENT

An essential goal of treatment of severe community-acquired pneumonia is to ensure adequate activity against *Str. pneumoniae*, the most common cause of death in such patients. The rapid dissemination of penicillin-non-susceptible *Str. pneumoniae* has raised concern about the role of penicillins and cephalosporins in the treatment of disease due to this organism. However, high-dose intravenous therapy with many β-lactams provides serum levels well in excess of the minimum inhibitory concentrations (MICs) of non-susceptible strains of *Str. pneumoniae*, and (with the exception of rare strains for which the MIC of penicillin is greater than 4 mg/L) cure rates for non-susceptible strains are comparable to those seen with susceptible strains. At present, therefore, it does not appear necessary to include vancomycin in empirical regimens for the treatment of severe community-acquired pneumonia.

Because *L. pneumophila* may cause severe community-acquired pneumonia, treatment with a macrolide (e.g. erythromycin, clarithromycin or azithromycin) or a 'respiratory' fluoroquinolone (e.g. levofloxacin, gatifloxacin or moxifloxacin) is widely considered an essential component of the initial antimicrobial regimen.[20,21] Both of these classes of antimicrobial agent possess the advantages of providing activity against other common respiratory pathogens. Macrolides have useful activity against *Str. pneumoniae*, *Mycoplasma pneumoniae*, *Chlamydophila* (*Chlamydia*) *pneumoniae* and, to a variable degree, *H. influenzae*, while the 'respiratory' quinolones are active against *Str. pneumoniae* (including penicillin non-susceptible strains), *M. pneumoniae*, *C. pneumoniae* and enteric Gram-negative bacilli. Two recent North American guidelines have recommended a combination of a group 4 (third-generation) cephalosporin (e.g. ceftriaxone or cefotaxime) or a penicillin with a penicillinase inhibitor (e.g. amoxicillin–clavulanate or ampicillin–sulbactam), together with a macrolide or a 'respiratory' quinolone for most patients in the ICU with community-acquired pneumonia.[20,21] It seems likely that a group 3 (second-generation) cephalosporin (such as cefuroxime), given in high doses, would provide comparable efficacy for pneumococcal pneumonia and only marginally less efficacy against enteric Gram-negative bacilli. Units that wish to limit their use of group 4 cephalosporins may consider replacing this component of the regimen with high-dose cefuroxime. Patients whose initial sputum (or tracheal aspirate)

Gram stain suggests infection due to enteric Gram-negative bacilli should be treated with a regimen with enhanced antipseudomonal activity (e.g. ceftazidime or gentamicin, combined with a fluoroquinolone). Patients with suspected or proven anaerobic infection should be treated with clindamycin or a penicillin with a penicillinase inhibitor.

NOSOCOMIAL PNEUMONIA

Ventilator-associated pneumonia (VAP) is a common nosocomial infection in the ICU:[1-5] in patients ventilated for more than 48 h the incidence of pneumonia is approximately 20% with an associated mortality of 40–60%.[22-24] Ventilator-associated pneumonia remains a diagnostic and therapeutic dilemma, pneumonia can be diagnosed with certainty in a minority of patients in whom it is suspected, the pathogen(s) responsible for pneumonia are often uncertain, and the outcome is poor despite aggressive investigation and antibiotic treatment.[22] Furthermore, ventilator-associated pneumonia is frequently a marker of terminal illness rather than an independently important cause of death, and most of the deaths associated with this condition cannot be attributed to it.[25,26]

Aspiration of oropharyngeal secretions is the usual route of acquiring lung infection. Impaired consciousness, immobility, the presence of endotracheal and nasogastric tubes, and tracheostomies all increase the risk of aspiration and the incidence of pneumonia. The organisms aspirated into the lungs reflect those present in the oropharynx and stomach. Following admission to the ICU, the oropharynx and stomach become increasingly colonized with enteric Gram-negative bacilli. Thus, aspiration of oropharyngeal secretions at the onset of the illness or injury which leads to ICU admission commonly result in pneumonia due to methicillin-sensitive *Staph. aureus*, *Str. pneumoniae* or *H. influenzae*, while aspiration occurring 3 or more days after admission to the unit is more likely to be due to enteric Gram-negative bacilli or MRSA.[27,28]

DIAGNOSIS

Diagnosis of pneumonia in patients in the ICU, particularly those who are being ventilated, may be difficult. Although fever, leukocytosis, hypoxemia, purulent sputum and the presence of pathogenic bacteria in the tracheobronchial secretions will raise concerns about the possibility of pneumonia, these clinical features are more commonly present in the absence of pneumonia. A simple assessment based on these clinical features can effectively identify patients with a low risk of pneumonia who do not require intensive or prolonged antimicrobial therapy.[29]

Because the organisms responsible for causing nosocomial pneumonia in ICU patients are commonly derived from those colonizing the oropharynx, the use of sputum or tracheal aspirates to identify the causative organism(s) is hampered by the problem of distinguishing between contaminants and true pathogens. A variety of techniques, including transthoracic aspiration and bronchoscopy with sampling by bronchoalveolar lavage or protected specimen brush, have been evaluated, but none has been shown consistently to lower mortality rates.[24,27,30]

Gram-negative enteric bacilli, *Staph. aureus*, *Str. pneumoniae* and *H. influenzae* are the pathogens most commonly responsible for ventilator-associated pneumonia. In one study of 168 patients with bacteremic nosocomial pneumonia, the organisms isolated from blood cultures were members of the *Klebsiella–Enterobacter–Serratia* family (26%), *Ps. aeruginosa* (13%), *Escherichia coli* (8%), other aerobic Gram-negative organisms (8%), *Staph. aureus* (23%), *Str. pneumoniae* (11%) and other Gram-positive organisms (10%).[31] Polymicrobial bacteremia, most commonly with *Staph. aureus*, *K. pneumoniae* or *Ps. aeruginosa*, occurred in 10% of episodes.

TREATMENT

Nosocomial pneumonia should be treated with an agent or combination of agents that covers this spectrum of pathogens. Occasionally, previous consistent isolation of a pathogen from surveillance cultures of the patient's sputum will assist with selection of an antibiotic regimen. Similarly, the knowledge that *H. influenzae* and *Staph. aureus* are much more likely to cause pneumonia in a patient who has not recently received antibiotic therapy, and that *Ps. aeruginosa* is a particularly common cause in patients who have received prior antibiotic therapy,[32] can assist with antibiotic selection. Finally, the occurrence of endemic or epidemic transmission of a nosocomial pathogen within the ICU may need to be considered.

The combination of an aminoglycoside plus a third-generation cephalosporin or a broad-spectrum penicillin have been most commonly recommended for initial treatment of nosocomial pneumonia in the ICU.[33,34] These regimens have been selected on the basis of having adequate activity against the usual spectrum of pathogens plus *Ps. aeruginosa* because of the especially high mortality associated with pneumonia due to this organism. In ICUs where *Ps. aeruginosa* and other multiresistant organisms are unusual causes of ventilator-associated pneumonia, a less broad-spectrum regimen may be used (e.g. a combination of an aminoglycoside with cefuroxime or amoxicillin–clavulanic acid). Concern about the nephrotoxicity and ototoxicity associated with aminoglycoside therapy has led to the use of regimens in which ciprofloxacin or aztreonam is substituted for the aminoglycoside. However, aztreonam lacks activity against Gram-positive organisms and generally should be used in combination with another agent with Gram-positive activity such as clindamycin, vancomycin or flucloxacillin.

Ceftazidime, imipenem–cilastatin, ciprofloxacin and a number of other agents have been evaluated as monotherapy for nosocomial pneumonia. Ceftazidime, imipenem–cilastatin and ticarcillin–clavulanic acid have all given high cure rates in patients with ventilator-associated pneumonia.[33–39] In contrast, monotherapy with ciprofloxacin or pefloxacin has been associated with unacceptably high failure rates.[40,41] None of the monotherapy regimens evaluated was adequate treatment for pneumonia due to *Pseudomonas* spp. Persistent infection during treatment, development of resistance to the agent used, and clinical failure of monotherapy, occasionally with an improved response when a second agent was added to the regimen, were common problems when *Pseudomonas* pneumonia was treated with any of the monotherapy regimens. Although the overall outcome of monotherapy is similar to that of combination therapy,[42] pneumonia known or suspected to be caused by *Ps. aeruginosa* (or by *Enterobacter* or *Serratia* spp.) should be treated with a combination regimen.

The patient in the ICU with a nosocomial pneumonia should usually be treated initially with a broad-spectrum cephalosporin (e.g. cefuroxime, ceftriaxone or cefotaxime) or penicillin (e.g. amoxicillin–clavulanate) plus an aminoglycoside. In patients in whom infection with *Pseudomonas* is more likely (e.g. those who have had a prolonged ICU stay plus prior antibiotic therapy), an aminoglycoside plus a β-lactam with activity against *Pseudomonas* (e.g. ceftazidime) should be used. A macrolide or quinolone should be a component of the regimen in hospitals experiencing epidemic or endemic infection with *Legionella* spp. Treatment should be modified on the basis of the microbiology results, for example to flucloxacillin or vancomycin in patients with staphylococcal infection, or to amoxicillin or cefuroxime alone in patients with infection due to a sensitive *Esch. coli*. Treatment can often be discontinued after 5–7 days but ventilator-associated pneumonia due to *Ps. aeruginosa* should be treated for at least 14 days.

INTRA-ABDOMINAL INFECTION

Intra-abdominal infection (Ch. 39) is a common important cause of sepsis in the ICU, especially in those units with surgical patients. Although the overall mortality of patients with severe generalized peritonitis or abdominal abscess(es), the most common intra-abdominal infections in the ICU, has variously been reported as being between 30% and 60%,[43,44] our recent experience (*see* Table 41.1) suggests that this is now overly pessimistic.

MICROBIOLOGY

The organisms responsible for intra-abdominal sepsis vary with the source of infection. Peritonitis secondary to contamination by intestinal contents usually results in a polymicrobial mixed aerobic and anaerobic infection, with *Bacteroides fragilis* and *Esch. coli* the most commonly isolated species.[45] Spontaneous bacterial peritonitis is usually a monomicrobial infection. *Esch. coli*, *K. pneumoniae* and Gram-positive cocci are the usual pathogens. Anaerobes are rarely present.[46] Tertiary peritonitis, which occurs in severely ill patients following laparotomy, and which is not usually associated with peritoneal contamination by intestinal contents, is often monomicrobial and commonly due to *Staph. epidermidis*, *Enterococcus* spp., *Enterobacter* spp., *Pseudomonas* spp. or *Candida albicans*.[47]

 ## TREATMENT

Antimicrobial therapy, other than brief perioperative prophylaxis, is not necessary either in patients with peritoneal contamination without infection (e.g. gastroduodenal ulcer perforation operated on within 24 h of onset) or in patients in whom a localized infectious process is treated by excision (e.g. acute suppurative appendicitis, simple acute cholecystitis and ischemic bowel without perforation). Peritonitis following contamination of the peritoneal cavity usually should be treated with a regimen active against enteric Gram-negative bacilli and anaerobes. An agent active against *Staph. aureus* should be used in patients with peritonitis following gastric perforation. A combination of an aminoglycoside (e.g. gentamicin or tobramycin) with an anti-anaerobic agent (e.g. metronidazole or clindamycin) are established regimens for patients with intra-abdominal sepsis. Aztreonam is widely used as an alternative to an aminoglycoside for those patients at significant risk from the nephrotoxicity of aminoglycosides. Aztreonam plus clindamycin was found to have similar efficacy to tobramycin (or gentamicin) plus clindamycin in five clinical trials reviewed by DiPiro and Fortson.[48] Monotherapy with imipenem–cilastatin, piperacillin–tazobactam, cefotetan or cefoxitin is as effective as combination treatment with an aminoglycoside plus an anti-anaerobic drug,[49–51] and is associated with significantly less nephrotoxicity. These data have led Gorbach to suggest that aminoglycoside-containing regimens should not be used routinely for the initial treatment of uncomplicated intra-abdominal infection.[45] Enterococci are frequently present in polymicrobial intra-abdominal infections but are seldom found alone. Treatment with an agent active against enterococci (e.g. amoxicillin) is not routinely required.[45,52] Monotherapy with cefoxitin, combination therapy with cefuroxime plus metronidazole or gentamicin plus metronidazole (or clindamycin) are cheap, widely used alternatives for treatment of intra-abdominal infection. More expensive alternatives such as imipenem–cilastatin or piperacillin–tazobactam should be reserved for patients with complicated infections. Patients with generalized peritonitis or localized abdominal abscess should ordinarily be treated for 5–7 days.[53] Runyon et al[54] treated spontaneous bacterial peritonitis with cefotaxime 2 g every 8 h for 5 days, with no deaths due to infection and a 93% microbiological cure rate. As spontaneous bacterial peritonitis is usually due to community-acquired infection with relatively sensitive organisms, it seems likely that very similar results could be achieved with cefuroxime or amoxicillin–clavulanate.

Tertiary peritonitis should initially be treated with amoxicillin, gentamicin and metronidazole, but treatment should be modified when appropriate microbiology results are available. When infection is due to *Candida* spp. other antimicrobial agents should be discontinued, foreign bodies removed if possible, and treatment with amphotericin given for at least 4 weeks.[55]

Infection is a common complication of severe acute pancreatic necrosis. It usually occurs 2 or 3 weeks after the onset of acute pancreatitis and is commonly due to enteric Gram-negative bacilli, *Staph. aureus*, streptococci or *B. fragilis*. Antimicrobial prophylaxis (e.g. monotherapy with imipenem–cilastatin or cefuroxime, or combination therapy with ceftazidime, metronidazole and amikacin) appears to be useful in preventing infection in high-risk patients, i.e. those with necrosis of more than one-third of the pancreas. However, no trial has shown a significant benefit in mortality. It seems reasonable to treat patients with severe acute pancreatic necrosis with cefuroxime for 14 days in the expectation that preventing infection will reduce morbidity, if not mortality.[56]

URINARY TRACT INFECTION

Urinary tract infections are the third most common cause of admissions to ICUs for sepsis and are present in approximately 10% of such patients.[57,58] Mortality from urinary tract sepsis is lower than for the two more common sources (intra-abdominal infections and pneumonia) and has been reported as around 30%,[59,60] but is less in our recent experience (*see* Table 41.1). Most patients with urinary tract sepsis who are admitted to an ICU have infections that are complicated, i.e. they are associated with obstruction in association with structural abnormalities of the urinary tract (usually urolithiasis, less commonly malignancy or congenital abnormalities). Rarely, and most often in patients with diabetes, there may be an associated perinephric abscess[61] or emphysematous pyelonephritis.[62]

 ## MICROBIOLOGY

The organisms most commonly responsible for complicated urinary infections are *Esch. coli*, *Proteus* and *Klebsiella* spp., other enteric Gram-negative bacilli, and less commonly enterococci. *Staph. aureus*, *Candida* spp. and other fungi are sometimes responsible, particularly in patients with a renal abscess. Azotemia should not be assumed to be acute as underlying chronic renal impairment is often present. Initial empirical antibiotic therapy should include amoxicillin and either an aminoglycoside or aztreonam. Immediate investigation should include imaging of the urinary tract with ultrasonography or CT scan to define the site and nature of any obstruction and detect the presence of an abscess or free gas in the tissues. Initial diagnostic radiology should be combined with either percutaneous nephrostomy or ureteric stenting (performed following the first dose of antibiotics). Treatment of perinephric abscess(es) should include an anti-staphylococcal antibiotic (e.g. (flucl)oxacillin or vancomycin)[63] and consideration of operative drainage. Nephrectomy is usually recommended in emphysematous pyelonephritis.[62]

Colonization and infection of the urinary tract occur in 6–18% of ICU patients.[1,2] In most of these patients urinary tract infection is a relatively insignificant complication of urinary catheterization, which usually resolves on removal of the catheter; however, in a minority it is the cause of systemic illness and in a few it may contribute to mortality. Antimicrobial treatment is not indicated in the majority of patients and should be reserved for those with evidence of systemic sepsis.

 ## TREATMENT

A variety of different antimicrobials have been evaluated in the treatment of hospital patients with serious urinary tract infection. The most important requirement of a regimen is adequate activity against aerobic Gram-negative bacilli, including *Pseudomonas* spp. Gentamicin, or another aminoglycoside, has long been considered the standard parenteral treatment for pyelonephritis, but concerns about nephrotoxicity and ototoxicity have prompted the assessment of other agents.

Aztreonam, ceftazidime, imipenem–cilastatin, ciprofloxacin and a host of other agents have demonstrated generally similar efficacy to the aminoglycosides.[64–66] The selection of initial empirical therapy is influenced more by the relative costs of these agents than by any differences in clinical efficacy. Once the urinary pathogen has been identified, treatment can often be modified to use a cheaper narrow-spectrum agent. Pyelonephritis should be treated for 7–10 days but colonized patients can usually be managed by observation until removal of the catheter. The management of urinary tract infection is discussed in Chapter 54.

INTRAVASCULAR CATHETER-ASSOCIATED INFECTIONS

Infections of intravascular cannulas may range in severity from asymptomatic colonization of the cannula hub or skin insertion site to suppurative thrombophlebitis. Bacteremia is a common complication of severe catheter-associated infection, and in ICU patients is associated with a significantly increased mortality.[67] The incidence of intravascular catheter-associated sepsis is particularly affected by the spectrum and density of bacterial colonization of the skin at the insertion site, the duration of catheterization and the type of catheter used. The rate of cannula-related bacteremia is approximately 0.2% for peripheral intravenous cannulas, 1% for arterial

catheters used for hemodynamic monitoring and 3–5% for short-term non-cuffed central venous catheters.[68] Infection rates in patients with burns are commonly much higher.[69] The organisms most commonly responsible for cannula-related sepsis in ICU patients are *Staph. epidermidis*, enteric Gram-negative bacilli, *Staph. aureus*, *Enterococcus* spp. and *Candida* spp.[70–72] (Table 41.4).

Catheter-associated infection should be suspected in all febrile patients who lack an identified source of sepsis. Infection of central venous catheters is not usually associated with any signs of sepsis at the insertion site. In contrast, insertion-site inflammation may be a useful sign of infection associated with peripheral venous and arterial catheters. However, most patients with peripheral catheter insertion-site inflammation do not have significant infection. Furthermore, sepsis may occur in the absence of local inflammation. In one study of 130 arterial catheters, bacteremia occurred in 3 of 14 patients with inflammation at the site of catheter insertion and 2 of 116 patients without local inflammation.[73]

The management of catheter-associated infection is discussed in detail in Chapter 42.

All patients with intravascular catheter-associated sepsis, especially those with infection due to *Staph. aureus*, should be carefully evaluated for the development of distant foci of infection (e.g. endocarditis, epidural abscess, septic arthritis). While these complications most commonly occur during the first 14 days after onset of the catheter-associated infection,[74] they may present as late as 2 months after the completion of antibiotic treatment.[75] Patients who have clinical evidence of suppurative thrombophlebitis or perivascular abscess may need adjunctive treatment with heparin, surgical removal of the infected vein or drainage of a perivascular abscess.[76]

The optimal duration of treatment for apparently uncomplicated intravascular catheter-associated sepsis is uncertain. Jernigan and Farr[75] reviewed 11 studies of short-course therapy of catheter-related *Staph. aureus* bacteremia and concluded that treatment should be for more than 2 weeks. Fowler et al[77] have suggested that patients with cannula-related *Staph. aureus* bacteremia who have no indwelling prosthetic devices, clinical resolution within 3 days of removal of the infected cannula, sterile blood cultures at 2–4 days after

Table 41.4 Etiology of primary bacteremia in patients in intensive care units

	Richards et al[5]	Richards et al[7]
Total no. of isolates	2971	4394
Organisms (%)		
Staphylococcus aureus	13	12
Staph. epidermidis	36	39
Enterococci	16	11
Enteric Gram-negative bacilli	17	20
Candida spp.	11	12

starting appropriate therapy and a normal transesophageal echocardiogram after 5–7 days of therapy should be treated for only 7 days. The duration of treatment for patients with cannula-related bacteremia due to other organisms is even less certain.

Use of central venous cannulas, coated with either chlorhexidine and silver sulfadiazine or rifampicin (rifampin) and minocycline has a significant benefit in the prevention of cannula-associated bacteremia.[78] Dramatic reductions in cannula-associated bacteremia can be achieved by consistent application of a bundle of infection-prevention procedures: handwashing and using full barrier precautions during the insertion of central venous catheters, cleaning the insertion site with chlorhexidine, avoiding the femoral site if possible and removal of unnecessary catheters.[79,80]

SINUSITIS

Sinusitis (Ch. 44), particularly affecting the maxillary sinuses, is an occasional cause of fever in ICU patients.[81,82] Complications of sinusitis include bronchopneumonia, septicemia and subdural empyema.

Sinusitis should be suspected in febrile patients who have endotracheal and gastric tubes inserted through the nares. Purulent rhinorrhea and middle ear effusion(s) (detected by pneumatic otoscopy) are useful clinical associations with sinusitis.[83] Partial or complete opacification of the sinuses has been demonstrated in 30–60% of patients admitted to an ICU for at least 7 days.[81,82] However, in approximately half of these patients the maxillary sinus fluid does not grow significant numbers ($>10^3$ cfu/mL) of organisms. The demonstration of fluid in the sinuses (by CT, radiography or ultrasonography) should not therefore be regarded as proof of the presence of purulent sinusitis. In patients who do have purulent sinusitis the infection is commonly polymicrobial, with Gram-negative bacilli present in most. *Candida* spp. and anaerobes are occasional causes of sinusitis.

The initial treatment of sinusitis should include removal of any nasal tubes and treatment with a broad-spectrum antibiotic such as cefoxitin. In patients with persistent fever, radiological evidence of significant sinus opacification and no other focus of infection, the affected sinuses should be surgically drained and lavaged, and treatment modified on the basis of culture results.

SOLID ORGAN TRANSPLANTATION

Solid organ transplant recipients are admitted to an ICU under two circumstances – immediately postoperatively or at some later time following transplantation. Infection is the most common reason for such admission.

Prophylactic perioperative antimicrobial therapy in solid organ transplant recipients should be effective against the common bacterial and fungal pathogens responsible for infection during this period of maximal immunosuppression. The regimen should represent the consensus views of transplant clinicians, intensivists and infectious disease physicians and should be in the form of a written protocol. Prophylaxis should begin immediately preoperatively so as to provide high blood levels during surgery. The agents used should be appropriate to the (site and organ-specific) infective risks and should be given for short periods only (<24 h). Finally, account should be taken of co-morbidity such as renal impairment so as to minimize iatrogenic complications. These recommendations are consistent with the general principles for the prevention of surgical site infections.[84]

Common regimens in abdominal organ transplantation include either a group 3 cephalosporin (cefuroxime or cefoxitin) or a combination of an antistaphylococcal penicillin (or vancomycin) and either an aminoglycoside or aztreonam. A short course of prophylactic systemic antifungal therapy is recommended in high-risk patients undergoing liver transplantation.[85]

Perioperative regimens in heart transplantation should be similar to those used in non-transplant cardiac surgery (e.g. cefuroxime). Lung transplant recipients with cystic fibrosis or bronchiectasis are frequently colonized with multiresistant enteric Gram-negative bacilli and should receive prophylaxis with a dual antipseudomonal regimen (e.g. ceftazidime and an aminoglycoside). Other lung transplant patients, for example those with pulmonary hypertension, should have similar prophylaxis to heart transplant recipients.

Bacterial infections in critically ill transplant recipients early after transplantation should be treated according to protocols designed for other critically ill patients, bearing in mind the local microbial flora, the nature of the putative septic site and the state of immunosuppression. Empirical treatment may consist of a group 3 cephalosporin (perhaps in combination with an aminoglycoside) in pneumonia or urinary tract infection; an anti-staphylococcal penicillin (or vancomycin) with an aminoglycoside and perhaps amphotericin[86,87] in clinical sepsis without an identified site; and either triple combination therapy (aminoglycoside, metronidazole and amoxicillin or vancomycin) or monotherapy with a carbapenem in intra-abdominal infection. *Enterococcus faecium*, including vancomycin-resistant strains, is a particular problem in biliary and intra-abdominal infection after liver transplantation, as are multiresistant organisms after lung transplantation.[88]

Serious fungal infections are particularly problematic[89–91] and constitute the most common unsuspected finding at autopsy in transplant recipients who die in the ICU.[92] Early recourse to liposomal amphotericin is recommended in life-threatening fungal infections in transplant recipients, although successful use of caspofungin or voriconazole has been reported for invasive aspergillosis (Ch. 60).[93,94]

Infections occurring more than a month after transplantation are more likely to be due to opportunistic organisms[95] and invasive means should be used if necessary to establish the nature of the causative organisms.

The prophylaxis and therapy of viral and other opportunistic infections in transplant patients is covered in Chapter 40.

SEPSIS MODULATORS

Sepsis (i.e. the clinical syndrome usually associated with severe life-threatening infections) has a complex pathophysiology that has proved difficult to elucidate.[96] Although understanding of many of the underlying mediators and mechanisms of disease (e.g. the inflammatory and coagulation cascades) is increasing,[97,98] attempts to convert this understanding into effective therapeutic strategies have so far been largely unsuccessful.[57,99,100] In large part this is because of the extreme heterogeneity of clinical sepsis with respect to patient factors (e.g. co-morbidity), quality of clinical care (e.g. the appropriateness of surgical and antimicrobial therapy),[101,102] the nature of the septic process (e.g. abscess or bacteremia), the timing of intervention with respect to the stage of evolution of the underlying pathophysiology, and the redundancy of disease mechanisms which limit the possible efficacy of a 'single magic bullet' intervention strategy.

The lack of specific clinical correlates of underlying disease mechanisms has prompted calls for a reappraisal of the utility of the clinical definition of sepsis and for a classification of septic patients in ways that ensure more homogeneity with respect to these mechanisms.[103] However, despite these formidable methodological difficulties, a meta-analysis[104] of 18 trials of a variety of anti-inflammatory therapies showed a small but statistically significant reduction in absolute mortality (from around 39% to 36%) in the 'active' arm. This suggests that such therapies may indeed have therapeutic benefit. It seems likely that some of these agents may be less effective than others and that the size of the 'benefit' in the meta-analysis may be an underestimate of the efficacy of a few 'strong performers'. Nevertheless, very large trial sizes (c. 6000 patients) would be required to detect such small (3%) benefits, unless trial design improved. After initial trials of antithrombin III suggested that this agent might be beneficial,[105] a large multicenter study was unfortunately confounded by the adverse effects in the antithrombin III arm of simultaneous heparin administration and the future of this agent is unclear.[106] Another agent with both anti-inflammatory and anti-thrombotic activity, recombinant human activated protein C or drotrecogin-alfa, was shown to reduce all-cause 28-day mortality from 30.8% to 24.7% in another large trial (PROWESS).[58] However, two subsequent trials with different protocols – one in adults (ADDRESS),[107] the other in children (RESOLVE)[108] – did not show benefit and

a fourth trial (PROWESS-SHOCK)[109] is currently recruiting, while the place of this expensive agent continues to be debated (*see* Ch. 38).[110]

PREVENTION OF INFECTION IN THE ICU

SELECTIVE DECONTAMINATION OF THE DIGESTIVE TRACT

The use of selective decontamination of the digestive tract (SDD) to reduce the incidence of infection in multiple trauma patients was first reported by Stoutenbeek et al.[111] The regimen used for SDD is commonly a mixture of polymyxin, tobramycin (or gentamicin) and amphotericin. This mixture is applied as a paste to the oral mucosa, and a liquid suspension is swallowed or administered via a nasogastric tube four times daily. The regimen is intended to eliminate fungi and aerobic Gram-negative bacteria from the gastrointestinal tract but to have little effect on the predominant anaerobic flora, thus maintaining 'colonization resistance' due to their continued growth. The purpose of SDD is to reduce the rate of pneumonia and other serious infections caused by pathogenic organisms originating from the gastrointestinal tract. In a modification of SDD the topical oral and enteric regimen used throughout a patient's stay in the ICU has been supplemented by the addition of a systemic broad-spectrum antibiotic (usually cefotaxime) for the first 4 days of the stay. This selective parenteral and enteral antisepsis regimen (SPEAR) is intended to improve upon the efficacy of SDD by treating occult or incubating infections present at admission to the ICU. Whether or not regimens have included an initial period of systemic antimicrobial therapy, the acronym SDD is most frequently used to describe this form of chemoprophylaxis.

Colonization of the oropharynx, stomach and rectum is dramatically affected by SDD regimens. Aerobic Gram-negative bacilli are eliminated from the oropharynx and stomach within 3–4 days of starting SDD. In contrast, they continue to be isolated from these sites in 20–50% of control patients not given SDD. The proportion of patients with aerobic Gram-negative bacilli present in rectal swabs also declines from approximately 60–90% to 10–20% over a period of 10–14 days.[102–114]

A meta-analysis of the results from 51 randomized controlled trials (including 8065 patients) of SDD regimens showed a 61% reduction in the incidence of bacteremia due to aerobic Gram-negative bacilli, no effect on bacteremia due to Gram-positive bacteria, and a 20% reduction in mortality.[115] The analysis suggested that approximately 22 patients would need to be treated to prevent one death. The adverse effects of SDD regimens include the significantly increased expenditure on antibiotics, the potential for increased antibiotic resistance in the endemic bacterial flora of the ICU due to the selective pressure exerted by the SDD regimen, and the toxicity of the agents used. Opinion is divided between those who consider SDD of proven benefit and those who consider that further study is required to determine whether it is cost-effective in selected subgroups (e.g. trauma and burn patients).[27,28]

OTHER STRATEGIES TO PREVENT VENTILATOR-ASSOCIATED PNEUMONIA

Semirecumbent positioning, enteral rather than gastric feeding, use of sucralfate rather than antacids, H_2 antagonists or proton pump inhibitors as prophylaxis against stress-induced gastric ulceration, continuous subglottic aspiration and removal of nasogastric and endotracheal tubes at the earliest opportunity have all been shown to reduce the incidence of ventilator-associated pneumonia.[28]

HAND HYGIENE

Despite clear evidence that micro-organisms are disseminated within the ICU on the hands of staff,[116] and increasing concern about nosocomial infection with ever more resistant organisms, ICU staff wash their hands on approximately only one-third of the occasions when they should do so. The level of compliance with handwashing guidelines in ICUs tends to be lower than it is in other parts of the hospital, perhaps because of heavier staff workloads in the ICU. Placing labels on ICU equipment that remind staff to wash their hands, provision of easily accessible handbasins and dispensers, and use of an antiseptic handrub rather than handwashing, have all been found to improve hand hygiene in the ICU.[117] Maintaining high levels of hand hygiene requires adequate staffing and continuous education and motivation of staff. While these actions may appear mundane, improvements in hand hygiene are likely to dramatically reduce nosocomial infection.

POLICIES TO MAXIMIZE THE EFFECTIVENESS OF ANTIMICROBIAL USE IN THE ICU

The prevalence of infection with antibiotic-resistant organisms is rising in ICUs,[118] as it is in hospitals generally. Such infections are difficult and costly to treat.[119] ICUs are often accused of indiscriminate use of antibiotics and of creating antibiotic-resistant organisms, which then spread to the rest of the hospital. While it is evident that the patients with the most severe infections in the hospital are often admitted to the ICU as a result of their infection, there is much that can be done in the ICU to limit the inappropriate use of antibiotics and the selection of resistant microbial strains.[120]

Crucial to the success of these endeavors, however, is the creation of a conservative culture with respect to the use of antibiotics, both prophylactically and therapeutically. This requires the cooperation of all clinicians practicing within the ICU. This culture should be expressed in an antibiotic management program. Infectious disease physicians and clinical microbiologists have a detailed knowledge of the local microbiological flora, both in hospital and in the surrounding community, and can provide evidence-based advice and facilitate consensus among other clinicians on appropriate antibiotic use.[120]

Antibiotic management programs should be specific and applicable to the clinical situation, where decisions often need to be made without supporting microbiological information. They should specifically cover 'surgical prophylaxis' and should specify the indications, agent, dose and duration of therapy.[121] They should also explicitly prohibit the use of antibiotic prophylaxis in situations where it is not indicated and should specify initial empirical therapy based on presenting clinical syndromes (i.e. before microbiological information comes to hand). Once again, the agents, dose and duration should be specified. Certain agents (e.g. perhaps expanded-spectrum cephalosporins, amphotericin, carbapenems, amikacin, streptogramins, linezolid) could be designated as mandating either prior approval or early review by an infectious disease physician. A policy commitment by the treating clinicians to reserve empirical antibiotic therapy for 'clinical sepsis' and not to treat 'colonization' is crucial to the success of an antibiotic management program in reducing unnecessary and probably harmful antibiotic use. Finally, these policies should also stipulate a commitment to rationalize antibiotics (narrower spectrum, less 'reserved', cheaper) in the light of appropriate definitive microbiological information.

Specifying the most appropriate investigation strategy for common syndromes of clinical infection[22] may reduce mortality, improve the quality of microbiological information and reduce unnecessary investigation, antibiotic use and cost.

INFECTIONS DUE TO UNUSUALLY RESISTANT BACTERIA

Colonization and infection with bacteria resistant to commonly used antibiotics is a rapidly growing problem in ICUs. Recent reports have described resistance to methicillin in 65% of infections due to *Staph. aureus*, gentamicin resistance in 46% of infection due to *Ps. aeruginosa* in European ICUs,[122] resistance to cefotaxime, ceftriaxone and aztreonam in 20–30% of isolates of *K. pneumoniae* from ICUs in France,[123] and resistance to vancomycin in 17% of enterococcal isolates from ICUs in the USA.[124] Potential adverse consequences of colonization or infection with multiresistant strains include failure of antimicrobial therapy, increased expense of antimicrobial therapy, spread of infection to other patients and transfer of resistance to other bacterial species. Epidemics of multiresistant bacteria in ICU patients are often followed by spread to patients in other parts of the hospital and then to the community, or back to the ICU. When formulating policies for antibiotic use in the ICU, doctors should be influenced by the distant effects of their antibiotic choices and avoid unnecessary prescription of those agents most likely to facilitate the selection of multiresistant strains (*see* Ch. 3).

Colonization and infection with multiresistant bacteria is usually the result of acquisition of endemic or epidemic strains following admission to the ICU.[125] A variety of factors (including greater severity of the underlying illness, prolonged stay in the ICU, the use of invasive devices and prolonged use of broad-spectrum antimicrobial therapy) increase the rate of infection with these organisms.[126] Resistance of a bacterial isolate to commonly tested antibiotics (e.g. methicillin resistance in *Staph. aureus*, vancomycin resistance in enterococci, aminoglycoside and group 4 cephalosporin resistance in Gram-negative bacilli) frequently serves as a marker of an epidemic of nosocomial infection, which might otherwise remain unsuspected. Such epidemics are not only of importance in themselves, but should also be regarded as the visible tip of an iceberg of undetected nosocomially transmitted infection.

Pseudomonas, Klebsiella, Enterobacter, Serratia and *Acinetobacter* spp., MRSA and enterococci are the most commonly reported causes of epidemics of nosocomial bacteremia in ICU patients.[127] Such epidemics usually last less than 3 months, affect an average of 10 patients per outbreak, commonly arise from contaminated medical equipment, and often depend on transmission of infection by the hands of ICU staff. Similar factors no doubt contribute to the much larger problem of endemic nosocomial infection, but are less easily identified because the organisms responsible often lack unusual antibiotic resistance patterns.

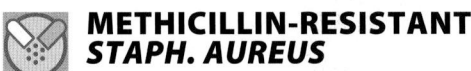 ## METHICILLIN-RESISTANT *STAPH. AUREUS*

Methicillin-resistant *Staph. aureus* (MRSA) is a common cause of epidemics of infection in ICUs. Burns, surgical wounds, prolonged stay in the unit and prolonged courses of multiple antibiotics all increase the risk of MRSA infection. Although persistent colonization of hospital staff has been suspected as the source of infection in some MRSA outbreaks, this is not found in most outbreaks. However, transient contamination of the hands is common in staff directly involved in the care of patients with MRSA infection, and is presumed to be the most common mode of transmission of infection between patients. Control and, not infrequently, termination of epidemics of MRSA can be achieved by surveillance of patients for MRSA colonization or infection, strict isolation of colonized or infected patients, consistent use of hand hygiene between each patient contact and appropriate treatment to minimize colonization or eradicate infection in affected patients and staff.

MRSA colonization may be reduced or eliminated by stopping antibiotic treatment whenever possible, effective treatment of underlying skin disorders, application of mupirocin ointment to colonized sites, and washing with an antiseptic.[128] Infection with MRSA is usually treated with intravenous vancomycin or linezolid, or oral clindamycin or fusidic acid supplemented by oral rifampicin.

 ## RESISTANT ENTEROCOCCI

Enterococci (especially *E. faecalis* and *E. faecium*) resistant to gentamicin, ampicillin or vancomycin have emerged as an important cause of nosocomial infection in ICUs. Prolonged stay in the unit, persistent intra-abdominal infection and prolonged broad-spectrum antimicrobial therapy with agents inactive against enterococci are common features in patients with enterococcal infection. Feces and urine of colonized patients are the usual sources of infection, and transmission on the hands of hospital staff is presumed to be the major route of cross-infection. The urinary tract, bloodstream and surgical wounds are the most common sites of infection.[7]

Bacteremia due to enterococci highly resistant to gentamicin (MIC >1000 mg/L) but susceptible to ampicillin or vancomycin may be successfully treated with amoxicillin (or ampicillin) or vancomycin monotherapy.[129,130] This is in contrast to enterococcal endocarditis, which requires combination treatment with amoxicillin or vancomycin plus an aminoglycoside for cure. Optimal treatment of infection with enterococci resistant to ampicillin, vancomycin and aminoglycosides is at present unclear, but linezolid and quinupristin–dalfopristin show some promise.

The rapid emergence of multiresistant enterococci, the difficulties posed by treatment of these infections and the specter of transfer of resistance to *Staph. aureus* are important reasons to limit the use of vancomycin as much as possible. Vancomycin should not ordinarily be used for perioperative prophylaxis, initial treatment of antibiotic-associated colitis, initial empirical treatment of febrile neutropenic patients, selective decontamination of the digestive tract or eradication of MRSA colonization.[131]

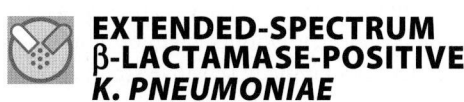 ## EXTENDED-SPECTRUM β-LACTAMASE-POSITIVE *K. PNEUMONIAE*

Extended spectrum β-lactamases (ESBL) providing resistance to broad-spectrum cephalosporins were first detected in *K. pneumoniae* in 1983.[132] Resistance is due to readily transmissible plasmids which encode for ESBL and for aminoglycoside and quinolone resistance. The β-lactamases are usually susceptible to inhibitors such as clavulanic acid and sulbactam, which may assist with identification of these strains in the laboratory.[125] Approximately 14% of *K. pneumoniae* and 6% of *Esch. coli* isolated from patients in ICUs in the USA in 2002 were ESBL positive.[132]

Infection with ESBL-positive *K. pneumoniae* usually involves the urinary tract, the respiratory tract or wounds.[132] Enteric colonization and transmission on the hands of hospital staff appear to contribute to epidemic spread. Treatment is with a carbapenem such as imipenem–cilastatin, meropenem or ertapenem.

GRAM-NEGATIVE BACILLI WITH INDUCIBLE β-LACTAMASES

Another important source of infection due to multiresistant Gram-negative bacilli is the selection of organisms with chromosomally encoded class I β-lactamase production. *Pseudomonas*, *Enterobacter*, *Citrobacter* and *Serratia* spp. are the organisms that most frequently produce class I β-lactamase (*see* Ch. 15). Induction of enzyme production or selection of stably depressed mutant cells which constitutively manufacture class I β-lactamase at a high level may lead to development of resistance to β-lactams during treatment.[133,134] Enzyme production is strongly induced when organisms are exposed to cephalosporins of groups 1 and 2 (*see* Ch. 13), cefoxitin or imipenem–cilastatin, but is only weakly induced by exposure to groups 3 and 4 cephalosporins, ureidopenicillins and monobactams. Induced enzyme production ceases promptly when treatment with the inducing antibiotic is stopped. Selection of stably depressed mutants constitutively producing large amounts of β-lactamase occurs when inducible strains (especially *Ps. aeruginosa* and *Enterobacter cloacae*) are exposed to broad-spectrum cephalosporins, ureidopenicillins or monobactams. Resistance persists even when treatment with the antibiotic responsible for selecting the mutant strain is stopped. Development of resistance during treatment occurs in approximately 10–20% of patients,[134] and spread within the ICU may result in multiresistance in 30% of ICU isolates of *Ent. cloacae*.[133]

Imipenem–cilastatin, despite being a strong inducer of class I β-lactamase, is not susceptible to the enzyme's action. Alternative regimens include imipenem–cilastatin monotherapy or combination therapy using imipenem–cilastatin plus an aminoglycoside or a fluoroquinolone selected on the basis of careful susceptibility testing.[135] Patients treated with a broad-spectrum cephalosporin, ureidopenicillin or monobactam for an infection due to an initially sensitive strain should be carefully observed for the emergence of resistant mutants during treatment.

MULTIRESISTANT *ACINETOBACTER BAUMANNII*

Multiresistant *A. baumannii* is an occasional cause of epidemics of infection in ICU patients. Epidemic strains are resistant to many broad-spectrum cephalosporins, and resistance to quinolones, carbapenems and aminoglycosides is also common. Colonization and infection of the respiratory tract in artificially ventilated patients is a common feature of epidemics, and improvements in the methods used to sterilize ventilator equipment has led to termination of epidemics.[136] In most patients *A. baumannii* merely colonizes the respiratory tract; however, it may be responsible for pneumonia and other serious infections. Imipenem–cilastatin alone, or in combination

with an aminoglycoside, is often appropriate treatment. Polymyxin B, colistin and tigecycline may be effective in the treatment of strains with multidrug resistance.

A frequent theme for many epidemics caused by multiresistant bacteria has been the widespread use of antibiotics in response to increased resistance in other commonly isolated bacterial species. For example, vancomycin resistance in enterococci has emerged following increased use of vancomycin to treat suspected or proven MRSA (or methicillin-resistant *Staph. epidermidis*) infections. Similarly, epidemics of infection due to multiresistant *K. pneumoniae* and *A. baumannii* have followed increased use of group 4 cephalosporins and imipenem–cilastatin.[135] Thus the increased use of potent antibiotics with ever broader spectra of activity acts as a stimulus to the evolution of new epidemics of ever more resistant pathogens. The effect is to mortgage the future of antibiotic treatment to pay for our present practices. While there is no one solution to this problem that can be applied to all ICUs, the use of prescribing guidelines which encourage the use of older narrow-spectrum antibiotics and limit the use of new broad-spectrum antibiotic agents should prolong the utility of new drugs, delay the emergence of resistant strains and set a better example for prescribing patterns in the rest of the hospital[137] (*see* Ch. 11).

References

1. Brown RB, Hosmer D, Chen HC, et al. A comparison of infections in different ICUs within the same hospital. *Crit Care Med.* 1985;13:472–476.
2. Vincent J-L, Bihari DJ, Suter PM, et al. The prevalence of nosocomial infection in intensive care units in Europe – the results of the EPIC study. *JAMA.* 1995;274:639–644.
3. Rivers E, Nguyen B, Havstad S, et al. Early goal-directed therapy in the treatment of severe sepsis and septic shock. *N Engl J Med.* 2001;345:1368–1377.
4. Marshall JC, Maier RV, Jimenez M, Dellinger EP. Source control in the management of severe sepsis and septic shock: an evidence-based review. *Crit Care Med.* 2004;32(suppl):S513–S526.
5. Richards MJ, Edwards JR, Culver DH, Gaynes RP; the National Nosocomial Infections Surveillance System. Nosocomial infections in medical intensive care units in the United States. *Crit Care Med.* 1999;27:887–892.
6. Khoo SH, Creagh-Barry P, Wilkins EGL, Pasvol G. Fulminant community acquired infections admitted to an intensive care unit. *Q J Med.* 1992;NS83:381–388.
7. Richards MJ, Edwards JR, Culver DH, Gaynes RP; the National Nosocomial Infections Surveillance System. Nosocomial infections in combined medical–surgical intensive care units in the United States. *Infect Control Hosp Epidemiol.* 2000;21:510–515.
8. Chandrasekar PH, Kruse JA, Mathews MF. Nosocomial infection among patients in different types of intensive care units at a city hospital. *Crit Care Med.* 1986;14:508–510.
9. Craven DE, Kunches LM, Lichtenberg DA, et al. Nosocomial infection and fatality in medical and surgical intensive care unit patients. *Arch Intern Med.* 1988;148:1161–1168.
10. Kollef MH, Sherman G, Ward S, Fraser VJ. Inadequate antimicrobial treatment of infections. A risk factor for hospital mortality among critically ill patients. *Chest.* 1999;115:462–474.
11. British Thoracic Society and the Public Health Laboratory Service. Community-acquired pneumonia in adults in British hospitals in 1982–1983: a survey of aetiology, mortality, prognostic factors and outcome. *Q J Med.* 1987;NS62:195–220.
12. American Thoracic Society. Guidelines for the initial management of adults with community-acquired pneumonia; diagnosis, assessment of severity, and initial antimicrobial therapy. *Am Rev Respir Dis.* 1993;148:1418–1426.

13. Lim WS, Badouin SV, George RC, et al. British Thoracic Society guidelines for management of community acquired pneumonia in adults. *Thorax*. 2009;64(suppl 3):iii1–iii55.

14. Moine P, Vercken JB, Chevret S, Gajdos P. and The French Study Group of Community-Acquired Pneumonia in ICU. Severe community-acquired pneumococcal pneumonia. *Scand J Infect Dis*. 1995;27:201–206.

15. Leroy O, Santre C, Beuscart C, et al. A five-year study of severe community-acquired pneumonia with emphasis on prognosis in patients admitted to an intensive care unit. *Intensive Care Med*. 1995;21:24–31.

16. Oleacha PM, Quintana JM, Gallardo MS, Insausti J, Maravi E, Alvarez B. A predictive model for the treatment approach to community-acquired pneumonia in patients needing ICU admission. *Intensive Care Med*. 1996;22:1294–1300.

17. Ortqvist A, Sterner G, Nilsson JA. Severe community-acquired pneumonia: factors influencing need of intensive care treatment and prognosis. *Scand J Infect Dis*. 1985;17:377–386.

18. Torres A, Serra-Batlles J, Ferrer A, et al. Severe community-acquired pneumonia. *Am Rev Respir Dis*. 1991;144:312–318.

19. Potgieter PD, Hammond JMJ. Etiology and diagnosis of pneumonia requiring ICU admission. *Chest*. 1992;101:199–203.

20. Mandell LA, Wunderink RG, Anzueto A, et al. Infectious Diseases Society of America/American Thoracic Society consensus guidelines on the management of community-acquired pneumonia in adults. *Clin Infect Dis*. 2007;44(suppl 2):S27–S72.

21. Mandell LA, Marrie TJ, Grossman RF, Chow AW, Hyland RH; the Canadian Community-Acquired Pneumonia Working Group. Canadian guidelines for the initial management of community-acquired pneumonia: an evidence-based update by the Canadian Infectious Diseases Society and the Canadian Thoracic Society. *Clin Infect Dis*. 2000;31:383–421.

22. Craven DE, Kunches LM, Kilinsky V, Lichtenberg DA, Make BJ, McCabe WR. Risk factors for pneumonia and fatality in patients receiving continuous mechanical ventilation. *Am Rev Respir Dis*. 1986;133:792–796.

23. Rello J, Quintana E, Ausina V, et al. Incidence, etiology and outcome of nosocomial pneumonia in mechanically ventilated patients. *Chest*. 1991;100:439–444.

24. Fagon JY, Chastre J, Wolff M, et al. Invasive and noninvasive strategies for management of suspected ventilator-associated pneumonia. A randomized trial. *Ann Intern Med*. 2000;132:621–630.

25. Fagon J-Y, Chaistre J, Hance AJ, Montravers P, Novara A, Gibert C. Nosocomial pneumonia in ventilated patients: a cohort study evaluating attributable mortality and hospital stay. *Am J Med*. 1993;94:281–288.

26. Kollef MH, Silver P, Murphy DM, Trovillion E. The effect of late-onset ventilator-associated pneumonia in determining patient mortality. *Chest*. 1995;108:1655–1662.

27. American Thoracic Society. Hospital-acquired pneumonia in adults: diagnosis, assessment of severity, initial antimicrobial therapy, and preventative strategies. *Am J Respir Crit Care Med*. 1995;153:1711–1725.

28. Kollef MH. The prevention of ventilator-associated pneumonia. *N Engl J Med*. 1999;340:627–634.

29. Singh N, Rogers P, Atwood CW, Wagener MM, Yu VL. Short-course empiric antibiotic therapy for patients with pulmonary infiltrates in the intensive care unit. A proposed solution for indiscriminate antibiotic prescription. *Am J Respir Crit Care Med*. 2000;162:505–511.

30. Grossman RF. Evidence-based assessment of diagnostic tests for ventilator-associated pneumonia. *Chest*. 2000;117:77S–181S.

31. Bryan CS, Reynolds KL. Bacteremic nosocomial pneumonia. Analysis of 172 episodes from a single metropolitan area. *Am Rev Respir Dis*. 1984;129:668–671.

32. Rello J, Ausina V, Ricart M, Castella J, Prats G. Impact of previous antimicrobial therapy on the etiology and outcome of ventilator-associated pneumonia. *Chest*. 1993;104:1230–1235.

33. Scheld WM, Mandell GL. Nosocomial pneumonia: pathogenesis and recent advances in diagnosis and therapy. *Reviews of Infectious Diseases*. 1991;13(suppl 9):S743–S751.

34. La Force FM. Lower respiratory tract infections. In: Bennett JV, Brachman PS, eds. *Hospital infections*. 3rd ed. Brown, Boston: Little; 1992:611–639.

35. Cone LA, Woodard DR, Stoltzman DS, Byrd RG. Ceftazidime versus tobramycin–ticarcillin in the treatment of pneumonia and bacteremia. *Antimicrob Agents Chemother*. 1985;28:33–36.

36. Salata RA, Gebhart RL, Palmer DL, et al. Pneumonia treated with imipenem/cilastatin. *Am J Med*. 1985;78(suppl 6A):104–109.

37. Schwigon CD, Hulla FW, Schulze B, Maslak A. Timentin in the treatment of nosocomial bronchopulmonary infections in intensive care units. *J Antimicrob Chemother*. 1986;17(suppl C):115–122.

38. Mandell LA, Nicolle LE, Ronald AR, et al. A prospective randomized trial of ceftazidime versus cefazolin/tobramycin in the treatment of hospitalized patients with pneumonia. *J Antimicrob Chemother*. 1987;20:95–107.

39. Norrby SR, Finch RG, Glauser M. European Study Group. Monotherapy in serious hospital-acquired infections: a clinical trial of ceftazidime versus imipenem/cilastatin. *J Antimicrob Chemother*. 1993;31:927–937.

40. Martin C, Gouin F, Fourrier F, Junginger W, Prieur BL. Pefloxacin in the treatment of nosocomial lower respiratory tract infections in intensive care patients. *J Antimicrob Chemother*. 1988;21:795–799.

41. Peloquin CA, Cumbo TJ, Nix DE, Sands MF, Schentag JJ. Evaluation of intravenous ciprofloxacin in patients with nosocomial lower respiratory tract infections. *Arch Intern Med*. 1989;149:2269–2273.

42. La Force FM. Systemic antimicrobial therapy of nosocomial pneumonia: monotherapy versus combination therapy. *Eur J Clin Microbiol Infect Dis*. 1989;8:61–68.

43. Bohnen J, Boulanger M, Meakins JL, McLean APH. Prognosis in generalized peritonitis. Relation to cause and risk factors. *Arch Surg*. 1983;118:285–290.

44. Bohnen JMA, Mustard RA, Oxholm SE, Schouten BD. APACHE II score and abdominal sepsis. A prospective study. *Arch Surg*. 1988;123:225–229.

45. Gorbach SL. Treatment of intra-abdominal infections. *J Antimicrob Chemother*. 1993;31(suppl A):67–78.

46. Mbopi Keou F-X, Bloch F, Buu Hoi A, et al. Spontaneous peritonitis in cirrhotic hospital in-patients: retrospective analysis of 101 cases. *Q J Med*. 1992;NS 83:401–407.

47. McClean KL, Sheehan GJ, Harding GKM. Intra-abdominal infection: a review. *Clin Infect Dis*. 1994;19:100–116.

48. DiPiro JT, Fortson NS. Combination antibiotic therapy in the management of intra-abdominal infection. *Am J Surg*. 1993;165(suppl 2A):82S–88S.

49. Ho JL, Barza M. Role of aminoglycoside antibiotics in the treatment of intra-abdominal infection. *Antimicrob Agents Chemother*. 1987;31:485–491.

50. Solomkin JS, Dellinger EP, Christou NV, Busutti RW. Results of a multi-center trial comparing imipenem/cilastatin to tobramycin/clindamycin for intra-abdominal infections. *Ann Surg*. 1990;212:581–591.

51. Eklund A-E, Nord CE; Swedish Study Group. A randomized multicenter trial of piperacillin/tazobactam versus imipenem/cilastatin in the treatment of severe intraabdominal infections. *J Antimicrob Chemother*. 1993;31(suppl A):79–85.

52. Nichols RL, Muzik AC. Enterococcal infections in surgical patients: the mystery continues. *Clin Infect Dis*. 1992;15:72–76.

53. Bohnen JMA, Solomkin JS, Dellinger EP, Bjornson HS, Page CP. Guidelines for clinical care: anti-infective agents for intra-abdominal infection. *Arch Surg*. 1992;127:83–89.

54. Runyon BA, McHutchison JG, Antillon MR, Akriviadis EA, Montano AA. Short-course versus long-course antibiotic treatment of spontaneous bacterial peritonitis. *Gastroenterology*. 1991;100:1737–1742.

55. British Society for Antimicrobial Chemotherapy Working Party. Management of deep *Candida* infection in surgical and intensive care unit patients. *Intensive Care Med*. 1994;20:522–528.

56. Kramer KM, Levy H. Prophylactic antibiotics for severe acute pancreatitis: the beginning of an era. *Pharmacotherapy*. 1999;19:592–602.

57. Opal SM, Fisher Jr CJ, Dhainaut JF, et al. Confirmatory interleukin-1 receptor antagonist trial in severe sepsis: a phase III, randomized, double-blind, placebo-controlled, multicenter trial. The Interleukin-1 Receptor Antagonist Sepsis Investigator Group. *Crit Care Med*. 1997;25:1115–1124.

58. Bernard GR, Vincent JL, Laterre PF, et al. Recombinant human protein C Worldwide Evaluation in Severe Sepsis (PROWESS) study group. Efficacy and safety of recombinant human activated protein C for severe sepsis. *N Engl J Med*. 2001;344:699–709.

59. Knaus WA, Sun X, Nystrom O, Wagner DP. Evaluation of definitions for sepsis. *Chest*. 1992;101:1656–1662.

60. Buisson C, Doyon F, Carlet J. Bacteremia and severe sepsis in adults: a multicenter prospective survey in ICUs and wards of 24 hospitals. French Bacteremia-Sepsis Study Group. *Am J Respir Crit Care Medi*. 1996;154:617–624.

61. Hutchison FN, Kaysen GA. Perinephric abscess: the missed diagnosis. *Med Clin North Am*. 1988;72:993–1014.

62. Huang JJ, Tseng CC. Emphysematous pyelonephritis: clinicoradiological classification, management, prognosis, and pathogenesis. *Arch Intern Med*. 2000;160:797–805.

63. Dembry LM, Andriole VT. Renal and perirenal abscesses. *Infect Dis Clin North Am*. 1997;11:663–680.

64. Sattler FR, Moyer JE, Schramm M, Lombard JS, Appelbaum PC. Aztreonam compared with gentamicin for treatment of serious urinary tract infections. *Lancet.* 1984;i:1315–1318.

65. Fang G, Brennen C, Wagener M, et al. Use of ciprofloxacin versus use of aminoglycosides for therapy of complicated urinary tract infection: prospective, randomized clinical and pharmacokinetic study. *Antimicrob Agents Chemother.* 1991;35:1849–1855.

66. Cox CE. Comparison of intravenous fleroxacin with ceftazidime for treatment of complicated urinary tract infections. *Am J Med.* 1993;94 (suppl 3A):118S–125S.

67. Renaud B, Brun-Buisson C. Outcomes of primary and catheter-related bacteremia. A cohort and case-controlled study in critically ill patients. *Am J Respir Crit Care Med.* 2001;163:1584–1590.

68. Maki DG. Infections due to infusion therapy. In: Bennett JV, Brachman PS, eds. *Hospital infections.* 3rd ed. Brown, Boston: Little; 1992:849–898.

69. Pruitt BA, McManus WF, Kim SH, Treat RC. Diagnosis and treatment of cannula-related intravenous sepsis in burn patients. *Ann Surg.* 1980;191:546–554.

70. Richet H, Hubert B, Nitemberg G, et al. Prospective multicenter study of vascular-catheter-related complications and risk factors for positive central-catheter cultures in intensive care unit patients. *J Clin Microbiol.* 1990;28:2520–2525.

71. Pittet D, Tarara D, Wenzel RP. Nosocomial bloodstream infection in critically ill patients. *JAMA.* 1994;271:1598–1601.

72. Hidron AI, Edwards JR, Patel J, et al. Antimicrobial-resistant pathogens associated with healthcare-associated infections: annual summary of data reported to the National Healthcare Safety Network at the Centers for Disease Control and Prevention, 2006–2007. *Infect Control Hosp Epidemiol.* 2008;29:996–1011.

73. Band JD, Maki DG. Infections caused by arterial catheters used for hemodynamic monitoring. *Am J Med.* 1979;67:735–741.

74. Arnow PM, Quimosing EM, Beach M. Consequences of intravascular catheter sepsis. *Clin Infect Dis.* 1993;16:778–784.

75. Jernigan JA, Farr BM. Short-course therapy of catheter-related *Staphylococcus aureus* bacteremia: a meta-analysis. *Ann Intern Med.* 1993;119:304–311.

76. Verghese A, Widrich WC, Arbeit RD. Central venous septic thrombophlebitis – the role of medical therapy. *Medicine.* 1985;64:394–400.

77. Fowler Jr VG, Sanders LL, Sexton DJ, et al. Outcome of *Staphylococcus aureus* bacteremia according to compliance with recommendations of infectious diseases specialists: experience with 244 patients. *Clin Infect Dis.* 1998;27:478–486.

78. Darouiche RO, Raad II, Heard SO, et al. A comparison of two antimicrobial-impregnated central venous catheters. *N Engl J Med.* 1999;340:1–8.

79. Provonost P, Needham D, Berenholtz S, et al. An intervention to decrease catheter-related bloodstream infections in the ICU. *N Engl J Med.* 2006;355:2725–2732.

80. Galpern D, Guerrero A, Tu A, Fahoum B, Wise L. Effectiveness of a central line bundle campaign on line-associated infections in the intensive care unit. *Surgery.* 2008;144:492–495.

81. Holzapfel L, Chevret S, Madinier G, et al. Influence of long-term oro- or nasotracheal intubation on nosocomial maxillary sinusitis and pneumonia: results of a prospective, randomized, clinical trial. *Crit Care Med.* 1993;21:1132–1138.

82. Rouby J-J, Laurent P, Gosnach M, et al. Risk factors and clinical relevance of nosocomial maxillary sinusitis in the critically ill. *Am J Respir Crit Care Med.* 1994;150:776–783.

83. Borman KR, Brown PM, Mezera KK, Jhaveri H. Occult fever in surgical intensive care unit patients is seldom caused by sinusitis. *Am J Surg.* 1992;164:412–416.

84. Mangram AJ, Horan TC, Pearson ML, Silver LC, Jarvis WR. Guideline for prevention of surgical site infection, 1999. Hospital Infection Control Practices Advisory Committee. *Infect Control Hosp Epidemiol.* 1999;20:250–278.

85. Singhal S, Ellis RW, Jones SG, et al. Targeted prophylaxis with amphotericin B lipid complex in liver transplantation. *Liver Transpl.* 2000;6:588–595.

86. Wagener MM, Yu VL. Bacteremia in transplant recipients: a prospective study of demographics, etiologic agents, risk factors, and outcomes. *Am J Infect Control.* 1992;20:239–247.

87. Palmer SM, Alexander BD, Sanders LL, et al. Significance of blood stream infection after lung transplantation: analysis in 176 consecutive patients. *Transplantation.* 2000;69:2360–2366.

88. Metras D, Viard L, Kreitmann B, et al. Lung infections in pediatric lung transplantation: experience in 49 cases. *Eur J Cardiothorac Surg.* 1999; 15:490–494.

89. Paradowski LJ. Saprophytic fungal infections and lung transplantation – revisited. *J Heart Lung Transplant.* 1997;16:524–531.

90. Mehrad B, Paciocco G, Martinez FJ, Ojo TC, Lannettoni MD, Lynch JP. Spectrum of *Aspergillus* infection in lung transplant recipients: case series and review of the literature. *Chest.* 2001;19:169–175.

91. Grossi P, Farina C, Fiocchi R, Dalla Gasperina D. Prevalence and outcome of invasive fungal infections in 1,963 thoracic organ transplant recipients: a multicenter retrospective study. Italian Study Group of Fungal Infections in Thoracic Organ Transplant Recipients. *Transplantation.* 2000;70:112–116.

92. Mort TC, Yeston NS. The relationship of pre mortem diagnoses and post mortem findings in a surgical intensive care unit. *Crit Care Med.* 1999;27:299–303.

93. Linden P, Williams P, Chan KM. Efficacy and safety of amphotericin B lipid complex injection (ABLC) in solid-organ transplant recipients with invasive fungal infections. *Clin Transplant.* 2000;14:329–339.

94. Denning DW, Ribaud P, Milpied N, et al. Efficacy and safety of voriconazole in the treatment of acute invasive aspergillosis. *Clin Infect Dis.* 2002;34:563–571.

95. Fishman JA, Rubin RH. Infection in organ-transplant recipients. *N Engl J Med.* 1998;338:1741–1751.

96. Bone RC, Balk RA, Cerra FB, et al. Definitions for sepsis and organ failure and guidelines for the use of innovative therapies in sepsis. The ACCP/SCCM Consensus Conference Committee. American College of Chest Physicians/ Society of Critical Care Medicine. *Chest.* 1992;101:1644–1655.

97. Glauser MP. Pathophysiologic basis of sepsis: considerations for future strategies of intervention. *Crit Care Med.* 2000;28:S4–S8.

98. Wanecek M, Weitzberg E, Rudehill A, Oldner A. The endothelin system in septic and endotoxin shock. *Eur J Pharmacol.* 2000;407:1–15.

99. Angus DC, Birmingham MC, Balk RA, et al. E5 murine monoclonal antiendotoxin antibody in gram-negative sepsis: a randomized controlled trial. E5 Study Investigators. *JAMA.* 2000;283:1723–1730.

100. Abraham E, Anzueto A, Gutierrez G, et al. Double-blind randomised controlled trial of monoclonal antibody to human tumour necrosis factor in treatment of septic shock. NORASEPTII Study Group. *Lancet.* 1998;351:929–933.

101. Clark MA, Plank LD, Connolly AB, et al. Effect of a chimeric antibody to tumor necrosis factor-alpha on cytokine and physiologic responses in patients with severe sepsis – a randomized, clinical trial. *Crit Care Med.* 1998;26:1650–1659.

102. Streat SJ, Plank LD, Hill GL. An overview of modern management of patients with critical injury and severe sepsis. *World J Surg.* 2000;24:655–663.

103. Abraham E, Matthay MA, Dinarello CA, et al. Consensus conference definitions for sepsis, septic shock, acute lung injury, and acute respiratory distress syndrome: time for a reevaluation. *Crit Care Med.* 2000;28:232–235.

104. Natanson C. Anti-inflammatory therapies to treat sepsis and septic shock: a reassessment. *Crit Care Med.* 1997;25:1095–1100.

105. Eisele B, Lamy M, Thijs LG, et al. Antithrombin III in patients with severe sepsis. A randomized, placebo-controlled, double-blind multicenter trial plus a meta-analysis on all randomized, placebo-controlled, double-blind trials with antithrombin III in severe sepsis. *Intensive Care Med.* 1998;24:663–672.

106. Warren BL, Eid A, Singer P, et al. High-dose antithrombin III in severe sepsis. A randomized controlled trial. *JAMA.* 2001;286:1869–1878.

107. Abraham E, Laterre PF, Garg R, et al. Drotrecogin alfa (activated) for adults with severe sepsis and a low risk of death. *N Engl J Med.* 2005;353:1332–1341.

108. Nadel S, Goldstein B, Williams MD, et al. Drotrecogin alfa (activated) in children with severe sepsis: a multicentre phase III randomised controlled trial. *Lancet.* 2007;369:836–843.

109. Finfer S, Ranieri VM, Thompson BT, et al. Design, conduct, analysis and reporting of a multi-national placebo-controlled trial of activated protein C for persistent septic shock. *Intensive Care Med.* 2008;34:1935–1947.

110. Costa V, Brophy JM. Drotrecogin alfa (activated) in severe sepsis: a systematic review and new cost-effectiveness analysis. *BMC Anesthesiology.* 2007;7:5.

111. Stoutenbeek CP, van Saene HKF, Miranda DR, Zandstra DF. The effect of selective decontamination of the digestive tract on colonisation and infection rate in multiple trauma patients. *Intensive Care Med.* 1984;10:185–192.

112. Ledingham IM, Alcock SR, Eastaway AT, McDonald JC, McKay IC, Ramsay G. Triple regimen of selective decontamination of the digestive tract, systemic cefotaxime, and microbiological surveillance for prevention of acquired infection in intensive care. *Lancet.* 1988;i:785–790.

113. Hammond JMJ, Potgieter PD, Saunders GL, Forder AA. Double-blind study of selective decontamination of the digestive tract in intensive care. *Lancet*. 1992;340:5–9.

114. Hamer DH, Barza M. Prevention of hospital-acquired pneumonia in critically ill patients. *Antimicrob Agents Chemother*. 1993;37:931–938.

115. Silvestri L, van Saene HKF, Milanese M, Gregori D, Gullo A. Selective decontamination of the digestive tract reduces bacterial bloodstream infection and mortality in critically ill patients. Systematic review of randomized, controlled trials. *J Hosp Infect*. 2007;65:187–203.

116. Paterson DL, Yu VL. Extended-spectrum beta-lactamases: a call for improved detection and control. *Clin Infect Dis*. 1999;29:1419–1422.

117. Boyce JM. It is time for action: improving hand hygiene in hospitals. *Ann Intern Med*. 1999;130:153–155.

118. Fridkin SK. Increasing prevalence of antimicrobial resistance in intensive care units. *Crit Care Med*. 2001;29:N64–N68.

119. Niederman MS. Impact of antibiotic resistance on clinical outcomes and the cost of care. *Crit Care Med*. 2001;29:N114–N120.

120. DeLisle S, Perl TM. Antimicrobial management measures to limit resistance: a process-based conceptual framework. *Crit Care Med*. 2001;29:N121–N127.

121. Namias N, Harvill S, Ball S, McKenney MG, Salomone JP, Civetta JM. Cost and morbidity associated with antibiotic prophylaxis in the ICU. *J Am Coll Surg*. 1999;188:225–230.

122. Vincent J-L. Microbial resistance: lessons from the EPIC study. *Intensive Care Med*. 2000;26:S3–S8.

123. Sirot DL, Goldstein FW, Soussy CJ, et al. Resistance to cefotaxime and seven other β-lactams in members of the family Enterobacteriaceae: a 3-year survey in France. *Antimicrob Agents Chemother*. 1992;36:1677–1681.

124. National Nosocomial Infections Surveillance System. National Nosocomial Infections Surveillance (NNIS) System report, data summary through June 2003, issued August 2003. *Am J Infect Control*. 2000;31:481–498.

125. Warren DK, Fraser VJ. Infection control measures to limit antimicrobial resistance. *Crit Care Med*. 2001;29:N128–N134.

126. Pittet D, Herwaldt LA, Massanari RM. The intensive care unit. In: Bennett JV, Brachman PS, eds. *Hospital infections*. 3rd ed. Boston: Little, Brown; 1992:405–439.

127. Pittet D. Nosocomial bloodstream infections. In: Wenzel RP, ed. *Prevention and control of nosocomial infections*. 2nd ed. Baltimore: Williams & Wilkins; 1993:512–555.

128. Duckworth G. Revised guidelines for the control of epidemic methicillin-resistant *Staphylococcus aureus*. *J Hosp Infect*. 1990;16:351–377.

129. Watanakunakorn C, Patel R. Comparison of patients with enterococcal bacteremia due to strains with and without high-level resistance to gentamicin. *Clin Infect Dis*. 1993;17:74–78.

130. Graninger W, Ragette R. Nosocomial bacteraemia due to *Enterococcus faecalis* without endocarditis. *Clin Infect Dis*. 1992;15:49–57.

131. Hospital Infection Control Practices Advisory Committee. Recommendations for preventing the spread of vancomycin resistance. *Infect Control Hosp Epidemiol*. 1995;16:105–113.

132. Brun-Buisson C, Legrand P, Philippon A, Montravers F, Ansquer M, Duval J. Transferable enzymatic resistance to third-generation cephalosporins during nosocomial outbreak of multi-resistant *Klebsiella pneumoniae*. *Lancet*. 1987;ii:302–306.

133. Livermore DM. Mechanisms of resistance to β-lactam antibiotics. *Scand J Infect Dis*. 1991;(suppl 78):7–16.

134. Snydman DR. Clinical implications of multi-drug resistance in the intensive care unit. *Scand J Infect Dis*. 1991;(suppl 78):54–63.

135. Meyer KS, Urban C, Eagan JA, Berger BJ, Rahal JJ. Nosocomial outbreak of *Klebsiella* infection resistant to late-generation cephalosporins. *Ann Intern Med*. 1993;119:353–358.

136. Munoz-Price LS, Weinstein RA. Acinetobacter infection. *N Engl J Med*. 2008;358:1271–1281.

137. Neu HC. Antimicrobial agents: role in the prevention and control of nosocomial infections. In: Wenzel RP, ed. *Prevention and control of nosocomial infections*. 2nd ed. Baltimore: Williams & Wilkins; 1993:406–419.

42 Infections associated with implanted medical devices

Michael Millar and David Wareham

There is a wide variety of implanted medical devices in use. This diversity is reflected in the range of infections associated with these devices. Device-associated infections account for 50% of hospital-acquired infections which have considerable economic and health costs.[1] Some of the more common and serious infections are covered in this chapter. These include infections associated with orthopedic implants, prosthetic heart valves, cardiac pacemakers, intravascular devices, cerebrospinal fluid drainage and pressure monitoring devices, urinary drainage catheters and peritoneal dialysis catheters. Ventilator-associated pneumonia is covered in Chapter 41.

PATHOGENESIS OF IMPLANT-ASSOCIATED INFECTIONS

Medical implants may be exposed to micro-organisms prior to, or at the time of, placement of the implant, through spread of bacteria from a contiguous site, via the bloodstream from a distant site or through a breach in the natural barrier to infection (such as the skin). Implants predispose to infections through a wide range of mechanisms including local tissue damage, compromise to local vascular perfusion, by providing both protected niches for microbial proliferation and surfaces for microbial attachment and biofilm formation, and by compromising local immunity. The majority of implanted medical devices in use today elicit a local immune response which depletes complement and reduces phagocytic and oxidative burst-dependent bactericidal activity of neutrophils.[2]

A biofilm consists of micro-organisms adherent to a surface often in a secreted polymer matrix. Biofilms on clinical implants almost always form within a complex matrix of both microbial secreted, polymer and host-derived molecules. Adhesion to conditioned surfaces is facilitated in some bacteria by specific adhesins, for example *Staphylococcus aureus* has both fibronectin- and fibrinogen-binding surface proteins. Biofilm forming *Staph. epidermidis* strains may produce an extracellular polysaccharide known as polysaccharide intercellular adhesin (PIA). This promotes the development and maturation of the biofilm and is under complex regulatory

control, enabling the organism to respond to the local environment.[3] Adhesion and biofilm formation are probably both prerequisites for the development of implant-associated infections.

Almost all infections associated with implants are caused by bacteria or fungi (most frequently *Candida* spp.). Bacteria associated with implant infections include not only Gram-positive bacteria, particularly staphylococci, but also enterococci, corynebacteria and Gram-negative bacteria such as Enterobacteriaceae, *Pseudomonas* spp. and *Acinetobacter* spp. Viruses, protozoa or helminths are rarely associated with implant infections. In the natural world and at sites of microbial colonization, such as the human oral cavity, biofilms usually consist of polymicrobial consortia. Biofilms associated with implant infection may be polymicrobial but more frequently consist of single strains of bacteria. Once a biofilm has formed, the micro-organisms within the biofilm are relatively resistant to both host defense factors and antimicrobial drugs.[4] As a consequence, infections are difficult to treat and device removal is frequently required to cure the infection.

Understanding the molecular biology of biofilm formation and stabilization has the potential to inform the development of new strategies for the prevention and treatment of biofilm-associated infections.[5–8]

DETERMINANTS OF BIOFILM ANTIBIOTIC RESISTANCE

Bacterial biofilms tend to show much higher levels of resistance to antimicrobial agents than planktonic cells.[9] There are many potential mechanisms to explain this. Growth phase and growth rate are key determinants of antimicrobial susceptibility.[10] Slowly growing bacteria are much less susceptible to the bactericidal activity of antimicrobials such as β-lactams. A proportion of micro-organisms in a biofilm are nutrient deprived and grow very slowly.[11] Binding of antimicrobials to extracellular matrix macromolecules and dead bacteria, protection of viable bacteria deep in the matrix by inactivating enzyme activity from surrounding bacteria[12] and changes in ionic gradients leading to changes in antimicrobial diffusion may also give some protection to biofilm bacteria. Alterations in microbial physiology associated with the biofilm mode of growth probably also contribute to reducing antimicrobial susceptibility. A recent report suggests that binding of antimicrobials to periplasmic glucans may be an important mechanism of resistance of biofilm bacteria to some antibiotics in *Pseudomonas aeruginosa*.[13] Microelectrode analysis of oxygen concentrations in *Ps. aeruginosa* biofilms[14] suggests that only the bacteria at the air–biofilm interface have sufficient oxygen for growth, and so it may be that oxygen utilization and poor diffusion are at least as important as the diffusion of antimicrobial agents in determining antimicrobial resistance. A genetic locus has been described in *Ps. aeruginosa* which is important in regulating phenotype (slow-growing, small colony variants), propensity to biofilm formation and antibiotic resistance.[15]

Cell-to-cell interactions in surface-associated bacterial populations are determined by quorum-sensing molecules. Interference with bacterial cell signaling mechanisms has the potential to control microbial colonization of implants;[8,16] for example, RNA III inhibiting peptide (RIP) inhibits biofilm formation by *Staph. aureus* and when combined with antibiotics can inhibit biofilm formation on implants in rats.[17] Eukaryotic cells may also respond to bacterial signaling molecules,[18] and this is an important consideration should targeted disruption of bacterial signaling become a therapeutic strategy for patients with implant infections. Much of the human commensal flora is biofilm associated and could also be disrupted by therapeutic strategies targeting bacterial intercellular signaling.

USE OF ANTIBIOTICS FOR THE PREVENTION OR TREATMENT OF IMPLANT-ASSOCIATED INFECTIONS

Basic principles for the prevention of implant-associated infections include the control of patient risk factors for infection (e.g. diabetes and obesity), optimization of the conditions under which devices are implanted, and ensuring that those who insert and care for medical devices are appropriately trained and experienced.

One of the simplest and most cost-effective strategies for the prevention of infections associated with some types of medical implant has been the use of perioperative antimicrobial prophylaxis following the principles that supra-inhibitory concentrations of an antimicrobial (with an appropriate spectrum of activity) are present at the site of surgery at the time the operative procedure starts. Further details are given in the sections on specific implant-associated infections.

Some antibiotics reach high concentrations and retain antimicrobial activity in biofilms, such as quinolones and rifampicin (rifampin). Both in-vitro[19] and clinical studies support the use of rifampicin as adjunctive treatment, particularly for

staphylococcal infections associated with medical implants. Vancomycin has a place in the treatment of infections caused by methicillin-resistant staphylococci but is probably inferior to β-lactam antibiotics for implant-associated infections caused by methicillin-susceptible strains.[1] Among the newer agents for the treatment of Gram-positive infections, daptomycin and tigecycline have demonstrated activity in vitro against organism-embedded biofilms.[20] With the exception of catheter-associated urinary tract infection, the empirical treatment of the majority of implant-associated infections discussed in this chapter would include the use of a glycopeptide such as vancomycin ± rifampicin ± an agent with activity against Gram-negative bacteria (such as a fluoroquinolone). Further details of antibiotic selection and duration of treatment are given in the sections describing treatment of infections associated with specific types of medical implant.

Use of antibiotics is not without adverse consequences; for example, administration of a single dose of a semisynthetic penicillin poses a risk of anaphylaxis of approximately 0.04%, of skin rash of 5% and of *C. difficile* antibiotic-associated colitis of >0.01%.[21] Antibiotic exposure may promote the formation of biofilms by some organisms. In *Ps. aeruginosa*, subinhibitory concentrations of aminoglycosides facilitate adhesion to plastic surfaces via induction of a transmembrane signaling system which modulates cell-surface adhesiveness.[22]

Recommendations in this chapter are based on the principle that antibiotics should only be used when there is evidence that the benefits of use outweigh the risks.

INFECTIONS ASSOCIATED WITH SPECIFIC TYPES OF MEDICAL IMPLANT

INFECTIONS ASSOCIATED WITH ORTHOPEDIC IMPLANTS

The mean cost of hip replacement across nine European countries reported in 2008 was over €5000 (~US$7200).[23] The number of hip and knee replacements carried out each year is increasing both in Europe and North America.[24] Infection of implanted joints adds substantial additional economic costs and morbidity.[25]

The risk of infection is probably highest in the first 2–3 years, with combined rates of hip and knee implant infection of 6.5 per 1000 joint-years for the first postoperative year, 3.2 per 1000 joint-years during the second year and 1.4 per 1000 in subsequent years. The risk of prosthetic joint infection varies with a number of factors, including the type of prosthesis, operator experience and duration of procedure(s), together with host-dependent risk factors including old age, immune compromise, obesity and diabetes mellitus.[1,26,27] In the UK National Health Service, hip and knee implant surgery has been subject to mandatory surveillance of surgical site infection since April 2004. There were over 140 000 primary prosthetic hip or knee implant procedures in England and Wales in the year 2007–8, and an additional 10 000 revision hip or knee procedures.[28] Rates of infection for hip and knee arthroplasty of 3.3% have been recorded over the 4-year period from April 2004, of 0.8% for total hip prostheses and 0.4% for knee prostheses.[28] Approximately one-quarter of infections involve the deep tissues. The infections that have been recorded are those which present in hospital. A proportion of orthopedic implant infections present weeks or even in some cases years after the initial procedure so rates of infection may be underestimated by short durations of follow-up. In the UK surveillance is being improved to try to capture infections that develop following hospital discharge.

Comparison of rates of infection by center requires risk adjustment. In the UK a risk index is used to measure variation in risk factors which comprise measures of the likely microbial contamination of the wound, determination of the degree of severity of underlying systemic disease and the duration of the operation.[29] In part, the differences between the rates of infection for different types of orthopedic implant procedure reflect the frequency and severity of risk factors in patients undergoing the various procedures.

 ## CLASSIFICATION OF PROSTHETIC JOINT INFECTIONS

Several staging systems have been proposed for prosthetic joint sepsis but consensus is lacking. The most widely accepted system is that formulated originally by Coventry[30] and modified by Gillespie:[31]

- *Stage 1* infections are defined as those occurring within 1 month of surgery. Patients with stage 1 infections typically present with signs of sepsis as well as local signs of infection, with local erythema and wound discharge. The organisms most commonly recovered from stage 1 infections derive from the patient's skin, bacteria in operating room air, or the skin of members of the surgical team.[32,33]
- *Stage 2* infections are defined as those that occur after 1 month but within 2 years of surgery. The infections are also thought to derive from the introduction of organisms of low pathogenicity, such as coagulase-negative staphylococci and *Propionibacterium* spp., at the time of surgery. Patients typically exhibit gradual impairment of prosthetic function (i.e. early loosening of the prosthesis and increasing joint pain).
- *Stage 3* infections are arbitrarily defined as infections that occur more than 2 years after surgery and are assumed to derive from hematogenous seeding of the joint.

In practice there is considerable variation in presentation and it is difficult to definitively identify a source of infection. The majority of infections can be prevented by measures that target the perioperative period and this observation is consistent with colonization at the time of operation being the major determinant of the risk of subsequent infection.

 ## MICROBIOLOGY

Gram-positive organisms, particularly staphylococci, are the most frequent isolates. Streptococci, corynebacteria, propionibacteria and enterococci are found less frequently, and rarely Gram-negative bacilli, anaerobes or fungi, particularly following gross contamination of the operation site or in association with sinus formation or other lesions, leading to a breakdown in natural barriers to infection.[25]

 ## DIAGNOSIS

The clinical presentation ranges from an acute illness with systemic signs of infection of varying severity to insidious illness associated with local pain and perhaps joint loosening. *Staph. aureus* bloodstream infection can lead to seeding of prosthetic joints and an acute onset of joint infection.[34] When a patient with an implant and few other risk factors for infection develops signs and symptoms of infection associated with inflammation at the site of the implant, then the diagnosis may be relatively straightforward. A more frequent scenario is the insidious development of non-specific signs and symptoms of infection.[35]

Diagnostic problems arise because of the difficulty in sampling the surface of the implant. Joint infection with coagulase-negative staphylococci, which are the most frequent cause of prosthetic joint infection, is rarely associated with bacteremia. There may be leukocytosis and raised non-specific markers of infection such as C-reactive protein. Ultrasound may show evidence of an effusion and may be used to facilitate aspiration. Conventional radiography is usually normal but may reveal bone loss and loosening around a chronically infected prosthesis. Newer radiological approaches, such as positron emission tomography and the use of labeled antimicrobial peptides, have the potential to improve the diagnostic sensitivity of radiological methods.

Identifying causative agents of infection has important implications for both treatment and prognosis. It is important to try to optimize the chance of a positive culture result by avoiding the use of antimicrobial agents in the period immediately preceding joint aspiration or open tissue biopsy. Multiple samples (up to six) should be sent to the laboratory for culture. The isolation of identical organisms from three such specimens is highly predictive of infection.[36] Histopathological analysis of tissue samples as well as the white cell count in aspirated synovial fluid can also be helpful. The place of molecular microbiological methods in the diagnosis of prosthetic joint infections remains unclear at the present time.

 ## TREATMENT

The treatment of prosthetic joint infections requires the integrated use of antimicrobials with surgical management, and tailoring the overall management strategy to the patient's particular circumstances, taking account of co-morbidities and life expectancy.[27,36] Traditionally infections associated with prosthetic joints have been managed by a two-stage exchange arthroplasty in which the colonized device is removed and the site debrided. The patient is then treated for an extended period with antibiotics based on the results of culture samples collected at the time of the surgery. When clinical signs of infection have resolved and the non-specific markers of infection such as C-reactive protein have normalized, then a new device is implanted.

A number of other approaches have been tried, including initial irrigation and debridement with retention of the device, one-stage exchange arthroplasty (in both of these cases combined with prolonged antimicrobial therapy), and the use of prolonged suppressive antimicrobial therapy.[37] There is evidence that each of these approaches can be appropriate and successful in selected patients. Debridement with retention of the colonized prosthesis followed by indefinite durations of suppressive antimicrobial therapy has also been used in patients where exchange arthroplasty is not feasible or where the quality of life associated with prolonged immobilization is unacceptable to the patient.[38]

The optimum antimicrobial treatment for infections associated with prosthetic devices is not known. Staphylococci are the most frequent infecting organisms and there is a wide range of drugs available, including isoxazole penicillins (such as flucloxacillin), clindamycin, linezolid, vancomycin, sodium fusidate, rifampicin, trimethoprim, tetracycline and quinolones, depending upon the antimicrobial susceptibility of isolates and clinical indications.

Animal models and clinical data[39,40] support the inclusion of rifampicin in treatment regimens. Rifampicin cannot be used as a single agent because of the risk of mutational resistance and should not be used if the infecting organism is shown to be resistant in vitro. For strains susceptible to methicillin, an isoxazole penicillin is recommended in combination with rifampicin; for patients with methicillin-resistant organisms or with a history of allergy to penicillin, then vancomycin can be combined with rifampicin.

Fluoroquinolones are highly bioavailable when administered orally and attain high joint fluid concentrations in experimental animal models of staphylococcal prosthetic joint infection and in clinical trials of oral therapy in chronic osteomyelitis, so may have a place in oral treatment, particularly after a period of treatment with intravenous antibiotics.[37] When used for staphylococcal infections in particular, antimicrobial susceptibility should be confirmed in vitro, and treatment with fluoroquinolones should be combined with another agent to limit the possibility of quinolone resistance developing during treatment. Fluoroquinolones generally have excellent activity against Gram-negative bacteria and may be the drugs of choice for susceptible Gram-negative infections. Carbapenems, cephalosporins and aminoglycosides may also have a place depending upon the laboratory findings and clinical picture.

Liposomal amphotericin preparations are the drugs of choice for fungal prosthetic joint infections. Rifampicin, sodium fusidate and fluoroquinolones such as ciprofloxacin are well absorbed orally and have been use in combinations for oral treatment or suppression of infection.[41]

The optimum duration of antibiotic therapy is unknown. Durations of 4–6 weeks are usually given for revision arthroplasty and longer durations (>3 months) for retained prostheses.[38]

There are a number of newer antimicrobial agents, including linezolid, daptomycin and tigecycline, but their role in the treatment of orthopedic implant infections is yet to be defined.[27,42]

 ## PREVENTION

Pooled analysis of four randomized placebo-controlled trials of antibiotic prophylaxis in prosthetic joint surgery demonstrates a 76% reduction in infection (odds ratio 0.24; 95% CI, 0.15–0.37).[32] The classic study by Hill et al[43] shows that the cumulative benefit of prophylaxis increases the further out the patient is from surgery; 99.5%, 99.3% and 99% of patients randomized to antibiotic prophylaxis remained free of prosthetic joint infection at 12, 24 and 36 months, respectively, compared with 97.5%, 97% and 96% in the control group during the same periods. The duration of perioperative prophylaxis in these trials ranged from 24 h to 2 weeks. Subsequent studies of antibiotic prophylaxis in orthopedic and other types of surgery have shown unequivocally that no added benefit is gained by extending prophylaxis beyond 24 h.[44,45]

Giving prophylactic antibiotics by other routes, such as incorporation into the polymethyl methacrylate (PMMA) cement, has been examined in several studies. A randomized trial in a large number of primary total hip arthroplasties demonstrated that the use of antibiotic-impregnated cement was equivalent to systemic antibiotic therapy alone; 13 late infections occurred in the systemic antibiotic prophylaxis group and nine in the antibiotic-impregnated cement group.[46] An analysis of 10 905 cemented primary hip arthroplasties in the Norwegian Arthroplasty Register suggests that combined use of systemic prophylactic antibiotics and antibiotic-impregnated cement is associated with a lower range of infection than either intervention alone (5-year incidence of infection 0.2% in the combined prophylaxis group vs 0.8% with systemic prophylaxis alone, $p = 0.001$);[47] however, a randomized trial comparing systemic prophylactic antibiotics alone with combined systemic antibiotic/antibiotic-impregnated cement regimens is lacking.

The use of late antibiotic prophylaxis after successful joint implantation to prevent hematogenous prosthetic joint infection, particularly with invasive dental procedures, is a routine practice of most orthopedic surgeons.[48] However, this has come under scrutiny, given the very low rates of late hematogenous infection seen in large series (7–11% of all prosthetic joint infections)[49,50] and the absence of studies demonstrating efficacy or cost benefit.[51,52] A decision analysis study of antibiotic prophylaxis for dental procedures to prevent prosthetic joint infections concluded that US$480 000 would need to be spent to prevent a single case of late prosthetic joint infection and that adoption of routine penicillin prophylaxis would actually result in more deaths than not using prophylaxis because of adverse effects from the prophylactic drugs.[53] A retrospective study of 3490 patients with prosthetic joints found that only seven developed prosthetic joint infection temporally related to a dental procedure.[50] Five of these seven had underlying co-morbidity that predisposed them to infection, such as diabetes mellitus or rheumatoid arthritis. Based on these data, recent recommendations for the use of antibiotic prophylaxis in patients with prosthetic joints undergoing invasive procedures include patients with rheumatoid arthritis with a prosthesis implanted within the past year, an overt oral infection, a prolonged dental procedure (>115 min) and, possibly, diabetes mellitus or chronic corticosteroid therapy.[54]

The prevention of infections with troublesome pathogens such as methicillin-resistant *Staph. aureus* (MRSA) has been attempted by decontamination of colonized individuals before surgery[55] and by the use of selective admission policies to beds ring-fenced for elective orthopedic surgery.[56] In addition to the use of prophylactic antibiotics, many orthopedic procedures are carried out in theatres supplied with ultra-filtered air over the operating field. The benefits of ultra-filtered air are much reduced when antimicrobial prophylaxis is used. The use of ultraviolet light to sterilize operating room air has also been shown to be effective. There is insufficient evidence to support the cost-effectiveness of use of impermeable clothing or ventilation suits in orthopedic implant surgery.

INFECTIONS ASSOCIATED WITH PROSTHETIC HEART VALVES

Prosthetic valve endocarditis is harder to diagnose and to treat than native valve endocarditis. Prosthetic valve endocarditis develops in 3–6% of patients within 5 years of valve implantation.[57] The risk of prosthetic valve endocarditis is highest within the first 2–3 months after surgery and then falls to 0.1–0.7% per patient-year thereafter. Prosthetic valve endocarditis has high associated mortality (in excess of 30%) which is highest when endocarditis develops within 60 days of operation.[57,58] Mitral and aortic valve replacements seem to have similar levels of risk of associated endocarditis. Mechanical valves have a higher incidence of infection in the first 12 months after implantation, whereas bioprosthetic valves have a higher incidence than mechanical valves after 12 months post operation. The overall 5-year risk of infection associated with mechanical and bioprosthetic valves is similar.[59]

 CLASSIFICATION

Prosthetic valve endocarditis (PVE) is usually defined as early or late. Many currently favor a cut-off of 12 months post surgery. Infections presenting in the first 2 months after surgery are usually the result of infection during surgery, whilst those occurring up to 12 months may be nosocomial or community acquired. Coagulase-negative staphylococci, *Staph. aureus* and *Enterococcus* spp. are the commonest causes of early PVE.[58,60] After 12 months, causes of PVE are more likely to be from the same groups of organisms that cause native valve endocarditis. The type of organism causing PVE probably contributes to the worst outcomes associated with early prosthetic valve endocarditis.

 DIAGNOSIS

Signs and symptoms associated with PVE are similar to those seen with native valve endocarditis and include fever, new or changing murmur, congestive heart failure, petechiae, splenomegaly, embolic phenomena including strokes or transient ischemic attacks, shock and conduction abnormalities. Osler's nodes, Janeway lesions and Roth's spots are relatively infrequent. The features of presentation are in part related to the causative agent of infection; for example, *Staph. aureus* endocarditis is associated with a neurological event in 25–67% of cases and septic shock in 30%.[61]

Blood cultures are the key to identification of the etiological agents of endocarditis. Endocarditis is one of the few conditions associated with continuous bacteremia. A large volume of blood should be collected from the patient (>30 mL from an adult) as soon as the diagnosis is considered and before antimicrobial therapy has been started. When blood cultures remain negative despite strong clinical suspicion of endocarditis, then it is important to consider the possibility of infection with fastidious micro-organisms which require the use of special cultures, molecular or serological tests.

Transthoracic echocardiography detects larger vegetations (>10 mm) and has a sensitivity of <40% compared with a sensitivity of 77–100% for transesophageal echocardiography for the diagnosis of PVE.[62] Transesophageal echocardiography is also much more sensitive for the detection of perivalvular abscess and valvular dysfunction. There may be advantages of using both transesophageal and transthoracic echocardiography.[63] The combination of clinical, laboratory and echocardiographic findings enables a decision on the likelihood of endocarditis to be made by comparison with the Duke criteria scoring system.[64]

 TREATMENT

There are many uncertainties with respect to the optimal treatment for PVE with the surgical approach, antimicrobial choices and the role of anticoagulation.[61] Effective intervention strategies often require a combined medical and surgical approach,[65] particularly when endocarditis is caused by *Staph. aureus*.[66] Guidelines on the treatment of PVE are given by both the British Society for Antimicrobial Chemotherapy[67] and the American Heart Association.[68]

When there is evidence of complicated PVE, such as a new or worsening murmur, progressive congestive heart failure due to valvular dysfunction or abscess, new echocardiographic conduction abnormalities or evidence of intracardiac abscess or fulminant abscess, then treatment should be started as soon as blood cultures have been collected. Empirical treatment of early PVE should include vancomycin to take account of methicillin-resistant staphylococci. In patients who suffered nosocomial bacteremia around the time of prosthetic valve implantation, consideration should be given to covering the microbes associated with bacteremia at that time.[69]

A decision to replace a prosthetic valve requires that a wide range of different factors are taken into account, including cardiac and valvular functional status, evidence of persistent bloodstream infection despite antibiotic treatment, relapse of endocarditis following cessation of treatment, evidence of persistent sepsis despite appropriate antimicrobial treatment for 10 days, and co-morbidities.

The duration of antimicrobial therapy for PVE is longer than for native valve endocarditis as is the duration of combination therapy. The addition of rifampicin to treatment regimens for staphylococcal infection based on experience in osteomyelitis and prosthetic joint infections may be of value. The place of newer agents such as linezolid, a bacteristatic drug,[70] and daptomycin remains unclear at the present time.

Fungal PVE frequently requires valve replacement and prolonged antifungal therapy. Liposomal amphotericin combined with 5-flucytosine has been recommended for PVE caused by *Candida* spp. and there is some evidence that prolonged suppressive therapy with oral azoles may reduce the risk of recurrent infection.[71]

PREVENTION

Prosthetic valves may be contaminated at the time of surgery or shortly thereafter with seeding as a consequence of bacteremia.[69] Strategies to reduce the use of invasive medical devices in these patients, such as intravascular catheters and urinary catheters, would be expected to reduce the risk of PVE. Antimicrobial prophylaxis makes an important contribution to reducing the risk of microbial colonization associated with surgery, using antimicrobials with activity against staphylococci such as isoxazole penicillins, cephalosporins and/or aminoglysides. Surgical technique is also a major factor in determining the risk of PVE.

There is little evidence that use of antibiotic prophylaxis for dental or non-dental procedures reduces the overall risk of endocarditis, so recent guidelines do not recommend the use of prophylactic antibiotics for patients with prosthetic valves undergoing dental or non-dental surgical interventions, unless the operation is at a site of suspected active infection[72] (*see* Ch. 46).

PACEMAKER DEVICE INFECTIONS

Cardiac pacemakers are increasingly used to control heart function. The reported incidence of pacemaker-associated infection varies from 0.1% to 20%, with a mortality of up to 70%.[73] Although pacemaker-associated infections can present years after implantation, 25% of infections present within 2 months of implantation. The risk of pacemaker infection may be higher when pacemakers have been replaced than following first implantation. Infections can arise around the pulse generator, along the pacing leads or within an intravascular compartment when there are transvenous endocardial tracking leads. Co-morbidities which predispose to pacemaker infection include diabetes mellitus, malignancy, corticosteroids and skin diseases.[74] Multiple pacemaker insertions and inexperienced operators are also associated with higher rates of infection.[75]

MICROBIOLOGY

Although the most frequent isolates in pacemaker-associated infections are staphylococci, a wide range of other microorganisms have been reported, including in particular Gram-negative bacilli, propionibacteria and fungi.[73]

DIAGNOSIS

The clinical presentation of pacemaker infection depends on whether it involves the pulse-generator pocket or the pacing leads. Infection of the pulse-generator pocket typically occurs shortly following implantation or battery exchange, and manifests with localized erythema, pain and fluctuance, occasionally with erosion of the overlying skin.[74,75] Rarely, migration of infection from the pocket produces pericardial involvement when epicardial pacing leads are used, or bloodstream infection with the use of endocardial pacing leads. Infection of endocardial pacing leads typically presents as a primary bloodstream infection that varies in severity, depending on the causative organism. Coagulase-negative staphylococci tend to cause an indolent febrile illness in contrast to fulminant sepsis with *Staph. aureus*. In either case, signs and symptoms of right-sided endocarditis are often present, including fever and chills (>80%), septic pulmonary emboli (20–45%) and tricuspid regurgitation (25%).[76,77]

A presumptive diagnosis of a pulse-generator pocket infection can usually be made on clinical grounds alone and is confirmed by a percutaneous aspirate from the pocket that shows micro-organisms on Gram stain or in culture. Diagnosing infection of an epicardial pacing lead can be more challenging unless bloodstream infection is present. Pericarditis or mediastinitis can usually be diagnosed by CT or MRI. Patients with endocardial pacing lead infections, in addition to manifesting signs of right-sided endocarditis, frequently have persistent bloodstream infection, despite appropriate antimicrobial therapy.[64,76] Echocardiography shows vegetations on the endocardial leads and/or the tricuspid valve, and is valuable for confirming infection. Transesophageal echocardiography, with a sensitivity that ranges from 90% to 96% (compared with a 22–43% sensitivity seen with transthoracic echocardiography) is preferred.[76–79]

 ## TREATMENT

Treatment usually requires combined medical and surgical management.[73] The overwhelming evidence is that for pacemaker-associated endocarditis the entire pacemaker system should be removed. Recent studies suggest that a new system can be implanted at a different site at the time of removal of the old system without an increase in recurrence rate by comparison with delayed replacement. Open heart surgery may be required to remove endocardial leads that have been in place for long periods.

There are no randomized comparative studies of antibiotic treatment protocols for pacemaker-associated infections. Most recommend treatment durations similar to those used for endocarditis, with antibiotic choice determined by in-vitro testing of isolates. Drugs with activity against methicillin-resistant staphylococci should be used when no organism can be cultured. The American Heart Association recommends 14 days of antimicrobial treatment after device removal and the first negative blood culture and 4 weeks of therapy when there is evidence of *Staph. aureus* bloodstream infection.[68]

 ## PREVENTION

The basic principles for reducing the risk of prosthetic device-associated infection apply to pacemakers (see introductory section). Perioperative antibiotic prophylaxis significantly reduces the risk of pacemaker-associated infection[80] both for primary procedures and for replacement of infected devices.[81]

INTRAVASCULAR DEVICE-ASSOCIATED INFECTIONS

The majority of patients admitted to acute hospitals will have an intravenous catheter placed to facilitate medical care. This may be for administration of fluids, electrolytes, blood products, drugs, nutritional support and for hemodynamic monitoring. Widespread use of peripheral and central venous access devices have led to these devices becoming the major risk factor for hospital-acquired bloodstream infection.[82–85] The attributable mortality for these bloodstream infections is up to 25%.[86]

The central vascular catheter infection rate varies from <1 to 15 episodes/1000 days of central line use, depending upon the patient population, type of device and a range of other factors.[87] The cost of a central vascular catheter-associated infection can be many thousands of dollars per episode, depending upon the virulence of the infecting agent. Complications of vascular access device infections include septic thrombophlebitis, endocarditis, septic shock and the dissemination of septic emboli.

 ## PATHOGENESIS

Vascular access device-associated infections can develop as a consequence of contamination of infusates, contamination of the luminal surface of the catheter from hubs and other connections, through migration of micro-organisms from the skin surface along the outside of the catheter, or through bloodstream spread from a distant site[77,88–90] (Fig. 42.1). There is some evidence that infections which develop in the first 2 weeks after implantation of the device are most frequently derived from migration of bacteria along the outside of the catheter, while those that present 2 weeks or more after implantation are more frequently intraluminal.[91–93] This is important when considering the potential benefits associated with the use of antimicrobial locks for the treatment of vascular access device-associated infections.

 ## MICROBIOLOGY

Although staphylococci are the most frequent cause of intravascular device-associated infection, there are a wide range of other bacteria (including particularly Gram-negative bacilli and yeasts) that may be associated with intravascular access device-associated infection.

 ## DIAGNOSIS

Diagnostic methods for vascular access device-associated infections have been subject to a recent review by the Infectious Diseases Society of America.[94] These include recommendations on blood cultures and catheter tip cultures. Clinical findings that point to vascular access device-associated infection include evidence of inflammation at the exit site (particularly when inflammation extends subcutaneously), fever and rigors associated with catheter manipulations, and septic shock in a patient with an intravascular device and without other risk factors for septic shock (e.g. immunocompetent

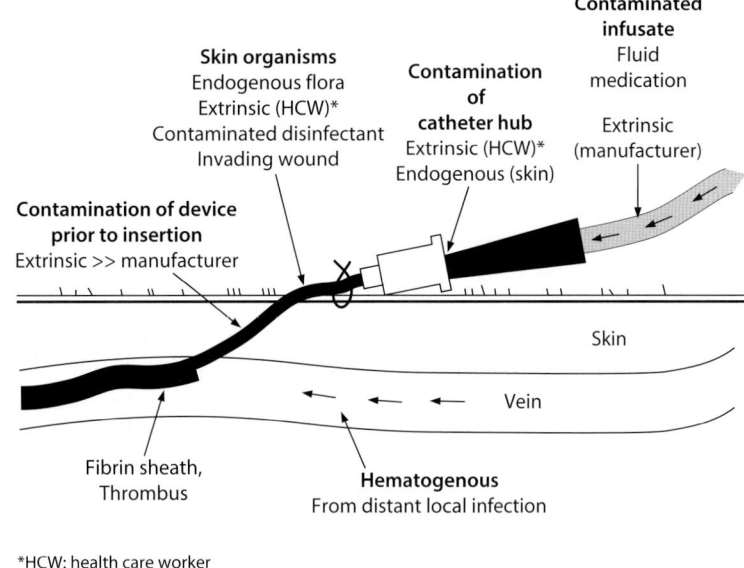

Fig. 42.1 Routes of microbial colonization in the pathogenesis of intravascular device-related bloodstream infection.

individuals receiving long-term intravenous feeding following bowel resection for trauma).[95] The isolation of staphylococci or other skin bacteria from multiple blood cultures, *Bacillus* spp. or fungi would also point to a potential vascular access device source of infection. Semiquantitative culture methods can be used to identify colonization of a device once it has been removed (>15 cfu/mL from a 5 cm segment of the catheter tip).[89,96] Culture of indistinguishable isolates from blood and from the device is strong evidence implicating the intravascular device in the etiology of bacteremia.[89,97,98]

In many groups of patients, particularly those with longer-term surgically implanted devices such as Hickman and Broviac catheters, hemodialysis catheters and venous ports, device removal and replacement may carry substantial risks as well as costs. In these groups, since less than half of the episodes of bloodstream infection are related to the intravascular device,[99,100] considerable emphasis is given to trying to improve diagnostic methods, and even if the intravascular device is thought to be the source of infection frequently attempts will be made to eradicate infection without device removal.

Numerous studies have shown quantitative differences in the concentration of micro-organisms in blood collected through intravascular devices compared with blood collected from a peripheral vein when there is a device-associated infection.[101–103] A relatively cost-effective way of estimating the differences in microbial numbers between blood collected from a vascular access device and peripheral blood is to use the differential time to positivity.[104] When a blood culture bottle is continuously monitored using an automated microbial growth detection device (as is widely used in diagnostic laboratories) the time to detection of positivity is a function of microbial numbers in the inoculated blood. Assuming that the blood volumes are similar, then detection of positivity in the blood drawn from the intravascular device more than 2 h

before positivity in the blood drawn from the peripheral site is highly predictive of an intravascular device-associated infection. This technique is particularly appropriate for longer-term devices in which infection is frequently intraluminal but probably less effective for short-term intravascular devices where infection may be on the outside of the catheter, or in patient populations in whom antimicrobial substances may be present in samples. When there are large numbers of bacteria in blood drawn through an intravascular catheter these can be visualized using techniques such as acridine orange leukocyte cytospin staining and this technique can provide a rapid diagnosis.[99,105] When peripheral blood cultures cannot be obtained, cultures may be drawn through different catheter lumens. A three-fold difference in quantitative blood cultures obtained from different lumens is suggestive of device infection in this instance; the value of differential time to positivity in this setting is uncertain.[106] Other methods that have been used to diagnose intravascular device-associated infection include luminal brushing[107,108] and quantitative microbial DNA detection.[109]

 TREATMENT

When a vascular catheter is suspected of being a source of infection and the catheter is no longer strictly required, it should be removed as soon as possible. Short-term vascular catheters can often be removed relatively easily and a new catheter inserted at another site. Long-term central venous devices should be removed when there is evidence of device-associated infection and also persistent exit site infection, infection extending along the tunnel, evidence of endocarditis, septic thrombosis or septic pulmonary emboli, persistent bacteremia or candidemia despite appropriate antimicrobial chemotherapy, or when infection is caused by

Staph. aureus-resistant species such as JK corynebacteria, *Stenotrophomonas* spp., *Burkholderia* spp., *Pseudomonas* spp., *Mycobacterium* spp., filamentous fungi or *Malassezia* spp. There are significant rates of recurrent bloodstream infection; for example for coagulase-negative staphylococcal vascular access device-associated infection, the risk of recurrent bacteremia is *c*. 20%.[110] Studies have shown an increased mortality rate in patients with vascular access device-associated candidemia when the catheter is left in place compared with prompt removal. This is a particular concern in infants.[111,112]

If the vascular access device is left in place, it is mandatory that the patient receives antibiotics through the infected line. There is some evidence that antibiotic locks can improve the outcome for patients, in particular by reducing the risk of recurrent infection.[113–117] Although there is a lower risk of infection associated with venous ports, there is also evidence that treatment of port-associated infections is less likely to be effective (without device removal) than infections associated with transcutaneous venous catheters.[118,119] Initial therapy for suspected intravascular device-associated infection should usually incorporate an agent with activity against methicillin-resistant staphylococci (probably a glycopeptide) and an agent with activity against Gram-negative bacilli. Initial therapy can be modified based on microbial isolates and their susceptibilities. The duration of treatment for uncomplicated intravascular device-associated infections is usually in the range of 7–10 days. Complications such as endocarditis may require much longer durations of treatment. *Staph. aureus* vascular access device-associated infection requires a longer duration of treatment. In immunocompetent patients and when the device has been removed it may be possible to restrict the duration of antibiotic treatment to 14 days. In immunocompromised patients, or where there is evidence of complications such as endocarditis, treatment should be given for a minimum of 4 weeks.[120,121]

Fluconazole can be used for candida vascular access device-associated infection in non-neutropenic patients[122] following removal of the intravascular device. In immunocompromised patients, those with complicated infections or those with infections caused by fluconazole-resistant species or strains, current evidence favors the use of amphotericin preparations.[123,124] The place of newer antifungal agents such as caspofungin and voriconazole is yet to be defined.

Patients may develop recurrent bloodstream infection weeks or months after treatment for vascular device-associated bloodstream infection and this may be associated with other complications such as endocarditis, retinitis and vertebral osteomyelitis.[123,125,126]

 PREVENTION

Widespread recognition of the costs and consequences of infection associated with intravascular devices has led to the development of practices which reduce these risks

and these have been included within strategies to improve patient safety such as the 'Saving 100 000 Lives' campaign in the USA.[127] Risk reduction measures include the use of barrier precautions for central venous catheter insertion (such as sterile gloves), chlorhexidine-based skin disinfection pre-implantation of the device, improved device designs such as Hickman or Broviac catheters which incorporate a Dacron cuff (which provides a mechanical barrier to microbial migration from the skin surface along the outside of the intravascular device), use of novel dressings, and the use of antimicrobial locks. Chlorhexidine preparations have been shown to be superior to povidone–iodine for skin decontamination prior to device insertion and are also now recommended for decontamination of hubs and connections.[128,129] Two percent chlorhexidine may be more effective than lower concentrations.[130]

Trial data suggest that chlorhexidine-impregnated sponge dressings reduce the risk of vascular access device-associated bloodstream infection in patients with short-term central venous catheters.[131–133]

Antimicrobial venous catheters

A number of antimicrobial impregnated venous catheters have been marketed over the last 10 years. The antimicrobials that have been incorporated have included silver sulfadiazine with chlorhexidine,[134,135] minocycline–rifampicin,[98] microdispersed silver[136,137] and silver–platinum.[138,139] Heparin bonded to venous catheters with benzalkonium chloride has also been shown to reduce microbial colonization.[140–142] A recent systematic review concluded that heparin-coated or antibiotic-impregnated central venous catheters are more effective at preventing bloodstream infection than those using chlorhexidine and silver sulfadiazine or silver impregnation.[143]

Antimicrobial locks

It is not clear that prophylactic use of systemic antibiotics at the time of vascular access device implantation reduces the risk of device-associated infection.[129] Continuous infusion of vancomycin in intravenous feeding solutions has been shown to reduce the rates of coagulase-negative staphylococcal bacteremia in low birth weight infants[144] but runs the theoretical risk of promotion of antibiotic resistance.

A number of randomized controlled trials have shown that rates of bloodstream infection can be greatly reduced by using antimicrobial lock solutions. Recent meta-analyses support the use of antimicrobial locks to prevent infection in patients with long-term devices.[145,146] These lock solutions have both anticoagulant and antimicrobial activities. Solutions that have been used include heparin with vancomycin 25 μg/mL ± ciprofloxacin (2 μg/mL), minocycline EDTA, taurolidine citrate and trisodium citrate. The benefits of use of antimicrobial locks is increasingly recognized within best practice guidelines.[129]

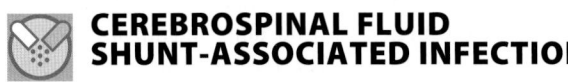

INFECTIONS ASSOCIATED WITH CEREBROSPINAL FLUID SHUNTS AND EXTERNAL DRAINAGE DEVICES

The pathological consequences of an excess of cerebrospinal fluid (CSF) within the ventricles of the brain can be ameliorated by draining the CSF to the exterior or to a distant body cavity from which it can be reabsorbed. Types of CSF shunt are shown in Figure 42.2.

CEREBROSPINAL FLUID SHUNT-ASSOCIATED INFECTION

Implantation of a CSF shunt is amongst the most frequent of neurosurgical procedures.[147] Although infection is a common complication associated with shunts,[148,149] rates may have declined in recent years.[150–153] The highest risks of infection are at the extremes of age (preterm infants and the elderly).[154,155] There is a significant mortality associated with CSF shunt infections[156,157] in addition to the other adverse consequences of prolongation of hospital stay and associated morbidities such as an increased risk of seizure disorders.[158] Internalized shunt systems may have a reservoir to allow access to the CSF such as an Omaya reservoir and may also have valve systems to regulate pressure and flow. The rates of infection between ventriculoatrial and ventriculoperitoneal shunts are similar.[159]

A number of risk factors have been identified for shunt-associated infections and these include CSF leak, infant maturity and breaches in surgical technique.[160,161] The pathogenesis of CSF shunt infections is probably similar to that of other implant-associated infections, micro-organisms being derived from intraoperative colonization, hematogenous seeding[162] or retrograde spread of infection along the catheter from a distant site.[148–150,163] The benefits of prophylactic intraoperative antibiotics suggest a significant proportion of infections arise at the time of the implantation of the device (see Prevention, *below*).

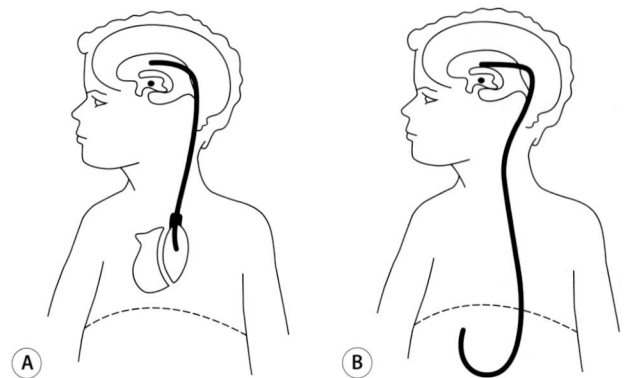

Fig. 42.2 Schematic of (A) ventriculoatrial (VA) and (B) ventriculoperitoneal (VP) cerebrospinal fluid shunts.

Microbiology

The great majority of shunt infections are caused by staphylococci[148,164,165] and, more rarely, Gram-negative bacilli. The latter are associated with high rates of morbidity and mortality.[166] A wide variety of microbes have been associated with shunt infections, reflecting the various potential routes of infection and individual patient risk factors.[167–169]

Diagnosis

Clinical signs and symptoms of CSF shunt-associated infections may be non-specific and include fever, headaches and lethargy. Classic signs of meningitis such as neck stiffness are present in a minority of patients.[170,171] There may be signs and symptoms related to the drainage site, so there may be intracardiac lesions and complications associated with intracardiac infections with ventriculoatrial shunts[172,173] and signs and symptoms of abdominal disease with those with ventriculoperitoneal shunts.[174,175] Blood cultures are frequently positive in patients with ventriculoatrial shunt-associated infections but infrequently positive in those with ventriculoperitoneal-associated infections.[149,176]

CSF changes may not be dramatic, with median CSF white cells counts of <100 cells/mm³.[149] The classic CSF findings of a high white cell count, raised CSF protein and low CSF:serum glucose ratio are often not seen in external ventricular drain (EVD) infections.[177] There are some data suggesting that levels of CSF lactate or serum procalcitonin may be useful in identifying individuals with bacterial EVD infections.[178] CSF culture may also be negative, particularly when collected by lumbar puncture. Positive microbial cultures are more frequent when CSF is directly aspirated from the shunt.[179] Radiological imaging can be helpful, particularly when there is involvement of the drainage site.

Treatment

The optimum approach to treatment of CSF shunt infection is complete removal of the shunt system with or without external CSF drainage through a ventriculostomy catheter if required.[148,156,176,180] Attempted treatment of shunt-associated infections without removal of the shunt is associated with much lower cure rates, extended hospital stay and a greater risk of patient death. Bacterial meningitis following bloodstream invasion of meninges can be successfully treated without shunt removal.[159] The optimum therapy for shunt-associated infections is not defined. As the majority of agents of infection are methicillin-resistant staphylococci, vancomycin is appropriate both for empirical treatment and following determination of microbial susceptibility. Rifampicin is frequently added because of its high levels of CSF penetration and its activity against biofilm-associated microbes.[37,181–183] For Gram-negative infections, imipenem is best avoided because of the risk of seizures.[184] Fourth-generation cephalosporins and meropenem are usually well-tolerated and reach supra-inhibitory concentrations in the CSF.

It is unclear the extent to which intraventricular antibiotics improve outcomes for patients. Intrathecal aminoglycosides and glycopeptides have been widely used in the treatment of shunt infections but there are no randomized controlled trials that have confirmed the benefit. A study in neonates with Gram-negative meningitis showed a higher mortality in infants given intrathecal gentamicin than in those given systemic gentamicin.[185] Many centers which use intrathecal aminoglycosides also measure drug levels in the CSF but, again, the relationship between levels and toxicity or patient outcome have not been defined.[186–188] When vancomycin is used intrathecally it is usually administered in doses of 5–20 mg every 24 h and again there are no trial data on the relationship between drug concentrations in the CSF and either toxicity or outcome.

Infection with multiresistant Gram-negatives can present particular challenges; for example, carbapenem-resistant *Acinetobacter baumanii* is an increasingly common cause of infection following intensive care unit admission for head trauma. Isolates may be resistant to a wide range of agents with few available options for treatment. Combined use of intrathecal and intravenous polymixins may be the only available treatment options in addition to removal of colonized device components.[189] Linezolid achieves high levels in the CSF and there are increasing reports of success in the treatment of multidrug-resistant Gram-positive ventriculitis where conventional approaches have failed.[190]

Prevention

Attempts to reduce the frequency of shunt-associated infection have included extreme measures to avoid contamination of the shunt or components[191] and a variety of changes to perioperative protocols.[192] There is evidence that preoperative shaving increases the risk of shunt-related infections.[193] Recent systematic reviews have concluded that systematic antibiotic prophylaxis does reduce the incidence of shunt-associated infection.[194] Antibiotics used in prophylaxis studies have included trimethoprim with sulfamethoxazole, trimethoprim with rifampicin and cephalosporins such as cefuroxime which achieves superinhibitory CSF concentrations. The use of antibiotic-impregnated shunts has also been associated with a reduction in the frequency of shunt infection.[195,196]

 ## EXTERNAL VENTRICULAR DRAIN (EVD)-ASSOCIATED INFECTION

Infection at the exit site is the most frequent infective complication of an EVD followed in decreasing order of frequency by ventriculitis, cerebritis, subdural empyema, osteomyelitis and complications consequent on the dissemination of infection.[196] Over 8% of patients with an EVD will develop positive CSF cultures.[197] Risk factors for infection include prolonged duration (>5 days) and irrigation.[198,199] Although algorithms describing the management of EVD-related ventriculitis have

been published,[196] it is important to base antibiotic choices on the prevalent causes of infection in a local context.

 ## CATHETER-ASSOCIATED URINARY TRACT INFECTIONS

Twenty-five percent of patients will have a urinary catheter inserted at some time during their hospital stay.[200] Rates of colonization of urinary catheters approach 100% by 30 days of catheterization and consequent urinary tract infection is a major cause of morbidity and mortality in individuals with long-term urinary catheters. The risk of catheter-associated urinary tract infection is higher in females than in males, in patients with co-morbidities (e.g. diabetes) that predispose to infection, when other foreign bodies are associated with the urinary drainage systems such as stents, and with increasing duration of catheterization. The costs associated with catheter-associated urinary tract infection are relatively low by comparison with many other hospital-acquired infections;[201] however, the aggregated costs are considerable. Urinary tract infections accounted for nearly 20% of hospital-acquired infections in a recent UK prevalence study[202] and catheterization was the major risk factor in that study.

Silver alloy-coated urinary catheters have lower rates of catheter-associated infection than non-coated catheters.[203] Although triclosan has been shown to reduce biofilm formation on urinary catheters,[204] intrinsic and acquired triclosan resistance preclude the use of triclosan as a routine preventive strategy.[205] Shanks et al have reported that heparin may promote biofilm formation by *Staph. aureus*.[206,207] Whether or not this is an important effect in patients is not known at this time.

Pathogenesis

Micro-organisms may contaminate the urinary catheter at the time of insertion or may migrate extraluminally from the periurethral area or intraluminally as the result of contamination of connections. Catheter-associated urinary tract infections are usually associated with the formation of biofilm on the catheter but can occasionally arise, particularly if there is back-flow of urine from a catheter drainage bag allowing inoculation of the bladder with large numbers of micro-organisms.

Microbiology

Patients with long-term urinary catheters who receive repeated courses of antibiotics for suspected catheter-associated infection or for other reasons are frequently colonized with antibiotic-resistant Enterobacteriaceae, *Ps. aeruginosa*, enterococci, staphylococci and/or fungi.

Diagnosis

Clinical criteria are an unreliable basis for the diagnosis of catheter-associated urinary tract infection. A patient with a transurethral catheter will not have dysuria and frequency, and suprapubic tenderness may be attributable to the irritating effects of the catheter on the bladder. Elderly patients particularly may not be febrile even in the presence of life-threatening infections.[208]

Bacteriuria may be a consequence of catheter colonization with or without associated infection. Pyuria has a high specificity for symptomatic catheter-associated urinary tract infection but may not be present in a large proportion of patients with symptomatic bacteriuria,[209] particularly when there is infection with Gram-positive cocci or yeasts.[210] Tests that may be useful in non-catheterized patients, such as for leukocyte esterase and bacterial nitrite, perform poorly in the catheterized patients.[211]

Treatment

Bacteriuria is common in patients with long-term urinary catheters, yet in the majority treatment is rarely required.[209] Treatment of asymptomatic catheter-associated bacteriuria has not been shown to be of benefit and may actually be detrimental to patients[212,213] other than in the context of pregnancy or urological procedures.[214] Unnecessary antibiotic treatment promotes colonization with antimicrobial-resistant species and increases the risk of antibiotic-associated complications such as *C. difficile* diarrhea.

In patients with signs and symptoms that may be attributable to urinary tract infection, and in the absence of other sources of infection, it may be reasonable to initiate antibiotic therapy which can be modified if required following the results of in-vitro sensitivity testing. In a recent study[215] in a large teaching hospital in the USA, it was found that over 30% of patients treated with antibiotics for catheter-associated bacteriuria did not have symptoms or signs consistent with infection, and were considered to have been inappropriately treated with antibiotics. It may be appropriate to treat asymptomatic catheter-associated bacteriuria in some specific groups of patients such as those who are immunocompromised[216] but these groups are exceptional. Recent guidelines have advocated that urine samples should not be routinely sent for microbiological testing from asymptomatic catheterized patients[217] because of the tendency of clinicians to prescribe on the basis of microbiological findings.

Prevention

There are few randomized controlled trials of prevention strategies for catheter-associated urinary tract infection. Avoiding unnecessary catheterizations, ensuring that trained professionals insert and care for urinary catheter systems, use of closed and dependent drainage systems, and avoidance of prolonged periods of catheterization all probably contribute to reducing the risk of catheter-associated urinary tract infection though with little support from randomized controlled trials.

Antimicrobial prophylaxis may reduce the frequency of catheter-associated urinary tract infection in patients with short periods of catheterization but this practice may lead to infections with difficult to treat antibiotic-resistant bacteria and yeasts and is probably best avoided.[218] Other practices which are best avoided because of lack of benefit or detriment to patients[200] include the use of anti-infective lubricants for catheter insertion, soaking the catheter in antimicrobial agents before insertion, use of topical agents of disinfection to the urethral meatus, continuous irrigation of the bladder and periodic instillation of anti-infectives into the bladder or collection system,[219] and closed catheter drainage systems with sealed connections.[220]

A number of antimicrobial urethral catheters have been developed and evaluated, several of which have been shown to be associated with a lower risk of catheter-associated urinary tract infection, including in particular silver hydrogel catheters.[221,222] A recent systematic review[223] concludes that antimicrobial urinary catheters can prevent or delay the onset of catheter-associated bacteriuria. The systematic review suggested that there may have been systematic overestimation of the effect sizes in many of the randomized and quasi-randomized trials reviewed because of drop-outs and exclusions. The effects of antimicrobial catheters on substantive outcomes such as bloodstream infection are also not known.

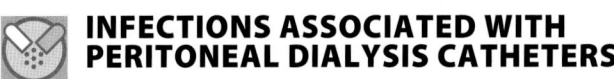

INFECTIONS ASSOCIATED WITH PERITONEAL DIALYSIS CATHETERS

Over the last 30 years dialysis through peritoneal catheters has become the treatment of choice for many patients with end-stage renal disease. The major complication associated with peritoneal dialysis is peritonitis. Sixty percent of patients undergoing peritoneal dialysis will develop an episode of peritonitis within the first 12 months following initiation of dialysis.[224] Recurrent episodes of peritonitis compromise the ability of the peritoneum to act as the dialysis membrane and is the common reason for patients being transferred to hemodialysis.

Peritonitis is a more frequent complication than catheter exit site or tunnel infection, suggesting that spread of microorganisms from connections along the lumen of the catheter is the most important route of infection.[225] Nasal carriers of *Staph. aureus* are more likely than non-carriers to develop both exit site infections and peritonitis.[226] Dilution of host defense elements such as immunoglobulin and complement and the relatively high osmolality and low pH of the dialysate probably increase the risk of dialysis-associated peritonitis.[227]

Microbiology

Although the majority of peritonitis cases are associated with isolation of coagulase-negative staphylococci from peritoneal fluid samples, a wide range of other microbes have been associated with peritonitis, as has been reported with other transcutaneous devices. *Staph. aureus* is particularly associated with exit site and tunnel infections.[228]

Diagnosis

Signs and symptoms include cloudy dialysate and abdominal pain or tenderness and fever.[228] Shock is unusual in association with coagulase-negative staphylococcal peritonitis but may be a feature of peritonitis caused by Gram-negatives and *Staph. aureus*.

Exit site and tunnel infection may be diagnosed by local signs and symptoms. Laboratory findings include a raised dialysate white cell count of >100 cells/mm³. White cells are usually predominantly neutrophils but may be dominated by other cell types when peritonitis is caused by unusual pathogens such as mycobacteria or fungi.[228]

Treatment

Current guidelines suggest that overall >80% of peritoneal dialysis-associated peritonitis should be cured without removal of the peritoneal catheter.[229] Intraperitoneal antibiotics achieve suprainhibitory concentrations both in the peritoneal cavity and in the bloodstream. A recent systematic review of treatment of peritoneal dialysis-associated peritonitis showed that intraperitoneal antibiotics were effective and (based on the results of one study) perhaps more effective than intravenous antibiotics in reducing treatment failures. A number of different intraperitoneal antibiotic regimens were effective.[230] Empirical regimens can include cephalosporins with or without an aminoglyside.[231] It is probably not necessary to use a glycopeptide unless there is evidence to support infection with MRSA or resistance to the empirical regimen is reported by the laboratory. Aminoglycosides are probably best avoided in patients with residual function (urine output >100 mL per day).[232]

Removal of the dialysis catheter may be necessary to control infection or to prevent recurrent infection which is particularly likely with *Staph. aureus*, *Ps. aeruginosa* and fungal infection. The optimal antimicrobial therapy for fungal peritonitis has not been defined. Fluconazole combined with flucytosine can be effective for susceptible strains.[228] The role of newer antifungals such as voriconazole, caspofungin and liposomal amphotericin preparations is ill-defined.

Prevention

The 2005 International Society for Peritoneal Dialysis guidelines[229] make specific recommendations for the prevention of peritoneal dialysis-related peritonitis. These emphasize the importance of surveillance of infection rates, the use of prophylactic antibiotics at the time of insertion of the device, recommendations for minimizing exit site care that target the control of *Staph. aureus* and requirements for training, including training

in practical methods (particularly for connection and disconnection), minimizing the risk of translocation of micro-organisms from the bowel and criteria for use of antifungal prophylaxis.

The use of a Y connection allows simultaneous connection of the drainage and infusion bags, minimizing the number of connections and disconnections that have to be made. Randomized trials have shown a reduction in the rate of peritoneal dialysis-related peritonitis when these Y connections are used.[225] These types of system have become further refined.[233]

Application of antimicrobials around the cannula exit site has been shown to reduce the risk of *Staph. aureus* exit site and tunnel infections but there are some concerns about the long-term consequences of this strategy, particularly with respect to the selection of antibiotic resistance.[234] Strategies involving anti-staphylococcal immunizations have so far been unsuccessful in reducing either exit site infections or peritonitis.[235]

 References

1. Darouiche RO. Treatment of infections associated with surgical implants. *N Engl J Med*. 2004;350:1422–1429.
2. Anderson JM, Rodriguez A, Chang DT. Foreign body reaction to biomaterials. *Semin Immunol*. 2008;20:86–100.
3. Heilmann C, Schweitzer O, Gerke C, Vanittanakom N, Mack D, Gotz F. Molecular basis of intercellular adhesion in the biofilm forming *Staphylococcus epidermidis*. *Mol Microbiol*. 1996;20:1083–1091.
4. Kristian SA, Birkenstock TA, Sauder U, Mack D, Götz F, Landmann R. Biofilm formation induces C3a release and protects *Staphylococcus epidermidis* from IgG and complement deposition and from neutrophil-dependent killing. *J Infect Dis*. 2008;197:1028–1035.
5. Hentzer M, Riedel K, Rasmussen TB, et al. Inhibition of quorum sensing in *Pseudomonas aeruginosa* biofilm bacteria by a halogenated furanone compound. *Microbiology*. 2002;148(Pt 1):87–102.
6. Rasmussen TB, Givskov M. Quorum-sensing in the pathogenicity of the cunning aggressor *Pseudomonas aeruginosa*. *Anal Bioanal Chem*. 2006;387:409–414.
7. Laux DC, Corson JM, Givskov M, et al. Lysophosphatidic acid inhibition of the accumulation of *Pseudomonas aeruginosa* PAO1 alginate, pyoverdin, elastase and LasA. *Microbiology*. 2002;148:1709–1723.
8. Costerton JW, Montanaro L, Arciola CR. Bacterial communications in implant infections: a target for an intelligence war. *Int J Artif Organs*. 2007;30:757–763.
9. Hoyle BD, Costerton WJ. Bacterial resistance to antibiotics: the role of biofilms. *Prog Drug Res*. 1991;37:91–105.
10. Cozens RM, Tuomanen E, Tosch W, Zak O, Suter J, Tomasz A. Evaluation of the bactericidal activity of beta-lactam antibiotics on slowly growing bacteria cultured in the chemostat. *Antimicrob Agents Chemother*. 1986;29:797–802.
11. Anderl JN, Zahller J, Roe F, Stewart PS. Role of nutrient limitation and stationary-phase existence in *Klebsiella pneumoniae* biofilm resistance to ampicillin and ciprofloxacin. *Antimicrob Agents Chemother*. 2003;47:1251–1256.
12. Ciofu O. Pseudomonas aeruginosa chromosomal beta-lactamase in patients with cystic fibrosis and chronic lung infection. Mechanism of antibiotic resistance and target of the humoral immune response. *Apmis*. 2003;116(suppl):1–47.
13. Mah TF, Pitts B, Pellock B, Walker GC, Stewart PS, O'Toole GA. A genetic basis for *Pseudomonas aeruginosa* biofilm antibiotic resistance. *Nature*. 2003;426:306–310.
14. Walters III MC, Roe F, Bugnicourt A, Franklin MJ, Stewart PS. Contributions of antibiotic penetration, oxygen limitation, and low metabolic activity to tolerance of *Pseudomonas aeruginosa* biofilms of ciprofloxacin and tobramycin. *Antimicrob Agents Chemother*. 2003;47:317–323.
15. Drenkard E, Ausubel FM. *Pseudomonas* biofilm formation and antibiotic resistance are linked to phenotypic variation. *Nature*. 2002;416:740–743.

16. Hentzer M, Givskov M. Pharmacological inhibition of quorum sensing for the treatment of chronic bacterial infections. *J Clin Invest*. 2003;112:1300–1307.

17. Giacometti A, Cirioni O, Gov Y, et al. RNA III inhibiting peptide inhibits in vivo biofilm formation by drug-resistant *Staphylococcus aureus*. *Antimicrob Agents Chemother*. 2003;47:1979–1983.

18. Mathesius U, Mulders S, Gao M, et al. Extensive and specific responses of a eukaryote to bacterial quorum-sensing signals. *Proc Nat Acad Sci U S A*. 2003;100:1444–1449.

19. Pelroth J, Kuo M, Tan J, Bayer AS, Miller LG. Adjunctive use of rifampin for the treatment of *Staphylococcus aureus* infections. *Arch Intern Med*. 2008;168:805–819.

20. Raad I, Hanna H, Jiang Y, et al. Comparative activities of daptomycin, linezolid, and tigecycline against catheter-related meticillin-resistant *Staphylococcus* bacteremic isolates embedded in biofilm. *Antimicrob Agents Chemother*. 2007;51:1656–1660.

21. Norden C, Gillespie WJ, Made S. Infections in total joint replacement. In: *Infections in Bones and Joints*. Boston: Blackwell; 1994:291–319.

22. Hoffmann LR, D'Argenio DA, MacCoss MJ, Zhang Z, Jones RA, Miller SA. Aminoglycoside antibiotics induce bacterial biofilm formation. *Nature*. 2005;436:1171–1175.

23. Stargardt T. I lealth service costs in Europe: costs and reimbursement of primary hip replacements in nine countries. *Health Econ*. 2008;17:S9–S20.

24. Kurtz S, Mowat F, Ong K, Chan N, Lau E, Halpern M. Prevalence of primary and revision total hip and knee arthroplasty in the United States from 1990 through 2002. *J Bone Joint Surg Am*. 2005;87:1487–1497.

25. Steckelberg JM, Osmon DR. Prosthetic joint infection. In: Bisno AL, Waldvogel FA, eds. *Infections Associated with Indwelling Medical Devices*. 3rd ed. Washington, DC: ASM Press; 2001:173–209.

26. Jameson E, Huhtala H, Puolakka T, Moilanen T. Risk factors for infection after knee arthroplasty. A register-based analysis of 43149 cases. *J Bone Joint Surg Am*. 2009;91:38–47.

27. Trampuz A, Widmer AF. Infections associated with orthopedic implants. *Curr Opin Infect Dis*. 2006;19:349–356.

28. Health Protection Agency. In: Fourth Report of the Mandatory Surveillance of Surgical Site Infection in Orthopaedic Surgery. April 2004–March 2008; London: HPA; 2008. Online Available at http://www.hpa.org.uk/web/HPAweb&HPAwebStandard/HPAweb_C/1257260303150.

29. National Joint Registry Newsletter. *Winter Edition*. 2008/9. Online Available at http://www.njrcentre.org.uk.

30. Coventry MB. Treatment of infections occurring in total hip surgery. *Orthop Clin North Am*. 1975;6:991–1003.

31. Gillespie WJ. Prevention and management of infection after total joint replacement. *Clin Infect Dis*. 1997;25:1310–1317.

32. Charnley J. Postoperative infection after total hip replacement with special reference to air contamination in the operating room. *Clin Orthop Relat Res*. 1972;87:167–187.

33. Lidwell OM, Lowbury FJ, Whyte W, Blowers R, Stanley SJ, Lowe D. Bacteria isolated from deep joint sepsis after operation for total hip or knee replacement and the sources of the infections with *Staphylococcus aureus*. *J Hosp Infect*. 1983;4:19–29.

34. Murdoch DR, Roberts SA, Fowler Jr VG, et al. Infection of orthopedic prostheses after *Staphylococcus aureus* bacteremia. *Clin Infect Dis*. 2001;32:647–649.

35. Matthews PC, Berendt AR, McNally MA, Byren I. Diagnosis and management of prosthetic joint infections. *Br Med J*. 2009;338:1378–1383.

36. Atkins BL, Athanasou N, Deeks JJ, et al. Prospective evaluation of criteria for microbiological diagnosis of prosthetic joint infection at revision arthroplasty. The OSIRIS Collaborative Study Group. *J Clin Microbiol*. 1998;36:2932–2939.

37. Zimmerli W, Trampuz A, Ochsner PE, et al. Prosthetic joint infections. *N Engl J Med*. 2004;351:1645–1654.

38. Betsch BY, Eggli S, Siebenrock KA, Tauber MG, Muhlemann K. Treatment of joint prosthesis infection in accordance with current recommendations improves outcomes. *Clin Infect Dis*. 2008;46:1221–1226.

39. Zimmerli W, Widmer AF, Blatter M, Frei R, Ochsner PE. Role of rifampin for treatment of orthopedic implant-related staphylococcal infections: a randomized controlled trial. Foreign-Body Infection (FBI) Study Group. *J Am Med Assoc*. 1998;279:1537–1541.

40. Choong PF, Dowsey MM, Carr D, Daffy J, Stanley P. Risk factors associated with acute hip prosthetic joint infections and outcome of treatment with a rifampin based regime. *Acta Orthop*. 2007;78:755–765.

41. Matthews PC, Conlon CP, Berendt AR, Kayley J, Jefferies L. Outpatient parenteral antimicrobial therapy (OPAT): is it safe for selected patients to administer at home? A retrospective analysis of a large cohort over 13 years. *J Antimicrob Chemother*. 2007;60:356–362.

42. John A-K, Baldoni D, Haschke M, et al. Efficacy of daptomycin in implant-associated infection due to methicillin-resistant *Staphylococcus aureus* (MRSA): the importance of combination with rifampin. *Antimicrob Agents Chemother*. 2009;53(7):2719–2724.

43. Hill C, Flamant R, Mazas F, Evrard J. Prophylactic cefazolin versus placebo in total hip replacement. Report of a multicentre double-blind randomised trial. *Lancet*. 1981;1:795–796.

44. Conte JE, Cohen SN, Roe BB, Elashoff RM. Antibiotic prophylaxis and cardiac surgery. A prospective double-blind comparison of single-dose versus multiple-dose regimens. *Ann Intern Med*. 1972;76:943–949.

45. Nelson CL, Green TG, Porter RA, Warren RD. One day versus seven days of preventive antibiotic therapy in orthopedic surgery. *Clin Orthop Relat Res*. 1983;176:258–263.

46. Josefsson G, Kolmert L. Prophylaxis with systematic antibiotics versus gentamicin bone cement in total hip arthroplasty. A ten-year survey of 1,688 hips. *Clin Orthop Relat Res*. 1993;292:210–214.

47. Espehaug B, Engesaeter LB, Vollset SE, Havelin LI, Langeland N. Antibiotic prophylaxis in total hip arthroplasty. Review of 10,905 primary cemented total hip replacements reported to the Norwegian arthroplasty register, 1987 to 1995. *J Bone Joint Surg Br*. 1997;79:590–595.

48. Shrout MK, Scarbrough F, Powell BJ. Dental care and the prosthetic joint patient: a survey of orthopedic surgeons and general dentists. *J Am Dent Assoc*. 1994;125:429–436.

49. Glynn MK, Sheehan JM. An analysis of the causes of deep infection after hip and knee arthroplasties. *Clin Orthop Relat Res*. 1983;178:202–206.

50. Waldman BJ, Mont MA, Hungerford DS. Total knee arthroplasty infections associated with dental procedures. *Clin Orthop Relat Res*. 1997;343:164–172.

51. Norden CW. Antibiotic prophylaxis in orthopedic surgery. *Rev Infect Dis*. 1991;13(suppl 10):S842–S846.

52. Deacon JM, Pagliaro AJ, Zelicof SB, Horowitz HW. Prophylactic use of antibiotics for procedures after total joint replacement. *J Bone Joint Surg Am*. 1996;78:1755–1770.

53. Jacobson JJ, Schweitzer S, DePorter DJ, Lee JJ. Antibiotic prophylaxis for dental patients with joint prostheses? A decision analysis. *Int J Technol Assess Health Care*. 1990;6:569–587.

54. Segreti J, Levin S. The role of prophylactic antibiotics in the prevention of prosthetic device infections. *Infect Dis Clin North Am*. 1989;3:357–370.

55. Wilcox MH, Hall J, Pike H, Templeton PA, Fawley WN, Parnell P, et al. Use of perioperative mupirocin to prevent meticillin-resistant Staphylococcus aureus (MRSA) orthopaedic surgical site infections. *J Hosp Infect*. 2003;54:196–201.

56. Nixon M, Jackson B, Varghese P, Jenkins D, Taylor G. Meticillin-resistant *Staphylococcus aureus* on orthopaedic wards: incidence, spread, mortality, cost and control. *J Bone Joint Surg*. 2006;88(6):812–817.

57. Vongpatanasin W, Hillis LD, Lange RA. Prosthetic heart valves. *N Engl J Med*. 1996;335:407–416.

58. Wang A, Athan E, Pappas PA, et al. Contemporary clinical profile and outcome of prosthetic valve endocarditis. *J Am Med Assoc*. 2007;297:1354–1361.

59. Blackstone EH, Kirklin JW. Death and other time-related events after valve replacement. *Circulation*. 1985;72:753–767.

60. Hill EE, Herijgers P, Herregods MC, Peetermans WE. Evolving trends in infective endocarditis. *Clin Microbiol Infect*. 2006;12:5–12.

61. Habib G, Thuny F, Avierinos J-F. Prosthetic valve endocarditis: current approach and therapeutic options. *Prog Cardiovasc Dis*. 2008;50:274–281.

62. Daniel WG, Mugge A, Grote J, et al. Comparison of transthoracic and transesophageal echocardiography for detection of abnormalities of prosthetic and bioprosthetic valves in the mitral and aortic positions. *Am J Cardiol*. 1993;71:210–215.

63. Ryan EW, Bolger AF. Transesophageal echocardiography (TEE) in the evaluation of infective endocarditis. *Cardiol Clin*. 2000;18:773–787.

64. Durack DT, Lukes AS, Bright DK. New criteria for diagnosis of infective endocarditis: utilization of specific echocardiographic findings. Duke Endocarditis Service. *Am J Med*. 1994;96:200–209.

65. Tomos P, Almirante B, Olona M, et al. Clinical outcome and long-term prognosis of late prosthetic valve endocarditis: a 20-year experience. *Clin Infect Dis*. 1997;24:381–386.

66. John MD, Hibberd PL, Karchmer AW, Sleeper LA, Calderwood SB. *Staphylococcus aureus* prosthetic valve endocarditis: optimal management and risk factors for death. *Ann Thorac Surg.* 1998;26:1302–1309.

67. Elliott TSJ, Foweraker J, Gould FK, Perry JD, Sandoe JAT. Guidelines for the antibiotic treatment of endocarditis in adults: report of the working party of the British Society for Antimicrobial Chemotherapy. *J Antimicrob Chemother.* 2004;54:971–981.

68. Baddour LM, Wilson WR, Bayer AS, et al. Infective endocarditis: diagnosis, antimicrobial therapy, and management of complications. *Circulation.* 2005;111:e394–e434.

69. Fang G, Keys TF, Gentry LO, et al. Prosthetic valve endocarditis resulting from nosocomial bacteremia. A prospective, multicenter study. *Ann Intern Med.* 1993;119:560–567.

70. Falagas ME, Manta KG, Ntziora F, Vardakas KZ. Linezolid for the treatment of patients with endocarditis: a systematic review of the published evidence. *J Antimicrob Chemother.* 2006;58:273–280.

71. Nguyen MH, Nguyen ML, Yu VL, McMahon D, Keys TF, Amidi M. *Candida* prosthetic valve endocarditis: prospective study of six cases and review of the literature. *Clin Infect Dis.* 1996;22:262–267.

72. Brooks N. Prophylactic antibiotic treatment to prevent infective endocarditis: new guidance from the National Institute for Health and Clinical Excellence. *Heart.* 2009;95:774–780.

73. Gandelman G, Frishman W, Wiese C, et al. Intravascular device infections. Epidemiology, diagnosis, and management. *Cardiol Rev.* 2007;15:13–23.

74. Chua JD, Wilkoff BL, Lee I, et al. Diagnosis and management of infections involving implantable electrophysiologic cardiac devices. *Ann Intern Med.* 2000;133:604–608.

75. Harcomber AA, Newell SA, Ludman PF, et al. Late complications following permanent pacemaker implantation or elective unit replacement. *Heart.* 1998;80:240–244.

76. Klug D, Lacroix D, Savoye C, et al. Systemic infection related to endocarditis on pacemaker leads: clinical presentation and management. *Circulation.* 1997;95:2098–2107.

77. Cacoub P, Leprince P, Nataf P, et al. Pacemaker infective endocarditis. *Am J Cardiol.* 1998;82:480–484.

78. Arber N, Pras E, Copperman Y, et al. Pacemaker endocarditis. Report of 44 cases and review of the literature. *Medicine.* 1994;73:299–305.

79. Victor F, De Place C, Camus C, et al. Pacemaker lead infection: echocardiographic features, management, and outcome. *Heart.* 1999;81:82–87.

80. Da Costa A, Kirkorian G, Cusherat M, et al. Antibiotic prophylaxis for permanent pacemaker implantation: a meta-analysis. *Circulation.* 1998;97:1796–1801.

81. Baddour LM, Bettmann MA, Bolger AF, et al. Non-valvular cardiovascular device-associated infections. *Circulation.* 2003;108:2015–2031.

82. Brun-Buisson C, Doyon F, Carlet J. Bacteremia and severe sepsis in adults: a multicenter prospective survey in ICUs and wards of 24 hospitals. French Bacteremia-Sepsis Study Group. *Am J Respir Crit Care Med.* 1996;154:617–624.

83. Waghorn DJ. Intravascular device associated systemic infections: a 2-year analysis of cases in a district general hospital. *J Hosp Infect.* 1994;28:91–101.

84. Fletcher SJ, Bodenham AR. Catheter-related sepsis: an overview – Part 1. *Br Med J.* 1999;92:46–53.

85. Nosocomial Infection National Surveillance Scheme. *Surveillance of Hospital-Acquired Bacteraemia in English Hospitals 1997–2002.* London: Public Health Laboratory Service; 2002.

86. Veenstra DL, Saint S, Sullivan SD. Cost-effectiveness of antiseptic-impregnated central venous catheters for prevention of catheter-related bloodstream infection. *J Am Med Assoc.* 1999;282:554–560.

87. Maki DG, Kluger DM, Crnich CJ. The risk of blood stream infection in adults with different intravascular devices: a systematic review of 200 published prospective studies. *Mayo Clin Proc.* 2006;81:1151–1152.

88. Marrie TJ, Costerton JW. Scanning and transmission electron microscopy of in situ bacterial colonization of intravenous and intraarterial catheters. *J Clin Microbiol.* 1984;19:687–693.

89. Maki DG, Jarrett F, Sarafin HW. A semiquantitative culture method for identification of catheter-related infection in the burn patient. *J Surg Res.* 1977;22:513–520.

90. Maki DG. Nosocomial bacteremia. An epidemiologic overview. *Am J Med.* 1981;70:719–732.

91. Cooper GL, Hopkins CC. Rapid diagnosis of intravascular catheter-associated infection by direct Gram staining of catheter segments. *N Engl J Med.* 1988;312:1142–1147.

92. Mermel LA, McCormick RD, Springman SR, Maki DG. The pathogenesis and epidemiology of catheter-related infection with pulmonary artery Swan-Ganz catheters: a prospective study utilizing molecular subtyping. *Am J Med.* 1991;91:197S–205S.

93. Cheesbrough JS, Finch RG, Burden RP. A prospective study of the mechanisms of infection associated with hemodialysis catheters. *J Infect Dis.* 1986;154:579–589.

94. Mermel LA, Allon M, Bouza E, et al. Clinical practice guidelines for the diagnosis and management of intravascular catheter-related infection: 2009 Update by the Infectious Diseases Society of America. *Clin Infect Dis.* 2009;49:1–45.

95. O'Grady NP, Barie PS, Bartlett J, et al. Practice parameters for evaluating new fever in critically ill adult patients. Task Force of the American College of Critical Care Medicine of the Society of Critical Care Medicine in collaboration with the Infectious Diseases Society of America. *Crit Care Med.* 1998;26:392–408.

96. Brun-Buisson C, Abrouk F, Legrand P, Huet Y, Larabi S, Rapin M. Diagnosis of central venous catheter-related sepsis: critical level of quantitative tip cultures. *Arch Intern Med.* 1987;147:873–877.

97. Maki DG, Stolz SS, Wheeler S, Mermel LA. A prospective, randomized trial of gauze and two polyurethane dressings for site care of pulmonary artery catheters: implications for catheter management. *Crit Care Med.* 1994;22:1729–1737.

98. Raad I, Darouiche R, Dupuis J, et al. Central venous catheters coated with minocycline and rifampin for the prevention of catheter-related colonization and bloodstream infections. A randomized, double-blind trial. The Texas Medical Center Catheter Study Group. *Ann Intern Med.* 1997;127:267–274.

99. Gowardman JR, Montgomery C, Thirlwell S, et al. Central venous catheter-related bloodstream infections: an analysis of incidence and risk factors in a cohort of 400 patients. *Intensive Care Med.* 1998;24:1034–1039.

100. Tacconelli E, Tumbarello M, Pittiruti M, et al. Central venous catheter-related sepsis in a cohort of 366 hospitalised patients. *Eur J Clin Microbiol Infect Dis.* 1997;16:203–209.

101. Telenti A, Steckelberg JM, Stockman L, Edson RS, Roberts GD. Quantitative blood cultures in candidemia. *Mayo Clin Proc.* 1991;66:1120–1123.

102. Siegman-Igra Y, Anglim AM, Shapiro DE, Adal KA, Strain BA, Farr BM. Diagnosis of vascular catheter-related bloodstream infection: a meta-analysis. *J Clin Microbiol.* 1997;35:928–936.

103. Sherertz RJ, Raad II, Belani A, et al. Three-year experience with sonicated vascular catheter cultures in a clinical microbiology laboratory. *J Clin Microbiol.* 1990;28:76–82.

104. Blot F, Nitenberg G, Chachaty E, et al. Diagnosis of catheter-related bacteremia: a prospective comparison of the time to positivity of hub-blood versus peripheral-blood cultures. *Lancet.* 1999;354:1071–1077.

105. Kite P, Dobbins BM, Wilcox MH, McMahon MJ. Rapid diagnosis of central-venous-catheter-related bloodstream infection without catheter removal. *Lancet.* 1999;354:1504–1507.

106. Gaur AH, Flynn PM, Heine DJ, Giannini MA, Shenep JL, Hayden RT. Diagnosis of catheter-related bloodstream infections among pediatric oncology patients lacking a peripheral culture, using differential time to detection. *Pediatr Infect Dis J.* 2005;24:445–449.

107. Kite P, Dobbins BM, Wilcox MH, et al. Evaluation of a novel endoluminal brush method for in situ diagnosis of catheter related sepsis. *J Clin Pathol.* 1997;50:278–282.

108. van Heerden PV, Webb SA, Fong S, Golledge CL, Roberts BL, Thompson WR. Central venous catheters revisited – infection rates and an assessment of the new Fibrin Analysing System brush. *Anaesth Intensive Care.* 1996;24:330–333.

109. Warwick S, Wilks M, Hennessy E, et al. Diagnosis of central vascular catheter associated bacterial infection using quantitative 16S rDNA detection. *J Clin Microbiol.* 2004;42:1402–1408.

110. Raad I, Davis S, Khan A, Tarrand J, Elting L, Bodey GP. Impact of central venous catheter removal on the recurrence of catheter-related coagulase-negative staphylococcal bacteremia. *Infect Control Hosp Epidemiol.* 1992;13:215–221.

111. Dato VM, Dajani AS. Candidemia in children with central venous catheters: role of catheter removal and amphotericin B therapy. *Pediatr Infect Dis J.* 1990;9:309–314.

112. Rex JH, Bennett JE, Sugar AM, et al. Intravascular catheter exchange and duration of candidemia. NIAID Mycoses Study Group and the Candidemia Study Group. *Clin Infect Dis.* 1995;21:994–996.

113. Anthony TU, Rubin LG. Stability of antibiotics used for antibiotic-lock treatment of infections of implantable venous devices (ports). *Antimicrob Agents Chemother*. 1999;43:2074–2076.

114. Rijnders BJ, Van Wijngaerden E, Vandecasteele SJ, et al. Treatment of long-term intravascular catheter-related bacteremia with antibiotic lock: randomized, placebo-controlled trial. *J Antimicrob Chemother*. 2005;55:90–94.

115. Messing B, Man F, Colimon R, Thuillier F, Beliah M. Antibiotic lock technique is an effective treatment of bacterial catheter-related sepsis during parenteral nutrition. *Clin Nutr*. 1990;19:220–224.

116. Krzywda EA, Andris DA, Edmiston Jr CE, Quebbeman EJ. Treatment of Hickman catheter sepsis using antibiotic lock technique. *Infect Control Hosp Epidemiol*. 1995;16:596–598.

117. Fernandez-Hidalgo N, Almirante B, Calleja R, et al. Antibiotic-lock therapy for long-term intravascular catheter-related bacteremia: results of an open, non-comparative study. *J Antimicrob Chemother*. 2006;57:1172–1180.

118. Champault G. Totally implantable catheters for cancer chemotherapy: French experience on 325 cases. *Cancer Drug Deliv*. 1986;3:131–137.

119. Brothers TE, Von Moll LK, Niederhuber JE, Roberts JA, Walker-Andrews S, Ensminger WD. Experience with subcutaneous infusion ports in three hundred patients. *Surg Gynecol Obstet*. 1988;166:295–301.

120. Raad II, Luna M, Khalil SA, Costerton JW, Lam C, Bodey GP. The relationship between the thrombotic and infectious complications of central venous catheters. *J Am Med Assoc*. 1994;271:1014–1016.

121. Fowler VG, Li J, Corey GR, et al. Role of echocardiography in evaluation of patients with *Staphylococcus aureus* bacteremia: experience in 103 patients. *J Am Coll Cardiol*. 1997;30:1072–1078.

122. Phillips P, Shafran S, Garber G, et al. Multicenter randomized trial of fluconazole versus amphotericin B for treatment of candidemia in non-neutropenic patients. Canadian Candidemia Study Group. *Eur J Clin Microbiol Infect Dis*. 1997;16:337–345.

123. Rose HD. Venous catheter-associated candidemia. *Am J Med Sci*. 1978;275:265–269.

124. Lecciones JA, Lee JW, Navarro EE, et al. Vascular catheter-associated fungemia in patients with cancer: analysis of 155 episodes. *Clin Infect Dis*. 1992;14:875–883.

125. Verghese A, Widrich WC, Arbeit RD. Central venous septic thrombophlebitis – the role of medical therapy. *Medicine*. 1985;64:394–400.

126. Lee YH, Kerstein MD. Osteomyelitis and septic arthritis. A complication of subclavian venous catheterization. *N Engl J Med*. 1971;285:1179–1180.

127. Centers for Disease Control and Prevention (CDC). Monitoring hospital-acquired infections to promote patient safety – United States, 1990–1999. *MMWR Morb Mortal Wkly Rep*. 2000;49:149–153.

128. Maki DG, Ringer M, Alvarado CJ. Prospective randomized trial of povidone–iodine, alcohol, and chlorhexidine for prevention of infection associated with central venous and arterial catheters. *Lancet*. 1991;338:339–343.

129. O'Grady NP, Alexander M, Dellinger EP, et al. HICPAC guidelines for the prevention of intravascular catheter-related infection. *Clin Infect Dis*. 2002;282:554–560.

130. Pratt RJ, Pellowe CM, Wilson JA, Loveday HP, Harper PJ, Jones S.R.L.J., et al. EPIC-2: national evidence-based guidelines for preventing healthcare-associated infection in NHS hospitals in England. *J Hosp Infect*. 2007;65(S1):S40–S41.

131. Levy I, Katz J, Solter E, et al. Chlorhexidine-impregnated dressing for prevention of colonization of central venous catheters in infants and children: a randomized controlled study. *Pediatr Infect Dis J*. 2005;24:676–679.

132. Timsit JF, Schwebel C, Bouadma L, et al. Chlorhexidine-impregnated sponges and less frequent dressing changes for prevention of catheter-related infections in critically ill adults: a randomized controlled trial. *J Am Med Assoc*. 2009;301:1231–1241.

133. Crnich CJ, Maki DG. The promise of novel technology for the prevention of intravascular device-related bloodstream infection. 1. Pathogenesis and short-term devices. *Clin Infect Dis*. 2002;34:1232–1242.

134. Maki DG, Stolz SM, Wheeler S, Mermel LA. Prevention of central venous catheter-related bloodstream infection by use of an antiseptic-impregnated catheter. A randomized, controlled trial. *Ann Intern Med*. 1997;127:257–266.

135. Hanley EM, Veeder A, Smith T, Drusano G, Currie E, Venezia RA. Evaluation of an antiseptic triple-lumen catheter in an intensive care unit. *Crit Care Med*. 2000;28:366–370.

136. Boswald M, Lugauer S, Regenfus A, et al. Reduced rates of catheter-associated infection by use of a new silver-impregnated central venous catheter. *Infection*. 1999;27(suppl 1):S56–S60.

137. Carbon RT, Lugauer S, Geitner U, et al. Reducing catheter-associated infections with silver-impregnated catheters in long-term therapy of children. *Infection*. 1999;27(suppl 1):S69–S73.

138. Ramritu P, Halton K, Collignon P, et al. A systematic review comparing the relative effectiveness of antimicrobial-coated catheters in intensive care units. *Am J Infect Control*. 2008;36:104–117.

139. Fraenkel D, Rickard C, Thomas P, et al. A prospective, randomized trial of rifampin–minocycline-coated and silver–platinum–carbon-impregnated central venous catheters. *Crit Care Med*. 2006;34:668–675.

140. Pierce CM, Wade A, Mok Q. Heparin bonded central venous lines reduce thrombotic and infective complications in critically ill children. *Intensive Care Med*. 2000;26:967–972.

141. Appelgren P, Ransjo U, Bindslev L. Surface heparisation of central venous catheters reduces microbial colonization in vitro and in vivo: results from a prospective, randomized trial. *Crit Care Med*. 1996;24:1482–1489.

142. Abdielkefi A, Achour W, Ben OT, et al. Use of heparin coated central venous lines to prevent catheter-related bloodstream infection. *J Support Oncol*. 2007;5:273–278.

143. Gilbert RE, Harden M. Effectiveness of impregnated central venous catheters for catheter related blood stream infection: a systematic review. *Curr Opin Infect Dis*. 2008;21:235–245.

144. Spafford PS, Sinkin RA, Cox C, Reubens L, Powell KR. Prevention of central venous catheter-related coagulase-negative staphylococcal sepsis in neonates. *J Pediatr*. 1994;125:259–263.

145. Safdar N, Maki DG. Use of vancomycin-containing lock or flush solutions for prevention of bloodstream infection associated with central venous access devices: a meta-analysis of prospective, randomized trials. *Clin Infect Dis*. 2006;43:474–484.

146. Yahav D, Rozen-Zvi B, Gafter-Gvili A, et al. Antimicrobial lock solutions for the prevention of infections associated with intravascular catheters in patients undergoing hemodialysis: systematic review and meta-analysis of randomized, controlled trials. *Clin Infect Dis*. 2008;47:83–93.

147. Guertin S.R. Cerebrospinal fluid shunts. Evaluation, complications, and crisis management. *Pediatr Clin North Am*. 34: 203–217.

148. Schoenbaum SC, Gardner P, Shillito J. Infections of cerebrospinal fluid shunts: epidemiology, clinical manifestations, and therapy. *J Infect Dis*. 1975;131:543–552.

149. Forward KR, Fewer HD, Stiver HG. Cerebrospinal fluid shunt infections. A review of 35 infections in 32 patients. *J Neurosurg*. 1983;59:389–394.

150. George R, Leibrock L, Epstein M. Long-term analysis of cerebrospinal fluid shunt infections. A 25-year experience. *J Neurosurg*. 1979;51:804–811.

151. Rieder MJ, Frewen TC, Del Maestro RF, Coyle A, Lovell S. The effect of cephalothin prophylaxis on postoperative ventriculoperitoneal shunt infections. *Can Med Assoc J*. 1987;136:935–938.

152. Rotim K, Miklic P, Paladino J, Melada A, Marcikic M, Scap M. Reducing the incidence of infection in pediatric cerebrospinal fluid shunt operations. *Childs Nerv Syst*. 1997;13:584–587.

153. Davis SE, Levy ML, McComb JG, Masri-Lavine L. Does age or other factors influence the incidence of ventriculoperitoneal shunt infections? *Pediatr Neurosurg*. 1999;30:253–257.

154. James HE, Bejar R, Gluck L, et al. Ventriculoperitoneal shunts in high risk newborns weighing under 2000 grams: a clinical report. *Neurosurgery*. 1984;15:198–202.

155. Little JR, Rhoton AL, Mellinger JF. Comparison of ventriculoperitoneal and ventriculoatrial shunts for hydrocephalus in children. *Mayo Clin Proc*. 1972;47:396–401.

156. James HE, Walsh JW, Wilson HD, Connor JD, Bean JR, Tibbs PA. Prospective randomized study of therapy in cerebrospinal fluid shunt infection. *Neurosurgery*. 1980;7:459–463.

157. Walters BC, Hoffman HJ, Hendrick EB, Humphreys RP. Cerebrospinal fluid shunt infection. Influences on initial management and subsequent outcome. *J Neurosurg*. 1984;60:1014–1021.

158. Chadduck W, Adametz J. Incidence of seizures in patients with myelomeningocele: a multifactorial analysis. *Surg Neurol*. 1988;30:281–285.

159. Lam CH, Villemure JG. Comparison between ventriculoatrial and ventriculoperitoneal shunting in the adult population. *Br J Neurosurg*. 1997;11:43–48.

160. Kulkarni AV, Drake JM, Lamberti-Pasculli M. Cerebrospinal fluid shunt infection: a prospective study of risk factors. *J Neurosurg*. 2001;94:195–201.

161. Bayston R. Epidemiology, diagnosis, treatment, and prevention of cerebrospinal fluid shunt infections. *Neurosurg Clin North Am*. 2001;36:703–708.

162. Stern S, Bayston R, Hayward RJ. *Haemophillus influenzae* meningitis in the presence of cerebrospinal fluid shunts. *Childs Nerv Syst.* 1988;4:164–165.

163. Sathyanarayana S, Wylen EL, Baskaya MK, Nanda A. Spontaneous bowel perforation after ventriculoperitoneal shunt surgery: case report and a review of 45 cases. *Surg Neurol.* 2000;54:388–396.

164. Odio C, McCracken Jr GH, Nelson JD. CSF shunt infections in pediatrics. A seven-year experience. *Am J Dis Child.* 1984;138:1103–1108.

165. Shapiro S, Boaz J, Kleiman M, Kalsbeck J, Mealey J. Origin of organisms infecting ventricular shunts. *Neurosurgery.* 1988;22:868–872.

166. Sells CJ, Shurtleff DB, Loeser JD. Gram-negative cerebrospinal fluid shunt-associated infections. *Pediatrics.* 1977;59:614–618.

167. Greene KA, Clark RJ, Zabramski JM. Ventricular CSF shunt infections associated with *Corynebacterium jeikeium*: report of three cases and review. *Clin Infect Dis.* 1993;16:139–141.

168. Snow RB, Lavyne MH, Fraser RA. Colonic perforation by ventriculoperitoneal shunts. *Surg Neurol.* 1986;25:173–177.

169. Chiou CC, Wong TT, Lin HH, et al. Fungal infection of ventriculoperitoneal shunts in children. *Clin Infect Dis.* 1994;19:1049–1053.

170. Yogev R. Cerebrospinal fluid shunt infections: a personal view. *Pediatr Infect Dis J.* 1985;4:113–118.

171. Ronan A, Hogg GG, Klug GL. Cerebrospinal fluid shunt infections in children. *Pediatr Infect Dis J.* 1995;14:782–786.

172. Valk PE, Morris JG, McRae J. Pulmonary embolism as a complication of ventriculoatrial shunt. *Australas Radiol.* 1970;14:272–274.

173. Bellamy CM, Roberts DH, Ramsdale DR. Ventriculo-atrial shunt causing tricuspid endocarditis: its percutaneous removal. *Int J Cardiol.* 1990;28:260–262.

174. Salomao JF, Leibinger RD. Abdominal pseudocysts complicating CSF shunting in infants and children. Report of 18 cases. *Pediatr Neurosurg.* 1999;31:274–278.

175. Egelhoff J, Babcock DS, McLaurin R. Cerebrospinal fluid pseudocysts: sonographic appearance and clinical management. *Pediatr Neurosci.* 1985;12:80–86.

176. Morissette I, Gourdeau M, Francoeur J. CSF shunt infections: a fifteen-year experience with emphasis on management and outcome. *Can J Neurol Sci.* 1993;20:118–122.

177. Schade RP, Schinkel J, Roelandse FW, et al. Lack of value of routine analysis of cerebrospinal fluid for prediction and diagnosis of external drainage-related bacterial meningitis. *J Neurosurg.* 2006;104:101–108.

178. Berger C, Schwarz S, Schaebitz WR, Aschoff A, Schwab S. Serum procalcitonin in cerebral ventriculitis. *Crit Care Med.* 2002;30:1778–1781.

179. Noetzel MJ, Baker RP. Shunt fluid examination: risks and benefits in the evaluation of shunt malfunction and infection. *J Neurosurg.* 1984;61:328–332.

180. Wang KC, Lee HJ, Sung JN, Cho BK. Cerebrospinal fluid shunt infection in children: efficiency of management protocol, rate of persistent shunt colonization, and significance of 'off-antibiotics' trial. *Childs Nerv Syst.* 1999;15:38–43; discussion 43–44.

181. Widmer AF, Frei R, Rajacic Z, Zimmerli W. Correlation between in vivo and in vitro efficacy of antimicrobial agents against foreign body infections. *J Infect Dis.* 1990;162:96–102.

182. Chuard C, Herrmann M, Vaudaux P, Waldvogel FA, Lew DP. Successful therapy of experimental chronic foreign-body infection due to meticillin-resistant *Staphylococcus aureus* by antimicrobial combinations. *Antimicrob Agents Chemother.* 1991;35:2611–2616.

183. Drancourt M, Stein A, Argenson JN, Zannier A, Curvale G, Raoult D. Oral rifampin plus ofloxacin for treatment of *Staphylococcus*-infected orthopedic implants. *Antimicrob Agents Chemother.* 1993;37:1214–1218.

184. Wong VK, Wright Jr HT, Ross LA, Mason WH, Inderlied CB, Kim KS. Imipenem/cilastatin treatment of bacterial meningitis in children. *Pediatr Infect Dis J.* 1991;10:122–125.

185. McCracken GH, Mize SG, Threlkeld N. Intraventricular gentamicin therapy in gram-negative bacillary meningitis of infancy. Report of the Second Neonatal Meningitis Cooperative Study Group. *Lancet.* 1980;1:787–791.

186. Rahal JJ, Simberkoff MS. Host defense and antimicrobial therapy in adult gram-negative bacillary meningitis. *Ann Intern Med.* 1982;96:468–474.

187. Kourtopoulos H, Holm SE. Intraventricular treatment of *Serratia marcescens* meningitis with gentamicin. Pharmacokinetic studies of gentamicin concentration in one case. *Scand J Infect Dis.* 1976;8:57–60.

188. Olsen L, Grotte G, Nordbring F. Successful treatment of *Pseudomonas aeruginosa*-ventriculitis with intraventricular gentamicin in a child with hydrocephalus. *Scand J Infect Dis.* 1977;9:243–245.

189. Baek-Nam K, Peleg AY, Lodise TP, et al. Management of meningitis due to antibiotic resistant *Acinetobacter* species. *Lancet.* 2009;9:245–255.

190. Ntziora F, Falagas ME. Linezolid for the treatment of central nervous system infection. *Ann Pharmacother.* 2007;41:296–308.

191. Faillace WJ. A no-touch technique protocol to diminish cerebrospinal fluid shunt infection. *Surg Neurol.* 1995;43:344–350.

192. Choux M, Genitori L, Lang D, Lena G. Shunt implantation: reducing the incidence of shunt infection. *J Neurosurg.* 1992;77:875–880.

193. Horgan MA, Piatt Jr JH. Shaving of the scalp may increase the rate of infection in CSF shunt surgery. *Pediatr Neurosurg.* 1997;26:180–184.

194. Ratilal B, Costa J, Sampaio C. Antibiotic prophylaxis for surgical introduction of intracranial ventricular shunts. *Cochrane Database Syst Rev.* 2006;3:CD005365.

195. Bayston R, Lambert E. Duration of protective activity of cerebrospinal fluid shunt catheters impregnated with antimicrobial agents to prevent bacterial catheter-related infection. *J Neurosurg.* 1997;87:247–251.

196. Beer R, Lackner P, Pfausler B, Schmutzhard E. Nosocomial ventriculitis and meningitis in neurocritical care patients. *J Neurol.* 2008;255:1617–1624.

197. Lozier AP, Sciacca RR, Romagnoli MF, Connolly Jr ES. Ventriculostomy-related infections: a critical review of the literature. *Neurosurgery.* 2002;51:170–181.

198. Lyke KE, Obsanjo OO, Williams MA, O'Brien M, Chotani R, Perl TM. Ventriculitis complicating use of intra-ventricular catheters in adult neurosurgical patients. *Clin Infect Dis.* 2001;33:2028–2033.

199. Aucoin PJ, Kotilainen HR, Gantz NM, Davidson R, Kellogg P, Stone B. Intracranial pressure monitors. Epidemiologic study of risk factors and infections. *Am J Med.* 1986;80:369–376.

200. Warren JW. Catheter-associated urinary tract infections. *Infect Dis Clin North Am.* 1997;11:609–622.

201. Tambyah PA, Knasinski V, Maki DG. The direct costs of nosocomial catheter-associated urinary tract infection in the era of managed care. *Infect Control Hosp Epidemiol.* 2002;23:27–31.

202. Smyth ET, McIlvenny G, Enstone JE. Four country healthcare associated infection prevalence survey 2006: overview of the results. *J Hosp Infect.* 2008;69:230–248.

203. Davenport K, Keeley FX. Evidence for the use of silver-alloy-coated urethral catheters. *J Hosp Infect.* 2005;60:298–303.

204. Williams GJ, Stickler DJ. Effect of triclosan on the formation of crystalline biofilms by mixed communities of urinary tract pathogens on urinary catheters. *J Med Microbiol.* 2008;57:1135–1140.

205. Stickler DJ, Jones GL. Reduced susceptibility of *Proteus mirabilis* to triclosan. *Antimicrob Agents Chemother.* 2008;52:991–994.

206. Shanks RM, Donegan NP, Graber ML, et al. Heparin stimulates *Staphylococcus aureus* biofilm formation. *Infect Immun.* 2005;78:4596–4606.

207. Shanks RM, Sargent JL, Martinez RM, et al. Catheter lock solutions influence staphylococcal biofilm formation on abiotic surfaces. *Nephrol Dial Transplant.* 2006;21:2247–2255.

208. Kunin CM, Chin QF, Chambers S. Morbidity and mortality associated with indwelling urinary catheters in elderly patients in a nursing home – confounding due to the presence of associated diseases. *J Am Geriatr Soc.* 1987;35:1001–1006.

209. Tambyah PA, Maki DG. The relationship between pyuria and infection in patients with indwelling urinary catheters: a prospective study of 761 patients. *Arch Intern Med.* 2000;160:673–677.

210. Huang CT, Leu HS, Ko WC. Pyuria and funguria. *Lancet.* 1995;346:582–583.

211. Mimoz O, Bouchet E, Edouard A, Costa Y, Samii K. Limited usefulness of urinary dipsticks to screen out catheter-associated bacteriuria in ICU patients. *Anaesth Intensive Care.* 1995;23:706–707.

212. Harding G, Zhanel G, Nicolle L, Cheang M. Antimicrobial treatment in diabetic women with asymptomatic bacteriuria. *N Engl J Med.* 2002;347:1576–1583.

213. Kaufmann C, Vazquez J, Sobel J, et al. Prospective multicenter surveillance study of funguria in hospitalized patients. *Clin Infect Dis.* 2000;30:14–18.

214. Nicolle I, Bradley S, Colgan R, et al. Infectious Diseases Society of America guidelines for the diagnosis and treatment of asymptomatic bacteriuria in adults. *Clin Infect Dis.* 2005;40:643–654.

215. Cope M, Cevallos ME, Cadle RM, et al. Inappropriate treatment of catheter-associated asymptomatic bacteriuria in a tertiary care hospital. *Clin Infect Dis.* 2009;48:1182–1188.

216. Quintiliani R, Klimek J, Cunha BA, Maderazo EG. Bacteremia after manipulation of the urinary tract. The importance of pre-existing urinary tract disease and compromised host defences. *Postgrad Med J.* 1978;54:668–671.

217. US Preventive Services Task Force. Screening for asymptomatic bacteriuria in adults: US Preventive Services Task Force reaffirmation recommendation statement. *Ann Intern Med*. 2008;149:43–47.

218. van der Wall E, Verkooyen RP, Mintjes-de Groot J, et al. Prophylactic ciprofloxacin for catheter-associated urinary-tract infection. *Lancet*. 1992;339:946–951.

219. Warren JW, Platt R, Thomas RJ, Rosner B, Kass EH. Antibiotic irrigation and catheter-associated urinary-tract infections. *N Engl J Med*. 1978;299:570–573.

220. Huth TS, Burke JP, Larsen RA, Classen DC, Stevens LE. Clinical trial of junction seals for the prevention of urinary catheter-associated bacteriuria. *Arch Intern Med*. 1992;152:807–812.

221. Maki DG, Tambyah PA. Engineering out the risk for infection with urinary catheters. *Emerg Infect Dis*. 2001;7:342–347.

222. Karchmer TB, Giannetta ET, Muto CA, Strain BA, Farr BM. A randomized crossover study of silver-coated urinary catheters in hospitalized patients. *Arch Intern Med*. 2000;160:3294–3298.

223. Johnson JR, Kuskowski MA, Wilt TJ. Systematic review: antimicrobial urinary catheters to prevent catheter-associated urinary tract infection in hospitalized patients. *Ann Intern Med*. 2006;144:116–126.

224. Peterson PK, Matzke G, Keane WF. Current concepts in the management of peritonitis in patients undergoing continuous ambulatory peritoneal dialysis. *Rev Infect Dis*. 1987;9:604–612.

225. Port FK, Held PJ, Nolph KD, Turenne MN, Wolfe RA. Risk of peritonitis and technique failure by CAPD connection technique: a national study. *Kidney Int*. 1992;42:967–974.

226. Luzar MA, Coles GA, Faller B, et al. *Staphylococcus aureus* nasal carriage and infection in patients on continuous ambulatory peritoneal dialysis. *N Engl J Med*. 1990;322:505–509.

227. Brulez HF, Verbrugh HA. First-line defense mechanisms in the peritoneal cavity during peritoneal dialysis. *Perit Dial Int*. 1995;15(suppl 7):S24–S33; discussion S33–S34.

228. Burkart JM. Peritoneal dialysis. In: Brenner BM, ed. *Brenner and Rector's The Kidney*. 6th ed. Philadelphia: Saunders; 2000:2454–2517.

229. Piraino B, Bailie GR, Bernardini J, et al. ISPD guidelines/recommendations. *Perit Dial Int*. 2005;25:107–131.

230. Wiggins KJ, Craig JC, Johnson DW, Stripolli GF. Treatment for peritoneal dialysis-associated peritonitis. *Nat Clin Pract Nephrol*. 2008;4:356–357.

231. Gucek A, Bren AF, Hergouth V, Lindic J. Cefazolin and netilmycin versus vancomycin and ceftazidime in the treatment of CAPD peritonitis. *Adv Perit Dial*. 1997;13:218–220.

232. Shemin D, Maaz D, St Pierre D, Kahn SI, Chazan JA. Effect of aminoglycoside use on residual renal function in peritoneal dialysis patients. *Am J Kidney Dis*. 1999;34:14–20.

233. Harris DC, Yuill EJ, Byth K, Chapman JR, Hunt C. Twin- versus single-bag disconnect systems: infection rates and cost of continuous ambulatory peritoneal dialysis. *J Am Soc Nephrol*. 1996;7:2392–2398.

234. Lobbedez T, Gardam M, Dedier H, et al. Routine use of mupirocin at the peritoneal catheter exit site and mupirocin resistance: still low after 7 years. *Nephrol Dial Transplant*. 2004;19:3140–3143.

235. Poole-Warren LA, Hallett MD, Hone PW, Burden SH, Farrell PC. Vaccination for prevention of CAPD associated staphylococcal infection: results of a prospective multicentre clinical trial. *Clin Nephrol*. 1991;35:198–206.

43 Antiretroviral therapy for HIV

Anton Pozniak

Before 1988 the management of HIV was primarily the treatment and prevention of opportunistic infections. When zidovudine became available on compassionate grounds to those patients with AIDS, the era of antiviral therapy for HIV began. Early studies with zidovudine monotherapy showed short-term benefits in symptomatic patients in delaying disease progression[1] and the results of one of the first AIDS treatment trials, ACTG 019, suggested that even asymptomatic patients with a CD4 count of less than 500 cells/mm^3 should be treated.[2] However, by 1993, the usefulness of HIV treatment was questioned. The results of the Concorde trial indicated little benefit in early intervention[3] and ACTG 155[4] showed no advantage of dual therapy with zidovudine and zalcitabine over zidovudine or zalcitabine monotherapy, generating a mood of therapeutic pessimism.

All that changed by mid-1995, when the results of several large-scale prospective studies proved that dual nucleoside analog regimens, especially zidovudine–didanosine, effectively delayed disease progression and prolonged life. Both the Delta and ACTG 175 trials[5,6] established the superiority of dual therapy over monotherapy and paved the way for the understanding of the importance of the use of surrogate markers, particularly viral load and CD4 levels, in measuring the efficacy of a regimen as well as the role of resistance in virological failure. At the same time, phase II studies of another dual nucleoside regimen with zidovudine and lamivudine demonstrated impressive CD4$^+$ and viral load benefits up to 1 year of follow-up.[7] Dual nucleoside-reverse transcriptase inhibitor (NRTI)-based regimens became commonplace, and AIDS-related mortality began to decrease.

In 1996, treatment of HIV changed dramatically for several reasons:

- First, there was an improved understanding of the pathogenesis of HIV infection.
- Second, tests became available to measure plasma HIV RNA levels down to below 1000 copies/mL.
- Third, a new and powerful class of drugs, the protease inhibitors, was introduced which, when added to the two nucleoside 'backbone' analogs, were capable of completely suppressing plasma HIV RNA levels. At the 10th International Conference on AIDS in 1996, the optimism surrounding the results of these triple drug regimens led to a belief that eradication of the virus and a cure was possible.

As a result of increasing use of this highly active antiretroviral therapy (HAART), hospital admission rates for HIV-related complications and mortality rates decreased dramatically, AIDS hospice units closed and patients returned to work. Opportunistic infections, such as those caused by cytomegalovirus (CMV), *Mycobacterium avium* complex (MAC) and toxoplasmosis became exceedingly rare.[8] Published data in the late 1990s estimated the mortality rate in patients with CD4 counts of less than 100×10^6/L had fallen by nearly two-thirds to less than 8 per 100 patient-years. In stark contrast at this time of hopes and expectations the epidemic rose exponentially in the resource-poor world where there was little access to HIV therapies and diagnostics. The global pandemic of HIV was established.

Further pathogenesis studies documented reservoirs of HIV in latently infected resting T lymphocytes and other long-lived cell populations, making it unlikely that HIV could be eradicated by antiretroviral therapy alone.[9] Strategies to sustain suppression of viral replication in the long term were required. Drug development concentrated on therapy that was potent, simple to adhere to, and could be used against resistant strains. The non-nucleoside analogs with their low pill burden, lack of food requirements and a perceived lack of long-term toxicity made them an increasingly common first-line treatment option. New classes of drugs blocking HIV entry such as fusion inhibitors, chemokine receptor antagonists and HIV integrase inhibitors preventing HIV from being integrated into host DNA are now available in the clinic.

In addition to drugs that inhibit targets in the viral replication cycle, immunotherapeutic approaches have been assessed using the cytokine interleukin (IL)-2 which results in increases in CD4 counts but had no impact on clinical outcome in trials where it was used in combination with antiretroviral regimens as the CD4 cells were non-functional.[10–12]

Therapeutic vaccines are also being pursued, which might improve specific immune responses and assist immunological control of HIV replication. Their clinical effectiveness remains unknown.

Sustained inhibition of viral replication results in partially reconstituting the immune system and substantially reducing the risk of clinical progression and death. The long-term efficacy of current antiretroviral regimens is becoming clearer and patients who have successful control of HIV therapy can live relatively normal life spans; for example, a 20-year-old individual starting HAART can expect to live for another 43 years on average, and a 35-year-old can expect 32 more years of life.

Mortality rates become similar to that of the general population after the sixth year of follow-up among patients whose CD4 counts reach 500 cells/mm[3].[13] It appears that patients have to take therapy lifelong and that interruptions in therapy are associated with an increased risk of cardiovascular events.[14,15] Patients' adherence to current regimens has to be very high to ensure virological success and limit the risk of resistance emerging.

Although antiretroviral therapy is extremely successful, there are still many challenges and problems, some of which are emerging, such as long-term metabolic, bone and cardiovascular complications of therapy.[16–18] For parts of the world with the highest HIV rates the problem is still access to therapy, monitoring and medical care.

INITIATING ANTIRETROVIRAL THERAPY

AIMS OF TREATMENT

With currently available antiretroviral agents, eradication of HIV infection is not likely to be possible;[19] thus, the aim of treatment is to prolong and improve quality of life by maintaining suppression of virus replication for as long as possible.

The objective of antiretroviral therapy is to reduce and sustain plasma viral load levels to below the level of detectability (<50 copies/mL). If patients are adherent to therapy, the likelihood of a viral load rebound and drug resistance is minimal. However, in spite of inhibition of viral replication in plasma, lymph nodes and other sites, reservoirs of HIV infection in latently infected resting macrophages and T lymphocytes remain. Bursts of viral replication from these reservoirs can be detected in patients with long-term viral suppression but whether or not new cells continue to be infected as a result of these bursts is still an area of debate. However, even in patients who have sustained, undetectable levels of plasma viral load for several years, discontinuation of antiretroviral therapy results in rapid rebound of plasma viral load to pretreatment levels.[20]

The three groups of treatment-naive patients for whom treatment might be considered are patients with primary HIV infection, patients with asymptomatic HIV infection and patients with symptomatic HIV disease or AIDS.

 PRIMARY HIV INFECTION

The burst of viremia in acute primary HIV infection usually resolves in 2 months and this period is the focus of research into giving early treatment. There is a rationale for treatment during the 2- to 6-month period after this, so-called recent primary HIV infection, and it is based on the probability that virus replication in lymphoid tissue is still not controlled during this time.[21]

Clinical trials information regarding treatment of acute HIV infection is limited.[22] Multiple studies have shown conflicting results of therapy with varying short-term effects on immunological markers.[23] A randomized prospective study is needed to weigh the risks and long-term benefit of treatment regimens initiated during acute infection. This strategy is being examined by the Medical Research Council (MRC) SPARTAC study and results are anticipated in 2010.

The rationale for starting treatment during or shortly after infection is to attempt to maintain specific and robust CD4 helper HIV responses,[24–27] which are generally lost, with the exception of long-term non-progressors[26] with chronic HIV infection.[28] Such immune responses appear to be maintained in people treated with potent antiretroviral therapy shortly after primary HIV infection. Some data suggest that there is more rapid and complete immune reconstitution in patients starting therapy during primary infection than in those starting treatment later.[29] There is, however, no evidence to date that any of these immunological benefits persist indefinitely with continuing treatment or after treatment is withdrawn.

Potential benefits of treating acute HIV infection

Decrease the severity of acute disease and reduce morbidity associated with high viraemia and CD4 depletion during acute infection
Reduce the risk of onward transmission of HIV
Limit loss of CD4-rich gastrointestinal lymphoid tissue that occurs during the first weeks of infection, although data are limited and the clinical relevance is unclear[30,31]

The possible benefits of treatment during primary infection with HIV should be considered against the known risks of drug toxicity,[32,33] the associated risk of development of drug resistance and the difficulties of long-term adherence. The optimal duration or optimal drugs to use in therapy for patients with acute or recent HIV infection is unknown. The potential need for lifelong treatment should be a consideration in making the decision to treat or not. As non-nucleoside reverse transcriptase inhibitor (NNRTI) transmitted resistance is more commonly seen than protease inhibitor (PI) transmitted resistance, a protease inhibitor-based regimen should be given until drug resistance test results are available.

While data are lacking a pragmatic approach would be to consider treatment of primary infection outside a prospective study when patients have neurological involvement, any AIDS-defining illness or a CD4 cell count persistently <200 cells/mm[3] (i.e. for 3 months or more).[34]

 CHRONIC HIV INFECTION

The aims of antiretroviral therapy are to reduce the viral load which will lead to improved and/or preserved immune function and consequently reduce HIV-associated morbidity and mortality. Another possible benefit that is being explored is the potential to reduce HIV transmission, especially if there are continued high-risk behaviors.[35]

Delaying therapy until the CD4 cell count is <200 cells/mm³ is associated with a substantially greater risk of disease progression and death. As the risk persists for a significant period after treatment is started, every effort should be made to start treatment before the CD4 cell count has fallen to <200 cells/mm³.

Symptomatic HIV infection

International guidelines recommend initiation of antiretroviral therapy in patients with a history of AIDS-defining illness or symptomatic HIV infection. One exception to this might be someone with tuberculosis who presents with a high CD4 count when the TB may be not a manifestation of immune suppression.

Asymptomatic disease

The timing of antiviral therapy in patients who are asymptomatic is an area of active debate and research. Until we have the results of a controlled, prospective study comparing early and deferred therapy (START trial), treatment guidelines rely largely on data from observational cohort studies.[6,7] Currently, these guidelines state that the optimal time to start therapy for an asymptomatic patient is around a CD4⁺ count of 350 cells per cubic millimeter (mm³).

Most physicians will use this 350 CD4 cell threshold as the main criterion for starting, but should patients or subgroups of patients start earlier than that? One of the driving forces for considering starting earlier is the impact of non-AIDS-related morbidity and mortality because of the effect of viremia on driving inflammatory and neoplastic processes independent of the CD4 count.

The SMART study helped us to understand this concept of viremia being harmful. SMART was a prospective, randomized, multicenter, cohort study, comparing treatment being discontinued when the CD4 T-cell count exceeded 350 cells/mm³ and reinitiated when the CD4 T-cell count fell to <250 cells/mm³ with continuous antiretroviral therapy. Mortality was largely due to causes other than AIDS, and several non-AIDS-defining conditions such as hepatic failure, renal disease, cardiovascular disease and non-AIDS malignancy were greater in participants randomized to treatment interruption than in those who received continuous therapy.[36,37]

When a subgroup analysis of the SMART study (in which treatment-naive patients with CD4 T-cell counts of >350 cells/mm³ were randomized to receive antiretroviral therapy either immediately or after the CD4 T-cell count dropped to <250 cells/mm³) was analyzed, the risk of opportunistic diseases and serious non-AIDS events was higher in the deferred-therapy arm than in the treatment arm, suggesting that delaying therapy until the CD4 T-cell count decreases to <350 cells/mm³ should be avoided.[38]

A large observational cohort, the North American AIDS Cohort Collaboration on Research and Design (NA-ACCORD),[39] showed that in the 8362 patients with a CD4⁺ count of 351–500 cells/mm³, deferral of therapy until the CD4⁺ count had fallen to 350 cells/mm³ or less was associated with an increase of 69% in the risk of death, as compared with patients who initiated therapy when their CD4⁺ count was within the designated range. The majority of deaths for which cause was available were from 'non-AIDS-defining' causes and thought to be due to the inflammatory effect of HIV itself.

Other data sets support the notion of starting earlier but consider that the advantage of starting above 500 cells/mm³ rather than somewhere between 500 and 350 cells/mm³ may be small.[40]

Other reasons for starting HAART early

Patients with a rapidly falling CD4 count (e.g. falling by >80 cells/mm³ per year on repeated testing) should be considered for initiation of therapy relatively earlier within the CD4 count range 350–500 cells/mm³

AIDS diagnosis (or any HIV-related co-morbidity)

– hepatitis B and C infection, where treatment is indicated or contemplated

– low CD4 percentage (e.g. <14%, where *Pneumocystis jirovecii* prophylaxis would be indicated)

– established cardiovascular disease (CVD) or a very high risk of cardiovascular events (e.g. Framingham risk of CVD more than 20% over 10 years)

Pregnant women

Persons with HIV-associated nephropathy

Potential benefits and risks of early therapy

Potential benefits

· Maintain a higher count and potentially prevent further irreversible damage to the immune system

· Decrease the risk for HIV-associated complications that occur even at high CD4 counts (e.g. tuberculosis, lymphoma, peripheral human papillomavirus-associated malignancies, neuropathy)

· Decrease the risk of non-AIDS-associated diseases such as cardiovascular disease, renal disease, liver disease, and non-AIDS-associated malignancies and infections

· Decrease the risk of HIV transmission to others

Potential risks

· Development of side effects and toxicities of treatment

· Development of drug resistance which may result in loss of future treatment options

· Treatment fatigue because of increased total time on medication

· Transmission of drug-resistant virus in patients who do not maintain full virological suppression

THERAPEUTIC STRATEGIES IN THE TREATMENT-NAIVE PATIENT

The very dramatic fall in AIDS-related mortality and frequency of AIDS events in the developed world coincided with the introduction of HAART.[41] Any HAART regimen should be individualized in order to achieve the best potency, adherence[42] and tolerability, to minimize potential toxicity, and to avoid any likely drug–drug interactions. A measurement of a regimen's success is achieving a viral load of <50 HIV-1 RNA copies/mL within 6–9 months of starting treatment.

BASELINE ASSESSMENT

Before starting treatment patients should be counseled about adherence and given appropriate information on the drugs they may be taking and their side effects.

A baseline assessment should be performed and should include HIV resistance testing to detect transmitted resistance screening for hepatitis B and C co-infection, routine hematology and biochemistry tests, a sexually transmitted infection screen and other tests as appropriate including co-receptor tropism and HLA B5701.

In addition, a full cardiovascular risk assessment should be undertaken and patients should be screened for diabetes and renal problems. A psychosocial history should also be taken to identify psychiatric problems, alcohol use and recreational drug use as well as safer sex knowledge and practice. A social and adherence assessment is essential.

In women of childbearing age, a discussion around plans for pregnancy and the use of contraception is important.

WHICH REGIMEN TO START?

When choosing a HAART regimen the advantages and disadvantages in terms of potency, adherence, toxicity and potential drug–drug interactions should be considered for each patient and therapy individualized accordingly.

Drug regimens that might be considered for a patient initiating antiretroviral therapy for the first time are listed below:

- A low-dose ritonavir 'boosted' protease inhibitor and two nucleo(t)sides
- A non-nucleoside reverse transcriptase inhibitor (NNRTI) such as efavirenz and two nucleo(t)sides
- Others include nucleo(t)side-sparing or integrase-based regimens, but these have been rarely used to date outside clinical trials.

TWO NRTIs PLUS A BOOSTED PROTEASE INHIBITOR

Protease inhibitors have a long history of clinical and surrogate marker efficacy in clinical practice.

Protease inhibitors are usually used in combination with low-dose ritonavir to provide a pharmacokinetic boosting effect. The rationale for this is that these drugs are extensively metabolized by the cytochrome P_{450} system, resulting in short half-lives and low trough concentrations. Ritonavir is a potent inhibitor of cytochrome P_{450} CYP3A and enhances plasma concentrations of other protease inhibitors, raising trough levels and extending the half-life. This improves

potency and is associated with a reduced risk of resistance development. In addition, a boosted protease inhibitor regimen can improve convenience by reducing dosage frequency and pill burden, and facilitating adherence. However, some toxicities (e.g. gastrointestinal upset) and lipid abnormalities may occur more commonly with some boosted protease inhibitor regimens.[43]

Which boosted protease inhibitor?

The three main boosted protease inhibitors currently used in the treatment of naive patients are lopinavir, atazanavir and darunavir. Other boosted protease inhibitors include fosamprenavir and saquinavir:

- Lopinavir boosted with ritonavir is currently the only co-formulated protease inhibitor and is available in a heat-stable Meltrex tablet form. The other protease inhibitors are given with ritonavir separately. Lopinavir has a tendency to cause gastrointestinal intolerance, notably diarrhea.
- Atazanavir causes unconjugated hyperbilirubinemia by competitive inhibition of the uridine diphosphate-glucuronosyl transferase (UGT) 1A1 enzyme. This is only rarely of clinical significance.
- Darunavir can cause a mild rash.

There have been two recent randomized trials of boosted lopinavir, one versus boosted atazanavir (Castle study) and one versus darunavir (Artemis study). In essence, in terms of overall efficacy, the comparator arms both outperformed the lopinavir arm, mainly based on discontinuations due to higher toxicity rates of the lopinavir arms, especially gastrointestinal effects. Lipid abnormalities were also higher in the lopinavir arms in both of the studies.[44,45]

NNRTI-BASED REGIMENS

These have gained much popularity in antiviral-naive patients because of the large clinical trial data available, lower pill burden, drug interactions and safety profile, as well as cost.

Which NNRTI?

Two NNRTIs are currently licensed for use in treatment-naive patients, nevirapine and efavirenz.

The 2NN study compared nevirapine with efavirenz. Both drugs were given in combination with stavudine and lamivudine in treatment-naive individuals. At 48 weeks of the study the difference in virological suppression did not reach criteria necessary to demonstrate non-inferiority of nevirapine. However, two patients taking nevirapine died, one from hepatic toxicity and one from septicemia related to Stevens–Johnson syndrome.[46]

Nevirapine

The toxicities and side effects of nevirapine are well known and are substantially higher in those with higher CD4 counts and in women, hence it is recommended that nevirapine is not started in men with CD4 counts of >400 cells/mm³ and in women with CD4 counts of >250 cells/mm³.

Efavirenz

Efavirenz has demonstrated potent viral suppression in large randomized, controlled trials and cohort studies of treatment-naive patients at up to 7 years of follow-up.[47–49]

Efavirenz-based regimens have demonstrated superior virological responses to lopinavir protease inhibitor-based regimens, and comparable activity to atazanavir-based regimens.[50] The potency of efavirenz is independent of baseline viral load and CD4 cell count.

Efavirenz is associated with neuropsychiatric effects including dizziness, abnormal dreams, insomnia, hallucination and euphoria. These side effects are more pronounced in the first 1–2 weeks of treatment. Occasionally patients report disabling side effects which persist beyond this induction period, necessitating switching from efavirenz.

Congenital abnormalities have been observed in cynomolgus monkeys whose mothers were treated with efavirenz during pregnancy. While prospective studies of its use in pregnant women have failed to demonstrate an excess risk of congenital abnormalities, it remains the recommendation that alternatives are used in women trying to conceive or in those at higher risk of unplanned pregnancy.

 ## NNRTI OR PI

There is still much discussion over which is the best regimen on which to start patients. Until recently we only had cohort data but the randomized trial ACTG A5142 compared efavirenz with lopinavir–ritonavir, plus two NRTIs. There was also a third arm with the boosted protease inhibitor and NNRTI in combination but without nucleosides. This ACTG A5142 study showed better virological responses with an efavirenz-based regimen compared with a lopinavir–ritonavir-based regimen, but it showed better CD4 cell responses and less resistance after virological failure with lopinavir–ritonavir plus two NRTIs.[50]

A smaller randomized trial in Mexico, which compared the same agents (efavirenz versus lopinavir–ritonavir) in treatment-naive participants who had CD4 cell counts of <200/mm³, also suggested a virological advantage among efavirenz recipients.[51]

Recently ACTG A5202 compared efavirenz with ritonavir boosted atazanavir (combined with 2 different NRTI backbones) and showed similar efficacy.[51a]

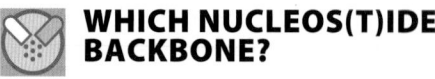 ## WHICH NUCLEOS(T)IDE BACKBONE?

Dual nucleos(t)ide combinations form the backbone of initial therapy regimens with either boosted protease inhibitors or non-nucleosides. In reality, although there are several possible different combinations, there are only four combinations in common use. Three of these combinations have been co-formulated to simplify dosing. However, one combination (tenofovir and emtricitabine) is preferred by most physicians.

Tenofovir and emtricitabine

Tenofovir, when used with emtricitabine as part of an efavirenz-based regimen in treatment-naive patients, has demonstrated potent virological suppression and was superior to zidovudine–lamivudine in virological efficacy up to 144 weeks. Renal impairment, with increases in serum creatinine, glycosuria, hypophosphatemia and Fanconi syndrome, has been reported with tenofovir use.

Renal function, urinalysis and electrolytes should be monitored in patients who are on tenofovir and alternative agents used in renal impairment. Tenofovir with emtricitabine has also been studied in combination with several different boosted protease inhibitors in randomized clinical trials; all such trials demonstrate good virological benefit.

Tenofovir plus either emtricitabine or lamivudine is the preferred NRTI combination for patients co-infected with both HIV and HBV, as these drugs have activity against both viruses.

Abacavir and lamivudine

Abacavir has the potential for serious hypersensitivity reactions which are observed in 5–8% of patients who start this drug. The risk for this reaction is highly associated with the presence of the HLA-B*5701 allele. Studies have shown that a negative HLA-B*5701 test is not associated with this reaction. Routine testing for HLA-B*5701 is recommended if abacavir is contemplated as part of the regimen.

Unfortunately there have been evolving issues with the use of abacavir:

- Data suggest that regimens given to patients with a starting viral load of >100 000 copies/mL showed a significantly shorter time to virological failure in an abacavir–lamivudine arm compared with a tenofovir–emtricitabine arm.
- The D:A:D and other cohort studies have suggested a link between abacavir use and myocardial infarction.[52] These data have been supported by some but not all studies and the mechanism is unknown. No such association has been seen with tenofovir.

Didanosine and lamivudine

Didanosine has to be taken fasting and has been linked to increased risk of pancreatitis and non-cirrhotic portal hypertension. In the ACTG 5175 study an inferior virological outcome was seen when it was used with lamivudine and a protease inhibitor.

The D:A:D study group have also implicated didanosine with the risk of myocardial infarction.

Zidovudine–lamivudine

Zidovudine–lamivudine is now considered an alternative rather than a preferred NRTI option, mainly because of the greater toxicity of zidovudine compared with tenofovir.

Bone marrow suppression, with macrocytic anemia and/ or neutropenia, is seen in some patients. Zidovudine is also associated with gastrointestinal toxicity, fatigue, lipoatrophy and abnormal lipids.

PROTEASE INHIBITOR/NNRTI COMBINATIONS

The interest in protease inhibitor/NNRTI-based ('nucleoside-sparing') regimens has arisen out of concern over the long-term toxicities of NRTIs (such as lipodystrophy, pancreatitis and lactic acidosis). Although these combinations should be highly effective, dosing schedules tend to be complicated as both NNRTIs and protease inhibitors are substrates of the cytochrome P_{450} system and have complex drug interactions. In ACTG 5142 the combination of efavirenz and lopinavir–ritonavir was as efficacious as the efavirenz nucleoside arms but had a higher rate of side effects and toxicities.

OTHER NOVEL COMBINATIONS

Nucleoside-sparing regimens combining a boosted protease inhibitor and an integrase inhibitor are under investigation.

Raltegravir-based regimen

An integrase inhibitor has been studied in phase III trials using a raltegravir-based regimen versus efavirenz in treatment-naive patients. There were similar viral load data at 48 weeks but a faster rate of becoming virologically undetectable on the raltegravir regimen, the significance of which is unknown. The overall toxicity rate, especially for neuropsychiatric events, was lower in the raltegravir arm.

Maraviroc-based regimen

A randomized, double-blind study (MERIT) compared the CCR5 antagonist maraviroc with efavirenz, both in combination with zidovudine–lamivudine, in treatment-naive participants.[53]

Only participants who had CCR5 virus and no evidence of resistance to any drugs used in the study were enrolled at 48 weeks. The HIV RNA (<50 copies/mL) results did not meet the set criteria to demonstrate non-inferiority for maraviroc (65.2% vs 69.2% for efavirenz patients). CD4 counts increased by an average of 170 cells/mm³ in the maraviroc arm and by an average of 143 cells/mm³ in the efavirenz arm. Toxicity of maraviroc was low. The result was influenced by the lack of sensitivity of the tropism test used in determining whether patients had R5 tropic virus and underestimated the number with dual X4 R5 tropic virus, leading to virological failure in such subjects.

MONITORING TREATMENT

Patients on HAART should have their CD4 count and plasma viral load levels monitored at regular intervals. Laboratory evaluations are usually performed at 2- to 4-week intervals initially and then eventually about 3 monthly, unless specifically needed. On effective therapy, plasma viral load falls rapidly as viral replication is inhibited. By 4 weeks a fall of greater than 1 log, and by 3–6 months a fall to <50 copies/mL, in viral load should be expected.

TOXICITY OF ANTIVIRAL AGENTS

All antiviral agents can cause side effects and toxicities. Some are more linked to a class of drug, such as rash and hepatitis which are commoner with NNRTIs or dyslipidaemia with protease inhibitors. The thymidine analogs AZT (zidovudine) and D4T (stavudine) are both associated with the development of lipoatrophy which can lead to significant changes in body shape and is only slowly reversible once the drug is stopped. One proposed mechanism is drug-induced damage to mitochondria. Other side effects are more drug specific, such as anemia with AZT, neuropathy with stavudine, hypersensitivity with abacavir and jaundice with atazanavir. The latter two problems are genetically linked. In the case of abacavir, by screening out patients who are HLA-B★5701 positive, hypersensitivity reactions can be prevented completely. Efavirenz, which is commonly used in first-line therapy, causes short-lived neuropsychiatric symptoms. Occasionally these can be severe and the drug needs to be stopped. In some patients these are linked to very high drug levels. Again a genetic basis for high drug levels can often be found in patients who have a cytochrome P_{450} 2B6 enzyme deficiency. Enfuvirtide had an almost 100% rate of injection-site reactions but the other new drugs raltegravir and maraviroc have good tolerability profiles.

Tenofovir is associated with decreases in renal tubular function which are usually clinically benign. It has, however, been linked to cases of Fanconi syndrome.

An association between an increased cardiovascular risk and the use of antivirals has been found for abacavir and more recently for lopinavir–ritonavir.

The most common reason for stopping antiretroviral agents is toxicity. These are often short lived and are usually gastrointestinal, but anemia, neuropathy and rash are also important. Long-term toxicities such as lipodystrophy are becoming less common in resource-rich countries as physicians have a choice of drugs other than thymidine analogs. The situation is worsening in many resource-poor countries where no such choice exists. As most antiviral regimens in drug-naive populations have similar efficacy, the advantages of one drug over another can be its side effect profile.

TREATMENT FAILURE AND SALVAGE THERAPY

FIRST TREATMENT FAILURE

One measure of treatment success is whether complete viral suppression is achieved; any evidence of ongoing viral replication indicates treatment failure. Once treatment failure is suspected, a repeat confirmatory viral load should be performed. There are several reasons why the viral load may increase on therapy and not all are the result of the development of viral resistance.

Causes of treatment failure

> **Major causes of treatment failure**
> - Insufficient drug exposure due to poor adherence
> - Drug–drug interactions leading to poor pharmacokinetics
> - Drug toxicity leading to cessation of the regimen
>
> **Less common causes of treatment failure**
> - Lack of potency
> - Inadequate drug absorption
> - Inability of the agents to penetrate viral reservoirs
> - Primary drug resistance acquisition at the time of infection

Starting treatment at a late stage of HIV disease (high HIV RNA levels[54] and/or CD4+ count <100 cells/mm³) has also been strongly associated with early virological failure.[55] Lifelong adherence to therapy is crucial, as demonstrated in studies of adherence. Counseling and directly observed therapy, rather than self-administered therapy, result in significantly better viral load and CD4 responses.

 TRANSIENT INCREASE IN VIRAL LOAD

If a patient's viral load rises to just above detectable (50–500 copies/mL), the viral load count should be repeated as soon as possible, preferably within 2 weeks. The patient should be clinically assessed to determine any contributing factors such as drug–drug interactions, poor adherence, coexisting infections and/or vaccinations, which can all increase the viral load transiently. Rises in viral load to just above detectable levels occur in a significant proportion of patients on treatment.[56,57] Those whose viral load is transiently detectable because of laboratory assay-related problems or other factors will show no further rise or revert to undetectable, and are called 'blips'. Patients who develop virological failure show further increases in viral load. Whether viral 'blips' are associated with an increased future risk of virological failure is unclear for those who have already achieved viral suppression. One study showed no such association,[56] but another suggested that, although a low-level viral 'blip' was not a predictor of failure, those with repeated episodes or sustained low-level viral rebound were more likely to experience future virological failure.[57] Patients with frequent 'blips' should be monitored more regularly than others.

 SUSTAINED VIRAL LOAD REBOUND

Falls in CD4 count and clinical disease progression is the usual outcome in patients whose viral load continues to rise towards pretreatment levels.[58] Although resistance to all drugs in a treatment regimen may not be detected in patients experiencing virological failure, a persistently high viral load on treatment will lead to the accumulation of resistance mutations. For some drugs, such as lamivudine and NNRTIs, mutations at one position in the reverse transcriptase gene usually emerge at low levels of viral load rebound and result in significant phenotypic resistance. Reduced susceptibility to other drugs usually requires the accumulation of two or more mutations, as can occur with ongoing viral replication. Thus, changing therapy should be considered if viral replication persists and other therapeutic options exist to completely suppress it. However, a decision to switch to a second regimen is complicated, and depends on several factors, including addressing the etiology of virological failure. A change of therapy should be considered if HIV load has never become undetectable or after being undetectable on antiviral therapy has subsequently becomes consistently detectable.

CHOICE OF SUBSEQUENT REGIMEN

 PROTEASE INHIBITOR FAILURE

Optimal virological responses to a second or subsequent regimen will be obtained only when adherence is maximized and ineffective drugs are eliminated from the regimen. Resistance testing and a history of drug exposure will help guide drug choices. Patients who begin therapy with a combination of two NRTIs and a protease inhibitor retain susceptibility to NNRTI as long as baseline resistance tests show wild-type virus.

Patients failing on unboosted protease inhibitor therapy are often difficult to treat because of broad cross-resistance within this class.[55,59,60] In recent years, use of low-dose ritonavir-based boosted protease inhibitor regimens have changed this and if treatment failure is due to poor adherence, primary protease mutations will usually not be found on resistance testing.

Newer protease inhibitors such as tipranavir and, especially, darunavir usually have good activity, even when several primary protease mutations are present, and can be used in case of prior protease inhibitor failure dependent on the genotype.

 NNRTI FAILURE

Patients who begin therapy with a combination of two NRTIs and an NNRTI retain susceptibility to protease inhibitors. Unfortunately, there is broad cross-resistance between efavirenz and nevirapine. Thus, they cannot be used reliably after failure of other drugs in the same class. The second-generation NNRTI etravirine has activity against some NNRTI-resistant strains but activity depends on the genotypic resistance that has developed to the existing agents. Fortunately it has excellent activity against the common K103N mutation often seen as a lone NNRTI mutant in early efavirenz failure.

SUBSEQUENT VIROLOGICAL FAILURE

Virological failure on treatment can be defined as a confirmed HIV RNA level >400 copies/mL after 24 weeks of prior therapy or >50 copies/mL after 48 weeks, or a repeated detectable HIV RNA level after prior suppression of viremia.

In the past, for those who had experienced virological failure on two or more HAART regimens (often referred to as 'salvage therapy'), the therapeutic approach and goal of therapy were very different as, with the drugs then available, complete viral suppression was rarely achievable. Partial viral suppression became the goal of therapy; even viral load reductions of >0.5 $\log_{10}$ copies/mL which resulted in clinical improvement implied that such salvage regimens were worth pursuing.[61] However, continuing viral replication on antiretroviral therapy selects for further resistance, limiting future options; eventually the viral load will rise, CD4 will fall and patients will progress to AIDS and death.

 ## ASSESSMENT OF THE HIGHLY EXPERIENCED PATIENT

Any new therapeutic regimen should have the optimal chance of success. Adherence problems should be carefully explored and the impact of the patient's social and psychological condition on adherence explored.

The following should all be considered prior to changing treatment:

- A detailed history of prior antiretroviral therapy and the reasons why the patient changed drugs.
- A resistance test, preferably while still on failing treatment.
- Data from prior resistance tests as mutations may have been lost over time because of lack of drug pressure (e.g. 184V mutation and protease inhibitor mutations).
- Retrospective resistance testing of stored plasma taken at the time of previous treatment failure in patients who have interrupted therapy.
- An assessment of any potential current and future drug–drug interactions and conditions that might lead to drug malabsorption.

With the development of next-generation boosted protease inhibitors and NNRTIs active against viruses with key mutations and new classes of entry/fusion drugs and integrase inhibitors, the aim of treatment in highly treatment experienced patients is to achieve undetectable viral loads. This can be achieved in the majority but there remains a small minority in whom an effective suppressive regimen cannot be constructed. These patients are the new 'salvage' group.

Over the last 5 years several studies (Torro, Power, Duet, Resist, Motivate and Benchmark) have defined an effective antiretroviral strategy for managing highly treatment-experienced patients. The principles of treatment are that new regimens should contain, whenever possible, three fully active drugs based on patient history and resistance testing. If three fully active drugs are not available, data suggest that most patients will still respond using two fully active drugs plus drugs with partial activity, with at least one of these drugs coming from a new class. If possible, the regimen should also contain an active boosted protease inhibitor.[62–66]

It should be noted that when agents from new classes are used in a regimen where they are, in effect, the only active drug, then resistance to that drug usually occurs within weeks. This phenomenon is seen with the integrase inhibitor raltegravir, the NNRTI etravirine, the entry inhibitor enfuvirtide and the CCR5 inhibitor maraviroc.

Patients who have few options based on history and resistance testing are difficult to manage and have limited choices. Options include the following:

- *Treatment interruption.* Treatment interruption, however, has not been shown to be associated with any durable benefit and may be associated with a rapid increase in viral load and decrease in CD4 count, with or without clinical progression, and an increase in non-HIV complications such as cardiovascular, renal or hepatic problems.[67–69]
- *A nucleoside-only regimen.* Cohort studies suggest continued immunological and clinical benefits if the HIV RNA level is maintained at <20 000 copies/mL.[70,71] There is evidence from cohort studies that continuing therapy, in the presence of viremia, decreases the risk of disease progression.[72]

Switching patients to a nucleosides-only regimen may be of benefit as not only will this strategy reduce the amount of drug taken but also decrease some of the toxicity, preventing further resistance mutations occurring to the other classes of drug.[73]

Monotherapy with or continuing nucleosides, including lamivudine, are strategies that have been used when there are few options available. Data suggest that lamivudine may reduce viral fitness and reduce viral load by maintaining the M184V mutation.[74,75]

 ## OTHER PATIENT POPULATIONS

Pregnant women and children require special consideration as far as antiviral therapy is concerned but the principle of using antiviral therapy to reduce the viral load to below detectability remains the same. Detailed guidance for their management can be found at http://aidsinfo.nih.gov/ContentFiles/Pediatric Guidelines.pdf and at http://aidsinfo.nih.gov/ContentFiles/PerinatalGL.pdf, and as published by the British HIV Association.[76]

Hepatitis C (HCV)

In patients co-infected with hepatitis C, treatment can be considered at any CD4 cell count for HCV genotypes 1a, 1b or 4, as it will potentially slow the progression of liver disease. Starting HAART should also be considered for those with HCV genotypes 2 or 3 who do not clear the virus with HCV therapy or who are intolerant to the HCV treatment.

For some patients with CD4 counts of <200 cells/mm³, it may be preferable to initiate antiretroviral therapy and delay HCV therapy.

Important drug interactions occur between ribavirin and didanosine, leading to pancreatitis and lactic acidosis. This means that they should not be used together. Zidovudine should also be avoided because both it and ribavirin can cause anemia. There are also some concerns with abacavir and ribavirin at lower doses.

Hepatitis B (HBV)

HAART should be started in those with active HBV co-infection irrespective of CD4 cell count to try to reduce the rate of liver disease progression. It is important that the HAART regimen contains two antiretroviral drugs that are active against HBV. Tenofovir and either emtricitabine or lamivudine are the preferred drugs for initial treatment of HBV in co-infection as they have activity against both HBV and HIV. Discontinuation of these drugs may potentially cause serious hepatocellular damage resulting from reactivation of HBV.

Tuberculosis co-infection

Rifamycins are essential drugs for the treatment of tuberculosis. Rifampicin (rifampin) is the most potent inducer of hepatic enzymes, especially CYP3A4, which then results in significant decreases in exposure to ritonavir-boosted or unboosted protease inhibitors. This can lead to antiretroviral treatment failure. Co-administration of rifampicin and nevirapine or efavirenz is associated with lower NNRTI drug exposures and greater variability in plasma NNRTI drug levels. This does not have such an impact on efavirenz, especially in patients of low body weight. In most patients, adjusting the dose of efavirenz and then performing drug levels can allow safe co-administration. Nevirapine dosing cannot be increased without substantially increasing the risk of hypersensitivity reactions. Nevirapine use in tuberculosis co-infection has been associated with an increased risk of virological failure compared to its use in non-tuberculosis-infected patients.

Rifabutin is a less potent inducer of cytochrome enzymes and has fewer and less severe drug interactions with antiretroviral drugs. Rifabutin has been successfully used instead of rifampicin in treating tuberculosis in HIV-negative patients. It can be regarded as an alternative in HIV-positive patients, especially to avoid drug interactions with rifampicin.

 References

1. Fischl MA, Richman DD, Hansen N, et al. The safety and efficacy of zidovudine (AZT) in the treatment of subjects with mildly symptomatic human immunodeficiency virus type 1 (HIV) infection. A double-blind, placebo-controlled trial. *Ann Intern Med.* 1990;112:727–737.
2. Volberding PA. Zidovudine in asymptomatic HIV infection: a controlled trial in persons with fewer than 500 CD4-positive cells per cubic millimeter. *N Engl J Med.* 1990;322:941–949.
3. Concorde Coordinating Committee. Concorde: MRC/ANRS randomised double-blind controlled trial of immediate and deferred zidovudine in symptom-free HIV infection. *Lancet.* 1994;343:871–881.
4. Fischl MA, Stanley K, Collier AC, et al. Combination and monotherapy with zidovudine and zalcitabine in patients with advanced HIV disease. *Ann Intern Med.* 1995;122:24–32.
5. Delta Coordinating Committee. Delta: a randomized double-blind controlled trial comparing combinations of zidovudine plus didanosine or zalcitabine with zidovudine alone in HIV-infected individuals. *Lancet.* 1996;348:283–291.
6. Hammer SM, Katzenstein DA, Hughes MD, et al. A trial comparing nucleoside monotherapy with combination therapy in HIV-infected adults with CD4 cell counts from 200 to 500 per cubic millimeter. *N Engl J Med.* 1996;335:1081–1090.
7. CAESAR Coordinating Committee. Randomized trial of addition of lamivudine plus loviride to zidovudine-containing regimens for patients with HIV-1 infection: the CAESAR trial. *Lancet.* 1997;349:1413–1421.
8. Kovacs JA, Masur H. Prophylaxis against opportunistic infections in patients with human immunodeficiency virus infection. *N Engl J Med.* 2000;342:1416–1429.
9. Finzi D, Blankson J, Siliciano JD, et al. Latent infection of CD4+ T cells provides a mechanism for lifelong persistence of HIV-1, even in patients on effective combination therapy. *Nat Med.* 1999;5:512–525.
10. Losso M, Abrams D, the INSIGHT ESPRIT Study Group. 16th Conference on Retroviruses and Opportunistic Infections (CROI 2009). Montreal, Canada; February 8–11, 2009. Abstract 90aLB.
11. Levy Y, the SILCAAT Scientific Committee. 16th Conference on Retroviruses and Opportunistic Infections (CROI 2009). Montreal, Canada; February 8–11, 2009. Abstract 90bLB.
12. Babiker AG, for the INSIGHT ESPRIT Study Group and the SILCAAT Scientific Committee. An analysis of pooled data from the ESPRIT and SILCAAT studies: findings by latest CD4+ count 5th International AIDS Society Conference on HIV Pathogenesis, Treatment and Prevention. July 2009:19–22.
13. Lewden C, Chene G, Morlat P, et al. HIV-infected adults with a CD4 cell count greater than 500 cells/mm³ on long-term combination antiretroviral therapy reach same mortality rates as the general population. *J Acquir Immune Defic Syndr.* 2007;46(1):72–77.
14. Lundgren JD, Babiker A, El-Sadr W. Strategies for Management of Antiretroviral Therapy (SMART) Study Group. Inferior clinical outcome of the CD4+ count-guided antiretroviral treatment interruption strategy in the SMART study: role of CD4+ cell counts and HIV RNA levels during follow-up. *J Infect Dis.* 2008;197(8):1145–1155.
15. El-Sadr WM, Lundgren JD, Neaton JD, et al. CD4+ count-guided interruption of antiretroviral treatment. *N Engl J Med.* 2006;355:2283–2296.
16. Brinkman K, Smeitink JA, Romijn J, Reiss P. Mitochondrial toxicity induced by nucleoside-analogue reverse transcriptase inhibitors is a key factor in the pathogenesis of antiretroviral-therapy-related lipodystrophy. *Lancet.* 1999;354:1112–1115.
17. Carr A, Samaras K, Thorisdottir A, et al. Diagnosis, prediction, and natural course of HIV-1 protease-inhibitor-associated lipodystrophy, hyperlipidemia, and diabetes mellitus: a cohort study. *Lancet.* 1999;353:2093–2099.
18. Sabin CA, Worm SW, Weber R, et al. Use of nucleoside reverse transcriptase inhibitors and risk of myocardial infarction in HIV-infected patients enrolled in the D:A:D study: a multi-cohort collaboration. *Lancet.* 2008;371:1417–1426.
19. Gazzard B, Hill A, Gartland M, for the AVANTI Study Group. Different analyses give highly variable estimates of HIV-1 RNA undetectability and log₁₀ reduction in clinical trials. *AIDS.* 1998;12(suppl 4):S36 [Abstract P77].
20. Ruiz L, Martinez-Picada J, Romeu J, et al. Structured treatment interruption in chronically HIV-1 infected patients after long-term viral suppression. *AIDS.* 2000;14:397–403.
21. Pantaleo G, Cohen OJ, Schacker T, et al. Evolutionary pattern of human immunodeficiency virus (HIV) replication and distribution in lymph nodes

following primary infection: implications for antiviral therapy. *Nat Med.* 1998;4(3):341–345.

22. Kinloch de Loes S, Hirschel BJ, Hoen B, et al. A controlled trial of zidovudine in primary human immunodeficiency virus infection. *N Engl J Med.* 1995;333:408–413.

23. Fidler S, Fox J, Porter K, et al. Primary HIV infection: to treat or not to treat? *Curr Opin Infect Dis.* 2008;21:4–10.

24. Koup RA, Safrit JT, Cao Y, et al. Temporal association of cellular immune responses with the initial control of viremia in primary human immunodeficiency virus type 1 syndrome. *J Virol.* 1994;68:4650–4655.

25. Borrow P, Lewicki H, Hahn BH, Shaw GM, Oldstone MB. Virus-specific CD8+ cytotoxic T-lymphocyte activity associated with control of viremia in primary human immunodeficiency virus type 1 infection. *J Virol.* 1994;68:6103–6110.

26. Rosenberg ES, Billingsley JM, Caliendo AM, et al. Vigorous HIV-1-specific CD4+ T cell responses associated with control of viremia. *Science.* 1997;278:1447–1450.

27. Rosenberg ES, Altfeld M, Poon SH, et al. Immune control of HIV-1 after early treatment of acute infection. *Nature.* 2000;407:523–526.

28. Walker BD, Rosenberg ES, Hay CM, Basgoz N, Yang OO. Immune control of HIV-1 replication. *Adv Exp Med Biol.* 1998;452:159–167.

29. Kaufmann GR, Bloch M, Zaunders JJ, Smith D, Cooper DA. Long-term immunological response in HIV-1-infected subjects receiving potent antiretroviral therapy. *AIDS.* 2000;14:959–969.

30. Mehandru S, Poles MA, Tenner-Racz K, et al. Primary HIV-1 infection is associated with preferential depletion of CD4+ T lymphocytes from effector sites in the gastrointestinal tract. *J Exp Med.* 2004;200(6):761–770.

31. Guadalupe M, Reay E, Sankaran S, et al. Severe CD4+ T-cell depletion in gut lymphoid tissue during primary human immunodeficiency virus type 1 infection and substantial delay in restoration following highly active antiretroviral therapy. *J Virol.* 2003;7(21):11708–11717.

32. Miller J, Finlayson R, Smith D, et al. *The occurrence of lipodystrophic phenomena in patients with primary HIV infection (HIV) treated with antiretroviral therapy (ARV).* 7th European Conference on Clinical Aspects and Treatment of HIV Infection. Lisbon, Portugal; October. 1999 Abstract 519.

33. Goujard C, Boufassa F, Deveau C, Laskri D, Meyer L. Incidence of clinical lipodystrophy in HIV-infected patients treated during primary infection. *AIDS.* 2001;15:282–284.

34. British HIV. Association guidelines for the treatment of HIV-1-infected adults with antiretroviral therapy 2008. *HIV Med.* 2008;9:563–608.

35. Porco TC, Martin JN, Page-Shafer KA, et al. Decline in HIV infectivity following the introduction of highly active antiretroviral therapy. *AIDS.* 2004;18(1):81–88.

36. Strategies for Management of Antiretroviral Therapy (SMART) Study Group, El-Sadr WM, Lundgren JD, et al. CD4+ count-guided interruption of antiretroviral treatment. *N Engl J Med.* 2006;355(22):2283–2296.

37. Silverberg MJ, Neuhaus J, Bower M, et al. Risk of cancers during interrupted antiretroviral therapy in the SMART study. *AIDS.* 2007;21(14):1957–1963.

38. Strategies for Management of Antiretroviral Therapy (SMART) Study Group, Emery S, Neuhaus JA, Phillips AN, et al. Major clinical outcomes in antiretroviral therapy (ART)-naive participants and in those not receiving ART at baseline in the SMART study. *J Infect Dis.* 2008;197(8):1133–1144.

39. Kitahata MM, Gange SJ, Abraham AG, et al. Effect of early versus deferred antiretroviral therapy for HIV on survival. *N Engl J Med.* 2009;360:1815–1826.

40. Sterne J. 16th Conference on Retroviruses and Opportunistic Infections (CROI 2009). Montreal, Canada; February 8–11, 2009. Abstract 72LB.

41. Palella FJ, Delaney KM, Moorman AC, et al. Declining morbidity and mortality among patients with advanced human immunodeficiency virus infection. *N Engl J Med.* 1998;338:853–860.

42. Haubrich RH, Little SJ, Currier JS, et al. The value of patient-reported adherence to antiretroviral therapy in predicting virologic and immunologic response. *AIDS.* 1999;130:1099–1107.

43. Gatell JM, Lange J, Arnaiz JA, et al. A randomized study comparing continued indinavir (800 mg tid) vs switching to indinavir/ritonavir (800/100 mg bid) in HIV patients having achieved viral load suppression with indinavir plus two nucleoside analogues: the BID Efficacy and Safety Trial (BEST). 12th World AIDS Conference. Durban, South Africa, July 2000. Abstract WeOrB484.

44. Ortiz R, Dejesus E, Khanlou H, et al. Efficacy and safety of once-daily darunavir/ritonavir versus lopinavir/ritonavir in treatment-naive HIV-1-infected patients at week 48. *AIDS.* 2008;22(12):1389–1397.

45. Molina JM, Andrade-Villanueva J, Echevarria J, et al. Once-daily atazanavir/ritonavir versus twice-daily lopinavir/ritonavir, each in combination with tenofovir and emtricitabine, for management of antiretroviral-naive HIV-1-infected patients: 48 week efficacy and safety results of the CASTLE study. *Lancet.* 2008;372(9639):646–655.

46. van Leth F, Phanuphak P, Ruxrungtham K, et al. Comparison of first-line antiretroviral therapy with regimens including nevirapine, efavirenz, or both drugs, plus stavudine and lamivudine: a randomised open-label trial, the 2NN Study. *Lancet.* 2004;363(9417):1253–1263.

47. Gulick RM, Ribaudo HJ, Shikuma CM, et al. Three- vs four-drug antiretroviral regimens for the initial treatment of HIV-1 infection: a randomized controlled trial. *J Am Med Assoc.* 2006;296(7):769–781.

48. Gallant JE, Staszewski S, Pozniak AL, et al. Efficacy and safety of tenofovir DF vs stavudine in combination therapy in antiretroviral-naive patients: a 3-year randomized trial. *J Am Med Assoc.* 2004;292(2):191–201.

49. Cassetti I, Madruga JV, Etzel A, et al. The safety and efficacy of tenofovir DF (TDF) in combination with lamivudine (3TC) and efavirenz (EFV) in antiretroviral-naive patients through seven years. 17th International AIDS Conference. Mexico City, Mexico; August 3–8, 2008. Abstract TUPE0057.

50. Riddler SA, Haubrich R, DiRienzo AG, et al. Class-sparing regimens for initial treatment of HIV-1 infection. *N Engl J Med.* 2008;358(20):2095.

51. Sierra Madero J, Villasis A, Mendez P, et al. A prospective, randomized, open label trial of efavirenz versus lopinavir/ritonavir based HAART among antiretroviral therapy naive, HIV infected individuals presenting for care with CD4 cell counts <200/mm³. 17th International AIDS Conference. Mexico City, Mexico; August 3–8, 2008. Abstract TUAB0104.

51a. Daar E, Tierney C, Fischl M, et al. ACTG 5202: Final Results of ABC/3TC or TDF/FTC with either EFV or ATV/r in Treatment-naive HIV-infected Patients. 17th Conference on Retroviruses & Opportunistic Infections (CROI 2010). San Francisco. February 16–19, 2010. Abstract 59LB.

52. D:A:D Study Group, Sabin CA, Worm SW, et al. Use of nucleoside reverse transcriptase inhibitors and risk of myocardial infarction in HIV-infected patients enrolled in the D:A:D study: a multi-cohort collaboration. *Lancet.* 2008;371(9622):1417–1426.

53. Saag M, Ive P, Heere J, et al. A multicenter, randomized, double blind, comparative trial of a novel CCR5 antagonist, maraviroc versus efavirenz, both in combination with combivir (zidovudine/lamivudine), for the treatment of antiretroviral-naive subjects infected with R5 HIV: week 48 results of the MERIT study. 4th IAS Conference on HIV Pathogenesis; Treatment and Prevention. Sydney, Australia; July 22–25 2007. Abstract MOPEB016.

54. Deeks SG, Barbour J, Martin J, Swanson M, Grant RM. Sustained CD4+ T cell response after virologic failure of protease inhibitor-based regimens in patients with human immunodeficiency virus infection. *J Infect Dis.* 2000;181(3):946–953.

55. Deeks SG, Hecht FM, Swanson M, et al. Virologic outcomes with protease inhibitor therapy in an urban AIDS clinic: relationship between baseline characteristics and response to both initial and salvage antiretroviral therapy. *AIDS.* 1999;13:F35–F44.

56. Greub G, Cozzi Lepri A, Ledergerber B, et al. Lower level HIV viral rebound and blips in patients receiving potent antiretroviral therapy. 8th Conference on Retroviruses and Opportunistic Infections. Chicago, IL; February 4–8, 2001. Abstract 522.

57. Havlir D, Levitan D, Bassett R, Gilbert P, Richman D, Wong J. Prevalence and predictive value of intermittent viraemia in patients with viral suppression. *Antivir Ther.* 2000;5(suppl 3):89.

58. Deeks SG, Barbor JD, Martin JN, Grant RM. Delayed immunological deterioration among patients who virologically fail protease inhibitor therapy. 7th Conference on Retroviruses and Opportunistic Infections. San Francisco, CA; 30 January–2 February 2000. Abstract 236.

59. Gallant JE, Hall C, Barnett S, Raines C. Ritonavir/saquinavir (RTV/SQV) as salvage therapy after failure of initial protease inhibitor (PI) regimen. 5th Conference on Retroviruses and Opportunistic Infections. Chicago IL; 1998:427.

60. Deeks SG, Grant RM, Beatty G, Horton C, Detmer J, Eastman S. Activity of a ritonavir plus saquinavir-containing regimen in patients with virologic evidence of indinavir or ritonavir failure. *AIDS.* 1998;12:F97–F102.

61. Deeks S, Barbour J, Grant R, et al. Incidence and predictors of clinical progression among HIV-infected patients experiencing virologic failure of protease inhibitor-based regimens. 8th Conference on Retroviruses and Opportunistic Infections Chicago IL; February 2001:428.

62. Lazzarin A, Clotet B, Cooper D, et al. Efficacy of enfuvirtide in patients infected with drug-resistant HIV-1 in Europe and Australia. *N Engl J Med.* 2003;348(22):2186–2195.

63. Lalezari JP, Henry K, O'Hearn M, et al. Enfuvirtide, an HIV-1 fusion inhibitor, for drug-resistant HIV infection in North and South America. *N Engl J Med.* 2003;348(22):2175–2185.

64. Clotet B, Bellos N, Molina JM, et al. Efficacy and safety of darunavir–ritonavir at week 48 in treatment-experienced patients with HIV-1 infection in POWER 1 and 2: a pooled subgroup analysis of data from two randomised trials. *Lancet.* 2007;369(9568):1169–1178.

65. Steigbigel RT, Cooper DA, Kumar PN, et al. Raltegravir with optimized background therapy for resistant HIV-1 infection. *N Engl J Med.* 2008;359(4):339–354.

66. Hicks CB, Cahn P, Cooper DA, et al. Durable efficacy of tipranavir–ritonavir in combination with an optimised background regimen of antiretroviral drugs for treatment-experienced HIV-1-infected patients at 48 weeks in the Randomized Evaluation of Strategic Intervention in multi-drug reSistant patients with Tipranavir (RESIST) studies: an analysis of combined data from two randomised open-label trials. *Lancet.* 2006;368(9534):466–475.

67. Deeks SG, Wrin T, Liegler T, et al. Virologic and immunologic consequences of discontinuing combination antiretroviral-drug therapy in HIV-infected patients with detectable viremia. *N Engl J Med.* 2001;344(7):472–480.

68. Lawrence J, Mayers DL, Hullsiek KH, et al. Structured treatment interruption in patients with multidrug-resistant human immunodeficiency virus. *N Engl J Med.* 2003;349(9):837–846.

69. Ghosn J, Wirden M, Ktorza N, et al. No benefit of a structured treatment interruption based on genotypic resistance in heavily pretreated HIV-infected patients. *AIDS.* 2005;19(15):1643–1647.

70. Ledergerber B, Lundgren JD, Walker AS, et al. Predictors of trend in CD4-positive T-cell count and mortality among HIV-1-infected individuals with virological failure to all three antiretroviral-drug classes. *Lancet.* 2004;364(9428):51–62.

71. Raffanti SP, Fusco JS, Sherrill BH, et al. Effect of persistent moderate viremia on disease progression during HIV therapy. *AIDS.* 2004;37(1):1147–1154.

72. Miller V, Sabin C, Hertogs K, et al. Virological and immunological effects of treatment interruptions in HIV-1 infected patients with treatment failure. *AIDS.* 2000;14(18):2857–2867.

73. Bonjoch A, Buzon MJ, Llibre JM, et al. Transient treatment exclusively containing nucleoside analogue reverse transcriptase inhibitors in highly antiretroviral-experienced patients preserves viral benefit when a fully active therapy was initiated. *HIV Clin Trials.* 2008;9(6):387–398.

74. Campbell TB, Shulman NS, Johnson SC, et al. Antiretroviral activity of lamivudine in salvage therapy for multidrug resistant HIV-1 infection. *Clin Infect Dis.* 2005;41:236–242.

75. Castagna A, Danise A, Menzo S, et al. Lamivudine monotherapy in HIV-1-infected patients harbouring a lamivudine-resistant virus: a randomized pilot study (E-184V Study). *AIDS.* 2006;20:795–803.

76. de Ruiter A, Mercey D, Anderson J, et al. British HIV Association and Children's HIV Association guidelines for the management of HIV infection in pregnant women 2008. *HIV Med.* 2008;9:452–502.

44 Infections of the upper respiratory tract

Nicholas A. Francis and Christopher C. Butler

Upper respiratory tract infections (URTI) are the most common symptomatic human infections in developed countries[1] and the most common reason for patients to consult a healthcare professional.[2,3] The vast majority are managed by self-care, with annual consulting rates in primary care varying from 125 to 1110 per 1000 registered patients.[4] As only complicated cases are generally seen in hospitals, this chapter will focus mainly on primary care and community perspectives.

Despite their high incidence, there are major gaps in the evidence base underpinning management. For example, although most of these infections are self-limiting with a low incidence of complications, there are limited tools to predict accurately which few will go on to develop a prolonged course or become complicated. Similarly, distinguishing those patients who are likely to benefit from antibiotic treatment from the majority who do not benefit remains a major challenge in everyday clinical practice. Faced with this uncertainty, clinicians frequently follow what they consider a cautious approach and prescribe antibiotics, even when they know the average patient is unlikely to benefit.[5–8] However, many patients are satisfied with non-antibiotic management if they feel they have been examined thoroughly and received a full explanation.[9] Nevertheless, antibiotics continue to be widely used for these infections.[10,11] Indeed, URTI are the most common reason for antibiotics to be prescribed. Widespread unnecessary antibiotic prescribing not only wastes healthcare resources and leads to a cycle that encourages further consulting in the future,[12] it is also the main driver of increasing antibiotic resistance.[13] Antibiotic prescribing for these infections varies widely between countries[14] and within primary care settings in countries,[10] suggesting there remains considerable scope for rationalizing their use.

Improving the quality of antibiotic prescribing for URTI depends on enhanced diagnosis, better communication within the consultation, empowering healthcare consumers to confidently self-manage their illness, and behavior-change interventions aimed at clinicians and the public so that the emerging evidence is translated into changes in the real world.

Here, we focus on the evidence supporting management for the four commonest URTIs.

THE COMMON COLD (CORYZA)

The common cold (coryza), which is often also called an acute URTI, is defined as inflammation in the nasal or pharyngeal mucosa, in the absence of any other defined upper respiratory tract infection. The common cold needs to be distinguished from other causes of rhinitis, such as allergic rhinitis. Common colds are almost invariably caused by viruses, with rhinoviruses, adenoviruses, influenzae, parainfluenzae and respiratory syncitial virus (RSV) the main causes.[1]

EFFECTIVENESS OF ANTIBIOTICS

Antibiotics are not effective in shortening or reducing symptom severity.[15] There is some evidence of benefit for people with purulent nasal discharge[15] and in children with persistent nasal discharge (10 days or more).[16] However, only one in every four to eight will receive benefit from treatment, and this comes at a cost of risk for side effects. Given the infrequency of serious complications, the lack of long-term benefits and the minimal short-term benefits, it is hard to justify treatment with antibiotics for these conditions.

OTHER TREATMENTS

Antihistamines are not effective by themselves, but oral decongestants in adults,[17] and the combination of oral decongestants and antihistamines in adults,[18] produce some symptomatic benefit. There is no evidence of benefit from steam[19] or from vitamin C initiated after the onset of symptoms.[20] However, prophylactic vitamin C may result in a shorter duration of illness.[20]

ACUTE SORE THROAT

Acute sore throat is one of the most common presentations in primary care. Controversies in management relate mainly to the place of antibiotic treatment, prognosis and diagnostic testing.

ANTIBIOTIC TREATMENT

A Cochrane review included 27 studies with a total of 12 835 patients with sore throat and found that spontaneous resolution was common, with 82% of those taking placebo being symptom-free by 1 week.[21] Antibiotics marginally reduced symptom duration. Six patients need to be treated with antibiotics for one fewer person to be symptomatic at day three, and 21 need to be treated for one to benefit by day seven. On average, antibiotics reduce symptom duration by around 16 h. Analysis of 1839 patients from 11 studies found that those who had positive throat cultures for group A streptococcus are more likely to benefit from treatment (number needed to treat [NNT] of 3.7 for one more patient to be pain-free at 3 days).

ACUTE RHEUMATIC FEVER

One of the main arguments for antibiotic treatment is that it reduces the risk of acute rheumatic fever (ARF). The Cochrane review and a recent meta-analysis[22] found evidence for a protective effect from antibiotic treatment. However, the studies contributing to both of these analyses were all conducted in the 1950s and early 60s when the incidence of ARF was much higher. Indeed, none of the trials reporting since 1961 had a single case of ARF. A retrospective cohort study of respiratory tract infections between 1991 and 2001, which included more than a million cases of sore throat, found virtually no cases of acute rheumatic fever or acute glomerulonephritis after sore throat.[23] Furthermore, the incidence of ARF started declining before antibiotic use became widespread. Therefore, while there is historical evidence for a relative benefit from treatment with antibiotics in the prevention of ARF, the absolute benefit in Western societies, where the incidence of ARF is now vanishingly small, is minimal. Clinicians need to take this context into account when making prescribing decisions. Those working in developing countries and with other populations at higher risk of developing ARF should consider prescribing antibiotics more readily, while clinicians working in Western countries should not prescribe antibiotics to prevent ARF.

QUINSY

The evidence for a preventive effect from antibiotics for quinsy largely comes from a study in the 1950s which used intramuscular penicillin.[24] More recent studies have included only nine cases of quinsy between them,[25] and therefore it is difficult to draw conclusions from them.

A UK case-control study found that around two-thirds of cases of quinsy presented without prior consultation for sore throat. In those that did consult with sore throat before the development of quinsy, antibiotic treatment did not appear to protect against the development of quinsy. Risk factors for quinsy include smoking, male gender and aged 21–40.[25] Another retrospective analysis of 1 065 088 cases of sore throat in a UK general practice database found that antibiotic use for sore throat was associated with a reduction in quinsy within the month following diagnosis. However, the incidence of quinsy is so low that 4300 patients need to be treated to prevent one case.[23]

IDENTIFICATION OF STREPTOCOCCAL INFECTION

A number of approaches are available for identifying those individuals with sore throat who have an infection caused by group A streptococcus (GAS), including clinical scoring systems, rapid antigen detection tests (RADTs) and throat culture. All have pitfalls and costs and therefore decisions about uptake need to include consideration of the benefit of identifying those with a GAS infection. There is no international consensus on the advantage of identifying and treating those with GAS.[26] North American, French and Finnish guidelines stress the importance of treating patients with GAS in order to prevent ARF. However, this is not the case with many other European guidelines. A review of international guidelines found considerable inconsistency in studies cited, with North American guidelines more likely to cite North American authors.[27]

Regardless of interpretation of the evidence for preventing ARF, it may still be worth identifying those with a GAS infection as these patients derive greater symptomatic benefit from antibiotic treatment. Clinical scoring systems clearly have the greatest potential utility, as they are generally simple and cheap. The most widely used scoring system, developed by Centor and colleagues, awards one point for each of the following: temperature >38°C, no cough, tender anterior cervical adenopathy, and tonsillar swelling or exudate.[28] This system was modified by McIsaac et al to increase its performance by adding one point for those aged 3–14 years and subtracting one point for those aged 45 years or more.[29] When combined with use of throat culture for those with mid-range scores, this clinical score achieved a sensitivity of 83–85% and a specificity of 92–94%.[30] However, many have argued that it is not sufficiently valid to be used on its own for detecting GAS. In a recent study in children, the modified Centor scoring system was found to produce an area under the receiver operating curve (ROC) of only 0.65–0.7.[26] This is clearly not adequate when detection of GAS is critical. However, it may have some value for identifying those who are at a greater likelihood of benefiting from antibiotic treatment.

RADTs are a potentially useful tool. However, one of the challenges in using both RADTs and throat swab culture is that up to 20% of the healthy population carries GAS in their throat. As asymptomatic carriers will also get viral throat infections, the presence of GAS does not confirm active infection. That being said, using a RADT in patients with McIsaac's modification of the Centor score >2 gives a sensitivity of 78% and a specificity of 97% for detecting GAS.[26] These tests are likely to play an increasing role, but before widespread uptake into everyday care, further research is needed that evaluates their impact on antibiotic use, symptoms and their cost-effectiveness.

Throat culture is the most accurate way of detecting the presence of GAS, but its use involves cost of transporting the specimen, plating, culture and the communication of results – both to the practitioner and then ultimately to the patient. Furthermore, its use may involve a delay of treatment (or unnecessary initiation of treatment in many patients), which may negate the benefit of identifying the organism. If accuracy of identification is the main aim, as those in the ARF prevention camp contend it is, then it is hard to argue for anything but throat culture. However, if one believes that reducing antibiotic use is not likely to result in a resurgence of ARF, then throat culture may be less of an important clinical tool.

 ANTIBIOTIC CHOICE

When a decision to prescribe antibiotics is made, an agent active against GAS should be selected. In most countries penicillin V continues to be the therapy of first choice, and erythromycin for those allergic to penicillin.

DIPTHERIA

Antibiotics are an essential but adjunctive part of treatment, and do not obviate the need for antitoxin.

Corynebacterium diphtheriae is moderately susceptible to penicillin and also susceptible to amoxicillin, erythromycin and clindamycin. Erythromycin remains active, apart from a few strains of the *mitis* biotype, and is preferred for the treatment of the index case as well as household contacts or known carriers.[31]

ACUTE EPIGLOTTITIS

This rapidly progressive and life-threatening illness is encountered mainly in children, but is increasingly being recognized in adults. It is caused by infections with *Haemophilus influenzae* type b, which may often be cultured from the blood as well as from the local lesion. The favorable impact of conjugate vaccines on *H. influenzae* meningitis has also fortunately reduced the incidence of acute epiglottitis in childhood. Treatment is as much concerned with maintaining the airway as with control of the infection. Ampicillin has been widely used in the past but the relative rarity of the condition does not allow objective judgment of its continued benefit. Ampicillin resistance is now widespread in *H. influenzae*, and a cephalosporin, such as cefotaxime or ceftriaxone, is now preferred on account of β-lactamase stability, high potency and excellent safety records.

Acute croup (laryngotracheobronchitis) is largely viral in etiology (RSV, parainfluenza), but may also occasionally be bacterial in nature (*M. pneumoniae*). The differential diagnosis of croup includes acute epiglottitis, diphtheria, and many non-infectious conditions. Pseudomembranous croup is a severe bacterial tracheitis.[32] *Staphylococcus aureus* is most commonly involved, although sometimes with other organisms,[33] and treatment should include a β-lactamase-resistant penicillin.

ACUTE SINUSITIS

Acute sinusitis is an acute inflammation of the paranasal air spaces that is usually the result of a viral or bacterial infection. In the USA, sinusitis affects one in seven adults and is the fifth most common reason for antibiotic prescription.[34] As most cases of sinusitis are caused by viral infections,[35] the benefit from antibiotic treatment for most of these infections is marginal. However, antibiotics continue to be widely used; in the USA, 96% of pediatricians report treating sinusitis with antibiotics 'always' or 'frequently'.[36]

ANTIBIOTIC TREATMENT

The effectiveness of antibiotics for acute sinusitis has been assessed in three recent systematic reviews and one meta-analysis of individual patient data.[37–40] All of these reviews found overall benefit from antibiotic treatment. However, the benefits are small, and therefore of questionable clinical relevance, and the rate of spontaneous improvement is high. Both effect size and rate of spontaneous resolution depend on the inclusion criteria of the studies selected. Those using clinical criteria had a lower effect size (NNT of 15 for one additional cure at 8–15 days in the meta-analysis of individual patient data) and higher rate of spontaneous improvement (80%), while those that included studies using radiological or microbiological definitions of sinusitis had slightly larger effect sizes and a slightly lower rate of spontaneous resolution (68%).

Patients diagnosed with 'acute sinusitis' clearly have a widely differing clinical course and will vary in their response to antibiotic treatment. As such, diagnostic criteria are important. The vast majority of patients are managed in primary care and therefore the use of microbiological culture or imaging studies is not feasible and clinical criteria must be used. A systematic review examining the predictive value of signs and symptoms found that purulent nasal discharge as a symptom, purulent nasal discharge as a sign, pain in teeth, pain on bending forward, and two phases to illness, were predictive in one or more studies.[41] However, they found that the studies used different 'gold standards' and their results were inconsistent. Bacterial sinusitis appears to be unlikely in those who have had symptoms for less than 7 days, and, as such, duration of illness of a week or more is a common diagnostic criterion in guidelines.[42] However, the most recent meta-analysis found that, although those with a longer prior duration of illness were more likely to have a prolonged course, those who had been unwell for a week or more were no more likely to benefit from antibiotic treatment.[39] The only factor found to predict a greater response to antibiotics in this study was purulent discharge seen in the pharynx (NNT = 8 in this group). In a secondary analysis of data from 300 participants feeling generally unwell and feeling unable to work were predictive of prolonged duration of sinusitis. No factors predicted response to antibiotics.[43]

So where does this leave clinicians faced with a patient with sinusitis-like symptoms? No systematic review has demonstrated a significant reduction in complications from antibiotic treatment and symptomatic improvement for most patients is modest. Conversely, those who receive antibiotics are more likely to experience adverse effects.[38] Therefore, antibiotic therapy should not be given to most people with suspected acute sinusitis. However, it is still not clear whether certain subgroups of patients will benefit from antibiotic treatment. Patients with signs of serious illness are intuitively more likely to benefit from treatment, and are usually excluded or do not agree to be randomized into placebo-controlled studies. Treatment should therefore not be withheld in this group. Another factor that may be helpful in identifying those more likely to benefit, and importantly in reducing prescribing for the majority, is the use of point of care testing. Use of a C-reactive protein point of care test has been shown to be associated with reduced antibiotic prescribing for acute sinusitis in an observational study,[44] but its use for sinusitis has not yet been evaluated in a trial. Until further improvements in diagnostics become available it seems sensible to broadly follow the advice of major guidelines and consider antibiotic treatment primarily in those with purulent nasal secretions (and particularly those with purulent secretions seen in the pharynx) or who have a 'double worsening', who have been unwell for 10 days or more and have moderate to severe symptoms.[40,42]

For those in whom antibiotic therapy is initiated, there is no evidence of superiority for one agent over another. Choices should provide coverage for the most common causative organisms, *Streptococcus pneumoniae*, *H. influenzae* and *Moraxella catarrhalis*. Most guidelines recommend amoxicillin as first-line therapy.[40,45] There is also no clear evidence over optimal duration of therapy. Most trials have used relatively long courses (10 days) and so this duration has therefore been adopted by many guidelines. However, a recent meta-analysis of data from 12 randomized controlled trials found no significant benefit from longer courses compared with shorter courses (3–7 days). This may simply reflect the lack of benefit from treatment for most patients and may not be representative of the optimal duration for selected patients with more severe symptoms.

OTHER THERAPIES

All patients with sinusitis should be given advice about analgesics. Intranasal corticosteroids appear to offer marginal benefit,[46] with those having milder symptoms possibly benefiting more.[47] No other therapies have been shown to have clear benefits, although topical saline appears to have some beneficial effects for those with more chronic symptoms.[48]

ACUTE OTITIS MEDIA

Acute otitis media (AOM) is one of the most common disorders of childhood – by the age of 3 years 80% of children have had at least one episode.[49] Nearly 40% of older children eventually have six or more episodes.[50] AOM is also the most common reason for antibiotic prescription for children, accounting for 45–53% of antibiotics prescribed for children in one US study.[51]

The most common bacterial pathogens implicated in causing AOM are *Str. pneumoniae*, non-encapsulated *H. influenzae*, *Mor. catarrhalis* and group A streptococcus.[52] However, viral respiratory pathogens can be isolated from up to 75% of children with AOM and can be detected in the middle ear fluid of 48%.[53]

Risk factors for AOM are: use of a pacifier, attendance in a day-care centre, not being breastfed, presence of siblings, passive smoking, craniofacial abnormalities and presence of adenoids.[54]

DIAGNOSIS

Diagnosis of AOM on clinical grounds is not accurate.[55,56] By definition, a middle ear effusion (MEE) is a prerequisite to the diagnosis, and most guidelines recommend using evidence of an MEE and evidence of inflammation in the middle ear to make the diagnosis.[57] An MEE is not easy to assess using simple otoscopy, but can be improved through the use of pneumatic otoscopy, which has a high sensitivity (94%) and specificity (80%) in diagnosing MEE.[50] Although this technique requires some training, it is simple and cheap and has the potential to improve diagnostic accuracy in community settings. Tympanometry is another method for diagnosing MEE that is simple and objective. It has a similar sensitivity to pneumatic otoscopy, but a slightly lower specificity.[50]

EFFECTIVENESS OF ANTIBIOTIC TREATMENT

Most children (80%) with AOM spontaneously recover within a week.[58] The most recent systematic review from the Cochrane Collaboration found that antibiotics had no overall effect on pain at 24 h, but a slight reduction in pain at 2–7 days, with an NNT of 15.[58] A subsequent meta-analysis

of individual patient data from 1643 children found that the subgroups most likely to benefit were children under 2 years of age with bilateral otitis media (NNT = 4) and those with otorrhea (NNT = 3).[59]

PREVENTING MASTOIDITIS

Treating AOM with antibiotics may prevent serious complications such as mastoiditis. However, a recent retrospective cohort study from the UK has called this into question. The records of over 2.5 million children were examined, identifying 854 cases of mastoiditits.[60] Most (two-thirds) had not seen their general practitioner prior to the development of the mastoiditis, and therefore could not have benefited from antibiotic treatment. There was a reduction in the risk of developing mastoiditis following AOM in those treated with antibiotics, but the number needed to treat was impractically large (NNT = 4831). The costs of increased microbial resistance from widespread antibiotic use may outweigh any symptomatic benefits. Furthermore, antibiotic prescribing results in increased re-consultations.[61,62]

OTHER TREATMENTS

A systematic review examined decongestants and antihistamines for AOM and found a small reduction in persistent AOM in those who took both decongestants and antihistamines. There were no benefits in terms of early cure rates, symptom resolution, prevention of surgery or other complications. There was also a large increase in side effects from both interventions and the authors concluded that the marginal benefits were outweighed by these adverse effects.[63]

REDUCING ANTIBIOTIC USE

We have outlined the evidence supporting reduced antibiotic prescribing for most upper respiratory tract infections. However, reducing antibiotic use is not always easy to achieve. One of the main approaches is to try to improve diagnostic accuracy. Clinical diagnostic criteria and clinical prediction rules have already been mentioned, and their use can make a significant contribution to improving management. Near-patient tests are likely to play an increasing role. A near-patient C-reactive protein test is already widely used in Scandinavian countries, and use of this test has been shown to reduce antibiotic prescribing for lower respiratory tract infections safely.[64]

Interventions aimed at changing clinician behavior tend to be more effective if they are interactive rather than didactic.[65] From behavior-change theories we also know that they are more likely to be effective if they addresses the 'why' of change (i.e. the importance of change, outcome expectations and beliefs about consequences) as well as the 'how' (i.e. confidence in making changes, self-efficacy and beliefs

about control).[66] New approaches that address these issues using blended learning (combination of online and face-to-face learning) are being developed.[67]

Education of patients through mass-media campaigns achieves important effects.[65,68] Parental education at the time of the consultation has been shown to reduce antibiotic use and consulting for AOM.[69,70] Training clinicians to provide parents with an 'interactive' booklet on respiratory tract infections reduces antibiotic prescribing for a range of such infections.[71] Multifaceted interventions that combine professional and patient education have consistently been shown to have some (generally modest) effect on prescribing.[65,68,72–75]

Finally, the use of a delayed antibiotic prescribing approach has been shown to safely reduce prescribing for sore throat,[76] otitis media,[77,78] common cold[79] and uncomplicated cough,[80] and has been promoted as a useful technique for managing respiratory tract infections in primary care by the UK National Institute for Health and Clinical Excellence (NICE) guidelines.[81,82]

 References

1. Monto AS. Epidemiology of viral respiratory infections. *Am J Med.* 2002;112(suppl 6A):4S–12S.
2. McCormick A, Fleming D, Charlton J. Morbidity statistics from general practice. *Fourth National Study 1991–1992.* London: HMSO; 1995.
3. Fleming DM, Cross KW, Barley MA. Recent changes in the prevalence of diseases presenting for health care. [See comment.]. *Br J Gen Pract.* 2005;55(517):589–595.
4. Ashworth M, Charlton J, Ballard K, Latinovic R, Gulliford M. Variations in antibiotic prescribing and consultation rates for acute respiratory infection in UK general practices 1995–2000. *Br J Gen Pract.* 2005;55(517):603–608.
5. McIsaac WJ, Butler CC. Does clinical error contribute to unnecessary antibiotic use? *Med Decis Making.* 2000;20(1):33–38.
6. Butler CC, Rollnick S, Pill R, Maggs-Rapport F, Stott N. Understanding the culture of prescribing: qualitative study of general practitioners' and patients' perceptions of antibiotics for sore throats. [See comment.] *Br Med J.* 1998;317(7159):637–642.
7. Simpson SA, Wood F, Butler CC. General practitioners' perceptions of antimicrobial resistance: a qualitative study. *J Antimicrob Chemother.* 2007;59(2):292–296.
8. Wood F, Simpson S, Butler CC. Socially responsible antibiotic choices in primary care: a qualitative study of GPs' decisions to prescribe broad-spectrum and fluoroquinolone antibiotics. *Fam Pract.* 2007;24(5):427–434.
9. Hamm RM, Hicks RJ, Bemben DA. Antibiotics and respiratory infections: are patients more satisfied when expectations are met? *J Fam Pract.* 1996;43(1):56–62.
10. Ashworth M, Charlton J, Ballard K, Latinovic R, Gulliford M. Variations in antibiotic prescribing and consultation rates for acute respiratory infection in UK general practices 1995–2000. *Br J Gen Pract.* 2005;55:603–608.
11. Shapiro E. Injudicious antibiotic use: an unforeseen consequence of the emphasis on patient satisfaction? *Clin Ther.* 2002;24(1):197–204.
12. Little P, Gould C, Williamson I, Warner G, Gantley M, Kinmonth AL. Reattendance and complications in a randomised trial of prescribing strategies for sore throat: the medicalising effect of prescribing antibiotics. [See comment.]. *Br Med J.* 1997;315(7104):350–352.
13. Butler CC, Hillier S, Roberts Z, Dunstan F, Howard A, Palmer S. Antibiotic-resistant infections in primary care are symptomatic for longer and increase workload: outcomes for patients with *E. coli* UTIs. *Br J Gen Pract.* 2006;56(530):686–692.
14. Goossens H, Ferech M, Vander Stichele R, Elseviers M. Group EP. Outpatient antibiotic use in Europe and association with resistance: a cross-national database study. [See comment.] *Lancet.* 2005;365(9459):579–587.

15. Arroll B, Kenealy T. Antibiotics for the common cold and acute purulent rhinitis. *Cochrane Database Syst Rev.* 2005;3: CD000247.

16. Morris P, Leach A. Antibiotics for persistent nasal discharge (rhinosinusitis) in children. *Cochrane Database Syst Rev.* 2002;(4) CD001094. [Update in: Cochrane Database of Systematic Reviews 2008;(2):CD001094; Cochrane Database of Systematic Reviews 2007;(3):CD001094].

17. Taverner D, Latte J. Nasal decongestants for the common cold. *Cochrane Database Syst Rev.* 2004;(3): CD001953. [Update in: Cochrane Database of Systematic Reviews 2007(1):CD001953].

18. De Sutter AI, Lemiengre M, Campbell H, Mackinnon HF. Antihistamines for the common cold. *Cochrane Database Syst Rev.* 2003;(3): CD001267.

19. Singh M. Heated, humidified air for the common cold. *Cochrane Database Syst Rev.* 2004;(2): CD001728. [Update in: Cochrane Database of Systematic Reviews 2006;3:CD001728.].

20. Hemila H, Douglas RM, Chalker E, Treacy B. Vitamin C for preventing and treating the common cold. *Cochrane Database Syst Rev.* 2004;(4): CD000980. [Update in: Cochrane Database of Systematic Reviews 2007(3):CD000980.].

21. Del Mar C, Glasziou Paul P, Spinks A. Antibiotics for sore throat. *Cochrane Database Syst Rev.* 2006;(4): CD000023.

22. Robertson KA, Volmink JA, Mayosi BM. Antibiotics for the primary prevention of acute rheumatic fever: a meta-analysis. *BMC Cardiovasc Disord.* 2005;5(1):11.

23. Petersen I, Johnson AM, Islam A, Duckworth G, Livermore DM, Hayward AC. Protective effect of antibiotics against serious complications of common respiratory tract infections: retrospective cohort study with the UK General Practice Research Database. *Br Med J.* 2007;335(7627):982.

24. Bennike T, Brochner-Mortensen K, Kjaer E, Skadhauge K, Trolle E. Penicillin therapy in acute tonsillitis, phlegmonous tonsillitis and ulcerative tonsillitis. *Acta Med Scand.* 1951;139(4):253–274.

25. Dunn N, Lane D, Everitt H, Little P. Use of antibiotics for sore throat and incidence of quinsy. *Br J Gen Pract.* 2007;57(534):45–49.

26. Tanz RR, Gerber MA, Kabat W, Rippe J, Seshadri R, Shulman ST. Performance of a rapid antigen-detection test and throat culture in community pediatric offices: implications for management of pharyngitis. *Pediatrics.* 2009;123(2):437–444.

27. Matthys J, De Meyere M, van Driel ML, De Sutter A. Differences among international pharyngitis guidelines: not just academic. *Ann Fam Med.* 2007;5(5):436–443.

28. Centor RM, Witherspoon JM, Dalton HP, Brody CE, Link K. The diagnosis of strep throat in adults in the emergency room. *Med Decis Making.* 1981;1(3):239–246.

29. McIsaac WJ, White D, Tannenbaum D, Low DE. A clinical score to reduce unnecessary antibiotic use in patients with sore throat. *Can Med Assoc J.* 1998;158(1):75–83.

30. McIsaac WJ, Goel V, To T, Low DE. The validity of a sore throat score in family practice. *Can Med Assoc J.* 2000;163(7):811–815.

31. Wilson AP. Treatment of infection caused by toxigenic and non-toxigenic strains of *Corynebacterium diphtheriae. J Antimicrob Chemother.* 1995;35(6):717–720.

32. Donnelly B, McMillan J, Weiner L. Bacterial tracheitis: report of eight new cases and review. *Rev Infect Dis.* 1990;12(5):729–735.

33. Henry R, Mellis C, Benjamin B. Pseudomembranous croup. *Arch Dis Child.* 1983;58(3):180–183.

34. Rosenfeld RM, Andes D, Bhattacharyya N, et al. Clinical practice guideline: adult sinusitis. *Otolaryngol Head Neck Surg.* 2007;137(suppl 3):S1–S31.

35. Hickner JM, Bartlett JG, Besser RE, Gonzales R, Hoffman JR, Sande MA. Principles of appropriate antibiotic use for acute rhinosinusitis in adults: background. *Ann Intern Med.* 2001;134(6):498–505.

36. McQuillan L, Crane LA, Kempe A. Diagnosis and management of acute sinusitis by pediatricians. *Pediatrics.* 2009;123(2):e193–e198.

37. Ahovuo-Saloranta A, Borisenko OV, Kovanen N, et al. Antibiotics for acute maxillary sinusitis. *Cochrane Database Syst Rev.* 2008;2: CD000243.

38. Falagas ME, Giannopoulou KP, Vardakas KZ, Dimopoulos G, Karageorgopoulos DE. Comparison of antibiotics with placebo for treatment of acute sinusitis: a meta-analysis of randomised controlled trials. *Lancet Infect Dis.* 2008;8(9):543–552.

39. Young J, De Sutter A, Merenstein D, van Essen GA, Kaiser L, Varonen H, et al. Antibiotics for adults with clinically diagnosed acute rhinosinusitis: a meta-analysis of individual patient data. [See comment.] *Lancet.* 2008;371(9616):908–914.

40. Rosenfeld RM, Singer M, Jones S. Systematic review of antimicrobial therapy in patients with acute rhinosinusitis. *Otolaryngol Head Neck Surg.* 2007;137(suppl 3):S32–S45.

41. Lindbaek M, Hjortdahl P. The clinical diagnosis of acute purulent sinusitis in general practice – a review. *Br J Gen Pract.* 2002;52(479):491–495.

42. Snow V, Mottur-Pilson C, Hickner JM. American Academy of Family Practitioners, American College of Physicians, American Society of Internal Medicine, Centers for Disease Control, Infectious Diseases Society of America. Principles of appropriate antibiotic use for acute sinusitis in adults. *Ann Intern Med.* 2001;134(6):495–497.

43. De Sutter A, Lemiengre M, Van Maele G, et al. Predicting prognosis and effect of antibiotic treatment in rhinosinusitis. *Ann Fam Med.* 2006;4(6):486–493.

44. Bjerrum L, Gahrn-Hansen B, Munck AP. C-reactive protein measurement in general practice may lead to lower antibiotic prescribing for sinusitis. *Br J Gen Pract.* 2004;54(506):659–662.

45. Clinical Knowledge Summaries. Sinusitis management, 2009: Online. Available at http://www.patient.co.uk/showdoc/50000019.

46. Zalmanovici A, Yaphe J. Steroids for acute sinusitis. *Cochrane Database Syst Rev.* 2007;(2) CD005149.

47. Williamson IG, Rumsby K, Benge S, et al. Antibiotics and topical nasal steroid for treatment of acute maxillary sinusitis: a randomized controlled trial. [See comment.] *J Am Med Assoc.* 2007;298(21):2487–2496.

48. Harvey R, Hannan SA, Badia L, Scadding G. Nasal saline irrigations for the symptoms of chronic rhinosinusitis. *Cochrane Database Syst Rev.* 2007;3: CD006394.

49. Teele DW, Klein JO, Rosner B. Epidemiology of otitis media during the first seven years of life in children in greater Boston: a prospective, cohort study. [See comment.]. *J Infect Dis.* 1989;160(1):83–94.

50. Rovers MM, Schilder AG, Zielhuis GA, Rosenfeld RM. *Otitis media Lancet.* 2004;363(9407):465–473.

51. Halasa NB, Griffin MR, Zhu Y, Edwards KM. Differences in antibiotic prescribing patterns for children younger than five years in the three major outpatient settings. *J Pediatr.* 2004;144(2):200–205 [Erratum in: Journal of Pediatrics 2004 Jun;144(6):838.].

52. Vergison A. Microbiology of otitis media: a moving target. *Vaccine.* 2008;26(suppl 7):G5–G10.

53. Pitkaranta A, Virolainen A, Jero J, Arruda E, Hayden FG. Detection of rhinovirus, respiratory syncytial virus, and coronavirus infections in acute otitis media by reverse transcriptase polymerase chain reaction. [See comment.] *Pediatrics.* 1998;102(2 Pt 1):291–295.

54. Lubianca Neto JF, Hemb L, Silva DB. Systematic literature review of modifiable risk factors for recurrent acute otitis media in childhood. *J Pediatr (Rio J).* 2006;82(2):87–96.

55. Asher E, Leibovitz E, Press J, Greenberg D, Bilenko N, Reuveni H. Accuracy of acute otitis media diagnosis in community and hospital settings. *Acta Paediatr.* 2005;94(4):423–428.

56. Legros JM, Hitoto H, Garnier F, Dagorne C, Parot-Schinkel E, Fanello S. Clinical qualitative evaluation of the diagnosis of acute otitis media in general practice. *Int J Pediatr Otorhinolaryngol.* 2008;72(1):23–30.

57. American Academy of Pediatrics Subcommittee on Management of Acute Otitis Media. Diagnosis and management of acute otitis media. *Pediatrics.* 2004;113(5):1451–1465.

58. Glasziou PP, Del Mar C, Sanders S, Hayem M. Antibiotics for acute otitis media in children. *Cochrane Database Syst Rev.* 2004;(1): CD000219.

59. Rovers MM, Glasziou P, Appelman CL, et al. Antibiotics for acute otitis media: a meta-analysis with individual patient data. *Lancet.* 2006;368(9545):1429–1435.

60. Thompson PL, Gilbert RE, Long PF, Saxena S, Sharland M, Wong ICK. Effect of antibiotics for otitis media on mastoiditis in children: a retrospective cohort study using the United Kingdom General Practice Research Database. *Pediatrics.* 2009;123(2):424–430.

61. Li J, De A, Ketchum K, Fagnan LJ, Haxby DG, Thomas A. Antimicrobial prescribing for upper respiratory infections and its effect on return visits. *Fam Med.* 2009;41(3):182–187.

62. Little P, Gould C, Williamson I, Warner G, Gantley M, Kinmonth AL. Reattendance and complications in a randomised trial of prescribing strategies for sore throat: the medicalising effect of prescribing antibiotics. [See comment.]. *Br Med J.* 1997;315(7104):350–352.

63. Coleman C, Moore M. Decongestants and antihistamines for acute otitis media in children. *Cochrane Database Syst Rev.* 2008;3: CD001727.

64. Cals JW, Butler CC, Hopstaken RM, Hood K, Dinant GJ. Effect of point of care testing for C reactive protein and training in communication skills on

antibiotic use in lower respiratory tract infections: cluster randomised trial. *Br Med J.* 2009;338:b1374.

65. Arnold SR, Straus SE. Interventions to improve antibiotic prescribing practices in ambulatory care. *Cochrane Database Syst Rev.* 2005;(4) CD003539.

66. Cosby JL, Francis N, Butler CC. The role of evidence in the decline of antibiotic use for common respiratory infections in primary care. *Lancet Infect Dis.* 2007;7(11):749–756.

67. Simpson SA, Butler CC, Hood K, et al. Stemming the tide of antibiotic resistance (STAR): a protocol for a trial of a complex intervention addressing the 'why' and 'how' of appropriate antibiotic prescribing in general practice. *BMC Fam Pract.* 2009;10:20.

68. Wutzke SE, Artist MA, Kehoe LA, Fletcher M, Mackson JM, Weekes LM. Evaluation of a national programme to reduce inappropriate use of antibiotics for upper respiratory tract infections: effects on consumer awareness, beliefs, attitudes and behaviour in Australia. *Health Promot Int.* 2007;22(1):53–64.

69. Pshetizky Y, Naimer S, Shvartzman P. Acute otitis media – a brief explanation to parents and antibiotic use. *Fam Pract.* 2003;20(4):417–419.

70. McWilliams DB, Jacobson RM, Van Houten HK, Naessens JM, Ytterberg KL. A program of anticipatory guidance for the prevention of emergency department visits for ear pain. [See comment.] *Arch Pediatr Adolesc Med.* 2008;162(2):151–156.

71. Francis N, Butler C, Hood K, Simpson S, Wood F, Nuttall J. Use of an interactive booklet on childhood respiratory tract infections in primary care consultations: a cluster randomised controlled trial. *Br Med J.* 2009;339:b2885.

72. Hickman DE, Stebbins MR, Hanak JR, Guglielmo BJ. Pharmacy-based intervention to reduce antibiotic use for acute bronchitis. *Ann Pharmacother.* 2003;37(2):187–191.

73. Welschen I, Kuyvenhoven MM, Hoes AW, Verheij TJ. Effectiveness of a multiple intervention to reduce antibiotic prescribing for respiratory tract symptoms in primary care: randomised controlled trial. *Br Med J.* 2004;329(7463):431.

74. Rubin MA, Bateman K, Alder S, Donnelly S, Stoddard GJ, Samore MH. A multifaceted intervention to improve antimicrobial prescribing for upper respiratory tract infections in a small rural community. *Clin Infect Dis.* 2005;40(4):546–553.

75. Gonzales R, Corbett KK, Leeman-Castillo BA, et al. The 'Minimizing Antibiotic Resistance in Colorado' project: impact of patient education in improving antibiotic use in private office practices. *Health Serv Res.* 2005;40(1):101–116.

76. Little P, Williamson I, Warner G, Gould C, Gantley M, Kinmonth AL. Open randomised trial of prescribing strategies in managing sore throat. *Br Med J.* 1997;314(7082):722–727.

77. Little P, Gould C, Williamson I, Moore M, Warner G, Dunleavey J. Pragmatic randomised controlled trial of two prescribing strategies for childhood acute otitis media. *Br Med J.* 2001;322(7282):336–342.

78. Spiro DM, Tay KY, Arnold DH, Dziura JD, Baker MD, Shapiro ED. Wait-and-see prescription for the treatment of acute otitis media: a randomized controlled trial. [See comment.] *J Am Med Assoc.* 2006;296(10):1235–1241.

79. Arroll B, Kenealy T, Kerse N. Do delayed prescriptions reduce the use of antibiotics for the common cold? A single-blind controlled trial. [See comment.] *J Fam Pract.* 2002;51(4):324–328.

80. Dowell J, Pitkethly M, Bain J, Martin S. A randomised controlled trial of delayed antibiotic prescribing as a strategy for managing uncomplicated respiratory tract infection in primary care. *Br J Gen Pract.* 2001;51(464):200–205.

81. Tan T, Little P, Stokes T. on behalf of the Guideline Development Group. Antibiotic prescribing for self limiting respiratory tract infections in primary care: summary of NICE guidance. *Br Med J.* 2008;337:a437.

82. Butler CC, Francis N. Commentary: Controversies in NICE guidance on antibiotic prescribing for self limiting respiratory tract infections in primary care. *Br Med J.* 2008;337:a656.

45 Infections of the lower respiratory tract

Lionel A. Mandell and Robert C. Read

Respiratory infections are usually divided into those involving the upper and those involving the lower respiratory tract. The former typically include infections of the sinuses, the tonsillopharyngeal area and the middle ear. Lower respiratory tract infections include acute bronchitis, acute exacerbations of chronic bronchitis and pneumonia. Pneumonia is further subdivided into community-acquired, healthcare-associated and hospital-acquired infections.

Acute lower respiratory tract infections are a significant cause of morbidity and mortality worldwide and most occur in developing countries where poverty and inadequate medical care contribute to the high mortality rates. Pneumonia continues to be the most common cause of death from infectious diseases worldwide. Although our understanding of the various etiological agents and the pathogenic mechanisms involved in various respiratory infections has increased, our ability to diagnose accurately the causative agent(s) has not kept pace. This means that often the physician initiates treatment on an empirical basis and in far too many situations antibiotics are used when the infection is viral in nature.

ACUTE BRONCHITIS

Lower respiratory tract infections are typically divided into either bronchitis or pneumonia. These can also be thought of as infections involving the airways and the pulmonary parenchyma, respectively. Acute bronchitis is very common and can be viewed as one end of a continuum that extends from bronchitis to pneumonia. While it is generally not a particularly serious infection, it still has a considerable economic impact because of the frequency of physician visits and the fact that despite the lack of any compelling evidence supporting antimicrobial therapy, physicians who diagnose acute bronchitis prescribe antibiotics for 66% of such patients.[1]

In the USA it is estimated that acute bronchitis results in approximately 12 000 000 visits to physicians per year at a cost of $200–300 million.[2]

ETIOLOGY AND EPIDEMIOLOGY

The most common infectious agents are viruses, and typically respiratory viruses such as rhinovirus, corona virus, adenovirus and influenza virus are implicated. Other viral agents include respiratory syncytial virus (RSV), parainfluenza virus, measles virus and herpes simplex virus.[3–5]

While the term 'atypical respiratory pathogens' can include a large and diverse number of etiological agents, by convention they usually refer to *Mycoplasma pneumoniae*, *Chlamydophila pneumoniae* and *Legionella* species. *Mycoplasma* and *Ch. pneumoniae* and the etiological agent of whooping cough, *Bordetella pertussis*, are the most commonly encountered non-viral causes of acute bronchitis.[6]

Like many other respiratory infections, acute bronchitis is most common during the winter months. The mean attack rate in developed countries is 87 cases per 100 000 persons per week, reaching a peak of 150 cases per 100 000 during the winter season.[7]

PATHOGENESIS

In cases of acute bronchitis the disease process is limited to the mucous membrane lining the tracheobronchial tree. The mucous membrane becomes edematous and hyperemic and increased bronchial secretion is typically seen. Epithelial injury is usually mild to moderate but in cases of influenza virus infection there may be fairly significant epithelial damage.

Studies of pulmonary function during attacks of acute bronchitis have demonstrated abnormal findings in both airway resistance and reactivity. Such results are in keeping with the association that has been described between an increased incidence of mild asthma and patients with a history of recurrent episodes of acute bronchitis.[8]

The increased airway reactivity and resistance may manifest themselves clinically as a persistent cough lasting up to several weeks following the initial infection.

CLINICAL MANIFESTATIONS

The predominant symptom is cough. This may last up to several weeks and, depending upon the etiological agent, may be non-productive or productive of either mucoid or purulent sputum. In some cases the sputum may be mucoid initially, but if secondary bacterial infection results it may become purulent. Patients may also experience a burning retrosternal sensation on inspiration.

Physical examination may reveal the presence of rhonchi or coarse rales but bronchial breath sounds should not be heard.

The patient may be febrile but usually does not appear particularly ill. The exceptions to this are herpes simplex infection or bronchitis complicating influenza, which can produce marked malaise.

DIAGNOSIS

The diagnosis of acute bronchitis in an otherwise well adult is usually obvious from the clinical features. If there is any question of pneumonia, a chest radiograph will exclude the presence of a pulmonary infiltrate.

In general, it is not worth obtaining blood samples for serology or sputum for Gram stain and culture.

TREATMENT

Acute bronchitis is a common condition and most patients are managed at home. The treatment of acute bronchitis can be symptomatic or specific. Symptomatic treatment relies primarily upon maintenance of adequate hydration and cough suppression in those unable to sleep. If bronchospasm is a problem, then inhaled β_2-adrenergic bronchodilators may be used. At present there is no evidence to support the routine use of oral or inhaled steroids. Smokers should be encouraged to stop.

In patients with underlying cardiopulmonary disease, an episode of acute bronchitis may precipitate cardiac failure and the patient may need to be admitted to hospital for appropriate ventilatory and cardiac support.

Antimicrobial chemotherapy is generally not recommended: a number of placebo-controlled trials have evaluated the role of antibiotics in acute bronchitis and there is minimal benefit at best. Antibiotics might be considered in patients with persistent, prolonged and worsening symptoms.

In such situations, doxycycline, or a macrolide (erythromycin, azithromycin or clarithromycin) should be considered.

ACUTE EXACERBATION OF CHRONIC BRONCHITIS

Chronic bronchitis is defined as the presence of a productive cough for at least 3 months of the year for 2 consecutive years. Chronic bronchitis itself constitutes a common component of chronic obstructive pulmonary disease (COPD), a clinical entity characterized by reduced expiratory air flow that is relatively stable over several months of observation. The prognosis for COPD correlates best with the forced expiratory volume in one second (FEV_1), and when this falls below 50% of predicted value the prognosis worsens.

Most physicians do not differentiate among COPD, acute bronchitis and acute exacerbation of chronic bronchitis (AECB). In fact, even pneumonia is often simply included as part of the designation 'lower respiratory tract infections'. It is difficult to obtain accurate data on the exact economic impact of such entities, although COPD has been estimated to afflict one-fifth of the population of the USA.[9] In the UK around 30 million working days are lost every year because of bronchitis, and the disease accounts for approximately 5% of deaths annually.[10]

ETIOLOGY AND EPIDEMIOLOGY

Chronic bronchitis is the result of a variety of insults to the lung over time. These include predominantly cigarette smoke, infection, and environmental pollutants and irritants. Once chronic bronchitis is established, the episodic worsening referred to as acute exacerbations of chronic bronchitis can be triggered by similar causes. For the purposes of this chapter, however, we will focus on infectious triggers.

Viruses account for up to 50% of acute exacerbations of chronic bronchitis and a variety of agents have been implicated: RSV, rhinovirus, influenza virus and parainfluenza virus. The remaining 50% of acute exacerbations are bacterial in nature, with the most common pathogens being *Haemophilus influenzae*, *Streptococcus pneumoniae* and *Moraxella catarrhalis*. The role of atypical pathogens such as *M. pneumoniae* and *Ch. pneumoniae* is unclear but it is thought that they may account for a small percentage of infections.

Infection results in the release of inflammatory mediators and further impairment of mucociliary clearance. This in turn alters the local milieu, making it easier for pathogens to further colonize the airways. Progressive airway damage is thought to occur as the result of injury caused either by the pathogens themselves or by the host response to the various infective agents.

CLINICAL MANIFESTATIONS

The clinical manifestations of patients with AECB represent a common pathway of underlying pulmonary disease in the form of chronic bronchitis or emphysema and the acute exacerbation triggered by infection or environmental pollutants. Patients may present with any or all of the following: increase in dyspnea, sputum volume or sputum purulence. In 1987, Anthonisen and colleagues demonstrated that patients with at least two of these three findings experienced better clinical outcomes when treated with antibiotics than with placebo.[11]

The Anthonisen classification refers to patients with one of these findings as type 3, two of the findings as type 2 and three of the findings as type 1. Other symptoms that may be noted during an exacerbation include wheezing, elevated temperature and a feeling of malaise.

The duration of an exacerbation can vary from a few days to several weeks. On average, most patients experience approximately three exacerbations annually, although significant variation has been described.

DIAGNOSIS

The diagnosis of AECB is usually clinical. Patients with a known history of chronic bronchitis who suffer periodic flare-ups are usually well aware of the signs and symptoms heralding the onset of an exacerbation. Increasing dyspnea, sputum volume and purulence are the main clues that an exacerbation has occurred.

One of the difficulties in defining etiology is that many, if not most, individuals with chronic bronchitis normally have bacteria in their respiratory secretions. These bacteria colonize the airways but during an exacerbation are present in higher numbers. *H. influenzae*, *Str. pneumoniae* and *Mor. catarrhalis* are the predominant pathogens. However, among those with severe exacerbations requiring admission to an intensive care unit (ICU) and mechanical ventilation, these pathogens seem to be present less frequently and organisms such as *H. parainfluenzae* and *Pseudomonas aeruginosa* are more frequently found, and bacteria in this context are often resistant to antibiotics.[12,13]

In most patients treatment is begun empirically. In those with more severe underlying disease or in whom the exacerbations appear to be more serious, it may be worthwhile obtaining sputum samples for culture and susceptibility testing in order to rule out the presence of a resistant pathogen. Data are available suggesting that as the severity of the illness increases (as indicated by markers such as illness lasting longer than 10 years, more than four exacerbations per year, steroid therapy, recent antibiotics, and severe airway obstruction [FEV_1 <35% predicted]) the microbiology becomes more complex.[14,15]

On the basis of a clinical examination, it may be impossible to differentiate between an acute exacerbation of chronic bronchitis and pneumonia. In such cases, a chest radiograph is necessary.

TREATMENT

Anthonisen was the first to assess response to treatment based upon stratification of patients according to their symptoms.[11] A meta-analysis of nine randomized placebo-controlled trials of patients treated for AECB demonstrated a statistically significant improvement in outcomes in those treated with antibiotics.[16] The effect size favored antibiotics in seven of the nine studies.

Despite such data, however, it is clear that routine antibiotic treatment fails in 13–25% of exacerbations.[17] Such failures carry an economic burden because they require additional visits to physicians, additional treatment regimens and more days lost from work.

A number of risk factors have been defined for treatment failure. These include the presence of cardiopulmonary disease and increased frequency of pulmonary infections during the previous year (>4).[17] A subgroup of patients is at risk, not only of treatment failure but also of respiratory failure. Mortality rates in hospital inpatients of 10–30% have been described, typically in patients older than 65 years, those with co-morbid respiratory and extrapulmonary organ dysfunction, and those residing in hospital before transfer to the ICU.[18,19]

It has been suggested that stratification of patients according to risk factors will allow physicians to treat more appropriately. No single stratification scheme has been agreed upon but those that do exist attempt to rank patients according to increased risk factors for treatment failure and possibly admission to hospital. Three schema have been published to date: Lode – Germany (1991), Balter – Canada (1994), and Wilson – UK (1995).[20–22] Their recommendations are summarized in Table 45.1.

Patients with AECB should be considered as being possibly infected with a 'core' group of pathogens such as *H. influenzae*, *Str. pneumoniae* and *Mor. catarrhalis*; those who are more complicated (such as elderly patients, patients with more frequent exacerbations and those with reduced lung function) may be infected not only by the core pathogens but also by Gram-negative bacilli such as the Enterobacteriaceae and *Ps. aeruginosa* or possibly resistant core pathogens.

The advantage of such an approach lies in the fact that they identify patients at increased risk of failure so that treatment may be initiated with antibiotic regimens most likely to be effective against all of the potential etiological pathogens.

Table 45.1 Stratification and treatment of acute exacerbations of chronic obstructive pulmonary disease[20]

Category	Characteristics	Suggested treatment
Group 1	Postviral tracheobronchitis; previously healthy person	None
Group 2	Simple chronic bronchitis; young person; mild–moderate impairment of lung function (FEV_1 >50% predicted); fewer than 4 exacerbations/year	No treatment or β-lactam antibiotic
Group 3	'Chronic bronchitis plus risk factors' older person; FEV_1 50% predicted or FEV_1 50–60% predicted but concurrent medical illnesses; CHF, diabetes mellitus, chronic renal disease, chronic liver disease, more than 4 exacerbations/year	Fluoroquinolone, amoxicillin–clavulanic acid, group 3 or 4 cephalosporin,[a] azithromycin or clarithromycin
Group 4	'Chronic bronchial sepsis', bronchiectasis, chronic airway colonization	Tailor antimicrobial treatment to airway pathogens

[a]See Ch. 13 for classification of cephalosporins.
CHF, congestive heart failure; FEV_1, forced expiratory volume in 1 second.
From Lode H. Respiratory tract infections: when is antibiotic therapy indicated? **Clin Ther.** 1991;13:149–156.

A variety of adjunctive or supportive measures, including the use of bronchodilators, steroids (oral and/or inhaled) and oxygen therapy, may be necessary. Preventive measures such as cessation of smoking, annual influenza vaccination and administration of the pneumococcal vaccine should be emphasized.

COMMUNITY-ACQUIRED PNEUMONIA

Community-acquired pneumonia (CAP) has a significant impact on both individual patients and society, and pneumonia is currently the sixth leading cause of death in the USA with an estimated 3–4 million cases annually, accounting for more than 600 000 hospital admissions and 64 million days of restricted activity.[23]

CAP is not a reportable disease so exact figures are not available. It is clear, however, that it has a significant impact on the individual patient and society as a whole. Most (80%) patients are treated as outpatients while 20% are admitted to hospital; it is these 20% who generate most of the costs. The annual costs of treatment are US$4.8 billion (patients older than 65 years) and $3.6 billion (patients under 65 years).[24]

ETIOLOGY AND EPIDEMIOLOGY

As with many other infections, the incidence rates of CAP are greatest at the extremes of age. Although the overall annual rate of pneumonia in the USA is 12 cases per 1000 the rate is 12–18 cases per 1000 in children below 4 years of age and 20 cases per 1000 in people over 60 years age.[25,26] Between the ages of 5 and 60 years, the annual rate ranges from one to five cases per 1000 and the incidence of CAP requiring admission to hospital in adult patients is 2.6 cases per 1000.[27]

Risk factors for pneumonia have been defined and include the following: alcoholism, asthma, immunosuppression, institutionalization, and age greater than or equal to 70 years versus age 60–69 years.[28] Specific risk factors for pneumococcal infection include dementia, seizure disorders, congestive heart failure, cerebrovascular disease, COPD and HIV infection.[29]

Numerous microbial pathogens are potential etiological agents, and patients may be infected with more than one agent. Such mixed infections are well described in hospital-acquired pneumonia, where multiple pathogens are present in more than half of the nosocomial pneumonia patients studied.[30] In CAP, the incidence of mixed infections is lower, ranging from 2.7% to 13% in well-defined studies of inpatients with CAP.[31–33]

The single most important etiological agent is undoubtedly *Str. pneumoniae*. In a meta-analysis covering a 30-year period and including 7000 cases of pneumonia in which an etiological diagnosis was made, *Str. pneumoniae* accounted for two-thirds of all cases and for two-thirds of fatalities.[34]

At one time it was thought that atypical pathogens such as *M. pneumoniae*, *Ch. pneumoniae* and *Legionella* species were

not important causes of pneumonia and that if they did cause infection they were usually mild and affected primarily the young. A study in 1997 of more than 2700 patients admitted to hospital with CAP ranked these pathogens second, third and fourth of all etiological agents meeting the criteria for a 'definite' diagnosis.[35] Another study described three outbreaks of *Ch. pneumoniae* in nursing homes with high attack and mortality rates.[36] These two studies have helped to dispel the earlier misconceptions surrounding infection with the atypical pathogens.

Gram-negative rods such as *Escherichia coli* and *Klebsiella* spp. are not particularly common causes of CAP but are nevertheless important to consider, particularly in elderly people or in those with co-morbid illness, especially if they are ill enough to require hospital treatment.[31,37] There has been considerable debate about whether or not *Ps. aeruginosa* is a significant pathogen requiring treatment. The consensus is that, while it is certainly not common, it can occur in selected patients if risk factors such as a recent course of antibiotics or steroids or a prolonged stay in hospital are present.

PATHOGENESIS

The various etiological pathogens can gain access to the lower respiratory tract by a number of possible routes. These include inhalation, aspiration and hematogenous spread. For bacterial pneumonia, aspiration of organisms colonizing the oropharynx appears to be the most important route.[38] Pneumonia results when innate immunity, including macrophage phagocytosis, fails to eradicate the infecting pathogen, and a neutrophilic infiltrate is recruited.[6]

CLINICAL MANIFESTATIONS

Until relatively recently, physicians tended to divide cases of CAP into typical or atypical pneumonia based upon their clinical presentation. Typical or classic pneumonia refers to infection caused by bacterial pathogens such as *Str. pneumoniae* or *H. influenzae*, whereas atypical pneumonia refers to infection caused by the atypical pathogens (*M. pneumoniae*, *Ch. pneumoniae* and *Legionella* spp.). It was thought that those with classic bacterial pneumonia presented with fairly sudden onset of signs and symptoms with cough productive of purulent sputum, pleuritic chest pain and rigors. In contrast, those with atypical infection presented with an illness of undefined duration, a non-productive cough and often a frontal headache. It has become clear, however, that it is not possible to determine the etiological agent from a careful history, physical examination, and non-specific laboratory tests and chest radiographs.

The symptoms of CAP may be constitutional and non-specific or they may be localized to the respiratory tract and be fairly specific for respiratory infection. The former category includes such findings as malaise, anorexia, myalgias and arthralgias, chills and rigors; the latter includes shortness of breath, pleuritic chest pain, cough and sputum production.

In elderly patients the findings may be imprecise because constitutional symptoms such as confusion may predominate and there may be fewer findings related to the respiratory tract.

DIAGNOSIS

The problem of the diagnosis of CAP has generated much debate among physicians. Unfortunately, despite extensive testing even in university medical centers, no specific etiological agent may be found in up to one-half of the cases. In routine clinical practice, the etiological agent is determined in approximately 25% of cases but results in a change in antimicrobial therapy in less than 10% of cases.[39] Furthermore, an improvement in clinical outcome does not always result from identification of the etiological agent.

Generally, diagnostic tests fall into two categories: clinical and invasive/quantitative. Clinical testing relies on information obtained from the patient history, physical examination, and selected tests or procedures such as chest radiography, sputum Gram stain, and blood and sputum cultures. Invasive/quantitative methods include bronchoscopic techniques, pleural fluid aspiration and (in selected cases) lung biopsy. As a rule, the clinical method is too sensitive and lacks specificity while the invasive/quantitative methods require special expertise and laboratory support, and are more costly.

CLINICAL EVALUATION

The first step is to determine whether the patient has pneumonia rather than some other infective process such as bronchitis, or whether a non-infectious etiology (e.g. congestive heart failure, pulmonary embolism) is the cause of the patient's problem. If a diagnosis of pneumonia is made, the next step is to determine the etiological agent if possible. Unfortunately, it is impossible to accurately identify the pathogen based on clinical findings, even when multiple clinical variables are used.[31,40] There is significant intraobserver variation in the ability to elicit abnormal physical findings and the sensitivity and specificity of the history and physical examination are currently undetermined.[41]

CHEST RADIOGRAPH

The presence of an infiltrate on the chest radiograph can help to establish the diagnosis of pneumonia but does not determine the causative pathogen. However, the radiograph is important in defining the presence of a lobar or multilobar infiltrate and in assessing the severity of illness and prognosis.

LABORATORY ASSESSMENT

Routine laboratory assessment is unnecessary for ambulatory patients with CAP, who are likely to be managed as outpatients. However, for those ill enough to require admission to hospital (or even for those considered for admission), a complete blood and differential count, serum electrolytes, liver function tests, serum creatinine and an oxygen saturation assessment should be obtained. Significant abnormalities have been identified as risk factors for a complicated course or increased mortality. These abnormalities can be used to assess mortality risk and to help in the site of care decision.[42]

MICROBIOLOGICAL ASSESSMENT

Sputum Gram stain and culture

Of the two tests, the sputum Gram stain is more reliable, but is regarded as neither sensitive nor specific, though in some laboratories the test has made a positive contribution to early diagnosis.[43] Many patients are unable to produce a sputum sample, and of those samples produced a significant percentage may not be adequate. Although current data suggest that atypical pathogens are responsible for 20–25% of all CAP cases, none is detectable by the sputum Gram stain. There is also considerable inter- and intraobserver variation in Gram stain interpretation.[44] The sputum culture also lacks sensitivity and specificity. Even in patients with confirmed pneumococcal pneumonia based upon positive blood cultures, a simultaneously obtained sputum culture tested positive in only one-half of patients.[45]

Blood cultures

The incidence of positive blood cultures in ambulatory patients with CAP is less than 1%.[46] In hospital inpatients it ranges from 6.6% to 17.6% but may reach 27% in patients in ICUs.[32] The most common pathogen is *Str. pneumoniae*, and pneumococcal pneumonia is complicated by bacteremia more frequently than pneumonia caused by other pathogens. It is generally recommended that blood cultures be obtained from all patients who are admitted with CAP but not from those treated in the community.

Serology

To determine the role of a specific micro-organism as a pathogen, serological assessments should be based on the results of paired (acute and convalescent) serum samples. Unfortunately, such results are never available at the time the initial treatment decision is being made. Therefore, other than helping to define the epidemiological role of selected pathogens, serological testing is not helpful and is not recommended for routine use.

Legionella urinary antigen

This test is easy to perform and yields rapid results with a sensitivity of 70% and specificity of 100%. It is limited by the fact that it identifies only *Legionella pneumophila* serogroup 1. However, this serogroup accounts for most *Legionella* infections.

DNA probes and amplification

Polymerase chain reaction-based methods are being used increasingly.[47] Unfortunately, rapid diagnostic techniques are not generally available and simply identifying the presence of a particular micro-organism does not confirm infection. There are, however, a few micro-organisms whose mere presence indicates infection. These include *M. tuberculosis*, *Coxiella burnetii* and *Pneumocystis jirovecii* (formerly *Pn. carinii*).

INVASIVE PROCEDURES

For most patients with CAP, invasive tests such as bronchoscopy, bronchoalveolar lavage, protected specimen brush and percutaneous lung needle aspiration are not required. However, they may be appropriate in certain situations (e.g. patients with fulminant pneumonia or those unresponsive to a standard course of antimicrobials), when it may be necessary to identify a resistant or fastidious pathogen or to rule out a non-infectious cause.

Thoracocentesis should be performed in CAP patients with a significant pleural effusion defined as a collection of greater than 10 mm thickness on the lateral decubitus view. The incidence of pleural effusion with pneumonia varies from 36% to 57% and is most common in patients with pneumococcal infection.[48]

TREATMENT

Therapy can be directed or empirical. Directed therapy implies that the etiological agent is known and that therapy is aimed specifically at that pathogen. Empirical therapy is the more usual; it is, in effect, an educated guess and the physician institutes a course of treatment aimed at the most likely causes. Of these two options, directed therapy is clearly more desirable because it limits the breadth of spectrum required of the treatment agent(s), it may limit the number of drugs, reduces the adverse reactions associated with antibiotics, reduces antibiotic selection pressure and may result in less antimicrobial resistance.

Before discussing the various regimens, it is important to consider how the decision is made in terms of outpatient versus inpatient therapy and the problem of antimicrobial resistance.

SITE OF CARE DECISION

This decision is an important one, with considerable economic implications. The cost of inpatient care exceeds that of outpatient treatment by a factor of 15–20, and the cost of hospital management accounts for most of the money spent annually on CAP in the USA.[49]

In some cases it is immediately obvious that a patient can be treated outside the hospital; in other situations it is equally apparent that a patient requires hospital treatment and possibly admission to an ICU.

Effective prognostic scoring and outcome assessment tools are necessary to help physicians make the site of care decision. Such tools provide objective methods to assess the risk of adverse outcomes, including death.

Studies by Fine and others have attempted to identify patients at increased risk for adverse outcomes and to define independent predictors of mortality or poor outcome.[34,42] However, weaknesses or design flaws were found in each of them.[49]

The use of prediction rules may minimize unnecessary hospital admissions and help to identify patients who will benefit from care and intervention in the hospital and the ICU. The best known and most widely used prognostic tool is that of Fine.[42] This is a two-step rule designed to identify patients at low risk for mortality. Points are given based on age, coexisting disease, and abnormal physical and laboratory findings, and patients are assigned to classes 1–5 based on the total number of points assigned. This scoring system has been used to triage low-risk patients towards outpatient therapy with a high degree of success.[50] Fine's rule has been adopted into recommendations published by the Infectious Diseases Society of America (IDSA), the American Thoracic Society (ATS) and the European Respiratory Society.[51–53]

An alternative system of assessing severity, the CURB score, has been recommended by the British Thoracic Society[54] and the European Respiratory Society.[53] This score incorporates assessments of pulse rate, respiratory rate, renal function and mental status for the initial evaluation of patients, assigning 1 point for each abnormal feature (plus 1 for patients over 65 years of age in the CURB65 variation) and is much easier to use than the Fine score.

In assessing patients for severity, such scoring systems can only be a guide. Ultimately the physician must decide on grounds of clinical experience whether an individual patient with pneumonia warrants intravenous therapy, admission to hospital or management in an intensive care facility.

ANTIMICROBIAL RESISTANCE

Antimicrobial resistance among respiratory pathogens has become a major concern and it is important that clinicians understand and appreciate the general mechanisms and implications of this phenomenon. The emergence of resistance to penicillin among *Str. pneumoniae* isolates represents a gradual reduction in in-vitro susceptibility. The National Committee for Clinical Laboratory Standards defines strains for which the minimum inhibitory concentration (MIC) of penicillin is <1 mg/L as sensitive, 1.0–2.0 mg/L as intermediate and ≥ 4 mg/L as resistant.[55] With *Str. pneumoniae*, the DNA incorporation and remodeling that results in resistance is from the DNA of closely related oral commensal bacteria (*see* Ch. 3). By such a process, our own flora can develop resistance when we are treated with antibiotics and pathogens such as *Str. pneumoniae* can subsequently acquire resistance coding DNA from our own colonizing microflora.[56] Pneumococcal resistance to β-lactams is due solely to the presence of low-affinity penicillin-binding proteins. Macrolide resistance, however, can occur either by target site modification or by an efflux pump (*see* Chs 3 and 22). The relative frequencies of the two mechanisms vary internationally but in North America account for approximately 45% and 55%, respectively, of resistant isolates. Reports of breakthrough pneumococcal bacteremia in patients treated with macrolides have highlighted concerns about resistance to this class of agents.[57,58]

Resistance to ciprofloxacin and to newer fluoroquinolones among pneumococcal isolates has been reported.[59] Pneumococcal resistance to fluoroquinolones may be mediated by changes in one or both target sites (topoisomerase II and IV), usually resulting from mutations in the *gyrA* and *parC* genes, respectively, and possibly also by an efflux pump (*see* Ch. 3).[60] Of greatest concern, however, are the multidrug-resistant isolates, those that are resistant to two or more antibiotics having different mechanisms of action. In the USA, between 1995 and 1998, the proportion of invasive pneumococcal isolates that were resistant to three or more classes of drugs increased from 9% to 14%; there also were increases in the proportions of isolates that were resistant to penicillin (21% to 25%), cefotaxime (10% to 15%), meropenem (10% to 16%), erythromycin (11% to 16%) and trimethoprim–sulfamethoxazole (25% to 29%). These increases in frequency of resistance to multiple antimicrobial agents occurred in penicillin-resistant isolates only.[61] Drug-resistant *Str. pneumoniae* is associated with various risk factors including the presence of co-morbidities, such as chronic heart, lung, liver or renal disease, diabetes, alcoholism, immunosuppression or use of antimicrobials within the previous 3 months.[62] Infection with drug-resistant pneumococci results in invasive disease with higher mortality rates amongst hospitalized individuals.[63]

Pathogens such as *H. influenzae* and the Enterobacteriaceae are also important to consider. *H. influenzae* is the third most common cause of CAP requiring admission to hospital and, while the Enterobacteriaceae are not particularly common, they are important because of the high mortality rates associated with them. Among such pathogens resistance is usually mediated by β-lactamases, and the highest prevalence of β-lactamase genes is found on plasmids rather than chromosomes. Members of the TEM and SHV families are the most successful of the plasmid-encoded β-lactamases, and the TEM-1 β-lactamase accounts for almost 80% of all plasmid-encoded β-lactamases.[64] The extended-spectrum β-lactamases include oxyimino enzymes that are TEM and SHV mutants and cephalosporinases unrelated to TEM and SHV enzymes (*see* Ch. 15).

THERAPEUTIC REGIMENS

Once the diagnosis of pneumonia has been made, the physician must decide whether to treat the patient outside or inside the hospital and this in turn will help to determine the appropriate therapeutic regimen. In most patients an empirical choice must be made; however, where the infecting pathogen is known, antibiotic choice can be guided by local knowledge of antimicrobial sensitivities and policies. The correct choice of antimicrobial(s) for empirical therapy has generated considerable discussion, and a number of societies have produced guidelines to help physicians with the initial management of patients with CAP.[51–54]

Guidelines have served a number of useful functions. They have codified our management of patients with CAP and (at the very least) they have highlighted the gaps in our knowledge and have helped to direct future studies and research. Adherence to guidelines has had a significant pharmaco-economic effect, lowered mortality rates and shortened hospital stay.[65,66]

The joint guidelines of the IDSA and the ATS[51] make recommendations for outpatient and inpatient treatment of pneumonia, and draw a distinction between those individuals who do or do not have risk factors for drug-resistant *Str. pneumoniae* (DRSP) (Table 45.2). For outpatient treatment of previously healthy individuals with no risk factors for DRSP, these guidelines recommend a macrolide (azithromycin, clarithromycin or erythromycin) or doxycycline. In the presence of risk factors for DRSP, outpatients are recommended a 'respiratory' fluoroquinolone (moxifloxacin, gemifloxacin or levofloxacin [750 mg]) or a high dose β-lactam plus a macrolide or doxycycline. This latter recommendation also pertains to all inpatients (non-ICU). For inpatients requiring ICU treatment the IDSA/ATS guidelines recommend a β-lactam (cefotaxime, ceftriaxone or ampicillin–sulbactam) plus either azithromycin or a fluoroquinolone, except where *Pseudomonas* infection is suspected, in which case an antipneumococcal, antipseudomonal β-lactam (piperacillin–tazobactam, cefepime, imipenem or meropenem) plus either ciprofloxacin or levofloxacin (750 mg) is the recommended first-line regimen. Where community-acquired methicillin-resistant *Staphylococcus aureus* infection is suspected to be the cause of the pneumonia, these guidelines recommend the addition of vancomycin or linezolid to the regimen.

The recommendation for the use of macrolides in these guidelines relates to the coverage of atypical pathogens. A β-lactam would be the agent of choice for *Str. pneumoniae* but it would be ineffective against any of the atypicals. However, a macrolide provides good-to-excellent coverage for all these likely pathogens.

In North America the fluoroquinolones have assumed an important role in the management of CAP coinciding with rising resistance to β-lactams and macrolides, the appreciation of the potential importance of Gram-negative rods in selected CAP patients and the availability of the 'respiratory' fluoroquinolones which offer once-daily monotherapy, compared with the multiple dosing required if a β-lactam and macrolide regimen is used.[51]

Table 45.2 Empirical antimicrobial selection for community-acquired pneumonia (IDSA/ATS guidelines)

Outpatient treatment

1. Previously healthy and no use of antimicrobials within the previous 3 months
   - A macrolide
   - Doxycycline
2. Presence of co-morbidities such as chronic heart, lung, liver or renal disease; diabetes mellitus; alcoholism; malignancies; asplenia; immunosuppressing conditions or use of immunosuppressing drugs; or use of antimicrobials within the previous 3 months (in which case an alternative from a different class should be selected)
   - A respiratory fluoroquinolone (moxifloxacin, gemifloxacin or levofloxacin [750 mg])
   - A β-lactam plus a macrolide
3. In regions with a high rate (>25%) of infection with high-level (MIC ≥16 μg/mL) macrolide-resistant *Streptococcus pneumoniae*, consider use of alternative agents listed above in (2) for patients without co-morbidities

Inpatients, non-ICU treatment

A respiratory fluoroquinolone
A β-lactam plus a macrolide

Inpatients, ICU treatment

A β-lactam (cefotaxime, ceftriaxone, or ampicillin–sulbactam) plus either azithromycin or a respiratory fluoroquinolone (for penicillin-allergic patients, a respiratory fluoroquinolone and aztreonam are recommended)

Special concerns

If *Pseudomonas* is a consideration
   - An antipneumococcal, antipseudomonal β-lactam (piperacillin–tazobactam, cefepime, imipenem or meropenem) plus either ciprofloxacin or levofloxacin (750 mg), *or*
   - The above β-lactam plus an aminoglycoside and azithromycin, or
   - The above β-lactam plus an aminoglycoside and an antipneumococcal fluoroquinolone (for penicillin-allergic patients, substitute aztreonam for above β-lactam)
If CA-MRSA is a consideration, add vancomycin or linezolid

CA–MRSA, community-acquired methicillin-resistant *Staphylococcus aureus*; ICU, intensive care unit.
Adapted from Mandell LA , Wunderink RG , Anzueto A , et al. Infectious Diseases Society of America; American Thoracic Society. Infectious Diseases Society of America/American Thoracic Society consensus guidelines on the management of community acquired pneumonia in adults. **Clin Infect Dis.** 2007;44(suppl 2): S27–S72.

Many experts feel that penicillin still has a role to play in the treatment of pneumococcal pneumonia and that it is effective against infections caused by susceptible organisms. For strains of *Str. pneumoniae* with intermediate levels of resistance to penicillin higher doses may be used, as recommended in the IDSA/ATS guidelines. Unfortunately, the identity or susceptibility of the etiological agent is unknown in most cases at the time of initial antibiotic treatment.

Efflux resistance to macrolides results in low-level resistance, whereas the target change mechanism results in high-level resistance. Low-level resistance predominates in North America, while the latter is more frequent in Europe. In the USA and Canada, therefore, macrolides are still seen as having a significant role to play in the management of many patients with CAP.

For those treated in hospital, the guidelines divide patients into those treated on a medical ward and those treated in the ICU, and use the risk of infection with *Ps. aeruginosa* as a means of further subdividing ICU patients, reflecting the enhanced mortality rate and constitutive antimicrobial resistance associated with this organism.

The recent British Thoracic Society (BTS) guidelines (Table 45.3) provide an exhaustive evidence-based approach to the management of CAP patients.[54] They differ from the IDSA/ATS guidelines quite extensively. For outpatients, the BTS does not consider that atypical pathogens such as *M. pneumoniae* or *Ch. pneumoniae* are important enough to warrant routine coverage, and therefore treatment is aimed primarily at *Str. pneumoniae*, for which the drug of choice is amoxicillin. For hospital inpatients, the North American document divides patients into those managed on a ward or in the ICU, whereas the British guidelines consider hospital-treated patients under three categories: (1) not severe and admitted for non-clinical reasons or previously treated in the community (CURB65 0–1); (2) moderate severity

Table 45.3 British Thoracic Society recommendations for initial empirical treatment of community-acquired pneumonia

Type of patient	First choice	Second choice
Low severity (i.e. CURB65 = 0–1), home treated	Amoxicillin 500 mg p.o. every 8 h	Doxycycline 200 mg loading dose then 100 mg/day or clarithromycin 500 mg p.o. every 12 h
Hospital treated, not severe (i.e. CURB65 = 0–1)	Amoxicillin 500 mg p.o. or i.v. every 8 h	Doxycycline 200 mg loading dose then 100 mg/day or clarithromycin 500 mg p.o. every 12 h
Hospital treated, moderately severe (i.e. CURB65 = 2)	1. Amoxicillin 500 mg–1 g p.o. every 8 h + clarithromycin 500 mg p.o. every 12 h 2. If oral treatment not possible, amoxicillin 500 mg –1 g i.v. every 8 h or benzylpenicillin 1.2 g i.v. every 6 h + clarithromycin 500 mg i.v. every 12 h	Doxycycline 200 mg loading dose then 100 mg/day or levofloxacin 500 mg p.o. every 12 h or moxifloxacin 400 mg p.o. every 12 h
Hospital treated, severe (i.e. CURB65 = 3–5); consider critical care review	Amoxicillin–clavulanate 1.2 g i.v. every 8 h + clarithromycin 500 mg i.v. every 12 h (if *Legionella* strongly suspected, consider adding levofloxacin)	Benzylpenicillin 1.2 g i.v. every 6 h + either levofloxacin 500 mg i.v. every 12 h or ciprofloxacin 400 mg i.v. every 12 h *or* Cefuroxime 1.5 g i.v. every 8 h or cefotaxime 1 g i.v. every 8 h or ceftriaxone 2 g i.v. per day + clarithromycin 500 mg i.v. every 12 h (if *Legionella* strongly suspected, consider adding levofloxacin)

Adapted from Lim WS , Baudouin SV , George RC , et al. Pneumonia Guidelines Committee of the BTS Standards of Care Committee. BTS guidelines for the management of community acquired pneumonia in adults: update 2009. **Thorax.** 2009;64(suppl 3):iii1–iii55.

(CURB65 = 2); and (3) severe (CURB65 3–5). The first group is treated with amoxicillin, the second is given amoxicillin plus a macrolide (erythromycin or clarithromycin) and the third group is given a β-lactam (amoxicillin–clavulanate) plus intravenous erythromycin or clarithromycin. Fluoroquinolones are recommended as an alternative only for the second and third categories. In general, the potency and breadth of intravenous antibiotics recommended increases as severity increases. In moderately ill hospitalized patients treated in the UK, a simple β-lactam in combination with a macrolide is likely to be used, if clinicians follow the BTS guidelines. Individual hospital policies will be tailored to balance the requirement for potent therapy, with the need to keep antimicrobial activity as narrow spectrum as possible to avoid potential impacts on hospital ecology.

Initiation of treatment should not be delayed, particularly when dealing with patients over 65 years of age. A study of elderly patients presenting to emergency departments with CAP showed that those who received antibiotics within 8 h of presentation had a significantly lower 30-day mortality rate than those who waited longer for initiation of treatment.[67]

Intravenous to oral sequential treatment is strongly recommended because it reduces costs, encourages patient mobility and allows earlier discharge from hospital. Ancillary measures such as supplemental oxygen, drainage of significant pleural effusions and hydration are also important.

The patient should be followed and objective parameters monitored. These include the resolution of cough, shortness of breath and elevated temperature and (for those in hospital) improvement in the oxygen saturation, C-reactive protein and white blood cell count.

UNUSUAL PATHOGENS

Staphylococcal pneumonia can be associated with a necrotizing pneumonitis, particularly when stains expressing Panton–Valentine leukocidin toxin are implicated. If such organisms are strongly suspected in patients with severe pneumonia, a combination of intravenous linezolid (600 mg every 12 h), intravenous clindamycin (1.2 g every 6 h) and intravenous rifampicin (rifampin) (600 mg every 12 h) should be added to the initial antibiotic regimen.[54]

HEALTHCARE-ASSOCIATED PNEUMONIA

'Healthcare-associated pneumonia' refers to pneumonia in patients who have recently been hospitalized, had hemodialysis or received intravenous chemotherapy, or reside in a nursing home or long-term care facility.[68] They are distinguished by having a different pattern of microbial flora associated with the pneumonia (often Gram-positive organisms with a higher tendency towards antimicrobial resis-

tance) and also more severe disease, longer hospital stay and higher mortality rates. The dominant group in this class of patients generally comprises residents of nursing homes. Nursing home pneumonia or pneumonia in elderly residents of long-term care facilities is an important entity and is only now becoming the subject of serious clinical investigation. Pneumonia is the main cause of death among residents of such facilities, with acute mortality rates ranging from 5% to 40% per infection. It is the most common reason for transfer of nursing home residents to an acute care hospital, with approximately one-third of pneumonia patients requiring hospital admission.[69]

ETIOLOGY AND EPIDEMIOLOGY

The incidence of pneumonia among residents of nursing homes is considerably higher than among persons living in the community, ranging from 1.2 to 2.5 episodes per 1000 resident days with a median incidence of 1 per 1000 resident days.[69] One of the difficulties in establishing the etiology of nursing home pneumonia is the fact that studies in this area have depended almost exclusively on results of sputum cultures. Such studies are compromised from the outset because over half the elderly patients do not produce any sputum. The likely pathogens are somewhat different from those in patients with CAP. In cases of CAP, the predominant etiological agents are *Str. pneumoniae* and the atypicals (in selected cases Gram-negative rods may be encountered). In nursing home pneumonia, *Str. pneumoniae* is still a significant pathogen, but (it is important to note that age >65 years and residence in a nursing home have been identified as risk factors for penicillin-resistant *Str. pneumoniae* infection) there is a greater proportion of cases caused by *Staph. aureus*, *H. influenzae* and Gram-negative rods in this population than in a younger cohort, and a disconcertingly high percentage of the *Staph. aureus* isolates are methicillin resistant.[70] Atypicals are more common in younger patients.

The role of anaerobes is still not definitely settled and appropriately designed studies to substantiate their role as pathogens in the elderly do not appear to have been undertaken.

In addition to aerobic and possibly anaerobic bacterial pathogens, viruses and *M. tuberculosis* must also be considered. Epidemics of influenza, RSV and parainfluenza have been described in such populations, and must always be considered if an institutional outbreak is encountered. The incidence of tuberculosis is substantially higher in the institutionalized elderly and must be included in the assessment of such patients.

PATHOGENESIS

A number of risk factors have been defined in a prospective cohort study of respiratory tract infections in nursing home residents.[69] Older age, male sex, inability to take oral medications and swallowing difficulties were identified as independent risk factors for the development of pneumonia. Swallowing difficulty, confusion and altered levels of consciousness have often been evoked as surrogate markers for aspiration and by inference as indicators of infection with anaerobes.

Nasogastric tube feeding and tracheostomy have also been identified as potential risk factors for pneumonia, presumably because of the increased risk of aspiration.

CLINICAL MANIFESTATIONS AND DIAGNOSIS

The physician must be aware that in an elderly patient with pneumonia rather than a history of elevated temperature, chills and cough with purulent sputum, the story may be that of confusion, weakness, anorexia and falls. The difficulty in making a diagnosis of pneumonia in a nursing home population is enhanced by the fact that nursing homes lack laboratory and radiographic facilities and many often do not have a physician in attendance on a full-time basis.

Ideally, if a patient presents with findings suggestive of pneumonia, he or she should be evaluated by a physician and a chest radiograph obtained. If feasible, an expectorated sputum sample should be sent for Gram stain and culture, and for people with more serious illness in whom parenteral therapy or transfer to a hospital is contemplated, the following additional tests should be done: blood samples for culture and susceptibility testing, complete blood count and differential, serum creatinine, urine for *Legionella* antigen.

If pneumonia occurs in the setting of an influenza outbreak or if a particular case is suggestive of influenza infection, a nasopharyngeal swab should be obtained for rapid detection of viral antigen by polymerase chain reaction. Similarly, if tuberculosis is a possibility, sputum samples for microscopy and rapid culture should be obtained. In both of these circumstances respiratory precautions must be instituted and the patient should be isolated to prevent spread of the disease.

TREATMENT

As with any patient, the use of an antimicrobial directed at a known pathogen is the ideal; however, at the time that the treatment decision is made it is unlikely that a definitive etiological agent will have been identified. As with most cases of pneumonia, an empirical regimen is usually selected, based upon local epidemiology and susceptibility patterns and risk stratification of the patient.

The site of care decision is an important one and nursing home residents with pneumonia can be evaluated using the same prediction rules for hospital admission as are used for other patients with CAP.[42] For most patients who can be treated in the nursing home setting, with no other risk factors for multidrug-resistant pathogens, a 'respiratory fluoroquinolone' such as moxifloxacin, gatifloxacin or levofloxacin

(according to availability), or a combination regimen consisting of amoxicillin–clavulanate, is generally recommended as first choice.[70,71]

Influenza outbreaks in an institutional setting can be associated with high attack rates and mortality rates. Annual immunoprophylaxis using vaccines offers protection and is recommended for all residents. Zanamivir and oseltamivir are neuraminidase inhibitors with activity against both influenza A and influenza B. Both of these agents are approved for treatment of uncomplicated influenza and if given within 48 h of onset of symptoms may decrease the severity and duration of the symptoms.

HOSPITAL-ACQUIRED PNEUMONIA

Hospital-acquired or nosocomial pneumonia is by definition infection that occurs 48 h or more after admission to hospital. Although it is the second most common nosocomial infection in the USA, accounting for 13–18% of all hospital-acquired infections, it is the one most frequently associated with a fatal outcome, and is associated with significant morbidity and mortality.[71]

Current figures are based on estimates from hospital records because nosocomial pneumonia is not a reportable disease. It is considered, however, that currently more than 300 000 cases occur annually in the USA, resulting in an average increase in length of hospital stay of 8 days.[71]

Mortality figures range from 15% to 70%; however, the more relevant attributable mortality figures are estimated at 33–50%.

ETIOLOGY AND EPIDEMIOLOGY

The estimated rate of occurrence is 4–8 episodes per 1000 hospital admissions in non-teaching hospitals and 8 per 1000 in teaching hospitals.[71] In patients who are intubated, the rate is up to 20 times higher than in non-intubated patients. Rates of ventilator-associated pneumonia are reported to be approximately 15 per 1000 ventilator days.[72]

Risk factors for nosocomial pneumonia include increasing age, COPD, neuromuscular disease, decreased consciousness, aspiration, endotracheal intubation, thoracic and upper abdominal surgery, and nasogastric intubation. Of the various pathogens, perhaps the most important with defined risk factors are *Staph. aureus* (head injury, coma longer than 24 h and intravenous drug use) and *Ps. aeruginosa* (prior antibiotics, structural lung disease and steroid treatment).[71,73]

The most common pathogens encountered in nosocomial pneumonia are the Gram-negative bacilli, which have been reported in up to 60% of cases, and *Staph. aureus*, which has been reported in up to 40% of patients. In infections occurring during the first 4 days of hospital stay, bacteria typically associated with CAP, such as *Str. pneumoniae* and *H. influenzae*, have also been reported.

The Gram-negative rods of interest are *Esch. coli*, *Klebsiella* spp., *Enterobacter* spp., *Proteus* spp. and *Serratia marcescens*. *Esch. coli* is the third most common coliform isolated from patients with nosocomial pneumonia and appears to affect predisposed hosts such as the critically ill. *K. pneumoniae* is the most commonly isolated of the *Klebsiella* species and may cause severe necrotizing lobar pneumonia in the elderly, in alcoholics and in diabetics. *K. pneumoniae* and *Esch. coli* are the bacteria that most commonly carry the extended-spectrum β-lactamases, rendering them resistant to oxyimino β-lactams such as cefotaxime, ceftazidime and aztreonam.

Among *Enterobacter* spp., *E. cloacae* and *E. aerogenes* are the primary cause of nosocomial pneumonia and frequently colonize patients who have received a course of antibiotics. Resistance to group 4 cephalosporins among these pathogens may develop within days of treatment.

Proteus mirabilis and *Proteus vulgaris* can act as opportunistic respiratory pathogens in a manner similar to that of the *Enterobacter* spp. Indole-positive species such as *Pr. vulgaris* may undergo a single-step mutation to become constitutive high-level producers of β-lactamase enzymes, which is manifested as resistance to group 4 cephalosporins. *Ser. marcescens* preferentially colonizes the respiratory and urinary tracts and has been associated with common source outbreaks of pneumonia in the setting of inhalation therapy and contaminated bronchoscopes. Like all Enterobacteriaceae, this organism may spread to patients by hand transfer from healthcare personnel.

The non-fermentative Gram-negative bacilli of importance are *Ps. aeruginosa* and *Acinetobacter* spp. *Ps. aeruginosa* is one of the leading causes of Gram-negative pneumonia. The most common mechanism of infection is direct contact with environmental reservoirs, including respiratory devices such as contaminated nebulizers or humidifiers. *Acinetobacter* spp. can also result in serious nosocomial infection and has been shown to be an important cause of ventilator-associated pneumonia.

H. influenzae frequently colonizes the upper respiratory tract of individuals with predisposing conditions such as COPD. Most adult infections are caused by non-typeable strains and *H. influenzae* (along with *Str. pneumoniae*) can often be isolated from tracheal secretions following intubation. *Str. pneumoniae*, like *H. influenzae*, colonizes the oropharynx and, although it is predominantly a pathogen associated with CAP, *Str. pneumoniae* is being recognized with increasing frequency as a cause of hospital-acquired infection.[71]

Anaerobes may be found as pathogens in patients predisposed to aspiration. The anaerobes that have been implicated in nosocomial pneumonia are those that colonize the oropharynx, such as *Fusobacterium* spp., *Prevotella melaninogenica* and *Bacteroides ureolyticus*.

Legionella pneumophila serogroup 1 is the most common of the *Legionella* spp. to be associated with both CAP and hospital-acquired pneumonia. The exact mode of transmission is controversial and there is evidence for both aspiration and inhalation. Contaminated potable water and contaminated aerosols have been reported as sources of infection in hospitals.

It is important to realize that nosocomial pneumonia may be caused by multiple pathogens in any one patient, emphasizing the need for broad coverage when empirical treatment is initiated. Bartlett and colleagues demonstrated that more than one pathogen could be documented in over half of the cases studied.[30]

PATHOGENESIS

The pathogenesis of nosocomial pneumonia is complex. Pathogens may gain access to the lower respiratory tract by inhalation, microaspiration or silent aspiration of oropharyngeal secretions, gross aspiration of gastric contents, hematogenous spread, translocation from the gastrointestinal tract, spread from a contiguous focus (e.g. pleural space) and direct inoculation during surgery.

For certain pathogens, such as *Mycobacteria* and *Aspergillus* spp., inhalation of aerosols is important. In patients being mechanically ventilated, contamination of a humidification reservoir may result in aspiration of potential pathogens directly into the airways. The most important mechanism, however, particularly for Gram-negative rods, is the microaspiration of bacteria colonizing the oropharynx.

Studies have shown that while oropharyngeal colonization by Gram-negative rods is unusual in healthy people, it occurs with increasing frequency in those with underlying disease.[71] Once oropharyngeal colonization is established, the silent aspiration of these potentially virulent bacteria eventually results in the overwhelming of host defenses in the lung and the development of pneumonia.

In addition to the oropharyngeal–pulmonary route, the gastropulmonary route has also been suggested as a means of introducing pathogens to the distal airways. Normally, the acidic pH of the stomach provides a hostile environment to bacteria, rendering the stomach contents virtually sterile, but above pH 4 bacterial overgrowth may occur. However, studies of stress ulcer prophylaxis have failed to demonstrate a definitive correlation between colonization of the stomach by bacteria and pneumonia.[74,75] A review of the literature concluded that the stomach should be regarded as an amplifier but not as the primary source of pathogens causing pneumonia and that the oropharyngeal–pulmonary route is more important than the gastropulmonary route.[76]

In patients who are being mechanically ventilated, the endotracheal tube plays an important role in the pathogenesis of ventilator-associated pneumonia. The tube itself breaches the upper airway defenses, and the inflated cuff allows the oropharyngeal secretions containing various pathogens to collect until they eventually pass the inflated cuff to the distal airways. In addition, the tube acts as a template upon which a layer of biofilm is deposited.[77] Pieces of this biofilm containing millions of bacteria may subsequently break off and reach the distal airways, thereby seeding remote sites of the lung.

CLINICAL MANIFESTATIONS

Much of what has been said in the discussion of the clinical manifestations of CAP and nursing home-acquired pneumonia applies to nosocomial pneumonia. The findings will vary, depending upon the age of the patient and the severity of the illness. As with CAP and nursing home-acquired infection, the symptoms may be constitutional and non-specific or localized to the respiratory tract.

DIAGNOSIS

As with CAP, two approaches may be used: clinical and invasive/quantitative.

With the clinical approach, pneumonia is defined as the presence of a new pulmonary infiltrate unexplained by other obvious causes plus one of a number of additional features, such as elevated temperature, production of purulent sputum or leukocytosis. While the clinical approach is relatively easy and straightforward and is not associated with significant costs, it is overly sensitive and does not reliably discriminate among the various causes. The invasive/quantitative approach, on the other hand, generally has greater precision but requires special training and laboratory support, is associated with significant costs, and has the potential for serious adverse effects.

Whichever approach is used, every patient with nosocomial pneumonia requires a careful history, including risk factors for specific pathogens, a physical examination, postero-anterior and lateral chest radiographs, complete blood count, blood chemistry, blood cultures, and either oximetry or arterial blood gases.

Chest radiography is useful in helping to determine the extent of the pneumonia and the presence of a pleural effusion. Multilobar involvement, cavitation or rapid radiographic progression indicates the presence of a severe infection.

Routine blood counts and chemistry may indicate evidence of end-organ dysfunction and can be helpful in adjusting treatment regimens. Blood cultures may be useful in identifying the pathogen in up to 20% of patients with nosocomial pneumonia. The presence of a pathogen in blood indicates not only that it is the etiological agent but also that the patient is at increased risk for a complicated course.

Serology is not normally useful in the management of individual patients with nosocomial pneumonia. It may, however, be helpful for epidemiological purposes, although this is more likely to be the case in patients with CAP.

The value of sputum Gram stain and culture is controversial as there are significant problems with both the sensitivity and specificity of these tests. Most studies have been carried out in patients with CAP; however, the results can be extrapolated to patients with nosocomial pneumonia. In selected cases direct staining of sputum samples for fungi or mycobacteria, or direct fluorescent antibody staining for *Legionella pneumophila*, may help in directing therapy.

Invasive techniques are not performed routinely in patients with nosocomial pneumonia. However, invasive techniques should be considered in selected cases, such as:
- patients receiving appropriate empirical antimicrobial coverage but who are failing to respond
- certain immunocompromised patients
- patients in whom an alternative diagnosis (e.g. carcinoma) is suspected.

A number of methods have been developed to obtain samples of lower respiratory tract secretions that are not contaminated by oropharyngeal micro-organisms. They are endotracheal aspirate, protected catheter aspirate, protected specimen brush and bronchoalveolar lavage. The studies that claim to support these techniques suffer from a lack of standardization, which makes comparison difficult at best. The discordant findings among the investigators studying these techniques make it difficult for practitioners to determine the most effective method.

Other invasive tests include transthoracic needle aspiration, transbronchial biopsy, thoracoscopy and open lung biopsy. One study comparing invasive and non-invasive strategies for management of suspected ventilator-associated pneumonia showed that there was a statistically significant reduction in mortality, sepsis-related organ failure and antibiotic-free days in the cohort managed with invasive diagnostic tests.[78]

TREATMENT

When devising an antimicrobial regimen, the patient, the pathogen and the drug should all be considered individually and the interactions among them taken into account.

 ## PATIENT-RELATED FACTORS

These include any previous history of adverse reactions (and, in particular, anything suggesting type 1 hypersensitivity to any antimicrobial) and increasing age (since adverse drug effects are more common in elderly people). Macrolides, lincosamides, chloramphenicol and metronidazole are eliminated via the liver, while most other antibiotics are eliminated by the kidney. When treating women of childbearing age, it is important to determine if the patient is pregnant because teratogenicity and fetotoxicity must be considered.

 ## PATHOGEN-RELATED FACTORS

Ideally, the narrowest spectrum agent associated with the least toxicity and lowest cost should be administered if the pathogen is known. Unfortunately, empirical therapy is usually the norm, and one must consider the likely pathogens based upon local epidemiology, risk factors for pneumonia and for specific pathogens, and severity of illness. The prevalence of resistance among pathogens to various antimicrobials must also be considered.

DRUG-RELATED FACTORS

When selecting any antibiotic, the first step is to select an agent to which the pathogen is known or likely to be susceptible. Other considerations include pharmacokinetic and pharmacodynamic properties, toxicity, drug interactions and cost. Depending upon the class of antibiotic being used, different pharmacokinetic/pharmacodynamic parameters correlate more or less closely with clinical or therapeutic efficacy. For β-lactam drugs, macrolides and clindamycin, the time during which the antibiotic concentration at the site of action in the tissues is above the MIC for the organism correlates best with efficacy. However, for aminoglycosides, fluoroquinolones and vancomycin, the 24 h area-under-the-curve/MIC ratio correlates best. Higher ratios of peak serum concentrations to MIC (C_{max}/MIC) have been shown to prevent the emergence of resistance during treatment with fluoroquinolones and aminoglycosides. Furthermore, aminoglycosides do not achieve high levels in lung tissue, and this problem is compounded by the fact that they are also relatively inactivated by the acidic pH present at the site of infection in the lung.

The approach to the management of patients with nosocomial pneumonia should take into account the risk factors, severity of illness and time of onset of the illness.[79,80] The risk factors are for infection with specific pathogens; severity of illness is either mild to moderate or severe; time of onset refers to early versus late (i.e. <5 or ≥5 days, respectively). Based upon these variables, a hierarchical approach to the patient with nosocomial pneumonia has been developed. While it is recognized that a large number of bacteria are potential pathogens, there is a 'core' group of organisms that must be considered for each patient for whom antimicrobial coverage must be provided (Table 45.4). This group consists of Gram-negative bacilli (such as *Enterobacter* spp., *Esch. coli*, *Klebsiella* and *Proteus* spp., *Ser. marcescens*), *H. influenzae*, *Staph. aureus* and *Str. pneumoniae*. Depending upon the risk factors present and the severity of illness, anaerobes, methicillin-resistant *Staph. aureus*, *Legionella* spp., *Ps. aeruginosa* and *Acinetobacter* spp. should also be considered.

The American Thoracic Society regimens are presented in Tables 45.4, 45.5 and 45.6.[71] Other countries have produced guidelines for local use which reflect variation in the target pathogens and choice of therapy. Until the evidence base surrounding nosocomial pneumonia improves, variations in practice are likely to continue. The decision to select an agent should be based upon the host, pathogen and drug-related issues outlined earlier. A few specific issues, however, deserve comment. Single-agent therapy is recommended in many situations. Although two drugs should be used to achieve synergistic or additive activity against *Ps. aeruginosa*, there are no

Table 45.4 Initial empirical antibiotic therapy for hospital-acquired pneumonia or ventilator-associated pneumonia in patients with no known risk factors for multidrug-resistant pathogens, early onset and any disease severity

Potential pathogen	Recommended antibiotic[a]
Streptococcus pneumoniae[b] *Haemophilus influenzae* Methicillin-sensitive *Staphylococcus aureus* Antibiotic-sensitive enteric gram-negative bacilli *Escherichia coli* *Klebsiella pneumoniae* *Enterobacter* spp. *Proteus* spp. *Serratia marcescens*	Ceftriaxone *or* Levofloxacin, moxifloxacin, or ciprofloxacin *or* Ampicillin–sulbactam *or* Ertapenem

[a]See Table 45.6 for recommended initial doses of antibiotics.
[b]The frequency of penicillin-resistant *Str. pneumoniae* and multidrug-resistant *Str. pneumoniae* is increasing; levofloxacin or moxifloxacin is preferred to ciprofloxacin. The role of other new quinolones, such as gatifloxacin, has not been established. Adapted from the American Thoracic Society.[71]

Table 45.5 Initial empirical therapy for hospital-acquired pneumonia, ventilator-associated pneumonia and healthcare-associated pneumonia in patients with late-onset disease or risk factors for multidrug-resistant pathogens and all disease severity

Potential pathogens	Combination antibiotic therapy[a]
Pathogens listed in Table 45.4 and multidrug-resistant pathogens	Antipseudomonal cephalosporin (cefepime, ceftazidime) *or*
Pseudomonas aeruginosa *Klebsiella pneumoniae* (ESBL⁺)[b]	Antipseudomonal carbapenem (imipenem or meropenem) *or*
Acinetobacter species[b]	β-Lactam/β-lactamase inhibitor (piperacillin–tazobactam) *plus* Antipseudomonal fluoroquinolone[h] (ciprofloxacin or levofloxacin) *or* Aminoglycoside (amikacin, gentamicin or tobramycin) *plus*
Methicillin-resistant *Staphylococcus aureus* (MRSA) *Legionella pneumophila*[b]	Linezolid or vancomycin[c]

[a]See Table 45.6 for adequate initial dosing of antibiotics. Initial antibiotic therapy should be adjusted or streamlined on the basis of microbiological data and clinical response to therapy.
[b]If an extended spectrum β-lactamase-positive (ESBL⁺) strain, such as *K. pneumoniae*, or an *Acinetobacter* species is suspected, a carbapenem is a reliable choice. If *L. pneumophila* is suspected, the combination antibiotic regimen should include a macrolide (e.g. azithromycin), or a fluoroquinolone (e.g. ciprofloxacin or levofloxacin) should be used rather than an aminoglycoside.
[c]If MRSA risk factors are present or there is a high incidence locally. Reproduced from the American Thoracic Society. From American Thoracic Society. Guidelines for the management of adults with hospital-acquired, ventilator-associated, and healthcare-associated pneumonia. **Am J Respir Crit Care Med.** 2005;171:388–416.

data to support the routine use of combination therapy for other bacterial pathogens in non-neutropenic patients.[81]

In patients who are either severely ill with risk factors and early onset or severely ill without risk factors but with late onset, combination therapy should be instituted. If the patient was not receiving any prior antibiotics and deep suction

Table 45.6 Initial intravenous, adult doses of antibiotics for empirical therapy of hospital-acquired pneumonia, including ventilator-associated pneumonia and healthcare-associated pneumonia in patients with late-onset disease or risk factors for multidrug-resistant pathogens

Antibiotic	Dosage[a]
Antipseudomonal cephalosporin	
Cefepime	1–2 g every 8–12 h
Ceftazidime	2 g every 8 h
Carbapenems	
Imipenem	500 mg every 6 h or 1 g every 8 h
Meropenem	1 g every 8 h
β-Lactam/β-lactamase inhibitor	
Piperacillin–tazobactam	4.5 g every 6 h
Aminoglycosides	
Gentamicin	7 mg/kg per day[b]
Tobramycin	7 mg/kg per day[b]
Amikacin	20 mg/kg per day[b]
Antipseudomonal quinolones	
Levofloxacin	750 mg/day
Ciprofloxacin	400 mg every 8 h
Vancomycin	15 mg/kg every 12 h[c]
Linezolid	600 mg every 12 h

[a] Dosages are based on normal renal and hepatic function.
[b] Trough levels for gentamicin and tobramycin should be <1 μg/mL; for amikacin they should be <4–5 μg/mL.
[c] Trough levels for vancomycin should be 15–20 μg/mL.
Reproduced from the American Thoracic Society. From American Thoracic Society. Guidelines for the management of adults with hospital-acquired, ventilator-associated, and healthcare-associated pneumonia. **Am J Respir Crit Care Med.** 2005;171:388–416.

aspirates or bronchoscopy samples fail to yield *Ps. aeruginosa* or other often-resistant pathogens such as *Acinetobacter* spp., treatment may be modified to a single-drug regimen.

Enterobacter spp. are among the most common causes of Gram-negative bacillary hospital-acquired pneumonia. A major concern with infection caused by this organism is that in the presence of a group 4 cephalosporin it can become a hyperproducer of β-lactamase.[82]

The final issue is that of duration of therapy. Unfortunately, there are no appropriately designed randomized controlled trials that specifically address this issue. The general consensus, however, is that patients with severe infection caused by pathogens such as *Ps. aeruginosa* or *Acinetobacter* spp. should be treated for a minimum of 14 days, whereas patients with less severe infection may only require 7–10 days of treatment.

 # References

1. Gonzales R, Steiner JF, Sande MA. Antibiotic prescribing for adults with colds, upper respiratory tract infections, and bronchitis by ambulatory care physicians. *J Am Med Assoc.* 1997;278:901–904.
2. Rodnick JE, Gude JK. The use of antibiotics in acute bronchitis and acute exacerbations of chronic bronchitis. *West J Med.* 1988;149:347–351.
3. Fleming DM, Elliot AJ. The management of acute bronchitis in children. *Expert Opin Pharmacother.* 2007;8(4):415–426.
4. Brodzinski H, Ruddy RM. Review of new and newly discovered respiratory tract viruses in children. *Pediatr Emerg Care.* 2009;25(5):352–360; quiz 361–363.
5. Smith CB, Golden CA, Kanner RE, et al. Association of viral and *Mycoplasma pneumoniae* infections with acute respiratory illness in patients with chronic obstructive pulmonary diseases. *Am Rev Respir Dis.* 1980;121:225–232.
6. Read RC. Bacterial infections of the respiratory tract. In: Borriello SP, Murray PR, Funke G, eds. *Topley and Wilson's microbiology and microbial infections.* 10th ed. London: Hodder Arnold; 2005:622–657.
7. Ayres JG. Seasonal pattern of acute bronchitis in general practice in the United Kingdom. *Thorax.* 1986;41:106–110.
8. Reynolds HY. Chronic bronchitis and acute infectious exacerbations. In: Mandell GL, Bennett JE, Dolin R, eds. *Mandell, Douglas and Bennett's Principles and Practice of Infectious Diseases.* 4th ed. Edinburgh: Churchill Livingstone; 1995:608.
9. US Bureau of the Census. In: *Statistical Abstract of the United States.* 14th ed. Washington, DC: US Bureau of the Census; 1994:95.
10. García Rodríguez LA, Wallander MA, Tolosa LB, Johansson S. Chronic obstructive pulmonary disease in UK primary care: incidence and risk factors. *COPD.* 2009;6(5):369–379.
11. Anthonisen NR, Manfreda J, Warren CPW, et al. Antibiotic therapy in exacerbations of chronic obstructive lung disease. *Ann Intern Med.* 1987;106:196–204.
12. Nseir S, Di Pompeo C, Cavestri B, et al. Multiple-drug-resistant bacteria in patients with severe acute exacerbation of chronic obstructive pulmonary disease: prevalence, risk factors, and outcome. *Crit Care Med.* 2006;34(12):2959–2966.
13. Soler N, Torres A, Ewig S, et al. Bronchial microbial patterns in severe exacerbations of chronic obstructive pulmonary disease (COPD) requiring mechanical ventilation. *Am J Respir Crit Care Med.* 1998;157:1498–1505.
14. Eller J, Ede A, Schaberg T, et al. Infective exacerbations of chronic bronchitis: relation between bacteriologic etiology and lung function. *Chest.* 1998;113:1542–1548.
15. Miravitlles M, Espinosa C, Fernandez-Laso E, et al. Relationship between bacterial flora in sputum and functional impairment in patients with acute exacerbations of COPD. *Chest.* 1999;116:40–46.
16. Saint S, Vittinghoff E, Grady D. Antibiotics in chronic obstructive pulmonary disease exacerbations. A meta-analysis. *J Am Med Assoc.* 1995;273:957–960.
17. Ball P, Harris JM, Lowson D, et al. Acute infective exacerbations of chronic bronchitis. *Q J Med.* 1995;88:61–68.
18. Derenne JP, Fleury B, Parienta R. Acute respiratory failure of chronic obstructive lung disease. *Am Rev Respir Dis.* 1998;138:1006–1033.
19. Seneff MG, Wagner DP, Wagner RP, et al. Hospital and 1-year survival of patients admitted to intensive care units with acute exacerbation of chronic obstructive lung disease. *J Am Med Assoc.* 1999;274:1852–1857.
20. Lode H. Respiratory tract infections: when is antibiotic therapy indicated? *Clin Ther.* 1991;13:149–156.
21. Balter NS, Hyland RH, Low DE, et al. Recommendations on the management of chronic bronchitis. *Can Med Assoc J.* 1994;151(suppl):7–23.
22. Wilson R. Outcome predictors in bronchitis. *Chest.* 1995;108(suppl):53–57.
23. National Center for Health Statistics. National hospital discharge survey: annual summary 1990. *Vital Health Statistics.* 1998;13:1–225.
24. Niederman MS, McCombs JS, Unger AN, et al. The cost of treating community-acquired pneumonia. *Clin Ther.* 1998;20:820–837.
25. Foy HM, Cooney MK, Allan I, et al. Rates of pneumonia during influenza epidemics in Seattle, 1964 to 1975. *J Am Med Assoc.* 1979;241:253–258.
26. Jokinen C, Heiskanen L, Juvonen H, et al. Incidence of community-acquired pneumonia in the population of four municipalities in eastern Finland. *Am J Epidemiol.* 1993;137:977–988.
27. Koivula I, Sten M, Makela PH. Risk factors for pneumonia in the elderly. *Am J Med.* 1994;96:313–320.
28. Sankilampi U, Herva E, Haikala R, et al. Epidemiology of invasive *Streptococcus pneumoniae* infections in adults in Finland. *Epidemiol Infect.* 1997;118:7–15.
29. Nielsen SV, Henrichsen J. Incidence of invasive pneumococcal disease and distribution of capsular types of pneumococci in Denmark, 1989–94. *Epidemiol Infect.* 1996;117:411–416.
30. Bartlett JG, O'Keefe P, Tally FP, et al. Bacteriology of hospital-acquired pneumonia. *Arch Intern Med.* 1986;146:868–871.
31. de Roux A, Ewig S, García E, et al. Mixed community-acquired pneumonia in hospitalised patients. *Eur Respir J.* 2006;27(4):795–800.
32. Marrie TJ. Community-acquired pneumonia. *Clin Infect Dis.* 1994;18:501–515.
33. Moine P, Vercken J-B, Chevret S, et al. Severe community-acquired pneumonia: etiology, epidemiology and prognostic factors. *Chest.* 1994;105:1487–1495.
34. Fine MJ, Smith MA, Carson CA, et al. Prognosis and outcomes of patients with community-acquired pneumonia. *J Am Med Assoc.* 1996;275:134–141.

35. Marston BJ, Plouffe JF, File TM, et al. Incidence of community-acquired pneumonia requiring hospitalization. *Arch Intern Med*. 1997;157:1709–1718.

36. Troy CJ, Peeling RW, Ellis AG, et al. *Chlamydia pneumoniae as* a new source of infectious outbreaks in nursing homes. *J Am Med Assoc*. 1997;277:1214–1218.

37. Pachon J, Prados MD, Capote F, et al. A. Severe community-acquired pneumonia: etiology, prognosis and treatment. *Am Rev Respir Dis*. 1990;142:369–373.

38. Johanson Jr WG, Pierce AK, Sanford JP, Thomas GD. Nosocomial respiratory infections with gram-negative bacilli. *Ann Intern Med*. 1972;77:701–706.

39. Woodhead MA, Arrowsmith J, Chamberlain-Webber R, et al. The value of routine microbial investigation in community-acquired pneumonia. *Respir Med*. 1991;85:313–317.

40. Farr BM, Kaiser DL, Harrison BDW, et al. Prediction of microbial aetiology at admission to hospital for pneumonia from the presenting clinical features. *Thorax*. 1989;44:1031–1035.

41. Spiteri MA, Cook DG, Clarke SW. Reliability of eliciting physical signs in examination of the chest. *Lancet*. 1988;1:873–875.

42. Fine MJ, Auble TE, Yealy DM, et al. A prediction rule to identify low-risk patients with community-acquired pneumonia. *N Engl J Med*. 1997;336:243–250.

43. Anevlavis S, Petroglou N, Tzavaras A, et al. A prospective study of the diagnostic utility of sputum Gram stain in pneumonia. *J Infect*. 2009;59(2):83–89.

44. Geckler RW, McAllister K, Gremillion DH, et al. Clinical value of paired sputum and transtracheal aspirates in the initial management of pneumonia. *Chest*. 1985;87:631–635.

45. Barrett-Connor E. The nonvalue of sputum culture in the diagnosis of pneumococcal pneumonia. *Am Rev Respir Dis*. 1971;103:845–848.

46. Woodhead. Prospective study of the aetiology and outcome of pneumonia in the community. *Lancet*. 1987;1(8534):671–674.

47. Chan YR, Morris A. Molecular diagnostic methods in pneumonia. *Curr Opin Infect Dis*. 2007;20(2):157–164.

48. Sahn SA. Management of complicated parapneumonic effusions. *Am Rev Respir Dis*. 1993;148:813–817.

49. Auble TE, Yealy DM, Fine MJ. Assessing prognosis and selecting an initial site of care for adults with community-acquired pneumonia. *Infect Dis Clin North Am*. 1998;12:741–759.

50. Carratalà J, Fernández-Sabé N, Ortega L, et al. Outpatient care compared with hospitalization for community-acquired pneumonia: a randomized trial in low-risk patients. *Ann Intern Med*. 2005;142(3):165–172.

51. Mandell LA, Wunderink RG, Anzueto A, et al. Infectious Diseases Society of America; American Thoracic Society. Infectious Diseases Society of America/American Thoracic Society consensus guidelines on the management of community-acquired pneumonia in adults. *Clin Infect Dis*. 2007;44(suppl 2): S27–S72.

52. Woodhead M, Blasi F, Ewig S, et al. European Respiratory Society; European Society of Clinical Microbiology and Infectious Diseases. Guidelines for the management of adult lower respiratory tract infections. *Eur Respir J*. 2005;26(6):1138–1180.

53. American Thoracic Society. Guidelines for the management of adults with community-acquired pneumonia: diagnosis, assessment of severity, antimicrobial therapy and prevention. *Am J Respir Crit Care Med*. 2001;163:1730–1754.

54. Lim WS, Baudouin SV, George RC, et al. Pneumonia Guidelines Committee of the BTS Standards of Care Committee. BTS guidelines for the management of community acquired pneumonia in adults: update 2009. *Thorax*. 2009;64(suppl 3):iii1–iii55.

55. CLSI. *Performance standards for antimicrobial susceptibility testing, 16th informational supplement*. Document M100-S15. Wayne, PA: Clinical and Laboratory Standards Institute; 2008.

56. Ferrandiz MJ, Fernoll A, Linares J, de La Campa AG. Horizontal transfer of parC and parA in fluoroquinolone-resistant clinical isolates of *Streptococcus pneumoniae*. *Antimicrob Agents Chemother*. 2000;44:840–847.

57. Johnston NJ, deAzavedo JC, Kellner JD, et al. Prevalence and characterization of the mechanisms of macrolide, lincosamide, and streptogramin resistance in *Streptococcus pneumoniae* from across Canada. In: Program and abstracts of the 37th Interscience Conference on Antimicrobial Agents and Chemotherapy, Toronto, Ontario, Canada, Sept 28–Oct 1, 1997. Abstract C–77a; 1997.

58. Kelley MA, Weber DJ, Gilligan P, et al. Breakthrough pneumococcal bacteremia in patients being treated with azithromycin and clarithromycin. *Clin Infect Dis*. 2000;31:1008–1011.

59. Wise R, Brenwald N, Gill M, et al. *Streptococcus pneumoniae* resistance to fluoroquinolones [letter]. *Lancet*. 1996;348:1660.

60. Kohler T, Pechere JC. Bacterial resistance to quinolones. In: Andriole VT, ed. *The Quinolones*. San Diego: Academic Press; 1998:117–142.

61. Whitney CG, Farley MM, Hadler J, et al. Active Bacterial Core Surveillance Program of the Emerging Infections Program Network. Increasing prevalence of multidrug-resistant *Streptococcus pneumoniae* in the United States. *N Engl J Med*. 2000;343(26):1917–1924.

62. Vanderkooi OG, Low DE, Green K, Powis JE, McGeer A. Toronto Invasive Bacterial Disease Network. Predicting antimicrobial resistance in invasive pneumococcal infections. *Clin Infect Dis*. 2005;40(9):1288–1297.

63. Tleyjeh IM, Tlaygeh HM, Hejal R, Montori VM, Baddour LM. The impact of penicillin resistance on short-term mortality in hospitalized adults with pneumococcal pneumonia: a systematic review and meta-analysis. *Clin Infect Dis*. 2006;42(6):788–797.

64. Livermore DM. Beta-lactamases in laboratory and clinical resistance. *Clin Microbiol Rev*. 1995;8:557–584.

65. Brown PD. Adherence to guidelines for community-acquired pneumonia: does it decrease cost of care? *Pharmacoeconomics*. 2004;22(7):413–420.

66. Arnold FW, LaJoie AS, Brock GN, et al. Community-Acquired Pneumonia Organization (CAPO) Investigators. Improving outcomes in elderly patients with community-acquired pneumonia by adhering to national guidelines: Community-Acquired Pneumonia Organization International cohort study results. *Arch Intern Med*. 2009;169(16):1515–1524.

67. Meehan TP, Fine MJ, Krumholz HM, et al. Quality of care, process and outcomes in elderly patients with pneumonia. *J Am Med Assoc*. 1997;278:2080–2084.

68. Venditti M, Falcone M, Corrao S, Licata G, Serra P. Study Group of the Italian Society of Internal Medicine. Outcomes of patients hospitalized with community-acquired, health care-associated, and hospital-acquired pneumonia. *Ann Intern Med*. 2009;150(1):19–26.

69. Loeb M, McGeer A, McArthur M, Walter S, et al. Risk factors for pneumonia and other lower respiratory tract infections in elderly residents of long-term care facilities. *Arch Intern Med*. 1999;159:2058–2064.

70. Mills K, Graham AC, Winslow BT, Springer KL. Treatment of nursing home-acquired pneumonia. *Am Fam Physician*. 2009;79(11):976–982.

71. American Thoracic Society. Guidelines for the management of adults with hospital-acquired, ventilator-associated, and healthcare-associated pneumonia. *Am J Respir Crit Care Med*. 2005;171:388–416.

72. Craven DE, Steger KA, LaForce FM. Pneumonia. In: Bennett JV, Brachman PS, eds. *Hospital Infections*. 4th ed. Philadelphia: Lippincott-Raven Press.

73. Loeb M, Mandell LA. Microbiology of hospital-acquired pneumonia. *Semin Respir Crit Care Med*. 1997;18:111–120.

74. Reusser P, Zimmerli W, Scheidegger D, et al. Role of gastric colonization in nosocomial infections and endotoxemia: a prospective study in neurosurgical patients on mechanical ventilation. *J Infect Dis*. 1989;160:414–421.

75. Bonten MJM, Gaillard CA, van der Geest S, et al. The role of intragastric acidity and stress ulcer prophylaxis on colonization and infection in mechanically ventilated ICU patients: a stratified, randomized double-blind study of sucralfate versus antacids. *Am J Respir Crit Care Med*. 1997;152:1825–1834.

76. Stoutenbeek CP, van Saene HKF. Nonantibiotic measures in the prevention of ventilator-associated pneumonia. *Semin Respir Infect*. 1997;12:294–299.

77. Inglis TJJ, Millar MR, Jones JG, et al. Tracheal tube biofilm as a source of bacterial colonization of the lung. *J Clin Microbiol*. 1989;27:2014–2018.

78. Fagen J. Invasive and noninvasive strategies for management of suspected VAP. *Ann Intern Med*. 2000;132:621–630.

79. American Thoracic Society. Hospital-acquired pneumonia in adults: diagnosis, assessment of severity, initial antimicrobial therapy, and preventative strategies. *Am J Respir Crit Care Med*. 1996;153:1711–1725.

80. Mandell LA, Marrie TJ, Niederman MS, the Canadian Hospital Acquired Pneumonia Consensus Conference Group. Initial antimicrobial treatment of hospital-acquired pneumonia in adults: a conference report. *Can J Infect Dis*. 1993;4:317–321.

81. Hilf M, Yu VL, Sharp J, et al. Antibiotic therapy for *Pseudomonas aeruginosa* bacteremia: outcome correlations in a prospective study of 200 patients. *Am J Med*. 1989;87:540–546.

82. Chow JW, Fine MJ, Shlaes DM, et al. *Enterobacter* bacteremia: clinical features and emergence of antibiotic resistance during therapy. *Ann Intern Med*. 1991;115:585–590.

Endocarditis

Kate Gould

Endocarditis is traditionally defined as an inflammation of the endothelial lining of the heart which usually results in the formation of 'vegetations' – platelet and fibrin aggregates which can enlarge to several centimeters in diameter. Endocarditis is most frequently infective in origin, and the definition has been expanded to include infection of intracardiac prosthetic material such as valves, patches, conduits, pacemaker/defibrillator leads and ventricular assist devices.

Estimates of the incidence of this condition vary but recent estimates based on Duke criteria[1] suggest that it is approximately 1 case per million of the population per year. The epidemiology of the condition is changing with a shift away from native valve endocarditis secondary to rheumatic heart disease cause by α-hemolytic streptococci to prosthetic endocarditis caused by staphylococci.

Treatment outcome and the requirement from surgery are also variable, depending on the patient, site of infection and the infecting organism. The most successful outcomes tend to be in right-sided endocarditis and the worst with fungal or enterococcal endocarditis.

William Osler first described 'malignant endocarditis' during the Gulstonian lecture in 1885.[2] At that time, the only treatment that could be offered was bed rest and serum from horses injected with the infecting bacteria. Following the discovery of penicillin there was hope of a cure, but it became clear that very high doses were needed, and even then there was a high risk of relapse when the antibiotic was stopped.

There followed an era of in-vitro and in-vivo experimentation from which the fundamental principles of therapy were determined.

The pathophysiology of endocarditis is such that the infecting micro-organisms are situated in the middle of a vegetation attached to a structure that has no blood supply. Thus, in order to reach these organisms, any therapeutic agent has to diffuse into the vegetation from the blood passing over it. In order to eradicate the infection, the therapeutic agent must also be bactericidal, since the body's usual host defence mechanisms may not penetrate into the vegetation.

The in-vivo experiments[3] determined that in a rabbit model at least four times the minimum bactericidal concentration (MBC) of an agent was required in the serum to diffuse into a vegetation, and that antibiotic peaks and troughs were more successful than continuous dosing.

In-vitro experiments demonstrated that for some Gram-positive bacteria, penicillin, although having a minimum inhibitory concentration (MIC) well within the sensitive range, was not cidal.[4] This phenomenon was labeled as 'tolerance', but further work determined that in the majority of cases kill could be achieved by adding streptomycin and, latterly, gentamicin.

Current endocarditis treatment guidelines[5,6] are still centered on these basic principles since very few evidence-based studies have been performed. This is despite the availability of newer agents which have superior pharmacokinetics to benzylpenicillin. Similarly, oral therapies with agents which have good bioavailability and achieve satisfactory serum levels are rarely recommended outwith pediatrics.

Recommendations for duration of therapy vary. For right-sided endocarditis, and for left-sided endocarditis with small vegetations, 14-day regimens have been used successfully, but there is little evidence to support why longer treatments are necessary in other cases.

LABORATORY INVESTIGATIONS

Full identification of all isolates – if necessary with the assistance of a reference laboratory – is mandatory in endocarditis. Routine antibiotic testing for a wide range of agents should be followed by formal MIC testing. The method by which the MIC is determined is not important so long as it is adequately controlled.

Unfortunately, although the MBC is important in endocarditis, it is technically difficult to perform in a routine diagnostic setting, creating problems with reproducibility.

The ability to perform high-level susceptibility testing for gentamicin and streptomycin is also important.

ANTIBIOTICS

β-LACTAMS

Traditionally, if sensitive, penicillin has been the β-lactam of choice to treat endocarditis. The advantage is that it is narrow spectrum and MICs are generally very low. The disadvantages are that it has a short serum half-life (<4 h), necessitating 4-hourly dosing regimens which are impracticable outside the intensive care arena. Benzylpenicillin also has a high sodium load which can be an issue in the elderly or patients with concomitant heart failure. It should also be remembered that given in high dose, especially in patients with renal impairment, penicillin can be neurotoxic.

There is no logical reason why other β-lactams such as ampicillin/amoxicillin or cephalosporins cannot be used in preference to benzylpenicillin.

GLYCOPEPTIDES

Glycopeptides are used as an alternative to β-lactams for patients with hypersensitivity to penicillin or who are infected with resistant bacteria. Glycopeptides are only slowly bactericidal, if at all, so must always be used in combination with another agent. Vancomycin is currently the glycopeptide of choice and in patients with normal renal function 1 g every 12 h should be used initially. Dosage can then be modified according to trough level, normally 10–15 mg/L, but increasing to 15–20 mg/L for staphylococcal isolates with an MIC ≥2 mg/L. Teicoplanin may be considered for streptococcal endocarditis but at an initial dosage of at least 10 mg/kg every 12 h, then 10 mg/kg per day. As pharmacokinetics are unpredictable, levels must be measured at least weekly to ensure trough levels of at least 20 mg/L.

The role of the newer long-acting glycopeptides in the treatment of endocarditis has yet to be determined.

AMINOGLYCOSIDES

Animal studies have demonstrated the efficacy of combination therapy based on the traditional 8-hourly or 12-hourly regimens at a dose of 1 mg/kg. There is no evidence to suggest that once-daily gentamicin would be less effective but authorities are reluctant to recommend it on the basis that in some patients there may be a significant time period when serum levels are below 1 mg/L. Either way, levels should be monitored at least twice weekly, and more frequently in patients with renal impairment or who are on concomitant therapy with other nephrotoxic drugs.

OTHER ANTIBIOTICS

Guideline recommendations are just that: recommendations which may need to be modified for individual patients. Controlled trials are few but a recent study of daptomycin[7] to treat staphylococcal bacteremia did include some patients with endocarditis. There are numerous case reports which have documented the successful use of quinolones, linezolid, rifampicin (rifampin), clindamycin and co-trimoxazole for a range of infecting bacteria.

EMPIRICAL THERAPY (Table 46.1)

For some patients who have an indolent presentation, it may be possible to delay antibiotics until the results of blood cultures are available. In practice this is rarely possible and therapy must be commenced immediately.

Table 46.1 Empirical therapy

Acute presentation	Flucloxacillin (8–12 g i.v. per day in 4–6 divided doses), *plus* gentamicin (1 mg/kg i.v. every 8 h, modified according to renal function)
Indolent presentation	Penicillin (7.2 g i.v. per day in six divided doses) or ampicillin/amoxicillin (2 g i.v. every 6 h), *plus* gentamicin (1 mg/kg i.v. every 8 h, modified according to renal function)
Penicillin allergy Intracardiac prosthesis Suspected methicillin-resistant *Staphylococcus aureus*	Vancomycin (1 g i.v. every 12 h, modified according to renal function), *plus* rifampicin (300–600 mg p.o. every 12 h), *plus* gentamicin (1 mg/kg i.v. every 8 h, modified according to renal function)

PROSTHETIC DEVICE ENDOCARDITIS

Prosthetic device endocarditis presents the greatest challenge for medical therapy since not only is it necessary to combat micro-organisms within a vegetation, they may also form part of a biofilm. Surgical intervention may need to be considered early, treatment may need to be more prolonged and antibiotic combinations that include agents active in biofilms may be more effective. Unfortunately, owing to the lack of robust clinical data, recommendations are based on the 'best guess' approach and expert advice should be sought for individual cases.

STAPHYLOCOCCAL ENDOCARDITIS (Table 46.2)

The choice of antibiotic will depend on the sensitivity of the infecting strain. There is no evidence that adding gentamicin to flucloxacillin offers any benefit when treating methicillin-sensitive strains of *Staph. aureus* and is associated with an increase in adverse events. The addition of sodium fusidate or rifampicin is also not recommended.

Table 46.2 Antibiotic therapy for staphylococcal endocarditis

Methicillin sensitive	Flucloxacillin (2 g i.v. every 4–6 h)
Methicillin resistant/ penicillin allergy	Vancomycin (1 g i.v. every 12 h, modified according to renal function), *plus* rifampicin (300–600 mg p.o. every 12 h), *or* gentamicin (1 mg/kg i.v. every 8 h, modified according to renal function), *or* sodium fusidate (500 mg p.o. every 8 h)
Endocarditis in presence of intracardiac prosthesis	Flucloxacillin (2 g i.v. every 4–6 h) or vancomycin (1 g i.v. every 12 h, modified according to renal function), *plus* rifampicin (300–600 mg p.o. every 12 h), *and/or* gentamicin (1 mg/kg i.v. every 8 h, modified according to renal function), *and/or* sodium fusidate (500 mg p.o. every 8 h)

If vancomycin is used, the addition of a second agent is required. The choice depends on the sensitivity profile of the infecting organism. Teicoplanin is not recommended for staphylococcal endocarditis.

There are published case series which suggest that right-sided endocarditis can be successfully treated with either 14 days of intravenous therapy or 28 days of oral therapy. Examples of regimens include flucloxacillin alone, flucloxacillin plus rifampicin and quinolones.

STREPTOCOCCAL ENDOCARDITIS (Table 46.3)

With a few provisos (size of vegetation, septic emboli, intracardiac prosthetic material), endocarditis caused by streptococci with an MIC ≤0.1 mg/L for penicillin can be successfully treated with 14 days of combination therapy of a β-lactam plus gentamicin. For less sensitive strains, 14 days of combination therapy followed by a further 14 days of a β-lactam is recommended.

Endocarditis caused by *Streptococcus pneumoniae* is associated with a high mortality and has been ascribed to patient factors rather than antibiotic failure. Penicillin-resistant strains should be managed in the same way as enterococcal endocarditis.

Group B streptococcal endocarditis is frequently associated with diabetes and has a high mortality. Tolerance has been described in some strains, so 28 days of treatment, including 14 days of combination therapy with gentamicin, is recommended.

Str. gallolyticus (*bovis*) endocarditis is associated with underlying gut pathology and liver disease and so a potential source should be sought. It should be treated according to its MIC for penicillin.

Nutritionally dependent streptococci are difficult to grow and appear tolerant to β-lactams, thus 28 days of combination therapy is usually advocated. For especially slow-growing isolates, treatment may need to be extended to 6 weeks.

For patients with documented penicillin allergy, a glycopeptide is generally advocated, but a carbapenem or daptomycin may also be considered.

ENTEROCOCCAL ENDOCARDITIS

Enterococci are usually tolerant to antibiotics and the range of available agents is more limited (Table 46.4), particularly for glycopeptide resistant strains. The use of new agents such as linezolid or daptomycin could potentially be life-saving in these circumstances.

Prolonged therapy (6–12 weeks) may be necessary, and relapse is not uncommon. For isolates with high-level gentamicin resistance, streptomycin should be used as an alternative if the organism is sensitive. For glycopeptide-resistant isolates, daptomycin should be used.

 ## OTHER BACTERIA

Choice of agents and duration of therapy will vary according to the infecting organism. Difficulties obviously arise when the diagnosis is made by serology, as sensitivity testing cannot be performed.

Table 46.3 Antibiotic therapy of streptococcal endocarditis[a]

Penicillin MIC (mg/L)	Penicillin or vancomycin and gentamicin 4 weeks	Penicillin 4 weeks	Ceftriaxone 4 weeks	Vancomycin or penicillin 4 weeks and gentamicin 2 weeks	Penicillin 4–6 weeks and gentamicin 4–6 weeks	Vancomycin 4–6 weeks and gentamicin 4–6 weeks
≤0.1	✓	✓	✓			
≥0.1–<0.5				✓		
0.5–<16					✓	✓
≥16						✓

[a]For dosages please refer to Tables 46.1, 46.2 and 46.4.

Table 46.4 Treatment of enterococcal endocarditis

Antimicrobial regimen	Dose and route	Duration (weeks)	Comments
Ampicillin or penicillin, *plus* gentamicin	2 g i.v. every 4 h (2.4 g every 4 h) 1 mg/kg i.v. every 8–12 h	≥4 ≥4	
Vancomycin, *plus* gentamicin, *or* streptomycin	1 g i.v. every 12 h 1 mg/kg i.v. every 8–12 h 7.5 mg/kg every 12 h	≥4	Alternative for penicillin-allergic patient provided isolate is vancomycin susceptible (MIC ≤4 mg/L)
Daptomycin	4–8 mg once daily	≥4	For glycopeptide-resistant strains

For fastidious Gram-negative bacteria, known as the 'HACEK'[8] group, initial therapy with ampicillin/amoxicillin plus gentamicin would be appropriate. If the infecting organism is ampicillin/amoxicillin resistant, consider ceftriaxone, a carbapenem, or another class of antibiotic according to sensitivity.

It has been estimated that *Coxiella burnetii* accounts for up to 5% of cases of endocarditis worldwide. A combination of doxycycline and a quinolone is recommended as first-line treatment, and this must be continued until titers return to normal. Patients should be followed up for at least 2 years.

FUNGAL ENDOCARDITIS

Fungal endocarditis is a rare and devastating condition which usually requires surgical intervention.

Ideally the antifungal agent(s) should be cidal, and as with bacterial endocarditis, the choice of agent will depend on the sensitivity of the strain of fungus implicated.

Amphotericin B plus flucytosine are traditionally the agents of first choice for *Candida*, although both are toxic. High-dose fluconazole (400 mg every 12 h) could be considered as second-line therapy, but it is only fungistatic. Caspofungin is fungicidal, but experience with its use in endocarditis is limited.

For other fungal species voriconazole or caspofungin should be considered as first-line empirical therapy.

PREVENTION OF ENDOCARDITIS

The role of antibiotics in the prevention of endocarditis is controversial. Over the past 5 years there has been a paradigm shift away from universal prophylaxis for at-risk patients undergoing dentistry due to lack of evidence for its efficacy.[9] Some authorities (UK and USA) have taken a more cautious approach, limiting prophylaxis to only those patients for whom endocarditis would carry a higher mortality, for example those who have had previous endocarditis or who have intracardiac prostheses.[10,11] For these reasons, readers should refer to their local guidelines for further information.

Nevertheless, it should not be forgotten that individuals with structural cardiac abnormalities or devices are at higher risk of endocarditis than those with 'normal' hearts. When undergoing surgical procedures requiring antibiotic prophylaxis for surgical site infection, special consideration should be given to the risk of enterococcal bacteremia and the prophylactic regimen adjusted accordingly.

 ## References

1. Durack DT, Lukes AS, Bright DK. New criteria for diagnosis of infective endocarditis: utilization of specific echocardiographic findings. Duke Endocarditis Service. *Am J Med.* 1994;96:200–209.
2. Pruitt RD. William Osler and his Gulstonian lectures on malignant endocarditis. *Mayo Clin Proc.* 1982;57:4–9.
3. Wright AJ, Wilson WR. Experimental animal endocarditis. *Mayo Clin Proc.* 1982;57:10–14.
4. Fantin B, Carbon C. In vivo antibiotic synergism: contribution of animal models. *Antimicrob Agents Chemother.* 1998;36:907–912.
5. Elliott TSJ, Foweraker J, Gould FK, Perry JD, Sandoe JAT. Guidelines for the antibiotic treatment of endocarditis in adults: report of the Working Party of the British Society for Antimicrobial Chemotherapy. *J Antimicrob Chemother.* 2004;54:971–981.
6. Nishimura RA, Carabello BA, Faxon DP, et al. Guideline update on valvular heart disease: focused update on infective endocarditis. A report of the American College of Cardiology/American Heart Association Task Force on Practice Guidelines. *J Am Coll Cardiol.* 2008;52:676–685.
7. Fowler Jr VG, Boucher HW, Corey GR, et al. Daptomycin versus standard therapy for bacteremia and endocarditis caused by Staphylococcus aureus. *N Engl J Med.* 2006;355(7):653–665.
8. Wilson WR, Karchmer AW, Dajani AS, et al. Antibiotic treatment of adults with infective endocarditis due to streptococci, enterococci, staphylococci and HACEK microorganisms. *J Am Med Assoc.* 1995;274(21):1706–1713.
9. National Institute for Health and Clinical Excellence. *Prophylaxis against infective endocarditis. Antimicrobial prophylaxis against infective endocarditis in adults and children undergoing interventional procedures.* NICE Clinical Guideline 64 Online. Available at. London: NICE; 2008. http://www.nice.org.uk/nicemedia/pdf/CG64NICEguidance.pdf.
10. Gould FK, Elliott TSJ, Foweraker J, et al. Guidelines for the prevention of endocarditis: report of the Working Party of the British Society for Antimicrobial Chemotherapy. *J Antimicrob Chemother.* 2006;57:1035–1042.
11. Wilson W, Taubert KA, Gewitz M, et al. American Heart Association Rheumatic Fever, Endocarditis and Kawasaki Disease Committee. Prevention of endocarditis: a guideline from the American Heart Association. *Circulation.* 2007;116(15):736–754.

47 Infections of the gastrointestinal tract

Peter Moss

Infectious diseases may affect any part of the gastrointestinal tract from the mouth to the anus. Most infections of the mouth, oropharynx and esophagus are caused either by commensal organisms or by opportunist pathogens. These infections are usually secondary to underlying problems, either local (e.g. poor oral hygiene, malignancy) or systemic (particularly immunosuppression). Infections of the stomach are relatively unusual, with the exception of *Helicobacter pylori*, which is associated with peptic ulceration and gastric neoplasms. It is infections of the lower gastrointestinal tract, the small and large bowel, which are of the greatest clinical significance.

Intestinal infections usually present with diarrhea, sometimes accompanied by vomiting, abdominal pain and fever. In severe cases there may be dehydration, hypovolemic shock and renal failure. Persistent infection may cause anorexia and weight loss. Gastroenteritis may be caused by viruses, bacteria, protozoa or (rarely) by helminths. Symptoms and signs may be produced by one or more of a number of different pathological mechanisms. The clinical presentation of gastroenteritis rarely allows a specific diagnosis, and it is not usually possible to identify the causative organism, at least in the early stages of illness. Management is therefore usually empirical and is based on the recognition of common clinical syndromes. These include acute watery diarrhea, dysentery, persistent diarrhea with or without malabsorption, and enteric fever. Identification of these patterns, along with a knowledge of the likely pathogens in a particular location and patient population, will guide treatment in most cases.

EPIDEMIOLOGY

Gastroenteritis causing diarrhea with or without vomiting is the second most common infectious cause of death worldwide (behind lower respiratory tract infection). Although oral rehydration programs have cut the death toll significantly, it is estimated that over 2 million people die every year as a direct result of diarrheal disease.[1] Gastroenteritis is a major cause of morbidity as well as mortality, with a disease burden of 160 million disability-adjusted life years (DALY) worldwide.[1] The main burden falls on the poorest countries, where children can expect on average 3–6 bouts of infective diarrhea every year, and 15–20% of deaths under the age of 5 are due to diarrheal disease.[2] In the Western world gastroenteritis is both less common and less likely to cause death, but it remains an important cause of morbidity and mortality. In Europe diarrheal disease is responsible for 39 000 deaths per year, and results in a burden of over three million DALY annually.[1]

Viral gastroenteritis is a common cause of diarrhea and vomiting in young children in both developed and developing countries, but is less often seen in adults. The viruses responsible (principally rotavirus, norovirus and enteric adenoviruses) are spread from person to person, mainly by the feco-oral route, but also as an aerosol. Seasonal outbreaks are seen in developed countries, and in comparison with other diarrheal diseases there is less association with poverty and poor hygiene.

The main cause of adult gastroenteritis is bacterial infection. In developed countries this is often related to food poisoning, a problem exacerbated by modern methods of food production and the globalization of food supply. In less developed areas transmission is frequently by the direct feco-oral route or from a contaminated water supply. Massive water-borne outbreaks may occur, especially in association with natural disasters or war. Protozoal and helminthic gut infections are rare in the West but are widespread in developing countries.

In all parts of the world it is children who are at most risk of catching diarrheal disease and at most risk of dying from it. Mortality is mainly related to dehydration, although other factors such as malnutrition are important in developing countries. Elderly people are also at increased risk of complications from gastroenteritis. In the developed world certain other groups have a higher incidence of diarrheal disease: these include travelers to developing countries, the immunocompromised (especially in HIV infection) and infants in daycare facilities.

PATHOGENESIS OF ENTERIC INFECTION

Micro-organisms with the potential to cause enteric infection are ubiquitous, and the development of disease depends on a number of host and microbial factors:

- Host factors include age and general health, personal hygiene, specific and non-specific immunity, and composition of normal intestinal microflora.
- Microbial factors include a number of virulence traits which determine the pathogenic mechanisms responsible for causing gastrointestinal infection.

Bacteria can cause diarrhea in three different ways: mucosal adherence, toxin production and mucosal invasion (Table 47.1). Many species employ more than one of these methods. In most cases the first step in the pathogenic process is adherence to the intestinal mucosa, the exception being those bacteria which secrete toxin in food before consumption. A number of different molecular adhesion mechanisms have been elaborated, typically involving microbial cell surface proteins (often located on pili or fimbriae) which bind to specific host glycoproteins. Expression of many of these adhesion proteins is encoded by transmissible plasmids. Usually attachment to the mucosa is merely the prelude to invasion or toxin production, but a few organisms such as enteropathogenic *Escherichia coli* can produce mucosal damage and secretory diarrhea directly as a result of adherence.[3]

Some bacteria, having attached to the intestinal mucosa, simply colonize the surface epithelium. Others, such as *Shigella* species and the invasive strains of *Esch. coli*, penetrate and destroy the cells of the intestinal mucosa. Many different mechanisms may be involved in the invasive process, including attachment to transmembrane glycoproteins, production of cytotoxic exotoxins, and deliberate induction of host inflammatory response.[4] Invasion leads to destruction of the epithelial cells and produces the typical symptoms of dysentery: low volume bloody diarrhea with abdominal pain.

Many bacterial enteric pathogens produce symptoms by means of toxin production. Gastroenteritis can be caused by three different types of bacterial toxin:

- Enterotoxins induce excessive fluid secretion into the bowel lumen without physically damaging the mucosa.
- Neurotoxins affect the autonomic nervous system, causing diarrhea and vomiting.
- Cytotoxins damage the intestinal mucosa and, in some cases, vascular endothelium as well.

Usually these toxins are produced by bacteria adhering to the intestinal epithelium, but neurotoxins (often stable to heat and gastric acid) may be elaborated exogenously by pathogens in poorly prepared food.

The pathogenic mechanisms underlying viral gastroenteritis are less well understood. The initial event is again adhesion, a viral capsid protein binding to specific glycolipid receptors in the mucosal cell membrane. This is followed by invasion, mainly of mature villus epithelial cells in the small intestine. A direct cytopathic effect leads to cell death, causing villus shortening, relative loss of absorptive epithelial cells relative to secretory crypt cells, and decreased production of intestinal disaccharidases.[5] In some cases (such as infection with Norwalk virus) there is significant mucosal inflammation, while in others (including rotavirus infection) there is little host inflammatory response. Diarrhea is probably produced by a combination of secretory/resorptive imbalance and disaccharide/fat malabsorption (which may persist for some time following acute infection).

Protozoa can cause diarrhea by both invasive and non-invasive mechanisms. *Entamoeba histolytica* (and probably *Balantidium coli*) attaches to the colonic mucosa by specific binding proteins. It then causes local destruction of the epithelium by a combination of lytic enzyme release and phagocytosis, leading to the clinical symptoms of dysentery.[6] *Giardia lamblia* (*intestinalis*), by contrast, is very rarely invasive. The parasite attaches to the duodenal and jejunal mucosa using a combination of mechanical and molecular bonds. Local disruption of the brush border ensues, with disaccharidase deficiency. There may also be more extensive damage to the epithelium with partial villous atrophy and inflammatory infiltrates; this is probably due to a cellular immune response to infection.[7] Several different pathogenic mechanisms may be important in the production of diarrhea by *Cryptosporidium parvum* (depending in part on the integrity of the host immune system), while the role of other parasites such as *Dientamoeba fragilis* and *Blastocystis hominis* in causing gastroenteritis remains unclear.

Although helminthic infection of the gut is very common, it rarely causes significant enteric symptoms. Schistosomal colitis can result from the inflammatory response to parasite eggs lodged in the bowel wall, and some nematodes (notably *Trichuris trichiura*) may cause symptoms due to superficial invasion of the colonic mucosa. Heavy worm infestations may cause mechanical problems such as obstruction or prolapse.

Table 47.1 Pathogenic mechanisms of bacterial gastroenteritis

Mechanism	Mode of action	Clinical presentation	Examples
Mucosal adherence	Effacement of intestinal mucosa	Moderate watery diarrhea	Enteropathogenic *Esch. coli*
Toxin production			
Neurotoxin	Paralysis of autonomic nervous system	Short-lived, profuse watery diarrhea and vomiting	*Bacillus cereus*
Enterotoxin	Fluid secretion without mucosal damage	Variable diarrhea ± vomiting	*Vibrio cholerae*
Cytotoxin	Damage to mucosa	Bloody diarrhea	Enterohemorrhagic *Esch. coli*
Mucosal invasion	Penetration and destruction of mucosa	Dysentery	*Shigella* spp.

SYNDROMIC MANAGEMENT OF GASTROENTERITIS

SYNDROMES

ACUTE WATERY DIARRHEA

Acute, self-limiting, watery diarrhea is the most common form of gastroenteritis. It is produced by direct or toxin-mediated damage to the secretory and absorptive gut mucosal cells, and may be caused by a number of different pathogens (Table 47.2). Specific microbiological diagnosis is rarely necessary, as antimicrobial therapy is not usually required. The morbidity and mortality of acute watery diarrhea is largely related to dehydration (especially in children), and by far the most important component of management is adequate rehydration. In most cases this can be achieved by oral rehydration solutions (ORS), although intravenous fluids may occasionally be needed. Antimotility agents are rarely helpful, and should definitely not be used in young children.

Dehydration is assessed clinically (Table 47.3) and treatment depends on the degree of fluid loss. Mildly dehydrated individuals should be given increased fluids; infants and children should continue feeding normally if possible. For moderate dehydration, ORS 75–100 mL/kg is given within the first 4 h, followed by further fluids to replace loss. Children should continue feeding once initial rehydration is completed. Intravenous rehydration is required only for severely dehydrated individuals with features of collapse. Several liters of intravenous fluid are usually required to overcome the features of shock: adults and older children should be given 30 mL/kg in the first 30 min, then 70 mL/kg over the next 2.5 h; the rates

should be halved for infants under 12 months.[8] Maintenance of hydration can usually be achieved with ORS. In moderate and severe dehydration the patient must be reassessed regularly to ensure that adequate fluid is being given. Attention should also be paid to nutrition, acid–base status and electrolytes, especially if the diarrhea is prolonged. Oral zinc (20 mg/day for 14 days; 10 mg/day age <6 months) should be given to children with acute diarrhea, at least in developing countries, as this decreases both the severity of the acute episode and the incidence of diarrhea in the following 2–3 months.[9]

Antimicrobial therapy is rarely indicated in the empirical management of acute watery diarrhea. Antibiotics may lead to a decrease in the duration and severity of symptoms in some cases, but the improvement is small, and the condition is usually mild and self-limiting anyway.[10] Even in situations where acute watery diarrhea is life threatening (e.g. in malnourished infants) there is little evidence that antibiotics are beneficial except in the case of cholera. In cases in which there is strong clinical suspicion of cholera (or another infection that does require specific treatment) antibiotics should be started empirically while awaiting confirmation. Occasionally acute watery diarrhea may be the presenting symptom of an enteric infection which develops into persistent diarrhea (e.g. giardiasis) or dysentery (shigellosis or *Campylobacter* infection). In these cases antibiotic therapy may be necessary when the diagnosis becomes clear.

DYSENTERY

Dysentery is a clinical syndrome of bloody, usually low volume, diarrhea often associated with abdominal pain and fever. It is caused by infection with invasive enteropathogens (*see* Table 47.2). Fluid and electrolyte loss is not as great as in watery

Table 47.2 Clinical syndromes of gastroenteritis and typical causative organisms

	Acute watery diarrhea	Bloody diarrhea	Persistent diarrhea
Viruses	Rotavirus Enteric adenoviruses Caliciviruses (including norovirus) Astroviruses		Recurrent infections with rotavirus
Bacteria	*Salmonella enterica* serotypes *Campylobacter jejuni* Enteropathogenic *Esch. coli* Enterotoxigenic *Esch. coli* Enteroaggregative *Esch. coli* *Vibrio cholerae* *V. parahaemolyticus* *Clostridium difficile* *Staphylococcus aureus* (toxin b) *Bacillus cereus*	*Salmonella enterica* serotypes *Campylobacter jejuni* *Shigella* spp. Enteroinvasive *Esch. coli* Enterohemorrhagic *Esch. coli* *Yersinia enterocolitica* *C. difficile*	*Mycobacterium tuberculosis* Recurrent or relapsing infections with other bacterial pathogens
Protozoa	*Giardia lamblia* *Cryptosporidium parvum* *Isospora belli* *Cyclospora cayetanensis* *Dientamoeba fragilis*	*Entamoeba histolytica* *Balantidium coli*	*Giardia lamblia* *Entamoeba histolytica* *Cryptosporidium parvum* *Isospora belli* *Cyclospora cayetanensis*
Miscellaneous		*Schistosoma mansoni* *Trichuris trichiura*	Postinfectious irritable bowel syndrome Disaccharidase deficiency

Table 47.3 Assessment of dehydration in acute diarrhea in children

Symptom/sign	No/minimal dehydration	Moderate dehydration	Severe dehydration
Mental state	Alert	Restless, irritable	Lethargic or unconscious; floppy infant
Eyes	Normal	Sunken	Very sunken, dry
Tears	Present	Absent	Absent
Tongue	Moist	Dry	Very dry
Thirst	Drinks normally	Drinks very eagerly	Unable to drink
Skin pinch	Goes back rapidly	Goes back slowly	Goes back very slowly
Probable fluid deficit	<2.5% body weight	2.5–10% body weight	>10% body weight
Management	Increased fluids	Oral rehydration	Intravenous fluids

diarrhea, although ORS may still be important, especially in children. Morbidity and mortality are often due to complications other than dehydration, including perforation, sepsis and hemolytic–uremic syndrome (HUS). In most cases of bacillary dysentery, antibiotics significantly reduce the severity and duration of illness, and in some instances decrease mortality.[8] Antimicrobials should always be used in shigellosis and amebic dysentery, and may be helpful in other forms of bacillary dysentery. In developed countries the empirical therapy for dysentery (when amebiasis is not suspected) is either a fluoroquinolone or azithromycin. In developing countries bacillary dysentery is presumptively treated as shigellosis (p. 600). However, in dysentery caused by verotoxigenic *Esch. coli*, antibiotic treatment increases the risk of toxin-mediated HUS and antibiotics should be used with caution if this is suspected.[11]

 ## PERSISTENT DIARRHEA

Infective diarrhea that continues for more than 14 days is defined as persistent, and may occur with or without malabsorption. It may be continuous, but is frequently intermittent, varying from day to day. Persistent diarrhea is often associated with weight loss and malnutrition, and accounts for most diarrheal deaths in children. It may be due to recurrent or relapsing infection with common and usually self-limiting bacterial or viral pathogens, especially in malnourished individuals. In other cases, such as giardiasis, Whipple's disease and intestinal tuberculosis, chronic diarrhea is the normal presentation in the absence of specific treatment (*see* Table 47.2). Immunocompromised patients, especially those infected with HIV, are susceptible to a variety of pathogens causing persistent diarrhea.

It is important to identify the infecting organism as specific treatment is often required. If this is not possible, empirical treatment based on local patterns of infection in relevant patients should be used. This is particularly important in people with HIV/AIDS. If malnutrition is either contributing to or resulting from infection, nutritional supplements should be given. Antimotility agents may give symptomatic relief when the underlying cause cannot be diagnosed or treated.

In some cases persistent diarrhea may be triggered by an acute and self-limiting infection. A number of pathogens, including rotavirus, can cause villus damage and disaccharidase deficiency, leading to malabsorption. This is managed by temporary withdrawal of the malabsorbed nutrient. Postinfectious irritable bowel may follow infection with some gastrointestinal pathogens.

 ## ENTERIC FEVER

Enteric fever is primarily a systemic illness, although the spread is feco-oral and the portal of entry gastrointestinal. The diagnosis is based on typical features and confirmed by isolation of the organism from blood or bone marrow. Treatment is with specific antimicrobial therapy (p. 600).

 ## ANTIBIOTIC-ASSOCIATED DIARRHEA

Diarrhea associated with antibiotic use can present from 1 day to several weeks after taking the antibiotic. Symptoms can vary from mild watery diarrhea to a dysenteric syndrome with severe colitis. In many cases (especially at the milder end of the spectrum) diarrhea is due to a direct effect of the antibiotic on the gut (commonly associated with macrolides and clavulanic acid) or to changes in the normal intestinal microflora. However, in 10–25% of patients with antibiotic-associated diarrhea (and 50–75% of those with antibiotic-associated colitis),[12] the symptoms are attributable to *Clostridium difficile* infection (p. 602).

 ## TRAVELERS' DIARRHEA

Travelers' diarrhea is defined as the passage of three or more unformed stools per day in a resident of an industrialized country traveling in or recently returned from a developing nation. Infection is usually food- or water-borne, and younger travelers are most often affected (probably reflecting behavior patterns). Reported attack rates vary from country to country, but approach 50% for a 2-week stay in many tropical countries. It may be caused by a wide variety of pathogens, the most common being enterotoxigenic *Esch. coli*.[13] The severity and duration of symptoms can be reduced by antibiotic treatment,[14,15] but the illness is usually relatively mild and self-limiting. ORS should be used to prevent dehydration. The decision to treat with antibiotics should be based on individual circumstances, bearing in mind the cost, potential side effects and the possible effects on antimicrobial resistance.

SOLUTIONS FOR ORAL AND INTRAVENOUS REHYDRATION

The use of oral rehydration solutions is based on the observation that glucose and other carbohydrates enhance sodium absorption in the small intestine, even in the presence of secretory loss due to toxins. The recognition of this principle, and the widespread promotion of the use of ORS by the World Health Organization (WHO) and other organizations, has saved millions of lives over the past 20 years. The composition of currently recommended (lower osmolarity) WHO/UNICEF and other ORS are shown in Table 47.4.

Although the original standard WHO/UNICEF ORS was effective in replacing fluid loss, it did not have any impact on the duration and severity of diarrhea. Other forms of ORS have been developed in an attempt to address this. ORS based on cereal carbohydrate (usually rice) rather than glucose has been shown significantly to decrease stool volume and length of illness in cholera, both in adults and in children.[16] In other forms of acute diarrhea it is at least as good as glucose ORS in replacing fluid loss (even in infants under 6 months), but does not have such a marked impact on the course of the illness.[16,17] Hypo-osmolar ORS has been shown to decrease stool fluid loss in children,[18] although this effect has not been demonstrated in adults and may be affected by other factors such as concurrent breast feeding.[19] Because of the significant benefits in children (who are at most risk from diarrhea) the WHO and UNICEF now recommend that the hypo-osmolar formulation should be the first choice ORS.[9]

Several other supplements have been added to ORS in an attempt to improve efficacy. The addition of lactobacilli has been shown to improve outcomes in children with rotavirus and non-rotavirus diarrhea, although this has not become standard practice.[20,21] Supplementation of ORS with zinc significantly decreases fluid requirements in malnourished children with persistent diarrhea,[22,23] but other nutritional supplements such as folic acid have not been shown to help.[24] It is important to keep the preparation and administration of ORS simple: community-based studies have shown that despite instruction a high proportion of mothers are unable to prepare even standard ORS correctly.[25]

In severely dehydrated patients intravenous fluids may be needed for initial resuscitation. The fluid used should contain electrolytes to replace those lost, and bicarbonate or lactate to correct any acid–base imbalance. Examples of suitable commercial and generic solutions are shown in Table 47.4. If these are not available, isotonic (0.9%) saline can be used but it does not contain base or potassium. Simple dextrose solutions should not be used as they contain no electrolytes.[8]

Table 47.4 Solutions for oral and intravenous rehydration

Solution	Components (mmol/L)		Substance added (grams/L of water)	
Oral				
WHO/UNICEF reduced osmolarity	Na	75	NaCl	2.6
	Cl	65	Trisodium citrate	2.9
	K	20	KCl	1.5
	Citrate	10	Glucose (anhydrous)	13.5
	Glucose	75		
Household (salt based)			Salt	2.5 (½ teaspoon)
			Sugar	30 (6 teaspoons)
UK/Europe	Na	35–60	Commercial	
	K	20–40	preparations	
	Glucose	90–200		
Intravenous				
Ringer's lactate	Na	130	Commercial	
	Cl	109	preparation	
	K	4		
	Lactate	28		
Dhaka solution	Na	133	NaCl	5
	Cl	98	NaHCO$_3$	4
	Lactate	48		
	K	13	KCl	1

DRUGS IN SYNDROMIC MANAGEMENT

ANTIBIOTICS

Antibiotics are often prescribed for acute watery diarrhea in developed countries, even though the disease is usually mild and self-limiting (Table 47.5). Quinolones have been shown to decrease slightly the duration and severity of symptoms in adults in industrialized countries;[10] there is little information on children (in whom viral diarrhea is much more common), or from the developing world. By decreasing fluid loss, antibiotic therapy should help to prevent dehydration, but there is no good evidence that the use of antimicrobials decreases mortality from dehydration or other complications of acute watery diarrhea. It may occasionally be justified on symptomatic grounds in adults with particularly severe or prolonged symptoms; in these cases either azithromycin 500 mg/day or ciprofloxacin 500 mg every 12 h for 3 days is the best choice. Any benefit from antibiotic therapy has to be balanced against cost, the risk of side effects and the possibility of inducing resistance.

Treatment with antibiotics is definitely indicated in shigellosis, which is the most common cause of dysentery in the developing world. The benefits are less marked in dysentery due to other organisms such as *Salmonella* and *Campylobacter*, which account for a large proportion of bloody diarrhea in industrialized countries. In general, in countries where shigellosis is relatively rare antibiotic therapy should be reserved for those with more serious or prolonged symptoms of bloody diarrhea; azithromycin or ciprofloxacin are again the drugs of choice. In developing countries adults and children should receive antibiotics for presumed shigellosis (p. 600).

Enteric fever should always be treated with antibiotics, and if clinical suspicion is high treatment should be started empirically while results are awaited.

A variety of different antibiotics have been shown to decrease the severity and duration of symptoms in travelers' diarrhea, including trimethoprim–sulfamethoxazole, erythromycin, azithromycin and quinolones.[15] Ciprofloxacin is effective in a single dose of 750 mg, and is the best choice if antimicrobial therapy is needed. Antibiotic prophylaxis may be appropriate in some cases, especially in immunocompromised individuals. New options for prophylaxis are becoming available with the use of non-absorbed antibiotics such as rifaximin, and vaccines are under development.[26]

ANTIMOTILITY AND ANTISECRETORY AGENTS

A number of antimotility agents are available for the symptomatic relief of diarrhea. The most widely used are codeine phosphate, loperamide, diphenoxylate and kaolin/opiate preparations: proprietary formulations of these are available over the counter in many countries. None is recommended for use in infants or young children with acute diarrhea because of the risk of precipitating respiratory depression or paralytic ileus. In adults antimotility agents may be useful for short-term relief of the symptoms of acute watery diarrhea (e.g. during a journey), although they can cause abdominal bloating. The use of these agents in dysentery is controversial. There is some evidence that they do provide symptomatic relief, but concerns exist about both increased risk of toxic dilatation and prolonged excretion of pathogens. If antimotility agents are used in more severe diarrhea and dysentery, they should be given in conjunction with appropriate antimicrobial therapy. Loperamide and codeine have a role in the management of chronic infective diarrhea, particularly in HIV-associated diarrhea where definitive treatment of the infection may be impossible.

Table 47.5 Antibiotics in the empirical treatment of acute gastroenteritis[a]

Condition	Drug of choice	Alternatives	Indications	Benefits
Acute watery diarrhea	Ciprofloxacin 500 mg every 12 h (15 mg/kg every 12 h) or azithromycin 500 mg per day for 3 days	Clarithromycin 500 mg every 12 h Trimethoprim–sulfamethoxazole 960 mg every 12 h (30 mg/kg every 12 h)	Severe symptoms, prolonged illness, immunosuppressed patient	Relieves symptoms, shortens illness
Dysentery[b]	Ciprofloxacin 500 mg every 12 h (15 mg/kg every 12 h) or azithromycin 500 mg/day for 3 days	Ofloxacin 200 mg every 12 h (15 mg/kg in two divided doses) Ceftriaxone 2 g per day	Most patients	Relieves symptoms, shortens illness Decreases mortality in children
Travelers' diarrhea	Ciprofloxacin 750 mg single dose	Trimethoprim–sulfamethoxazole 960 mg every 12 h (30 mg/kg every 12 h) Azithromycin 1 g single dose	Rarely needed	Relieves symptoms, shortens illness

Treatment is for 5 days unless otherwise stated.
[a]The doses indicated are for adults; when provided, children's doses are given in parentheses (not to exceed adult dose). Fluoroquinolones are not licensed for children under 12 years old, although they are widely used and appear safe.
[b]Antibiotics should be used with caution if enterohemorrhagic *Esch. coli* is suspected.

MANAGEMENT OF SPECIFIC INFECTIONS

BACTERIAL INFECTIONS
(Table 47.6)

Cholera

Cholera is characterized by watery diarrhea that is often profuse and may be life-threatening. It is caused by secretory enterotoxins (principally cholera toxin) produced by *Vibrio cholerae*. The main pathogenic strain of *V. cholerae* worldwide is O1 El Tor, which first appeared in South East Asia in 1961 (the start of the seventh pandemic), and is now endemic in Africa, Asia, and Central and South America. A smaller number of cases are caused by the O1 (classical) and O139 biotypes. The mainstay of treatment for cholera is rehydration, and with appropriate and effective rehydration therapy mortality can be reduced to less than 1%. Oral rehydration with ORS is usually adequate, but severely dehydrated individuals may need intravenous fluids. Several liters of intravenous fluid may be required initially, and fluids must be continued to keep up with ongoing loss. As in other forms of watery diarrhea, zinc supplementation is beneficial in children.[27]

Antibiotics reduce the duration and volume of diarrhea, and may limit transmission by reducing the infectivity of the stools.[28] Treatment should be started as soon as possible in order to decrease the fluid requirement. The standard treatment in children is a 12-dose course of erythromycin. In adults doxycycline (300 mg single dose) remains the antibiotic of choice in most cases but resistance is becoming a major problem in many parts of the world.[29,30] Plasmid-mediated multidrug resistance is common, but unlike shigellosis, cholera does not tend to accrue resistance over time, and resistance patterns fluctuate rapidly even in the same region.[31] For this reason in an outbreak situation samples should be obtained for sensitivity testing as soon as possible. *V. cholerae* is generally sensitive to fluoroquinolones, and a single dose of ciprofloxacin has been shown to be as effective as doxycycline (in adults)[32,33] and erythromycin (in children)[34] in treating cholera. Recently, however, some resistance to fluoroquinolones has been reported.[35] Azithromycin, another possible alternative, is effective as single-dose therapy in children and adults, but is more expensive and less widely available than the other drugs.[36]

Effective surveillance and improvements in hygiene and sanitation are the main factors in limiting the spread of cholera. Antibiotic prophylaxis should not be given to asymptomatic contacts: this practice promotes the development of resistance and is not cost-effective.[37] A number of cholera vaccines are available or under development.

Table 47.6 Antibiotic treatment of specific bacterial causes of acute gastroenteritis[a]

Condition	Drug of choice	Alternatives	Indications	Benefits
Cholera	Ciprofloxacin 1 g single dose (20 mg/kg single dose) or doxycycline 300 mg single dose	Erythromycin 250 mg every 6 h (12.5 mg/kg every 6 h) for 3 days Azithromycin 1 g single dose (20 mg/kg single dose)	All patients	Relieves symptoms, shortens illness Reduces transmission
Enteric fever	Ciprofloxacin 500 mg every 12 h (15 mg/kg every 12 h) for 7 days	Ofloxacin 15mg/kg/day in 2 divided doses for 3 days Azithromycin 500 mg once daily (10 mg/kg once daily) for 5–7 days Chloramphenicol 500 mg every 6 h (12.5 mg/kg every 6 h) for 7 days Ceftriaxone 2 gm daily	All patients	Reduces morbidity and mortality
Non-typhoidal salmonellosis	Ciprofloxacin 500 mg every 12 h (15 mg/kg every 12 h)	Trimethoprim–sulfamethoxazole 960 mg every 12 h (30 mg/kg every 12 h) Azithromycin 500 mg/day	Prolonged illness; severe symptoms; immunosuppressed	Relieves symptoms, shortens illness *May* decrease complications in selected groups
Shigellosis	Ciprofloxacin 500 mg every 12 h (15 mg/kg every 12 h)	Ofloxacin 200 mg every 12 h (15 mg/kg in two divided doses only) Azithromycin 500 mg on day one then 250 mg/day for 4 days (10 mg/kg per day) Ceftriaxone 2 g per day	All patients	Relieves symptoms, shortens illness Decreases morbidity and mortality
Campylobacter	Azithromycin 500 mg/day (10 mg/kg per day)	Clarithromycin 500 mg every 12 h	Immunosuppressed; severe symptoms (rarely needed)	

Treatment is for 5 days unless otherwise stated. Therapy should be guided by local antimicrobial sensitivities where known.
[a] The doses indicated are for adults; when provided, children's doses are given in parentheses (not to exceed adult dose). Fluoroquinolones are not licensed for children under 12 years old.

ENTERIC FEVER

The enteric fever syndrome is an acute systemic illness characterized by fever, headache and abdominal discomfort. Typhoid, the typical form of enteric fever, is caused by *Salmonella enterica* serotype Typhi. A similar but generally less severe illness known as paratyphoid is due to infection with *Salmonella enterica* serotypes Paratyphi A, B or C. Untreated typhoid carries a mortality of up to 30%, but this can be reduced dramatically with appropriate therapy. After clinical recovery, 5–10% of patients will continue to excrete *S. Typhi* for several months: these are termed convalescent carriers. Between 1% and 4% will continue to carry the organism for more than a year: this is chronic carriage.

Chloramphenicol has long been the drug of choice in enteric fever, but from the late 1980s onwards isolates resistant not only to chloramphenicol but also to ampicillin and co-trimoxazole have been reported from many parts of the world[38,39] (multiple antibiotic resistance is mediated by a transmissible plasmid).[40] As a result, quinolones are now widely used to treat typhoid and paratyphoid. Although many strains remain fully sensitive to all quinolones, decreased susceptibility has been reported in a number of countries.[41] Such isolates, although apparently ciprofloxacin susceptible on disc testing, often show in-vitro resistance to nalidixic acid and are associated with increased clinical failure rates when treated with ciprofloxacin.[42] Newer quinolones such as gatifloxacin appear to have better activity against these nalidixic acid resistant strains.[43]

Wherever possible the treatment of enteric fever should be based on individual or local antibiotic susceptibility patterns. With decreased usage chloramphenicol resistance rates have actually fallen in India and Bangladesh, and many isolates are now once again sensitive to this drug[44,45] (which is cheap and widely available). However, fluoroquinolones give better outcomes than chloramphenicol even in fully susceptible strains,[46] and are the drug of choice in most situations. Where there is no decreased fluoroquinolone sensitivity, ciprofloxacin gives a clinical cure rate of 98%, fever clearance time of 4 days, and relapse and chronic carriage rates of less than 2% (better in all respects than chloramphenicol).[42] No one drug of this class has been shown to be better than others; ciprofloxacin is the most widely used, and short courses of both ofloxacin and fleroxacin have proved effective in children.[47–49] Despite concerns about the use of these agents in children (because of the risk of damage to developing cartilage) there is now considerable evidence to suggest that ciprofloxacin is sufficiently safe to be used in the treatment of childhood typhoid.[50,51] Studies using cephalosporins have produced variable results: one study showed good a cure rate with ceftriaxone[52] but others have demonstrated less efficacy with ceftriaxone and with cefixime than with other drugs, especially in short-course regimens.[48,53]

Several trials in adults and children have shown excellent results using a 5- or 7-day course of azithromycin.[54–57] Studies directly comparing ciprofloxacin, azithromycin and ceftriax-

one have produced mixed results and are difficult to interpret because of variations in study design and populations.[58] Where there is known to be decreased susceptibility to quinolones, azithromycin appears to be the most effective agent,[59] but the use of this drug (and the cephalosporins) is limited by cost and availability. Another potential option in this situation is a quinolone such as gatifloxacin.[43]

Most of these studies have been carried out in patients with mild or moderate typhoid. Patients with hypotension, impaired mental function or evidence of decreased organ perfusion have a worse prognosis, and the impact of newer antibiotics in this group has not been assessed. The role of steroids in severe typhoid remains controversial: one trial (with relatively small numbers) demonstrated increased survival in patients treated with high-dose dexamethasone,[60] but there is little corroborating evidence for this. Complications such as intestinal perforation and renal failure should be managed aggressively, with surgical intervention and intensive care support where necessary.

Chronic carriage of *S. Typhi* may be difficult to eradicate, especially in the presence of gallbladder disease or urinary schistosomiasis. Prolonged courses of amoxicillin or trimethoprim–sulfamethoxazole are sometimes effective, and quinolones appear to have a higher success rate.[61,62] Treating underlying gallbladder or parasitic disease may help, but cholecystectomy is not justified on public health grounds alone.

 ## SHIGELLOSIS

Infection with *Shigella* species can cause either watery diarrhea (clinically indistinguishable from other causes of acute watery diarrhea) or, more typically, dysentery. Four species can cause enteritis in humans: *Shigella dysenteriae* produces the most severe dysentery and may also secrete a toxin which can induce hemolytic–uremic syndrome. Antibiotic treatment of shigella dysentery leads to a reduction in the severity and duration of symptoms, as well as a decrease in mortality in children.[8] In theory the use of antibiotics in toxigenic *S. dysenteriae* could lead to an increased risk of hemolytic–uremic syndrome (as has been demonstrated in infections with verotoxigenic *Esch. coli*), but this remains to be confirmed.

Shigella spp. can rapidly develop resistance to antimicrobials, due to their ability to acquire plasmid-borne resistance genes from other species such as *Esch. coli*.[63] Multiresistance is common, and some of the older and cheaper antibiotics such as ampicillin and trimethoprim–sulfamethoxazole are now ineffective in many developing and developed countries.[64,65] Most isolates remain sensitive to quinolones, although it is now recognized that quinolone resistance too can be acquired through horizontal plasmid transfer,[66] and clinical fluoroquinolone resistance is being reported.[67,68] The group 1 quinolone nalidixic acid has been used extensively for the treatment of shigellosis in the past. However, resistance to this drug develops rapidly and predisposes to more extensive quinolone resistance.[69] Nalidixic acid dosing regimens are more complicated than those of more modern quinolones, it is no longer the cheapest option, and its use in shigellosis is no longer recommended.[70]

A number of studies have demonstrated the clinical efficacy of ciprofloxacin, norfloxacin and ofloxacin in both adults and children.[71,72] Short courses of quinolones (e.g. ofloxacin 15 mg/kg in two divided doses in children) appear to be effective in many cases, making their use more economically viable. Ceftibuten, cefixime and ceftriaxone have all been shown to be effective in various regimens,[73,74] as has azithromycin (500 mg, followed by 250 mg/day for 4 days),[75] but the data on these drugs are less complete and their use is limited by cost and availability. Ideally, the choice of antibiotic for shigellosis should be guided by current local resistance patterns. In the absence of these, a fluoroquinolone is the drug of choice in most areas,[70] with ciprofloxacin being the cheapest and most widely available.

Although dehydration is not usually a major feature of shigella dysentery ORS should be given, especially to children.

NON-TYPHOIDAL SALMONELLOSIS

Salmonella serotypes other than Typhi and Paratyphi most commonly cause self-limiting gastroenteritis, which is usually watery but may be dysenteric. Bacteremia is documented in about 5% of cases: this may be transient and benign, but can lead to serious complications such as metastatic infection. Clinical trials suggest that fluoroquinolones may reduce the duration and severity of gastrointestinal symptoms in salmonella infection, but the effect is small (1–2 days reduction).[10] In general, antibiotics are not recommended for people with mild or moderate salmonella enteritis: even the presence of bacteremia in an otherwise healthy person is not a definite indication. Treatment is justified in patients with severe or prolonged symptoms, in neonates, and for those at increased risk of invasive disease (in particular the immunocompromised and patients with significant underlying disease). Some authorities recommend a short (48–72 h) 'pre-emptive' course of antibiotics in those who have other risk factors for metastatic disease (e.g. elderly people and people with known atherosclerotic lesions or aortic aneurysm),[76] while others suggest a 10- to 14-day course in the same group:[77] the clinical efficacy of either approach is unproven.

If antibiotic treatment is indicated, then fluoroquinolones are the best choice. Ceftriaxone, azithromycin and aztreonam are also effective; trimethoprim–sulfamethoxazole may be used although resistance is increasing. A number of studies have looked at the effect of quinolone treatment on fecal excretion of *Salmonella* spp., which typically persists for several weeks after infection. Treated patients usually have negative stool cultures immediately after treatment, but overall antibiotics have little effect on the time taken to clear the organism.[78] Even this limited response may be effective in interrupting spread of the disease in institutional outbreaks.[79] The management of symptomatic salmonella bacteremia (which is common in HIV-positive patients in developing countries) is difficult: antibiotics may help, but eradication often proves impossible. Metastatic salmonella infection, which typically affects atheromatous endothelium, also requires prolonged antibiotic therapy, often in conjunction with surgery.

ESCHERICHIA COLI INFECTION

Esch. coli infection of the gut with enterotoxigenic (ETEC), enteropathogenic (EPEC), enteroinvasive (EIEC), enterohemorrhagic (EHEC) or enteroaggregative (EAggEC) strains can cause human disease, but these pathogens are not routinely identified in most microbiological laboratories. Consequently information about these infections is limited, and there are few therapeutic trials.

Verotoxin-secreting strains of EHEC (principally O157:H7) can cause hemolytic–uremic syndrome (HUS) and thrombotic thrombocytopenic purpura (TTP), especially in children, and have therefore been the focus of much attention in industrialized countries. Several large food-borne outbreaks of *Esch. coli* O157 have been reported; most patients had a mild self-limiting bloody diarrhea, but 2.5–14% of children (and occasional adults) developed HUS.[11,80] Antibiotic treatment appears to increase the risk of HUS, presumably by increasing toxin release from dying bacteria,[11] and antibiotics should generally be avoided in *Esch. coli* O157 enteritis. EHEC has also been reported as a cause of gastroenteritis in adults and children in Africa.[81]

ETEC, which can produce both heat-stable and heat-labile toxins, is an important cause of acute watery diarrhea in children and adults throughout the world.[81,82] It has been responsible for large food- and water-borne outbreaks, and is the most commonly confirmed cause of travelers' diarrhea.[83,84] Widespread antibiotic resistance has been reported, with isolates from many parts of the world showing resistance to multiple drugs, including trimethoprim–sulfamethoxazole and amoxicillin.[83] The majority of ETEC remain sensitive to fluoroquinolones, but a survey in Thailand showed 1% of isolates to be ciprofloxacin resistant; 15% of isolates in the same study were azithromycin resistant.[85] The illness caused by ETEC is usually mild and self-limiting; however, if treatment is deemed necessary, then a fluoroquinolone should be used if available.

EIEC causes bacillary dysentery indistinguishable from shigellosis. It is rarely isolated and most cases are probably treated empirically as shigellosis. If EIEC is cultured, treatment should be guided by sensitivities.

EPEC is now recognized as a cause of acute watery diarrhea in infants and children worldwide, although it appears to be more common in developing countries.[81,86,87] Relatively little is known about antibiotic sensitivities of EPEC: resistance to trimethoprim–sulfamethoxazole has been reported, but it is generally sensitive to quinolones.[87,88] Antibiotic treatment is rarely indicated.

EAggEC can be isolated from healthy people, but it also appears to be responsible for episodes of travelers' diarrhea,[89] persistent diarrhea in children[87,90] and HIV-associated diarrhea.[91] The symptoms of both travelers' diarrhea and HIV-related chronic diarrhea caused by EAggEC can be alleviated by ciprofloxacin,[89,91] although in the former case this is not usually necessary. The epidemiology and treatment of EAggEC diarrhea in developing countries remains unclear.

CAMPYLOBACTER INFECTION

Infection with *Campylobacter jejuni* can cause acute watery diarrhea or, less commonly, dysentery. The illness is usually relatively mild and self-limiting, although there may occasionally be more severe dysenteric or systemic features. *Campylobacter coli* causes a similar but generally less severe illness. *Campylobacter* spp., which are widespread in livestock animals, have considerable potential to develop antibiotic resistance. This is usually plasmid mediated and has been associated with the use of antibiotics in both humans and animals. Resistance to fluoroquinolones has become a major problem in many countries, with up to 70–80% of human isolates being resistant in some areas (notably Spain and Thailand).[92] This has been linked to the veterinary use of these drugs,[93] but resistance has also been shown to develop in humans during a course of treatment.[94] Macrolide resistance is also increasing.[92]

Most cases of campylobacter enteritis resolve without specific treatment. More severe cases are likely to be treated empirically, but if campylobacter is suspected then azithromycin is the best choice. If a *Campylobacter* species is grown and significant symptoms persist (especially in patients with HIV/AIDS), then antibiotic treatment should be guided by in-vitro sensitivities.

YERSINIA INFECTION

Yersinia enterocolitica is a relatively unusual cause of enteric infection in all ages. The spectrum of illness is very variable, and includes severe dysentery, septicemia and extraintestinal manifestations such as lymphadenopathy and reactive arthritis. More severe cases should be treated with antibiotics: fluoroquinolones appear to be the most effective agents, although data are limited.[95]

NON-CHOLERA VIBRIO, AEROMONAS AND PLESIOMONAS SPECIES

These organisms are being isolated with increasing frequency from patients with gastroenteritis, although whether this represents a genuine increase in prevalence or simply better laboratory techniques is unclear. *Vibrio parahaemolyticus* has caused major food- and water-borne outbreaks in Asia,[96] while *Aeromonas* and *Plesiomonas* species are common causes of diarrhea in children and travelers in some parts of the world.[77,84,97]

All three usually cause self-limiting watery diarrhea. Almost all of these organisms are sensitive to fluoroquinolones in vitro; there is widespread and variable resistance to other antibiotics.[98] Clinical data are very limited.

TOXIN-SECRETING BACTERIA

Some bacteria, notably *Clostridium perfringens*, *Bacillus cereus* and strains of *Staphylococcus aureus*, can produce heat-stable neurotoxins that affect the autonomic nervous system to cause diarrhea and vomiting. If toxin is ingested in contaminated food, symptoms start within a few hours. Although diarrhea may be profuse, the illness is usually short lived (24–48 h) and no specific treatment is required. Bacterial toxins are a common cause of food poisoning in Europe and the USA; the prevalence in developing countries is unknown. Ingestion of preformed toxins of *Clostridium botulinum* (especially from inadequately processed canned food) is a rarer but potentially fatal form of food poisoning.

CLOSTRIDIUM DIFFICILE

C. difficile has been recognized as a cause of antibiotic-associated diarrhea and of pseudomembranous colitis since the 1970s. In the last decade, however, it has attracted increased attention as a major cause of morbidity and mortality, especially in the healthcare setting. The overall incidence has increased, and mortality has risen since the emergence of the hypervirulent 027 ribotype in 2000.[99] The epidemiology of *C. difficile* as a healthcare-associated infection (HCAI) is well documented in the developed world, but there is a paucity of information on the prevalence and behavior in developing countries.

A spore-forming bacterium, *C. difficile* is widespread in the environment. It is occasionally found in asymptomatic individuals (especially neonates), but is usually prevented from colonizing the human gut by the presence of normal intestinal microflora. If the normal commensals are eradicated by antibiotic treatment, *C. difficile* is able to move into the vacant niche: this is especially likely in the immunocompromised and the elderly. The propensity for antibiotics to precipitate *C. difficile*-associated diarrhea (CDAD) depends on: (1) the effect of the antibiotic on the normal bowel flora, and (2) the resistance of *C. difficile* itself to the drug. Although almost any antibiotic can be associated with CDAD, cephalosporins, clindamycin and aminopenicillins have been the most frequently implicated in the past. More recently fluoroquinolones have emerged as an important predisposing factor because of increasing *C. difficile* resistance to quinolones.[100,101]

Although antibiotics are important in the acquisition of *C. difficile* infection, there are complex organism and host factors involved in the development and course of CDAD. Once the gut is colonized the organism produces cytopathic toxins (of which CDT A and B are the most important). These are responsible for the symptoms, which can range from mild watery diarrhea to potentially fatal pseudomembranous colitis.

The most obvious first step in managing CDAD is to stop or simplify antibiotic therapy. However, symptoms often do not start for days or weeks after the offending course, and if the patient is still on antibiotics it is often not clinically appropriate to stop them. The majority of patients with symptomatic *C. difficile* infection will require specific antimicrobial treatment. Metronidazole remains the most widely used agent, although the use of vancomycin is increasing. In mild or moderate CDAD the two drugs have similar efficacy, with cure rates of >90% (although recurrence is common). Some recent studies have shown poorer results with metronidazole; this may be related to the emergence of metronidazole-resistant *C. difficile*, although this relationship is unproven.[12,102] In more severe disease vancomycin is more effective, with a better cure rate and faster time to cure,[103] and there is some evidence that higher doses (2 g per day) may be better still.[99] However, these benefits have to be weighed against the potential for increasing the rate of vancomycin resistance in other pathogens. Suggested treatment regimens are shown in Table 47.7.

Data on intravenous vancomycin and metronidazole in CDAD are limited. There is some evidence supporting the use of intravenous metronidazole in patients who are unable to take oral therapy;[12] vancomycin enemas have also been used in this situation. Relapse following treatment is common: this is usually due to reinfection with the same or a different strain rather than failure to clear the original infection. It is common practice to treat relapses with an antibiotic other than that originally used, but there are no data to support this.

Other drugs have been used to treat CDAD. Teicoplanin and fusidic acid have been shown to have similar efficacy to metronidazole and vancomycin, but neither seems to offer significant advantages. Nitazoxanide (an antiprotozoal drug) and rifaximin (used for prophylaxis of travelers' diarrhea) have been used successfully for treating CDAD; neither is approved for this indication, but further assessment is underway. A number of new antimicrobials with activity against *C. difficile* are under development.[104,105]

Other potential therapeutic measures include antimotility agents, probiotics, immunoglobulins and steroids. Antimotility agents have traditionally been contraindicated in CDAD, but recent evidence suggests that they may sometimes be helpful.[106] Further clinical trial data are needed before they can be recommended. The evidence on probiotics is extensive and confusing. For secondary prophylaxis in patients at high risk of recurrent disease, *Saccharomyces boulardii* may be protective.[107] There is not yet sufficient evidence that primary prophylaxis with probiotics has a role. Probiotics should be used with caution in immunocompromised patients as there is a risk of bacteremia and metastatic infection. Methylprednisolone and pooled human immunoglobulin have each been used with variable success to treat refractory CDAD.[12] These may be tried in intractable cases, although there is no real evidence of their efficacy. Severe CDAD is life-threatening, and surgical intervention (with colectomy) should be considered if there is no response to medical treatment. All severe cases should have regular surgical assessment, especially if there is significant cecal dilatation.[108]

C. difficile is principally a healthcare-associated infection, and preventive measures include good antimicrobial stewardship, scrupulous attention to hand washing and hygiene, and contact isolation of affected patients.[109]

 WHIPPLE'S DISEASE

Whipple's disease (caused by infection with *Tropheryma whipplei*) is a multisystem disorder, but the most commonly affected site is the small intestine. It is extremely rare, with an estimated incidence of less than 1 per million. Antibiotic treatment may be curative, but relapse after treatment is common, especially in the central nervous system (CNS). There have been no randomized prospective trials comparing different drug therapy. A reasonable regimen is to give 2 weeks of intravenous therapy with either benzylpenicillin (2.4 g per day) and streptomycin (15 mg/kg per day) or ceftriaxone (2 g per day), followed by 1 year of trimethoprim–sulfamethoxazole 960 mg every 12 h.[109] Resistance to trimethoprim has been reported, and if possible isolates should be tested for resistance genotypes.[110] Longer courses may be needed for CNS infection, and lumbar puncture should be performed in all cases to exclude CNS involvement.[109]

Table 47.7 Suggested management path for CDAD

	Antimicrobial treatment	Alternative/additional treatment
First episode		
General measures		Stop antibiotics if possible Fluid and electrolyte replacement Isolate; strict hygiene
Mild	Metronidazole 400 mg p.o. or 500 mg p.o. every 8 h[a]	Vancomycin 125 mg p.o. every 6 h
Severe[b,c]	Vancomycin 125 mg p.o. every 6 h[d]	Metronidazole 500 mg i.v. every 8 h[e] Vancomycin enema[e]
Recurrence	Metronidazole 400 mg or 500 mg p.o. every 8 h[a]	Vancomycin 250 mg p.o. every 6 h
Second recurrence	Vancomycin 500 mg p.o. every 6 h	*Saccharomyces boulardii* probiotic[f] Methylprednisolone[g] Immunoglobulins[g]

[a]Switch to vancomycin after 72 h if condition worsens.
[b]Criteria for severe CDAD[98] include white blood cell count >15 × 10⁹, >50% rise in serum concentration of creatinine, severe diarrhea, temperature >38.3°C, albumin <25 mg/dL.
[c]Consider surgery for megacolon or severe colitis.
[d]May be increased to 250 mg.
[e]If unable to take by mouth.
[f]Caution in immunocompromised.
[g]Consider in severe or refractory cases.

INTESTINAL MYCOBACTERIAL INFECTION

Intestinal tuberculosis should be treated with standard antituberculosis chemotherapy (Ch. 58).

SMALL BOWEL OVERGROWTH

Colonization of the small intestine with exogenous bacteria may occur in patients with structural abnormalities of the small bowel (such as strictures or diverticula), bypassed surgical loops, or in conditions associated with hypomotility such as scleroderma. Bacterial overgrowth may lead to diarrhea and malabsorption. Clinical improvement is usually seen after treatment with metronidazole, tetracycline or a fluoroquinolone, but repeated courses are often required if the underlying abnormality remains.

HELICOBACTER PYLORI

Infection with *H. pylori* is common throughout the world. It is characterized by a mild chronic active gastritis, but this is usually asymptomatic. However, *H. pylori* gastritis is implicated in the pathogenesis of duodenal and gastric ulcers, mucosa-associated lymphoid tissue (MALT) lymphomas and some gastric adenocarcinomas.[111] Eradication of *H. pylori* virtually abolishes duodenal ulcer relapse, and all patients with peptic ulcer disease in association with *H. pylori* infection should receive antibiotics. Eradication therapy should also be used in the treatment of gastric lymphomas. Non-ulcer dyspepsia is commonly associated with *H. pylori* infection, but the evidence for a causal connection is limited. Some patients do get symptomatic improvement after clearance of *H. pylori*, but expert opinion is divided on who should be treated.[111,112]

Several different therapeutic regimens have been used for treating *H. pylori* infection, including various combinations of antibiotics, proton pump inhibitors (PPI), H$_2$-receptor antagonists and bismuth compounds. The recommended first-line therapy in Europe remains PPI, plus clarithromycin (500 mg every 12 h), plus either metronidazole (400–500 mg every 12 h) or amoxicillin (1 g every 12 h) for 7–14 days.[112] The longer course is more effective, but not necessarily more cost-effective. The success rate of this regimen has fallen from >90% to <80%, largely due to increasing clarithromycin resistance. Various alternative treatment strategies have been proposed, both as primary therapy and as second line or rescue therapy. These include bismuth-based quadruple therapy, regimens substituting either fluoroquinolones or rifabutin for clarithromycin, and sequential treatment with different combinations.[111] The European Helicobacter Study Group continue to recommend bismuth-based treatment for people who fail to respond to first-line therapy[112] (PPI, bismuth, metronidazole 400–500 mg every

8 h, and tetracycline 500 mg every 6 h. A number of bismuth salts are available commercially, and dosage will depend on which preparation is in use locally.) This recommendation may change as more data on new regimens become available.[111]

In children, *H. pylori* is associated with gastric and duodenal ulcer disease, as well as chronic gastritis. Eradication of the infection leads to long-term resolution of these conditions. However, there is a lack of data on treatment regimens and no clear consensus on optimal management.[113]

VIRAL INFECTIONS

Viral gastroenteritis is extremely common throughout the world, especially in children. It can be caused by several different organisms, notably rotavirus, enteric adenovirus (types 40 and 41), Caliciviridae and Astroviridae. Norovirus, a genus of closely related RNA viruses in the calicivirus family, is highly transmissible and is responsible for large outbreaks of gastroenteritis both in the community and in healthcare institutions.

All these viruses cause self-limiting watery diarrhea and require only supportive treatment and rehydration. Occasionally mucosal damage or disaccharidase deficiency caused by the infection may result in more prolonged diarrhea. Viral gastroenteritis, often in association with malnutrition, is a major cause of morbidity and mortality in children in the developing world.

Some viruses, notably cytomegalovirus and herpes simplex, can cause severe ulcerating infection of the gastrointestinal tract in patients with HIV/AIDS or other immunosuppressing conditions.

PROTOZOAL INFECTIONS

GIARDIASIS

Infection with *Giardia lamblia* (*intestinalis*) can produce a variety of responses including acute watery diarrhea, persistent diarrhea (often associated with nausea, anorexia and belching) and asymptomatic colonization. Most people recover spontaneously and treatment is often unnecessary. Treatment of symptomatic patients probably accelerates parasitological and clinical cure, and is definitely indicated in patients with a more protracted illness. There is little point in treating people with asymptomatic infection in endemic areas, as reinfection rates are high, but those living in non-endemic areas should be treated. The most commonly used drugs are metronidazole and tinidazole.[114] Treatment regimens are discussed in more detail in Chapter 63.

AMEBIASIS

Infection with *Entamoeba histolytica* can be divided into three clinical pictures: asymptomatic cyst passage, dysentery and liver abscess. The management of asymptomatic carriage has been complicated by the recognition that there are at least two species of ameba, *E. histolytica* and *E. dispar*, which are indistinguishable by microscopy of the cysts. Only the former is potentially pathogenic. The importance of a third species, *E. moshkovskii*, remains uncertain.[115] In endemic areas attempts to eradicate cyst carriage are of limited value due to the high rate of reinfection. In non-endemic areas people with proven *E. histolytica* in the gut should be treated, because of the potential pathogenicity and the risk of transmission. However, tests to distinguish *E. histolytica* from *E. dispar* are still not widely available, and treatment of asymptomatic cyst carriers based on microscopy alone is not recommended (unless there is other reason to suspect *E. histolytica*).[116] The drug of choice for treating cyst carriage is diloxanide furoate, a non-absorbed luminal amebicide; paromomycin is also effective.

Proven amebic dysentery and amebic liver abscess should always be treated. The best agents are nitroimidazoles, either metronidazole or tinidazole, although nitazoxanide is an alternative for amebic dysentery. In non-endemic areas systemic treatment should always be followed with a luminal amebicide. Appropriate regimens are described in Chapter 63.

OTHER PROTOZOAL INFECTIONS

The treatment of cryptosporidiosis, microsporidiosis, isosporiasis and infection with *Cyclospora cayetanensis* is described in Chapter 63.

Carriage of *Balantidium coli* is usually asymptomatic, but it can cause a syndrome similar to amebic dysentery. Tetracycline and metronidazole are effective, although there are no good clinical trials to guide therapy.[117]

Dientamoeba fragilis is often found in association with other gut parasites, but there is evidence that isolated *D. fragilis* infection can cause gastrointestinal symptoms.[118] Treatment with tetracycline or metronidazole may be effective.

The role of *Blastocystis hominis* in human disease remains uncertain. It may occasionally be associated with clinical features (possibly related to a particular genetic subtype of the parasite),[119] but in general the presence of this organism should not be accepted as a cause of symptoms.

INTESTINAL HELMINTHS

See Chapter 64.

References

1. World Health Organization. *Health statistics and information systems.* Online. Available at www.who.int/healthinfo/global_burden_disease/estimates_regional/en/index.html
2. World Health Organization. *World Health Statistics 2009.* Online. Available at http://www.who.int/whosis/whostat/2009/en/index.html
3. Fleckenstein JM, Kopecko DJ. Breaching the mucosal barrier by stealth: an emerging pathogenic mechanism for enteroadherent bacterial pathogens. *J Clin Invest.* 2001;107(1):27–30.
4. Pizarro-Cerdá J, Cossart P. Bacterial adhesion and entry into host cells. *Cell.* 2006;124(4):715–727.
5. Greenberg HG, Estes MK. Rotaviruses: from pathogenesis to vaccination. *Gastroenterology.* 2009;136(6):1939–1951.
6. Baxt LA, Singh U. New insights into *Entamoeba histolytica* pathogenesis. *Curr Opin Infect Dis.* 2008;21(5):489–494.
7. Muller N, von Allman N. Recent insights into the mucosal reactions associated with *Giardia lamblia* infections. *Int J Parasitol.* 2005;35(13):1339–1347.
8. World Health Organization (Department of Child and Adolescent Health and Development). *The treatment of diarrhoea. A manual for physicians and other senior health workers.* Geneva: WHO; 2005.
9. WHO/UNICEF. *Joint statement on the clinical management of acute diarrhoea.* Geneva: WHO; 2004. Online. Available at http://whqlibdoc.who.int/hq/2004/WHO_FCH_CAH_04.7.pdf
10. Moss PJ, Read RC. Empiric antibiotic therapy for acute diarrhoea in the developed world. *J Antimicrob Chemother.* 1995;35:903–913.
11. Wong CS, Jelacic S, Habeeb RL, Watkins SL, Tarr PI. The risk of the hemolytic–uremic syndrome after antibiotic treatment of *Escherichia coli* O157:H7 infections. *N Engl J Med.* 2000;342:1930–1936.
12. Aslam S, Hamill RJ, Musher DM. Treatment of *Clostridium difficile*-associated disease: old therapies and new strategies. *Lancet Infect Dis.* 2005;5(9):549–557.
13. Jiang Z-D, Lowe B, Verenkar MP, et al. Prevalence of enteric pathogens among international travelers with diarrhea acquired in Kenya (Mombasa), India (Goa), or Jamaica (Montego Bay). *J Infect Dis.* 2002;185(4):497–502.
14. Du Pont HL, Ericsson CD, Farthing MJ, et al. Expert review of the evidence base for self-therapy of travelers' diarrhoea. *J Travel Med.* 2009;16:161–171.
15. De Bruyn G, Hahn S, Borwick A. Antibiotic treatment for travellers' diarrhoea. *Cochrane Database Syst Rev.* 2001;3: CD002242.
16. Fontaine O, Gore SM, Pierce NF. Rice-based oral rehydration solution for treating diarrhoea. *Cochrane Database Syst Rev.* 2000;2: CD001264.
17. Iynkaran N, Yadav M. Rice-starch oral rehydration therapy in neonates and young infants. *J Trop Pediatr.* 1998;44:199–203.
18. Dutta P, Mitra U, Dutta S. Hypo-osmolar oral rehydration salts (ORS) solution in dehydrating persistent diarrhoea in children: double-blind, randomised, controlled, clinical trial. *Acta Paediatr.* 2000;89:411–416.
19. Alam NH, Majumder RN, Fuchs GJ. Efficacy and safety of oral rehydration solution with reduced osmolarity in adults with cholera: a randomised double-blind clinical trial. *Lancet.* 1999;354:296–299.
20. Simakachorn N, Pichaipat V, Rithipornpaisarn P. Clinical evaluation of the addition of lyophilised heat-killed *Lactobacillus acidophilus* LB to oral rehydration therapy in the treatment of acute diarrhea in children. *J Pediatr Gastroenterol Nutr.* 2000;30:68–72.
21. Guandalini S, Pensebene L, Zikri MA, et al. *Lactobacillus* GG administered in oral rehydration solution to children with acute diarrhea: a multicenter European trial. *J Pediatr Gastroenterol Nutr.* 2000;30:54–60.
22. Dutta P, Mitra U, Datta A, et al. Impact of zinc supplementation in malnourished children with acute watery diarrhea. *J Trop Pediatr.* 2000;46:259–263.
23. Bhutta ZA, Black RE, Brown KH, et al. Prevention of diarrhoea and pneumonia by zinc supplementation in children in developing countries: pooled analysis of randomized controlled trials. Zinc Investigators' Collaborative Group. *J Paediatr.* 1999;135(6):689–697.
24. Ashref H, Rahman MM, Fuchs GJ, et al. Folic acid in the treatment of acute watery diarrhoea in children: a double-blind, randomised controlled trial. *Acta Paediatr.* 1998;87:1113–1115.
25. Ahmed FU, Rahman ME, Mahmood CB. Mothers' skill in preparing oral rehydration salt solution. *Indian J Pediatr.* 2000;67:99–102.
26. DuPont HL. Systematic review: prevention of travellers' diarrhoea. *Aliment Pharmacol Ther.* 2008;27(9):741–751.
27. Roy SK, Hossain MJ, Khatun W, et al. Zinc supplementation in children with cholera in Bangladesh: randomised controlled trial. *Br Med J.* 2008;336(7638):266–268.
28. Roy SK, Islam A, Ali R, et al. A randomised clinical trial to compare the efficacy of erythromycin, ampicillin and tetracycline for the treatment of cholera in children. *Trans R Soc Trop Med Hyg.* 1998;92:460–462.
29. Ranjit K, Nurahan M. Tetracycline resistant cholera in Kelantan. *Med J Malaysia.* 2000;55:143–145.
30. Garg P, Chakraborty S, Basu I, et al. Expanding multiple antibiotic resistance among clinical strains of *Vibrio cholerae* isolated from 1992–7 in Calcutta, India. *Epidemiol Infect.* 2000;124:393–399.
31. Sack DA, Lyke C, McLaughlin C, Suwanvanichkij V. *Antimicrobial resistance in shigellosis, cholera and campylobacteriosis.* Geneva: WHO; 2001.

32. Gotuzzo E, Seas C, Echeverria J, et al. Ciprofloxacin for the treatment of cholera: a randomised double-blind controlled clinical trial of a single daily dose in Peruvian adults. *Clin Infect Dis*. 1995;20:1485–1490.

33. Khan WA, Bennish M, Seas C, et al. Randomised controlled trial of single-dose ciprofloxacin and doxycycline for cholera caused by *Vibrio cholerae*, O1 or O139. *Lancet*. 1996;348:296–300.

34. Saha D, Khan WA, Karim MM, Chowdhury HR, Salam MA, Bennish ML. Single-dose ciprofloxacin versus 12-dose erythromycin for childhood cholera: a randomised controlled trial. *Lancet*. 2005;366:1085–1093.

35. Garg P, Sinha S, Chakraborty R, et al. Emergence of fluoroquinolone-resistant strains of *Vibrio cholerae* O1 biotype El Tor among hospitalized patients with cholera in Calcutta, India. *Antimicrob Agents Chemother*. 2001;45:1605–1606.

36. Khan WA, Saha D, Rahman A, Salam MA, Bogaerts J, Bennish ML. Comparison of single-dose azithromycin and 12-dose, 3-day erythromycin for childhood cholera: a randomised, double-blind trial. *Lancet*. 2002;360:1722–1727.

37. Sack RB. Prophylactic antibiotics? The individual versus the community. *N Engl J Med*. 1979;300:1107–1108.

38. Kabra SK, Madhulika, Talati A, Soni N, Patel S, Modi RR. Multidrug resistant typhoid fever. *Trop Doct*. 2000;30:195–199.

39. Ackers ML, Puhr ND, Tauxe RV, Mintz ED. Laboratory based surveillance of *Salmonella* serotype Typhi infections in the United States: antimicrobial resistance on the rise. *J Am Med Assoc*. 2000;283:2668–2673.

40. Le TA, Lejay-Collin M, Grimont PA, et al. Endemic, epidemic clone of *Salmonella enterica* serovar Typhi harboring a single multidrug-resistant plasmid in Vietnam between 1995 and 2002. *J Clin Microbiol*. 2004;42:3094–3099.

41. Threlfall EJ, Skinner JA, Ward LR. Detection of decreased in vitro susceptibility to ciprofloxacin in *Salmonella enterica* serotypes Typhi and Paratyphi A. *J Antimicrob Chemother*. 2001;48:740–741.

42. Parry CM. The treatment of multidrug-resistant and nalidixic acid-resistant typhoid fever in Viet Nam. *Trans R Soc Trop Med Hyg*. 2004;98:413–422.

43. Dolecek C, La TTP, Rang NN, et al. A multi-center randomised controlled trial of gatifloxacin versus azithromycin for the treatment of uncomplicated typhoid fever in children and adults in Vietnam. *PLoS ONE*. 2008;3(5):e2188.

44. Rahman M, Ahmad A, Shoma S. Decline in epidemic of multidrug resistant *Salmonella typhi* is not associated with increased incidence of antibiotic-susceptible strain in Bangladesh. *Epidemiol Infect*. 2002;129:29–34.

45. Sood S, Kapil A, Das B, Jain Y, Kabra SK. Re-emergence of chloramphenicol-sensitive *Salmonella typhi*. *Lancet*. 1999;353:1241–1242.

46. Gasem MH, Keuter M, Dolmans WM, et al. Persistence of Salmonellae in blood and bone marrow: randomized controlled trial comparing ciprofloxacin and chloramphenicol treatments against enteric fever. *Antimicrob Agents Chemother*. 2003;47:1727–1731.

47. Duong NM, Vinh Chau NV, Van Anh DC, et al. Short course fleroxacin in the treatment of typhoid fever. *JAMA (Southeast Asia)*. 1995;11:6–11.

48. Cao XT, Kneen R, Nguyen TA, Truong DL, White NJ, Parry CM. A comparative study of ofloxacin and cefixime for the study of typhoid fever in children. *Pediatr Infect Dis J*. 1999;18:245–248.

49. Hien TT, Bethell DB, Hoa NT, et al. Short course of ofloxacin for treatment of multidrug resistant typhoid. *Clin Infect Dis*. 1995;20:917–923.

50. Bethell DB, Hien TT, Phi LT, et al. The effects on growth of single short courses of fluoroquinolones. *Arch Dis Child*. 1996;74:44–64.

51. Doherty CP, Saha SK, Cutting WA. Typhoid fever, ciprofloxacin, and growth in young children. *Ann Trop Paediatr*. 2000;20:297–303.

52. Girgis NJ, Kilpatrick ME, Farid Z, Mikhail IA, Bishay E. Ceftriaxone versus chloramphenicol in the treatment of typhoid fever. *Drugs Exp Clin Res*. 1990;16:607–609.

53. Bhutta ZA, Khan IA, Shadmani M. Failure of short course ceftriaxone chemotherapy for multidrug resistant typhoid fever in children: a randomised controlled trial in Pakistan. *Antimicrob Agents Chemother*. 2000;44:450–452.

54. Frenck Jr RW, Mansour A, Nakhla I, et al. Short-course azithromycin for the treatment of uncomplicated typhoid fever in children and adolescents. *Clin Infect Dis*. 2004;38:951–957.

55. Effa EE, Bukirwa H. Azithromycin for treating uncomplicated typhoid and paratyphoid fever (enteric fever). *Cochrane Database Syst Rev*. 2008;(4) CD006083.

56. Frenck RW, Nakhla I, Sultar Y, et al. Azithromycin versus ceftriaxone for the treatment of uncomplicated typhoid fever in children. *Clin Infect Dis*. 2000;31:1134–1138.

57. Chinh N, Parry CM, Ly NT, et al. A randomised controlled comparison of azithromycin and ofloxacin for the treatment of multidrug resis-tant or nalidixic acid resistant enteric fever. *Antimicrob Agents Chemother*. 2000;44:1855–1859.

58. Thaver D, Zaidi AK, Critchley JA, Azmatullah A, Madni SA, Bhutta ZA. Fluoroquinolones for treating typhoid and paratyphoid fever (enteric fever). *Cochrane Database Syst Rev*. 2008;(4) CD004530.

59. Girgis NI, Butler T, Frenck RW, et al. Azithromycin versus ciprofloxacin for treatment of uncomplicated typhoid fever in a randomized trial in Egypt that included patients with multidrug resistance. *Antimicrob Agents Chemother*. 1999;43:1441–1444.

60. Hoffman SL, Punjabi NH, Kumala S. Reduction of mortality of chloramphenicol-treated severe typhoid fever by high dose dexamethasone. *N Engl J Med*. 1984;310:82–88.

61. Ferrecio C, Morris JG, Valdirieso C, et al. Efficacy of ciprofloxacin in the treatment of chronic typhoid carriers. *J Infect Dis*. 1988;157:1235–1239.

62. Gotuzzo E, Guerro JG, Benavente L, et al. Use of norfloxacin to treat chronic typhoid carriage. *J Infect Dis*. 1998;157:1221–1225.

63. Bratoeva MP, John JF. In vivo R plasmid transfer in a patient with a mixed infection of *Shigella* dysentery. *Epidemiol Infect*. 1994;112:247–252.

64. Zafar A, Hasan R, Nizami S.Q, et al. Frequency of isolation of various subtypes and antimicrobial resistance of *Shigella* from urban slums of Karachi, Pakistan. *Int J Infect Dis*. 13(6):668–72.

65. Lewis HC, Ethelberg S, Olsen KE, et al. Outbreaks of *Shigella sonnei* infections in Denmark and Australia linked to consumption of imported raw baby corn. *Epidemiol Infect*. 2009;137(3):326–334.

66. Robicsek A, Jacoby GA, Hooper DC. The worldwide emergence of plasmid-mediated quinolone resistance. *Lancet Infect Dis*. 2006;6:629–640.

67. Von Seidlein L, Deok RK, Ali M, et al. A multicentre study of *Shigella* diarrhoea in six Asian countries: disease burden, clinical manifestations, and microbiology. *PLoS Med*. 2006;3(9):1556–1569.

68. Pazhani GP, Niyogi SK, Singh AK, et al. Molecular characterization of multidrug-resistant *Shigella* species isolated from epidemic and endemic cases of shigellosis in India. *J Med Microbiol*. 2008;57(7):856–863.

69. Engels D, Madaras T, Nyandwi S, Murray J. Epidemic dysentery caused by *Shigella dysenteriae* type 1: a sentinel site surveillance of antimicrobial resistance patterns in Burundi. *Bull World Health Org*. 1995;73:787–791.

70. Anonymous. Antibiotics in the management of shigellosis. *Wkly Epidemiol Rec* 2004;79:349–356. Online. Available at http://www.who.int/wer.

71. Vinh H, Wain J, Chinh MT, et al. Treatment of bacillary dysentery in Vietnamese children: two doses of ofloxacin versus 5 days nalidixic acid. *Trans R Soc Trop Med Hyg*. 2000;94:323–326.

72. Salam MA, Dhar U, Khan WA, Bennish ML. Randomised comparison of ciprofloxacin suspension and pivmecillinam for childhood shigellosis. *Lancet*. 1998;352:522–527.

73. Martin JM, Pitetti R, Maffei F, Tritt J, Smail K, Wald ER. Treatment of shigellosis with cefixime: two days versus five days. *Pediatr Infect Dis J*. 2000;19:522–526.

74. Moolasart P, Eampokalap B, Ratanasrithong M. Comparison of the efficacy of ceftibuten and norfloxacin in the treatment of acute gastrointestinal infection in children. *Southeast Asian J Trop Med Public Health*. 1999;30:764–769.

75. Khan WA, Seas C, Dhar U, Salam MA, Bennish ML. Treatment of shigellosis: comparison of azithromycin and ciprofloxacin. A double-blind, randomised, controlled trial. *Ann Intern Med*. 1997;26:697–703.

76. Hohmann EL. Nontyphoidal salmonellosis. *Clin Infect Dis*. 2001;32:263–269.

77. Montes M, DuPont HL. Enteritis, enterocolitis and infectious diarrhea syndromes. In: Cohen J, Powderley W, eds. *Infectious diseases*. London: Mosby; 2004:477–490.

78. Barbara G, Stanghellini V, Berti-Ceroni C, et al. Role of antibiotic therapy on long term germ excretion in faeces and digestive symptoms in *Salmonella* infection. *Aliment Pharmacol Ther*. 2000;14:1127–1131.

79. Dyson C, Ribeiro CD, Westmoreland D. Large scale use of ciprofloxacin in the control of a *Salmonella* outbreak in a hospital for the mentally handicapped. *J Hosp Infect*. 1995;29:287–296.

80. Fukushima H, Hashizume T, Morita T, et al. Clinical experiences in Sakai City Hospital during the massive outbreak of enterohemorrhagic *Escherichia coli* O157 infections in Sakai City 1996. *Pediatr Int*. 1999;41:213–217.

81. Akinyemi KO, Oyefolu AO, Opere B, Otunba-Payne VA, Oworu AO. *Escherichia coli* in patients with acute gastroenteritis in Lagos, Nigeria. *East Afr Med J*. 1998;75:512–515.

82. Jain S, Chen L, Dechet A, et al. An outbreak of enterotoxigenic *Escherichia coli* associated with sushi restaurants in Nevada, 2004. *Clin Infect Dis*. 2008;47(1):1–7.

83. Vila J, Vargas M, Ruiz J, Corachan M, De Anta MTJ, Gascon J. Quinolone resistance in enterotoxigenic *Escherichia coli* causing diarrhea in travelers to India in comparison with other geographical areas. *Antimicrob Agents Chemother.* 2000;44(6):1731–1733.

84. Shah N, DuPont HL, Ramsey DJ. Global etiology of travelers' diarrhea: systematic review from 1973 to the present. *Am J Trop Med Hyg.* 2009;80(4):609–614.

85. Hoge CW, Gambel JM, Srijan A, Pitarangsi C, Echeverria P. Trends in antibiotic resistance among diarrheal pathogens isolated in Thailand over 15 years. *Clin Infect Dis.* 1998;26:341–345.

86. Asrat D. Screening for enteropathogenic *Escherichia coli* in paediatric patients with diarrhoea and controls using pooled antisera. *Ethiop Med J.* 2001;39:23–28.

87. Obi CL, Coker AO, Epoke J, Ndip RN. Distributional patterns of bacterial diarrhoeagenic agents and antibiograms of isolates from diarrhoeaic and non-diarrhoeaic patients in urban and rural areas of Nigeria. *Cent Afr J Med.* 1998;44:223–229.

88. Dow MA, Tóth I, Malik A, et al. Phenotypic and genetic characterization of enteropathogenic *Escherichia coli* (EPEC) and enteroaggregative *E. coli* (EAEC) from diarrhoeal and non-diarrhoeal children in Libya. *Comp Immunol Microbiol Infect Dis.* 2006;29(2–3):100–113.

89. Glandt M, Adachi JA, Mathewson JJ, et al. Enteroaggregative *Escherichia coli* as a cause of travellers' diarrhoea: clinical response to ciprofloxacin. *Clin Infect Dis.* 1999;29:335–338.

90. Huppertz HI, Rutkowski S, Aleksic S, Karch H. Acute and chronic diarrhoea and abdominal colic associated with enteroaggregative *Escherichia coli* in young children living in western Europe. *Lancet.* 1997;349:1660–1662.

91. Wanke CA, Gerrior J, Blais V, Mayer H, Acheson D. Successful treatment of diarrheal disease associated with enteroaggregative *Escherichia coli* in adults infected with human immunodeficiency virus. *J Infect Dis.* 1998;178:1369–1372.

92. Engberg J, Aarestrup FM, Taylor DE, Gerner-Smidt P, Nachamkin I. Quinolone and macrolide resistance in *Campylobacter jejuni* and *C. coli*: resistance mechanisms and trends in human isolates. *Emerg Infect Dis.* 2001;7(1):24–34.

93. Endtz HP, Ruijs GJ, van Klingeren B, Jansen WH, van der Ryden T, Moulton RP. Quinolone resistance in campylobacter isolated from man and poultry following the introduction of fluoroquinolones in veterinary medicine. *J Antimicrob Chemother.* 1991;27:199–208.

94. Adler-Mosca H, Luthy-Hottehstein J, Martinetti Lucchini G, Burnens A, Altwegg M. Development of resistance to quinolones in five patients with campylobacteriosis treated with ciprofloxacin or norfloxacin. *Eur J Clin Microbiol Infect Dis.* 1991;10:953–959.

95. Zheng H, Sun Y, Lin S, Mao Z, Jiang B. *Yersinia enterocolitica* infection in diarrheal patients. *Eur J Clin Microbiol Infect Dis.* 2008;27(8):741–752.

96. Wootipoom N, Bhoopong P, Pomwised R, et al. A decrease in the proportion of infections by pandemic *Vibrio parahaemolyticus* in Hat Yai Hospital, Southern Thailand. *J Med Microbiol.* 2007;56(12):1630–1638.

97. Gomez Campdera J, Munoz P, Lopez Prieto F, et al. Gastroenteritis due to *Aeromonas* in pediatrics. *An Esp Pediatr.* 1996;44:548–552.

98. Ahmed A, Hafiz S, Ahmed QT, et al. Sensitivity pattern and beta-lactamase production in clinical isolates of *Aeromonas* strains. *J Pak Med Assoc.* 1998;48:158–161.

99. Kuipers EJ, Surawicz CM. *Clostridium difficile* infection. *Lancet.* 2008;371:1486–1488.

100. Owens Jr RC, Donskey CJ, Gaynes RP, Loo VG, Muto CA. Antimicrobial-associated risk factors for *Clostridium difficile* infection. *Clin Infect Dis.* 2008;46(suppl 1):S19–S31.

101. Muto CA, Pokrywka M, Shutt K, et al. A large outbreak of *Clostridium difficile*-associated disease with an unexpected proportion of deaths and colectomies at a teaching hospital following increased fluoroquinolone use. *Infect Control Hosp Epidemiol.* 2005;26(3):273–280.

102. Baines SD, O'Connor R, Freeman J, et al. Emergence of reduced susceptibility to metronidazole in *Clostridium difficile*. *J Antimicrob Chemother.* 2008;62(5):1046–1052.

103. Zar FA, Bakkanagari SR, Moorthi KMLST, Davis MB. A comparison of vancomycin and metronidazole for the treatment of *Clostridium difficile*-associated diarrhea, stratified by disease severity. *Clin Infect Dis.* 2007;45(3):302–307.

104. Musher DM, Logan N, Bressler AM, Johnson DP, Rossignol J-F. Nitazoxanide versus vancomycin in *Clostridium difficile* infection: a randomized, double-blind study. *Clin Infect Dis.* 2009;48(4):e41–e46.

105. Gerding DN, Muto CA, Owens Jr RC. Treatment of *Clostridium difficile* infection. *Clin Infect Dis.* 2008;46(suppl 1):S32–S42.

106. Koo HL, Koo DC, Musher DM, Dupont HL. Antimotility agents for the treatment of *Clostridium difficile* diarrhea and colitis. *Clin Infect Dis.* 2009;48(5):598–605.

107. Parkes GC, Sanderson JD, Whelan K. The mechanisms and efficacy of probiotics in the prevention of *Clostridium difficile*-associated diarrhoea. *Lancet Infect Dis.* 2009;9(4):237–244.

108. Health Protection Agency. *Clostridium difficile infection: how to deal with the problem*. London: Health Protection Agency; 2009. Online. Available at http://www.hpa.org.uk/web/HPAwebFile/HPAweb_C/1232006607827.

109. Puéchal X. Whipple's disease [Maladie de Whipple]. *Rev Med Interne.* 2009;30(3):233–241.

110. Fenollar F, Rolain J-M, Alric L, et al. Resistance to trimethoprim/sulfamethoxazole and *Tropheryma whipplei*. *Int J Antimicrob Agents.* 2009;34(5):467–470.

111. Chey WD, Wong BCY. American College of Gastroenterology guideline on the management of *Helicobacter pylori* infection. *Am J Gastroenterol.* 2007;102:1808–1825.

112. Malfertheiner P, Megraud F, O'Morain C, et al. The European Helicobacter Study Group (EHSG). Current concepts in the management of *Helicobacter pylori infection*: the Maastricht III Consensus Report. *Gut.* 2007;56:772–781.

113. Khurana R, Fischbach L, Chiba N, Veldhuyzen van Zanten S. An update on anti-*Helicobacter pylori* treatment in children. *Can J Gastroenterol.* 2005;19(7):441–445.

114. Zaat JOM, Mank TG, Assendelft WJJ. Drugs for treating giardiasis. *Cochrane Database Syst Rev.* 2000;(2)CD000217. [Update in: *Cochrane Database of Syst Rev.* 2007;(2):CD000217]

115. Pritt BS, Clark G. Amebiasis. *Mayo Clin Proc.* 2008;83(10):1154–1160.

116. WHO/PAHO/UNESCO report. A consultation with experts on amoebiasis: Mexico City, Mexico 28–29 January, 1997. *Epidemiol Bull.* 1997;18(1):13–14.

117. Schuster FL, Ramirez-Avila L. Current world status of *Balantidium coli. Clin Microbiol Rev.* 2008;21(4):626–638.

118. Johnson EH, Windsor JJ, Clark CG. Emerging from obscurity: biological, clinical, and diagnostic aspects of *Dientamoeba fragilis. Clin Microbiol Rev.* 2004;17(3):553–570.

119. Stensvold CR, Lewis HC, Hammerum AM, et al. Blastocystis: unravelling potential risk factors and clinical significance of a common but neglected parasite. *Epidemiol Infect.* 2009;137(11):1655.

48 Hepatitis

Janice Main and Howard C. Thomas

Acute and chronic viral hepatitis continue to cause significant morbidity and mortality worldwide. While many viruses cause hepatitis this chapter concentrates on the hepatotropic viruses, particularly those associated with chronic hepatitis.

HEPATITIS A VIRUS INFECTION

Hepatitis A virus (HAV) is a member of the Picornaviridae family and a major cause of acute hepatitis. HAV is transmitted by the feco-oral route. Although most cases of acute HAV infection are subclinical, life-threatening fulminant hepatitis can occur and is particularly seen in older patients in the setting of significant alcohol consumption or pre-existing chronic liver disease such as chronic hepatitis B or C or non-alcoholic fatty liver disease (NAFLD).

There are anecdotal reports of interferon-β being used in severe cases[1] but this is an experimental approach and referral to a transplant center is recommended for those with life-threatening disease.

PREVENTION

A major advance in the prevention of HAV infection has been the development of a safe and effective vaccine.[2] Prior to this the only approach was the administration of 'normal human immunoglobulin', also known as gamma globulin, as passive prophylaxis. The efficacy of this depended on the presence of protective anti-HAV antibodies in the pool of blood donors, but the seroprevalence of IgG anti-HAV has declined with improved sanitation in many countries and failures of prophylaxis have occurred. There are also increasing concerns regarding the safety of immunoglobulin products with potential risk of new variant Creutzfeldt–Jakob disease.

HAV vaccine has also been combined with hepatitis B vaccine and, in a preparation particularly targeted towards travelers, with typhoid vaccine.

Different countries have used varying strategies for the administration of HAV vaccine. Some have included the vaccine as part of the normal childhood vaccination program and others have recommended a more targeted approach. The vaccine is recommended for those who travel to areas of poor sanitation, for those with underlying liver disease such as chronic hepatitis B or C and those involved in food preparation where the infection could be passed on to many individuals.

HEPATITIS B VIRUS INFECTION

EPIDEMIOLOGY

Hepatitis B virus (HBV) can be transmitted sexually, by blood, blood products or vertically (mother to child). There are an estimated 350 million cases of chronic HBV worldwide. In some areas of South East Asia approximately 20% of the population have chronic HBV infection, with many infected vertically. Already vaccination programs are reducing the prevalence in some countries, but it will be many years before the disease can be eradicated. In the Western world chronic hepatitis B (CHB) is mainly seen in high-risk individuals such as men who have sex with men (MSM) or intravenous drug users (IDU).

NATURAL HISTORY

HBV is a small (3.2 kb), partially double-stranded DNA virus and a member of the hepadnavirus group.

The incubation period is 2–6 months and although many cases are subclinical, fulminant hepatitis can occur.

Chronic HBV infection is defined by ongoing viral replication 6 months or more after the initial infection. Chronic infection is seen in approximately 5% of healthy adults, with higher rates in those with underlying immunodeficiency.

With perinatal infection the risk of chronicity is much higher (95%), and it is thought that this may be related to the immaturity of the neonatal immune system, circulating hepatitis B e antigen (HBeAg) inducing immune tolerance and possibly host genetic factors.[3]

More severe disease is seen in men and it is estimated that 40% of infected men, if untreated, will die because of the subsequent complications which include the development of cirrhosis, liver failure and the development of hepatocellular carcinoma (HCC).[4,5]

WILD-TYPE VIRUS AND VIRAL VARIANTS

Patients infected with wild-type HBV have circulating hepatitis B surface antigen (HBsAg) and HBeAg. HBV variants are increasingly recognized and many have implications for diagnosis, management and vaccination programs. For example, a subgroup of patients who are HBsAg positive and HBeAg negative, with anti-HBe antibodies, have active viral replication with HBV DNA levels of more than 10^5 genomes/mL in the blood and active liver damage with raised transaminase levels and inflammation and often fibrosis on liver biopsy. Viral sequencing in these patients revealed a mutation in the pre-core gene[6] which resulted in a stop codon which limited production of HBeAg. These viral variants are known as pre-core variants or HBe-negative variants and can develop in patients with wild-type virus, during antiviral therapy or, alternatively, patients can be infected de novo with these variants.

GENOTYPES

There are several genotypes of HBV and these were originally thought mainly to be of epidemiological interest. It is also recognized that the response to treatment may additionally be determined by the genotype. Patients infected with genotype A, for example, are more likely to respond to interferon therapy by HBe antigen/antibody seroconversion than those with other genotypes.

ANIMAL MODELS

Hepadnavirus infections with similar outcomes are seen in several animal species, including woodchucks, Beechey ground squirrels and Pekin ducks.

ACUTE HEPATITIS B

The development of acute hepatic illness appears to coincide with the host immune response and the detection of anti-hepatitis core (anti-HBc) IgM antibodies. Although fatigue is not uncommon for some months following infection, it does not necessarily correlate with ongoing viral replication. Large multicenter trials would be required to determine whether immunomodulatory or antiviral therapy could limit the acute illness and reduce the risk of chronicity. There are theoretical risks that the immune stimulant effects of interferons could be detrimental in this setting. This has not been seen in practice.[7] Small studies support the use of nucleoside analogs, particularly lamivudine, in severe cases.[8]

CHRONIC HEPATITIS B

The risks of developing decompensated liver disease or HCC have been shown to be positively correlated with viremia levels of more than 10^5 genomes/mL. The aims of antiviral therapy are to clear or suppress the infection and to reduce the risks of developing life-threatening liver disease. Viral clearance also reduces the risk of viral transmission to others.

CANDIDATES FOR THERAPY

Chronic infection is defined as the presence of ongoing viral replication (HBV DNA in blood) for more than 6 months. Those infected with wild-type virus will be HBsAg and HBe Ag positive and those with HBe-negative variants will be HBsAg positive, HBeAg negative and anti-HBe antibody positive. HBe antigen positive and negative patients with viremia levels of more than 10^5 genomes/mL with evidence of hepatic necroinflammatory activity and fibrosis are candidates for therapy.[9]

ASSESSING THE RESPONSE TO ANTIVIRAL THERAPY

In patients with wild-type infection, a response is defined as:
1. sustained clearance of HBV DNA
2. sustained clearance of HBeAg and the development of anti-HBe antibodies (known as HBeAg/anti-HBe seroconversion)
3. sustained clearance of HBsAg and the development of anti-HBs antibodies (this can occur many years after (1)).

In patients infected with HBe-negative variants, only (1) and (3) are applicable.

In a successfully treated patient the clearance of virus is associated with a biochemical response (normalization of the elevated transaminase value) and a histological response (decreased hepatic inflammation and fibrosis).

With the available treatments only a minority of patients achieve a sustained virological response after 1 year of therapy, and long-term suppressive therapy has become an increasingly popular strategy for patients most at risk of the life-threatening complications of chronic HBV infection.

TREATMENTS

Interferons

Interferon-α has been administered for chronic HBV infection since 1976 and is now licensed therapy in many countries. Standard interferon-α was given thrice weekly for 3–6 months but has now been phased out in preference to the more long-acting pegylated interferons (peginterferons) which are administered weekly for 6–12 months.

It is thought that the successful response to interferon therapy is from its combination of antiviral and immunostimulatory effects.

Interferons induce intracellular enzymes which inhibit viral protein synthesis. They stimulate the production of about 30 host proteins including 2',5'-oligoadenylate synthetase which leads to activation of ribonuclease enzymes that cleave viral mRNA. Protein kinases are also induced which can have an inhibitory effect on viral protein synthesis.

Hepatocytes have very little major histocompatibility complex (MHC) class I display and it is thought that this limits host immune recognition of infected cells. Interferons enhance the MHC class I display and it is thought that this encourages immune lysis of infected cells, which sometimes manifests as an elevation of the transaminase values in patients successfully treated with interferon. In patients with HIV and HBV infection, a similar phenomenon is seen with the immune restoration that follows effective antiretroviral therapy.[10] This 'transaminitis' (Fig. 48.1) is generally asymptomatic; in those with advanced liver disease, however, a brisk hepatitic response can lead to hepatic decompensation. Particular care is therefore required when treating patients with cirrhosis with interferon-based regimens.

In successfully treated patients with wild-type virus, an HBeAg/anti-HBe seroconversion occurs. Patients may continue to be HBsAg positive for some years but eventually this is often cleared.[11] Follow-up studies have shown an improvement in the level of inflammation and fibrosis in the liver and this has been associated with a reduced risk of HCC in these patients.[12]

The original studies were with standard interferon given thrice weekly subcutaneously and success rates of 25–40% were reported in those with adult acquired disease.[13–16] Similar results have been seen with peginterferon.[17]

Lower sustained response rates (approximately 20%) are seen with treatment of patients with anti-HBe variants.[18]

Patients with an existing active immune response with high transaminase levels, or active inflammation on a liver biopsy and low HBV DNA levels, are more likely to respond to therapy than those with immunodeficiency such as HIV infection or vertically acquired disease.

The main adverse effects of interferon-α are listed in Box 48.1. In view of the potential myelotoxicity, careful monitoring of the blood count is advised, with dose alteration as required. Patients with advanced liver disease and leukopenia or thrombocytopenia at baseline require particularly careful monitoring. Influenza-like symptoms with malaise, fever and myalgia are particularly troublesome with the initiation of therapy. These can be minimized by administration of the interferon in the late evening and by prescribing paracetamol (acetaminophen) or non-steroidal anti-inflammatory drugs as required.

Depression is another major side effect and may limit therapy for some individuals. Patients with mild depressive symptomatology often find antidepressants helpful but expert psychiatric help is advised for those with more severe symptoms.

The immunostimulatory effects of interferon can also result in the exacerbation of underlying autoimmune conditions.

OTHER IMMUNOMODULATORY APPROACHES

Trials with thymic hormones, thymic peptides,[19] levamisole and inosine pranobex have generally shown no benefit and the use of adjuvant vaccines remains experimental.

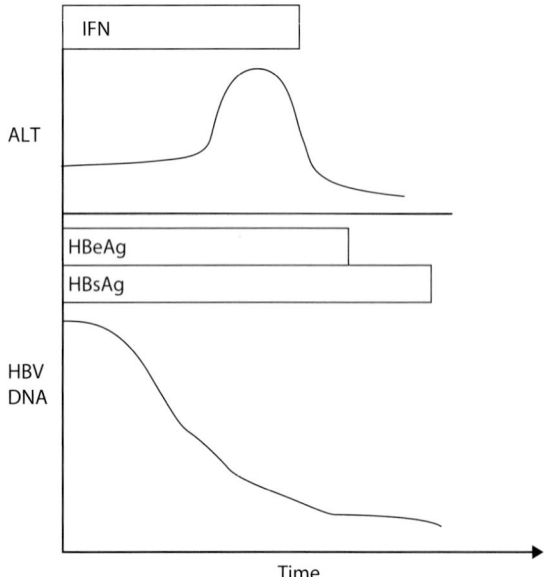

Fig. 48.1 Chronic hepatitis B; successful response to interferon (IFN). ALT, alanine transaminase.

Box 48.1 Side effects of interferon-α

Fever and chills (less with subsequent doses)
Myalgia
Fatigue
Myelotoxicity (regular monitoring of full blood count required)
Impaired concentration
Altered mood (particularly depression – can be severe)
Exacerbation or development of underlying autoimmune disease, e.g. hyperthyroidism or hypothyroidism
Alopecia
Arthralgia
Hypersensitivity reactions (rare)
Pulmonary infiltrates (very rare)

There are case reports of patients with CHB with hematological conditions who have been given bone marrow transplants from HBV immune donors and subsequently cleared HBV.[20] This has led to considerable interest in the potential for lymphocyte transfer or modulation of the host immune response by ex-vivo stimulation of host lymphocytes.

NUCLEOSIDE/NUCLEOTIDE ANALOGS (NUCS)

There are three classes of NUCs used as therapy for HBV infection.

L-Nucleosides

Lamivudine

Lamivudine (3′-thiacytidine, 3TC) was one of the first of the new generation of agents to be shown to have a significant effect on HBV replication.[21–23] Its low toxicity, even with long-term use, is thought to relate to its minus enantiomer configuration.

After 1 year of therapy in one study 17% of patients cleared HBeAg and the response rate increased to 27% after a second year of therapy.[24] An incremental increase is seen with longer treatment periods and a success rate of up to 66% has been reported with 4 years of therapy.[25]

Viral resistance was initially reported in the setting of liver transplantation[26,27] and was noted to involve the YMDD motif (the equivalent of the 184 mutation in the HIV reverse transcriptase gene).

After 1 year of therapy approximately 20% of patients have resistant virus and this increases over time to around 70% at 5 years.

Although the YMDD variant is thought to be less replication competent,[28] there have been 'flares' in hepatitis[29,30] reported with its emergence.

Although lamivudine in combination with interferon or other NUCs has not been shown to result in increased clearance rates, the emergence of resistance appears to be decreased by combination therapy.[31]

Lamivudine monotherapy appears effective for viral prophylaxis in patients at risk of HBV reactivation who are about to receive immunosuppressive therapy for co-existent morbidities.[32] Lamivudine monotherapy is also occasionally used in pregnant mothers with high levels of viremia to reduce the risk of mother-to-baby transmission,[33] but otherwise, having been recognized as having a low genetic barrier, it is now rarely used as monotherapy.

Emtricitabine

As an antiviral agent, emtricitabine (FTC) appears very similar to lamivudine.[34,35] Abnormal dreams are reported by some patients. It is mainly prescribed in combination with tenofovir and as both agents also have activity against HIV, this has proved very useful for the management of patients with HIV/HBV co-infection.

Telbivudine

Although telbivudine appeared more effective than lamivudine in a large controlled trial,[36] there were reports of elevated creatine kinase levels and concerns regarding peripheral neuropathy with more prolonged therapy.

Acyclic nucleoside phosphonates

Adefovir

Adefovir as monotherapy has been shown to be effective in patients with HBeAg positive and negative chronic hepatitis B.[37,38] More prolonged therapy appears more advantageous in HBeAg-negative chronic hepatitis.[39] There have been concerns regarding nephrotoxicity.[40] It has activity against lamivudine-resistant HBV and has therefore been mainly used in combination with lamivudine as a 'de novo' therapy or as an 'add-on' agent for patients on lamivudine monotherapy[41,42] and emerging resistance.

Tenofovir

Tenofovir is more potent than adefovir.[43] It is increasingly used in patients with HBV infection as it has potent anti-HBV activity and low rates of resistance compared to lamivudine monotherapy. Reports suggest that patients with the anti-HBe variant may be more at risk of resistance than those infected with wild-type virus.[44] There are some concerns regarding the potential for nephrotoxicity, with reports of elevated creatinine, renal tubular dysfunction and risks of osteomalacia,[44–48] and monitoring (creatinine, calcium and phosphate levels) is recommended. It is only with longer-term follow-up that the risk of this will be clarified.

Deoxyguanosine analogs

Entecavir

Entecavir has potent activity against HBV[49,50] and low rates of resistance have been reported.[51] It appears more potent than adefovir.[52] It has been suggested that with low toxicity, high potency and low rates of resistance it is useful as a first-line agent as minimal monitoring is required in the outpatient clinic. It is less useful for patients with lamivudine-resistant virus[53] and also has limited efficacy in patients with a partial response to adefovir therapy.[54] There were concerns in animal studies regarding development of tumors but this has not been observed in humans.

PLANNING THERAPY FOR THE PATIENT

Overall it is possible to offer a sustained HBeAg/anti-HBe seroconversion rate of 30–40% of immunocompetent adults with adult acquired disease. Treatment can be stopped 6 months after HBe clearance.

Many patients, however, have only minimal liver disease and the risks of therapy with side effects of drugs and emergence of resistance have to be weighed against the clinical benefit and the healthcare costs.

Studies such as the REVEAL study[55,56] have been helpful in determining which patients are most likely to benefit from therapy and this is acknowledged in guidelines.

This study showed that a worse disease outcome is seen in those with higher levels of HBV replication. Guidelines generally recommend targeting therapy to those with active viral replication and evidence of progressive liver disease.[57,58] The potential risks and benefits of therapy have to be carefully assessed for the individual patient and guidelines are being frequently updated[59] with the development of new agents and the results of more long-term studies. Interferon is often recommended as a first-line therapy, particularly in those with a reasonable chance of response (genotype A, high transaminase level, low HBV DNA levels) as it is a 'one-off therapy'.

In a subgroup of patients treated with NUCs it is possible to discontinue therapy after a finite course of therapy; however, NUCs are increasingly being used as long-term suppressive therapy. The potency and high genetic barrier of tenofovir and entecavir have encouraged their use as monotherapy. These approaches should not be embarked on lightly as antiviral treatment requires monitoring, is expensive and there are risks of potentially fatal flares of hepatitis if the patient discontinues medication.

PREVENTION

Safe and effective vaccines have now been developed against HBV.[60] Passive prophylaxis with HBV immune globulin continues to be used to help prevent vertical transmission and in the setting of transplantation if nucleoside NUCs are ineffective.

HEPATITIS C VIRUS INFECTION

Hepatitis C virus (HCV), a member of the Flaviviridae family, was discovered in 1989,[61] although its existence was suspected for many years as some patients who had been exposed to blood products developed acute or chronic hepatitis but had negative tests for HAV or HBV infection. The terms 'post-transfusion' or 'parenterally transmitted' non-A, non-B hepatitis evolved and on retrospective testing the majority were found to be caused by HCV.

EPIDEMIOLOGY

HCV is mainly transmitted via blood. The screening of blood products has limited new cases but the infection remains common in those with a background of exposure to blood products before screening was introduced and in those with a history of intravenous drug use. Mother-to-baby transmission can occur but, in contrast to HBV, sexual transmission among heterosexuals is rare. An outbreak of HCV infection among HIV-positive men has, however, raised the possibility that sexual transmission is a potential route of transmission in men who have sex with men (MSM).[62]

In many patients there is no clear source of infection. It is estimated that there are 170 million people with hepatitis C worldwide.[63] The seroprevalence is low (0.07%)[64] in UK blood donors but thought to be 0.7% in the general UK population.[65]

Higher seroprevalence rates are reported elsewhere. In some areas of Egypt, for example, 25% of the adult population have HCV infection.[66]

There are six main genotypes of HCV:[67] genotypes 1, 2 and 3 are the predominant genotypes in Europe and the USA,[68] with genotype 4 predominating in Egypt.[69]

NATURAL HISTORY

The incubation period of HCV infection is 6–12 weeks. Acute hepatitis is generally subclinical and therefore often undiagnosed unless the patient is being monitored following a needlestick injury. Chronic infection follows in 60–80% of patients which can, over decades, lead to the development of cirrhosis and HCC.[70,71] More rapid progression is associated with male gender, older age at time of infection, heavy alcohol consumption[72] and immunosuppression such as HIV infection.[73]

It is also recognized that many patients with often only mild liver disease complain of significant fatigue and it has been postulated that HCV may cause CNS infection and/or dysfunction.[74]

TREATMENT

 ### ACUTE HEPATITIS

Although acute HCV is often undiagnosed, a number of studies have assessed the benefits of antiviral therapy with interferon monotherapy[75] or in combination with ribavirin. One study showed a response rate of more than 95% with standard interferon monotherapy.[76] Even in the setting of HIV infection, response rates of 60%[77] are recorded, apparently undetermined by the viral genotype.[78] These rates are much higher than those seen in established chronic infection.

Overall, early diagnosis and treatment are beneficial and this is important when dealing with a patient or with a healthcare worker, for example, who has sustained a needlestick injury from an infected patient.

The optimal regimen and, indeed, timing have yet to be determined but most clinicians would recommend treatment within 3 months, particularly if monitoring has shown no decline in HCV RNA levels.

CHRONIC HEPATITIS

Chronic hepatitis is when infection has been present for 6 months or more. Spontaneous clearance thereafter is highly unusual. Just as with HBV infection, the main aims of therapy are to clear the infection and to reduce the risks of fatal liver disease. There is no vaccine for HCV infection so treatment is also important in limiting potential spread of the disease.

The initial studies were before the discovery of HCV and the response limited to the transaminase levels and the liver biopsy appearances. Molecular virological advances have led to increased use of HCV RNA levels in determining the response to antiviral therapy.

Some patients when treated with antiviral therapy show no response or only a partial decline in the level of HCV RNA. Some patients who respond initially, subsequently 'breakthrough', and some patients show a favorable response and then relapse following cessation of therapy

A sustained virological response (SVR) is defined as a negative HCV RNA test 6 months after cessation of therapy (Fig. 48.2). Relapse thereafter is highly unusual.

Detailed monitoring of the viral load during the first few weeks of therapy helps tailor the antiviral regimen.

The rapid virological response (RVR) is the response of the HCV RNA level to undetectable levels after 4 weeks of therapy, and the early virological response (EVR) is the response to negativity at 12 weeks. It is generally recommended, for example, that patients who fail to demonstrate an EVR should discontinue therapy as it is very unlikely that they will achieve an SVR.

Interferon-α

Interferon-α has been used in trials since 1986[79] and is licensed in many countries. Initially it was given as monotherapy thrice weekly, and SVR rates of 10–20% were seen

with this approach. With the introduction of peginterferons and combination therapy with ribavirin, however, overall SVR rates of 45–55% are now seen.[80,81] SVR rates are 70–80% in patients with genotype 2 or 3 infection and 40–50% in patients with genotype 1 infection. The Hadziyannis study[81] demonstrated that 48 weeks of therapy and full dose ribavirin was required to treat genotype 1 infection (SVR 52%), whereas 24 weeks of therapy and low dose ribavirin was sufficient for patients with genotypes 2 or 3 infection. The main side effects of interferon are listed in the Box 48.1 (p. 610).

Ribavirin

Ribavirin is a guanosine analog with broad-spectrum antiviral activity. In initial monotherapy studies a reduction was seen in transaminase levels during therapy[82] but subsequent studies showed very little effect on HCV replication[83] and its mode of action in hepatitis C therapy is therefore unclear. It is given orally in combination with interferon for HCV infection. Side effects (Box 48.2) include anemia (mainly secondary to hemolysis), skin rash, pruritus and, more rarely, hypersensitivity. There are concerns regarding its potential for teratogenicity and prospective patients and their partners should be carefully counseled regarding this. It is recommended that both men and women avoid conception whilst on therapy and for several months thereafter in view of the long half-life.

Combination therapy

Peginterferon and ribavirin combination therapy has been generally shown to be cost-effective. Older patients in particular should be carefully assessed prior to commencing therapy as they may risk cardiac decompensation if they develop significant anemia with ribavirin-associated hemolysis. Low

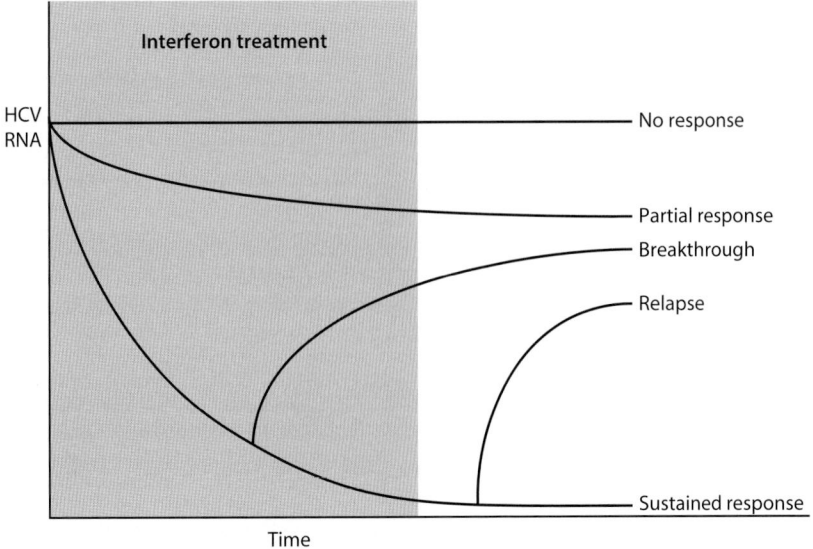

Fig. 48.2 Schematic representation of the influence of interferon treatment on hepatitis C virus RNA levels.

Box 48.2 Side effects of ribavirin

Hemolysis – caution in patients with cardiac problems
Risk of teratogenicity – males and females to avoid conception
Rash – continue therapy if transient or mild
Pruritus – may limit continuation of therapy
Acute hypersensitivity – rare

response rates in genotype 1 infection suggest that it is not cost-effective to treat older patients with genotype 1 infection and mild liver damage[84] or cirrhosis.[85]

Newer agents

Protease, polymerase and helicase inhibitors are being developed.

Telaprevir, for example, is a peptidomimetic. It resembles the HCV polypeptide which is cleaved by HCV protease. With monotherapy significant reductions were seen in HCV RNA levels[86] but viral resistance was observed early in the treatment course. Treatment courses (12–24 weeks) of telaprevir in combination with peginterferon and ribavirin (24–48 weeks) appear promising, with SVR rates of 61–67% in patients with genotype 1 infection.[87,88] Rashes, pruritus, nausea and diarrhea were more common in patients given the triple therapy and this may limit longer treatment regimens with triple therapy.

Boceprevir is a protease inhibitor with activity against genotype 1 HCV,[89] and trials are underway with the drug in combination therapy with peginterferon and ribavirin.

PLANNING THERAPY FOR THE PATIENT

Initially antiviral therapy was considered only for patients with more severe liver disease as determined by liver biopsy. The improved success rates with more effective combination therapy and analysis of viral load responses have encouraged more patients to embark on antiviral therapy. The standard guidelines recommend 24 weeks of peginterferon and ribavirin for patients with genotype 2 or 3 infection.[90]

A 48-week treatment course is recommended for patients with genotype 1 infection but treatment should only be continued beyond the first 12 weeks if there is a favorable response ($2 \log_{10}$ or more reduction in HCV RNA or undetectable HCV RNA). This early virological response is helpful in stopping ineffective therapy at an early stage. Those patients with genotype 1 infection who have undetectable levels of HCV RNA at 4 weeks (rapid virological response) may only require 24 weeks of therapy.

 References

1. Yoshiba M, Inoue K, Sekiyama K, et al. Interferon for hepatitis A. *Lancet.* 1994;343:288–289.
2. Lemon SD, Thomas D. Vaccines to prevent viral hepatitis. *N Engl J Med.* 1997;336:196.
3. Thursz MR, Thomas HC, Greenwood BM, Hill AV. Heterozygote advantage for HLA class-II type in hepatitis B virus infection. *Nat Genet.* 1997;17:11–12.
4. De Jongh FE, Jamssea HL, De Man RA, Hopw WC, Schalm SW, Blankenstein MV. Survival and prognostic indicators in hepatitis B surface antigen-positive cirrhosis of the liver. *Gastroenterology.* 1992;103:1630–1635.
5. Liaw YF, Tai DI, Chu CM, Chen TJ. The development of cirrhosis in patients with chronic type B hepatitis: a prospective study. *Hepatology.* 1988;8:493–496.
6. Carman WF, Jacyna MR, Hadziyannis S, et al. Mutation preventing formation of hepatitis B e antigen in chronic hepatitis B virus infection. *Lancet.* 1989;ii:588–591.
7. Kundu SS, Kundu AK, Pal NK. Interferon-alpha in the treatment of acute prolonged hepatitis B virus infection. *J Assoc Physicians India.* 2000;48:671–673.
8. Reshef R, Sbeit W, Tur-Kaspa R. Lamivudine in the treatment of acute hepatitis. *N Engl J Med.* 2000;343:1123–1124.
9. Thomas HC. Best practice in the treatment of chronic hepatitis B: a summary of the European Viral Hepatitis Educational Initiative (EVHEI). *J Hepatol.* 2007;47(4):588–597.
10. Carr A, Cooper DA. Restoration of immunity to chronic hepatitis B infection in HIV-infected patient on protease inhibitor. *Lancet.* 1997;349:995–996.
11. Korenman J, Baker B, Waggoner J, et al. Long term remissions of chronic hepatitis B after alpha interferon. *Ann Intern Med.* 1991;114:629–634.
12. Lin SM, Yu ML, Lee CM, et al. Interferon therapy in HBeAg positive chronic hepatitis reduces progression to cirrhosis and hepatocellular carcinoma. *J Hepatol.* 2007;46:45–52.
13. Anderson MG, Harrison TJ, Alexander GJM, et al. Randomised controlled trial of lymphoblastoid interferon for chronic active hepatitis B. *J Hepatol.* 1986;3(suppl):S225–S227.
14. Brook MG, Chan G, Yap I, et al. Randomised controlled trial of lymphoblastoid interferon alfa in Europid men with chronic hepatitis B virus infection. *Br Med J.* 1989;299:652–656.
15. Perrillo RP, Schiff ER, Davis GL, et al. A randomised controlled trial of interferon alfa 2-b alone and after prednisone withdrawal for the treatment of chronic hepatitis B. *N Engl J Med.* 1990;323:295–301.
16. Wong DK, Cheung AM, O'Royurke K, Naylor CD, Detsky AS, Heathcote J. Effect of alpha interferon treatment in patients with hepatitis B e antigen positive chronic hepatitis B. A meta analysis. *Ann Intern Med.* 1993;119:312–323.
17. Lau GK, Piratvisuth T, Luo KX, et al. Peginterferon alfa-2a, lamivudine, and the combination for HBeAg-positive chronic hepatitis B. *N Engl J Med.* 2005;352(26):2682–2695.
18. Marcellin P, Lau GK, Bonino F, et al. Peginterferon alfa-2a alone, lamivudine alone, and the two in combination in patients with HBeAg-negative chronic hepatitis B. *N Engl J Med.* 2004;351(12):1206–1217.
19. Fattovich G, Giustina G, Alberti A, et al. A randomised controlled trial of thymopentin therapy in patients with chronic hepatitis B. *J Hepatol.* 1994;21:361–366.
20. Ilan Y, Nagler A, Adler R, Tur-Kaspa R, Slavin S, Shouval D. Ablation of persistent hepatitis B by bone marrow transplantation from a hepatitis B-immune donor. *Gastroenterology.* 1993;104:1818–1821.
21. Dienstag JL, Perrillo RP, Schiff ER, Bartholomew M, Vicary C, Rubin M. A preliminary trial of lamivudine for chronic hepatitis B infection. *N Engl J Med.* 1995;333:1657–1661.
22. Nevens F, Main J, Honkoop P, et al. Lamivudine therapy for chronic hepatitis B: a six-month randomized dose-ranging study. *Gastroenterology.* 1997;113:1258–1263.
23. Lai CL, Chien RN, Leung NW, et al. A one-year trial of lamivudine for chronic hepatitis B. Asia Hepatitis Lamivudine Study Group. *N Engl J Med.* 1998;339:61–68.
24. Liaw YF, Leung NW, Chang TT, et al. Effects of extended lamivudine therapy in Asian patients with chronic hepatitis B. Asia Hepatitis Lamivudine Study Group. *Gastroenterology.* 2000;119:172–180.
25. Chang TT, Lai CL, Liaw YF, et al. Incremental increases in HBeAg seroconversion and continued ALT normalization in Asian chronic HBV patients treated with lamivudine for four years. *Antivir Ther.* 2000;5(suppl 1):44.
26. Ling R, Mutimer D, Ahmed M, et al. Selection of mutations in the hepatitis B virus polymerase during therapy of transplant recipients with lamivudine. *Hepatology.* 1996;24:711–713.
27. Bartholomew MM, Jansen RW, Jeffers LJ, et al. Hepatitis B virus resistance to lamivudine given for recurrent infection after orthotopic liver transplantation. *Lancet.* 1997;349:20–22.

28. Melegari M, Scaglioni PP, Wands JR. Hepatitis B mutants associated with 3TC and famciclovir administration are replication defective. *Hepatology*. 1998;27:628–633.

29. Mutimer D, Pillay D, Shields P, et al. Outcome of lamivudine resistant hepatitis B virus infection in the liver transplant recipient. *Gut*. 2000;46:107–113.

30. Peters MG, Singer G, Howard T, et al. Fulminant hepatic failure resulting from lamivudine-resistant hepatitis B virus in a renal transplant recipient: durable response after orthotopic liver transplantation on adefovir dipivoxil and hepatitis B immune globulin. *Transplantation*. 1999;68:1912–1914.

31. Sung JJ, Lai JY, Zeuzem S, et al. Lamivudine compared with lamivudine and adefovir dipivoxil for the treatment of HBeAg-positive chronic hepatitis B. *J Hepatol*. 2008;48:728–735.

32. Shibolet O, Ilan Y, Gillis S, Hubert A, Shouval D, Safadi R. Lamivudine therapy for prevention of immunosuppressive-induced hepatitis B virus reactivation in hepatitis B surface antigen carriers. *Blood*. 2002;100:391–396.

33. van Zonneveld M, van Nunen AB, Niesters HG, de Man RA, Schalm SW, Janssen HL. Lamivudine treatment during pregnancy to prevent perinatal transmission of hepatitis B virus infection. *J Viral Hepat*. 2003;10:294–297.

34. Lim SG, Ng TM, Kung N, et al. A double-blind placebo-controlled study of emtricitabine in chronic hepatitis B. *Arch Intern Med*. 2006;166:49–56.

35. Gish RG, Trinh H, Leung N, et al. Safety and antiviral activity of emtricitabine (FTC) for the treatment of chronic hepatitis B infection: a two-year study. *J Hepatol*. 2005;43:60–66.

36. Lai CL, Gane E, Liaw YF, et al. Telbivudine versus lamivudine in patients with chronic hepatitis B. *N Engl J Med*. 2007;357:2576–2588.

37. Marcellin P, Chang TT, Lim SG, et al. Long-term efficacy and safety of adefovir dipivoxil for the treatment of hepatitis e antigen-positive chronic hepatitis B. *Hepatology*. 2008;48:750–758.

38. Hadziyannis SJ, Tassopoulos NC, Heathcote EJ, et al. Long-term therapy with adefovir dipivoxil for HBeAg-negative chronic hepatitis B. *N Engl J Med*. 2005;352:2673–2681.

39. Hadziyannis SJ, Tassopoulos NC, Heathcote EJ, et al. Long-term therapy with adefovir dipivoxil for HBeAg-negative chronic hepatitis B for up to 5 years. *Gastroenterology*. 2006;131:1743–1751.

40. Ha NB, Ha NB, Garcia RT, et al. Renal dysfunction in chronic hepatitis B patients treated with adefovir dipivoxil. *Hepatology*. 2009;50:727–734.

41. Lampertico P, Viganò M, Manenti E, Iavarone M, Sablon E, Colombo M. Low resistance to adefovir combined with lamivudine: a 3-year study of 145 lamivudine-resistant hepatitis B patients. *Gastroenterology*. 2007;133:1445–1451.

42. Rapti I, Dimou E, Mitsoula P, Hadziyannis SJ. Adding-on versus switching-to adefovir therapy in lamivudine-resistant HBeAg-negative chronic hepatitis B. *Hepatology*. 2007;45:307–313.

43. Marcellin P, Heathcote EJ, Buti M, et al. Tenofovir disoproxil fumarate versus adefovir dipivoxil for chronic hepatitis B. *N Engl J Med*. 2008;359:2442–2455.

44. Amini-Bavil-Olyaee S, Herbers U, Sheldon J, Luedde T, Trautwein C, Tacke F. The rtA194T polymerase mutation impacts viral replication and susceptibility to tenofovir in hepatitis B e antigen-positive and hepatitis B e antigen-negative hepatitis B virus strains. *Hepatology*. 2009;49:1158–1165.

45. Fontana RJ. Side effects of long-term oral antiviral therapy for hepatitis B. *Hepatology*. 2009;49(suppl 5):S185–S195.

46. Kinai E, Hanabusa H. Progressive renal tubular dysfunction associated with long-term use of tenofovir DF. *AIDS Res Hum Retroviruses*. 2009;25:387–394.

47. Goicoechea M, Liu S, Best B, et al. Greater tenofovir-associated renal function decline with protease inhibitor-based versus nonnucleoside reverse-transcriptase inhibitor-based therapy. *J Infect Dis*. 2008;197:102–108.

48. Fux CA, Rauch A, Simcock M, et al. Tenofovir use is associated with an increase in serum alkaline phosphatase in the Swiss HIV Cohort Study. *Antivir Ther*. 2008;13:1077–1082.

49. Gish RG, Lok AS, Chang TT, et al. Entecavir therapy for up to 96 weeks in patients with HBeAg-positive chronic hepatitis B. *Gastroenterology*. 2007;133:1437–1444.

50. Chang TT, Gish RG, de Man R, et al. A comparison of entecavir and lamivudine for HBeAg-positive chronic hepatitis B. *N Engl J Med*. 2006;354:1001–1010.

51. Tenney DJ, Rose RE, Baldick CJ, et al. Long-term monitoring shows hepatitis B virus resistance to entecavir in nucleoside-naive patients is rare through 5 years of therapy. *Hepatology*. 2009;49:1503–1514.

52. Leung N, Peng CY, Hann HW, et al. Early hepatitis B virus DNA reduction in hepatitis B e antigen-positive patients with chronic hepatitis B: a randomized international study of entecavir versus adefovir. *Hepatology*. 2009;49:72–79.

53. Sherman M, Yurdaydin C, Sollano J, et al. Entecavir for treatment of lamivudine-refractory, HBeAg-positive chronic hepatitis B. *Gastroenterology*. 2006;130:2039–2049.

54. Reijnders JG, Pas SD, Schutten M, de Man RA, Janssen HL. Entecavir shows limited efficacy in HBeAg-positive hepatitis B patients with a partial virologic response to adefovir therapy. *J Hepatol*. 2009;50:674–683.

55. Chen CJ, Iloeje UH, Yang HI. Long-term outcomes in hepatitis B: the REVEAL-HBV study. *Clin Liver Dis*. 2007;11:797–816 viii.

56. Chen CJ, Yang HI, Iloeje UH. REVEAL-HBV Study Group. Hepatitis B virus DNA levels and outcomes in chronic hepatitis B. *Hepatology*. 2009;49(suppl 5):S72–S84.

57. European Association for the Study of the Liver. EASL Clinical Practice Guidelines: management of chronic hepatitis B. *J Hepatol*. 2009;50:227–242.

58. Lok AS, McMahon BJ, Practice Guidelines Committee, American Association for the Study of Liver Diseases (AASLD). Chronic hepatitis B: update of recommendations. *Hepatology*. 2004;39:857–861.

59. Kennedy PT, Lee HC, Jeyalingam L, et al. NICE guidelines and a treatment algorithm for the management of chronic hepatitis B: a review of 12 years experience in west London. *Antivir Ther*. 2008;13:1067–1076.

60. Zuckerman JN, Zuckerman AJ. Current topics in hepatitis B. *J Infect*. 2000;41:130–136.

61. Choo QL, Kuo G, Weiner AJ, et al. Isolation of a cDNA clone derived from blood-borne non-A, non-B viral hepatitis genome. *Science*. 1989;244:359–362.

62. van de Laar T, Pybus O, Bruisten S, et al. Evidence of a large, international network of HCV transmission in HIV-positive men who have sex with men. *Gastroenterology*. 2009;136:1609–1617.

63. World Health Organization. Hepatitis C global prevalence. *Wkly Epidemiol Rec*. 1997;72:341–344.

64. Ryan KW, McLennan S, Barbara JA, Hewitt PE. Follow-up of blood donors positive for antibodies to hepatitis C. *Br Med J*. 1994;308:696–697.

65. Sallie R, King R, Silva E, Tibbs C, Johnson P, Williams R. Community prevalence of hepatitis C viraemia: a polymerase chain reaction study. *J Med Virol*. 1994;43:111–114.

66. Abdel-Aziz F, Habib M, Mohamed MK, et al. Hepatitis C virus (HCV) infection in a community in the Nile Delta: population description and HCV prevalence. *Hepatology*. 2000;32:111–115.

67. Simmonds P. Viral heterogeneity of the hepatitis C virus. *J Hepatol*. 1999;31(suppl 1):54–60.

68. Alter HJ, Purcell RH, Shih JW, et al. Detection of antibody to hepatitis C virus in prospectively followed transfusion recipients with acute and chronic non-A, non-B hepatitis. *N Engl J Med*. 1989;321:1494–1500.

69. Ray SC, Arthur RR, Carella A, Bukh J, Thomas DL. Genetic epidemiology of hepatitis C virus throughout Egypt. *J Infect Dis*. 2000;182:698–707.

70. Seeff LB, Buskell-Bales Z, Wright EC, et al. Long term mortality after transfusion-associated non-A, non-B hepatitis. *N Engl J Med*. 1992;327:1906–1911.

71. Tong MJ, El-Farra NS, Reikes AR, et al. Clinical outcomes after transfusion associated hepatitis C. *N Engl J Med*. 1995;332:1463–1466.

72. Poynard T, Ratziu V, Benhamou Y, Opolon P, Cacoub P. Natural history of HCV infection. *Baillieres Clin Gastroenterol*. 2000;14:211–218.

73. Poynard T, Redossa P, Opolon P. Natural history of liver fibrosis progression in patients with chronic hepatitis C. *Lancet*. 1997;349:825–832.

74. Forton DM, Allsop JM, Main J, Foster GR, Thomas HC, Taylor-Robinson SD. Evidence for a cerebral effect of the hepatitis C virus. *Lancet*. 2001;358:38–39.

75. Wiegand J, Buggisch P, Boecher W, et al. German HEP-NET Acute HCV Study Group. Early monotherapy with pegylated interferon alpha-2b for acute hepatitis C infection: the HEP-NET acute-HCV-II study. *Hepatology*. 2006;43:250–256.

76. Jaeckel E, Cornberg M, Wedemeyer H, et al. Treatment of acute hepatitis C with interferon alfa-2b. *N Engl J Med*. 2001;345:1452–1457.

77. Vogel M, Nattermann J, Baumgarten A, et al. Pegylated interferon-alpha for the treatment of sexually transmitted acute hepatitis C in HIV-infected individuals. *Antivir Ther*. 2006;11:1097–1101.

78. Gilleece YC, Browne RE, Asboe D, et al. Transmission of hepatitis C virus among HIV-positive homosexual men and response to a 24-week course of pegylated interferon and ribavirin. *J Acquir Immune Defic Syndr*. 2005;40:41–46.

79. Hoofnagle JH, Mullen KD, Jones DB, et al. Treatment of chronic non-A, non-B hepatitis with recombinant human alpha interferon. A preliminary report. *N Engl J Med*. 1986;315:1575–1578.

80. Fried MW, Shiffman ML, Reddy KR, et al. Peginterferon alfa-2a plus ribavirin for chronic hepatitis C virus infection. *N Engl J Med*. 2002;347:975–982.

81. Hadziyannis SJ, Sette Jr H, Morgan TR, et al. Peginterferon-alpha2a and ribavirin combination therapy in chronic hepatitis C: a randomized study of treatment duration and ribavirin dose. *Ann Intern Med*. 2004;140:346–355.

82. Reichard O, Andersson J, Schvarcz R, Weiland O. Ribavirin treatment for chronic hepatitis C. *Lancet*. 1991;337:1058–1061.

83. Dusheiko G, Main J, Thomas H, et al. Ribavirin treatment for patients with chronic hepatitis C: results of a placebo-controlled study. *J Hepatol*. 1996;25:591–598.

84. Grieve R, Roberts J, Wright M, et al. Cost effectiveness of interferon alpha or peginterferon alpha with ribavirin for histologically mild chronic hepatitis C. *Gut*. 2006;55:1332–1338.

85. Grishchenko M, Grieve RD, Sweeting MJ, et al. Cost-effectiveness of pegylated interferon and ribavirin for patients with chronic hepatitis C treated in routine clinical practice. *Int J Technol Assess Health Care*. 2009;25:171–180.

86. Reesink HW, Zeuzem S, Weegink CJ, et al. Rapid decline of viral RNA in hepatitis C patients treated with VX-950: a phase Ib, placebo-controlled, randomized study. *Gastroenterology*. 2006;131:997–1002.

87. McHutchison JG, Everson GT, Gordon SC, et al. Telaprevir with peginterferon and ribavirin for chronic HCV genotype 1 infection. *N Engl J Med*. 2009;360:1827–1838.

88. Hézode C, Forestier N, Dusheiko G, et al. Telaprevir and peginterferon with or without ribavirin for chronic HCV infection. *N Engl J Med*. 2009;360:1839–1850.

89. Sarrazin C, Rouzier R, Wagner F, et al. SCH 503034, a novel hepatitis C virus protease inhibitor, plus pegylated interferon alpha-2b for genotype 1 nonresponders. *Gastroenterology*. 2007;132:1270–1278.

90. Ghany MG, Strader DB, Thomas DL, Seeff LB. American Association for the Study of Liver Diseases. Diagnosis, management, and treatment of hepatitis C: an update. *Hepatology*. 2009;49:1335–1374.

Skin and soft-tissue infections

Anita K. Satyaprakash, Parisa Ravanfar and Stephen K. Tyring

The skin and underlying soft tissues form a formidable defensive barrier against infection despite the fact that the skin's surface is normally colonized by a variety of organisms. Disruption of the integrity of the integument, immunocompromised conditions, or spread of an organism via the circulation can lead to a variety of skin and soft-tissue infections. Diagnosis may rely solely upon the appearance of the skin lesions or on simple diagnostic tests such as cultures or skin biopsies. Isolation of the causative organism may be difficult, in many cases due to contamination by normal commensal skin flora. Treatment with systemic antiviral or antibacterial agents offers excellent tissue penetration and rapid recovery. Topical antimicrobial therapy is limited by lack of adequate tissue penetration and skin hypersensitivity; however, the advantage of topical therapy is its lack of systemic toxicity and ease of application.

CHILDHOOD EXANTHEMS

Viral exanthems are common in children. In some cases the morphology of the rash and associated findings may allow for a specific diagnosis and treatment, although many cases are non-specific and not pathognomonic for a specific virus. There are now more than 50 specific agents known to cause viral exanthems. The classic six childhood exanthems are not all caused by viruses (Table 49.1).

Most childhood exanthems cause a rather non-specific generalized rash that occurs in a predictable pattern. Most are benign and self-limiting viral diseases with no specific treatment except for supportive care; however, when these diseases

Table 49.1 Classic childhood exanthems

First disease	Rubeola (measles)
Second disease	Scarlet fever
Third disease	Rubella
Fourth disease	Filatov–Duke's disease
Fifth disease	Erythema infectiosum
Sixth disease	Exanthem subitum (roseola infantum)

occur during pregnancy and affect the fetus, they can have serious sequelae. For example, rubella (German measles) is a benign disease but the effects of congenital rubella can be very serious. If a pregnant woman is afflicted in the first trimester, the incidence of fetal damage approaches 50%.[1] Likewise, if erythema infectiosum (fifth disease; caused by parvovirus B19 infection) is acquired during pregnancy, the risk of spontaneous abortion or hydrops fetalis in a surviving offspring is increased. Some viral exanthems are known for the unique skin lesions they produce; measles (rubeola) causes the characteristic Koplik's spots and erythema infectiosum is known for the erythematous 'slapped cheek' appearance.

Treatment for viral exanthems is supportive, although childhood vaccination remains the most effective means of prevention in the case of measles and rubella.

ENTEROVIRAL INFECTIONS

Enteroviral infections such as hand, foot and mouth disease, herpangina, and echovirus 9 are the leading cause of childhood exanthems in the summer and fall. Enteroviruses enter through the gastrointestinal tract and are thought to account for two-thirds of all exanthems in August, September and October in the USA. More than 30 have been identified to cause exanthems. Enteroviral infections are spread by the oral–oral or fecal–oral route, and the typical incubation period is 3–5 days. The cutaneous manifestations are quite pleomorphic and include rubelliform, morbilliform, roseola-like, scarlatiniform, urticarial, pustular, petechial, purpuric and hemangioma-like eruptions. A specific enteroviral diagnosis is not possible for most exanthems. Hand, foot and mouth disease is characterized by vesicular lesions in the mouth and on the extremities associated with a mild fever. Herpangina is a specific infectious disease characterized by sudden onset of fever, headache and neck pain, and gray–white papulovesicular lesions on the anterior pillars, soft palate, uvula and tonsils. No specific treatment is available; only supportive care is recommended for enteroviral infections.

HERPESVIRUSES

HERPES SIMPLEX (HSV)

HSV-1 and HSV-2 are double-stranded DNA viruses. Both types are characterized by a primary infection, which may or may not be symptomatic, followed by the establishment of a latent infection in the spinal ganglion.

HSV-1 commonly causes herpes labialis, also known as cold sores. Primary infection is more severe than recurrences, and may be associated with fever and lymphadenopathy. Infection usually recurs on or near the vermilion border of the lip and is triggered by sunlight, emotional stress, trauma to the lips, fatigue or fever. Recurrence is heralded by a typical prodrome of itching or burning at the site, followed by the classic appearance of an erythematous macule, followed by a papule, vesicle and finally a crust.

Genital herpes is most commonly caused by HSV-2, generally acquired through sexual contact; however, HSV-1 has been increasingly associated with genital herpes. Over 50% of persons with asymptomatic HSV-2 actively shed the virus; 70–80% of cases of genital herpes are thought to be spread by asymptomatic viral shedding.[2] Like herpes labialis, a prodrome occurs in 40–50% of episodes.

Both oral and genital herpes infections appear as vesicles on an inflamed base. The vesicles erode quickly or become pustular before crusting over. Healing usually occurs in about 9 days for recurrent lesions and up to 3 weeks for primary infections.

Herpetic lesions such as herpetic whitlow are caused by primary or recurrent HSV infection on the fingers due to digital contact with infected oral or genital tissues.

Herpes gladiatorum, caused by direct skin-to-skin contact, is seen among wrestlers and rugby players and may affect the head, trunk and extremities.

Eczema herpeticum is a widespread cutaneous infection with HSV, which occurs in patients with skin disorders such as atopic dermatitis, Darier's disease and pemphigus. It is frequently superinfected with bacteria and is associated with fever, lymphadenopathy and malaise.

DIAGNOSIS

Diagnosis of herpes can be made by identifying multinucleated balloon keratinocytes on a Tzanck smear taken from the floor of an early vesicle stained with Wright or Giemsa stain. Culture is the gold standard for diagnosis, and serology via ELISA or Western blot can be used to distinguish between HSV-1 and HSV-2.

TREATMENT

HSV-1 and HSV-2 infections can be treated with oral aciclovir, famciclovir or valaciclovir, and are treated differently depending on whether the patient presents with a first episode of infection, recurrence of infection or a need for suppressive therapy (more than six recurrences yearly). Table 49.2 lists the recommended treatment regimens for both herpes labialis and genital herpes. Both famciclovir and valaciclovir, which are equally effective, are more conveniently dosed and better absorbed than the prototype aciclovir (acyclovir).

Penciclovir and aciclovir creams are approved for herpes labialis; however, their effectiveness is limited by poor tissue penetration and by the frequent inconvenient dosing regimen.

VARICELLA ZOSTER VIRUS (HHV-3)

Varicella (chickenpox) and herpes zoster (shingles) are both caused by a single member of the herpesvirus family (human herpesvirus-3; HHV-3). Varicella results from a primary infection in a susceptible person, whereas zoster is a reactivation in persons who have had varicella. Varicella is highly contagious and usually transmitted via the respiratory route or by direct contact. The clinical manifestations of primary varicella include an occasional prodrome; in children, low-grade fever and malaise may proceed or occur simultaneously with the onset of the rash. In adults, a headache, myalgia, nausea, vomiting and anorexia can precede the rash. The rash is characterized by small erythematous macules that initially appear on the face and trunk, spread to the proximal upper limbs, and somewhat spare the distal lower limbs. The skin lesions rapidly evolve in crops over 12–14 h. The rash progresses in a predictable manner: first papules, next vesicles and, finally, crusts. Vesicles may have slightly hemorrhagic bases and have the characteristic

Table 49.2 Oral treatment regimens for herpes infections

Clinical disease	Treatment
Herpes labialis	
First episode	Aciclovir 400 mg every 8 h for 7–10 days (children and adults)
	Famciclovir 500 mg every 12 h for 7 days (adults)
	Valaciclovir 1 g every 12 h for 7 days (adults)
Recurrences	Aciclovir 400 mg every 8 h for 5 days
	Famciclovir 1.5 g once
	Valaciclovir 2 g every 12 h for 1 day
Suppressive therapy	Aciclovir 400 mg every 12 h
	Famciclovir 500 mg every 12 h
	Valaciclovir 500 mg once daily
Genital herpes	
First episode	Aciclovir 400 mg every 8 h for 7–10 days
	Aciclovir 200 mg five times daily for 7–10 days
	Famciclovir 250 mg every 8 h for 7–10 days
	Valaciclovir 1 g every 12 h for 7–10 days
Recurrences	Aciclovir 400 mg every 8 h for 5 days
	Aciclovir 800 mg every 8 h for 2 days
	Aciclovir 800 mg every 12 h for 5 days
	Famciclovir 125 mg every 12 h for 5 days
	Famciclovir 1 g every 12 h for 1 day
	Valaciclovir 500 mg every 12 h for 3 days
Suppressive therapy	Aciclovir 400 mg every 12 h
	Famciclovir 250 mg every 12 h
	Valaciclovir 500 mg once daily (≤9 outbreaks a year)
	Valaciclovir 1 g once daily (>9 outbreaks a year)

appearance of 'dewdrops on a rose petal'. Infection tends to be more severe in older children and adults.

For primary varicella in healthy children, treatment has traditionally been symptomatic, using only calamine lotion, cool compresses, tepid baths and non-aspirin antipyretics. Healthy children with primary varicella virus infection may also be treated with oral aciclovir.

Treatment of primary varicella in older children, adults and immunocompromised patients is mandatory. If the patient is an adult or of adult size, the dosage of acyclovir is 800 mg five times a day for 7 days; in smaller children the recommendation is 10 mg/kg four times a day for 5 days. Although neither famciclovir nor valaciclovir has been approved for treatment of primary varicella, zoster-equivalent doses are effective.

Herpes zoster is an acute inflammatory unilateral dermatosis having both dermatological and neurological manifestations. It is estimated to afflict 15–20% of the population, with incidence rising with increasing age.[3] Immune senescence, resulting in a decline in T-cell-mediated immunity, is suspected to contribute to the reactivation of the varicella zoster virus lying dormant in the spinal cord dorsal root ganglia.[4] The patient may experience prodromal symptoms of low-grade fever, pain, numbness, pruritus and paresthesia several days before cutaneous involvement. These signs foreshadow the appearance of the classic rash, most often described as unilateral grouped vesicles on an erythematous and edematous base along a dermatomal distribution. Frequently, there are a few scattered non-dermatomal lesions, and rarely a generalized eruption may occur. Complete cutaneous healing is expected in 3–4 weeks and patients are considered contagious until the lesions are crusted.

Varicella and herpes zoster are generally diagnosed clinically. The Tzanck smear is positive in 80–100% of zoster cases. The current recommendation for treatment of herpes zoster is famciclovir 500 mg every 8 h for 7 days or valaciclovir 1 g every 8 h for 7 days. These medications are more conveniently dosed and achieve higher plasma concentrations than oral aciclovir, for which the recommended dosing is 800 mg five times daily for 7 days.

EPSTEIN–BARR VIRUS (HHV-4)

Epstein–Barr virus (EBV) is a double-stranded DNA virus with an envelope and is a member of the herpesvirus family (HHV-4). Humans acquire infection through contact with salivary secretions. EBV persists for life as a latent infection in B cells. It is the etiological agent of infectious mononucleosis, and is associated with oral hairy leukoplakia and B-cell lymphoma in patients with AIDS, Burkitt's lymphoma, nasopharyngeal carcinoma, Hodgkin's disease and some T-cell lymphomas.

The triad of fever, sore throat and lymphadenopathy characterizes infectious mononucleosis.[5] The monospot test is used to diagnose EBV. Mononucleosis is often self-limiting and management consists of rest and antipyretics. Severe cases may result in splenomegaly and subsequent splenic rupture after trauma.

Oral hairy leukoplakia is a non-malignant hyperplasia of the epithelial cells due to active replication of EBV, most commonly seen in HIV-positive individuals.[6,7] Lesions are usually present on the lateral tongue and appear slightly raised and white with a corrugated or hairy appearance. Oral hairy leukoplakia resolves with oral aciclovir, but will recur 2 weeks to 2 months after stopping therapy.

CYTOMEGALOVIRUS (HHV-5)

Cytomegalovirus (CMV) is an enveloped, double-stranded DNA virus of the herpes family, also known as HHV-5. It is ubiquitous, with nearly everyone infected by adulthood. After primary infection, which is usually asymptomatic and subclinical, the virus remains present for life in a latent stage. Immunocompromised patients and neonates are at the highest risk of danger from CMV infection. Transmission occurs via intimate contact with body fluids such as saliva, vaginal secretions, semen, breast milk, feces or blood. Cutaneous lesions associated with CMV are rare and non-specific, and usually occur only in immunocompromised states. The most specific manifestation of cutaneous CMV is ulceration of the perianal area.

Treatment is generally not needed in immunocompetent individuals. Immunocompromised patients may be treated with ganciclovir, valganciclovir, foscarnet or cidofovir. Fomivirsen is also approved for treatment of CMV retinitis.

HUMAN HERPESVIRUS 6 (ROSEOLA)

Roseola (also known as exanthem subitum) is a very common childhood exanthem in which HHV-6 has been shown to play a causal role. Roseola is characterized by a prodrome of high fever (102–105°F) for 3–5 days, followed by an abrupt decrease in fever and sudden appearance of an exanthem (hence 'subitum') that occurs almost exclusively in children under 2 years old. Ganciclovir and foscarnet may be helpful in cases with severe complications, but are not approved for this purpose in the USA. Primary infections confer lasting immunity.

HUMAN HERPESVIRUS 7

This virus is also known to cause roseola, but much less commonly than HHV-6. It is also thought to be the causative agent of pityriasis rosea, a benign skin disease characterized by the appearance of a large, scaly, oval 'herald patch' followed by smaller patches on the trunk and extremities. The rash is self-limiting, with resolution in 6–14 weeks. Although HHV-7 is susceptible to ganciclovir and foscarnet and minimally susceptible to aciclovir, these agents are not routinely used since only supportive care is needed in most cases.

HUMAN HERPESVIRUS 8 (KAPOSI's SARCOMA)

Kaposi's sarcoma is a malignancy associated with HHV-8 infection.[8] It presents as violaceous, red–dark-brown firm macules or papules, irregularly oval-shaped and parallel to skin tension lines. Systemic therapy should be restricted to patients with disseminated disease or with massive involvement of visceral organs. In HIV-positive patients therapy should be postponed until the patient has had time to respond to highly active antiretroviral therapy (HAART), as the lesions may improve with HAART only. Therapies for Kaposi's sarcoma include radiotherapy, interferon-α, cidofovir, conventional chemotherapy, and topical and systemic retinoids.[9]

POXVIRUSES

SMALLPOX

Smallpox is caused by a DNA virus known as variola. The last known case occurred in October 1977 and worldwide eradication was announced in 1979. Smallpox had a 25–30% mortality rate and was generally managed with supportive care; no treatment was ever found during its prevalence.

CONTAGIOUS ECTHYMA (CONTAGIOUS PUSTULAR DERMATITIS, ORF)

Contagious ecthyma is a member of the *Parapox* genus. It is acquired from infected sheep or goats with crusted lesions on the lips. The lesions appear as flat or dome-shaped bullae with minimal fluid and a central umbilicated crust. They bleed easily and heal without scarring. During a period of approximately 35 days the lesions pass through six clinical stages, each lasting about 6 days.[10] The diagnosis is based on history and physical examination, viral culture on sheep cells, fluorescent antibody tests, electron microscopy and complement fixation test.[11] No treatment is usually necessary as the lesions resolve in 4–6 weeks. Liquid nitrogen or shave excision may be used to speed recovery; antibiotics are indicated for superinfection.

MILKER'S NODULE

Milker's nodule (caused by the paravaccinia virus) is similar to orf. The virus is endemic in cattle and is transmitted by direct contact with them.[12] Lesions have been described as passing through six clinical stages similar to the orf virus. Milker's nodule resolves without therapy.

MOLLUSCUM CONTAGIOSUM

Molluscum contagiosum is caused by a double-stranded DNA virus of the poxvirus group. It affects mainly children,

sexually active adults and immunocompromised individuals, and is spread by direct inoculation between humans. The lesions are small, discrete waxy, flesh-colored, dome-shaped papules with a central umbilication that are 3–6 mm in size. In patients with AIDS, several systemic fungal infections commonly mimic molluscum contagiosum, including cryptococcosis, histoplasmosis and *Penicillium marneffei* infection.

Histologically, molluscum bodies are present. The stratum corneum disintegrates in the center of the lesion, releasing the molluscum bodies and creating a central crater.

Treatment options include cryosurgery, curettage, incision and expression of the molluscum body; cantharidin, topical podophyllotoxin cream, salicylic acid preparations, imiquimod and topical cidofovir.

HUMAN PAPILLOMAVIRUSES

Warts are caused by papillomaviruses, members of the family Papillomaviridae. Papillomaviruses are double-stranded DNA viruses that do not have an envelope and thus can remain infectious for long periods of time after drying. More than 100 different types of human papillomavirus (HPV) have been identified by their separate DNA genotypes as detected by polymerase chain reaction.[13] Incubation period is 2–9 months (average 3 months). Table 49.3 lists the various HPV types and their common lesions.

Table 49.3 Human papillomaviruses and their common lesions

Human papillomaviruses type	Wart type
HPV-1, HPV-2, HPV-4	Palmoplantar warts
HPV-2, HPV-4, HPV-27, HPV-29	Common warts
HPV-3, HPV-10, HPV-28, HPV-49	Flat warts
HPV-6, HPV-11	Condyloma (low risk of carcinoma)
HPV-16, HPV-18, HPV-31, HPV-33–35, HPV-40, HPV-51–60	Squamous cell carcinoma (high risk of carcinoma)
HPV-6, HPV-11	Laryngeal papillomas
HPV-30	Laryngeal carcinoma
HPV-13, HPV-32	Oral focal epithelial hyperplasia (Heck's disease)
HPV-16, HPV-18, HPV-31, HPV-33–35, HPV-39, HPV-40, HPV-51–60	Bowenoid papulosis
HPV-7	Butcher's warts
HPV-5, HPV-8, HPV-9, HPV-12, HPV-14, HPV-15, HPV-17, HPV-19–26, HPV-36, HPV-47, HPV-50	Epidermodysplasia verruciformis
HPV-6, HPV-11	Giant condyloma of Buschke and Loewenstein

Palmoplantar warts usually occur on the palms, soles and the lateral aspects of the fingers and toes. They can be painful on pressure and look similar to a callus, but are differentiated by their loss of skin lines and multiple black dots (which represent punctate hemorrhages from thrombosed dermal capillaries). Common warts (verruca vulgaris) can occur on any skin surface and are described as scaly, rough, spiny papules. Flat warts (verruca plana) are most common on the face, lower legs and dorsal hands.

Epidermodysplasia verruciformis (EV) represents a unique susceptibility to cutaneous HPV infection, especially types that are not generally responsible for human infection, such as HPV-5, -8, -9, -12, -14, -15, -17, -19, -25, -36, -38, -47 and -50.[14] Approximately 50% of cases are inherited, usually with an autosomal recessive pattern. Recent findings have shown mutations in the EVER1 and EVER2 genes to be associated with this disease. Patients suffer from extensive infection with warts that resemble verruca plana.[15]

Condyloma acuminatum commonly occurs on the penis, vulva and anal region. The lesions appear as soft verrucous papules that coalesce into cauliflower-like masses.

Giant condyloma acuminata of Buschke and Loewenstein has been associated with HPV-6 and HPV-11 DNA, and is regarded as a low-grade verrucous carcinoma that resembles a large aggregate of condyloma acuminata. It is most common on the glans penis, vulva and anal region.

Bowenoid papulosis is described as multiple, small, reddish-brown flat-topped papules of the genitalia of men and women. Squamous cell carcinoma may arise in a Bowenoid papule, and is most commonly associated with HPV-16.

Oral focal epithelial hyperplasia (Heck's disease) is a rare condition described in Native Americans and Eskimos. Heck's disease is a chronic disease associated with HPV-13 and HPV-32. Lesions commonly present on the oral mucosa of the lower lip, buccal and gingival mucosa.

Therapy depends on the type of lesion seen clinically:

- For common and palmoplantar warts, daily topical salicylic acid preparations, cryotherapy, curettage, electrodesiccation, cantharidin, intralesional bleomycin and CO_2 laser ablation are routine therapies.
- Genital warts respond to imiquimod, sinecatechin cream, cryotherapy, trichloroacetic acid 50–80%, electrosurgery, excision, laser ablation and interferon-α intralesionally. Imiquimod induces interferon-α and is the most effective treatment with the lowest recurrence rate. Podophyllin is contraindicated because it contains mutagens which are potential carcinogens.
- Flat warts may respond to topical treatment with the vitamin A derivative tretinoin or 5-fluorouracil, cryotherapy and imiquimod.
- Epidermodysplasia verruciformis may also respond to systemic retinoids.
- Radiation of verrucas is contraindicated due to its association with the development of malignancy.

GRAM-POSITIVE ORGANISMS

STAPHYLOCOCCAL INFECTIONS

 ### IMPETIGO

Both bullous and non-bullous forms of impetigo exist; however, non-bullous impetigo caused by *Staphylococcus aureus* accounts for the majority of cases. A prodrome of itching and pain heralds the appearance of a vesicle or pustule, after which the classic honey-colored crusted plaque with surrounding erythema appears.

Treatment with topical mupirocin or bacitracin every 8 h for 7–10 days or retapamulin every 12 h for 5 days is generally sufficient for localized involvement, although a course of oral antibiotics with a penicillinase-resistant semisynthetic penicillin may be needed (Table 49.4). Oral dicloxacillin

Table 49.4 Common penicillin doses (for adults) used in skin and soft-tissue infections

Penicillin	Route	Dose
Natural penicillins		
Aqueous penicillin G	i.v.	8–24 MU every 2–6 h
Procaine benzylpenicillin G	i.m.	0.6–1.2 MU once
Benzathine penicillin G	i.m.	1.2–2.4 MU once
Procaine + benzathine penicillin	i.m.	2.4 MU once
Penicillin V	oral	250–500 mg every 6 h
Penicillin-resistant penicillins		
Dicloxacillin	oral	125–500 mg every 6 h before meals
Cloxacillin	oral	250–500 mg every 6 h
Flucloxacillin	oral	250–500 mg every 6 h before meals
	i.m.	250–500 mg every 6 h
	i.v.	250–1 g every 6 h
Nafcillin	i.m.	500 mg every 4 h
	i.v.	500–2000 mg every 4–6 h
Oxacillin	oral	500–1000 mg every 6 h
	i.m., i.v.	250–2000 mg every 4–6 h
Aminopenicillins		
Amoxicillin	oral	250–500 mg every 8 h
	i.m.	500–1000 mg every 6 h
	i.v.	1–2 g every 4–6 h
Ampicillin	oral	250–1000 mg every 6 h
	i.m.	500–1000 mg every 6 h
	i.v.	1–2 g every 4 h
Ampicillin–sulbactam	i.v.	1.5–3 g every 6 h
Amoxicillin–clavulanate	oral	250/125 mg every 8 h
		500/125 mg every 12 h
		875/125 mg every 12 h
Antipseudomonal penicillins		
Piperacillin–tazobactam	i.v.	3.375 g every 6 h
		4.5 g every 8 h
Ticarcillin–clavulanate	i.v.	3.1–3.2 g every 4–6 h
Ticarcillin	i.v.	3 g every 4 h or 4 g every 6 h
Mezlocillin	i.v., i.m.	3 g every 4 h or 4 g every 6 h
Piperacillin	i.m., i.v.	6–24 g per day in divided doses

MU, megaunit (1 megaunit = 600 mg).

125–500 mg every 6 h, flucloxacillin 250–500 mg every 6 h or oxacillin 500–1000 mg every 4–6 h (Table 49.4) are recommended. A first-generation cephalosporin such as oral cefalexin 250–500 mg every 6 h (Table 49.5) may also be used. Alternatives include ampicillin plus clindamycin and either azithromycin, erythromycin or clarithromycin (Tables 49.4 and 49.6).

ECTHYMA

Impetigo can evolve into ecthyma if left untreated. Either *Staph. aureus* or *Streptococcus pyogenes* causes ecthyma (Table 49.7). The lesions of ecthyma penetrate the epidermis, creating a yellow–gray crusted ulcer up to 3 cm in diameter. The lesions most commonly affect the lower extremities in neglected debilitated patients with poor hygiene. Healing can take

Table 49.5 Common cephalosporin doses (for adults) used in skin and soft-tissue infections

Cephalosporin	Route	Dose
First generation		
Cefalexin	oral	250–500 mg every 6 h
Cefadroxil	oral	1–2 g per day
Cefamandole	i.v., i.m.	500–1000 mg every 4–8 h
Cefazolin	i.m., i.v.	500–2000 mg every 8 h
Second generation		
Cefaclor	oral	250–1000 mg every 8 h
Cefuroxime	i.m., i.v.	750–1500 mg every 8 h
Loracarbef	oral	400 mg every 12 h
Cefoxitin	i.v.	2 g every 6 h
Cefotetan	i.v.	2 g every 12 h
Third generation		
Cefotaxime	i.v., i.m.	1–2 g every 6–12 h
Ceftriaxone	i.m., i.v.	1–2 g per day
Cefixime	oral	400 mg/day or 200 mg every 12 h
Ceftazidime	i.m., i.v.	1–2 g every 8–12 h
Cefoperazone	i.v., i.m.	2–4 g every 12 h
Cefpodoxime	oral	200 mg every 12 h
Fourth generation		
Cefepime	i.v.	500–2000 mg every 12 h

Table 49.6 Common macrolide doses (for adults) used in skin and soft-tissue infections

Macrolide	Route	Dose
Erythromycin base	oral	250–500 mg every 6 h
Erythromycin ethyl succinate	oral	400 mg every 6 h
Erythromycin estolate	oral	250 mg every 6 h
Erythromycin lactobionate	i.v.	15–20 mg/kg every 6 h (maximum dose, 1 g every 6 h; 4 g per day)
Azithromycin	oral	500 mg for one day followed by 250 mg/day for 4 days or 1–2 g single dose
	i.v.	500 mg/day
Clarithromycin	oral	250–500 mg every 12 h

several weeks, despite antibiotic therapy. Topical antibiotics plus the same oral antibiotic regimens as used in impetigo, coupled with warm compresses 3–4 times daily, are recommended.

FOLLICULITIS

Folliculitis is most commonly caused by *Staph. aureus* (Table 49.7). The two common types of folliculitis are superficial and deep. The superficial types are referred to as follicular or Bockhart's impetigo and commonly are located on the beard area, axilla, buttocks and extremities. The deep form of folliculitis typically occurs in the beard areas and involves perifollicular inflammation. Treatment with topical mupirocin, clindamycin 1% or erythromycin 2% along with an antibacterial wash or soap is usually sufficient; systemic treatment with antibiotics is reserved for deep extensive cases. Left untreated, folliculitis can evolve into a furuncle or carbuncle.

FURUNCLES AND CARBUNCLES

A furuncle, also known as a boil, is a deep, firm, erythematous painful inflammatory nodule, which occurs around hair follicles and gradually enlarges to form a fluctuant abscess. *Staph. aureus* is the etiological agent (Table 49.7), and increasing numbers of infections are found to be due to methicillin-resistant *Staph. aureus* (MRSA), which may be hospital or community acquired. Following rupture of a furuncle, pus is expressed along with a core of necrotic material and the lesion begins to heal. Several furuncles can coalesce into a deeper network of more extensive lesions and form a carbuncle.

Carbuncles are usually more erythematous and indurated than furuncles. Carbuncles and furuncles can evolve into more serious diseases such as cellulitis and bacteremic spread.

Treatment is aimed at incision and drainage of the pus. If a carbuncle or furuncle is complicated by fever or cellulitis, treatment with a semisynthetic penicillin is indicated: oral dicloxacillin, flucloxacillin, cefalexin, clindamycin or erythromycin, or intravenous nafcillin/oxacillin 2 g every 6 h (Table 49.4). Alternatively, intravenous cefazolin 1–2 g every 8 h or vancomycin 1 g every 12 h may be used. When MRSA infection is suspected, oral tetracyclines, trimethoprim–sulfamethoxazole, clindamycin or linezolid (400 mg every 12 h) may be used.

PARONYCHIA

Paronychia are infections caused predominately by *Staph. aureus* entering a break in the skin around the fingernails in persons exposed to hand trauma or chronic moisture[16] (Table 49.7). Other organisms causing paronychia include *Streptococcus*, *Candida*, *Pseudomonas* spp., oral anaerobes

Table 49.7 Skin and soft-tissue infections, causative organisms and primary and secondary treatment regimens

Disease	Causative organism	Primary treatment	Secondary treatment
Acne	*Propionibacterium acnes*	Doxycycline Minocycline Tetracycline	Erythromycin base Clindamycin
Actinomycosis	*Actinomyces israelii,* *Actinomyces gerencseriae*	Penicillin V	Clindamycin
Anthrax	*Bacillus anthracis*	Penicillin G (aqueous) Ciprofloxacin Levofloxacin	Erythromycin base Doxycycline
Bacillary angiomatosis	*Bartonella henselae,* *Bartonella quintana*	Erythromycin base	Doxycycline
Blistering distal dactylitis	*Staphylococcus aureus,* *Streptococcus pyogenes*	Dicloxacillin Penicillin V	Cephalosporin (2nd generation) Erythromycin base Clindamycin
Boils (carbuncles, furuncles)	*Staphylococcus aureus*	Dicloxacillin	Cephalosporin (2nd generation) Erythromycin base Clindamycin Levofloxacin
Cat bite	*Pasteurella multocida,* *Staphylococcal aureus*	Amoxicillin–clavulanate	Doxycycline Cefuroxime Penicillin G (aqueous) Penicillin V
Cat-scratch disease	*Bartonella henselae*	Ciprofloxacin	Trimethoprim–sulfamethoxazole
Cellulitis	*Streptococcus pyogenes,* *Staphylococcus aureus*	Nafcillin Oxacillin Dicloxacillin Cefazolin	Cephalosporin (2nd generation) Erythromycin base Azithromycin or clarithromycin Clindamycin Levofloxacin Linezolid
Clostridium cellulitis	*Clostridium perfringens*	Penicillin G (aqueous)	Clindamycin Metronidazole Tetracycline Chloramphenicol Imipenem
Diphtheria	*Corynebacterium diphtheriae*	Erythromycin base	Penicillin V Benzylpenicillin
Dog bites	*Pasteurella multocida,* *Viridans group streptococci,* *Staphylococcus aureus*	Amoxicillin–clavulanate	Clindamycin plus: 1. fluoroquinolone (adults) 2. trimethoprim–sulfamethoxazole (children)
Ecthyma	*Staphylococcus aureus*	Dicloxacillin	Cephalosporin (2nd generation) Erythromycin Clindamycin
Ehrlichiosis	*Ehrlichia* spp.	Doxycycline	Chloramphenicol
Erysipelas	*Streptococcus pyogenes*	Penicillin G (benzathine) Nafcillin Oxacillin Dicloxacillin	Erythromycin base Azithromycin Clarithromycin Cephalosporin (2nd generation)
Erysipeloid	*Erysipelothrix rhusiopathiae*	Penicillin G (aqueous) Ampicillin	Erythromycin base Fluoroquinolones Cephalosporin (4th generation) Clindamycin
Erythema gangrenosum	*Pseudomonas aeruginosa*	Ceftazidime Amikacin	Piperacillin Tobramycin Ciprofloxacin
Erythrasma	*Corynebacterium* *minutissimum*	Erythromycin base	Topical benzoyl peroxide Topical clindamycin

(Continued)

Table 49.7 Skin and soft-tissue infections, causative organisms and primary and secondary treatment regimens—cont'd

Disease	Causative organism	Primary treatment	Secondary treatment
Folliculitis	*Staphylococcus aureus*	Topical mupirocin	Dicloxacillin Penicillin V Oxacillin Penicillin G (benzathine) Erythromycin base
Gangrenous cellulitis (necrotizing fasciitis)	*Peptostreptococcus* spp. *Bacteroides* spp. *Enterobacter* spp. *Proteus* spp.	Ampicillin–sulbactam Imipenem–cilastatin Ticarcillin–clavulanate	Cephalosporin (3rd generation) Clindamycin Metronidazole + aminoglycoside
Gangrenous cellulitis (streptococcal gangrene)	*Streptococcus* group A/B/C/G	Penicillin G (aqueous) Penicillin V	Erythromycin base Cephalosporin Vancomycin Clarithromycin Azithromycin Clindamycin
Gas gangrene	*Clostridium perfringens*	Penicillin G (aqueous) Clindamycin	Doxycycline Erythromycin base Chloramphenicol Cefazolin Cefoxitin
Human bites	Viridans group streptococci *Staphylococcus epidermidis* *Bacteroides* spp. *Corynebacterium* spp. *Eikenella corrodens*	Amoxicillin–clavulanate	Amoxicillin–sulbactam Cefoxitin Ticarcillin–clavulanate Piperacillin–tazobactam Clindamycin + ciprofloxacin or trimethoprim–sulfamethoxazole
Impetigo	*Staphylococcus aureus*, *Streptococcus pyogenes*	Dicloxacillin Penicillin V Oxacillin Penicillin G (benzathine)	Cephalosporin (2nd or 3rd generation) Erythromycin base Clindamycin Azithromycin Clarithromycin Mupirocin
Kawasaki syndrome	*Staphylococcus aureus* superantigens	Intravenous immunoglobulin + aspirin	None
Listeriosis	*Listeria monocytogenes*	Ampicillin Penicillin G (aqueous)	Trimethoprim–sulfamethoxazole
Lyme disease (erythema migrans)	*Borrelia burgdorferi*	Ceftriaxone Ceftizoxime Doxycycline Amoxicillin	Penicillin G (aqueous) Azithromycin Clarithromycin
Meningococcemia	*Neisseria meningitidis*	Penicillin G (aqueous)	Ceftriaxone Chloramphenicol Minocycline
Nocardiosis	*Nocardia asteroides*	Trimethoprim–sulfamethoxazole	Minocycline
Paronychia	*Staphylococcus aureus*	Clindamycin	Erythromycin
Plague	*Yersinia pestis*	Gentamicin Streptomycin	Doxycycline Chloramphenicol Fluoroquinolones
Pseudomonal infection	*Pseudomonas aeruginosa*	Meropenem Cefepime Piperacillin–tazobactam plus amikacin	Gentamicin Tobramycin
Rat bite fever	*Streptobacillus moniliformis*	Penicillin G (aqueous) Doxycycline	Erythromycin base Chloramphenicol
Rocky Mountain spotted fever	*Rickettsia rickettsii*	Doxycycline	Chloramphenicol Fluoroquinolones

(Continued)

Table 49.7 Skin and soft-tissue infections, causative organisms and primary and secondary treatment regimens—cont'd

Disease	Causative organism	Primary treatment	Secondary treatment
Rosacea	Unknown	Minocycline Doxycycline Tetracycline Erythromycin Metronidazole (topical 1%) Ampicillin	Trimethoprim–sulfamethoxazole Metronidazole (oral) Dapsone
Saltwater contaminated wound	*Vibrio vulnificus*, *Vibrio damsela*	Ceftazidime + doxycycline	Cefotaxime Ciprofloxacin
Scarlet fever	*Streptococcus pyogenes*	Penicillin (all)	Cephalosporins (all) Macrolides (all)
Staphylococcal scalded skin syndrome	*Staphylococcus aureus* exotoxin	Nafcillin	Oxacillin
Toxic shock syndrome	*Staphylococcus aureus* exotoxin	Nafcillin or Oxacillin + intravenous immunoglobulins	Cephalosporin (1st generation)
Tularemia	*Francisella tularensis*	Streptomycin	Gentamicin Doxycycline Chloramphenicol
Wound infection postoperative	*Staphylococcus aureus*, *Streptococcus*, Enterobacteriaceae	Cephalosporin (2nd generation) Amoxicillin–clavulanate	Doxycycline Cephalosporin (2nd and 3rd generation) Levofloxacin Linezolid

Note: Flucloxacillin can be substituted for nafcillin, oxacillin or dicloxacillin in countries in which it is available.

and dermatophytes. Paronychia usually presents as red-hot, tender, proximal and lateral nail-fold inflammation.

Treatment of bacterial paronychia includes both topical and oral antibiotic therapy plus incision and drainage of any abscess formation. Oral amoxicillin–clavulanate (375–625 mg every 8 h) or clindamycin (300 mg every 6 h) are the suggested regimens (Table 49.6). Fungal paronychia may be treated with topical antifungal preparations or oral ketoconazole (200 mg/day).

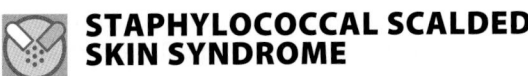

STAPHYLOCOCCAL SCALDED SKIN SYNDROME

Staphylococcal scalded skin syndrome is a severe skin exfoliation caused by a staphylococcal exotoxin (Table 49.7). Children under the age of 5 years are most commonly affected due to their immature immune systems; however, immunocompromised adults can also be afflicted.

The generalized syndrome can begin with an upper respiratory tract, eye or ear infection.[17] Areas around the mouth and axilla initially become tender and slightly erythematous; this heralds the appearance of the generalized blisters that evolve into large flaccid bullae. Next, large sheets of epidermis are shed, leaving an erythematous, denuded base exposed. Uniquely, the mucous membranes are spared. Healing of the lesions can be expected in 5–7 days. Culture and biopsy confirm diagnosis.

Treatment with an intravenous penicillinase-resistant antibiotic and subsequent substitution with an oral agent within a few days is appropriate (Table 49.4). Diligent management of electrolytes and supportive skin care will speed recovery; however, despite all efforts the mortality rate is approximately 2–3% (rates are higher in adults than in children). Care must be taken to avoid epidemics in neonatal care units by eradicating *Staph. aureus* from healthcare workers who are nasal carriers and by implementing strict handwashing policies.

The recommended penicillinase-resistant antibiotic is intravenous nafcillin, oxacillin or flucloxacillin (2 g every 4 h in adults; 150 mg/kg every 6 h in children). Treatment should last 5–7 days (Table 49.4).

STAPHYLOCOCCAL TOXIC-SHOCK SYNDROME

Staphylococcal toxic-shock syndrome, like staphylococcal scalded skin syndrome, is an illness that results from an exotoxin produced by *Staph. aureus* (Table 49.7). In addition, it is a multisystem disease involving at least three organ systems, with hypotension, fever, and a rash resembling that of scarlet fever followed by skin desquamation.

Menstruating women using tampons for a prolonged period of time account for up to 90% of cases. The conjunctiva may become infected; the oral mucosa and vagina may appear intensely erythematous. Palmar and plantar desquamation occurs between 1 and 2 weeks later.

Initial treatment is aimed at controlling the hypotension and shock with fluid replacement. The tampon must be removed and intravenous penicillinase-resistant antibiotics started. If therapy is instituted early, intravenous γ-globulins and fresh-frozen plasma containing immunoglobulins will expedite recovery.[16] Treatment with intravenous clindamycin 600–900 mg every 8 h is recommended. Intravenous nafcillin, oxacillin or flucloxacillin 2 g every 4 h or a first-generation cephalosporin such as cefazolin 1–2 g every 8 h may also be used (Tables 49.4 and 49.5).

 ## KAWASAKI SYNDROME

Kawasaki syndrome is an acute multisystem vasculitis of infancy and childhood associated with high fever, mucocutaneous inflammation and the development of coronary artery abnormalities.[18] The etiology of Kawasaki syndrome is unknown; however, it is suspected that *Staph. aureus* superantigens may trigger the disease (Table 49.7).

Treatment should begin with intravenous immunoglobulin 2 g/kg over 12 h, plus oral aspirin 80–100 mg/kg per day in four divided doses, followed by aspirin 3–5 mg/kg per day for 6–8 weeks. If the patient remains febrile after the first dose of immunoglobulin, a second dose may be administered.

STREPTOCOCCAL INFECTIONS

 ### IMPETIGO

Streptococcal impetigo is often indistinguishable from the staphylococcal variant (Table 49.7). Patients may be infected with both staphylococcal and streptococcal impetigo. Treatment of the streptococcal form with mupirocin ointment is effective, but more severe forms of group A streptococcal impetigo should be treated with oral or intramuscular penicillin. Oral penicillin V 250–500 mg/day is the recommended regimen (Table 49.4). If an intramuscular dose of penicillin is preferred, then benzathine penicillin G(0.6–1.2 million units) is advocated (Table 49.4). An alternative oral antibiotic is a second-generation cephalosporin (Table 49.5). Second-line treatment consists of a macrolide antibiotic or a third-generation cephalosporin (Tables 49.5 and 49.6).

 ### BLISTERING DISTAL DACTYLITIS

Blistering distal dactylitis is caused most commonly by *Str. pyogenes* (Table 49.7). Mostly children and adolescents are affected.[19] The lesion is described as a seropurulent blister on an erythematous base that develops on the distal palmar or plantar aspect of the fingers and toes. Treatment with oral penicillin or erythromycin base is appropriate (Tables 49.4 and 49.6).

 ## ERYSIPELAS

Erysipelas is a form of superficial cellulitis with lymphatic vessel involvement, caused mainly by group A β-hemolytic streptococci (Table 49.7). The lesions may be precursors to a more invasive cellulitis. The painful lesions are well demarcated and the plaques appear very erythematous and edematous, with an advancing raised border.[20] The diagnosis is usually clinical; however, Gram stain and culture will confirm the organism. It is important to differentiate between the more superficial erysipelas and the deeper cellulitis so that appropriate treatment can be instituted.

Treatment is with either oral or intramuscular penicillin; erythromycin base can be used in the penicillin-allergic patient (Tables 49.4 and 49.6). A penicillin-resistant semisynthetic penicillin such as oral dicloxacillin or flucloxacillin 500 mg every 6 h or, for a more severe infection, intravenous nafcillin, oxacillin or flucloxacillin 2 g every 4 h is preferred. Second-line agents include macrolide antibiotics, first-generation cephalosporins or ampicillin and clindamycin (Tables 49.5 and 49.6). Improvement can be expected in 24–28 h with antibiotic therapy.

 ## CELLULITIS

Cellulitis is caused most commonly by *Staph. aureus* and group A streptococci (Table 49.7). Other pathogens involved include group B streptococci, cryptococci, pneumococci and Gram-negative bacilli. Unlike erysipelas, the deep dermis and subcutaneous soft tissues are affected, and the margins are indistinct, not raised and are indurated. However, like erysipelas, cellulitis is very painful. Diagnosis is clinical and confirmed with Gram stain and culture.

Treatment must be implemented rapidly to avoid any complications such as superinfections, bacteremia, necrotizing fasciitis and amputations. Treatment can be customized depending on the offending pathogen (if cultures are available). Realistically, when patients present with cellulitis, cultures are not immediately available and therefore empirical treatment with an intravenous penicillinase-resistant penicillin should be initiated to treat both staphylococcal and streptococcal infections. Intravenous nafcillin or oxacillin 2 g every 4 h is appropriate (Table 49.4). Subsequent culture results can help guide specific therapy. For moderately complicated infections oral levofloxacin 500–750 mg every 12 h is acceptable (Table 49.8). Treatment with intravenous vancomycin (1 g every 12 h) or linezolid is preferred for methicillin-resistant cases of cellulitis.[21] Linezolid is available in intravenous and oral preparations and is 100% orally bioavailable so patients may be switched from intravenous preparations to oral preparations without dose changes. Linezolid is available in 600 mg tablets, an oral suspension containing 100 mg/mL and an intravenous solution. The recommended oral dose for uncomplicated skin infections is 400 mg every 12 h.[21] Immobilization and elevation of the affected limb will aid in reducing edema and pain.

Table 49.8 Common fluoroquinolones doses (for adults) used in skin and soft-tissue infections

Fluoroquinolones	Route	Dose
Nalidixic acid	oral	1 g every 6 h
Ciprofloxacin	oral i.v.	250–750 mg every 12 h 200–400 mg every 12 h
Ofloxacin	oral, i.v.	200–400 mg every 12 h
Levofloxacin	oral, i.v.	200–750 mg once daily or every 12 h
Trovafloxacin/ alatrofloxacin	oral	100–200 mg once daily
	i.v.	300 mg once daily
Sparfloxacin	oral	400 mg first day, followed by 200 mg once daily
Gatifloxacin	i.v., oral	400 mg once daily
Moxifloxacin	oral	400 mg once daily

Frequent dressing changes with sterile saline will keep the lesion clean. Oral analgesics may be necessary for pain management.

 ## GANGRENOUS CELLULITIS

Necrotizing fasciitis is a type of gangrenous cellulitis. The various forms of necrotizing fasciitis include a non-streptococcal gangrene, streptococcal gangrene, synergistic necrotizing cellulitis and Fournier's gangrene. Gangrenous cellulitis usually begins on an extremity, the perineum, or postoperative wound or trauma site and initially appears as a cellulitis infection. As the infection evolves, gangrenous changes become apparent within 36–72 h. The area becomes purple, followed by formation of vesicles and bullae that quickly rupture, producing sharply demarcated areas of necrotic eschar and crepitus that destroy all soft tissues, including vessels and nerves. A foul-smelling discharge and palpable gas in the tissues can sometimes be detected.

Streptococcal gangrene is caused principally by group A streptococci.

Non-streptococcal gangrene is a type of necrotizing fasciitis caused by pathogens other than group A streptococci, such as anaerobes plus at least one facultative species.[20] These same pathogens can also cause Fournier's gangrene, which involves the scrotum and penis.[22]

Another type of highly lethal necrotizing fasciitis is the polymicrobial synergistic necrotizing cellulitis, which involves necrosis of all layers of soft tissues and commonly involves the perineum. The diagnosis is based on Gram stain, culture and clinical findings. Treatment with broad-spectrum antibiotics (with aerobic, anaerobic and antipseudomonal coverage) plus wide surgical debridement of the gangrenous tissue is recommended. Despite therapy, mortality remains high.

 ## SCARLET FEVER

Scarlet fever is usually caused by a pharyngeal infection with group A streptococci and subsequent elaboration of a pyrogenic exotoxin occurring in children under 10 years of age (Table 49.7). Between 24 and 48 h after the appearance of the fever and pharyngitis, the unique cutaneous manifestations of scarlet fever, including the characteristic diffuse erythematous 'sandpaper' like rash, and 'strawberry' red tongue appear. Diagnosis is confirmed by the presence of a positive group A streptococcal throat culture.

Following treatment with penicillin the symptoms improve quickly; however, a desquamation may persist for a few weeks. If untreated, uncomplicated infection may last 4–5 days.

CORYNEBACTERIUM MINUTISSIMUM

 ## ERYTHRASMA

Erythrasma caused by *Corynebacterium minutissimum* is a common disease, occurring more often in men and with a predilection for the intertriginous areas (Table 49.7). The organism possesses keratolytic properties and lesions cause thick lamellated plaques on affected areas. The toe web spaces are commonly affected; a Wood's lamp examination revealing a striking bright coral red–pink fluorescence will confirm the diagnosis, as will a culture. Recommended treatment for widespread involvement is oral erythromycin (250 mg every 6 h or 500 mg every 12 h for 14 days) and, for more localized involvement, benzoyl peroxide (Table 49.7).

BACILLUS ANTHRACIS (ANTHRAX)

Anthrax is caused by infection with *Bacillus anthracis*, an aerobic, encapsulated, square rod (Table 49.7). Although primarily a disease of animals, humans can be infected by contact with infected carcasses during animal product handling. Other means of infection include aerosolized spores, which may cause pulmonary infection. A painless malignant pustule occurring on an exposed surface of the body is the hallmark of cutaneous anthrax.

Treatment of choice is aqueous penicillin G 20 million units a day intravenously in four divided doses (Table 49.4). For aerosolized anthrax, fluoroquinolones and doxycycline are effective alternatives (Table 49.8).

ERYSIPELOTHRIX RHUSIOPATHIAE (ERYSIPELOID)

E. rhusiopathiae is a rod-shaped Gram-positive organism (Table 49.7), which occurs most commonly in people handling raw fish, poultry or other meat products. The organism is inoculated through a break in the skin.[23]

The macular and plaque-like lesions appear violaceous with sharply defined borders. A culture may confirm the presence of *E. rhusiopathiae*; however, the clinical history is usually enough to suggest the diagnosis.

Treatment with oral or intramuscular penicillin 2–3 million units (1.2–1.8 g) per day for 7–10 days is recommended (Table 49.4). In the penicillin-allergic patient, a fourth-generation cephalosporin, imipenem or ciprofloxacin would be adequate; however, most isolates are resistant to vancomycin[24] (Tables 49.5 and 49.8).

BARTONELLA HENSELAE (CAT-SCRATCH DISEASE)

Cat-scratch disease caused by *B. henselae* is the most common cause of localized chronic lymphadenopathy in children and young adults (Table 49.7).[25] Infection is typically benign and is caused by a bite or scratch from a cat. The initial inoculation may start as a papule and evolve into a vesicle and subsequent crust within 5 days.[26] The gold standard for diagnosis is the cat-scratch disease skin test.

Treatment with antibiotics remains controversial, because most cases of this disease spontaneously resolve. *B. henselae* is sensitive to fluoroquinolones, macrolides, tetracyclines, and third- or fourth-generation cephalosporins (Tables 49.6, 49.8 and 49.9). A recommended regimen would be oral azithromycin 500 mg for 1 day followed by 250 mg for 4 additional days (Table 49.6); oral ciprofloxacin 500–750 mg every 12 h is also effective (Table 49.8).

BARTONELLA QUINTANA (BACILLARY ANGIOMATOSIS)

Either *B. henselae* or *B. quintana* may cause bacillary angiomatosis (Table 49.7). Bacillary angiomatosis typically affects severely immunocompromised patients, such as advanced cases of HIV with CD4+ lymphocytes <50 cells/mm³.[27] Symptoms of bacillary angiomatosis include fever, lymphadenopathy, abdominal pain, and the classic grouped dark-red and violaceous papules and nodules that are friable and painful. The lesions of bacillary angiomatosis appear similar to Kaposi's sarcoma and pyogenic granulomas, and should be distinguished from these conditions.

Erythromycin (500 mg every 6 h) is the drug of choice; oral macrolide antibiotics (clarithromycin 500 mg every

12 h or azithromycin 250 mg/day) may also be used (Table 49.6). Ciprofloxacin (oral 500–750 mg every 12 h) (Table 49.8) and oral doxycycline (100 mg every 12 h) are also recommended (Table 49.9). Treatment must continue for up to 6 months.

PROPIONIBACTERIUM ACNES (ACNE)

Acne is an inflammatory condition caused by the accumulation of free fatty acids in the follicles of the skin, produced by the action of bacterial lipolytic enzymes on triglycerides (Table 49.7). Acne begins with the formation of a comedone, sometimes papules, pustules and nodules. The ensuing inflammation is a result of the presence of *P. acnes* which is the target of the inflammatory response. The accumulation of sebum in the follicles of the face, chest, shoulders and back produces nutrients on which *P. acnes* thrives.

The disruption in keratinization is a fundamental component of acne for which therapy is directed. Topical agents include use of products containing benzoyl peroxide, salicylic acid, vitamin A derivatives, the synthetic retinoids adapalene and tazarotene, and dapsone. Topical antibacterial agents such as clindamycin and erythromycin are effective (Table 49.10). Another cream intended to affect the keratinization process is azelaic acid. Cleansing is of limited value because soaps will not remove bacteria or lipids from inside the follicle. Intralesional steroid injection of larger nodular lesions will decrease inflammation and avoid potential scar formation. Daily oral tetracycline, erythromycin, clindamycin, doxycycline and minocycline decrease the concentration of free fatty acids and suppress *P. acnes* (Tables 49.6 and 49.9). Oral contraceptives containing estrogen will decrease sebum production and therefore decrease acne lesions. Isotretinoin, a synthetic oral retinoid that produces profound decreases in sebum production, has several side effects, including pronounced dryness of the skin and mucous membranes. A dose of 0.5–1.0 mg/day is recommended for a 20-week treatment. Baseline complete blood cell counts, liver function tests and triglyceride levels should be checked and repeated at 3–4 weeks and 6–8 weeks of therapy. As isotretinoin is teratogenic, women of childbearing age should start contraception 1 month before therapy.

CLOSTRIDIUM PERFRINGENS (CLOSTRIDIUM CELLULITIS)

Clostridium perfringens infection can cause a crepitant cellulitis of the subcutaneous tissue, possibly muscle, following traumatic tissue injury associated with soil contamination (Table 49.7). The crepitus present is caused by gas in the underlying tissues (gas gangrene). Pure clostridial infections do not emit foul odors; however, mixed and non-clostridial infections will produce foul-smelling hydrogen compounds through incomplete oxidation produced by anaerobic organisms.[28]

Table 49.9 Common tetracycline doses (for adults) used in skin and soft-tissue infections

Tetracycline	Route	Dose
Short-acting tetracyclines		
Tetracycline	oral	250–500 mg every 6 h
Long-acting tetracyclines		
Doxycycline	oral, i.v.	200 mg initially then 50–100 mg every 12 h
Minocycline	oral, i.v.	200 mg initially then 100 mg every 12–24 h

Table 49.10 Topical antimicrobial agents

Antibiotic/strength	Indications	Bacterial coverage	Available forms
Azelaic acid 20%	Acne	Gram-positive	Cream
Bacitracin	Impetigo, furunculosis	Gram-positive	Ointment
Chloramphenicol 1%	Minor skin infections	Gram-positive and negative	Cream
Clindamycin 1%	Acne	Gram-positive	Solution, gel, pledget, lotion
Clioquinol	Tinea pedis	Broad spectrum	Cream, ointment
Demeclocycline	Skin infections	Gram-positive	Cream
Erythromycin 1.5–2%	Acne	Gram-positive and negative	Solution, gel, pledget, ointment solution
Fusidic acid	Skin infections	Gram-positive	Cream, ointment, impregnated gauze
Gentamicin 0.01%	Prophylaxis of malignant otitis externa	Gram-negative	Cream, ointment
Gramicidin	Skin infections	Gram-positive	Ointment
Metronidazole 0.75%	Rosacea	Anaerobes	Gel, cream
Mupirocin 2%	Impetigo, antimicrobial prophylaxis, and eliminating *Staph. aureus* nasal carriage	Gram-positive	Ointment
Neomycin	Abrasions, burns	Gram-negative	Ointment
Neomycin + polymyxin	Abrasions	Gram-negative	Cream
Neomycin + polymyxin + bacitracin	Abrasions	Gram-positive and negative	Ointment
Nitrofurazone 0.2%	Burns	Gram-positive and negative	Cream, solution
Paromomycin	Cutaneous leishmaniasis	Broad-spectrum antibacterial and antiparasitic	
Polymyxin B	Infected atopic, nummular, stasis dermatitis and swimmer's ear	Gram-negative	Ointment
Retapamulin 1%	*Staph. aureus*	Gram-positive	Ointment
Silver sulfadiazine	Burns	Broad spectrum	Cream
Tetracycline	Acne	Gram-positive and negative	Ointment, solution

The pain of a clostridium cellulitis is often mild and infection appears superficial, although tissue damage may be extensive. Treatment requires surgery and adjunct penicillin G, with possibly clindamycin and hyperbaric oxygen therapy (Table 49.4).

LISTERIA MONOCYTOGENES (LISTERIOSIS)

Listeria monocytogenes is found in the feces of wild animals, birds and soil; however, infection cannot usually be associated with exposure to any of the common sources (Table 49.7). Treatment is with either ampicillin or penicillin (Table 49.4). For adults the dosage of aqueous penicillin G is 12–24 million units (7.2–14.4 g) intravenously daily in divided doses every 2–4 h; the dose of ampicillin is 12 g intravenously in divided doses every 3–4 h (Table 49.4). In non-pregnant adults allergic to penicillin, trimethoprim–sulfamethoxazole is an alternative.[29]

ACTINOMYCES (ACTINOMYCOSIS)

Either *Actinomyces israelii* or *Actinomyces gerencseriae* can cause actinomycosis (Table 49.7). Infection typically involves the cervicofacial anatomy following a traumatic procedure such as a dental extraction. Infection can result in a painful indurated soft-tissue swelling around the oral mucosa known as 'woody fibrosis'. As the lesion enlarges at the angle of the jaw it is referred to as 'lumpy jaw'. Direct extension to adjacent thoracic structures may occur.

Diagnosis is based on clinical suspicion and detection of the organism on Gram stain, culture, exudates or biopsy.

Treatment is with intravenous aqueous penicillin G 10–20 million units (6–12 g) per day in divided doses every 4 h for 4–6 weeks (Table 49.4) or intravenous ampicillin 50 mg/kg per day in divided doses every 12 h for 4–6 weeks, followed by amoxicillin 500 mg/day for 6–12 additional months to prevent relapse (Table 49.4).

GRAM-NEGATIVE ORGANISMS

NEISSERIA MENINGITIDIS (MENINGOCOCCEMIA)

Neisseria meningitidis is an obligate aerobic, encapsulated Gram-negative coccus (Table 49.7). Humans are the only known host. Asymptomatic exposure to *N. meningitidis* can elicit protective bactericidal antibodies; thus immunity increases with age.[30] A brief upper respiratory tract infection and subsequent nausea, vomiting, myalgia, fever, meningismus, stupor, hypotension and hemorrhagic rash can precede acute meningococcemia. The hemorrhagic rash is a result of the pathogen damaging the small dermal blood vessels. The rash may transiently appear macular and papular with an erythematous hue with evolving purpura, and sometimes there are large red–black geographic-appearing areas of tissue infarction with a gray center.

Polymorphonuclear leukocytosis is observed in the peripheral blood and cerebrospinal fluid. The organism may be seen on Gram stain and is easily cultured in cases of meningococcemia.

Untreated infection with *N. meningitidis* is fatal. Adults should be given aqueous penicillin G, 4 million units (2.4 g) intravenously every 4 h for 7 days after the temperature has returned to normal (Table 49.4); in the penicillin-allergic patient, chloramphenicol 1 g intravenously every 6 h is the recommended regimen. In parts of the world where meningococcal resistance to penicillin has been isolated (e.g. Spain or the UK), a third-generation cephalosporin should be used[31] (Table 49.5). The recommended prophylactic dose of rifampicin (rifampin) is 600 mg orally every 12 h for 2 days.[32] In cases of rifampicin resistance, a fluoroquinolone is an effective oral single-dose substitute (Table 49.8). Ceftriaxone is an alternative parenteral single dose for children and adults[31,33] (Table 49.5). Immunization with polysaccharide vaccines is safe and effective in preventing disease in adults and children over the age of 2 years.[32,34]

PSEUDOMONAS AERUGINOSA

Pseudomonas aeruginosa is an obligate aerobic Gram-negative bacillus (Table 49.7). Some strains produce the characteristic blue pigment pyocyanin or the yellow–green pigment fluorescein, which will fluoresce under Wood's ultraviolet lamp. An odor of grapes, characteristic of trimethylamine, is typical of pseudomonal infection.[35] Healthy people infected with *Pseudomonas* will typically be affected in areas exposed to increased humidity and moisture, such as the toe webs, fingernails (green nail syndrome) and the ear canal (swimmer's ear). People utilizing public swimming pools or hot tubs (hot tub folliculitis) can also be affected.[36] Local infections will improve with topical therapy and drying of the affected area. Superficial skin infections such as toe web infections respond to acetic acid, silver nitrate and gentian violet each applied 2–3 times per day. Paronychia responds well to 4% thymol in chloroform, surgical drainage and nail trimming. For external ear infection, acetic acid in 50% alcohol, 0.1% polymyxin in acetic acid, or glucocorticoids with neomycin are effective. Systemic infection is rare in the immunocompetent host.

Patients with *Pseudomonas* infections are typically immunocompromised and may be afflicted with gangrenous cellulitis or possibly ecthyma gangrenosum. Ecthyma gangrenosum lesions are painless and begin with an area of erythema surrounding a gray region of infarcted tissue. The lesions evolve to become black necrotic eschars. Treatment for systemic infections requires intravenous antibiotic therapy; meropenem, cefepime and piperacillin–tazobactam plus amikacin are recommended as first-line agents. The aminoglycosides gentamicin and tobramycin are also recommended (Table 49.11).

BORRELIA BURGDORFERI (LYME BORRELIOSIS)

Lyme disease is caused by a tick vector that transmits the offending Gram-negative bacterial spirochete *Borrelia burgdorferi* to humans (Table 49.7). Lyme borreliosis is common throughout the northern hemisphere. Lyme disease can be classified into three stages: the first stage is called the early localized stage, the second the early disseminated and the last stage the late or chronic stage of Lyme disease.

The hallmark cutaneous manifestation of Lyme disease, erythema migrans, begins at the site of a tick bite. Initially, the lesion appears as a confluent erythematous macule or patch; however, as the lesion spreads centrifugally the center of the lesion fades, leaving an annular area of erythema. The rash may be asymptomatic; however, systemic symptoms such as lymphadenopathy, headache, fever, malaise, myalgia, arthralgia and gastrointestinal symptoms may be present.

Diagnosis is based on the history of exposure to a tick bite plus the appearance and evolution of the characteristic rash and serology.

Amoxicillin (1 g every 8 h) or doxycycline (200 mg every 12 h) for 14 days, as well as intravenous ceftriaxone or ceftizoxime, have all been suggested for treatment (Tables 49.4–49.6 and 49.9).

Table 49.11 Adult doses of aminoglycosides for treatment of skin and soft-tissue infections

Aminoglycoside	Route	Dose
Amikacin	i.m., i.v.	15 mg/kg daily every 8–12 h
Gentamicin	i.m., i.v.	1.7–5.0 mg/kg daily every 8 h
Spectinomycin	i.m.	2 g once
Tobramycin	i.m., i.v.	3–5 mg/kg daily every 8 h
Streptomycin	i.m., i.v.	15 mg/kg daily or 25–30 mg/kg 2–3 times per week

YERSINIA PESTIS (PLAGUE)

The plague is an infection in humans caused by *Yersinia pestis*, which is endemic in wild rodents and spread to humans via flea bites (*see* Ch. 61). Bubonic plague is the most common form of plague in the USA. Treatment is with intravenous gentamicin 2 mg/kg loading dose then 1.7 mg/kg every 8 h, or intramuscular streptomycin 1 g every 12 h for 10 days[37] (Table 49.11). Chloramphenicol, doxycycline and fluoroquinolones are alternative treatments and preferred if streptomycin-resistant strains are present (Table 49.9).

FRANCISELLA TULARENSIS (TULAREMIA)

Tularemia is an infection of humans that typically follows direct inoculation by animals or by insect vectors with *Francisella tularensis* (*see* Ch. 61). Treatment is with streptomycin 1–2 g per day for 7–10 afebrile days. Gentamicin, tetracycline and chloramphenicol are alternatives (Tables 49.9 and 49.11).

STREPTOBACILLUS MONILIFORMIS (RAT BITE FEVER)

Rat bite fever is acquired from rodents and is characterized by fever, polyarthralgia, and a rash[38] (Ch. 61). Treatment is with intravenous penicillin G 4 million units every 4 h; therapy can be switched to oral amoxicillin 1 g every 8 h for total treatment course of 14 days. Doxycycline, erythromycin and chloramphenicol are alternatives in the penicillin-allergic patient[37] (Tables 49.6 and 49.9).

PASTEURELLA MULTOCIDA

Pasteurella multocida infection typically follows an animal bite (Ch. 61); *P. multocida* can be isolated from the upper respiratory tract of healthy dogs, cats, rats and mice. Treatment of choice is intravenous penicillin G 2–4 million units every 4 h or oral penicillin V 500–750 mg every 6 h (Table 49.4). For the penicillin-allergic patient, amoxicillin, doxycycline, chloramphenicol and trimethoprim–sulfamethoxazole (Table 49.9) are alternatives. Fourth-generation cephalosporins are also effective (Table 49.5); alternatively, oral clindamycin 150–300 mg every 6 h plus a fluoroquinolone may be effective (Table 49.8).

VIBRIO VULNIFICUS

Vibrio vulnificus is the most pathogenic of the *Vibrio* species. The soft-tissue infection and septicemia caused by *V. vulnificus* is fatal 50% of the time (Table 49.7). *V. vulnificus* produces a toxin and lytic enzymes that contribute to its pathogenicity. Gastroenteritis and saltwater wound injuries are common clinical findings. Septicemia following consumption of raw oysters can develop within 24 h.

Treatment of septicemia initially involves fluid replacement for shock followed by treatment with ceftazidime 2 g intravenously every 8 h plus doxycycline 100 mg (intravenously or orally) every 12 h (Tables 49.5 and 49.9). Alternative regimens include cefotaxime 2 g intravenously every 8 h or ciprofloxacin (oral 750 mg every 12 h or intravenous 400 mg every 12 h) (Tables 49.5 and 49.8). Surgical debridement of necrotic lesions is indicated.[37]

RICKETTSIA RICKETTSII

Rickettsiae are obligate intracellular parasites transmitted to humans by arthropod vectors. The most common rickettsial disease in the USA is Rocky Mountain spotted fever. Others include typhus, trench fever and Q fever. Rocky Mountain spotted fever can range from virtually asymptomatic disease to fulminant, fatal disease.[39] The disease begins with abrupt fever, chills, headache, myalgias and arthralgias, followed by a characteristic rash. The rash is a result of diffuse vasculitis that often begins first on the wrist, ankles and forearms, progresses to involve the palms and soles, and then spreads centrally to involve the trunk, arms, thighs and face. The lesions initially appear as blanchable macules and papules, which become hemorrhagic with time. Treatment is with oral or intravenous doxycycline 200 mg every 12 h for 3 days and then 100 mg once daily for 4 days or for 2 days after the temperature returns to normal (Table 49.9). An alternative is oral or intravenous quinolones or chloramphenicol for 7 days or 2 days after the temperature reaches normal.

PARASITES

SCABIES

Scabies is caused by the mite *Sarcoptes scabiei* var. *humanus*. The scabies mite is transmitted by skin-to-skin contact between sexual partners or family members. Infestation is usually bilateral and commonly involves the finger web spaces, wrists, elbows, and genital and axillary folds. Diagnosis is made by identifying the mite, eggs or fecal pellets.

Treatment is permethrin 5% cream, applied to the entire body from the neck down, paying special attention to the commonly infested areas. The cream must be washed off approximately 10 h after application. A second application may be used a week later if necessary. Lindane 1% (discontinued in several countries, but still available in the USA) is equally effective, and since low levels of systemic absorption may occur, central nervous system toxicity has been reported. Permethrin and lindane must not be used on children under 2 years of age. Sulfur 6% in petrolatum, applied nightly for three nights and washed off in the morning, is safe and effective for infants (and pregnant mothers). Symptomatic therapy of pruritus that may persist for weeks after effective therapy should include oral and topical antihistamines, and low to mid-potency topical steroids.

In serious cases, systemic treatment with ivermectin 18 mg as a single dose may be effective.[40]

PEDICULOSIS (LICE)

Lice are blood-sucking insects. Their bites are painless and a person would be unaware of infestation if it were not for the body's immune system recognizing the foreign saliva and anticoagulant produced by the bite of the insect feeding on the underlying dermis. Head lice (*Pediculus humanus* var. *capitis*) are typically isolated to the scalp. Crab lice or pubic lice (*Phthirus pubis*) are typically sexually transmitted. Body lice (*Pediculus humanus*) are found on people with poor hygiene.

Head lice are treated with synthetic pyrethroids: permethrin 5% shampoo applied to a previously shampooed and rinsed hair and scalp, allowed to set for 10 minutes and then rinsed off with water. Alternatives include synergized pyrethrins applied in a similar manner. A second application of the medication 7–10 days later will kill any surviving eggs or nymphs that were not killed with the first treatment.

Crab lice are treated similarly with either synergized pyrethrins or lindane shampoo. The pubic area and the surrounding abdomen and thighs should be treated, especially if the patient is hairy. All undergarments and linens should be washed in hot water and dried on a high heat dryer cycle.

Body lice should be treated with a single application of permethrin 5% cream, exactly as one would treat scabies. Clothing and bed linens should be discarded or washed thoroughly in hot water.

OTHER INFECTIONS

- **Fungal infections** are discussed in detail in Chapter 60.
- **Mycobacterial infections** are discussed in detail in Chapter 58.
- **Sexually transmitted diseases** are discussed in detail in Chapter 56.
- **Protozoal infections** are discussed in detail in Chapter 63.
- **Helminthic infections** are discussed in detail in Chapter 64.
- **Hepatitis infection** is discussed in detail in Chapter 48.
- **HIV infection** is discussed in detail in Chapter 43.
- **Leprosy** is discussed in detail in Chapter 57.

 References

1. Freedberg IM, Eisen AZ, Wolff K, et al, eds. *Fitzpatrick's Dermatology in General Medicine*. 5th ed. New York: McGraw-Hill; 1999: Chapter 210.
2. Wald A, Zeh J, Selke S, et al. Reactivation of genital herpes simplex virus type 2 infection in asymptomatic HSV-2 seropositive persons. *N Engl J Med*. 2000;342:844–850.
3. Hope Simpson RE. The nature of herpes zoster: a long term study and new hypothesis. *Proc R Soc Lond B*. 1965;58:9–20.
4. Weksler ME. Immune senescence. *Ann Neurol*. 1994;35:S35–S37.
5. Straus SE. Epstein–Barr virus infections: biology, pathogenesis, and management. *Ann Intern Med*. 1993;118:45–58.
6. Epstein JB. Hairy leukoplakia-like lesions in immunosuppressed patients following bone marrow transplantation. *Transplantation*. 1998;46:462–464.
7. Schmidt-Westhausen A. Oral hairy leukoplakia in an HIV seronegative heart transplant patient. *J Oral Pathol Med*. 1990;19:192–194.
8. Chang Y, Cesarman E, Pessin MS, et al. Identification of herpes-like DNA sequences in AIDS-associated Kaposi's sarcoma. *Science*. 1994;266:1865–1869.
9. Vander Straten MR, Carrasco DA, Tyring SK. Treatment of human herpesvirus 8 infections. *Dermatological Therapy*. 2000;13:2277–2284.
10. Leavell Jr UW. Ecthyma contagiosum (Orf). *South Med J*. 1965;58:238.
11. Nagington J. The structure of the orf virus. *Virology*. 1964;23:461.
12. Moscovici C. Isolation of a viral agent from pseudocowpox disease. *Science*. 1963;141:915.
13. de Villiers EM, Fauquet C, Broker TR, Bernard HU, zur Hausen H. Classification of papillomaviruses. *Virology*. 2004;324:17–27.
14. Gewirtzman A, Bartlett B, Tyring S. Epidermodysplasia verruciformis and human papilloma virus. *Curr Opin Infect Dis*. 2008;21:141–146.
15. Ramoz N, Rueda LA, Bouadjar B, Montoya LS, Orth G, Favre M. Mutations in two adjacent novel genes are associated with epidermodysplasia verruciformis. *Nat Genet*. 2002;32:579–581.
16. Freedberg IM, Eisen AZ, Wolff K, et al, eds. *Fitzpatrick's Dermatology in General Medicine*. 5th ed. New York: McGraw-Hill; 1999: Chapter 35.
17. Freedberg IM, Eisen AZ, Wolff K, et al, eds. *Fitzpatrick's Dermatology in General Medicine*. 5th ed. New York: McGraw-Hill; 1999: Chapter 196.
18. Leung DY, Meissner C, Fulton D, Schlievert PM. The potential role of bacterial superantigens in the pathogenesis of Kawasaki syndrome. *J Clin Immunol*. 1995;15(suppl 6):11S–17S.
19. McCray MK, Esterly NB. Blistering distal dactylitis. *J Am Acad Dermatol*. 1981;5:592–594.
20. Freedberg IM, Eisen AZ, Wolff K, et al, eds. *Fitzpatrick's Dermatology in General Medicine*. 5th ed. New York: McGraw-Hill; 1999: Chapter 197.
21. Abramowicz M. Linezolid (Zyvox). *Medical Letter*. 2000;14:45–46.
22. Laucks SS. Fournier's gangrene. *Surg Clin North Am*. 1994;74:1339–1352.
23. Reboli AC, Farrar WE. *Erysipelothrix rhusiopathiae*. An occupational pathogen. *Clin Microbiol Rev*. 1989;2:354–359.
24. Venditti M, Gelfusa V, Tarasi A, Brandimarte C, Serra P. Antimicrobial susceptibilities of *Erysipelothrix rhusiopathiae*. *Antimicrob Agents Chemother*. 1990;34:2038–2040.
25. Midani S, Ayoub EM, Anderson B. Cat-scratch disease. *Adv Pediatr*. 1996;43:387–422.
26. Carithers HA. Cat scratch disease: and overview based on a study of 1200 patients. *Am J Dis Child*. 1985;139:1124–1133.
27. Maurin M, Raoult D. *Bartonella* (*Rochalimaea*) *quintana* infections. *Clin Microbiol Rev*. 1996;9:273–292.
28. Feingold DS. Gangrenous and crepitant cellulitis. *J Am Acad Dermatol*. 1982;6:289–299.
29. Lorber B. Listeriosis. *Clin Infect Dis*. 1997;24:1–9 quiz 10–11.
30. Goldschneider I, Gotschlich EC, Artenstein MS. Human immunity to the meningococcus: development of natural immunity. *J Exp Med*. 1969;129:1327–1348.
31. Oppenheim BA. Antibiotic resistance in *Neisseria meningitidis*. *Clin Infect Dis*. 1997;24(suppl 1):S98–S101.
32. Centers for Disease Control. Control and prevention of meningococcal disease. *MMWR Morb Mortal Wkly Rep*. 1997;46(RR-5):1.
33. Gilja OH, Halstensen A, Digranes A, Mylvaganam H, Aksnes A, Høiby EA. Use of single dose of ofloxacin to eradicate tonsillopharyngeal carriage of *Neisseria meningitidis*. *Antimicrob Agents Chemother*. 1993;37:2024–2026.
34. Fass RJ, Saslaw S. Chronic meningococcemia. Possible pathogenic role of IgM deficiency. *Arch Intern Med*. 1972;130:943–946.
35. Freedberg IM, Eisen AZ, Wolff K, et al, eds. *Fitzpatrick's Dermatology in General Medicine*. 5th ed. New York: McGraw-Hill; 1999: Chapter 198.
36. Agger WA, Mardan A. Pseudomonas aeruginosa infection of intact skin. *Clin Infect Dis*. 1995;20:302–308.
37. Freedberg IM, Eisen AZ, Wolff K, et al, eds. *Fitzpatrick's Dermatology in General Medicine*. 5th ed. New York: McGraw-Hill; 1999: Chapter 200.
38. Brown TMP, Nunemaker JC. Ratbite fever. A review of the American cases with reevaluation of etiology. *Bulletin of the Johns Hopkins Hospital*. 1942;70:210.
39. Freedberg IM, Eisen AZ, Wolff K, et al, eds. *Fitzpatrick's Dermatology in General Medicine*. 5th ed. New York: McGraw-Hill; 1999: Chapter 227.
40. In: Cunha BA, ed. *Antibiotic Essentials*. 6th ed. Michigan: Physician's Press; 2007.

50 Bacterial infections of the central nervous system

Jeffrey Tessier and W. Michael Scheld

Bacterial meningitis remains an important cause of mortality and morbidity despite the widespread availability of effective antimicrobials.[1] Bacterial meningitis was nearly always a fatal disease in the pre-antimicrobial era. However, following the introduction of penicillin, mortality fell to 15–30%. Today, despite the availability of potent antimicrobials, the overall mortality from bacterial meningitis in adults has not decreased, averaging 25% over the past three decades.[2] In children, major progress was achieved in the 1990s following the successful implementation of immunization against *Haemophilus influenzae* type b. However, in the neonate bacterial meningitis remains a serious disease; while the incidence has changed little in the past 30 years, the mortality rate has declined in industrialized countries from almost 50% in the 1970s to ~10% in 2001.[3] Nevertheless, neurological sequelae remain problematic in spite of improvements in treatment.

BACTERIAL MENINGITIS

Epidemiological data are largely derived from developed countries, in which the most common infecting organisms are *Streptococcus pneumoniae*, *Neisseria meningitidis*, Group B streptococci, *Escherichia coli* and *Listeria monocytogenes*. In contrast, Gram-negative bacilli such as *Klebsiella pneumoniae* and *Pseudomonas aeruginosa* are important but occasional pathogens, both in the context of nosocomial and community-acquired meningitis. In the latter, the elderly and those individuals with chronic diseases such as diabetes mellitus, cirrhosis and malignancy are at risk from Gram-negative meningitis. *Str. pneumoniae* is numerically now the most important cause of community-acquired meningitis; strains resistant to penicillin and cephalosporins are increasingly recognized worldwide and have led to significant changes in management. Despite the widespread use of the conjugated 7-valent pneumococcal vaccine among children in developed countries, the pneumococcus continues to be the most common cause of pediatric bacterial meningitis in these settings, with at least half of the cases caused by serotypes not included in the PCV7 vaccine (especially 19A).[4]

The etiology of bacterial meningitis varies by age and region of the world. One million cases of bacterial meningitis are estimated to occur worldwide; of these, ~200 000 people die annually. Case-fatality rates vary by age and the causative organism, ranging from 3% to 19% in developed countries, and rates of 37–60% have been reported from developing countries.[5] Up to 54% of survivors are left with disability due to bacterial meningitis, especially following meningitis caused by *Str. pneumoniae* or *Str. suis*. These include deafness, mental retardation and other neurological sequelae.[6,7]

The etiology of bacterial meningitis has changed substantially since the introduction of conjugate *Haemophilus influenzae* (Hib) vaccine in the early 1990s. In addition, the frequency of neonatal group B streptococcal meningitis has declined in some countries because of the implementation of screening and treatment protocols in obstetric patients.[8] *Str. pneumoniae* is a well-recognized cause of meningitis following fracture of the skull. Nosocomial cases of bacterial meningitis are commonly associated with neurosurgery and are caused by Gram-positive (coagulase-negative staphylococci, *Staphylococcus aureus*) and Gram-negative bacteria (Enterobacteriaceae, *Ps. aeruginosa*). Mixed infections, sometimes involving anaerobic organisms, are also found (Table 50.1).

Community-acquired bacterial meningitis exhibits seasonal variation. The lowest incidence is in the summer months while pneumococcal infections are most common in the winter and meningococcal infections in the spring. Epidemic meningococcal infections are uncommon in developed countries but still occur in parts of Africa, India and other emerging nations.

PRINCIPLES OF DIAGNOSIS AND TREATMENT

Early diagnosis of bacterial meningitis is essential for successful treatment. The age of the patient is of some value in indicating which of the common bacteria might be responsible. However, the only helpful physical sign is the characteristic

Table 50.1 Recommended empirical antimicrobials for patients with meningitis according to age

Empirical therapy	Frequent pathogens	Recommended antimicrobials	
Patients <3 months	Group B streptococci *Escherichia coli* *Listeria monocytogenes*	Cefotaxime 50 mg/kg every 12 h in <1 month age 50 mg/kg every 6 h in >1 month age	*plus* ampicillin 200 mg/kg per day
Patients 3 months to 50 years	*Streptococcus pneumoniae* *Neisseria meningitidis*	Ceftriaxone 100 mg/kg per day (children), 2 g every 12 h (adult) *or* cefotaxime 300 mg/kg per day (children), 2 g every 6 h (adult) *plus* vancomycin 60 mg/kg per day (children) *or* 30–45 mg/kg per day (adult)	
Adults over 50 years	*Str. pneumoniae* *L. monocytogenes* Gram-negative bacilli	Ceftriaxone 2 g every 12 h *or* cefotaxime 2 g every 6 h *plus* ampicillin 2 g every 4 h *plus* vancomycin 30–45 mg/kg total daily dose	
Immunocompromised adults	*L. monocytogenes* *Str. pneumoniae* Gram-negative bacilli (*Pseudomonas aeruginosa*)	Ceftazidime 2 g every 8 h *or* cefepime 2 g every 8 h *plus* ampicillin 2 g every 4 h *plus* vancomycin 30–45 mg/kg total daily dose	
Head trauma, postneurosurgery patient (adult dosing)	Enteric Gram-negative bacilli, Staphylococci, including *Staphylococcus aureus* and coagulase-negative staphylococci; *Pseudomonas aeruginosa*	Ceftazidime 1–2 g every 8–12 h *or* cefepime 2 g every 8 h *or* meropenem 2 g every 8 h *plus* vancomycin 30–45 mg/kg total daily dose	

rash found in some patients with severe meningococcal infection. Because of this paucity of clinical evidence, early bacteriological diagnosis is of the utmost importance, and identification of bacteria on a Gram-stained film of cerebrospinal fluid (CSF) should be regarded as a medical emergency. One of the most important factors contributing to delayed diagnosis and therapy is the decision to perform a head CT scan prior to lumbar puncture and therapy (Table 50.2). In patients with papilledema, age >60 years, an immunocompromised state, altered level of consciousness, focal neurological symptoms or a seizure, a CT scan should be obtained;[9] a lumbar puncture should not be performed immediately due to the risk of herniation. If cranial imaging is deemed necessary, patients should have blood cultures drawn and empirical antimicrobials administrated before CT evaluation. Administering 1 or 2 h of antimicrobial therapy before lumbar puncture does not decrease diagnostic sensitivity as long as CSF culture is performed in conjunction with additional CSF analysis and blood culture.[10] A prospective study of adults with pneumococcal meningitis admitted to an intensive care unit found that a delay in the administration of antimicrobials greater than 3 h from the time of presentation is a major predictor (odds ratio [OR] 14.12, CI 3.93–50.9) of mortality 3 months after diagnosis.[11] This and other data support the rapid diagnosis and administration of antimicrobial therapy when bacterial meningitis is suspected.

Other methods to supplement Gram stain and culture are now becoming more widely available. Rapid methods can be used to detect microbial antigens in CSF, blood or urine using specific sera against the common causal pathogens. These methods enable a rapid causal diagnosis to be made in some patients (especially those who have received antimicrobial treatment before lumbar puncture or when no bacteria can be seen in the Gram-stained CSF). Countercurrent immunoelectrophoresis and other methods such as enzyme-linked immunosorbent assays have been supplanted by commercially prepared latex agglutination kits which are easy to use and give results in a few minutes, although they vary in their sensitivity

Table 50.2 Guidelines for the role of CT scans and lumbar puncture in suspected intracranial infection

Urgent CT scan indicated, lumbar puncture contraindicated	Urgent CT scan indicated, followed by lumbar puncture if CT satisfactory	Lumbar puncture contraindicated, urgent CT scan may not alter management, antimicrobials should not be delayed

1. Raised intracranial pressure
  (a) focal neurological signs
  (b) definite papilledema
2. CT findings
  (c) lateral shift of midline structures
  (d) loss of suprachiasmic or context of suspected basilar cisterns
  (e) obliteration of fourth ventricle
  (f) obliteration of superior cerebellar/quadrigeminal plate cisterns with sparing of ambient cisterns
	(a) Altered level of consciousness, confusion, Glasgow Coma Scale <13
	(b) Seizures (recent or upon presentation)
	(c) When abscess suspected in view of ear/sinus or other focus of infection ± a subacute onset
	(d) Immunocompromised patient
	(e) Age >60 years
	(f) Papilledema
	(g) Focal neurological findings
		Fulminant presentation ± purpuric rash ± coagulopathy ± hypotension

Lumbar puncture must be performed without preceding CT scan in the absence of all of the above.

and specificity.[12] Obtaining a CSF sample for polymerase chain reaction (PCR) assay between 24 and 72 h after admission is now standard practice in many centers and is reported to have increased the diagnostic rate and led to improved management.[13] For patients treated with antimicrobials prior to lumbar puncture, the CSF culture may remain negative but the PCR may still reveal the causative pathogen. A recent Danish study described the development and use of a multiplex PCR to detect the eight most common pathogens causing meningitis in Denmark (*Str. pneumoniae*, *N. meningitidis*, *Esch. coli*, *L. monocytogenes*, group B streptococci, *Staph. aureus*, HSV-1/2 and VZV).[14] When compared to the 'gold standard' of Gram stain microscopy and bacterial culture for the two most common pathogens, *Str. pneumoniae* and *N. meningitidis*, the PCR assay had excellent sensitivity (95% and 100%, respectively) and specificity (99.1% and 99.7%, respectively) while providing an accurate result in less than 1 workday.

No organism can be isolated from the CSF in some cases of purulent meningitis; the proportion varies between 12% and 25% in different series. The major reason for this is the pre-admission administration of an antimicrobial, which reduces the number of positive CSF Gram-stained films and cultures. One large study of pediatric patients with bacterial meningitis found that antimicrobial therapy >12–72 h prior to lumbar puncture was associated with higher CSF glucose levels and lower CSF protein levels, but not with changes in the CSF leukocyte or absolute neutrophil count compared to those receiving no pre-treatment or treatment <12 h prior to the lumbar puncture.[15] The low CSF glucose concentration normally found in pyogenic meningitis tends to persist and in the presence of a predominantly lymphocytic reaction suggests tuberculous meningitis. A variety of studies have investigated the use of various biochemical markers as a means of differentiating between bacterial and viral meningitis; elevated CSF lysozyme, β-glucuronidase, complement C3, factor B

and serum procalcitonin levels have all been advocated as useful diagnostically, but none is used routinely for this purpose pending further data.[16–19]

PHARMACOKINETIC FACTORS

FACTORS AFFECTING ANTIMICROBIAL PENETRATION INTO CSF

The factors affecting penetration of antimicrobials into CSF include molecular size and configuration, lipophilicity, plasma protein binding, the degree of meningeal inflammation, molecular charge and active efflux from the CSF.[20]

Numerous studies have focused on the penetration of antimicrobials into CSF, brain tissues and brain abscess pus. Most measurements were performed with lumbar CSF and consist of a single determination in several individuals, either after a single dose or repeated bolus doses. The available data on CSF levels vary greatly from drug to drug (Table 50.3), but it is possible to make a clinical classification (Box 50.1) into four groups:

1. Therapeutic CSF concentrations may be reached by standard dosage and route of administration.
2. A high therapeutic ratio allows adequate CSF concentrations to be achieved by high intravenous or intramuscular doses; the CSF concentration is usually higher when the meninges are inflamed.
3. Drug toxicity precludes an increase in dose, and the CSF concentration may reach therapeutic levels only when meninges are inflamed.
4. Little or no drug is found in the CSF with or without meninges; intrathecal administration may be needed.

Table 50.3 Penetration of some agents into human CSF in relation to MIC$_{90}$ for selected meningeal pathogens

Agent	Dose (route/ frequency)	Concentration in CSF (mg/L)	CSF:serum ratio (%)	MIC$_{90}$ against common meningeal pathogen					
				NM	HI	PSSP	PRSP	EC	PA
Penicillin G	1.5 × 10^5 i.v./M	0.8	8	0.03	1–256	≤0.06	4	NA	NA
Ampicillin	15 mg/kg i.v./S	0–0.9	3.4	0.004–32	0.5–256	0.06	4	≥8	NA
Ceftriaxone	100 mg/kg i.v./M	2–42	8.6	≤0.06	≤0.125	≤0.06	16	≤0.06	≥16
Cefotaxime	40 mg/kg i.v./M	3.7–5.5	18	≤0.06	≤0.06	≤0.05	0.5	0.125	≥32
Ceftazidime	2.0 g i.v./M	2–56	23.5	≤0.125	0.125–0.5	≤0.125	4	0.25–4	≥8
Meropenem	40 mg/kg i.v./S	0.3–6.5	21	≤0.06	0.015–0.25	≤0.06	16	0.015–4	0.015–16
Gentamicin	1.5 mg/kg i.m./S	0–0.10	2.5	NA	1–4	32	32	≥0.5	≥4
Ciprofloxacin	500 mg oral/S	0.3–0.5	25	≤0.06	≤0.06	1–2	12	0.03–0.125	0.5–4
Chloramphenicol	100 mg/kg i.v./M	2.0–15.6	38	0.06–8	0.5–8	1	16	4	NA

M, multiple; S, single; I, inflamed; U, non-inflamed; NA, not available; NM, *Neisseria meningitidis*; HI, *Haemophilus influenzae*; PSSP, Penicillin-sensitive *Streptococcus pneumoniae*; PRSP, penicillin-resistant *Streptococcus pneumoniae*; EC, *Escherichia coli*; PA, *Pseudomonas aeruginosa*.

Box 50.1 Penetration of antimicrobial agents into CSF

---

1. Therapeutic CSF concentrations achieved by standard doses and routes of administration

Chloramphenicol
Sulfonamides
Trimethoprim
Fluoroquinolones
Metronidazole
Doxycycline
Isoniazid
Rifampicin
Pyrazinamide
Ethionamide

2. Therapeutic CSF concentrations achieved by high intravenous or intramuscular doses, especially in meningitis

Penicillins
Cephalosporins

3. Therapeutic CSF concentrations may be achieved by standard doses and routes in meningitis

Clindamycin
Vancomycin
Tetracycline
Erythromycin
Ethambutol

4. Therapeutic CSF concentrations cannot be reliably achieved except where intrathecal route is possible

Aminoglycosides
Polymyxin
Fusidic acid

Logical decisions regarding antimicrobial dosing depend not only on knowledge of drug penetration but also on knowledge of the pharmacokinetic and pharmacodynamic properties of the antimicrobial.

Because of the general limitation in antimicrobial penetration into the CSF, the use of oral antimicrobials is discouraged since the dose and tissue levels tend to be considerably lower than with parenteral agents. An exception can be made for rifampicin (rifampin), given either as a synergistic drug or for eradication of mucosal carriage of *H. influenzae* or *N. meningitidis*.

Because of erratic distribution within the CSF, and failure of antimicrobials injected into lumbar theca to become distributed throughout the ventricular system, intrathecal therapy is discouraged by many physicians as risks outweigh the doubtful therapeutic advantage. There are, nevertheless, some situations in which intrathecal treatment is indicated, when the ventricular route must be used. Doses and preparations for intrathecal injection should be determined carefully.

CONTRIBUTION OF EXPERIMENTAL STUDIES

Although much information has been gathered about antimicrobial concentrations in serum and CSF in humans with meningitis, ethical and practical limitations make it difficult to achieve a full picture of the conditions necessary for successful treatment. Many factors contribute to the poor results of treatment in neonatal meningitis and in Gramnegative bacillary meningitis in older age groups, but recent studies indicate that failure to achieve the appropriate concentration of the correct antimicrobial at relevant sites correlates with poor results. As elsewhere in the body, local foci of infection remain important and, in neonatal meningitis especially, persistent ventriculitis results in treatment failure. General principles apply here: the antimicrobial regimen used must be active and, in this situation, bactericidal against the causal organism at concentrations regularly achieved in CSF. Additional factors related to success or failure have been clarified in experimental animals, especially in a rabbit model of experimental meningitis, in which repeated estimations of bacterial counts and of antimicrobial concentrations can be made. McCracken has shown that, for some agents, the pharmacokinetic factors can be quite similar in the rabbit and the human infant.[21] McCracken concludes that measurement of the ratio of CSF area under curve to serum area under curve (CSF AUC:serum AUC × 100) after single doses and the mean relative concentrations after 9 h infusions are good predictors for CSF penetration in infants and children. Both in rabbits and in children, best results are achieved if the bactericidal titer of the CSF for the relevant organism is at least 1:8, but the rate of decline in the CSF bacterial population is no greater even if this titer is much exceeded. Measurements of this type, both in experimental animals and in humans, are helpful in the initial evaluation of new putative agents for treating meningitis, but are impractical clinically once pharmacokinetic features of the drug have been well established.

SPECIFIC FEATURES OF ANTIMICROBIALS COMMONLY USED IN THE TREATMENT OF MENINGITIS

BENZYLPENICILLIN AND AMPICILLIN

As a general rule, most β-lactams, including penicillins, ampicillin and amoxicillin, penetrate into the CSF poorly. Their low toxicity, however, enables this disadvantage to be overcome by high systemic dosages which normally require intravenous therapy. Where conditions make this impracticable or hazardous, intramuscular injections can be used but the large injection volumes are painful. CSF concentrations appropriate for the treatment of penicillin-susceptible meningococcal or pneumococcal meningitis can be achieved with a dosage of 150 mg/kg (250 000 units/kg) daily divided into 4-hourly intravenous doses.[22] The same general points apply to ampicillin and its congeners. The range of doses in controlled trials has varied from 150 to 400 mg/kg per day. The highest doses are unnecessary, and a standard dose of 200 mg/kg per day is recommended. Notably, none of the oral forms of penicillin or ampicillin is suitable for treating meningitis. CSF penetration diminishes even further as meningeal inflammation begins to resolve. The short half-lives of these compounds make it unwise to prolong the dose interval beyond 4–6 h.

Neurological toxicity from penicillin presents a danger only when excessively high blood or CSF concentrations are reached. This sometimes occurs when very large doses are given intravenously in the presence of renal failure, but was especially associated with incorrectly high intrathecal dosage at a time when this form of administration was commonly used.

CEPHALOSPORINS

The extended-spectrum cephalosporins (cefotaxime, ceftriaxone and cefepime) are characterized by excellent antibacterial activity against common meningitis-causing bacteria, and are currently the drugs of choice for the empirical therapy of bacterial meningitis. Cephalosporins, like other antimicrobials, are not known to be metabolized in the CSF; thus, their concentrations in CSF depend on the balance between penetration and elimination. In most clinical trials, the penetration of cephalosporins through the blood–brain barrier is expressed as the ratio of CSF to blood concentration at a particular time-point (Table 50.3, p. 635). Because of the slow entry of cephalosporins secondary to low lipophilicity, their concentration–time curves in CSF lag behind those in blood.[23] Furthermore, the most important determinant predicting efficacy in meningitis is the relationship between the antimicrobial concentration in CSF and the minimum bactericidal concentration (MBC) of the common organisms causing meningitis. The wide variability and occasional low CSF concentrations are worth noting because higher dosages are well tolerated and therapeutic concentrations in the CSF can still be achieved. Goldwater measured the concentration of ceftriaxone or cefotaxime in the CSF of children with bacterial meningitis caused by *Str. pneumoniae*, *H. influenzae* or *N. meningitidis*.[24] Though there was significant variability in the CSF concentrations of these antimicrobials, the concentrations exceeded the minimum inhibitory concentrations (MICs) for these organisms by 45- to 8750-fold. During the 1980s many controlled trials evaluated different cephalosporins in treating meningitis. The largest groups studied were children with *H. influenzae* meningitis. In most trials the compound under investigation was compared with ampicillin and chloramphenicol in combination, the prevailing standard of treatment for community-acquired childhood meningitis at the time. These trials gave results generally similar to, but not better than, the standard regimen. Of the many compounds available, cefotaxime and ceftriaxone have been especially well studied.

In addition to clinical comparisons with the standard regimens, many trials included measurements of the rate of decline of bacterial counts in the CSF, and time to negative CSF cultures, which were again generally comparable in the two groups. In one trial comparing twice-daily ceftriaxone with chloramphenicol and ampicillin, repeat lumbar puncture 10–18 h after the start of treatment showed similar reductions of bacterial counts, but the median bactericidal titer in the CSF was 1:1024 in the ceftriaxone group, compared with 1:4 in the conventional therapy group.[25] Ceftriaxone concentrations in the CSF were 3–24% (mean 11.8%) of the serum concentration. These generally good results emboldened investigators to study once-daily ceftriaxone dosing, allowing the possibility of outpatient treatment in patients who were well enough after the initial diagnostic assessment and initiation of treatment. Again, results were satisfactory;[26] diarrhea, the main adverse effect, was not severe enough to necessitate a change of treatment. Duration of treatment has also been studied, with Lin et al[27] showing that the results with 7 days of ceftriaxone were as good as those after 10 days. Roine et al[28] found that 4 days of ceftriaxone therapy proved to be almost as safe as a 7-day course, especially in patients with rapid initial recovery from bacterial meningitis.

Cefotaxime has also been studied extensively and shown to be effective in the common forms of bacterial meningitis, usually at a dose of 50 mg/kg every 6 h. Cefotaxime may be administered at a dose of 300 mg/kg per day (maximum dose, 24 g per day) in treating resistant pneumococci.[29] A large study of 285 children prospectively randomized to receive cefotaxime or meropenem showed similar progress in the two groups.[30]

The increasing importance of drug resistance in *H. influenzae* infection, and the possible antagonism between ampicillin and chloramphenicol, led Finnish investigators to conduct an important multicenter comparison in 220 children with meningitis (146 with *H. influenzae*) of chloramphenicol, ampicillin (initially with chloramphenicol), cefotaxime or ceftriaxone.[31] Results were similar in the four treatment groups, but all four bacteriological failures were with chloramphenicol and treatment had to be changed more frequently in this group. Use of ampicillin was limited by the problem of resistance. Results were equivalent between groups receiving either cephalosporin. Cefotaxime has fewer adverse effects, but the cost of both drugs limits their potential in developing countries.

Although cefotaxime and ceftriaxone are the most widely used cephalosporins for meningitis, other β-lactam compounds have also been studied in *Haemophilus* meningitis, including ceftazidime, ceftizoxime and aztreonam – again, usually in comparison with ampicillin and chloramphenicol. Other cephalosporins currently available or under development for clinical use are ceftobiprole, cefpirome, cefepime, cefoselis, cefclidin, cefozopran and cefluprenam. Cefepime is active against a broader spectrum of bacteria than earlier cephalosporins. This cephalosporin penetrates inflamed meninges to produce CSF concentrations ±20% of the serum concentrations.[32] This concentration is two- to four-fold greater than that achieved by ceftriaxone or cefotaxime. In 1995, Saez-Llorens et al compared the use of cefepime and cefotaxime in 90 children with bacterial meningitis aged between 2 months and 15 years, randomized to receive cefepime 50 mg/kg every

8 h or cefotaxime 50 mg/kg every 6 h.[33] CSF concentrations of cefepime varied from 55 to 95 times greater than the MIC of the causative pathogens. Clinical response, CSF sterilization, complications and hospital stay were similar for the two treatment regimens, leading to the conclusion that cefepime is safe and therapeutically equivalent.[33] This study has been confirmed by the same group in 345 pediatric patients in two randomized trials that compared cefepime with either ceftriaxone or cefotaxime.[34] However, non-convulsive status epilepticus and reversible severe encephalopathy have been observed as unwanted side effects, especially if given in high doses or in patients with renal failure.[35]

CARBAPENEMS

Carbapenems (meropenem, imipenem–cilastatin, ertapenem and doripenem) have a spectrum of antimicrobial activity that exceeds most other antimicrobial classes, which includes organisms resistant to many other antimicrobials, including other β-lactam agents. The mean CSF concentration of meropenem following a single dose of 40 mg/kg in patients with inflamed meninges who had received dexamethasone (which markedly reduces the CSF concentrations of β-lactam antimicrobials) has been reported to be 3.28 mg/L at 2.5–3.5 h after administration.[36]

Meropenem has been extensively evaluated in treating bacterial meningitis in children but few studies have been comparative. Schmutzhard et al randomized 56 adults with bacterial meningitis to meropenem ($n = 28$), cefotaxime ($n = 17$) or ceftriaxone ($n = 11$).[37] The dose of meropenem was 40 mg/kg, up to a maximum of 2 g, every 8 h. The causative pathogens included meningococci, pneumococci, *Ps. aeruginosa* and *H. influenzae*. All bacterial isolates were eliminated, regardless of the drug used. Among evaluable patients at the end of treatment, all patients on meropenem, 9 of 12 on cefotaxime, and 8 of 10 on ceftriaxone were classified as cured.[37] Klugman and Dagan randomized 98 children with bacterial meningitis to meropenem 40 mg/kg every 8 h and 98 children to cefotaxime 75–100 mg/kg every 8 h.[38] Two cefotaxime-treated patients died while receiving therapy and one meropenem-treated patient died of trauma 26 days after therapy. None of the deaths was judged to be related to the study drug. In evaluable patients, cure without sequelae was reported in 54 of 75 (72%) patients on meropenem and 52 of 64 (81%) randomized to cefotaxime; 21 patients (28%) on meropenem and 10 on cefotaxime (16%) had neurological and/or audiological sequelae. Seizures after the start of therapy were seen in five patients randomized to meropenem and three given cefotaxime.[38] Meropenem would appear to be as effective as cefotaxime for this indication.

Imipenem–cilastatin has been evaluated for the treatment of bacterial meningitis in children.[39] Although highly effective at eradicating bacteria from the CSF, 33% of the children developed seizures after administration of this drug. As a consequence, the clinical trial was terminated; neurological

toxicity limits enthusiasm for the use of imipenem–cilastatin in the treatment of bacterial meningitis.

The latest carbapenems, ertapenem and doripenem, have not been evaluated for the treatment of bacterial meningitis. Ertapenem has a significantly longer half-life than the other carbapenems but lacks activity against *Ps. aeruginosa*, while doripenem has an antimicrobial spectrum similar to meropenem.

GLYCOPEPTIDES

Vancomycin is approximately 55% bound to serum proteins. It does not diffuse well into CSF, especially in the absence of inflamed meninges. Therapeutic concentrations can be achieved when higher dosages (15 mg/kg) are administered every 6 h or by continuous infusion.[40] Animal studies reveal that maximal bacterial killing rate is achieved with C_{max}:MBC ratios of 5:1 to 10:1; any further increases in vancomycin CSF concentration does not increase bacterial killing.[41] Vancomycin in combination with a cephalosporin is recommended to treat pneumococcal meningitis caused by strains with diminished susceptibility to the cephalosporin, especially in children older than 1 month.[42,43]

Although vancomycin (and teicoplanin) has not been systematically evaluated for the treatment of meningitis caused by methicillin-resistant *Staph. aureus* (MRSA), multiple case reports and series describe its successful use for this disease.[44,45] While *Staph. aureus* is not a common cause of community-acquired bacterial meningitis, this pathogen must be considered in specific scenarios, such as intravenous drug use, post-neurosurgical patients, and patients at risk for *Staph. aureus* bacteremia (e.g. hemodialysis, long-term intravenous catheters). In these settings, empirical use of vancomycin pending antimicrobial susceptibility testing is warranted.

CHOICES OF EMPIRICAL ANTIMICROBIALS

All adults in whom a diagnosis of bacterial meningitis is suspected should receive antimicrobials as rapidly as possible, even if in the community while awaiting transport to the hospital. There is little published evidence to indicate that the diagnosis is obscured by preadmission antimicrobials. In view of the serious nature of this disease, it is strongly recommended that primary care physicians should give 2 g of ceftriaxone or cefotaxime intravenously without delay upon suspicion of possible bacterial meningitis.

For patients admitted to hospital with suspected bacterial meningitis, empirical antimicrobial therapy is indicated if the lumbar puncture is to be delayed or if the CSF findings are compatible with bacterial meningitis with or without a diagnostic Gram stain. Antimicrobial therapy should be started as soon as possible. Early antimicrobial administration does not hinder microbiological diagnosis when PCR testing is used. The concern that early antimicrobial administration may aggravate the clinical condition by causing antimicrobial-induced endotoxin release[46,47] has not been confirmed clinically.[48] In contrast, delayed antimicrobial therapy will simply result in an increase in bacterial biomass and the damaging effects of a more severe inflammatory response.

Because the CNS is an immunologically defective site, optimal therapy for bacterial meningitis depends on using antimicrobials with bactericidal activity in vivo. Empirical treatment must cover the full spectrum of possible causative pathogens, based on the patient's age, co-morbidities, and whether infection is community or hospital acquired (Table 50.1, p. 634). It is also important to note any history of drug allergy, recent travel, exposure to someone with meningitis, recent infections (especially respiratory and otic), use of antimicrobials, injection drug use, and the presence of a petechial or ecchymotic rash.

Currently a cephalosporin (usually cefotaxime or ceftriaxone) is recommended for the empirical treatment of community-acquired meningitis in adults and children older than 3 months. Empirical therapy for children younger than 3 months of age consists of ampicillin and cefotaxime (in preference to ceftriaxone, which can bind albumin and alter bilirubin metabolism), though often ampicillin plus gentamicin is used in resource-limited settings. Cefotaxime and ceftriaxone have emerged as the β-lactams of choice in the empirical treatment of meningitis in all other age groups. These drugs have potent activity against the major pathogens, with the notable exception of *Listeria*. They are clinically equivalent to, or better than, penicillin and ampicillin owing to their consistent CSF penetration. Their activity also includes most strains of penicillin-resistant *Str. pneumoniae*. Furthermore, synergistic activity has been reported between ceftriaxone and vancomycin in vitro and in experimental meningitis with strains for which the MIC of ceftriaxone was >4 mg/L.[49-51] These findings have led most authorities to recommend vancomycin and ceftriaxone as empirical therapy for patients with meningitis in areas with a high incidence of cephalosporin-resistant pneumococci.

ROLE OF CORTICOSTEROIDS IN MANAGING (NON-TUBERCULOUS) BACTERIAL MENINGITIS

A variety of host inflammatory factors involved in the complex pathophysiology of bacterial meningitis have been identified that may serve as targets for adjunctive therapy. Dexamethasone has been the most widely evaluated since benefit was observed in experimental bacterial meningitis. Early administration of corticosteroids such as dexamethasone in childhood meningitis, although showing no survival advantage, reduced the incidence of severe neurological complications and deafness in *H. influenzae* infection.[52] A meta-analysis of five studies in children showed a relative risk of bilateral deafness of 4.1 and of late neurological sequelae of 3.9 in controls compared with children treated with steroids.[53] Concerns over the adjunctive use of steroids include gastrointestinal bleeding, secondary fever, difficulties in the clinical assessment of bacteriological cure due to quicker defervescence, and reduced penetration

of antimicrobials through the blood–brain barrier, particularly in penicillin-resistant pneumococcal meningitis.[54] Children with bacterial meningitis may be in septic shock and the role of steroids in septic shock and viral infections is unclear.[55] Sterilization of CSF by ampicillin and gentamicin in the presence of steroids also needs clarification. Not much is known about the use of dexamethasone in malnourished patients or those with HIV infection or other serious illness.

In 2002 a prospective, randomized clinical trial of dexamethasone therapy in adults with bacterial meningitis was published.[56] This trial randomized 301 adults to receive either placebo ($n = 144$) or 10 mg of dexamethasone every 6 h for 4 days ($n = 157$), with the dexamethasone administered before or with the first antimicrobial dose. Approximately one-third of the patients were infected with *Str. pneumoniae*, one-third with *N. meningitidis*, and the remainder with other bacteria or negative CSF cultures. The group receiving dexamethasone had a lower risk of an unfavorable clinical outcome (relative risk [RR] 0.59, CI 0.37–0.94, $p = 0.03$), based on the Glasgow Outcome Scale at 8 weeks, and a reduction in mortality (RR 0.48, CI 0.24–0.96, $p = 0.04$) compared to the placebo group. Subgroup analysis based on causative organism demonstrated particular benefit for those infected with *Str. pneumoniae*.

For pediatric meningitis, the evidence from recent meta-analyses confirms benefit from dexamethasone in *H. influenzae* type b meningitis and efficacy in pneumococcal meningitis only if given early (before or during initial parenteral antimicrobials). The American Academy of Pediatrics recommends that adjunctive therapy with dexamethasone should be considered for infants and children 6 weeks of age and older; the potential benefits and risks must be carefully weighed. An important concern is that the administration of steroids in combination with vancomycin may be disadvantageous. Vancomycin does not penetrate well into non-inflamed CSF and the addition of steroids has been shown to decrease CSF vancomycin concentrations in adults, but this concern may be moot as vancomycin should not be used alone to treat pneumococcal meningitis.[57] This effect has not been observed in children. Ricard et al measured vancomycin concentrations in the CSF of 14 adult patients with bacterial meningitis (13 with *Str. pneumoniae*, 1 with *N. meningitidis*) who were being treated with dexamethasone 10 mg every 6 h.[58] The vancomycin was dosed as a continuous infusion of 60 mg/kg per day after a loading dose of 15 mg/kg. The mean serum concentration was 25.2 mg/L with a mean CSF concentration of 7.2 mg/L (~29% of mean serum levels). This mean CSF concentration is above the MBCs for the vast majority of pneumococci, so it appears safe to use steroids during concomitant vancomycin administration with an extended-spectrum cephalosporin.

Two prospective, randomized, double-blind trials examining the use of adjunctive dexamethasone in the treatment of bacterial meningitis were published in 2007, one conducted among 465 adults in sub-Saharan Africa and one among 435 adolescents and adults in Vietnam. In the African study, the majority (90%) of patients were HIV infected. When compared to placebo, dexamethasone had no effect on 40-day mortality, the main outcome measure of this trial.[59] Additionally, no difference was observed between dexamethasone- and placebo-treated patients in the secondary outcomes of disability or death, hearing impairment and adverse events. In the Vietnamese study, patients >14 years old with suspected bacterial meningitis were randomized to receive adjunctive dexamethasone or placebo, with the main outcome measures being death at 1 month and the risk of death or disability at 6 months.[60] Intention-to-treat analysis of all suspected bacterial meningitis cases indicated no difference between the dexamethasone- and placebo-treated groups with respect to death at 1 month or death/disability at 6 months. However, among the randomized patients with confirmed (by CSF culture) bacterial meningitis, dexamethasone significantly reduced the risk of death at 1 month (OR 0.43, 95% CI 0.20–0.94) and death/disability at 6 months (OR 0.56, 95% CI 0.32–0.98) compared to placebo.

A prospective, randomized, double-blind study comparing adjuvant dexamethasone or glycerol with placebo was performed among children (2 months to 16 years) with bacterial meningitis in Latin America.[61] The study included 654 patients infected mainly with *H. influenzae* type b, *Str. pneumoniae* and *N. meningitidis*, and the primary endpoints were death or severe neurological sequelae (as a composite) or deafness. Dexamethasone (0.15 mg/kg every 6 h for 48 h, first dose 15 min prior to ceftriaxone) was given to 166, glycerol (1.5 g/kg orally every 6 h, first dose 15 min prior to ceftriaxone) to 166, both dexamethasone and glycerol to 159, and placebo to 163. None of the adjuvant therapies affected death or deafness as individual outcomes, but the groups receiving either glycerol (OR 0.31, CI 0.13–0.76, $p = 0.01$) or dexamethasone plus glycerol (OR 0.39, CI 0.17–0.93, $p = 0.033$) had a reduced risk of severe neurological sequelae. Based on this trial, glycerol appears to be a safe adjunct to ceftriaxone therapy in pediatric bacterial meningitis and has the advantage of oral administration in many patients.

Agents other than dexamethasone that are capable of intervening with inflammatory mediators such as nitric oxide synthase inhibitors, peroxynitrite scavengers, endothelin antagonists and matrix metalloproteinase inhibitors are beneficial in experimental bacterial meningitis and await clinical trials in humans.

DURATION OF THERAPY

The duration of antimicrobial therapy in patients with bacterial meningitis has traditionally been 10–14 days for non-meningococcal isolates (Table 50.4). Further information is presented later when each pathogen is discussed.

Table 50.4 Recommended antimicrobial regimens for patients with culture proven meningitis

Organism	Antimicrobial therapy	Dosage in children>1 month age (mg/kg/day), dose interval	Dosage in adults	Duration of treatment (days)
Streptococcus pneumoniae				
Penicillin MIC <0.1 mg/L	Penicillin G	300 000–400 000 U[a] every 4–6 h	2.4 g every 4 h	10–14
Penicillin MIC 0.1–1.0 mg/L	Cefotaxime or	225–300 mg every 6–8 h	2 g every 6 h	
	ceftriaxone ±	100 mg every 12–24 h	2 g every 12 h	
	vancomycin	60 mg every 6 h	30–45 mg/kg per day in 2–3 divided doses or by continuous infusion	
Penicillin MIC >1.0 mg/L	Cefotaxime or	300 mg every 6–8 h	2 g every 6 h (up to 24 g)	
	ceftriaxone ±	100 mg every 12–24 h	2 g every 12 h	
	vancomycin	60 mg every 6 h	30–45 mg/kg per day in 2–3 divided doses or by continuous infusion	
Ceftriaxone or cefotaxime MIC ≥1.0 mg/L	Cefotaxime or	300 mg every 6–8 h	2 g every 6 h (up to 24 g)	
	ceftriaxone plus	100 mg every 12–24 h	2 g every 12 h	
	vancomycin ±	60 mg every 6 h	30–45 mg/kg per day in 2–3 divided doses or by continuous infusion	
	rifampicin	20 mg every 12 h	300–600 mg every 12 h	
Haemophilus influenzae				7
β-lactamase negative	Ampicillin	300 mg every 6 h	2 g every 4 h	
β-lactamase positive	Cefotaxime or	225–300 mg every 6–8 h	2 g every 6 h	
	ceftriaxone	100 mg every 12–24 h	2 g every 12 h	
Neisseria meningitidis	Penicillin G	300 000–400 000 U[a] every 4–6 h (maximum dose, 12 MU per day)	2.4 g every 4 h	5–7
Listeria monocytogenes	Ampicillin plus aminoglycoside	300 mg every 6 h / Depends on aminoglycoside	2 g every 4 h / Depends on aminoglycoside	14–21
Str. agalactiae	Ampicillin ± aminoglycoside	300 mg every 6 h / Depends on aminoglycoside	2 g every 4 h / Depends on aminoglycoside	14–21
Enterobacteriaceae	Ceftriaxone or cefotaxime ± aminoglycoside	100 mg every 2–24 h / 300 mg every 6–8 h / Depends on aminoglycoside	2 g every 12 h / 2 g every 4 h / Depends on aminoglycoside	21
Pseudomonas aeruginosa	Ceftazidime (or cefepime) + aminoglycoside	150 mg every 8 h / Depends on aminoglycoside	2 g every 8 h / Depends on aminoglycoside	21

[a]300 000–400 000 U penicillin G = 180–240 mg. MU, million units.

PATHOGEN-DIRECTED THERAPY

MENINGOCOCCAL MENINGITIS

Although meningococcal meningitis is a serious illness and meningococcal shock syndrome one of the most rapidly fatal of all infections, the organism itself is easily eliminated by appropriate chemotherapy. The mainstay of treatment is benzylpenicillin, administered as described earlier, though the Infectious Diseases Society of America recommends a third-generation cephalosporin with penicillin as an alternative.[62] Susceptibility testing is necessary because of the appearance of strains with reduced susceptibility to penicillin. In-vitro testing of 431 isolates of *N. meningitidis* (373 from the USA, 58 non-USA) demonstrated an elevated penicillin MIC (≥ 0.12 µg/mL) in 14.3%, though the MIC range for these organisms was ≤ 0.007 to 1 µg/mL.[63] These levels of reduced susceptibility are not clinically important if the correct dosage is used.

Ampicillin is also suitable for meningococcal disease. When the microbial diagnosis of pyogenic meningitis is uncertain, the cephalosporins (discussed above) are fully active against meningococci. Ceftriaxone has the added advantage of eradicating nasopharyngeal carriage (*see below*) in the index case, which is not true of benzylpenicillin.

In sharp contrast to the situation with many other forms of meningitis, eradication of the organism can be achieved rapidly and prolonged treatment is unnecessary. Treatment is often continued for 7 days, but 5 days suffices to eradicate infection and even shorter treatments have been effective. Viladrich et al[64] treated 50 patients with meningococcal meningitis with intravenous penicillin for 4 days. Even shorter regimens, such as 2 days of ceftriaxone[65] or single-dose therapy with a parenteral preparation of long-acting chloramphenicol, have been successful.[66] A randomized, open-label trial compared a single dose of long-acting oily chloramphenicol (100 mg/kg intramuscularly, up to 3 g) with a single dose of ceftriaxone (100 mg/kg intramuscularly, up to 4 g) in African patients with epidemic meningococcal meningitis.[67] This trial demonstrated clinical equivalence between these regimens, supporting a role for single-dose ceftriaxone in this resource-limited setting.

If meningococcal disease is suspected, the patient should be given parenteral penicillin or a third-generation cephalosporin and admitted to hospital immediately. All suspected cases should be reported to the relevant public health authority. Although formerly widely used, nasal or throat swabs are no longer routine practice. Chemoprophylaxis should be offered promptly to all household and mouth-kissing contacts, to patients before discharge, and anyone who has had contact with a patient's nasopharyngeal secretions (healthcare workers whose mouth or nose has been directly and heavily exposed to respiratory droplets/secretions from a case of meningococcal disease around the time of hospital admission).[68] Contacts should be advised about possible early symptoms and of the persisting risk, even if they have received prophylaxis. In epidemic situations the use of vaccine should be considered, although prevention of epidemics of meningococcal disease in developing countries will be difficult until long-lasting conjugate vaccines capable of interrupting transmission of *N. meningitidis* can be incorporated into routine infant immunization schedules.

Prophylaxis of meningococcal meningitis

Outbreaks of meningococcal meningitis in closed communities, especially military recruits, are well recognized, but spread within family groups may also occur, especially in conditions of overcrowding. Sulfadiazine has been very effective for chemoprophylaxis, but the emergence of sulfonamide-resistant strains has posed a problem and this agent is no longer used for this purpose. Rifampicin is much more effective than penicillin, ampicillin, tetracycline or erythromycin in controlling the carriage of sulfonamide-resistant strains. A number of trials in the early 1970s established the degree of efficacy of rifampicin (85–90%) in immediate reduction of the meningococcal carrier rate, but a substantial proportion of the residual strains isolated in the post-treatment period were rifampicin resistant; it is therefore possible that widespread use of rifampicin will be accompanied by an increase in strains resistant to this drug. The dosage of rifampicin is 600 mg every 12 h for four doses (10 mg/kg every 12 h for four doses for children). Moderate success in controlling meningococcal carriage has also been achieved with minocycline 200 mg followed by 100 mg every 12 h for 5 days. Total clearance of carriers was achieved using a combination of rifampicin and minocycline, but one-third of the patients given both drugs experienced unpleasant side effects. Sequential use of minocycline followed by rifampicin has also been employed. Single-dose oral ciprofloxacin, in a dose of either 500 or 750 mg, has proved notably effective, and is now the preferred agent for adult contacts. Cuevas et al conducted a randomized comparative study of rifampicin and ciprofloxacin for eradicating nasopharyngeal carriage of meningococci.[69] Ciprofloxacin proved a safe and effective alternative to rifampicin for eradication of meningococcal carriage in adults but remains contraindicated in children. Similarly, 46 persistent carriers were treated with 750 mg in a single oral dose in a placebo-controlled double-blind trial:[70] 20 of the 22 placebo recipients remained positive, whereas 20 of 23 recipients of active drug showed negative results on swabbing 7 and 21 days later. Adverse drug reactions occur rarely following a single dose of ciprofloxacin but have included hypersensitivity reactions. Single-dose injection treatment with ceftriaxone has also been successful in clearing nasopharyngeal carriage[71] and this is the agent of choice in pregnant contacts. The adult dose is 250 mg as a single intramuscular injection; children under 12 years should receive half this dose. Furthermore, single doses of ofloxacin or azithromycin were found to be 97.2%[72] and 95%[73] effective, respectively, in eradicating carriage of *N. meningitidis*.

Chemoprophylaxis may fail if given too late or given to the wrong person, or because of non-compliance. Rifampicin resistance, although rare, is another cause of failure.[74] The effect of chemoprophylaxis is further limited because it does not prevent reintroduction of the pathogenic strain from a carrier outside the group, and therefore late secondary cases may occur.

Based on the observation that approximately half of the secondary cases in families develop within 24 h in children under 15 years, the Norwegian health authorities have advised treating these possible co-primary cases with phenoxymethylpenicillin for 1 week. Although this strategy has substantially reduced the number of co-primary fatalities in families, no controlled studies are available and this strategy has not been widely adopted elsewhere.

 # PNEUMOCOCCAL MENINGITIS

Initially, all *Str. pneumoniae* isolates were exquisitely susceptible to penicillin (MIC ≤0.06 mg/L), and this antimicrobial served as the drug of choice. Today, drug-resistant *Str. pneumoniae* is recognized worldwide. Several reports of treatment failures related to pneumococcal isolates with decreased susceptibility to penicillin were published in the 1970s. In these cases, pneumococci with penicillin MICs between 0.1 and 1.0 mg/L were associated with microbiological and/or clinical treatment failures in patients given penicillin. These cases led to the conclusion that penicillin at routine doses did not result in high enough levels in the CSF (peak ~1.0 mg/L) to reliably treat meningitis caused by intermediately susceptible pneumococcal strains (penicillin MIC 0.1–1.0 mg/L). At that time, ampicillin and chloramphenicol were the standard empirical agents for suspected bacterial meningitis in children. Chloramphenicol was considered an acceptable alternative to complete therapy if a penicillin-resistant *Str. pneumoniae* isolate was recovered, which at that time was still an infrequent occurrence. However, by the early 1990s, as penicillin-resistant pneumococcal isolates became more common throughout the world, treatment failures associated with cefotaxime or ceftriaxone administration for pneumococcal meningitis were reported. Vancomycin has also been used, but the correct drug concentration is difficult to achieve and a number of failures have been recorded. It is suggested that vancomycin be used (in penicillin- and chloramphenicol-resistant pneumococcal meningitis) only when high-dose cephalosporins have failed.[75] Vancomycin may also have a place in combination with cephalosporins when diminished susceptibility to the cephalosporin has been demonstrated.[76] Although optimal therapy for infections caused by drug-resistant pneumococci is not known at present, several options are available. Where the majority of isolates remain sensitive to penicillin, this drug can continue to be used, although for empirical therapy ceftriaxone would be a more reliable choice. Where resistance rates are high, it seems prudent to treat all patients with purulent meningitis empirically with vancomycin combined with either cefotaxime or ceftriaxone while awaiting CSF culture and antimicrobial susceptibility test results. The recommended dose of vancomycin in cases resistant to other drugs is 60 mg/kg per day. Alternative combination regimens for penicillin- and cephalosporin-resistant pneumococcal meningitis include rifampicin with either ceftriaxone or cefotaxime, rifampicin and vancomycin, and vancomycin and chloramphenicol. Both cefepime and meropenem have been evaluated in clinical trials for the treatment of bacterial meningitis. Randomized comparative studies assessed the efficacy of cefepime as empirical monotherapy in the treatment of bacterial meningitis. This drug represents an important therapeutic option for the empirical treatment of bacterial meningitis in children based on the good clinical response and bacteriological eradication rates observed in this study.[34] However, no penicillin-resistant pneumococci were identified in the study; the effectiveness of cefepime for treating pneumococcal meningitis due to resistant strains could not be assessed and thus remains unknown.

Although meropenem is an alternative to extended-spectrum cephalosporins, much more experience with the drug is required before it can be reliably recommended as an effective antimicrobial for the treatment of antimicrobial-resistant pneumococcal meningitis.

Daptomycin, a lipopeptide antimicrobial with excellent in-vitro activity against *Str. pneumoniae* (MIC_{90} range <0.125–0.5 mg/L), may become a useful agent for the treatment of pneumococcal meningitis.[77,78] Unlike β-lactams, daptomycin does not lyse pneumococci in experimental animal models of pneumococcal meningitis, despite having bactericidal activity in the CSF.[79,80] Importantly, daptomycin does not cause release of pneumolysin from dead or dying pneumococci; pneumolysin is a critical virulence factor for pneumococci and has been shown to induce apoptosis in neurons.[81,82] Daptomycin is more rapidly bactericidal than ceftriaxone in experimental pneumococcal meningitis and retains antimicrobial activity against penicillin- and quinolone-resistant pneumococci.[83] A rabbit model of experimental pneumococcal meningitis also demonstrated that a combination of daptomycin and ceftriaxone was more effective than vancomycin plus ceftriaxone after the addition of dexamethasone.[84] Clinical trials are needed to confirm the efficacy, safety and appropriate dosing of daptomycin in patients with pneumococcal meningitis.

In summary, the initial treatment of suspected pneumococcal meningitis should be altered especially in areas where resistant pneumococci have been encountered. Initial therapy with cefotaxime or ceftriaxone combined with vancomycin is recommended (Table 50.4), with administration of dexamethasone (10 mg every 6 h) before or with the initial antimicrobial agent. Once the results of susceptibility testing are available, modifications of therapy should be made. If the strain is susceptible to penicillin, vancomycin should be discontinued. Vancomycin plus cefotaxime or ceftriaxone should be used only if the organism is either intermediately or highly resistant to both penicillin and the cephalosporins. The addition of rifampicin or substitution of rifampicin for vancomycin after 24–48 h could be considered if the organism is susceptible to rifampicin or if there is evidence to suggest an inadequate clinical or microbiological response. It is prudent to perform a repeat CSF examination and culture at 24–48 h, until more experience is gained in treating meningitis caused by penicillin-resistant pneumococci.

HAEMOPHILUS MENINGITIS

With the widespread addition of conjugate *H. influenzae* type b vaccine in developed countries, very few cases of meningitis from this organism now occur in childhood. *H. influenzae* meningitis, although very much less common overall, is now encountered more frequently in adults.

The treatment for *Haemophilus* meningitis over the years illustrates the progressive limitation of therapeutic choice that results from the spread of antimicrobial resistance. For many years chloramphenicol was unquestionably the drug of choice: it is bactericidal at concentrations that can readily be achieved in the CSF and is superior to ampicillin in that respect. Ampicillin appeared to be equally effective, and being free from possible hematological toxicity, it became the preferred drug, especially in the USA.

In 1974, the situation changed when resistant strains of *H. influenzae* type b emerged. Resistance of *H. influenzae* is most commonly due to plasmid-mediated β-lactamase production. Ampicillin resistance in *H. influenzae* has increased globally and ranges from 0% to 94%, depending on the geographical area. Resistance to chloramphenicol, though reported in the early 1970s, has remained rare, the incidence being about 0.5%. These changing resistance patterns have led to the widespread use of cephalosporins as initial treatment of *Haemophilus* meningitis. It is important to note that there is no evidence that cephalosporins give better results; the sole reason for their use is the presence of antimicrobial resistance. Treatment with chloramphenicol or ampicillin is entirely appropriate when isolates are susceptible, an especially important consideration in resource-poor countries. Practice in the USA, before ampicillin resistance became common, favored the initial use of chloramphenicol together with high-dose ampicillin. The antagonism between ampicillin (or penicillin) and chloramphenicol makes it likely that this form of combined treatment effectively relies on the chloramphenicol component,[85] and equivalent results are obtained whether chloramphenicol is used alone or in combination with penicillin.[86]

A number of choices are available when cephalosporins are indicated for the treatment of *Haemophilus* meningitis. In many countries cefotaxime or ceftriaxone is chiefly used but, as indicated, many other extended-spectrum cephalosporins are equally suitable for *Haemophilus* meningitis. The generally low toxicity of β-lactams permits high parenteral dosage and this, together with their high intrinsic activity against common bacterial causes of meningitis, overcomes their poor CSF penetration. CSF concentrations and CSF:serum ratios for these compounds are summarized in Table 50.3. The wide variability and occasional low concentrations in CSF are worth noting.

Protection of contacts

The risk of child contacts of patients with *Haemophilus* meningitis (and possibly other systemic *Haemophilus* infections) is of a similar order to that experienced by contacts of meningococcal disease. The overall risk is about 0.5% but nearer 2% in household contacts under 5 years of age. The high rate of nasopharyngeal carriage of the organism in contacts suggests the need for chemoprophylaxis. As with meningococcal infections, many agents that are effective in vitro or in vivo are ineffective in reducing nasopharyngeal carriage. Rifampicin, given in a dose of 20 mg/kg once daily for 4 days, has been shown to reduce carriage rates by 90% and the effect persists, to a lessening extent, for several weeks. Resistance to rifampicin has been documented, although most re-isolates are still susceptible. These findings provided the basis for a number of trials, which showed a significant reduction of risk in contacts given rifampicin. The importance of correct dosage emerged clearly; in one study, carriage was reduced by 97% in children given 20 mg/kg of rifampicin but only by 63% in those given half that dose (and by 28% in the placebo group). Current recommendations have been influenced by the success of vaccination against invasive *Haemophilus* disease. Rifampicin chemoprophylaxis is now offered to all contacts in households in which there are any unvaccinated or incompletely vaccinated children less than 4 years old. The index case should also be given rifampicin, because persistent nasopharyngeal carriage may re-emerge after the acute infection has been treated. Chemoprophylaxis is also given to adult and child contacts in preschool age groups if two or more cases of disease have occurred within 120 days.

Chemoprophylaxis does not obviate the need for careful observation of all contacts, because a workable policy for chemoprophylaxis cannot include all those at risk. Rifampicin may fail to eradicate carriage, and the risk of rifampicin resistance is as yet uncertain. Moreover, although the re-colonization rate is reduced, it does still occur. Failure of rifampicin prophylaxis has been reported a number of times. Rifampicin chemoprophylaxis, although marginally effective, will have negligible effect on the total number of patients with invasive *H. influenzae* disease and is much less important than vaccination as a control measure.

STAPHYLOCOCCAL MENINGITIS

Staphylococcus aureus meningitis is usually encountered as a component of a generalized hematogenous infection, commonly in the elderly or in patients with serious underlying disease[87] such as post-neurosurgical or post-trauma patients and those with CSF shunts; other underlying conditions include diabetes mellitus, alcoholism, chronic renal failure requiring hemodialysis, injection drug use and malignancies. Other sources of community-acquired *Staph. aureus* meningitis include patients with sinusitis, osteomyelitis and pneumonia. Mortality rates have ranged from 14% to 77% in various series. The course of the illness is difficult to modify, even with appropriate therapy. Vancomycin is a suitable choice pending information from susceptibility tests. Meningitis caused by methicillin-sensitive *Staph. aureus* (MSSA) may be treated with a penicillinase-resistant penicillin (nafcillin, oxacillin, flucloxacillin). Results in the series quoted gave a suggestion that prognosis might be improved by the use of fusidic acid in conjunction with a penicillin. Meningitis due to MRSA should be treated with vancomycin; daptomycin may be an alternative, but linezolid or quinupristin–dalfopristin is not recommended. *Staph. epidermidis* is the most common cause of meningitis in patients with CSF shunts (discussed in detail in Ch. 42).

STREPTOCOCCUS SUIS MENINGITIS

Streptococcus suis meningitis has a strong occupational association with pigs or pork production. Arthritis, endocarditis and other septic manifestations have been reported, and deafness is a common sequel. Importantly, 6–31% of patients infected with *Str. suis* develop skin findings similar to purpura fulminans seen with meningococcemia.[7] Kay et al, in a review that included 25 of their own cases,[88] indicated that *Str. suis* is susceptible to penicillin, ampicillin, cephalosporins, trimethoprim–sulfamethoxazole and vancomycin. Although 2–3 weeks' treatment with penicillin or ampicillin is usually satisfactory, relapses sometimes occur and require further treatment.

GRAM-NEGATIVE BACILLARY MENINGITIS

Meningitis caused by organisms such as *Esch. coli*, *Klebsiella* and *Proteus* spp. is mainly encountered in neonates. It has become less unusual in older patients and those with immunosuppression or other conditions such as chronic renal failure. Cephalosporins (notably ceftriaxone and cefotaxime) have revolutionized the approach to their management, with reported recovery rates of 78–94%. Ceftazidime is active in vitro against *Ps. aeruginosa* and has demonstrated clinical efficacy in infected patients. It is recommended that ceftazidime be combined with a parenteral aminoglycoside for the treatment of *Ps. aeruginosa* meningitis. Concomitant intraventricular aminoglycoside therapy should be considered in patients who fail to respond.[89] Other cephalosporins such as cefepime have been successful in the treatment of patients with Gram-negative enteric bacillary meningitis. However, although the MICs of these drugs for many Gram-negative bacilli found in

meningitis are low and greatly exceeded by attainable serum and CSF concentrations, MICs for some organisms such as *Enterobacter cloacae* and *Acinetobacter baumannii* may be relatively high and treatment may fail for this reason.

The fluoroquinolones (e.g. ciprofloxacin) have also been used to treat these infections but are contraindicated in infants and children because of concerns about cartilage damage. Fluoroquinolones are most useful against multiresistant Gram-negative organisms or when the response to conventional β-lactam therapy is slow.[90] The fluoroquinolones penetrate well into the CSF, producing CSF:serum ratios of 20–30% for ciprofloxacin and ofloxacin.[91] Hence, they find occasional utility in the treatment of Gram-negative bacillary meningitis, especially for organisms resistant to standard regimens.[92]

The carbapenems (e.g. meropenem) are logical choices for the treatment of Gram-negative bacterial meningitis, particularly for carbapenem-sensitive strains of extended-spectrum or AmpC β-lactamase-expressing organisms (e.g. *Esch. coli*, *K. pneumoniae*, *Enterobacter* spp.). These agents may also be used to treat meningitis caused by *A. baumannii*, though there has been a worldwide increase in carbapenem-resistant strains of this organism. Very few options exist for the treatment of meningitis caused by broadly resistant strains of *A. baumannii*. A comprehensive review of therapies for *Acinetobacter* meningitis suggested the combination of intravenous meropenem with an aminoglycoside (intrathecal or intraventricular, depending on the presence of ventriculitis) for those isolates susceptible to a carbapenem.[93] These authors suggest the use of an intravenous polymyxin (colistin methanesulphonate, polymyxin B) with an aminoglycoside (intrathecal or intraventricular, depending on the presence of ventriculitis) and optional rifampicin. As these infections are commonly nosocomially acquired in the post-neurosurgical setting, removal of all potentially infected hardware is also recommended.

NEONATAL MENINGITIS

Meningitis often complicates neonatal sepsis, and carries both a high mortality and risk of residual neurological damage. The organisms responsible are summarized in Table 50.1. Among these, *Esch. coli* and *Str. agalactiae* (group B streptococcus) predominate. Factors predisposing to neonatal meningitis are low birthweight, a complicated labor and maternal puerperal infection. Other causes include meningomyelocele or other neurological defects. Gram-negative bacilli causing meningitis often demonstrate a varied antimicrobial susceptibility pattern, and prompt laboratory guidance on positive CSF and blood cultures is essential.

Historically, neonatal meningitis was often treated empirically with a penicillin, usually ampicillin, and an aminoglycoside, usually gentamicin, as initial treatment. The poor penetration of aminoglycosides into CSF led to frequent supplementary administration of daily intrathecal injections of gentamicin. The erratic distribution of drug into the ventricular system following administration led to the introduction of ventricular reservoirs, allowing repeated CSF sampling and drug administration. The achievement of adequate ventricular concentrations of antimicrobial is not merely a theoretical requirement. However, successive trials have also shown that addition of gentamicin by the lumbar intrathecal route to a parenteral regimen of ampicillin and gentamicin does not improve the outlook, and that intraventricular administration carries a substantial risk.

The most appropriate initial regimen, if no organism is seen on Gram stain of the CSF deposit, is a combination of ampicillin and an appropriate cephalosporin, usually cefotaxime or ceftriaxone. If Gram-negative bacilli are seen, the cephalosporin can be used as sole initial agent. The former regimen of ampicillin and gentamicin (or other aminoglycoside) is still widely employed, especially when health budgets are low. However, failure to achieve adequate concentrations in the CSF and increasing resistance among Gram-negative bacilli account for some treatment failures with persistent meningitis.

LISTERIA MONOCYTOGENES

Listeria monocytogenes meningitis is less uncommon than previously thought. When it occurs in the newborn, it appears to result from maternal genital tract infection. It is also encountered in adults and is especially associated with lymphoreticular disease, immune suppression (as in transplant patients), pregnancy, diabetes mellitus and alcoholism.[94] Some patients have no underlying disease.

Ampicillin or penicillin G should be used as therapy for meningitis caused by *L. monocytogenes*. Many add an aminoglycoside for proven infection due to documented in-vitro synergy, even though a controlled trial comparing ampicillin with ampicillin plus gentamicin has never been performed in humans. Ceftriaxone, cefotaxime and cefepime are inactive against *L. monocytogenes* and should not be used alone as an empirical regimen in neonates or when this organism is considered a likely pathogen.

Trimethoprim–sulfamethoxazole is increasingly used in patients who are allergic to penicillin, despite the in-vitro activity of chloramphenicol against *Listeria*, because the latter drug has an unacceptably high failure rate. Intraventricular vancomycin has been successful in one patient with recurrent *L. monocytogenes* meningitis. Meropenem, which is active in vitro and in experimental animal models of *Listeria* meningitis, may be a further useful alternative.[95]

STREPTOCOCCUS AGALACTIAE

Neonatal infections caused by *Str. agalactiae* (group B streptococcus) have come to prominence in recent years, especially in the USA. Much is now known of their epidemiology and pathogenesis. Two syndromes are seen: an early septic variety of rapid course and high mortality (50%) closely simulating the respiratory distress syndrome, and a meningitic syndrome developing somewhat later in the neonatal period. Group B streptococcal meningitis carries a high mortality (20%), as do other forms of neonatal meningitis. The median MICs of benzylpenicillin and ampicillin are 0.02 and 0.04 mg/L, respectively, with conventional inocula (10^5 colony forming units), but rise appreciably with larger inocula. Since the CSF may contain 10^6–10^8 bacteria/mL, treatment with high doses of penicillin, in excess of 150 mg/kg per day by intravenous injection, is recommended.

In most patients treated with high-dose penicillin or ampicillin alone, the CSF rapidly becomes and remains sterile. In some patients, however, poor response or relapse has been noted. One reason may be failure to eradicate the organisms from focal sites such as the ventricles or cardiac valves; another possibility is infection by a penicillin-tolerant strain, showing a high MBC:MIC ratio. These difficulties, together with the demonstration of synergy in vitro and in animal models between penicillin and aminoglycosides against group B streptococci, suggest the initial use of benzylpenicillin in high dosage with an aminoglycoside. The latter drug may be withdrawn if clinical progress and further laboratory data on the causal organism are satisfactory. Some units, following the recommendation of the American Academy of Pediatrics,[96] use penicillin or ampicillin as single agents.

Prophylaxis

Acquisition of these organisms by neonates is highly correlated with maternal carriage, although nosocomial transmission acts as an additional source. Attempts to reduce the risk of neonatal group B streptococcal disease are discussed elsewhere (*see* Ch. 55).

BRAIN ABSCESS

The mortality from brain abscess is high and has changed little in the antimicrobial era. The reasons for this are complex, but particularly important among them is the dangerously rapid rise of intracranial pressure which so often accompanies the development of brain abscess during the early stage of cerebritis. Discussion here is confined to antimicrobial aspects of treatment, but other aspects of management are of crucial importance, notably the control of raised intracranial pressure, and drainage (using stereotactic CT scanning) or excision of the abscess. As in other forms of abscess, bacteria may be found in the abscess contents after many days of systemic chemotherapy. Surgical intervention may not be possible with multiple abscesses, and the advent of modern scanning has increased the frequency of non-surgical treatment if the condition can be recognized early and treatment closely monitored.

The causal organisms differ to some extent in their order of frequency with the origins of the abscess, but several studies have confirmed the importance of anaerobic Gram-negative bacteria, especially *Bacteroides* and *Fusobacterium* spp., and of aerobic and anaerobic streptococci. Enterobacteria of various genera are also commonly found, and staphylococci are important in infection associated with trauma and in spinal epidural abscess. Several species are often isolated from a single specimen when suitable selective techniques are used, especially in abscesses of middle ear origin. De Louvois et al stressed the strong association of *Bacteroides* spp. with temporal lobe abscess and the general importance of streptococci,[97] especially streptococci of the *anginosus* group (formerly *Str. milleri*). Streptococci were the most prominent single pathogen in non-temporal lobe abscesses but, as Grace and Drake-Lee point out,[98] *Bacteroides* spp. may also be found in abscesses of sinus origin. A similar distribution of causal organisms is found in cerebral abscess in childhood, common associations of which are cyanotic congenital heart disease, otitis, sinusitis, head injuries and cystic fibrosis. It has to be remembered that, although the dominant organisms in cerebral abscesses are well documented, other less common agents are sometimes encountered, including species of *Actinomyces*, *Nocardia* and fungi. A recent study utilized 16S ribosomal DNA sequencing to identify the bacteria in pus from patients with brain abscesses in France.[99] This technique identified a much larger number of bacterial species than culture and confirms that the vast majority of brain abscesses are polymicrobial infections.

An appropriate antimicrobial regimen must take into account not only this diverse flora, but also the characteristics of potentially effective drugs in penetrating brain tissue, CSF and abscess cavities. Data on these aspects may be found in the work of Black et al,[100] Picardi et al,[101] De Louvois et al[97,102] and a report by the British Society for Antimicrobial Chemotherapy.[103] Microbiological data are occasionally available at the time chemotherapy is started (e.g. when brain abscess is diagnosed during the course of sepsis of known etiology). Generally, however, no such information is available and initial antimicrobial policy must be based on the organisms known to be dominant in the etiology of cerebral abscess (Table 50.5), as described above, bearing in mind that the common forms of brain abscess are polymicrobial. Some

authors recommend variations of regimens based on the different frequency of various species found in cerebral abscess associated with different parameningeal or pulmonary sources. These differences are not big enough to allow this sort of fine tuning; a single-unit policy for brain abscess associated with parameningeal or pulmonary sepsis is preferable.

High-dose ampicillin and penicillin retain an important role as they are effective against streptococci, including the microaerophilic species not susceptible to metronidazole, and against most of the relevant anaerobes. The recognition of anaerobes as an important component of the flora of many brain abscesses led to the use of metronidazole, especially relevant as *Bacteroides fragilis* and perhaps some strains of *Prevotella melaninogenica*[104] are penicillin resistant but susceptible to metronidazole. This has led to the widespread use of metronidazole, together with ampicillin or penicillin (or ceftriaxone or cefotaxime), as agents of first choice. Good results in otogenic abscess were reported by Ingham et al,[105] who found that metronidazole, given orally or intravenously, achieved high concentrations in pus or ventricular fluid. In addition to high-dose ampicillin or penicillin and metronidazole, it is now customary to include a cephalosporin such as cefotaxime, ceftriaxone or ceftazidime in the treatment of patients with intracranial infections. Sjölin et al successfully treated 15 patients with a combination of cefotaxime (3 g every 8 h) and metronidazole (500 mg every 8 h) for a minimum of 3 weeks.[106] There are also a number of other reports of the successful use of cefotaxime to treat patients with brain abscess. Both ceftriaxone and ceftazidime achieve therapeutic concentrations in intracranial pus. However, to date, the numbers of patients treated with these cephalosporins are small.[107] Cerebral abscesses in neonates caused by *Proteus mirabilis*, *Esch. coli* or *Serratia marcescens* have been successfully treated with combinations of cefotaxime and gentamicin or, with an even higher success rate, ceftriaxone and amikacin.[108] Chloramphenicol was formerly widely used but now remains a reserve agent because of toxicity concerns. There is very little information on the efficacy of more recently introduced antimicrobials, such as the carbapenems, in the treatment of brain abscess.

Table 50.5 Initial empirical antimicrobial therapy for patients with brain abscess

Infective source	Intracerebral location	Antimicrobial regimen[a]
Paranasal sinuses	Frontal lobe	Cefotaxime 2 g every 6 h or ceftriaxone 2 g every 12 h and metronidazole 7.5 mg/kg every 6 h
Teeth	Frontal lobe	Penicillin G 2.4 g every 4–6 h and metronidazole 7.5 mg/kg every 6 h
Middle ear (less often, sphenoidal sinuses)	Temporal lobe, cerebellum	Ceftazidime (or cefepime) 2 g every 8 h plus metronidazole 7.5 mg/kg every 6 h
Penetrating trauma	Depends on site of wound	Vancomycin 30–45 mg/kg every 8–12 h plus ceftazidime (or cefepime) 2 g every 8 h plus metronidazole 7.5 mg/kg every 6 h
Metastatic and cryptogenic	Multiple lesions (usually in area supplied by middle cerebral artery)	Depends on source: penicillin G 2.4 g every 6 h plus metronidazole 7.5 mg/kg every 6 h if endocarditis or cyanotic congenital heart disease; ceftriaxone 2 g every 12 h or cefotaxime 2 g every 6 h plus metronidazole 7.5 mg/kg every 6 h

[a]Adult daily dosages.

Causal organisms in subdural empyema are generally similar to those in brain abscess and a similar antimicrobial policy may be used. For methicillin-sensitive staphylococcal brain abscess a combination of nafcillin or flucloxacillin (or a similar isoxazolyl penicillin) and fusidic acid is suggested. MRSA is a growing problem globally and has been isolated from brain abscesses in both community and nosocomial settings. The optimal management of MRSA brain abscess is unclear at this time. Vancomycin continues to be the mainstay of antimicrobial therapy for infections caused by MRSA; the role of newer MRSA-active agents such as daptomycin and linezolid remains undefined. Other abscesses of hematogenous origin may require specific chemotherapy different from those recommended for the common types associated with paramengineal sources in the ear or sinuses; these must be tailored to the particular organism.

EPIDURAL ABSCESS

SPINAL EPIDURAL ABSCESS

Spinal epidural abscess is a rare but potentially devastating condition. Many abscesses begin as a focal pyogenic infection involving the vertebral disk or the junction between the disk and the vertebral body (pyogenic infectious diskitis); in such cases the abscesses are often located in the anterior aspect of the spinal canal. However, hematogenous spread was identified in 26% of cases, primarily located in the posterior aspect of the spinal canal. Reihsaus et al performed a meta-analysis of 915 patients with spinal epidural abscesses, 753 of which were bacterial in nature.[109] Of these bacterial abscesses, *Staph. aureus* accounted for 73%, with the remainder caused by other staphylococcal species, streptococci, Gram-negative pathogens and anaerobes. In children, Auletta and John reviewed the literature over 15 years and confirmed that *Staph. aureus* is the predominant pathogen in spinal epidural abscess and community-acquired MRSA has been recognized in pediatric populations.[110] For this reason, empirical therapy should be broad spectrum, including a combination of drugs with bactericidal activity against staphylococci, anaerobes and Gram-negative organisms. The vast majority of spinal epidural abscesses should be drained, either surgically or via image-guided methods, and intraoperative cultures obtained for identification of the causative organism(s). If methicillin-sensitive *Staph. aureus* is isolated, successful treatment is possible with a penicillinase-resistant penicillin, first-generation cephalosporin or vancomycin (in the case of a penicillin-allergic patient). Vancomycin should be used for the treatment of abscesses caused by MRSA as experience is limited with other agents active against this pathogen. Parenteral treatment should be continued for at least 4 weeks and may be prolonged for 8 weeks or longer if vertebral osteomyelitis is suspected. When no pathogen is isolated, broad 'best-guess' bactericidal cover is safest and best.

INTRACRANIAL EPIDURAL ABSCESS

Intracranial epidural abscesses are less common than spinal epidural abscesses, and less acute in their evolution. They are usually associated with frontal sinusitis, prior craniotomy or mastoiditis. The morbidity and mortality of intracranial epidural abscesses in isolation are low. However, the great majority of patients have an associated brain abscess (up to 17%), subdural empyema (up to 81%) or meningitis (up to 38%). Treatment usually consists of surgical drainage of the abscess and associated infected sinus in addition to intravenous antimicrobial therapy. Empirical antimicrobial therapy should be chosen based upon the probable infection. The regimens listed above for the treatment of spinal epidural abscesses when the etiology is unknown are also appropriate here.

 References

1. Quagliarello V, Scheld WM. Bacterial meningitis: pathogenesis, pathophysiology, and progress. *N Engl J Med.* 1992;327(12):864–872.
2. Durand ML, Calderwood SB, Weber DJ, et al. Acute bacterial meningitis in adults. A review of 493 episodes. *N Engl J Med.* 1993;328(1):21–28.
3. Heath PT, Yusoff NK, Baker CJ. Neonatal meningitis. *Arch Dis Child Fetal Neonatal Ed.* 2003;88(3):F173–F178.
4. Nigrovic LE, Kuppermann N, Malley R. Children with bacterial meningitis presenting to the emergency department during the pneumococcal conjugate vaccine era. *Acad Emerg Med.* 2008;15(6):522–528.
5. Salih MA, Khaleefa OH, Bushara M, et al. Long term sequelae of childhood acute bacterial meningitis in a developing country. A study from the Sudan. *Scand J Infect Dis.* 1991;23(2):175–182.
6. Ciana G, Parmar N, Antonio C, Pivetta S, Tamburlini G, Cuttini M. Effectiveness of adjunctive treatment with steroids in reducing short-term mortality in a high-risk population of children with bacterial meningitis. *J Trop Pediatr.* 1995;41(3):164–168.
7. Wertheim HF, Nghia HD, Taylor W, Schultsz C. *Streptococcus suis*: an emerging human pathogen. *Clin Infect Dis.* 2009;48(5):617–625.
8. Centers for Disease Control and Prevention. Prevention of perinatal group B streptococcal disease: a public health perspective. *MMWR Recomm Rep.* 1996;45(RR-7):1–24.
9. Hasbun R, Abrahams J, Jekel J, Quagliarello VJ. Computed tomography of the head before lumbar puncture in adults with suspected meningitis. *N Engl J Med.* 2001;345(24):1727–1733.
10. Coant PN, Kornberg AE, Duffy LC, Dryja DM, Hassan SM. Blood culture results as determinants in the organism identification of bacterial meningitis. *Pediatr Emerg Care.* 1992;8(4):200–205.
11. Auburtin M, Wolff M, Charpentier J, et al. Detrimental role of delayed antibiotic administration and penicillin-nonsusceptible strains in adult intensive care unit patients with pneumococcal meningitis: the PNEUMOREA prospective multicenter study. *Crit Care Med.* 2006;34(11):2758–2765.
12. Landgraf IM, Alkmin M, Vieira M. Bacterial antigen detection in cerebrospinal fluid by the latex agglutination test. *Revista di Instituto de Medicina Tropical de Sao Paolo.* 1995;37(3):257–260.
13. Carrol ED, Thomson AP, Shears P, Gray SJ, Kaczmarski EB, Hart CA. Performance characteristics of the polymerase chain reaction assay to confirm clinical meningococcal disease. *Arch Dis Child.* 2000;83(3):271–273.
14. Boving MK, Pedersen LN, Moller JK. Eight-plex PCR and liquid-array detection of bacterial and viral pathogens in cerebrospinal fluid from patients with suspected meningitis. *J Clin Microbiol.* 2009;47(4):908–913.
15. Nigrovic LE, Malley R, Macias CG, et al. Effect of antibiotic pretreatment on cerebrospinal fluid profiles of children with bacterial meningitis. *Pediatrics.* 2008;122(4):726–730.
16. Bohuon C, Assicot M, Raymond J, Gendrel D. [Procalcitonin, a marker of bacterial meningitis in children]. *Bull Acad Natl Med.* 1998;182(7):1469–1475.
17. Gendrel D, Raymond J, Assicot M, et al. Measurement of procalcitonin levels in children with bacterial or viral meningitis. *Clin Infec Dis.* 1997;24(6):1240–1242.

18. Stahel PF, Nadal D, Pfister HW, Paradisis PM, Barnum SR. Complement C3 and factor B cerebrospinal fluid concentrations in bacterial and aseptic meningitis. *Lancet*. 1997;349(9069):1886–1887.

19. Beratis NG, Eliopoulou MI, Syrogiannopoulos GA. Beta-glucuronidase in the diagnosis of bacterial meningitis and response to treatment. *Acta Paediatr*. 2003;92(11):1272–1276.

20. Nau R, Sorgel F, Prange HW. Pharmacokinetic optimisation of the treatment of bacterial central nervous system infections. *Clin Pharmacokinet*. 1998;35(3):223–246.

21. McCracken Jr GH. Pharmacokinetic and bacteriological correlations between antimicrobial therapy of experimental meningitis in rabbits and meningitis in humans: a review. *J Antimicrob Chemother*. 1983;12(suppl D):97–108.

22. Hieber JP, Nelson JD. A pharmacologic evaluation of penicillin in children with purulent meningitis. *N Engl J Med*. 1977;297(8):410–413.

23. Trang JM, Jacobs RF, Kearns GL, et al. Cefotaxime and desacetylcefotaxime pharmacokinetics in infants and children with meningitis. *Antimicrob Agents Chemother*. 1985;28(6):791–795.

24. Goldwater PN. Cefotaxime and ceftriaxone cerebrospinal fluid levels during treatment of bacterial meningitis in children. *Int J Antimicrob Agents*. 2005;26(5):408–411.

25. Barson WJ, Miller MA, Brady MT, Powell DA. Prospective comparative trial of ceftriaxone vs. conventional therapy for treatment of bacterial meningitis in children. *Pediatr Infect Dis*. 1985;4(4):362–368.

26. Scholz H, Hofmann T, Noack R, Edwards DJ, Stoeckel K. Prospective comparison of ceftriaxone and cefotaxime for the short-term treatment of bacterial meningitis in children. *Chemotherapy*. 1998;44(2):142–147.

27. Lin TY, Chrane DF, Nelson JD, McCracken Jr GH. Seven days of ceftriaxone therapy is as effective as ten days' treatment for bacterial meningitis. *J Am Med Assoc*. 1985;253(24):3559–3563.

28. Roine I, Ledermann W, Foncea LM, Banfi A, Cohen J, Peltola H. Randomized trial of four vs. seven days of ceftriaxone treatment for bacterial meningitis in children with rapid initial recovery. *Pediatr Infect Dis J*. 2000;19(3):219–222.

29. Viladrich PF, Cabellos C, Pallares R, et al. High doses of cefotaxime in treatment of adult meningitis due to *Streptococcus pneumoniae* with decreased susceptibilities to broad-spectrum cephalosporins. *Antimicrob Agents Chemother*. 1996;40(1):218–220.

30. Odio CM, Puig JR, Feris JM, et al. Prospective, randomized, investigator-blinded study of the efficacy and safety of meropenem vs. cefotaxime therapy in bacterial meningitis in children. Meropenem Meningitis Study Group. *Pediatr Infect Dis J*. 1999;18(7):581–590.

31. Peltola H, Anttila M, Renkonen OV. Randomised comparison of chloramphenicol, ampicillin, cefotaxime, and ceftriaxone for childhood bacterial meningitis. Finnish Study Group. *Lancet*. 1989;1(8650):1281–1287.

32. Blumer JL, Reed MD, Knupp C. Review of the pharmacokinetics of cefepime in children. *Pediatr Infect Dis J*. 2001;20(3):337–342.

33. Saez-Llorens X, Castano E, Garcia R, et al. Prospective randomized comparison of cefepime and cefotaxime for treatment of bacterial meningitis in infants and children. *Antimicrob Agents Chemother*. 1995;39(4):937–940.

34. Saez-Llorens X, O'Ryan M. Cefepime in the empiric treatment of meningitis in children. *Pediatr Infect Dis J*. 2001;20(3):356–361.

35. Martinez-Rodriguez JE, Barriga FJ, Santamaria J, et al. Nonconvulsive status epilepticus associated with cephalosporins in patients with renal failure. *Am J Med*. 2001;111(2):115–119.

36. Dagan R, Velghe L, Rodda JL, Klugman KP. Penetration of meropenem into the cerebrospinal fluid of patients with inflamed meninges. *J Antimicrob Chemother*. 1994;34(1):175–179.

37. Schmutzhard E, Williams KJ, Vukmirovits G, Chmelik V, Pfausler B, Featherstone A. A randomised comparison of meropenem with cefotaxime or ceftriaxone for the treatment of bacterial meningitis in adults. Meropenem Meningitis Study Group. *J Antimicrob Chemother*. 1995;36(suppl A):85–97.

38. Klugman KP, Dagan R. Randomized comparison of meropenem with cefotaxime for treatment of bacterial meningitis. Meropenem Meningitis Study Group. *Antimicrob Agents Chemother*. 1995;39(5):1140–1146.

39. Wong VK, Wright Jr HT, Ross LA, Mason WH, Inderlied CB, Kim KS. Imipenem/cilastatin treatment of bacterial meningitis in children. *Pediatr Infect Dis J*. 1991;10(2):122–125.

40. Albanese J, Leone M, Bruguerolle B, Ayem ML, Lacarelle B, Martin C. Cerebrospinal fluid penetration and pharmacokinetics of vancomycin administered by continuous infusion to mechanically ventilated patients in an intensive care unit. *Antimicrob Agents Chemother*. 2000;44(5):1356–1358.

41. Ahmed A, Jafri H, Lutsar I, et al. Pharmacodynamics of vancomycin for the treatment of experimental penicillin- and cephalosporin-resistant pneumococcal meningitis. *Antimicrob Agents Chemother*. 1999;43(4):876–881.

42. Pneumococcal infection. In: Pickering LK, Baker CJ, Long SS, McMillan JA, eds. *AAP Committee on Infectious Diseases*. Elk Grove Village, IL: Red Book of the American Academy of Pediatrics, AAP; 2006.

43. Klugman KP, Feldman C. Penicillin- and cephalosporin-resistant *Streptococcus pneumoniae*. Emerging treatment for an emerging problem. *Drugs*. 1999;58(1):1–4.

44. Arda B, Yamazhan T, Sipahi OR, Islekel S, Buke C, Ulusoy S. Meningitis due to methicillin-resistant *Staphylococcus aureus* (MRSA): review of 10 cases. *Int J Antimicrob Agents*. 2005;25(5):414–418.

45. Naesens R, Ronsyn M, Druwe P, Denis O, Ieven M, Jeurissen A. Central nervous system invasion by community-acquired methicillin-resistant *Staphylococcus aureus*: case report and review of the literature. *J Med Microbiol*. 2009;58(Pt 9):1247–1251.

46. Kirikae T, Nakano M, Morrison DC. Antibiotic-induced endotoxin release from bacteria and its clinical significance. *Microbiol Immunol*. 1997;41(4):285–294.

47. Morrison DC. Antibiotic-mediated release of endotoxin and the pathogenesis of gram-negative sepsis. *Prog Clin Biol Res*. 1998;397:199–207.

48. Horn DL, Opal SM, Lomastro E. Antibiotics, cytokines, and endotoxin: a complex and evolving relationship in gram-negative sepsis. *Scand J Infect Dis*. 1996;101(suppl):9–13.

49. Desbiolles N, Piroth L, Lequeu C, Neuwirth C, Portier H, Chavanet P. Fractional maximal effect method for in vitro synergy between amoxicillin and ceftriaxone and between vancomycin and ceftriaxone against *Enterococcus faecalis* and penicillin-resistant *Streptococcus pneumoniae*. *Antimicrob Agents Chemother*. 2001;45(12):3328–3333.

50. Ribes S, Taberner F, Domenech A, et al. Evaluation of ceftriaxone, vancomycin and rifampicin alone and combined in an experimental model of meningitis caused by highly cephalosporin-resistant *Streptococcus pneumoniae* ATCC 51916. *J Antimicrob Chemother*. 2005;56(5):979–982.

51. Friedland IR, Paris M, Ehrett S, Hickey S, Olsen K, McCracken Jr GH. Evaluation of antimicrobial regimens for treatment of experimental penicillin- and cephalosporin-resistant pneumococcal meningitis. *Antimicrob Agents Chemother*. 1993;37(8):1630–1636.

52. Schaad UB, Lips U, Gnehm HE, Blumberg A, Heinzer I, Wedgwood J. Dexamethasone therapy for bacterial meningitis in children. Swiss Meningitis Study Group. *Lancet*. 1993;342(8869):457–461.

53. Prasad K, Haines T. Dexamethasone treatment for acute bacterial meningitis: how strong is the evidence for routine use? *J Neurol Neurosurg Psychiatry*. 1995;59(1):31–37.

54. Paris MM, Hickey SM, Uscher MI, Shelton S, Olsen KD, McCracken Jr GH. Effect of dexamethasone on therapy of experimental penicillin- and cephalosporin-resistant pneumococcal meningitis. *Antimicrob Agents Chemother*. 1994;38(6):1320–1324.

55. Warrell DA, Looareesuwan S, Warrell MJ, et al. Dexamethasone proves deleterious in cerebral malaria. A double-blind trial in 100 comatose patients. *N Engl J Med*. 1982;306(6):313–319.

56. de Gans J, van de BD. Dexamethasone in adults with bacterial meningitis. *N Engl J Med*. 2002;347(20):1549–1556.

57. Quagliarello VJ, Scheld WM. Treatment of bacterial meningitis. *N Engl J Med*. 1997;336(10):708–716.

58. Ricard JD, Wolff M, Lacherade JC, et al. Levels of vancomycin in cerebrospinal fluid of adult patients receiving adjunctive corticosteroids to treat pneumococcal meningitis: a prospective multicenter observational study. *Clin Infect Dis*. 2007;44(2):250–255.

59. Scarborough M, Gordon SB, Whitty CJ, et al. Corticosteroids for bacterial meningitis in adults in sub-Saharan Africa. *N Engl J Med*. 2007;357(24):2441–2450.

60. Nguyen TH, Tran TH, Thwaites G, et al. Dexamethasone in Vietnamese adolescents and adults with bacterial meningitis. *N Engl J Med*. 2007;357(24):2431–2440.

61. Peltola H, Roine I, Fernandez J, et al. Adjuvant glycerol and/or dexamethasone to improve the outcomes of childhood bacterial meningitis: a prospective, randomized, double-blind, placebo-controlled trial. *Clin Infect Dis*. 2007;45(10):1277–1286.

62. Tunkel AR, Hartman BJ, Kaplan SL, et al. Practice guidelines for the management of bacterial meningitis. *Clin Infect Dis*. 2004;39(9):1267–1284.

63. Jorgensen JH, Crawford SA, Fiebelkorn KR. Susceptibility of *Neisseria meningitidis* to 16 antimicrobial agents and characterization of resistance mechanisms affecting some agents. *J Clin Microbiol*. 2005;43(7):3162–3171.

64. Viladrich PF, Pallares R, Ariza J, Rufi G, Gudiol F. Four days of penicillin therapy for meningococcal meningitis. *Arch Intern Med*. 1986;146(12):2380–2382.

65. Marhoum F, Noun M, Chakib A, Zahraoui M, Himmich H. Ceftriaxone versus penicillin G in the short-term treatment of meningococcal meningitis in adults. *Eur J Clin Microbiol Infect Dis*. 1993;12(10):766–768.

66. Pecoul B, Varaine F, Keita M, et al. Long-acting chloramphenicol versus intravenous ampicillin for treatment of bacterial meningitis. *Lancet*. 1991;338(8771):862–866.

67. Nathan N, Borel T, Djibo A, et al. Ceftriaxone as effective as long-acting chloramphenicol in short-course treatment of meningococcal meningitis during epidemics: a randomised non-inferiority study. *Lancet*. 2005;366(9482):308–313.

68. Stuart JM, Gilmore AB, Ross A, et al. Preventing secondary meningococcal disease in health care workers: recommendations of a working group of the PHLS meningococcus forum. *Commun Dis Public Health*. 2001;4(2):102–105.

69. Cuevas LE, Kazembe P, Mughogho GK, Tillotson GS, Hart CA. Eradication of nasopharyngeal carriage of *Neisseria meningitidis* in children and adults in rural Africa: a comparison of ciprofloxacin and rifampicin. *J Infect Dis*. 1995;171(3):728–731.

70. Dworzack DL, Sanders CC, Horowitz EA, et al. Evaluation of single-dose ciprofloxacin in the eradication of *Neisseria meningitidis* from nasopharyngeal carriers. *Antimicrob Agents Chemother*. 1988;32(11):1740–1741.

71. Schwartz B, Al Tobaiqi A, Al Ruwais A, et al. Comparative efficacy of ceftriaxone and rifampicin in eradicating pharyngeal carriage of group A *Neisseria meningitidis*. *Lancet*. 1988;1(8597):1239–1242.

72. Halstensen A, Gilja OH, Digranes A, et al. Single dose ofloxacin in the eradication of pharyngeal carriage of *Neisseria meningitidis*. *Drugs*. 1995;49(suppl 2):399–400.

73. Girgis N, Sultan Y, Frenck Jr RW, El Gendy A, Farid Z, Mateczun A. Azithromycin compared with rifampin for eradication of nasopharyngeal colonization by *Neisseria meningitidis*. *Pediatr Infect Dis J*. 1998;17(9):816–819.

74. Yagupsky P, Ashkenazi S, Block C. Rifampicin-resistant meningococci causing invasive disease and failure of chemoprophylaxis. *Lancet*. 1993;341(8853):1152–1153.

75. Viladrich PF, Gudiol F, Linares J, et al. Evaluation of vancomycin for therapy of adult pneumococcal meningitis. *Antimicrob Agents Chemother*. 1991;35(12):2467–2472.

76. Klugman KP. Management of antibiotic-resistant pneumococcal infections. *J Antimicrob Chemother*. 1994;34(2):191–193.

77. Piper KE, Steckelberg JM, Patel R. In vitro activity of daptomycin against clinical isolates of Gram-positive bacteria. *J Infect Chemother*. 2005;11(4):207–209.

78. Malli E, Spiliopoulou I, Kolonitsiou F, et al. In vitro activity of daptomycin against Gram-positive cocci: the first multicentre study in Greece. *Int J Antimicrob Agents*. 2008;32(6):525–528.

79. Stucki A, Cottagnoud M, Winkelmann V, Schaffner T, Cottagnoud P. Daptomycin produces an enhanced bactericidal activity compared to ceftriaxone, measured by [3H]choline release in the cerebrospinal fluid, in experimental meningitis due to a penicillin-resistant pneumococcal strain without lysing its cell wall. *Antimicrob Agents Chemother*. 2007;51(6):2249–2252.

80. Grandgirard D, Schurch C, Cottagnoud P, Leib SL. Prevention of brain injury by the nonbacteriolytic antibiotic daptomycin in experimental pneumococcal meningitis. *Antimicrob Agents Chemother*. 2007;51(6):2173–2178.

81. Braun JS, Hoffmann O, Schickhaus M, et al. Pneumolysin causes neuronal cell death through mitochondrial damage. *Infect Immun*. 2007;75(9):4245–4254.

82. Spreer A, Kerstan H, Bottcher T, et al. Reduced release of pneumolysin by *Streptococcus pneumoniae* in vitro and in vivo after treatment with nonbacteriolytic antibiotics in comparison to ceftriaxone. *Antimicrob Agents Chemother*. 2003;47(8):2649–2654.

83. Cottagnoud P, Pfister M, Acosta F, et al. Daptomycin is highly efficacious against penicillin-resistant and penicillin- and quinolone-resistant pneumococci in experimental meningitis. *Antimicrob Agents Chemother*. 2004;48(10):3928–3933.

84. Egermann U, Stanga Z, Ramin A, et al. Combination of daptomycin plus ceftriaxone is more active than vancomycin plus ceftriaxone in experimental meningitis after addition of dexamethasone. *Antimicrob Agents Chemother*. 2009;53(7):3030–3033.

85. Asmar BI, Dajani AS. Ampicillin–chloramphenicol interaction against enteric Gram-negative organisms. *Pediatr Infect Dis*. 1983;2(1):39–42.

86. Kumar P, Verma IC. Antibiotic therapy for bacterial meningitis in children in developing countries. *Bull World Health Org*. 1993;71(2):183–188.

87. Jensen AG, Espersen F, Skinhoj P, Rosdahl VT, Frimodt-Moller N. *Staphylococcus aureus* meningitis. A review of 104 nationwide, consecutive cases. *Arch Intern Med*. 1993;153(16):1902–1908.

88. Kay R, Cheng AF, Tse CY. *Streptococcus suis* infection in Hong Kong. *Q J Med*. 1995;88(1):39–47.

89. Saha V, Stansfield R, Masterton R, Eden T. The treatment of *Pseudomonas aeruginosa* meningitis – old regime or newer drugs? *Scand J Infect Dis*. 1993;25(1):81–83.

90. Modai J. Potential role of fluoroquinolones in the treatment of bacterial meningitis. *Eur J Clin Microbiol Infect Dis.*. 1991;10(4):291–295.

91. Scheld WM. Quinolone therapy for infections of the central nervous system. *Rev Infect Dis*. 1989;11(suppl 5):S1194–S1202.

92. Wolfson JS, Hooper DC. Pharmacokinetics of quinolones: newer aspects. *Eur J Clin Microbiol Infect Dis*. 1991;10(4):267–274.

93. Kim BN, Peleg AY, Lodise TP, et al. Management of meningitis due to antibiotic-resistant *Acinetobacter* species. *Lancet Infect Dis*. 2009;9(4):245–255.

94. Mylonakis E, Hohmann EL, Calderwood SB. Central nervous system infection with *Listeria monocytogenes*. 33 years' experience at a general hospital and review of 776 episodes from the literature. *Medicine (Baltimore)*. 1998;77(5):313–336.

95. Nairn K, Shepherd GL, Edwards JR. Efficacy of meropenem in experimental meningitis. *J Antimicrob Chemother*. 1995;36(suppl A):73–84.

96. American Academy of Pediatrics Committee on Infectious Diseases. Treatment of bacterial meningitis. *Pediatrics*. 1988;81(6):904–907.

97. De Louvois J, Gortavai P, Hurley R. Bacteriology of abscesses of the central nervous system: a multicentre prospective study. *Br Med J*. 1977;2(6093):981–984.

98. Grace A, Drake-Lee A. Role of anaerobes in cerebral abscesses of sinus origin. *BMJ (Clinical Research ed.)*. 1984;288(6419):758–759.

99. Al Masalma M, Armougom F, Scheld WM, et al. The expansion of the microbiological spectrum of brain abscesses with use of multiple 16S ribosomal DNA sequencing. *Clin Infect Dis*. 2009;48(9):1169–1178.

100. Black P, Graybill JR, Charache P. Penetration of brain abscess by systemically administered antibiotics. *J Neurosurg*. 1973;38(6):705–709.

101. Picardi JL, Lewis HP, Tan JS, Phair JP. Clindamycin concentrations in the central nervous system of primates before and after head trauma. *J Neurosurg*. 1975;43(6):717–720.

102. De Louvois J. Antimicrobial chemotherapy in the treatment of brain abscess. *J Antimicrob Chemother*. 1983;12(3):205–207.

103. Infection in Neurosurgery Working Party of the British Society for Antimicrobial Chemotherapy. The rational use of antibiotics in the treatment of brain abscess. *Br J Neurosurg*. 2000;14(6):525–530.

104. Nau R, Behnke-Mursch J. [Diagnosis and treatment of brain abscesses]. *Ther Umsch*. 1999;56(11):659–663.

105. Ingham HR, Selkon JB, Roxby CM. Bacteriological study of otogenic cerebral abscesses: chemotherapeutic role of metronidazole. *Br Med J*. 1977;2(6093):991–993.

106. Sjölin J, Lilja A, Eriksson N, Arneborn P, Cars O. Treatment of brain abscess with cefotaxime and metronidazole: prospective study on 15 consecutive patients. *Clin Infect Dis*. 1993;17(5):857–863.

107. Mathisen GE, Johnson JP. Brain abscess. *Clin Infect Dis*. 1997;25(4):763–779.

108. Renier D, Flandin C, Hirsch E, Hirsch JF. Brain abscesses in neonates. A study of 30 cases. *J Neurosurg*. 1988;69(6):877–882.

109. Reihsaus E, Waldbaur H, Seeling W. Spinal epidural abscess: a meta-analysis of 915 patients. *Neurosurg Rev*. 2000;23(4):175–204.

110. Auletta JJ, John CC. Spinal epidural abscesses in children: a 15-year experience and review of the literature. *Clin Infect Dis*. 2001;32(1):9–16.

51 Viral infections of the central nervous system

Kevin A. Cassady

Viral infections of the central nervous system (CNS) occur infrequently and most often result in relatively benign, self-limited disease. Nevertheless, these infections have tremendous importance because of the potential for death and neurological damage. Neural tissues are exquisitely sensitive to metabolic derangements and injured brain tissue recovers slowly and often incompletely. The diseases discussed in this chapter include viral meningitis, encephalitis and transmissible spongiform encephalopathies (TSEs). The definitions of viral CNS disease are often based on both virus tropism and disease duration. Inflammation occurs at multiple sites within the CNS and accounts for the myriad of clinical descriptors of viral neurological disease. *Aseptic meningitis* is a misnomer frequently used to refer to a benign, self-limited, viral infection causing inflammation of the leptomeninges. *Encephalitis* refers to inflammation of parenchymal brain tissue and is usually accompanied by a depressed level of consciousness, altered cognition and frequently focal neurological signs. Slow progressive neurological deterioration, gliosis, abnormal accumulation of prion proteins in the brain and the lack of CNS inflammation characterize the TSEs. Meningitis and encephalitis represent separate clinical entities; however, a continuum exists between these distinct forms of disease. A change in a patient's clinical condition can reflect disease progression with involvement of different regions in the CNS. Therefore, in many cases, it is difficult to accurately and prospectively predict the etiology and extent of CNS infection. To provide organization for this chapter, viral meningitis and encephalitis will be discussed as discrete entities.

EPIDEMIOLOGY

Acute viral meningitis and meningoencephalitis represent the majority of viral CNS infections and frequently occur in epidemics or in seasonal distribution.[1,2] The etiology and frequency differ based on geography and immunization practices. Enteroviruses cause an estimated 90% of cases (in countries that immunize against mumps), while arboviruses constitute the majority of the remaining reported cases in the USA.[1,3–5] Mumps virus is also an important cause of viral CNS disease in countries that do not immunize against this virus. Mumps infection was the second leading cause of aseptic meningitis, accounting for ~30% of the cases in regions that do not routinely vaccinate against the virus.[6] A retrospective survey performed in the 1980s found that the annual incidence of 'aseptic meningitis' was approximately 10.9/100 000 persons or at least four times the incidence passively reported to the Centers for Disease Control and Prevention (CDC) during the period.[2] Virus was identified in only 11% of patients in this study. This low viral isolation rate likely reflects the technological limits of the period, the infrequency with which viral cultures were performed, and the decreased incidence of viral CNS disease resulting from widespread vaccination against mumps and polio viruses. With the advent of improved nucleic acid-based diagnostic methods, these data have changed. Isolation rates now approach 50–86%.[1,7,8]

Similar to viral meningitis, passive reporting systems underestimate the incidence of viral encephalitis.[1,2] For example, an estimated 20 000 cases of encephalitis occur each year in the USA; however, the CDC received only 740 (0.3/100 000) to 1340 (0.54/100 000) annual reports of persons with encephalitis from 1990 to 1994.[1,9] A prospective multicenter study in Finland, a region with a low incidence of arboviral encephalitis, found the incidence of encephalitis to be 10.5/100 000.[10] Although nucleic acid-based diagnostic tests have enhanced the detection of viral pathogens, the tests fail to identify a pathogen in the majority (83%) of cases.[7,11] While the etiology of encephalitis has changed with alterations in the viral reservoirs in North America, the overall death rates from encephalitis have not changed since the late 1970s and 1980s.[12] Herpes simplex virus (HSV) CNS infections occur without seasonal variation, affect all ages, and constitute the majority of fatal cases of endemic encephalitis in the USA.[1] Arboviruses, a group of over 500 arthropod-transmitted RNA viruses, are the leading cause of encephalitis worldwide.[1,13,14] Arboviral infections occur in epidemics and show a seasonal predilection, reflecting the prevalence of the transmitting vector. Encephalitis occurs in a minority of persons with arboviral infections, but the case fatality rate varies widely, from 5% to 70%, depending upon viral etiology and age of the patient. Based on passive reporting to the CDC, neuroinvasive West Nile virus infections now far outnumber other arboviral causes of encephalitis in the USA.[15] It is unknown if this is a function of improved testing and more active surveillance for this disease. Historically, La Crosse encephalitis was the most commonly reported arboviral disease in the USA.[16,17]

Japanese B encephalitis and rabies constitute the majority of cases of encephalitis outside of North America. Japanese encephalitis virus, a member of the flavivirus genus, occurs throughout Asia and causes epidemics in China despite routine immunization.[1,18] In warmer locations, the virus occurs endemically.[1,19] The disease typically affects children, although adults with no history of exposure to the virus are also susceptible.[20] The disease has a high case fatality rate and leaves half of the survivors with a significant degree of neurological morbidity.[1] Rabies virus remains endemic around much of the world. Human infections in the USA decreased over the past few decades to 1–3 cases per year due to the immunization of domesticated animals. Bat exposure is increasingly recognized as the source of infection. Fifteen percent (685 of 4470) of bats tested carried the rabies virus in one study analyzing the risk of bat exposure and rabies.[21] Since 1990, bat-associated variants of the virus have accounted for 24 of the 32 cases recorded. In most cases (22 of 24) there was no evidence of bite; however, in half of the cases direct contact (handling of the bats) was documented.[22] In areas outside the USA, human cases of rabies encephalitis number in the thousands and are caused by unvaccinated domestic animals following contact with infected wild animals.

Postinfectious encephalitis, an acute demyelinating process, has also been referred to as acute disseminated encephalomyelitis (ADEM) or autoimmune encephalitis. ADEM accounts for approximately 100–200 additional cases of encephalitis annually in the USA and is associated with antecedent upper respiratory virus (notably influenza virus) and varicella infections.[1,23] In locations that do not immunize against measles and mumps, ADEM produces approximately one-third of the encephalitis cases and remains associated with the exanthematous viruses.[1,24] Measles continues to be the leading cause of postinfectious encephalitis worldwide and is estimated to occur in 1 of every 1000 measles infections.[20]

The slow viral brain infections (TSEs) occur sporadically. Creutzfeldt–Jakob disease (CJD), a prototypical TSE, occurs worldwide with an estimated incidence of 0.5–1.5 cases per million population, with high rates of familial occurrence.[25] In 1986, cases of a TSE in cattle, bovine spongiform encephalopathy (BSE), were reported in the UK. In addition to affecting other livestock throughout Europe that were fed supplements containing meat and bone meal, cross-species transmission of BSE has been documented, leading to a ban on the use of bovine offal in fertilizers, pet food or other animal feed.[25] A decrease in the recognized cases of BSE has occurred since the institution of these restrictions. Concomitant with increased cases of BSE in Europe, an increase in cases of atypical CJD also occurred, suggesting animal-to-human transmission. The report of atypical CJD (unique clinical and histopathological findings) affecting young adults (an age at which CJD has rarely been diagnosed) and a characteristic methionine at the polymorphic codon 129 led to the designation of a new disease, new variant Creutzfeldt-Jacob disease (nvCJD). As of 2006, a total of 160 cases of nvCJD were diagnosed in the UK and 28 cases outside of the UK.[26]

PATHOGENESIS

Viruses use two basic pathways to gain access to the CNS: hematogenous and neuronal spread. Most cases of viral meningitis occur following a high titer secondary viremia. A combination of host and viral factors, combined with seasonal, geographical and epidemiological probabilities, influence the proclivity to develop viral CNS infection. Enteroviral meningitis occurs with greater frequency during the summer and early autumn months, reflecting the seasonal increase in enteroviral infections. Enteroviral infections also exemplify the difference that host physiology plays in determining the extent of viral disease. In children less than 2 weeks of age, enterovirus infections can produce a severe systemic infection, including meningitis or meningoencephalitis.[5] Ten percent of neonates with systemic enteroviral infections die, while as many as 76% are left with permanent sequelae. In children over 2 weeks of age, however, enteroviral infections are rarely associated with severe disease or significant morbidity.[5]

Viral hematogenous dissemination to the CNS involves initial inoculation, local spread and replication, often in regional lymph nodes (e.g. measles, influenza). The virus then enters the circulatory system (primary viremia), enabling virus to seed distant locations of the body. In rare circumstances, such as disseminated neonatal HSV infection, viruses can infect the CNS during primary viremia; however, most viruses infect an intermediate tissue such as the liver and spleen, replicate and then infect the CNS during a prolonged high titer secondary viremia.[27,28] The pathophysiology of viral transport from blood to brain and viral endothelial cell tropism is poorly understood. Virus infects endothelial cells, leaks across damaged endothelia, passively channels through endothelium (pinocytosis or colloidal transport) or bridges the endothelium within migrating leukocytes.[1,29,30]

Historically, the peripheral neural pathway was considered the only pathway of viral neurological infection. Contemporary data, however, demonstrate that the circulatory system provides the principal pathway for most CNS infections in humans.[16] Herpes simplex virus and rabies provide examples of viruses that infect the CNS by neuronal spread. Rabies classically infects by the myoneural route and provides a prototype for peripheral neuronal spread.[1,31] Rabies virus replicates locally in the soft tissue following a rabid animal bite. After primary replication, the virus enters the peripheral nerve by acetylcholine receptor binding. Once in the muscle the virus buds from the plasma membrane, crosses myoneural spindles or enters across the motor end plate.[31] The virus travels by anterograde and retrograde axonal transport to infect neurons in the brainstem and limbic system. Eventually the virus spreads from the diencephalic and hippocampal structure to the remainder of the brain, killing the animal.[31]

Viruses exhibit differences in neurotropism and neurovirulence. For example, reovirus types 1 and 3 produce different CNS diseases in mice based on differences in receptor affinities. Viral hemagglutinin receptors on reovirus type 3 bind to neuronal receptors, enabling fatal encephalitis. Reovirus type 1 has a distinct hemagglutinin antigen and binds to ependymal cells, producing hydrocephalus and ependymitis.[16] Receptor difference is only one determinant of viral neurotropism. For example, enteroviruses with similar receptors produce very different diseases. Five Coxsackie B viruses (B1–B5) readily produce CNS infections, whereas type B6 rarely produces neurological infection.[32,33] Viral genes have been discovered that influence the neurovirulence of HSV-1.[34] Mutant HSV-1 viruses with either γ134.5 gene deletions or stop codons inserted into the gene have a decreased ability to cause encephalitis and death following intracerebral inoculation in mice as compared to wild-type virus.[34,35]

In patients with acute encephalitis, the parenchyma exhibits neuronophagia and cells containing viral nucleic acids or antigens.[20,36] The pathological findings are unique for different viruses and reflect differences in pathogenesis and virulence. For example, in cases of typical HSE, a hemorrhagic necrosis occurs in the inferomedial temporal lobe with evidence of perivascular cuffing, lymphocytic infiltration and neuronophagia.[1,37] Pathological specimens in animals with rabies encephalitis demonstrate microglial proliferation, perivascular infiltrates and neuronal destruction.

Some viruses do not directly infect the CNS but produce immune system changes that result in parenchymal damage. Patients with postinfectious encephalitis (ADEM) exhibit focal neurological deficits and altered consciousness associated temporally with a recent (1–2 week) viral infection or immunization.[24] Pathological specimens, while they show evidence of demyelination by histological or radiographic analysis, do not demonstrate evidence of viral infection in the CNS by culture or antigen tests. Patients with postinfectious encephalitis have subtle differences in their immune system and some authors have proposed an autoimmune reaction as the pathogenic mechanism of disease.[20,24] Postinfectious encephalitis occurs most commonly following measles, varicella zoster virus (VZV), mumps, influenza and parainfluenza infections. With immunization the incidence of postinfectious encephalitis has decreased in the USA; however, measles continues to be the leading cause of postinfectious encephalitis worldwide.[16]

The TSEs are non-inflammatory CNS diseases involving the accumulation of an abnormal form of a normal glycoprotein, the prion protein (PrP).[38] These encephalopathies differ in mode of transmission. While most of the TSEs are experimentally transmissible by direct inoculation in the CNS, this mode rarely occurs except for iatrogenic transmission.[25] The scrapie agent spreads by contact and lateral transmission.

There is no evidence for lateral transmission in the case of BSE or nvCJD and all cases appear to have occurred following parenteral inoculation or ingestion of affected materials. The transmissible agents remain infectious after treatments that would normally inactivate viruses or nucleic acids (detergent formalin, ionizing radiation, nucleases).[38] Most of the experimental work on TSEs has involved analysis of the scrapie agent. The current working model is that post-translational alteration of the normally α-helical form of the prion protein results in a protease resistant β-pleated sheet structure that accumulates in neurons, leading to progressive dysfunction, cell death and subsequent astrocytosis. In studies on the scrapie agent and recently with nvCJD, gastrointestinal tract involvement with infection of abdominal lymph nodes occurs first, followed by hematogenous spread throughout the reticuloendothelial system and brain involvement a year or more later.[39] Experimental subcutaneous inoculation in mice and goats also leads to local lymph node involvement, followed by splenic spread and then CNS involvement. Cases of nvCJD by blood transfusion have also occurred.[40] Based on animal studies, there is an equal distribution of the agent associated with leukocytes and free in the plasma with negligible levels associated with the red blood cells and platelets.[41]

DIAGNOSIS

Establishing a diagnosis requires a meticulous history, knowledge of epidemiological factors and a systematic evaluation of possible treatable diseases. In the past, investigators failed 50–75% of the time to identify an etiology for encephalitis depending on the study and diagnostic tests used.[16,42,43] The techniques for identifying viral CNS infection were invasive and often insensitive as they relied on viral culture.[42] A CSF pleocytosis usually occurs in encephalitis but is not necessary for the diagnosis. White blood cell counts typically number in the tens to hundreds in viral encephalitis, although higher counts also occur.[1] Cerebrospinal glucose levels are usually normal, although some viral etiologies (Eastern equine encephalitis) produce CSF studies consistent with acute bacterial meningitis.[1] With the advent of PCR, reliable diagnosis has improved the timely management of patients with viral CNS infections. The demonstration of viral nucleic acid in the CSF of patients with symptoms of meningitis or encephalitis has replaced viral culture and serological diagnosis for many CNS infections.[23,44]

For many viruses – HSV, enterovirus, Epstein–Barr virus (EBV), VZV, JC virus, human herpesvirus-6 (HHV-6) – detection of viral nucleic acids by PCR or reverse transcription PCR (RT-PCR) from the CSF has replaced culture and brain biopsy as the standard for diagnosing encephalitis.[1,45,46] In the case of herpes simplex encephalitis, CSF PCR has a sensitivity of >95% and a specificity approaching 100%.[47,48] Investigators are increasingly using these sensitive PCR-based diagnostic techniques to correlate treatment response and predict clinical outcomes.[48]

As with any PCR-based technique, nucleic acid contamination of the laboratory area is a concern and results must always be interpreted within a clinical context. While PCR-based assays exist for many viruses, there are still some for which (notably the arthropod-borne viral infections) universal primers are still being developed.[49] In other cases (cytomegalovirus, HHV-6) the presence of latent virus or a virus associated with inflammatory cells can produce positive results of unknown significance. Molecular diagnostic techniques have greatly improved the speed, sensitivity and specificity of the diagnosis of enterovirus infections.[3,7] PCR and other molecular biological assays provide rapid and reliable tests for verifying the etiology of certain types of meningitis and can detect low copy numbers of viral RNA in patients with agammaglobulinemia or hyper IgM syndrome. Enterovirus is the cause of ~90% of aseptic meningitis cases for which a pathogen is detected.[5] These techniques provide results within 24–36 h and therefore may limit the duration of hospitalization, antibiotic use and excessive diagnostic procedures.[3,44]

Magnetic resonance imaging (MRI) can provide supportive evidence for encephalitis but is rarely diagnostic alone. The increased sensitivity of MRI to alterations in brain water content and the lack of bone artifacts make this the neuroradiological modality of choice for CNS infections.[50,51] MRI, and especially diffusion-weighted imaging, detects parenchymal changes earlier than CT scan and better defines the extent of a lesion.[52] Furthermore, MRI is more sensitive for detecting evidence of demyelinating lesions in the periventricular and deep white matter, thus allowing the differentiation of para-infectious from acute viral encephalitis.

TSEs are currently only diagnosed by histological examination, characteristic electroencephalographic (EEG) changes and the clinical context. The clinical diagnosis of a TSE is supported by detection of characteristic EEG changes (periodic sharp and slow wave complexes), the presence of 14-3-3 protein in the CSF, and characteristic MRI findings (increased signal in the basal ganglia in sporadic CJD [sCJD] or evidence of increased signal in the posterior pulvinar in nvCJD).[53] Most laboratory tests are of little value in the diagnosis in humans. CSF examination shows normal values or slightly elevated protein levels. The EEG in classic CJD reveals generalized slowing early in the disease, punctuated by biphasic or triphasic peaks late in the disease with the onset of myoclonus. MRI changes late in the illness reveal global atrophy with a hyperintense signal from the basal ganglia.[25] Diffusion-weighted imaging and fluid attenuation inversion recovery (FLAIR) remain the most reliable and sensitive imaging techniques for CJD.[53,54] Histopathological examination of the brain using a specific antibody to the protease-resistant prion protein (PrP-res) confirms the disease. In addition, evidence of gliosis, neuronal loss and spongiform changes support the diagnosis. In cases of nvCJD, characteristic amyloid plaques (so-called florid plaques) microscopically define the disease. The florid plaques are not seen in other TSEs and consist of flower-like amyloid deposits surrounded by vacuolar halos. The detection of PrP-res in the tonsillar tissue by immunohistochemical staining is also strongly supportive of nvCJD diagnosis.[25]

GENERAL THERAPY

The approach to a patient with a presumed CNS viral infection must be tailored to the severity and distribution of neurological involvement. After establishing the degree of CNS disease by history and physical examination, and stabilizing the patient (airway, breathing, circulation), the clinician must next ascertain a diagnosis. With the advent of highly sensitive and less invasive diagnostic techniques (CSF PCR), identification of treatable forms of viral CNS disease (notably HSE) is essential in preventing further CNS damage. Potentially treatable diseases (fungal CNS infections, partially treated bacterial meningitis, tuberculous meningitis, parameningeal infection, mycoplasma, fastidious bacterial infections) can mimic viral CNS disease and should be vigorously investigated before attributing the illness to an untreatable viral etiology. The same logic applies to treatable viral infections and non-infectious etiologies. In the normal host, viral meningitis is a relatively benign self-limited disease and does not usually warrant specific antiviral treatment.[55] In certain cases (e.g. neonate or agammaglobulinemic patient), therapy may be required. After establishing a presumptive diagnosis and instituting therapy, the clinician must anticipate and treat complications (seizures, syndrome of inappropriate antidiuretic hormone secretion, cerebral edema, cardiac arrhythmias or respiratory arrest from brainstem inflammation). Patients in a coma from encephalitis can recover after long periods of unconsciousness. The physician should limit the amount of iatrogenic damage and vigorously support the patient during the acute phase of the illness.

A limited number of antiviral medications are available to treat CNS infections. Prevention remains the mainstay of therapy. Historically the most frequent cause of viral CNS disease, mumps, has largely been eliminated through vaccination. Live attenuated vaccines against measles, mumps and rubella have resulted in a dramatic decrease in the incidence of encephalitis and postinfectious encephalitis in industrialized countries. Vaccination has also changed the character of previously common viral CNS disease. In 1952, poliomyelitis affected 57 879 Americans. Widespread vaccination has eliminated disease in the Western hemisphere and reduced the incidence worldwide.[56] Vaccines exist for some arboviral infections. Vaccination against Japanese encephalitis virus has reduced the incidence of encephalitis in Asia; however, in China where 70 million children are immunized for this virus, cases still occur annually.[57,58]

In order to reduce the potential exposure to TSE agents in the blood supply, the US Food and Drug Administration (FDA) has implemented guidelines eliminating whole blood or blood components prepared from individuals who later developed CJD or nvCJD. Changes in agricultural practices in Europe and bans on infected cattle have been associated with a decline in cases of nvCJD. In North America no cases of nvCJD have been reported and the Department of Agriculture has programs in place to monitor for TSEs in livestock. Further discussion will be limited to those infections for which therapies exist (HSV-1, HSV-2, VZV, cytomegalovirus, HIV, B-virus and enterovirus infection).

CHEMOTHERAPEUTICS

HSV INFECTION – ENCEPHALITIS

The introduction of aciclovir has resulted in a sharp decline in mortality and morbidity from herpes infections. For example, neonatal mortality from disseminated HSV disease and HSE has declined from 70% to 40% since the development of aciclovir and vidarabine.[1] Aciclovir (9-[2-hydroxyethoxymethyl] guanine) is a nucleoside analog that is selectively phosphorylated by the HSV-1 and HSV-2 thymidine kinase gene product and then incorporated into the viral genome during DNA synthesis, resulting in premature DNA chain termination. The Collaborative Antiviral Study Group randomized controlled trials in the 1980s established that 81% of adults with biopsy-proven HSE who received aciclovir at 10 mg/kg every 8 h for 10–14 days survived and 38% of the aciclovir recipients regained normal neurological function.[59] Early initiation of antiviral therapy is essential for optimal recovery. Patients with encephalitis lasting longer than 4 days had a worse outcome. For HSE, intravenous administration of aciclovir is the treatment of choice and oral antivirals should not be used.

In cases of neonatal HSV infection, aciclovir dosage, treatment duration and toxicities differ from adult HSE therapy. Encephalitis occurs in 33% of neonates perinatally infected with HSV. Neonates with evidence of CNS dysfunction or cutaneous manifestations of HSV infection should be empirically started on high-dose aciclovir until HSV neurological infection can be excluded. In neonates with localized cutaneous or mucocutaneous disease, intravenous aciclovir 15 mg/kg every 8 h (45 mg/kg per day) for a minimum of 14–21 days is the treatment of choice. Neonates demonstrate a much lower rate of viral clearance than do immunocompromised adults, thus justifying the longer duration of treatment.[1] Higher dose therapy, 20 mg/kg intravenously every 8 h (60 mg/kg per day), is used for neonates with disseminated disease or evidence of neurological involvement. A minimum of 14–21 days of therapy is indicated for the treatment of neonatal HSE. In patients who have evidence of viral DNA in the CSF after a standard course of aciclovir, therapy should be extended until virus is no longer detectable. Studies are currently ongoing evaluating the utility of aciclovir therapy for reactivations and suppressive therapy during the first 6 months of life.[50,60]

Aciclovir is associated with few adverse effects. In patients receiving large doses of aciclovir by rapid infusion, a dose-related nephrotoxicity from crystal deposition has been reported but is readily reversible with slower infusion times and improved hydration.[61] CNS disturbances (hallucinations, disorientation, tremors) have also been reported with aciclovir therapy.[62,63] Neutropenia is well documented in children receiving prolonged aciclovir therapy.

HSV INFECTION – MENINGITIS

Although no definitive clinical trials have been conducted, most authors recommend the use of intravenous aciclovir (10 mg/kg every 8 h) for HSV meningitis associated with primary HSV-2 infection, as it decreases the duration of primary herpes disease and may limit meningeal involvement.[64] Recurrent HSV-2 meningitis occurs rarely and recently a single case of meningitis associated with HSV-1 reactivation was reported. At this time there are no data on the benefit of antiviral treatment or on suppressive therapy for recurrent HSV CNS disease.[65]

VARICELLA ZOSTER VIRUS

Varicella immunoglobulin (VZIG) and aciclovir have reduced the complications from primary VZV infection and herpes zoster in the neonate and immunocompromised patient. VariZIG is no longer produced by the Red Cross but is available under an investigational new drug (IND) protocol through FFF Enterprises. Although controlled trials have not evaluated the efficacy of aciclovir in VZV CNS infections, the medication is routinely used to treat this complication.[66,67] Varicella can produce cerebral vasculitis, postinfectious encephalitis, ventriculitis, meningitis, and, historically, encephalopathy (Reye's syndrome). Other than postinfectious encephalitis, most of the VZV CNS manifestations are rare and occur most frequently in immunocompromised patients. Empirical therapy using intravenous aciclovir 10–15 mg/kg every 8 h for 10 days, combined with prednisone 60–80 mg for 3–5 days, is recommended for patients with large vessel cerebral vasculitis. Small vessel encephalitis should also be treated with aciclovir 5–10 mg/kg every 8 h for a minimum of 10 days.[67] Myelitis can complicate acute VZV or zosteriform reactivation, especially in immunocompromised patients, and presents as paraparesis 1–2 weeks after the development of a rash. MRI studies demonstrate significant spinal cord involvement, while the CSF from patients frequently demonstrates an inflammatory infiltrate or increased protein levels. The demonstration of VZV in the CSF by PCR or the demonstration of specific antibodies in the CSF confirms the diagnosis. Aggressive treatment with intravenous aciclovir as described above for small vessel encephalitis can produce clinical improvements.[68]

CONGENITAL CYTOEGALOVIRUS INFECTION

Ganciclovir and foscarnet have been used for the treatment of cytomegalovirus encephalitis, although controlled clinical trials have not confirmed the efficacy of treatment. In the case of congenital cytomegalovirus infection, a multicenter study demonstrated slight protection against hearing loss for a subset of congenitally infected neonates receiving intravenous ganciclovir during the first 6 months of life. The children enrolled in this study were severely affected (CNS calcifications, microcephalic) and were closely monitored for development of hepatitis or neutropenia.[69] A follow-up randomized controlled trial is evaluating the oral prodrug (valganciclovir) and the effect of duration of therapy (6 months vs 6 weeks) upon neurodevelopmental outcome and hearing in symptomatic congenitally infected infants (D Kimberlin, personal communication).

CERCOPITHECINE HERPES INFECTION (B VIRUS)

B virus is indigenous in old world monkeys (rhesus, cynologous and Asian species of the *Macaca* genus) and causes a frequently fatal disease in humans if not treated. Infection has been documented in most cases following direct inoculation (bites), although cases exist following exposure to infected materials (animal bedding) as well as human-to-human spread. In humans bitten by an infected animal, the risk of transmission is low, as the frequency of virus excretion is only 2–3% in infected animals at any given time.[70] Nonetheless, because of the severity of infection, therapy should be instituted immediately. B virus infection in humans produces a rapid infection with evidence of a vesicular rash and an ascending myelitis in most cases within days and progression within a month.[71,72] Ultimately, 90% of the documented infected persons progressed to develop encephalomyelitis and 70% died.

Management of potential B virus exposure is controversial but guidelines set up by the 2002 B Virus Working Group provide a framework for post-exposure management. Similar to post-exposure rabies treatment, rapid wound decontamination minutes after the injury is the most important component and the only way of preventing infection. Thorough irrigation for 15 min with water or sterile saline (mucosal surfaces), along with washing with detergent or a povidone–iodine-containing solution (non-mucosal surfaces), is critical in preventing infection.[71,73] In persons bitten by a known infected or seropositive animal, cultures should be obtained from the animal (buccal mucosa of the biting monkey, urogenital area for urine exposure, swab from the cage for infected bedding). Some authors recommend culturing the patient after thorough cleansing and irrigation have been completed. Even more controversial are the recommendations for instituting prophylactic antiviral therapy. In order to be most effective, antiviral therapy must be initiated before the onset of neurological symptoms;

however, few exposed cases progress to disease. The 2002 B Virus Working Group recommended antiviral prophylaxis based upon the likely risk of virus exposure or infection. The likelihood of infection is influenced by: (1) the type of primate exposure (macaque highest risk); (2) timeliness and adequacy of irrigation and first aid; (3) the type, depth and location of the wound; and (4) the type of infectious materials in cases of indirect exposure. Based on the guidelines from the 2002 B Virus Working Group, prophylaxis should be considered or is recommended except for contact with skin where there is no break in the skin or after exposure to a non-macaque species. For high-risk exposures (infected shedding monkeys, monkeys of unknown B-virus serology, ill macaques or a high titer fluid source) prophylaxis is indicated, especially if the wound was not immediately cleansed/irrigated for 15 min, or if the wound is a deep laceration or puncture. Because the inhibitory concentration of aciclovir for B-virus is ~10-fold higher than that for HSV-1, high-dose prophylaxis should be administered. Because valaciclovir and famciclovir achieve higher antiviral bloodstream concentrations, they are considered superior to aciclovir or penciclovir. While recent in-vitro data suggest that the B virus TK gene has lower affinity for the acyclonucleosides (aciclovir, ganciclovir, 5-bromovinyldeoxyuridine) when compared with penciclovir, in-vitro susceptibility studies showed that inhibition of replication of B virus in cell culture did not consistently correlate with substrate affinity.[74]

The 2002 B Virus Working Group recommended the use of the highly bioavailable prodrug valaciclovir (1 g orally every 8 h) because the prodrug provides higher serum levels of aciclovir and, unlike famciclovir, has been evaluated in in-vivo studies.[73] If valaciclovir is unavailable, high-dose aciclovir (varicella dose regimen five times per day) was recommended by the 2002 B Virus Working Group. In-vitro data suggest that famciclovir (500 mg orally every 8 h) could be used for B-virus prophylaxis and has higher affinity for the TK gene; however, in-vivo studies are not currently available.[71,73,74] If B virus is cultured from the wound culture, from the monkey, or if the bitten worker develops cutaneous or peripheral nervous system signs or symptoms of B-virus infection, immediate hospitalization (with body fluid precautions) is required and intravenous aciclovir or ganciclovir instituted until symptoms resolve and three consecutive culture sets are negative.[73] Patients with central neurological signs or symptoms of B-virus infection should receive intravenous ganciclovir 5 mg/kg every 12 h according to the 2002 B Virus Working Group recommendations.[73]

It is equally important in the management of these patients to obtain acute and convalescent serological studies. In patients with B-virus infection (seroconversion or clinical disease), long-term management is essential. Be aware that antiviral prophylaxis, however, can interfere with humoral response and diagnostic studies. Experts at the CDC should be consulted for more detailed information on this subject. In general, long-term management requires monitoring the patient for evidence of virus shedding and in most instances long-term oral antiviral prophylaxis (minimum of 6 months, although some authors recommend lifelong suppression).

ENTEROVIRUS INFECTION

Currently antibody preparations and an antiviral agent, pleconaril, showed activity against enterovirus in case reports and animal studies. Randomized controlled trials, however, have not supported their use in routine enterovirus meningitis.[75,76]

RABIES VIRUS INFECTION

Pre- and immediate post-exposure prophylaxis are the only ways known to prevent death in rabies-exposed individuals.[31] Case reports exist of patients surviving symptomatic rabies without prior vaccination.[77-82] Other case reports, however, indicate that therapeutic pharmacological coma is not universally effective.[77,79] Most patients who survive rabies have prior immunity or received post-exposure prophylaxis prior to developing symptoms. Both of the surviving patients in the literature developed neutralizing antibodies in the CSF at or shortly after presentation.[83] An investigation is currently underway to evaluate the role of pharmacological coma in rabies after one patient without prior immunity survived after receiving this therapy.

Individuals exposed to rabies require vigorous cleansing of the wound, passive immunization with direct administration of rabies hyperimmunoglobulin at the site of the animal bite, and post-exposure intramuscular vaccination with human diploid cell vaccine or rhesus diploid cell vaccine on the first day of treatment and repeat doses on days 3, 7, 14 and 28 after the initial dose. Individuals with frequent contact with potentially rabid animals (veterinarians, animal control staff, workers in rabies laboratories and travelers to rabies-endemic areas) should receive pre-exposure vaccination.

ADEM/POSTINFECTIOUS ENCEPHALITIS

In cases of postinfectious encephalitis or ADEM, no randomized controlled trial has confirmed the benefit of immunomodulatory drugs. In practice, clinicians often treat ADEM with different immunomodulators (corticosteroids, intravenous immunoglobulin preparations, plasmapheresis) in an attempt to limit immune-mediated destruction of the CNS.[24,84-86] It must be emphasized, however, that no placebo-controlled studies have been performed and immunomodulatory therapy is based simply on isolated case reports. As with most case reports, clinical failures and iatrogenic morbidity from a therapeutic modality are rarely ever reported.

CONCLUSION

Central nervous system infections must be examined in a geographic, cultural and environmental context as well as at the cellular, molecular and genetic levels. The development of improved diagnostic and molecular biological studies should improve our understanding of viral pathogenesis and the development of targeted therapeutics for viral CNS infection.

 References

1. Cassady KA, Whitley RJ. Viral central nervous system infections. In: Richman DD, Whitley RJ, Hayden FG, eds. *Clinical virology*. 3rd ed. Washington, DC: ASM Press; 2009:29–44.
2. Nicolosi A, Hauser WA, Beghi E, Kurland LT. Epidemiology of central nervous system infections in Olmsted County, Minnesota, 1950–1981. *J Infect Dis*. 1986;154(3):399–408.
3. Nigrovic LE, Chiang VW. Cost analysis of enteroviral polymerase chain reaction in infants with fever and cerebrospinal fluid pleocytosis [see comments]. *Arch. Pediatr. Adolesc. Med*. 2000;154(8):81721.
4. Pozo F, Casas I, Tenorio A, Trallero G, Echevarria JM. Evaluation of a commercially available reverse transcription-PCR assay for diagnosis of enteroviral infection in archival and prospectively collected cerebrospinal fluid specimens. *J Clin Microbiol*. 1998;36(6):1741–1745.
5. Sawyer MH. Enterovirus infections: diagnosis and treatment [review]. *Pediatr Infect Dis J*. 1999;18(12):1033–1039.
6. Hosoya M, Honzumi K, Sato M, Katayose M, Kato K, Suzuki H. Application of PCR for various neurotropic viruses on the diagnosis of viral meningitis. *J Clin Virol*. 1998;11(2):117–124.
7. Kupila L, Vuorinen T, Vainionpaa R, Hukkanen V, Marttila RJ, Kotilainen P. Etiology of aseptic meningitis and encephalitis in an adult population. *Neurology*. 2006;66(1):75–80.
8. Kupila L, Vuorinen T, Vainionpaa R, Marttila RJ, Kotilainen P. Diagnosis of enteroviral meningitis by use of polymerase chain reaction of cerebrospinal fluid, stool, and serum specimens. *Clin Infect Dis*. 2005;40(7):982–987.
9. Johnson RT. Acute encephalitis. *Clin Infect Dis*. 1996;23(2):219–224 quiz 25-6.
10. Koskiniemi M, Korppi M, Mustonen K, et al. Epidemiology of encephalitis in children. A prospective multicentre study. *Eur J Pediatr*. 1997;156(7):541–545.
11. Glaser CA, Honarmand S, Anderson LJ, et al. Beyond viruses: clinical profiles and etiologies associated with encephalitis. *Clin Infect Dis*. 2006;43(12):1565–1577.
12. Khetsuriani N, Holman RC, Lamonte-Fowlkes AC, Selik RM, Anderson LJ. Trends in encephalitis-associated deaths in the United States. *Epidemiol Infect*. 2007;135(4):583–591.
13. Ho DD, Hirsch MS. Acute viral encephalitis. *Med Clin North Am*. 1985;69(2):415–429.
14. Vernet G. Diagnosis of zoonotic viral encephalitis. *Arch Virol Suppl*. 2004;(18):231–244.
15. McNabb SJ, Jajosky RA, Hall-Baker PA, et al. Summary of notifiable diseases – United States, 2005. *MMWR Morb Mortal Wkly Rep*. 2007;54(53):1–92.
16. Cassady KA, Whitley RJ. Viral central nervous system infections. In: Richman DD, Whitley RJ, Hayden FG, eds. *Clinical virology*. 2nd ed. Washington, DC: ASM Press; 2002:27–44.
17. Sejvar JJ. The evolving epidemiology of viral encephalitis. *Curr Opin Neurol*. 2006;19(4):350–357.
18. Ayukawa R, Fujimoto H, Ayabe M, et al. An unexpected outbreak of Japanese encephalitis in the Chugoku district of Japan, 2002. *Jpn J Infect Dis*. 2004;57(2):63–66.
19. Handy R, Lang S. Flavivirus encephalitis. *N Engl J Med*. 2004;351(17):1803–1804 author reply 1804.
20. Johnson RT. The pathogenesis of acute viral encephalitis and postinfectious encephalomyelitis. *J Infect Dis*. 1987;155(3):359–364.
21. Pape WJ, Fitzsimmons TD, Hoffman RE. Risk for rabies transmission from encounters with bats, Colorado, 1977–1996. *Emerg Infect Dis*. 1999;5(3):433–437.
22. CDC. Human Rabies – California, Georgia, Minnesota, New York, and Wisconsin, 2000. *MMWR Morb Mortal Wkly Rep*. 2000;49(49):1111–1115.
23. Kennedy PG. Viral encephalitis. *J Neurol*. 2005;252(3):268–272.
24. Stuve O, Zamvil SS. Pathogenesis, diagnosis, and treatment of acute disseminated encephalomyelitis [review]. *Curr Opin Neurol*. 1999;12(4):395–401.
25. Whitley RJ, Macdonald N, Ascher DM. Technical Report. Transmissible spongiform encephalopathies: a review for pediatricians. *Pediatrics*. 2000;106(5):1160–1165.

26. Collee JG, Bradley R, Liberski PP. Variant CJD (vCJD) and bovine spongiform encephalopathy (BSE): 10 and 20 years on: part 2. *Folia Neuropathol.* 2006;44(2):102–110.

27. Kimura H, Futamura M, Kito H, et al. Detection of viral DNA in neonatal herpes simplex virus infections: frequent and prolonged presence in serum and cerebrospinal fluid. *J Infect Dis.* 1991;164(2).289–293.

28. Stanberry LR, Floyd-Reising SA, Connelly BL, et al. Herpes simplex viremia: report of eight pediatric cases and review of the literature. *Clin Infect Dis.* 1994;18(3):401–407.

29. German AC, Myint KS, Mai NT, et al. A preliminary neuropathological study of Japanese encephalitis in humans and a mouse model. *Trans R Soc Trop Med Hyg.* 2006;100(12):1135–1145.

30. Wiestler OD, Leib SL, Brustle O, Spiegel H, Kleihues P. Neuropathology and pathogenesis of HIV encephalopathies. *Acta Histochemica Suppl.* 1992;42:107–114.

31. Mrak RE, Young L. Rabies encephalitis in humans: pathology, pathogenesis and pathophysiology. *J Neuropathol Exp Neurol.* 1994;53(1):1–10.

32. Rotbart HA, Brennan PJ, Fife KH, Romero JR, Griffin JA, McKinlay MA, et al. Enterovirus meningitis in adults. *Clin Infect Dis.* 1998;27:896–898.

33. Scheld WM, Whitley RJ, Marra CM. *Infections of the central nervous system.* 3rd ed. Philadelphia: Lippincott Williams & Wilkins; 2004.

34. Chou J, Kern ER, Whitley RJ, Roizman B. Mapping of herpes simplex virus-1 neurovirulence to gamma 134.5, a gene nonessential for growth in culture. *Science.* 1990;250(4985):1262–1266.

35. Markovitz NS, Baunoch D, Roizman B. The range and distribution of murine central nervous system cells infected with the gamma(1)34.5 mutant of herpes simplex virus 1. *J Virol.* 1997;71(7):5560–5569.

36. Bouffard JP, Riudavets MA, Holman R, Rushing EJ. Neuropathology of the brain and spinal cord in human West Nile virus infection. *Clin Neuropathol.* 2004;23(2):59–61.

37. Whitley RJ, Kimberlin DW. Herpes simplex encephalitis: children and adolescents. *Semin Pediatr Infect Dis.* 2005;16(1):17–23.

38. Pruisner SB. Novel proteinaceous infectious particles cause scrapie. *Science.* 1982;216:136–144.

39. Hilton DA. Pathogenesis and prevalence of variant Creutzfeldt–Jakob disease. *J Pathol.* 2006;208(2):134–141.

40. Hewitt P. vCJD and blood transfusion in the United Kingdom. *Transfus Clin Biol.* 2006;13(5):312–316.

41. Dobra SA, Bennett PG. vCJD and blood transfusion: risk assessment in the United Kingdom. *Transfus Clin Biol.* 2006;13(5):307–311.

42. Whitley RJ, Cobbs CG, Alford Jr CA, et al. Diseases that mimic herpes simplex encephalitis. Diagnosis, presentation, and outcome. NIAD Collaborative Antiviral Study Group. *J Am Med Assoc.* 1989;262(2):234–239.

43. Ahmed A, Brito F, Goto C, et al. Clinical utility of the polymerase chain reaction for diagnosis of enteroviral meningitis in infancy. *J Pediatr.* 1997;131(3):393–397.

44. Ramers C, Billman G, Hartin M, Ho S, Sawyer MH. Impact of a diagnostic cerebrospinal fluid enterovirus polymerase chain reaction test on patient management. *J Am Med Assoc.* 2000;283(20):2680–2685.

45. Steiner I, Budka H, Chaudhuri A, et al. Viral encephalitis: a review of diagnostic methods and guidelines for management. *Eur J Neurol.* 2005;12(5):331–343.

46. Debiasi RL, Tyler KL. Molecular methods for diagnosis of viral encephalitis. *Clin Microbiol Rev.* 2004;17(4):903–925 table of contents.

47. Al-Shekhlee A, Kocharian N, Suarez JJ. Re-evaluating the diagnostic methods in herpes simplex encephalitis. *Herpes.* 2006;13(1):17–19.

48. Domingues RB, Lakeman FD, Mayo MS, Whitley RJ. Application of competitive PCR to cerebrospinal fluid samples from patients with herpes simplex encephalitis. *J Clin Microbiol.* 1998;36(8):2229–2234.

49. Kuno G. Universal diagnostic RT-PCR protocol for arboviruses. *J Virol Methods.* 1998;72(1):27–41.

50. Fonseca-Aten M, Messina AF, Jafri HS, Sanchez PJ. Herpes simplex virus encephalitis during suppressive therapy with acyclovir in a premature infant. *Pediatrics.* 2005;115(3):804–809.

51. Deresiewicz RL, Thaler SJ, Hsu L, Zamani AA. Clinical and neuroradiographic manifestations of eastern equine encephalitis [see comments]. *N Engl J Med.* 1997;336(26):1867–1874.

52. Maschke M, Kastrup O, Forsting M, Diener HC. Update on neuroimaging in infectious central nervous system disease. *Curr Opin Neurol.* 2004;17(4):475–480.

53. Krasnianski A, Meissner B, Heinemann U, Zerr I. Clinical findings and diagnostic tests in Creutzfeldt–Jakob disease and variant Creutzfeldt–Jakob disease. *Folia Neuropathol.* 2004;42(suppl B):24–38.

54. Tschampa HJ, Kallenberg K, Urbach H, et al. MRI in the diagnosis of sporadic Creutzfeldt–Jakob disease: a study on inter-observer agreement. *Brain.* 2005;128(Pt 9):2026–2033.

55. Rorabaugh ML, Berlin LE, Heldrich F, et al. Aseptic meningitis in infants younger than 2 years of age: acute illness and neurologic complications. *Pediatrics.* 1993;92(2):206–211.

56. Progress toward interruption of wild poliovirus transmission – worldwide, 2008. *MMWR Morb Mortal Wkly Rep.* 2009;58(12):308–312.

57. Lam K, Tsang OT, Yung RW, Lau KK. Japanese encephalitis in Hong Kong. *Hong Kong Med J.* 2005;11(3):182–188.

58. Liu W, Clemens JD, Yang JY, Xu ZY. Immunization against Japanese encephalitis in China: a policy analysis. *Vaccine.* 2006;24(24):5178–5182.

59. Whitley RJ, Alford CA, Hirsch MS, et al. Vidarabine versus acyclovir therapy in herpes simplex encephalitis. *N Engl J Med.* 1986;314(3):144–149.

60. Kimberlin D, Powell D, Gruber W, et al. Administration of oral acyclovir suppressive therapy after neonatal herpes simplex virus disease limited to the skin, eyes and mouth: results of a phase I/II trial. *Pediatr Infect Dis J.* 1996;15(3):247–254.

61. Mihara A, Mori T, Nakazato T, Ikeda Y, Okamoto S. Acute renal failure caused by intravenous acyclovir for disseminated varicella zoster virus infection. *Scand J Infect Dis.* 2007;39(1):94–95.

62. Yang HH, Hsiao YP, Shih HC, Yang JH. Acyclovir-induced neuropsychosis successfully recovered after immediate hemodialysis in an end-stage renal disease patient. *Int J Dermatolo.* 2007;46(8):883–884.

63. Das V, Peraldi MN, Legendre C. Adverse neuropsychiatric effects of cytomegalovirus prophylaxis with valaciclovir in renal transplant recipients. *Nephrology, Dialysis. Transplantation.* 2006;21(5):1395–1401.

64. Whitley RJ, Gnann JWJ. Acyclovir: a decade later. *N Engl J Med.* 1992;327:782–793.

65. Conway JH, Weinberg A, Ashley RL, Amer J, Levin MJ. Viral meningitis in a preadolescent child caused by reactivation of latent herpes simplex (type 1). *Pediatr Infect Dis J.* 1997;16(6):627–629.

66. Arvin AM. Antiviral therapy for varicella and herpes zoster. *Semin Pediatr Infect Dis.* 2002;13(1):12–21.

67. Gilden DH, Kleinschmidt-DeMasters BK, LaGuardia JJ, Mahalingam R, Cohrs RJ. Neurologic complications of the reactivation of varicella-zoster virus. *N Engl J Med.* 2000;342(9):635–645.

68. de Silva SM, Mark AS, Gilden DH, et al. Zoster myelitis: improvement with antiviral therapy in two cases. *Neurology.* 1996;47:929–931.

69. Kimberlin DW, Lin CY, Sanchez P, et al. Ganciclovir (GCV) treatment of symptomatic congenital cytomegalovirus (CMV) infections: results of a phase III randomized trial. *40th Interscience Conference on Antimicrobial Agents and Chemotherapy, September 17–20.* Canada Toronto; 2000.

70. Keeble SA, Christofinis GJ, Wood W. Natural virus B infection in rhesus monkeys. *J Patholo Bacteriol.* 1958;76:189–199.

71. Huff JL, Barry PA. B-virus (Cercopithecine herpesvirus 1) infection in humans and macaques: potential for zoonotic disease. *Emerg Infect Dis.* 2003;9(2):246–250.

72. Ritchey JW, Payton ME, Eberle R. Clinicopathological characterization of monkey B virus (Cercopithecine herpesvirus 1) infection in mice. *J Comp Pathol.* 2005;132(2–3):202–217.

73. Cohen JI, Davenport DS, Stewart JA, Deitchman S, Hilliard JK, Chapman LE. Recommendations for prevention of and therapy for exposure to B virus (cercopithecine herpesvirus 1). *Clin Infect Dis.* 2002;35(10):1191–1203.

74. Focher F, Lossani A, Verri A, et al. Sensitivity of monkey B virus (Cercopithecine herpesvirus 1) to antiviral drugs: role of thymidine kinase in antiviral activities of substrate analogs and acyclonucleosides. *Antimicrob Agents Chemother.* 2007;51(6):2028–2034.

75. Desmond RA, Accortt NA, Talley L, Villano SA, Soong SJ, Whitley RJ. Enteroviral meningitis: natural history and outcome of pleconaril therapy. *Antimicrob Agents Chemother.* 2006;50(7):2409–2414.

76. Abzug MJ, Cloud G, Bradley J, et al. Double blind placebo-controlled trial of pleconaril in infants with enterovirus meningitis. *Pediatr Infect Dis J.* 2003;22(4):335–341.

77. McDermid RC, Saxinger L, Lee B, et al. Human rabies encephalitis following bat exposure: failure of therapeutic coma. *Can Med Assoc J.* 2008;178(5):557–561.

78. Watson NF, Woo D, Doherty MJ, et al. Humoral immune responses after rabies infection. *Arch Neurol.* 2007;64(9):1355–1356.

79. Hemachudha T, Sunsaneewitayakul B, Desudchit T, et al. Failure of therapeutic coma and ketamine for therapy of human rabies. *J Neurovirol.* 2006;12(5):407–409.

80. Hemachudha T, Wilde H. Survival after treatment of rabies. *N Engl J Med*. 2005;353(10):1068–1069 author reply 1069.

81. Jackson AC. Recovery from rabies. *N Engl J Med*. 2005;352(24):2549–2550.

82. Willoughby Jr RE, Tieves KS, Hoffman GM, et al. Survival after treatment of rabies with induction of coma. *N Engl J Med*. 2005;352(24):2508–2514.

83. Wilde H, Hemachudha T, Jackson AC. Viewpoint: Management of human rabies. *Trans R Soc Trop Med Hyg*. 2008;102(10):979–982.

84. Pradhan S, Gupta RP, Shashank S, Pandey N. Intravenous immunoglobulin therapy in acute disseminated encephalomyelitis. *J Neurol Sci*. 1999;165(1):56–61.

85. Aronica E, Boer K, van Vliet EA, et al. Complement activation in experimental and human temporal lobe epilepsy. *Neurobiol Dis*. 2007;26(3):497–511.

86. Nishikawa M, Ichiyama T, Hayashi T, Ouchi K, Furukawa S. Intravenous immunoglobulin therapy in acute disseminated encephalomyelitis. *Pediatr Neurol*. 1999;21(2):583–586.

52 Bone and joint infections

Werner Zimmerli

The different bone and joint infections vary in regard to pathogenesis, diagnostic investigation and treatment. Whereas acute hematogenous osteomyelitis can generally be treated with antibiotics alone, implant-associated osteomyelitis needs careful surgical debridement combined with long-term antibiotics.[1] The presence of infected implant material requires different treatment principles since bacteria adhere to the foreign surface by forming a biofilm.[2,3] As most antibiotics have no effect on biofilm bacteria, treatment needs to be for as long as a stable internal fixation is required, or an antibiotic should be used with efficacy on stationary phase and adherent bacteria.[1,2,4]

In the case of diabetic foot ulcers, it is important to know whether the patient has superficial infection or osteomyelitis. Microbiological diagnosis usually requires the culture of invasive biopsies, due to the poor correlation between superficial cultures and bone cultures.[5] Septic native arthritis and periprosthetic joint infection are different diseases. Whereas the former generally responds to antibiotics and non-invasive joint lavage, periprosthetic arthritis always needs long-term antibiotics combined with careful debridement, surgery and sometimes even joint replacement.[6]

In studies of antimicrobial therapy of bone and joint infection, results are often presented at the end of treatment without adequate follow-up. In a meta-analysis of 167 studies of antibiotic treatment of different types of bone and joint infection, only 37 were randomized and 22 remained eligible.[7] In 771 out of 927 patients, a 1-year follow-up was reported. In the eligible patients, an eradication rate of 78.6% (95% CI, 66–94%) was found. There were no differences between comparative antibiotic treatment groups, except for rifampicin (rifampin) in device-associated infection.[4] Interestingly, standard intravenous therapy and oral fluoroquinolones were equivalent in seven studies published between 1987 and 1999.[7] These data may be outdated because of increasing resistance; Staphylococcus aureus is the most frequent micro-organism in bone and joint infection and treatment with fluoroquinolones alone is compromised by the rapid emergence of resistance during therapy.[4,8] In summary, the following apply to the analysis of antimicrobial therapy of bone and joint infection: (1) end of treatment analysis is useless; 1-year follow-up is adequate; (2) 2-year follow-up is required in device-associated infection; (3) concomitant adequate surgical management is needed in chronic osteomyelitis and periprosthetic joint infection; and (4) when analyzing older studies, the current resistance pattern of bone and joint pathogens should be considered.

CLASSIFICATION OF OSTEOMYELITIS

There are several classifications of osteomyelitis that consider pathogenesis, duration of infection, localization, presence or absence of an implant, or anatomic type and local host factors. Cierny and Mader developed a classification system which is especially useful for orthopedic surgeons treating patients with chronic osteomyelitis.[9] For infection specialists, a more useful approach considers the pathogenesis of bone infection.[10] Hematogenous osteomyelitis bacterial seeding in bone mainly occurs in the metaphysis of long bones of prepubertal children and in the vertebral column of adults.[11] Exogenous osteomyelitis spreading from a contiguous source mainly follows thorax surgery (sternum osteomyelitis), bite wounds, deep perforating lesions (mainly on feet), chronic ear, nose and throat infections (sinusitis, otitis media), open bone fractures, joint replacement or internal fixation.[12] Another type of exogenous osteomyelitis results from deep soft-tissue infections mainly in diabetic patients with vascular insufficiency and/or neuropathy.[13]

HEMATOGENOUS OSTEOMYELITIS

Hematogenous infection of the metaphysis of long bones is seen in young children. It is mainly caused by Staphylococcus aureus, group-B streptococci and various other streptococci. Haemophilus influenzae group b has almost disappeared due to widely used vaccination. The main symptoms are fever, local pain, signs of inflammation and sinus tracts in untreated chronic cases. In cases of unclear bone pain after a bacterial infection, osteomyelitis should be sought.

In adults, hematogenous osteomyelitis mainly involves vertebral bodies. The risk of infection rises with increasing age.[14] In almost 60% of cases, spondylodiskitis is in the lumbar or lumbosacral region. It is mainly caused by *Staph. aureus* (~50%), Gram-negative bacilli (~25%) and streptococci (~10%).[14,15] Tuberculous or brucellar spondylitis is still prevalent in endemic regions (e.g. Southern Europe), whereas it has almost disappeared in Central and Northern Europe. The predominant symptoms are fever, backache and local pain in the involved vertebrae. Local signs of infection are generally not present. Severe local pain is a classic sign of spinal epidural abscess; neurological signs have to be looked for and emergency MRI evaluation is required.[16] Diagnosis comprises blood cultures, C-reactive protein and white cell differential counts. Imaging procedures include ^{99m}Tc-methylene diphosphonate (MDP) bone scan, antigranulocyte antibody scan, CT scan and MRI.[14,17] MRI has the highest sensitivity and specificity. However, it should not be used for monitoring progress because of the low correlation between image improvement and healing.[18]

Acute hematogenous osteomyelitis can usually be successfully treated with antibiotics alone. Surgery is mainly required for diagnostic purposes (open biopsy) if blood cultures remain negative which occurs in 22–70% of cases.[14,19] In addition, surgery is also needed in patients with spinal epidural abscesses or paravertebral extension (e.g. psoas abscess).

Table 52.1 summarizes the antibiotic treatment according to the micro-organism isolated. The duration of therapy is not standardized; controlled studies are missing. A 6-week course of high-dose antibiotics is generally recommended for acute hematogenous osteomyelitis.[14,20] Treatment is generally started by the intravenous route. However, oral bactericidal drugs with excellent bioavailability are equally effective and allow early switch to the oral route. β-Lactams should not be commenced by the oral route because of their low bioavailability.

Staphylococcal osteomyelitis can be treated with a combination of quinolones (e.g. levofloxacin 750 mg orally per day) plus rifampicin (300 mg orally every 12 h). In a prospective randomized study in patients with deep-seated or bacteremic staphylococcal infection, the quinolone–rifampicin

Table 52.1 Antibiotic therapy for adults with hematogenous osteomyelitis (excludes patients with implant devices)

Micro-organism	Antimicrobial agent[a]	Dose[b]	Route
Staphylococcus aureus or coagulase-negative staphylococci			
Methicillin-susceptible	(Flu)cloxacillin[c] *followed by*	2 g every 6 h	i.v.
	rifampicin, *plus*	300 mg every 12 h	p.o.
	levofloxacin	750 mg every 24 h	p.o.
Methicillin-resistant	Vancomycin* *or*	1 g every 12 h	i.v.
	teicoplanin[e] *followed by*	400 mg (6 mg/kg) every 24 h	i.v., i.m.
	rifampicin *plus*	300 mg every 12 h	p.o.
	levofloxacin *or*	750 mg every 24 h	p.o.
	fusidic acid *or*	500 mg every 8 h	p.o.
	co-trimoxazole	960 mg every 8 h	p.o.
Streptococcus spp.	Penicillin G[c] *or*	5 million U (3g) every 6 h	i.v.
	ceftriaxone for 4 weeks, *followed by*	2 g every 24 h	i.v.
	amoxicillin	750–1000 mg every 8 h	p.o.
Enterococcus spp. (penicillin-susceptible)	Penicillin G *or*	5 million U (3g) every 6 h	i.v.
	ampicillin or amoxicillin *plus*	2 g every 4–6 h	i.v.
	aminoglycoside[f]		i.v.
Enterobacteriaceae (quinolone-susceptible)	Ciprofloxacin	750 mg every 12 h	p.o.
Non-fermenters (e.g. *Pseudomonas aeruginosa*)	Cefepime or ceftazidime *plus*	2 g every 8 h	i.v.
	aminoglycoside[f] for 2–4 weeks, *followed by*		i.v.
	ciprofloxacin	750 mg every 12 h	p.o.
Anaerobes[g]	Clindamycin for 2–4 weeks, *followed by*	600 mg every 6–8 h	i.v.
	clindamycin	300 mg every 6 h	p.o.
Mixed infections (without methicillin–resistant staphylococci)	piperacillin–tazobactam *or*	4.5 g every 8 h	i.v.
	imipenem *or*	500 mg every 6 h	i.v.
	meropenem	1 g every 8 h	i.v.
	for 2–4 weeks, followed by individual regimens according to antimicrobial susceptibility		

*Vancomycin trough level should exceed 15 mg/litre
[a]In the absence of an implant the total duration of antimicrobial treatment is generally 6 weeks.
[b]All dosages are for adults assuming normal renal function.
[c]In patients with delayed hypersensitivity to penicillins, cefuroxime (1.5 g i.v. every 6–8 h) can be administered. In patients with immediate hypersensitivity to penicillins, vancomycin (1 g i.v. every 12 h) is recommended.
[d]Trough blood levels should be monitored regularly during treatment.
[e]A loading dose of 800 mg i.v. in one or two doses should be given on day 1. Trough level should exceed 20 mg/litre
[f]Aminoglycosides can be administered in a single daily dose.
[g]Alternatively, penicillin G (5 million U (3g) i.v. every 6 h) or ceftriaxone (2 g i.v. every 24 h) can be used for Gram-positive anaerobes (e.g. *Propionibacterium acnes*), and metronidazole (500 mg i.v. or p.o. every 8 h) for Gram-negative anaerobes (e.g. *Bacteroides* spp.).
i.m., intramuscular, i.v., intravenous, p.o. orally.
[h]Note: Formulations of amoxicillin-clavulanic acid differ internationally, therefore dose should be checked.

combination was equivalent to standard intravenous therapy.[21] Clindamycin has good bioavailability, but is only bacteriostatic against staphylococci. Therefore, it is adequate for long-term therapy of chronic osteomyelitis, and should not be given in acute spondylodiskitis caused by *Staph. aureus*. Nowadays, it is no longer adequate to treat staphylococcal osteomyelitis with a quinolone alone, even with newer fluoroquinolones; because of the risk of emergence of resistance, quinolones should always be combined with rifampicin in the treatment of susceptible staphylococci.[21]

OSTEOSYNTHESIS-ASSOCIATED OSTEOMYELITIS

Infections associated with internal fracture fixation generally occur exogenously as a result of the penetrating trauma (preoperatively), during insertion of the fixation device (intraoperatively) or during disturbed wound healing (postoperatively).[22] The most common micro-organisms causing implant-associated infections are *Staph. aureus* (30%), coagulase-negative staphylococci (22%) and Gram-negative bacilli (10%).[23]

Infections after internal fixation are classified as early (<2 weeks), delayed (2–10 weeks) and late onset (>10 weeks).[22,24] Leading clinical signs of early infection are persistent local pain, erythema, edema, wound healing disturbance, large hematoma and fever. Highly virulent organisms (e.g. *Staph. aureus*, Gram-negative bacilli) are frequent agents of early infections. In cases of wound healing disturbance, necrosis of the wound edges or postoperative hematoma and infection must be actively sought.[25,26]

Persistent or increasing pain, pseudarthrosis, implant loosening and occasionally development of a sinus tract are hallmarks of delayed infection. However, clinical signs and symptoms of infection may be entirely lacking. Delayed and late infections are mainly caused by micro-organisms of low virulence (e.g. coagulase-negative staphylococci). Alternatively, manifestation of infection due to any micro-organism may be delayed because initial antimicrobial treatment was insufficient for complete microbial eradication. Late infections may be caused by a low inoculum or low virulence micro-organisms introduced during penetrating trauma or perioperatively with an insidious onset of systemic or local symptoms.

A combination of clinical, laboratory, histopathological, microbiological and imaging studies is required to diagnose infection. Blood leukocyte count and differential are neither sufficiently sensitive nor specific to confirm osteomyelitis. Repeated postoperative measurements of C-reactive protein, or a secondary increase after an initial postoperative fall, are highly suggestive of infection. Preoperative aspiration of accumulated fluid and intraoperative tissue cultures provide the most accurate microbiological specimens. At least three intraoperative tissue areas should be sampled. Swabs should be avoided because of low sensitivity. It is important to discontinue any antimicrobial therapy at least 2 weeks before collecting tissue cultures.[27] If the implanted material is removed,

the use of sonication to dislodge micro-organisms from the surface of explanted devices has the best sensitivity.[28] Imaging lacks sensitivity in early infection, but is useful in delayed and late infections to assess the extent of infection.[29]

Treatment includes both surgery and antibiotic therapy. The goals of treating infection associated with internal fixation devices are to consolidate the fracture and prevent chronic osteomyelitis. Complete eradication of infection is not the primary goal, since the device can be removed once consolidated. If the implant is stable, debridement with retention of the fracture-fixation device combined with long-term antibiotic treatment is reasonable.[4] In cases of chronic osteomyelitis associated with a fixation device, surgical therapy should always include both orthopedic and plastic reconstructive surgery.

Antimicrobial therapy should ideally be based on clear microbiological evidence. Suggested antimicrobial treatment according to pathogen and its antimicrobial susceptibility has recently been published[1,6] and is similar to the recommendations for infection without an implant (Table 52.1). A controlled study in patients with device-associated staphylococcal infection supports initial intravenous treatment for 2 weeks, followed by rifampicin (450 mg orally every 12 h) once there is no more wound secretion. The dose of rifampicin in these patients is higher than in the absence of an implant.[4,21] The suggested treatment duration is 3 months in cases of device retention, but only 6 weeks if the infected device is removed. Except for quinolone-susceptible Gram-negative bacilli, intravenous treatment should be given initially and followed by oral therapy to complete the treatment course.

FOOT OSTEOMYELITIS

Diabetic foot infection is frequent due to the increasing prevalence of diabetes mellitus. Risk factors are: (1) peripheral motor, sensory and autonomic neuropathy; (2) neuro-osteoarthropathic deformities (Charcot foot); (3) arterial insufficiency; (4) uncontrolled hyperglycemia; (5) patient disabilities, such as reduced vision; and (6) maladaptive patient behaviors.[30] Diabetics have a 25% lifetime risk of foot complications. Fifteen percent have a risk of infected foot wounds, of which 20–66% involve bone.

Due to the importance of correct therapy, foot osteomyelitis must be diagnosed as early as possible. Most clinicians now rely on the 'probe-to-bone' test which has a positive predictive value of 89% which is comparable to MRI.[31] With this test, touching bone with a metallic instrument is indicative of osteomyelitis. Lavery et al[32] reported a lower positive predictive value of only 62%, because of a lower prevalence of osteomyelitis (20% vs 66%). Thus, probe to bone is an excellent test in patients with high pretest probability. Otherwise, MRI should be performed due to its high sensitivity (80–100%) and specificity (80–90%).[31]

The correlation between cultures from bone biopsy and wound biopsy is poor.[33] Identical pathogens were found in less than 20%.[34,35] Therefore, treatment of diabetic foot osteomyelitis should be based either on bone culture or empirically on the most frequent micro-organisms. Treatment according to wound biopsy culture results may be inadequate, since coagulase-negative staphylococci, *Corynebacterium* spp. and Gram-negative bacilli are heavily overestimated.[33]

According to newer treatment concepts, wound debridement with a 4- to 6-week antibiotic course should replace early amputation. In a review of 11 studies with 546 patients undergoing debridement and 1–6 months of antibiotics, the median remission rate was 65% (29–88%).[36] Thus, in about two-thirds of patients, early amputation can be avoided. If the patient can be treated with antimicrobial agents with excellent bioavailability, there is no need for intravenous therapy. However, there are a few exceptions. Patients with *Staph. aureus* infection should be treated initially with a bactericidal agent such as flucloxacillin (2 g intravenously every 6 h) or ampicillin-sulbactam (3 g intravenously every 8 h – see footnote[h] in Table 52. 1) in case of mixed infection with anaerobes. After about 2 weeks, this regimen can be switched to oral clindamycin (300 mg every 6 h). Similarly, *Pseudomonas aeruginosa* should be treated with an initial 2-week intravenous course (e.g. cefepime or ceftazidime 2 g every 8 h or piperacillin–tazobactam 4.5 g every 6-8 h) in order to diminish the bacterial density before starting the only possible oral therapy (ciprofloxacin 750 mg every 12 h). This may avoid the emergence of resistance to ciprofloxacin. Other micro-organisms should be treated according to susceptibility testing of bone cultures (Table 52.1). Oral therapy with linezolid (600 mg every 12 h) can be considered.[37] However, this option should be restricted to experienced clinicians alert to the myelotoxicity and neurotoxicity of this agent[38].

If no bone biopsy is available, empirical treatment should be given. In treatment of naive patients, clindamycin is a good option (300 mg orally every 6 h) since *Staph. aureus*, streptococci and anaerobes are the most frequent micro-organisms in diabetic osteomyelitis.[33] In pretreated patients, Gram-negative bacilli may be selected. Here a combination of clindamycin plus ciprofloxacin (750 mg orally every 12 h) is preferred.

The Infectious Diseases Society of America (IDSA) guidelines[30] recommend the following duration of treatment:

- If the patient requires amputation, a postoperative course of 2–5 days is sufficient.
- If there is residual infected soft tissue, a 2- to 4-week course is suggested.
- In case of residually infected but viable bone, a treatment course of 4–6 weeks is recommended.
- In chronic bone infections in which debridement is not possible, or residual bone sequestration is present, at least 3 months' treatment is required.

SEPTIC ARTHRITIS

Rapid diagnosis and prompt local and systemic therapy are key to a good prognosis in acute arthritis. With purulent arthritis, empirical antimicrobial therapy should be started immediately. Since surgical and antimicrobial treatment differ in the presence of an artificial joint, periprosthetic joint infections are discussed separately.

Bacterial arthritis is caused by either hematogenous seeding or direct exogenous inoculation. In an analysis of 2407 cases, the most common micro-organisms were *Staph. aureus* (44%), group A streptococci (8%), *Streptococcus pneumoniae* (6%) and *Escherichia coli* (4%).[39] In intravenous drug users, *Ps. aeruginosa* and *Candida* spp. are frequent pathogens, while in infants below 2 years *Kingella kingae* are encountered.[40] *Pasteuralla multocida* or *Captocytophaga* spp. are commonly found after cat or dog bites, while after human bites (e.g. fist-to-mouth trauma) bacteria from the HACEK group should be considered. Gonococcal arthritis should be suspected after sexual exposure, especially if the patient has oligoarthritis and a macular exanthem.[41] Patients with meningococcal arthritis share the same clinical picture.

Signs and symptoms of acute bacterial arthritis include pain, signs of inflammation (redness, heat) and impaired function due to pain and joint inflammation. The pain is present in the neutral position and increases with movement. In 90% of cases, a single joint is affected, predominantly the knee (45–55%) or the hip (15–25%). Septic arthritis is rare in other joints, but can occur even in syndesmoses (symphysis, sacroiliac and sternoclavicular joints).[42] Careful history may reveal rare diagnoses such as *Brucella* spp. (travel to Mediterranean region), *Salmonella* spp. (food history), *Pasteurella multocida*, *Capnocytophaga canimorsus* (animal bite), *Neisseria gonorrhoeae* (sexual exposure), *Mycoplasma hominis* (gynecological intervention) and *Ps. aeruginosa* (intravenous drug use).

The most important diagnostic investigations are blood cultures (positive in only 50%) and joint puncture. Leukocyte counts in synovial fluid can differentiate between inflammatory and culture-positive infectious arthritis where they exceed 20 000/μL. This value has a sensitivity of >80%;[43] however, patients with rheumatoid arthritis or crystal synovitis may also have leukocyte counts above this threshold. The culture is positive in 80–90% of patients with bacterial arthritis. The sensitivity increases by using pediatric blood cultures.[44] In most cases, imaging is unnecessary in acute septic arthritis. Ultrasound may be useful to detect synovial fluid, and bone scan (or CT scan) in sacroiliac arthritis. CT scan is preferred when concomitant psoas abscess is suspected.

Treatment of septic arthritis includes joint decompression and antibiotic therapy. The aim of local treatment is the elimination of granulocytes and their products (proteases) which can rapidly destroy the joint cartilage. Initial empirical antimicrobial therapy should be guided according to the history (see above). In general, an intravenous cephalosporin such as cefazolin (2 g every 8 h), or cefuroxime (1.5 g every 6–8 h) is appropriate. In the case of staphylococcal infection, therapy can be rapidly switched to an oral fluoroquinolone plus rifampicin[21] which is equivalent to classic intravenous therapy. This is not the case with oral β-lactams due to the inadequate joint drug concentrations. With fluoroquinolone-resistant strains, rifampicin can be combined with co-trimoxazole or fusidic acid. The total duration of therapy is 4 weeks.[21] Pneumococci and other streptococci should be treated with penicillin G for 3–4 weeks. Ceftriaxone is an alternative for outpatient therapy. Arthritis due to Enterobacteriaceae, gonococci or meningococci can be treated with an oral fluoroquinolone, once susceptibility is confirmed. The former needs 4 weeks, the latter 2–3 weeks of therapy.

PERIPROSTHETIC JOINT INFECTION

Periprosthetic joint infections (PJIs) are classified as early (<3 months), delayed (3–24 months) and late (>2 years after surgery).[1] In early infection, typical signs and symptoms include fever, shivering and tachycardia. In addition, local signs of postoperative wound infection such as erythema, warmth, a wet or gaping wound, as well as prolonged wound secretion are suspicious for surgical site infection. Early infections are mainly caused by *Staph. aureus* or Gram-negative bacilli. Delayed or low-grade infection is characterized by subtle or absent signs and symptoms. Persistent pain after implantation indicates inflammation and/or early loosening. This type of infection is mainly caused by low-virulence micro-organisms, such as coagulase-negative staphylococci and *Propionibacterium acnes*. Late infection is caused by hematogenous seeding. Hallmarks are sudden local joint pain due to inflammation or increasing pain due to loosening. The main sources of bacteremia are skin, respiratory tract, dental and urinary tract infection.[45] However, hematogenous infection can also occur after primary *Staph. aureus* sepsis without a detectable focus.[46]

PJI is confirmed if at least one of the following criteria is present: (1) growth of an identical micro-organism in two or more cultures of synovial fluid or periprosthetic tissue; (2) purulence of synovial fluid or the implant site; (3) presence of granulocytes on histopathological examination of periprosthetic tissue; or (4) presence of a sinus tract communicating with the device.[47]

For diagnosis of PJI, blood leukocyte count and differential are neither sensitive nor specific. C-reactive protein (CRP) is elevated after surgery and returns to normal within weeks;[48] as such, repeat measurements are more informative than a single value in the postoperative period. Procalcitonin or interleukin-6 are no better than CRP for diagnosing PJI.[49] Synovial fluid leukocyte count and differential allow differentiation of PJI from aseptic failure. The cut-off value of synovial leukocytes is much lower for diagnosing PJI than septic arthritis in native joints. In patients without inflammatory joint disease and PJI of a knee, a synovial fluid leukocyte count of >1.7 × 10^9/L and differential of >65% neutrophils has a sensitivity for diagnosing PJI of 94% and 97%, and specificity of 88% and 98%, respectively.[50] In total hip arthroplasty, the optimal cut-off is at 4.2 × 10^9 leukocytes/L.[51]

The diagnosis of infection by plain radiography includes rapid prosthetic migration, rapidly progressive periprosthetic osteolysis and/or irregular periprosthetic osteolysis.[52] CT scan is more sensitive than plain radiography in the imaging of joint space. It allows detection of joint effusion, sinus tracts, soft-tissue abscesses, bone erosion and periprosthetic lucency. The main drawbacks are metallic artifacts reducing image quality. MRI can be used safely in patients with non-ferromagnetic implants and has a better resolution for soft-tissue abnormalities than CT. The main disadvantages of MRI are imaging interferences in the vicinity of metal implants. Bone scintigraphy with ^{99m}Tc has a good sensitivity, but a low specificity to diagnose prosthetic joint infection. Scintigraphy with ^{99m}Tc-labeled monoclonal antibodies demonstrates an accuracy in the detection of prosthetic joint infection of 81%.[53] Fluorine-18-fluorodeoxyglucose (FDG) positron emission tomography (PET) has a sensitivity of 91% and a specificity of 87% for detecting PJI.[54]

Superficial wound or sinus tract cultures often yield skin micro-organisms and should be avoided. The yield from synovial fluid culture varies from 45% to 100%. Sensitivity may be improved by inoculation into a pediatric blood culture bottle.[44] The most reliable specimens for detecting micro-organism(s) are samples from periprosthetic tissue during surgery. At least three intraoperative tissue specimens should be sampled.[1] Swabs have a low sensitivity and should be avoided. It is important to discontinue antimicrobial therapy at least 2 weeks prior tissue sampling for culture.[27] Since implant-associated infection involves microbial biofilms, the yield of implant culture may be higher than the one of tissue specimens. Sonication of implants with the appropriate frequency, power density and time improves the yield of positive cultures in patients pretreated with antibiotics.[28]

In order to reach the goal of successful therapy, namely a long-term, pain-free, functional joint following complete eradication of infection, a combination of an appropriate surgical procedure and antimicrobial treatment acting on adherent bacteria is needed.[1,2,4,6,55] The cornerstone of successful treatment is early diagnosis; since treatment is less invasive in patients with a short history of infection (see Fig. 52.1). This requires a high degree of suspicion and strict avoidance of empirical antibiotics where the diagnosis is equivocal.

The choice of antimicrobial agents by pathogen and its susceptibility is summarized in Table 52.1.[1,6] Based on a controlled trial in patients with orthopedic implant-associated infection, 3 months for hip prostheses and 6 months for knee prostheses is suggested.[1,4] Intravenous treatment should be administered for the first 2 weeks, followed by oral therapy if a drug with good oral bioavailability is available.

The treatment course can be shortened to 6 weeks after explantation, if all foreign material is removed and no spacer is implanted. In this situation, persistence of a device-associated biofilm can be avoided. After 6 weeks of treatment, reimplantation should be delayed a further 2 weeks in order to obtain tissue specimens for culture and to confirm treatment success. After reimplantation, antimicrobial therapy is reinstated. If cultures of intraoperative specimens remain negative, antibiotic treatment is stopped. Otherwise it is continued for 3 and 6 months, respectively.

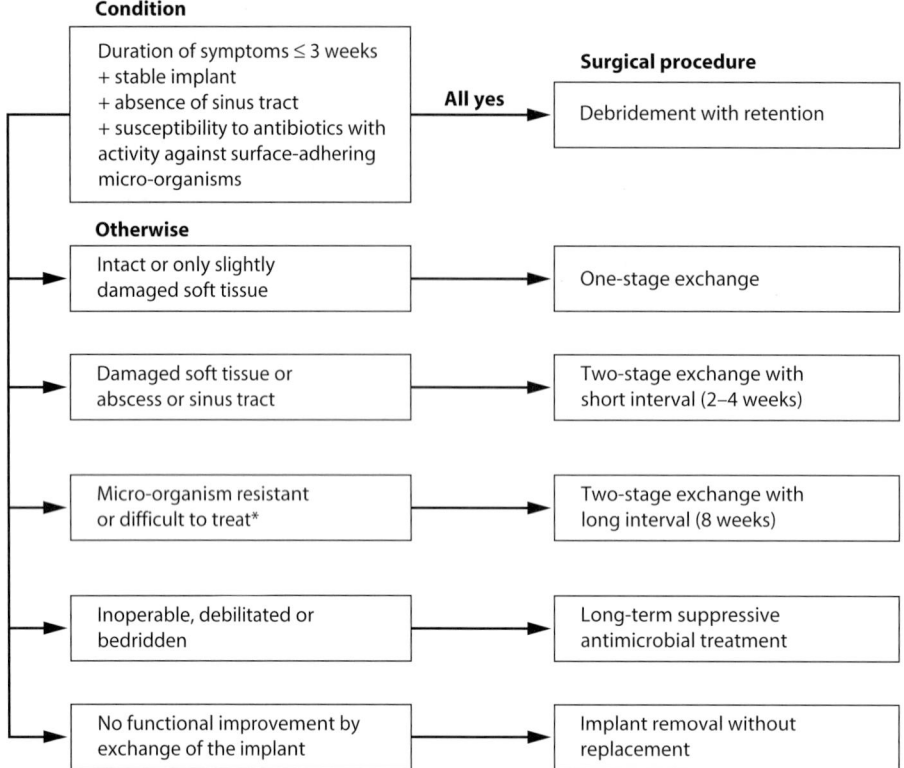

Fig. 52.1 Surgical treatment algorithm for prosthetic joint infections. * Difficult-to-treat micro-organisms include methicillin-resistant *Staph. aureus* (MRSA), small-colony variants of staphylococci,[68] enterococci, quinolone-resistant *Ps. aeruginosa* and fungi. (Modified from Trampuz A, Zimmerli W. Prosthetic joint infections: update in diagnosis and treatment. **Swiss Med Wkly.** 2005;135:243–251.)

Optimal antimicrobial therapy is best defined in staphylococcal implant infections. Rifampicin combination regimens have excellent activity on susceptible slow-growing and adherent staphylococci.[2] Rifampicin has proven activity in vitro, in animal models and in several clinical studies.[1,2,4,56,57] It must always be combined with another drug to prevent emergence of resistance in staphylococci. Quinolones are excellent drugs for combination therapy because of their good bioavailability, activity and safety. Newer quinolones have been studied in experimental bone infections,[58] but only anecdotal clinical data exist.[59] Since resistance of staphylococci to quinolones is an increasing problem, other anti-staphylococcal drugs have been combined with rifampicin, such as co-trimoxazole, minocycline, fusidic acid[60] or linezolid.[61] Linezolid is active against most Gram-positive cocci, including methicillin-resistant staphylococci and vancomycin-resistant enterococci (VRE). However, the success rate in patients with orthopedic infections is modest, with clinical cure rates of 55% and clinical improvement rates of 35%.[62] Unfortunately, adverse events such as reversible myelosuppression (40%) and irreversible peripheral neuropathy (5%) occur.[38] Experimentally, a combination of linezolid with rifampicin is more efficacious.[63] Daptomycin is active against several Gram-positive bacteria, including methicillin-resistant *Staph. aureus* (MRSA), vancomycin-resistant *Staph. aureus* and VRE. Its efficacy has been tested in an animal model of implant-associated infections, where it proved better in combination with rifampicin than vancomycin.[64]

In implant-associated infection, antimicrobial treatment without any surgical intervention usually fails. Figure 52.1 provides a treatment algorithm for surgery in PJI.

Debridement with retention has a success rate >80%[4,65–67] if the patients fulfill the following conditions: (1) stable implant; (2) pathogen with susceptibility to antimicrobial agents active against surface-adhering micro-organisms; (3) absence of a sinus tract or an abscess; and (4) duration of symptoms of infection of not more than 3 weeks.

Direct exchange includes the removal and implantation of a new prosthesis during the same surgical procedure. Patients with intact or only slightly compromised soft tissues qualify for this procedure. A success rate of 86–100% can be expected in appropriately selected patients.[1] If resistant or difficult-to-treat micro-organisms are causing the infection, such as MRSA, small-colony variants of staphylococci,[68] enterococci, quinolone-resistant *Ps. aeruginosa* or fungi, a two-stage revision is preferred. Two-stage exchange includes removal of the prosthesis with implantation of a new prosthesis during a later surgical procedure. In the absence of difficult-to-treat micro-organisms, a short interval until reimplantation (2–4 weeks) and a temporary antimicrobial-impregnated bone cement spacer may be used. If difficult-to-treat micro-organisms are isolated, a longer interval (8 weeks) without a spacer is preferred. The two-stage procedure can be used for every patient and has success rates exceeding 90%.[1] However, the expenditure for the patient and the surgeon is higher than for other surgical options.

Permanent removal of the device is usually reserved for patients with a high risk of reinfection (e.g. severe immunosuppression, active intravenous drug use) or when no functional improvement after reimplantation is expected. Alternatively, long-term antimicrobial suppression may be chosen, if the patient is inoperable, bedridden or debilitated. However, suppressive therapy only controls clinical symptoms rather than curing the infection. Therefore, infection relapses occur in most patients (>80%) when antimicrobials are discontinued.

CONCLUSION

Antimicrobial therapy of bone and joint infection should ideally be based on positive microbiological evidence. As an exception, diabetic foot osteomyelitis may be treated empirically if no debridement surgery is needed. Generally, prolonged treatment courses are required in order to avoid recurrence.

References

1. Zimmerli W, Trampuz A, Ochsner PE. Prosthetic-joint infections. *N Engl J Med.* 2004;351:1645–1654.
2. Zimmerli W, Frei R, Widmer AF, Rajacic Z. Microbiological tests to predict treatment outcome in experimental device-related infections due to *Staphylococcus aureus. J Antimicrob Chemother.* 1994;33:959–967.
3. Del Pozo JL, Patel R. The challenge of treating biofilm-associated bacterial infections. *Clin Pharmacol Ther.* 2007;82:204–209.
4. Zimmerli W, Widmer AF, Blatter M, Frei R, Ochsner PE. Role of rifampin for treatment of orthopedic implant-related staphylococcal infections: a randomized controlled trial. Foreign-Body Infection (FBI) Study Group. *JAMA.* 1998;279:1537–1541.
5. Senneville E, Morant H, Descamps D, et al. Needle puncture and transcutaneous bone biopsy cultures are inconsistent in patients with diabetes and suspected osteomyelitis of the foot. *Clin Infect Dis.* 2009;48:888–893.
6. Zimmerli W. Infection and musculoskeletal conditions: prosthetic-joint-associated infections. *Best Pract Res Clin Rheumatol.* 2006;20:1045–1063.
7. Stengel D, Bauwens K, Sehouli J, Ekkernkamp A, Porzsolt F. Systematic review and meta-analysis of antibiotic therapy for bone and joint infections. *Lancet Infect Dis.* 2001;1:175–188.
8. Coskun-Ari FF, Bosgelmez-Tinaz G. grlA and gyrA mutations and antimicrobial susceptibility in clinical isolates of ciprofloxacin–methicillin-resistant *Staphylococcus aureus. Eur J Med Res.* 2008;13:366–370.
9. Mader JT, Shirtliff M, Calhoun JH. Staging and staging application in osteomyelitis. *Clin Infect Dis.* 1997;25:1303–1309.
10. Lew DP, Waldvogel FA. Osteomyelitis. *Lancet.* 2004;364:369–379.
11. Waldvogel FA, Medoff G, Swartz MN. Treatment of osteomyelitis. *N Engl J Med.* 1970;283:822.
12. Patzakis MJ, Zalavras CG. Chronic posttraumatic osteomyelitis and infected nonunion of the tibia: current management concepts. *J Am Acad Orthop Surg.* 2005;13:417–427.
13. Armstrong DG, Lipsky BA. Diabetic foot infections: stepwise medical and surgical management. *Int Wound J.* 2004;1:123–132.
14. Zimmerli W. Vertebral osteomyelitis. *N Engl J Med* 2010;362:1022–1029.
15. McHenry MC, Easley KA, Locker GA. Vertebral osteomyelitis: long-term outcome for 253 patients from 7 Cleveland-area hospitals. *Clin Infect Dis.* 2002;34:1342–1350.
16. Sendi P, Bregenzer T, Zimmerli W. Spinal epidural abscess in clinical practice. *Q J M.* 2008;101:1–12.
17. Stumpe KD, Strobel K. Osteomyelitis and arthritis. *Semin Nucl Med.* 2009;39:27–35.
18. Kowalski TJ, Berbari EF, Huddleston PM, Steckelberg JM, Osmon DR. Do follow-up imaging examinations provide useful prognostic information in patients with spine infection? *Clin Infect Dis.* 2006;43:172–179.
19. Mylona E, Samarkos M, Kakalou E, Fanourgiakis P, Skoutelis A. Pyogenic vertebral osteomyelitis: a systematic review of clinical characteristics. *Semin Arthritis Rheum.* 2009;39(1):10–17.
20. Roblot F, Besnier JM, Juhel L, et al. Optimal duration of antibiotic therapy in vertebral osteomyelitis. *Semin Arthritis Rheum.* 2007;36:269–277.
21. Schrenzel J, Harbarth S, Schockmel G, et al. A randomized clinical trial to compare fleroxacin–rifampicin with flucloxacillin or vancomycin for the treatment of staphylococcal infection. *Clin Infect Dis.* 2004;39:1285–1292.
22. Trampuz A, Zimmerli W. Diagnosis and treatment of infections associated with fracture-fixation devices. *Injury* 2006;37 Suppl 2:S59–S66.
23. Trampuz A, Gilomen A, Flueckiger U 2005: Treatment outcome of infections associated with internal fixation devices: results from a 5-year retrospective study (1999–2003). 45th ICAAC, American Society for Microbiology; Washington, DC. 2005 December 16–19, 2005. No K-882.
24. Gustilo RB, Gruninger RP, Davis T. Classification of type III (severe) open fractures relative to treatment and results. *Orthopedics.* 1987;10:1781–1788.
25. Gustilo RB, Merkow RL, Templeman D. The management of open fractures. *J Bone Joint Surg Am.* 1990;72:299–304.
26. Zych GA, Hutson Jr JJ. Diagnosis and management of infection after tibial intramedullary nailing. *Clin Orthop Relat Res.* 1995;315:153–162.
27. Spangehl MJ, Masri BA, O'Connell JX, Duncan CP. Prospective analysis of preoperative and intraoperative investigations for the diagnosis of infection at the sites of two hundred and two revision total hip arthroplasties. *J Bone Joint Surg Am.* 1999;81:672–683.
28. Trampuz A, Piper KE, Jacobson MJ, et al. Sonication of removed hip and knee prostheses for diagnosis of infection. *N Engl J Med.* 2007;357:654–663.
29. Schiesser M, Stumpe KD, Trentz O, Kossmann T, Von Schulthess GK. Detection of metallic implant-associated infections with FDG PET in patients with trauma: correlation with microbiologic results. *Radiology.* 2003;226:391–398.
30. Lipsky BA, Berendt AR, Deery HG, et al. Diagnosis and treatment of diabetic foot infections. *Clin Infect Dis.* 2004;39:885–910.
31. Grayson ML, Gibbons GW, Balogh K, Levin E, Karchmer AW. Probing to bone in infected pedal ulcers. A clinical sign of underlying osteomyelitis in diabetic patients. *J Am Med Assoc.* 1995;273:721–723.
32. Lavery LA, Armstrong DG, Peters EJ, Lipsky BA. Probe-to-bone test for diagnosing diabetic foot osteomyelitis: reliable or relic? *Diabetes Care.* 2007;30:270–274.
33. Tan JS, Friedman NM, Hazelton-Miller C, Flanagan JP, File Jr TM. Can aggressive treatment of diabetic foot infections reduce the need for above-ankle amputation? *Clin Infect Dis.* 1996;23:286–291.
34. Lavery LA, Sariaya M, Ashry H, Harkless LB. Microbiology of osteomyelitis in diabetic foot infections. *J Foot Ankle Surg.* 1995;34:61–64.
35. Newman LG, Waller J, Palestro CJ, et al. Unsuspected osteomyelitis in diabetic foot ulcers. Diagnosis and monitoring by leukocyte scanning with indium in 111 oxyquinoline. *J Am Med Assoc.* 1991;266:1246–1251.
36. Jeffcoate WJ, Lipsky BA. Controversies in diagnosing and managing osteomyelitis of the foot in diabetes. *Clin Infect Dis.* 2004;39(suppl 2):115–122.
37. Majcher-Peszynska J, Haase G, Sass M, et al. Pharmacokinetics and penetration of linezolid into inflamed soft tissue in diabetic foot infections. *Eur J Clin Pharmacol.* 2008;64:1093–1100.
38. Bressler AM, Zimmer SM, Gilmore JL, Somani J. Peripheral neuropathy associated with prolonged use of linezolid. *Lancet Infect Dis.* 2004;4:528–531.
39. Ross JJ, Saltzman CL, Carling P, Shapiro DS. Pneumococcal septic arthritis: review of 190 cases. *Clin Infect Dis.* 2003;36:319–327.
40. Yagupsky P, Dagan R. *Kingella kingae:* an emerging cause of invasive infections in young children. *Clin Infect Dis.* 1997;24:860–866.
41. Rice PA. Gonococcal arthritis (disseminated gonococcal infection). *Infect Dis Clin North Am.* 2005;19:853–861.
42. Ross JJ, Shamsuddin H. Sternoclavicular septic arthritis: review of 180 cases. *Medicine (Baltimore).* 2004;83:139–148.
43. Punzi L, Oliviero F. Arthrocentesis and synovial fluid analysis in clinical practice: value of sonography in difficult cases. *Ann N Y Acad Sci.* 2009;154:152–158.
44. Hughes JG, Vetter EA, Patel R, et al. Culture with BACTEC Peds Plus/F bottle compared with conventional methods for detection of bacteria in synovial fluid. *J Clin Microbiol.* 2001;39:4468–4471.
45. Maderazo EG, Judson S, Pasternak H. Late infections of total joint prostheses. A review and recommendations for prevention. *Clin Orthop Relat Res.* 1988;229:131–142.
46. Murdoch DR, Roberts SA, Fowler Jr VG, et al. Infection of orthopedic prostheses after *Staphylococcus aureus* bacteremia. *Clin Infect Dis.* 2001;32:647–649.
47. Berbari EF, Hanssen AD, Duffy MC, et al. Risk factors for prosthetic joint infection: case-control study. *Clin Infect Dis.* 1998;27:1247–1254.

48. Shih LY, Wu JJ, Yang DJ. Erythrocyte sedimentation rate and C-reactive protein values in patients with total hip arthroplasty. *Clin Orthop Relat Res*. 1987;225:238–246.

49. Bottner F, Wegner A, Winkelmann W, Becker K, Erren M, Gotze C. Interleukin-6, procalcitonin and TNF-alpha: markers of peri-prosthetic infection following total joint replacement. *J Bone Joint Surg Br*. 2007;89:94–99.

50. Trampuz A, Hanssen AD, Osmon DR, Mandrekar J, Steckelberg JM, Patel R. Synovial fluid leukocyte count and differential for the diagnosis of prosthetic knee infection. *Am J Med*. 2004;117:556–562.

51. Schinsky MF, Della Valle CJ, Sporer SM, Paprosky WG. Perioperative testing for joint infection in patients undergoing revision total hip arthroplasty. *J Bone Joint Surg Am*. 2008;90:1869–1875.

52. Stumpe KD, Notzli HP, Zanetti M, et al. FDG PET for differentiation of infection and aseptic loosening in total hip replacements: comparison with conventional radiography and three-phase bone scintigraphy. *Radiology*. 2004;231:333–341.

53. Ivancevic V, Perka C, Hasart O, Sandrock D, Munz DL. Imaging of low-grade bone infection with a technetium-99m labelled monoclonal anti-NCA-90 Fab' fragment in patients with previous joint surgery. *Eur J Nucl Med Mol Imaging*. 2002;29:547–551.

54. Kwee TC, Kwee RM, Alavi A. FDG-PET for diagnosing prosthetic joint infection: systematic review and metaanalysis. *Eur J Nucl Med Mol Imaging*. 2008;35:2122–2132.

55. Trampuz A, Zimmerli W. Prosthetic joint infections: update in diagnosis and treatment. *Swiss Med Wkly*. 2005;135:243–251.

56. Schwank S, Rajacic Z, Zimmerli W, Blaser J. Impact of bacterial biofilm formation on in vitro and in vivo activities of antibiotics. *Antimicrob Agents Chemother*. 1998;42:895–898.

57. Widmer AF, Frei R, Rajacic Z, Zimmerli W. Correlation between in vivo and in vitro efficacy of antimicrobial agents against foreign body infections. *J Infect Dis*. 1990;162:96–102.

58. Shirtliff ME, Calhoun JH, Mader JT. Comparative evaluation of oral levofloxacin and parenteral nafcillin in the treatment of experimental methicillin-susceptible *Staphylococcus aureus* osteomyelitis in rabbits. *J Antimicrob Chemother*. 2001;48:253–258.

59. Frippiat F, Meunier F, Derue G. Place of newer quinolones and rifampicin in the treatment of Gram-positive bone and joint infections. *J Antimicrob Chemother*. 2004;54:1158.

60. Drancourt M, Stein A, Argenson JN, Roiron R, Groulier P, Raoult D. Oral treatment of *Staphylococcus* spp. infected orthopaedic implants with fusidic acid or ofloxacin in combination with rifampicin. *J Antimicrob Chemother*. 1997;39:235–240.

61. Trampuz A, Zimmerli W. Antimicrobial agents in orthopaedic surgery: Prophylaxis and treatment. *Drugs*. 2006;66:1089–1105.

62. Razonable RR, Osmon DR, Steckelberg JM. Linezolid therapy for orthopedic infections. *Mayo Clinic Proceedings*. 2004;79:1137–1144.

63. Baldoni D, Haschke M, Rajacic Z, Zimmerli W, Trampuz A. Linezolid alone or combined with rifampin against methicillin-resistant *Staphylococcus aureus* in experimental foreign-body infection. *Antimicrob Agents Chemother*. 2009;53:1142–1148.

64. John AK, Baldoni D, Haschke M, et al. Efficacy of daptomycin in implant-associated infection due to methicillin-resistant *Staphylococcus aureus* (MRSA): the importance of combination with rifampin. *Antimicrob Agents Chemother*. 2009;53(7):2719–2724.

65. Byren I, Bejon P, Atkins BL, et al. One hundred and twelve infected arthroplasties treated with 'DAIR' (debridement, antibiotics and implant retention): antibiotic duration and outcome. *J Antimicrob Chemother*. 2009;63:1264–1271.

66. Giulieri SG, Graber P, Ochsner PE, Zimmerli W. Management of infection associated with total hip arthroplasty according to a treatment algorithm. *Infection*. 2004;32:222–228.

67. Laffer RR, Graber P, Ochsner PE, Zimmerli W. Outcome of prosthetic knee-associated infection: evaluation of 40 consecutive episodes at a single centre. *Clin Microbio Infect*. 2006;12:433–439.

68. Sendi P, Rohrbach M, Graber P, Frei R, Ochsner PE, Zimmerli W. *Staphylococcus aureus* small colony variants in prosthetic joint infection. *Clin Infect Dis*. 2006;43:961–967.

53 Infections of the eye

David V. Seal, Stephen P. Barrett and Linda Ficker

DEFENSE OF THE OCULAR SURFACE

The commensals of the ocular surface are chiefly Gram-positive bacteria (coagulase-negative staphylococci, diphtheroids and *Propionibacterium acnes*), with occasional Gram-negative bacteria, especially in elderly people. They are found with greater frequency on the lid margin than in the conjunctival sac. *Staphylococcus aureus* colonizes up to 10% of normal lids where it can have both a pathogenic and commensal role; this rate is increased to as much as 70% in atopic individuals.[1,2]

The cornea and conjunctiva are protected by a tear film with an outer lipid, a middle aqueous and an inner mucin layer. The aqueous layer is of lacrimal origin and contains several antibacterial proteins. Non-specific defense mechanisms in the tears include lysozyme, lactoferrin and the defensins, while specific mechanisms involve IgA antibodies directed against a wide range of organisms. There is cooperation between specific and non-specific mechanisms. At the ocular surface potent antimicrobials (such as lysozyme and IgA) are entrained in the mucus film and maintain an antimicrobial presence in the surface microenvironment. With age, tear secretion and the concentration of protective lacrimal proteins falls. This situation is magnified in the dry eye, including Sjögren's syndrome, where lacrimal secretion is compromised and surface defenses are lowered.

Infection at the ocular surface involves binding of organisms by bacterial ligands or adhesins to specific surface molecules, which initiate the process of invasion. For example, *Pseudomonas aeruginosa* lipopolysaccharide binds to the lectin galectin-3 present on corneal epithelial cells; experimental infection can be inhibited passively by antibodies against either molecule or by active immunization against lipopolysaccharide.

PHARMACOKINETICS

The bulbar conjunctiva and corneal epithelium are relatively impermeable to water-soluble drugs, which penetrate poorly into the anterior chamber. Water-soluble, proprietary ophthalmic preparations, such as gentamicin sulfate, are available as eye drops or ointments at high concentration (e.g. 0.3%) relative to their effective antimicrobial concentration and are thus active in the treatment of surface ocular infections such as conjunctivitis. In contrast, agents with a relatively high lipid-water solubility (such as the fluoroquinolones, fusidic acid, chloramphenicol and the sulfonamides) readily penetrate the conjunctiva and cornea to enter the tissues of the anterior segment.

If the surface epithelium is breached, as by corneal ulceration, water-soluble drugs can diffuse more readily into the anterior segment in high concentration. This can be enhanced using antibiotic concentrations exceeding those of commercially available preparations (fortified drops). The topical route is unable to produce therapeutic concentrations in the posterior segment of the eye because of diffusion barriers across the lens and zonule and the vitreous. Also, drug is lost from the vitreous and aqueous to the systemic circulation across the iris and retina or by aqueous drainage.

The surface epithelial barrier can be circumvented by delivering a bolus of drug under the conjunctiva (subconjunctival injection) or close to the surface of the globe (sub-Tenon's injection). These periocular routes deliver effective antimicrobial concentrations into the anterior segment of the eye (e.g. cornea and anterior chamber) and, less often, the posterior segment (e.g. the vitreous). Drugs may, however, be injected directly into the vitreous to treat infections of the vitreous and retina and controlled-release devices may be implanted in the scleral wall or suspended in the vitreous to provide long-term drug delivery.

THE BLOOD–OCULAR BARRIERS

In the uninflamed eye, barriers exist to the transfer of antibiotic from the circulation into the eye. A blood–aqueous barrier inhibits the entry of water-soluble drugs across the epithelium of the ciliary body into newly formed aqueous, and a blood–retinal barrier limits the entry of such drugs into the vitreous humor. Although drugs may reach a high concentration within the choroid via its fenestrated capillaries, diffusion across the outer retina is obstructed by tight junctions between the cells of the retinal pigment epithelium (the outer blood–retinal barrier), and across the retinal capillaries by endothelial tight junctions (the inner blood–retinal barrier).

In addition, anionic drugs (such as penicillins, cephalosporins and quinolones) present in the vitreous are actively transported out of the eye by the iris and ciliary epithelia, the retinal capillary endothelial cells and the retinal pigment epithelium (RPE), giving a half-life of about 8 h for such drugs injected into the vitreous. There is also a passive route for outflow of the drugs, regardless of charge, by forward diffusion into the aqueous.

These barriers affect the potential for drugs to enter the vitreous space after systemic administration, as well as their retention after direct injection into the vitreous. In the uninflamed eye, the highest aqueous concentrations using the systemic route are achieved by lipid-soluble drugs such as chloramphenicol or the fluoroquinolones. Negligible concentrations are achieved using water-soluble drugs, particularly those in anionic form (such as the penicillins and cephalosporins), which are actively transported out of the eye.

In the inflamed eye, breakdown of the blood–ocular barriers allows higher concentrations of antibiotic to be achieved in the ocular compartments following systemic therapy. Effective antimicrobial concentrations may be reached in the aqueous, but concentrations in the vitreous are still too low to provide adequate therapeutic levels, for instance in the treatment of endophthalmitis. Vitreous concentrations after high-dose systemic therapy in such situations will be subtherapeutic (0.5–2 mg/L) and much lower than those achievable by direct injection into the vitreous (up to 1000 mg/L). The latter route is always favored in the treatment of endophthalmitis and reliance should not be made on intravenous therapy alone.

The above barriers (Fig. 53.1) do not exist for other orbital structures. Thus, infections within the orbit or ocular adnexae (the eyelids, lacrimal gland and nasolacrimal system) are readily accessible to systemic antibiotics.

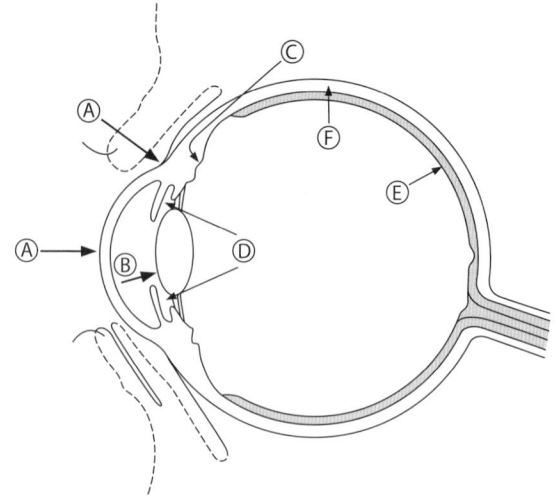

Fig. 53.1 (A) Epithelial barrier (breached by an ulcer; negotiated by topical drops or subconjunctival injection). (B) Aqueous–vitreous barrier. (C) Blood–aqueous barrier limits entry into the aqueous from the blood. (D) Iris pigment epithelial pump removes anions from the aqueous. (E) Blood–retinal barrier; external, pigment–epithelial barrier. (F) Internal, capillary–endothelial barrier. There is an outward pumping of anions across the retina.

MODES OF DELIVERY OF ANTIBIOTICS TO THE EYE

Some modes of delivery discussed here are outside the specifications of the product license and should be used at the clinician's discretion. Infections of the eye are treated primarily with antimicrobials administered topically, or as local injections, which may be supplemented by the systemic route. This leads to some differences in practice from the treatment of infections in other body sites; for example, resistance to antibacterials has to be assessed in the context of the higher concentrations that can be achieved by local administration, and antimicrobial prophylaxis for procedures such as cataract surgery routinely continues for 7 days postoperatively, in contrast to the single preoperative dose that is normal in most branches of surgery.

TOPICAL PREPARATIONS

Drops and ointments are the standard means of administering antibiotics to the surface of the eye, either for prophylaxis or treatment. Ointments (Box 53.1) prolong contact and permit less frequent instillation but should not be mixed with aqueous drops. Prior to the availability of commercial topical quinolone drugs (0.3–0.5%), the preparation of fortified antibiotic eye drops was advocated for the treatment of suppurative keratitis. Their use still has a place. Fortified drops are prepared by combining commercially available parenteral preparations with artificial tear preparations or sterile water to widen the range and concentration of agents used (Table 53.1).[3–6]

Various studies in the past have tried to increase the concentration of antibiotics in the anterior chamber to levels in excess of minimum inhibitory concentrations (MICs) of common ocular pathogens, either for prophylaxis or for treatment. This can be achieved with systemic dosage of lipophilic antibiotics such as chloramphenicol or Septrin (Bactrim, co-trimoxazole) but both are considered to be too toxic to the bone marrow for routine use in prophylaxis. Azithromycin and clarithromycin given systemically accumulate in the aqueous humor well in excess of MICs of Gram-positive cocci and bacilli but may not have good activity against Gram-negative bacteria. Others have tried to increase diffusion from the corneal surface into the anterior chamber, either by iontophoresis or by removing the corneal epithelium.

Box 53.1 Topical antimicrobial ointments

Antibacterial eye ointments	
Chloramphenicol[a]	1%
Chlortetracycline	1%
Erythromycin	0.5% (not commercially available)
Framycetin	0.5%
Gentamicin	0.3%
Neomycin	0.5%
Rifampicin	2.5% (not commercially available)
Sulfacetamide	2.5–10%
Tetracycline	1%
Antibacterial ointment combinations	
Graneodin:	
Neomycin	0.25%
Gramicidin	0.025%
Polyfax:	
Bacitracin	500 U/g
Polymyxin B	10 000 U/g
Polytrim:	
Trimethoprim	0.5%
Polymyxin B	10 000 U/g
Antiprotozoal eye ointment	
Dibromopropamidine	0.15%

[a]There is no evidence from new studies that topical chloramphenicol use in the eye contributes to bone marrow toxicity.[4]

Table 53.1 Selected topical antimicrobial drops: commercially available and fortified extemporaneous preparations

Antibacterial eye drops	Fortified[a] preparation	Commercial
Amikacin	25/50 mg/mL	
Bacitracin		10 000 U/mL (Not in UK)
Cefuroxime	50 mg/mL	
Chloramphenicol[b]		5 mg/mL
Ciprofloxacin		3 mg/mL (0.3%)
Gentamicin	15 mg/mL	3 mg/mL
Fusidic acid gel		10 mg/mL
Levofloxacin[c]		5 mg/mL (0.5%)
Ofloxacin		3 mg/mL (0.3%)
Penicillin G	5000 U/mL (0.3%)	
Piperacillin	50 mg/mL	
Propamidine isethionate		1 mg/mL (1%)
Sulfacetamide		100–300 mg/mL
Tetracycline		10 mg/mL, oil vehicle
Tobramycin	15 mg/mL	3 mg/mL
Vancomycin	50 mg/mL	

Combinations

Neosporin:		
Polymyxin B		5000 U/mL
Gramicidin		25 U/mL
Neomycin		2.5 mg/mL
Polytrim:		
Polymyxin B		10 000 U/mL
Trimethoprim		1 mg/mL

Antifungal eye drops

Amphotericin[d]	1.5–3.0 mg/mL
Clotrimazole and other azoles	1% in arachis oil
Flucytosine	1%
Natamycin[d]	50 mg/mL

Antiprotozoal eye drops[e]

Propamidine isethionate	0.1% (1 mg/mL)
Chlorhexidine digluconate and polyhexamethylene biguanide	0.02% (200 mg/L)

[a]Produced in hospital pharmacy.
[b]There is no evidence from new studies that topical chloramphenicol use in the eye contributes to bone marrow toxicity.[4]
[c]Used for pulse dosing to achieve high levels in the anterior chamber.[3]
[d]Aqueous suspension.
[e]For the treatment of *Acanthamoeba* keratitis.[5,6]

In studies using aqueous drops of quinolones such as levofloxacin, ofloxacin and ciprofloxacin in humans, these have been given twice to four times preoperatively, sometimes with added oral dosing, but sampling has only taken place at the start of cataract surgery.[3] Such studies have produced levels of 0.4–1.6 µg/mL against an expected MIC required to inhibit the growth of 90% of organisms (MIC_{90}) for common ocular pathogens up to 1.0 µg/mL. While the concentration on the ocular surface will be bactericidal, the levels achieved within the anterior chamber will be subinhibitory.

A new technique of pulsed dosing was introduced for the European Society of Cataract and Refractive Surgeons' (ESCRS) prophylaxis study of endophthalmitis following cataract surgery (*see* p. 682) using levofloxacin 0.5% preserved with benzalkonium chloride. Two drops were given before surgery – 60 and 30 min preoperatively – and three drops postoperatively, once immediately at the end of surgery, then 5 min later and finally 5 min later again. Sampling took place in 30 volunteers at the start of surgery, after the first two doses as for other studies, withdrawing 50 µL of aqueous humor. Volunteers were later sampled at 5, 15, 30, 45, 60 or 90 min, each on one occasion only following the fifth postoperative dose, aspirating separate 50 µL samples with a needle and tuberculin syringe.[3] All samples were stored at –20°C and transported on ice to Santen Oy in Finland for high-performance liquid chromatographic analysis of levofloxacin levels.

It was found that pulsed dosing with levofloxacin 0.5%, a quinolone that is water and lipid soluble, increases the concentration in the anterior chamber by 10-fold from 0.4 µg/mL at the time of surgery (after two doses) to a maximum of 4.4 µg/mL 60 min after the fifth dose (Fig. 53.2).[3] This level is four times in excess of the MIC_{90} for common ocular pathogens including *Staph. aureus*, *Streptococcus pneumoniae*, *Ps. aeruginosa* and *Haemophilus influenzae*. At 90 min after the fifth dose, the mean level was still 3.1 µg/mL. The half-life was estimated to be approximately 60 min.[3] It can be speculated, but not proven, that repeat dosing at 2-hourly intervals will maintain levels of levofloxacin in the anterior chamber close to 4 µg/mL.

The possible benefits of using this new pulsed dosing regimen are discussed below under refractive surgery and endophthalmitis prophylaxis following cataract surgery (p. 681). The recent introduction of single-dose 0.5 mL containers of unpreserved levofloxacin 0.5% (in the UK, Germany and Nordic countries) is particularly suitable for pulsed dosing at the time of surgery as it removes any possible toxicity of the preservative (benzalkonium chloride).

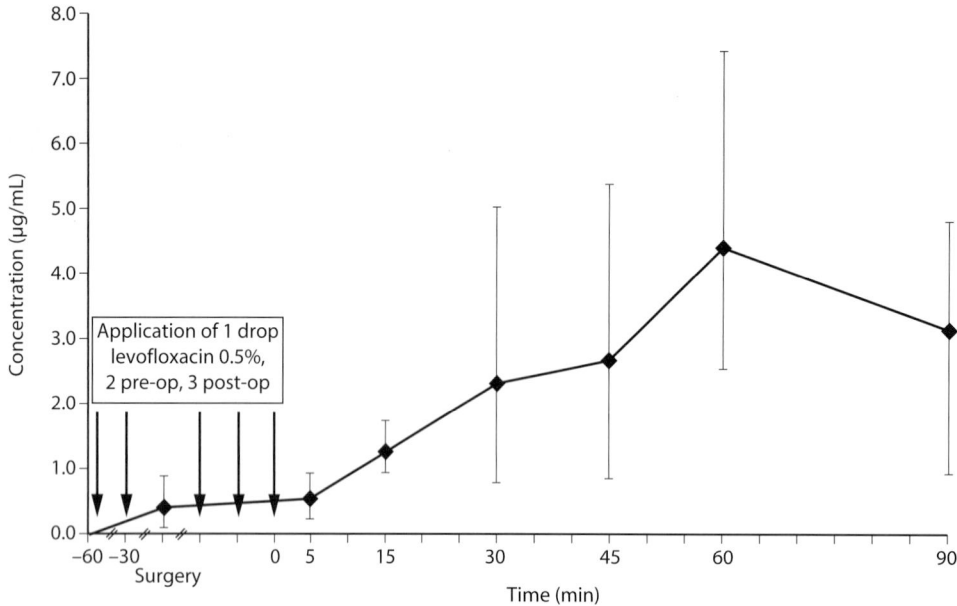

Fig. 53.2   Pulsed dosing of aqueous levofloxacin drops (0.5%) twice preoperatively (60 and 30 min) and three times postoperatively (0, 5 and 10 min) in cataract surgery showing the concentrations achieved in the anterior chamber up to 90 min after the 5th dose.[3] From Sundelin K , Seal D , Gardner S, et al. Increased anterior chamber penetration of topical levofloxacin 0.5% after pulsed dosing in cataract patients. **Acta Ophthalmol (Copenh).** 2009;87:173–178.

Ofloxacin aqueous solution is marketed at a concentration of 0.3% rather than at 0.5% and is absorbed similarly to levofloxacin. However, 50% of ofloxacin is virtually inactive. This means that use of 0.5% levofloxacin will achieve a concentration of active antibiotic inside the anterior chamber that is four-fold higher than that of ofloxacin. To inhibit and kill bacteria, a level of antibiotic is needed that is at least four times and preferably 10 times in excess of the MIC_{90}.

Unit doses of moxifloxacin are produced at a concentration of 0.5% and without preservative. Animal data only are available, but peak concentrations similar to levofloxacin can occur, although the half-life of moxifloxacin in the anterior chamber appears much shorter than that of levofloxacin. Moxifloxacin has an advantage of increased activity against streptococci and methicillin-resistant *Staph. aureus* (MRSA). As such, it is better retained for therapy rather than routine prophylaxis unless a surgical unit has a particular problem with a moxifloxacin-sensitive, levofloxacin-resistant bacterium when its possible use for prophylaxis may be justified. However, moxifloxacin-resistant bacteria do occur and are discussed in the section on endophthalmitis (p. 681).

PERIOCULAR INJECTION

Subconjunctival delivery involves the injection of 0.25–1.0 mL of antibiotic solution under the conjunctiva. There is some leakage of antibiotic back into the conjunctival sac, but the bolus chiefly acts as a depot for diffusion which will produce transient high levels of antibiotic in cornea, sclera, choroid and aqueous and, to a lesser and variable extent, the vitreous. Vitreous levels are lower because of the absorption of drug into the choroidal and retinal circulations, and because of the natural barriers to penetration into the vitreous across the retina (see above). Doses for subconjunctival injection include 125 mg for cefuroxime, 40 mg for gentamicin, 34 mg for clindamycin and 25 mg for vancomycin.

Peak aqueous levels are achieved in the first hour and effective levels are maintained for about 6 h. Inclusion of adrenaline (epinephrine) in the subconjunctival injection prolongs antibiotic activity for 24 h or more, so that injections may be repeated less frequently. This is contraindicated in patients with cardiac disease, and caution must be exercised in the elderly, or when patients are receiving general anesthesia with halothane. Where possible, the injection is delivered close to the site of infection, since tissue levels are highest near the injection site.

A sub-Tenon's injection is delivered in a similar volume but more deeply into the orbit, beneath Tenon's capsule and close to the sclera. Care must be taken to avoid penetration of the globe. It is said to achieve higher levels in the posterior eye than the more anterior, subconjunctival route.

Periocular injections require local anesthesia, and are not without complications. Conjunctival ischemia and necrosis may occur locally and orbital hemorrhage and penetration of the globe have been reported. Although high aqueous levels can be achieved, they are not sustained.

INTRAVITREAL INJECTION

Intravitreal antibiotic injection is the standard treatment for endophthalmitis. Injected antibiotic persists in the vitreous in effective concentrations for up to 96 h. Only a small volume

Table 53.2   Selected intravitreal and parenteral antibiotics

Intravitreal injection[a] agent	Dose (µg)	Effective duration (h)	Intravenous injection, dose
Amikacin	400	24–28	15 mg/kg every 24 h[c]
Amphotericin	5–10	–	0.25–1.0 mg/kg every 24 h[c]
Cefuroxime	2000	16–24	0.75 g every 8 h
Ceftazidime	2000	–	1–2 g every 8–12 h
Chloramphenicol[b]	–	–	1 g every 6–8 h
Clindamycin	1000	16–24	0.3–0.6 g every 8 h
Gentamicin	100–200	48	5 mg/kg every 24 h[c]
Vancomycin	1000	25	1 g every 12 h

[a]Maximum intravitreal injection volume is usually 0.2 mL, i.e. 0.1 mL of each agent used in combination.
[b]Chloramphenicol given systemically penetrates into the vitreous to treat acute bacterial endophthalmitis satisfactorily providing the organism is sensitive to it; it should be reserved for therapy when intravitreal antibiotics cannot be given, but must be used within 48 h of the start of endophthalmitis if useful vision is to be saved.
[c]Administered in three divided doses.

is injected (up to 0.2 mL), and an equal volume of vitreous withdrawn, to minimize ocular pressure elevation and to provide a specimen for culture. The retina is sensitive to toxic damage; amounts injected are based on animal toxicity studies. Selected doses are indicated in Table 53.2.

The vitreous is entered via the pars plana to avoid retinal injury. Sampling may be combined with a total vitrectomy to reduce the infective load and facilitate drug diffusion. The injection can be repeated at 48–72 h intervals according to clinical response. Subsequent vitreous samples can be used to assay the vitreous level of antibiotic.

Cationic drugs such as gentamicin have longer half-lives in the vitreous than anionic drugs such as penicillin, which are actively transported out of the vitreous space. This effect is less in the inflamed eye. Persistence of drug can be prolonged if the same drug is given systemically, since the outward diffusion gradient is decreased. In the case of certain anionic drugs, such as the penicillins, cephalosporins and ciprofloxacin, levels can be further increased by parenteral probenecid. This raises plasma levels by inhibiting renal tubular excretion and blocks active transport out of the eye.

THE SYSTEMIC ROUTE

Systemic medication may be used to treat preseptal and orbital cellulitis, dacryoadenitis, acute dacryocystitis and the rare condition of ocular 'erysipelas' (necrotizing fasciitis of the eyelids), which may need surgical debridement. In the management of chronic blepharitis, tetracyclines used in low dose (e.g. oxytetracycline 250 mg every 12 h) may act by an effect on meibomian oil composition through inhibition of bacterial lipases. In rosacea-associated blepharitis, oral tetracycline 250 mg every 12 h or doxycycline 100 mg once daily will be effective in 50% of patients.[7] Minocycline has also been found effective.[8]

Systemic medication may be combined with local therapy in the treatment of ophthalmia neonatorum due to *Neisseria gonorrhoeae*, *Chlamydia* spp. or, rarely, *Pseudomonas* spp. It is also used in the treatment of adult chlamydial or gonococcal eye disease.

Systemic chemotherapy has no place in the management of uncomplicated bacterial keratitis. It is often employed in high dosage as adjunctive treatment of bacterial endophthalmitis but must not be used alone without intravitreal injection. It is essential in the management of metastatic endophthalmitis associated with septicemia. High-dose regimens should be closely monitored.

THE ROLE OF BIOFILMS IN OCULAR INFECTION

Many serious ocular infections are caused by virulent organisms invading a compromised eye. Increasingly, however, indolent infections result from organisms harbored in biofilms, carried by a therapeutic device, including contact lenses, lens cases, sutures and explants, keratoprostheses and intraocular lens implants. Similar infections occur on prosthetic heart valves, joint prostheses and indwelling catheters. The polymer becomes a physical vector, conveying the biofilm to the eye.

THE BIOFILM

 ## MICRO-ORGANISMS RESPONSIBLE

A biofilm is an association of replicating micro-organisms within their polysaccharide glycocalyx. Certain strains of *Staph. epidermidis* or *Pseudomonas* spp. secrete a glycocalyx, which will attach to and encase the biopolymer, dividing slowly and colonizing the device. Attachment may be enhanced for *Staph. epidermidis* and *Staph. aureus* by the presence of fibronectin.

Free-swimming organisms such as *Ps. aeruginosa* are ideally suited to the formation of biofilms. Having formed a glycocalyx they divide at a slower rate than in the planktonic conditions (5–15 times slower). Bacteria within the biofilm are relatively inaccessible to antibiotics, biocides, surfactants, antibodies, bacteriophages and neutrophils, and are consequently better able to survive attack. The levels of antibiotics required to inhibit growth within the biofilm may be 20–1000 times higher than that required to inhibit planktonic growth. Antigens expressed at the biofilm surface can activate complement.

Biofilm-related infections tend to be chronic, resistant to antibiotics, polymicrobial and culture negative, since treatment may effectively free tissue fluids from planktonic forms, and shedding may be intermittent. The sensitivity to antibiotics of shed bacteria is usually higher than those within the biofilm. To obtain positive cultures it may be necessary to sample directly from the device and to release the bacteria with ultrasound. Simple or non-nutrient agar should be used in addition to normal cultural procedures.

Antibiotic resistance within the biofilm results in part from binding of the antibiotic, with a variable effect on sensitivity. Thus ciprofloxacin is inhibited more than tobramycin. In addition, antibacterial enzymes, such as β-lactamases produced by resistant staphylococci, are concentrated within the biofilm and reduce the antibiotic action of some penicillins and cephalosporins.

BIOFILMS ON OPHTHALMIC BIOMATERIALS

Silicone polymers, polymethylmethacrylate, hydrogels, nylon, polypropylene, aluminum oxide ceramics and Teflon may be non-specifically colonized. Biofilms are encountered in the following situations causing ocular infection.[9]

 ## CONTACT LENSES

The incidence of contact lens-associated keratitis increased greatly with the introduction of hydrogel lenses, particularly for extended wear and to a lesser extent with daily wear. Risk is associated with overnight wear and poor lens hygiene. A number of studies have demonstrated the same strains of organism in the lens case and in saline dispensers used for lens care.

The sequence of events leading to infection is as follows:

1. Organisms, such as staphylococci, are transferred to the surface of a contact lens from the commensal population of the eye or by lens handling when there is poor lens hygiene.
2. Overnight wet storage of a soft hydrogel lens provides an environment which encourages the glycocalyx formation.
3. Homemade storage solutions from a saline dispenser increase the bacterial load by adding organisms from the dispenser nozzle.
4. Organisms within an established biofilm are relatively protected from storage preservatives, although the

preservatives may kill organisms shed from the biofilm. Lens storage cases tend to be washed in tap water, contaminating the case with coliforms, *Ps. aeruginosa* and *Acanthamoeba* spp. The lens and its case become a reservoir for organisms and a physical vector from which organisms or their products can be transferred to the ocular surface on the lens to establish an infection.

The risk of infection is multiplied five times when there is extended, overnight wear of the lens because of the increased exposure time and because conditions at the ocular surface are altered during prolonged eye closure.[10] During sleep, the ocular surface is in a proinflammatory state and the tears are rich in polymorphonuclear neutrophils and their digestive enzymes. Tear flow is almost at a standstill and IgA makes up the major fraction of the tear proteins. The new extended-wear silicone hydrogel lenses provide greater oxygen transmission and reduce the risk of hypoxia and corneal edema, but microbial keratitis still occurs similarly to other extended-wear lenses.[10] In addition, the risk of microbial keratitis with daily disposable lenses has not been found to be reduced but vision loss is less likely to occur.[10]

 ## CONTACT LENS-ASSOCIATED KERATITIS

Ps. aeruginosa is the most common cause of contact lens-associated keratitis followed by *Staph. aureus* and coagulase-negative staphylococci. Those coagulase-negative strains with virulence factors for contact lens-associated keratitis adhere more effectively to biomaterials and resist disinfection.

Acanthamebae are of particular interest because their growth is encouraged by the presence of other organisms and they feed on bacterial products. The trophozoite and cyst stages are introduced from tap water, showers and hot tubs. In the USA and the UK about 85% of infections have been contact-lens associated; in South India most of the infections arise from corneal trauma to the eyes of paddy-field workers.

Mycotic keratitis in soft lens wearers occurs most frequently in relation to extended-wear therapeutic lenses, when yeasts predominate, or with aphakic lenses, when filamentous fungi are more frequent.

Prevention of biofilm-related, contact-lens-associated keratitis

Preventive measures include:

1. Good hygiene and removal of proteinaceous contact lens deposits.
2. The use of cleaners and surfactants to remove adherent micro-organisms or 'multipurpose solutions' that clean and disinfect (polyhexamethylene biguanide or polyquat) with little toxic residual activity.
3. Avoidance of home-prepared saline.

Hydrogen peroxide within 10 min is an effective microbicide against bacteria and within 60 min against some filamentous fungi. Hydrogen peroxide 3% is effective against the trophozoites and cysts of *Acanthamoeba* spp. over a period of 6 h. Catalytic neutralization of hydrogen peroxide allows microbial contamination and is not recommended. The 'gold standard' for soft lenses is 3% hydrogen peroxide overnight followed by neutralization with a thiosulfate/catalase solution made up from tablets in the morning.

SUTURES

Biofilms can form around unburied sutures with a sequence of events including attachment to the hydrophobic polymer, colonization and biofilm formation. Once formed, a suture biofilm may give rise to a stitch abscess, corneal abscess or infectious crystalline keratopathy.

Infectious crystalline keratopathy is an indolent corneal infection when bacterial multiplication occurs within a biofilm within the stroma, in which the close packing of microorganisms and disturbance of stromal lamellae give rise to a crystalline appearance on biomicroscopy.[11] Most cases occur as a complication of surgery or keratitis. The organism responsible for infectious crystalline keratopathy is usually an α-hemolytic streptococcus, although other bacteria and, rarely, fungi or amebae have been incriminated. For streptococci, intensive treatment with topical vancomycin or bacitracin is recommended, although penetration is poor in the absence of an epithelial defect.

PUNCTAL PLUGS

Punctal plugs are used to provide long-term occlusion of the lacrimal puncta, in order to conserve tears in dry eye states. Biofilms around punctal plugs occasionally give rise to canaliculitis or dacryocystitis.

EXPLANTS FOR RETINAL SURGERY

Both solid and sponge explants cause infection by means of a biofilm, although bacteria adhere more readily to sponge explants, presumably because of their greater surface area. Organisms include *Staph. aureus*, coagulase-negative staphylococci, *Ps. aeruginosa*, *Proteus* spp., *Moraxella* spp. and *Branhamella catarrhalis*; coagulase-negative staphylococci predominate. The frequency of infection has been estimated to be 0.6%.

INTRAOCULAR LENS IMPLANTS

While 15–40% of aqueous samples at the end of cataract surgery contain bacteria, endophthalmitis is not an inevitable consequence. Lens implantation can nonetheless be associated with a chronic, saccular or capsular-bag-associated endophthalmitis due to coagulase-negative staphylococci, diphtheroids and *P. acnes* from a biofilm around the implant or due to macrophage-associated bacteria within the capsule remnant.[12] The non-purulent inflammatory reaction is thought to be due to anterior-chamber-associated immune deviation. Systemic azithromycin or clarithromycin can provide effective therapy and high intracellular concentrations.[13,14]

MICROBIAL INFECTIONS OF THE EYE

BLEPHARITIS

Blepharitis is an inflammation of the lid margins involving either the lash line (anterior blepharitis) or the meibomian oil glands (posterior blepharitis). Both forms are often associated with skin diseases such as seborrheic and atopic dermatitis and rosacea.

ANTERIOR BLEPHARITIS

'Staphylococcal' blepharitis implies an anterior blepharitis with lash collarettes, crusting, lid ulceration and folliculitis, and a positive culture for *Staph. aureus*. This is an indication for antimicrobial treatment. However, a positive culture alone does not warrant treatment since the lid margins are colonized with *Staph. aureus* in 6–15% of normal persons, rising to 50% in atopes.[1,2] Coagulase-negative staphylococci are isolated from over 80% of normal lid margins as commensals.

Chronic anterior blepharitis is common and requires regular cleansing of the lid margins with dilute bicarbonate or baby lotion to remove adherent scales. Misdirected lashes must also be removed. Culture of the lid margin requires 'scrubbing' with a swab soaked in sterile broth, and plating directly onto blood agar and a selective medium for *Staph. aureus*. Blepharitis due to *Staph. aureus* is treated with topical ophthalmic fusidic acid gel 1%, 2–4 times daily, or with ocular Polytrim or ocular tetracycline. A highly active staphylococcal blepharitis merits a course of systemic antistaphylococcal therapy, such as flucloxacillin (oxacillin) or erythromycin (500 mg every 6 h for 4 days). Patients should be encouraged to wash with antiseptic soaps such as chlorhexidine to suppress the carriage of *Staph. aureus* at other skin sites.

Anterior blepharitis may respond to short courses of 0.5% hydrocortisone lotion or ointment applied sparingly to the lid margin.

POSTERIOR BLEPHARITIS

The most common form is obstructive meibomian gland dysfunction (MGD), which is highly symptomatic. Lid margins are thickened and red, there is plugging of the meibomian gland orifices and lid oil is poorly expressible. MGD is treated by daily heat to the lids to increase oil fluidity, and firm massage to express retained secretions.

Generally, MGD is not an infective condition but both anterior and posterior blepharitis are accompanied by an increase in commensals, which produce lipases capable of releasing fatty acids from the lipid esters of the tear oils. These contribute to the inflammation. Lipases are inhibited by sub-antimicrobial levels of tetracycline, given intermittently as oxytetracycline (250 mg every 12 h) or doxycycline (50 mg/day), for 3 months which can be repeated after a 3-month interval. Minocycline has been proposed for recalcitrant staphylococcal blepharitis[8] or erythromycin in children to avoid dental abnormalities.

 ## ATOPY

Atopic blepharitis should not be confused with staphylococcal blepharitis, although they may coexist. Non-inflamed lids in patients with atopic dermatitis are colonized with *Staph. aureus*,[1,2] as are the conjunctivae, nasal mucosae and skin. While tear IgE levels are high, they are not directed against *Staph. aureus* antigens.[1] Anterior and posterior blepharitis occurring in association with atopic dermatitis are treated as for non-atopes.

 ## ROSACEA

Rosacea is also associated with blepharitis and the lids are often colonized by *Staph. aureus*. Although cell-mediated immunity to *Staph. aureus* is enhanced, it is not known whether this is cause or effect. In a randomized, placebo-controlled crossover trial, symptomatic improvement of blepharitis in mild rosacea occurred in 90% of patients receiving topical fusidic acid (Fucithalmic) compared with 50% in those on oral oxytetracycline.[7] This improvement did not occur in non-rosacea blepharitis. The non-infective keratitis of rosacea is treated with topical steroid.

STYES

Styes are painful microabscesses of the lid margin, at the base of a lash follicle. Colonization of the lash base with *Staph. aureus* is well recognized. Styes may respond to the application of heat, combined with a topical antibiotic with good tissue penetration, every 4–6 h (e.g. ofloxacin, ciprofloxacin, chloramphenicol or fusidic acid gel). Resistant cases may require treatment with a systemic antistaphylococcal agent.

CHALAZIA

A chalazion is a granuloma within the meibomian glands, associated with obstruction of the gland orifices. It usually forms a painless swelling, which may resolve without treatment or may require incision and curettage. Secondary infection with pain can occur which responds to systemic antimicrobials.

CONJUNCTIVITIS

Conjunctivitis can be due to bacteria, chlamydia, viruses, fungi, protozoa and helminths (Box 53.2). Non-infective causes include allergy or toxicity. Toxicity may be due to preservatives, such as benzalkonium chloride, associated with tear substitutes or occasionally to circulating bacterial toxins.

 ## CLINICAL PRESENTATION

Bacterial conjunctivitis presents with an acute purulent discharge, which frequently becomes bilateral. Viral conjunctivitis is usually associated with a watery discharge and in both

Box 53.2 Microbial and other causes of conjunctivitis

Bacteria
- *Staphylococcus aureus*, associated with blepharitis
- *Streptococcus pneumoniae*, associated with sinus disease
- *Str. pyogenes*, associated with throat infections
- *Listeria monocytogenes*, associated with rural and farmyard dust (farmer's eye)
- *Corynebacterium diphtheriae*, associated with a pseudomembrane
- *Neisseria meningitidis/gonorrhoeae*, associated with throat/genital infection
- *Pseudomonas aeruginosa*, associated with contact lens wear
- *Klebsiella pneumoniae* and other Enterobacteriaceae, associated with contact lens wear
- *Proteus* spp., associated with old age (more in men than women)
- *Moraxella* spp., associated with damaged ocular surface
- *Haemophilus influenzae*, associated with intrinsic throat flora

Chlamydia
- *Chlamydia trachomatis*, associated with overcrowding, poor hygiene and flies (encouraged by cattle dung) in the Near and Middle East and tropics
- Trachoma/inclusion conjunctivitis, associated with genital infection in Western countries

Viruses
- *Herpes simplex*, associated with corneal disease
- *Herpes zoster*, associated with affection of the fifth nerve
- Adenovirus, associated with epidemics from shipyards, close-living quarters, and eye clinics (via tonometers and staff handling of patients); early diagnosis is required to bring outbreaks to a quick halt
- Acute hemorrhagic conjunctivitis: enterovirus 70, poliovirus and Coxsackie A24v are associated with epidemics and occasional paralysis; it is associated with foreign travel, especially tropical areas of Asia
- Conjunctivitis occurs with systemic infection in measles, mumps and dengue, glandular fever and hepatitis A infection

Fungi
- Fungal conjunctivitis is uncommon, but may complicate fungal keratitis

Helminths
- *Thellazia capillaris* and *Thellazia californensis*, associated with birds in the Middle East and the USA
- *Loa loa*, subconjunctival worm occurring in tropical countries

Protozoa
- Protozoa include *Acanthamoeba* spp., associated with contact lens wear, or rural corneal trauma and keratitis

viral and chlamydial conjunctivitis there is often a follicular conjunctival response. Bacterial conjunctivitis may sometimes be confused with viral or chlamydial disease but an associated urethritis or proctitis points to chlamydial infection.

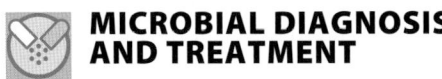

MICROBIAL DIAGNOSIS AND TREATMENT

The patient's history will often give a clue to the organism responsible.

Presumed bacterial conjunctivitis

Swabs should be collected for smears (for Gram and acridine orange stains) and for culture on blood and chocolate agars (and a selected gonococcal agar if relevant). Culture should take place in carbon dioxide at 37°C for 48 h. Treatment is listed in Table 53.1 and Box 53.1 (p. 669).

Presumed chlamydial conjunctivitis

The diagnosis is confirmed by polymerase chain reaction (PCR) or using a monoclonal antibody (e.g. the 'Syvamicrotrak' test). Conjunctival cells are scraped using a spatula and placed on special slides provided in the kit.

The older and cheapest method involved Giemsa staining for intracytoplasmic (Bedson) bodies (complete chlamydial cells lacking a traditional bacterial cell wall). Under ultraviolet light the stained chlamydiae fluoresce yellow, a non-specific reaction which renders the method more sensitive.

Presumed viral conjunctivitis

Diagnosis is carried out by PCR tests on conjunctival scrapings.

THERAPY

Bacterial conjunctivitis

Therapy requires antibacterial drops or ointment for 5 days. If a primary culture is not collected, treatment with a broad-spectrum antibiotic should be given, such as chloramphenicol,[4] levofloxacin or another quinolone or Polytrim. If treatment fails, conjunctival specimens should be collected after stopping drop therapy, including specimens for chlamydia where appropriate.

Ophthalmia neonatorum

Ophthalmia neonatorum is defined as any purulent discharge from the eyes during the first 28 days of life. The presentation may be hyperacute and infection may progress rapidly to keratitis and perforation, leading to blindness. It is an important cause of blindness in low-income countries. Ophthalmia neonatorum in the UK occurs in up to 12% of live births but gonococcal infection is now rare. Elsewhere, the incidence of gonococcal conjunctivitis varies from 0.04% of live births in the West to 1.0% in parts of Africa. The incidence of neonatal chlamydial ophthalmia in London has been estimated at less than 1%.

Neonatal prophylaxis is not used in Western countries. If needed, topical tetracycline protects against both gonococcal and chlamydial ophthalmia, without the toxicity of silver nitrate drops (Créde's solution).

Systemic treatment for gonococcal keratoconjunctivitis is essential, with 30 mg of benzylpenicillin/kg in every 12 h for 7 days. Isolation of penicillin-resistant strains has led to the use of β-lactamase-stable cephalosporins such as ceftriaxone 25–40 mg/kg intravenously every 12 h for 3 days, combined with topical saline lavage and antibiotic ointment (e.g. ocular gentamicin). Single-dose intramuscular therapy may be appropriate when there is no corneal involvement. As is the case with neonatal chlamydial ophthalmia, the infection must be treated systemically as well as topically.

TRACHOMA AND OTHER CHLAMYDIAL DISEASE

Ocular infection by *Chlamydia trachomatis* takes three forms: trachoma, adult chlamydial ophthalmia and neonatal chlamydial ophthalmia.

Trachoma affects 500 million people in developing countries and accounts for 5–10 million blind patients. It is caused by the chlamydial serovars A, B and C, and is transmitted by 'eye-seeking' flies. In hyperendemic areas 30–50% of the population have active disease and 10% exhibit blinding sequelae. Although infection may be encountered as early as the second month of life, active inflammatory disease is most common in preschool children, when the infection leads to conjunctival scarring, entropion and trichiasis, causing recurrent microbial keratitis from repeated corneal infection and trauma. Blinding sequelae occur after the age of 40 years. Public health intervention is required to prevent spread of the infection and reinfection during childhood. The World Health Organization program for the elimination of trachoma (GET 2020) has adopted the SAFE strategy of control measures (**S**urgery for ectropion and entropion, **A**ntibiotics for infectious trachoma, **F**acial cleanliness to reduce transmission by the fly vector and **E**nvironmental improvements, such as control of disease-spreading flies, improved access to clean water and provision of latrines).[15]

Adult chlamydial ophthalmia, also known as inclusion conjunctivitis, and neonatal chlamydial ophthalmia result from sexual transmission. They are caused by serotypes D–K. The adult disease has its greatest prevalence between the ages of 15 and 20 years. The neonatal form may rarely occur immediately after birth, but presents most commonly in the first week or up to 6 weeks later. Treatment of maternal genital *C. trachomatis* infection during pregnancy, usually with erythromycin, is an important preventive measure.

TREATMENT

C. trachomatis is unresponsive to aminoglycosides and only partially susceptible to chloramphenicol and penicillin, which adversely affect growth in culture media. For this reason, transport media for chlamydial culture do not contain penicillin. The organism is fully sensitive to the tetracyclines, erythromycin and other macrolides including azithromycin, rifampicin (rifampin) and the quinolones. Some authorities regard quinolones as second-line treatment. It is also sensitive to chlorhexidine.

Topical treatment of trachoma with tetracycline or erythromycin ointment or quinolone drops can be effective given every 8–12 h for 6 weeks. In trachoma, treatment of other family members or whole villages is necessary to prevent reinfection. Treatment of the early active inflammatory stages is effective with a single oral dose of azithromycin, which is now the preferred therapy, but the cost is higher.[16]

Mass treatment of villagers with single-dose azithromycin has been shown to reduce the prevalence and intensity of infection in a Tanzanian community when infective levels remained low for 2 years after treatment.[16] However, more recent work has found that trachoma and ocular *C. trachomatis* were not eliminated 3 years after two rounds of mass treatment with azithromycin in a trachoma hyperendemic village, again in Tanzania, which is disappointing.[17] Continued implementation of the SAFE strategy is needed in this environment to eradicate the infection.

Systemic therapy is necessary for the treatment or prophylaxis of systemic manifestations such as cervicitis, uveitis, upper respiratory or ear disorders and Reiter's disease in adult chlamydial ophthalmia, and for pharyngitis, vaginitis and a potentially fatal pneumonitis in the neonatal disease.

Adult chlamydial ophthalmia treatment with oral tetracycline, erythromycin or rifampicin for 2 weeks has been recommended but long-acting tetracyclines, such as doxycycline and minocycline, offer convenience and improved compliance, as fewer doses are required and dietary constraints are not necessary. Oral azithromycin therapy is effective with a single dose. The patient and partner(s) should be checked for genital carriage and treated with erythromycin or azithromycin if positive.

A suitable treatment for neonatal chlamydial ophthalmia is oral erythromycin 50 mg/kg per day in four divided doses for 2–3 weeks. Topical therapy may be used adjunctively, but is inadequate on its own (see also Ch. 56).

VIRAL CONJUNCTIVITIS

Primary herpes simplex causes a watery blepharoconjunctivitis, which responds well to aciclovir ointment 3% five times daily.

Adenovirus conjunctivitis may begin unilaterally, but commonly becomes bilateral and may cause a disabling punctate keratitis. In its acute form it lasts up to 21 days, but full recovery from visual sequelae may take several months. No commercial agent is currently available for treatment. Current management is palliative; samples should be collected to confirm the diagnosis by PCR and to highlight the risk of potential epidemics.

Acute hemorrhagic conjunctivitis may occur in epidemics and is due to enterovirus 70; mild paralysis occasionally ensues. Diagnosis is usually clinical. Viral culture should be performed if possible for epidemiological reasons. No specific antiviral therapy is available and treatment is symptomatic.

OTHER FORMS OF CONJUNCTIVITIS

Treatment of *Acanthamoeba* conjunctivitis and episcleritis is dealt with in section on keratitis (p. 677).

CANALICULITIS

Recurrent unilateral conjunctivitis due to an antibiotic-sensitive bacterium such as *H. influenzae* can be the presenting symptom of a canaliculitis due to *Actinomyces* spp. (formerly *Streptothrix* or *Leptothrix* spp.) or *Arachnia propionica*. The organism does not usually invade the canaliculus wall but forms a 'fungal' ball that obstructs the lumen. The canaliculus provides a microaerophilic environment, which supports the growth of non-fastidious anaerobic bacteria, and becomes infected with endogenous flora.

Pus, massaged along the canaliculus to the punctum, can be Gram stained to show typical, branching Gram-positive bacilli. Prolonged anaerobic culture on blood agar plates is necessary to demonstrate actinomycetes. Thioglycolate broth should also be inoculated. Sensitivity tests should be performed.

Actinomycetes and *Arachnia* spp. are usually sensitive to penicillin, tetracycline and erythromycin but resistant to aminoglycosides. Initial treatment involves irrigating the canaliculus with penicillin. If this fails, the canaliculus is opened and debrided and material removed is Gram stained and cultured. The canaliculus should be treated with 5% povidone–iodine for 5 min as an effective antiseptic and syringed daily for 7 days with penicillin.

DACRYOCYSTITIS

Acute dacryocystitis is caused by nasolacrimal stasis, with *Staph. aureus* or streptococci as the usual causes. Infection may respond to systemic chemotherapy or require drainage of a lacrimal sac abscess and ultimately dacryocystorhinostomy.

Chronic dacryocystitis, commonly involving Gram-negative organisms, can only be treated effectively by relieving the nasolacrimal duct obstruction.

The postoperative infection rate in patients undergoing dacryocystorhinostomy is greatly reduced by a single dose of intraoperative cefuroxime intravenously (750 mg).

MICROBIAL KERATITIS

Suppurative bacterial keratitis presents clinically with acute pain, globe redness, lid swelling, watering and visual loss, accompanying a corneal stromal infiltrate or abscess with an overlying ulcer. Common causes are given in Box 53.3. It is usually central, but can be peripheral, particularly if traumatic. Because the cornea is only about 0.5 mm thick, such an ulcer may rapidly progress to perforation within 24 h of onset. In this case, in the aphakic or in the pseudophakic eye with a capsulotomy, there is access to the vitreous space and a secondary endophthalmitis may supervene. There is an urgent need to treat bacterial keratitis with high doses of effective antibiotic. Corneal transplantation may be required later to deal with corneal scarring or perforation.

In northern climates bacteria account for over 80% of cases, with 60% in the south, where fungal keratitis is more common. In tropical regions the risk of fungal infection is even higher,[18] and mixed bacterial and fungal infections are common.

Box 53.3   Bacteria causing bacterial keratitis

Gram-positive cocci

Staphylococcus aureus
Coagulase-negative staphylococci (in the compromised eye)
Streptococcus pneumoniae
Streptococcus pyogenes
Viridans streptococci (in the compromised eye)
Anaerobic streptococci (rare)

Gram-negative coccobacilli

Moraxella spp.
Neisseria gonorrhoeae
Neisseria meningitidis

Gram-positive rods

Corynebacterium diphtheriae (rare)
Diphtheroids (rare)

Gram-negative rods

Pseudomonas aeruginosa (associated with contact lens wear)
Proteus spp.
Klebsiella pneumoniae
Escherichia coli
Serratia marcescens
Acinetobacter spp.
Morganella morganii
Other enteric bacteria

Acid-fast bacteria

Mycobacterium chelonei
Nocardia asteroides

In the past, suppurative keratitis was due chiefly to trauma, or occurred in compromised eyes with existing corneal disease. In recent years, however, there has been a rapid increase in contact-lens-associated keratitis, most of which is bacterial. In general, the risk is much lower for wearers of hard lenses than soft-lens wearers and is greater with extended wear than daily wear. The risk has not been removed by the introduction of 'daily disposable' contact lenses or oxygen-permeable silicone hydrogels.[10]

In previous and current multicenter case-controlled studies, the overall risk for ulcerative keratitis with extended-wear lenses was four times greater than that for daily wear.[10] In addition, overnight wear of contact lenses increased the risk of keratitis to five times that occurring with daily wear alone.[10,19] Wearing soft contact lenses in corneal graft patients also increases the risk of microbial keratitis.

The incidence of contact-lens-associated microbial keratitis has been estimated to be 1 in 500 for extended-wear patients and 1 in 2500 in daily-wear patients.[10,19] The bacteria responsible for contact lens-associated keratitis include those usually associated with suppurative keratitis, but Gram-negative bacteria are more common than Gram-positive, with *Ps. aeruginosa* the most frequent. Contamination of contact lens care solutions is an important potential source of keratitis, with homemade solutions a major risk factor. The number of contact lens wearing patients infected with *Acanthamoeba* spp. has reduced considerably since the introduction of multipurpose solutions based on polyhexamethylene biguanide (PHMB).

 ## DIAGNOSIS

Diagnosis depends on smears and cultures from direct scrapes of the corneal ulcer (Fig. 53.3). The base and edge of the ulcer are most likely to yield organisms.

One drop of unpreserved amethocaine or benoxinate is instilled. The first scrape should be discarded. The second scrape should be taken for microscopy, using a platinum spatula, large-gauge needle or surgical blade. A fresh sterile instrument is used for each sample and the material gathered is spread onto a clean glass slide and air dried. A third scrape should be cultured by plating out directly onto blood, chocolate and Sabouraud agars; then a fluid medium, preferably brain–heart infusion, should be inoculated with the same instrument. In addition, a mycobacterial culture medium should be inoculated if the keratitis is chronic, although the atypical *Mycobacterium chelonae* will grow on blood agar if incubated for 1 week at 37°C. With chronic ulcers, blood agar should be incubated for 1 week in 4% CO_2 in order to culture *Nocardia* spp.

When keratitis due to *Acanthamoeba* spp. is suspected, an appropriate specimen should be taken (*see* p. 667–679).

Media should be inoculated directly at the slit lamp or operating microscope. If possible, duplicate specimens should be taken, to culture at different temperatures. Transport media

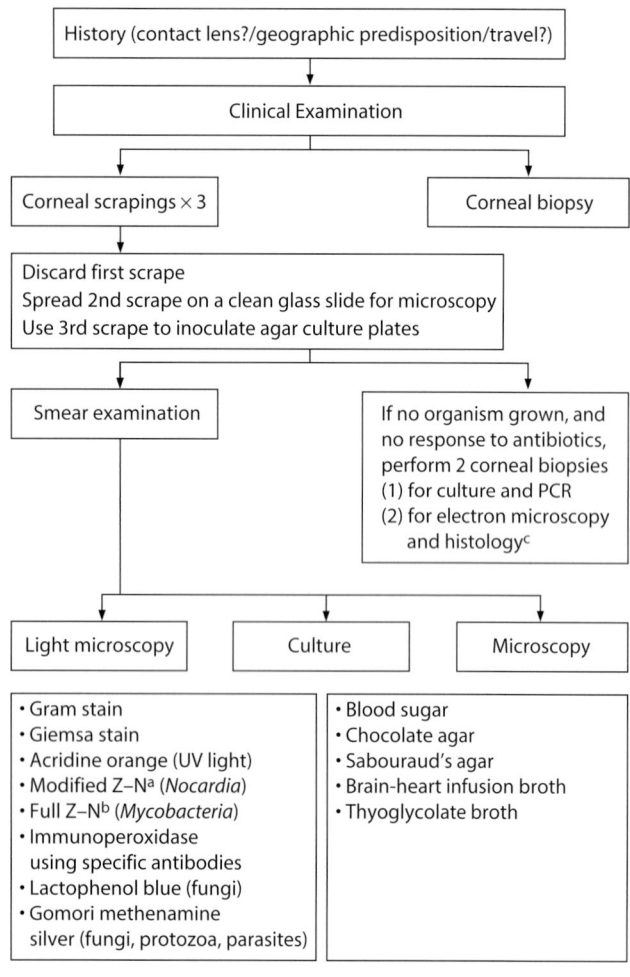

aModified Ziehl-Neelsen stain: use hot carbol fuchsin, rinse with weak (acetic) acid (5%) and no alcohol for *Nocardia* spp., *M.leprae*.
bFull Ziehl-Neelsen stain: use hot carbol fuchsin, rinse with concentrated acid and 95% alcohol for 15 seconds for mycobacteria
cCollect sample in gluteraldehyde

Fig. 53.3 Flow chart for investigating microbial keratitis. PCR, pulsed chain reaction.

should not be necessary. Culture of agar plates should always take place at 37°C for 1 week. The fluid media should be incubated at 30°C in 4% CO_2 for at least 3 weeks. Anaerobic cultures should be considered when there is an unsatisfactory response to therapy.

Stains include Gram stain and acridine orange for common bacteria, modified Ziehl–Neelsen stain (decolorizing with 5% acetic acid only) for *Nocardia* and mycobacteria, full Ziehl–Neelsen stain for mycobacteria and periodic–acid Schiff (PAS) or methenamine silver (Grocott) stains for fungi and protozoal cysts. Selective stains include the use of labeled polyclonal or monoclonal antibodies. Acridine orange and Gram stains together will identify organisms in about 80% of cases. It is also possible to maximize the available material by decolorizing and restaining the same slide with a further intermediate stain and finally an end stain.

TREATMENT OF SUPPURATIVE KERATITIS

Treatment is initiated with a commercial preparation of levofloxacin 0.5%, ofloxacin 0.3% or ciprofloxacin 0.3%, or, alternatively, with combination drop therapy using fortified preparations prepared in the hospital pharmacy. A common empirical combination is gentamicin or tobramycin 1.5% (15 mg/mL) with cefazolin or 5% cefuroxime (50 mg/mL).

Trials have demonstrated that monotherapy with fluoroquinolones is as effective as combination therapy in the treatment of bacterial keratitis,[20–23] with greater toxicity in the combined group. Fortified preparations may have an advantage in the management of advanced disease. The growing recognition of bacterial resistance to the fluoroquinolones[24,25] suggests that there should be caution in adopting monotherapy as a universal approach.

Drops are given every 15–30 min, day and night, and then hourly for the first 3 days, then 2-hourly by day and night, weaning according to response and cultural findings. It is unusual to modify therapy on the basis of the smear report alone, unless fungi are identified. An exception is the identification of *Str. pneumoniae*, when penicillin drops should be substituted. Successful eradication of bacterial infection is reported in about 90% of patients treated in this way.

Unpreserved levofloxacin 0.5% is now available in the UK, Germany and Nordic countries; other countries and the above have levofloxacin 0.5% preserved with benzalkonium chloride. Levofloxacin has the advantage of twice the activity of ofloxacin, half of which is inert, and is marketed at the higher concentration. Ofloxacin treatment causes less irritation than ciprofloxacin, which can leave microcrystalline corneal deposits.

Moxifloxacin (0.5% unpreserved)[26] and gatifloxacin (0.3% preserved) are available in some countries; moxifloxacin has the advantage of increased activity against streptococci but should be reserved for this purpose and not used for prophylaxis. Fortified gentamicin drops cause an inferior, perilimbal conjunctival necrosis which resolves on withdrawing therapy.

If monotherapy is used, a loading dose of one drop every minute for five doses can be initiated, and repeated hourly, to achieve high initial levels in the cornea. In the USA, a regimen of fortified drops every 15–30 min day and night is recommended on an outpatient basis for 3 days in the first instance. In the UK it is usual to admit patients to hospital. Systemic antibiotics have no place in the management of bacterial keratitis in the absence of limbal involvement or perforation.

Where frequent application is not possible, as in a child or a disturbed individual, subconjunctival injections of gentamicin 40 mg and cefazolin 100 mg can be delivered under general anesthetic. In the absence of cardiac disease, inclusion of adrenaline (epinephrine) 0.3 mL (of 1:1000) in 1 mL of solution prolongs the tissue concentration of antibiotic from 6 to 24 h. Other regimens are given in Box 53.4.

Box 53.4 Suppurative bacterial keratitis: specific antibiotic regimens for topical or periocular therapy

Initial therapy

To treat unknown organism(s) (new case or no growth on presentation):
- levofloxacin 0.5% or, if unavailable, ofloxacin 0.3%

These therapies will treat the following organisms:
- *Staphylococcus aureus*
- Coagulase-negative staphylococci
- *Streptococcus* spp.
- *Pseudomonas aeruginosa*
- *Klebsiella* spp.
- *Proteus* spp. and other Enterobacteriaceae
- *Haemophilus influenzae*

MRSA keratitis

Moxifloxacin 0.5% or, if non-responsive, vancomycin* 5%

Pseudomonas aeruginosa infection (culture-proven)

Levofloxacin 0.5% or a combination of piperacillin* (5%) + gentamicin* (1.5%) and/or ceftazidime* (5%)

Mycobacterial keratitis

Amikacin* 5% and/or levofloxacin or other quinolone

Nocardial keratitis

Amikacin* 5% and/or vancomycin* 5% and trimethoprim* 0.1% ± azithromycin*

See text.

Fungal keratitis (hyphae or yeasts seen on smear or fungus cultured)

Hyphal infection (*Aspergillus* spp., *Fusarium* spp.): natamycin* (5%) or amphotericin* B (0.15–0.3%).

Yeast infection (*Candida* spp.): clotrimazole* (or other imidazole*) at 1% in arachis oil eye drops or flucytosine* 1% drops.

*Needs to be prepared by local hospital pharmacy.

Antibiotics should be modified according to the results of cultures and clinical response. If there is a clear clinical response, the same regimen should be continued. Susceptibility tests may be misleading because they assume lower tissue antibiotic levels than achievable in the cornea during topical therapy. Therapy is reduced by increasing the time interval between drops every 3–4 days and not by reducing their concentration. The decision to terminate therapy is based on the clinical response and the nature of the causative organism.

If there is no response, topical therapy should be stopped and the clinical condition reappraised after 24 or 48 h when the cornea is scraped again. A full search must be made for fastidious organisms.

If no organism is identified, a second-line broad-spectrum empirical antibiotic regimen should be started, to include antimicrobial action against resistant streptococci, *Nocardia* and mycobacteria. This may include drop therapy with topical vancomycin 50 mg/mL (5%) plus amikacin 50 mg/mL (5%) and trimethoprim 0.1% (given as Polytrim), substituting erythromycin (0.5%) or rifampicin (2.5%) ointment at

night. This is less likely to be necessary since the introduction of topical quinolone therapy, since quinolones are effective against *Nocardia* and mycobacteria, although not against resistant streptococci.

Special cases

Treatment of *M. chelonae* infection requires topical amikacin or a quinolone. This mycobacterium, which causes a chronic keratitis and may follow radial keratotomy, is resistant to the common antituberculosis drugs.

Nocardia spp. cause a refractory keratitis. Therapy usually demands surgery to debulk the infectious load plus antibiotics. Antibiotics alone often fail despite apparent full invitro sensitivity. A combination of topical amikacin (always) plus erythromycin and/or vancomycin and/or trimethoprim has been used successfully. Isolates are resistant to penicillin but may be sensitive to sulfonamides. The new generation of macrolides (azithromycin and clarithromycin) may prove useful.

ACANTHAMOEBA INFECTION

Acanthamebae are free-living protozoa, found in fresh-water ponds, lakes, domestic water supplies, swimming pools and soil. Subclinical exposure occurs frequently and antibodies against *Acanthamoeba* are common. *Acanthamoeba* keratitis was first recognized between 1973 and 1975 and this was followed in the 1980s by a virtual epidemic of cases, related to the expansion of contact lens use: in various series, 71–85% of patients have been contact lens wearers.[27] In the UK, this infection has occurred in 1 in 6750 contact lens wearers but the figure has reduced since multipurpose solutions were introduced for lens storage and disinfection. In Asia it is associated with rural, traumatic eye disease and presentation is often late.

Persons who present with an unusual keratitis after exposure to hot tubs or natural springs may have *Acanthamoeba* keratitis. A high index of suspicion must be maintained for all contact-lens-related keratopathies presenting with epithelial infiltrations, especially with a 'snowstorm' appearance, multiple superficial abscesses or dendritiform ulcers. Keratoneuritis (corneal nerve infiltration) is diagnostic and *Acanthamoeba* cysts may be visible in vivo by confocal microscopy. Suppurative keratitis that is 'culture-negative' and resistant to standard therapy may be due to infection with *Acanthamoeba* spp.

Diagnosis

Early diagnosis, when the infection is confined to epithelium or anterior stroma, is important for successful outcome. Sheets of cells should be removed for both culture and microscopy. Identification of cysts in wet mounts may establish the diagnosis within 10 min of collection. The epithelial material is placed in a conical tube containing 2 mL saline, agitated on a vibrator, centrifuged and the deposit inspected by wet-field microscopy at × 100.

If the disease has progressed to a stromal ring abscess, epithelial scrapes may not yield viable organisms. Cysts from the midst of the abscess may fail to excyst, and results may be delayed. Corneal biopsy allows sampling of the deep infiltrate for viable trophozoites. Both culture and electron microscopy are useful to demonstrate stromal amebae.

For culture, scrapes are inoculated onto non-nutrient agar, ideally made up in Page's amebal saline. If non-nutrient agar without Page's saline is used, then the plate should be pre-inoculated with a suspension of heat-killed *Klebsiella pneumoniae* or other Enterobacteriaceae as a nutrient source for the amebae. The plate is incubated at 32°C for 4 weeks. Amebae are usually visible by light microscopy after 1 week; after 2 weeks the whole plate is covered by the typical double-walled, star-shaped cysts. Isolates should be sent to a reference laboratory for in-vitro drug sensitivity testing and genotyping.

Treatment

Acanthamoeba spp. exist in two forms: the free-living trophozoite is relatively responsive to therapy, whereas cysts may be highly resistant. Cysts form in response to adverse conditions and may remain viable for years. Acanthamebae do not invade the epithelial cells themselves but are found between them, where host defense depends on phagocytosis by macrophages. Drugs are therefore targeted to the stroma, to amebae internalized within cysts, rather than to the epithelial cells. Thus the cationic antiseptics chlorhexidine[5] and PHMB,[6] which do not penetrate the epithelial cell, are highly effective in the treatment of *Acanthamoeba* keratitis and other forms of amebic keratitis.

Treatment should begin with either 0.02% (200 mg/L) chlorhexidine in physiological saline[5,6] or with PHMB (0.02%);[6] however, the latter is less available and not licensed for use as a drug. Both agents are highly effective against the trophozoite and cystic forms of the organism. The diamidines – propamidine isethionate (Brolene) 0.1% or hexamidine isethionate (Desmodine) 0.1% – are usually used in combination with the above biguanide drugs.[5] Propamidine has been used effectively in combination with neomycin but most cysts are resistant to neomycin, and propamidine is moderately toxic with intensive use.

Drops are given hourly day and night for the first 3 days, reducing to 2-hourly by day only. This requires admission to hospital. Adjunctive therapy includes oral flurbiprofen, for both non-steroidal anti-inflammatory and analgesic effects, and a topical mydriatic. Thereafter, combination therapy (chlorhexidine or PHMB and a diamidine) should be given 3-hourly by day for 1 month and then 4-hourly by day for up to one further month. Chlorhexidine and PHMB should not be used together because of the increased toxic effect and lack of synergy. Eradication of the *Acanthamoeba* trophozoites and cysts should then be complete but considerable inflammation can persist.

However, Lim et al[6] have found that live cysts can persist with either chlorhexidine or PHMB therapy in approximately 7% of patients; outcomes were similar when treating with monotherapy of either guanide when the majority of patients were satisfactorily treated. Prolonged treatment for more than 2 months should not be used with either chlorhexidine or PHMB. PHMB is a much larger molecule than chlorhexidine and is less likely to be absorbed into the anterior chamber. If treatment fails, combination therapy with either chlorhexidine or PHMB and a diamidine should be given.

If infection is diagnosed early, cure is possible with complete recovery of vision. Therapy can be limited to 1 month. One week after starting therapy, however, there may be a corneal reaction to the lysis of dead amebae, with localized stromal edema and anterior chamber activity, which lasts up to 3 weeks.[5] Although this may be suppressed with steroids, their use is not encouraged. Steroid treatment, necessary in cases presenting late with considerable pain, ring abscess and episcleritis, prolongs treatment but can relieve intolerable pain. Steroids appear to have a role in controlling the late immunoinflammatory responses, when the amebae have been killed and antigens remain bound to the corneal stroma or sclera. Adjunctive immunosuppression has been advocated for *Acanthamoeba* scleritis. Steroids suppress the host macrophage response needed for successful treatment so should be restricted as far as possible.

Rapid progressive (mature) cataract and iris atrophy were not seen in the original series of 12 patients treated with chlorhexidine and propamidine in 1996.[5] They have since been reported anecdotally with chlorhexidine treatment, with two cases published in 2004[28] and 6 cases out of 81 patients with laboratory-confirmed diagnosis published in 2008.[29] All cases had been treated with prolonged therapy with chlorhexidine, the latter six for 6 months. Cataract may occur and progress during the management of *Acanthamoeba* keratitis in association with anterior segment inflammation, iris atrophy and secondary glaucoma. This is likely due to the toxic effect of chlorhexidine, in particular its absorption into the anterior chamber to damage the lens epithelium. This was an original concern when introducing chlorhexidine therapy for *Acanthamoeba* keratitis.[5] Chlorhexidine is approximately 50 000 times more active against the membrane of the *Acanthamoeba* cell than the human cell but all epithelial cells are sensitive to it at high concentration. It is well known to delay wound healing at a concentration of 0.5% as exemplified in a pig model.[30] Chlorhexidine accumulates in tissues with an ever-increasing concentration, when absorption into the anterior chamber may occur with resulting damage to the epithelia of the lens and iris.

Prevention

Contact-lens storage cases become contaminated with *Acanthamoeba* spp. from the domestic water supply and airborne dust.[31] Prevention involves use of acanthamebicidal disinfectants in storage and cleaning solutions, of which the best is hydrogen peroxide 3%; if PHMB is included as the disinfectant, the minimum concentration for an acanthame-bicidal effect is 1 mg/L (0.0001%) but needs 5 mg/L for a full cysticidal effect. Chlorine is ineffective against cysts. Storage cases should never be washed in tap water, but with boiled water only, and should be stored dry. This is important because Enterobacteriaceae die quickly in dry conditions, and amebae cannot then multiply.

REFRACTIVE SURGERY-ASSOCIATED INFECTIOUS KERATITIS

A steadily increasing number of infections following laser in situ keratomileusis (LASIK) and photorefractive keratectomy (PRK) have been reported recently, leading to moderate to severe reductions in visual acuity in some eyes.[32] The incidence is best provided by a study of 12 668 USA navy and army personnel with a total of 25 337 PRK procedures;[33] infectious keratitis developed in 5 eyes (1 in 5067 procedures) within 2–7 days due to Gram-positive bacteria (GPB). GPB (*Staph. aureus*, coagulase-negative staphylococci, *Str. pneumoniae* and viridans streptococci,[33–35] MRSA,[36,37] *Actinomyces* spp.[38]), mycobacteria (*M. chelonae*[39–43]) and *Nocardia*[44] are the common causative organisms. Gram-positive infections are more likely to present within 7 days of LASIK and to be associated with pain, discharge, epithelial defects and anterior chamber reactions. Mycobacterial infections are more likely to present 10 or more days after LASIK surgery. Fungal infections are associated with redness and tearing on presentation and can cause severe reduction in visual acuity; isolates include *Candida parapsilosis*,[45,46] *Aspergillus fumigatus*,[47] *Alternaria* spp.,[48] *Aureobasidium pullulans*,[49] *Exophiala dermatitidis*[50] and *Exophiala jeanselmei*.[51] *Acanthamoeba* spp. have been reported recently following refractive surgery for the first time.[52] An early flap lift and repositioning within 3 days of symptoms has been recommended for better visual outcome.[32]

 ## DIAGNOSIS AND TREATMENT

Early diagnosis, appropriate laboratory testing and aggressive antimicrobial therapy can result in good outcomes. Antibiotics are given as for suppurative keratitis above. Topical quinolones are suitable for most GPB except MRSA, when topical vancomycin should be used, and will treat some but not all mycobacteria, when amikacin should be used. Therapy for *Nocardia* spp. and *Acanthamoeba* spp. are given above.

 ## PROPHYLAXIS

Topical quinolones are well suited for this purpose, in particular levofloxacin 0.5%, which should be given at least twice in the 1 hour preoperatively and every 6 h postoperatively for 1 week to suppress contaminating conjunctival bacteria.

The newer 'fourth-generation' quinolones – moxifloxacin and gatifloxacin – should be reserved for therapy only.

ENDOPHTHALMITIS

Endophthalmitis implies infection of the vitreous, retina and uveal coats of the eye. It is commonly exogenous and encountered as a complication of intraocular surgery or refractive surgery, or following suture removal after cataract or corneal graft surgery. Alternatively, it may be caused by penetrating eye injury. Organisms introduced into the anterior chamber at the time of cataract surgery may give rise to an acute endophthalmitis. Less pathogenic organisms may induce chronic infection. Some cases of endophthalmitis result from contaminated irrigation fluids, which may lead to an epidemic of infections. The formation of thin-walled drainage blebs after glaucoma operations using mitomycin C may predispose to late infections. The risk of infection is reduced by application of 5% povidone–iodine to the cornea and conjunctiva immediately before surgery.[53]

Less commonly, endogenous or metastatic endophthalmitis may arise in association with septicemia. This may result from bacterial endocarditis, infusion of contaminated fluids, the presence of infected intravenous lines or in intravenous drug users using contaminated needles or syringes commonly associated with *Candida albicans* infection. In children, pneumonia due to *Ps. aeruginosa* may be the cause of a bilateral endophthalmitis which rapidly leads to blindness.

Patients can present with a fulminant endophthalmitis within 5 days of cataract surgery, often leading to permanent loss of vision. Alternatively, a subacute or chronic endophthalmitis may occur within 12 weeks of surgery, often presenting as a hypopyon uveitis. Risk factors include duration of surgery, iris manipulation, torn posterior capsule with vitreous loss, lens fragments in the vitreous and type of intraocular lens, with silicone intraocular lenses being more commonly associated with infection.[53]

Causes of acute endophthalmitis include *Str. pyogenes*, *Staph. aureus* and Enterobacteriaceae and, with penetrating injury, *Bacillus* spp. and clostridia. Acute endophthalmitis occasionally follows squint surgery, when infection is usually due to *Staph. aureus*. Surgeons should use appropriate prophylaxis against *Staph. aureus* in atopic or allergic patients. Causes of chronic endophthalmitis include coagulase-negative staphylococci, *P. acnes* and, occasionally, viridans streptococci. Polymicrobial endophthalmitis is also reported, particularly after injury.

 ## DIAGNOSIS AND TREATMENT

Acute endophthalmitis

Endophthalmitis is potentially blinding from irreversible retinal damage occurring within 24–48 h of onset. Early diagnosis and prompt treatment are essential. Bacterial endophthalmitis is treated with a combination of intravitreal and systemic antibiotic therapy. Subconjunctival therapy currently has no place in treatment and reliance should not be placed on intravenous therapy alone.

The clinical diagnosis of endophthalmitis is based on the presence of pain, vision loss, lid swelling and redness of the eye, including chemosis. A hypopyon uveitis may be present and, most importantly, loss of the red reflex. The vitreous is often opaque.

Microbiological diagnosis requires a vitreous biopsy for smears and cultures. PCR is useful for diagnosis and may yield a higher positive rate than direct culture, especially for Gram-negative organisms.[53-56] A simultaneous intravitreal injection of an antibiotic combination is given at the time of sampling and repeated at intervals (e.g. 48–72 h) depending on the expected intravitreal persistence of the selected drug and the clinical response (see Table 53.2, p. 671, for dosages); empirical combinations include vancomycin and ceftazidime or vancomycin and amikacin, with restricted use of intravitreal gentamicin due to the macular infarction that it can cause. Unpreserved dexamethasone (400 µg) is given by intravitreal injection to reduce the vitreous inflammatory response and subsequent vitreous organization.[57]

Additional systemic therapy with the same antibiotic as used for intravitreal therapy will maintain effective intravitreal levels for longer by reducing outward diffusion through the retina. High doses are required and there is a need to be aware of the risks of systemic toxicity.

Antibiotic therapy is modified after 24–48 h according to the clinical response and to the antibiotic sensitivity profile of the cultured organism.

Chronic endophthalmitis

A diagnosis of chronic endophthalmitis should be considered in patients presenting late, several days or weeks after surgery, with a 'hypopyon uveitis' that has failed to respond to routine topical antibiotic and steroid therapy. Symptoms are less marked than in acute endophthalmitis. Vision loss may be more evident than pain. Chronic endophthalmitis is usually caused by indolent organisms such as coagulase-negative staphylococci or *P. acnes*, capable of forming a biofilm on the lens implant and causing a granular or saccular endophthalmitis.[12,57]

Diagnosis may be established as late as 1 year after surgery, by an aqueous or vitreous tap, followed by Gram stain and culture or PCR. Microbiological diagnosis may await explanation of the implant and histological examination of the implant and capsular bag.[12]

Initial treatment should commence with oral clarithromycin 500 mg every 12 h for 1 week, followed by 250 mg every 12 h for 3 weeks, as a 'trial of therapy'.[13,14] A good response, when it occurs, may be due to concentration of the drug within macrophages containing bacteria.[12,13] If this treatment fails, then further intravitreal therapy should be given, with emphasis on drugs against Gram-positive organisms, such as vancomycin. Capsulectomy, vitrectomy and removal of the intraocular lens, with or without lens exchange, may be necessary to eradicate the organism.

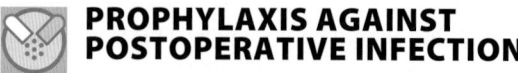

PROPHYLAXIS AGAINST POSTOPERATIVE INFECTION

Several approaches can reduce the risk of endophthalmitis following intraocular surgery:

- Meticulous preoperative preparation with occlusive drapes
- Irrigation of the operative field with povidone–iodine (5%)
- Avoidance of contamination of the intraocular lens during insertion
- Use of antimicrobials

Postoperative infection is the most common form of exogenous bacterial endophthalmitis. Sources of organisms include the patients themselves (conjunctiva, cornea and nasolacrimal duct), surgeon (hands, gloves, nose, technique), contaminated instruments, implants, drugs, irrigations and infusions, and environmental sources. Phako machines, vitrectomy machines and viscoelastic materials may all be sources of infection. Metastatic endophthalmitis occurs after contaminated intravenous infusions and blood transfusions.

Eyelid and conjunctival sac commensals are responsible for 80% of postcataract surgery endophthalmitis. Since eyelid cultures vary from day to day, preoperative cultures are no longer performed, and reliance is placed on preoperative antiseptic preparation with povidone–iodine and an aseptic technique.[53]

CATARACT SURGERY

The rate of endophthalmitis following modern cataract surgery is 0.1–0.7%. While this rate is low, the risk of blindness presents a challenge to reduce infection.

Some bacteria (predominantly coagulase-negative staphylococci or *P. acnes*) enter the chamber during cataract surgery. Re-entry of the anterior chamber increases this risk. DNA typing of postoperative staphylococcal cultures from lids and those causing endophthalmitis has shown similarity in 85% of cases, suggesting that most patients become infected by their own bacterial flora. To combat this, some surgeons add an antibiotic, such as gentamicin 5 mg/L or vancomycin 10 mg/L, to the irrigant fluid. While this is controversial, there is anecdotal evidence that this approach may reduce the incidence of postoperative endophthalmitis.

Intracameral injection with 1 mg cefuroxime (0.1 mL of 10 mg/mL) around the intraocular lens at the end of surgery has been associated with an incidence of endophthalmitis as low as 0.06%.[58] This technique was evaluated in the ESCRS Endophthalmitis Study which compared prophylaxis of phakoemulsification cataract surgery prospectively in 16 000 patients with intracameral cefuroxime 1 mg versus topical levofloxacin 0.5% in a ×5 pulsed dose, as described in the pharmacokinetic section, with the combination and with neither.[53] The overall rate of postcataract surgery endophthalmitis was reduced by five times, from 0.3% to 0.06%, in the groups given intracameral cefuroxime. In addition, seven patients developed severe streptococcal infection, with loss of vision in three, in the group of 8000 patients not receiving cefuroxime. However, there was a trend, but not statistically significant, for use of topical levofloxacin drops as well as intracameral cefuroxime. Unfortunately, in the trial design, dosing with the levofloxacin drops was not continued from the pulsed dose regime given at the time of surgery (*see* Fig. 53.2) until the following morning. This allowed drug levels to fall in the important first 12 h after contamination of the anterior chamber had taken place at the time of the intraocular lens insertion. It is now recommended that dosing with topical levofloxacin should be continued on a 2-hourly basis from the time of surgery until the patient sleeps at night, recommencing 6-hourly on waking for 1 week.

Newer generation fluoroquinolones (moxifloxacin, gatifloxacin) have been promoted as a potential substitute for intracameral cefuroxime. Recent reports, however, describe steadily increasing resistance among endophthalmitis isolates to these fluoroquinolones. Over the period 1990–2004, in 111 ocular endophthalmitis isolates of coagulase-negative staphylococci (CNS), 67.6% being *Staph. epidermidis*, the percentage of strains sensitive to moxifloxacin declined significantly from 96.6% (1990–1994) to 65.4% (2000–2004) ($p = 0.03$), a 32.2% decline over a relatively short period of time.[59]

A significant increase in the prevalence of resistant isolates was also documented for moxifloxacin over this time period ($p = 0.007$), with the MIC_{90} for moxifloxacin increasing by a factor of 266. The concentrations required to inhibit or kill 90% (the MIC_{90}) rose from 0.12 µg/mL (for 93.2% of isolates) during 1990–1994, to 4 µg/mL (for 100% of isolates) during 1995–1999, and to 32 µg/mL (for 100% of isolates) during 2000–2004.[59] Overall, only 72.1% of 111 CNS isolates recovered from patients with clinical endophthalmitis were sensitive to moxifloxacin (sensitivity defined as susceptible to 0.5 µg/mL or less).

In the ESCRS study, two of the five *Staph. epidermidis* isolates tested showed reduced susceptibility to moxifloxacin.[56] This trend – together with reports describing postoperative endophthalmitis after peri- and postoperative use of moxifloxacin and gatifloxacin,[60] the potentially unresolved question of safe dosage (especially for intracameral use of moxifloxacin)[61] and cautionary statements that moxifloxacin should not be injected directly into the eye[62] – suggests that large scale randomized trials are needed to validate either prophylaxis with topical moxifloxacin or gatifloxacin, or for intracameral injection of moxifloxacin.

Subconjunctival antibiotics (cefuroxime 125 mg or gentamicin 20 mg) have been given at the end of surgery for many years. Cefuroxime provides good antibiotic prophylaxis against *Staph. aureus*, *Str. pyogenes*, coagulase-negative staphylococci and *P. acnes*. Gentamicin gives poor coverage

against streptococci and *P. acnes*. The subconjunctival route of prophylaxis is not proven to be effective and has been given to many patients who suffer from postoperative infectious endophthalmitis.

Contact between the intraocular lens implant and conjunctiva during insertion can be avoided using injectable foldable lenses. Careful wound closure is also important. It has been suggested that if just one suture was used to close the clear corneal incision made at the time of surgery, then there would be no need for prophylactic antibiotics but surgeons prefer to try to close the wound with an injection of saline into the open edges of the corneal wound to avoid astigmatism from scarring around the suture. However, this wound is known to leak for several days postoperatively, during which time bacteria can egress back through the wound from the conjunctiva into the anterior chamber to cause infection.

Management of surgery in atopy

In the atope *Staph. aureus* colonizes the skin, including the lids and nasal mucosa, to a high degree.[1,2] Care is needed when planning intraocular surgery, particularly in the presence of blepharitis. The following additional regimen is suggested:

- Whole-body bathing, including shampooing with 4% chlorhexidine soap, for 72 h before surgery
- Topical antistaphylococcal prophylaxis with fusidic acid (Fucithalmic) for 24 h before surgery
- Intracameral cefuroxime 1 mg around the intraocular lens if having cataract surgery
- Fusidic acid 750 mg every 8 h postoperatively (enteric-coated capsules) or trimethoprim for 5 days.

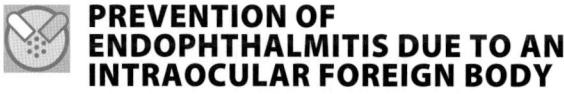 **PREVENTION OF ENDOPHTHALMITIS DUE TO AN INTRAOCULAR FOREIGN BODY**

An intraocular foreign body represents a medical emergency, especially metal fragments arising from hammering farmyard equipment, soil-contaminated items and machinery. Seal and Kirkness[63] found that 8% of patients with an intraocular foreign body developed endophthalmitis, and half became blind.

Bacillus spp. are the most common virulent pathogens carried by an intraocular foreign body, while *Staph. aureus*, Enterobacteriaceae, streptococci and, occasionally, *Clostridium perfringens* are equally likely to cause sight-threatening endophthalmitis. All patients undergoing removal of a foreign body require intravitreal antibiotic prophylaxis. Any delay, or dependence on intravenous antibiotics alone, will risk blindness.[64] Intravitreal dexamethasone may reduce early inflammatory signs but may not influence visual outcome.[65]

The regimen shown in Box 53.5 is suggested; cephalosporins are excluded because *Bacillus* spp. produce β-lactamases that inactivate them.

Box 53.5 Prophylaxis against endophthalmitis following intraocular foreign body

Essential prophylaxis

Intravitreal gentamicin 200 μg (or amikacin 400 μg) + vancomycin 1 mg (or clindamycin 1 mg)

Adjunctive prophylaxis

Subconjunctival gentamicin 40 mg + clindamycin 34 mg

Levofloxacin 0.5% (or other quinolone) + clindamycin 20 mg/mL

Intravenous therapy (with same drugs as given intravitreally) – give adequate dosage for weight but assay to avoid systemic toxicity, especially to the kidney and eighth nerve

ORBITAL CELLULITIS

Orbital cellulitis is an extraocular infection presenting with pain, proptosis and diplopia. A few cases follow penetrating injury or panophthalmitis, but most are secondary to sinusitis. The condition commonly affects children, spreading to the orbit across the thin orbital plate of the ethmoid bone. Delayed or inadequate treatment may lead to blindness or death. Retroseptal infection requires multidisciplinary management because of the risk of extension to the eye or cranial cavity. Loculated pus must be drained.

The lid swelling of preseptal cellulitis may resemble orbital cellulitis, but ocular movements are normal and globe inflammation absent in preseptal disease. Diagnosis can be resolved by MRI. It is associated with sinusitis, ocular infection and infected wounds.

Parenteral therapy is directed against common causative organisms: *H. influenzae, Staph. aureus, Str. pneumoniae* and *Str. pyogenes. H. influenzae* is the prominent cause of orbital cellulitis in young children and in this age group amoxicillin–clavulanic acid or cefuroxime are the drugs of choice. Due to the emergence of multiresistant strains of *H. influenzae*, cefotaxime should be given particularly when the clinical response is poor or resistant organisms are isolated from nasal swabs. In adults, therapy is directed against streptococci and *Staph. aureus*, with high-dose intravenous benzylpenicillin and flucloxacillin, clindamycin or vancomycin.

INFECTIONS DUE TO METHICILLIN-RESISTANT *STAPHYLOCOCCUS AUREUS*

Methicillin-resistant *Staph. aureus* (MRSA) has become a prominent cause of antimicrobial-resistant infections, and this includes those involving the eye. MRSA causes the same spectrum of ophthalmic infections as methicillin-sensitive *Staph. aureus* (MSSA), and it is not clear that they are of greater virulence;[66] however, they are frequently resistant to multiple antibiotics and so may be more difficult to treat.

MRSA conjunctivitis is particularly common in elderly patients in residential care and has been found increasingly in some community settings.[67] Although originally primarily healthcare associated, recent years have witnessed an upsurge in community-acquired MRSA (CA-MRSA), which has been reflected in their isolation from infections such as keratitis[37] and endophthalmitis[68] following photorefractive and cataract surgery. Although CA-MRSA frequently remains susceptible to the antibiotics favored in ophthalmological practice, such as chloramphenicol and quinolones, healthcare-associated strains are often resistant to the earlier quinolones. Experimental work has suggested that the newer quinolones with enhanced activity against Gram-positive bacteria, such as moxifloxacin, may have superior activity in MRSA endophthalmitis.[69] However, serious endophthalmitis due to MRSA should be treated with vancomycin by the intravitreal route and keratitis due to MRSA with vancomycin by the topical route. For less serious MRSA eye infections, such as conjunctivitis, other antimicrobials that can be administered include tetracyclines, linezolid and mupirocin which are active against most MRSA infections.

LYME DISEASE

Although ocular manifestations are rare in this tick-borne disease, the spirochete *Borrelia burgdorferi* invades the eye early and remains dormant, accounting for both early and late ocular manifestations. A follicular conjunctivitis occurs in approximately 10% of patients with early Lyme disease, and an interstitial keratitis within a few months of onset. Inflammatory events include orbital myositis, episcleritis, vitritis, uveitis and retinal vasculitis. When serology is negative, a vitreous tap may be required for diagnosis. Neuro-ophthalmic manifestations include bilateral mydriasis, neuroretinitis, pigmentary retinopathy, involvement of multiple cranial nerves, optic atrophy and disc edema. Seventh nerve paresis can lead to neuroparalytic keratitis. In endemic areas, Lyme disease may be responsible for approximately 25% of presenting Bell's palsy.

Diagnosis is based on a history of exposure in an endemic area, positive serology and response to treatment. Antibodies may be measured by ELISA and Western blot. PCR has been used successfully for vitreous and cerebrospinal fluid. Serum reagin tests are non-reactive in Lyme borreliosis, but false-positive specific tests for syphilis (e.g. fluorescent treponemal antibody) can occur. The spirochetes have been identified in the vitreous of a seronegative patient with vitritis and choroiditis and cultured from an iris biopsy in a treated patient.

Therapy with doxycycline or amoxicillin is effective in the early stages but serious late complications require high doses of intravenous penicillin or ceftriaxone.

WHIPPLE's DISEASE

Whipple's disease is a rare systemic disorder with malaise, fever, migrating arthralgias, fatigue, abdominal discomfort, diarrhea and weight loss. Ocular signs include uveitis, vitritis and retinal vasculitis. Small bowel biopsy shows diastase-resistant PAS-positive macrophages in the mucosal lamina propria. The cause is a Gram-positive actinomycete called *Tropheryma whipplei*. There may be a predisposing immunodeficiency.

Antibiotics that penetrate the blood–brain barrier minimize central nervous system (CNS) complications. Relapse is common. Combination therapy is recommended – e.g. parenteral streptomycin and benzylpenicillin for 2 weeks followed by sulfamethoxazole (800 mg) and trimethoprim (160 mg) (co-trimoxazole) orally twice daily for 1 year.

TOXOPLASMA RETINOCHOROIDITIS

The intracellular protozoan *Toxoplasma gondii* can enter the fetal retina during intrauterine life to cause retinochoroiditis in the second and third decades, when it is the most common cause of posterior uveitis. However, primary toxoplasmosis, which may be subclinical or cause a glandular fever-like syndrome with lymph node enlargement, can produce an acute primary retinochoroiditis. Evidence from Brazil, where the prevalence of ocular toxoplasmosis is high, suggests that the condition is most commonly acquired postnatally.[70]

Therapy is directed against the dividing organism and the inflammatory host response. Small peripheral retinal lesions may be allowed to run their course but lesions near the macula, optic disc or maculopapular nerve fiber bundle, or those associated with severe vitritis, should be treated. Treatment is complicated because tissue cysts, multiplying within retinal cells, are impervious to drug penetration, so that recurrence can be expected. *Toxoplasma* infection is encountered in immunocompromised patients.

TREATMENT

Pyrimethamine and sulfadiazine act synergistically to interfere with folic acid synthesis. They should be commenced early in the course of the disease and continued for 4–6 weeks (Box 53.6). Pyrimethamine therapy should be avoided in early pregnancy and monitored to exclude bone marrow depression. Folinic acid supplements reduce this risk, but platelet and white cell counts should be performed weekly.

Clindamycin has also been shown effective in the treatment of ocular toxoplasmosis but does carry the risk of pseudomembranous colitis.

OCULAR TOXOCARA (LARVA MIGRANS) INFECTION

Toxocara canis is a worm whose natural hosts are the cat and the dog. Humans are accidental hosts, infected by ingesting the ova from contaminated soil. The larval stage causes visceral and ocular larva migrans, but adult worms are not found. These larvae migrate and are deposited in the CNS, including

---

Box 53.6 Treatment of *Toxoplasma* retinochoroiditis

Regimen

Pyrimethamine[a] 100 mg immediately then 25 mg orally per day for 4–6 weeks
and
Sulfadiazine 2 g immediately then 1 g orally every 6 h for 4–6 weeks
and
Folinic acid 3 mg orally or i.m. twice weekly.

Alternative regimen

Clindamycin[b] 300 mg orally every 6 h for 4–6 weeks
and
Sulfadiazine 2 g immediately then 1 g orally every 6 h for 4–6 weeks.

[a]Pyrimethamine may cause bone marrow depression; leukocyte and platelet counts should be monitored weekly.
[b]Clindamycin may cause pseudomembranous colitis.

---

the retina. Here they can present as a possible tumor, usually unilateral, for which eyes have been enucleated in the past.

Serological tests only confirm previous exposure and may be negative when a choroidal lesion is present. Fine-needle biopsy in a reference center with cytology for tumor cells and PCR for *Toxocara* antigen is the best approach.

If the retinal lesion is close to the macula, treatment is warranted, with oral diethylcarbamazine 3 mg/kg for 3 weeks. There may be symptoms of allergic reaction to the dying larvae, for which prednisolone is given. Alternative therapies include albendazole or a single dose of ivermectin.

OCULAR ONCHOCERCIASIS

Ocular onchocerciasis, or 'river blindness', results from infection with the filarial parasite *Onchocerca volvulus*. The disease is endemic in areas of Africa and Central and South America, where it is a major cause of blindness. The ocular manifestations include keratitis, anterior uveitis, glaucoma, chorioretinitis and optic neuritis.

For several decades diethylcarbamazine and sumarin have been used systemically and have a positive effect on keratitis and uveitis; they are, however, less beneficial in posterior segment disease. The use of diethylcarbamazine may be followed by a severe systemic reaction, which is largely prevented by the use of systemic corticosteroids.

Ivermectin (single 12 mg dose) represents an important advance in the mass therapy of onchocerciasis in endemic areas. It inhibits reproduction by adult female worms so that no new microfilariae are produced for several months. It also kills microfilariae in tissues, including skin and the eye, slowly eliminating them from the anterior chamber with minimal ocular inflammation and little systemic reaction. It has to be given yearly so that the eradication program is a continuous one. Ivermectin should not be given to children under 5 years, to pregnant women or to patients with other severe infections such as trypanosomiasis.

Recently it has been recognized that onchocercal oocytes contain endosymbiotic organisms (*Wolbachia* spp.), which are passed on to the microfilaria and are essential to embryogenesis in the female worm. *Wolbachia* spp. are sensitive to tetracyclines, rifampicin, chloramphenicol and azithromycin. In a trial where doxycycline 200 mg/day for 4–6 weeks was combined with ivermectin, embryogenesis was disrupted for 24 months (1 year longer than ivermectin alone), and microfilaria were absent from the skin after 18 months.[71,72]

Oral corticosteroid therapy is indicated in vision-threatening disease, but should not be used without concurrent, specific antiprotozoal therapy or in immunocompromised patients.

OCULOMYCOSIS

Fungal infections of the eye are invariably sight-threatening and include keratomycosis, exogenous or endogenous endophthalmitis and orbital mycosis. Although oculomycosis is rare in the UK, it may account for one-third or more of infective corneal ulcers in some rural settings and in developing countries.[18] The management of keratomycosis is summarized in Figure 53.4.

The fungi responsible for keratomycosis, with the exception of *Candida* spp. (common in the UK and northern climates), are mainly filamentous. The species most frequently

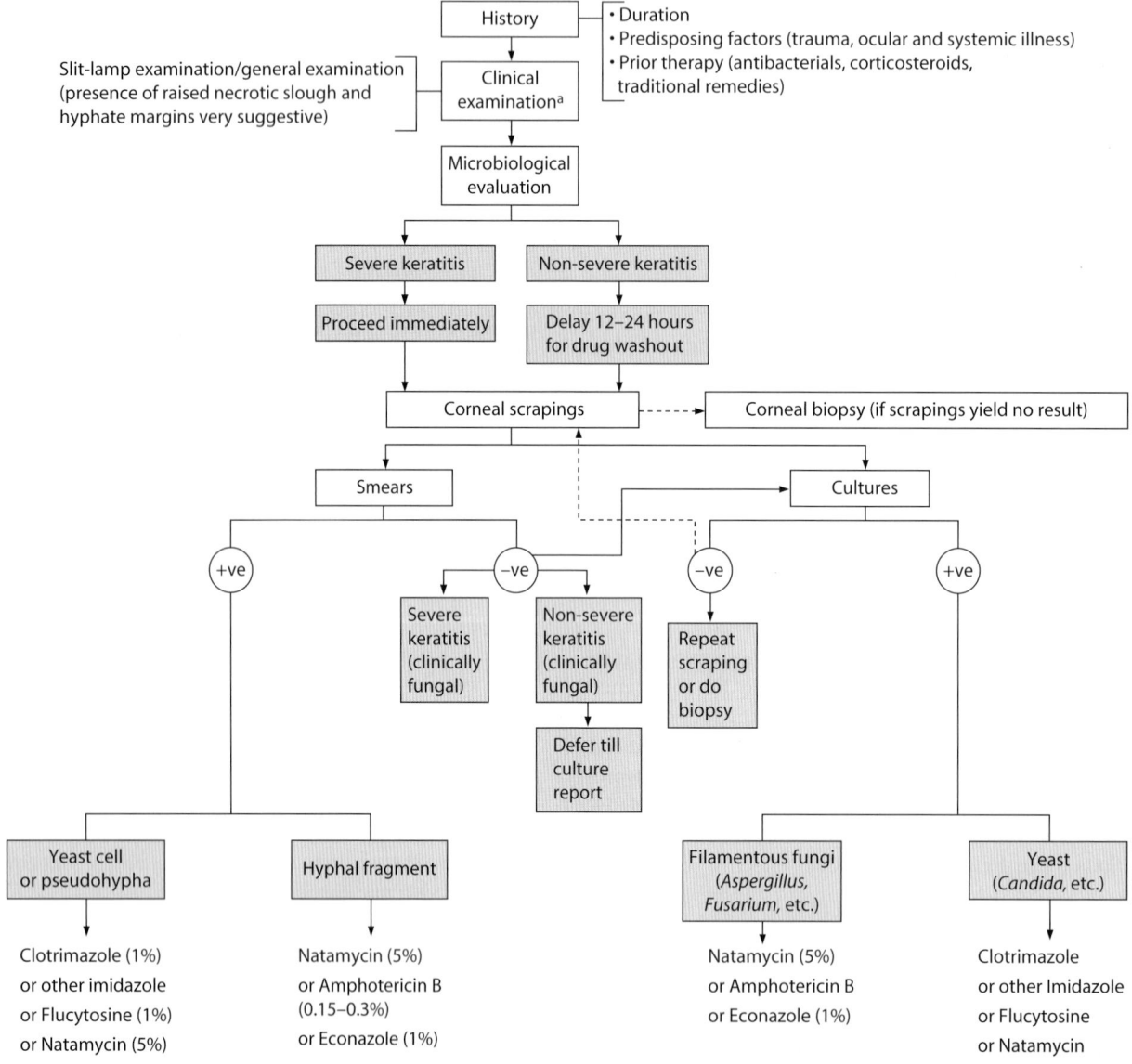

aNon-severe keratitis: slow, moderate progression; <6mm diameter; ulceration and suppuration involves superficial 2/3; perforation unlikely; scleral suppuration absent.
Severe keratitis: rapid progression; >6mm diameter ulceration; ulceration and suppuration involves deep 1/3; perforation present or imminent, scleral suppuration present.

Fig. 53.4 Flow chart for investigating keratomycosis.

encountered are *Aspergillus*, *Fusarium* and *Curvularia*, but prevalence varies geographically. *Candida* spp. are an important cause of endogenous endophthalmitis in intravenous drug users and immunocompromised individuals.[57] Penetration of drugs such as natamycin and amphotericin B in the treatment of a fungal ulcer is greatly enhanced by the absence of an epithelial barrier.

Because of the toxicity of the most effective antifungal agents, the relatively narrow activity spectrum of some and the difficulties of clinical diagnosis, treatment is rarely instituted in the absence of direct evidence of fungal etiology, based at least on the results of smears. Filamentous fungi such as *Fusarium* spp. can be detected in the cornea in vivo by confocal microscopy, observing hyphal density and morphology, inflammatory and corneal cells,[69] or by histology of corneal biopsies (Fig. 53.4).

Effective therapy requires mycological identification and, preferably, information about drug sensitivity. The number of drugs available for local ocular use is limited, not only by problems of local and systemic toxicity, but also by poor solubility and ocular penetration. No commercial antifungal preparations are available in the UK for local ocular use; eye drops are formulated from parenteral preparations.

Amphotericin B is active against a wide range of fungal organisms causing oculomycosis including *Aspergillus* spp., *Fusarium* spp. (most but not all isolates) and *Candida* spp. It may be given topically as drops, subconjunctivally or intravitreally. Although it is toxic when used topically at high concentration, in part due to the presence of deoxycholate in the parenteral preparation, the 0.15% formulation is virtually non-toxic. Amphotericin B is given parenterally by slow intravenous infusion in the management of endophthalmitis, often in a background of more widespread systemic infection, in addition to intravitreal therapy. Renal and hematological status must be kept under surveillance and drug levels monitored.

Natamycin (pimaricin) is a tetraene antifungal agent which has been used in the topical treatment of a wide range of filamentous fungi that cause keratitis such as *Fusarium* spp. (particularly *F. solani*) and, to a lesser extent, *Aspergillus* spp. A 5% suspension is available commercially in the USA. It has some topical toxicity.

Imidazoles have also been used effectively in the topical treatment of keratomycosis: clotrimazole, miconazole and econazole are effective against *Candida* spp. and *Aspergillus* spp. but not against the majority of *Fusarium* spp. Generally they have been considered less effective than amphotericin B in clinical use. They can be locally toxic. Ketoconazole is well absorbed after oral administration and is generally well tolerated, although there is a risk of hepatotoxicity. It has been used effectively in oculomycosis caused by *Fusarium* spp., combined with another antifungal agent to prevent the emergence of resistance.

Topical fluconazole is effective in animal models and patients in the treatment of *Candida* keratitis and shows less protein binding than the imidazoles. Itraconazole also has an enhanced therapeutic index compared to the imidazoles. *Candida* endophthalmitis can be effectively treated with oral fluconazole combined with intravitreal amphotericin B, but vitrectomy and fluconazole alone have also been reported to be successful. Aqueous levels of fluconazole 2 h after oral treatment with 20 mg were 2.7–5.4 mg/L and vitreous levels were up to 1.7 mg/L. Corneal levels were low (0.031 mg/L).

5-Fluorocytosine is active only against *Candida* spp. It is well absorbed by the oral route and achieves high blood and tissue levels. It has been used effectively in the treatment of *Candida* endophthalmitis, in combination with systemic or intravitreal amphotericin to prevent the otherwise rapid emergence of resistant strains. 5-Fluorocytosine has also been used topically (1% suspension) in the treatment of *Candida albicans* keratomycosis.

Thomas, reviewing the results of treating 318 patients with culture-proven keratitis,[73] found oral and/or topical ketoconazole and itraconazole useful in treating severe keratitis, especially that due to *Aspergillus* spp.

Fungal keratitis usually responds slowly to antifungal therapy over a period of weeks. Signs of toxicity (conjunctival chemosis and injection, recurrent corneal erosions) should also be observed. Negative scrapings during treatment do not always indicate that the fungus has been eradicated, since it may become deep seated; hence therapy should be maintained for 6 weeks or more. Confocal microscopy has proven valuable for managing treatment, observing morphological changes versus drug application.[74]

Patients who respond most poorly to topical antifungal therapy are those with deep corneal infections and those who have received corticosteroids prior to diagnosis. Fungal growth is aided by corticosteroids and argues against their use alone, or in combination with antifungal agents. Voriconazole, one of the more recent triazoles, has been found effective for treatment of refractory *Aspergillus fumigatus* keratitis[75] as well as for a broad range of fungal pathogens.[76] Like voriconazole, caspofungin, which similarly covers a wide range of yeasts and molds, has been used with success in the treatment of endophthalmitis due to *Candida* spp.[77]

Therapeutic surgery may be required for cases which respond poorly to medical therapy. However, therapy should be prolonged, to render the infecting fungus non-viable prior to surgery.

VIRAL INFECTIONS OF THE EYE

HERPES SIMPLEX EYE DISEASE

Herpes simplex keratitis (HSK) affects some 500 000 patients in the USA alone with about 50 000 episodes per annum and is the commonest cause of corneal opacification in the developed world. It is thus a major indication for corneal transplantation[78] with reported survival rates varying between 14% and 61%.

Primary ocular herpes simplex viral (HSV) infection is a self-limiting disease, expressed as blepharitis, conjunctivitis or punctate keratitis. Zosteriform spread along the fifth cranial nerve axons can then establish latency in the trigeminal ganglion; reactivation, with peripheral viral shedding, causes 'recurrent' disease expressed as epithelial keratitis (dendritic and geographic), stromal keratitis (disciform and necrotizing), limbitis, keratouveitis (and secondary glaucoma) or, rarely, acute retinal necrosis.

Ocular disease may be caused by two types of HSV: type 1 causes non-genital disease and has direct or indirect non-sexual transmission whereas type 2 is primarily sexually transmitted. Thus neonatal disease is usually acquired during birth and is caused by HSV-2 which has shown drug resistance.

An epidemic increase in genital herpes has been observed, hence it is expected that increased neonatal ocular herpes is likely, including delayed acute retinal necrosis syndrome.[79] Oral–genital transmission has become more common, hence HSV-1 is more frequently caused by sexual transmission. In childhood, herpetic keratitis is more frequently bilateral than when disease develops in adulthood. Children are more likely to suffer recurrent disease and significant visual loss including amblyopia.[80] Patients with severe atopic disease appear to be at greater risk of herpetic disease[81] and atopy is also increasingly common in children.

 ## HERPES ANTIVIRAL THERAPY

Epithelial keratitis

Early clinical trials established that trifluorothymidine (F3T) was more effective than idoxuridine (IDU) or debridement of the infected corneal epithelium, and that debridement added no adjunctive benefit to F3T alone. These early drugs were incorporated into host DNA and caused toxicity. They have been superseded by more effective non-toxic agents such as aciclovir and the prodrug valaciclovir. Systematic review has confirmed these are equivalent to F3T and IDU but do not cause toxicity.[82,83] Oral aciclovir (200 mg five times daily) and topical 3% aciclovir (five times daily) are equally effective;[84] however, oral therapy is more expensive and two randomized controlled trials have demonstrated that 3% aciclovir is equivalent to either 0.05% or 0.15% ganciclovir.[85] Topical interferon may have additional benefit but as yet there is no evidence base for this.[86] It is expected that therapy will achieve healing within a week of commencement.[87]

Aciclovir resistance has been documented with cross-resistance to ganciclovir and foscarnet.[88]

Disciform keratitis

This describes a circular focus of corneal edema and is considered to be an immunological response to a viral antigen, hence it requires topical steroid therapy (G Predsol 0.5% five times daily). Antivirals are required to prevent viral shedding and aciclovir combined with topical steroids has been shown to accelerate disease resolution. The HEDS project (Herpetic Eye Disease Study) addressed the need for steroids by double-blind, placebo-controlled, randomized controlled trial and demonstrated that steroids resulted in resolution of disciform disease at a median 27 days compared with 72 days for the placebo group; topical and oral aciclovir were equivalent both for disease control and recurrence rates.[89] Intraocular inflammation may be caused by stromal keratitis and is manifest by iritis with aqueous cells, flare and keratic precipitates.

Stromal keratitis

Stromal inflammation may cause progressive stromal lysis and corneal perforation and may be associated with dendritic ulceration. There is randomized controlled trial evidence that antiviral prophylaxis is effective during steroid management of stromal keratitis but no evidence that oral aciclovir influences the development of stromal keratitis in patients treated for epithelial disease.[90] In patients using long-term topical steroids, those with steroid-dependent stromal keratitis or those with corneal transplants, there is evidence that aciclovir prophylaxis is effective, but the duration of prophylaxis is not established.[78,91]

Necrotizing retinopathies

These may be caused by either HSV-1 or HSV-2, the latter being a relatively rare but serious infection, usually among neonates. Visual loss occurs due to retinal necrosis or ischemic optic neuropathy and treatment is with high-dose antiviral therapy (Box 53.7) and high-dose oral prednisolone (at least 20 mg/day). Laser therapy or surgery may be indicated for the management of retinal detachment.

 ## PROPHYLACTIC ANTIVIRAL THERAPY

The risk of recurrent HSK is 25% in the year following a first episode and 72% in 10 years,[92] but this risk is reduced by prophylactic oral aciclovir 400 mg every 12 h.[93] It is especially effective for atopic patients.[94]

Box 53.7 Systemic therapy for necrotizing herpetic retinopathy

Intravenous aciclovir 13 mg/kg per day in three divided doses for 14 days, *then*	
Oral aciclovir 800 mg five times a day	
Oral famciclovir 500 mg every 8 h for 3 months	More effective in immunocompromised patients
Intravitreal ganciclovir 400 mg twice a week, *combined with* intravenous foscarnet 60 mg/kg three times a week	May delay progress in immunocompromised patients

The risk of corneal transplant failure is determined in part by minimizing the risk of recurrent HSK; prophylactic aciclovir is effective in achieving this[95] and remains effective beyond 12 months.[96] Although valaciclovir is equally effective, the dosing may be more acceptable, thereby increasing compliance.[97]

HERPES ZOSTER VIRUS

Involvement of the first division of the fifth cranial nerve by varicella zoster virus (VZV) is associated with ocular features ranging from blepharitis, to persistent conjunctivitis, keratouveitis, glaucoma, papillitis, ocular nerve palsy and neuralgic ocular pain. This is termed herpes zoster ophthalmicus (HZO).

Oral administration of aciclovir is now standard treatment for HZO at a dose of 600–800 mg five times daily, initiated within 72 h of the onset of skin lesions. It is well tolerated and reduces the incidence and severity of epithelial and stromal keratitis and uveitis. Treatment reduces pain in the acute phase, but not neurotrophic keratitis or postherpetic neuralgia. The higher bioavailability of valaciclovir and famciclovir has allowed their use in more convenient dosing schedules at 1 g every 8 h and 500 mg every 8 h for 7 days, respectively, with faster resolution of acute pain in herpes zoster infection. Placebo-treated patients in a trial of intravenous aciclovir therapy suffered progression until topical aciclovir was started.

Intravenous aciclovir has replaced vidarabine as the treatment of choice in the management of HZO in AIDS and other immunocompromised patients, and intravenous foscarnet has been used effectively for the treatment of those patients with aciclovir-resistant HZO.

Although the use of topical ocular steroids to suppress the inflammation does not have the dire consequences seen with HSV eye disease (e.g. induction of dendritic or geographic ulceration), outcome in those treated with aciclovir alone may be better than in those receiving steroids alone (aciclovir 3% ointment vs betamethasone 0.1% ointment, five times daily). No recurrence occurred in the aciclovir-treated group, whereas the recurrence rate was 63% in the steroid-only group. Such recurrences were more difficult to suppress than the initial disease features. Corneal epithelial disease healed significantly more quickly in the aciclovir patients.

ADENOVIRUS KERATOCONJUNCTIVITIS

Adenovirus (ADV) infection causes epidemic forms of clinical disease, including pharyngeal conjunctival fever (ADV-3, -4 and -7), follicular conjunctivitis (ADV-1–11 and ADV-19) and epidemic keratoconjunctivitis (EKC). EKC is a self-limiting disorder characterized by a follicular conjunctivitis and a multifocal keratitis, with subepithelial features developing at 10–14 days after the onset of the disease. These infiltrates can be confused with *Acanthamoeba* keratitis but with

Acanthamoeba infection they occur within the first 7 days after onset. These infiltrates may persist for weeks or months, giving rise to disabling symptoms of glare and discomfort. Although subepithelial infiltrates may be suppressed by topical steroids, they reappear on steroid withdrawal, with a return of symptoms. Therefore, in practice, steroids are used only for selected, highly symptomatic patients and are weaned slowly, over a period of months. It appears that topical ciclosporin (cyclosporin) can be used in a similar fashion. Nosocomial, hospital outbreaks of EKC may be reduced by establishing appropriate infection control policies.

No antiviral agents are available commercially for the treatment of adenovirus infection.

OTHER VIRAL INFECTIONS

Most cases of measles are associated with conjunctivitis. Measles keratitis is a major cause of blindness in developing nations where secondary infection and vitamin A deficiency are compounding factors. Although there is no specific antiviral agent available, topical antibiotics and systemic vitamin A supplements improve the prognosis.

ACQUIRED IMMUNE DEFICIENCY SYNDROME

Human immunodeficiency virus (HIV) has been identified in tear fluid, conjunctiva, corneal epithelium and retina, and can give rise to a retinal microangiopathy, but the principal ophthalmic manifestations of acquired immune deficiency syndrome (AIDS) relate to florid opportunistic infections and to conjunctival and orbital involvement with Kaposi's sarcoma and other neoplasms. Therapy is directed against the relevant organism and generally is more intense and prolonged than is required in immunocompetent individuals. Highly active antiretroviral therapy (HAART) in AIDS patients leads to a striking fall in HIV load and substantial improvements in immune functions, including increases in total CD4 and CD8 cell counts, in memory and naive T-cell subsets, and in antigen responses to certain opportunistic pathogens. HAART leads to improved survival and reduced progression of HIV disease, with complete or partial resolution of infections or malignancies.

CYTOMEGALOVIRUS

Cytomegalovirus (CMV) is the most common of the ocular opportunists and produces a hemorrhagic, necrotizing retinitis. Because the onset of retinitis is often asymptomatic, it is recommended that in patients with AIDS with blood CD4+ counts below 50 cells/μL, ophthalmological examinations are carried out on a monthly basis. The onset or reactivation of CMV retinitis is heralded by elevated or rising blood CMV DNA levels.

During the first 7 years after infection, fewer than 1% of HIV-infected persons present with CMV retinopathy as the initial manifestation of AIDS, but CMV retinitis is found in approximately 18% of terminal AIDS patients, bilateral in about 17%. The delay from presentation with HIV infection is shorter in bilateral cases. HSV, Epstein–Barr virus and *Toxoplasma* occasionally cause a clinically similar retinitis.

In a study of CMV retinitis in AIDS patients, 58% presented with unilateral disease and 15% of these developed contralateral infection, despite treatment with ganciclovir. The risk factors for progression or involvement of the fellow eye have been reviewed.[98]

The incidence of CMV disease and of CMV relapse has fallen significantly since the introduction of HAART,[99,100] including the frequency of CMV-related retinal detachment. However, subclinical infections may be awakened at the initiation of HAART, and CMV retinitis may be activated when it is necessary to interrupt HAART for reasons of toxicity. At present, with the use of nucleoside and non-nucleoside analogs and protease inhibitors, CMV retinitis does not frequently pose an immediate threat to vision, but it may do so with development of retinal detachment, in association with peripapillary disease or by affecting the central retina. Retinal detachment, an important cause of blindness from CMV retinitis, can be treated successfully by vitrectomy, silicone oil and endolaser.

In patients with AIDS receiving HAART and treated additionally for CMV retinitis, it has been possible to withdraw anti-CMV therapy without major risk of reactivation of the retinitis for at least 48 weeks after ceasing antiviral therapy.[101] Reactivation, if it occurs, is more likely in those patients whose CD4[+] counts fall below 50 cells/µL and in whom there are signs of virological failure. At the time when CMV retinitis has become inactive, patients receiving HAART are at risk of developing a visually symptomatic 'immune recovery' vitritis or uveitis and macular edema, thought to represent a T-cell-mediated reaction to latent CMV antigens. The vitritis responds to treatment with periocular steroids without reactivation of the retinitis.

CMV retinitis occurring in AIDS patients implies a high risk for the development of CMV encephalitis. Vice versa, in patients with AIDS without CMV retinitis, CNS symptoms are unlikely to be attributable to CMV infection.

 ## SYSTEMIC THERAPY

Progression of CMV retinitis may be delayed in the short term by intravenous ganciclovir or foscarnet.[102] Repeated, local intravitreal therapy is more effective and particularly valuable when there are no signs of disseminated CMV disease. Ganciclovir, a virustatic drug similar in structure to aciclovir and foscarnet, improves or temporarily stabilizes the retinitis in the majority of patients receiving long-term maintenance therapy. Ganciclovir and foscarnet are equally effective in controlling CMV retinitis, but foscarnet is less well tolerated. Repeated therapy is indicated because of the high relapse rate. Ganciclovir is given by intravenous infusion over

1 h in a dose of 5 mg/kg every 12 h. Valganciclovir, the oral prodrug of ganciclovir, has excellent oral bioavailability, giving high ganciclovir blood levels without the need for prolonged intravenous access.

Intravenous administration of ganciclovir results in intravitreal concentrations which are subtherapeutic (0.93 ± 0.39 mg/mL) for many CMV isolates, which explains the difficulty of long-term complete suppression of CMV retinitis by this route.

Combined daily therapy with ganciclovir and foscarnet has been shown to be beneficial, with prolonged intervals between progression without increased toxicity. Such therapy may halt the progress of peripheral outer retinal necrosis in AIDS patients.

Improved results have been achieved with cidofovir treatment with 5 mg/kg once weekly for 2 weeks, then 5 mg/kg every other week, which retarded the progression of retinitis in AIDS patients compared to delayed therapy. Toxicity to cidofovir may occur in the form of proteinuria (23%), neutropenia (15%) and uveitis, and may lead to discontinuation of the drug.

 ## INTRAOCULAR DELIVERY

Intravitreal injection of antiviral agents is effective in the treatment of CMV retinitis, and avoids the risk of systemic toxicity. Intravitreal ganciclovir or foscarnet has been given on a weekly basis with little local ocular complication and no greater risk of retinal detachment. An intravitreal dose of ganciclovir (0.2–0.4 mg) is as effective as intravenous therapy, and a dose of 2 mg in 0.05–0.1 mL probably provides adequate intravitreal levels (0.25–1.22 µg/L) for up to 7 days. Levels at 24 h have been recorded as 143.4 µg/L and at 72 h as 23.4 µg/L. This higher dose (2 mg) has been used effectively to produce prolonged remission, with a low relapse rate (5% at 44 weeks).[103] The intravitreal dose of foscarnet is 2.4 mg in 0.1 mL. A lower dose of these agents has been given in patients whose eyes contain silicone oil in relation to retinal surgery.

Intravitreal cidofovir, together with oral probenecid, has also been effective in halting progression of CMV retinitis. Fomivirsen is an antisense oligonucleotide newly approved for intravitreal use.

More recently, the development of intraocular controlled-release devices has provided the opportunity to deliver drugs for prolonged periods with minimum local toxicity. Rhegmatogenous detachments can occur in CMV retinitis, with or without systemic treatment or ganciclovir implant therapy, but implants do not appear to increase the risk of detachment.[104]

TOXOPLASMA

Ocular toxoplasmosis in patients with AIDS is less common than CNS involvement. It may be the cause of presentation, with blurred vision and floaters, or pronounced visual loss from macular, papillomacular bundle or optic nerve head involvement.

The retinochoroiditis is unassociated with a pre-existing retinochoroidal scar, suggesting that the lesions are a manifestation of acquired rather than congenital disease. Lesions may be single or multifocal, in one or both eyes, or consist of massive areas of retinal necrosis. They may resemble those of CMV retinitis and may occur concurrently in the same eye. In comparison, toxoplasmic lesions tend to be thick and opaque, with smooth borders and a relative lack of hemorrhage.

Treatment of toxoplasmic ocular infection with pyrimethamine, clindamycin and sulfadiazine is effective in over 75% of patients. Once resolution is observed, maintenance therapy is continued, as relapses occur in the absence of treatment. Corticosteroid treatment is unnecessary and its use has been associated with the development of CMV retinitis.

PNEUMOCYSTIS JIROVECII

Pneumocystis jirovecii (formerly *Pneumocystis carinii*) can cause a choroidopathy as a result of systemic spread from primary lung infections. Multiple yellow placoid fundus lesions are seen.

CANDIDA ALBICANS AND CRYPTOCOCCUS NEOFORMANS

These can also produce retinal lesions or endophthalmitis, particularly in AIDS patients who are intravenous drug users. A bilateral epithelial keratopathy caused by *Encephalitozoon* has been described in an HIV-positive patient with cryptococcal meningitis, which responded to itraconazole given for the meningitis.

HERPES ZOSTER OPHTHALMICUS

This occurs in a more severe and chronic form in AIDS and may require prolonged systemic penciclovir therapy.

MICROSPORIDIA

Microsporidial keratoconjunctivitis in a patient with AIDS has responded to treatment with dibromopropamidine isethionate ointment.

OTHER INFECTIONS

VIBRIO SPECIES

In the coastal regions of the Gulf of Mexico, infections with *Vibrio* spp. are responsible for gastroenteritis, wound infections and septicemia. Penland et al[105] reported *Vibrio* spp. as a cause of conjunctivitis, keratitis and endophthalmitis on the Texas Gulf Coast, often following eye trauma with contaminated water containing shellfish or exposure to brackish sea water. Responsible organisms include *V. vulnificus*, *V. albensis*, *V. fluvialis* and *V. parahaemolyticus*. Jung et al reported a case of endogenous endophthalmitis from South Korea caused by *V. vulnificus* after ingestion of raw seafood.[106]

References

1. Tuft SJ, Ramakrishnan M, Seal DV, Kemeney DM, Buckley RJ. Role of *Staphylococcus aureus* in chronic allergic conjunctivitis. *Ophthalmology*. 1992;99:180–184.
2. Nakata K, Inoue Y, Harada J, et al. A high incidence of *Staphylococcus aureus* colonization in the external eyes of patients with atopic dermatitis. *Ophthalmology*. 2000;107:2167–2171.
3. Sundelin K, Seal D, Gardner S, et al. Increased anterior chamber penetration of topical levofloxacin 0.5% after pulsed dosing in cataract patients. *Acta Ophthalmol (Copenh)*. 2009;87:173–178.
4. Walker S, Diaper CJ, Bowman R, Sweeney G, Seal DV, Kirkness CM. Lack of evidence for systemic toxicity following topical chloramphenicol use. *Eye*. 1998;12:875–879.
5. Seal DV, Hay J, Kirkness CM, et al. Successful medical therapy of *Acanthamoeba* keratitis with chlorhexidine and propamidine. *Eye*. 1996;10:413–421.
6. Lim N, Goh D, Bunce C, et al. Comparison of polyhexamethylene biguanide and chlorhexidine as monotherapy agents in the treatment of *Acanthamoeba* keratitis. *Am J Ophthalmol*. 2008;145:130–135.
7. Seal DV, Wright P, Ficker L, Hagan K, Troski M, Menday P. Placebo controlled trial of fusidic acid gel and oxytetracycline for recurrent blepharitis and rosacea. *Br J Ophthalmol*. 1995;79:42–45.
8. Ta CN, Shine WE, McCulley JP, Pandya A, Trattler W, Norbury JW. Effects of minocycline on the ocular flora of patients with acne rosacea or seborrheic blepharitis. *Cornea*. 2003;22:545–548.
9. Behlau I, Gilmore MS. Microbial biofilms in ophthalmology and infectious disease. *Arch Ophthal*. 2008;126:1572–1581.
10. Dart JK, Radford CF, Minassian D, Verma S, Stapleton F. Risk factors for microbial keratitis with contemporary contact lenses: a case-control study. *Ophthalmology*. 2008;115:1647–1654.
11. Fulcher TP, Dart JK, McLaughlin-Borlace L, Howes R, Matheson M, Cree I. Demonstration of biofilm in infectious crystalline keratopathy using ruthenium red and electron microscopy. *Ophthalmology*. 2001;108:1088–1092.
12. Warheker PT, Gupta SR, Mansfield DC, Seal DV, Lee WR. Post-operative saccular endophthalmitis caused by macrophage-associated staphylococci. *Eye*. 1998;12:1019–1021.
13. Warheker PT, Gupta SR, Mansfield DC, Seal DV. Successful treatment of saccular endophthalmitis with clarithromycin. *Eye*. 1998;12:1017–1019.
14. Okhravi N, Guest S, Matheson MM, et al. Assessment of the effect of oral clarithromycin on visual outcome following presumed bacterial endophthalmitis. *Curr Eye Res*. 2000;21:691–702.
15. Wright HR, Turner A, Taylor HR. Trachoma. *Lancet*. 2008;371:1945–1954.
16. Solomon AW, Holland MJ, Alexander ND, et al. Two doses of azithromycin to eliminate trachoma in a Tanzanian community. *N Engl J Med*. 2004;351:1962–1971.
17. West SK, Munoz B, Mkocha H, Gaydos C, Quinn T. Trachoma and ocular *Chlamydia trachomatis* were not eliminated three years after two rounds of mass treatment in a trachoma hyperendemic village. *Invest Ophthalmol Vis Sci*. 2007;48:1492–1497.
18. Houang E, Lam D, Fan D, Seal D. Microbial keratitis in Hong Kong – relationship to climate, environment and contact lens disinfection. *Trans R Soc Trop Med Hyg*. 2001;95:361–367.
19. Lam DS, Houang E, Fan DS, Lyon D, Seal D, Wong E; Hong Kong Microbial Keratitis Study Group. Incidence and risk factors for microbial keratitis in Hong Kong: comparison with Europe and North America. *Eye*. 2002;16:608–618.
20. O'Brien TP, Maguire MG, Fink NE, Alfonso E, McDonnell P. Efficacy of ofloxacin vs cefazolin and tobramycin in the therapy for bacterial keratitis. Report from the Bacterial Keratitis Study Research Group. *Arch Ophthal*. 1995;113:1257–1265.

21. Hyndiuk RA, Eiferman RA, Caldwell DR. Comparison of ciprofloxacin ophthalmic solution 0.3% to fortified tobramycin–cefazolin in treating bacterial corneal ulcers. Ciprofloxacin Bacterial Keratitis Study Group. *Ophthalmology.* 1996;103:1854–1862.

22. Ofloxacin Study Group. Ofloxacin monotherapy for the primary treatment of microbial keratitis: a double-masked, randomized, controlled trial with conventional dual therapy. *Ophthalmology.* 1997;104:1902–1909.

23. Khokhar S, Sindhu N, Mirdha BR. Comparison of topical 0.3% ofloxacin to fortified tobramycin–cefazolin in the therapy of bacterial keratitis. *Infection.* 2000;28:149–152.

24. Alexandrakis G, Alfonso EC, Miller D. Shifting trends in bacterial keratitis in south Florida and emerging resistance to fluoroquinolones. *Ophthalmology.* 2000;107:1497–1502.

25. Kresken M, Behrens-Baumann W. Resistance to anti-bacterial agents amongst pathogens causing superficial ocular infection. *J Chemother.* 2007;16:49–59.

26. Schlech BA, Alfonso E. Overview of the potency of moxifloxacin ophthalmic solution 0.5% (Vigamox). *Surv Ophthalmol.* 2005;50(suppl 1):S7–S15.

27. Thebpatiphat N, Hammersmith KM, Rocha FN, et al. *Acanthamoeba* keratitis: a parasite on the rise. *Cornea.* 2007;26:701–706.

28. Ehlers N, Hjortdal J. Are cataract and iris atrophy toxic complications of medical treatment of *Acanthamoeba* keratitis? *Acta Ophthalmol Scand.* 2004;82:228–231.

29. Herz NL, Matoba AY, Wilhelmus KR. Rapidly progressive cataract and iris atrophy during treatment of *Acanthamoeba* keratitis. *Ophthalmology.* 2008;115:866–869.

30. Archer HG, Barnett S, Irving S, Middleton KR, Seal DV. A controlled model of moist wound healing: comparison between semi-permeable film, antiseptics and sugar paste. *J Exp Pathol.* 1990;71:155–170.

31. Shoff ME, Rogerson A, Kessler K, Schatz S, Seal DV. Prevalence of *Acanthamoeba* and other naked amoeba in South Florida domestic water. *J Water Health.* 2008;6:99–104.

32. Chang MA, Jain S, Azar DT. Infections following laser in situ keratomileusis: an integration of the published literature. *Surv Ophthalmol.* 2004;49:269–280.

33. Wroblewski KJ, Pasternak JF, Bower KS, et al. Infectious keratitis after photorefractive keratectomy in the United States army and navy. *Ophthalmology.* 2006;113:520–525.

34. Donnenfeld ED, O'Brien TP, Solomon TP, Perry HD, Speaker MG, Wittpenn J. Infectious keratitis after photorefractive keratectomy. *Ophthalmology.* 2003;110:743–747.

35. Karimian F, Baradaran-Rafi A, Javadi MA, Nazari R, Rabei HM, Jafarinasab MR. Bilateral bacterial keratitis in three patients following photorefractive keratectomy. *J Refract Surg.* 2007;23:312–315.

36. Solomon R, Donnenfeld ED, Perry HD, Biser S. Bilateral methicillin-resistant *Staphylococcus aureus* keratitis in a medical resident following an uneventful bilateral photorefractive keratectomy. *Eye.* 2003;29:187–189.

37. Solomon R, Donnenfeld ED, Perry HD, Maloney RK. Methicillin-resistant *Staphylococcus aureus* infectious keratitis following refractive surgery. *Am J Ophthalmol.* 2007;143:629–634.

38. Karimian F, Feizi S, Nazari R, Zarin-Bakhsh P. Delayed-onset *Actinomyces* keratitis after in situ keratomileusis. *Cornea.* 2008;27:843–846.

39. Daines BS, Vroman DT, Sandoval HP, Steed LL, Solomon KD. Rapid diagnosis and treatment of mycobacterial keratitis after laser in situ keratomileusis. *J Cataract Refract Surg.* 2003;29:1014–1018.

40. Freitas D, Alvarenga L, Sampaio J, Mannis M, Belfort R. An outbreak of *Mycobacterium chelonae* infection after LASIX. *Ophthalmology.* 2003;110:276–285.

41. Moshirfar M, Meyer JJ, Espandar L. Fourth-generation fluoroquinolone-resistant mycobacterial keratitis after laser in situ keratomileusis. *J Cataract Refract Surg.* 2007;33:1978–1981.

42. de la Cruz J, Behlau I, Pindela R. Atypical mycobacteria keratitis after laser in situ keratomileusis unresponsive to fourth-generation fluoroquinolone therapy. *J Cataract Refract Surg.* 2007;33:1318–1321.

43. de la Cruz J, Pindela R. LASIX-associated atypical mycobacteria keratitis: a case report and review of the literature. *Int Ophthalmol Clin.* 2007;47:73–84.

44. Garg P, Sharma S, Vemuganti GK, Ramamurthy B. A cluster of *Nocardia* keratitis after LASIK. *J Refract Surg.* 2007;23:309–312.

45. Muallem MS, Alfonso EC, Romano AC, Miller D, Kurstin J, Yoo SH. Bilateral *Candida parapsilosis* interface keratitis after laser in situ keratomileusis. *J Cataract Refract Surg.* 2003;29:2022–2025.

46. Chen WL, Tsai YY, Lin JM, Chiang CC. Unilateral *Candida parapsilosis* interface keratitis after laser in situ keratomileusis: case report and review of the literature. *Cornea.* 2009;28:105–107.

47. Sun Y, Jain A, Ta CN. *Aspergillus fumigatus* keratitis following laser in situ keratomileusis. *J Cataract Refract Surg.* 2007;33:1806–1807.

48. Kocaturk T, Pineda R, Green LK, Azar DT. Post-LASIK epithelial dendritic defect associated with *Alternaria*. *Cornea.* 2007;26:1144–1146.

49. Maverick KJ, Conners MS. *Aureobasidium pullulans* fungal keratitis following LASEK. *J Refract Surg.* 2007;23:727–729.

50. Patel SR, Hammersmith KM, Rapuano CJ, Cohen EJ. *Exophiala dermatitidis* keratitis after laser in situ keratomileusis. *J Cataract Refract Surg.* 2006;32:681–684.

51. Leung EH, Moskalewicz R, Parada JP, Kovach KJ, Bouchard C. *Exophiala jeanselmei* keratitis after laser in situ keratomileusis. *J Cataract Refract Surg.* 2008;34:1809–1811.

52. Balasubramanya R, Garg P, Sharma S, Vemuganti GK. *Acanthamoeba* keratitis after LASIK. *J Refract Surg.* 2006;22:616–617.

53. ESCRS Endophthalmitis Study Group. Prophylaxis of post-operative endophthalmitis following cataract surgery. *J Cataract Refract Surg.* 2007;33:978–988.

54. Lohmann CP, Linde HJ, Reischl U. Improved detection of microorganisms by polymerase chain reaction in delayed endophthalmitis after cataract surgery. *Ophthalmology.* 2000;107:1047–1051 1051–1052.

55. Okhravi N, Adamson P, Carroll N. PCR-based evidence of bacterial involvement in eyes with suspected intraocular infection. *Invest Ophthalmol Vis Sci.* 2000;41:3474–3479.

56. Seal D, Reischl U, Behr A, et al. the ESCRS Endophthalmitis Study Group. Laboratory diagnosis of endophthalmitis: comparison of microbiology and molecular methods in the European Society of Cataract & Refractive Surgeons multicenter study and susceptibility testing. *J Cataract Refract Surg.* 2008;34:1439–1450.

57. Seal D, Pleyer U. *Ocular infection.* 2nd ed. New York: Informa Healthcare; 2007.

58. Lundstrom M, Wejde G, Stenevi U, Montan P. Endophthalmitis after cataract surgery. A nationwide prospective study evaluating incidence in relation to incision type and location. *Ophthalmology.* 2007;114:866–870.

59. Miller D, Flynn PM, Scott IU. In vitro fluoroquinolone resistance in staphylococcal endophthalmitis isolates. *Arch Ophthal.* 2006;124:479–483.

60. Deramo VA, Lai JC, Fastenberg DM, Udell IJ. Acute endophthalmitis in eyes treated prophylactically with gatifloxacin and moxifloxacin. *Am J Ophthalmol.* 2006;142:721–725.

61. Kernt M, Neubauer AS, Ulbig MW, Kampik A, Welge-Lussen U. In vitro safety of intravitreal moxifloxacin for endophthalmitis treatment. *J Cataract Refract Surg.* 2008;34:480–488.

62. Vigamox (moxifloxacin) product insert. *Alcon Laboratories.* Texas: Fort Worth; 2008.

63. Seal DV, Kirkness CM. Criteria for intravitreal antibiotics during surgical removal of intraocular foreign bodies. *Eye.* 1992;6:465–468.

64. Jonas JB, Knorr HL, Budde WM. Prognostic factors in ocular injuries caused by intraocular or retrobulbar foreign bodies. *Ophthalmology.* 2000;107:823–882.

65. Das T, Jalali S, Gothwal VK, Sharma S, Naduvilath TJ. Intravitreal dexamethasone in exogenous bacterial endophthalmitis: results of a prospective randomised study. *Br J Ophthalmol.* 1999;83:1050–1055.

66. Freidlin J, Acharya N, Lietman TM, Cevallos V, Whitcher JP, Margolis TP. Spectrum of eye disease caused by methicillin-resistant *Staphylococcus aureus*. *Am J Ophthalmol.* 2007;144:313–315.

67. Blomquist PH. Methicillin-resistant *Staphylococcus aureus* infections of the eye and orbit. *Transactions of the American Society of Ophthalmology.* 2006;104:322–345.

68. Deramo VA, Lai JC, Winokur J, Luchs J, Udell IJ. Visual outcome and bacterial sensitivity after methicillin-resistant *Staphylococcus aureus*-associated acute endophthalmitis. *Am J Ophthalmol.* 2008;145:413–417.

69. Kowalski RP, Romanowski EG, Mah FS, Sasaki H, Fukuda M, Gordon YJ. A comparison of moxifloxacin and levofloxacin topical prophylaxis in a fluoroquinolone-resistant *Staphylococcus aureus* rabbit model. *Jpn J Ophthalmol.* 2008;52:211–216.

70. Jones JL, Muccioli C, Belfort R, Holland GN, Roberts JM, Silveira C. Recently acquired *Toxoplasma gondii* infection, Brazil. *Emerg Infect Dis.* 2006;12:582–587.

71. Hoerauf A, Büttner DW, Adjei O. Onchocerciasis. *Br Med J.* 2003;326:207–210.

72. Hoerauf A, Specht S, Büttner DW, Adjei O, Fimmers R. Effect of 5-week doxycycline treatment on adult *Onchocerca volvulus*. *Parasitol Res.* 2009;104:437–447.

73. Thomas PA. Current perspectives on ophthalmic mycoses. *Clinical Microbiological Reviews.* 2003;16:730–797.

74. Shi W, Li S, Liu M, Jin H, Xie L. Antifungal chemotherapy for fungal keratitis guided by *in vivo* confocal microscopy. *Graefe's Archives of Clinical and Experimental Ophthalmology.* 2008;246:581–586.

75. Mehta H, Mehta HB, Garg P, Kodial H. Voriconazole for the treatment of refractory *Aspergillus fumigatus* keratitis. *Indian J Ophthalmol.* 2008;56:243–245.

76. Hariprasad SM, Mieler WF, Lin TK, Sponsel WE, Graybill JR. Voriconazole in the treatment of fungal eye infections: a review of current literature. *Br J Ophthalmol.* 2008;92:871–878.

77. Breit SM, Hariprasad SM, Mieler WF, Shah GK, Mills MD, Grand MG. Management of endogenous fungal endophthalmitis with voriconazole and caspofungin. *Am J Ophthalmol.* 2005;139:135–140.

78. Foster CS, Barney NP. Systemic acyclovir and penetrating keratoplasty for herpes simplex keratitis. *Doc Ophthalmol.* 1992;80:363–369.

79. Pepose JS, Keadle TL, Morrison LA. Ocular herpes simplex: changing epidemiology, emerging disease patterns, and the potential of vaccine prevention and therapy. *Am J Ophthalmol.* 2006;141:547–557.

80. Chong EM, Wilhelmus KR, Matoba AY, Jones DB, Coats DK, Paysse EA. Herpes simplex virus keratitis in children. *Am J Ophthalmol.* 2004;138:474–475.

81. Prabriputaloong T, Margolis TP, Lietman TM, Wong IG, Mather R, Gritz DC. Atopic disease and herpes simplex eye disease: a population-based case-control study. *Am J Ophthalmol.* 2006;142:745–749.

82. McCulley JP, Binder PS, Kaufman HE, O'Day DM, Poirier RH. A double-blind, multi-center clinical trial of acyclovir versus idoxuridine for treatment of epithelial herpes simplex corneal ulceration. *Ophthalmology.* 1982;89:1195–1200.

83. Wilhelmus KR. Interventions for herpes simplex virus epithelial keratitis. *Cochrane Database Syst Rev.* 2003;(3): CD002898.

84. Collum LM, Akhtar J, McGettrick P. Oral acyclovir in herpetic keratitis. *Trans Ophthalmol Soc U K.* 1985;104(Pt 6):629–632.

85. Colin J, Hoh HB, Easty DL, et al. Ganciclovir ophthalmic gel (Virgan; 0.15%) in the treatment of herpes simplex keratitis. *Cornea.* 1997;16(4):393–399.

86. Guess S, Stone DU, Chodosh J. Evidence-based treatment of herpes simplex virus keratitis: a systematic review. *Ocul Surf.* 2007;5:240–250.

87. Wilhelmus KR. Therapeutic interventions for herpes simplex virus epithelial keratitis. *Cochrane Database Syst Rev.* 2008;1:CD002898.

88. Duan R, de Vries RD, Osterhaus AD, Remeijer L, Verjans GM. Acyclovir-resistant corneal HSV-1 isolates from patients with herpetic keratitis. *J Infect Dis.* 2008;198:659–663.

89. Barron BA, Gee L, Hauck WW. Herpetic Eye Disease Study. A controlled trial of oral acyclovir for herpes simplex stromal keratitis. *Ophthalmology.* 1994;101:1871–1882.

90. Herpetic Eye Disease Study Group. A controlled trial of oral acyclovir for the prevention of stromal keratitis or iritis in patients with herpes simplex virus epithelial keratitis. The Epithelial Keratitis Trial. *Arch Ophthal.* 1997;115:703–712.

91. Barney NP, Foster CS. A prospective randomized trial of oral acyclovir after penetrating keratoplasty for herpes simplex keratitis. *Cornea.* 1994;13:232–236.

92. Liesegang TJ. Epidemiology of ocular herpes simplex. Natural history in Rochester, Minn, 1950 through 1982. *Arch Ophthal.* 1989;107:1160–1165.

93. HEDS Group. Acyclovir for the prevention of recurrent herpes simplex virus eye disease. *N Engl J Med.* 1998;339:300–306.

94. Rezende RA, Bisol T, Hammersmith K, et al. Efficacy of oral antiviral prophylaxis in preventing ocular herpes simplex virus recurrences in patients with and without self-reported atopy. *Am J Ophthalmol.* 2006;142:563–567.

95. Garcia DD, Farjo Q, Musch DC, Sugar A. Effect of prophylactic oral acyclovir after penetrating keratoplasty for herpes simplex keratitis. *Cornea.* 2007;26:930–934.

96. Uchoa UB, Rezende RA, Carrasco MA, Rapuano CJ, Laibson PR, Cohen EJ. Long-term acyclovir use to prevent recurrent ocular herpes simplex virus infection. *Arch Ophthal.* 2003;121:1702–1704.

97. Goldblum D, Bachmann C, Tappeiner C, Garweg J, Frueh BE. Comparison of oral antiviral therapy with valacyclovir or acyclovir after penetrating keratoplasty for herpetic keratitis. *Br J Ophthalmol.* 2008;92:1201–1205.

98. Holbrook JT, Davis MD, Hubbard LD. Risk factors for advancement of cytomegalovirus retinitis in patients with acquired immunodeficiency syndrome. Studies of Ocular Complications of AIDS Research Group. *Arch Ophthal.* 2000;118:1196–1204.

99. Accorinti M, Pirraglia MP, Corradi R. Changing patterns of ocular manifestations in HIV seropositive patients treated with HAART. *Eur J Ophthalmol.* 2006;16:728–732.

100. Jabs DA, van Natta ML, Holbrook JT. Longitudinal study of the ocular complications of AIDS 2. Ocular examination results at enrollment. *Ophthalmology.* 2007;114:787–793.

101. Jouan M, Saves M, Tubiana R. Discontinuation of maintenance therapy for cytomegalovirus retinitis in HIV-infected patients receiving highly active anti-retroviral therapy. *AIDS.* 2001;15:23–31.

102. Hoffman VF, Skiest DJ. Therapeutic developments in cytomegalovirus retinitis. *Expert Opin Investig Drugs.* 2000;9:207–220.

103. Cochereau I, Diraison MC, Mousalatti H. High-dose intravitreal ganciclovir in CMV retinitis. *J Fr Ophtalmol.* 2000;23:123–126.

104. Kempen JH, Jabs DA, Dunn JP, West SK, Tonascia J. Retinal detachment risk in cytomegalovirus retinitis related to the acquired immunodeficiency syndrome. *Arch Ophthal.* 2001;119:33–40.

105. Penland RL, Boniuk M, Wilhelmus KR. Vibrio ocular infections on the U.S. Gulf Coast. *Cornea.* 2000;19:26–29.

106. Jung SI, Shin DH, Park KH, Shin JH, Seo MS. *Vibrio vulnificus* endophthalmitis occurring after ingestion of raw seafood. *J Infect.* 2005;51:281–283.

54 Urinary tract infections

S. Ragnar Norrby

This chapter deals with cystitis, pyelonephritis, prostatitis and urethritis caused by pathogens other than sexually transmitted ones such as *Neisseria gonorrhoeae*, *Chlamydia trachomatis*, *Trichomonas vaginalis* and *Ureaplasma urealyticum*. Cystitis and pyelonephritis are characterized by significant bacteriuria, which was originally defined by Kass as 10^5 colony forming units (cfu) or more per mL in each of two voided urine samples or any bacterial count in urine obtained by catheterization or bladder puncture.[1] This concept has now been redefined (Table 54.1), based on studies showing that by lowering the bacterial counts and including pyuria, the diagnostic sensitivity can be increased without marked loss of specificity.[2–4]

Both cystitis and pyelonephritis can be classified as symptomatic or asymptomatic, complicated or uncomplicated, and sporadic or recurrent. This classification is meaningful because etiology, choice of antibiotics, treatment times and needs for follow-up differ considerably between the various types of infection. The approximate frequencies of the various types are outlined in Table 54.2.

Asymptomatic bacteriuria is common in girls and occurs in 1–7% of adult women, depending on age. All patients with long-term urinary catheters have significant bacteriuria, which in most cases is asymptomatic. Many patients with cystitis who do not respond bacteriologically to antibiotic treatment but have persistent bacteriuria are also asymptomatic.

Complicated cystitis or pyelonephritis is defined as infections in patients with anatomical or functional defects which facilitate establishment of bacteriuria and/or make elimination of bacteriuria difficult. Examples of such defects are congenital anomalies of the urethra, ureters or kidneys, foreign bodies (stones, catheters), residual bladder urine due to obstruction or neurological disease, tumors and obstructions of the urethra by strictures, prostate hyperplasia, prostate cancer or prostatitis. Diseases that may aggravate the course of pyelonephritis (e.g. diabetes mellitus with nephropathy and malignant hypertension) are sometimes considered complicating factors. However, these conditions do not increase the risk of establishment of bacteriuria. Significant bacteriuria in a man should always be considered a complicated urinary tract infection; the length of the male urethra prevents ascending infections and establishment of bacteriuria in a healthy man.

Cystitis and pyelonephritis are often recurrent infections, both in patients with uncomplicated and complicated infections but more commonly in the latter. Recurrent urinary tract infections can be subclassified into relapse, when the same bacterial strain that caused the previous episode is isolated, or reinfection, when the causative pathogen is a new strain. There is no internationally accepted definition of a recurrent urinary tract infection. In clinical trials it is often defined as more than one episode in 6 months or more than two episodes in 1 year. Consequently, sporadic infections occur less than twice per 6 months or less than three times per year. It should be noted that this classification does not include chronic infections; chronic pyelonephritis and chronic glomerulonephritis are inflammatory diseases, albeit often aggravated by infections.

Urethritis is an inflammation of the urethra without concomitant significant bacteriuria. In patients with sexually transmitted diseases, urethritis is a well-defined concept (see Ch. 56). However, when such organisms are not identified and significant bacteriuria is not present, the 'urethral syndrome' becomes a microbiologically poorly defined disease, usually without identified etiology.

Prostatitis is an inflammation of the prostate gland, which often also involves the seminal vesicles. When prostatitis is caused by bacterial pathogens it is subdivided into acute and chronic bacterial prostatitis, which may or may not be associated with significant bacteriuria.

Table 54.1 Definitions of bacteriuria in midstream urine samples. Note that in all patients with symptomatic infections, pyuria must also be present[4]

Type of infection	Definition
Acute uncomplicated cystitis in women	
Infections caused by Gram-negative bacteria	$\geq 10^3$ cfu/mL
Infections caused by staphylococci	$\geq 10^2$ cfu/mL
Acute uncomplicated pyelonephritis	
Infections caused by Gram-negative bacteria	$\geq 10^4$ cfu/mL
Infections caused by staphylococci	$\geq 10^3$ cfu/mL
Complicated infections and infections in men	$\geq 10^4$ cfu/mL
Patients with asymptomatic bacteriuria	$\geq 10^5$ cfu/mL in two samples

From Rubin EH, Shapiro ED, Andriole VT, Davis RJ, Stamm WE. Evaluation of new anti-infective drugs for the treatment of urinary tract infections. **Clin Infect Dis.** 1992; 15(suppl 1): S216–S227.

Table 54.2 Approximate frequencies of various types of symptomatic urinary tract infections in an unselected material of outpatients with significant bacteriuria

Type of urinary tract infection	Approximate frequency (%)
Cystitis	90
Pyelonephritis	10
Uncomplicated infections	98
Complicated infections	2
Sporadic infections	75
Recurrent infections	25

EPIDEMIOLOGY AND PATHOGENESIS

Urinary tract infections occur in all ages and are most common in sexually active women. Below the age of 3 years, symptomatic cystitis or pyelonephritis is somewhat more common in boys than in girls due the higher frequency of congenital defects of the male urethra. In very old people bacteriuria is more common in men than in women due to the high frequency of prostate disease.

Cystitis and pyelonephritis are infections resulting from the aerobic fecal flora.[5] The pathogenesis of these infections should be considered from two aspects: host factors and virulence factors of the infecting organisms.

HOST FACTORS

Host factors of importance for establishment of bacteriuria are the ones mentioned above defining a complicated cystitis or pyelonephritis. In addition, the short length of the female urethra explains the higher frequency of bacteriuria in adult women than in adult men. Also in women without urinary tract defects bacteria can ascend the urethra and reach the bladder. In postmenopausal women atrophy of the vaginal mucosa constitutes an important and usually treatable (with topical or systemic estrogen) complicating factor, which is surprisingly often overlooked.

Establishment of significant bacteriuria in a woman is facilitated by a high number of bacteria in the periurethral area. This is achieved during sexual intercourse, which often leads to bacteriuria if the bladder is not emptied post-coitus.

In men, especially those who are sexually active, the source of a bacteriuria may be prostatitis. Otherwise a prerequisite for bacteria to reach the bladder in sufficient amounts to establish bacteriuria is a turbulent urine flow, which may result from strictures or obstruction of the urethra.

Irrespective of age and gender, pyelonephritis almost invariably results from bacteria ascending the ureters. This is facilitated by defects in the ureteral bladder sphincters causing ureteric reflux during micturition. Such defects may be congenital but are also common in pregnant women during the latter half of pregnancy due to the pressure of the uterus on the bladder. Pyelonephritis is also common in patients with ureteral stones or stones in the renal pelvis. Pyelonephritis and renal abscesses resulting from hematogenous dissemination of bacteria from other infectious foci is extremely rare but may be seen in patients with endocarditis.

VIRULENCE FACTORS

Virulence factors of the organisms causing cystitis and pyelonephritis have been extensively studied. With the most common etiological agent, *Escherichia coli*, it has been demonstrated that an important virulence factor is the ability of the bacterial cells to adhere to epithelial cells in the urinary tract mucosa.[6] This is achieved by antigens located on the fimbriae of the bacteria, which adhere to glycosphingolipid receptors on the epithelial cells. As a result of adherence, transportation of bacteria in the urethra and the ureters is facilitated. Another consequence of adherence is that cytokines (e.g. interleukins 1, 6 and 8) are released and that invasive infections are facilitated.[6–8] Adherence is important in patients without complicating factors but seems less important when such factors are present.[9] Other defined bacterial virulence factors are the antigenic structures of Enterobacteriaceae, the O, H and K antigens and the polysaccharide capsules. Virulence factors in Gram-positive organisms of importance in urinary tract infections are less extensively studied. In some situations (e.g. after treatment of bacteriuria caused by Gram-negative bacteria) the pathogenicity of Gram-positives in an asymptomatic patient should be questioned.[10]

ETIOLOGY

Bacteriuria is acquired by the fecal–genital route, often via periurethral colonization in women. With the exception of patients who have rectovesical fistulas or other abnormal communications between the bladder and the intestines or vagina, anaerobic bacteria rarely cause bacteriuria. The most common organisms causing bacteriuria are listed in Table 54.3.

In women with sporadic uncomplicated cystitis or pyelonephritis, the etiology is quite predictable; about 85% of these patients will have infections caused by *Esch. coli*. The second most common organism is *Staphylococcus saprophyticus*, which accounts for about 10% of the infections. However, in north Europe *Staph. saprophyticus* has a seasonal pattern:[11] it is normally not found between November and March and reaches a peak in July and August, when it causes up to 40% of all uncomplicated infections. The reason for this variation is unknown and it is not seen in the Southern Hemisphere.[12]

Esch. coli is also the most common etiology in recurrent and/or complicated cystitis and pyelonephritis but other Gram-negatives as well as enterococci become increasingly frequent. Of importance in these patients is the antibiotic treatment given for the preceding episode, which is likely to have

Table 54.3 Etiology of cystitis and pyelonephritis

Bacterial species	Dominating type of infection
Escherichia coli	All types
Staphylococcus saprophyticus	Uncomplicated cystitis and pyelonephritis in women during April to September
Klebsiella spp.	Recurrent/complicated infections
Enterobacter spp.	Recurrent/complicated infections
Enterococcus spp.	Recurrent/complicated infections
Proteus spp.	Tumors or stones
Morganella morganii	Recurrent/complicated infections
Pseudomonas spp.	Recurrent/complicated infections, bladder catheters
Other organisms	Recurrent infections

selected resistant organisms. Organisms such as *Enterobacter* spp., *Pseudomonas aeruginosa*, *Pseudomonas* spp., *Acinetobacter* spp., *Burkholderia* spp. and *Citrobacter* spp. typically appear in patients who have received repeated antibiotic courses or who have acquired their bacteriuria in hospital.

Proteus spp., *Morganella morganii* and *Providencia* spp., which all grow in alkaline pH, are common findings in patients with kidney or bladder stones or tumors. Since *Proteus* spp. is also common in the preputial flora, it is often a contaminant in urine samples from young boys.

Fungal growth in the urine is in most cases due to *Candida albicans* or other *Candida* spp. The clinical importance of funguria is uncertain or doubtful in patients with bladder catheters. In patients without catheters growth of *Candida* may reflect a renal infection resulting from hematological dissemination of the organisms. In rare cases candiduria is also seen as a result of the formation of a mycelial ball in the bladder.

DIAGNOSIS

CLINICAL DIAGNOSIS

Patients with cystitis are afebrile and the dominating symptoms are dysuria, frequent micturition and/or suprapubic pain. Sometimes macroscopic hematuria is present, especially in infections caused by *Staph. saprophyticus*.[11] With the exception of hematuria these symptoms are difficult or impossible to differentiate from those of urethritis unless the patient has a urethral discharge.

Pyelonephritis is a systemic infection; the patients develop fever and may have signs of septicemia, which occurs in up to 30% of patients with this infection.[9] Other symptoms are chills and flank pain. Differential diagnoses are urinary stones, cholecystitis, appendicitis and basal pneumonia. The clinical symptoms of pyelonephritis are often masked by patients taking drugs with analgesic and/or antipyretic activity.

In children urinary tract infections often present with few clinical symptoms and fever may be the only symptom of pyelonephritis.

Acute prostatitis is characterized by symptoms similar to those of cystitis but the patient also has a distinct tenderness and enlargement of the prostate at rectal palpation. In chronic prostatitis the symptoms may be more diffuse and the prostate is often normal at rectal examination.

RADIOLOGICAL DIAGNOSIS

Radiological examinations are rarely indicated in the acute phase of a urinary tract infection. An exception is when an obstruction of a ureter is suspected in a patient with signs of pyelonephritis. In children with pyelonephritis or with recurrent cystitis, radiological examinations for identification of congenital anatomical defects and/or ureteral reflux should be performed after treatment of the acute infection. For detection of vesicoureteral reflux in children, contrast-enhanced ultrasound is recommended as a better alternative to micturating cystourethrography.[13]

In adults who have recovered from pyelonephritis it is recommended that ultrasound or a radiological examination is performed to exclude renal scars from childhood episodes of pyelonephritis.[14,15]

LABORATORY DIAGNOSIS

The keystone in the diagnosis of cystitis and pyelonephritis is the demonstration of significant bacteriuria. The reference technique is the quantitative urine culture. The sample can be obtained as a clean-catch (midstream) urine or by bladder puncture or catheterization. Bladder puncture is the preferred technique in small children, especially boys. After sampling, the urine must be kept chilled (but not frozen) until analyzed. If there is likely to be a delay in transportation to a laboratory, a dip-slide culture can be used. With this technique an agar-covered slide is dipped in urine and incubated overnight at room temperature or a small incubator. It provides results in terms of quantity of bacteria and differentiation of Gram-negative and Gram-positive organisms. The slide can then be sent to a microbiological laboratory for determination of species and antibiotic susceptibility.

In patients with infections caused by Gram-negative bacteria other than *Pseudomonas* spp. bacteriuria can also be demonstrated by the nitrite test, a rapid paper-strip test. Nitrite is formed by bacterial metabolism of nitrate and is not normally present in urine. A positive nitrite test has a very high specificity. The sensitivity, however, is low because the method requires bladder incubation and because Gram-positive bacteria and *Pseudomonas* do not form nitrite.

Urine cultures should always be obtained in patients with complicated infections, recurrent infections or pyelonephritis. In patients with sporadic uncomplicated cystitis, etiological diagnosis should be optional, especially when the local antibiotic susceptibility pattern is known.

A marker for significant bacteriuria is pyuria. Demonstration of pyuria is best achieved by microscopy of unspun urine using a Bürker counting chamber and defining pyuria as $>10 \times 10^6$ leukocytes per liter of urine. The second-best method is to use a leukocyte esterase paper-strip test. Sediment microscopy has a low reliability because it is a technique that cannot be standardized.[10] Marked pyuria in a patient with negative bacteriological cultures should lead to a suspicion of renal tuberculosis (see Ch. 58).

There is no specific laboratory test for the differentiation of cystitis from pyelonephritis. Patients with pyelonephritis normally have increased serum concentrations of C-reactive protein and peripheral white blood cell counts may be increased. Erythrocyte sedimentation rate is not always increased when the patient is first seen but is likely to rise during the following days. A regular finding in patients with acute pyelonephritis is that the concentration ability of the kidneys is reduced. This can be measured as urine osmolality after 12 h of no fluid intake or, more easily, by a subcutaneous (not nasal) challenge with antidiuretic hormone. However, this test cannot be used when the patient is febrile and it is therefore a confirmatory test, which can be done once the patient's condition has improved.

Bacteria causing pyelonephritis form complexes with antibodies. Therefore, detection of antibody-coated bacteria by immunofluorescence has been used as a method to differentiate cystitis and pyelonephritis. However, this test has tended to show a high frequency of false-positive results if a reasonable sensitivity is strived for, or too many false-negative results if the specificity of the test is high.

The etiological diagnosis of prostatitis is difficult. The most ambitious technique is to culture four samples:

- The first portion of a voided urine sample
- A midstream urine portion
- Prostate secretion obtained by rectal massage of the prostate
- The first portion of new voided urine sample.[16,17]

Patients with acute or chronic bacterial prostatitis should be culture positive with the same organism in all four of these samples.

ANTIBIOTIC TREATMENT

Antibiotic treatment of cystitis and pyelonephritis is normally empirical. Women with acute cystitis are rarely willing to wait 24 h for treatment and patients with acute pyelonephritis should be treated as soon as possible to avoid damage to the kidneys and reduce the risk of serious systemic manifestations of the infections.

PHARMACOKINETIC REQUIREMENTS

All antibiotics used for treatment of urinary tract infections with significant bacteriuria should be excreted via the kidneys. This makes drugs such as chloramphenicol and the tetracyclines less suitable because they are lipid soluble, with elimination mainly via liver metabolism resulting in low urine concentrations. In patients with pyelonephritis it is also important that the antibiotic achieves serum concentrations sufficiently high to eliminate bacteremia. With renally excreted antibiotics therapeutic concentrations are normally achieved in the renal parenchyma.

In patients with prostatitis special pharmacokinetic requirements apply. The prostate tissue is a difficult-to-penetrate compartment. Moreover, the pH of the prostatic and vesicular fluid varies and is often altered by infection. Hence, the drugs used must be active at a wide range of pH values. Finally, in chronic prostatitis calculi may be present, which reduce the efficacy of antibiotic treatment.

SAFETY CONSIDERATIONS

Uncomplicated cystitis is an infection that constitutes no threat to the patient if adequately treated. When such infections are treated it is a prerequisite that the antibiotics used have the highest possible degree of safety; serious or life-threatening adverse effects cannot be accepted even if they appear in very low frequencies. On the other hand, in patients with pyelonephritis the infection per se constitutes a considerable risk to the patient, which makes adverse effects to the treatment given more acceptable if a high degree of efficacy can be expected.

CHOICE OF ANTIBIOTICS

Of paramount importance in this respect is the local antibiotic resistance pattern: it is not possible to extrapolate susceptibility data generated in one country to another. In the hospital environment there may be marked differences between hospitals in the same country in the frequency of resistance to commonly used antibiotics. The local microbiological laboratories must provide data from regular resistance surveillance studies performed on clinically relevant collections of bacterial strains. Results obtained in outpatients should be considered separately from hospital-generated data. Preferably, resistance surveillances should be prospective and denominator driven. If they are made (as is often the case) on routine samples sent to a diagnostic laboratory, they are likely to overestimate frequencies of resistance because cultures are more often taken in patients with recurrent infections or treatment failures.

Due to high frequencies of antibiotic use, antibiotic resistance in urinary isolates is becoming an increasing problem, especially since more and more isolates are multiresistant.[18-21]

DOCUMENTATION OF ANTIBIOTIC EFFICACY

Treatment of urinary tract infections with antibiotics aims at eliminating the symptoms and, most importantly in patients with cystitis or pyelonephritis, the bacteriuria. Systematic

Table 54.4 Requirements of clinical trials of antibiotic treatment of urinary tract infections

Criterion	Requirements
Type of infection	Only one – e.g. uncomplicated cystitis in women or complicated infections in either sex
Sample size	For trials in cystitis at least 200 patients with confirmed bacteriuria per treatment group; smaller samples for complicated infections and pyelonephritis
Entry criteria	Verified pyuria and/or positive nitrite test, typical symptoms, urine for culture
Control	Well-documented regimen
Design	Always prospective, controlled and randomized. Preferably double-blind
Endpoints	Bacteriological efficacy, clinical efficacy and safety. Efficacy to be analyzed 5–9 days and 4–6 weeks after treatment
Analyses	Both intention-to-treat analysis of outcome in all patients randomized and per-protocol analysis of patients fulfilling defined criteria (e.g. minimum treatment time, bacteriuria pretreatment and at least one follow-up visit)

evaluation of antibiotic efficacy is made in clinical trials. Table 54.4 lists minimal requirements on clinical trials of antibiotic treatment of cystitis and pyelonephritis. Most trials initiated by pharmaceutical companies today fulfill these criteria. However, before the mid-1980s many clinical trials often included too few patients to allow any conclusions to be drawn.

TREATMENT OF CYSTITIS

Cystitis accounts for approximately 90% of all infections with significant bacteriuria. Typically, about 75% of women with cystitis have sporadic infections and 25% recurrent infections in an unselected sample. Complicated infections are seen in only about 2% of unselected patients. Most of the patients with cystitis are women aged 15–50 years.

In addition to antibiotic treatment, it is important to provide advice to the patient on how to prevent recurrences. Sexually active women should be told that emptying of the bladder after intercourse will reduce the risk of recurrences.

Although cystitis is a self-limiting benign infection in most patients, antibiotic treatment is recommended,[22] the most important reason being to prevent ascending infections and pyelonephritis.

A large number of antibiotics are used for treatment of uncomplicated cystitis. A general rule is that oral β-lactam antibiotics (ampicillin, amoxicillin, carbapenems, cephalosporins, amoxicillin–clavulanic acid and other β-lactam–β-lactamase inhibitor combinations and pivmecillinam) seem to be considerably less efficacious in eradicating bacteriuria than trimethoprim–sulfonamide combinations, trimethoprim or fluoroquinolones (Table 54.5).[10,23] This is not due to more

Table 54.5 Bacteriological efficacy in a study comparing a β-lactam (ritipenem acoxil) with a fluoroquinolone (norfloxacin) for 5 days' treatment of uncomplicated cystitis in women[10]

Follow-up and outcome	Treatment	
	Ritipenem acoxil	Norfloxacin
5–9 days post-treatment		
No bacteriuria	51/122 (42%)[a]	77/114 (68%)
Superinfection	22/122 (18%)	20/114 (18%)
Persistence	41/122 (34%)[a]	12/114 (11%)
Not assessable	8/122 (7%)	5/114 (4%)
3–4 weeks post-treatment		
No bacteriuria	31/59 (53%)	52/82 (63%)
Recurrence	17/59 (29%)	16/82 (20%)
Reinfection	11/59 (19%)	8/82 (10%)
Not assessable	0/59	6/82 (7%)

[a]$p < 0.001$.

From The Swedish Urinary Tract Infection Study Group. Interpretation of the bacteriological outcome of antibiotic treatment for uncomplicated cystitis: impact of the definition of significant bacteriuria in a comparison of ritipenem axetil with norfloxacin. **Clin Infect Dis.** 1995;20:507–1503.

frequent resistance to β-lactams than to other antibiotics in bacteria causing bacteriuria: a possible explanation is that β-lactam antibiotics are rapidly eliminated (i.e. the urine becomes free from antibacterial drug about 12 h after the last treatment dose). On the other hand, with trimethoprim, trimethoprim–sulfamethoxazole and fluoroquinolones, high concentrations of drug are maintained in the urine for 24 h or more after the end of treatment. Another possibility is that the latter drugs reduce the periurethral inoculum more effectively than β-lactams, thereby reducing the risk of recurrences.

There are no major differences in clinical efficacy between antibiotics used for the treatment of uncomplicated cystitis. Irrespective of whether the bacteriuria is eliminated or not, symptoms tend to disappear after 3 days. Thus, there is a poor correlation between clinical efficacy and bacteriological efficacy.

The treatment time in uncomplicated cystitis is a controversial issue. Recommendations range from a large single dose to 7 days or more of treatment. A short treatment time offers better patient compliance, reduces costs and minimizes risks of adverse effects; however, all antibiotics tested in sufficiently

Table 54.6 Comparative efficacy of trimethoprim–sulfonamide combinations and β-lactam antibiotics when used for different treatment times in patients with uncomplicated cystitis[18]

Treatment time	Rate of eradication of bacteriuria and treatment	
	Trimethoprim–sulfonamide	β-Lactam
Single-dose	267/300 (89%)	58/60 (66%)
3-day	139/147 (95%)	282/343 (82%)
>5-day	294/308 (96%)	370/423 (88%)

From Karlowsky JA, Hoban DJ, DeCorby MR, Laing NM, Zhanel GG. Fluoroquinoloneresistant isolates of **Escherichia coli** from outpatients are frequently multidrug resistant: results from the North American Urinary Tract Infection Collaborative Alliance–Quinolone Resistance Study. **Antimicrob Agents Chemother.** 2006;50:2251–2254.

Table 54.7 Frequencies of adverse events reported after treatment of uncomplicated cystitis[18]

| Treatment time | No. of patients with adverse events and treatment | |
	Trimethoprim–sulfonamide	β-Lactam
Single-dose	30/404 (7%)	23/212 (11%)
3-day	13/195 (7%)	55/630 (9%)
>5-day	101/406 (25%)	126/934 (14%)

From Karlowsky JA, Hoban DJ, DeCorby MR, Laing NM, Zhanel GG. Fluoroquinoloneresistant isolates of **Escherichia coli** from outpatients are frequently multidrug resistant: results from the North American Urinary Tract Infection Collaborative Alliance–Quinolone Resistance Study. **Antimicrob Agents Chemother.** 2006; 50:2251–2254.

large trials have been found to be less effective if used as a single dose than in a longer treatment time (Table 54.6).[23] Differences exist between antibiotics. For trimethoprim–sulfamethoxazole and other combinations of trimethoprim and sulfonamides, high cure rates could be demonstrated after administration of a single dose. Treatment for 3 days improved the efficacy but no further benefits were achieved with longer treatment times. However, with prolonged treatment the frequencies of adverse events increased markedly in patients receiving trimethoprim-sulfonamide combinations whereas the safety of β-lactam antibiotics was far less affected by the treatment time (Table 54.7). Fluoroquinolones also seem to be relatively effective if used for 3 days or less and probably little is gained by increasing the treatment time to 5 days or more.

It is recommended that a short course (3 days or less) of trimethoprim–sulfamethoxazole, another trimethoprim–sulfonamide combination or trimethoprim alone is used as first-line treatment of sporadic uncomplicated cystitis when the local susceptibility pattern so allows. The documentation of efficacy is less comprehensive for trimethoprim because for many years trimethoprim–sulfamethoxazole was the gold standard in clinical trials. In pregnant women nitrofurantoin or a β-lactam antibiotic for 5–7 days should be used. β-Lactam antibiotics should otherwise generally be used restrictively due to their poor bacteriological efficacy.

Older, non-fluorinated quinolones should not be used for treatment of any type of urinary tract infection because they are considerably less active than the fluorinated quinolones and resistance emerges in high frequencies with these antibiotics. Moreover, resistance to older quinolones increases the risk of resistance to fluoroquinolones. Resistance to these antibiotics is chromosomal. With the non-fluorinated derivatives a single mutation of one the bacterial genes coding for the DNA gyrase (topoisomerase I), which is the main target for quinolones, will result in resistance (*see* Ch. 3). Such mutations occur in a frequency of about 10^{-8}. The new fluoroquinolones are 100–1000 times more active and require two consecutive mutations in species such as *Esch. coli* before the organisms become resistant, which is likely to occur at a frequency of 10^{-16}. If an old quinolone is used, the first mutation is often initiated, and the risk for mutation to resistance against the fluoroquinolones (if they are used) then increases from 10^{-16} to 10^{-8}.

Patients with recurrent uncomplicated cystitis are more likely to have bacteriuria caused by organisms other than *Esch. coli* or *Staph. saprophyticus.* Pathogens that should be covered are enterococci and *Klebsiella* spp. The choice of antibiotics will depend on the treatment used for the preceding episode. Fluoroquinolones, if they have not been used in the same patient recently, are very likely to be effective. To preserve the usefulness of the fluoroquinolones for treatment of these more serious infections and patients with pyelonephritis, these antibiotics are not recommended as first-line drugs for treatment of uncomplicated sporadic cystitis.

In women with frequently recurring cystitis and in whom underlying complicating factors have been excluded, short-term self-treatment has been proven to be effective.[24,25]

No follow-up procedures are warranted following treatment of uncomplicated sporadic cystitis. The patient should be told to come back if she again experiences clinical symptoms. However, advice should always be given about ways to avoid recurrences – e.g. double- or triple-voiding, generous fluid intake and (as mentioned above) post-coital bladder emptying.

Antibiotics for treatment of uncomplicated sporadic cystitis can often be chosen without urine cultures, based on knowledge of the local antibiotic susceptibility pattern. In patients with complicated infections (which are typically recurrent), and in patients with uncomplicated infections that recur, urine cultures should be performed routinely.

Antibiotics used for treatment of complicated and recurrent cystitis are the same as those used in sporadic uncomplicated infections. However, β-lactams tend to perform even less well than in sporadic cases and treatment must last 5 days or longer. In these patients the urine should be cultured after treatment to identify and eliminate any complicating factors.

TREATMENT OF PYELONEPHRITIS

Pyelonephritis may be a life-threatening infection. In adults, septicemia may lead to septic shock. In children, there is a marked risk for developing renal scars, which may lead to permanent renal damage if the patient develops recurrent urinary tract infections involving the affected kidney.[14,15] Correct choice of empirical antibiotic treatment is therefore essential.[22,23] The first therapeutic decision to be taken is whether or not the patient needs parenteral treatment. If an injectable antibiotic is needed, there are several alternatives for empirical treatment. In patients with community-acquired sporadic infections, a group 3 (second-generation) cephalosporin (e.g. cefuroxime), an aminoglycoside or, in some countries, trimethoprim–sulfamethoxazole is likely to be effective; ampicillin, amoxicillin and groups 1 and 2 (first-generation) cephalosporins (cephalotin, cefazolin, cefadine and others), against which more than 10% of *Esch. coli* strains are resistant, are not recommended.

In patients with hospital-acquired infections a group 4 or group 6 (third-generation) cephalosporin such as ceftazidime, cefotaxime or ceftriaxone, a carbapenem (imipenem or meropenem), an aminoglycoside or a fluoroquinolone (e.g. ciprofloxacin or levofloxacin) are effective in most countries.

In the acute phase of pyelonephritis, renal function is always reduced. This, together with the fact that β-lactams, aminoglycosides and quinolones all achieve high concentrations in urine, blood and renal tissues, allows the use of low doses (e.g. cefuroxime 750 mg every 8 h, 3 mg/kg per day of gentamicin, netilmicin or tobramycin, and 200 mg every 12 h of intravenous ciprofloxacin). Some patients with pyelonephritis may be given oral antibiotics throughout the course of treatment. Preferred antibiotics are the fluoroquinolones, which are more efficacious than oral β-lactam antibiotics.[26] Because quinolones are not recommended for pregnant women, and since the therapeutic efficacy of oral (but not parenteral) β-lactams must be questioned, oral treatment is not recommended initially in pregnant women with signs of pyelonephritis.

An insufficiently studied problem is what to use when a patient started on parenteral treatment is to be switched to an oral regimen. Clinical trials of antibiotics have traditionally not been directed towards this problem and few studies have evaluated the normal clinical situation – i.e. that a patient is treated parenterally for 24–48 h and then continued on an oral antibiotic. At present the best choice for oral follow-up to an injectable antibiotic in a patient with pyelonephritis seems to be a fluoroquinolone.

The treatment time is traditionally 2 weeks in pyelonephritis. Longer periods seem not to increase the cure rates but are likely to result in higher frequencies of adverse reactions to the antibiotics used. One study comparing ciprofloxacin for 7 days with trimethoprim–sulfamethoxazole for 14 days showed equally good results in the two groups.[27] Further studies are needed in this field. The efficacy of treatment for pyelonephritis should be followed up with urine cultures at least once after treatment.

ASYMPTOMATIC BACTERIURIA

Most patients with asymptomatic bacteriuria should not be treated. This is certainly true for patients with bladder catheters: in such cases treatment will only result in selection of increasingly resistant bacterial strains and, if the patient should develop a systemic infection, it may be difficult to find an active antibiotic. Early studies indicated that asymptomatic bacteriuria in elderly people was correlated to an increased mortality; however, more recent investigations have not shown that bacteriuria per se is an independent risk factor for increased mortality.[28–30] In one such study antimicrobial treatment of asymptomatic bacteriuria did not affect mortality. Exceptions to this rule are pregnant women and patients who are to undergo urogenital tract surgery: both these categories should be screened for bacteriuria and treated if positive. Antibiotics recommended are those used for treatment of uncomplicated cystitis. In other categories of patients (e.g. elderly people and those with diabetes mellitus), screening for bacteriuria is not recommended because treatment of asymptomatic bacteriuria has not been proven to have beneficial effects.

PROPHYLAXIS AND LONG-TERM TREATMENT

Antibiotic prophylaxis of cystitis and pyelonephritis should be used very restrictively. Patients with frequent recurrences of these infections should be investigated in order to find and eradicate complicating factors leading to the recurrences. In some patients episodes of cystitis or pyelonephritis may require prolonged treatment to prevent recurrence before surgery is performed. An important group in which such prophylaxis is indicated is children with congenital anatomical defects. Several studies have indicated that reflux and pyelonephritis in young children are correlated with renal cortical damage and scarring.

In a small fraction of patients with recurrent cystitis or pyelonephritis, mainly girls and young women, no complicating factor can be identified. Such patients benefit from prophylaxis and should be given nitrofurantoin or trimethoprim once daily at bedtime to ensure high bladder concentrations of drug during sleep. The treatment time is normally 6 months but several years of treatment may be required.

As mentioned above, cystitis in older women is often due to atrophic changes of the vaginal mucosa, increasing the periurethral bacterial inoculum. Elderly women should therefore be examined for vaginal atrophy; if present, atrophy should be treated with estrogen to prevent recurrence. Intravaginal treatment with estriol seems to give the lowest frequencies of adverse reactions.[31,32] In a randomized trial in older women, trimethoprim prophylaxis was only marginally better than cranberry juice for prevention of recurrences of urinary tract infections.[33]

TREATMENT OF PROSTATITIS

Antibiotic treatment of prostatitis differs from that of cystitis and pyelonephritis, both in choice of antibiotic and in treatment time. In patients in whom gonorrhea and chlamydial infection have been excluded, identification of the etiology can be attempted using segmented urine culture (*see above*). However, in most cases this procedure is too cumbersome and treatment is started without etiological verification. Drugs frequently used and well documented are trimethoprim–sulfamethoxazole, tetracyclines (e.g. doxycycline) and fluoroquinolones. Treatment should last 3 weeks or longer.

TREATMENT OF FUNGURIA

When *Candida* sp. is isolated in the urine and considered clinically relevant, treatment should be given. Amphotericin B is generally active against *Candida* and resistance has never been reported. However, the drug is difficult to administer and has considerable nephrotoxicity. One alternative in selected patients is local instillation of amphotericin B.[34] The azole derivatives (e.g. fluconazole and itraconazole) are liver metabolized and achieve low urine concentrations. Resistance to these drugs may occur; *Candida krusei* and *Candida glabrata* are normally fluconazole resistant. An alternative choice for treatment of candiduria, if the isolated organisms are susceptible, is 5-fluorocytosine (flucytosine) which is excreted by the kidneys and achieves high concentrations in renal tissue. However, caution should be taken not to use too high a dose of this drug, which may lead to adverse reactions. Optimally, serum concentrations of flucytosine should be kept between 25 and 75 mg/L during the entire dose period.

 # References

1. Kass EH. Bacteriuria and diagnosis of infections of the urinary tract: with observations on the use of methenamine as a urinary antiseptic. *Arch Intern Med*. 1957;100:709–714.

2. Stamm WE, Counts GW, Running KR, Fihn S, Turck M, Holmes KK. Diagnosis of coliform infection in acutely dysuric women. *N Engl J Med*. 1982;307:463–468.

3. Stamm WE. Measurement of pyuria and its relation to bacteriuria. *Am J Med*. 1983;75:53–58.

4. Rubin EH, Shapiro ED, Andriole VT, Davis RJ, Stamm WE. Evaluation of new anti-infective drugs for the treatment of urinary tract infections. *Clin Infect Dis*. 1992;15(suppl 1):S216–S227.

5. Moreno E, Andreu A, Pigrau C, Kuskowski MA, Johnson JR, Prats G. Relationship between *Escherichia coli* strains causing acute cystitis in women and the fecal *E. coli* population of the host. *Antimicrob Agents Chemother*. 2008;46:2529–2534.

6. Svanborg-Edén C, Hanson L, Jodal U, Sohl-Åkelund A. Variable adherence to normal urinary tract epithelial cells of *Escherichia coli* strains associated with various forms of urinary tract infections. *Lancet*. 1976;1:490–492.

7. Wullt B, Bergsten G, Samuelsson M, Gebretsadik N, Hull R, Svanborg C. The role of *P. fimbriae* for colonization and host response induction in the human urinary tract. *J Infect Dis*. 2001;183(suppl 1):S43–S46.

8. Frendelis B, Godaly G, Hang L, Karpman D, Svanborg C. Interleukin-8 receptor deficiency confers susceptibility to acute pyelonephritis. *J Infect Dis*. 2001;183(suppl 1):S43–S46.

9. Otto G, Sandberg T, Marklund BI, Ulleryd P, Svanborg C. Virulence factors and pap genotype in *Escherichia coli* isolates from women with acute pyelonephritis, with or without bacteremia. *Clin Infect Dis*. 1993;17:448–456.

10. The Swedish Urinary Tract Infection Study Group. Interpretation of the bacteriological outcome of antibiotic treatment for uncomplicated cystitis: impact of the definition of significant bacteriuria in a comparison of ritipenem axetil with norfloxacin. *Clin Infect Dis*. 1995;20:507–1503.

11. Hovelius B, Mårdh PA. *Staphylococcus saprophyticus* as a common cause of urinary tract infections. *Rev Infect Dis*. 1984;6:328–337.

12. Schneider PF, Riley TV. *Staphylococcus saprophyticus* urinary tract infections: epidemiological data from Western Australia. *Eur J Epidemiol*. 1996;12:51–54.

13. Westwood ME, Whiting PF, Cooper J, Watt JS, Kleijnen J. Further investigations of confirmed urinary tract infection (UTI) in children under five years: a systematic review. *BMC Pediatr*. 2005;5:1–10.

14. Ditchfield MR, Decampo JF, Nolan TM, et al. Risk factors in the development of early renal cortical defects in children with urinary tract infections. *Am J Roentgenol*. 1994;162:1393–1397.

15. Smellie JM, Poulton A, Prescod NP. Retrospective study of children with renal scarring associated with reflux and urinary infection. *Br Med J*. 1994;308:1193–1196.

16. Domingue Sr GR, Hellstrom WJ. Prostatitis. *Clinical Microbiological Reviews*. 1998;11:604–613.

17. Krieger JN, Jacobs R, Ross SO. Detecting urethral and prostatic inflammation in patients with chronic prostatitis. *Urology*. 2000;55:186–191.

18. Karlowsky JA, Hoban DJ, DeCorby MR, Laing NM, Zhanel GG. Fluoroquinolone-resistant isolates of *Escherichia coli* from outpatients are frequently multidrug resistant: results from the North American Urinary Tract Infection Collaborative Alliance–Quinolone Resistance Study. *Antimicrob Agents Chemother*. 2006;50:2251–2254.

19. Bean DC, Krahe D, Wareham DW. Antimicrobial resistance in community and nosocomial *Escherichia coli* urinary tract isolates, London 2005–2006. *Ann Clin Microbiol Antimicrob*. 2008;7:13.

20. Colgan R, Johnson JR, Kuskowski M, Gupta K. Risk factors for trimethoprim-sulfamethoxazole resistance in patients with acute uncomplicated cystitis. *Antimicrob Agents Chemother*. 2008;52:846–851.

21. Oteio J, Campos J, Lazaro E, et al. Increased amoxicillin–clavulanic acid resistance in *Escherichia coli*. *Emerg Infect Dis*. 2008;14:1259–1262.

22. Warren JW, Abrutyn E, Hebel JR, Johnson JR, Schaeffer AJ, Stamm WE. Guidelines for antimicrobial treatment of uncomplicated acute bacterial cytitis and acute pyelonephritis in women. *Clin Infect Dis*. 1999;29:745–758.

23. Norrby SR. Short-term treatment of uncomplicated urinary tract infections in women. *Rev Infect Dis*. 1990;12:458–467.

24. Wong ES, McKevitt M, Running K, Counts GW, Turck M. Management of recurrent urinary tract infections with patient-administered single-dose therapy. *Ann Intern Med*. 1985;102:301–307.

25. Schaeffer AJ, Stuppy BA. Efficacy and safety of self-start therapy in women with recurrent urinary tract infections. *Urology*. 1999;161:207–211.

26. Sandberg T, Englund K, Lincoln K, Nilsson LG. Randomized double-blind study of norfloxacin and cefadroxil in the treatment of acute pyelonephritis. *Eur J Clin Microbiol Infect Dis*. 1990;9:317–322.

27. Talan DA, Stamm WE, Hooton TM, et al. Comparison of ciprofloxacin (7 days) and trimethoprim–sulfamethoxazole (14 days) for acute uncomplicated pyelonephritis in women. *J Am Med Assoc*. 2000;283:1583–1590.

28. Abrutyn E, Mossey J, Berlin JA, Levison M, Pitsakis P, Kaye D. Does asymptomatic bacteriuria predict mortality and does antimicrobial treatment reduce mortality in elderly ambulatory women? *Ann Intern Med*. 1994;120:827–833.

29. Nicolle LE, Mayhew WJ, Bryan L. Prospective randomized comparison of therapy or no therapy for asymptomatic bacteriuria in institutionalized elderly women. *Am J Med*. 1987;83:27–33.

30. Nicolle LE, Bjornson J, Harding GK, MacDonell JA. Bacteriuria in elderly institutionalized men. *N Engl J Med*. 1983;309:1420–1425.

31. Raz R, Stamm WE. A controlled trial of intravaginal estriol in post-menopausal women with recurrent urinary tract infections. *N Engl J Med*. 1993;329:753–756.

32. Raz R. Hormone replacement therapy or prophylaxis in postmenopausal women with recurrent urinary tract infection. *J Infect Dis*. 2001;183(suppl 1): S74–S76.

33. McMurdo MET, Argo I, Phillips G, Daly F, Davey P. Cranberry or trimethoprim for prevention of recurrent urinary tract infections? A randomized controlled trial in older women. *J Antimicrob Chemother*. 2009;63:389–395.

34. Fisher FJ. Candiduria: when and how to treat it. *Current Infectious Disease Report*. 2000;2:523–530.

 # Further information

Butler CC, Hillier S, Roberts Z, Dunstan F, Howard A, Palmer S. Antibiotic-resistant infections in primary care are symptomatic for longer and increase workload: outcomes for patients with *E. coli* UTIs. *Br J Gen Pract*. 2006;56:686–692.

Cendron M. Antibiotic prophylaxis in the management of vesicoureteral reflux. *Advances in Urology*. 2008; 825475.

Huppert JS, Biro F, Lan D, et al. Urinary symptoms in adolescent females: STI or UTI? *J Adoles Health*. 2007;40:418–424.

Kwok W-Y, de Kwaadsteniet MCE, Harmsen M, van Suijlekom-Smit LWA, Schellevis FG, van der Wouden J. Incidence rates and management of urinary tract infections among children in Dutch general practice: results from a nation-wide registration study. *BMC Pediatr*. 2006;6:10.

Moorthy I, Easty M, McHugh K, Ridout D, Biassoni L, Gordon I. The presence of vesicoureteric reflux does not identify a population at risk of renal scarring following a first urinary tract infection. *Arch Dis Child*. 2005;90:733–736.

Welsh A, ed. *Urinary tract infection in children*. London: RCOG Press at the Royal College of Obstetricians and Gynaecologists; 2007.

55 Infections in pregnancy

Phillip Hay and Rüdiger Pittrof

On a global scale, infection during or after pregnancy is an important public health problem and a leading cause of pregnancy-related health loss. The prevention and appropriate treatment of infection in pregnancy must have a high priority in any health service. Healthcare interventions during pregnancy, the puerperium and the lactational period differ from those occurring at other times as they may affect the health of both mother and fetus/baby.

Possible outcomes of pregnancy-related infections are shown in Table 55.1. The US Food and Drug Administration (FDA) categories for prescribing antimicrobials are shown in Table 55.2.

While treating infections in pregnancy can improve the health of mother and fetus/baby, it may result in congenital or neonatal health problems or litigation. In affluent countries approximately 1 in 400 babies is affected by a birth defect with a teratogenic etiology. If nutritional supplements are excluded, medication to treat infection constitutes the largest single group of prescribed drugs. As patients often assume that congenital malformations are secondary to a drug taken in pregnancy[1] and attorneys offer 'no-cost litigation', litigation following antimicrobial treatment is a real risk of prescribing in pregnancy.

GENERAL PRINCIPLES OF DRUG USE IN PREGNANCY AND THE PUERPERIUM

As for any medical intervention, antimicrobial treatment in pregnancy aims to maximize expected benefits while minimizing expected harms. The frequency of harmful outcomes of treatment or its omission is uncertain for most conditions and drugs. When estimating the risks of a treatment, teratology studies in non-human primates offer the best predictors of human teratogenicity as they have a sensitivity and specificity of >90%.[2]

When treating infection in pregnancy and the puerperium the prescriber has to decide:

1. when to initiate treatment; when the diagnosis is suspected, as in possible maternal pyelonephritis.

2. when the diagnosis is confirmed, for example maternal tuberculosis, or when the risk of congenital or neonatal problems is minimized as in maternal HIV infection after the first trimester of pregnancy.

3. which medication to use – whether scientific data is available regarding the safety of various treatments options in pregnancy. Unfortunately, little information is available to assess the frequency of maternal side effects.

4. how the physiological changes in normal and abnormal pregnancy (Table 55.3) affect the pharmacokinetics, dose regimen and side effects of the treatment chosen.

While there is little information as to how these changes affect the pharmacokinetics of antimicrobial medication, it is reasonable to assume that, for a given dose and dose interval, serum levels of antimicrobial agents will be 10–15% lower than in a similar non-pregnant patient.[3]

SPECIAL CONSIDERATIONS FOR ANTIMICROBIAL TREATMENT IN PREGNANCY OR DURING LACTATION

ANTIBACTERIALS

 ### AMINOGYCOSIDES

Aminoglycosides readily cross the placenta, and fetal blood concentrations reach 20–60% of maternal blood levels. Following the long-term use of streptomycin for the treatment of maternal tuberculosis, eighth nerve damage has been reported in the neonate, but short-term use of aminoglycosides at therapeutic dose is extremely unlikely to result in fetal ototoxicity.[4] The physiological changes in pregnancy may make it very difficult to maintain therapeutic levels of aminoglycosides in mother (or fetus) and regular monitoring of serum is indicated.

Table 55.1 Theoretically possible outcomes of pregnancy-related infections

Outcome	Example
Healthy mother and healthy fetus	Common cold (most infections)
Mother without apparent health problems, congenital infection with abortion, stillbirth or long-term morbidity of the child	Untreated latent syphilis infection
Maternal infection causing minimal maternal illness but resulting in congenital infection	Cytomegalovirus infection causing mental retardation Parvovirus infection causing non-immune hydrops fetalis, toxoplasmal congenital eye disease
Maternal infection causing (preterm) delivery of non-infected child	Urinary tract infection with high maternal fever, malaria
Maternal infection causing (preterm) delivery of an infected child	Chorioamnionitis secondary to ascending lower genital tract infection (group B streptococcus, bacterial vaginosis, toxoplasmosis, rubella)
Maternal death or long-term morbidity following inadequate treatment (this may also affect the health of the fetus/baby)	Postabortion or puerperal sepsis leading to maternal death or infertility
Treatment of maternal illness causing fetal problems	Treatment of maternal infection with aminoglycosides resulting in 8th cranial nerve damage of the fetus
Treatment of maternal illness causing neonatal problems	Neonatal gray syndrome following maternal chloramphenicol treatment Neonatal kernicterus following maternal long-acting sulfonamides
Litigation of the prescribing physician (not uncommon)	Treatment of maternal illness and birth of a child with congenital abnormalities not related to the infection or treatment

Table 55.2 US Food and Drug Administration (FDA) categories for prescribing antimicrobials in pregnancy

	FDA pregnancy category		
	B	**C**	**D**
FDA definition	Animal reproduction studies fail to demonstrate a risk to the fetus and adequate and well-controlled studies of pregnant women have not been conducted	Safety in human pregnancy has not been determined, animal studies are either positive for fetal risk or have not been conducted, and the drug should not be used unless the potential benefit outweighs the potential risk to the fetus	Positive evidence of human fetal risk based on adverse reaction data from investigational or marketing experiences, but the potential benefits from the use of the drug in pregnant women may be acceptable despite its potential risks
Antimicrobials	Amoxicillin, ampicillin, azithromycin, carbenicillin, cefazolin, cefotaxime, cefoxitin, ceftriaxone, cefuroxime, cefalexin, cefalotin, clindamycin, cloxacillin, dicloxacillin, erythromycin, metronidazole, nafcillin, nitrofurantoin, sulfonamides, vancomycin	Aciclovir, amikacin, chloramphenicol, ciprofloxacin, clarithromycin, fluconazole, gentamicin, imipenem, trimethoprim	Tetracyclines, tobramycin

Antiretroviral agents Shown in Table 55.4
Source: Perinatal HIV Guidelines Working Group. Public Health Service Task Force recommendations for use of antiretroviral drugs in pregnant HIV-infected women for maternal health and interventions to reduce perinatal HIV transmission in the United States. April 29, 2009; pp 1–90. Available at http://aidsinfo.nih.gov/ContentFiles/PerinatalGL.pdf, table 2, pp 23–25.

Group A
FDA definition: Adequate and well-controlled studies of pregnant women fail to demonstrate a risk to the fetus during the first trimester of pregnancy (and there is no evidence of risk during later trimesters).
Antimicrobials: there are no antimicrobials in this group.

Group X
FDA definition: Studies in animals or reports of adverse reactions have indicated that the risk associated with the use of the drug for pregnant women clearly outweighs any possible benefit.
Antimicrobials: there are no antimicrobials in this group.

CEPHALOSPORINS

The cephalosporins are the most commonly prescribed antibiotics in pregnancy. All cephalosporins cross the placenta and no adverse fetal effects have been reported in humans.

However, testicular damage has been observed in male rats following intrauterine exposure to *N*-methylthiotetrazole cephalosporins. Many group 3 and group 4 (second- and third-generation) cephalosporins contain this side chain (*see* Ch. 13) and should be used with caution in pregnancy. Cefoxitin (a group 3 cephalosporin) does not contain the side chain.

Table 55.3 Implications of physiological changes in pregnancy

Physiological effects in pregnancy	Therapeutic implications
Increased blood volume (>40% at term) and total body water	Possibly larger loading dose
Decreased serum albumin concentration	Possible underestimation of free active drug
Increased hepatic metabolism, increased creatinine clearance	Possible increased drug clearance and need for higher doses and/or shorter dose intervals
Decreased gastrointestinal motility	Unpredictable absorption of oral medication. Possibly increased frequency of gastrointestinal side effects
Pathophysiological changes in pre-eclampsia (proteinuric hypertension in pregnancy). Compared with normal pregnancy: reduced intravascular volumes and total body water, serum albumin and creatinine clearance	Use high doses for drugs with a wide safety margin (such as penicillins) and/or monitor therapeutic levels of drugs with narrow safety margin (such as aminoglycosides) frequently

 CLINDAMYCIN

Cord blood levels of clindamycin are only 15–50% of those in maternal blood. Clindamycin has not been linked to congenital abnormalities. However, this is based on limited data and in a recent review by Nahum and colleagues[5] clindamycin, together with gentamicin and vancomycin, was classified as undetermined.

 CHLORAMPHENICOL

Chloramphenicol has not been associated with an increased risk of congenital malformation. However, when given in late pregnancy there is a theoretical risk of 'gray baby syndrome' (cyanosis, vascular collapse and death in premature neonates).

 MACROLIDES

The most commonly used macrolides are erythromycin, azithromycin and clarithromycin. Placental transfer of these antibiotics is low and no fetal problems have been reported.

While there is considerable evidence of the safety of azithromycin in pregnancy it is still labeled as a category B drug by the manufacturer.

Clarithromycin is usually used for the treatment or prophylaxis of *Mycobacterium avium* complex in HIV-positive patients. There are no large studies of this drug in pregnancy and its manufacturer rates it as category C.

Erythromycin has been used extensively in pregnancy but may be associated with an increased risk of cardiovascular malformations and pyloric stenosis.[6]

 METRONIDAZOLE

Metronidazole is the treatment of choice for trichomoniasis and anaerobic infections. It crosses the placenta readily and cord blood levels are similar to maternal blood levels. In mice and bacteria it is tumorigenic and mutagenic, but no such observations have been made in humans, and administration to over 1000 women during the first trimester of pregnancy did not result in an increased rate of malformations.[7] A possible association between vaginal treatment with metronidazole during the first trimester of pregnancy and congenital hydrocephalus has been described.[8] Metronidazole should be used during the first trimester only if the benefits outweigh the potential risks. Metronidazole concentrates in breast milk, causing it to taste bitter and may thus cause problems with breastfeeding.

 NITROFURANTOIN

Nitrofurantoin is commonly used for the treatment of urinary tract infections in pregnancy. As it crosses the placenta, it could cause hemolysis in a fetus with glucose-6-phosphate dehydrogenase deficiency. With our current knowledge, 'treatment with nitrofurantoin during pregnancy does not present detectable teratogenic risk to the fetus'.[9]

 PENICILLINS

Although all penicillins cross the placenta rapidly and result in cord blood concentrations that may be higher than those observed in maternal blood, there is good evidence of their safety in pregnancy[5] and no evidence that they are teratogenic.

 QUINOLONES

In a study of 549 pregnancies exposed to quinolones during the first trimester, no increased rate of malformations was observed.[10] However, quinolones are not recommended in pregnancy as they can cause lesions of the cartilage leading to lameness and arthropathy in immature dogs.

SULFONAMIDES AND TRIMETHOPRIM

Sulfonamides inhibit folate synthesis and may thus be associated with an increased risk of congenital malformations. Sulfonamides cross the placenta readily and compete for fetal and neonatal bilirubin binding sites. In the neonate this could cause hyperbilirubinemia. An association between folic acid antagonist treatment in early pregnancy and neural tube defects has been reported.[11]

TETRACYCLINES

Tetracyclines readily cross the placenta and when given in the second half of pregnancy are deposited in the long bones (no adverse effects) and deciduous teeth (causing yellow–brown discoloration) of the fetus. The impact of pregnancy on the frequency or severity of adverse side effects of tetracyclines in the mother is unknown but gastrointestinal problems appear to be more frequent. Except for the treatment of penicillin-allergic patients for whom desensitization is not available, tetracyclines are rarely indicated in pregnancy or during lactation.

GLYCOPEPTIDE ANTIBIOTICS (VANCOMYCIN AND TEICOPLANIN)

There are insufficient data to comment on the safety of vancomycin and teicoplanin in pregnancy. Vancomycin can be ototoxic and nephrotoxic and, as it crosses the placenta, similar effects could also occur in the fetus. Manufacturers advise use only if potential benefit outweighs risk, and monitoring of levels of vancomycin to minimize the risks of fetal toxicity.

OTHER ANTIBIOTICS

There are insufficient data to comment on the safety of aztreonam, imipenem, linezolid or daptomycin in pregnancy. Fusidic acid is not known to be harmful.

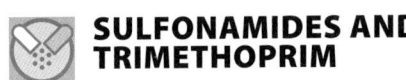

ANTITUBERCULOSIS DRUGS

There is good evidence that antituberculosis drugs do not increase the frequency of congenital malformations. Rifampicin (rifampin), ethambutol and isoniazid have no apparent adverse effects and, therefore, are considered safe throughout pregnancy. As pyridoxine requirements in pregnancy are likely to be increased, pregnant women taking isoniazid should also take 50 mg pyridoxine per day. Insufficient

human data are available for pyrazinamide, which may best be avoided during the first trimester. Streptomycin and kanamycin are associated with eighth cranial nerve damage in the fetus.

ANTIFUNGALS

Nystatin, clotrimazole and miconazole are frequently used for the treatment of candidiasis. There are no reports of increases in malformations from their use and they can be regarded as safe to take in pregnancy. Butoconazole, terconazole and ketoconazole are unlikely to cause malformations, but have not been adequately investigated in large studies.

Fluconazole has been associated with multiple congenital abnormalities at doses of 400 mg/day or greater. The published experience with the use of smaller doses, such as those prescribed for vaginal fungal infections, suggests that the risk for adverse outcomes is low, if it exists at all.[12] In those instances in which continuous, high-dose fluconazole is the only therapeutic choice during the first trimester, the patient should be informed of the potential risk to her fetus.

The available human data suggest that itraconazole is unlikely to cause major anomalies in humans.

There are also serious risks of fetal malformations associated with the use of griseofulvin, ketoconazole, voriconazole and flucytosine. Caspofungin is classified as pregnancy category C; it is not genotoxic or mutagenic, but is embryotoxic in rats and rabbits. No controlled studies have evaluated the safety of amphotericin B in pregnancy but case reports do not suggest teratogenicity.

SPECIFIC THERAPEUTIC PROBLEMS IN PREGNANCY

INTRODUCTION

During the 19th century maternal death from puerperal sepsis was a feared and common outcome of delivery. It is now rare in industrialized countries, but infections continue to present more subtle problems for pregnant women. The unique vulnerability of the developing fetus to infection and the role of subclinical infections in preterm birth (and possibly cerebral palsy) are being unraveled.

CHORIOAMNIONITIS AND INTRA-AMNIOTIC INFECTION

Premature delivery is a continuing and serious neonatal problem. Most neonatal deaths and morbidity (in the form of chronic lung disease and neurological impairment) occur in preterm births. Algorithms have been produced to enable obstetricians to estimate the risk of preterm birth for a particular pregnancy.

A history of previous preterm birth is the greatest risk factor; this, and most of the other risk factors, are not easily modified during pregnancy. Few interventions have been shown to reduce the incidence of preterm birth, and the incidence has changed little in the last 40–50 years in Europe and the USA.[13] Currently the incidence of birth at less than 37 weeks' gestation is 5–7% in Europe and 11% in North America. Most of the mortality and morbidity occurs in babies born before 34 weeks' gestation.

Histological chorioamnionitis and subsequent amniotic fluid infection are associated with preterm birth; this association is strongest in very preterm birth (<29 weeks). Animal models have demonstrated putative mechanisms through which infection leads to the release of proinflammatory cytokines such as interleukin-6 and tumor necrosis factor-α.[14] These cytokines in turn stimulate production of arachidonic acid metabolites, including prostaglandins, leading to cervical ripening, uterine contractions and preterm birth. This process is often subclinical, but in its most acute forms is associated with maternal fever, a raised C-reactive protein and an elevated erythrocyte sedimentation rate (ESR) in the mother. Recent studies have implicated elevated levels of proinflammatory cytokines with adverse sequelae in the neonate, including the pathogenesis of fetal cerebral white matter damage and bronchopulmonary dysplasia, precursors of cerebral palsy and chronic lung disease, respectively. This has been reviewed in more detail elsewhere.[15]

Most chorioamnionitis is due to ascending spread of bacteria from the lower genital tract either during or before pregnancy. The organisms found most frequently in association with chorioamnionitis and amniotic fluid infection include mycoplasmas (*Ureaplasma urealyticum* and *Mycoplasma hominis*), *Bacteroides* (*Prevotella*) species, *Gardnerella vaginalis*, peptostreptococci and group B streptococci.[16] Most of these organisms are found in high concentrations in the vaginal fluid of women with bacterial vaginosis, but also make up part of the normal flora in healthy women.

Bacterial vaginosis (BV) is the most common cause of vaginal discharge in women of childbearing age. The principal symptom is an offensive, fishy-smelling vaginal discharge that is often more apparent during menstruation or following unprotected intercourse. BV may resolve and occur spontaneously. In some populations its prevalence is greater than 50%, although in the UK it occurs in only 10–15% of women. It is thought to represent a disturbance of the vaginal ecosystem in which the usually dominant lactobacilli are overwhelmed by an overgrowth of predominantly anaerobic organisms including *Gardnerella vaginalis*, *Bacteroides* spp. *Mycoplasma hominis* and *Mobiluncus* spp. There is an increase in the vaginal pH from a normal below 4.5 to up to 7.0. BV is not a sexually transmitted infection and there is no benefit from treating male partners. Many observational studies have confirmed that women with BV have an increased risk of second trimester loss and preterm birth, with odds ratios between 1.4 and 6.9;[17] indeed, it may be the most important cause of idiopathic preterm birth.

Several studies have evaluated the use of antibiotics to treat women in pregnancy with BV to prevent preterm birth. Some studies of selected women at high risk have shown a benefit from treatment with metronidazole, or with a combination of erythromycin and metronidazole. The largest study, however, used short courses of metronidazole orally and showed no benefit in unselected asymptomatic women, or the subgroup with a previous preterm delivery.[18] Further studies are being performed, but at present no definitive conclusions can be reached on the value of such treatment. In 2007 a Cochrane review[19] found that antibiotic therapy for bacterial vaginosis during pregnancy did not reduce the risk of delivery before 37 weeks. However, treatment before 20 weeks' gestation may reduce the risk of preterm birth less than 37 weeks. In women with a previous preterm birth it may decrease the risk of premature preterm rupture of membranes.

Current guidelines from the USA (Centers for Disease Control and Prevention guidelines) and the UK (British Association for Sexual health and HIV, Clinical Effectiveness Group) do not suggest screening for bacterial vaginosis in pregnancy. A Cochrane review in 2008, however, found that screening for lower genital tract infection (BV, *Trichomonas vaginalis* and candidiasis) resulted in a 'lower incidence of preterm birth for low birth weight preterm infants with a weight equal to or below 2500 g and very low birth weight infants with a weight equal to or below 1500 g were significantly lower in the intervention group than in the control group'.[20]

Standard treatment in the UK for BV is metronidazole 400 mg every 12 h for 5 days, resulting in resolution within a few days; however, relapse occurs in as many as 30% of women within 1 month. Alternative treatments include intravaginal 0.75% metronidazole gel, 2% clindamycin cream and oral clindamycin 300 mg every 12 h for 5 days. Physicians have been wary of prescribing metronidazole during pregnancy because of reputed teratogenicity, but this has not been proven by human experience. If a woman requires treatment, it is sensible to discuss the potential risks and weigh them against the benefits. Both oral and intravaginal clindamycin have been associated with pseudomembranous colitis, a potentially fatal condition. Women who develop diarrhea following such treatment, particularly with blood, should cease treatment and seek medical advice.

PRETERM LABOR AND PRETERM PREMATURE RUPTURE OF MEMBRANES

Many of the infections that trigger preterm premature rupture of membranes and preterm birth are subclinical, without accompanying fever, maternal tachycardia, raised white cell count or raised ESR. A large multicenter UK-based study (ORACLE) of antibiotic treatment for women presenting in preterm labor has been completed recently. There was a reduction in adverse neonatal outcome for the use of erythromycin, but not amoxicillin–clavulanic acid, compared with the placebo group. There was an increase in neonatal morbidity with amoxicillin–clavulanic acid, with 2.3% of infants whose mothers received it developing necrotizing enterocolitis (compared with 0.8% in the other groups).[21]

A Cochrane review (last updated in 2004)[22] confirmed a statistically significant reduction in chorioamnionitis, numbers of babies born within 48 h and 7 days of randomization, neonatal infection and abnormal cerebral ultrasound scan prior to discharge from hospital. Symptomatic intrauterine infection should be managed by delivery and intrapartum antibiotics, as described for postpartum infection.

Antibiotics should not, however, be given in preterm labor in the absence of ruptured membranes or evidence of infection.[23]

ANTIBIOTIC PROPHYLAXIS AND CESAREAN SECTION

Randomized trials provide conflicting evidence as to the value of antibiotic prophylaxis on the prevention of postoperative febrile illness and wound infection following cesarean section. While the most recent and largest study[24] showed no significant benefit, a Cochrane review found that prophylactic antibiotics 'reduce the risk of endometritis by two-thirds to three-quarters and a decrease in wound infections justifies a policy of recommending prophylactic antibiotics to women undergoing elective or non-elective caesarean section'.[25] In a 'litigation-friendly environment' obstetricians are currently advised to follow local or national guidelines. If antibiotic prophylaxis is used, ampicillin or a group 1 (first-generation) cephalosporin is a reasonable choice.

URINARY TRACT INFECTION

Asymptomatic bacteriuria occurs in 5–10% of all pregnancies. If it is left untreated, 20–30% of mothers will develop acute pyelonephritis.[26] A Cochrane review compared antibiotic treatment with placebo or no treatment. It found that antibiotic treatment was effective in clearing asymptomatic bacteriuria (risk ratio (RR) 0.25, 95% confidence interval (CI) 0.14–0.48), reducing the incidence of pyelonephritis (RR 0.23, 95% CI 0.13–0.41) and the incidence of low birth weight babies (RR 0.66, 95% CI 0.49–0.89) but a difference in preterm delivery was not seen.[27] Furthermore, screening for and treatment of asymptomatic bacteriuria in pregnancy has been shown to be cost-effective.[28]

It is uncertain whether single-dose therapy is as effective as longer conventional antibiotic treatment[29] (*see* Ch. 54).

POSTPARTUM INFECTION

Following pregnancy the genital tract offers ideal culture conditions for many bacteria. The presence of virulent bacteria (group A and B streptococci, aerobic Gram-negative rods,

Neisseria gonorrhoeae, organisms associated with bacterial vaginosis or *Mycoplasma hominis*) increases the risk of endometritis,[30] as do prolonged rupture of membranes and multiple vaginal examinations.

A Cochrane review of antibiotic regimens for endometritis after delivery concluded: 'The combination of gentamicin and clindamycin is appropriate for the treatment of endometritis. Regimens with activity against penicillin-resistant anaerobic bacteria are better than those without. There is no evidence that any one regimen is associated with fewer side effects. Once uncomplicated endometritis has clinically improved with intravenous therapy, oral therapy is not needed.'[31]

SPECIFIC INFECTIONS

BACTERIAL INFECTIONS

 ### SYPHILIS

Syphilis is a sexually transmitted infection caused by the spirochete *Treponema pallidum*. It can also be spread nosocomially through contact with infected secretions, occasionally through blood products, and transplacentally. Syphilis is common in many developing countries, where up to 10% of pregnant women may have positive serological tests. In Western Europe and the USA the incidence fell progressively over the course of the second half of the 20th century. An increase in incidence in the USA during the late 1980s was linked to substance abuse, particularly 'crack' cocaine, as was a small epidemic in Bristol in the UK in 1998. Such outbreaks, including the epidemic reported in Russia and Eastern Europe during the 1990s, reinforce the importance of continued vigilance and surveillance against this infection. Syphilis is described fully in Chapter 56, so only the aspects relevant to pregnancy are reviewed here.

Syphilis may infect the fetus at any time during gestation and can be transmitted during any stage of maternal disease; at least two-thirds of all babies born to untreated women with syphilis are infected.[32] The spectrum of congenital syphilis varies, from a severe fetal infection causing intrauterine death to a neonate with symptomatic disease (early congenital syphilis), late congenital syphilis presenting after more than 2 years of age, or asymptomatic infection.

Penicillin is the treatment of choice for syphilis. Current UK guidelines recommend treating early syphilis (primary, secondary or early latent) with benzathine penicillin 2.4 million units intramuscularly as a single dose. This should be repeated after 7 days in the third trimester of pregnancy when the levels of penicillin may be reduced. Procaine penicillin G 600 000 units intramuscularly daily for 10 days can also be used. Later stages of syphilis require three doses of benzathine penicillin at weekly intervals, or 21 days of procaine penicillin. Particularly during early syphilis, a Jarisch–Herxheimer reaction may occur. This is mediated by the release of proinflammatory cytokines in response to dying organisms, and presents as a worsening of symptoms with fever for 12–24 h after starting treatment. It does not represent an allergic reaction and may be associated with uterine contractions and preterm labor.

Women who are allergic to penicillin represent a problem. Ceftriaxone 500 mg/day intramuscularly for 10 days is now recommended as an alternative regimen. Tetracycline, a more established second-line treatment, is relatively contraindicated in pregnancy. Erythromycin is less reliable, and resistance has been reported. If erythromycin is to be used, it is best administered intravenously. Azithromycin 500 mg/day can be an option, but there are few data on its use in pregnancy. The neonate should receive treatment with penicillin. One further alternative if the risk of fetal infection is high, is to perform penicillin desensitization with assistance from a clinical allergist. Current and recent sexual partners of women with syphilis must be screened, as well as older children in the family, if the date of acquisition is unknown.

Treatment in pregnancy should be instituted before 20 weeks' gestation to prevent the development of the stigmata of congenital syphilis.[33] In one population studied in the USA, one-third of the cases of syphilis diagnosed in pregnant women were acquired during the course of the index pregnancy, suggesting that rescreening may be an appropriate policy in some populations.[34]

The ideal treatment for syphilis in pregnancy is currently uncertain. A Cochrane review (last updated in 2009) found that none of the 29 studies included met the predetermined criteria but that none included comparisons between randomly allocated groups of pregnant women. The author concluded: 'While there is no doubt that penicillin is effective in the treatment of syphilis in pregnancy and the prevention of congenital syphilis, uncertainty remains about what are the optimal treatment regimens.'[35] Further studies are needed to evaluate the impact of HIV on the effectiveness of the currently recommended treatment regimens.

Stoll comprehensively reviewed the management of an infant born to a mother with reactive serological tests for syphilis.[36] In principle, if the mother has not received definitive treatment with penicillin, the infant *should* be treated with penicillin. The infant should be evaluated clinically, through serological tests and examination of the cerebrospinal fluid (CSF).

 # GONORRHEA

Neisseria gonorrhoeae is a sexually transmissible agent causing cervicitis, urethritis, endometritis, salpingitis and perihepatitis in women. In men it causes urethritis and epididymitis. In both men and women it causes proctitis and pharyngitis. Gonorrhea is common worldwide, although the incidence has decreased in developed countries since the Second World War. Infection in both sexes may be asymptomatic (*see* Ch. 56). Like chlamydia, gonorrhea is most common in young, sexually active women, with the incidence declining over the age of 25. Its importance in obstetrics is due to a neonatal eye

infection that, if untreated, can progress to blindness due to corneal scarring. The introduction of silver nitrate drops as prophylaxis produced a dramatic decline in the incidence of this complication.

The diagnosis is confirmed by culture. DNA detection-based tests are available and might be used for screening, but do not currently provide information about antibiotic sensitivity. *N. gonorrhoeae* has demonstrated a great ability to acquire resistance to antibiotics. It readily exchanges plasmids with other bacterial species and plasmid-mediated resistance to penicillin and tetracycline appear rapidly under selection pressure with such antibiotics. In many developing countries the price of antibiotics is prohibitive for most individuals, so that suboptimal doses are used; this encourages the development of resistant strains, which are then exported worldwide.

Chromosomal mutation has also produced moderate levels of penicillin resistance and is responsible for resistance to quinolones. Quinolones are contraindicated in pregnancy because of potential damage to developing cartilage and therefore in a penicillin-allergic woman or a woman with penicillin-resistant infection a cephalosporin such as ceftriaxone 500 mg in a single intramuscular dose, or cefixime 400 mg in a single oral dose, should be administered. Cephalosporin resistance has been reported in Japan and it is almost inevitable that further resistance will develop worldwide. A Cochrane review[37] (last updated 2009) found that little difference between different treatment options (amoxicillin plus probenecid, spectinomycin, ceftriaxone, ceftriaxone and cefixime) and, depending on resistance pattern, treatment with any of these antibiotics would be appropriate.

Neonates may present with ophthalmia neonatorum due to gonorrhea a few days after birth. If *N. gonorrhoeae* is cultured, topical and systemic treatment should be administered according to antibiotic sensitivities (*see* Ch. 53). In a similar way to *Chlamydia trachomatis* infection, gonorrhea is associated with chorioamnionitis and preterm birth.

Chlamydia trachomatis

Chlamydia trachomatis is important in pregnancy because it causes neonatal eye infection (ophthalmia neonatorum) and infant pneumonitis. Its role in miscarriage, chorioamnionitis and preterm birth is unclear, with some studies finding associations and others none. Nevertheless, chlamydia infections need to be treated at whatever stage of pregnancy they are diagnosed.

Estimates of the prevalence of genital *C. trachomatis* infection vary between 2% and 10% of women in the UK. The organism is detected much more commonly in young sexually active women, particularly those under the age of 25. The spectrum of disease varies from chronic asymptomatic infection to cervicitis, endometritis, salpingitis (pelvic inflammatory disease) and intraperitoneal spread leading to perihepatitis (Fitz-Hugh–Curtis syndrome). In men it causes non-gonococcal urethritis, which may present with urethral discharge and dysuria.

Approximately 15–25% of babies born to women with chlamydial infection develop ophthalmia neonatorum. The treatment of choice for *C. trachomatis* in the non-pregnant woman is tetracycline, usually doxycycline or azithromycin. Tetracycline should be avoided in the second and third trimesters of pregnancy because it binds to developing bones and deciduous teeth in the fetus, causing yellow–brown staining of the teeth. A Cochrane review (last updated in 2009) concluded that amoxicillin is an acceptable therapy of genital chlamydial infections in pregnancy when compared with erythromycin and that clindamycin and azithromycin may be considered if erythromycin and amoxicillin are contraindicated or not tolerated.[38]

The treatments suggested in UK guidelines are erythromycin 500 mg every 6 h for 7 days or erythromycin 500 mg every 12 h for 14 days, or amoxicillin 500 mg every 8 h for 7 days or azithromycin 1 g as a single dose.[39] Amoxicillin or azithromycin is also recommended by the US Centers for Disease Control (CDC)[40] and the draft World Health Organization (WHO) guidance for Europe.[41]

A test of cure should therefore be performed 3 weeks after completing treatment. It is essential that male partners are screened and treated before sexual intercourse is resumed. Neonates with ophthalmia neonatorum should be treated with tetracycline eye ointment. Because there is a risk of subsequent chlamydial pneumonitis they should also be treated with a 2-week course of erythromycin syrup.

Chlamydophila abortus

This organism, formerly classified as a strain of *Chlamydia psittaci*, causes epidemic abortion in ewes. In humans it causes an atypical pneumonia. Exposure to lambing ewes and the products of conception can lead to infection of pregnant women, resulting in intrauterine infection and abortion. It occurs most commonly in veterinarians and farm workers. All pregnant women should be advised to avoid sheep during the lambing season. Treatment is as for *C. trachomatis*.

 ## LISTERIOSIS

Listeria monocytogenes is commonly found in the stool samples of pregnant women; however, invasive disease in pregnancy is very rare. Most maternal disease results in influenza-like symptoms and does not usually require treatment.

Vertical transmission can occur transplacentally or, more frequently, during birth from cervicovaginal secretions. Intrauterine infection often leads to premature labor, fetal distress and meconium-stained amniotic fluid. Infection with *L. monocytogenes* responds to treatment with high-dose penicillin, ampicillin or trimethoprim–sulfamethoxazole (not a first-choice drug in the first trimester or in late pregnancy). While most causes of chorioamnionitis call for the early termination of pregnancy (delivery), chorioamnionitis caused by *L. monocytogenes* can be treated medically.[42]

 ## GROUP B STREPTOCOCCI

Colonization of the vagina with group B streptococci (GBS) is very common in pregnancy.[43] The importance of this is, however, uncertain and guidelines on the screening for GBS colonization are conflicting. While CDC 2002 guidance recommends universal screening,[44] current UK guidance states that 'routine screening (either bacteriological or risk based) for antenatal GBS carriage is not recommended'.[45] Bergeron and colleagues[46] used the polymerase chain reaction (PCR) in labor. In their hands the test had a sensitivity of 97% and a specificity of 100% and yielded results within 30–45 min.

While GBS do not usually cause morbidity in mothers, they are a common cause of neonatal infection. A Cochrane review (2009)[47] concluded that intrapartum antibiotic treatment reduces the rate of early onset GBS infection, but has no effect on other outcomes including overall morbidity and mortality.

VIRAL INFECTIONS

Specific therapeutic agents to treat viral infections systemically have not been available for more than a few years, with the exception of aciclovir for herpes simplex virus. Their role and safety in pregnancy is not fully established. The potential harm caused by intrauterine or congenital infections means that clinicians must consider the use of many such agents in pregnancy. Nevertheless, for many viral infections that can harm a fetus specific treatments are either not available (e.g. parvovirus and rubella) or have not been studied sufficiently in pregnancy (e.g. cytomegalovirus).

 ## CYTOMEGALOVIRUS

Cytomegalovirus (CMV) is a herpes virus with the ability to establish latency. In the UK approximately 40% of pregnant women are susceptible. The incidence of primary infection in pregnancy is unknown, but estimated to be about 1%. In healthy women reactivation of latent CMV infection is unusual, but may occur in pregnancy. The exposed fetus is less likely to have severe manifestations than in primary maternal infection: the principal features are microcephaly, blindness and deafness but some affected children have sensorineural hearing loss as the only sign of congenital CMV infection. A definitive diagnosis of congenital CMV infection can be made by isolating the virus in cell culture from throat swabs, urine, blood or CSF in the first 3 weeks of life. Serological diagnosis is made by the demonstration of a rising titer of IgG antibody or specific CMV IgM antibody.

Specific antiviral agents such as ganciclovir, valganciclovir, foscarnet and cidofovir are available for CMV; however, none should be used routinely. These agents are used in immunosuppressed individuals with AIDS or following transplantation.

A trial of intravenous ganciclovir in infected infants has shown some benefit in reducing deafness, but no role for treatment in pregnancy has been established.

 ## HERPES SIMPLEX VIRUS

Herpes is important in pregnancy because a devastating neonatal infection can occur with involvement of skin, liver and central nervous system (CNS). Neonatal mortality may reach 75%, but can be reduced to 40% if aciclovir is administered rapidly to the neonate. This syndrome is more common in the USA than the UK, with rates of 1 in 5000 and 1 in 33 000 live births, respectively. The vast majority of these cases are associated with a primary herpes infection in the mother in the weeks before delivery. The baby has no protective antibody and is vulnerable to disseminated infection or localized herpes encephalitis. The incidence of neonatal herpes is remarkably low considering the high prevalence of both symptomatic and asymptomatic genital herpes in these populations. The risk of neonatal herpes is greatest if primary infection occurs shortly before delivery, when there is no maternal IgG to cross the placenta, providing partial protection to the neonate.

In adults herpes is initially a clinical diagnosis. Typical vesicles or ulcers are seen on the genital mucosa. In primary infection lesions may be widespread, and persist for up to 3 weeks; secondary or recurrent episodes are usually localized and resolve in 3–7 days. In pregnancy recurrences may resemble primary infections, making clinical staging more difficult. Type-specific serological tests are becoming available, which may help to clarify the diagnosis. If IgG antibody to the same type of virus as is isolated on culture is present in the serum, then it is not a primary infection.

In the non-pregnant woman primary herpes is treated with a 5-day course of aciclovir 200 mg five times a day. This prevents further lesions from developing and allows current ulcers to heal. Recurrent episodes do not usually require treatment, as use of antivirals has not been shown to usefully reduce the time to healing.

For aciclovir, extensive reproductive toxicology studies in animal models before drug approval did not show a teratogenic effect.[48] Subsequent studies using a newer model showed head and tail abnormalities in rats at higher doses. It crosses the placenta. There was no evidence of teratogenicity in the prospective Acyclovir in Pregnancy Registry.[49] Less information is available for famciclovir and its active metabolite penciclovir, and valaciclovir, a prodrug for aciclovir. None is teratogenic in animal studies, and there is currently no excess of birth defects reported from their registries. The authors have used aciclovir to control symptoms in pregnant women with primary herpes following such discussions. Like any febrile illness, primary herpes may be associated with early miscarriage. Use of continuous aciclovir to suppress recurrent herpes throughout pregnancy is inadvisable.

Neonatal infection usually follows exposure to active lesions in the mother during delivery. When lesions are present the risk increases in proportion to the time between rupture of the membranes and delivery. The risk of intrapartum mother-to-child transmission can be reduced by cesarean section provided that the amniotic membranes are ruptured for less than 4 h. Current USA guidelines[50] recommend that 'women with active recurrent genital herpes should be offered suppressive viral therapy at or beyond 36 weeks of gestation and that cesarean delivery is indicated in women with active genital lesions or prodromal symptoms, such as vulval pain or burning at delivery, because these symptoms may indicate an impending outbreak'. Current UK guidelines do not recommend suppressive treatment and only advise cesarean section for symptomatic primary herpes infection.[51] In the Netherlands cesarean section for recurrent herpes was abandoned in 1987 and there was no subsequent increase in neonatal herpes.[52]

If primary herpes presents around the time of delivery, the pediatrician should be informed and genital swabs should be cultured from the mother and throat swabs from the baby within 24 h of birth. Intravenous aciclovir should be administered to the neonate.

 ## HUMAN IMMUNODEFICIENCY VIRUS

The acquired human immunodeficiency virus (HIV) pandemic has been spreading around the world since before the original descriptions of AIDS in 1981. Worldwide, approximately equal numbers of men and women are infected; most affected women are of childbearing age. In some cities in sub-Saharan Africa more than 30% of pregnant women are HIV infected. In London some hospitals have a prevalence of 1% of antenatal attendees. In the UK, nearly 1000 children are born to HIV-infected women annually. Since the vast majority of HIV-infected children acquire the infection by perinatal transmission, the prevention of vertical transmission is of paramount importance in reducing the prevalence of pediatric HIV.

Vertical transmission

Mother-to-child (vertical) transmission of HIV may occur during pregnancy, during childbirth or through breastfeeding. In the absence of intervention, vertical transmission of HIV infection is reported in 15–20% of babies born to HIV-positive women in European/American populations and in 25–35% in Africa and Asia.[53,54] Transmission is more likely if the mother has advanced HIV disease, as shown by a high viral load and a low CD4 count. Other risk factors include prolonged rupture of membranes and exposure to events that brings the fetus into contact with maternal blood such as vaginal/instrumental delivery, the use of fetal scalp electrodes and episiotomy.[54] Premature birth, low birth weight and breastfeeding are also established risk factors associated with increased risk of vertical transmission.

The exact mechanisms for perinatal transmission of HIV and the gestational age of greatest risk have not yet been determined. Viral DNA has been detected in fetal tissues as early as 12 weeks of gestation.[55] At birth, the virus can be detected in 30–50% of infected children,[56] suggesting that the remaining 50–70% of infected infants without viral markers at birth may have been infected late in pregnancy, during delivery or after birth, mainly through breastfeeding. The additional risk of transmission through breastfeeding in infants of infected mothers, over and above transmission in utero or during birth, is estimated to be 16%.[57]

The duration of breastfeeding is important and correlates with the risk of transmission. Nevertheless, in developing countries, the negative nutritional impact on overall infant morbidity and mortality of not breastfeeding may outweigh the benefit of avoiding HIV transmission from breast milk.

Preventing vertical transmission

Three interventions have been shown to reduce the risk of vertical transmission: elective cesarean section; bottle feeding; and antiretroviral treatment for the mother and neonate. In Europe and the USA the rate is currently below 2% in pregnancies in which the mother undertakes the recommended regimens to reduce the risk of transmission. A recent audit from the UK and Ireland reported an overall transmission rate of 1.2%, and it was 0.1% in women taking triple therapy with a viral load <50 copies/mL.[58]

Antiretroviral therapy

The aims of antiretroviral therapy in pregnancy are to prevent vertical transmission and maintain maternal health. Current UK guidelines for treatment of adults recommend starting combination antiretroviral therapy if there are clinical indications, or if the CD4 count is below 350 cells/mL (British HIV Association guidelines).

The safety of antiretrovirals in pregnancy has not been assessed adequately. The US FDA guidelines (Table 55.4), available at http://www.apregistry.com/forms/interim_report.pdf, rate them all as category B or C, with the exception of efavirenz which is category D. Among nucleoside/tide analogs, didanosine, emtricitabine and tenofovir are category B. Four protease inhibitors are category B: atazanavir, nelfinavir, ritonavir and saquinavir. The non-nucleoside analog drugs etravirine

Table 55.4 FDA categories for antiretroviral agents in pregnancy

Antiretroviral drug	FDA pregnancy category[a]	Placental passage (newborn:mother drug ratio)	Long-term animal carcinogenicity studies	Animal teratogen studies
Nucleoside and nucleotide analog reverse transcriptase inhibitors				
Abacavir (Ziagen, ABC)	C	Yes (rats)	Positive (malignant and non-malignant tumors of liver, thyroid in female rats, and preputial and clitoral gland of mice and rats)	Positive (rodent anasarca and skeletal malformations at 1000 mg/kg [35× human exposure based on AUC during organogenesis; not seen at 8.5× human exposure in rabbits])
Didanosine (Videx, ddl)	B	Yes (human) (0.5)	Negative (no tumors, lifetime rodent study at 0.7–3× maximum human exposure)	Negative (at 12× and 14.2× the human exposure in rabbits and rats, respectively)
Emtricitabine (Emtriva, FTC)	B	Yes (mice and rabbits) (0.4–0.5)	Negative (no tumors, lifetime rodent study at 26–31× human exposure at the recommended dose)	Negative (at 60×, 60× and 120× the human exposure in rats, mice and rabbits, respectively)
Lamivudine (Epivir, 3TC)	C	Yes (human) (~1.0)	Negative (no tumors, lifetime rodent study at 10–58× human exposure at the recommended dose)	Negative (at 35× the plasma levels of humans in both the rat and rabbit; however, embryolethality seen in rabbits with 1× human exposure)
Stavudine (Zerit, d4T)	C	Yes (rhesus monkey) (0.76)	Positive (mice and rats, at very high-dose exposure, liver and bladder tumors [rats only] at 250× and 732× the human exposure in mice and rats, respectively)	Negative (at 399× [rats] and 183× [rabbits] human exposure based on C_{max}, although sternal bone ossification is decreased and rat neonatal mortality increased at 399× human exposure in rats)
Tenofovir DF (Viread)	B	Yes (human) (0.95–0.99)	Positive (hepatic adenomas [female mice only] at 16× human exposure)	Negative (14× and 19× the human dose based on body surface area in rats and rabbits, respectively)
Zidovudine (Retrovir, AZT, ZDV)	C	Yes (human) (0.85)	Positive (non-metastasizing vaginal epithelial tumors at 3× to 24× human exposure in mice and rats, respectively)	Positive (increased fetal malformations associated with maternal toxicity at 300× human exposure in rats. Increased fetal resorptions at 66–226× and 12–87× human exposure in rats and rabbits, respectively, with no developmental abnormalities)

(Continued)

Table 55.4   FDA categories for antiretroviral agents in pregnancy—cont'd

Antiretroviral drug	FDA pregnancy category[a]	Placental passage (newborn:mother drug ratio)	Long-term animal carcinogenicity studies	Animal teratogen studies
Non-nucleoside reverse transcriptase inhibitors				
Efavirenz (Sustiva)	D	Yes (cynomolgus monkey, rat, rabbit) (~1.0)	Positive (hepatocellular adenomas and carcinomas and pulmonary alveolar/bronchiolar adenomas in female but not male mice at 1.7× human exposure; no increases in tumors in rats at 0.2× human exposure)	Positive (anencephaly, anophthalmia, micro-ophthalmia, and cleft palate in cynomolgus monkeys at drug concentrations comparable to humans; no reproductive toxicities in pregnant rabbits at 0.5–1× human exposure)
Etravirine (Intelence)	B	Unknown	Carcinogenicity studies in rodents are ongoing. Not mutagenic or clastogenic in in-vitro and in-vivo assays	Negative (rats and rabbits at exposures comparable to humans)
Nevirapine (Viramune)	B	Yes (human) (~1.0)	Positive (hepatocellular adenomas and carcinomas in mice and rats at systemic exposures lower than human)	Negative (rats and rabbits at 1–1.5× human exposure. However, decreased fetal body weight in rats at 1.5× human exposure)
Protease inhibitors				
Atazanavir (Reyataz)	B	Minimal/variable (human)	Positive (benign hepatocellular adenomas in female mice at 7.2× the human exposure)	Negative (2× and 1× the human exposure in rats and rabbits, respectively)
Darunavir (Prezista)	C	Unknown	Positive (hepatic adenomas, carcinomas [male mice], thyroid neoplasms [rats only] at 0.1–0.3× and 0.7–1× human exposure in mice and rats, respectively)	Negative (at 0.5× and 0.05× human exposure in rats/mice and rabbits, respectively)
Fosamprenavir (Lexiva)	C	Unknown	Positive (hepatic adenomas and carcinomas [mice and rats]; thyroid adenomas, interstitial cell hyperplasia, and uterine endometrial adenocarcinoma [rat only]; relative human exposures varied from 0.1–0.7× [mouse] to 0.3–1.4× [rat] depending on the human dosing regimen)	Negative (at 0.8× and 2× human exposure in rabbits and rats respectively; increased incidence of abortions in rabbits at 0.8× human exposure)
Indinavir (Crixivan)	C	Minimal (human)	Positive (thyroid adenomas in male rats at 1.3× human exposure)	Negative (however, extra ribs in rats at exposures below or slightly above those in humans)
Lopinavir–ritonavir (Kaletra)	C	Yes (human) (0.20 ± 0.13)	Positive (hepatic adenomas and carcinomas at 1.6–2.2× and 0.5× human exposure in mice and rats, respectively)	Positive (no effects in rabbits and dogs [~1× human exposure]; decreased fetal viability, body weight, delayed skeletal ossification and increase in skeletal variations in rats at maternally toxic doses [lopinavir 0.7×/ritonavir 1.8× human exposure])
Nelfinavir (Viracept)	B	Minimal/variable (human)	Positive (thyroid follicular adenomas and carcinomas in rats at 1–3× human exposure in rats)	Negative (in rats with comparable exposure to humans and rabbits at significantly lower exposure than humans)
Ritonavir (Norvir)	B	Minimal (human)	Positive (liver adenomas and carcinomas in male mice at 0.3× human exposure)	Positive (early resorptions, decreased fetal body weight, ossification delays, and developmental variations in the rat at maternally toxic dose [~0.3× human exposure]; cryptorchidism in rats [0.22× human exposure])

(Continued)

Table 55.4 FDA categories for antiretroviral agents in pregnancy—cont'd

Antiretroviral drug	FDA pregnancy category[a]	Placental passage (newborn:mother drug ratio)	Long-term animal carcinogenicity studies	Animal teratogen studies
Saquinavir (Invirase)	B	Minimal (human)	Negative (at 0.29× and 0.65× human exposure [co-administration with ritonavir] in rats and mice, respectively)	Negative (at 0.29× and 0.21× human exposure [co-administration with ritonavir] in the rat and the rabbit, respectively)
Tipranavir (Aptivus)	C	Unknown	In progress	Negative (decreased ossification and pup weights in rats associated with fetal toxicity at dose exposure 0.8× human exposure)
Entry inhibitors				
Enfuvirtide (Fuzeon)	B	None based on very limited human data	Not conducted	Negative
Maraviroc (Selzentry)	B	Unknown	Negative (transgenic mice; rats at 11× human exposure)	Negative (no evidence of harm to fetus at 20× and 5× human exposure in rats and rabbits, respectively)
Integrase inhibitors				
Raltegravir (Isentress)	C	Yes (rats [1.5–2.5], rabbits [0.02])	In progress	Negative (however, supernumerary ribs at 3× human exposure in rats)

AUC, area under the curve; C_{max}, maximum concentration.
[a]See Table 55.2 for an explanation of pregnancy categories.

and nevirapine are category B. The newer agents that block viral entry – enfuvirtide and maraviroc – are category B, while raltegravir, an integrase inhibitor, is category C. A discussion of the choice of agents in a standard triple-therapy regimen is beyond the scope of this chapter, but is discussed fully in the FDA guidelines and updated by the perinatal HIV working group at http://www.hivatis.org. Efavirenz is associated with congenital abnormalities in Rhesus macaque monkeys and its use is not recommended, particularly in the first trimester. To date, when used in human pregnancy, no increased rate of birth defects has been reported, and the upper 95% confidence interval for the rate of reported neonatal defects is now 4.9% compared to a background rate of 2.7%.

Potential hazards for the mother and fetus include the usual side effects of triple therapy, such as increased insulin resistance and diabetes mellitus, mitochondrial toxicity and lactic acidosis. Lactic acidosis is most common with stavudine and didanosine regimens, and a fatality in the third trimester has been reported. Tenofovir has been associated with osteopenia in animal studies, but it has not been reported in exposed children. In animals it resolves after exposure stops.

A further hazard is the risk of resistant virus emerging if monotherapy is used. If monotherapy is prescribed to women with low viral loads, CD4 counts >350 cells/mL and who are clinically well, the risk of developing zidovudine resistance mutations is low. A study from London reported no new resistance developing in 80 women prescribed zidovudine monotherapy with low viral loads and high CD4 counts.[59] Many antiretroviral drugs are potent inducers and inhibitors of cytochrome P_{450} enzymes. This leads to many potential drug interactions. Many should be taken with food to achieve adequate levels. A particular caution is to avoid co-administration of proton pump inhibitors with the protease inhibitor atazanavir. Heartburn is common in pregnant women. If an antacid is needed it should be taken at least 2 h after atazanavir.

The role of single agent (mono-) therapy

The efficacy of zidovudine monotherapy in reducing vertical transmission was demonstrated in a landmark randomized, double-blind, placebo-controlled trial.[60] Treatment was started at between 14 and 34 weeks of gestation, administered intravenously during delivery, and the neonate received oral treatment for 6 weeks. The rate of vertical transmission was reduced by 67% in women treated with zidovudine (25.5% placebo versus 8.3% zidovudine). Apart from a mild self-limiting anemia, no adverse effects were observed after a 4-year follow-up.

Nevirapine is the only other single drug (other than zidovudine) that has been shown in a randomized controlled trial to significantly reduce vertical transmission. In the HIVNET 012 trial,[61] 600 pregnant women were randomized to receive zidovudine during and at the onset of labor followed by 1 week of neonatal treatment, or a single 200 mg dose of nevirapine at the onset of labor with a single dose administered to the neonate within 3 days of delivery. At 14–16 weeks of age, 13.1% of the nevirapine-treated group were HIV infected, compared with 25.1% in the zidovudine group, a 47% reduction in transmission. Nevirapine monotherapy is relatively inexpensive, easy to administer and has immense potential for use in developing countries. There are concerns about the risk of resistance developing, as occurred in 23% of women in a small substudy. Current WHO guidance[62] does not recommend monotherapy (zidovudine for 7 days) in any setting other than for infants of mothers on established triple antiretroviral therapy.

Combination therapy

Triple therapy is recommended for pregnant women with advanced HIV disease, high viral load or low CD4 counts because the risk of mother-to-infant transmission correlates with these parameters.[61] Nevertheless, the marked reduction in viral load produced by triple therapy, and the resultant reduction in transmission, may be outweighed by potential and unquantified risks of these interventions on the neonate. For women with advanced HIV disease who are reluctant to expose their babies to combination therapy, zidovudine monotherapy plus an elective cesarean section is recommended.[63]

For women who present too late in pregnancy to allow formal virological/immunological assessment, the consensus guidelines recommend a zidovudine regimen with the possible addition of lamivudine and/or nevirapine. In women who conceive while on antiretroviral therapy treatment, it should be continued, although a change to (or the addition of) zidovudine should be considered while it remains the main agent of proven efficacy and safety in human pregnancy.

A randomized controlled trial comparing breastfeeding with formula feeding under study conditions with access to clean water showed no improvement of HIV-free survival for the formula group.[57] Outside such study setting, formula or mixed feeding leads to higher overall mortality than exclusive breastfeeding. Studies are underway exploring the reduction associated with continuing maternal triple therapy after delivery to allow breastfeeding, or continuing treatment for the baby if the mother does not require treatment herself. Initial studies report a transmission rate of approximately 2% through breastfeeding with antiretroviral treatment.

 ## HEPATITIS

In pregnancy the liver appears to be particularly vulnerable to infectious agents. Thus, hepatitis A, for which there is no specific antiviral agent, may cause fulminant, fatal infection in pregnancy, as may hepatitis E. Vaccination against hepatitis A and the use of human immunoglobulin may provide some protection if initiated in the incubation period. In non-pregnant adults ribavirin and interferon are used to treat hepatitis C, but their effects have not been studied in pregnancy. The risk of vertical transmission is low (<3%), but increases if there is a high level of maternal viremia.

Hepatitis B

Hepatitis B is a more severe infection, which may be followed by chronic carriage and disease ending in cirrhosis. Infection is transmitted sexually through blood or blood products or vertically to the fetus from an infected mother. The majority of acute infections are not clinically recognized, as only 20% of individuals develop jaundice. The earlier in life the infection occurs, the more likely the person

is to become a carrier: 80% of infants infected perinatally become carriers. Infection is particularly common in China and South-East Asia but prevalent in most tropical countries (*see* Ch. 48).

Pregnant women are screened for hepatitis B at booking. Treatment is available with interferon under the guidance of a liver specialist, and antiviral drugs with specific activity against hepatitis B are being introduced. However, the safety of interferon in pregnancy has not been adequately evaluated.[64] Vertical transmission can be reduced by vaccination of neonates born to mothers with hepatitis B. Hepatitis B immune globulin is also given at birth if the mother is antigen e positive. Many countries have a policy of universal vaccination of all infants.

PROTOZOAL AND FUNGAL INFECTIONS

 ### TOXOPLASMOSIS

Maternal infection with the intracellular protozoan parasite *Toxoplasma gondii* is usually asymptomatic and the risk to an immunocompetent mother is minimal. Transplacental fetal infection occurs in 20–50% of primary infections and may cause chorioretinitis, intracranial calcifications and hydrocephalus. Diagnosis of primary infection during pregnancy depends on serological screening for *Toxoplasma*-specific IgG in pregnant women followed by confirmatory testing and, ultimately, amniocentesis or cordocentesis. Where the incidence of primary toxoplasmosis in pregnancy is low (e.g. in the USA and UK) screening is currently not recommend. Women who seroconvert during pregnancy should be treated with spiramycin (a macrolide that does not cross the placenta) and, if fetal infection is confirmed, treatment should be changed to pyrimethamine and sulfadiazine plus folate supplements (after 18 weeks' gestation).[65]

Mothers should be informed that: (1) such treatment will not always prevent transmission but will reduce the risk of severe congenital malformations developing; and (2) maternal side effects and congenital abnormalities may occur as a result of the treatment.

 ### TRICHOMONIASIS

Trichomonas vaginalis causes a severe vulvovaginitis in susceptible women. It is generally sexually transmitted, although infection may persist asymptomatically for many months in women and in some men. In men it causes urethritis but is frequently asymptomatic. Male partners should be screened for sexually transmitted diseases and treated with metronidazole.

Transient infection may be transmitted to newborn female infants who have stratified squamous epithelium in the vagina, similar to that of an adult, due to the influence of high levels of maternal estrogen in utero. These infants are susceptible to infection and may present with purulent vaginal discharge. As the influence of maternal estrogen wanes over the first few weeks of life, infection usually resolves spontaneously and specific treatment is rarely necessary.

The only established treatments for trichomoniasis are metronidazole and tinidazole. As discussed above, there is no evidence of teratogenicity from metronidazole use, and it should be used to treat symptomatic infection whatever the stage of pregnancy. Treatment of asymptomatic trichomoniasis with metronidazole did not prevent preterm birth and may cause harm.[66] A Cochrane review[67] 'found no evidence to support the use of metronidazole in pregnant asymptomatic women with *Trichomonas vaginalis*. It is not clear why metronidazole should cause adverse pregnancy outcomes when it is effective in clearing the infection.'

MALARIA

Malaria is prevalent throughout the tropics and is a major cause of mortality in both children and adults. *Plasmodium falciparum* causes the most severe type of malaria, which can present with hepatic and cerebral manifestations. It is transmitted between human hosts by the female *Anopheles* mosquito. *P. falciparum* has been able to develop resistance to most antimalarials, creating a need for new agents. The other strains of malaria seldom cause fatal disease, but cause considerable morbidity; they are virtually always chloroquine sensitive (*see* Ch. 62).

Pregnant and puerperal women are at increased risk of malaria infection. If they become infected with malaria, complications – particularly hypoglycemia and lactic acidosis – are more frequent. Infection may also trigger a miscarriage or premature labor. In hyperendemic areas the disease may present as severe anemia, with a negative blood film.

In women at risk of malaria, regular or intermittent chemoprophylaxis reduces the risk of several maternal anemia, perinatal death and low birth weight.[68] Even non-falciparum malaria has been associated with intrauterine growth retardation. Congenital malaria has been described.

The diagnosis should be suspected in anyone who has been to the tropics and presents with a febrile illness. A history of taking prophylaxis does not exclude the diagnosis, as no prophylaxis is 100% effective. A blood film should be requested and stained for malaria parasites. Repeated blood films should be taken during episodes of fever if the initial test is negative. As well as anemia there may be thrombocytopenia and elevation of liver enzymes. Fever in the tropics or in people recently returned may be caused by many other infections, including typhoid, food poisoning organisms and viral infections such as dengue fever.

In affluent countries pregnant women with suspected malaria should be admitted to hospital and monitored closely as sudden deterioration requiring intensive care may occur.

Confirmed or possible falciparum malaria is usually treated with quinine sulfate. The dose regimen and mode of administration are not affected by pregnancy. Quinine does not cause abortion or preterm labor (unless massively overdosed), but can induce hypoglycemia and lactic acidosis. Malariae, vivax and ovale malaria should be treated with standard doses of chloroquine. Vivax and ovale malaria can develop persisting forms (hypnozoites). The best method of eradication therapy in pregnancy is currently controversial and expert advice should be obtained. A treatment course of pyrimethamine–sulfadoxine may be appropriate.

Individuals living in endemic areas acquire immunity to malaria, but lose it within a few months of moving away. Therefore, anyone traveling from a non-malarial country to an endemic area should take prophylaxis (*see* Ch. 62 for recommendations). A randomized controlled trial in Kenya found that intermittent sulfadoxine–pyrimethamine (Fansidar) was safe and prevented severe anemia secondary to malaria in pregnancy.[69]

The choice of prophylactic agent should be made after consulting current recommendations giving details of resistance patterns. Chloroquine is probably the least toxic prophylactic agent for pregnant women. Those traveling to areas of chloroquine resistance must balance the risk of malaria against the potential toxicity of prophylactic agents. It is safest to avoid travel to such areas when pregnant, but if the mother cannot be persuaded to delay travel the potential risks and benefits of chemoprophylaxis (and/or standby treatment) must be discussed. The role of artemether/lumefantrine in pregnancy is currently uncertain but we expect that initial reports about its safety in pregnancy[70] will be confirmed. The reader is strongly advised to consult the most recent local guidelines.

VAGINAL CANDIDIASIS

Over three-quarters of women have at least one episode of vaginal candidiasis during their lifetime. The organism is carried in the gut, under the nails, in the vagina and on the skin. The yeast *Candida albicans* is implicated in more than 80% of cases; *Candida glabrata*, *Candida krusei* and *Candida tropicalis* account for most of the rest (*see* Ch. 60). *Candida* is an opportunist, growing under favorable conditions. Symptomatic episodes are common in pregnancy; its growth is favored by the high levels of estrogen, increased availability of sugars, and subtle alterations in immunity.

In general it is better to use a topical treatment rather than a systemic one. This minimizes the risk of systemic side effects and exposure of the fetus. Vaginal creams and pessaries can be prescribed at a variety of doses and duration of treatment. For uncomplicated candidosis, a single dose treatment, such as clotrimazole 500 mg, is not adequate in pregnancy, and a longer course (e.g. 100 mg/day for 7 days) is recommended.

References

1. Brent LB. Legal considerations of drug use in pregnancy. In: Gilstrap LC, Little BB, eds. *Drugs and pregnancy*. New York: Chapman and Hall; 1998:33–42.

2. Little BB, Gilstrap LC. Human teratology principles. In: Gilstrap LC, Little BB, eds. *Drugs and pregnancy*. New York: Chapman and Hall; 1998:7–24.

3. Gilstrap LC, Little BB. Antimicrobial agents during pregnancy. In: Gilstrap LC, Little BB, eds. *Drugs and pregnancy*. New York: Chapman and Hall; 1998:77–102.

4. Donald PR, Sellars SL. Streptomycin ototoxicity in the unborn child. *S Afr Med J*. 1981;60:316–318.

5. Nahum GG, Uhl K, Kennedy DL. Antibiotic use in pregnancy and lactation: what is and is not known about teratogenic and toxic risks. *Obstet Gynecol*. 2006;107:1120–1138.

6. Källén BA, Otterblad Olausson P, Danielsson BR. Is erythromycin therapy teratogenic in humans? *Reprod Toxicol*. 2005;20:209–214.

7. Rosa FW, Baum C, Shaw M. Pregnancy outcomes after first-trimester vaginitis drug therapy. *Obstet Gynecol*. 1987;69:751–755.

8. Kazy Z, Puhó E, Czeizel AE. Teratogenic potential of vaginal metronidazole treatment during pregnancy. *Eur J Obstet Gynecol Reprod Biol*. 2005;123:174–178.

9. Czeizel AE, Rockenbauer M, Sørensen HT, Olsen J. Nitrofurantoin and congenital abnormalities. *Eur J Obstet Gynecol Reprod Biol*. 2001;95:119–126.

10. Schaefer C, Amoura-Elefant E, Vial T, et al. Pregnancy outcome after prenatal quinolone exposure. Evaluation of a case registry of the European Network of Teratology Information Services (ENTIS). *Eur J Obstet Gynecol Reprod Biol*. 1996;69:83–89.

11. Hernandez-Diaz S, Werler MM, Walker AM, Mitchell AA. Neural tube defects in relation to use of folic acid antagonists during pregnancy. *Am J Epidemiol*. 2001;153:961–968.

12. King CT, Rogers PD, Cleary JD, Chapman SW. Antifungal therapy during pregnancy. *Clin Infect Dis*. 1998;27:1151–1160.

13. Gibbs RS, Romero R, Hillier SL, Eschenbach DA, Sweet RL. A review of premature birth and subclinical infection. *Am J Obstet Gynecol*. 1992;166:1515–1528.

14. Gravett MG, Witkin SS, Haluska GJ, Edwards JL, Cook MJ, Novy MJ. An experimental model for intraamniotic infection and preterm labor in rhesus monkeys. *Am J Obstet Gynecol*. 1994;171:1660–1667.

15. Hay PE, Ugwumadu A, Sharland M. Infections in obstetrics. In: Chamberlain G, Steer P, eds. *Turnbull's obstetrics*. 3rd ed. London: Churchill Livingstone; 2001:356–381.

16. Hillier SL, Martius J, Krohn M, Kiviat N, Holmes KK, Eschenbach DA. A case control study of chorioamnionic infection and histologic chorioamnionitis in prematurity. *N Engl J Med*. 1998;319:972–978.

17. Hillier SL, Nugent RP, Eschenbach DA, et al. Association between bacterial vaginosis and preterm delivery of a low-birth-weight infant. The Vaginal Infections and Prematurity Study Group. *N Engl J Med*. 1995;333:1737–1742.

18. Carey JC, Klebanoff MA, Hauth JC, et al. Metronidazole to prevent preterm delivery in pregnant women with asymptomatic bacterial vaginosis. *N Engl J Med*. 2000;342:534–540.

19. McDonald HM, Brocklehurst P, Gordon A. Antibiotics for treating bacterial vaginosis in pregnancy. *Cochrane Database Syst Rev*. 2007; CD000262.

20. Swadpanich U, Lumbiganon P, Prasertcharoensook W, Laopaiboon M. Antenatal lower genital tract infection screening and treatment programs for preventing preterm delivery. *Cochrane Database Syst Rev*. 2008; CD006178.

21. Kenyon SL, Taylor DJ, Tarnow-Mordi W, ORACLE Collaborative Group. Broad-spectrum antibiotics for spontaneous preterm labour: the ORACLE II randomised trial. ORACLE Collaborative Group. *Lancet*. 2001;357:989–994.

22. Kenyon S, Boulvain M, Neilson JP. Antibiotics for preterm rupture of membranes. *Cochrane Database Syst Rev*. 2003; CD001058.

23. ACOG Committee Opinion No. 445. Antibiotics for preterm labor. *Obstet Gynecol*. 2009;114:1159–1160.

24. Bagratee JS, Moodley J, Kleinschmidt I, Zawilski W. A randomised controlled trial of antibiotic prophylaxis in elective caesarian delivery. *Br J Obstet Gynaecol*. 2001;108:143–148.

25. Hofmeyr GJ, Smaill FM. Antibiotic prophylaxis for cesarean section. *Cochrane Database Syst Rev*. 2002; CD000933.

26. Whalley P. Bacteriuria of pregnancy. *Am J Obstet Gynecol*. 1967;97:723–738.

27. Smaill FM, Vazquez JC. Antibiotics for asymptomatic bacteriuria in pregnancy. *Cochrane Database Syst Rev*. 2007; CD000490.

28. Rouse DJ, Andrews WW, Goldenberg RL, Owen J. Screening and treatment of asymptomatic bacteriuria of pregnancy to prevent pyelonephritis: a cost-effectiveness and cost-beneficial analysis. *Obstet Gynecol*. 1995;86:119–123.

29. Villar J, Lydon-Rochelle MT, Gülmezoglu AM, Roganti A. Duration of treatment for asymptomatic bacteriuria during pregnancy. *Cochrane Database Syst Rev*. 2000; CD000491.

30. Newton ER, Prihoda TJ, Gibbs RS. A clinical and microbiologic analysis of risk factors for puerperal endometritis. *Obstet Gynecol*. 1990;75:402–406.

31. French LM, Smaill FM. Antibiotic regimens for endometritis after delivery. *Cochrane Database Syst Rev*. 2007; CD001067.

32. Zenker PN, Rolfs RT. Treatment of syphilis, 1989. *Rev Infect Dis*. 1990;12(suppl 6):S590–S609.

33. Wendel GD. Gestational and congenital syphilis. *Clin Perinatol*. 1988;15:287–303.

34. Goldmeier D, Hay P. A review and update on adult syphilis with particular reference to its treatment. *Int J STD AIDS*. 1993;4:70–82.

35. Walker GJA. Antibiotics for syphilis diagnosed during pregnancy. *Cochrane Database Syst Rev*. 2001; CD001143.

36. Stoll BJ. Congenital syphilis: evaluation and management of neonates born to mothers with reactive serologic tests for syphilis. *Pediatr Infect Dis J*. 1994;13:845–853.

37. Brocklehurst P. Antibiotics for gonorrhoea in pregnancy. *Cochrane Database Syst Rev*. 2002; CD000098.

38. Brocklehurst P, Rooney G. Interventions for treating genital Chlamydia trachomatis infection in pregnancy. *Cochrane Database Syst Rev*. 1998; CD000054.

39. British Association for Sexual Health and HIV. *UK national guideline for the management of genital tract infection with Chlamydia trachomatis*. London: BASSH; 2006. Online. Available at http://www.bashh.org/documents/61/61.pdf.

40. Centers for Disease Control and Prevention. *Chlamydial infections in adolescents and adults*. Atlanta: CDC; 2007. Online. Available at http://www.cdc.gov/STD/treatment/2006/urethritis-and-cervicitis.htm#uc4.

41. International Union against Sexually Transmitted Infections/World Health Organization. *Draft European guideline (IUSTI/WHO) for the management of Chlamydia trachomatis infections*. Geneva: WHO; 2009. Online. Available at http://www.iusti.org/regions/europe/Draft_Euroguideline_chlamydial_infections0809.

42. Silver HM. Listeriosis in pregnancy. *Obstet Gynecol Surv*. 1998;53:737–740.

43. Campbell JR, Hillier SL, Krohn MA, Ferrieri P, Zaleznik DF, Baker CJ. Group B streptococcal colonization and serotype-specific immunity in pregnant women at delivery. *Obstet Gynecol*. 2000;6:498–503.

44. Centers for Disease Control and Prevention. *Prevention of perinatal group B streptococcal disease*. Atlanta: CDC; 2002. Online. Available at http://www.cdc.gov/mmwr/preview/mmwrhtml/rr5111a1.htm.

45. Royal College of Obstetricians and Gynaecologists. *Prevention of early onset neonatal Group B streptococcal disease*. London: RCOG; 2003. Online. Available at http://www.rcog.org.uk/files/rcog-corp/uploaded-files/GT36GroupBStrep2003.pdf.

46. Bergeron MG, Ke D, Menard C, et al. Rapid detection of group B streptococci in pregnant women at delivery. *N Engl J Med*. 2000;343:175–179.

47. Ohlsson A, Shah VS. Intrapartum antibiotics for known maternal Group B streptococcal colonization. *Cochrane Database Syst Rev*. 2009; CD007467.

48. Moore HL Jr, Szczech GM, Rodwell DE, et al. Preclinical toxicology studies with acyclovir: teratologic, reproductive and neonatal tests. *Fundam Appl Toxicol*. 1983;3:560–568.

49. Stone KM, Reiff-Eldridge R, White AD, et al. Pregnancy outcomes following systemic prenatal acyclovir exposure: conclusions from the international acyclovir pregnancy registry, 1984–1999. *Birth Defects Res A Clin Mol Teratol*. 2004;70:201–207.

50. American Congress of Obstetricians and Gynecologists. Clinical management guidelines for obstetrician-gynecologists. Practice Bulletin No. 82, June 2007. Management of herpes in pregnancy. ACOG Committee on Practice Bulletins. *Obstet Gynecol*. 2007;109:1489–1498.

51. Royal College of Obstetricians and Gynaecologists. *Management of genital herpes in pregnancy*. London: RCOG; 2007. Online. Available at http://www.rcog.org.uk/files/rcog-corp/uploaded-files/GT30GenitalHerpes2007.pdf.

52. van Everdingen JJ, Peeters MF, ten Have P. Neonatal herpes policy in the Netherlands. Five years after a consensus conference. *J Perinat Med*. 1993;21:371–375.

53. Peckham C, Gibb D. Mother-to-child transmission of the human immunodeficiency virus. *N Engl J Med*. 1995;333:298–302.

54. Newell ML, Gray G, Bryson YJ. Prevention of mother-to-child transmission of HIV-1 infection. *AIDS*. 1997;11(suppl A):S165–S172.

55. Backe E, Unger M, Jimenez E, Siegel G, Schafer A, Vogel M. Fetal organs infected by HIV-1. *AIDS*. 1993;7:896–897.

56. Burgard M, Mayaux MJ, Blanche S, et al. The use of viral culture and p24 antigen testing to diagnose human immunodeficiency virus infection in neonates. The HIV Infection in Newborns French Collaborative Study Group. *N Engl J Med*. 1992;327:1192–1197.

57. Nduati R, John G, Mbori-Ngacha D, et al. Effect of breastfeeding and formula feeding on transmission of HIV-1: a randomized clinical trial. *JAMA*. 2000;283:1167–1174.

58. Townsend CL, Cortina-Borja M, Peckham C, et al. Low rates of mother-to-child transmission of HIV following effective pregnancy interventions in the United Kingdom and Ireland, 2000–2006. *AIDS*. 2008;22:973–981.

59. Larbalestier N, Mullen J, O'Shea S, et al. Drug resistance is uncommon in pregnant women with low viral loads taking zidovudine monotherapy to prevent perinatal HIV transmission. *AIDS*. 2003;17:2665–2667.

60. Connor EM, Sperling RS, Gelber R, et al. Reduction of maternal–infant transmission of human immunodeficiency virus type 1 with zidovudine treatment. Pediatric AIDS Clinical Trials Group Protocol 076 Study Group. *N Engl J Med*. 1994;331:1173–1180.

61. Guay LA, Musoke P, Fleming T, et al. Intrapartum and neonatal single-dose nevirapine compared with zidovudine for prevention of mother-to-child transmission of HIV-1 in Kampala, Uganda: HIVNET 012 randomised trial. *Lancet*. 1999;354:795–802.

62. World Health Organization. *Antiretroviral drugs for treating pregnant women and preventing HIV infection in infants: towards universal access. Recommendations for a public health approach. – 2006 version*. Geneva: WHO; 2006. Online. Available at http://www.who.int/entity/hiv/pub/mtct/arv_guidelines_mtct.pdf.

63. Taylor GP, Lyall EG, Mercey D, et al. British HIV Association guidelines for prescribing antiretroviral therapy in pregnancy (1998). *Sex Transm Infect*. 1999;75:90–97.

64. Watanabe M, Kohge N, Akagi S, Uchida Y, Sato S, Kinoshita Y. Congenital anomalies in a child born from a mother with interferon-treated chronic hepatitis B. *Am J Gastroenterol*. 2001;96:1668–1669.

65. Jones JL, Lopez A, Wilson M, Schulkin J, Gibbs R. Congenital toxoplasmosis: a review. *Obstet Gynecol Surv*. 2001;56:296–305.

66. Klebanoff MA, Carey JC, Hauth JC, et al. Failure of metronidazole to prevent preterm delivery among pregnant women with asymptomatic *Trichomonas vaginalis* infection. *N Engl J Med*. 2001;345:487–493.

67. Gülmezoglu AM. Interventions for trichomoniasis in pregnancy. *Cochrane Database Syst Rev*. 2002; CD000220.

68. Garner P, Gülmezoglu AM. Drugs for preventing malaria in pregnant women. *Cochrane Database Syst Rev*. 2006; CD000169.

69. Shulman CE, Dorman EK, Cutts F, et al. Intermittent sulphadoxine–pyrimethamine to prevent severe anaemia secondary to malaria in pregnancy: a randomised placebo-controlled trial. *Lancet*. 1999;353:632–636.

70. Falade C, Manyando CJ. Safety profile of Coartem®: the evidence base. *Malaria J*. 2009;8(suppl 1):S6.

 ## Further information

Antiretroviral drug interactions at http://www.hiv-druginteractions.org.
Antiretroviral pregnancy registry at http://www.apregistry.com/who.htm.
Clinical Effectiveness Group (Association of Genitourinary Medicine and the Medical Society for the Study of Venereal Diseases). *National guidelines*. Available at http://www.bashh.org/guidelines.
United States Centers for Disease Control (CDC) Guidelines. 2006. Available at http://www.cdc.gov/std/treatment/.

56

Sexually transmitted diseases

Sheena Kakar and Adrian Mindel

Many infections are sexually transmitted (Table 56.1). Some, including HIV, hepatitis B and C, are also transmitted by blood or blood products. Others, like human papillomavirus (HPV), herpes simplex virus (HSV) and molluscum contagiosum are also transmitted by close bodily contact.

In 2005, the World Health Organization (WHO) estimated there were 448 million cases of the four major curable sexually transmitted infections (STIs), trichomoniasis, chlamydia, gonorrhea and syphilis, among people aged 15–49.[1] Ninety percent of cases occur in developing countries. In recent years the viral STIs, in particular HIV, have become increasingly important. The joint United Nations program on HIV/AIDS estimated that at the end of 2007 there were 33 million people living with HIV/AIDS, most in developing countries.[2]

The rate of spread of STIs within a community depends on several factors, including the size of the susceptible population, exposure to an infected individual, efficiency of transmission and duration of infectiousness. Epidemiological patterns of individual infections depend on the interplay between these factors and the social, economic and political environment. One of the major reasons why STIs are more common in developing nations is that a large proportion of these populations is aged 18–35, the age group considered to be at greatest risk for STI acquisition.

An example of the effect of social, economic and political changes on STIs is the epidemic growth of these infections in the former USSR. Profound social and economic changes, and a partial collapse of the health system, have been contributory. The epidemic has been fuelled by growth in the commercial sex industry, unsafe intravenous drug use and exchange of sex for drugs.

At an individual level, risk factors include early coitarche, multiple sexual partners, partners from high-risk groups, poor condom usage and drug use.

STIs have important health, social and economic consequences for the individual and the community. These include pelvic inflammatory disease (PID) leading to infertility and ectopic pregnancy; congenital, perinatal and postnatal infections; and a variety of genital tract cancers. In addition, STIs, in particular genital ulcer disease (GUD), increase the transmission of HIV.

CHLAMYDIA

These obligate intracellular bacteria have several species, two of which infect humans as their primary host – *Chlamydia trachomatis* and *Chlamydophila* (formerly *Chlamydia*) *pneumoniae*. *C. trachomatis* can be further divided into biovars, distinct groups of biological variants, each producing a different disease spectrum. Serovariants or serovars of the trachoma biovar result in trachoma (serovars A–C) or STIs (serovars D–K). Lymphogranuloma venereum comprises the serovars L1, L2 and L3 and forms the second biovar in the *C. trachomatis* species.

EPIDEMIOLOGY

C. trachomatis has the highest prevalence of any bacterial STI in developed countries. In 2005, the WHO estimated that there were 102 million new cases of *C. trachomatis* infection in people aged 15–49 worldwide,[1] second only to trichomoniasis as the leading cause of curable STIs. In both sexes, the prevalence of infection ranges from 3–5% in low-prevalence general medical settings to 15–20% in high-prevalence STI clinics.

Since 1998, diagnoses of uncomplicated chlamydia infections in genitourinary medicine (GUM) clinics in the UK have increased by 150% from 48 726 in 1998 to 121 986 in 2007.[3]

In common with other STIs, risk factors include age below 25, one or more sexual partner in the recent past, inconsistent condom use, oral contraceptive use, termination of pregnancy and non-white race.

Chlamydia may result in significant complications, including PID, with resultant infertility and ectopic pregnancy, neonatal infection, epididymo-orchitis and reactive arthritis. In the UK the annual cost of chlamydia, including complications, is estimated to be at least £100 million and in the USA in 2007 the annual cost was estimated at US$624 million.[4,5]

Table 56.1 Sexually transmitted infections

Disease	Causative organism	Complications
Bacterial		
Gonorrhea	*Neisseria gonorrhoeae*	Pelvic inflammatory disease, bartholinitis and Bartholin's abscess, systemic dissemination, epididymo-orchitis
Chlamydia	*Chlamydia trachomatis*	Pelvic inflammatory disease, bartholinitis and Bartholin's abscess, epididymo-orchitis
Syphilis	*Treponema pallidum*	Central nervous system, cerebrovascular system and gummatous infection
Chancroid	*Haemophilus ducreyi*	Local genital destruction
Lymphogranuloma venereum	*Chlamydia trachomatis*	Local abscesses, fistulae, strictures and genital destruction, rarely meningoencephalitis, hepatitis, pneumonitis
Donovanosis (granuloma inguinale)	*Klebsiella granulomatis*	Local genital destruction, genital lymphedema, squamous cell carcinoma, bone and liver dissemination
Viral		
Genital warts	Human papillomaviruses	Genital tract tumor (mainly cervical cancer – with 'high risk' types)
Genital herpes	Herpes simplex virus type 1 and 2	Acute systemic viremia with primary HSV-2, local recurrences
Molluscum contagiosum	Molluscum contagiosum virus	
HIV	Human immunodeficiency virus types 1 and 2	Severe immune suppression, opportunistic infections
Hepatitis B	Hepatitis B virus	Fulminant hepatitis, chronic infection, cirrhosis, hepatocellular carcinoma
Hepatitis A	Hepatitis A virus	Fulminant hepatitis
Hepatitis C	Hepatitis C virus	Fulminant hepatitis, chronic infection, cirrhosis, hepatocellular carcinoma
Other infections and miscellaneous conditions		
Candidiasis	*Candida albicans* *Candida glabrata*	
Bacterial vaginosis	Reduced lactobacilli, high-concentration anaerobic bacteria	Pelvic inflammatory disease, and chorioamnionitis, prematurity, premature rupture of membranes, low birthweight
Trichomoniasis	*Trichomonas vaginalis*	Premature rupture of membranes, low birthweight
Non-specific genital infections	*Mycoplasma genitalium, Ureaplasma urealyticum, Mycoplasma hominis*	

PATHOGENESIS

The developmental cycle of Chlamydiae is unique. The bacterium infects eukaryotic cells, depending on these cells for many of the nutrients required for its growth and replication. The infectious particle of chlamydia is a metabolically inactive elementary body which attaches to epithelial cells, induces phagocytosis and, avoiding lysosomal fusion, enters the reticulate system. Within the phagosome the elementary body undergoes morphological change to form the reticulate body, the metabolically active, replicating form of chlamydia. Over the next 48–72 h the reticulate body replicates, increasing in numbers, reorganizing into elementary bodies: a mature inclusion body may contain thousands of elementary bodies. When cell death is imminent, lysosomal fusion occurs, the cell ruptures and elementary bodies are released. The disease process is thought to result from a combination of direct tissue damage secondary to chlamydial replication, local inflammatory responses and the body's humoral and cell-mediated immune responses.

Immune responses to chlamydia control the acute infection. However, the infection evolves into a low-grade chronic infection which, unless treated, persists. One hypothesis regarding the pathogenesis postulates a delayed hypersensitivity reaction to chlamydia heat shock protein (hsp 60) which shares extensive amino acid sequence with human hsp 60. Chlamydial hsp 60 shares some antigenic sites with mycobacteria and *Escherichia coli*. These infections could presensitize patients, resulting in a primed response to chlamydial infection and greater disease severity.

DIAGNOSIS

 ### CLINICAL

Most women with uncomplicated chlamydia are asymptomatic. Those who have symptoms present with vaginal discharge, intermenstrual or postcoital bleeding and occasionally lower abdominal pain. On examination, mucopurulent cervicitis and/or contact bleeding may be noted. Men present with dysuria and urethral discharge. Rectal infection may result in proctitis. Pharyngeal infections are usually asymptomatic.

 ### INVESTIGATIONS

Diagnostic options include culture, antigen testing and nucleic acid amplification tests (NAATs). Although culture has the highest specificity, sensitivity is low. It requires endocervical or urethral swabs and is expensive. NAATs are cheap, have relatively easy specimen collection and transport conditions. However, sensitivities are variable and positive predictive value low (<5%) in low-prevalence populations. NAATs such as the polymerase chain reaction (PCR) and ligase chain reaction (LCR) are highly specific and sensitive but more expensive. PCR and LCR have gained popularity in male diagnosis due to non-invasive specimen collection (urine instead of urethral swab) and are comparable with other test methods.[6] Urine may also be a suitable sample in women.[7] Serology is available but of little diagnostic value in genital disease as it fails to differentiate between previous and current infections.

MANAGEMENT[5,8,9]

Uncomplicated infection:
- Azithromycin 1 g orally (single dose)
- Doxycycline 100 mg orally every 12 h for 7 days.

Alternative regimens:
- Erythromycin 500 mg orally every 12 h for 7 days or every 12 h for 14 days
- Ofloxacin 200 mg orally every 12 h for 7 days
- Amoxicillin 500 mg orally every 8 h for 7 days in pregnancy.

A meta-analysis of 12 randomized controlled trials (RCTs) demonstrated equal efficacy of azithromycin and doxycycline.[10] Azithromycin has a very long half-life, a large volume of distribution with excellent tissue and cellular penetration (*see* Ch. 22), and can be given as a single dose. It has fewer side effects than doxycycline, the most common being mild gastrointestinal disturbance. Doxycycline can also cause gastrointestinal disturbance, particularly esophagitis. Another common side effect is photosensitivity (*see* Ch. 30). When compliance is taken into account, though expensive, azithromycin is more cost-effective than doxycycline.[11]

Alternative therapies have broadly comparable cure rates, but use is limited by side effects or cost. Erythromycin has been studied at 500 mg every 6 h or 500 mg every 12 h for 7–14 days. Higher dose regimens are slightly more efficacious but less effective because of gastrointestinal intolerance, with up to 50% of patients not completing the course. Ofloxacin (a fluoroquinolone) is as effective as doxycycline, with a better side effect profile, but is considerably more expensive and does not share the advantage of single-dose therapy (with azithromycin).[12] Tetracyclines are as efficacious, but have more side effects than doxycycline and have to be taken every 6 h.

Rifalazil, a new rifamycin compound, has been found to be highly active against chlamydia in cell cultures. A recent RCT demonstrated a dose-dependent microbiological and clinical cure rate comparable to azithromycin.[13] Moxifloxacin also demonstrates activity against chlamydia in vitro. Both agents may be useful in chlamydia infections.[14,15]

To minimize transmission, abstinence for a week after treatment completion is recommended.

 ### PREGNANCY AND BREASTFEEDING

Doxycycline and ofloxacin are contraindicated in pregnancy, but azithromycin appears to be safe.[8,16,17] Amoxicillin has also been evaluated in pregnancy and provides microbiological clearance despite some resistance detected in vitro. It has a better side effect profile than erythromycin, with a similar cure rate. However, it is not clear whether amoxicillin eliminates the organism or temporarily suppresses replication.

While erythromycin remains effective, its use may be limited by gastrointestinal side effects.[8] Erythromycin estolate is contraindicated in pregnancy because of possible drug-related hepatoxicity.

Due to concerns over efficacy of therapy in pregnancy, and possible sequelae in the neonate and mother in the event of persistent infection, a test of cure is advised 3 weeks following treatment.[5] Data on neonatal outcomes are limited.

Amoxicillin and azithromycin may be used during breastfeeding. Erythromycin is best avoided in the early postnatal period (risk of neonatal pyloric stenosis) but is safe for use thereafter.[18]

 ### RESISTANCE

There are case reports of clinically significant, multidrug-resistant chlamydial infections, causing relapse or persistence. Resistance to azithromycin, doxycycline, ofloxacin, erythromycin and josamycin has been documented in vitro.[19,20] While this does not seem to be a widespread phenomenon, it highlights the need for increased surveillance to monitor treatment failures, and in vitro resistance of isolates.

Resistance of *C. trachomatis* depends on its ability to proliferate within the host cell, in the presence of varying concentrations of antibiotics. Consequently, resistance is usually not absolute and described as being 'heterotypic'. This implies that all organisms may be capable of resistance. However, only a small proportion will show resistance at any given time. It is hypothesized that this heterotypic resistance may be a by-product of undefined alterations in the growth phase or life cycle in some bacteria, rendering them refractory to antimicrobial agents. An alternative theory is that resistance may be mediated through mechanisms that exclude drugs from chlamydial cells or inclusions (e.g. an efflux pump). Further research is required in this area.[19]

SEXUAL PARTNERS

All sexual contacts of the index case (within 4 weeks if symptomatic or up to 6 months if asymptomatic) should be traced, screened and treated if necessary. Studies have demonstrated the advantages of partner-delivered therapy for contacts. To optimize partner notification, counseling and written information may be helpful.

SCREENING

As many infections with chlamydia are asymptomatic and sequelae can be devastating, screening programs should be implemented. Screening criteria are normally age related (18–24 years) and can include behavioral and clinical measures. Where screening programs have been implemented, prevalence has decreased. They are epidemiologically effective and cost-effective in areas with prevalence as low as 3%.[21,22]

GONORRHEA

Neisseria gonorrhoeae is an aerobic, Gram-negative diplococcus of the genus *Neisseria*. In common with other members of this genus, its primary site of infection is mucous membranes. Gonococci and meningococci are the two major pathogenic species seen in humans. Gonococcal infections can lead to urethritis, cervicitis, proctitis or pharyngitis. Co-infection with chlamydia has been reported in 20–40% of people.

EPIDEMIOLOGY

In 2005 the WHO estimated that, worldwide, there were 88 million cases of gonorrhea in adults aged 15–49, the majority in the developing world.[1] The incidence declined in most developed countries in the 1980s; however, the incidence increased in the late 1990s and early 2000s with a recent stabilization of rates.

Gonorrhea is the second most common bacterial STI (after chlamydia) in the UK. In 2007, a total of 18 710 diagnoses were made in UK GUM clinics, a decrease of 1% from 18 898 diagnoses in 2006, in line with the trend since 2002.[15]

Following a 75% decline in gonorrhea incidence in the USA, the rate now seems to have reached a plateau. In 2007, the rate was 118.9/100 000 population, with the highest rate in the South (156/100 000), only slightly higher than 2006 when the rate was 119.7/100 000.[23]

Risk factors for gonorrhea are similar to most STIs. However, gonorrhea also shows a distinct ethnic minority bias in the USA and Europe, which is partly explained by accessibility to healthcare, poverty and socioeconomic status. However, differences still exist in studies attempting to control for these factors.[24]

Men have a 20% risk of acquiring urethral infection after one episode of vaginal intercourse with an infected partner. In women the risk of acquisition is higher (50–90%). Pharyngeal to urethral infection is increasingly recognized with the growing popularity of orogenital sex. Asymptomatic infection is reported in up to 35% of women and 1–3% of men.

PATHOGENESIS

N. gonorrhoeae has two main patterns of infection. Most bacteria are limited to the mucosal surface, where they cause marked tissue damage. Some bacteria can resist the killing activity of antibodies and complement in human serum, causing disseminated infection with little or no mucosal damage. Within each infection pattern, there exists a spectrum of pathogenicity. The severity and pattern of the infection are determined by molecules expressed on the surface, including those responsible for adherence, metabolite transport and tissue toxicity, against which various antibodies are formed. Two surface molecules, pilus and opacity proteins, are responsible for adherence to cells. Both show antigenic variation, allowing them to attach to different niches and escape the host's immune responses, and show phase variation, which alters the pathogenicity of the gonococci. Once adhered to the cell, gonococci must evade neutrophil phagocytosis to survive. Pili surface proteins increase resistance to phagocytosis and killing.[25] Even following phagocytosis, 2% of gonococci survive.[26] Gonococci adhere to and invade mucus-secreting, non-ciliated cells. Inside this immune privileged site they multiply, divide, and then exit from the basal surface by exocytosis. Tissue damage caused by gonococci is thought to be secondary to extracellular products such as enzymes (phospholipase, peptidase), lipo-oligosaccharides and peptidoglycans.

Gonococci have developed a number of mechanisms to avoid killing by serum antibodies and complement. For example, blocking antibodies against a surface molecule, reduction modifiable protein (RMP), appear to inhibit IgM complement-fixing antibodies from recognizing their target on lipo-oligosaccharides.[27] Blocking antibodies to RMP are not only important in the development of serum resistance, but also appear to play a part in mucosal immunity, and therefore transmission. Women with antibodies against RMP are more likely to acquire mucosal infection. Serum-resistant gonococci, however, lead to limited (if any) mucosal inflammation, correlating with their inability to trigger chemotactic response to neutrophils. Serum-sensitive gonococci, which are limited to mucosal surfaces, are thought capable of triggering a strong chemotactic response and marked mucosal inflammation.

DIAGNOSIS

CLINICAL[28]

Symptomatic women commonly present with vaginal discharge associated with cervical infection. Dysuria, but not frequency, is seen with urethral infection and is present in 70–90% of infections. Less commonly, patients will present with intermenstrual bleeding or menorrhagia. Clinical findings can include mucopurulent cervical discharge with contact cervical bleeding and ectopy. Frequently, no signs are evident in uncomplicated infection.

In men, the most common presentation is urethral discharge, which tends to be purulent, occurring up to 14 days after infection and often associated with meatal erythema. About half of these will have dysuria. Epididymitis occurs in 1% of infections. Asymptomatic infections are less common than with chlamydia. Rectal infection via direct inoculation occurs after receptive anal sex. In women it is often asymptomatic, but up to 50% of men will have discharge or proctitis. Pharyngeal infection is asymptomatic in most cases and spontaneously resolves in about 12 weeks.

Disseminated infection is rare and presents as an arthritis–dermatitis syndrome. The arthritis may be an acute, asymmetric, destructive monoarthritis or a reactive arthropathy. Classically, the rash appears as distal, tender, necrotic pustules. Meningitis and endocarditis are infrequently described.

INVESTIGATIONS

The gold standard investigation is culture on selective media containing antimicrobials to reduce contamination. This has a high sensitivity (80–95%) and specificity. In male urethral swabs, the sensitivity of microscopy and Gram stain alone in symptomatic individuals is 90–95%, which is comparable with culture. However, sensitivity falls to 50–75% in asymptomatic infections and 50–70% in cervical infections.[28] Microscopy and Gram stain, therefore, have a place in rapid diagnostic testing, but cannot supplant culture. NAATs are growing in popularity with sensitivity in the range of 87–98%, but with an organism that shows increasing antibiotic resistance, culture and antimicrobial testing will always be the gold standard. Sensitivity and specificity of serological testing is very low, limiting its use in screening, case finding or diagnosis.

MANAGEMENT[29-33]

UNCOMPLICATED INFECTIONS OF CERVIX, URETHRA AND RECTUM

Single-dose treatment with:
- cefixime 400 mg orally
- ceftriaxone 125–250 mg intramuscularly.

Alternative regimen: single-dose treatment with spectinomycin 2 g intramuscularly or other cephalosporin regimens such as:
- ceftizoxime 500 mg intramuscularly
- cefoxitin 2 g intramuscularly (with concurrent probenecid 1 g orally)
- cefotaxime 500 mg intramuscularly.

Possible oral alternatives:
- Cefpodoxime – 200 mg (British Association for Sexual Health and HIV [BASSH] recommendation) or 400 mg (US Centers for Disease Control and Prevention [CDC] recommendation)
- Cefuroxime axetil 1 g.

Patients with positive microscopy or culture, or a recent partner with confirmed gonorrhea, should receive treatment. The choice of antibiotics depends on local resistance patterns. The WHO and individual countries use sentinel surveillance systems to monitor susceptibility and guide treatment recommendations.

Since the 1950s, antibiotic resistance has been documented to several antibiotics, particularly penicillin, tetracycline and quinolones. Resistance is acquired through multiple chromosomal mutations or single-step plasmid acquisition. The antibiotics chosen should eliminate infection in 95% of those treated. Quinolone resistance has been increasingly documented worldwide, with highest levels in South East Asia and the Pacific. Quinolones are no longer recommended in these areas. In 2006, the Gonococcal Isolate Surveillance Project (GISP) in the USA recorded 22.3% of isolates resistant to penicillin, tetracycline or both, and also widespread fluoroquinolone resistance.[30] Consequently, fluoroquinolones are no longer recommended for gonorrhea in the USA.[29] Similarly in the UK, between 2006 and 2007, increased antimicrobial resistance to penicillin, tetracycline, ciprofloxacin and azithromycin was noted. None of these are currently recommended in the UK.

In the USA[30] and the UK[31] gonococci remain sensitive to ceftriaxone.

In the UK, few spectinomycin-resistant isolates have been noted since 1988; however, no isolate has demonstrated spectinomycin resistance since 2005.[31]

One systematic review of studies published between 1980 and 1993 looked at single-dose antimicrobial therapy (excluding β-lactamase-sensitive penicillin and tetracycline). A total of 21 antibiotics were considered, including cephalosporins, fluoroquinolones, azithromycin, rifampicin (rifampin) and spectinomycin. The best balance of efficacy and safety for uncomplicated gonococcal infection included ceftriaxone (125 mg), cefixime (400 mg), ciprofloxacin (500 mg) and ofloxacin (400 mg). However, the need to alter treatment depending on sensitivity patterns implies that only ceftriaxone and cefixime are currently recommended. The dose of ceftriaxone remains disputed. The Centers for Disease Control and Prevention (CDC) recommends 125 mg, but both Australian[34] and British guidelines[35] recommend 250 mg.

In general, all single-dose regimens recommended above have few side effects and are well tolerated. Disadvantages to using ceftriaxone and spectinomycin are that both have to be given intramuscularly. Many would prefer oral alternatives like cefixime. In a study regarding potential cost benefits of prescribing ceftriaxone versus cefixime, both were found to be equally cost-effective.[36] Given the prevalence and diversity of gonococcal resistance it is important to monitor local resistance patterns.

PHARYNGEAL INFECTION

Ceftriaxone 125 mg or 250 mg intramuscularly can be used for pharyngeal infections. Cefixime may also be used.[37] Spectinomycin and ampicillin have poor efficacy.

DISSEMINATED GONOCOCCAL INFECTION[29]

- Intravenous or intramuscular ceftriaxone 1 g per day.

Alternative regimens:

- Intravenous cefotaxime 1 g every 8 h
- Intravenous ceftizoxime 1 g every 8 h
- Intramuscular spectinomycin 2 g every 12 h.

There have been no recent studies on the treatment of disseminated gonococcal infection. The above regimens have been used in clinical practice with few reported adverse effects.

All patients should be hospitalized for initial treatment and examined for endocarditis and meningitis. Parenteral therapy should be continued for 24–48 h after signs of improvement are seen, followed by oral therapy (cefixime 400 mg every 12 h or cefpodoxime 400 mg orally every 12 h) to complete a full week's course. If meningitis is present, ceftriaxone is continued parenterally for up to 2 weeks. If endocarditis is present, the drug should be taken for at least 4 weeks. Local expert opinion is advised when treating disseminated infection.

PREGNANCY AND BREASTFEEDING[29,38]

- Intramuscular ceftriaxone 250 mg.
- Oral cefixime 400 mg.
- Oral amoxicillin 3 g given 30 min after oral probenecid 1 g.
- Intramuscular spectinomycin 2 g.

A Cochrane review of studies amongst pregnant women with gonorrhea suggests both ceftriaxone and spectinomycin are effective in microbiological clearance, while amoxicillin with probenecid may be less effective. However, study numbers were too small to state this with confidence.[38]

Two RCTs have studied the treatment of gonorrhea in pregnancy; one compared ceftriaxone with cefixime, the other evaluated ceftriaxone, amoxicillin and spectinomycin. Microbiological cure ranged from 89% to 97%. In these two trials, all antibiotics were efficacious and no serious side effects were reported. Fluoroquinolones are not recommended in pregnancy because of reported arthropathy in animal studies.

Ceftriaxone, cefixime and amoxicillin are safe for use in lactation.[18] It is unknown whether spectinomycin is secreted in breast milk and should be used with caution in nursing mothers.

SEXUAL PARTNERS

All sexual partners in the last 2–3 months should be evaluated and treated for gonococcal and chlamydial infection.

FURTHER MANAGEMENT

All patients should be screened for other STIs, particularly chlamydia, as some patients (20–40%) may have dual infection. At that co-infection level, the cost of routine dual therapy is less than testing for chlamydia. Therefore, chlamydia treatment should be routinely provided when treating gonorrhea.[5,35]

MYCOPLASMA GENITALIUM

Mycoplasma genitalium belongs to the family Mycoplasmataceae, class Mollicutes. These bacteria are phenotypically distinct. They lack cell walls and have the smallest known genome amongst cellular organisms that can be cultured.

EPIDEMIOLOGY

M. genitalium is increasingly recognized as an important STI. In men with acute chlamydia-negative non-specific urethritis (NGU), several studies have demonstrated that the prevalence of *M. genitalium* ranges from 18% to 46%.[39] Infection of the rectum may occur in individuals practicing anal sex.

In women, *M. genitalium* can cause cervicitis and urethritis.[39] It has been detected in the endometrium of women with PID[40] and has been isolated from fallopian tubes.[41] PID associated with *M. genitalium* is less likely to be symptomatic than gonococcal PID and appears clinically similar to chlamydial

PID.[42] Further, because symptoms may be mild, women with *M. genitalium* PID may not seek treatment.[42] Serological studies amongst women with tubal infertility indicate a possible relationship between past infection with *M. genitalium* and tubal damage.[43] Further studies are needed to fully understand the natural history of *M. genitalium* and its relationship with PID. It is noteworthy that most PID treatment regimens do not cover *M. genitalium*.[44]

PATHOGENESIS

M. genitalium can bind to human spermatozoa and potentially be carried up into the female genital tract.[45] The ability of *M. genitalium* to elicit pathological changes in the human host depends on a complex set of interactions between the organism and immune mechanisms. *M. genitalium*'s genome consists of at least seven proteins, two of which have been studied in detail: MgPa (aka MG191 and MG140) and P110. They are required for adherence to the host cell and are highly immunogenic. The organism has also developed 'gliding motility' and the ability to express antigenic variants and other virulence-associated phenotypes, enhancing its ability to evade human defense mechanisms. Additionally, *M. genitalium* can survive within epithelial cells and attach to mucin, further contributing to its virulence.[46]

DIAGNOSIS

CLINICAL

In men, the signs and symptoms are those of urethritis. In women, the clinical picture may be that of cervicitis, urethritis or PID. The infection may remain asymptomatic in both sexes.

INVESTIGATIONS

M. genitalium is difficult to culture, usually requiring complex media.[47] More commonly NAATs, particularly PCR, are used to diagnose infections.[48]

Suitable specimens include urethral, vaginal and endocervical swabs; urine samples; and rectal swabs, if infection at that site is suspected. For culture, a suitable transport medium is required. For NAATs, swabs may be transported in phosphate-buffered saline or 'dry'.

MANAGEMENT

As *M. genitalium* lacks a cell wall, it is resistant to the β-lactams and cephalosporins.

The following may be used in the treatment of *M. genitalium*:[39,44,49]

- Azithromycin 1 g orally (single dose)
- Moxifloxacin 400 mg orally every 12 h for 7–10 days.

Treatment failures have occurred with the use of azithromycin, with some strains showing resistance. This resistance is believed to have a genetic basis, with a mutation in the V region of the 23S rRNA. The basis for development of this mutation is induction of macrolide resistance by use of inappropriate dosages.[50] Consequently, patients treated with azithromycin should have a test of cure and treatment failures managed with moxifloxacin.[49]

PREGNANCY AND BREASTFEEDING

Azithromycin is safe for use in pregnancy and while breastfeeding. Quinolones are contraindicated in pregnancy and breastfeeding.

SEXUAL PARTNERS

Contact tracing and treatment of partners is recommended.

NON-SPECIFIC URETHRITIS

There are several infectious causes of urethritis other than gonorrhea, chlamydia and *M. genitalium*. These include *Trichomonas vaginalis*, HSV-2, *Ureaplasma urealyticum* and *Mycoplasma hominis*. Oral pathogens are also being increasingly implicated in urethritis, including adenovirus, HSV-1 and *Streptococcus pneumoniae*. However, once gonorrhea and chlamydia have been excluded, other organisms are seldom sought. Instead, the condition is usually managed empirically. Tetracyclines, erythromycin and azithromycin are all effective:[51,52]

- Azithromycin 1 g orally (single dose)
- Doxycycline 100 mg every 12 h for 7 days
- Erythromycin 500 mg every 6 h for 7–14 days
- Tetracycline 500 mg every 6 h for 7 days.

Moxifloxacin is active against *Ureaplasma* spp., *Mycoplasma* and *Chlamydia*, and is being evaluated as potential therapy.[14]

Urethritis caused by organisms such as *T. vaginalis* and HSV should be treated as detailed in subsequent sections.

PELVIC INFLAMMATORY DISEASE

There are many causes of PID and it is beyond the scope of this chapter to review these in detail. However, PID is a major complication of two sexually transmitted organisms (*Neisseria gonorrhoea* and *Chlamydia trachomatis*), together

Box 56.1 Treatment for pelvic inflammatory disease

Parenteral (inpatient) regimens

Regimen A[a]

Cefoxitin 2 g i.v. every 6 or 12 h, *or*

Cefotetan 2 g i.v. every 12 h, *plus*

Doxycycline 100 mg i.v. or p.o. every 12 h

Regimen B[a]

Clindamycin 900 mg intravenously every 8 h, *plus*

Gentamicin loading dose 2 mg/kg i.v. or i.m., followed by 1.5 mg/kg every 8 h maintenance dose. Single daily dosing may be substituted

Alternative regimen[a]

Ampicillin–sulbactam 3 g i.v. every 6 h, *plus*

Doxycycline 100 mg orally or i.v. every 12 h

Outpatient treatment

Regimen A

Ceftriaxone 250 mg i.m. in a single dose, *plus*

Doxycycline 100 mg orally every 12 h for 14 days, *with or without*

Metronidazole 400–500 mg every 12 h for 14 days

Regimen B

Cefoxitin 2 g i.m. plus probenecid 1 g p.o. administered concurrently in a single dose, *plus*

Doxycycline 100 mg p.o. every 12 h for 14 days, *with or without*

Metronidazole 400–500 mg p.o. every 12 h for 14 days

Regimen C

Other parental third-generation cephalosporin (e.g. ceftizoxime or cefotaxime), *plus*

Doxycycline 100 mg p.o. every 12 h for 14 days, *with or without*

Metronidazole 400–500 mg p.o. every 12 h for 14 days

[a]Oral therapy may be initiated 24 h after clinical improvement using doxycycline 100 mg every 12 h or clindamycin 450 mg/day for 14 days.

with anaerobic organisms. *M. genitalium* is increasingly implicated as a causative organism for PID.[53]

As a definitive diagnosis is dependent on laparoscopy, many individuals are treated presumptively. This may result in overdiagnosis of PID and underdiagnosis of other causes of pelvic pain.[54] As microbiological confirmation is seldom undertaken, treatment is directed at the most likely organism(s).

High cure rates (i.e. microbiological resolution and clearance of symptoms) are achieved with most regimens (Box 56.1). A meta-analysis showed that regimens with two or more antibiotics had a better than 90% success rate.[55] However, damage to the fallopian tubes and subsequent infertility are long-term consequences, particularly where infection occurs more than once.

A recent RCT showed that the efficacy of azithromycin 1 g orally weekly for 2 weeks was comparable to doxycycline in treating mild PID[56] and may be preferred in situations where compliance is questionable or there is evidence of *M. genitalium* infection.

Moxifloxacin is currently being evaluated for use in PID as it is active against organisms causing PID, including mycoplasmas,[14] and demonstrates uterine tissue concentrations sufficient to eradicate major pathogens. Other advantages are once-daily dosing and few side effects.

EPIDIDYMO-ORCHITIS

Epididymo-orchitis is a complication of gonorrhea and chlamydia, particularly in men under 35 years, and treatment should be directed at these organisms, i.e.:

- ceftriaxone 250 mg intramuscularly (single dose), plus
- doxycycline 100 mg every 12 h for 10 days.[29]

In men over 35 years, treatment should be directed at urinary tract infections.

LYMPHOGRANULOMA VENEREUM

EPIDEMIOLOGY

Lymphogranuloma venereum (LGV) is usually a disease of developing countries where it is often endemic. In developed countries, cases tend to occur in individuals with multiple sexual partners, low socioeconomic groups and urban areas. Traditionally, LGV occurred sporadically in developed countries, often secondary to sexual contact overseas. However, outbreaks have been described in several developed countries[57] amongst men who have sex with men (MSM), particularly in those with numerous casual partners. Where LGV is endemic, most patients are males in their twenties. The male-to-female ratio varies but can reach as high as 5:1 and may be due to a greater proportion of asymptomatic cases in women. However, late complications are reported more frequently in women.

PATHOGENESIS

LGV is a disease of the lymphatics. The organism induces a thrombolymphangitis and perilymphangitis in the drainage site of the primary infection. The endothelial cells lining the lymphatic vessels proliferate and central necrosis occurs. These areas coalesce to form abscesses from which fistulae or sinuses can develop. This acute inflammatory process lasts weeks to months, followed by fibrosis, resulting in further destruction of the lymphatics. Chronic edema develops secondary to lymphatic obstruction and the affected area often becomes indurated with breakdown of the overlying skin. In rectal involvement, a picture similar to Crohn's disease develops with transmural inflammation, mucosal ulceration and inflammatory strictures.

DIAGNOSIS

CLINICAL

LGV is divided into three stages:

- Stage 1 is the development of a painless non-scarring ulcer or papule, usually on the glans penis, vaginal wall or labia. It occurs 3–12 days after sexual contact and often heals unnoticed. Lesions can occur in the urethra, cervix or rectum, leading to urethritis, cervicitis or proctitis, respectively. Lymphangitis develops in the field of drainage.

- Stage 2 manifests as tender lymphadenopathy in the inguinal and/or femoral region. In two-thirds of cases this is unilateral. The area can feel matted, with ulceration and sinus formation. When inguinal and femoral regions are affected, the taut inguinal ligament forms a groove, which is said to be pathognomonic of LGV. This stage is often associated with fever. Meningoencephalitis, hepatitis, pneumonitis, erythema nodosum and erythema multiforme have been described. The time between the primary lesion and lymphadenopathy is 10–30 days, but may be up to 6 months.

- Not all cases progress to stage 3, where widespread destruction of surrounding areas results in proctocolitis, abscess formation, fistulae and strictures. This is more common in females and MSM. Alternatively, a lesion (esthiomene) develops when the primary infection has involved the lymphatics of the scrotum, penis or vulva. Lymphangitis, lymphatic obstruction and fibrosis result in induration, enlargement and ulceration of affected parts. This destructive process is most commonly seen in women.

INVESTIGATIONS

Investigations need to exclude other causes of GUD and other coexisting STIs. Various techniques can be used to assess lymph node aspirates or ulcer base exudates, including culture, immunofluorescence, enzyme immunoassay (EIA) and PCR. Alternatively, serological testing including micro-immunofluorescence, complement fixation or enzyme-linked immunosorbent assay (ELISA) may be used. Culture is the most specific method but its sensitivity is poor (50–85%). Culture and immunofluorescence are labor intensive and expensive. EIA is relatively easy but has poor sensitivity and requires confirmation by another method. PCR, used in non-LGV chlamydia, has not been used to any great extent in LGV. PCR has high sensitivity and specificity, but is expensive. Of the serological tests, microimmunofluorescence is one of the most sensitive and specific. It can distinguish serotypes, making it the diagnostic test of choice if available.

MANAGEMENT

Studies regarding the treatment of LGV are few. Assessment of treatment outcome is difficult because spontaneous resolution can occur. Various guidelines suggest the following:[5,58,59]

- first-line therapy: doxycycline 100 mg orally every 12 h for 21 days
- erythromycin base 500 mg orally every 6 h for 21 days.

Early treatment is essential to limit the chronic phase. Resolution of symptoms should occur within a few days, although healing may take several weeks. Complications such as fistulae, sinuses or strictures may require surgery, always under antibiotic cover.

Treatment of MSM remains the same as that for heterosexuals.

PREGNANCY AND BREASTFEEDING

Erythromycin base is safe for use in pregnancy and lactation. Doxycycline is contraindicated in pregnancy.[18]

SYPHILIS

The causative organism of syphilis is *Treponema pallidum*, subspecies *pallidum*, a spirochetal organism belonging to the genus *Treponema*. The genus includes three other human pathogens, *T. pallidum* subspecies *pertenue* (the cause of yaws), *T. pallidum* subspecies *endemicum* (the causative organism of bejel) and *Treponema carateum* (the causative organism of pinta).

EPIDEMIOLOGY

The incidence of syphilis in the developed world fluctuated dramatically during the 20th century. It was extremely common throughout Europe in the early part of the century. Following the First World War, social stability, improvements in living standards and healthcare resulted in a decline in incidence. However, this was short lived. During, and immediately after, the Second World War the incidence increased. The introduction of penicillin and improvements in healthcare resulted in a dramatic decline in syphilis in the 15 years following the Second World War. During the 1960s and 1970s, there was an increase in many parts of the world, particularly in MSM. However, as a consequence of the HIV epidemic, the 1980s saw widespread promotion of safer sex messages, leading to dramatic declines in syphilis, particularly in Europe, North America and Australia. In the late 1990s, Eastern Europe and some inner cities in North America saw an increase in incidence secondary to poverty, unemployment, poor healthcare and social breakdown.

In the USA, between 1990 and 2000, the rate of primary and secondary syphilis declined by 90%. However, from 2001 to 2007 the rates increased annually, predominantly among men (from 3/100 000 to 6.6/100 000).[23]

In sub-Saharan Africa and South and South East Asia, syphilis remains a major public health problem with an estimated 6 million new diagnoses in both regions in 2005.[1]

PATHOGENESIS

Treponemes enter the body via microabrasions caused by trauma during sexual intercourse and then migrate into the dermis where they attach to the surface of cells. They do not enter the cell, but penetrate the endothelial junctions and tissue layers. There is localized infection at the site of invasion, usually resulting in a local lesion (chancre). The organism then disseminates throughout the body. Late complications are due to a chronic inflammatory reaction which continues over many years. Cardiovascular syphilis is characterized by lymphocytic and perivascular infiltrates, resulting in an obliterative endarteritis. The pathological changes of neurosyphilis again reflect a chronic inflammatory reaction with lymphocytes and plasma cells infiltrating the meninges and perivascular areas, resulting in degeneration of neural cells. *T. pallidum* has an immune evasiveness, which is its key to success as a pathogen. This may partly be due to sequestration in immune sanctuary sites masking the organism's surface by host proteins, or paucity of outer membrane proteins acting as antigenic targets. Some immunogenic proteins appear to be under the cell surface and associated with the periplasmic leaflet. Additionally, the proteins are usually present in small numbers, further restricting their potential as immune targets.

DIAGNOSIS

 ## CLINICAL

The incubation varies from 9 to 90 days (average 21 days) and the clinical features can be divided into three stages:

- Primary infection (chancre) occurs at the site of local inoculation. Chancres are usually painless ulcers, accompanied by local lymphadenopathy, and heal within 3–10 weeks.
- The secondary stage corresponds with dissemination of the infection, characterized by skin and mucous membrane lesions and constitutional symptoms. In many individuals, latency is established without any signs or symptoms of early infection; they may go on to develop the late complications of infection.
- Late complications include cardiovascular, neurological or gummatous disease. Cardiovascular problems include aortitis, aortic incompetence and aortic aneurysms. The second major late complication is neurological syphilis involving the brain and/or spinal cord. Gummatous disease represents a hypersensitivity reaction characterized by nodules consisting of necrotic tissue surrounded by mononuclear cells and proliferating connective tissue. They can occur in any tissue or organ, but most commonly occur in skin or bone.

Infection is completely curable in the primary, secondary and early latent stages. However, cardiovascular and/or neurological damage is irreversible, although progression can be prevented with treatment. The natural history of untreated syphilis is variable: around 10% develop cardiovascular disease, 10% neurological disease and 10% gummatous disease.

INVESTIGATIONS

Syphilis can be diagnosed through direct visualization of the organism or by serological testing. Direct visualization may be possible in primary and secondary syphilis. Specimens may be obtained from primary chancres or mucous membrane lesions. The organism can be viewed under dark-field microscopy of serous exudate placed on a saline-moistened slide. Treponemes can be seen as motile spirochetes, characteristically said to display 'corkscrew' and 'angular' motion, with 15–20 coils. Specimens may also be examined with fluorescent antibody stains, a method that can also be used on biopsy and autopsy specimens.

The mainstay of syphilis diagnosis is serology. There are two types of serological tests: non-treponemal and treponemal.

Non-specific antibodies directed towards anticardiolipin, cholesterol and lecithin form the basis for the non-treponemal tests. They can be detected in serum and are related to disease activity. However, these tests also become positive in response to other conditions, including acute viral and mycoplasmal infection, vaccination, pregnancy, and connective tissue disorders. Two tests commonly used are the Venereal Disease Research Laboratory (VDRL) test and the rapid plasma regain (RPR) test.

Treponemal tests are specific. However, once positive they tend to remain so, and consequently detection of antibodies indicates past or present infection. Three tests are commonly used: fluorescent treponemal antibody absorption test (FTA), *Treponema pallidum* hemagglutination assay (TPHA)[60] and a variation of TPHA, the *Treponema pallidum* particle agglutination assay (TPPA). Antibodies can be detected in serum and cerebrospinal fluid (CSF). In early infection no antibodies are present and the first test to become positive is usually the FTA.

There has been an increase in availability of the treponemal EIA for the detection of IgM and IgG treponemal antibodies. EIA for treponemal IgM antibodies is particularly helpful in the diagnosis of suspected early syphilis as they are almost invariably detectable 2 weeks after infection. IgG antibodies become detectable by the fourth or fifth week of infection.[61]

MANAGEMENT

Treatment aims to eliminate infection and prevent complications and onward spread. Since its introduction in the late 1940s, penicillin has revolutionized the management of syphilis and remains the mainstay of treatment, although no RCTs have been conducted. Despite its widespread use, *T. pallidum* remains sensitive to penicillin. Treatment choices are predicated on convenience of dosage, CSF penetration, concomitant HIV infection and allergy. Benzathine penicillin is convenient to use, but has poor CSF penetration.[62] Some experts prefer procaine penicillin, particularly when used with probenecid, which delays renal excretion and prolongs the half-life of penicillin and has good CSF penetration.[63]

PRIMARY, SECONDARY OR EARLY LATENT SYPHILIS IF THE CSF IS NEGATIVE[5,61,64]

Treatment is procaine penicillin 1.2 g (600 000 units) intramuscularly daily for 10 days with probenecid 500 mg every 6 h. An alternative is single-dose benzathine penicillin G 1.8 g intramuscularly.

If the patient is allergic to penicillin the following regimens may be employed:
- Doxycycline 100 mg orally every 12 h for 21 days[65]
- Azithromycin 2 g orally[66] (single dose)
- Erythromycin 500 mg orally every 6 h for 14 days
- Ceftriaxone 500 mg intramuscularly daily for 10 days
- Amoxicillin 500 mg orally every 6 h for 14 days (with probenecid 500 mg every 6 h for 14 days).

Ceftriaxone should be used with caution in individuals with history of anaphylactic reaction to penicillin.

Patients treated with alternative regimens must be monitored carefully for treatment failure. There are few reports of treatment failure with azithromycin.[67] A Cochrane review comparing azithromycin with penicillin is currently underway.

In individuals whose compliance to alternative regimens is questionable or follow-up unlikely, desensitization and subsequent treatment with benzathine penicillin may be recommended.

CARDIOVASCULAR, GUMMATOUS OR NEUROSYPHILIS[5,61,64]

Choices include intramuscular procaine penicillin 1.2 g (600 000 units) daily and probenecid 500 mg every 6 h for 17 days, intramuscular benzathine penicillin G 1.8 g weekly for 3 weeks or doxycycline 100 mg orally every 12 h for 28 days.

THE JARISCH–HERXHEIMER REACTION

An influenza-like reaction with headache, myalgia and fever sometimes occurs within 24 h of starting therapy, believed to be due to rapid reduction in treponemal load which can be managed with simple antipyretics. Occasionally this reaction may cause severe complications in late syphilis, particularly where the cerebral vasculature or the aorta is involved. Systemic steroids such as prednisolone 30 mg/day for 3 days, commencing the day before treatment, are useful.

SYPHILIS IN HIV-POSITIVE PATIENTS[5,61,64]

Treatment of syphilis in HIV-positive individuals remains an area of dispute. Some experts believe all HIV-positive patients should be treated as for late syphilis. Others believe treatment remains the same as for HIV-negative patients.

PREGNANCY AND BREASTFEEDING

Procaine penicillin and benzathine penicillin are both suitable for treatment in pregnancy and while breastfeeding. Doxycycline is not recommended. Erythromycin 500 mg orally every 6 h for 21 days is suitable in patients allergic to penicillin. If erythromycin is used, the baby should be treated with procaine penicillin as erythromycin does not reliably ensure cure of an infected fetus.[5] There is little or no evidence to recommend a change in antibiotic treatment schedule amongst pregnant women.[64,68]

CONGENITAL SYPHILIS

Infants under 2 years should receive aqueous crystalline penicillin 100 000–150 000 U/kg per day, administered intravenously as 50 000 U/kg (30–60 mg) per dose, every 12 h for the first 7 days of life, and every 8 h thereafter for a total of 10 days, as recommended by the CDC. The BASSH also recommends intravenous benzyl penicillin sodium 100 000–150 000 U/kg per day as per the CDC regimen. Alternatively, procaine penicillin G may be administered in a daily single dose of 50 000 U/kg intramuscularly for 10 days.[5,69]

CHANCROID

Chancroid is an important cause of GUD in developing countries. The causative agent is *Haemophilus ducreyi*, a Gram-negative anaerobic coccobacillus.

EPIDEMIOLOGY

In 1995, the WHO estimated the annual incidence of chancroid to be 7 million.[70] The burden of this infection is predominantly in some developing countries where it is endemic. Several studies in the late 1990s suggested the prevalence of chancroid had decreased. A larger proportion of GUD is attributable to reactivation of HSV in HIV-positive populations. Mixed infections with HSV, syphilis or both are also common (17.4% [13.1–21.5% at 95% confidence intervals]).[71]

In developed nations, incidence and prevalence are low, with occasional outbreaks described in Canada and the southern states of the USA, often associated with exchange of sex for money or drugs and the use of crack cocaine or alcohol. Recently there has been a significant decline in prevalence in the USA, with only 23 reported cases in 2007.[72]

H. ducreyi is transmitted mainly through sexual contact, with lower socioeconomic groups at greatest risk. Infection is twice as common among uncircumcised men as in circumcised men. Commercial sex workers (CSWs) with subclinical disease form a reservoir of infection, but there is no evidence for asymptomatic carriage. If untreated, the infection is thought to last about 45 days.

The presence of GUD, particularly chancroid, is an important risk factor in transmission of HIV. The mechanism behind this is thought to be *H. ducreyi* recruiting CD4 cells and macrophages to the genital surface, providing an increased target population of cells for HIV to infect.

PATHOGENESIS

H. ducreyi penetrates the epidermis through an abrasion or trauma. It incites a predominantly Th1 response, with recruitment of CD4 and CD8 lymphocytes, macrophages and granulocytes to the infection site. The initial lesion is commonly intraepidermal and organisms can be found within polymorphs and the interstitium. More virulent strains of *H. ducreyi* can withstand phagocytosis and killing by neutrophils. In addition to cellular immune response, a humoral immune response is elicited, with antibodies targeted particularly against lipo-oligosaccharides. The role of these immune responses in the pathogenesis of chancroid is not fully understood.

DIAGNOSIS

CLINICAL

Chancroid has an incubation period of 3–10 days. Men usually present with a genital ulcer or tender inguinal lymphadenopathy. Women present with dysuria, dyspareunia, vaginal discharge and pain or bleeding on defecation, depending on the infection site.[73] The ulcer can be single or multiple. Women often have a number of discrete ulcers, whereas over half of affected men will only have a single ulcer. The ulcer classically has ragged, undermined edges, a necrotic base with purulent exudate and bleeds easily on contact. It is non-indurated with little surrounding inflammation. Pain is characteristic, but less common in women. Ulcers occur at sites of trauma: in men, either on the internal or external surface of the prepuce, frenulum or coronal sulcus; in women, on the fourchette, labia, vestibule or clitoris. Ulcers may extend into the vagina and have been described on the cervix.

Associated painful inguinal lymphadenopathy occurs in about 50% of cases, being unilateral and extensive. Buboes form, become fluctuant and rupture, leading to extensive ulceration. Superinfection of these and primary ulcers by anaerobic organisms can lead to phagedenic ulceration and extensive tissue destruction. In men, phimosis may occur as a late complication, often requiring circumcision.

INVESTIGATIONS

Currently the 'gold standard' for diagnosis is culture of swabs taken from the base of the ulcer. Pus aspirated from a bubo can also be cultured, but has a lower yield as the number of organisms is low. For optimum results, a selective culture medium is required, for example gonococcal agar base, supplemented with fetal calf serum or charcoal. With these methods, sensitivities of at least 80% are reached. Gram staining samples may reveal Gram-negative coccobacilli with occasional chains. However, this is only 50% sensitive when compared with culture. PCR is the most sensitive method (>95%) but is only commercially available as a combined test for *H. ducreyi*, *T. pallidum* and HSV. Some laboratories have developed in-house PCR tests, but these are not Food and Drug Administration (FDA) approved.

Serology is available in the form of an ELISA, although it is unable to distinguish between new and old infection. Other causes of GUD should be considered and excluded.

MANAGEMENT[5,74]

- Azithromycin 1 g orally (single dose)
- Erythromycin 500 mg orally every 6 h for 7 days
- Ciprofloxacin 500 mg orally every 12 h for 3 days
- Ciprofloxacin 500 mg orally (single dose)
- Ceftriaxone 250 mg intramuscularly (single dose)
- Spectinomycin 2 g intramuscularly (single dose).

With the emergence of plasmid-mediated antimicrobial resistance, tetracyclines, penicillins, streptomycin, chloramphenicol and sulfonamides are no longer reliable. Trimethoprim also shows widespread resistance, although the mechanism behind this has not been characterized. Intermittent resistance to ciprofloxacin and erythromycin has been described in several isolates worldwide, although in insufficient numbers to limit their use. If *H. ducreyi* is not eradicated from the ulcer within 72 h of commencing therapy, clinical failure can be anticipated.

All regimens recommended above have been proven effective in RCTs.[75,76] A small study demonstrated cure rates of 93.7% and 93.3% with ciprofloxacin and erythromycin, respectively, but only 53.3% with co-trimoxazole.[77] The advantage of azithromycin and ceftriaxone is they are single-dose regimens. The option of using ciprofloxacin in a single dose has also been evaluated, with cure rates of 92%, compared to erythromycin, with cure rates of 91%.[78] Some studies raised concern regarding single-dose regimens in HIV-positive patients. In one study 30% of patients administered ceftriaxone failed treatment.[79] Treatment failures have also been described with azithromycin.[75] Single-dose regimens should be used cautiously, particularly in HIV-positive patients. The CDC recommends that single-dose regimens should only be used in HIV-positive individuals if follow-up is ensured.[5] Fluctuant buboes are managed by repeated aspiration of pus through adjacent healthy skin, a safe and effective procedure.

PREGNANCY AND BREASTFEEDING

Fluoroquinolones cannot be used in pregnancy and lactation, or in children. Azithromycin, erythromycin or ceftriaxone is the treatment of choice.

FOLLOW-UP

Patients should be reassessed after treatment completion to ensure healing has occurred. Re-epithelialization will be evident by day 7, although complete healing depends on initial ulcer size. Failure to respond may be due to antibiotic resistance or the presence of a co-infection. Sensitivity testing and exclusion of syphilis and HSV are warranted.

CONTACT TRACING

Contact tracing is necessary for any sexual contact in the 10 days prior to symptom onset. Contacts should be examined and treated if necessary. Active tracing and treating contacts and condom promotion programs make eradication of *H. ducreyi* achievable, a goal with high priority due to the enhanced HIV transmission.

DONOVANOSIS (GRANULOMA INGUINALE)

Donovanosis is a form of GUD seen predominantly in tropical countries and caused by the Gram-negative bacillus *Klebsiella granulomatis* (formally classified as *Calymmatobacterium granulomatis*).[80]

EPIDEMIOLOGY

Recently, donovanosis has been seen in small endemic foci in only a few geographical areas; in particular, Papua New Guinea (PNG), southern Africa, North East Brazil, French Guyana and remote Australian aboriginal communities. Outbreaks have also been identified in parts of South Africa.[81] However, the numbers of cases in PNG[82] and in Australia have decreased dramatically following successful elimination programs.[83] Most cases occur via sexual transmission, with men outnumbering women by up to 6:1,[84] and are associated with poor personal hygiene.[85] Vertical transmission has been reported, as has primary infection, in children. There appears to be a genetic component to donovanosis, with individuals with HLA-B57 being more susceptible and those with HLA-A23 having some resistance to infection.[86]

PATHOGENESIS

Organisms gain entry via trauma or abrasions. A small firm nodule containing 'Donovan bodies' occurs at the site of inoculation and is considered classic for the disease. 'Donovan bodies' consist of large mononuclear cells in which intracytoplasmic inclusion bodies contain the bacteria. These inclusion bodies rupture, releasing infective organisms.

DIAGNOSIS

CLINICAL

At the site of primary inoculation, a small, non-tender papule or subcutaneous nodule forms; this either ulcerates or becomes a hypertrophic growth. The ulcer can become necrotic and destructive, leading to the formation of extensive scar tissue. The primary ulcer, in contrast to chancroid, is painless and can be single or multiple; however, like chancroid, it bleeds easily on contact and often has a distinctive odor. Genitals are affected in 90% of cases. Extragenital ulcers are found in 6% of cases, usually associated with primary disease. Sites include the oropharynx, neck and chest. Inguinal lesions occur in 10% of cases secondary to spread of infection from lymph nodes to overlying skin.

Some cases may resolve, but others develop into a chronic form leading to extensive tissue destruction. Other complications include hemorrhage, genital elephantiasis secondary to lymphoedema, squamous cell carcinoma and, rarely, dissemination to bone and liver. Disseminated disease is seen more frequently in pregnancy.

INVESTIGATIONS

Suitable samples include swabs or scrapings from the base of ulcers or tissue biopsy. These are stained with Giemsa or Gram stain and studied under a direct microscope. Donovan bodies (Gram-negative with bipolar staining) are found within histiocytes and are characteristic of infection (seen in 60–80% of suspected cases). *K. granulomatis* has been cultured but culture is not yet used in routine practice; neither is PCR nor serology.[87]

MANAGEMENT

All patients with proven or clinically suspected donovanosis from endemic areas should be treated, with therapy continuing until the ulcer has healed.

The following regimens have been evaluated in prospective studies:[5,84,87–91]

- Azithromycin orally 1 g weekly or 500 mg daily
- Erythromycin orally 500 mg every 6 h
- Doxycycline orally 100 mg every 12 h
- Trimethoprim–sulfamethoxazole orally 160/800 mg every 12 h
- Norfloxacin orally 400 mg every 12 h
- Gentamicin (intramuscular or intravenous) 1 mg/kg every 8 h
- Ceftriaxone (intramuscular or intravenous) 1 g daily.

Australian antibiotic guidelines recommend azithromycin. As lengthy therapy is often required, this may be one of the most cost-effective regimens. Like chancroid, there is some evidence that patients with HIV may not respond to first-line therapy and may require longer courses of antibiotics.[81]

Sexual contacts of the index case should be assessed and treated in order to reduce transmission of donovanosis, as well as HIV, in endemic areas.

PREGNANCY AND BREASTFEEDING

Azithromycin, erythromycin and ceftiaxone are safe for use in pregnancy and while breastfeeding. Doxycline and ciprofloxacin and contraindicated. Pregnancy is a relative contraindication to the use of sulfonomides.

BACTERIAL VAGINOSIS

Bacterial vaginosis (BV) is a syndrome characterized by alteration in normal bacterial flora found in the vagina, from a predominance of lactobacilli, to high concentrations of anaerobic bacteria (*Gardnerella vaginalis*, *Prevotella* spp., *Mycoplasma hominis*, *Mobiluncus* spp.). It presents with an offensive vaginal discharge and is believed to be associated with PID, and an increased risk of preterm labor and chorioamnionitis in pregnant women.

EPIDEMIOLOGY

The infection is common in most countries, with highest reported rates in women in rural parts of sub-Saharan Africa (over 50%), followed by CSWs and women attending STI clinics (24–37%).[92,93] Higher prevalence appears to be related to ethnicity, being sexually active and having symptoms.[94] A recent UK study indicated a prevalence of BV amongst asymptomatic pregnant women of 3.54%[95] and a study in Burkina Faso indicated a prevalence of 6.4% amongst women attending antenatal clinics.[96] BV appears to double women's risk of HIV acquisition.[97]

PATHOGENESIS

The pathogenesis of BV is unclear. Inoculation studies in human and animal models, together with epidemiological data, suggest that sexual intercourse may introduce a set of bacteria that in some women set in motion a chain of events leading to alteration in bacterial flora and subsequent BV. Lack of inflammation in vaginal epithelial cells suggests that BV is due to a change in bacterial flora and composition of vaginal fluid rather than a true infection. Practices like 'douching' of the vagina are associated with BV and may play a role in pathogenesis.[98] Another factor thought to influence the host's susceptibility to infection is the predominant strain of lactobacillus present. Some strains produce hydrogen peroxide, which may inhibit growth of anaerobic rods, *Gardnerella*, *Mobiluncus* and *Mycoplasma*. These lactobacilli are found more frequently colonizing the vagina of normal women than those with BV and women with these strains are less likely to develop BV.

DIAGNOSIS

CLINICAL

BV is asymptomatic in many women. The characteristic symptom is a malodorous thin, white, homogeneous vaginal discharge, coating the walls of the vagina.

BV is associated with chorioamnionitis, preterm labor, low birthweight, premature rupture of membranes,[99] postpartum PID (following cesarean and vaginal delivery), post-abortion PID and PID following gynecological surgery. It is not clear if treating women with asymptomatic BV reduces their risk of developing PID.

INVESTIGATIONS

The diagnosis of BV is based on the presence of symptoms and signs. Cultures for specific bacteria are of limited use as these form part of normal vaginal flora. Diagnostic criteria consist of three of the following four signs:

1. Characteristic, white adherent vaginal discharge
2. Vaginal pH <4.5
3. Fishy odor (from release of amines) when vaginal fluid is mixed with 10% potassium hydroxide
4. Presence of clue cells.[100]

Clue cells are vaginal squamous cells covered with bacteria giving them a stippled appearance. They can be visualized by placing a drop of vaginal fluid and normal saline on a slide and viewed microscopically. Gram staining vaginal fluid will also reveal clue cells, in addition to large numbers of Gram-negative or Gram-variable coccobacilli.

Commercially available diagnostic kits have not been validated for diagnosis.

MANAGEMENT

BV can remit spontaneously. Even with treatment, it may recur in up to one-third of women. Consequently, women with BV who are symptomatic, undergoing surgical procedures or are pregnant should be treated to reduce anaerobic flora.[101,102]

 ## RECOMMENDED REGIMENS

- Metronidazole 400–500 mg orally every 12 h for 7 days
- Metronidazole 2 g orally (single dose)
- Metronidazole gel (0.75%) intravaginally daily for 5 days
- Clindamycin cream (2%) intravaginally daily for 7 days
- Clindamycin 300 mg orally every 12 h for 7 days
- Tinidazole 2 g orally (single dose).

Metronidazole and clindamycin (oral and intravaginal preparations) have been evaluated in several RCTs and appear to have similar efficacy with cure rates at 1 month of 71–89%. A systematic review of oral and intravaginal preparations in non-pregnant women showed that at 4 weeks post therapy, cumulative cure rates were 78% for oral metronidazole, 82% for intravaginal clindamycin and 71% for intravaginal metronidazole.[103] One RCT comparing oral metronidazole with clindamycin showed no difference in short-term cure rates (94–96% at 7–10 days).[104] Comparison of metronidazole 2 g statim with 500 mg every 12 h for 7 days suggests that the single dose may be less effective.[105] Both metronidazole and clindamycin (intravaginal applications) have demonstrated similar efficacy in restoring lactobacilli at 21–30 days after initiation of therapy.[106]

Clindamycin has few side effects but has been associated with pseudomembranous colitis and vaginal candidiasis. Up to two-thirds of women treated with oral metronidazole will experience side effects, mainly gastrointestinal. Intravaginal metronidazole preparations are equally effective, have fewer side effects, but may be more expensive.[107]

The UK guidelines recommend tinidazole 2 g (single dose). An RCT found tinidazole 2 g per day for 2 days or 1 g per day for 5 days to be significantly more effective than placebo,[96] though more expensive than metronidazole.[101]

Although the recurrence rate among women treated for BV is high, there is no evidence from several placebo-controlled trials to support treatment of male sexual partners.

 ## TREATMENT OF BV IN PREGNANCY AND BREASTFEEDING

Several RCTs regarding treatment of BV in pregnant women with a history of preterm labor indicate that this group should receive oral metronidazole or clindamycin early in the second trimester as both drugs are efficacious and safe.[108–110]

Evidence does not support the use of intravaginal clindamycin to prevent preterm labor in women with BV. In fact, its use in the latter half of pregnancy has been associated with low birthweight and neonatal infections.[111]

There is a suggestion that treating BV in the first 20 weeks of pregnancy may have a beneficial effect on preterm labor.[112] However, there are insufficient data to support treatment of all asymptomatic pregnant women.

Metronidazole enters breast milk and high doses should be avoided. Small amounts of clindamycin enter breast milk. It is prudent therefore to use intravaginal treatment during lactation.

 ## TEST OF CURE

Only pregnant women with BV require test of cure. They should be retested after 1 month to assess requirement for further treatment.

 ## PROPHYLACTIC THERAPY

Data on the use of prophylactic treatment before gynecological procedures and insertion of intrauterine contraceptive devices are limited. Currently there is insufficient evidence to support its use.

 ## ALTERNATIVE MEDICATIONS

Various alternative treatments are currently available, including acidifiers, yoghurt and lactobacillus preparations but data supporting their use are limited.

GENITAL HERPES

EPIDEMIOLOGY

Genital herpes is caused by infection with one of the two herpes simplex viruses (HSV): HSV-1 or HSV-2. Most genital infections are caused by HSV-2 as a consequence of direct genital-to-genital spread. In some countries, particularly in the developed world, HSV-1 accounts for a considerable proportion of cases.[113] HSV-1 is spread to the genitals during orogenital sex. Individuals infected genitally with HSV-1 or HSV-2 may remain asymptomatic,[114] although most shed the virus sporadically and can infect their sexual partners.[115]

Several seroepidemiological studies have been conducted. These showed that among pregnant women, HSV-2 seroprevalence ranged from 7% to 50%,[116] in STI clinics from 15% to 75%[116,117] and among CSWs from 74% to 96%.

The presence of HSV-2 antibodies is related to age at coitarche, number of lifetime sexual partners, increasing age, ethnic origin, socioeconomic status, gender (women more commonly infected than men) and previous STIs.[118,119]

PATHOGENESIS

HSV enters the body via the skin or mucous membranes of the genital tract. The virus is then taken up by sensory nerve cells and transported retrogradely to sensory or autonomic ganglia. The virus remains in the sensory neurons, where it may reactivate, and then be taken via anterograde transport to the cutaneous surface, where viral replication occurs. This results in either asymptomatic viral excretion or clinical recurrence of the disease.[120] The nature of the latent virus and cause of recurrences remain to be fully elucidated.

DIAGNOSIS

 ### CLINICAL

Most individuals exposed to HSV remain asymptomatic.[121] Amongst individuals who do develop symptoms, the first episode is usually more severe than recurrences. Individuals may present with symptoms suggestive of viremia with headache, fever and myalgia.[122] Local symptoms include genital pain, dysuria and sometimes vaginal or rectal discharge. The first sign of infection is erythema followed by vesicles, which soon rupture to superficial ulcers that eventually heal. The lesions are often excruciatingly painful and the entire illness may last 2–4 weeks. The lesions may occur anywhere on the genitalia and draining lymph glands are often painfully enlarged.[122]

Recurrences are usually shorter, often consisting of a single lesion or small group of lesions on the external genitalia, usually healing within 7–10 days.[122] Many individuals with recurrent herpes have prodromal or warning symptoms consisting of neuralgia-type pain. Frequency of recurrences is variable: HSV-2 infections tend to recur more often than HSV-1 and lesions recur more often in the first year of infection. Some individuals may have 12 or more recurrences per year.[123]

 ### INVESTIGATIONS

HSV may be grown in cell culture from specimens such as vesicle fluid or material from the base of ulcers. Additional methods of identification include direct immunofluorescence, cytology (where typical cytological changes can be seen) and PCR. The use of PCR for the diagnosis of HSV has many advantages, including increased sensitivity, less dependency on collection and transport conditions, as well as stage of the outbreak. It can also be potentially quicker than viral culture.[124,125]

Serological tests can be divided into group-specific and type-specific. Group-specific serological tests will indicate whether the individual has previously been exposed to either of the two HSV viruses, whereas type-specific serology will differentiate between the two viruses. A number of EIA tests are currently available for type-specific serology. However, the most reliable technology is Western blot.[126] IgG antibodies take approximately 6–8 weeks to develop and consequently are of little use in primary infection. However, as many individuals are asymptomatic, type-specific serological tests should be used cautiously.

MANAGEMENT

Several nucleoside analogs are available for the management of genital herpes. These include aciclovir, valaciclovir (prodrug of aciclovir) and famciclovir (prodrug of penciclovir, converted to the active agent in the liver). Both aciclovir and penciclovir have similar modes of action[127,128] (*see* Ch. 2). However, pharmacokinetic differences exist between these agents (*see* Ch. 37).

 ### FIRST-EPISODE GENITAL HERPES

All three nucleoside analogs have been evaluated for treatment of first-episode genital herpes. Numerous RCTs of intravenous, oral and topical aciclovir have demonstrated considerable efficacy in reducing constitutional symptoms, preventing new lesion formation and reducing the duration of lesions by many days.[129–131] Intravenous and oral therapy appear to be better than topical. Oral valaciclovir and famciclovir have similar efficacy to aciclovir.

Recommended regimens are:

- aciclovir 200 mg five times daily for 5–10 days
- aciclovir 400 mg every 12 h for 5–10 days
- valaciclovir 500 mg every 12 h for 5–10 days
- famciclovir 250 mg every 8 h for 5–10 days.

Note: Although the 400 mg dose of aciclovir can be administered every 8 h, rather than every 12, this has not been the subject of any randomized controlled trial.

Treatment should be initiated as early as possible, resulting in a significant reduction in the duration of lesions, symptoms and viral shedding. None of the drugs has any effect on the likelihood of frequency of subsequent recurrences. The efficacy of all three agents appears to be similar, although the superior bioavailability of valaciclovir and famciclovir allows for less-frequent dosing schedules.

 ### RECURRENT GENITAL HERPES

There are two approaches to managing recurrent genital herpes. Drugs can be used intermittently to treat each episode (intermittent therapy) or continuously over a period of time to prevent episodes from occurring (suppressive therapy).

Intermittent therapy

Intermittent therapy reduces the duration of each episode and may be useful for individuals with severe but infrequent recurrences. It may also be beneficial during the prodrome when it may abort episodes. All three available drugs have been evaluated in RCTs and have demonstrated similar efficacy.[132–135]

Doses for intermittent treatment

- Aciclovir 200 mg five times daily for 5 days.
- Valaciclovir 500 mg every 12 h for 5 days.
- Famciclovir 125 mg every 12 h for 5 days.

Recently, the trend is to use shorter regimens (1–3 days) for intermittent therapy.[136–138] The efficacy of these regimens appears similar to that of the 5-day regimens with the advantage of fewer days of treatment without increased toxicity.

Suppressive therapy

Suppressive therapy is particularly useful for individuals having frequent recurrences. Most individuals on suppressive therapy will have no recurrences. All three drugs have similar efficacy,[139–141] although the superior bioavailability of valaciclovir and famciclovir allows for less-frequent dosing schedules. Many patients treated with suppressive therapy will also have an improvement in psychosexual morbidity.[134]

Doses for suppressive therapy

- Aciclovir 200 mg every 6 h or 400 mg every 12 h.
- Valaciclovir 500 mg once daily for individuals with 10 or fewer recurrences per year; 500 mg every 12 h for individuals with more than 10 recurrences per year.[141]
- Famciclovir 250 mg every 12 h.

Treatment should continue for a year and then stopped to see if recurrences are occurring with similar frequency and to determine the need for further therapy. Suppressive therapy does not appear to affect the natural history of recurrences. Individuals on treatment should be advised that viral shedding may still occur, and consistent condom use will reduce the risk of transmission.

 ## PREGNANCY

None of the drugs has been formally evaluated during pregnancy. However, the inadvertent use of aciclovir during pregnancy did not demonstrate any adverse events.[142,143]

Primary herpes in pregnancy

Women acquiring primary herpes during pregnancy should be treated with aciclovir or valaciclovir as described above. If the mother has primary herpes, the risk of mother-to-child transmission is 30–50%.[144] The risk increases significantly if the outbreak occurs in the third trimester.[145] Neonatal herpes is a devastating infection (*see* Ch. 55).

Cesarean birth before membrane rupture significantly reduces the risk of intrapartum transmission to the infant.[5,146]

Recurrent herpes during pregnancy

The risk of transmission from mother to child with recurrent genital herpes is very low (<1%).[145] However, women with recurrent genital herpes are often extremely anxious about the risk and may request antiviral therapy or even elective cesarean section. Suppressive therapy in the last month of pregnancy decreases the risk of recurrences during that period[147,148] and may be more cost-effective when compared to cesarean delivery.[149] If lesions or prodromal symptoms occur at the onset of labor, cesarean section is recommend to minimize the risk of viral exposure to the infant, even if suppressive therapy has been used.[5]

GENITAL WARTS

EPIDEMIOLOGY

Over 40 human papillomavirus (HPV) infections can involve the genital tract. These may be divided into those with low oncogenic transforming potential and those with high transforming potential. Types with low transforming potential are associated with condylomata acuminata (genital warts), whereas those with high transforming potential are associated with subsequent development of cervical cancer and other genital tract tumors. All HPV types found in the genital tract are transmitted by sexual intercourse.[150]

The true prevalence of these infections is unknown, as a large number of individuals are asymptomatic with no reliable serological tests available currently. However, the incidence of genital warts has increased in Europe, North America and Australia.[151] Using PCR-based methods, HPV infection has been detected in 1.5–44.3% of women with normal Papanicolaou (Pap) smears and 3.5–46.4% of men.[152] These data are difficult to interpret as many of the studies were small, detection techniques varied and the population groups were different. Finally, recent studies suggest that genital warts and HPV infection may be more common in HIV-positive populations.[153,154]

PATHOGENESIS

HPV infects the stratified squamous epithelium of the genital tract. The infection does not result in cell lysis; rather, infected cells are shed from the surface of the skin or mucous membranes. This means that no viral proteins are released, and consequently immune response is limited. It takes approximately 6 months after infection for natural immunity to develop.[155] T-cell function appears to be critical in modifying the effects of HPV and allows for persistence or spontaneous regression. Individuals with depressed cellular immunity often have persistent and proliferative lesions.[156]

In benign lesions, HPV remains extrachromosomal. However, in cervical and other genital tract tumors, viral DNA is incorporated into the host chromosome.[155]

DIAGNOSIS

CLINICAL

Most individuals infected with genital tract HPV remain asymptomatic. Some will develop genital warts which, in women, can occur on the vulva, vagina or cervix; in men, they occur on the penis, scrotal skin and occasionally within the urethra. In both sexes, perianal and anal warts can occur. Internal warts in women tend to be asymptomatic. HPV infections associated with cervical intraepithelial neoplasia are usually asymptomatic.

INVESTIGATIONS

No routine diagnostic tests are available for detecting HPV. While DNA amplification tests have been used in research and epidemiological studies, their use in routine clinical management is yet to be fully evaluated.

MANAGEMENT

There are no agents that specifically eradicate HPV or limit its replication. Treatments are directed at obliterating genital warts or removing dysplastic lesions. Several ablative techniques can be used, including cryotherapy, electrocautery, laser therapy or surgical removal.

Choice of treatment depends on the site and number of warts, availability of individual methods, operator expertise, cost and side effects. Success rates for all these treatments appear to be similar, with initial removal of warts achievable in most cases, although relapse is common.

Several chemical treatments are also used, including the anti-mitotic drug podophyllin and its purified counterpart, podophyllotoxin. The advantage of podophyllotoxin is that it does not contain any of the toxic ligands present in podophyllin, its consistency and strength can be guaranteed, and it is suitable for self-application on external warts. Podophyllin should be applied once or twice weekly for 3–6 weeks. Podophyllotoxin is applied every 12 h for 3 days, repeated in 7-day cycles. Complete clearance occurs in 50–90% of cases.[157,158] Relapses occur in up to 38% of cases.[159,160] Neither drug is recommended during pregnancy nor for treatment of lesions on the cervix.

Use of imiquimod, an immune-modulating agent that acts by inducing interferon-α and -γ and recruitment of CD4$^+$ T lymphocytes, results in 'immune-induced' regression of warts and HPV DNA.[161,162] The 5% cream should be applied three times a week[163] for up to 16 weeks. Clearance occurs in 56–62% of cases.[161,164] An RCT suggested that use of imiquimod for 4 weeks may be just as effective in lesion clearance as the 8- to 16-week regimen, as well as being more cost-effective.[165] Imiquimod sometimes causes local irritation[161,164] and recurrences do occur.

There is limited evidence to suggest recurrences may be less in individuals treated with imiquimod than with other treatment modalities.[164] A meta-analysis of RCTs comparing curative effects of 5% imiquimod and 0.5% podophyllotoxin on genital warts demonstrated a similar curative effect.[166]

Finally, trichloracetic acid (TCA) or bichloracetic acid in 80–90% solutions may be used. It is recommended these solutions be applied to warts weekly for up to 6 weeks. These methods carry a risk of local irritation due to low viscosity of the solutions and are best applied by trained healthcare workers.[152]

MOLLUSCUM CONTAGIOSUM

Molluscum contagiosum is an infectious skin condition characterized by umblicated papules of up to 5–10 mm. The infective agent is a pox virus, but little is known about its life cycle and pathogenesis due to its inability to grow in tissue culture. Infection is mainly found in two population groups: children and young adults. Transmission of the virus is via skin-to-skin contact, which is reflected in the distribution of lesions in these two groups: most lesions in children are on the trunk and upper limbs and in adults on the buttocks, thighs and perineal area. The exception to this is HIV-positive adults where lesions are widespread, larger and often affect the face. Adults with atypical lesions should be offered HIV testing.

Diagnosis of molluscum contagiosum is clinical. Lesions may resolve spontaneously over a period of months and treatment can leave residual scarring. The decision to treat must therefore be discussed carefully with the patients. Options include extrusion or chemical ablation of the central core of the papule; topical creams including podophyllotoxin, TCA, acidified nitrite, an imiquimod analog; or physical ablation with cryotherapy.[167,168]

VIRAL HEPATITIS

Hepatitis A and B (and occasionally C) can be acquired sexually. These infections are discussed in Chapter 48.

TRICHOMONAS VAGINALIS

This flagellated protozoan is found in the genitourinary tract of both sexes. It is transmitted primarily by sexual intercourse and in women is often found in association with other STIs. HIV is thought to have a two- to four-fold increased transmission rate in the presence of trichomoniasis.[169] Also, vaginal trichomoniasis has a demonstrated association with HIV seroconversion.[170] Finally, trichomoniasis has several adverse pregnancy outcomes including premature rupture of membranes and/or delivery and low birthweight.[171,172]

EPIDEMIOLOGY

In 2005, the WHO estimated the worldwide incidence of trichomoniasis in adults at 248.5 million.[1] The infection is very common in CSWs (up to 60% prevalence) and in individuals with multiple sex partners, poor personal hygiene, previous STIs and from low socioeconomic groups.

The incubation period is from 5 to 28 days. Transmission from men to women is greater than from women to men: 67–100% and 14–60%, respectively.[173]

PATHOGENESIS

Infection with *T. vaginalis* elicits a cellular and humoral immune response. An initial event is the influx of polymorphonuclear leukocytes. There is evidence that molecules of the organism act as a chemoattractant for these cells.[174] Leukocytes can then kill these organisms and the fragments are phagocytosed by macrophages. A second line of attack is complement mediated: C3 binds to the organism, activating the alternative complement pathway leading to its death.[175] Multiple environmental factors are thought to influence susceptibility of *T. vaginalis* to complement-mediated lysis. Iron has been shown to induce resistance to lysis, probably by induction of cysteine protease, which degrades C3.[176] Antibodies (IgA, IgG, IgM) against a number of different surface molecules are found both locally and in serum. The level of protection in resolving the initial infection and protecting against future reinfection has not been defined.

DIAGNOSIS

CLINICAL

The main site of infection in women is the vaginal epithelium. The urethra is often involved. Paraurethral glands may also be infected but endocervical infection is rare. In men, the urethra is the most common site infected, although the organism has also been isolated from external genitalia, epididymal aspirates and the prostate. Between 20% and 50% of infected women are asymptomatic. Symptoms include vaginal discharge, which can be malodorous, and vulval itch. Abdominal pain is described but may be secondary to co-infection with other organisms. On examination, patients may have vulval and vaginal erythema, with a small percentage having erythematous cervicitis, sometimes described as a 'strawberry' appearance; 5–15% of women will have no signs of infection.[175,177] Men often present on contact tracing and, like women, up to half will have no symptoms. Symptoms include dysuria and/or urethral discharge. Some men may have balanitis. Spontaneous resolution and prolonged asymptomatic infections often occur in men.

INVESTIGATIONS

Direct microscopy of a 'wet' preparation (saline and vaginal discharge) in 50–70% of cases in women and 30% in men will demonstrate characteristic jerky movements caused by the beating of the organism's anterior flagella, and an increased number of polymorphonuclear leukocytes. Microscopy must be performed within 10–20 minutes of collection or the organisms will lose viability. Culture remains the 'gold standard' and can diagnose up to 95% of cases in women and 60–80% in men.[178,179]

PCR tests have been developed to detect *T. vaginalis*; however, their commercial availability is limited.

MANAGEMENT[5,180]

- Metronidazole 2 g orally (single dose).
- Metronidazole 400 mg (or 500 mg) orally every 12 h for 5–7 days.
- Tinidazole 2 g orally (single dose).

Metronidazole or its related compounds remain the mainstay of treatment with a 95% cure rate if both partners are treated.[181] Reasons for failure include reinfection, non-compliance and co-infections. Some organisms are capable of living under aerobic conditions, but there are currently no effective treatments for these organisms. Prolonged courses, higher doses and parenteral administration have all been tried with some reports of success.

In individuals reporting hypersensitivity to nitroimidazoles, desensitization with antihistamines and/or steroids may be employed prior to treatment.[182,183]

Treating asymptomatic trichomoniasis during pregnancy does not appear to reduce the incidence of preterm labor. However, women with symptoms should always be treated.[184] Metronidazole is safe in pregnancy and during lactation.

CANDIDIASIS

Up to 89% of genital tract candidal infections are caused by *Candida albicans*. The remainder are caused by non-*albicans* species, the most common being *Candida glabrata*.[185]

EPIDEMIOLOGY

Over 70% of women will have one or more episodes of vulvovaginal candidiasis in their lifetime, half of whom will have a recurrence.[186] However, frequent recurrences are uncommon. Factors predisposing women to infection include pregnancy, diabetes mellitus, the oral contraceptive pill, intrauterine contraceptive devices, steroids and HIV infection.[187,188] Candidiasis is not usually sexually transmitted and is uncommon in circumcised men.

PATHOGENESIS

C. albicans is a common bowel commensal, gaining access to the vagina via the perianal area. Whether it is ever a vaginal commensal is disputed.[189] How and why the organism causes inflammation is unclear, although there are a number of recognized predisposing factors. A possible mechanism relates to the production of proteases and phospholipases by *Candida* organisms.[190]

DIAGNOSIS

CLINICAL

In women, candida causes a vulvovaginitis, characterized by vulval pruritus and a white curdy vaginal discharge. On examination there may be vulval and/or vaginal erythema. Discharge is white and often adheres to the vaginal walls.[190] However, many women present with atypical features and laboratory confirmation is important, particularly if other STIs are possible. Infected males usually present with an acute balanoposthitis.

INVESTIGATIONS

A 'wet mount' microscopic examination of vaginal fluid may reveal yeast cells and mycelia.[190] On Gram staining, the cells and mycelia stain Gram-positive. *Candida* species can readily be cultured on Sabouraud's medium. Newer diagnostic methods are being developed for rapid diagnosis of vaginitis by *Trichomonas vaginalis*, *Candida* spp. and *Gardnerella vaginalis*. They are based on the principle of visual aggregation of latex particles bound to specific antibodies to surface antigens.[191]

MANAGEMENT

Topical agents with activity against *Candida* include imidazole agents and nystatin. They are available in the form of creams or pessaries for intravaginal and vulval use. Imidazole agents commonly used are miconazole, clotrimazole or econazole. Several dosing options are available with apparently similar efficacy (over 80%) and a low relapse rate. Nystatin is used less as it is less effective and messy. Recommended topical agents for vulvovaginal candidiasis are listed below:

- Clotrimazole vaginal tablet 500 mg (single dose)
- Clotrimazole pessaries or 200 mg/day for 3 days
- Clotrimazole pessaries 100 mg/day for 6 days
- Clotrimazole cream 5 g (single dose)
- Miconazole pessaries 200 mg/day for 3 days
- Miconazole pessaries 100 mg/day for 7 days
- Miconazole pessaries 100 mg/day for 14 days

- Miconazole vaginal ovule 1200 mg (single dose)
- Econazole pessaries 150 mg/day for 3 days
- Fenticonazole pessary 600 mg (single dose).

The oral azole agents (ketoconazole, fluconazole and itraconazole; doses below) have efficacy similar to topical agents[192–195] and are preferred by many women. Also, single-dose oral fluconazole has been shown to be cost-effective:

- Fluconazole★ 150 mg (single dose)
- Itraconazole★ 200 mg every 12 h for 1 day.

RECURRENT VULVOVAGINAL CANDIDIASIS

Recurrent candidiasis is defined as four or more episodes of symptomatic vulvovaginal candidiasis with positive microscopy and/or culture, documented on two such occasions with partial resolution of symptoms in between episodes.[196,197] While RCT evidence is lacking, the following regimens may be used to manage the condition.

Recommended treatment[196,198,199]

- Fluconazole 150 mg orally every 72 h (3 doses) followed by a maintenance dose of 150 mg weekly for 6 months
- Clotrimazole 500 mg pessary twice weekly for 2 weeks ± clotrimazole 1% vaginal cream every 12 h or clotrimazole 200 mg nocturnally for 6–12 nights followed by a maintenance regimen of clotrimazole 500 mg pessary weekly.

Alternative regimens:

- Clotrimazole pessary 500 mg weekly
- Fluconazole★ 50 mg orally daily
- Itraconazole★ – suppression: 100 mg orally daily; maintenance: 100–200 mg orally weekly
- Ketoconazole★ 100 mg orally daily.

CANDIDAL BALANITIS

Topical use of azoles is usually successful.

TREATMENT OF NON-*ALBICANS CANDIDA* SPECIES

Most are usually susceptible to available azoles. *Candida krusei* may demonstrate an intrinsic resistance to fluconazole.[200]

Although there are no RCTs, it is generally believed that longer courses of azoles may be needed.

★Avoid in pregnancy/risk of pregnancy/breastfeeding.
★Avoid in pregnancy/risk of pregnancy/breastfeeding.

References

1. Schmid G, Rowley J, Samuelson J, et al.; World Health Organization (WHO). *Global estimates of the incidence and prevalence of sexually transmitted infections (STIs)*. Paper presented at: 18th ISSTDR - London 2009; Queen Elizabeth II Conference Centre, London: 28 June–1 July 2009; 2005.

2. UNAIDS/WHO. *AIDS epidemic update: December*. Online. Available at http://data.unaids.org/pub/EPISlides/2007/2007_epiupdate_en.pdf; 2007.

3. Health Protection Agency. http://www.hpa.org.uk/web/HPAwebFile/HPAweb_C/1204619473757.

4. Taylor-Robinson D. *Chlamydia trachomatis* and sexually transmitted disease. *Br Med J*. 1994;308(6922):150–151.

5. Centers for Disease Control and Prevention. Sexually transmitted disease treatment guidelines. *MMWR Morb Mortal Wkly Rep*. 2006;55:33–40.

6. Chernesky MA, Lee H, Schachter J, et al. Diagnosis of *Chlamydia trachomatis* urethral infection in symptomatic and asymptomatic men by testing first-void urine in a ligase chain reaction assay. *J Infect Dis*. 1994;170(5):1308–1311.

7. Lee HH, Chernesky MA, Schachter J, et al. Diagnosis of *Chlamydia trachomatis* genitourinary infection in women by ligase chain reaction assay of urine. *Lancet*. 1995;345(8944):213–216.

8. Brocklehurst P, Rooney G. Interventions for treating genital *Chlamydia trachomatis* infection in pregnancy. *Cochrane Database Syst Rev*. 2000;(2):CD000054.

9. Kropp RY, Latham-Carmanico C, Steben M, et al. What's new in management of sexually transmitted infections? Canadian Guidelines on Sexually Transmitted Infections, 2006 Edition. *Can Fam Physician*. 2007;53(10):1739–1741.

10. Lau CY, Qureshi AK. Azithromycin versus doxycycline for genital chlamydial infections: a meta-analysis of randomized clinical trials. *Sex Transm Dis*. 2002;29(9):497–502.

11. Magid D, Douglas Jr JM, Schwartz JS. Doxycycline compared with azithromycin for treating women with genital *Chlamydia trachomatis* infections: an incremental cost-effectiveness analysis. *Ann Intern Med*. 1996;124(4):389–399.

12. Hooton TM, Batteiger BE, Judson FN, et al. Ofloxacin versus doxycycline for treatment of cervical infection with *Chlamydia trachomatis*. *Antimicrob Agents Chemother*. 1992;36(5):1144–1146.

13. Stamm WE, Batteiger BE, McCormack WM, et al. A randomized, double-blind study comparing single-dose rifalazil with single-dose azithromycin for the empirical treatment of nongonococcal urethritis in men. *Sex Transm Dis*. 2007;34(8):545–552.

14. Bebear CM, de Barbeyrac B, Pereyre S, et al. Activity of moxifloxacin against the urogenital mycoplasmas *Ureaplasma* spp., *Mycoplasma hominis* and *Mycoplasma genitalium* and *Chlamydia trachomatis*. *Clin Microbiol Infect*. 2008;14(8):801–805.

15. Health Protection Agency. *All new STI episodes seen at GUM clinics in the UK: 1998–2007*. Online. Available at http://www.hpa.org.uk/web/HPAwebFile/HPAweb_C/1215589014474.

16. Jacobson GF, Autry AM, Kirby RS, et al. A randomized controlled trial comparing amoxicillin and azithromycin for the treatment of *Chlamydia trachomatis* in pregnancy. *Am J Obstet Gynecol*. 2001;184(7):1352–1356.

17. Kacmar J, Cheh E, Montagno A, et al. A randomized trial of azithromycin versus amoxicillin for the treatment of *Chlamydia trachomatis* in pregnancy. *Infect Dis Obstet Gynecol*. 2001;9(4):197–202.

18. Hale TW. *Medication and mother's milk*. 11th ed. Texas: Pharmasoft Publishing; 2004.

19. Somani J, Bhullar VB, Workowski KA, et al. Multiple drug-resistant *Chlamydia trachomatis* associated with clinical treatment failure. *J Infect Dis*. 2000;181(4):1421–1427.

20. Samra Z, Rosenberg S, Soffer Y, et al. In vitro susceptibility of recent clinical isolates of *Chlamydia trachomatis* to macrolides and tetracyclines. *Diagn Microbiol Infect Dis*. 2001;39(3):177–179.

21. Howell MR, Quinn TC, Gaydos CA. Screening for *Chlamydia trachomatis* in asymptomatic women attending family planning clinics. A cost-effectiveness analysis of three strategies. *Ann Intern Med*. 1998;128(4):277–284.

22. Gift TL, Blake DR, Gaydos CA, et al. The cost-effectiveness of screening men for *Chlamydia trachomatis*: a review of the literature. *Sex Transm Dis*. 2008;35(suppl 11):S51–S60.

23. Centers for Disease Control and Prevention. *Sexually transmitted disease surveillance*. Division of STD Prevention December 2008. National Center for HIV/AIDS, Viral; Hepatitis, STD and TB Prevention. Online. Available at http://www.cdc.gov/std/stats07/tables/41.htm; 2007.

24. Ellen JM, Kohn RP, Bolan GA, et al. Socioeconomic differences in sexually transmitted disease rates among black and white adolescents, San Francisco, 1990 to 1992. *Am J Public Health*. 1995;85(11):1546–1548.

25. Densen P, Mandell GL. Gonococcal interactions with polymorphonuclear neutrophils: importance of the phagosome for bactericidal activity. *J Clin Invest*. 1978;62(6):1161–1171.

26. Casey SG, Shafer WM, Spitznagel JK. *Neisseria gonorrhoeae* survive intraleukocytic oxygen-independent antimicrobial capacities of anaerobic and aerobic granulocytes in the presence of pyocin lethal for extracellular gonococci. *Infect Immun*. 1986;52(2):384–389.

27. Rice PA, Kasper DL. Characterization of serum resistance of *Neisseria gonorrhoeae* that disseminate. Roles of blocking antibody and gonococcal outer membrane proteins. *J Clin Invest*. 1982;70(1):157–167.

28. Hook EWI, Handsfield HH. Gonococcal infections in the adult. In: Holmes KK, Sparling PF, Mardh P.-A., et al., eds. *Sexually Transmitted Diseases*. 3rd ed. New York: McGraw-Hill; 1999:451–466.

29. Centers for Disease Control and Prevention. *Updated recommended treatment regimens for gonococcal infections and associated conditions – United States*. Online. Available at http://www.cdc.gov/std/Treatment/2006/GonUpdateApril2007.pdf; 2007.

30. Centers for Disease Control and Prevention. *Sexually Transmitted Disease Surveillance 2006 Supplement*. Gonococcal Isolate Surveillance Project (GISP) Annual Report 2006. Online. Available at http://www.cdc.gov/std/gisp2006/GISPSurvSupp2006Short.pdf.

31. Health Protection Agency. *The Gonococcal Resistance to Antimicrobials Surveillance Programme (GRASP)*. Annual Report 2007. Online. Available at http://www.hpa.org.uk/web/HPAwebFile/HPAweb_C/1221117895841; 2007.

32. Handsfield HH, McCormack WM, Hook 3rd EW, et al. A comparison of single-dose cefixime with ceftriaxone as treatment for uncomplicated gonorrhea. The Gonorrhea Treatment Study Group. *N Engl J Med*. 1991;325(19):1337–1341.

33. Novak E, Paxton LM, Tubbs HJ, et al. Orally administered cefpodoxime proxetil for treatment of uncomplicated gonococcal urethritis in males: a dose–response study. *Antimicrob Agents Chemother*. 1992;36(8):1764–1765.

34. CDI. *Annual report of the Australian Gonococcal Surveillance Programme, 2006*. Online. Available at http://www.health.gov.au/internet/main/publishing.nsf/content/cda-cdi3102-pdf-cnt.htm/$FILE/cdi3102b.pdf; 2006.

35. British Association for Sexual Health and HIV (BASHH). *National guideline on the diagnosis and treatment of gonorrhoea in adults 2005*. Online. Available at http://www.bashh.org/documents/116/116.pdf; 2005.

36. Friedland LR, Kulick RM, Biro FM, et al. Cost-effectiveness decision analysis of intramuscular ceftriaxone versus oral cefixime in adolescents with gonococcal cervicitis. *Ann Emerg Med*. 1996;27(3):299–304.

37. McMillan A, Young H. The treatment of pharyngeal gonorrhoea with a single oral dose of cefixime. *Int J STD AIDS*. 2007;18(4):253–254.

38. Brocklehurst P. 2009; Antibiotics for gonorrhoea in pregnancy. *The Cochrane Library*. (1).

39. Ross JD, Jensen JS. *Mycoplasma genitalium* as a sexually transmitted infection: implications for screening, testing, and treatment. *Sex Transm Infect*. 2006;82(4):269–271.

40. Cohen CR, Manhart LE, Bukusi EA, et al. Association between *Mycoplasma genitalium* and acute endometritis. *Lancet*. 2002;359(9308):765–766.

41. Cohen CR, Mugo NR, Astete SG, et al. Detection of *Mycoplasma genitalium* in women with laparoscopically diagnosed acute salpingitis. *Sex Transm Infect*. 2005;81(6):463–466.

42. Short VL, Totten PA, Ness RB, et al. Clinical presentation of *Mycoplasma genitalium* infection versus *Neisseria gonorrhoeae* infection among women with pelvic inflammatory disease. *Clin Infect Dis*. 2009;48(1):41–47.

43. Svenstrup HF, Fedder J, Kristoffersen SE, et al. *Mycoplasma genitalium*, *Chlamydia trachomatis*, and tubal factor infertility – a prospective study. *Fertil Steril*. 2008;90(3):513–520.

44. Haggerty CL, Totten PA, Astete SG, et al. Failure of cefoxitin and doxycycline to eradicate endometrial *Mycoplasma genitalium* and the consequence for clinical cure of pelvic inflammatory disease. *Sex Transm Infect*. 2008;84(5):338–342.

45. Svenstrup HF, Fedder J, Abraham-Peskir J, et al. *Mycoplasma genitalium* attaches to human spermatozoa. *Hum Reprod*. 2003;18(10):2103–2109.

46. Totten PA, Taylor-Robinson D, Jensen JS. Genital mycoplasmas. In: Holmes KK, Sparling PF, Stamm WE, et al., eds. *Sexually Transmitted Diseases*. 4th ed.New York: McGraw Hill Medical; 2008:709–736.

47. Razin S, Yogev D, Naot Y. Molecular biology and pathogenicity of mycoplasmas. *Microbiol Mol Biol Rev*. 1998;62(4):1094–1156.

48. Jensen JS, Bjornelius E, Dohn B, et al. Use of TaqMan 5′ nuclease real-time PCR for quantitative detection of *Mycoplasma genitalium* DNA in males with and without urethritis who were attendees at a sexually transmitted disease clinic. *J Clin Microbiol*. 2004;42(2):683–692.

49. Jernberg E, Moghaddam A, Moi H. Azithromycin and moxifloxacin for microbiological cure of *Mycoplasma genitalium* infection: an open study. *Int J STD AIDS*. 2008;19(10):676–679.

50. Jensen JS, Bradshaw CS, Tabrizi SN, et al. Azithromycin treatment failure in *Mycoplasma genitalium*-positive patients with nongonococcal urethritis is associated with induced macrolide resistance. *Clin Infect Dis*. 2008;47(12):1546–1553.

51. Lauharanta J, Saarinen K, Mustonen MT, et al. 1993; Single-dose oral azithromycin versus seven-day doxycycline in the treatment of non-gonococcal urethritis in males. *J Antimicrob Chemother*. 31(suppl E):177–183.

52. Stamm WE, Hicks CB, Martin DH, et al. Azithromycin for empirical treatment of the nongonococcal urethritis syndrome in men. A randomized double-blind study. *J Am Med Assoc*. 1995;274(7):545–549.

53. Ross JD. Is *Mycoplasma genitalium* a cause of pelvic inflammatory disease? *Infect Dis Clin North Am*. 2005;19(2):407–413.

54. Marks C, Tideman RL, Estcourt CS, et al. Diagnosing PID – getting the balance right. *Int J STD AIDS*. 2000;11(8):545–547.

55. Walker CK, Kahn JG, Washington AE, et al. Pelvic inflammatory disease: metaanalysis of antimicrobial regimen efficacy. *J Infect Dis*. 1993;168(4):969–978.

56. Savaris RF, Teixeira LM, Torres TG, et al. Comparing ceftriaxone plus azithromycin or doxycycline for pelvic inflammatory disease: a randomized controlled trial. *Obstet Gynecol*. 2007;110(1):53–60.

57. Van de Laar MJ, Fenton KA, Ison C. Update on the European lymphogranuloma venereum epidemic among men who have sex with men. *Euro Surveill*. 2005;10(6): E050602.1.

58. McLean CA, Stoner BP, Workowski KA. Treatment of lymphogranuloma venereum. *Clin Infect Dis*. 2007;44(suppl 3):S147–S152.

59. World Health Organization. *Guidelines for the Management of Sexually Transmitted Infections*. Online. Available at http://www.emro.who.int/aiecf/web79.pdf; 2003.

60. Jaffe HW, Larsen SA, Jones OG, et al. Hemagglutination tests for syphilis antibody. *Am J Clin Pathol*. 1978;70(2):230–233.

61. Kingston M, French P, Goh B, et al. UK national guidelines on the management of syphilis 2008. *Int J STD AIDS*. 2008;19(11):729–740.

62. Dunlop EM. Survival of treponemes after treatment: comments, clinical conclusions, and recommendations. *Genitourin Med*. 1985;61(5):293–301.

63. Goh BT, Smith GW, Samarasinghe L, et al. Penicillin concentrations in serum and cerebrospinal fluid after intramuscular injection of aqueous procaine penicillin 0.6 MU with and without probenecid. *Br J Vener Dis*. 1984;60(6):371–373.

64. Thin RN, Barlow D, Bingham JS, et al. Investigation and management guide for sexually transmitted diseases (excluding HIV). *Int J STD AIDS*. 1995;6(2):130–136.

65. Wong T, Singh AE, De P. Primary syphilis: serological treatment response to doxycycline/tetracycline versus benzathine penicillin. *Am J Med*. 2008;121(10):903–908.

66. Hook EW III, Martin DH, Stephens J, et al. A randomized, comparative pilot study of azithromycin versus benzathine penicillin G for treatment of early syphilis. *Sex Transm Dis*. 2002;29(8):486–490.

67. Katz KA, Klausner JD. Azithromycin resistance in *Treponema pallidum*. *Curr Opin Infect Dis*. 2008;21(1):83–91.

68. Walker GJA. 2009; Antibiotics for syphilis diagnosed during pregnancy [review]. *The Cochrane Library*. (1):1–28.

69. Chakraborty R, Luck S. Managing congenital syphilis again? The more things change. *Curr Opin Infect Dis*. 2007;20(3):247–252.

70. World Health Organization. *1995 Press Release. WHO/64 Sexually transmitted diseases: 333 million new curable cases*. WHO: Geneva; 1995.

71. Spinola SM. Chancroid and *Haemophilus ducreyi*. In: Holmes KK, Sparling PF, Stamm WE, et al., eds. *Sexually Transmitted Diseases*. 4th ed. New York: McGraw Hill Medical; 2008:689–699.

72. Centers for Disease Control and Prevention. *Sexually transmitted diseases surveillance. Chancroid – reported cases and rates by state/area order: United States and outlying areas, 2003*. Online. Available at http://www.cdc.gov/STD/stats07/tables/41.htm; 2007.

73. Plummer FA, D'Costa LJ, Nsanze H, et al. Clinical and microbiologic studies of genital ulcers in Kenyan women. *Sex Transm Dis*. 1985;12(4):193–197.

74. British Association for Sexual Health and HIV (BASHH). *National guideline for the management of chancroid. Clinical Effectiveness Group (BASHH)*. Online. Available at http://www.bashh.org/documents/85/85.pdf; 2007.

75. Tyndall MW, Agoki E, Plummer FA, et al. Single dose azithromycin for the treatment of chancroid: a randomized comparison with erythromycin. *Sex Transm Dis*. 1994;21(4):231–234.

76. Martin DH, Sargent SJ, Wendel Jr GD, et al. Comparison of azithromycin and ceftriaxone for the treatment of chancroid. *Clin Infect Dis*. 1995;21(2):409–414.

77. D'Souza P, Pandhi RK, Khanna N, et al. A comparative study of therapeutic response of patients with clinical chancroid to ciprofloxacin, erythromycin, and co-trimoxazole. *Sex Transm Dis*. 1998;25(6):293–295.

78. Malonza IM, Tyndall MW, Ndinya-Achola JO, et al. A randomized, double-blind, placebo-controlled trial of single-dose ciprofloxacin versus erythromycin for the treatment of chancroid in Nairobi, Kenya. *J Infect Dis*. 1999;180(6):1886–1893.

79. Tyndall M, Malisa M, Plummer FA, et al. Ceftriaxone no longer predictably cures chancroid in Kenya. *J Infect Dis*. 1993;167(2):469–471.

80. Carter JS, Bowden FJ, Bastian I, et al. Phylogenetic evidence for reclassification of *Calymmatobacterium granulomatis* as *Klebsiella granulomatis* comb. nov. *Int J Syst Bacteriol*. 1999;49(Pt 4):1695–1700.

81. O'Farrell N. Donovanosis: an update. *Int J STD AIDS*. 2001;12(7):423–427.

82. World Health Organization. *Consensus Report on STI, HIV and AIDS epidemiology, Papua New Guinea 2000*. Online. Available at http://www.wpro.who.int/NR/rdonlyres/EEC64817-5D9F-4E72-9F7C-6014887E3483/0/consensus_Report_PNG_2000.pdf; 2000.

83. Bowden FJ. Donovanosis in Australia: going, going. *Sex Transm Infect*. 2005;81(5):365–366.

84. Maddocks I, Anders EM, Dennis E. Donovanosis in Papua New Guinea. *Br J Vener Dis*. 1976;52(3):190–196.

85. O'Farrell N. Clinico-epidemiological study of donovanosis in Durban, South Africa. *Genitourin Med*. 1993;69(2):108–111.

86. O'Farrell N, Hammond M. HLA antigens in donovanosis (granuloma inguinale). *Genitourin Med*. 1991;67(5):400–402.

87. Richens J. Donovanosis (granuloma inguinale). *Sex Transm Infect*. 2006;82(suppl 4):iv21–iv22.

88. British Association for Sexual Health and HIV (BASHH). *National guideline for the management of donovanosis (granuloma inguinale)*. Online. Available at http://www.bashh.org/documents/39/39.pdf; 2001.

89. Lal S, Garg BR. Further evidence of the efficacy of co-trimoxazole in granuloma venereum. *Br J Vener Dis*. 1980;56(6):412–413.

90. Ramanan C, Sarma PS, Ghorpade A, et al. Treatment of donovanosis with norfloxacin. *Int J Dermatol*. 1990;29(4):298–299.

91. Merianos A, Gilles M, Chuah J. Ceftriaxone in the treatment of chronic donovanosis in central Australia. *Genitourin Med*. 1994;70(2):84–89.

92. Hill LH, Ruparelia H, Embil JA. Nonspecific vaginitis and other genital infections in three clinic populations. *Sex Transm Dis*. 1983;10(3):114–118.

93. Cohen CR, Duerr A, Pruithithada N, et al. Bacterial vaginosis and HIV seroprevalence among female commercial sex workers in Chiang Mai, Thailand. *AIDS*. 1995;9(9):1093–1097.

94. Hillier S, Holmes KK. Bacterial vaginosis. In: Holmes KK, Sparling PF, Mardh P.-A., et al., eds. *Sexually Transmitted Diseases*. 3rd ed. New York: McGraw-Hill; 1999:563–586.

95. Akinbiyi AA, Watson R, Feyi-Waboso P. Prevalence of *Candida albicans* and bacterial vaginosis in asymptomatic pregnant women in South Yorkshire, United Kingdom. Outcome of a prospective study. *Arch Gynecol Obstet*. 2008;278(5):463–466.

96. Kirakoya-Samadoulougou F, Nagot N, Defer MC, et al. Bacterial vaginosis among pregnant women in Burkina Faso. *Sex Transm Dis*. 2008;35(12):985–989.

97. Atashili J, Poole C, Ndumbe PM, et al. Bacterial vaginosis and HIV acquisition: a meta-analysis of published studies. *AIDS*. 2008;22(12):1493–1501.

98. McClelland RS, Richardson BA, Graham SM, et al. A prospective study of risk factors for bacterial vaginosis in HIV-1-seronegative African women. *Sex Transm Dis*. 2008;35(6):617–623.

99. Leitich H, Bodner-Adler B, Brunbauer M, et al. Bacterial vaginosis as a risk factor for preterm delivery: a meta-analysis. *Am J Obstet Gynecol.* 2003;189(1):139–147.

100. Amsel R, Totten PA, Spiegel CA, et al. Nonspecific vaginitis. Diagnostic criteria and microbial and epidemiologic associations. *Am J Med.* 1983;74(1):14–22.

101. Livengood 3rd CH, Ferris DG, Wiesenfeld HC, et al. Effectiveness of two tinidazole regimens in treatment of bacterial vaginosis: a randomized controlled trial. *Obstet Gynecol.* 2007;110(2 Pt 1):302–309.

102. British Association for Sexual Health and HIV (BASHH). *The national guideline for the management of bacterial vaginosis (2006). Clinical Effectiveness Group.* British Association for Sexual Health and HIV. Online. Available at http://www.bashh.org/documents/62/62.pdf; 2006.

103. Joesoef MR, Schmid GP, Hillier SL. Bacterial vaginosis: review of treatment options and potential clinical indications for therapy. *Clin Infect Dis.* 1999;28(suppl 1):S57–S65.

104. Greaves WL, Chungafung J, Morris B, et al. Clindamycin versus metronidazole in the treatment of bacterial vaginosis. *Obstet Gynecol.* 1988;72(5):799–802.

105. Joesoef MR, Schmid GP. Bacterial vaginosis: review of treatment options and potential clinical indications for therapy. *Clin Infect Dis.* 1995;20 (suppl 1):S72–S79.

106. Nyirjesy P, McIntosh MJ, Gattermeir DJ, et al. The effects of intravaginal clindamycin and metronidazole therapy on vaginal lactobacilli in patients with bacterial vaginosis. *Am J Obstet Gynecol.* 2006;194(5):1277–1282.

107. Brandt M, Abels C, May T, et al. Intravaginally applied metronidazole is as effective as orally applied in the treatment of bacterial vaginosis, but exhibits significantly less side effects. *Eur J Obstet Gynecol Reprod Biol.* 2008;141(2):158–162.

108. McDonald HM, O'Loughlin JA, Vigneswaran R, et al. Impact of metronidazole therapy on preterm birth in women with bacterial vaginosis flora (*Gardnerella vaginalis*): a randomised, placebo controlled trial. *Br J Obstet Gynaecol.* 1997;104(12):1391–1397.

109. Morales WJ, Schorr S, Albritton J. Effect of metronidazole in patients with preterm birth in preceding pregnancy and bacterial vaginosis: a placebo-controlled, double-blind study. *Am J Obstet Gynecol.* 1994;171(2):345–347; discussion 348-349.

110. McGregor JA, French JI, Parker R, et al. Prevention of premature birth by screening and treatment for common genital tract infections: results of a prospective controlled evaluation. *Am J Obstet Gynecol.* 1995;173(1):157–167.

111. Joesoef MR, Hillier SL, Wiknjosastro G, et al. Intravaginal clindamycin treatment for bacterial vaginosis: effects on preterm delivery and low birth weight. *Am J Obstet Gynecol.* 1995;173(5):1527–1531.

112. McDonald HM, Brocklehurst P, Gordon A. Antibiotics for treating bacterial vaginosis in pregnancy. *Cochrane Database Syst Rev.* 2007;(1):CD000262.

113. Tayal SC, Pattman RS. High prevalence of herpes simplex virus type 1 in female anogenital herpes simplex in Newcastle upon Tyne 1983–92. *Int J STD AIDS.* 1994;5(5):359–361.

114. Koutsky LA, Stevens CE, Holmes KK, et al. Underdiagnosis of genital herpes by current clinical and viral-isolation procedures. *N Engl J Med.* 1992;326(23):1533–1539.

115. Wald A, Zeh J, Selke S, et al. Virologic characteristics of subclinical and symptomatic genital herpes infections. *N Engl J Med.* 1995;333(12):770–775.

116. Nahmias AJ, Lee FK, Beckman-Nahmias S. Sero-epidemiological and sociological patterns of herpes simplex virus infection in the world. *Scand J Infect Dis Suppl.* 1990;69:19–36.

117. Cowan FM, Johnson AM, Ashley R, et al. Relationship between antibodies to herpes simplex virus (HSV) and symptoms of HSV infection. *J Infect Dis.* 1996;174(3):470–475.

118. Cunningham AL, Taylor R, Taylor J, et al. Prevalence of infection with herpes simplex virus types 1 and 2 in Australia: a nationwide population based survey. *Sex Transm Infect.* 2006;82(2):164–168.

119. Tideman RL, Taylor J, Marks C, et al. Sexual and demographic risk factors for herpes simplex type 1 and 2 in women attending an antenatal clinic. *Sex Transm Infect.* 2001;77(6):413–415.

120. Stanberry LR, Jorgensen DM, Nahmias AJ. Herpes simplex viruses 1 and 2. In: Evans AS, Kaslow RA, eds. *Viral infection of humans: epidemiology and control.* 4th ed. New York: Plenum Press; 1997:419–454.

121. Langenberg A, Benedetti J, Jenkins J, et al. Development of clinically recognizable genital lesions among women previously identified as having 'asymptomatic' herpes simplex virus type 2 infection. *Ann Intern Med.* 1989;110(11):882–887.

122. Corey L, Adams HG, Brown ZA, et al. Genital herpes simplex virus infections: clinical manifestations, course, and complications. *Ann Intern Med.* 1983;98(6):958–972.

123. Benedetti J, Corey L, Ashley R. Recurrence rates in genital herpes after symptomatic first-episode infection. *Ann Intern Med.* 1994;121(11):847–854.

124. Gupta R, Warren T, Wald A. Genital herpes. *Lancet.* 2007;370(9605):2127–2137.

125. Ramaswamy M, McDonald C, Smith M, et al. Diagnosis of genital herpes by real time PCR in routine clinical practice. *Sex Transm Infect.* 2004;80(5):406–410.

126. Ho DW, Field PR, Irving WL, et al. Detection of immunoglobulin M antibodies to glycoprotein G-2 by western blot (immunoblot) for diagnosis of initial herpes simplex virus type 2 genital infections. *J Clin Microbiol.* 1993;31(12):3157–3164.

127. Elion GB. 1993;Acyclovir: discovery, mechanism of action, and selectivity. *J Med Virol.* (suppl 1):2–6.

128. Boyd MR, Safrin S, Kern ER. Penciclovir: a review of its spectrum of activity, selectivity and cross-resistance pattern. *Antivir Chem Chemother.* 1993;4 (suppl 1):3–11.

129. Mindel A, Adler MW, Sutherland S, et al. Intravenous acyclovir treatment for primary genital herpes. *Lancet.* 1982;1(8274):697–700.

130. Corey L, Nahmias AJ, Guinan ME, et al. A trial of topical acyclovir in genital herpes simplex virus infections. *N Engl J Med.* 1982;306(22):1313–1319.

131. Mertz GJ, Critchlow CW, Benedetti J, et al. Double-blind placebo-controlled trial of oral acyclovir in first-episode genital herpes simplex virus infection. *J Am Med Assoc.* 1984;252(9):1147–1151.

132. Spruance SL, Tyring SK, DeGregorio B, et al. A large-scale, placebo-controlled, dose-ranging trial of peroral valaciclovir for episodic treatment of recurrent herpes genitalis. Valaciclovir HSV Study Group. *Arch Intern Med.* 1996;156(15):1729–1735.

133. Sacks SL, Aoki FY, Diaz-Mitoma F, et al. Patient-initiated, twice-daily oral famciclovir for early recurrent genital herpes. A randomized, double-blind multicenter trial. Canadian Famciclovir Study Group. *J Am Med Assoc.* 1996;276(1):44–49.

134. Carney O, Ross E, Ikkos G, et al. The effect of suppressive oral acyclovir on the psychological morbidity associated with recurrent genital herpes. *Genitourin Med.* 1993;69(6):457–459.

135. Fife KH, Warren TJ, Justus SE, et al. An international, randomized, double-blind, placebo-controlled, study of valacyclovir for the suppression of herpes simplex virus type 2 genital herpes in newly diagnosed patients. *Sex Transm Dis.* 2008;35(7):668–673.

136. Aoki FY, Tyring S, Diaz-Mitoma F, et al. Single-day, patient-initiated famciclovir therapy for recurrent genital herpes: a randomized, double-blind, placebo-controlled trial. *Clin Infect Dis.* 2006;42(1):8–13.

137. Bodsworth N, Bloch M, McNulty A, et al. 2-day versus 5-day famciclovir as treatment of recurrences of genital herpes: results of the FaST study. *Sex Health.* 2008;5(3):219–225.

138. Leone PA, Trottier S, Miller JM. Valacyclovir for episodic treatment of genital herpes: a shorter 3-day treatment course compared with 5-day treatment. *Clin Infect Dis.* 2002;34(7):958–962.

139. Mindel A, Weller IV, Faherty A, et al. Prophylactic oral acyclovir in recurrent genital herpes. *Lancet.* 1984;2(8394):57–59.

140. Douglas JM, Critchlow C, Benedetti J, et al. A double-blind study of oral acyclovir for suppression of recurrences of genital herpes simplex virus infection. *N Engl J Med.* 1984;310(24):1551–1556.

141. Reitano M, Tyring S, Lang W, et al. Valaciclovir for the suppression of recurrent genital herpes simplex virus infection: a large-scale dose range-finding study. International Valaciclovir HSV Study Group. *J Infect Dis.* 1998;178(3):603–610.

142. Andrews EB, Yankaskas BC, Cordero JF, et al. Acyclovir in pregnancy registry: six years' experience. The Acyclovir in Pregnancy Registry Advisory Committee. *Obstet Gynecol.* 1992;79(1):7–13.

143. Reiff-Eldridge R, Heffner CR, Ephross SA, et al. Monitoring pregnancy outcomes after prenatal drug exposure through prospective pregnancy registries: a pharmaceutical company commitment. *Am J Obstet Gynecol.* 2000;182(1 Pt 1):159–163.

144. Corey L, Wald A. Genital herpes. In: Holmes KK, Sparling PF, Stamm WE, et al., eds. *Sexually Transmitted Diseases.* 4th ed. New York: McGraw Hill Medical; 2008:399–438.

145. Brown ZA, Selke S, Zeh J, et al. The acquisition of herpes simplex virus during pregnancy. *N Engl J Med.* 1997;337(8):509–515.

146. Brown ZA, Wald A, Morrow RA, et al. Effect of serologic status and cesarean delivery on transmission rates of herpes simplex virus from mother to infant. *J Am Med Assoc*. 2003;289(2):203–209.

147. Sheffield JS, Hollier LM, Hill JB, et al. Acyclovir prophylaxis to prevent herpes simplex virus recurrence at delivery: a systematic review. *Obstet Gynecol*. 2003;102(6):1396–1403.

148. Scott LL, Sanchez PJ, Jackson GL, et al. Acyclovir suppression to prevent cesarean delivery after first-episode genital herpes. *Obstet Gynecol*. 1996;87(1):69–73.

149. Randolph AG, Hartshorn RM, Washington AE. Acyclovir prophylaxis in late pregnancy to prevent neonatal herpes: a cost-effectiveness analysis. *Obstet Gynecol*. 1996;88(4 Pt 1):603–610.

150. Oriel JD. Natural history of genital warts. *Br J Vener Dis*. 1971;47(1):1–13.

151. Cunningham AL, Mindel A, Dwyer DE. Global epidemiology of sexually transmitted diseases. In: Stanberry LR, Bernstein DI, eds. *Sexually transmitted diseases, vaccines, prevention and control*. London: Academic Press; 2000:3–42.

152. Winer RL, Koutsky LA. Genital human papillomavirus infection. In: Holmes KK, Sparling PF, Stamm WE, et al., eds. *Sexually Transmitted Diseases*. 4th ed. New York: McGraw-Hill Medical; 2008:489–508.

153. Melbye M, Palefsky J, Gonzales J, et al. Immune status as a determinant of human papillomavirus detection and its association with anal epithelial abnormalities. *Int J Cancer*. 1990;46(2):203–206.

154. Palefsky JM, Gonzales J, Greenblatt RM, et al. Anal intraepithelial neoplasia and anal papillomavirus infection among homosexual males with group IV HIV disease. *J Am Med Assoc*. 1990;263(21):2911–2916.

155. Severson JL, Beutner KR, Tyring SK. Genital papillomavirus infection. In: Stanberry LR, Bernstein DI, eds. *Sexually transmitted diseases, vaccines, prevention and control*. London: Academic Press; 2000:259–272.

156. Kast W, Feltkamp M, Ressing M, et al. Cellular immunity against human papillomavirus associated cervical cancer. *Seminars in Virology*. 1996;7(2):117–123.

157. von Krogh G, Szpak E, Andersson M, et al. Self-treatment using 0.25%–0.50% podophyllotoxin-ethanol solutions against penile condylomata acuminata: a placebo-controlled comparative study. *Genitourin Med*. 1994;70(2):105–109.

158. Petersen CS, Agner T, Ottevanger V, et al. A single-blind study of podophyllotoxin cream 0.5% and podophyllotoxin solution 0.5% in male patients with genital warts. *Genitourin Med*. 1995;71(6):391–392.

159. Greenberg MD, Rutledge LH, Reid R, et al. A double-blind, randomized trial of 0.5% podofilox and placebo for the treatment of genital warts in women. *Obstet Gynecol*. 1991;77(5):735–739.

160. Kirby P, Dunne A, King DH, et al. Double-blind randomized clinical trial of self-administered podofilox solution versus vehicle in the treatment of genital warts. *Am J Med*. 1990;88(5):465–469.

161. Tyring SK, Arany I, Stanley MA, et al. A randomized, controlled, molecular study of condylomata acuminata clearance during treatment with imiquimod. *J Infect Dis*. 1998;178(2):551–555.

162. Miller RL, Gerster JF, Owens ML, et al. Imiquimod applied topically: a novel immune response modifier and new class of drug. *Int J Immunopharmacol*. 1999;21(1):1–14.

163. Gotovtseva EP, Kapadia AS, Smolensky MH, et al. Optimal frequency of imiquimod (Aldara) 5% cream for the treatment of external genital warts in immunocompetent adults: a meta-analysis. *Sex Transm Dis*. 2008;35(4):346–351.

164. Edwards L, Ferenczy A, Eron L, et al.; HPV Study Group. Self-administered topical 5% imiquimod cream for external anogenital warts. *Arch Dermatol*. 1998;134(1):25–30.

165. Garland SM, Waddell R, Mindel A, et al. An open-label phase II pilot study investigating the optimal duration of imiquimod 5% cream for the treatment of external genital warts in women. *Int J STD AIDS*. 2006;17(7):448–452.

166. Yan J, Chen SL, Wang HN, et al. Meta-analysis of 5% imiquimod and 0.5% podophyllotoxin in the treatment of condylomata acuminata. *Dermatology*. 2006;213(3):218–223.

167. Bikowski Jr JB. Molluscum contagiosum: the need for physician intervention and new treatment options. *Cutis*. 2004;73(3):202–206.

168. Ormerod AD, White MI, Shah SA, et al. Molluscum contagiosum effectively treated with a topical acidified nitrite, nitric oxide liberating cream. *Br J Dermatol*. 1999;141(6):1051–1053.

169. Wasserheit JN. Epidemiological synergy. Interrelationships between human immunodeficiency virus infection and other sexually transmitted diseases. *Sex Transm Dis*. 1992;19(2):61–77.

170. Laga M, Manoka A, Kivuvu M, et al. Non-ulcerative sexually transmitted diseases as risk factors for HIV-1 transmission in women: results from a cohort study. *AIDS*. 1993;7(1):95–102.

171. Sutton MY, Sternberg M, Nsuami M, et al. Trichomoniasis in pregnant human immunodeficiency virus-infected and human immunodeficiency virus-uninfected Congolese women: prevalence, risk factors, and association with low birth weight. *Am J Obstet Gynecol*. 1999;181(3):656–662.

172. Cotch MF, Pastorek 2nd JG, Nugent RP, et al. *Trichomonas vaginalis* associated with low birth weight and preterm delivery. The Vaginal Infections and Prematurity Study Group. *Sex Transm Dis*. 1997;24(6):353–360.

173. Krieger JN. Alderete JF. *Trichomonas vaginalis* and trichomoniasis. In: Holmes KK, Sparling PF, Mardh P.-A., et al., eds. *Sexually Transmitted Diseases*. 3rd ed. New York: McGraw-Hill; 1999:587–604.

174. Mason PR, Forman L. Polymorphonuclear cell chemotaxis to secretions of pathogenic and nonpathogenic *Trichomonas vaginalis*. *J Parasitol*. 1982;68(3):457–462.

175. Wolner-Hanssen P, Krieger JN, Stevens CE, et al. Clinical manifestations of vaginal trichomoniasis. *J Am Med Assoc*. 1989;261(4):571–576.

176. Alderete JF, Provenzano D, Lehker MW. Iron mediates *Trichomonas vaginalis* resistance to complement lysis. *Microb Pathog*. 1995;19(2):93–103.

177. Fouts AC, Kraus SJ. *Trichomonas vaginalis*: reevaluation of its clinical presentation and laboratory diagnosis. *J Infect Dis*. 1980;141(2):137–143.

178. Krieger JN, Verdon M, Siegel N, et al. Risk assessment and laboratory diagnosis of trichomoniasis in men. *J Infect Dis*. 1992;166(6):1362–1366.

179. Krieger JN, Tam MR, Stevens CE, et al. Diagnosis of trichomoniasis. Comparison of conventional wet-mount examination with cytologic studies, cultures, and monoclonal antibody staining of direct specimens. *J Am Med Assoc*. 1988;259(8):1223–1227.

180. British Association for Sexual Health and HIV (BASHH). *The UK national guideline on the management of Trichomoniasis vaginalis (2007)*. Online. Available at http://www.bashh.org/documents/87/87.pdf; 2007.

181. Hager WD, Brown ST, Kraus SJ, et al. Metronidazole for vaginal trichomoniasis. Seven-day vs single-dose regimens. *J Am Med Assoc*. 1980;244(11):1219–1220.

182. Kurohara ML, Kwong FK, Lebherz TB, et al. Metronidazole hypersensitivity and oral desensitization. *J Allergy Clin Immunol*. 1991;88(2):279–280.

183. Helms DJ, Mosure DJ, Secor WE, et al. Management of *Trichomonas vaginalis* in women with suspected metronidazole hypersensitivity. *Am J Obstet Gynecol*. 2008;198(4):370, e371–e377.

184. Gulmezoglu AM. 2009; Interventions for trichomoniasis in pregnancy [review]. *The Cochrane Library*. (1).

185. Holland J, Young ML, Lee O, et al. Vulvovaginal carriage of yeasts other than *Candida albicans*. *Sex Transm Infect*. 2003;79(3):249–250.

186. Reed BD. Risk factors for *Candida* vulvovaginitis. *Obstet Gynecol Surv*. 1992;47(8):551–560.

187. Chassot F, Negri MF, Svidzinski AE, et al. Can intrauterine contraceptive devices be a *Candida albicans* reservoir? *Contraception*. 2008;77(5):355–359.

188. Odds FC. Genital candidosis. *Clin Exp Dermatol*. 1982;7(4):345–354.

189. Soll DR. High-frequency switching in *Candida albicans* and its relations to vaginal candidiasis. *Am J Obstet Gynecol*. 1988;158(4):997–1001.

190. Sobel JD. Vulvovaginal candidiasis. In: Holmes KK, Sparling PF, Mardh P.-A., et al., eds. *Sexually Transmitted Diseases*. 3rd ed. New York: McGraw-Hill; 1999:629–639.

191. Bravo AB, Miranda LS, Lima OF, et al. Validation of an immunologic diagnostic kit for infectious vaginitis by *Trichomonas vaginalis*, *Candida* spp., and *Gardnerella vaginalis*. *Diagn Microbiol Infect Dis*. 2009;63(3):257–260.

192. Pitsouni E, Iavazzo C, Falagas ME. Itraconazole vs fluconazole for the treatment of uncomplicated acute vaginal and vulvovaginal candidiasis in nonpregnant women: a metaanalysis of randomized controlled trials. *Am J Obstet Gynecol*. 2008;198(2):153–160.

193. Nurbhai M, Grimshaw J, Watson M, et al. Oral versus intra-vaginal imidazole and triazole antifungal treatment of uncomplicated vulvovaginal candidiasis (thrush). *The Cochrane Library*. 2009;(1).

194. Kutzer E, Oittner R, Leodolter S, et al. A comparison of fluconazole and ketoconazole in the oral treatment of vaginal candidiasis; report of a double-blind multicentre trial. *Eur J Obstet Gynecol Reprod Biol*. 1988;29(4):305–313.

195. Osser S, Haglund A, Westrom L. Treatment of candidal vaginitis. A prospective randomized investigator-blind multicenter study comparing topically applied econazole with oral fluconazole. *Acta Obstet Gynecol Scand*. 1991;70(1):73–78.

196. British Association for Sexual Health and HIV (BASHH). *National guideline on the management of vulvovaginal candidiasis*. Online. Available at http://www.bashh.org/documents/50/50.pdf.

197. Sobel JD, Faro S, Force RW, et al. Vulvovaginal candidiasis: epidemiologic, diagnostic, and therapeutic considerations. *Am J Obstet Gynecol*. 1998;178(2):203–211.

198. Sobel JD, Wiesenfeld HC, Martens M, et al. Maintenance fluconazole therapy for recurrent vulvovaginal candidiasis. *N Engl J Med*. 2004;351(9):876–883.

199. Watson C, Calabretto H. Comprehensive review of conventional and non-conventional methods of management of recurrent vulvovaginal candidiasis. *Aust N Z J Obstet Gynaecol*. 2007;47(4):262–272.

200. Singh S, Sobel JD, Bhargava P, et al. Vaginitis due to *Candida krusei*: epidemiology, clinical aspects, and therapy. *Clin Infect Dis*. 2002;35(9):1066–1070.

57 Leprosy

Diana Lockwood, Sharon Marlowe and Saba Lambert

Leprosy is one of the oldest recorded diseases. In 1988 the World Health Organization (WHO) proposed to eliminate leprosy (i.e. <1 case per 10 000 population) by the year 2000; however, in 2007, 258 133 new cases were reported globally by the WHO.

In 1873 the Norwegian Armauer Hansen showed that leprosy was caused by *Mycobacterium leprae*, which invades the skin and nerves, causing a chronic granulomatous disease with peripheral neuropathy and skin lesions.

Outside endemic areas, doctors often fail to diagnose leprosy, with unfortunate consequences for the patients: for example, in the UK, 40% of new cases have severe neuropathy at diagnosis. Early recognition of leprosy is important because the infection is curable and prompt treatment can reduce nerve damage and associated stigma.

EPIDEMIOLOGY

Leprosy remains a public health problem in 24 countries, mainly in the tropics. The top seven endemic countries are India, Brazil, Indonesia, Democratic Republic of Congo, Madagascar, Bangladesh and Nepal: 54% of the detected cases worldwide are found in India[1] (Fig. 57.1).

M. leprae is transmitted via the nasal discharge of untreated lepromatous patients and enters another human subject through the nasal mucosa, with subsequent hematogenous spread to the skin and peripheral nerves. Some literature suggests transmission via broken skin[2,3] or blood-borne, or by way of soil as the mycobacteria are known to survive in the environment for up to 46 days.[4] Leprosy is a uniquely human disease with no animal reservoir except the nine-banded armadillo; although this animal is frequently infected or seropositive for *M. leprae*, there have been few reports of transmission from this animal to humans.

In England and Wales, where leprosy is a notifiable disease, a total of 1358 cases have been registered since 1951.[5] There are still 128 individuals who are on treatment or under surveillance. Since 1993 approximately nine new cases per year have been diagnosed. Half of the new cases in the UK are found in immigrants from the Indian subcontinent and there are a few cases in Caucasians who have lived in leprosy-endemic areas for prolonged periods (8–42 years).[6] Patients originating from Brazil have also been seen recently at the Hospital for Tropical Diseases. The epidemiological pattern of leprosy in the UK is influenced by both migration patterns and levels of leprosy in migrants' home countries. As leprosy has a long incubation period (2–10 years), patients can present long after leaving endemic areas.

PATHOGENESIS

Leprosy manifests in a spectrum of disease forms, ranging from the tuberculoid to the lepromatous (Fig. 57.2).[7] The varied clinical manifestations of leprosy are determined by the host's response to the leprosy bacillus: tuberculoid (TT) patients have a uniform clinical, histological and immunological response manifesting as limited clinical disease, granuloma formation and active cell-mediated immunity; lepromatous (LL) patients have multiple clinical signs, a high bacterial load and low cell-mediated immunity. Between these two extremes there is a range of variations in host response; these comprise borderline cases (BT, BB, BL)[8] (Table 57.1). Immunologically, borderline cases are unstable and polar tuberculoid and lepromatous cases are stable.

CLINICAL FEATURES AND SPECTRUM OF DISEASE

Patients present with skin or nerve lesions, or a combination of both. Leprosy affects only the peripheral nerves – *never* the central nervous system. A patient may present with a macular hypopigmented skin lesion, weakness or pain in the hand due to nerve involvement, facial palsy, acute foot drop or a painless burn or ulcer in an anesthetic hand or foot.

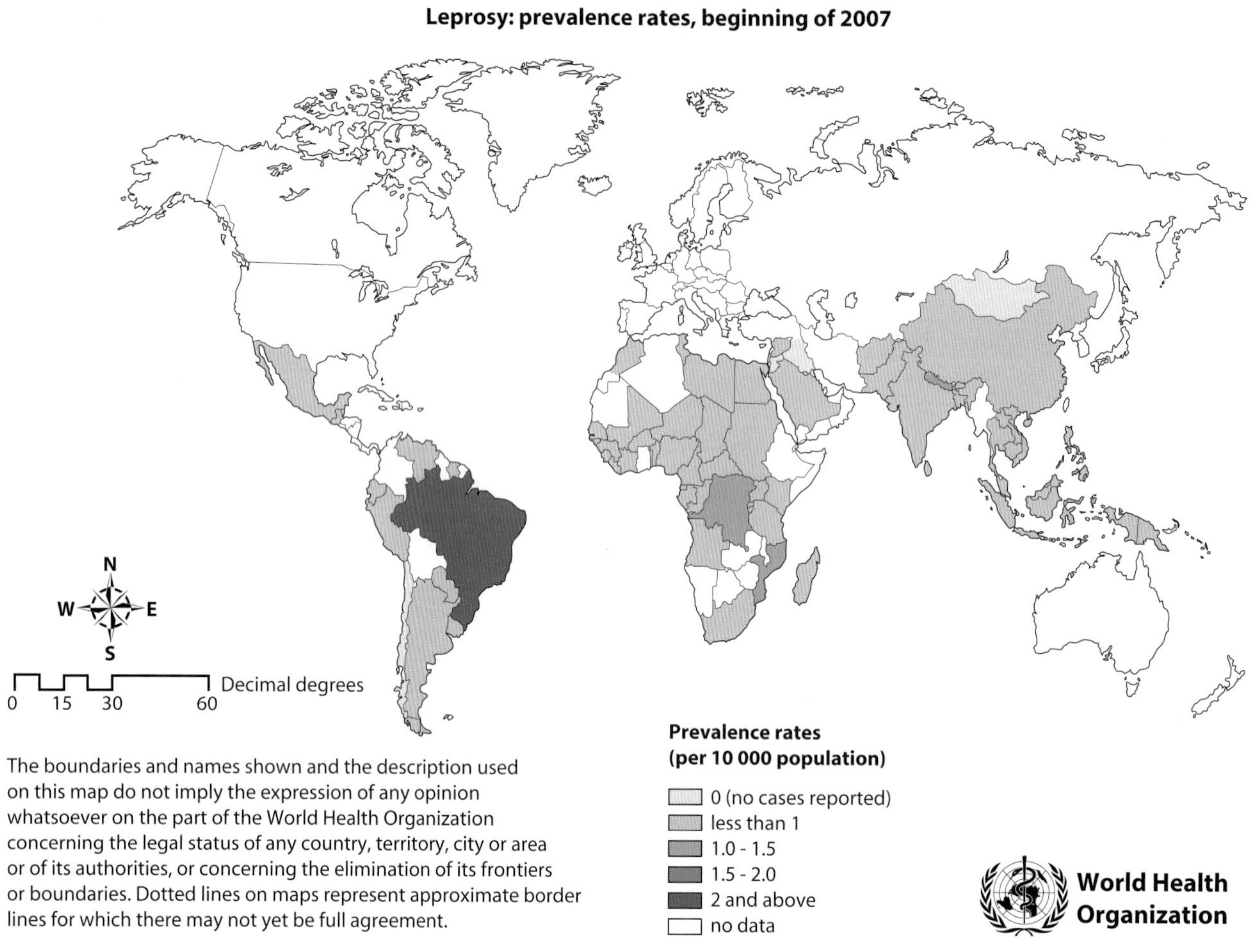

Leprosy: prevalence rates, beginning of 2007

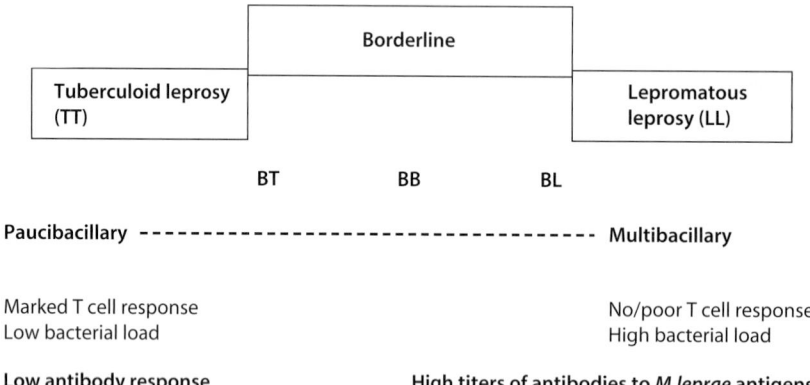

Decimal degrees
0 15 30 60

The boundaries and names shown and the description used on this map do not imply the expression of any opinion whatsoever on the part of the World Health Organization concerning the legal status of any country, territory, city or area or of its authorities, or concerning the elimination of its frontiers or boundaries. Dotted lines on maps represent approximate border lines for which there may not yet be full agreement.

Prevalence rates (per 10 000 population)
- 0 (no cases reported)
- less than 1
- 1.0 - 1.5
- 1.5 - 2.0
- 2 and above
- no data

World Health Organization

Fig. 57.1 Global leprosy prevalence, beginning of 2007.[1] Adapted from WHO. Leprosy – global situation. **Wkly Epidemiol Rec.** 2008; 83(33): 293–300 and 2008;83(50):459.

Borderline

Tuberculoid leprosy (TT)

Lepromatous leprosy (LL)

BT   BB   BL

Paucibacillary – Multibacillary

Marked T cell response
Low bacterial load

No/poor T cell response
High bacterial load

Low antibody response

High titers of antibodies to *M.leprae* antigens

Fig. 57.2 Leprosy – a spectrum of disease.

Table 57.1 Characteristic features of different types of leprosy

	TT	BT	BB	BL	LL
Skin lesions	Single, well-defined, hypopigmented, erythematous macule	Few, asymmetric, well-demarcated macules	Few asymmetric, less well-demarcated and shiny	Many symmetric shiny macules and plaques	Many symmetric erythematous, shiny macules, papules and nodules
Sensory impairment in lesions	Marked	Marked	Moderate	Slight neuropathy	Late 'glove and stocking'
Peripheral nerve involvement	Single peripheral nerve trunk	Several and asymmetric	Multiple	Multiple and symmetric	Multiple, late, symmetric

TT, tuberculoid; BT, borderline tuberculoid; BB, mid-borderline; BL, borderline lepromatous; LL, lepromatous.

Patients may also present with painful eyes as a first indication of lepromatous leprosy. The diagnosis of leprosy should be considered in anyone from an endemic area who presents with typical skin lesions, neuropathic ulcers or a peripheral neuropathy.

DIAGNOSIS

BACTERIOLOGICAL AND HISTOLOGICAL EXAMINATION

In a suspected case, slit skin smears are taken to look for acid-fast bacilli. *M. leprae* on the smears are counted and the bacterial index calculated on a logarithmic scale. A negative result does not exclude leprosy, as tuberculoid lesions may contain no detectable bacteria. *M. leprae* cannot be cultivated on artificial media, but can be grown with difficulty in nude mice and the nine-banded armadillo with a 14-day doubling time and at low temperatures (30–33°C). Sequencing of the *M. leprae* genome revealed that it has lost approximately one-third of the genes possessed by *M. tuberculosis*.[9]

Histopathological evaluation is essential for accurate classification of leprosy lesions and is the best diagnostic test in a well-resourced setting, both for confirming and for excluding the diagnosis of leprosy. The presence of granulomata and lymphocytic infiltration of dermal nerves in anesthetic skin lesions confirms the diagnosis. A nerve biopsy may be required in cases with no visible skin lesions.

SEROLOGICAL TESTS AND POLYMERASE CHAIN REACTION

Recent advances have been made in serological diagnostic tests. Antibodies to the *M. leprae*-specific antiphenolic glycolipid 1 (PGL-1) are present in 90% of patients with untreated lepromatous disease, but in only 40–50% of patients with paucibacillary disease and 1–5% of healthy controls.[10] An easy to use immunohistochromatographic assay, the ML Flow test, based on PGL-1 detection, is being assessed by a Brazilian team.[11] Polymerase chain reaction (PCR) for detection of *M. leprae* encoding specific genes or repeat sequences is potentially highly sensitive and specific, since it detects *M. leprae* DNA in 95% of multibacillary and 55% of paucibacillary patients. Currently PCR is not used in clinical practice.[10]

TREATMENT

The management of leprosy consists of treating the *M. leprae* infection with antibiotic chemotherapy, management of the immune-mediated reactions, prevention of nerve damage and education.

CHEMOTHERAPY

TREATMENT OF INFECTION

Multidrug therapy (MDT) with a combination of dapsone, rifampicin (rifampin) and clofazimine is the current treatment for infection with *M. leprae*. Following the resistance to dapsone-only regimens, the WHO introduced MDT in 1982. MDT is very successful, with a high cure rate, few side effects and low relapse rates (relapse is defined as the reappearance of signs of activity and/or appearance of new lesions and/or bacteriological positivity during or after surveillance). Relapse rates as low as 0.1% per annum have been recorded.[12] In a review of the outcome of MDT of more than 67 000 Indian patients from 1983 to 1992, Lobo showed that only 0.3% of all paucibacillary and multibacillary cases relapsed and that 2.7% of all patients were recorded as treatment failures.[13] Lobo also found that 92.2% of patients completed satisfactory treatment, were declared cured and released from treatment.

The benefits of MDT include the prevention of drug resistance and better patient compliance due to a fixed duration of therapy. Another advantage is that field workers review patients and supervise the taking of their monthly medication (Table 57.2). The WHO reduced the recommended treatment period for multibacillary disease from 24 to 12 months, but many advocate 24 months for patients with a BI (the logarithmic scale used to assess response to MDT in skin smears) of >4 at diagnosis.[14] One option would be to treat such patients until their skin smears are negative or to keep them under regular review. MDT is safe in pregnancy and in breastfeeding mothers.[15,16] Children should receive reduced doses of the drugs.

Dapsone

Dapsone is bacteristatic and effective against a wide range of bacteria and protozoa.[17] In 1947, Cochrane used 1.25 g of subcutaneous dapsone twice weekly to successfully treat leprosy patients.[18,19] This effectiveness was confirmed in

Table 57.2 Multidrug regimens for treatment of *M. leprae* infection

Regimen	Drug	Dosage	Frequency	Duration
Paucibacillary	Dapsone	100 mg	Daily (self-administered)	6 months
	Rifampicin	600 mg	Monthly (supervised)	
Multibacillary	Dapsone	100 mg	Daily (self-administered)	
	Clofazimine	50 mg	Daily (self-administered)	1 year
	Clofazimine	300 mg	Monthly (supervised)	
	Rifampicin	600 mg	Monthly (supervised)	

Malaysia with a reduced subcutaneous dose of 200–400 mg. At the same time, research in Calcutta,[20] Nigeria[21,22] and the French West Indies reported good results with an oral preparation.[23] By 1951, the standard treatment for leprosy was oral dapsone, 100 mg/day, and was used widely as monotherapy in the 1950s and 1960s. However, in the late 1960s two important problems developed: primary and secondary dapsone resistance:

- Primary resistance refers to resistance in patients who have never been exposed to dapsone.
- Secondary resistance refers to relapse in patients who have previously been treated with dapsone.

Dapsone acts as other sulfonamides, by competing with *para*-aminobenzoic acid for the enzyme dihydropteroate synthetase and therefore inhibiting the synthesis of dihydrofolic acid (*see* Ch. 2). A dose of 100 mg of dapsone is weakly bactericidal against *M. leprae* and after a few weeks of starting dapsone therapy active lesions start to improve.

Side effects are rare with dapsone and include mild hemolysis and dapsone allergy, occurring within the first few months of treatment. Dapsone allergy usually starts 3–6 weeks after starting the drug, with fever, pruritus and a dermatitic rash. Unless dapsone is stopped immediately, the syndrome may progress to exfoliative dermatitis; hepatitis, albuminuria, psychosis and death have also been recorded.[21] Treatment is to stop dapsone and treat with corticosteroids for several weeks. The incidence of dapsone allergy is estimated at one per several hundred patients. Although dapsone-induced peripheral neuropathy has been reported in some diseases, there have been few reports of it occurring in leprosy.

Clofazimine

Clofazimine was first used for the treatment of leprosy as monotherapy in the early 1960s and continued until the mid 1970s. To date there has been only one reported case of resistance.[24]

Clofazimine is bacteristatic and slowly bactericidal against *M. leprae*, similar to dapsone.[25] Clofazimine is active against other mycobacteria, this effect being more pronounced in vitro than in vivo, but the mechanism of its action against *M. leprae* is unknown. The speed of response is similar to that of dapsone but slower than that of rifampicin. At doses greater than 1 mg/kg per day, clofazimine exhibits increasing anti-inflammatory activity.[26]

The main problems encountered with clofazimine are increased skin pigmentation and dryness, which occur as the drug becomes clinically effective. This ichthyosis is reversible and slowly resolves on stopping the drug. Pigmentation can also be seen in the cornea and conjunctival and macular areas of the eyes. Clofazimine is lipophilic and is therefore deposited in fatty tissue and cells of the reticuloendothelial system. Autopsies carried out on patients who had been on clofazimine therapy revealed large quantities of the drug in mesenteric lymph nodes, adrenal glands, subcutaneous fat, liver, spleen, small intestine and skin but not in the central nervous system.[27]

Rifampicin (rifampin)

Rifampicin is used mainly for the treatment of tuberculosis and leprosy, although it also inhibits the growth of other bacteria[28] (*see* Ch. 27).

Rifampicin is bactericidal and the most effective anti-leprosy drug, rendering the patient non-infectious within days of commencing therapy.[29] Resistance has been shown to be due to tightly clustered mutations in a short region of the *rpoβ* gene.[30]

Few serious side effects have been related to rifampicin, which may be due to its monthly dosing regimen, and no cases of resistance have been recorded in leprosy patients. The most common reported side effect is hepatotoxicity, which has (rarely) resulted in death. Early symptoms are anorexia, vomiting and jaundice associated with a two- or three-fold increase in hepatic transaminases. The elevated transaminases may be transient and return to normal despite continuing therapy.

A 'flu-like' syndrome has been reported with intermittent rifampicin therapy and consists of chills, fever, headache, myalgia and arthralgia. This syndrome has a reported incidence of 0.3% in the WHO/MDT report of complications. Rifampicin also produces a red–brown discoloration of urine, feces, saliva, sputum, sweat and tears; patients should be informed that this is inconsequential and will last only 24–48 h.

Other regimens instead of MDT

Following the success of MDT there has been research into the use of other drugs that are more potent than, and as effective as, MDT, but which require a shorter duration of therapy. Other antibiotics currently available as second-line therapy to MDT are minocycline, ofloxacin, clarithromycin and moxifloxacin.

Minocycline

Minocycline has strong bactericidal activity against *M. leprae* due to its lipophilic properties, which allow it to penetrate the outer capsule and cell wall of the organism.[31] Data from a clinical trial carried out in Mali in 1992 showed that 100 mg minocycline daily caused marked clinical improvement by 1 month. After 2 months of treatment there was a significant decrease in bacterial index, indicating that minocycline was very effective at killing *M. leprae* bacilli.[32]

The main side effect observed in minocycline-treated leprosy patients is hyperpigmentation, presenting as a patchy blue–black color at the site of skin lesions, especially on the legs and feet.[33] Dizziness is a specific side effect of minocycline and other mild adverse effects include gastrointestinal symptoms of nausea, abdominal pain or diarrhea, and headache[34] (*see* Ch. 30).

Ofloxacin

Ofloxacin is a fluoroquinolone derivative with strong bactericidal activity against *M. leprae*.[35] A clinical trial in Côte d'Ivoire, studying the efficacy of a daily dose of 400 mg of ofloxacin,[36] showed definite clinical improvement after 22 doses, 99.9% of initially viable organisms being dead at day 22.

Clarithromycin

Clarithromycin is a macrolide with potent bactericidal activity against *M. leprae*, both in mice and in lepromatous patients. A study in Mali showed that 500 mg of daily clarithromycin was as effective as 100 mg of daily minocycline. Of the 12 patients treated with clarithromycin alone, 5 (42%) showed definite clinical improvement and 6 (50%) showed marked clinical improvement after 1 month of treatment. This treatment also resulted in significant reductions in bacterial index after 3 months.[32] Mouse studies have reported additive effects of clarithromycin and minocycline, but this has not been confirmed in human trials.[37]

Moxifloxacin

Moxifloxacin, another quinolone, was recently tested in the Philippines. Eight multibacillary leprosy patients were given a single 400 mg dose of moxifloxacin, which resulted in significant killing of *M. leprae*, ranging from 82% to 99%, mean 91%. No viable bacilli were detected with an additional 3 weeks of daily therapy.[38]

Single-dose therapy

A single-dose MDT is now available for single-lesion paucibacillary patients: rifampicin 600 mg, ofloxacin 400 mg and minocycline 100 mg (ROM). A large, multicentered, randomized controlled, double-blind trial carried out in India to test single-dose ROM versus 6 months of paucibacillary MDT in single-lesion cases demonstrated that 51.8% of patients treated with ROM showed marked clinical improvement compared with 57.3% of those on WHO/MDT for patients with paucibacillary disease. Although this result showed that the WHO regimen was statistically better than single-dose ROM for single-lesion cases, ROM may still be appropriate for field situations.[39] ROM given as a single monthly dose for 24 months was shown in a small Philippines study to be as effective as MDT in the treatment of multibacillary leprosy.[40]

Other drug regimens

In the mouse model, the combination of minocycline and ofloxacin has been found to be almost as bactericidal as rifampicin, and the combination of rifapentine, moxifloxacin and minocycline significantly more bactericidal than the ROM regimen.[41]

Urgent research is needed targeting patients with rifampicin-resistant leprosy. One proposed regimen was an initial 6-month intensive phase (moxifloxacin 400 mg, clofazimine 50 mg, clarithromycin 500 mg and minocycline 100 mg – daily for 6 months), followed by an additional 18-month continuation phase (moxifloxacin 400 mg, clarithromycin 1000 mg and minocycline 200 mg – once monthly for an additional 18 months).[42]

TREATMENT OF NERVE DAMAGE

Nerve damage refers to peripheral sensory or motor neuropathy. Patients may present with nerve damage or develop nerve function impairment during or after MDT.

A large field study in Ethiopia looked prospectively at 650 patients treated with WHO/MDT and followed them up for 11 years (1988–1999). In this study 55% of patients had some nerve function impairment at diagnosis and 12% developed new impairment after starting MDT; 33% had no initial impairment and never developed neuropathy. Patients with no initial nerve impairment who later developed nerve damage and were treated with corticosteroids within 6 months of symptoms (defined as acute neuropathy) had full recovery in 88% of nerves. Corticosteroids were also successful in treating 51% of patients who had chronic or recurrent nerve damage. Chronic neuropathy was defined as nerve function impairment occurring within 3 months of stopping corticosteroids and recurrent neuropathy as new nerve impairment occurring at least 3 months after stopping corticosteroids.[43]

Current treatment for patients presenting with new nerve damage of ≤6 months' duration is corticosteroids in addition to MDT. Oral prednisolone is started at 40 mg/day and reduced over 4–6 months depending on clinical response.

The Bangladesh Acute Nerve Damage Study (BANDS) showed that there was a delay in patients presenting for treatment, and this could be as long as 12 months after initial symptoms started. The prevalence of nerve function impairment was seven times greater in multibacillary than paucibacillary patients and twice as high in men as in women. Of the patients presenting with nerve damage, almost 12% had a sensory neuropathy and just over 7% had a motor neuropathy. The nerve most commonly affected was the posterior tibial nerve (sensory neuropathy), followed by the ulnar nerve.[44]

The TRIPOD trials (Trials in the Prevention of Disability in Leprosy) showed that the use of low-dose prophylactic prednisolone during the first 4 months of MDT for leprosy reduces the incidence of new reactions and nerve function impairment in the short term, but the effect is not sustained at 1 year.[45] A recent Cochrane review concluded that evidence from randomized controlled trials does not show a significant long-term effect for either long-standing nerve function impairment or mild sensory impairment. However, the evidence was very thin and better studies are needed. A 5-month corticosteroid regimen was significantly more beneficial than a 3-month corticosteroid regimen.[46]

TREATMENT OF REACTIONS

Leprosy is complicated by immunological phenomena called reactions: reversal reactions (type 1 reactions); ENL reactions (erythema nodosum leprosum, or type 2 reactions). The clinical features of these reactions are listed in Table 57.3.

Table 57.3 Clinical features of leprosy reactions

	Reversal reactions	ENL reactions
Immune response	T-cell mediated	Immune complex deposition
Type of leprosy affected	BT, BB and BL	BL and LL
Clinical features	*Skin lesions:* erythema, swelling, tenderness *Peripheral nerve lesions:* pain/tenderness, increased weakness, increased sensory loss	*Skin lesions:* transient crops of small, painful red nodules, lasting 2–3 days *Other signs:* fever, malaise, lymph node enlargement, arthritis, iritis, orchitis, neuritis

BB, mid-borderline; BL, borderline lepromatous; BT, borderline tuberculoid; ENL, erythema nodosum leprosum; LL, lepromatous.

These sudden episodes of acute inflammation occur in approximately 30% of leprosy patients. This is due to immune reactions against antigenic components liberated from the bacilli. Patients can present in reaction before MDT, and a significant proportion of patients develop reactions within the first 6 months of treatment. There is also an increase in the incidence of reactions in postpartum patients. However, reactions can also occur after successful MDT and are probably due to persistence of *M. leprae* antigens.

Patients may suffer from recurrent reactions or repeated reactions after treatment, resulting in increased suffering and disability.

Treatment of reversal reactions

Reversal reactions are characterized by edema, inflammation and an increase in lymphocytic infiltration in skin and/or nerves of borderline patients. Reversal reactions are due to delayed hypersensitivity at sites of localization of *M. leprae* antigens. They are characterized by CD4 cell activation and production of tissue-damaging T-cell and macrophage cytokines. Mild reactions can be treated with aspirin (600–1200 mg every 4 h). Moderate and severe reactions are treated with prednisolone.

Prednisolone

Oral prednisolone has proved to be an effective treatment for severe reactions. Steroid treatment should be started within the first 6 months of an episode of reaction or nerve function impairment to be effective.[47–49] Starting doses may be as high as 60 mg and tapered over several months to prevent further nerve damage; a starting dose of 40 mg is usually sufficient to suppress inflammation in the skin or nerves. The response to treatment can be seen by a decrease in skin inflammation over a few days. In a study looking at motor nerve conduction velocity, Naafs et al confirmed that there is a good response to several months of steroid therapy with remyelinization and nerve regeneration.[50]

Prednisolone has many effects on cytokines, but it down-regulates proinflammatory cytokines, mainly by inhibition of nuclear factor kappa B (NF-κB)-induced transcription of cytokine mRNA. Little et al assessed the in-vivo effects of prednisolone in reversal reaction (RR) patients: they found that 1 month of prednisolone treatment reduced cellularity, cytokine production (interferon-γ, interleukin-12) and inducible nitric oxide synthetase in skin lesions of RR patients.[51]

Prednisolone is the drug of choice for severe reversal reactions, although about 30% of patients do not respond to therapy or need a protracted course of corticosteroids. Other established immunosuppressant drugs might have a role in treating reactions. A pilot study in Nepal showed equivalent outcomes whether treated with an azathioprine–prednisolone combination or prednisolone alone.[52] Ciclosporin (cyclosporine) also showed a similar result and further trials are ongoing.[53]

Treatment of ENL

ENL presents as a systemic illness: a patient with ENL may be very sick with high temperatures, painful subcutaneous nodules, peripheral edema and inflammation of the nerves, eyes, joints, muscles, bones and testes. In ENL, antigen–antibody complexes are deposited in the tissues with the activation of complement and migration of neutrophils into lesions.

For mild cases aspirin may be used, but many cases require treatment with prednisolone and an increased dose of clofazimine (up to 300 mg) or thalidomide. Thalidomide is the treatment of choice for severe ENL but its availability and teratogenicity limit its use.

Thalidomide

Thalidomide was first synthesized in 1954 and marketed as a hypnotic in 1956. It is now being used for its anti-inflammatory properties in ENL[54] and other diseases.[55] Thalidomide has two main actions: a potent depressant effect on the central nervous system and an immunomodulatory effect in inflammatory disease. Sampaio et al showed that it selectively inhibits transcription of the inflammatory cytokine tumor necrosis factor-alpha (TNF-α)[56] by accelerating the degradation of mRNA encoding the protein.[57] Thalidomide also enhances cell-mediated immunity by directly stimulating cytotoxic T cells and increasing the production of interleukin-10.[58]

Thalidomide has been used for treatment of ENL since the early 1960s. In 1965, Sheskin[59] reported that six patients with ENL responded well to thalidomide, and this was confirmed with other studies.[60] It has also been shown that the raised serum TNF-α levels in ENL are lowered by thalidomide.[61] Thalidomide shortens the ENL reaction. It acts rapidly, with improvement occurring after 8 h, although it may take up to 48 h before the patient becomes afebrile. The dose used is 400 mg/day in 2–4 divided doses, with a gradual reduction to 50 mg/day. Thalidomide is the most effective drug for ENL but must be strongly discouraged in women of childbearing age unless using double contraception; it is absolutely contraindicated in pregnancy. All patients should be given specific advice (Box 57.1) before commencing thalidomide therapy. If thalidomide is either not available or contraindicated, prednisolone is used to treat ENL.

Box 57.1 Advice for female patients before commencing thalidomide therapy

- Do not share tablets with anyone else
- Use double contraception whilst on therapy
- Seek medical advice at the first sign of amenorrhea
- An abortion should be considered if pregnancy is confirmed

There have been no reports of thalidomide causing accelerated nerve damage in leprosy. However, when used in other conditions such as Behçet's disease, thalidomide is known to cause an axonal sensory neuropathy and there is evidence to suggest more widespread effects of the nervous system.[62-65] Other side effects that occur with thalidomide include a widespread rash developing 6–12 days after starting the drug, drowsiness, constipation, xerostomia, increased appetite, nausea and loss of libido.[66] It can also rarely result in menstrual abnormalities, increased urinary secretion of corticosteroids, myxedema and a euthyroid state in previous thyrotoxicosis.[67]

CHEMOPROPHYLAXIS AND IMMUNOTHERAPY

In the 1960s and 1970s chemoprophylaxis with dapsone and acedapsone was investigated. However, as dapsone showed varying protection to contacts of leprosy patients and there were anxieties about dapsone resistance, this regimen was curtailed. In the 1980s–1990s rifampicin, used either alone or in combination with other drugs, was found to have chemoprophylactic efficacy.[68] An intervention study in highly endemic Micronesia using a single dose of ROM as chemoprophylaxis showed an apparent reduced leprosy incidence in the first 3 years in the blanket group. Whether this is due to a delayed development of leprosy or a complete clearance of infection needs to be determined.[69] A recent study in Bangladesh[70] randomized 28 092 close contacts of newly diagnosed leprosy patients to a single dose of rifampicin or placebo with a follow up of 4 years. The overall reduction in incidence of leprosy using a single dose of rifampicin in the first 2 years was 57% (close to that achieved with longer dapsone treatment). However, the difference was no longer significant in the third and fourth years. Further studies are needed to raise the efficacy of rifampicin.

A meta-analysis of 14 trials showed that chemoprophylaxis gives approximately 60% protection against leprosy. Leprosy chemoprophylaxis may be an effective way of reducing incidence and is more cost-effective if it is given only to household contacts.[71] Current UK practice is for all childhood contacts of newly diagnosed patients to be given rifampicin prophylaxis (1 mg/kg). At present chemo- and immunoprophylaxis are not cost-effective measures for wide usage because there is no means of identifying all persons who are at high risk of developing leprosy and the prophylactic measures are not close to 100% efficacy.

To date no specific vaccine has been developed to prevent infection by *M. leprae*, although there is good evidence that bacille Calmette–Guérin (BCG) has protective efficacy. Large field trials in Uganda, Burma, Papua New Guinea and India have all demonstrated a protective efficacy varying from 20% to 80% with BCG vaccines. Adding *M. leprae* antigen to BCG does not increase the efficacy of the vaccine.[72]

ONGOING MANAGEMENT AND PREVENTION OF COMPLICATIONS

Education concerning factual information such as mode of transmission, treatment and complications is essential for all patients and health providers. Education is also important in equipping patients with knowledge on how to adapt their lifestyle to prevent the development of complications (e.g. comfortable footwear and cessation of smoking in order to care for the anesthetic limb).

LEPROSY AND HIV

There were concerns that an interaction between HIV and *M. leprae* infection would result in an increased incidence of leprosy cases. However, studies in Uganda, Mali, Ethiopia and South India have not shown an increased prevalence of leprosy cases associated with HIV infection.[73-75]

An association has been found between HIV infection and complications of leprosy. In a case-controlled study in Uganda, Kawuma et al[73] found that HIV seropositivity was a significant risk factor for developing reactions and neuritis; an unusual finding because reversal reactions are associated with an increase in CD4 cells. Similarly, Sampaio et al found that HIV-infected patients with low CD4 counts had normal granuloma formation with numerous CD4 cells.[76]

Treatment of a leprosy patient with concurrent HIV infection does not differ from that of a seronegative leprosy patient and reactions should be managed with corticosteroids or thalidomide as appropriate.

Since the introduction of highly active antiretroviral therapy (HAART) in the management of HIV, leprosy is being increasingly reported as part of the immune reconstitution inflammatory syndrome (IRIS).[77] It is possible that the immune response to *M. leprae* in an HIV-infected person is suppressed before starting HAART and that leprosy manifests as IRIS with the sudden reversal of this suppression and the rise in CD4 count.[78] Further studies are needed to understand the clinical and pathological features in HIV and leprosy co-infection.

CONCLUSION

MDT has been a success story in both the treatment of *M. leprae* infection and the mobilization of many people involved in treatment, surveillance and leprosy control programs. In 1982 MDT was implemented in endemic areas and since then more than 90% of registered cases have received treatment, 14 million patients have been cured and global prevalence has declined.

The current treatment for leprosy reactions is still not optimal, with a significant number of patients not responding to prednisolone and some ENL patients requiring chronic thalidomide therapy. Researchers are still looking for different immunosuppressant drugs with efficacy in the treatment of reactions (e.g. azathioprine and ciclosporin A).

The stigma associated with the diagnosis of leprosy is still a very real problem and the management of someone with the disease should include discussion of their psychosocial status and education for the patient and their family.

References

1. WHO. Leprosy – global situation. *Wkly Epidemiol Rec*. 2008;83(33):293–300 and 2008;83(50):459.
2. Job CK, Jayakumar J. Transmission of leprosy: a study of skin and nasal secretions of household contacts of leprosy patients using PCR. *American Society of Tropical Medicine and Hygiene*. 2008;78(3):518–521.
3. Girdhar BK. Skin to skin transmission of leprosy. *Indian J Dermatol Venereol Leprol*. 2005;71:223–225.
4. Desikan KV, Sreevatsa. Studies on viability of *M. leprae* outside the human body. *Lepr India*. 1979;51:588–589.
5. Van Buynder P, Eccleston J, Leese J, Lockwood DNJ. Leprosy in England and Wales. *Commun Dis Public Health*. 1999;2:119–121.
6. Lockwood DNJ, Reid AJ. The diagnosis of leprosy is delayed in the United Kingdom. *Q J Med*. 2001;94:207–212.
7. Hastings RC. *Leprosy*. 2nd ed. Edinburgh: Churchill Livingstone; 1994.
8. Evans M, Lockwood D. Leprosy: a clinical update. *Africa Health*. 1999;21:14–16.
9. Cole ST, Eiglmeier K, Parkhill J, et al. Massive gene decay in the leprosy bacillus. *Nature*. 2001;409:1007–1011.
10. Britton WJ, Lockwood DNJ. Leprosy. *Lancet*. 2004;363:1209–1219.
11. Lyon S, Lyon AC, Da Silva RC, et al. A comparison of ML flow serology and slit skin test smears to assess the bacterial load in newly diagnosed leprosy patients in Brazil. *Lepr Rev*. 2008;79:162–170.
12. World Health Organization. Chemotherapy of leprosy. Report of a WHO Study Group. *World Health Organ Tech Rep Ser*. 1994;847:1–24.
13. Lobo D. Treatment failures with multidrug therapy. *Lepr Rev*. 1992;63:93s–98s.
14. World Health Organization. *MDT: duration of treatment FAQ*. WHO: Geneva; Online. Available at http://www.who.int/lep/mdt/duration; 2010.
15. Maurus JN. Hansen's disease in pregnancy. *Obstet Gynaecol*. 1978;52:22–25.
16. Farb H, West DP, Pedvis-Leftick A. Clofazimine in pregnancy complicated by leprosy. *Obstet Gynaecol*. 1982;59:122–123.
17. Anonymous. In: Dollery C, ed. *Therapeutic drugs*. 2nd ed. Edinburgh: Churchill Livingstone; 1999:D13–D18.
18. Cochrane RG. A comparison of sulphone and hydnocarpus therapy of leprosy. In: (Portuguese –Brazil) *Memoria del V Congreso Internacional de la Lepra*. Editorial Cenit, Havana, Cuba. 1949:220–224.
19. Cochrane RG, Ramanujam K, Paul H, Russell D. Two and a half years' experimental work on the sulphone group of drugs. *Lepr Rev*. 1949;20:4–64.
20. Muir E. Preliminary report on 4:4'-diaminodiphenylsulphone (DDS) treatment of leprosy. *Int J Lepr*. 1950;18:299–308.
21. Lowe J, Smith M. The chemotherapy of leprosy in Nigeria, with an appendix on glandular fever and exfoliative dermatitis precipitated by sulphones. *Int J Lepr*. 1949;17:181–195.
22. Lowe J. Treatment of leprosy with diaminodiphenlysulphone by mouth. *Lancet*. 1950;1:145–150.
23. Floch H, Destomes R. Traitement de la lepre par la 'sulphone-mere' (diamino-diphenyl-sulphone). *Int J Lepr*. 1949;17:367–377.
24. Levy L, Shepard CC, Fasal P. Clofazimine therapy of lepromatous leprosy caused by dapsone-resistant *Mycobacterium leprae*. *Am J Trop Med Hyg*. 1972;21:315–321.
25. Warndorff-van Diepen T. Clofazimine-resistant leprosy, a case report. *Int J Lepr*. 1982;50:139–142.
26. Browne SG, Hogerzell L. B.663 in the treatment of leprosy. Preliminary report of a pilot trial. *Lepr Rev*. 1962;33:6–10.
27. Mansfield RE. Tissue concentrations of clofazimine (B663) in man. *Am J Trop Med Hyg*. 1974;50:139–142.
28. Anonymous. In: Dollery C, ed. *Therapeutic drugs*. 2nd ed. Edinburgh: Churchill Livingstone; 1999:R32–R36.
29. Levy L, Shepard CC, Fasal P. The bactericidal effect of rifampicin on *M. leprae* in man: a) single doses of 600, 900, and 1200 mg; and b) daily doses of 300 mg. *Int J Lepr*. 1976;44:183–187.
30. Honoré N, Cole ST. The molecular basis of rifampicin-resistance in *Mycobacterium leprae*. *Antimicrob Agents Chemother*. 1993;37:414–418.
31. Gelber RH. Activity of minocycline in *Mycobacterium leprae*-infected mice. *J Infect Dis*. 1987;156:236–239.
32. Ji B, Jamet P, Perani EG, Bobin P, Grosset JH. Powerful bactericidal activities of clarithromycin and minocycline against *Mycobacterium leprae* in lepromatous leprosy. *J Infect Dis*. 1993;168:188–190.
33. Rea TH. Trials of daily, long-term minocycline and rifampicin or clarithromycin and rifampicin in the treatment of borderline lepromatous and lepromatous leprosy. *Int J Lepr*. 2000;68:129–135.
34. Bernier C, Dreno B. Minocycline. *Ann Dermatol Venereol*. 2001;128:627–637.
35. Grosset JH, Geulpa-Lauras CC, Perani EG, Beoletto C. Activity of ofloxacin against *Mycobacterium leprae* in the mouse. *Int J Lepr*. 1988;56:259–264.
36. Grosset JH, Ji B, Geulpa-Lauras CC, Perani EG, N'Deli LN. Clinical trial of perfloxacin and ofloxacin in the treatment of lepromatous leprosy. *Int J Lepr*. 1990;58:281–295.
37. Ji B, Perani EG, Grosset JH. Effectiveness of clarithromycin and minocycline alone and in combination against experimental *Mycobacterium leprae* infection in mice. *Antimicrob Agents Chemother*. 1991;35:579–581.
38. Pardillo FE, Burgos J, Fajardo TT, et al. Powerful bactericidal activity of moxifloxacin in human leprosy. *Antimicrob Agents Chemother*. 2008;52(9):3113–3117.
39. Gupte MD. Field trials of a single dose combination of rifampicin–ofloxacin–minocycline (ROM) for the treatment of paucibacillary leprosy. *Lepr Rev*. 2000;71:S77–S80.
40. Villahermosa LG. Parallel assessment of 24 monthly doses of rifampin, ofloxacin, and minocycline versus two years of World Health Organization multi-drug therapy for multi-bacillary leprosy. *Am J Trop Med Hyg*. 2004;70(2):197–200.
41. Grosset L. The new challenges for chemotherapy research. *Lepr Rev*. 2000;71(suppl):100–104.
42. Sundar Rao PSS, Chandna R. Future research needs in leprosy: highlights of the pre Congress Workshop No 7 – Hyderabad. *Lepr Rev*. 2008;79:223–229.
43. Saunderson P, Gebre S, Desta K, Byass P, Lockwood DNJ. The pattern of leprosy-related neuropathy in the AMFES patients in Ethiopia: definitions, incidence, risk factors and outcome. *Lepr Rev*. 2000;71:285–308.
44. Croft IRP, Richardus JH, Nicholls PG, Smith WCS. Nerve function impairment in leprosy: design, methodology and intake status of a prospective cohort of 2664 new leprosy cases in Bangladesh. The Bangladesh Acute Nerve Damage Study. *Lepr Rev*. 1999;70:140–159.
45. Smith WC, Anderson A. Steroid prophylaxis for prevention of nerve function impairment in leprosy: randomized placebo controlled trial (TRIPOD!). *Br Med J*. 2004;328:1459.
46. Van Veen N, Nicholls P. Corticosteroids for treating nerve damage in leprosy. A Cochrane review. *Lepr Rev*. 2008;79:361–371.
47. Becx-Bleumink M, Berhe D, Mannetje W. The management of nerve damage in the leprosy control services. *Lepr Rev*. 1990;61:1–11.
48. Becx-Bleumink M, Berhe D. Occurrence of reaction, their diagnosis and management in leprosy patients with MDT; experience in the Leprosy Control Programme of the All Africa Leprosy and Rehabilitation Training Centre (ALERT) in Ethiopia. *Int J Lepr*. 1992;60:173–184.
49. Van Brakel WH, Kwasas IB. Nerve function impairment in leprosy: an epidemiological and clinical study – Part 2: Results of steroid treatment. *Lepr Rev*. 1996;67:104–118.
50. Naafs B, Pearson JMH, Baar AJM. A follow-up study of nerve lesions in leprosy during and after reactions using motor nerve conduction velocity. *Int J Lepr*. 1976;44:188–197.
51. Little D, Khanolkar-Young S, Coulthart A, Suneetha A, Lockwood DNL. Immunohistochemical analysis of cellular infiltrate and gamma-interferon, interleukin-12 and inducible nitric oxide synthetase expression in leprosy type 1 (reversal) reactions before and during prednisolone treatment. *Infect Immun*. 2001;69:3413–3417.

52. Marlowe SN, Hawksworth RA, Butlin CR, Nicholls PG, Lockwood DN. Clinical outcomes in a randomized controlled study comparing azathioprine and prednisolone versus prednisolone alone in the treatment of severe leprosy type 1 reactions in Nepal. *Trans R Soc Trop Med Hyg*. 2004;98:602–609.

53. Marlowe SN, Leekassa R, Bizuneh E, et al. Response to ciclosporin treatment in Ethiopian and Nepali patients with severe leprosy type 1 reactions. *Trans R Soc Trop Med Hyg*. 2007;101:1004–1012.

54. Walker SL, Waters MFR, Lockwood DNJ. The role of thalidomide in the management of erythema nodosum leprosum. *Lepr Rev*. 2007;78:197–215.

55. Anonymous. Dollery C, ed. *Therapeutic drugs*. 2nd ed. Edinburgh: Churchill Livingstone; 1999:T60–T74.

56. Sampaio EP, Sarno EN, Galilly R, Cohn ZA, Kaplan G. Thalidomide selectively inhibits tumour necrosis factor α production by stimulated human monocytes. *J Exp Med*. 1991;173:699–703.

57. Sarno EN, Grau GE, Vieira LMM, Nery JA. Serum levels of tumour necrosis factor-alpha and interleukin-1 beta during leprosy reactional states. *Clin Exp Immunol*. 1991;84:103–108.

58. Singhal S, Mehta J, Desikan R, et al. Antitumor activity of thalidomide in refractory multiple myeloma. *N Engl J Med*. 1999;341:1565–1571.

59. Sheskin J. Thalidomide in the treatment of lepra reactions. *Clin Pharmacol Ther*. 1965;6:303–306.

60. Leading Article. Thalidomide in leprosy reaction. *Lancet*. 1994;343:432–433.

61. Sampaio EP, Kaplan G, Miranda A, et al. The influence of thalidomide on the clinical and immunologic manifestations of erythema nodosum leprosum. *J Infect Dis*. 1993;168:408–414.

62. Fullerton PM, Kremer M. Neuropathy after intake of thalidomide (Distaval). *Br Med J*. 1961;ii:855–858.

63. Editorial. Thalidomide neuropathy. *Br Med J*. 1961;ii:876.

64. Fullerton PM, O'Sullivan DJ. Thalidomide neuropathy: an electrophysiological study. *Muscle Nerve*. 1968;9:837–844.

65. Harland CC, Steventon GB, Marsden JR. Thalidomide induced neuropathy and drug metabolite polymorphism. *Clin Res*. 1993;41:496A.

66. Gunzler V. Thalidomide in human immunodeficiency virus. A review of safety considerations. *Drug Safety*. 1992;7:116–134.

67. Mellin GW, Katzenstein M. The saga of thalidomide. *N Engl J Med*. 1962;267:1184–1193 1238–1244.

68. Cartel JL, Chanteau S, Moulia-Pelat JP, et al. Chemoprophylaxis of leprosy with a single dose of 25 mg/kg rifampicin in the Southern Marquesas: results after 4 years. *Int J Lepr*. 1992;60:416–420.

69. Bakker MI, Hatta M, Kwenang A, et al. Prevention of leprosy using rifampicin as chemoprophylaxis. *Am J Trop Med Hyg*. 2005;72:443–448.

70. Moet FJ, Pahan D, Oskam L, Richardus JH. Effectiveness of single dose rifampicin in preventing leprosy in close contacts of patients with newly diagnosed leprosy: cluster randomised controlled trial. *Br Med J*. 2008;336:761–764.

71. Smith CM, Smith WCS. Chemoprophylaxis is effective in the prevention of leprosy in endemic countries: a systematic review and meta-analysis. *J Infect*. 2000;41:137–142.

72. Nordeen SK. Prophylaxis – scope and limitations. *Lepr Rev*. 2000;71:S16–S20.

73. Kawuma HJS, Bwire R, Adatu-Engwau F. Leprosy and infection with the human immunodeficiency virus in Uganda: a case-control study. *Int J Lepr*. 1994;62:521–526.

74. Lienhardt C, Kamate B, Jamet P, et al. Effect of HIV infection on leprosy: a three year survey in Bamako, Mali. *Int J Lepr Other Mycobact Dis*. 1996;64:383–391.

75. Sekar B, Jayasheela M, Chattopadhya D, et al. Prevalence of HIV infection and high-risk characteristics among leprosy patients of South India; a case-control study. *Int J Lepr*. 1994;62:527–531.

76. Sampaio EP, Caneshi JRT, Nery JAC, et al. Cellular immune response to *Mycobacterium leprae* infection in human immunodeficiency virus infected individuals. *Infect Immun*. 1995;63:18848–18854.

77. Deps PD, Lockwood DNJ. Leprosy occurring as immune reconstitution syndrome. *Trans R Soc Trop Med Hyg*. 2008;102:966–968.

78. Ustianowski AP, Lawn SD, Lockwood DNJ. Interactions between HIV infection and leprosy: a paradox. *Lancet Infect Dis*. 2006;6:350–360.

58 Tuberculosis and other mycobacterial infections

L. Peter Ormerod

Tuberculosis (TB) has been increasing significantly on a worldwide basis over the last decade, to such an extent that the World Health Organization (WHO) proclaimed it a global emergency in 1995. The WHO 2007 estimates are that there are 9.27 million new clinical cases at a rate of 139/100 000 per annum, 1.3 million deaths each year, and two billion persons infected in the world as judged by a positive tuberculin skin test.[1] This increase has been seen both in the developing world and in developed countries, reversing the historical continuous decline seen since the Second World War. The reasons for the increase are different in the developing and developed worlds.

In developed countries, particularly in Europe, the increases are due to an increasing proportion of the cases of TB occurring in ethnic minority groups who have come from countries of high prevalence and who consequently have very high TB rates. The rates in the native population continue generally to decline. In England and Wales, incidence increased nearly 70% between 1987 and 2008, but only 21% of cases are now in the White ethnic population, with over 73% of cases being foreign born.[2] Rates in ethnic minority groups are 25–40 times higher than in the White ethnic group.[2] Similar trends have been seen in most European countries, with the increase being due to immigrants and refugees/asylum seekers from high-prevalence countries. In the USA the increase seen between 1985 and 1990, which was partly due to HIV co-infection, but also due to social factors and the dismantling of TB programs, has been significantly reversed but (as in Europe) an increasing proportion of cases are now in the foreign born.[3]

In developing countries the increase is largely due to the lack of funding, marked population increases and the associated economic and social deprivation. To this is now added the effect of HIV co-infection. Although first described in the USA,[4] its largest impact so far has been in sub-Saharan Africa where TB rates doubled between 1985 and 1991 in some countries (e.g. Malawi and Zambia[5]), and have continued to rise almost exponentially since. This dual epidemic, which has hit largely younger, economically active adults (and children), has further fuelled deprivation, social pressures and economic collapse. Although currently only 12% of TB worldwide is HIV associated,[1] this proportion is expected to rise over the next 5–10 years as dual infection increasingly occurs in South Asia, which, because of the much larger populations of these countries, will have a much greater numerical effect.[1]

In this chapter the principles underlying the development of short-course treatment will be set out, together with recommendations based on those principles for individual patients and sites of disease. The complexities of treatment of HIV-infected patients with particular relation to highly active antiretroviral treatment (HAART) are also discussed. Such treatments, as well as prophylactic therapy in both HIV-negative and HIV-positive individuals, need to be within the context of a monitored TB control program. Multidrug-resistant (MDR) and extensively drug-resistant (XDR) TB are challenging TB control, particularly in resource-poor settings, and their management will be discussed. Trials, including quinolones, are ongoing to see if 6-month short-course chemotherapy can be reduced to 4 months. New drugs are also in development and will be briefly summarized. Finally, treatment of the opportunist mycobacteria that cause human disease is also considered.

SCIENTIFIC BASIS OF SHORT-COURSE CHEMOTHERAPY

Each of the main antituberculosis drugs varies in its capacity to kill bacteria, to sterilize lesions and to prevent the emergence of drug resistance. Killing capacity is measured by early bactericidal activity,[6] sterilizing ability by a low relapse rate after cessation of treatment and a low culture-positive rate at 2 months of treatment.[7] The efficiency of a drug in preventing the emergence of drug resistance is more difficult to assess and is largely derived from the interpretation of clinical studies.[7]

Isoniazid (H) is the most potent bactericidal drug and kills more than 90% of bacilli within 7 days, acting on metabolically active bacilli. It is also quite effective at preventing the emergence of drug resistance. Rifampicin (rifampin; R) is another effective bactericidal drug, with a potent sterilizing effect and a good ability to prevent the emergence of drug resistance. In addition to acting on rapidly dividing bacilli it kills so-called 'persisters', which remain inactive for long periods but have intermittent periods of metabolism, with only a short drug exposure. This gives it its potent sterilizing efficiency. Although bactericidal, pyrazinamide (Z) is used mainly for its sterilizing ability; it is particularly effective at killing intracellular mycobacteria sequestered inside macrophages in an acid environment.[6] Streptomycin (S) and ethambutol (E) are less potent drugs, with ethambutol probably being bactericidal only at a high concentration. They are less effective at preventing the emergence of resistance to rifampicin and isoniazid.

The efficacy of regimens based on rifampicin, isoniazid and pyrazinamide has been extensively studied by many controlled trials of different durations and dosing schedules. With this type of regimen it is possible to convert over 90% of sputum smear-positive patients to culture-negative at 2 months, to cure greater than 95%, and to have a relapse rate of less than 5%. The studies from which various aspects of treatment can be deduced, and on which later chemotherapy recommendations are based, are set out in Table 58.1.[8–19]

A duration of 6 months seems to be the shortest period for a regimen based on isoniazid and rifampicin that will give an acceptably low relapse rate. If the duration is reduced below 6 months higher relapse rates and lower cure rates are found, which are not acceptable for developed countries. Studies in Singapore and Hong Kong comparing 2, 4 and 6 months of pyrazinamide with rifampicin and isoniazid for 6 months showed that pyrazinamide is needed only for the initial 2 months. Conversely, however, if pyrazinamide is not used or cannot be tolerated, then a 9-month regimen of rifampicin and isoniazid is required, supplemented by ethambutol for the initial 2 months.

The trials described in Table 58.1 covered a spectrum of dosing schedules from daily treatment throughout, a daily initial phase followed by a twice or thrice weekly continuation phase, or twice or thrice weekly dosing throughout. All of these schedules gave relapse rates of less than 5% during periods of follow-up between 6 and 30 months after cessation of treatment. The dosing schedule used therefore depends on a balance of cost, side effects and tolerance, drug availability and organizational aspects.

When rifampicin was omitted from the regimen in the continuation phase because of cost constraints, a 6-month total duration gave higher relapse rates and inadequate sterilization. Before the HIV epidemic regimens with an extended continuation phase of isoniazid for 6 months with either ethambutol or thiacetazone (Th) had been tested. A regimen of 2SHRZ/6HTh had been shown to be very effective when combined with admission to hospital for the initial 2 months.[20,21] This is no longer viable as a 'cheaper' regimen because of the rate of drug reactions to thiacetazone in HIV-positive patients (*see later*) and the costs of initial hospital care. If rifampicin is not used in the continuation phase then there is a significantly increased failure rate if the organism is found to have initial isoniazid resistance.

Regimens of various durations of between 2 and 4 months have been studied in sputum smear-negative tuberculosis.

Table 58.1 Six-month short course regimen trials for the treatment of pulmonary tuberculosis

	Regimen	No. of patients	Bacteriological relapse (%)	Reference
Daily throughout				
United Kingdom	2SHRZ/4HR	125	1	8
	2EHRZ/4HR	132	2	8
Hong Kong	2EHRZ/4EHRZ	163	1	9–11
US Trial 21	2HRZ/4HR	273	4	12
Singapore	2SHRZ/4HRZ	78	1	13–14
	2SHRZ/4HR	80	2	13–14
Daily initial phase and intermittent continuation phase				
Poland	2HRZ/4HR(3)	116	4	15
	2SHRZ/4HR(2)	56	2	15
Singapore	2SHRZ/4HR(3)	97	1	16–17
	1SHRZ/5HR(3)	94	1	16–17
	2HRZ/4HR(3)	109	1	16–17
Intermittent throughout				
Hong Kong	6SHRZE(3)	152	1	9–11
	6SHRZ(3)	151	1	9–11
	6HRZE(3)	160	2	9–11
	2SHRZ(3)/2SHR(3)/3HR(3)	149	3	18
	4SHRZ(3)/2HR(3)	133	6	18
	4SHRZ(3)/2HRZ(3)	142	1	18
	4HRZ(3)/4HRZ(3)	135	4	18
USA	0.5SHRZ/1.5SHRZ(2)/4HR(2)	125	2	19

E, ethambutol; H, isoniazid; R, rifampicin; S, streptomycin; Z, pyrazinamide. The number in front of the letters represents the duration of treatment in months. The number in brackets after the letters represents the number of doses per week.

For those with positive initial cultures, relapse rates of 32% with 2 months' treatment,[22] 7–13% with 3 months' treatment,[22,23] and 4% with 4 months' treatment have been reported.[22,23] The results of the 4-month regimen varied with the initial sensitivities of those with a positive culture. For initially sensitive organisms, the relapse rate was 2%, but rose to 8% for those with initial resistance to isoniazid and/or streptomycin.[23]

RECOMMENDED REGIMENS

The recommendations made by various expert bodies are founded on the substantial body of evidence for pulmonary tuberculosis, and take into account the likelihood of drug resistance in the target population. The recommendations of the National Institute for Health and Clinical Excellence are set out in Table 58.2.[24] Where there are variations between these recommendations and those of the European Respiratory Society,[25] the American Thoracic Society[26] and the World Health Organization,[27] these are also shown in Table 58.2.

In the UK, a 6-month regimen comprising isoniazid, rifampicin, pyrazinamide and ethambutol for 2 initial months, followed by rifampicin and isoniazid for a further 4 months, is recommended for adult respiratory tuberculosis, including isolated pleural effusion and mediastinal lymphadenopathy, irrespective of the bacteriological status of the sputum.[24] A 6-month regimen is therefore recommended for sputum smear-negative disease. Where a positive culture for *M. tuberculosis* has been obtained but susceptibility results are outstanding at 2 months, the initial four-drug phase should be continued until full susceptibility is known, but the total duration of treatment does not need to be extended. Ethambutol is included to cover the possibility of initial isoniazid resistance because of its increasing prevalence.[2]

If a patient cannot tolerate pyrazinamide, then the treatment required to give a suitably high cure rate is 9 months of rifampicin and isoniazid supplemented by 2 months of initial ethambutol.[28] Routine daily pyridoxine is not required but should be given to people at higher risk of peripheral neuropathy: those with diabetes mellitus, chronic renal failure, alcohol dependency, malnourishment and the HIV positive.[24]

NON-PULMONARY TUBERCULOSIS

Non-respiratory tuberculosis has been subject to fewer controlled clinical trials than respiratory tuberculosis, but there are sites where evidence-based advice can be obtained.

Table 58.2   Recommended regimens for treatment of tuberculosis

Type of tuberculosis	American Thoracic Society	European Respiratory Society	National Institute for Health and Clinical Excellence
Adult			
New smear positive pulmonary or New extensive smear-negative pulmonary Extensive non-respiratory	2RHZ(E/S)/4HR or 0.5RHZ(S/E)/1.5RHZ(E)(2)/4HR(2) (DOT) or 2RHZ(E/S)(3)/4RHZ(E/S)(3) DOT	2RHZ(E)/4HR or 2RHZ(E)/4HR(3)	2RHZ(E)/4HR or 2RHZS(3)/4HR(3) DOT
Non-extensive smear-negative pulmonary	2RHZ/4HR	As above	As above
Adult meningitis	Presumed as extensive non-respiratory but not specified	Presumed as extensive non-respiratory but not specified	2RHZ(E/S)/10HR
Children			
Pulmonary/lymph node	As adult	As adult	As adult
Central nervous system	2RHZ(S)/10HR	As adult	2RHZ(E)/10HR
Miliary	As above	As adult	2RHZ(E)/4HR
Bone/joint	As above	As adult	2RHZ(E)/4HR
Drug resistance			
Isoniazid	2RZE/4RZE or 2RE/10RE	Not specified	2RZES/7RE DOT or 2RZE/10RE
MDR-TB	Individualized	Individualized	Individualized
Other resistances	Not specified	Not specified	See Table 3

DOT, directly observed therapy; E, ethambutol; H, isoniazid; R, rifampicin; S, streptomycin; Z, pyrazinamide. The number in front of the letters represents duration in months. The number in parentheses after the letters represents the number of doses per week. The 2009 WHO guidelines recommend the use of 2RHZE/6HE should stop, and a weak recommendation to consider 4RHE as the continuation phase in areas with proven or suspected isoniazed resistance rates of over 5%.

LYMPH-NODE TUBERCULOSIS

The third British Thoracic Society lymph node trial showed that a 6-month regimen was just as effective as a 9-month regimen.[29,30] From this trial,[29,30] and from earlier lymph node studies,[31,32] the course of lymph node disease is variable. In 10–15% of cases nodes may enlarge, abscesses may form, and new nodes may develop, both during and after treatment. These are usually without any bacteriological evidence of relapse or recurrence, and in the absence of a positive culture should not in themselves be taken as failure of treatment[31] or relapse.[32] The 6-month regimen recommended for respiratory tuberculosis is therefore also recommended for lymph node disease.[24]

BONE/JOINT TUBERCULOSIS

Approximately half of all cases are in spinal sites. This form of tuberculosis has been the subject of a number of controlled clinical trials, with 6 months of therapy being shown to give good results.[33–36] These studies also showed that chemotherapy can be fully ambulant in nearly all cases of tuberculosis of the thoracic and lumbar spine, with surgery reserved for the few patients with evidence of spinal cord compression or instability.[33–36] The 6-month regimen recommended for respiratory tuberculosis is therefore advised for bone and joint tuberculosis.[24]

PERICARDIUM

A 6-month regimen of rifampicin and isoniazid supplemented by 3 months initial pyrazinamide and streptomycin has been shown to be highly effective.[37,38] The continuation of streptomycin and pyrazinamide after 2 months is not likely to confer additional benefit, so the 6-month regimen preferred for respiratory disease is recommended.[24] Trials have shown that corticosteroids confer additional benefit in this form of tuberculosis (*see later*).[37,38]

CENTRAL NERVOUS SYSTEM

There is lack of evidence from controlled trials but management in centers treating large numbers suggests that rifampicin and isoniazid for 12 months, supplemented by pyrazinamide and a fourth drug for at least the first 2 months, will give good results.[39] Isoniazid, pyrazinamide and prothionamide/ethionamide penetrate the cerebrospinal fluid well, but rifampicin penetrates less well.[40] Ethambutol and streptomycin penetrate the cerebrospinal fluid in adequate concentrations only when there is active meningeal inflammation early in the treatment. Although the risk of ethambutol ocular toxicity at the recommended dosage of 15 mg/kg is low,[41] ethambutol should be used with caution in unconscious patients (Stage III) as visual acuity cannot be tested. Intrathecal administration of streptomycin is unnecessary. The fourth drug in the initial phase of treatment can be ethambutol,[40] streptomycin[40] or ethion(prothion)amide.[42] In the UK a 12-month regimen of rifampicin and isoniazid, supplemented by 2 months initial pyrazinamide and ethambutol, is recommended for both meningitis and tuberculoma,[24] prolonged to 18 months if pyrazinamide is not given or cannot be tolerated. Additional corticosteroids are of benefit (*see later*).

OTHER SITES

There are few clinical trial data for other sites. In the UK, by extrapolation from respiratory disease and the more common non-respiratory data, the 6-month regimen recommended for respiratory disease is advised;[24] it is also advised for tuberculosis in multiple sites, or for miliary (classic or cryptic) disease.[43] Because of the high rates of blood-borne spread to the meninges in miliary tuberculosis, lumbar puncture is recommended in such cases so that the correct duration of therapy can be determined.[24]

CORTICOSTEROIDS AS AN ADJUNCT TO THERAPY

Clinical trial data support a beneficial effect of corticosteroids in addition to the recommended antituberculosis chemotherapy for pericarditis,[37,38] for TB meningitis[40,44] and for endobronchial disease in children.[45] There are clinical, but no clinical trial, data of possible benefit in pleural effusions,[46] in tuberculosis affecting the ureter,[47] in patients with extensive pulmonary disease[48] and in suppression of hypersensitivity reactions to antituberculosis drugs.[48]

TREATMENT IN PREGNANCY

Pregnancy in patients taking rifampicin is not an indication for termination. Standard treatment should be given to pregnant women, the risk to both mother and fetus being greater if suboptimal treatment is given.[49] None of the first-line drugs has been shown to be teratogenic in humans, but the reserve drugs (*see later*) ethionamide and prothionamide may be and are best avoided. Streptomycin and other aminoglycosides are potentially ototoxic to the fetus and should be avoided in pregnancy. Women may breastfeed normally whilst taking antituberculosis drugs. Patients on rifampicin-containing regimens should be told of the reduced effectiveness of oral contraceptives and be given contraceptive advice.

TREATMENT IN CHILDREN

Recommended dosages of isoniazid vary substantially. The British Thoracic Society,[50] the International Union against Tuberculosis and Lung Diseases,[51] and the WHO[27] recommend 5 mg/kg up to a maximum dose of 300 mg/day. Other organizations such as the American Thoracic Society[26] and the American Academy of Pediatrics[52] recommend 10 mg/kg up to a maximum of 300 mg. Pharmacokinetic studies[53] show that 5 mg/kg gives serum levels 60–100 times the minimum inhibitory concentration and satisfactory clinical outcome is achieved.[54] Dosages should generally be rounded up to easily given volumes of syrup or appropriate strengths of tablet.

The 6-month regimen advised for adults should be used for children with respiratory tuberculosis including hilar lymphadenopathy.[24] Ethambutol should also be included for the first 2 months. A recent literature review concluded that use of a 15 mg/kg dosage of ethambutol, in children aged 5 years or older, required no more precautions to be taken than for adults.[55] The same review also concluded that ethambutol could be used in younger children without undue fear of side effects.[55]

No controlled trials examining the treatment of extrapulmonary tuberculosis in children have been reported. Recommendations are therefore made by extrapolation from adult trials. Treatment of tuberculous lymphadenopathy, pericarditis, bowel disease, bone and joint disease and other end-organ disease using the 6-month regimen advised for adults is recommended.[24] For disseminated and congenital tuberculosis, treatment should also last 6 months unless there is evidence of any central nervous system involvement, when a 12-month regimen is advised.[24] Meningitis should be treated with 12 months of isoniazid and rifampicin supplemented by 2 months initial pyrazinamide plus either ethambutol or streptomycin.[24,26,40,51]

DRUG-RESISTANT TUBERCULOSIS

MOLECULAR BASIS

Advances in molecular genetics over the last 15 years have demonstrated the mechanisms of resistance to specific antituberculosis drugs, and in general these come about because of mutation at a small number of sites in the chromosome. Isoniazid resistance has been linked to mutations in either the *inhA* gene which codes for an enzyme involved in mycolic acid synthesis in the cell wall[56] or the catalase peroxidase gene (*katG*).[57] For streptomycin, resistance is due to changes in ribosomal S12 protein (*rpsL*) and 16S ribosomal RNA;[58] for fluoroquinolones the mutation is in the DNA gyrase A gene (*gyrA*);[59] rifampicin resistance is due to point mutations in the *rpoB* gene in the RNA polymerase B subunit[60] and has allowed the development of a molecular probe to detect this resistance, which is a key component of MDR-TB (*see below*). Pyrazinamide resistance is due to mutations in the *pncA* gene.[61] Ethambutol resistance is due to mutations in the *embB* region, specifically codon 306.[62]

EPIDEMIOLOGY

Drug resistance is an increasing problem in developed countries because an increasing proportion of cases come from people originally infected in underdeveloped countries. For underdeveloped countries themselves problems are increasing because of economic and population pressures on TB control services, variable drug availability, inadequate programs and the difficulties of service delivery.[63] The incidence of drug resistance has to be differentiated into primary resistance (that found in previously untreated patients) and secondary or acquired resistance (that found in those with a history of treatment). Resistance to first-line antituberculosis drugs is found in all countries, with higher rates in underdeveloped countries, in parts of countries where there is economic collapse, or in certain populations (e.g. the Russian prison population[63]). Resistance rates to isoniazid of >5% are now common in most underdeveloped countries, and the drug resistance rates of minority ethnic groups in developed countries often follows that of their country of origin. Drug resistance data in the UK are monitored by Mycobnet, a section of the Public Health Laboratory Service Communicable Disease Surveillance Centre, which has monitored trends prospectively since 1993. The current levels of isoniazid resistance are 6% (HPA 2009) overall.[2] Risk factors for drug resistance include prior treatment, HIV infection and foreign birth. In the UK, the national treatment guidelines[24] have been designed with these factors in mind.

Combined resistance to rifampicin and isoniazid, with or without additional drug resistances (so-called MDR-TB), is a particular concern and is found worldwide. Certain countries (such as the Baltic republics, Russia, the Dominican Republic and Côte d'Ivoire) are 'hotspots' with an incidence greater than 5%.[63] MDR-TB occurred infrequently in England and Wales between 1982 and 1991, being found in only 0.6% of isolates.[64] It rose to nearly 2% in the early 1990s but fell to 1.3% in 2005,[63] representing approximately 50 cases, two-thirds of which occurred in Greater London. In England and Wales the risk factors for MDR-TB are those for drug resistance in general, but are even more pronounced:[65]

- Previous treatment 12.63 (OR 8.20–19.45)
- HIV infection 3.52 (OR 2.48–5.01)
- Age younger than 65 years 2.53 (OR 1.74–4.83)
- Foreign born 2.46 (OR 1.86–3.24)
- Male sex 1.38 (OR 1.16–1.65).

Clinical suspicion of acquired resistance should also be raised by failure of clinical response to treatment or by prolonged sputum smear or culture positivity, particularly at 3 months or later, while on treatment.

Now added to problems of drug resistance is the recognition of XDR-TB, brought to prominence by the Tugela Ferry outbreak,[66] which is now described in more than 45 countries.[67] Initially defined as high-level resistance to three or more of the six classes of reserve drugs,[68] in addition to rifampicin and isoniazid, this definition has been revised to resistance to quinolones and one injectable other than streptomycin (kanamycin, amikacin or capreomycin).[69]

Because of the rates of drug resistance, every effort should be made to obtain bacteriological confirmation of the diagnosis. In addition to proving the diagnosis, drug susceptibility information comes only from positive culture. Three sputum samples, obtained on separate mornings, should be sent for pulmonary cases. In patients unable to produce sputum, fibreoptic bronchoscopy and washings from the appropriate lung segment(s) has a good yield.[70] Pus obtained from neck glands and other sites, and fluid from serous sites (pleura, peritoneum and pericardium) should also be sent for culture. Surgeons performing biopsies on lesions in which tuberculosis is suspected should be reminded that half of the sample should be sent for TB culture without preservative such as formalin.[24]

A risk assessment, using the factors above, should be made for the likelihood of drug resistance in all cases. If concerns are raised as to the possibility of MDR-TB or XDR-TB, rapid molecular tests for rifampicin resistance are available on either sputum microscopy-positive or culture-positive material. These can be performed rapidly and are >95% accurate. If a test reports rifampicin resistance in a patient with *M. tuberculosis*, the patient should be managed as if he or she has M(X)DR-TB, pending the results of full susceptibility tests, as 'isolated' rifampicin resistance accounts for less than 10% of rifampicin resistance, and rifampicin resistance for MDR-TB in more than 90%. Separate isolation criteria are also advised for suspected or proven MDR-TB.[71,72]

TREATMENT OF DRUG-RESISTANT TUBERCULOSIS

Various short-course chemotherapy studies have allowed assessment of the efficacy of 'standard' chemotherapy in patients with prior initial drug resistance.[73] In these trials, patients with initial isoniazid and/or streptomycin resistance had a failure rate of 17% when given a 6-month regimen of rifampicin and isoniazid; the failure rate was 12% in those treated in the 2-month initial phase. As the number of drugs given in the regimen and the duration of rifampicin treatment increased, the failure rate fell, reaching only 2% of those receiving 4–5 drugs, including rifampicin throughout, in a 6-month regimen. The key exception was that of rifampicin resistance, where the outcome was much poorer.[73]

Such a policy is appropriate in underdeveloped countries where routine drug susceptibility data are not available, but in developed countries it is thought preferable to modify treatment on the basis of the drug resistance data.[24] The recommendations are set out below and summarized in Table 58.3.

 ## SINGLE DRUG RESISTANCE

Streptomycin

Some of the drug resistance encountered, particularly in ethnic minority groups, is to streptomycin alone. Streptomycin is now seldom used, and the efficacy of the regimen recommended for both pulmonary and non-pulmonary disease is not affected.

Isoniazid

If isoniazid resistance is known about before treatment, a regimen of rifampicin, pyrazinamide, ethambutol and streptomycin for 2 months, followed by rifampicin and ethambutol for

Table 58.3 Management of drug resistance in tuberculosis

Resistance	Non-MDR-TB regimen	Comment
Streptomycin	2RHZ(E)/4RH	Standard treatment unaffected
Isoniazid	2RZSE/7RE if known pretreatment 2RZE/7-10RE	Fully supervised (DOT)
Pyrazinamide	Usually *M. bovis* If had 2RHZE: stop ZE then 7RH If had 2RHZ: then 2RHE/7HR	
Ethambutol	2RHE/7HR	Standard treatment unaffected
Rifampicin	Uncommon: see text. Manage as MDR-TB until full susceptibilities known; if true: 2HZE/16HE	
Streptomycin/isoniazid	As for isoniazid resistance during treatment	Fully supervised (DOT)
Other combination	Individual regimen needed	See text

E, ethambutol; H, isoniazid; R, rifampicin; S, streptomycin; Z, pyrazinamide. The number in front of the letters represents the duration of treatment in months.

7 months, has given good results when fully supervised.[74] For the usual scenario of isoniazid resistance being reported after treatment has started, isoniazid should be stopped and ethambutol and rifampicin given for 12 months, supplemented by 2 months initial pyrazinamide.[24]

Pyrazinamide

See *Mycobacterium bovis* infection later (p. 758).

Ethambutol

This is uncommon; the standard regimen minus ethambutol (2RHZ/4HR) should be used.

Rifampicin

Isolated rifampicin resistance accounts for less than 10% of rifampicin resistance, 90% or more being due to M(X) DR-TB. Rifampicin resistance should be managed as for M(X)DR-TB until full first- and second-line susceptibilities are available. If true isolated rifampicin resistance is shown, a regimen of 18 months of ethambutol and isoniazid, supplemented by 2 months initial pyrazinamide, is recommended.[24]

COMBINED NON-MDR RESISTANCE

Streptomycin and isoniazid

This is the most common dual resistance. Management should be as for isoniazid resistance found after treatment commencement but fully supervised throughout.[24]

Other combinations

These are uncommon. An individualized regimen is required and should be discussed with an experienced clinician.

MDR-TB AND XDR-TB

Where MDR-TB is suspected, using the risk criteria set out earlier, molecular methods are available for rapid detection of rifampicin resistance using genetic probes on culture material[75] and increasingly on direct microscopy-positive samples.[76] Treatment is complex, time-consuming, demanding on both the physician and the patient, must be individually planned[77,78] and is likely to need the inclusion of reserve drugs (Table 58.4). There are also additional infection control measures required to prevent nosocomial outbreaks.[71,72] Such treatment should be carried out only in the following circumstances:

- The physician has substantial experience in managing complex resistant cases
- Only in a hospital with appropriate isolation facilities
- In close liaison with the appropriate mycobacteriology service.

Table 58.4 Reserve drugs that may be needed for multidrug-resistant tuberculosis

Injectable	Tablet
Streptomycin	Ciprofloxacin, ofloxacin, levofloxacin, gatifloxacin, moxifloxacin
Amikacin	Ethionamide or prothionamide
Kanamycin	Clarithromycin or azithromycin
Capreomycin, linezolid, meropenem/co-amoxiclav	Cycloserine, rifabutin, thiacetazone, PAS sodium, clofazimine
PAS, *p*-aminosalicylic acid.	

For this to happen, the patient may need to be transferred to an appropriate unit. All treatment, both as an inpatient and as an outpatient, must be closely monitored because of increased toxicity, and must be directly observed throughout to prevent the emergence of further drug resistance. Consideration may also need to be given to resection of pulmonary lesions under drug cover.[79] Criteria for removal from isolation have been set out.[71,72]

The principles of treating such patients are to start treatment with five or more drugs to which the organism is (or is likely to be) susceptible, including one injectable if possible, and to continue these until cultures become negative. Drug treatment should then be continued with at least three drugs to which the organism is susceptible on in-vitro testing for a further minimum of 9 months. This may extend up to or beyond 24 months depending on the drug susceptibility profile, which drugs are available, and the patient's HIV status.[78]

MYCOBACTERIUM BOVIS

Infection with *M. bovis* cannot be differentiated clinically from *M. tuberculosis* infection, and can only be diagnosed on culture. In the UK, only some 40 cases per year are diagnosed, now accounting for less than 1% of bacteriologically confirmed *M. tuberculosis* complex cases.[2] Of 210 isolates reported, 200 were in patients of White ethnic origin, of whom over three-quarters were aged over 50 years, suggesting reactivation of disease acquired earlier in life.[80] Commercial molecular DNA- or RNA-based tests cannot differentiate between *M. bovis* and *M. tuberculosis*, emphasizing the role of culture. Non-commercial molecular methods exist for the identification of *M. bovis*, such as identification of mutations of the *pncA* gene.[81]

The main difference between *M. bovis* and *M. tuberculosis* is the presence of pyrazinamide resistance in the former. This influences recommended drug regimens because the inclusion of pyrazinamide is required for an effective 6-month regimen and is nullified by the presence of pyrazinamide resistance. If a four-drug initial phase has been given, then a 7-month continuation phase of rifampicin and isoniazid can be used (*see* Table 58.3).[24] Once the diagnosis has been made, the pyrazinamide should be stopped, 9 months of rifampicin and isoniazid given, supplemented by 2 months initial ethambutol (*see* Table 58.3).[24] If against national guidance a person has had only a three-drug initial regimen (2RHZ), then 2RHE/7HR will need to be given from that point.

Contact tracing of human contacts of human *M. bovis* disease should follow the recommendations given for human contacts of *M. tuberculosis*.[24] Where studies of human contacts of cattle with *M. bovis* disease have been undertaken, little evidence of transmission (as judged by tuberculin testing and no evidence of disease) has been found.[82] Recent advice on contact tracing of human contacts of cattle, largely based on first principles, has been published.[24]

BCG

Bacille Calmette-Guérin (BCG) is an attenuated strain of *M. bovis* and is therefore pyrazinamide resistant. There are differences between the UK[24,72] and the USA[26] in its use, with the USA putting a much lower emphasis on its use and efficacy. In the UK, BCG was advocated in unvaccinated children aged 10–13 years and in anyone thought to be at higher risk[72] such as:

- previously unvaccinated tuberculin-negative household contacts of pulmonary disease
- tuberculin-negative unvaccinated new immigrants from high-prevalence countries
- neonates of African–Asian ethnic origin
- tuberculin-negative previously unvaccinated healthcare workers.

The UK unselective BCG vaccination program for those aged 10–13 years stopped in 2005 following review by the Joint Committee on Vaccination and Immunisation and later supported by NICE,[24] whose economic appraisals showed it to be grossly uneconomic, either as a vaccination, even with a 15-year protective efficacy, or as a safety net vaccination system for those high-risk individuals who had missed prior BCG.[24]

The complications of BCG vaccination are local abscess and ulceration at the vaccination site and local lymph node disease. Complications are almost always due to faulty vaccination technique, with subcutaneous rather than intradermal administration. These may resolve spontaneously but over a prolonged period.

Antibiotic therapy with isoniazid,[83] rifampicin and isoniazid, and macrolides[84] have all been advocated. Surgical removal of regional nodes is rarely required. Disseminated BCG infection after vaccination is rare, but occurs in people with immune deficiency and has been reported in HIV infection. Prospective studies, however, have so far failed to show increased complications overall in asymptomatic neonates, and at the moment the WHO still recommends vaccination in developing countries for all neonates unless they have clinical evidence of AIDS.

Instillation of BCG into the bladder has been found to be very effective in the management of transitional cell carcinoma.

Complications can occur, with mycobacterial dissemination, and focal forms of disease localized to both the urinary tract and other sites.[85] These complications require treatment as for *M. bovis* because of the pyrazinamide resistance (*see* Table 58.3).

DELIVERY OF THERAPY

Adherence is the major determinant of outcome in treating tuberculosis,[86] both the compliance of the patient in taking medication as prescribed and the compliance of the physician in prescribing the correct regimen and monitoring it. Respiratory physicians are more likely to prescribe the standard chemotherapy than other clinicians, and drug reactions are more common with non-standard regimens.[87,88] In the UK it is advised that only physicians with full training and expertise in managing tuberculosis, and who have direct working access to TB nurses or health visitors, should manage respiratory tuberculosis.[24] It is further recommended that they also manage the drug treatment of non-respiratory tuberculosis, and manage children jointly with a general pediatrician, unless they are a specialist infectious disease pediatrician trained in tuberculosis.[24]

Tuberculosis cases should be managed by a team as part of a district policy that covers all aspects of management, including notification of disease to the proper authorities, chemotherapy, compliance and contact tracing.[89] A minimum of one full-time TB nurse or health visitor plus full clerical support is recommended for every 50 notifications per annum per district,[50] with a higher ratio of staff if there are significant numbers of 'hard to reach' individuals.

ADHERENCE MOTORING

Monitoring patient adherence with medication is a vital part of management, and is carried out by TB nurses or health visitors, together with checking on the accuracy and continuity of prescribing. An assessment of the likelihood of adherence should be made for all patients at the onset of treatment.[24] For patients not on directly observed therapy (DOT; *see below*) tablet checks and urine tests for rifampicin should be carried out at least monthly throughout chemotherapy. If non-compliance is detected in patients being allowed self-administered therapy, they should be switched to supervised (DOT) therapy, and an assessment made of the possibility of acquired drug resistance. This may require repeat cultures and susceptibility tests, and consideration of molecular tests for rifampicin resistance.

COMBINATION TABLETS

Combination tablets are extremely useful in patients taking daily therapy and prevent the deliberate or accidental consumption of a single drug, which in active disease can very easily lead to acquired drug resistance. They have the further advantage that compliance can be checked by using the orange/pink coloration of urine of the rifampicin component, which can be inspected for either visually or in the laboratory. Rifater (Hoechst Marion Roussel), for use in the initial phase of treatment, contains rifampicin, isoniazid and pyrazinamide, and Rifinah (Hoechst Marion Roussel) combine rifampicin and isoniazid for use in the continuation phase. In some studies of combined preparations, the dosages of isoniazid, rifampicin and pyrazinamide[90,91] have varied slightly from those in Rifater currently available in the UK (isoniazid 50 mg, rifampicin 120 mg, pyrazinamide 300 mg). The bioavailability of the drugs in combination tablets is similar to that of the same doses given individually,[90] and gives satisfactory clinical results.[91] The slight variations in dosage are therefore not thought to be important in combined preparations of proven bioavailability. Because of the similarity in name (rifampicin, Rifinah, Rimactazid, Rifadin, Rimifon and Rifater), care must be taken in writing and dispensing prescriptions. Care is also needed with computer-generated prescribing, because if the system does not recognize the name it may default to rifampicin alone, leading to monotherapy.

For the above reasons, for patients on daily therapy in the UK, combination tablets are recommended to aid compliance and to prevent monotherapy.[24]

PRETREATMENT SCREENING

Liver function should be checked before treatment of clinical cases: modest elevations of the hepatic transaminases (ALT/AST) are not uncommon in the pretreatment liver function tests of people with TB. Detailed advice on the monitoring of liver function and hepatotoxicity is available.[92]

Renal function should be checked before treatment with either streptomycin or ethambutol. If possible these drugs should be avoided in renal failure, but if their use is required serum concentrations should be monitored and substantial dosage reductions made unless dialysis is used.[24] Because of its rare, but possible, toxic effects on the optic nerve, visual acuity should be tested using a Snellen chart before ethambutol is given.[93] Patients should have reasonable visual acuity and ideally be able to report symptoms, although the use of ethambutol in children appears to be safe.[55] A patient should be told to stop the drug immediately if symptoms occur and report to the physician, and this should be documented. In those with language difficulties or in small children this advice should be given to carers and family members. With increasing evidence to support the use of third-generation quinolones (moxifloxacin and gatifloxacin) in TB from data from trials in Africa (*see later*), some clinicians are substituting moxifloxacin for ethambutol, where either renal or visual impairment makes the use of ethambutol as the fourth drug in the initial phase problematic. Such use, however, has not yet reached national/international guidance.[24–27]

DIRECTLY OBSERVED THERAPY

Concerns about patient adherence, its effects on relapse and the development of drug resistance, has lead to the WHO advocating directly observed therapy (DOT) in the form of short-course chemotherapy or DOTS. With this method of treatment, the ingestion of every dose is monitored by a nursing or lay observer. DOT can be given daily but an intermittent regimen, with appropriate dosage adjustments, is often more convenient as doses can be scheduled to avoid weekends. A regimen of rifampicin, isoniazid, pyrazinamide and either ethambutol or streptomycin thrice weekly for 2 months, followed by thrice-weekly rifampicin and isoniazid for a further 4 months, is advised in the UK.[24,50]

The strategy of universal DOT, although strongly advocated by the WHO[93] and bodies such as the International Union against Tuberculosis and Lung Diseases,[94] has not been tested by randomized controlled studies. Cohort studies against historical control groups receiving self-administered therapy in different countries have shown DOT to improve outcomes (e.g. cure rates).[95–97] Decision analyses have also suggested that both selective and universal DOT strategies are more cost-effective than conventional self-administered therapy.[98–100] However, when DOT was compared in a controlled way directly with self-administration it actually performed less well overall, although subgroups had differing results.[101] Critics of universal DOT, which they call 'supervised pill swallowing', say that the success of DOT programs is derived from the substantial financial and technical investment in tuberculosis programs that DOT represents and not the DOT element itself.[102] Even in the USA there have been dissenting analyses of DOT effectiveness.[103]

Authors who admitted initial prejudice in favor of DOT conceded that treatment completion rates of over 90% could be obtained with a much lower proportion of DOT than that proposed by the advocates of universal DOT.[103] The US Centers for Disease Control and Prevention (CDC) recommend that DOT treatment should be considered for all patients, but that if more than 90% of the patients in an area are completing self-administered therapy, selective DOT in unreliable patients is an alternative.[104]

In the UK, where tuberculosis is (or should be) treated by experienced physicians working in direct conjunction with tuberculosis nurses or health visitors[24] and as part of a district plan,[72,90] DOT is recommended for selective use in people with an adverse adherence assessment. This includes patients who are homeless, alcohol or other drug abusers, vagrants, seriously mentally ill, patients with multiple drug resistances and those with any history of non-compliance with antituberculosis medication, either previously or shown during treatment monitoring.[24,72]

NOTIFICATION AND CONTACT TRACING

All cases of tuberculosis, whether respiratory or non-respiratory, should be notified to the proper authorities. The purpose of notification is two-fold:

1. It allows proper epidemiological data to be collected and outbreaks detected, so that treatment services can be planned and monitored.
2. Contact tracing procedures are activated by notification, and so it is essential that all cases, including active cases diagnosed after death, are notified.

Failure to notify could lead to failure to screen appropriate close contacts, which could result in contacts requiring treatment for active disease, or those eligible for BCG vaccination or chemoprophylaxis being denied the appropriate intervention. Detailed guidance, recently updated, is available in the UK.[24] The emphasis on aspects of contact tracing in the UK, where BCG vaccination is more widely advised,[24] is different from that in the USA, where there is greater emphasis on chemoprophylaxis (*see below*) and less on BCG vaccination.[26]

TUBERCULOSIS IN HIV-POSITIVE PATIENTS

The incidence of tuberculosis in HIV-positive individuals is much higher than in those who are HIV negative,[24] and the mortality rate in such patients is also higher.[1] The classic type of tuberculosis with upper zone pulmonary disease tends to occur less commonly in patients as the CD4 lymphocyte count declines. In this context patients are more likely to have non-cavitatory disease, or mediastinal lymphadenopathy, disseminated disease, to be sputum smear-microscopy negative or even have a normal chest X-ray.[105,106] A high index of suspicion for TB needs to be maintained in symptomatic HIV-positive individuals, especially in those born in high TB prevalence settings.

Although small studies have suggested that standard 2RHZE/4RH regimens, particularly if adequately supervised, are equally effective in HIV-positive and HIV-negative patients,[107] there have been no controlled trials of adequate power in HIV-positive patients to show differences of efficacy between regimens. As HIV-positive individuals have the same drug resistance rates as the population that they come from, the four-drug initial phase should always be used, unless there are risk factors for MDR-TB (*see above*). If cultures remain positive at 3 months in HIV-positive patients, compliance and drug absorption should be assessed in detail.

In patients with dual infection there is no doubt that the priority is to treat the tuberculosis, especially in sputum smear-positive cases where there is also a public health element. TB treatment is also important in reversing the potentially deleterious effects of tuberculosis on the progress of the HIV infection suggested by in-vitro and in-vivo studies.[108] The treatment of TB in HIV-positive patients is becoming more complex because of:

- increased drug reactions to both TB drugs and highly active antiretroviral drugs in such patients
- a move to earlier treatment of HIV-positive individuals with HAART, at higher CD4 counts for the initiation of treatment, and an increasing number of drug treatment options[109]

- drug–drug interactions with TB drugs, HAART and other drugs, e.g. conazoles, particularly due to rifampicin interactions.[110]

These will be discussed briefly here and in Table 58.5; however, the complexities, with particular emphasis on drug interactions, are set out fully in reference 110:

1. Reactions to antituberculosis drugs are more common in HIV-positive individuals, in whom severe adverse reactions can occur to any drug. This has been the case particularly with thiacetazone, causing Stevens–Johnson syndrome in 10%, with a 10% mortality, leading to its withdrawal from routine use in Africa.[111,112]
2. The range of anti-HIV drugs is widening all the time. These now include:
   a. nucleoside reverse transcriptase inhibitors (NRTIs): abacavir, enteric-coated didanosine, emtricitabine, lamivudine, stavudine, tenofovir, zidovudine
   b. non-nucleoside reverse transcriptase inhibitors (NNRTIs): efavirenz, nevirapine, etravirine, TMC-278
   c. protease inhibitors (PIs), including boosted combinations with low-dose ritonavir: amprenavir, atazanavir, atazanavir–ritonavir, darunavir–ritonavir, fosamprenavir, fosamprenavir–ritonavir, indinavir, lopinavir–ritonavir, nelfinavir, ritonavir, saquinavir, saquinavir–ritonavir, tipranavir–ritonavir
   d. integrase inhibitors and entry inhibitors: elvitegravir, raltegravir, maraviroc, enfuvirtide (T-20).
3. Important drug interactions occur. Ketoconazole can inhibit rifampicin absorption if given at the same time, which could lead to TB treatment failure.[113] Rifampicin and isoniazid interact with the azole antifungal drugs, reducing serum concentrations of flu- and itraconazoles to suboptimal levels.[113–115] The most important area, however, is the interaction with rifampicin, the current key sterilizing drug in TB regimens, which is a potent inducer of the CYP3A P_{450} enzyme through which the PIs, NNRTIs and some other anti-HIV drugs are metabolized (Table 58.5). As a general rule, rifampicin can be used with all NRTIs and with efavirenz (with an increased dose of efavirenz), but not with other NNRTIs. Rifampicin cannot be used with PIs (single or boosted) or with integrase inhibitors, but can be used with T20 inhibitors and with maraviroc (doubled dose of maraviroc). Rifabutin in reduced dosage can be used with most PIs (except saquinavir).

The data to support rifabutin-containing regimens, as opposed to rifampicin-containing regimens, for TB are weak. If at all possible a 6-month rifampicin-based regimen should be used.[110] Treatment supervised for 5 days per week with conventional dosages, including at least 56 doses of pyrazinamide and 182 doses of rifampicin–isoniazid, is thought to be adequate.[110] Prolongation of the rifampicin–isoniazid continuation phase to 9 months is needed in HIV-positive individuals if there is pyrazinamide intolerance, and should be considered for those still culture-positive for *M. tuberculosis* after 2 months' treatment.[110] If rifamycins cannot be tolerated for

Table 58.5 Drug interactions between TB and antiretroviral drugs

Antiretroviral drug/class	Rifampicin	Rifabutin	Clarithromycin
Nucleoside reverse transcriptase inhibitors (NRTIs)			
	No interaction	No interaction	No interaction
	Dose as normal	Dose as normal	Dose as normal
Non-nucleoside reverse transcriptase inhibitors (NNRTIs)			
Efavirenz	Rifampicin standard dose Efavirenz 800 mg if >50 kg, 600 mg if ≤50 kg	Rifabutin 450 mg Efavirenz standard	No interaction Dose as normal
Nevirapine	Do not use	Few data, do not use	Dose as normal
Etravirine	Do not use	Few data, do not use	
TMC-278	Do not use	Double dose TMC-278	
Protease inhibitors (PIs), including boosted			
	Do not use	Some but not all can be used with reduced rifabutin dose (see ref. 111)	Dose as normal
Integrase inhibitors and entry inhibitors			
Elvitegravir/raltegravir	Do not use	No data	
Maraviroc	Double maraviroc dose	No data	
Enfuvirtide	Dose both as normal	Dose both as normal	

some reason, HIV-related TB can be treated with a non-rifamycin-containing regimen; however, this strategy has an inferior efficacy with high relapse rates[116,117] and should only be contemplated in patients with serious toxicity to rifamycins, and where desensitization or reintroduction has failed, or in those with rifamycin-resistant isolates.

Because of the complexities of managing such dually infected patients, detailed liaison between the TB and HIV services is needed, and drug levels of both antituberculosis and antiretroviral drugs may need monitoring. A detailed view on the complexities, with particular emphasis on drug interactions, is found in reference 110 (*see also* Ch. 6).

NEW TRIALS AND NEW DRUGS IN DEVELOPMENT

A 6-month regimen of rifampicin and isoniazid, supplemented by an initial 2 months of pyrazinamide and ethambutol, remains the 'gold standard' treatment.[24–27] It does, however, have unacceptably high relapse rates, at least by developed country standards, if the regimen is shortened in duration,[118] certainly for smear- and culture-positive disease. Moxifloxacin is highly active against *M. tuberculosis*, with activity equivalent to that of isoniazid[119] and early bactericidal activity exceeding that of isoniazid between days 2 and 7 of therapy.[120] These data and data on the murine model, showing that substitution of moxifloxacin for isoniazid, dramatically increasing sterilizing activity and allowing a 4-month regimen,[121] have led to the

potential role of it and other third-generation quinolones in shortening treatment duration coming under extensive investigation. Three phase IIb studies have now reported. The IIb study reported in 2006 only showed equivalence to ethambutol in the sterilizing ability of the regimen over 2 months[122] using the usual 2-month culture conversion method. A more recent analysis of the phase II Oflotub study data,[123] however, showed that the two newer fluoroquinolones, moxifloxacin and gatifloxacin, may have the ability to potentially shorten the duration of therapy to 4 months. This study also showed that serial sputum colony counts and the time to culture conversion have the potential to be quantitative predictive 'endpoints' in phase II trials of the newer antituberculosis medications (*see below*).[123] The most recent to report[124] from Brazil also showed superiority in culture conversion rates for the moxifloxacin-containing regimen.

Two phase III studies are underway to test the regimen shortening potential of moxifloxacin and gatifloxacin. These are actively recruiting in Africa and are soon to be expanded to other sites. The Oflotub study by the WHO[125] is comparing standard 6-month short course chemotherapy (2RHZE/4RH) with a 4-month regimen of rifampicin, isoniazid and gatifloxacin, supplemented with 2 months initial pyrazinamide (2RHZGati/2RHGati). This study of 1836 patients should have completed treatment by summer 2009, and report the 1-year outcome in mid-2010. The REMOX study[126] is comparing standard treatment (2RHZE/4RH) with a 6-month regimen substituting moxifloxacin for ethambutol (2RHZMoxi/4RH), and a further 4-month regimen of rifampicin, isoniazid and moxifloxacin, supplemented by 2 months initial pyrazinamide (2RHZMoxi/2HRMoxi). This is actively recruiting in multiple sites in Africa, with further sites being added.

Other novel agents are under development, some of which will shortly come to phase II and possibly phase III studies. These include the following:

- PA-824 (TB Alliance/Chiron) is a nitroimidazopyran that inhibits the synthesis of proteins and cell-wall lipids. This drug has a narrow spectrum of activity, no cross-resistance with current antituberculosis drugs and a unique mechanism of action. It has bactericidal activity against both replicating and static organisms,[127] and has good sterilizing activity.[128] It is currently in phase II testing.[129]
- OPC-67683 (Otsuka) is a further nitroimino-oxazole that has advanced to phase II testing. Cross-resistance with PA-824 is anticipated, but it may be up to 20 times more potent.[130] Preliminary data from the murine model suggest that substituting OPC-67683 for isoniazid in the standard treatment regimen resulted in greater activity and more rapid culture conversion.[130]
- TMC207 (Tibotec) is a diarylquinoline (previously R207910) that selectively inhibits mycobacterial F1F0 ATP synthetase. This is a new class of drug, without cross-resistance with other classes of antituberculosis drugs. TMC207 has time-dependent bactericidal activity in vivo and in vitro, and substitution for any of the three main first-line drugs increases potency. It has a particularly impressive synergy with pyrazinamide.[131] Although well absorbed orally, one potential drawback is that it has a drug–drug interaction with rifampicin which reduces the bioavailability of TMC207 by 50%.[132]
- Diamine SQ109 (Sequella) is a novel 1,2-ethylenediamine ethambutol analog that acts on cell-wall inhibition by a yet to be understood mechanism. In vitro it has activity against rifampicin- and isoniazid-resistant isolates, demonstrates synergy with isoniazid and rifampicin, and has a high sterilizing activity in the mouse model, with drug levels in the lungs and spleen exceeding the minimum inhibitory concentration.[133] It is currently in phase I testing.
- Pyrrole LL-3858 Sudoterb (Lupin) is a substituted pyrrole; early data suggest activity against both susceptible and MDR strains.[134] In the mouse model, used as a single drug it is bactericidal, and in combination significantly enhances the sterilizing ability of the standard RHZ regimen.[134] Less information is available than for some other drugs due to commercial considerations, but this drug is also in phase I testing.

These, and the other drugs which may follow them,[129] will need a series of controlled clinical trials, such as were done a generation ago by the British Medical Research Council[118] to establish the best regimens, durations and combinations. Their use will have to be strictly limited to such trials to prevent indiscriminate or uncontrolled use which could lead to an even worse version of XDR-TB emerging, until their utility and roles are established. The more recent data from the Oflotub study may give us additional 'endpoints' to monitor.[123]

TREATMENT OF LATENT TB INFECTION, FORMERLY KNOWN AS CHEMOPROPHYLAXIS

PRINCIPLES

A proportion of people with tuberculosis infection, as judged by a positive tuberculin skin reaction or now confirmed by an interferon-γ release assay (IGRA), are thought to have a small number of dormant bacilli, perhaps in the order of 10^3 or 10^4. The administration of one or two drugs for a shorter period of time than for disease – chemoprophylaxis or preventive therapy – is likely to kill these organisms and hence reduce the chance of progression to disease. It is therefore very important to differentiate between disease and infection:

- In tuberculosis infection, the tuberculin skin test (and IGRA test if available) is positive, the chest radiography is normal, and the patient is asymptomatic and has no clinical findings.
- In tuberculosis disease, the skin test is usually positive and there are clinical signs and symptoms or radiographic changes present. (*Note*: neither commercially available IGRA test is currently licensed for use in diagnosis.)

This matter is further complicated in HIV-positive individuals, where anergy to tuberculin does not necessarily mean tuberculosis infection has not occurred, and it becomes difficult to differentiate between disease and infection. Most latent TB infection (LTBI) treatment is secondary (i.e. after infection, as judged by a positive tuberculin test or IGRA, has occurred). Occasionally it may be given before evidence of infection, to prevent infection occurring (e.g. in the neonate of a sputum smear-positive mother); this is primary chemoprophylaxis.

REGIMENS

Although multiple drug regimens are required for the treatment of disease in order to prevent the emergence of drug resistance, it is not illogical to use a one- or two-drug regimen for prophylaxis. Individuals who are receiving chemoprophylaxis are thought to have a low organism burden, in the order of 10^3 to 10^4. The chance of spontaneous resistance developing to a single drug is in the order of 10^{-5} to 10^{-7}. The chance of drug resistance developing is therefore very low, particularly if a two-drug regimen is used. For instance, when mass isoniazid chemoprophylaxis was given to Inuit communities there was no increase in isoniazid-resistant disease.[135]

Many randomized placebo-controlled trials of isoniazid chemoprophylaxis have been conducted.[136] Alaskan studies showed that the maximal effect was achieved by durations up to 12 months and that there was no additional benefit from more extended treatment.[137] Where the rate of new infection was low, protection lasted for more than 15 years.[138] A multicenter study by the International Union against Tuberculosis and Lung Disease (IUATLD)[139] showed that for small radiographic lesions (<2 cm) 6 months of treatment with isoniazid was just as effective as 12 months, and for larger lesions (>2 cm) 6 months of isoniazid provided considerable protection. A later meta-analysis of 77 000 persons, in 11 different placebo-controlled studies (including reference 139), however, clearly shows no additional protective efficacy with isoniazid durations of over 6 months, only increased toxicity.[140]

As with chemotherapy for disease, compliance with therapy is important, particularly because individuals on chemoprophylaxis are clinically well and so have less incentive to complete medication: the Alaskan studies also showed that to obtain the full benefit from chemoprophylaxis, more than 60% of treatment must be taken.[137] There is also concern about increased isoniazid hepatotoxicity for durations over 6 months. In the later US Public Health Service studies the probable isoniazid hepatitis rate was approximately 1%.[136] There was, however, a clear relationship with age: no cases under 30 years, rising to 2.3% in patients over 50 years. The hepatitis rate was lower in the IUATLD trial[139] at 0.27% for 6H and 0.52% for 12H, but was still higher than the rate of 0.1% in the placebo-treated group.[139]

These concerns have led to a search for alternative and shorter regimens. Rifampicin has been shown to have a greater sterilizing effect in animal studies,[141] either alone or with pyrazinamide, than has isoniazid. A placebo-controlled prophylaxis study from Hong Kong in patients with silicosis suggested that rifampicin alone for 3 months had similar efficacy to rifampicin and isoniazid for 3 months or isoniazid alone for 6 months.[142] In UK studies the use of rifampicin and isoniazid combined for 3 months showed a significant decrease in childhood tuberculosis.[143,144] Using these data, and others from experimental studies, the American Thoracic Society/CDC recommended a regimen of rifampicin and pyrazinamide for 2 months (2RZ) rather than isoniazid alone for 6 months.[145] The predictable toxicity of the 2RZ regimen[72] led to severe hepatotoxic reactions and fatalities[146] and the withdrawal of this recommendation.[147]

In the USA either rifampicin for 4 months (4R) or isoniazid for 9 months (9H) is now recommended,[146] despite the meta-analysis on isoniazid preventive therapy showing no additional benefit of regimens longer than 6 months, only increased toxicity,[140] and there being no controlled trial data to support 4R. In the UK, either 6H or 3RH is recommended,[24] both having 'A' category data or SIGN 1+[148] evidence to support their use. There is also evidence to support 6R for contacts of isoniazid-resistant disease[149,150] and is recommended for this category in the UK.[24,72]

IN HIV-NEGATIVE PERSONS

In the UK, where there is greater emphasis on BCG, and where prior BCG vaccination modifies the tuberculin response, the following groups are recommended for consideration of treatment for LTBI, based on either incidence of active TB in persons with a positive tuberculin test or from selected clinical conditions (Box 58.1)[24] and for certain conditions with a high relative risk of tuberculosis (Box 58.2).

Treatment of LTBI should be offered in the following settings:

- Neonates of mothers with sputum-smear positive TB as a primary measure until shown to be tuberculin negative at age 6–8 weeks.
- Children aged between 4 weeks and 2 years of age in contact with sputum smear-positive TB, either as a primary measure (no prior BCG) or if inappropriately tuberculin positive (prior BCG).
- TB contacts aged up to 35 years with an inappropriately positive Mantoux test confirmed by a positive IGRA test.
- New entrants aged under 16 years from countries with a TB prevalence of 40/100 000 per annum or greater with a positive Mantoux test confirmed by a positive IGRA test.
- New entrants aged 16–35 years from sub-Saharan Africa, or countries with a TB rate of 500/100 000 per annum or greater, with a positive Mantoux test confirmed by a positive IGRA test.

Persons for whom chemoprophylaxis is recommended, but who do not receive it or decline to take it, should have radiographic follow-up at 3 and 12 months.[67]

Box 58.1 Consideration for treatment of LTBI in selected clinical conditions

	TB cases/10 000 person years
HIV infection	35–162
Intravenous drug use	10–76
Silicosis	68
Recent latent TB infection	1.6–12.9
Chest X-ray changes consistent with prior TB	2.0–13.6

Box 58.2 Consideration for treatment of LTBI in conditions with a high relative risk of tuberculosis

	Relative risk
Solid organ transplant (renal)	37
Solid organ transplant (heart)	20–74
Jejunoileal bypass	27–63
Silicosis	30
Chronic renal failure/hemodialysis	10–25.3
Gastrectomy	2.5
Diabetes mellitus	2–41
Anti-tumor necrosis factor-α treatment	4–8
Contact smear-positive TB	5–10

In the USA, preventive therapy with a positive tuberculin reaction[26] (>5 mm in persons with HIV infection, close contact of infectious disease and with fibrotic X-ray lesions; >10 mm in other at-risk persons, including infants and children younger than 4 years; and >15 mm in low-risk populations) is recommended for the following groups:

1. Close contacts of persons with newly diagnosed infectious tuberculosis.
2. Recent tuberculin skin test converters (defined as a 10 mm or greater increase within a 2-year period for those <35 years of age, and 15 mm or greater increase for those >35 years).
3. Persons with medical conditions that have been reported to increase the risk of tuberculosis:
   a. diabetes mellitus
   b. prolonged therapy with adrenocorticosteroids
   c. immunosuppressive therapy
   d. some hematological and reticuloendothelial diseases
   e. intravenous drug users known to be HIV negative
   f. end-stage renal disease
   g. clinical situations associated with substantial rapid weight loss or chronic undernutrition.
4. People under 35 years with a tuberculin test >10 mm, even in the absence of the above risk categories, if:
   a. foreign born from high-prevalence countries
   b. from medically under-served low-income populations, including high-risk racial or ethnic minority populations
   c. resident of a long-term care facility.

In the USA, the use of an IGRA test (QuantiFERON-TB Gold) is now recommended as a one-step test for screening for LTBI, rather than tuberculin testing.[151]

 ## IN HIV-POSITIVE PERSONS

The identification of individuals at high risk of developing tuberculosis in HIV infection is complicated by loss of response to tuberculin, and to some extent IGRA tests, and also the atypical radiological changes. Such therapy was recommended by the WHO and IUATLD.[152] When this policy has been examined in developing countries, short-term benefits have been shown but there are also logistical difficulties in implementing such a policy.[153,154] A more recent study in the USA did not support isoniazid prophylaxis in high-risk patients with anergy unless they had been exposed to active tuberculosis.[155]

For the above reasons, and because of concerns about the higher rates of drug resistance in HIV-infected persons in the UK, chemoprophylaxis in HIV-positive individuals is recommended only in contacts of sputum smear-positive pulmonary disease[24,110] and to be considered in others with HIV. Isoniazid treatment[111] is no longer recommended for people treated for TB disease after completion of chemotherapy.[42,110] In the USA[26] LTBI treatment for a tuberculin test of 5 mm (or a positive IGRA test) is advised in HIV-positive individuals as

it is thought that such patients have a high annual rate of disease.[156] It may also be considered for HIV-infected persons who are tuberculin negative but belong to groups in which the prevalence of tuberculosis infection is high.

 ## FOR MULTIDRUG-RESISTANT TUBERCULOSIS

There are no data on what preventive regimen is feasible in persons in contact with MDR-TB. Any LTBI regimen should include two (and ideally three) drugs to which the organism is known to be susceptible, although the resistance pattern can be so extensive that no preventive regimen is available. If the drug susceptibility pattern is not known then ofloxacin or ciprofloxacin with pyrazinamide might be effective.[157] The CDC suggest this combination, or ethambutol and pyrazinamide.[158]

The view in the UK is that, since only a minority of people infected with tuberculosis develop clinical disease, and because there are no data on which to base advice, long-term regular follow-up of individual cases is currently advised.[24]

OPPORTUNIST (NON-TUBERCULOUS) MYCOBACTERIA

Isolates of opportunist mycobacteria – also called atypical mycobacteria, mycobacteria other than tuberculosis (MOTT), non-tuberculous mycobacteria (NTM) or environmental mycobacteria – are increasing. Although this may be related to an increasing incidence, there has been a very significant rise in the isolation of rapidly growing mycobacteria (RGM), e.g. *M. chelonae*, *M. gordonae* and *M. abscessus*, with the increasing use of liquid culture, with its greater sensitivity, but many of these isolates appear to be commensal, rather than associated with clinical disease. NTM are ubiquitous in the environment and the significance of an isolate can be established only by considering the specimen type from which the organism was isolated, the number of isolates, the degree of growth and the species of *Mycobacterium*. In general, in non-sterile sites, multiple isolates are required to establish disease, whereas one positive culture from a sterile site, particularly if supported by histopathology, is usually sufficient.[159,160]

The management of opportunistic organisms was reviewed by the Joint Tuberculosis Committee of the British Thoracic Society (BTS) in 1999, and guidelines on their management produced,[159] although these are much less based on controlled trials than is the case for tuberculosis. The 5-year follow-up results of controlled trials in *M. avium intracellulare* (MAC), *M. malmoense* and *M. xenopi* with both quinolone- and macrolide-containing regimens have also recently been published.[161] Guidelines from the USA are much more recently updated.[160] These, and the earlier BTS advice, modified by reference 161, are summarized in Table 58.6, but for detailed recommendations the original references should be consulted.

Table 58.6 Treatment of opportunist mycobacteria[159–161]

Organism	Situation	UK advice	USA advice
HIV-negative			
Any	Cervical nodes in children	Excision	Excision
M. kansasii	Adult pulmonary disease	9RE; 15–24RE if recurrent	HR + E 15 mg/kg until culture negative for 1 year
M. avium intracellulare (MAC)	Adult pulmonary disease	24RHCipro/Clari or 24RHE	Clari/R/E 25 mg/kg three times weekly or daily Clari/R/E 15 mg/kg ± other until culture negative for 12 months (see text)
M. malmoense	Adult pulmonary disease	24RHCipro/Clari or 24RHE	Not covered
M. xenopi	Adult pulmonary disease	24RHCipro/Clari or 24RHE	Not covered
M. kansasii	Non-pulmonary disease	9RE initially; add macrolide or streptomycin/prothionamide depending on response	As for pulmonary disease
MAC	Non-pulmonary disease	24REClari	Excision/debridement + drugs as for adult pulmonary disease
M. malmoense	Non-pulmonary disease	24REClari	RHE ± Clari, quinolones Duration unspecified
M. xenopi	Non-pulmonary disease	24REClari	HEClariR or rifabutin ± initial streptomycin
Rapid growing organisms			
M. abscessus and other rapid growers	Disease	Pulmonary: resect if possible under drug cover. Use REClari; consider other drugs Non-pulmonary: wound debridement; Cipro/Clari, plus aminoglycoside or imipenem	Pulmonary: resect if possible under multidrug cover including Clari Non-pulmonary: surgical debridement; Clari-based treatment for 4–6 months Clari/amikacin + initial cefoxitin
M. fortuitum	Disease	As M. abscessus	Complex; see ref. 160
M. chelonae/gordonae	Disease	As M. abscessus	Complex; see ref. 160
M. marinum	Skin	Co-trimoxazole; tetracycline; R/E until resolved	Clari/ethambutol until resolved, then 2 months. Add rifampicin if deep structures involved
HIV-positive			
MAC	Treatment	HAART + 24R(Rifabutin)EClari	Clari/Azithro + E ± rifabutin until resolution of symptoms and reconstitution of cell-mediated immunity
MAC	Prophylaxis	1st Azithro 1200 mg/week 2nd Clari 500 mg every 12 h 3rd Azithro 1200 mg/week + rifabutin 300 mg/day	Azithro 1200 mg/week or Clari 1000 mg/day if CD4 below 50/mL. Rifabutin 300 mg/day effective but less well tolerated
M. kansasii	Treatment	HAART + 24R(Rifabutin)EClari	Not covered
M. malmoense	Treatment	HAART + 24R(Rifabutin)EClari	Not covered
M. xenopi	Treatment	HAART + 24E(Rifabutin)EClari	Not covered

Azithro, azithromycin; Cipro, ciprofloxacin; Clari, clarithromycin; E, ethambutol; H, isoniazid; HAART, highly active antiretroviral therapy; R, rifampicin. The number in front of the letters represents the duration in months.

Generally, in HIV-negative people, these opportunistic organisms cause disease in two main settings:

- In children, usually under the age of 5 years, isolated lymphadenopathy, usually cervical, occurs and should be managed by surgical excision.[159,160,162]
- In HIV-negative patients with underlying structural lung disease, often chronic obstructive pulmonary

disease, infection with *M. kansasii*, *M. avium* complex, *M. malmoense* or *M. xenopi* can all simulate conventional tuberculosis or bronchiectasis with nodularity. Unlike the management of tuberculosis where the drug susceptibility data must be scrupulously followed, the susceptibility to individual drugs in vitro does not correspond to clinical response and should largely be ignored, being of major utility only in *M. kansasii* disease, and for macrolide susceptibility. Laboratory studies also show that there is synergy between drugs, with rifampicin and ethambutol in particular, which are bactericidal in combination, although the organism has been reported as in-vitro resistant to them singly.[163] Clinical trials on pulmonary *M. kansasii* have shown that 9 months of treatment with rifampicin and ethambutol is adequate for most people, but that longer treatment may be needed in some cases.[164]

For the other mycobacteria which cause pulmonary infection, treatment with rifampicin and ethambutol, sometimes with isoniazid as well, gives cure rates of approximately 80%.[165] Unfortunately, results using either clarithromycin or ciprofloxacin, with rifampicin and ethambutol replacing isoniazid, have not shown much improvement.[161] Treatment of extra-pulmonary disease other than *M. marinum* disease in adults is more complex and detailed recommendations should be followed.[159,160]

In HIV-positive patients, restoring immune function with combinations of antiretroviral treatment is as important as, if not more so than, antimycobacterial treatment.[160] There are important interactions between macrolides, rifamycins and protease inhibitors and/or antiretroviral drugs (*see* Table 58.5) which may limit treatment. In those who require treatment for pulmonary or disseminated disease, rifampicin, ethambutol and clarithromycin on an indefinite basis are advised.[159,160] For prophylaxis against *M. avium* complex, the first-choice recommendation is azithromycin 1200 mg weekly, with clarithromycin 500 mg every 12 h as second, and azithromycin 1200 mg once weekly plus rifabutin 300 mg once daily as third choice.[160]

 ## References

1. World Health Organization. *Global tuberculosis control – epidemiology, strategy, financing.* WHO: Geneva; Online Available at http://www.who.int/tb/publications/global_report/2009/en/; 2009.

2. Health Protection Agency Centre for Infections. *Tuberculosis in the United Kingdom. Annual report on tuberculosis surveillance in the United Kingdom.* London: HPA; 2009.

3. Cain KP, Benoit SR, Winston CA, MacKenzie WR. Tuberculosis among foreign-born persons in the United States. *J Am Med Assoc.* 2008;300:405–412.

4. Pitchenik AE, Cole C, Russell BW, Fischl MA, Spira TJ, Snider DE. Tuberculosis, atypical mycobacteriosis and the acquired immunodeficiency syndrome among Haitian and non-Haitian patients in South Florida. *Ann Intern Med.* 1984;101:641–645.

5. Nunn P, Elliot AM, McAdam KPWJ. The impact of human immunodeficiency virus on tuberculosis in developing countries. *Thorax.* 1994;49:511–518.

6. Jindani A, Aber VR, Edwards EA, Mitchison DA. The early bactericidal activity of drugs in patients with pulmonary tuberculosis. *Am Rev Respir Dis.* 1980;121:139–148.

7. Mitchison DA. Basic concepts in the chemotherapy of tuberculosis. In: Gangadharam PRJ, Jenkins PA, eds. *Mycobacteria Vol II Chemotherapy.* New York: Chapman and Hall; 1998:15–50.

8. British Thoracic Society. A controlled trial of 6-month chemotherapy in pulmonary tuberculosis. Final report: results during 36 months after the end of chemotherapy and beyond. *Br J Dis Chest.* 1984;78:330–336.

9. Hong Kong Chest Service/British Medical Research Council. First report: controlled trial of four thrice-weekly regimens and a daily regimen all given for six months for pulmonary tuberculosis. *Lancet.* 1981;1:171–174.

10. Hong Kong Chest Service/British Medical Research Council. Second Report: controlled trial of four thrice-weekly regimens and a daily regimen all given for 6 months. The results up to 24 months. *Tubercle.* 1982;63:89–98.

11. Hong Kong Chest Service/British Medical Research Council. Five year follow-up of a controlled trial of five 6-month regimens of chemotherapy for pulmonary tuberculosis. *Am Rev Respir Dis.* 1987;136:1339–1342.

12. Combs DL, O'Brien R, Geiter L. USPHS tuberculosis short course chemotherapy trial 21. Effectiveness, toxicity and acceptability. The report of final results. *Ann Intern Med.* 1990;112:397–406.

13. Singapore Tuberculosis Service/British Medical Research Council. Clinical trial of 6-month and 4-month regimens of chemotherapy in the treatment of pulmonary tuberculosis. *Am Rev Respir Dis.* 1979;119:579–585.

14. Singapore Tuberculosis Service/British Medical Research Council. Clinical trial of 6-month and 4-month regimens of chemotherapy in the treatment of pulmonary tuberculosis. The results up to 30 months. *Tubercle.* 1981;61:95–102.

15. Snider DE, Graczyk J, Bek E, Rogowski J. Supervised six-months treatment of newly diagnosed pulmonary tuberculosis using isoniazid, rifampin and pyrazinamide with or without streptomycin. *Am Rev Respir Dis.* 1984;130:1091–1094.

16. Singapore Tuberculosis Service/British Medical Research Council. Clinical trial of three 6-month regimens of chemotherapy given intermittently in the continuation phase in the treatment of pulmonary tuberculosis. *Am Rev Respir Dis.* 1985;132:374–378.

17. Singapore Tuberculosis Service/British Medical Research Council. Five year follow-up of a clinical trial of three 6-month regimens of chemotherapy given intermittently in the continuation phase in the treatment of pulmonary tuberculosis. *Am Rev Respir Dis.* 1988;137:1147–1150.

18. Hong Kong Chest Service/British Medical Research Council. Controlled trial of 2, 4 and 6 months of pyrazinamide in 6-month, three-times-weekly regimens for smear-positive tuberculosis, including an assessment of a combined preparation of isoniazid, rifampicin and pyrazinamide. Results at 30 months. *Am Rev Respir Dis.* 1991;143:700–706.

19. Cohn DL, Catlin BJ, Peterson KL, et al. A 62 dose, 6 month therapy for pulmonary and extra-pulmonary tuberculosis. A twice weekly, directly observed, and cost-effective regimen. *Ann Intern Med.* 1990;112:407–415.

20. Third East African/British Medical Research Council Study. First report: Controlled clinical trial of four short course regimens of chemotherapy for two durations in the treatment of pulmonary tuberculosis. *Am Rev Respir Dis.* 1978;118:39–48.

21. Third East African/British Medical Research Council Study. Second report: controlled clinical trial of four short course regimens of chemotherapy for two durations in the treatment of pulmonary tuberculosis. *Tubercle.* 1980;61:59–69.

22. Hong Kong Chest Service/Tuberculosis Research Centre Madras/British Medical Research Council. A controlled trial of 2-month, 3-month and 12-month regimens of chemotherapy for sputum-negative pulmonary tuberculosis. The results at 30 months. *Am Rev Respir Dis.* 1981;124:138–142.

23. Hong Kong Chest Service/Tuberculosis Research Centre Madras/British Medical Research Council. A controlled trial of 3-month, 4-month and 6-month regimens of chemotherapy for sputum smear-negative pulmonary tuberculosis. Results at 5 years. *Am Rev Respir Dis.* 1989;139:871–876.

24. Royal College of Physicians. *Clinical diagnosis and management of tuberculosis, and measures for its prevention and control.* London: RCP; 2006.

25. Migliori GB, Raviglione MC, Schaberg T, et al. Tuberculosis management in Europe. Task Force of ERS, WHO and the Europe Region of IUATLD. *Eur Respir J.* 1999;14:978–992.

26. Recommendations from the American Thoracic Society, CDC and the Infectious Diseases Society of America. Controlling tuberculosis in the United States. *MMWR Morb Mortal Wkly Rep.* 2005;54:RR–12.

27. World Health Organization Tuberculosis Unit, Division of Communicable Disease. *Treatment of tuberculosis: guidelines for national programmes.* 4th edn. WHO/HTM/TB/2009.429.

28. British Thoracic and Tuberculosis Association. Short-course chemotherapy in pulmonary tuberculosis. *Lancet.* 1976;ii:1102–1104.

29. British Thoracic Society Research Committee. Six months versus nine months chemotherapy for tuberculosis of lymph nodes: preliminary results. *Respir Med.* 1992;86:15–19.

30. Campbell IA, Ormerod LP, Friend JR, et al. Six months versus nine months chemotherapy for tuberculosis of lymph nodes: final results. *Respir Med.* 1993;87:621–623.

31. Campbell IA, Dyson AJ. Lymph node tuberculosis: a comparison of various methods of treatment. *Tubercle*. 1977;58:171–179.

32. Campbell IA, Dyson AJ. Lymph node tuberculosis: a comparison of treatments 18 months after completion of chemotherapy. *Tubercle*. 1979;60:95–98.

33. Girling DJ, Darbyshire JH, Humphries MJ, et al. Extrapulmonary tuberculosis. *Br Med Bull*. 1988;44:738–756.

34. Medical Research Council Working Party on Tuberculosis of the Spine. A controlled trial of 6-month and 9-month regimens of chemotherapy in patients undergoing radical surgery for tuberculosis of the spine in Hong Kong. *Tubercle*. 1986;67:243–259.

35. Medical Research Council Working Party on Tuberculosis of the Spine. Controlled trial of short-course regimens of chemotherapy in ambulatory treatment of spinal tuberculosis. *J Bone Joint Surg*. 1993;75:240–248.

36. Indian Council of Medical Research/British Medical Research Council Working Party. A controlled trial of short-course regimens of chemotherapy in patients receiving ambulatory treatment or undergoing radical surgery for tuberculosis of the spine. *Indian Journal of Tuberculosis*. 1989;36(suppl):1–22.

37. Strang JIG, Kakaka HHS, Gibson DG, et al. Controlled trial of prednisolone as an adjuvant in treatment of tuberculous constrictive pericarditis in Transkei. *Lancet*. 1987;ii;1418–1422.

38. Strang JIG. Management of tuberculous constrictive pericarditis and tuberculous pericardial effusion in Transkei: results at 10 year follow-up. *Q J Med*. 2004;97:525–535.

39. Loenhout-Rooyakers JH, Keyser A, Laheji RJ, Veerbeck AL, van der Meer JW. Tuberculous meningitis: is a six-month treatment regimen sufficient? *Int J Tuberc Lung Dis*. 2001;5:1028–1035.

40. Humphries MJ. The management of tuberculous meningitis. *Thorax*. 1992;47:577–581.

41. Citron KM, Thomas GO. Ocular toxicity from ethambutol. *Thorax*. 1986;41:737–739.

42. Donald PR, Seifart HI. Cerebrospinal fluid concentrations of ethionamide in children with tuberculous meningitis. *J Pediatr*. 1989;115:383–386.

43. Ormerod LP, Watson JM, Pozniak A, et al. Notification of tuberculosis: an updated code of practice for England and Wales. *J R Coll Physicians Lond*. 1997;31:299–303.

44. Prasad K, Volmink J, Menon GR. Steroids for treating tuberculous meningitis. *The Cochrane Library*. 2003;2000(3):CD002244.

45. Toppet M, Malfroot A, Derde MP, et al. Corticosteroids in primary tuberculosis with bronchial obstruction. *Arch Dis Child*. 1990;65:1222–1226.

46. Lee CH, Wang WJ, Lan RS, et al. Corticosteroids in the treatment of tuberculous pleurisy. A double-blind, placebo-controlled, randomized study. *Chest*. 1988;94:1256–1259.

47. Home NW, Tulloch WS. Conservative management of renal tuberculosis. *Br J Urol*. 1973;47:481–487.

48. Home NW. A critical evaluation of corticosteroids in tuberculosis. *Adv Tuberc Res*. 1966;15:1–54.

49. Ormerod LP. Tuberculosis in pregnancy and the puerperium. *Thorax*. 2001;56:494–499.

50. Joint Tuberculosis Committee of the British Thoracic Society. Chemotherapy and management of tuberculosis in the United Kingdom: recommendations 1998. *Thorax*. 1998;53:536–548.

51. International Union against Tuberculosis and Lung Disease. Antituberculosis regimens of chemotherapy. Recommendations from the Committee on Treatment of IUATLD. *Bull Int Union Tuberc Lung Dis*. 1988;63:60–64.

52. American Academy of Pediatrics, Committee on Infectious Diseases. Chemotherapy for tuberculosis in infants and children. *Pediatrics*. 1992;89:161–165.

53. Roy V, Tekur U, Chopra K. Pharmacokinetics of isoniazid in pulmonary tuberculosis: a comparative study at two dose levels. *Indian Pediatr*. 1996;33:287–291.

54. Palma Beltran OR, Pelosi F, Budani H, et al. The treatment of child tuberculosis with isoniazid (H), rifampicin (R) and pyrazinamide (Z). *Bull Int Union Tuberc Lung Dis*. 1986;61:17.

55. Trebucq A. Should ethambutol be recommended for routine treatment of tuberculosis in children? A review of the literature. *Int J Tuberc Lung Dis*. 1997;1:12–15.

56. Banerjee A, Dubnau E, Quemard A, et al. InhA, a gene encoding a target for isoniazid and ethionamide in *Mycobacterium tuberculosis*. *Science*. 1994;263:227–230.

57. Zhang Y, Heym B, Allen B, Young D, Cole S. The catalase–peroxidase gene of *Mycobacterium tuberculosis*. *Nature*. 1992;358:591–593.

58. Finken M, Kirschner P, Meier A, Wrede A, Bottger EC. Molecular basis of streptomycin resistance in *Mycobacterium tuberculosis*: alterations in the ribosomal protein S12 gene and point mutations within a functional 16S ribosomal RNA pseudoknot. *Mol Microbiol*. 1993;9:1239–1246.

59. Takiff HE, Salazar L, Guerrero C, et al. Cloning and nucleotide sequence of the *Mycobacterium tuberculosis* gyrA and gyrB genes and detection of quinolone resistance mutations. *Antimicrob Agents Chemother*. 1994;38:773–780.

60. Telenti A, Imboden P, Marcheu F, et al. Detection of rifampicin resistance mutations in *Mycobacterium tuberculosis*. *Lancet*. 1993;341:647–650.

61. Somoskovi A, Dormandy J, Parsons LM, et al. Sequencing of the pncA gene in members of the *Mycobacterium tuberculosis* complex has important diagnostic implications: identification of a species-specific pncA mutation in *Mycobacterium canetti*, and the reliable and rapid predictor of pyrazinamide resistance. *J Clin Microbiol*. 2007;45:595–599.

62. Mikusova K, Slayden RA, Besra GS, Brennan PJ. Biogenesis of the mycobacterial cell wall and the site of action of ethambutol. *Antimicrob Agents Chemother*. 1995;39:2484–2489.

63. Aziz MA, Wright A, Laszlo A, et al. Epidemiology of anti-tuberculosis drug- resistance (the Global Project on Anti-tuberculosis Drug Resistance Surveillance): an updated analysis. *Lancet*. 2006;368:2142–2154.

64. Warburton AR, Jenkins PA, Waight PA, Watson JM. Drug resistance in initial isolates of *Mycobacterium tuberculosis* in England and Wales, 1982–1991. *Commun Dis Rep CDR Rev*. 1993;3:R175–179.

65. Faustini A, Hall AJ, Perucci CA. Risk factors for multi-drug resistant tuberculosis in Europe: a systematic review. *Thorax*. 2006;61:158–163.

66. Gandhi NR, Moll A, Sturm AW, et al. Extensively drug-resistant tuberculosis as a cause of death in patients co-infected with tuberculosis and HIV in a rural area of South Africa. *Lancet*. 2006;368:1575–1580.

67. World Health Organization. *Antituberculosis drug resistance in the world: fourth global report*. Geneva: WHO; 2008. Online Available at http://whqlibdoc.who.int/hq/2008/WHO_HTM_TB_2008.394_eng.pdf.

68. Anonymous. Emergence of *Mycobacterium tuberculosis* with extensive resistance to second-line drugs – worldwide, 2000–2004. *MMWR Morb Mortal Wkly Rep*. 2006;55:301–305.

69. Centers for Disease Control and Prevention. Extensively drug resistant tuberculosis in the United States: 1993–2006. *MMWR Morb Mortal Wkly Rep*. 2007;56(11):250–253.

70. Chawla R, Pant K, Jaggi OP, et al. Fibreoptic bronchoscopy in smear-negative pulmonary tuberculosis. *Eur Respir J*. 1998;1:804–806.

71. The Interdepartmental Working Group on Tuberculosis. *The prevention and control of tuberculosis in the United Kingdom: UK guidance on the prevention and control of transmission of: 1. HIV-related tuberculosis, 2. Drug resistant, including multiple drug-resistant, tuberculosis*. London: Department of Health, The Scottish Office, The Welsh Office; 1998.

72. Joint Tuberculosis Committee of the British Thoracic Society. Control and prevention of tuberculosis in the United Kingdom: Code of Practice 2000. *Thorax*. 2000;55:887–901.

73. Mitchison DA, Nunn AJ. Influence of initial drug resistance on the response to short-course chemotherapy in pulmonary tuberculosis. *Am Rev Respir Dis*. 1986;133:423–430.

74. Babu Swai O, Alnoch JA, Githui WA, et al. Controlled clinical trial of a regimen of two durations for the treatment of isoniazid resistant tuberculosis. *Tubercle*. 1988;69:5–14.

75. Drobniewski FA, Pozniak AL. Molecular diagnosis, detection of drug resistance and epidemiology of tuberculosis. *Br J Hosp Med*. 1996;56:204–208.

76. Goyal M, Shaw RJ, Banerjee DK, et al. Rapid detection of multi-drug resistant tuberculosis. *Eur Respir J*. 1997;10:120–124.

77. Goble M, Iseman M, Madsen LA, et al. Treatment of 171 patients with pulmonary tuberculosis resistant to isoniazid and rifampin. *N Engl J Med*. 1993;328:527–532.

78. Iseman M. Treatment of multidrug resistant tuberculosis. *N Engl J Med*. 1993;328:784–790.

79. Ormerod LP. The role of surgery for pulmonary multidrug-resistant tuberculosis. *Thorax*. 2007;62:377.

80. Public Health Laboratory Service. Enhanced surveillance of *Mycobacterium bovis* in humans. *Commun Dis Rep CDR Wkly*. 1998;8(32):281–284.

81. Scorpio A, Zhang Y. Mutations in pncA, a gene encoding pyrazinamidase/nicotinamidase causes resistance to the antituberculosis drug pyrazinamide in the tubercle bacillus. *Nat Med*. 1996;2:662–667.

82. Cawthorne D, Raashed M, Synnott M, et al. Contact tracing in bovine TB. *Eur Respir J*. 1997;11:P1388.

83. De Souza GRM, Sant'Anna CC, Silva JRL, Mano DB, Bethlem NM. Intradermal BCG vaccination complications – analysis of 51 cases. *Tubercle.* 1983;64:23–27.

84. Murphy PM, Maters DL, Brock NF, Wagner KF. Cure of bacille Calmette-Guérin vaccination abscesses with erythromycin. *Rev Infect Dis.* 1989;11:335–337.

85. Lamm DL, van der Meijden PM, Morales A, et al. Incidence and treatment of complications of bacillus Calmette-Guérin intravesical therapy in superficial bladder cancer. *J Urol.* 1992;147:596–600.

86. Ormerod LP, Prescott RJ. Interrelationships between compliance, regimen and relapse in tuberculosis. *Respir Med.* 1991;85:339–342.

87. Ormerod LP, Bentley C, for the Joint Tuberculosis Committee of the British Thoracic Society. The management of pulmonary tuberculosis in England and Wales in 1993. *J R Coll Physicians Lond.* 1997;31:662–665.

88. Ormerod LP, Bentley C, for the Joint Tuberculosis Committee of the British Thoracic Society. The management of lymph node tuberculosis in England and Wales in 1993. *J R Coll Physicians Lond.* 1997;31:666–668.

89. Interdepartmental Working Group on Tuberculosis. *Recommendations for the control and prevention of tuberculosis at a local level.* London: Department of Health and Welsh Office; 1996.

90. Ellard GA, Ellard DR, Allen BW, et al. The bioavailability of isoniazid, rifampicin and pyrazinamide in two commercially available combined formulations designed for use in short course chemotherapy in tuberculosis. *Am Rev Respir Dis.* 1986;133:1076–1080.

91. Geiter LJ, O'Brien RJ, Coombs DL, et al. Unites States Public Health Service tuberculosis therapy trial 21. Preliminary results of an evaluation of a combination tablet of isoniazid, rifampin and pyrazinamide. *Tubercle.* 1987;68:41–46.

92. Ormerod LP, Skinner C, Wales JM. Hepatotoxicity of antituberculosis drugs. *Thorax.* 1996;51:111–113.

93. World Health Organization, Global Tuberculosis Programme. *Treatment of tuberculosis.* Geneva: WHO; 1997 Report WHO/TB/97.220.

94. Chaulk CP, Kazanjjian VH. DOT for treatment completion of pulmonary tuberculosis: consensus statement of the Public Health Tuberculosis Guidelines Panel. *J Am Med Assoc.* 1998;27:943–945.

95. Morse DI. Directly observed therapy for tuberculosis. *Br Med J.* 1996;312:719–720.

96. China Tuberculosis Control Collaboration. Results of directly observed short-course chemotherapy in 112,842 Chinese patients with smear-positive tuberculosis. *Lancet.* 1996;347:358–362.

97. Caminero JA, Pavon JM, Rodriguez de Castro F, et al. Evaluation of a directly observed six month fully intermittent treatment regimen for tuberculosis in patients suspected of poor compliance. *Thorax.* 1996;51:1130–1133.

98. Moore RD, Chaulk CP, Griffiths R, et al. Cost-effectiveness of directly observed versus self administered therapy in tuberculosis. *Am J Respir Crit Care Med.* 1996;154:1013–1019.

99. Sbarbaro JA. The ultimate decision analysis: the confirmation of reality through theory. *Am J Respir Crit Care Med.* 1996;154:835–836.

100. Miller B, Palmer CS, Halpern MT, et al. Decision model to assess the cost-effectiveness of DOT for tuberculosis. *Tuber Lung Dis.* 1996;77(suppl 2):74–75.

101. Zwarenstein M, Schoeman JH, Vundule C, et al. Randomised controlled trial of self-supervised and directly observed therapy for tuberculosis. *Lancet.* 1998;352:1340–1343.

102. Volmink J, Garner P. Directly observed therapy for treating tuberculosis 2007. *Cochrane Database Syst Rev.* 2007;(4) CD003343.

103. Bayer R, Stayton C, Desvarieux M, et al. Directly observed therapy and treatment completion for tuberculosis in the United States: is universal supervised treatment necessary? *Am J Public Health.* 1998;88:1052–1058.

104. Centers for Disease Control. Initial therapy for tuberculosis in the era of multidrug resistance. Recommendations of the Advisory Council for the Elimination of Tuberculosis. *MMWR Morb Mortal Wkly Rep.* 1993;42:RR–R7.

105. Ackah AN, Coulibaly D, Digbeu H, et al. Response to treatment, mortality and CD4 lymphocyte counts in HIV-infected persons with tuberculosis in Abidjan, Côte d'Ivoire. *Lancet.* 1995;345:607–610.

106. Jones BE, Young SMM, Antoniskis D, Davidson PT, Kramer F, Barnes PF. Relationship of the manifestations of tuberculosis to CD4 cell counts in patients with human immunodeficiency virus infection. *Am Rev Respir Dis.* 1993;148:1292–1297.

107. Perriens JH, St Louis ME, Yiadiul B, et al. Pulmonary tuberculosis in HIV-infected patients in Zaire. *N Engl J Med.* 1995;332:779–784.

108. Goletti D, Weissman D, Jackson RW, et al. Effect of *Mycobacterium tuberculosis* in HIV replication: role of immune activation. *J Immunol.* 1996;157:1271–1278.

109. British HIV Association (BHIVA). *Treatment of HIV-1 infected adults with anti-retroviral treatment.* Online Available at http://www.bhiva.org/cmsl222226asp; 2008.

110. British HIV Association (BHIVA) Treatment of tuberculosis in HIV infected individuals. Online Available at http://www.bhiva.org/InDevelopment.aspx2010.

111. Dean GL, Edwards SG, Ives NJ, et al. Treatment of tuberculosis in HIV-1 infected persons in the era of highly active antiretroviral therapy. *AIDS.* 2002;16:75–83.

112. Small PM, Schecter GF, Goodman PC, et al. Treatment of tuberculosis in patients with advanced human immunodeficiency virus infection. *N Engl J Med.* 1990;324:289–294.

113. Englehard D, Stutman HR, Marks MI. Interaction of ketoconazole with rifampicin and isoniazid. *N Engl J Med.* 1994;311:1681–1683.

114. Lazar JD, Wilner KD. Drug interactions with fluconazole. *Rev Infect Dis.* 1990;12(suppl 3):S327–S333.

115. Heyden R, Miller R. Adverse effects and drug interactions of medications commonly used in the treatment of adult HIV positive patients. *Genitourin Med.* 1996;72:237–246.

116. Jindani A, Nunn AJ, Enarson DA. Two 8-month regimens of chemotherapy for treatment of newly diagnosed pulmonary tuberculosis: international multicentre randomized trial. *Lancet.* 2004;364:1244–1251.

117. Okwera A, Whalen C, Byekwaso F, et al. Randomised trial of thiacetazone and rifampicin containing regimens for pulmonary tuberculosis in HIV-infected Ugandans. *Lancet.* 1994;344:1323–1328.

118. Ormerod LP. Chemotherapy of tuberculosis [chapter]. *Eur Respir J.* 1997;2(4):273–297.

119. Alvirez-Frietes EJ, Carter JL, Cynamon MH. In vitro and in vivo of gatifloxacin against *Mycobacterium tuberculosis. Antimicrob Agents Chemother.* 2002;46:1875–1879.

120. Pietz MW, De Roux A, Roth A, et al. Early bactericidal activity of moxifloxacin in treatment of pulmonary tuberculosis. A prospective, randomized study. *Antimicrob Agents Chemother.* 2004;48:780–782.

121. Nuermberger EL, Yoshimatsu T, Tyagi S, et al. Moxifloxacin-containing regimens of reduced duration produce a stable cure in murine tuberculosis. *American Journal of Critical Care Medicine.* 2004;170:1131–1134.

122. Burman WJ, Goldberg S, Johnson JL, et al. Moxifloxacin versus ethambutol in the first two months of treatment for tuberculosis. *Am J Respir Crit Care Med.* 2006;174:331–338.

123. Rustomjee R, Lienhardt C, Kanyok T, et al. A phase II study of the sterilizing activities of ofloxacin, gatifloxacin and moxifloxacin in pulmonary tuberculosis. *Int J Tuberc Lung Dis.* 2008;12:128–138.

124. Conde MB, Efron A, De Souza GRM, et al. Moxifloxacin versus ethambutol in the initial treatment of tuberculosis: a double-blind, randomized, controlled phase II trial. *Lancet.* 2009;373:1183–1189.

125. World Health Organization. Oflotub study. Online Available at www.who.int/tdr/svc/research/evidence-treatment-tb-hiv/projects.

126. MRC Clinical Trials Unit. *REMOX TB: Controlled comparison of two moxifloxacin containing treatment shortening regimens in pulmonary tuberculosis.* London: MRC; 2010. Online Available at http://www.ctu.mrc.ac.uk/research_areas/study_details.aspx?s=29. *See also* RemoxTB_trial@ctu.mrc.ac.uk.

127. Lenaerts AJ, Gruppo V, Marietta KS, et al. Preclinical testing of nitroimidazopyran PA 824 for activity against *Mycobacterium tuberculosis* in a series of in vitro and in vivo models. *Antimicrob Agents Chemother.* 2005;49:2294–2301.

128. Tyagi S, Nuermberger E, Yoshimatsu T, et al. Bactericidal activity of the nitroimidazopyran PA-284 in a murine model of tuberculosis. *Antimicrob Agents Chemother.* 2005;49:2289–2293.

129. Global Alliance for TB Drug Development. Handbook of anti-tuberculosis agents. *Tuberculosis.* 2008;88:850–870.

130. Matsumoto M, Hashizume H, Tomishige T, et al. OPC-67683, a nitro-dihydro-imidazooxazole derivative with promising action against tuberculosis in vitro and in mice. *PLoS Med.* 2006;3:e466.

131. Andries K, Verhasselt P, Guillemont J, et al. A diarylquinoline drug active on the ATP synthetase of *Mycobacterium tuberculosis. Science.* 2005;307:223–227.

132. Rustomjee R, Diacon AH, Allen J, et al. Early bactericidal activity and pharmacokinetics of the diarylquinoline TMC207 in the treatment of pulmonary tuberculosis. *Antimicrob Agents Chemother.* 2008;52:2831–2835.

133. Jia L, Tomaszewski JE, Hanrahan C, et al. Pharmacodynamics and pharmacokinetics of SQ109, a new diamine based antitubercular drug. *Br J Pharmacol.* 2005;144:8087.

134. Arora S. Eradication of *Mycobacterium tuberculosis* infection in 2 months with LL3858: a pre-clinical study. *Int J TubercLung Dis*. 2004;8(suppl 1):S29.

135. Gryzbowski S, Ashley MJ, Pinkus G. Chemoprophylaxis in inactive tuberculosis: long term evaluation of a Canadian trial. *Can Med Assoc J*. 1976;114:607–611.

136. Ferebee SH. Controlled chemoprophylaxis trials in tuberculosis: a general review. *Adv Tuberc Res*. 1969;17:29–106.

137. Comstock GW, Ferebee SH. How much isoniazid is needed for chemoprophylaxis? *Am Rev Respir Dis*. 1970;101:780–782.

138. Comstock GW, Baum C, Snider DE. Isoniazid chemoprophylaxis amongst Alaskan Eskimos: a final report of the Bethel isoniazid studies. *Am Rev Respir Dis*. 1969;119:827–830.

139. Thompson NJ. Efficacy of various durations of isoniazid preventive therapy in tuberculosis: 5 years of follow-up in the IUATLD Trial. *Bull World Health Org*. 1982;60:555–564.

140. Smieja MJ, Marchetti CA, Cook DJ, Smaill FM. Isoniazid for preventing tuberculosis in non-HIV infected persons. *Cochrane Database of Sys Rev*. 2000;(2) CD001363.

141. Lecouer HF, Truffot-Pernot C, Grosset JH. Experimental short-course preventive therapy of tuberculosis with rifampicin and pyrazinamide. *Am Rev Respir Dis*. 1989;140:1189–1193.

142. Hong Kong Chest Service/Tuberculosis Research Centre Madras/British Medical Research Council. A double-blind placebo-controlled clinical trial of three antituberculosis chemoprophylaxis regimens in patients with silicosis in Hong Kong. *Am Rev Respir Dis*. 1992;145:36–41.

143. Ormerod LP. Reduced incidence of tuberculosis by prophylactic chemotherapy in children showing strong reactions to tuberculin testing. *Arch Dis Child*. 1987;62:1005–1008.

144. Ormerod LP. Rifampicin and isoniazid prophylactic chemotherapy for tuberculosis. *Arch Dis Child*. 1998;78:169–171.

145. American Thoracic Society and Centers for Disease Control and Prevention. Targeted tuberculin testing and treatment of latent tuberculosis infection. *Am J Respir Crit Care Med*. 2001;161:S221–S247.

146. American Thoracic Society, Centers for Disease Control and Prevention. Targeted tuberculin testing and treatment of latent tuberculosis infection. *Am J Respir Crit Care Med*. 2000;161:S221–S247.

147. American Thoracic Society, Centers for Disease Control and Prevention. Update: fatal and severe liver injuries associated with rifampicin and pyrazinamide for latent tuberculosis infection, and revisions in the American Thoracic Society/CDC recommendations – United Sates 2001. *Am J Respir Crit Care Med*. 2001;164:1319–1320.

148. National Institute for Health and Clinical Excellence. *Guideline development methods: information for National Collaborating Centres and Guideline Developers*. London: NICE. Online Available at http://www.nice.org; 2005.

149. Ploesky A, Farber HW, Gottlieb DJ, et al. Rifampin preventive therapy for tuberculosis in Boston's homeless. *Am J Respir Crit Care Med*. 1996;154:1473–1477.

150. Villarino ME, Ridszon R, Weismuller PC, et al. Rifampin preventive therapy for tuberculosis infection. Experience with 157 adolescents. *Am J Respir Crit Care Med*. 1997;155:1735–1738.

151. Mazurek GH, Jereb J, Lobue P, Iademarco MF, Metchcock B, Vernon A; Division of TB elimination. Centers for Disease Control and Prevention. Guidelines for using the QuantiFERON-TB Gold test for detecting *Mycobacterium tuberculosis* infection. United States. *MMWR Morb Mortal Wkly Rep*. 2005;54(RR-15):49–55.

152. IUATLD, GPA (WHO). Tuberculosis preventive therapy in HIV infected individuals; a joint statement of the IUATLD and GPA (WHO). *Tuber Lung Dis*. 1994;75:96–98.

153. Fitzgerald JM. The downside of isoniazid chemoprophylaxis. *Lancet*. 1995;305:404.

154. Aisu T, Raviglione MC, Van Praag E, et al. Preventive chemotherapy for HIV associated tuberculosis in Uganda: an operational assessment of a voluntary counselling and testing centre. *AIDS*. 1995;9:267–273.

155. Gordin FM, Matts JP, Miller C, et al. A controlled trial of isoniazid in persons with anergy and human immunodeficiency virus infection who are at high risk of tuberculosis. *N Engl J Med*. 1997;337:315–320.

156. Selwyn PA, Hartel D, Lewis VA, et al. A prospective study of the risk of tuberculosis among intravenous drug users with human immunodeficiency virus infection. *N Engl J Med*. 1989;320:545–550.

157. Gallagher CT, Passannante MR, Reichman LB. Preventive therapy for multidrug resistant tuberculosis (MDR-tuberculosis): a Delphi survey. *Am Rev Respir Dis*. 1992;145: abstract.

158. Anonymous Management of persons exposed to multi-drug resistant tuberculosis. *MMWR Morb Mortal Wkly Rep*. 1992;41:61–71.

159. Joint Tuberculosis Committee of the British Thoracic Society. Management of opportunist mycobacterial infections: Joint Tuberculosis Committee guidelines 1999. *Thorax*. 2000;55:210–218.

160. American Thoracic Society/Infectious Diseases Society of America. An official ATS/IDSA statement: diagnosis, treatment and prevention of nontuberculous mycobacterial diseases. *Am J Respir Crit Care Med*. 2007;175:367–415.

161. Jenkins PA, Campbell IA, Banks J, Gelder CM, Prescott RJ, Smith PA. Clarithromycin vs ciprofloxacin as adjuncts to rifampicin and ethambutol in the treatment of opportunist mycobacteria and an assessment of the value of immunotherapy with *M. vaccae*: a pragmatic, randomized trial by the British Thoracic Society. *Thorax*. 2008;63:627–634.

162. MacKellar A. Diagnosis and management of atypical mycobacterial lymphadenitis in children. *J Pediatr Surg*. 1976;11:85–89.

163. Banks J, Jenkins PA. Combined versus single antituberculosis drugs on the in vitro sensitivity patterns of non-tuberculous mycobacteria. *Thorax*. 1987;42:838–842.

164. British Thoracic Society. *Mycobacterium kansasii* pulmonary infection: a prospective controlled study of the results of nine months treatment with rifampicin and ethambutol. *Thorax*. 1994;49:442–445.

165. Research Committee of the British Thoracic Society. First randomised trial of treatments for pulmonary disease caused by *M. avium intracellulare, M. malmoense*, and *M. xenopi* in HIV negative patients: rifampicin, ethambutol and isoniazid versus rifampicin and ethambutol. *Thorax*. 2001;56:167–172.

59 Superficial and mucocutaneous mycoses

Roderick J. Hay

The most prevalent superficial mycoses are caused by different groups of pathogenic fungi, the dermatophytes or ringworm fungi, *Candida* and *Malassezia* species. These infections are very common, usually infecting otherwise healthy individuals, although the clinical pattern of infection and response to treatment will be affected if the patient is immunosuppressed. Dermatophyte infections include clinical disease states such as tinea capitis (scalp), cruris (groin), corporis (body) and pedis (feet). They are caused by filamentous fungi of the genera *Trichophyton*, *Microsporum* and *Epidermophyton* spp. *Malassezia* species are commensal yeasts on normal skin, but under certain conditions can cause human disease such as pityriasis versicolor. *Candida* species are the main cause of mucocutaneous infections, including oral and vaginal candidiasis (or thrush) as well as skin disease, particularly in the region of body folds. In addition there are other less common superficial fungal pathogens.

DERMATOPHYTOSIS

TINEA CAPITIS

Tinea capitis presents with a range of clinical features from alopecia (or hair loss) with little inflammation to the formation of a kerion, which is a pustular and inflammatory mass containing hair shafts and fungi. Tinea capitis is mainly a disease of childhood.[1] This is an infection that is difficult to diagnose on clinical grounds alone and it is important to confirm the diagnosis using mycological sampling. The mycological causes of tinea capitis vary geographically but it is useful to know whether the infection can be spread from child to child (anthropophilic) or whether it originates from an animal source (zoophilic) such as a cat or dog. Common organisms include *Trichophyton tonsurans* (anthropophilic), *T. violaceum* (anthropophilic) and *Microsporum canis* (zoophilic). In the UK, *T. tonsurans* is now more common than *M. canis* but in other countries in Europe the latter dominates. Whatever the cause, it is important to treat other infected individuals; in the case of anthropophilic infections this includes other family members and with zoophilic infections domestic pets such

as cats may be infected. In other parts of the world, *T. violaceum* and *T. soudanense* are more common. Identification of the cause is important as there are differences in response rates between *Trichophyton* and *Microsporum* species that may determine the medication used.[2]

Generally no topical therapy is effective long term for tinea capitis. For instance, ketoconazole shampoo may be effective clinically for *T. tonsurans* infection during the active treatment phase but there is a very high relapse rate.[3] The main alternatives are all oral therapies (Table 59.1). Griseofulvin (500–1000 mg/day with food) is given for 8 weeks or longer but has the disadvantage of being more protracted and having a higher relapse rate in some infections.[4] Griseofulvin in suspension form, for use in children, is also not available in all countries. Oral terbinafine 250 mg/day for 4 weeks (unless *M. canis* when double doses are needed)[5] or itraconazole 100 mg/day are appropriate but must be continued for 4 weeks, depending on severity[6] (Table 59.1 – see modified child dose regimen for terbinafine). Pediatric formulations of these drugs are also not universally available.

In children with tinea capitis caused by *M. canis*, a 6-week course of either itraconazole 100 mg or griseofulvin 500 mg/day exhibited equivalent efficacy of 88%, but itraconazole was better tolerated.[7] A longer course may be necessary in people with severe disease. Higher doses of itraconazole (200 mg/day or 3 mg/kg solution) may be advantageous, especially as only 40% of patients with *T. tonsurans* infection responded to 4 weeks of itraconazole 100 mg/day.[8] Corticosteroids, even in cases of kerion, are not recommended. An alternative approach is once-weekly fluconazole 6–8 mg/kg.[9]

TINEA CRURIS

Tinea cruris is more common in men than in women, producing a red, scaly rash with a prominent margin covering the groin, scrotum and thighs. It is caused by various dermatophytes, mainly *Epidermophyton floccosum* and *T. rubrum*. Topical imidazoles such as clotrimazole, miconazole

Table 59.1   Treatment of tinea infections

Condition	Agent	Daily dose	Duration
Tinea capitis	Griseofulvin	10 mg/kg	2–3 months
	Itraconazole	100 mg	2–6 weeks
	Terbinafine	250 mg[a]	2–4 weeks
Tinea cruris	Clotrimazole	Topical twice daily	2–3 weeks
	Miconazole	Topical twice daily	2–3 weeks
	Sulconazole	Topical twice daily	2–3 weeks
	Itraconazole	200 mg	1 week
	Terbinafine	250 mg	1 week
Tinea corporis	Itraconazole	200 mg	1 week
	Terbinafine	250 mg	1 week
	Terbinafine, 1% cream	Topical twice daily	1 week
Tinea pedis	Terbinafine, 1% cream	Topical twice daily	1 week
	Terbinafine film-forming solution	One application	
	Clotrimazole, 1% cream	Topical twice daily	1 week
Moccasin-type tinea pedis	Itraconazole	200 mg	2 weeks
	Terbinafine	250 mg	2 weeks

[a]Modified terbinafine dose in children <20 kg, 62.5 mg/day; 20–40 kg, 125 mg/day; >40 kg, 250 mg/day.

or sulconazole twice daily for at least 2 weeks are usually effective (Table 59.1). Oral itraconazole (200 mg/day)[10] or terbinafine (250 mg/day) for 7 days[11] are highly effective and may be preferred. An alternative topical therapy is terbinafine 1% cream applied once daily for 1 week which is effective in >90% of cases.[12]

TINEA CORPORIS

Tinea corporis (ringworm) tends to affect exposed areas of the extremities and may be treated systemically, as for tinea cruris, or with azole or terbinafine creams (Table 59.1). Topical therapy is usually used for infections of limited extent.

TINEA PEDIS

Tinea pedis (athlete's foot) affects about 16% of the population and is often recurrent. Terbinafine cream 1% twice daily for 1 week compares well with 1% clotrimazole cream twice daily for 4 weeks (97% vs 84% response)[13] (Table 59.1). However, topical azole creams (e.g. bifonazole, miconazole) or powders are effective. A single application of terbinafine, a film-forming solution, applied to the soles is also curative in many cases.[14] Moccasin-type tinea pedis affecting the soles is invariably due to *T. rubrum*: 2–4 weeks' therapy with either terbinafine 250 mg/day or itraconazole 200 mg/day are the best options.

SEBORRHEIC DERMATITIS, PITYRIASIS VERSICOLOR AND *MALASSEZIA* FOLLICULITIS

There is a range of superficial diseases related to superficial infection with, or sensitization by, *Malassezia* species. These are seborrheic dermatitis (dandruff is a form of the latter confined to the scalp), cradle cap, pityriasis versicolor and *Malassezia* folliculitis.

Pityriasis versicolor is a superficial skin infection of the upper trunk, mainly caused by *M. globosa*, which results in patchy hypo- or hyperpigmented scaly macules on the trunk. It can be treated with azole creams or ketoconazole shampoo applied daily for up to 7 days. Topical terbinafine cream is also effective. Topical treatments are often difficult to apply as the area affected is often extensive; oral itraconazole 200 mg/day for 7 days is 85% effective.[15] *Malassezia* folliculitis is less common, but causes itchy pustular lesions on the upper chest or back and is best treated with oral itraconazole.

Seborrheic dermatitis is characterized by excess scaling of the scalp, face and anterior chest associated with inflammation; dandruff or scaling of the scalp may be a manifestation of seborrheic dermatitis. Cradle cap in infants is thought to be a similar process. The mechanism by which *Malassezia* contributes to these conditions is not understood, but they are common problems: some authors have stated a lifetime incidence of seborrheic dermatitis of 10% for the normal population with an incidence of 50% in HIV-infected patients. Seborrheic dermatitis frequently accompanies symptomatic HIV infection and may be one of the first signs of infection.

Seborrheic dermatitis is a chronic disease that relapses rapidly after treatment. It may also be difficult to effect improvement despite antifungal therapy and anti-inflammatory agents. Topical corticosteroids have largely been supplanted by the use of topical azole creams with or without a steroid component. Lithium succinate 8% ointment is also effective. Patients with very inflammatory lesions benefit from combined hydrocortisone 1% and azole antifungal preparations. Oral itraconazole 200 mg/day is also effective.[16] By contrast, fluconazole is not very effective, especially in those with AIDS. Maintenance antifungal therapy is not recommended for seborrheic dermatitis, unless it is very severe.

FUNGAL NAIL DISEASE (PARONYCHIA AND ONYCHOMYCOSIS)

Fungi may affect the nail fold (paronychia) or the nail itself (onychomycosis). Paronychia is usually associated with *Candida albicans* and occasionally other *Candida* species. Confirmation by culture is desirable because many cases of paronychia are due to bacteria, especially *Staphylococcus aureus*, and irritant dermatitis also contributes to nail fold inflammation. Onychomycosis is caused by a variety of fungi: the most common is *T. rubrum*, which causes about 80% of cases in the UK; less common dermatophyte causes include *T. interdigitale*, *Epidermophyton floccosum*, *T. erinacei*, *T. soudanense*, *T. tonsurans*, *T. violaceum* and *M. canis*. Non-dermatophyte molds that occasionally cause onychomycosis, usually of the toenails, include *Fusarium* spp., *Aspergillus* spp., *Acremonium* spp., *Scytalidium dimidiatum*, *S. hyalinum*, *Scopulariopsis brevicaulis* and *Onychocola canadensis*. *Scytalidium* species can also infect the toe web spaces, soles and fingernails, mimicking dermatophytosis. Rarely true onychomycosis is caused by *C. albicans*.

CANDIDA PARONYCHIA

Candida paronychia, when mild and localized, will usually respond to imidazole lotions, applied topically for up to 12 weeks. In addition, patients should carefully dry their hands after washing, which is often the primary reason for the development of paronychia. Sometimes where irritant dermatitis is present a topical steroid cream is useful. For patients with extensive *Candida* paronychia or an immunodeficiency state, including chronic mucocutaneous candidosis, itraconazole 200 mg/day for 3–6 weeks is usually adequate, although some patients require longer therapy. Patients who also have onychomycosis require longer therapy. Fluconazole is also active against *Candida* spp., doses of 200 mg/day being effective depending on the severity of disease and the immune status of the patient.[17]

ONYCHOMYCOSIS

The treatment of onychomycosis depends on the species of infecting fungus, whether and how many fingernails or toenails are involved, the clinical pattern of nail involvement, and the age and immune status of the patient.[18]

 ### DISTAL SUBUNGUAL AND SUPERFICIAL ONYCHOMYCOSIS

In distal fingernail disease affecting less than 30% of the nail plate in non-immunocompromised patients, topical therapy can be used. Options include 28% tioconazole and amorolfine nail paint applied once or twice weekly.[19] Alternative strategies include bifonazole 1% combined with urea paste 40%, which softens the nail plate for subsequent ablation and has a reported response rate of up to 70%.[20]

However, the overall cure rate of topical therapy is only about 40% and many months of treatment are required. Failure is more likely if more than 30% of the nail is involved. Removal of the nail after application of 40% urea ointment alone[21] or surgical ablation is an alternative option for these patients.

 ### EXTENSIVE DISTAL OR PROXIMAL SUBUNGUAL, ENDONYX AND TOTALLY DYSTROPHIC ONYCHOMYCOSIS

For patients with proximal nail involvement or extensive distal nail disease, which may also include the skin around the nails, systemic therapy is appropriate. Both itraconazole 200 mg/day or 400 mg/day for 1 week per month and terbinafine 250 mg/day yield a response in excess of 75% for fingernail involvement with dermatophytes but terbinafine is more effective than intermittent itraconazole for toenail disease.[22] Treatment is usually given for 3 months for fingernails[23] and 6–12 months for toenails. Relapse may occur after discontinuation of therapy – 22% in one study.[24] Studies with itraconazole have shown lower efficacy rates than terbinafine, which is also more cost-effective,[25] but this depends on the infecting fungus. Despite these measures many nail infections are difficult to treat and other measures such as retreating with terbinafine[26] or using a combined treatment with itraconazole or terbinafine and amorolfine nail lacquer[27] may be successful. The presence of longitudinal streaks in the nail plate is often associated with relapse and removal of these areas using 40% urea ointment may be useful.

In patients with non-dermatophyte onychomycosis of the toenails, itraconazole or terbinafine may be appropriate for those caused by *Aspergillus* spp. However, these are less effective therapies for *Fusarium* or *Acremonium* onychomycosis and the data supporting use in *Scopulariopsis* and *Scytalidium* infections are limited. Response rates in toenails are <80% and disease-free nails 1 year after therapy are seen in only 35–50% of cases.[28] Nail plate ablation after urea treatment may be the preferred option.

In leukemic patients with onychomycosis it is important to ascertain whether *Fusarium* is the cause. Removal of the nail may prevent disseminated *Fusarium* infection, which carries a high mortality.[29]

Onychomycosis, including rapidly developing onychomycosis, caused by dermatophytes is common in people with AIDS. Although the normal treatment regimens for nail infection can be used, often it is necessary to double the dose and prolong treatment times.

Onychomycosis in children is usually due to dermatophyte infection. In very small children fluconazole syrup 2–3 mg/day may be preferable. In older children itraconazole or itraconazole are effective, although responses are often poorer than in adults.

MUCOSAL CANDIDOSIS

Mucosal fungal infections are extremely common. The vast majority are caused by *C. albicans* but occasionally by other yeasts, especially *C. glabrata*, and rarely by filamentous molds such as *Aspergillus* spp.

OROPHARYNGEAL CANDIDOSIS

Before the AIDS epidemic, oropharyngeal candidosis (OPC) was largely seen in patients at the extremes of age, those receiving inhaled steroids or antibiotic therapy, following oral cavity radiotherapy, after cytotoxic chemotherapy and in denture wearers. Chronic oral candidosis occurs in patients with chronic mucocutaneous candidosis (CMC). *C. albicans* is the primary pathogen and rarely *C. glabrata* and *C. krusei* (Table 59.2). The most common pattern of OPC is the pseudomembranous form, but an erythematous type is also found. Occasionally, denture-related candidosis or angular cheilitis is the primary manifestation. In untreated AIDS, the pseudomembranous or erythematous forms predominate.

Topical agents such as nystatin or amphotericin B oral suspension (1 mL every 6 h for 2–3 weeks) are effective in non-immunocompromised patients. Clotrimazole troches (available in the USA) are also effective. Miconazole oral gel in a dose of 10 mL every 6 h is particularly useful for denture-related candidosis or in infants.

Table 59.2 Intrinsically resistant fungi

Species	Antifungal agents
Candida krusei	Fluconazole, ketoconazole
Candida glabrata[a]	Fluconazole, ketoconazole, itraconazole
Candida parapsilosis	Echinocandins
Candida lusitaniae[a]	Amphotericin B
Malassezia spp.	Amphotericin B
Trichosporon spp.	Amphotericin B
Aspergillus spp.	Ketoconazole, fluconazole
Mucorales	Azoles, flucytosine, echinocandins
Scedosporium apiospermum (*Pseudallescheria boydii*)	Amphotericin B
Scedosporium prolificans	Amphotericin B, azoles, flucytosine
Paecilomyces spp.	Amphotericin B
Fusarium spp.	Azoles, flucytosine
Penicillium spp.	Ketoconazole

[a]A substantial proportion or majority of isolates.

In immunocompromised patients, fluconazole 100 mg/day is more effective than topical therapy and is the agent of first choice, with response rates in excess of 90%. Ketoconazole and itraconazole are also effective at doses of 200–400 mg/day but are less well absorbed in conditions of hypochlorhydria that complicate AIDS and bone marrow transplantation. Improved serum of levels of both itraconazole and ketoconazole are achieved by acid drinks such as orange juice or cola and food. Itraconazole oral solution overcomes this problem.

VULVOVAGINAL CANDIDOSIS

Vulvovaginal candidosis is common. By the age of 24 years, 60% of 76 women had suffered at least one episode of vulvovaginal candidosis.[30] Among these women, 36% had at least one episode a year and 3% had it 'almost all the time'. Certain conditions increase the incidence and possibly the severity of vulvovaginal candidosis. These include pregnancy, antibiotic use, diabetes mellitus and cystic fibrosis.[30] HIV-seropositive women are no more likely to develop vaginal candidiasis than controls,[31] but in these patients there is often a worse response to initial treatment and a shorter time to relapse. Over 90% of cases are caused by *C. albicans*, about 5% by *C. glabrata* and other species such as *C. tropicalis* can be isolated from the remainder.

Treatment may be local or systemic (Table 59.3). Topical treatment regimens with azoles yield response rates of 80–90%. Many different formulations are available, which vary primarily in cost. Women without predisposing factors, such as pregnancy, will usually prefer single-dose or 3-day treatments. Responses are slower in those with predisposing factors and 5- to 14-day treatment regimens are generally preferable if topical therapy is preferred. Nystatin, one to two pessaries inserted high into the vaginal vault nightly for 14 nights, has a lower response rate (80%) than the azoles and stains clothing, but is useful for azole-resistant organisms such as *C. glabrata*.

Oral therapy is preferred by many women; fluconazole as a single dose of 150 mg or itraconazole two 200 mg doses 8 h apart are effective in over 90% of patients. Itraconazole may be preferable for *C. glabrata* infections.

In pregnancy, local therapy with a clotrimazole 500 mg vaginal tablet is often effective and does not expose the fetus to an antifungal.[32] This is desirable in the first trimester, although there is no evidence that azoles are teratogenic in humans at the doses usually used.[33,34] However 4 days' therapy is more effective than single-dose therapy and 7 days' therapy even better.[35] Later in pregnancy, systemic therapy with fluconazole or itraconazole are accepted alternatives.[36] Treatment of vaginal candidiasis in pregnancy appears to reduce preterm birth.[37]

Suppressive treatment may be indicated for frequent recurrent infections. Continuous therapy for 3–6 months suppresses symptoms and reduces the subsequent frequency of relapse, and once monthly intermittent therapy with itraconazole 400 mg was partially successful.[38] If symptoms recur, local treatment

Table 59.3 Examples of treatment regimens for vulvovaginal candidosis

Antifungal agent	Formulation	Dose	Duration
Local therapy			
Clotrimazole	Vaginal tablet	1–200 mg	3–7 daily doses
Clotrimazole	Vaginal tablet	500 mg	1 dose
Econazole	Vaginal tablet	150 mg	3 daily doses
Miconazole	Pessary	100–200 mg	3–7 daily doses
Miconazole	Pessary	1200 mg	1 dose
Nystatin	Vaginal tablet	100 000 U	14 daily doses
Terconazole	Pessary	300 mg	1 dose
Terconazole	Vaginal tablet	80 mg	3 days
Butoconazole	2% cream	5 g	1–3 daily doses
Clotrimazole	1% cream	5 g	7–14 daily doses
Clotrimazole	10% cream	5 g	1 dose
Econazole	1% cream		Twice daily for 3–7 days
Fenticonazole	2% cream	5 g	7 daily doses
Miconazole	2% cream	5 g	7 daily doses
Terconazole	0.4–2% cream	5 g	3 daily doses
Tioconazole	2% cream	5 g	3 daily doses
Tioconazole	6.5% cream	5 g	1 dose
Systemic therapy			
Fluconazole	Capsule	150 mg	1 dose
Itraconazole	Capsule	200 mg	2 doses, or 3 days

with single-dose clotrimazole 500 mg fortnightly or intermittent single-dose oral treatment with fluconazole 150 mg may be helpful. There is no evidence to date of antifungal resistance resulting from such a regimen, although *C. glabrata* infections are more common in women who have received repeated courses of azole therapy.

OTOMYCOSIS (OTITIS EXTERNA)

Otomycosis is a relatively common problem in non-immunocompromised patients and is commoner in hot humid climates. The causative fungi include *Aspergillus niger* and *C. albicans*. The latter may form a blackish mat in the ear canal but many infections do not have characteristic features.

The vast majority of cases of otomycosis respond to a combination of cleaning of the ear canal and topical antifungal therapy. Clotrimazole solution or cream, applied at least twice daily for a minimum of a week, is probably the best primary therapy. Alternatives include cresyl acetate solution or topical ketoconazole, econazole or amphotericin B. Care should be taken in the application of any of these compounds if the tympanic membrane is perforated, as hearing loss has been reported.

Occasionally, invasive otomycosis of the bone, in particular of the mastoid, occurs usually in immunosuppressed patients. It is usually caused by *Aspergillus fumigatus*, but occasionally by other organisms. Many, but not all, patients are immunocompromised. These patients require systemic antifungal therapy according to the nature of the organism; surgical debridement is also often necessary.

 References

1. Elewski BE. Tinea capitis: a current perspective. *J Am Acad Dermatol.* 2000;42:1–20.
2. Dragos V, Lunder M. Lack of efficacy of 6-week treatment with oral terbinafine for tinea capitis due to *Microsporum canis* in children. *Pediatr Dermatol.* 1997;14:4–48.
3. Greer DL. Successful treatment of tinea capitis with 2% ketoconazole shampoo. *Int J Dermatol.* 2000;29:302–304.

4. Caceres-Rios H, Rueda M, Ballona R, Bustamante B. Comparison of terbinafine and griseofulvin in the treatment of tinea capitis. *J Am Acad Dermatol*. 2000;42:80–84.

5. Filho ST, Cuce LC, Foss NT, Marques SA, Santamaria JR. Efficacy, safety and tolerability of terbinafine for tinea capitis in children: Brazilian multicentric study with daily oral tablets for 1, 2 and 4 weeks. *J Eur Acad Dermatol Venereol*. 1998;11:141–146.

6. Jahangir M, Hussain I, Hasan MU, Haroon TS. A double-blind, randomised, comparative trial of itraconazole versus terbinafine for 2 weeks in tinea capitis. *Br J Dermatol*. 1998;139:672–674.

7. Lopez-Gomez S, Del Palacio A, Van Cutsem J, Soledad Cuetara M, Iglesias L, Rodriguez-Noriega A. Itraconazole versus griseofulvin in the treatment of tinea capitis: a double-blind randomized study in children. *Int J Dermatol*. 1994;33:743–747.

8. Abdel-Rahman SM, Powell DA, Nahata MC. Efficacy of itraconazole in children with *Trichophyton tonsurans* tinea capitis. *J Am Acad Dermatol*. 1998;38:443–446.

9. Gupta AK, Dlova N, Taborda P, et al. Once weekly fluconazole is effective in children in the treatment of tinea capitis: a prospective, multicentre study. *Br J Dermatol*. 2000;142:965–968.

10. Parent D, Decroix J, Heenen M. Clinical experience with short schedules of itraconazole in the treatment of tinea corporis and/or tinea cruris. *Dermatology*. 1994;189:378–381.

11. Farag A, Taha M, Halim S. One-week therapy with oral terbinafine in cases of tinea cruris/corporis. *Br J Dermatol*. 1994;131:684–686.

12. Bakos L, Brito AC, Castro LC, et al. Open clinical study of the efficacy and safety of terbinafine cream 1% in children with tinea corporis and tinea cruris. *Pediatr Infect Dis J*. 1997;16:545–548.

13. Evans EGV. A comparison of terbinafine (Lamisil) 1% cream given for one week with clotrimazole (Canesten) 1% cream given for four weeks, in the treatment of tinea pedis. *Br J Dermatol*. 1994;130(suppl 43):12–14.

14. de Chauvin MF, Viguie-Vallanet C, Kienzler JL, Larnier C. Novel, single-dose, topical treatment of tinea pedis using terbinafine: results of a dose-finding clinical trial. *Mycoses*. 2008;51:1–6.

15. Delescluse J. Itraconazole in tinea versicolor: a review. *J Am Acad Dermatol*. 1990;23:551–554.

16. Gupta A, Bluhm R, Cooper E, Summerbell R, Batra R. Seborrheic dermatitis. *Dermatol Clin*. 2003;21:401–412.

17. Tosti A, Piraccini B. Treatment of common nail disorders. *Dermatol Clin*. 2000;18:339–348.

18. Gupta A. Onychomycosis therapies: strategies to improve efficacy. *Dermatol Clin*. 2006;24:381–386.

19. Zaug M, Bergstraesser M. Amorolfine in the treatment of onychomycosis and dermatomycoses (an overview). *Clin Exp Dermatol*. 1992;17(suppl 1):61–70.

20. Bonifaz A, Ibarra G. Onychomycosis in children: treatment with bifonazole-urea. *Pediatr Dermatol*. 2000;17:310–314.

21. McInnes BD, Dockery BL. Surgical treatment of mycotic toenails. *J Am Podiatr Med Assoc*. 1997;87:557–564.

22. Evans EGV, Sigurgeirsson B. Double blind, randomised study of continuous terbinafine compared with intermittent itraconazole in treatment of toe-nail onychomycosis. The LION study group. *Br Med J*. 1999;318:1031–1035.

23. Tausch I, Brautigam M, Weidinger G, Jones TC. Evaluation of 6 weeks treatment of terbinafine in tinea unguium in a double blind trial comparing 6 and 12 weeks therapy. The Lagos V Study Group. *Br J Dermatol*. 1997;136:737–742.

24. Tosti A, Piraccini BM, Stinchi C, Colombo MD. Relapses of onychomycosis after successful treatment with systemic antifungals: a three-year follow-up. *Dermatology*. 1998;197:162–166.

25. Arikian SR, Einarson TR, Kobelt-Nguyen G, Schubert F. A multinational pharmacoeconomic analysis of oral therapies for onychomycosis. The Onychomycosis Study Group. *Br J Dermatol*. 1994;130:35–44.

26. Sigurgeirsson B, Ólafsson JH, Steinsson J, Paul C, Billstein S, Evans EGV. Long-term effectiveness of treatment with terbinafine vs itraconazole in onychomycosis. *Arch Dermatol*. 2002;138:353–357.

27. Bristow IR, Baran R. Topical and oral combination therapy for toenail onychomycosis. *J Am Podiatr Med Assoc*. 2006;96:116–119.

28. Epstein E. How often does oral treatment of toenail onychomycosis produce a disease-free nail? *Arch Dermatol*. 1998;134:1551–1554.

29. Nelson PE, Dignani MC, Anaissie EJ. Taxonomy, biology and clinical aspects of *Fusarium* species. *Clin Microbiol Rev*. 1994;7:479–504.

30. Sawyer SM, Bowes G, Phelan PD. Vulvovaginal candidiasis in young women with cystic fibrosis. *Br Med J*. 1994;308:1609.

31. Sobel JD. Vaginitis. *N Engl J Med*. 1998;337:1896–1903.

32. Lindeque BG, Van Niekerk WG. Treatment of vaginal candidiasis in pregnancy with a single clotrimazole 500 mg vaginal pessary. *S Afr Med J*. 1984;65:123–124.

33. Sobel JD. Use of antifungal drugs in pregnancy: a focus on safety. *Drug Safety*. 2000;23:77–85.

34. Czeizel AE, Toth M, Rochenbauer M. No teratogenic effect after clotrimazole therapy during pregnancy. *Epidemiology*. 1999;10:437–440.

35. Young GL, Jewell D. Topical treatment for vaginal candidiasis in pregnancy. *Cochrane Database Syst Rev*. 2000; CD000225.

36. Inman W, Pearce G, Wilton L. Safety of fluconazole in the treatment of vaginal candidiasis. A prescription-event monitoring study, with special reference to the outcome of pregnancy. *Eur J Clin Pharmacol*. 1994;46:115–118.

37. Czeizel AE, Rockenbauer M. A lower rate of preterm birth after clotrimazole therapy during pregnancy. *Paediatr Perinat Epidemiol*. 1999;13:58–64.

38. Spinillo A, Colonna L, Piazzi G, Baltaro F, Monaco A, Ferrari A. Managing recurrent vulvovaginal candidiasis. Intermittent prevention with itraconazole. *J Reprod Med*. 1997;42:83–87.

60 Systemic fungal infections

Paula S. Seal and Peter G. Pappas

The treatment of fungal disease has evolved significantly with the recent introduction of several new antifungal agents. The number of immunocompromised patients, including solid organ and stem cell transplant recipients and others on chronic immunomodulating therapy, continues to increase as has the population at risk of invasive fungal infection. New clinical trial data and treatment guideline recommendations have become available while emerging fungal pathogens pose a challenge with regard to the most appropriate antifungal regimens. In this chapter, we discuss the approach to treatment of the more common systemic mycoses.

INVASIVE CANDIDIASIS

CANDIDEMIA

Candidemia is the fourth most common cause of nosocomial bloodstream infections in the USA, with an attributable mortality ranging between 15% and 49% in adults.[1-3] Recent epidemiological studies have demonstrated the increase of non-*albicans Candida* spp. as a cause of invasive candidiasis.[4] Factors associated with mortality in invasive candidiasis include higher APACHE II scores, non-*parapsilosis* isolates, persistently positive blood cultures and significant underlying illness.

All patients with candidemia require systemic antifungal therapy. Specific recommendations are detailed in Table 60.1. The selection of an antifungal agent should be based on the *Candida* species, presumed susceptibility, a history of prior therapy including recent azole exposure, and a clinical suspicion of deep organ involvement, such as central nervous system, endocardial or hepatic/splenic involvement.[5,6] All patients with candidemia require a dilated fundoscopic examination to evaluate for endophthalmitis. Removal of central venous catheters is strongly recommended in non-neutropenic patients and may decrease the duration of candidemia.[7]

The standard therapy for many patients with candidemia without prior azole exposure is fluconazole (6 mg/kg per day).[8-11] In the first multicenter randomized trial comparing amphotericin B deoxycholate (AmB-d) with fluconazole as treatment for candidemia in non-neutropenic patients, no difference in outcome to therapy was found.[8] Based on these data and other studies, the recommended duration of therapy is 14 days after documented clearance of *Candida* bloodstream infection together with resolution of signs and symptoms of infection.[8-15] Recent data suggest that echinocandins are an effective first-line therapy for candidemia; most experts agree that patients who are moderately to severely ill should be treated initially with an echinocandin. Echinocandins are also the agents of choice for patients with prior azole exposure, allergy or intolerance to other antifungals, and those at high risk of infection with *C. glabrata* or *C. krusei*.[15] Current recommended therapy is at least 3–5 days of echinocandin therapy followed by fluconazole as stepdown therapy when the patient is clinically stable and candidemia has cleared. Among the more common species, *C. parapsilosis* has decreased susceptibility to the echinocandins, and initial treatment with fluconazole is recommended.[4]

Amphotericin B (AmB) is also effective for candidemia, but its role as initial therapy is restricted to resource-limited environments, echinocandin or azole intolerance, documented resistance to current therapy, or suspicion of a non-*Candida* yeast (e.g. *Cryptococcus*, *Histoplasma*, *Trichosporon*).

The role for the expanded spectrum triazoles (e.g. voriconazole and posaconazole) is very limited. They lack any clear advantage over conventional therapy with fluconazole, echinocandins or AmB. Currently, their role is limited to treatment of fluconazole-resistant *Candida* spp. which are susceptible to one of these agents (e.g. *C. krusei*).

Breakpoints for *Candida* spp. exist for susceptibility testing to fluconazole, itraconazole, voriconazole, flucytosine (5FC) and the echinocandins.[16,17] General susceptibility patterns of *Candida* species are detailed in Table 60.2. When there is concern about azole resistance, susceptibility testing should be performed. All *C. glabrata* isolates should ideally be tested for azole susceptibility.

Table 60.1 Treatment of invasive candidiasis

Condition	Primary therapy	Alternative therapy	Comments
Candidemia Non-neutropenic	Fluconazole 800 mg (12 mg/kg) loading dose then 400 mg (6 mg/kg) per day; or an echinocandin	LFAmB 3–5 mg/kg per day; or voriconazole 4 mg/kg every 12 h for 2 doses, then 3 mg/kg per day	Duration of therapy is 14 days from negative blood culture and resolution of clinical signs and symptoms An echinocandin is favored for patients with moderate to severe disease and among patients with risk factors for non-*albicans Candida* spp.
Neutropenic	LFAmB 3–5 mg/kg per day; or an echinocandin	Voriconazole 4 mg/kg every 12 h for 2 doses, then 3 mg/kg per day; or fluconazole 800 mg (12 mg/kg) loading dose, then 400 mg (6 mg/kg) per day	Duration of therapy is 14 days from negative blood culture, resolution of clinical signs and symptoms, *and* recovery from neutropenia
Endocarditis	LFAmB 3–6 mg/kg or AmB-d 0.6–1.0 mg/kg per day, ± 5FC 100 mg/kg per day; or an echinocandin	Fluconazole 400–800 mg (6–12 mg/kg) per day for stepdown therapy in stable patients, negative blood cultures and susceptible organisms	Surgical intervention is recommended Duration of induction therapy is 6 weeks, followed by lifelong suppressive therapy For echinocandins, higher than standard dosing is recommended: caspofungin 50–150 mg/day; micafungin 100–150 mg/day; anidulafungin 100–200 mg/day
Meningitis	LFAmB 3–6 mg/kg per day ± 5FC 100 mg/kg per day	Fluconazole 400–800 mg (6–12 mg/kg) per day	Duration of therapy is 4–6 weeks pending clinical improvement and resolution of CSF abnormalities; stepdown therapy with fluconazole 400–800 mg (6–12 mg/kg) per day
Chronic disseminated	LFAmB 3–6 mg/kg or fluconazole 400–800 mg (6–12 mg/kg) per day	An echinocandin	Stepdown fluconazole is appropriate following 1–2 weeks' induction with LFAmB or an echinocandin Antifungal therapy is indicated until radiographic resolution of lesions
Osteomyelitis	LFAmB 3–6 mg/kg or AmB-d 0.6–1.0 mg/kg per day; or fluconazole 6–12 mg/kg per day	An echinocandin	Duration of parenteral therapy is 3–6 weeks, followed by stepdown therapy with oral fluconazole for 6–12 months Surgical intervention may be indicated in selected cases
Endophthalmitis	AmB-d 0.7–1.0 mg/kg plus 5FC 100 mg/kg per day; and/or intravitreal AmB-d 5 μg plus 5FC; or fluconazole 400–800 mg (6–12 mg/kg) per day	LFAmB 3–6 mg/kg; or voriconazole 6 mg/kg every 12 h for 2 doses, then 3–4 mg/kg every 12 h	Duration of parenteral therapy is at least 4–6 weeks Vitrectomy may be necessary for sight preservation
Esophagitis	Fluconazole 200–400 mg (3–6 mg/kg) per day; or AmB-d 0.3–0.7 mg/kg per day; or an echinocandin (*see comments*)	Itraconazole solution 200 mg/day; or posaconazole 400 mg every 12 h; or voriconazole 200 mg every 12 h	Duration of therapy is 14–21 days Oral agents are preferred; intravenous agents are indicated in the setting of intolerance to oral agents For the echinocandins, the following dosing is recommended: caspofungin 50 mg/day; micafungin 150 mg/day; anidulafungin 200 mg/day

AmB, amphotericin B; AmB-d: amphotericin B deoxycholate; CSF, cerebrospinal fluid; 5FC, flucytosine; LFAmB, lipid formulation of amphotericin B.
Voriconazole standard dosing: loading dose of 400 mg every 12 h (6 mg/kg every 12 h) for 1 day, followed by a maintenance dose of 200 mg every 12 h (4 mg/kg every 12 h).
Posaconazole standard dosing: 200 mg every 6 h until stabilization of disease followed by maintenance dose of 400 mg bid.
Itraconazole standard dosing: loading dose of 200 mg every 8 h for 3 days followed by maintenance dose of 200 mg every 12 h.
Echinocandin loading dose: Caspofungin 70 mg loading dose, Anidulafungin 200 mg loading dose, Micafungin no loading dose.
Echinocandin standard dosing: Caspofungin 50 mg/day; Micafungin 100 mg/day; Anidulafungin 100 mg/day.

CANDIDA ENDOCARDITIS

Candida primarily causes prosthetic valve endocarditis, although native valve endocarditis may complicate candidemia, often as a consequence of illicit intravenous drug use. Mortality rates for *Candida* endocarditis are as high as 30%.[18] Both valvular replacement and antifungal therapy are required for the management of *Candida* endocarditis given the risk of embolism, difficulty in sterilizing blood cultures, and high mortality rate with medical therapy alone.[19]

Most of the data pertaining to treatment of *Candida* endocarditis are retrospective. Historically, the most common treatment is AmB-d (0.7–1.0 mg/kg per day), with or without flucytosine (25 mg/kg every 6 h), followed by stepdown therapy with an azole, usually fluconazole (6–12 mg/kg per day). Lipid

Table 60.2 General susceptibility patterns of *Candida* species

Species	Fluconazole	Itraconazole	Voriconazole	Posaconazole	5FC	AmB	Echinocandins
C. albicans	S	S	S	S	S	S	S
C. tropicalis	S	S	S	S	S	S	S
C. parapsilosis	S	S	S	S	S	S	S to R[a]
C. glabrata	S-DD to R	S-DD to R	S-DD to R	S-DD to R	S	S to I	S
C. krusei	R	S-DD to R	S	S	I to R	S to I	S
C. lusitaniae	S	S	S	S	S	S to R	S

I, intermediate susceptibility; R, resistant; S, susceptible; S-DD, susceptible dose-dependent.
[a]*C. parapsilosis* isolates resistant to echinocandins are uncommon.

formulation of amphotericin B (LFAmB) (3–6 mg/kg per day) is less nephrotoxic and generally preferred to AmB-d.[20,21]

Echinocandins at dosages higher than those used to treat candidemia have been used successfully to treat endocarditis. The suggested dose range for caspofungin is 50–150 mg/day, for micafungin 100–150 mg/day and for anidulafungin 100–200 mg/day. Successful treatment in the absence of vascular surgery with AmB-d–caspofungin induction or caspofungin–fluconazole induction, followed by suppressive therapy with either caspofungin or fluconazole, has been demonstrated in several cases.[21–26]

Prosthetic valve endocarditis requires chronic suppressive therapy with an azole due to the high risk of relapse. Lifelong suppressive therapy with fluconazole 400–800 mg/day is also recommended in patients who are not surgical candidates.[24,26]

CANDIDA MENINGITIS

Central nervous system (CNS) *Candida* infections are usually complications of candidemia or neurosurgical procedures in adults.[27–29] *C. albicans* is the most common cause of *Candida* meningitis. Disseminated candidiasis may be associated with cerebral microabscesses in close proximity to the vasculature and is a particularly common complication in neonates.[30]

In suspected CNS candidiasis in adults, the preferred first-line therapy is LFAmB. For neonates, AmB-d (1 mg/kg per day) is still generally used due to its proven efficacy and good tolerance. Echinocandins have poor CNS penetration and cannot be recommended.

In the absence of prospective trial data, current treatment regimens, based on retrospective data, support combination therapy with LFAmB (3–6 mg/kg per day) and flucytosine (25 mg/kg every 6 h). Combination therapy is also supported by in-vitro synergism and cerebrospinal fluid (CSF) penetration by flucytosine.[30] Liposomal AmB is less nephrotoxic and has greater CNS penetration, and may offer a therapeutic advantage in adults, but this is unproven. Upon evidence of significant clinical improvement after initial treatment with AmB, fluconazole (6–12 mg/kg per day) stepdown therapy

is recommended.[9,11–13,15] For fluconazole-resistant isolates such as *C. krusei*, *C. guilliermondii* or *C. glabrata*, voriconazole (3 mg/kg every 12 h) is an acceptable alternative, provided susceptibility is confirmed.[7] Duration of antifungal therapy is poorly defined, but most experts suggest at least 4–6 weeks. Significant improvement in the CSF findings and related symptoms should be demonstrated before considering stepdown therapy to an azole.[2–4,31] In patients with infected ventricular shunts, shunt removal is critical to clear infection. Instillation of AmB directly into the shunt has limited efficacy and is generally discouraged.

HEPATOSPLENIC (CHRONIC DISSEMINATED) CANDIDIASIS

Hepatosplenic candidiasis, also known as chronic disseminated candidiasis, is a distinctive clinical entity appearing during recovery from neutropenia. It is manifested by abdominal pain, hepatomegaly, with or without splenomegaly, and elevated alkaline phosphatase. Involvement of liver, spleen and kidneys is common. Biopsy is required for diagnosis which demonstrates granulomata surrounding yeasts and hyphae; cultures of biopsy material are usually negative. Historically, hepatosplenic candidiasis has been treated with AmB-d, LFAmB and fluconazole.[32–36] More recently, data have emerged supporting the use of echinocandins and voriconazole.[30,37,38] Duration of therapy is guided by improvement/resolution of lesions on radiographic imaging. Two weeks of parenteral therapy with LFAmB (3–5 mg/kg per day) or an echinocandin, followed by an oral azole (fluconazole 6 mg/kg per day) is a typical approach to therapy. Months of systemic antifungal therapy are usually required to achieve cure. Evidence of radiographic resolution is important to avoid relapse.

CANDIDA OSTEOMYELITIS

Up to 60% of *Candida* osteomyelitis cases are a consequence of candidemia, with intravenous drug use as the most important predisposing factor.[39] *Candida* osteomyelitis can occur as late as

14 months after the initial episode of candidemia.[40] Treatment recommendations for osteoarticular *Candida* infections are based on small series and case reports. Initial antifungal therapy with an AmB formulation or an echinocandin for 2–3 weeks, followed by surgical debridement and subsequent oral stepdown therapy to an azole is ideal. Success has also been documented with medical therapy with AmB for at least 6 weeks. Regardless of the initial regimen chosen, suppressive therapy with fluconazole (6 mg/kg per day) for 6–12 months should follow.[41]

OCULAR CANDIDIASIS

Up to 10% of patients with untreated candidemia develop ocular *Candida* infection, manifested as either chorioretinitis or endophthalmitis. The diagnosis is usually based on clinical findings, but can be confirmed by a positive culture or Gram stain from a vitreous aspirate. In most cases, ophthalmological consideration of partial vitrectomy and intravitreal AmB-d (5 μg) is recommended.[30] Conventional therapy is intravenous AmB in combination with flucytosine and/or intravitreal AmB-d. Systemic AmB has poor ocular penetration, combination therapy is usually recommended.[42–44] Fluconazole (6–12 mg/kg per day) has excellent intravitreal penetration, and can be used as initial treatment in selected cases and for salvage therapy.[43,45] In cases of fluconazole or AmB-d treatment failure, limited data support the use of treatment with LFAmB (3–6 mg/kg per day) or voriconazole.[46,47] Voriconazole has excellent vitreal penetration at dosages of 3–4 mg every 12 h; it may also be given topically.[48] Echinocandins have poor ocular penetration and are generally not recommended for *Candida* endophthalmitis. Duration of therapy is usually 4–6 weeks of systemic therapy until clinical infection has resolved.[30]

CANDIDA ESOPHAGITIS

Esophageal candidasis (EC) usually coexists with oropharyngeal disease, although in 30% of cases there are no oral lesions visible. It is an AIDS-defining illness and is common among patients receiving myeloablative chemotherapy. Rare reports of esophageal candidasis in immunocompetent individuals and after omeprazole therapy suggest that hypochlorhydria favors development of disease.

The majority of cases of oropharyngeal candidiasis are due to *C. albicans*; however, cases of *C. glabrata* and *C. krusei* are reported.[49–51] All cases of suspected or proven EC should be treated with systemic antifungals. In patients with suspected esophageal disease, empirical therapy with fluconazole 200–400 mg/day is a reasonable initial approach. Itraconazole solution (200 mg/day), posaconazole suspension (400 mg every 12 h) or voriconazole (200 mg every 12 h) can be used to treat fluconazole-refractory disease. Duration of therapy is 14–21 days. Intolerance to oral therapy or inability to swallow warrants treatment with intravenous fluconazole (400 mg/day), AmB-d (0.3–0.7 mg/kg per day) or an echinocandin.

ASPERGILLOSIS

Aspergillus species are important invasive fungal pathogens, causing considerable morbidity and mortality in immunocompromised hosts. They also cause chronic, saprophytic and allergic conditions in immunocompetent patients. *Aspergillus* species grow well on standard media; identification to species level is usually recommended. Pathology specimens reveal the characteristic angular dichotomously branching septate hyphae by direct microscopy or culture.[52] Diagnosis is based on a combination of culture, histopathology, radiographical imaging and serological studies. The use of serum enzyme immunoassay for galactomannan has remarkably enhanced the early diagnosis of invasive aspergillosis; its use in CSF and bronchoalveolar lavage (BAL) fluid remains investigational, as does the use of serial galactomannan for therapeutic monitoring.[53,54]

INVASIVE ASPERGILLOSIS

Invasive aspergillosis typically affects patients who are significantly immunocompromised. Untreated mortality approaches 100%.[55] Those at risk of invasive aspergillosis include patients with advanced HIV infection, prolonged neutropenia, allogeneic hematopoietic stem cell transplantation (HSCT) and inherited immunodeficiency.[52] Outcome depends in part on the potential for immune recovery, stage of disease when treatment is initiated and the rate of disease progression. Prompt initiation of antifungal therapy is important in highly immunocompromised patients. Thus, empirical therapy is appropriate for suspected disease in these patients. In contrast, in less immunocompromised patients, disease progression is often slower, allowing the diagnosis to be confirmed before treatment is given. Specific recommendations regarding therapy are detailed in Table 60.3.

In the USA, voriconazole and AmB-d are the only compounds licensed for the primary treatment of invasive aspergillosis, while LFAmB, itraconazole (200 mg tablets every 12 h) and caspofungin (50 mg/day) are approved for salvage therapy. Primary therapy with parenteral or oral voriconazole (4 mg/kg every 12 h) is recommended for the treatment of most forms of invasive aspergillosis. In the largest prospective, randomized trial for invasive pulmonary aspergillosis, voriconazole was superior to AmB-d (1.0–1.5 mg/kg per day) and other licensed antifungal therapy with significantly improved survival (53% vs 32%) and successful response at 12 weeks and at the end of the study period.[56] Parenteral voriconazole is recommended for seriously ill patients and those unable to tolerate oral medications. In the event of drug intolerance or disease progression, LFAmB is an acceptable alternative, and is preferable to AmB-d.[57–60] Optimal dosing of LFAmB for invasive aspergillosis is unclear. Many experts prescribe an initial dose of 5–6 mg/kg per day, although a recent randomized trial comparing two initial doses of LFAmB (3 mg/kg

Table 60.3 Treatment for aspergillosis

Condition	Primary therapy	Alternative therapy	Comments
Invasive aspergillosis	Voriconazole[a]	LFAmB 5–6 mg/kg per day or caspofungin 70 mg loading dose, 50 mg/day maintenance dose or posaconazole[b] or itraconazole[c]	Duration of therapy not defined Recommend treatment until resolution of symptoms and radiographic changes Initial monotherapy with voriconazole is preferred Alternative therapy with combination therapy or change in class is recommended in setting of treatment failure
Chronic necrotizing pulmonary aspergillosis	Voriconazole[a] or itraconazole[c]	LFAmB 5–6 mg/kg/day or caspofungin 70 mg loading dose, 50 mg/day maintenance dose or posaconazole[b]	Oral azole therapy is preferred Chronic azole suppressive therapy is required for months
Aspergilloma	Antifungal therapy is of minimal benefit. Surgical evaluation is recommended	Itraconazole[c] or voriconazole[a]	Oral ketoconazole and parenteral AmB are ineffective

[a]Voriconazole standard dosing: loading dose of 400 mg every 12 h (6 mg/kg every 12 h) for 1 day, followed by a maintenance dose of 200 mg every 12 h (4 mg/kg every 12 h).
[b]Posaconazole standard dosing: 200 mg every 6 h until stabilization of disease followed by maintenance dose of 400 mg bid.
[c]Itraconazole standard dosing: loading dose of 200 mg every 8 h for 3 days followed by maintenance dose of 200 mg every 12 h.

per day vs 10 mg/kg per day) showed similar efficacy (50% vs 46% success, respectively).[61]

Primary combination therapy remains investigational but may be useful in the context of salvage therapy. For salvage therapy, a change in therapeutic class is recommended using LFAmB or an echinocandin. Azole use as combination therapy should take into account prior therapy, host factors and pharmacokinetic considerations. Optional agents include LFAmB, posaconazole (200 mg every 6 h, followed by 400 mg every 12 h with stable disease), itraconazole (200 mg tablets every 12 h) and caspofungin (50 mg/day).[52] In one salvage study, caspofungin therapy was 40% successful, with less than 5% of patients experiencing drug-related nephrotoxicity or hepatotoxicity.[62] Oral itraconazole has had similar results (39%), but is a less attractive alternative and is rarely used in this setting.[63,64] Posaconazole is approved as salvage therapy in Europe for patients refractory to AmB or itraconazole. In an open-labeled salvage trial, 42% of posaconazole recipients vs 26% of control patients were successfully treated.[65]

The management of breakthrough invasive aspergillosis during azole prophylaxis or suppressive therapy has not been defined by clinical trial data, but changing drug class from the azoles is suggested. Medical management should always include reversal of the underlying condition, when feasible. Surgical resection of lesions contiguous with the great vessels or pericardium, those associated with hemoptysis, or lesions eroding into the pleural space or ribs is recommended.[52]

Resistance to itraconazole and the expanded-spectrum azoles is infrequent among *Aspergillus* spp. With the exception of *A. terreus*, few *Aspergillus* isolates demonstrate in-vitro resistance in to AmB. Based on clinical experience and in-vitro data, primary treatment of *A. terreus* infection should involve the use of an expanded spectrum triazole.[66]

Persistent neutropenia is often associated with a fatal outcome in invasive aspergillosis. In these patients granulocyte-colony stimulating factor or granulocyte macrophage-colony stimulating factor may be used to reverse immunosuppression, although the benefit is unproven. Case reports also suggest a potential role for the use of interferon-γ as adjunctive therapy for invasive aspergillosis in immunocompromised non-neutropenic patients, particularly those with chronic granulomatous disease.

Treatment of invasive aspergillosis should continue while the patient is immunocompromised and until there has been resolution of disease. In the neutropenic patient, treatment should continue until the neutrophil count recovers and there has been radiographic disease regression. In solid organ transplant recipients, therapy should be continued until there is a complete or near-complete clinical response.

CHRONIC NECROTIZING ASPERGILLOSIS

Chronic necrotizing pulmonary aspergillosis (CNPA) is a complex condition sharing features of invasive aspergillosis and pulmonary aspergillomata. CNPA is more common among patients with underlying lung disease or low-grade immunosuppression. It usually is not life threatening with appropriate treatment. All patients with CNPA have radiological evidence of one or more cavitary lesions in the lung, usually in the upper lobe. The cavities may contain aspergillomata. Serology is often positive for *Aspergillus* galactomannan and inflammatory markers are elevated. CNPA requires systemic antifungal therapy.[67,68]

Itraconazole (200 mg capsules every 12 h) and voriconazole (4 mg/kg intravenously every 12 h, or 200 mg orally every 12 h) appear to be the agents of choice for CNPA.[69,70]

Other options include intracavitary AmB and voriconazole.[71,72] Oral therapy of CNPA is generally preferred. Chronic suppressive therapy with an azole is essential to prevent relapse.

Surgery should be avoided if possible, as complications are common, including fungal empyema and significant intra- or postoperative bleeding. Embolization of involved vasculature may be preferable to surgery for hemoptysis.

ASPERGILLOMA

The vast majority of pulmonary fungus balls are due to *Aspergillus* spp., with rare cases due to *Scedosporium apiospermum* or the zygomycetes. A pulmonary aspergilloma is composed of *Aspergillus* hyphae, fibrin and mucus, consolidated within a pre-existing pulmonary cavity or ectatic bronchus.[73] Radiographically these can appear solid or as water density within a cavity but clearly demarcated from the wall of the cavity. Adjacent pleural thickening is common. Aspergillomata most commonly occur in patients with underlying lung disease such as cavitary tuberculosis or histoplasmosis, sarcoidosis, emphysema or fibrotic lung disease.

Approximately 10% of aspergillomata resolve spontaneously. Medical therapy is of limited benefit for the treatment of aspergillomata. Itraconazole (200 mg every 12 h) is of marginal symptomatic and little radiological benefit.[74]

Hemoptysis is the main indication for surgical intervention.[75] In non-surgical candidate patients with recurrent hemoptysis, bronchial artery embolization may be used as a temporizing measure until medical therapy or surgical resection can occur. Endobronchial or intracavitary instillation of the aspergilloma with AmB has been used with some success.[52] There are few published data for voriconazole, but many experts agree that this is a reasonable option for many patients with acute or intermittent hemoptysis due to aspergillomata.

MUCORMYCOSIS (ZYGOMYCOSIS)

Most human causes of zygomycosis belong to the genera *Rhizopus*, *Mucor*, *Rhizomucor*, *Cumminghamella* and *Absidia*. These organisms are found in soil and dust and infection is usually acquired by inhalation of the spores. Zygomycetes have a predilection to cause invasive sinusitis, cutaneous, pulmonary or disseminated infection in immunocompromised hosts such as diabetics and allogeneic stem cell transplant recipients. The clinical diagnosis can be difficult to distinguish from invasive aspergillosis. In a recent review of 929 cases of zygomycosis, rhinocerebral zygomycosis was more closely associated with diabetes, whereas pulmonary infection was more closely associated with malignancy.[76] Diagnosis is suggested histologically based on the presence of non-septate, broad-based hyphal structures with 90° branching.[77] Routinely obtained cultures of infected tissue are often negative.[78]

The drug of choice for zygomycosis is AmB. AmB-d (1.0–1.5 mg/kg per day) has been the cornerstone of therapy for decades. LFAmB is efficacious in doses of 5–10 mg/kg per day. Posaconazole, a newer triazole administered as an oral suspension, is an alternative drug for zygomycosis, but is not approved for primary therapy.[79,80] Posaconazole (400 mg every 12 h) has demonstrated success as salvage therapy after failure of AmB, with treatment success rates of 60% at 12 weeks of therapy.[80,81] Combination antifungal therapy with LFAmB and posaconazole or caspofungin has proven effective in several reports.[82] A recent retrospective analysis of rhino–orbital–cerebral mucormycosis in non-neutropenic patients demonstrated greater success with combination therapy of AmB plus caspofungin (50 mg/day) versus AmB monotherapy.[83] Antifungal therapy versus combination antifungal therapy plus surgical intervention has led to survival rates of 61–69% versus 70%, respectively.[76]

Deferasirox, a non-desferrioxamine iron-chelating agent with in-vitro activity against many zygomycetes, is being examined as a potential adjunctive agent in combination with more traditional antifungal agents. Prompt correction of the underlying disorder is necessary for optimal management of zygomycosis, i.e. control of hyperglycemia, neutropenia or modulation of immunosuppressive therapy.

ENDEMIC MYCOSES AND CRYPTOCOCCUS

CRYPTOCOCCOSIS

Human cryptococcal infections due to *C. neoformans* and *C. gattii* have increased in prevalence in immunocompromised hosts, with mortality rates of 10–25% in non-HIV patients.[84] *C. neoformans* is found ubiquitously in the soil and is frequently associated with birds, particularly pigeons and chickens. *C. gattii* is often associated with river red gum and forest red gum trees. Inhalation is the principal portal of entry. Although the organism is widely distributed, infection is uncommon in normal hosts. Immunosuppressed patients are at greatest risk of complicated infections. Diagnosis is made on the basis of culture, or microscopically by India-ink preparation. Histopathological findings demonstrate budding yeasts staining positive for capsular material (mucicarmine stain). Measurement of cryptococcal antigen (CrAg) in serum and CSF has become a standard for non-culture-based diagnosis among the deep mycoses, and its presence is considered indicative of invasive disease.

CRYPTOCOCCAL PNEUMONIA

The presentation of pulmonary cryptococcosis is dependent on the host's immune status, and ranges from asymptomatic infection to life-threatening acute respiratory distress syndrome (ARDS).[85] All immunocompromised and/or symptomatic patients with pulmonary disease require systemic therapy. However, the optimal antifungal therapy and its duration have yet to be clearly delineated. Recommendations regarding therapy are detailed in Table 60.4.

Asymptomatic immunocompetent patients with culture-proven disease, or those with mild-to-moderate pulmonary disease, should be treated with fluconazole (400 mg/day) for 3–6 months.[86–88] In a retrospective analysis of non-CNS cryptococcal disease in HIV-negative patients, fluconazole was found to have similar efficacy compared to AmB-d (0.5–1.0 mg/kg per day). Itraconazole (200 mg every 12 h) for 6–12 months is an acceptable alternative.[89] AmB can be used with progressive pulmonary involvement or azole intolerance.[85] Immunocompromised patients with moderate-to-severe pulmonary disease should undergo a 2-week course of induction with AmB (0.5–1.0 mg/kg per day) or LFAmB (3–6 mg/kg per day) plus flucytosine (25 mg/kg every 6 h) followed by consolidation with oral fluconazole (400–800 mg/day) for a minimum of 10 weeks. Between 6 and 12 months of suppressive therapy with fluconazole (200 mg/day) is recommended. Alternative therapy with AmB-d plus flucytosine in combination for a minimum of 6–10 weeks is less efficacous.[85,87] Lumbar puncture should be considered in all patients with cryptococcal pulmonary disease, regardless of symptoms or underlying disease. Only asymptomatic, non-immunocompromised patients with negative or low-titer serum CrAg can be safely excluded from undergoing lumbar puncture.

CNS CRYPTOCOCCAL DISEASE IN NON-HIV PATIENTS

Meningitis is the most common manifestation of cryptococcal CNS disease. CNS cryptococcomas are much less common and are more frequently associated with *C. gattii* infections.

Recommended therapy for immunocompetent patients is combination therapy for at least 4 weeks of AmB-d (0.7–1.0 mg/kg per day) plus flucytosine (25 mg/kg every 6 h).[86,90] An alternative regimen based on supporting data in HIV-infected patients is induction with AmB-d (0.7–1.0 mg/kg per day) plus flucytosine (25 mg/kg every 6 h) for 2 weeks, followed by consolidation with oral fluconazole (400–800 mg/day) for at least 10 weeks. The addition of flucytosine and fluconazole to consolidation therapy are each independently associated with CSF sterilization.[88,91,92] Monitoring of CSF pressure and sterilization of CSF after 2 weeks is recommended.

Current treatment guidelines for normal and non-HIV immunosuppressed patients are extrapolated from the experiences of CNS cryptococcosis in HIV patients. Recommended treatment is induction with combination AmB-d (0.7–1.0 mg/kg per day) plus flucytosine (25 mg/kg every 6 h) for 2 weeks, followed by consolidation with oral fluconazole

Table 60.4 Treatment of cryptococcosis

Condition	Primary therapy	Alternative therapy	Comments
Pneumonia Non-immunocompromised	Fluconazole 400 mg (6 mg/kg) per day	Itraconazole 400 mg/day; or LFAmB 3–6 mg/kg or AmB-d 0.5–1.0 mg/kg per day ± 5FC 100 mg/kg for 6 weeks	Duration of therapy is 6 months. LFAmB is indicated for moderate to severe disease or azole intolerance
Immunocompromised	LFAmB 3–6 mg/kg or AmB 0.5–1.0 mg/kg per day, ± 5FC 100 mg/kg induction; fluconazole 400–800 mg/day consolidation		Duration of parenteral therapy is 2 weeks. Consolidation with oral fluconazole 400 mg/day for 10 weeks is recommended, followed by suppressive fluconazole 200 mg/day for 6–12 months
Meningoencephalitis, non-immunocompromised	LFAmB 3–6 mg/kg or AmB-d 0.7–1.0 mg/kg per day, ± 5FC 100 mg/kg per day for 4–6 weeks	LFAmB 3–6 mg/kg or AmB 0.7–1.0 mg/kg per day, ± 5FC 100 mg/kg per day for 2 weeks, then fluconazole 400 mg/day for 8 weeks	All patients should receive suppressive fluconazole 200–400 mg/day for 6 months following induction/consolidation
Transplant recipient	LFAmB 3–6 mg/kg plus 5FC 100 mg/kg per day for 2 weeks, then fluconazole 400–800 mg/day for 8 weeks	LFAmB 3–6 mg/kg per day for 4–6 weeks, then fluconazole 400–800 mg/day for 8 weeks	Chronic suppressive therapy with fluconazole 200 mg/day for 6–12 months is recommended
HIV-positive	LFAmB 3–6 mg/kg or AmB 0.7–1.0 mg/kg ± 5FC 100 mg/kg per day for 2 weeks, then fluconazole 400 mg/day for 8 weeks	LFAmB 3–6 mg/kg per day for 4–6 weeks, then fluconazole 400 mg/day for 8 weeks; itraconazole 200 mg every 12 h is an alternative oral azole	Maintenance therapy with fluconazole 200 mg/day is recommended in AIDS patients; itraconazole 400 mg/day is an alternative suppressive regimen

AmB, amphotericin B; AmB-d, amphotericin B deoxycholate; 5FC, flucytosine; LFAmB, lipid formulation amphotericin B.

(400–800 mg/day) for a minimum of 10 weeks; suppression with fluconazole (200 mg/day) for 6–12 months is recommended.[85,88,91,92] This regimen is preferred to the combination regimen of AmB-d/flucytosine for 6 weeks.[86,91] Rarely, salvage therapy involves intrathecal and/or intraventricular administration of AmB. AmB-d can be replaced with LFAmB, 3–6 mg/kg per day, during induction.[93] Itraconazole (200 mg every 12 h) may be substituted for fluconazole if necessary, but may be associated with a higher relapse rate than fluconazole.[91]

Aggressive management of increased intracranial pressure is critical to a successful outcome in most patients with CNS cryptococcosis. Frequent lumbar punctures, sometimes daily, may be required for days or weeks until the opening pressure is consistently less than 250 mm/H$_2$O. The decision to place a drainage device (lumbar drain, ventriculostomy, ventriculoperitoneal shunt) is based on clinical considerations and patient preference.

CRYPTOCOCCOSIS IN HIV-INFECTED PATIENTS

All HIV-positive patients with suspected cryptococcal infection warrant evaluation with a serum CrAg and fungal blood cultures. Those with a CD4 count <200 cells/mm^3 and concurrent pneumonia also warrant sputum culture. Cryptococcal pneumonia should be treated regardless of symptoms to prevent dissemination of cryptococcal disease.[85]

Evaluation for cryptococcal meningitis in HIV-infected patients includes brain imaging and CSF CrAg titers, as well as CSF fungal culture with documentation of the opening pressure. In cryptococcal meningitis cases, 99% of serum CrAg will be positive.[85,91,92] Randomized trial data demonstrate faster CSF sterilization and decreased mortality rates with combination therapy of AmB-d (0.7–1.0 mg/kg per day) or LFAmB (3–6 mg/kg per day) plus flucytosine (100–150 mg/kg divided into four doses daily) compared to monotherapy with AmB.[91,94] Induction for a 2-week minimum is followed by consolidation with oral fluconazole (400 mg/day).[89,91,92,94,95] Other treatment options include fluconazole (400–800 mg/day) and flucytosine (100–150 mg/kg divided into four doses daily) for 6 weeks.[96] If salvage therapy is required, intrathecal or intraventricular AmB may be used.

Upon treatment for cryptococcal meningitis, patients with AIDS require maintenance therapy with antiretroviral therapy (ARV) and fluconazole (200 mg/day) to prevent relapse. Fluconazole is recommended for maintenance therapy of AIDS-associated cryptococcal meningitis as it is superior to AmB-d in this setting (relapse rates of 2% vs 17%, respectively).[97]

Fluconazole also demonstrated superiority to itraconazole for maintenance therapy (relapse rates of 4% and 24%, respectively).[98] Itraconazole (200 mg every 12 h) may be used as an alternative to fluconazole therapy when necessary in the treatment of both pulmonary and CNS cryptococcal infection. Chronic suppressive antifungal therapy can be

discontinued once there is clinical control of disease, CSF cultures are negative, and the CD4 count is consistently >150 cells/mm^3.

HISTOPLASMOSIS

Histoplasmosis due to *Histoplasma capsulatum* occurs in most regions of the world, but is most common in Midwestern and South Central USA. It is also highly endemic in parts of Central and South America. The organism is found in soil enriched by bat and bird droppings. Inhalation is the primary portal of entry. Disease manifestations are dependent on the host immune status and the intensity of the exposure.[99] Diagnosis is based on a combination of culture, histopathology and serological studies, of which culture is the gold standard. Histology reveals granulomata with small intracellular oval yeast forms with eccentric nuclei. Intracellular budding yeast cells are best visualized with a methenamine silver stain. Antigen assays performed on urine and blood specimens have a sensitivity of 90% and 70%, respectively. Cross-reactivity can occur in urine *Histoplasma* antigen assays with blastomycosis, coccidioidomycosis, paracoccidioidomycosis and, less commonly, penicilliosis.[100]

ACUTE PULMONARY HISTOPLASMOSIS

Presentation of acute exposure can range from asymptomatic infection to severe pulmonary pneumonitis with respiratory distress. Complications, although uncommon, include mediastinal lymphadenopathy, chronic cavitary histoplasmosis and fibrosing mediastinitis.[101] Other sequelae include persistent cough and focal inflammatory manifestations. Table 60.5 details treatment recommendations.

Acute pulmonary histoplasmosis usually resolves spontaneously within 1 month and does not require therapy. Persistent symptoms for more than 1 month may be indicative of complicated disease, signifying a need for therapy. Such patients should be treated with itraconazole (200 mg once or twice daily) for 6–12 weeks.[102]

Moderate-to-severe acute pulmonary histoplasmosis is treated with LFAmB (3–5 mg/kg per day) for 2 weeks, followed by stepdown therapy with itraconazole (200 mg every 12 h) for a total of 12 weeks.[100] AmB-d (0.7–1.0 mg/kg per day) can be substituted for LFAmB. Methylprednisolone (0.5–1 mg/kg per day) is recommended for concurrent hypoxemia and respiratory distress.[103] Duration of therapy has not been clearly defined, but treatment should continue until resolution of infiltrates on chest radiograph.[99]

COMPLICATIONS FROM ACUTE PULMONARY HISTOPLASMOSIS

Complications of pulmonary histoplasmosis include histoplasmomas, mediastinal granulomas, mediastinal fibrosis, and

Table 60.5 Treatment of histoplasmosis

Condition	Primary therapy	Alternative therapy	Comments
Acute pulmonary			
Mild	Symptoms <4 weeks do not warrant therapy Symptoms >4 weeks: itraconazole 200 mg every 12 h		Duration of therapy is 6–12 weeks
Moderate to severe	LFAmB 3–5 mg/kg per day; itraconazole 200 mg every 12 h	AmB-d 0.7–1.0 mg/kg per day	Duration of parenteral therapy is 2 weeks; itraconazole stepdown therapy for a 12-week duration Concomitant methylprednisolone is recommended for 2 weeks in the setting of hypoxemia
Chronic cavitary pneumonia	Itraconazole 200 mg every 12 h	AmB 0.7–1.0 mg/kg per day for induction (1–2 weeks), then itraconazole 200 mg every 12 h	Duration of therapy is 12–24 months
Disseminated	LFAmB 3–mg/kg per day	Itraconazole 200 mg every 12 h	Therapy for at least 12 months. For milder disease, initial itraconazole is acceptable. For more severe disseminated histoplasmosis, AmB is preferred for induction, followed by stepdown therapy to itraconazole Duration of parenteral of therapy is 2–6 weeks
Meningoencephalitis	LFAmB 5–6 mg/kg per day; or itraconazole 200 mg every 12 h		Duration of parenteral of therapy is 4–6 weeks; itraconazole stepdown therapy is for a minimum of 12 months

AmB, amphotericin B; AmB-d, amphotericin B deoxycholate; LFAmB:, lipid formulation amphotericin B.

mediastinal lymphadenitis, pericarditis and erythema nodosum. Most complications do not warrant antifungal therapy, only management of the complication itself. Associated inflammatory reactions should be treated with anti-inflammatory medications, including, but not limited to, steroids.[99,104]

CHRONIC PULMONARY HISTOPLASMOSIS

Chronic pulmonary histoplasmosis usually occurs in the setting of underlying baseline lung disease, often presenting radiographically as chronic cavitary lesions with surrounding inflammation.[101,102,105] Itraconazole (200 mg every 12 h) is recommended as first-line therapy for 12–24 months to avoid relapse. Duration of therapy is based on resolution of lesions on radiographic imaging, which should be performed every 4–6 months. As antigen tests are often negative in chronic cavitary histoplasmosis, serial antigen testing is not recommended.[99]

DISSEMINATED HISTOPLASMOSIS (DH)

Hematogenous spread of acute infection, occurring within the first few weeks of infection, is a consequence of defective cell-mediated immunity. Disseminated histoplasmosis can present with symptoms of pancytopenia, skin lesions, mucosal ulcers, hepatosplenomegaly and gastrointestinal disease. Symptoms are usually present for at least 3 weeks and are associated with radiographic and laboratory findings.[99] Antigen levels should be monitored during and 12 months after therapy to observe for relapse.

 DH IN HIV-NEGATIVE PATIENTS

Progressive disseminated histoplasmosis should be treated with either itraconazole (200 mg every 12 h) or LFAmB (3–5 mg/kg per day). Response rates of 80–100% have been documented for the treatment of mild-to-moderate disease with oral itraconazole, with relapse rates of 10–15%. Recommended duration of therapy is for at least 12 months.[102,106] Moderate to severe disease should be treated with LFAmB (3–5 mg/kg per day) or amphotericin B lipid complex (ABLC) (5 mg/kg per day) for 2 weeks, followed by stepdown therapy with itraconazole (200 mg every 12 h) for at least 12 months. Immunosuppressed patients should receive itraconazole (200 mg/day) suppressive therapy until reversal of the immunological disorder. Duration of therapy is based on resolution of symptoms, radiographic and laboratory abnormalities.[99]

 DH IN PATIENTS WITH AIDS

Higher success rates and lower mortality have been demonstrated with LFAmB (3–5 mg/kg per day) versus AmB-d (0.7–1.0 mg/kg per day) for 1–2 weeks as induction therapy for DH in patients with AIDS (2% vs 13%, respectively). Following induction with LFAmB, stepdown therapy with oral itraconazole (200 mg every 12 h) is recommended for 12 months.[107] Long-term response rates are higher in ARV recipients compared with non-recipients (100% vs 47%).[108,109]

Before stopping chronic suppressive antifungal therapy, immune function (CD4 count >150 cells/mm³) improvement associated with ARV therapy should be documented; blood cultures and urine *Histoplasma* antigen should be negative.[110] If the CD4 counts drop below 150 cells/mm^3, then suppressive (Itraconazole 200 mg/day) therapy should be restarted.[99]

DH IN NEONATES

Neonatal DH is a severe complication and is often accompanied by meningitis. It reflects an immature and underdeveloped cellular immune system. Untreated disease is rapidly fatal. AmB-d (1 mg/kg per day) is recommended for a 4-week induction course. LFAmB (3–5 mg/kg per day) may be substituted as necessary. Alternative therapy includes shorter duration of AmB-d completed with a course of azole therapy. These recommendations apply for infants with concurrent CNS involvement. Itraconazole (10 mg/kg per day) is favored over ketoconazole for stepdown therapy, although duration of antifungal therapy in neonates is unclear; most experts advise at least 12 months' therapy.

CNS HISTOPLASMOSIS

CNS histoplasmosis occurs in 5–10% of cases of disseminated disease, with neurological symptoms occurring in 25%, and is the most challenging complication to treat. Of the LFAmBs, liposomal AmB achieves the greatest concentration in brain tissue.[111] Recent experience has demonstrated greater efficacy with higher doses of LFAmB (5 mg/kg per day) for 4–6 weeks, followed by suppressive therapy with itraconazole stepdown therapy.[112] Compared to fluconazole (200–400 mg/day), itraconazole has greater efficacy in the treatment of CNS histoplasmosis in animal studies. Stepdown itraconazole therapy (200 mg every 12 h) is recommended for at least 1 year and until there is no clinical/laboratory evidence of active CNS infection and urine *Histoplasma* antigen titers are consistently negative.[113]

COCCIDIOIDOMYCOSIS

Coccidioides immitis (endemic to California) and *C. posadasii* (found in all other endemic areas) cause symptomatic infection usually within 1–3 weeks after inhalation of aerosolized arthroconidia. *Coccidioides* species, endemic in the southwestern United States and parts of Central and South America, cause acute and reactivation infections in persons living in an endemic area, in travelers, and especially among immunosuppressed persons.[114,115]

Acute symptoms, when present, include an influenza-like illness or acute/subacute pneumonia. Most cases are self-limited, resolving spontaneously. Pulmonary sequelae such as pulmonary nodules or cavitary pneumonia arise in 5–10% of cases. There is a strong propensity for extrapulmonary involvement among persons of African or Filipino descent,

pregnant women and immunosuppressed patients (30–50% of cases).[116–118] Diagnosis is confirmed by sputum culture or positive anticoccidioidal antibodies in serum via complement fixation.[119–121]

PRIMARY COCCIDIOMYCOSIS (VALLEY FEVER)

Most healthy patients with acute coccidioidomycosis do not require therapy. All immunosuppressed patients, including diabetics, those with poor pulmonary reserve, or women with newly diagnosed disease in the third trimester of pregnancy/postpartum period should receive treatment.[121]

Oral azole therapy with ketoconazole (400 mg/day), fluconazole (400–800 mg/day) or itraconazole (200 mg every 8–12 h) for 3–6 months is recommended for acute coccidioidal pneumonia. Patients should be monitored clinically, radiographically and serologically every 3 months for at least 1 year.

Miliary infiltrates or bilateral reticulonodular disease is more common in immunocompromised hosts and those exposed to a large inoculum of spores. In the setting of hypoxia, AmB-d (0.5–1.5 mg/kg per day) or LFAmB (3.0–5.0 mg/kg per day) is indicated until improvement in symptoms and stable radiographic imaging. Subsequent stepdown therapy with ketoconazole (400 mg/day), fluconazole (400–800 mg/day) or itraconazole (200 mg every 8–12 h) can be given for at least 12 months. Fungemia and extrapulmonary involvement should be excluded.[122]

CHRONIC PULMONARY COCCIDIOIDOMYCOSIS

Chronic coccidioidomycosis occurs in fewer than 10% of cases and is restricted to the lung in 50–70% of cases. Manifestations include asymptomatic nodules, small thin-walled and large thick-walled cavities, progressive destruction and consolidation. Close monitoring for progressive enlargement or pleural involvement is recommended in asymptomatic cases. A positive sputum culture does not always justify therapy, depending on the radiographic status. Surgical evaluation of lesions present for more than 2 years is recommended to minimize the risk of future complications.

Chronic infections often result in persistent cough with serological evidence of coccidioidomycosis. Chronic pulmonary coccidioidomycosis should be treated with ketoconazole (400 mg/day), fluconazole (400–800 mg/day) or itraconazole (200 mg every 8–12 h). Minimal duration of therapy is 12 months, with close monitoring every 3 months. Recurrence of symptoms may occur with cessation of azole therapy. Those patients with a negative coccidioidin skin test during therapy and a peak complement fixation titer of ≥256 have very high relapse potential, regardless of the therapy.[123] In the presence of clinical and/or radiographic disease progression, it is recommended to change azoles or commence AmB-d (0.5–1.5 mg/kg per day). In cases of recurrent pulmonary coccidioidomycosis, surgical resection may be beneficial.[122]

DISSEMINATED COCCIDIODOMYCOSIS

Disseminated coccidioidomycosis, involving lymphoreticular, cutaneous, CNS and osteoarticular sites, often responds better to antifungal therapy than pulmonary infection. Initial therapy with oral itraconazole (200 mg every 12h) or fluconazole (400 mg/day) is recommended. If necessary, dosing of itraconazole and fluconazole can be increased to 200 mg every 6 h and 2000 mg/day, respectively. Duration of therapy has not been clearly defined but treatment for months to years has a 90% response rate.[124] Itraconazole has greater efficacy in the treatment of skeletal lesions than fluconazole.[125] Alternative therapy with AmB-d (0.5–1.5 mg/kg per day) or LFAmB (3–5 mg/kg per day) is recommended for vertebral lesions or rapidly progressive disease. Although combination AmB-d and azole therapy is widely used to treat severe, progressive disease, there are no data that demonstrate superiority over single-agent therapy. Surgical debridement of abscesses or stabilization of spinal instability may be necessary if the response to antifungal therapy alone is poor.[122,126–129]

COCCIDIOIDAL MENINGITIS

Coccidioidal meningitis is a progressive lymphocytic meningitis with a 100% mortality when untreated. The clinical course may be indolent over months, or more rapid and fatal within weeks. Fluconazole is the preferred treatment of coccidioidal meningitis, but itraconazole can be used successfully. For fluconazole, initial daily doses of 800–1000 mg, followed by 400 mg/day is recommended. For itraconazole, 400–600 mg/day is recommended, followed by 400 mg/day. For most patients, lifelong suppression with fluconazole (200 mg/day) or itraconazole (200 mg every 12 h) is required. Chronic suppression with fluconazole is successful in approximately 80% of patients at 3 years.[129]

Recent experience with posaconazole is encouraging. Although not approved for this indication, the response of non-CNS coccidioidomycosis is impressive and deserves more detailed investigation. There is far less experience with voriconazole for coccidioidomycosis.

Recommendations for salvage therapy are based upon independent case reports. Intrathecal AmB-d is rarely administered for CNS coccidioidomycosis, being reserved for azole and intravenous AmB refractory disease. AmB (0.1–1.5 mg per dose) is prepared in 5 mL of 5% dextrose and is administered over 3–5 min. The patient should remain in the head-down position for 2 h after administration. The AmB-d dose can be escalated by 0.05 mg/day to a maximum of 1.5 mg.[122,130] Doses are usually administered 1–3 times weekly. Intrathecal hydrocortisone, 25 mg, can be given to ameliorate adverse effects. The response to therapy is based on the CSF findings and antibody titers.

COCCIDIOIDOMYCOSIS IN IMMUNOCOMPROMISED PATIENTS

Solid organ transplantation recipients in endemic areas have up to a 9% risk of coccidioidomycosis within 1 year after transplantation.[122,131] Fluconazole and ketoconazole doses of 100–200 mg and 200–400 mg/day have been used for primary and secondary prophylaxis, respectively. The risk of dissemination and associated complications following active disease warrants lifelong therapy in these patients.[132,133]

All HIV-positive patients with active coccidioidomycosis and CD4 counts <250 cell/mm^3 require antifungal treatment. Recommendations are based on demonstrated success using AmB-d (0.5–1.5 mg/kg per day) followed by stepdown therapy with fluconazole (400–800 mg/day) or itraconazole (200 mg every 8–12 h). Alternatively, combination AmB-d plus an azole may be used. Therapy is recommended until infection is controlled and a CD4 count of >250 cell/mm^3 is achieved in response to ARV.[134,135]

BLASTOMYCOSIS

Infection with the dimorphic fungus *Blastomyces dermatitidis* ranges from asymptomatic infection to pulmonary disease and disseminated disease. Blastomycosis occurs in Midwestern and South Central USA, central and eastern Canadian provinces, and parts of Africa. Primary infection results from inhalation of the conidia. Most infections are asymptomatic. Among clinically apparent infections, 60% are limited to the lungs and 40% involve extrapulmonary sites, particularly skin/subcutaneous tissues, osteoarticular, genitourinary and/ or CNS sites.[136] Risk factors for infection include activities along streams, excavation of soil enriched with decaying vegetation/wood, hunting and fishing, and outdoor occupation.[137]

Diagnosis is made by culture, histopathology, or by urine or blood antigen detection assays. Pulmonary cases are culture positive from respiratory samples in 86–100% of cases. Typical broad-based budding yeasts can be readily visualized in histological specimens.[138,139] The *Blastomyces* antigen assay cross-reacts with other fungi, particularly *H. capsulatum*.[140]

PULMONARY BLASTOMYCOSIS

Pulmonary blastomycosis infection varies from asymptomatic to chronic pulmonary disease. Symptomatic disease manifests as an acute community-acquired pneumonia which may spontaneously resolve, or progress to chronic pulmonary blastomycosis. Radiographic imaging reveals alveolar infiltrates, fibronodular interstitial infiltrates, one or more mass lesions and, rarely, diffuse bilateral pulmonary infiltrates.[141]

All symptomatic cases should be treated. Mild-to-moderate disease is effectively treated in 95% of cases with oral itraconazole (200–400 mg per day).[102] Alternative regimens include ketoconazole (400–800 mg/day) and fluconazole (400–800 mg/day), but these are generally less effective.[142–144] Moderate-to-severe pulmonary disease treated with AmB is cured in 70–90% of patients.[145] Current recommendations for severe disease include initial therapy with LFAmB (3–5 mg/kg per day) or AmB-d (0.7–1 mg/kg per day), followed by stepdown itraconazole therapy (200 mg every 12 h). AmB should be used for 1–2 weeks or until clinical symptoms improve. Total duration of treatment is generally 6–12 months, depending on clinical and radiographic improvement.[134]

EXTRAPULMONARY BLASTOMYCOSIS

Treatment for extrapulmonary blastomycosis is based upon organ system involvement. Itraconazole is successful in 90% of non-CNS cases.[102] Mild-to-moderate extrapulmonary disease can be treated with oral itraconazole (200 mg every 12 h). Duration of therapy is at least 6–12 months, depending on clinical improvement of skin or other lesions. Osteoarticular blastomycosis requires at least 12 months of therapy given the higher rate of relapse.[146] Fluconazole (400–800 mg/day) is an alternative agent but is less efficacious.[143] In the setting of progressive or refractory disease, LFAmB (3–5 mg/kg per day) should be administered.

Moderate-to-severe non-CNS disease is treated with LFAmB (3–5 mg/kg per day) or AmB-d (0.7–1 mg/kg per day) for 1–2 weeks and until clinical improvement is noted. Stepdown therapy with itraconazole (200 mg every 12 h) is recommended for at least 12 months.

CNS BLASTOMYCOSIS

CNS involvement is most common among immunocompromised patients, with rates up to 40% in patients with AIDS.[147] Manifestations of CNS blastomycosis include meningitis, epidural, brain or parenchymal abscesses, and mass lesions. LFAmB (5 mg/kg per day) for 4–6 weeks is recommended for induction therapy.[148] Maintenance therapy with an azole is recommended following clinical improvement with fluconazole (800 mg/day), itraconazole (200 mg every 8–12 h) or voriconazole (200–400 mg every 12 h) for at least 12 months.[136] Experience with voriconazole is promising, and may be the azole of choice for CNS blastomycosis.[149–153]

IMMUNOSUPPRESSED PATIENTS

Immunosuppressed patients are predisposed to severe disease with increased mortality.[148,154] Treatment recommendations, based upon small case series and case reports, support LFAmB (3–5 mg/kg per day) for at least 1–2 weeks. Stepdown

therapy with itraconazole (200 mg every 12 h) for at least 12 months is favored. Given the risk of relapsing disease in immunosuppressed patients, lifelong suppressive therapy with itraconazole (200 mg/day) is recommended. Based on experience of treating histoplasmosis in patients with AIDS, suppressive itraconazole therapy may be discontinued after 1 year in those with CD4 counts consistently >150 cells/mm³.

PARACOCCIDIOIDOMYCOSIS

Paracoccidioidomycosis, caused by *Paracoccidioides brasiliensis*, is endemic to parts of South America. Primary infection, acquired via inhalation of the conidia, results in pulmonary disease. Although often asymptomatic, reactivation of latent infection may occur decades following exposure. Dissemination involving the mucus membranes, lungs, skin, lymph nodes, adrenal glands and the CNS is common, as is chronic pulmonary disease, which may mimic malignancy or tuberculosis (coexists in 30% of patients).[155] Untreated infection can be fatal. A wet mount of sputum showing the 'pilot wheel' image of mother cell and multiple daughter cells or blastoconidia is diagnostic. Methenamine silver stain demonstrates yeast cells with granuloma formation. Culture requires 20–30 days for growth. Serological testing is limited to a few endemic areas.

Mild-to-moderate disease is treated with itraconazole (200 mg/day) for at least 6–12 months, with a response of approximately 90%.[156,157] Relapse associated with alcoholism, AIDS and subtherapeutic itraconazole levels occurs in 15% of cases.[158] Alternative therapy with ketoconazole (200–400 mg/day) for 12 months yields response rates of 90%.[159] Sulfadiazine (100–150 mg/kg per day) and fluconazole (200–40 mg/day) are other alternatives. A recent comparative study of voriconazole and itraconazole in chronic paracoccidioidomycosis demonstrated success in 89% versus 94% of patients, respectively.[160] Voriconazole is not recommended as first-line therapy. Refractory moderate-to-severe disease and intolerance to other agents should be managed with AmB-d (1.0 mg/kg per day) or LFAmB (3–5 mg/kg per day).

PENICILLIOSIS

Infection due to *Penicillium marneffei* is endemic in South East Asia. and largely affects HIV-infected patients with a CD4 count of <100 cells/mm³.[161–165] Untreated, the mortality rate is high.[166,167] Diagnosis is made by culture or histopathology and visualization of the organism. Disseminated disease is most common and typically involves lungs, heart, liver, intestine, lymph nodes and bone marrow. The disease resembles histoplasmosis clinically.

P. marneffei is highly susceptible to itraconazole, ketoconazole and flucytosine, and intermediately susceptible to AmB and fluconazole. Mild-to-moderate disease is treated with oral itraconazole (400 mg/day) for 8 weeks,[168] and moderate-to-severe disease with AmB-d (0.6 mg/kg per day) for 2 weeks, followed by stepdown therapy with oral itraconazole (400 mg/day) for an additional 10 weeks.[169] Long-term itraconazole (200 mg/day) is recommended to prevent recurrence among patients with persistently low CD4 counts (<200 cells/mm³).

SPOROTRICHOSIS

Sporotrichosis is caused by the dimorphic fungus *Sporothrix schenckii*, found globally in decaying soil, vegetation and moss. Transmission usually occurs by cutaneous inoculation via trauma or zoonotic spread, resulting in lymphocutaneous disease. Inhalation of the conidia rarely causes pulmonary or disseminated disease in immunosuppressed hosts.

LYMPHOCUTANEOUS SPOROTRICHOSIS

Most cases of lymphocutaneous infection are localized with proximal spread to the lymphatic circulation. Treatment response rates for lymphocutaneous/cutaneous disease are 90–100% with itraconazole (200 mg/day) and 60–70% with fluconazole (200–400 mg/day).[170–172] Therapy should be continued for at least 4 weeks beyond resolution of skin lesions. Terbinafine 500 mg or 1000 mg/day has been used successfully, with cure rates of 53% and 87%, respectively.[173] Treatment with potassium iodide saturated solution, 15–20 drops per day for 3–6 months, leads to cure in 80–100% of cases. Adverse effects are common, and include abdominal pain, nausea and rash.[174–177]

OSTEOARTICULAR SPOROTRICHOSIS

Osteoarticular sporotrichosis usually occurs in immunosuppressed patients and those with alcoholism.[178,179] Infection is chronic, resulting from either direct inoculation or hematogenous spread. Articular infection, tenosynovitis and bursitis are all manifestations of this form of disease.[180] Itraconazole (200 mg every 12 h) is recommended for at least 12 months. Unresponsive infection should be treated with AmB-d (0.7–1.0 mg/kg per day). Surgical intervention in combination with medical therapy is not routinely recommended.[181]

PULMONARY SPOROTRICHOSIS

Pulmonary sporotrichosis may present as chronic fibronodular cavitary disease and is more common in men with underlying lung disease.[182] Mild-to-moderate disease can be treated with oral itraconazole (200 mg every 12 h) for a total of 12 months.[183] Clinical experience supports the use of LFAmB-d (3–5 mg/kg per day) in severe disease. AmB-d (0.7–1.0 mg/kg per day) may be used as an alternative. Parenteral therapy is warranted until clinical improvement, followed by itraconazole (200 mg every 12 h) for at least 12 months. Surgical evaluation is recommended for localized disease.

DISSEMINATED SPOROTRICHOSIS

Current management of disseminated sporotrichosis is based on anecdotal experience. Traditionally, treatment of disseminated sporotrichosis requires AmB-d (0.7–1.0 mg/kg per day) or LFAmB (3–5 mg/kg per day) until a clinical response is noted. Subsequent therapy with itraconazole (200 mg every 12 h) for at least 12 months is recommended. Immunosuppressed patients warrant chronic suppressive therapy with itraconazole (200 mg/day) until resolution of the underlying condition.[183,184]

MENINGEAL SPOROTRICHOSIS

Meningeal sporotrichosis is a rare complication of disseminated infection. Anecdotal experience supports the use of AmB-d for the treatment of meningeal infection. However, LFAmB (5 mg/kg per day) for 4–6 weeks is the preferred agent. Following completion of LFAmB therapy, itraconazole (200 mg every 12 h) for at least 12 months is recommended.[183] Clinical experience does not support the use of combination therapy.[185]

OTHER MOLD INFECTIONS

FUSARIOSIS

Fusarium species are found globally in soil, plant debris and aquatic biofilms. Infection ranges from superficial to disseminated disease. The principal routes of transmission are through inhalation of the conidia and direct penetration of skin from breakdown in the normal skin barrier. Most human infections are due to *Fusarium solani* (50%), followed by *F. oxysporum* (20%) and *F. verticillioides* (10%) and *F. moniliforme* (10%).[186] In immunocompetent hosts, infection is more commonly manifested as keratitis and onychomycosis. Disseminated disease usually occurs in the setting of severe neutropenia complicating hematological malignancy, leukemia and stem cell transplantation.[187] Disseminated disease is manifest by positive blood cultures with concurrent skin lesions.[188]

Localized infection requires surgical debridement and antifungal therapy. Intravenous AmB, voriconazole (200 mg every 12 h) or posaconazole (400 mg every 12 h with meals) is appropriate for localized infection.[189] Keratitis is treated with topical natamycin 5% (1 drop 6–8 times/day).[190]

Treatment of invasive and disseminated infections is usually ineffective in the immunocompromised. AmB (1 mg/kg per day) or LFAmB (>4 mg/kg per day) is preferred for treating invasive fusariosis.[191,192] Recent data support the use of voriconazole (200 mg every 12 h) and posaconazole

(400 mg every 12 h with meals), in combination with AmB, as alternative treatment or as salvage therapy (63% vs 48%, for voriconazole and posaconazole, respectively).[193]

In addition to medical management, surgical debridement of necrotic tissue may be beneficial. Central venous catheters should be removed in cases of isolated fungemia.

SCEDOSPORIOSIS

Two *Scedosporium* species, *S. apiospermum* (*Pseudallescheria boydii*) and *S. prolificans*, are rare causes of opportunistic infections in humans. *S. apiospermum* causes a wide spectrum of infection from superficial skin disease and mycetomas to CNS and disseminated disease in immunocompromised patients.[194] *S. prolificans* infections in immunocompetent hosts include localized skin, soft tissue, joint and bone disease, usually occurring after trauma; in neutropenic patients, pulmonary disease, fungemia and widely disseminated disease are common.[195,196] In immunocompromised hosts, these organisms are associated with a 58–100% mortality rate.[197] Concern for breakthrough *Scedosporium* spp. infection has recently increased as a result of antifungal prophylaxis with little or no activity against *Scedosporium* spp. *Scedosporium* spp. have erratic susceptibilities to AmB; *S. apiospermum* has documented resistance to AmB in vitro and in vivo.[198]

The expanded spectrum triazoles demonstrate in-vitro activity against *S. apiospermum*. The greatest clinical experience is with voriconazole (4 mg/kg every 12 h), which compares favorably to AmB-d.[199] *S. apiospermum* also demonstrates in-vitro susceptibility to posaconazole, miconazole, ketoconazole and itraconazole.[60] Cerebral abscesses due to *S. apiospermum* are treated with voriconazole (4 mg/kg every 12 h) or itraconazole (200 mg every 12 h) in conjunction with surgical intervention.[200] Treatment should be continued for months.

S. prolificans is resistant to most antifungal agents. Voriconazole exhibits limited in-vitro activity against *S. prolificans* but has little to no in-vivo activity.[201–203] Voriconazole (4 mg/kg every 12 h) and itraconazole (200 mg every 12 h) have been used in combination with terbinafine (500 mg/day) or an echinocandin with some success, and currently offer the best therapeutic option.[204–208]

PHAEOHYPHOMYCOSES

 ### EUMYCETOMA (MADUROMYCOSIS)

Eumycetomas are chronic, granulomatous infections resulting in progressive infection of the subcutaneous tissue of the distal extremities, most commonly the legs and feet. Infections are due to soil fungi (*Eumycetoma* spp.) and higher bacteria (*Actinomycetoma* spp.). Transmission occurs via skin inoculation to produce subcutaneous nodules and draining sinus tracts, in which grains can be visualized. Untreated, eumycetoma can result in chronic disability and osteomyelitis.[209]

Eumycetomas are endemic in Latin American, Africa and the Indian subcontinent. Multiple fungi cause mycetomas that vary by locality. The more common causative organisms include *Madurella mycetomatis* (Africa and India), *Madurella grisea* (the Americas), *S. apiospermum* (Europe and the USA), and *Fusarium* spp. and *Acremonium* spp., found globally.[210] The causative organism must be identified to guide antimicrobial or antifungal therapy.

Eumycetomas, less responsive to therapy than actinomycetomas, often require surgical debulking. Clinical experience supports the use of itraconazole and ketoconazole (400 mg/day), for 18–24 months.[210–212] Fluconazole has proved less successful. The newer triazoles are efficacious but cost-prohibitive in resource-limited settings. Posaconazole (80% success) is dosed at 400 mg every 12 h for 24 months.[213] AmB, flucytosine and griseofulvin are not recommended.[214] Despite medical and surgical intervention, relapse rates as high as 90% have been documented. Fortunately, many eumycetomas remain relatively stable for long periods of time without therapy.

CHROMOBLASTOMYCOSIS

Chromoblastomycosis is a chronic infection of the skin and subcutaneous tissue of non-immunocompromised individuals caused by several dematiaceous fungi, including *Fonsecaea pedrosoi*, *Fonsecaea compacta*, *Phialophora verrucosa*, *Cladosporium* (or *Cladophialophora*) *carrionii*, *Rhinocladiella aquaspersa* and *Botryomyces caespitosus*. The disease occurs worldwide, but is more common in tropical and subtropical areas.

Although smaller lesions can be surgically excised, larger lesions require antifungal therapy. Resistance to standard antifungal therapy (fluconazole, flucytosine and AmB) is common and affects therapeutic response. Reasonable results have been observed with oral itraconazole (200 mg/day) with or without flucytosine (25 mg/kg every 6 h).[215] Posaconazole (400 mg every 12 h with meals) has demonstrated success in the treatment of disease refractory to fluconazole, flucytosine and AmB. Terbinafine (200–500 mg/day) demonstrates good clinical activity, with cure rates approaching 80%.[216] Thiabendazole (2 g/day), with or without flucytosine, is also effective.[217] Treatment is prolonged, up to 2 years in some cases. Response rates vary by causative organism and extent of disease. Conventional therapy involves cryotherapy and topical heat in conjunction with antifungal therapy. Cryotherapy with liquid-nitrogen-soaked cotton balls, swabs or spray has demonstrated success with negative cultures at 4 months. Historically, local heat (42–46°C) applied directly to the lesion for 2–12 months has been efficacious.[217,218]

PNEUMOCYSTOSIS

Pneumocystis pneumonia (PCP), caused by *Pneumocystis jirovecii*, occurs in immunocompromised patients. Primary infection is usually an unrecognized event in childhood.

Pneumonia occurs with either reactivation of latent disease or newly acquired infection.

Clinical manifestations of progressive dyspnea, fever, dry cough and progressive chest discomfort are most common. Radiographic imaging in early disease may be normal. As disease progresses, diffuse, bilateral, symmetrical interstitial infiltrates are consistent with PCP.[219]

Diagnosis is confirmed by identification of the organism in tissue, bronchoalveolar lavage fluid or induced sputum by histopathology.[220–222] Nucleic acid tests have lower specificity than immunological stains and limited availability.[223,224] First-line therapy for mild-to-moderate disease is oral trimethoprim–sulfamethoxazole (TMP–SMX; 15–20 mg/kg per day trimethoprim and 75–100 mg/kg per day sulfamethoxazole divided in 2–3 doses) for 21 days.[225,226] With TMP–SMX intolerance, alternative regimens include:

- dapsone 100 mg/day plus TMP 20 mg/kg orally or intravenously in 2–3 doses
- clindamycin 600 mg every 6 h combined with primaquine 15 mg/day
- atovaquone 750 mg every 12 h.

Prior to receiving dapsone, patients should be tested for glucose-6-phosphate dehydrogenase (G6PD) deficiency.

Moderate-to-severe disease necessitates adjunctive corticosteroids: prednisolone 40–60 mg/day for 5 days, followed by a 14-day taper.[227–230] If parental administration is required, methylprednisolone can be given at 75% of the prednisone dose. The recommended first-line treatment of moderate-to-severe PCP is TMP–SMX (see above dosing) for 21 days.[231] If an alternative regimen is required, intravenous pentamidine (4 mg/kg per day) or clindamycin plus primaquine, in order of preference, may be used for 21 days.[232,233] Response to therapy is multifactorial: severity of illness, degree of immunosuppression, prior history of PCP, medications used for therapy and timing of therapy. PCP prophylaxis is required in HIV patients until the CD4 count is consistently >200 cells/mm³.

Twenty to 85% of patients can develop intolerance to the high dose of TMP–SMX. Side effects to TMP–SMX consist of skin rash, including Stevens–Johnson syndrome, nausea, vomiting, fever, leukopenia, thrombocytopenia, renal insufficiency with hyperkalemia, and hepatitis.[234–238]

In the absence of a consensus regarding the appropriate time to initiate ARV in patients with severe PCP, current clinical practice includes delaying the initiation of ARV until after the completion of anti-PCP therapy, or holding ARV initiation until at least 2 weeks into therapy for PCP. Recent data suggest that initiating ARV therapy during initial PCP treatment may be beneficial.[239,240]

References

1. National Nosocomial Infections Surveillance (NNIS) System report, data summary from January 1990–May 1999, issued June 1999. *Am J Infect Control.* 1999;27:520–532.
2. Edmond MB, Wallace SE, McClish DK, et al. Nosocomial bloodstream infections in United States hospitals: a three-year analysis. *Clin Infect Dis.* 1999;29:239–244.
3. Gudlaugsson O, Gillespie S, Lee K, et al. Attributable mortality of nosocomial candidemia, revisited. *Clin Infect Dis.* 2003;37:1172–1177.
4. Pappas PG, Rex JH, Lee J, et al. A prospective observational study of candidemia: epidemiology, therapy and influences on mortality in hospitalized adult and pediatric patients. *Clin Infect Dis.* 2003;37:634–643.
5. Morrell M, Fraser VJ, Kollef MH. Delaying the empiric treatment of *Candida* bloodstream infection until positive blood culture results are obtained: a potential risk factor for hospital mortality. *Antimicrob Agents Chemother.* 2005;49:3640–3645.
6. Garey KW, Rege M, Pai MP, et al. Time to initiation of fluconazole therapy impacts mortality in patients with candidemia: a multi-institutional study. *Clin Infect Dis.* 2006;43:25–31.
7. Karlowicz MG, Hashimoto LN, Kelly Jr RE, Buescher ES. Should central venous catheters be removed as soon as candidemia is detected in neonates? *Pediatrics.* 2000;106:E63.
8. Rex JH, Bennett JE, Sugar AM, et al. A randomized trial comparing fluconazole with amphotericin B for the treatment of candidemia in patients without neutropenia. Candidemia Study Group and the National Institute. *N Engl J Med.* 1994;331:1325–1330.
9. Rex JH, Pappas PG, Karchmer AW, et al. A randomized and blinded multicenter trial of high-dose fluconazole plus placebo versus fluconazole plus amphotericin B as therapy for candidemia and its consequences in nonneutropenic subjects. *Clin Infect Dis.* 2003;36:1221–1228.
10. Reboli AC, Rotstein C, Pappas PG, et al. Anidulafungin versus fluconazole for invasive candidiasis. *N Engl J Med.* 2007;356:2472–2482.
11. Kullberg BJ, Sobel JD, Ruhnke M, et al. Voriconazole versus a regimen of amphotericin B followed by fluconazole for candidemia in nonneutropenic patients: a randomised non-inferiority trial. *Lancet.* 2005;366:1435–1442.
12. Kuse ER, Chetchotisakd P, da Cunha CA, et al. Micafungin versus liposomal amphotericin B for candidaemia and invasive candidosis: a phase III randomised double-blind trial. *Lancet.* 2007;369:1519–1527.
13. Mora-Duarte J, Betts R, Rotstein C, et al. Comparison of caspofungin and amphotericin B for invasive candidiasis. *N Engl J Med.* 2002;347:2020–2029.
14. Kullberg BJ, Sobel JD, Ruhnke M, et al. Voriconazole versus a regimen of amphotericin B followed by fluconazole for candidemia in nonneutropenic patients: a randomised non-inferiority trial. *Lancet.* 2005;366:1435–1442.
15. Pappas PG, Rotstein CM, Betts RF, et al. Micafungin versus caspofungin for treatment of candidemia and other forms of invasive candidiasis. *Clin Infect Dis.* 2007;45:883–893.
16. Pfaller MA, Diekema DJ, Sheehan DJ. Interpretive breakpoints for fluconazole and *Candida* revisited: a blueprint for the future of antifungal susceptibility testing. *Clin Microbiol Rev.* 2006;19:435–447.
17. Clinical and Laboratory Standards Institute (CLSI). *Reference method for broth dilution antifungal susceptibility testing of yeasts: Approved standard.* 3rd ed. CLSI document M27-A3. Wayne, PA: CLSI; 2008.
18. Baddley JW, Benjamin Jr DK, Patel M, et al. *Candida* infective endocarditis. *Eur J Clin Microbiol Infect Dis.* 2008;27:519–529.
19. Utley JR, Mills J, Roe BB. The role of valve replacement in the treatment of fungal endocarditis. *J Thorac Cardiovasc Surg.* 1974;69:255–258.
20. Steinbach WJ, Perfect JR, Cabell CH, et al. A meta-analysis of medical versus surgical therapy for *Candida* endocarditis. *J Infect.* 2005;51:230–247.
21. Ellis ME, Al-Abdely H, Sandrige A, Greer W, Ventura W. Fungal endocarditis: evidence in the world literature, 1965–1995. *Clin Infect Dis.* 2001;32:50–62.
22. Mrówczynski W, Wojtalik M. Caspofungin for *Candida* endocarditis. *Pediatr Infect Dis J.* 2004;23:376.
23. Moudgal V, Little T, Boikov D, Vazquez JA. Multiechinocandin and multiazole-resistant *Candida parapsilosis* isolates serially obtained during therapy for prosthetic valve endocarditis. *Antimicrob Agents Chemother.* 2005;49:767–769.
24. Lye DC, Hughes A, O'Brien D, Athan E. *Candida glabrata* prosthetic valve endocarditis treated successfully with fluconazole plus caspofungin without surgery: a case report and literature review. *Eur J Clin Microbiol Infect Dis.* 2005;24:753–755.
25. Lopez-Ciudad V, Castro-Orjales MJ, Leon C, et al. Successful treatment of *Candida parapsilosis* mural endocarditis with combined caspofungin and voriconazole. *BMC Infect Dis.* 2006;6:73.
26. Cornely OA, Lasso M, Betts R, et al. Caspofungin for the treatment of less common forms of invasive candidiasis. *J Antimicrob Chemother.* 2007;60:363–369.
27. Sanchez-Portocarrero J, Perez-Cecilia E, Corral O, Romero-Vivas J, Picazo JJ. The central nervous system and infection by *Candida* species. *Diagn Microbiol Infect Dis.* 2000;37:169–179.

28. Nguyen Mh, Yu VL. Meningitis caused by *Candida* species: an emerging problem in neurosurgical patients. *Clin Infect Dis*. 1995;21:323–327.

29. Voice RA, Bradley SF, Sangeorzan JA, Kauffman CA. Chronic candidal meningitis: an uncommon manifestation of candidiasis. *Clin Infect Dis*. 1994;19:60–66.

30. Pappas P, Kauffman C, Andes, D, et al. Clinical practice guidelines for the management of candidiasis: 2009. Update by the Infectious Diseases Society of America. *Clin Infect Dis*. 2009;48:503–535.

31. Smego Jr RA, Perfect JR, Durack DT. Combined therapy with amphotericin B and 5-fluorocytosine for *Candida* meningitis. *Rev Infect Dis*. 1984;6:791–801.

32. Thaler M, Pastakia B, Shawker TH, O'Leary T, Pizzo PA. Hepatic candidiasis in cancer patients: the evolving picture of the syndrome. *Ann Intern Med*. 1988;108:88–100.

33. Walsh TJ, Whitcomb PO, Revankar SG, Pizzo PA. Successful treatment of hepatosplenic candidiasis through repeated cycles of chemotherapy and neutropenia. *Cancer*. 1995;76:2357–2362.

34. Gokhale PC, Barapatre RJ, Advani SH, Kshirsagar NA, Pandya SK. Successful treatment of disseminated candidiasis resistant to amphotericin B by liposomal amphotericin B: a case report. *J Cancer Res Clin Oncol*. 1993;119:569–571.

35. Anaissie E, Bodey GP, Kantarjian H, et al. Fluconazole therapy for chronic disseminated candidiasis in patients with leukemia and prior amphotericin B therapy. *Am J Med*. 1991;91:142–150.

36. Kauffman CA, Bradley SF, Ross SC, Weber DR. Hepatosplenic candidiasis: successful treatment with fluconazole. *Am J Med*. 1991;91:137–141.

37. Sora F, Chiusolo P, Piccirillo N, et al. Successful treatment with caspofungin of hepatosplenic candidiasis resistant to liposomal amphotericin B. *Clin Infect Dis*. 2002;35:1135–1136.

38. Ostrosky-Zeichner L, Oude Lashof AM, Kullberg BJ, Rex JH. Voriconazole salvage treatment of invasive candidiasis. *Eur J Clin Microbiol Infect Dis*. 2003;22:651–655.

39. Hennequin C, Bouree P, Hiesse C, Dupont B, Charpentier B. Spondylodiskitis due to *Candida albicans*: report of two patients who were successfully treated with fluconazole and review of the literature. *Clin Infect Dis*. 1996;23:176–178.

40. Ferra C, Doebbeling BN, Hollis RJ, Pfaller MA, Lee KC, Gingrich RD. *Candida tropicalis* verterbral osteomyelitis: a late sequela of fungemia. *Clin Infect Dis*. 1994;19:697–703.

41. Sugar AM, Saunders C, Diamond RD. Successful treatment of *Candida* osteomyelitis with fluconazole: a noncomparative study of two patients. *Diagn Microbiol Infect Dis*. 1990;13:517–520.

42. Edwards JE Jr, Foos RY, Montgomerie JZ, Guze LB. Ocular manifestations of *Candida* septicemia: review of seventy-six cases of hematogenous *Candida* endophthalmitis. *Medicine (Baltimore)*. 1974;53:47–75.

43. Essman TF, Flynn Jr HW, Smiddy WE, et al. Treatment outcomes in a 10-year study of endogenous fungal endophthalmitis. *Ophthalmic Surg Lasers*. 1997;28:185–194.

44. Parke II DW, Jones DB, Gentry LO. Endogenous endophthalmitis among patients with candidemia. *Ophthalmology*. 1982;89:789–796.

45. Akler ME, Vellend H, McNeely DM, Walmsley SL, Gold WL. Use of fluconazole in the treatment of candidal endophthalmitis. *Clin Infect Dis*. 1995;20:657–664.

46. Breit SM, Hariprasad SM, Mieler WF, Shah GK, Mills MD, Grand MG. Management of endogenous fungal endophthalmitis with voriconazole and caspofungin. *Am J Ophthalmol*. 2005;139:135–140.

47. Varma D, Thaker HR, Moss PJ, Wedgwood K, Innes JR. Use of voriconazole in *Candida* retinitis. *Eye*. 2005;19:485–487.

48. Thiel MA, Zinkernagel AS, Burhenne J, Kaufmann C, Haefeli WE. Voriconazole concentration in human aqueous humor and plasma during topical or combined topical and systemic administration for fungal keratitis. *Antimicrob Agents Chemother*. 2007;51:239–244.

49. Sangeorzan JA, Bradley SF, He X, et al. Epidemiology of oral candidiasis in HIV-infected patients: colonization, infection, treatment, and emergence of fluconazole resistance. *Am J Med*. 1994;97:339–346.

50. Bonacini M, Young T, Laine L. The causes of esophageal symptoms in human immunodeficiency virus infection: a prospective study of 110 patients. *Arch Intern Med*. 1991;151:1567–1572.

51. Phillips P, Zemcov J, Mahmood W, Montaner JS, Craib K, Clarke AM. Itraconazole cyclodextrin solution for fluconazole-refractory oropharyngeal candidiasis in AIDS: correlation of clinical response with in vitro susceptibility. *AIDS*. 1996;10:1369–1376.

52. Walsh TJ, Anaissie EJ, Denning DW, et al. Treatment of aspergillosis: clinical practice guidelines of the Infectious Diseases Society of America. *Clin Infect Dis*. 2008;46:327–360.

53. Verweij PE, Brinkman K, Kremer HPH, Kullberg BJ, Meis J. *Aspergillus* meningitis: diagnosis by non-culture based microbiological methods and management. *J Clin Microbiol*. 1999;37:1186–1189.

54. Musher B, Fredricks D, Leisenring W, Balajee SA, Smith C, Marr KA. *Aspergillus* galactomannan enzyme immunoassay and quantitative PCR for diagnosis of invasive aspergillosis with bronchoalveolar lavage fluid. *J Clin Microbiol*. 2004;42:5517–5522.

55. Holding KJ, Dworkin MS, Wan P-CT, et al. Aspergillosis among people infected with human immunodeficiency virus: incidence and survival. *Clin Infect Dis*. 2000;31:1253–1257.

56. Herbrecht R, Denning DW, Patterson TF, et al. Voriconazole versus amphotericin B for primary therapy of invasive aspergillosis. *N Engl J Med*. 2002;347:408–415.

57. Bowden R, Chandrasekar P, White MH, et al. A double-blinded, randomized, controlled trial of amphotericin B for treatment of invasive aspergillosis in immunocompromised patients. *Clin Infect Dis*. 2002;21:240–248.

58. White MH, Anaissie EJ, Kusne S, et al. Amphotericin B colloidal dispersion vs. amphotericin B as therapy for invasive aspergillosis. *Clin Infect Dis*. 1997;24:635–642.

59. Leenders AC, Daenen S, Jansen RL, et al. Liposomal amphotericin B compared with amphotericin B deoxycholate in the treatment of documented and suspected neutropenia-associated invasive fungal infections. *Br J Haematol*. 1998;103:205–212.

60. Walsh TJ, Hiemenz JM, Seibel NH, et al. Amphotericin B lipid complex for invasive fungal infections: analysis of safety and efficacy in 556 cases. *Clin Infect Dis*. 1998;26:1383–1396.

61. Cornely OA, Maertens J, Bresnik M, et al. Liposomal amphotericin B as initial therapy for invasive mold infection: a randomized trial comparing a high-loading dose regimen with standard dosing (AmBiLoad trial). *Clin Infect Dis*. 2007;44:1289–1297.

62. Maertens J, Raad I, Petrikkos G, et al. Efficacy and safety of caspofungin for treatment of invasive aspergillosis in patients refractory to or intolerant of conventional antifungal therapy. *Clin Infect Dis*. 2004;39:1563–1571.

63. Caillot D. Intravenous itraconazole followed by oral itraconazole for the treatment of amphotericin-B-refractory invasive pulmonary aspergillosis. *Acta Haematologica*. 2003;109:111–118.

64. Steinbach WJ, Stevens DA, Denning DW. Combination and sequential antifungal therapy for invasive aspergillosis: review of published in vitro and in vivo interactions and 6281 clinical cases from 1966 to 2001. *Clin Infect Dis*. 2003;37(suppl 3):S188–S224.

65. Walsh TJ, Raad I, Patterson TF, et al. Treatment of invasive aspergillosis with posaconazole in patients who are refractory to or intolerant of conventional therapy: an externally controlled trial. *Clin Infect Dis*. 2007;44:2–12.

66. Steinbach WJ, Benjamin Jr DK, Kontoyiannis DP, et al. Infections due to *Aspergillus terreus*: a multicenter retrospective analysis of 83 cases. *Clin Infect Dis*. 2004;39:192–198.

67. Saraceno JL, Phelps DT, Ferro TJ, Futerfas R, Schwartz DB. Chronic necrotizing pulmonary aspergillosis. *Chest*. 1997;112:541–548.

68. Denning DW. Chronic forms of pulmonary aspergillosis. *Clin Microbiol Infect*. 2001;7(suppl 2):25–31.

69. Dupont B. Itraconazole therapy in aspergillosis: study in 49 patients. *J Am Acad Dermatol*. 1990;23:607–614.

70. Caras WE, Pluss JL. Chronic necrotizing pulmonary aspergillosis: pathologic outcome after itraconazole therapy. *Mayo Clin Proc*. 1996;71:25–30.

71. Camuset J, Nunes H, Dombret MC, et al. Treatment of chronic pulmonary aspergillosis by voriconazole in non-immunocompromised patients. *Chest*. 2007;131:1435–1441.

72. Sambatakou H, Dupont B, Lode H, Denning DW. Voriconazole treatment for subacute invasive and chronic pulmonary aspergillosis. *Am J Med*. 2006;119(527):e17–e24.

73. Judson MA, Stevens DA. The treatment of pulmonary aspergilloma. *Curr Opin Investig Drugs*. 2001;2:1375–1377.

74. Campbell JH, Winter JH, Richardson MS, Shankland GS, Banham SW. Treatment of pulmonary aspergilloma with itraconazole. *Thorax*. 1991;46:839–841.

75. Regnard JF, Icard P, Nicolosi M, et al. Aspergilloma: a series of 89 surgical cases. *Ann Thora Surg*. 2000;69:898–903.

76. Roden MM, Zaoutis TE, Buchanan WL, et al. Epidemiology and outcome of zygomycosis: a review of 929 reported cases. *Clin Infect Dis*. 2005;41:634–653.

77. Chamilos G, Luna M, Lewis RE, et al. Invasive fungal infections in patients with hematologic malignancies in a tertiary care cancer center: an autopsy study over a 15-year period (1989–2003). *Haematologica.* 2006;91:986–989.

78. Rogers R, Thomas. Treatment of zygomycosis: current and new options. *J Antimicrob Chemother.* 2008;61(suppl 1):i35–i39.

79. Greenberg RN, Multane K, VanBurik J-A, et al. Posaconazole as salvage therapy for zygomycosis. *Antimicrob Agents Chemother.* 2006;50:126–133.

80. Van Burik J-A, Hare RS, Solomon HF, et al. Posaconazole is effective as salvage therapy in zygomycosis: a retrospective summary of 91 cases. *Clin Infect Dis.* 2006;42:e61–e65.

81. Sedlacek M, Cotter JG, Suriawinata AA, et al. Mucormycosis peritonitis: more than 2 years of disease-free follow-up after posaconazole salvage therapy after failure of liposomal amphotericin B. *Am J Kidney Dis.* 2008;51:302–306.

82. Vazquez L, Mateos JJ, Sanz-Rodriquez C, et al. Successful treatment of rhinocerebral zygomycosis with a combination of caspofungin and liposomal amphotericin B. Haematologica. 2005;90(suppl 12):ECR39.

83. Reed C, Bryant R, Ibrahim AS, et al. Combination polyene-caspofungin treatment of rhino-orbital-cerebral mucormycosis. *Clin Infect Dis.* 2008;47:364–371.

84. Dromer F, Mathoulin S, Dupont B, et al. Comparison of the efficacy of amphotericin B and fluconazole in the treatment of cryptococcosis in human immunodeficiency virus-negative patients: retrospective analysis of 83 cases. *Clin Infect Dis.* 1996;22:S154–S160.

85. Saag MS, Graybill RJ, Larsen RA, Pappas PG, et al. Practice guidelines for the management of cryptococcal disease. *Clin Infect Dis.* 2000;30:710–718.

86. Dismukes WE, Cloud G, Gallis HA, et al. Treatment of cryptococcal meningitis with combination amphotericin B and flucytosine for four and compared with six weeks. *N Engl J Med.* 1987;317:334–341.

87. Yamaguchi H, Ikemoto H, Watanabe K, et al. Fluconazole monotherapy for cryptococcosis in non-AIDS patients. *Eur J Clin Microbiol Infect Dis.* 1996;15:787–792.

88. Pappas PG, Perfect J, Cloud GA, et al. Cryptococcosis in human immunodeficiency virus-negative patients in the era of effective azole therapy. *Clin Infect Dis.* 2001;33:690–699.

89. Denning DW, Tucker RM, Hanson LH, et al. Itraconazole therapy for cryptococcal meningitis and cryptococcosis. *Arch Intern Med.* 1989;149:2301–2308.

90. Bennett JE, Dismukes W, Duma RJ, et al. A comparison of amphotericin B alone and combined with flucytosine in the treatment of cryptococcal meningitis. *N Engl J Med.* 1979;301:126–131.

91. Van der Host C, Saag MS, Cloud GA, et al. Treatment of cryptococcal meningitis associated with the acquired immunodeficiency syndrome. *N Engl J Med.* 1997;337:15–21.

92. Saag MS, Powderly WG, Cloud GA, et al. Comparison of amphotericin B with fluconazole in the treatment of acute AIDS-associated cryptococcal meningitis. *N Engl J Med.* 1992;326:83–89.

93. Leenders AC, Reiss P, Portegies P, et al. Liposomal amphotericin B (Ambisome) compared with amphotericin B followed by oral fluconazole in the treatment of AIDS-associated cryptococcal meningitis. *AIDS.* 1997;11:1463–1471.

94. Larsen RA, Leal MAE, Chan LS. Fluconazole compared with amphotericin B plus flucytosine for the treatment of cryptococcal meningitis in AIDS: A randomized trial. *Ann Intern Med.* 1990;113:183–187.

95. de Gans J, Portegies P, Tiessens G, et al. Itraconazole compared with amphotericin B plus flucytosine in AIDS patients with cryptococcal meningitis. *AIDS.* 1992;6:185–190.

96. Larsen RA, Bozzette SA, Jones B, et al. Fluconazole combined with flucytosine for cryptococcal meningitis in persons with AIDS. *Clin Infect Dis.* 1994;19:741–745.

97. Powderly WG, Saag MS, Cloud GA, et al. A controlled trial of fluconazole or amphotericin B to prevent relapse of cryptococcal meningitis in patients with acquired immunodeficiency syndrome. *N Engl J Med.* 1991;324:580–584.

98. Saag MS, Cloud CG, Graybill JR, et al. A comparison of itraconazole versus fluconazole as maintenance therapy for AIDS-associated cryptococcal meningitis. *Clin Infect Dis.* 1999;28:291–296.

99. Wheat LJ, Freifeld AG, Kleiman MB, et al. Clinical practice guidelines for the management of patients with histoplasmosis: 2007 update by the Infectious Diseases Society of America. *Clin Infect Dis.* 2007;45:807–825.

100. Wheat LK. Improvements in diagnosis of histoplasmosis. *Expert Opin Biol Ther.* 2006;6:1207–1221.

101. Wheat LJ, Conces D, Allen SD, Blue-Hnidy D, Loyd J. Pulmonary histoplasmosis syndromes: recognition, diagnosis, and management. *Semin Respir Crit Care Med.* 2004;25:129–144.

102. Dismukes WE, Bradsher Jr RW, Cloud GC, et al. Itraconazole therapy for blastomycosis and histoplasmosis. NIAID Mycoses Study Group. *Am J Med.* 1992;93:489–497.

103. Kataria YP, Campbell PB, Burlingham BT. Acute pulmonary histoplasmosis presenting as adult respiratory distress syndrome: effect of therapy on clinical and laboratory features. *South Med J.* 1981;74:534–537.

104. Loyd JE, Tillman BF, Atkinson JB, Des Prez RM. Mediastinal fibrosis complicating histoplasmosis. *Medicine (Baltimore).* 1988;67:295–310.

105. Parker JD, Sarosi GA, Doto IL, Bailey RE, Tosh FE. Treatment of chronic pulmonary histoplasmosis. *N Engl J Med.* 1970;283:225–229.

106. Wheat J, Hafner R, Korzun AH, et al. Itraconazole treatment of disseminated histoplasmosis in patients with the acquired immunodeficiency syndrome. AIDS Clinical Trial Group. *Am J Med.* 1995;98:336–342.

107. Johnson PC, Wheat LJ, Cloud GA, et al. Safety and efficacy of liposomal amphotericin B compared with conventional amphotericin B for induction therapy of histoplasmosis in patients with AIDS. *Ann Intern Med.* 2002;137:105–109.

108. Tobon AM, Agudelo CA, Rosero DS, et al. Disseminated histoplasmosis: a comparative study between patients with acquired immunodeficiency syndrome and non-human immunodeficiency virus-infected individuals. *Am J Trop Med Hyg.* 2005;73:576–582.

109. Nacher M, Sarazin F, El Guedj M, et al. Increased incidence of disseminated histoplasmosis following highly active antiretroviral therapy initiation. *J Acquir Immune Defic Syndr.* 2006;41:468–470.

110. Goldman M, Zackin R, Fichtenbaum CJ, et al. Safety of discontinuation of maintenance therapy for disseminated histoplasmosis after immunologic response to antiretroviral therapy. *Clin Infect Dis.* 2004;38:1485–1489.

111. Wheat LJ, Batteiger BE, Sathapatayavongs B. *Histoplasma capsulatum* infections of the central nervous system: a clinical review. *Medicine (Baltimore).* 1990;69:244–260.

112. Groll AH, Giri N, Petraitis V, et al. Comparative efficacy and distribution of lipid formulations of amphotericin B in experimental *Candida albicans* infection of the central nervous system. *J Infect Dis.* 2000;182:274–282.

113. Haynes RR, Connolly PA, Durkin MM, et al. Antifungal therapy for central nervous system histoplasmosis, using a newly developed intracranial model of infection. *J Infect Dis.* 2002;185:1830–1832.

114. Fisher MC, Koenig GL, White TJ, Taylor JT. Molecular and phenotypic description of *Coccidioides posadasii* sp. Nov., previously recognized as the non-California population of *Coccidioides immitis.* Mycologia. 2002;94:73–84.

115. Galgiani JN. Coccidioidomycosis: a regional disease of national importance – rethinking approaches for control. *Ann Intern Med.* 1999;130:293–300.

116. Chiller TM, Galgiani JN, Stevens DA. Coccidioidomycosis. *Infect Dis Clin North Am.* 2003;17:41–57, viii.

117. Stevens DA. Current concepts: coccidioidomycosis. *N Engl J Med.* 1995;332:1077–1082.

118. Drutz DJ, Catanzaro A. Coccidioidomycosis: part II. *Am Rev Respir Dis.* 1978;117:727–771.

119. Panackal AA, Hajjeh RA, Cetron MS, Warnock DW. Fungal infections among returning travelers. *Clin Infect Dis.* 2002;35:1088–1095.

120. Feldman BS, Snyder LS. Primary pulmonary coccidioidomycosis. *Semin Respir Infect.* 2001;16:231–237.

121. Pappagianis D. Serologic studies in coccidioidomycosis. *Semin Respir Infect.* 2001;16:242–250.

122. Galgiani JN, Ampel NK, Blair JE, et al. Coccidioidomycosis. *Clin Infect Dis.* 2005;41:1217–1223.

123. Oldfield EC, Bone WD, Martin CR, Gray GC, Olson P, Schillaci RF. Prediction of relapse after treatment of coccidioidomycosis. *Clin Infect Dis.* 1997;25:1205–1210.

124. Tucker RM, Denning DW, Arathoon EG, Rinaldi MG, Stevens DA. Itraconazole therapy of non-meningeal coccidioidomycosis: clinical and laboratory observations. *J Am Acad Dermatol.* 1990;23:593–601.

125. Galgiani JN, Catanzaro A, Cloud GA, et al. Comparison of oral fluconazole and itraconazole for progressive, nonmeningeal coccidioidomycosis: a randomized, double-blind trial. Mycoses Study Group. *Ann Intern Med.* 2000;133:676–686.

126. Galgiani JN, Stevens DA, Graybill JR, Dismukes WE, Cloud GA. Ketoconazole therapy of progressive coccidioidomycosis: comparison of 400- and 800-mg doses and observations at higher doses. *Am J Med.* 1988;84:603–610.

127. Graybill JR, Stevens DA, Galgiani JN, Dismukes WE, Cloud GA. Itraconazole treatment of coccidioidomycosis. NAIAD Mycoses Study Group. *Am J Med*. 1990;89:282–290.

128. Catanzaro A, Galgiani JN, Levine BE, et al. Fluconazole in the treatment of chronic pulmonary and nonmeningeal disseminated coccidioidomycosis. NIAID Mycoses Study Group. *Am J Med*. 1995;98:249–256.

129. Galgiani JN, Catanzaro A, Cloud GA, et al. Fluconazole therapy for coccidioidal meningitis: the NIAID Mycoses Study Group. *Ann Intern Med*. 1993;119:28–35.

130. Stevens DA, Shatsky SA. Intrathecal amphotericin in the management of coccidioidal meningitis. *Semin Respir Infect*. 2001;16:263–269.

131. Hall KA, Sethi GK, Rosado LJ, Martinez JD, Huston CL, Copeland JG. Coccidioidomycosis and heart transplantation. *J Heart Lung Transplant*. 1993;12:525–526.

132. Canafax DM, Graves NM, Hilligoss DM, et al. Interaction between cyclosporine and fluconazole in renal allograft recipients. *Transplantation*. 1991;51:1014–1018.

133. Manez R, Martin M, Raman D, et al. Fluconazole therapy in transplant recipients receiving FK506. *Transplantation*. 1994;57:1521–1523.

134. Ampel NM. Coccidioidomycosis in persons infected with HIV-1. *Ann N Y Acad Sci*. 2007;1111:336–342.

135. Woods CW, McRill C, Plikaytis BD, et al. Coccidioidomycosis in human immunodeficiency virus-infected persons in Arizona, 1994–1997: incidence, risk factors, and prevention. *J Infect Dis*. 2000;181:1428–1434.

136. Chapman SW, Dismukes WE, Proria LA, et al. Clinical practice guidelines for the management of blastomycosis: 2008 update by the Infectious Diseases Society of America. *Clin Infect Dis*. 2008;46:1801–1812.

137. Klein BS, Vergeront JM, DiSalvo AF, Kaufman L, Davis JP. Two outbreaks of blastomycosis along rivers in Wisconsin: isolation of *Blastomyces dermatitidis* from riverbank soil and evidence of its transmission along waterways. *Am Rev Respir Dis*. 1987;136:1333–1338.

138. Martynowicz MA, Prakash UB. Pulmonary blastomycosis: an appraisal of diagnostic techniques. *Chest*. 2002;121:768–773.

139. Lemos LB, Guo M, Baliga M. Blastomycosis: organ involvement and etiologic diagnosis: a review of 123 patients from Mississippi. *Ann Diagn Pathol*. 2000;4:391–406.

140. Durkin M, Witt J, Lemonte A, Wheat B, Connolly P. Antigen assay with the potential to aid in diagnosis of blastomycosis. *J Clin Microbiol*. 2004;42:4873–4875.

141. Meyer KC, McManus EJ, Maki DG. Overwhelming pulmonary blastomycosis associated with the adult respiratory distress syndrome. *N Engl J Med*. 1993;329:1231–1236.

142. National Institute of Allergy and Infectious Diseases Mycoses Study Group. Treatment of blastomycosis and histoplasmosis with ketoconazole: results of a prospective randomized clinical trial. *Ann Intern Med*. 1985;103:861–872.

143. Pappas PG, Bradsher RW, Chapman SW, et al. Treatment of blastomycosis with fluconazole: a pilot study. The National Institute of Allergy and Infectious Diseases Mycoses Study Group. *Clin Infect Dis*. 1995;20:267–271.

144. Pappas PG, Bradsher RW, Kauffman CA, et al. Treatment of blastomycosis with higher doses of fluconazole. The National Institute of Allergy and Infectious Diseases Mycoses Study Group. *Clin Infect Dis*. 1997;25:200–205.

145. Bradsher RW. Histoplasmosis and blastomycosis. *Clin Infect Dis*. 1996;22(suppl 2):S102–S111.

146. Johnson MD, Perfect JR. Fungal infections of the bones and joints. *Current Infectious Disease Reports*. 2001;3:450–460.

147. Pappas PG, Pottage JC, Powderly WG, et al. Blastomycosis in patients with the acquired immunodeficiency syndrome. *Ann Intern Med*. 1992;116:847–853.

148. Groll AH, Giri N, Petraitis V, et al. Comparative efficacy and distribution of lipid formulations of amphotericin B in experimental *Candida albicans* infection of the central nervous system. *J Infect Dis*. 2000;182:274–282.

149. Panicker J, Walsh T, Kamani N. Recurrent central nervous system blastomycosis in an immunocompetent child treated successfully with sequential liposomal amphotericin B and voriconazole. *Pediatr Infect Dis J*. 2006;25:377–379.

150. Bakleh M, Aksamit AJ, Tleyjeh IM, Marshall WF. Successful treatment of cerebral blastomycosis with voriconazole. *Clin Infect Dis*. 2005;40:e69–e71.

151. Borgia SM, Fuller JD, Sarabia A, El-Helou P. Cerebral blastomycosis: a case series incorporating voriconazole in the treatment regimen. *Med Mycol*. 2006;44:659–664.

152. Lentnek AL, Lentnek IA. Successful management of *Blastomyces dermatitidis* meningitis. *Infect Med*. 2006;23:39–41.

153. Bariola J, Perry P, Pappas P, Shealey W, Bradsher R. Central nervous system blastomycosis: review of recent experience [abstract 162]. In: *Programs and abstracts of the 45th Annual Meeting of the Infectious Diseases Society of America (San Diego)*. Alexandria, VA: Infectious Diseases Society of America; 2007:81.

154. Pappas PG, Threlkeld MG, Bedsole GD, Cleveland KO, Gelfand MS, Dismukes WE. Blastomycosis in immunocompromised patients. *Medicine (Baltimore)*. 1993;72:311–325.

155. Brummer E, Castaneda E, Restrepo A. Paracoccidioidomycosis: an update. *Clin Microbiol Rev*. 1993;6:89–117.

156. Manns BJ, Baylis BW, Urbanski SJ, Gibb AP, Rabin HR. Paraccidioidomycosis: case report and review. *Clin Infect Dis*. 1996;23:1026–1032.

157. Naranjo MS, Trujillo M, Munera MI, Restrepo P, Gomez I, Restrepo A. Treatment of paracoccidioidomycosis with itraconazole. *J Med Vet Mycol*. 1990;28:67–76.

158. Shikanai-Yasuda MA, Benard G, Higaki Y, et al. Randomized trial with itraconazole, ketoconazole and sulfadiazine in paracoccidioidomycosis. *Med Mycol*. 2002;40:411–417.

159. Rios-Fabra A, Restrepo Moreno A, Isturiz RE. Fungal infection in Latin American countries. *Infect Dis Clin North Am*. 1994;8:129–154.

160. Queiroz-Telles F, Goldani LZ, Schlamm HT, Goodrich JM, Espinel-Ingroo A, Shikanai-Yasuda MA. An open-label comparative pilot study of oral voriconazole and itraconazole for long-term treatment of paracoccidioidomycosis. *Clin Infect Dis*. 2007;45:1462–1469.

161. Supparatpinyo K, Khamwan C, Baosoung V, Nelson KE, Sirisanthana T. Disseminated *Penicillium marneffei* infection in Southeast Asia. *Lancet*. 1994;344:110–113.

162. Clezy K, Sirisanthana T, Sirisanthana V, Brew B, Cooper DA. Late manifestations of HIV in Asia and the Pacific. *AIDS*. 1994;8(suppl 2):35–43.

163. Kantipong P, Panich V, Pongsurachet V, Watt G. Hepatic penicilliosis in patients without skin lesions. *Clin Infect Dis*. 1998;26:1215–1217.

164. Singh PN, Ranjana K, Singh YI, et al. Indigenous disseminated *Penicillium marneffei* infection in the state of Manipur, India: report of four autochthonous cases. *J Clin Microbiol*. 1999;37:2699–2702.

165. Ranjana KH, Priyokumar K, Singh TJ, et al. Disseminated *Penicillium marneffei* infection among HIV-infected patients in Manipur state, India. *J Infect Dis*. 2002;45:268–271.

166. Chariyalertsak S, Supparatpinyo K, Sirisanthana T, Nelson KE. A controlled trial of itraconazole as primary prophylaxis for systemic fungal infections in patients with advanced human immunodeficiency virus infection in Thailand. *Clin Infect Dis*. 2002;34:277–284.

167. Supparatpinyo K, Nelson KE, Merz WG, et al. Response to antifungal therapy by human immunodeficiency virus-infected patients with disseminated *Penicillium marneffei* infections and in vitro susceptibilities of isolates from clinical specimens. *Antimicrob Agents Chemother*. 1993;37:2407–2411.

168. Supparatpinyo K, Chiewchanvit S, Hirunsri P, et al. An efficacy study of itraconazole in the treatment of *Penicillium marneffei* infection. *J Med Assoc Thai*. 1992;75:688–691.

169. Sirisanthana T, Supparatpinyo K, Perriens J, Nelson KE. Amphotericin B and itraconazole for treatment of disseminated *Penicillium marneffei* infection in human immunodeficiency virus-infected patients. *Clin Infect Dis*. 1998;26:1107–1110.

170. Sharkey-Mathis PK, Kauffman CA, Graybill JR, et al. Treatment of sporotrichosis with itraconazole. NIAID Mycoses Study Group. *Am J Med*. 1993;95:279–285.

171. Restrepo A, Robledo J, Gomez I, Tabares AM, Gutierrez R. Itraconazole therapy in lymphangitic and cutaneous sporotrichosis. *Arch Dermatol*. 1986;122:413–417.

172. Conti Diaz IA, Civila E, Gezuele E, et al. Treatment of human cutaneous sporotrichosis with itraconazole. *Mycoses*. 1992;35:153–156.

173. Chapman SW, Pappas P, Kauffman C, et al. Comparative evaluation of the efficacy and safety of two doses of terbinafine (500 and 1000 mg/day) in the treatment of cutaneous or lymphocutaneous sporotrichosis. *Mycoses*. 2004;47:62–68.

174. Cabezas C, Bustamante B, Holgado W, Begue RE. Treatment of cutaneous sporotrichosis with one daily dose of potassium iodide. *Pediatr Infect Dis J*. 1996;15:352–354.

175. da Rosa AC, Scroferneker ML, Vettorato R, Gervini RL, Vettorato G, Weber A. Epidemiology of sporotrichosis: a study of 304 cases in Brazil. *J Am Acad Dermatol*. 2005;52:451–459.

176. Mahajan VK, Sharma NL, Sharma RC, Gupta ML, Garg G, Kanga AK. Cutaneous sporotrichosis in Himachal Pradesh, India. *Mycoses*. 2005;48:25–31.

177. Itoh M, Okamoto S, Kariya H. Survey of 200 cases of sporotrichosis. *Dermatologica*. 1986;172:209–213.

178. Bayer AS, Scott VJ, Guze LB. Fungal arthritis. III. Sporotrichal arthritis. *Semin Arthritis Rheum*. 1979;9:66–74.

179. Crout JE, Brewer NS, Tompkins RB. Sporotrichosis arthritis: clinical features in seven patients. *Ann Intern Med*. 1977;86:294–297.

180. Stratton CW, Lichtenstein KA, Lowenstein SR, Phelps DB, Reller LB. Granulomatous tenosynovitis and carpal tunnel syndrome caused by *Sporothrix schenckii*. *Am J Med*. 1981;71:161–164.

181. Kauffman CA, Bustamante B, Chapman SW, Pappas PG. Clinical practice guidelines for the management of sporotrichosis: 2007 update by the Infectious Diseases Society of America. *Clin Infect Dis*. 2007;45:1255–1265.

182. Pluss JL, Opal SM. Pulmonary sporotrichosis: review of treatment and outcome. *Medicine (Baltimore)*. 1986;65:143–153.

183. Bonifaz A, Peniche A, Mercadillo P, Saul A. Successful treatment of AIDS-related disseminated cutaneous sporotrichosis with itraconazole. *AIDS Patient Care STDS*. 2001;15:603–606.

184. Oscherwitz SL, Rinaldi MG. Disseminated sporotrichosis in a patient infected with human immunodeficiency virus. *Clin Infect Dis*. 1992;15:568–569.

185. Silva-Vergara ML, Maneira FR, De Oliveira RM, Santos CT, Etchebehere RM, Adad SJ. Multifocal sporotrichosis with meningeal involvement in a patient with AIDS. *Med Mycol*. 2005;43:187–190.

186. Nucci M. Anaissie E. *Fusarium* infections in immunocompromised patients. *Clin Microbiol Rev*. 2007;20:695–704.

187. Nucci M, Anaissie E. Cutaneous infection by *Fusarium* species in healthy and immunocompromised hosts: implications for diagnosis and management. *Clin Infect Dis*. 2002;35:909–920.

188. Guimera-Martin-Neda F, Garcia-Bustinduy M, Noda-Cabrera A, Sanchez-Gonzalez R, Montelongo RG. Cutaneous infection by *Fusarium*: successful treatment with oral voriconazole. *Br J Dermatol*. 2004;150:777–778.

189. Bunya VY, Hammersmith KM, Rapuano CJ, Ayres BD, Cohen EJ. Topical and oral voriconazole in the treatment of fungal keratitis. *Am J Ophthalmol*. 2007;143:151–153.

190. Doczi, I, Gyetvai T, Kredics L, Nagy E. Involvement of *Fusarium* spp. in fungal keratitis. *Clin Microbiol Infect*. 2004;10:773–776.

191. Lodato F, Tamé MR, Montagnani M, et al. Systemic fungemia and hepatic localization of *Fusarium solani* in a liver transplanted patient: an emerging fungal agent. *Liver Transpl*. 2006;12:1711–1714.

192. Jensen TG, Gahrn-Hansen B, Arendrup M, et al. *Fusarium* fungemia in immunocompromised patients. *Clin Microbiol Infect*. 2004;10:499–501.

193. Stanzani M, Tumietto F, Vianelli N, Baccarani M. Update on the treatment of disseminated fusariosis: focus on voricaonazole. *Therapeutics and Clinical Risk Management*. 2007;3:1165–1173.

194. Husain S, Patricia Munoz P, Forrest G, et al. Infections due to *Scedosporium apiospermum* and *Scedosporium prolificans* in transplant recipients: clinical characteristics and impact of antifungal agent therapy on outcome. *Clin Infect Dis*. 2005;40:89–99.

195. Idigoras P, Perez-Trallero E, Pineiro L, et al. Disseminated infection and colonization by *Scedosporium prolificans*: a review of 18 cases, 1990–1999. *Clin Infect Dis*. 2001;32:e158–e165.

196. Berenguer J, Diaz-Mediavilla J, Urra D, Munoz P. Central nervous system infection caused by *Pseudallescheria boydii*: case report and review. *Rev Infect Dis*. 1989;11:890–896.

197. Husain S, Alexander B, Munoz P, et al. Opportunistic mycelial fungi in organ transplant recipients: emerging importance of non-*Aspergillus* mycelial infections. *Clin Infect Dis*. 2003;37:221–229.

198. Walsh TJ, Peter J, McGough DA, Fothergill AW, Rinaldi MG, Pizzo PA. Activities of amphotericin B and antifungal azoles alone and in combination against *Pseudallescheria boydii*. *Antimicrob Agents Chemother*. 1995;39:1361–1364.

199. Meletiadis J, Meis JF, Mouton JW, et al. In vitro activities of new and conventional antifungal agents against clinical *Scedosporium* isolates. *Antimicrob Agents Chemother*. 2002;46:62–68.

200. Nesky MA, McDougal EC, Peacock Jr JE. *Pseudallescheria boydii* brain abscess successfully treated with voriconazole and surgical drainage: case report and literature review of central nervous system pseudallescheriasis. *Clin Infect Dis*. 2000;31:673–677.

201. Capilla J, Guarro J. Correlation between in vitro susceptibility of *Scedosporium apiospermum* to voriconazole and in vivo outcome of scedosporiosis in guinea pigs. *Antimicrob Agents Chemother*. 2004;48:4009–4011.

202. Meletiadis J, Meis JF, Mouton JW, Rodriquez-Tudela JL, Donnelly JP, Verweij PE. In vitro activities of new and conventional antifungal agents against clinical *Scedosporium* isolates. *Antimicrob Agents Chemother*. 2002;46:62–68.

203. Steinbach WJ, Perfect JR. *Scedosporium* species infections and treatments. *J Chemother*. 2003;15:16–27.

204. Meletiades J, Mouton JW, Meis JF, Verweij PE. In vitro drug interaction modeling of combinations of azoles with terbinafine against clinical *Scedosporiium prolificans* isolates. *Antimicrob Agents Chemother*. 2003;47:106–117.

205. Meletiadis J, Mouton JW, Meis JF, Verweij PE. Combination chemotherapy for the treatment of invasive infections *by Scedosporium prolificans*. *Clin Microbiol Infect*. 2000;6:336–337.

206. Bhat SV, Paterson DL, Rinaldi MG, Veldkamp PJ. *Scedosporium prolificans* brain abscess in a patient with chronic granulomatous disease: successful combination therapy with voriconazole and terbinafine. *Scand J Infect Dis*. 2007;39:87–90.

207. Howden BP, Slavin MA, Schwarer AP, Mijch AM. Successful control of disseminated *Scedosporium prolificans* infection with a combination of voriconazole and terbinafine. *Eur J Clin Microbiol Infect Dis*. 2003;22:111–113.

208. Steinbach WJ, Schell WA, Miller JL, Perfect JR. *Scedosporium prolificans* osteomyelitis in an immunocompetent child treated with voriconazole and caspofungin, as well as locally applied polyhexamethylene biguanide. *J Clin Microbiol*. 2003;41:3981–3985.

209. Ameen M, Areans R. Developments in the management of mycetomas. *Clin Exp Dermatol*. 2008;34:1–7.

210. Venugopal PV, Venugopal TV. Treatment of eumycetoma with ketoconazole. *Australas J Dermatol*. 1993;34:27–29.

211. Welsh O, Salinas MC, Rodriguez MA. Treatment of eumycetoma and actinomycetoma. *Curr Top Med Mycol*. 1995;6:47–71.

212. Estrada-Chavez GE, Vega-Memije ME, Arenas R, et al. Eumycotic mycetoma caused by *Madurella mycetomatis* successfully treated with antifungals, surgery and topical negative pressure therapy. *Int J Dermatol*. 2009;48:401–403.

213. Negroni R, Tobon A, Bustamante B, et al. Posaconazole treatment of refractory eumycetoma and chromoblastomycosis. *Rev Inst Med Trop São Paulo*. 2005;47:339–346.

214. N'Diaye B, Dieng MT, Perez A, et al. Clinical efficacy and safety of oral terbinafine in fungal mycetoma. *Int J Dermatol*. 2006;45:154–157.

215. Queiroz-Telles F, Purim KS, Fillus JN, et al. Itraconazole in the treatment of chromoblastomycosis due to *Fonsecaea pedrosoi*. *Int J Dermatol*. 1992;31:805–812.

216. Esterre P, Inzan CK, Rtasioharana M, et al. A multicenter trial of terbinafine in patients with chromoblastomycosis: effects on clinical and histological criteria. *J Dermatolog Treat*. 1998;9:529–534.

217. Esterre P, Queiroz-Telles. Management of chromoblastomycosis: novel perspectives. *Curr Opin Infect Dis*. 2006;19:148–152.

218. Tagami H, Ginoza M, Imaizumi S, et al. Successful treatment of chromoblastomycosis with topical heat therapy. *J Am Acad Dermatol*. 1984;10:615–619.

219. Selwyn PA, Pumerantz AS, Durante A, et al. Clinical predictors of *Pneumocystis carinii* pneumonia, bacterial pneumonia and tuberculosis in HIV-infected patients. *AIDS*. 1998;12:885–893.

220. Baughman RP, Dohn MN, Frame PT. The continuing utility of bronchoalveolar lavage to diagnose opportunistic infection in AIDS patients. *Am J Med*. 1994;97:515–522.

221. Stover DE, Zaman MB, Hajdu SI, et al. Bronchoalveolar lavage in the diagnosis of diffuse pulmonary infiltrates in the immunosuppressed host. *Ann Intern Med*. 1984;101:1–7.

222. Roger PM, Vandenbos F, Pugliese P, et al. Persistence of *Pneumocystis carinii* after effective treatment of *P. carinii* pneumonia is not related to relapse or survival among patients infected with human immunodeficiency virus. *Clin Infect Dis*. 1998;26:509–510.

223. Larsen HH, Masur H, Kovacs JA, et al. Development and evaluation of a quantitative, touch-down, real-time PCR assay for diagnosing *Pneumocystis carinii* pneumonia. *J Clin Microbiol*. 2002;40:490–494.

224. Torres J, Goldman M, Wheat LJ, et al. Diagnosis of *Pneumocystis carinii* pneumonia in human immunodeficiency virus-infected patients with polymerase chain reaction: a blinded comparison to standard methods. *Clin Infect Dis*. 2000;30:141–145.

225. Safrin S, Finkelstein DM, Feinberg J, et al. Comparison of three regimens for treatment of mild to moderate *Pneumocystis carinii* pneumonia in patients with AIDS: a double-blind, randomized, trial of oral trimethoprim-sulfamethoxazole, dapsone–trimethoprim, and clindamycin–primaquine. *Ann Intern Med*. 1996;124:792–802.

226. Centers for Disease Control and Prevention. Guidelines for prevention and treatment of opportunistic infections in HIV-infected adults and adolescents. Recommendations from CDC, the National Institutes of Health, and the HIV Medicine Association of the Infectious Diseases Society of America. *MMWR Morb Mortal Wkly Rep.* 2009;58(RR-4):1–207.

227. Nielsen TL, Eeftinck Schattenkerk JK, Jensen BN, et al. Adjunctive corticosteroid therapy for *Pneumocystis carinii* pneumonia in AIDS: a randomized European multicenter open label study. *J Acquir Immune Defic Syndr.* 1992;5:726–731.

228. Bozzette SA, Sattler FR, Chiu J, et al. A controlled trial of early adjunctive treatment with corticosteroids for *Pneumocystis carinii* pneumonia in the acquired immunodeficiency syndrome. *N Engl J Med.* 1990;323:1451–1457.

229. Montaner JS, Lawson LM, Levitt N, et al. Corticosteroids prevent early deterioration in patients with moderately severe *Pneumocystis carinii* pneumonia and the acquired immunodeficiency syndrome (AIDS). *Ann Intern Med.* 1990;113:14–20.

230. Briel M, Bucher HC, Boscacci R, Furrer H. Adjunctive corticosteroids for *Pneumocystis jiroveci* pneumonia in patients with HIV-infection. *Cochrane Database of Syst Rev.* 2006;3:CD006150.

231. Hughes W, Leoung G, Kramer F, et al. Comparison of atovaquone (566C80) with trimethoprim–sulfamethoxazole to treat *Pneumocystis carinii* pneumonia in patients with AIDS. *N Engl J Med.* 1993;328:1521–1527.

232. Smego Jr RA, Nagar S, Maloba B, Popara M. A meta-analysis of salvage therapy for *Pneumocystis carinii* pneumonia. *Arch Intern Med.* 2001;161:1529–1533.

233. Wharton JM, Coleman DL, Wofsy CB, et al. Trimethoprim–sulfamethoxazole or pentamidine for *Pneumocystis carinii* pneumonia in the acquired immunodeficiency syndrome: a prospective randomized trial. *Ann Intern Med.* 1986;105:37–44.

234. Medina I, Mills J, Leoung G, et al. Oral therapy for *Pneumocystis carinii* pneumonia in the acquired immunodeficiency syndrome: a controlled trial of trimethoprim–sulfamethoxazole versus trimethoprim–dapsone. *N Engl J Med.* 1990;323:776–782.

235. Toma E, Thorne A, Singer J, et al. Clindamycin with primaquine vs. trimethoprim–sulfamethoxazole therapy for mild and moderately severe *Pneumocystis carinii* pneumonia in patients with AIDS: a multicenter, double-blind, randomized trial. *Clin Infect Dis.* 1998;27:524–530.

236. Hughes WT, LaFon SW, Scott JD, Masur H. Adverse events associated with trimethoprim–sulfamethoxazole and atovaquone during the treatment of AIDS-related *Pneumocystis carinii* pneumonia. *J Infect Dis.* 1995;171:1295–1301.

237. Klein NC, Duncanson FP, Lenox TH, et al. Trimethoprim–sulfamethoxazole versus pentamidine for *Pneumocystis carinii* pneumonia in AIDS patients: results of a large prospective randomized treatment trial. *AIDS.* 1992;6:301–305.

238. Sattler FR, Frame P, Davis R, et al. Trimetrexate with leucovorin versus trimethoprim–sulfamethoxazole for moderate to severe episodes of *Pneumocystis carinii* pneumonia in patients with AIDS: a prospective, controlled multicenter investigation of the AIDS Clinical Trials Group Protocol 029/031. *J Infect Dis.* 1994;170:165–172.

239. Dworkin MS, Hanson DL, Navin TR. Survival of patients with AIDS, after diagnosis of *Pneumocystis carinii* pneumonia, in the United States. *J Infect Dis.* 2001;183:1409–1412.

240. Huang L, Quartin A, Jones D, Havlir DV. Intensive care of patients with HIV infection. *N Engl J Med.* 2006;355:173–181.

Zoonoses

Lucy Lamb and Robert Davidson

BRUCELLOSIS

Worldwide about 500 000 human cases of brucellosis occur annually with a patchy global distribution.[1] The disease is endemic in the Mediterranean basin, the Arabian Gulf, the Indian subcontinent and parts of Mexico, Central and South America. Brucellosis is a systemic disease that can involve any organ or system of the body. The responsible species are: *Brucella melitensis* (sheep, goats and camels); *B. abortus* (cattle, buffalo, yaks, camels); *B. suis* (pigs, wild hares, caribou, wild rodents and reindeer); *B. ovis* (sheep) and *B. canis* (dogs). *B. melitensis* remains the main cause of human brucellosis worldwide.[2] Disease from marine species have emerged (*B. pinnipediae* and *B. cetaceae*). Infected animals shed large numbers of bacilli in milk, urine and products of conception. Humans are infected by direct contact with infected animals or by ingestion of unpasteurized milk or milk products. The infective dose of *Brucella*, especially of *B. melitensis* is very low (10 organisms). The incubation period is usually 7 days to 3 months, although longer intervals have been reported.

In humans the disease manifests as an acute (<2 months) or subacute (2–12 months) febrile illness which may persist and progress to become chronic (>1 year). *Brucella* has been considered a potential biological weapon as it has a propensity for airborne transmission and induction of chronic debilitating disease with vague clinical characteristics. Nowadays its inclusion is of historical significance because of the emergence of new, more virulent weapons.[3]

ANTIBIOTIC THERAPY – DRUG COMBINATIONS

Treatment has been designed to shorten the duration of symptoms, prevent relapse and avert complications such as arthritis, sacroiliitis, spondylitis, encephalitis, endocarditis, epididymo-orchitis and abortion. Monotherapies have a high rate of relapse so a combination of two drugs is usually used.

The recommendations for specific drug combinations in published sources are very inconsistent. The regimen of choice recommended by the World Health Organization (WHO) Expert Committee is doxycycline 200 mg/day plus rifampicin (rifampin) 600–900 mg/day for 6 weeks; however, these guidelines were published in 1986 and are subject to debate.[4]

There are significant differences in effectiveness between currently recommended treatment regimens. A recent Systematic Review in the British Medical Journal summarizes the evidence-based treatment options.[1,5] The therapy of brucellosis is complicated by the location of the organism within an acid compartment in reticuloendothelial cells, where optimal concentrations and effects of antibiotics are difficult to achieve. Therefore regimens should include at least one agent with good intracellular penetration.

The main outcomes of trials indicate the following:

- Monotherapy is not recommended because of its high failure rates.
- The combination of tetracycline–streptomycin is significantly superior to tetracycline–rifampicin, mainly due to a reduced rate of relapse. The tetracycline recommended is doxycycline 200 mg/day. Doxycycline is central to treatment regimens as the minimum inhibitory concentrations (MICs) of tetracycline for *Brucella* are generally <1 mg/L. Streptomycin works synergistically with doxycycline and is recommended at a dose of 1 g/day for the first 14 days of treatment. Adverse events in general and discontinuation because of these events were similar in the two treatment groups.
- Comparing the aminoglycosides, there is a trend to support the use of gentamicin rather than streptomycin. Thus gentamicin could replace streptomycin for dual treatment regimens. This has the added advantage of allowing therapeutic drug monitoring, which is routinely available for gentamicin.
- A regimen consisting of a quinolone plus rifampicin or streptomycin is less effective than the above, although the adverse events are less in this group.

- The optimal treatment regimen includes triple combination therapy with tetracycline–aminoglycoside–rifampicin and this has been found to be significantly more effective than most dual regimens. The tetracycline–rifampicin combination is administered for 6–8 weeks and the aminoglycoside for 2 weeks. If this is not successful, then a regimen containing a tetracycline–aminoglycoside combination is recommended.
- It is recommended that patients are treated for ≥6 weeks to prevent relapse, with a tetracycline and an aminoglycoside being administered for the first 7–14 days.

CHILDREN WITH BRUCELLOSIS

The treatment of childhood brucellosis will vary according the child's age. Optimal treatment of brucellosis remains based on combinations of doxycycline with either rifampicin or streptomycin. Doxycycline is not recommended for children younger than 9 years. Instead, a regimen consisting of gentamicin 5 mg/kg (5 days) or streptomycin 20 mg/kg (14 days) and co-trimoxazole 8 mg/kg (6 weeks), or co-trimoxazole plus rifampicin 20 mg/kg (6 weeks), are shown to be effective with low relapses. Relapses could be treated with a triple drug regimen, such as co-trimoxazole–aminoglycoside–rifampicin. There is no evidence on the use of triple drug regimens in children at present but adult studies have shown that this is an area for possible further research.[6]

TREATMENT OF BRUCELLOSIS DURING PREGNANCY AND LACTATION

Brucellosis can cause fetal death at any stage of pregnancy, whether maternal infection is mild or severe. The natural history of brucellosis in pregnant women may be altered by the early institution of antimicrobial therapy, particularly prior to vaginal bleeding. An important consideration when treating brucellosis in pregnant women is the possibility of fetal toxicity of the drugs. Although the data are limited, it is known that the incidence of abortion observed in patients with active brucellosis exceeds that in patients with other micro-organisms. Treatment with either co-trimoxazole (although monotherapy is not recommended because of the high incidence of relapse) or co-trimoxazole plus rifampicin had a strong protective effect against abortion. The length of treatment is 6 weeks, similar to non-pregnant individuals.[7]

SPINAL BRUCELLOSIS

Brucellosis affects many organ systems, with septic arthritis and osteomyelitis being common, especially in the elderly. It is a destructive disease, often confused with tuberculosis, so a thorough history (particularly focusing on risk factors like prior unpasteurized milk consumption) and examination are essential. Early diagnosis and treatment are vital for patient prognosis. The evidence supports the classic treatment regimen of doxycycline 100 mg every 12 h for at least 12 weeks, with streptomycin 1 g/day for the first 2 weeks. Alternative therapies using fluoroquinolones and co-trimoxazole are only considered when adverse reactions are reported.[8]

Another study showed that triple therapy using a combination of streptomycin 1 g/day intramuscularly for 15 days, doxycycline 100 mg every 12 h and rifampicin 15 mg/kg per day for 45 days had good response rates and low relapse rates.[9]

NEUROBRUCELLOSIS

Central nervous system involvement is a serious complication of brucellosis.[10] The recommended treatment regimen should include doxycycline (which crosses the blood–brain barrier better than generic tetracycline), plus rifampicin plus ceftriaxone. High concentrations in the cerebrospinal fluid (CSF) offers significant efficacy against the pathogen.[11] Although the therapy should be individualized, the duration of therapy should be a minimum of 6 months with suitable antibiotics.[12] Treatment should be continued until the CSF analysis has returned to normal. Steroids may prevent early clinical deterioration following the commencement of antibiotics.[13]

BRUCELLA ENDOCARDITIS

This devastating condition has a higher mortality rate than endocarditis caused by other pathogens due to its rapid valvular destruction and the late diagnosis of cases. The aortic valve is most commonly involved. Optimal therapy is a combination of antibiotics and surgery, although medical therapy with close observation can be attempted in hemodynamically stable patients. The recommended antibiotic regimen is a combination of doxycycline 200 mg/day, rifampicin 900 mg/day and gentamicin (for the first 21 days). The addition of a third-generation cephalosporin instead of an aminoglycoside is an alternative.[14] Treatment should be continued for a year or more.[15–17]

BRUCELLOSIS IN PATIENTS INFECTED WITH HIV

Twelve patients with brucellosis and HIV co-infection have been reported from Spain; all were cured by the combination of doxycycline and streptomycin.[18] A case reported from India responded well to a regimen consisting of 6 weeks of tetracycline 250 mg every 6 h for 6 weeks and 3 weeks of streptomycin 1 g/day.[19]

PREVENTION OF LABORATORY-ACQUIRED BRUCELLOSIS

Brucellosis is one of the most common laboratory-acquired infections, as it has a potential for aerosolization. It is recommended that the organism should be handled according to Level 3 Biosafety Precautions. Aerosol-generating procedures should be avoided or minimized. Prophylaxis to laboratory workers exposed to *Brucella* is recommended: doxycycline 100 mg every 12 h plus rifampicin 450–600 mg/day. An alternative, e.g. in pregnancy, is co-trimoxazole plus rifampicin.[20] The duration of prophylaxis should be a minimum of 3 weeks, and usually continued for 6 weeks. Laboratory staff are followed up with serological testing for 3 months after exposure.[21]

ANTHRAX

Bacillus anthracis is a large, Gram-positive, non-motile, aerobic, spore-forming rod. The principal virulence factors are encoded on two plasmids: one is involved in synthesis of a capsule that inhibits phagocytosis of the vegetative forms; the other is involved in the production of the exotoxins that are important for its virulence. The exotoxins consist of the edema toxin and the lethal toxin which are divided into A (enzymatically active) protein and B (binding) protein necessary for entry into the host cell.[22]

Between 20 000 and 100 000 cases of anthrax are estimated to occur worldwide annually. Anthrax can exist in the soil as long-lived spores and cause infection in humans, and farm and wild animals. In 1979, it was recognized that anthrax could be used as a biological weapon after 66 people died from human exposure (by inhalation) to the accidental discharge of anthrax spores at a military biological facility in Sverdlovsk, Russia. Further evidence includes the deliberate use in the USA in the 1990s.[23]

Human anthrax has three major clinical forms: cutaneous, inhalation and gastrointestinal. Cutaneous anthrax is a result of introduction of the spore through the skin from animal hair or hides, inhalation anthrax (woolsorter's disease) through the respiratory tract, and gastrointestinal anthrax by ingestion. Anthrax meningitis may occur as a result of a bacteremia after inhalational anthrax; it is rare and has mortality close to 100%. If untreated, anthrax in all forms can lead to septicemia and death. Early treatment of cutaneous anthrax is usually curative.

POSTEXPOSURE PROPHYLAXIS

Postexposure prophylaxis is recommended to individuals by the public health authorities when there is an evident risk of exposure to anthrax. A long period of prophylaxis is required because of the latency period that may occur prior to the germination of spores. Recently there has been concern about antibiotic resistance, particularly to penicillin, doxycycline, chloramphenicol, macrolides and rifampicin. Ciprofloxacin is the drug of choice (500 mg every 12 h) (Table 61.1).

Table 61.1 Recommendations for anthrax postexposure prophylaxis

Type of therapy	Adults (including pregnant women)	Children
Recommended initial therapy	Ciprofloxacin 500 mg every 12 h[a]	Ciprofloxacin 10–15 mg/kg every 12 h[a]
Alternative initial therapy	Doxycycline 100 mg every 12 h	Doxycycline 100 mg every 12 h if >8 years and >45 kg
Optimal therapy (if strain susceptible)	Amoxicillin 500 mg every 8 h or doxycycline 100 mg every 12 h	Amoxicillin 500 mg every 8 h if >20 kg; 40 mg/kg divided into 3 doses if <20 kg

[a]Although fluoroquinolones are not recommended for use during pregnancy and in young children, the possibility of antibiotic resistance warrants their use in exposed pregnant women and children. This also applies to doxycycline in extreme circumstances. The total duration of treatment should be 60 days.

ANTHRAX VACCINE

An anthrax vaccine has been licensed for use in humans. Limited clinical data suggest that after completing a primary immunization course, protection against cutaneous and inhalation anthrax is afforded.[24] The vaccine is administered at 0, 2 and 4 weeks and again at 6, 12 and 18 months. Studies in rhesus monkeys have demonstrated complete protection against aerosol challenge at 8 weeks and 88% protection at 100 weeks. Annual boosters are required to maintain immunity. The vaccine has been given to the American Armed Forces since 1988 because of the concern of anthrax as a biological weapon. Contraindications to its use include sensitivity to vaccine components and a history of anthrax. No serious adverse side effects have been reported.

TREATMENT OF ANTHRAX

Penicillin is the drug of choice in sensitive strains, but alternative agents have been used because of reports of resistance (Table 61.2).

Surgical debridement of the black, necrotic eschar is contraindicated. Systemic steroids have been used for the extensive edema, but their efficacy is unproven.

ANIMAL BITES

Animal bites continue to pose major public health challenges.[25] Dogs represent the species most frequently responsible for bite-related injuries, followed by cats (~80% and <20%, respectively). Wildlife, farm animals, rodents and other pets are responsible for the remainder. Most wounds are contaminated with multiple strains of aerobic and anaerobic bacteria. The common bacteria involved are *Pasteurella multocida*, *Staphylococcus aureus*, *Staphylococcus intermedius*, alpha-hemolytic

Table 61.2 Recommendations for treatment of inhalational and cutaneous anthrax

| Type of therapy | Inhalational anthrax | | Cutaneous anthrax | |
	Adults	Children	Adults	Children
Initial therapy	Ciprofloxacin 400 mg iv every 12 h	Ciprofloxacin 20–30 mg/kg iv, divided into 2 doses	Mild: ciprofloxacin 500 mg p.o. every 12 h Severe: intravenous	Ciprofloxacin 20–30 mg/kg iv, divided into 2 doses
Optimal therapy if susceptible	Benzylpenicillin 2.4 g iv every 4 h Doxycycline 100 mg iv every 12 h	Benzylpenicillin 150 mg/kg per day in 4 divided doses for children <12 years; for children >12 years, use adult doses	Doxycycline 100 mg p.o. every 12 h Severe: ciprofloxacin 400 mg i.v. every 12 h Amoxicillin 500 mg p.o. every 8 h	As per inhalational doses Amoxicillin 500 mg every 8 h if >20 kg; 40 mg/kg divided into 3 doses if <20 kg

Note: Treatment should continue for 60 days in the context of bioterrorism and for 7–10 days for natural exposure.

streptococci, *Capnocytophaga canimorsus* (formerly called dysgonic fermenter 2, DF2) and other members of the oral flora of animals. Anaerobic bacteria including *Fusobacterium*, *Bacteroides*, *Porphyromonas* and *Prevotella* spp. are present in approximately one-third of bite wounds and are associated with the formation of abscesses and with relatively serious infections. *Past. multocida* is found in infections from cat bites. The bacteriology of bite wounds inflicted by exotic animals reflects the animals' oral flora.[26,27] Infection rates differ significantly between cat and dog bites (30–50% vs 2–4%). Risk factors for infection include patient age >50 years, puncture wounds, full-thickness wounds and wounds requiring debridement.

Animal bite wounds can be classified into three groups on the basis of the injury received: avulsion, lacerations or punctures. Avulsions and lacerations tend to be associated with dog bites whilst puncture wounds occur with cat bites. Ferrets are becoming more popular as pets and tend to bite children particularly on the face.

MANAGEMENT AND PROPHYLAXIS OF INFECTED ANIMAL BITES

The initial evaluation should include a thorough assessment of the wound and the patient's medical history and status, determination of the time that has elapsed before treatment was initiated, and identification of the animal responsible and the circumstances under which the bite occurred. The wound should be cleansed and debrided, and tetanus, rabies and antimicrobial prophylaxis should be considered. There is a debate regarding primary versus delayed repair. Most studies favor the use of primary surgical closure because of the improved cosmetic outcome. However, with certain wounds which present late or have an increased risk for complications, then primary closure is not recommended.

Prophylactic administration of antimicrobials should be considered in:

- moderate or severe injuries
- possible bone or joint penetration

- facial, genital and hand wounds
- those patients with underlying illnesses: liver disease, limb edema or prosthetic joints.

Amoxicillin–clavulanic acid has good activity against the likely organisms, and is the best choice both for prophylaxis of infection-prone bites and for empirical treatment of infected bites before the results of cultures become available. Other combinations include a second-generation cephalosporin that has anaerobic activity such as cefuroxime, a combination of penicillin with a first-generation cephalosporin such as cefradine or, for penicillin-allergic individuals, clindamycin plus a fluoroquinolone. For patients with a head injury who might have evidence of a skull fracture, then a combination of antimicrobials with good CSF penetration, such as vancomycin, ceftriaxone and metronidazole, is recommended.

There are an increasing number of methicillin-resistant *Staph. aureus* (MRSA) infections from animal bites. A newly released article in the *Lancet Infectious Disease* journal has suggested that additional steps should be taken in managing these patients:[28]

- Consider radiological imaging in case of fracture or bone penetration.
- Consider prophylactic antibiotics to cover MRSA (trimethoprim–sulfamethoxazole, doxycycline, minocycline and clindamycin).
- Consider admission if the patient is immunocompromised or septic.

RAT-BITE FEVER

The term 'rat-bite fever' refers to two similar diseases caused by different Gram-negative facultative anaerobes: streptobacillary rat-bite fever, caused by infection with *Streptobacillus moniliformis* (a pleomorphic fastidious Gram-negative bacillus) is more common in North America, and spirochetal rat-bite fever, caused by *Spirillum minus* also known as sodoku (a short, thick, Gram-negative spirochete with darting motility) is more common in Asia.[29] Both organisms are common inhabitants of the pharynx of wild, pet and laboratory rats in all parts of the world. Humans usually acquire the disease through the bite of a rat, though a history of a bite is sometimes absent in *S. moniliformis* infections, which may be acquired by oral ingestion. An example was illustrated by a milk-associated outbreak in Haverhill in 1926.[30] Cases of *S. moniliformis* rat-bite fever have been associated with the bites of mice, squirrels and gerbils, and exposure to animals that prey on these rodents. The reported incidence of rat-bite fever caused by *S. moniliformis* from laboratory rat bites is low. The efficacy of prophylaxis against rat-bite fever has yet to be assessed in practice.

STREPTOBACILLUS MONILIFORMIS INFECTION

The clinical syndrome is characterized by fever, rigors and migratory polyarthralgias. After exposure, the incubation period is usually <7 days, and ranges from 3 days to more than 3 weeks. If a bite occurs it usually heals quickly with minimal residual inflammation. Other reported clinical features include headache, nausea, vomiting, myalgia, minimal regional lymphadenopathy, anemia, endocarditis, myocarditis, meningitis, pneumonia, focal abscesses and a rash (75% of patients). Most cases resolve spontaneously, but if untreated has a mortality of 10% (ranging from 7% to 13%). It is therefore important to initiate antibiotic treatment early. Diagnosis is made from blood cultures; however, as the organism is fastidious, the growth time may be prolonged. Other methods used for diagnosis include fatty acid profiles, high-resolution polyacrylamide gel electrophoresis and polymerase chain reaction (PCR) assays.

Penicillin is the treatment of choice for proven or highly suspected cases of rat-bite fever. Only one penicillin-resistant strain has been reported, over 50 years ago.[31] Tests of *S. moniliformis* antibiotic susceptibility usually demonstrate sensitivity to penicillins, cephalosporins, carbapenems, aztreonam, clindamycin, erythromycin, nitrofurantoin, bacitracin, tetracycline, teicoplanin and vancomycin. Adults with uncomplicated *S. moniliformis* should receive 400 000–600 000 IU/day (240–360 mg) of intravenous penicillin G for at least 7 days and the dose should be doubled if no response is seen in 2 days. Children should receive 20 000–50 000 IU/kg per day (12–30 mg/kg per day) of intravenous penicillin for 5–7 days, followed by oral penicillin V, 25–50 mg/kg per day (maximum 3 g/day) divided into four doses. For penicillin-allergic patients both streptomycin and tetracycline appear to be effective; erythromycin has been associated with treatment failures. Cephalosporins have also been shown to be effective.

Complications such as septic arthritis, meningitis and pneumonia require more intensive treatment with intravenous penicillin. Endocarditis due to *S. moniliformis* is rare and generally occurs on previously damaged valves. It will probably respond to standard regimens used to treat endocarditis caused by other penicillin-sensitive organisms.

SPIRILLUM MINUS INFECTION (SODOKU)

Sodoku differs from streptobacillary rat-bite fever both clinically and geographically; it is more common in Asia. After a longer incubation period (14–18 days), the bite site becomes indurated and may ulcerate, and is associated with regional lymphadenopathy. Fevers regularly relapse and may be separated by afebrile periods lasting 3–7 days. Fifty percent of patients develop a violaceous red–brown macular rash which has occasional plaques and urticarial lesions. Joint manifestations are rare. Sodoku is highly sensitive to penicillin but a Jarisch–Herxheimer reaction may occur following the initiation of treatment.

TULAREMIA

Francisella tularensis is an extremely virulent aerobic, Gram-negative coccoid, facultative intracellular bacterium, which does not form spores but can survive in water, soil, hay and animal carcasses for up to 6 months. There are two types:

- Type A is found mostly in North America and is transmitted from the rabbit tick to humans. It is highly virulent, causing disease in humans with an inoculum of <25 bacteria.
- Type B is widespread throughout the Northern Hemisphere and is the only subspecies in Europe. It is associated with rodents and hares; humans contract the disease by inhalation, direct contact, insect bites or ingestion. Type B is generally non-lethal in humans but may cause a prolonged complicated disease.[32]

Tularemia is considered to be a category A bioterrorist threat by the US Centers for Disease Control and Prevention (CDC) as it is easy to acquire, weaponize and is transmissible by aerosol, although there have been no confirmed cases of its use in this situation. After exposure, ulceroglandular, oculoglandular and glandular disease are common manifestations, accompanied by fever, chills, myalgias and cough. Other forms may occur such as pulmonary disease and a typhoidal form. Rare complications include meningitis, pericarditis and endocarditis. The main difference between type A and type B is the ability of the former to replicate faster and cause necrosis. Diagnosis relies on clinical suspicion, serological testing, blood cultures and now PCR.

TREATMENT OF TULAREMIA

Aminoglycosides are the mainstay of treatment and whilst streptomycin has been used historically, gentamicin is also active against tularemia. Relapses have been seen with doxycycline. There are encouraging reports of quinolones showing activity against the bacteria. There is no currently licensed vaccine. Streptomycin is the antibiotic of choice, at a dose of 7.5–15 mg/kg intramuscularly every 12 h for 7–14 days, the higher doses being used for more severe illness. Gentamicin is an acceptable alternative to streptomycin; the recommended dose is 3–5 mg/kg per day in divided doses.

PLAGUE

Yersinia pestis is a Gram-negative, non-spore-forming bacillus. It is transmitted by the oriental rat flea, *Xenopsylla cheopis.* There are three main forms: bubonic, septicemic and pneumonic plague. Pneumonic plague is rare, highly transmissible between humans and has a high mortality rate. Its presence should alert authorities to the deliberate release of *Y. pestis.*[33] Diagnosis is made by culture of the organism from blood, sputum or aspiration of the buboes with special staining. Some laboratories can perform specific IgM testing and PCR.

TREATMENT OF PLAGUE

Early treatment is essential to prevent fatal pneumonic plague. Patients must be nursed in isolation with negative pressure (48 h for bubonic and 4 days for pneumonic). The CDC guidelines recommend streptomycin (15 mg/kg intravenously every 12 h) for 10 days or gentamicin with doxycycline or ciprofloxacin.[34] In a recent study in New Mexico it was found that gentamicin alone (5 mg/kg intravenously every 24 h) or in combination with a tetracycline (intravenous doxycycline 200 mg/day or 100 mg every 12 h) was as efficacious as streptomycin for treating human plague.[35] This study was supported by a clinical trial in Tanzania which showed gentamicin 2.5 mg/kg intramuscularly every 12 h for 7 days and doxycycline 100 mg every 12 h for 7 days (2.2 mg/kg in children) to be effective treatments for adult and pediatric plague.[36] Penicillins and cephalosporins are considered to be ineffective against plague, although in-vitro and animal studies have shown ceftriaxone to have variable activity.

Trimethoprim–sulfamethoxazole is recommended for plague when tetracyclines are contraindicated. Chloramphenicol is used in cases of plague meningitis as it penetrates the blood–brain barrier.

PROPHYLAXIS OF PLAGUE

Any person within 2 meters of a confirmed case of plague should receive postexposure prophylaxis with ciprofloxacin 500 mg every 12 h or doxycycline 100 mg every 12 h for 7 days.

BARTONELLA-ASSOCIATED INFECTIONS

The genus *Bartonella* comprises 19 distinct species, at least eight of which are responsible for human disease; some examples are shown below:[37,38]

- *Bartonella bacilliformis* causes bartonellosis (Carrion's disease).
- *Bartonella henselae* causes cat-scratch disease, peliosis hepatis and bacillary angiomatosis.
- *Bartonella quintana* causes trench fever, endocarditis, bacillary angiomatosis and chronic or recurrent bacteremia.
- *Bartonella vinsonii* is isolated from blood of small rodents.
- *Bartonella elizabethae* (*Rattus* rats have been shown to be a reservoir) causes endocarditis.
- *Bartonella clarridgeiae* (isolated from blood of 5% of pet cats and 17% of stray cats) may be responsible for some cases of cat-scratch disease.
- *Bartonella grahamii* causes cases of retinitis.
- *Bartonella washoensis* causes myocarditis.

Bartonellae are small, fastidious, intracellular Gram-negative bacilli that are aerobic and oxidase negative. The diagnosis of these diseases is complicated as there is no optimal procedure for the isolation of the organism.

RECOMMENDATIONS FOR TREATMENT

 ### BARTONELLOSIS (CARRION'S DISEASE)

Oroya fever

B. bacilliformis is a Gram-negative intraerythrocytic organism transmitted by the *Lutzomyia* sandfly and is limited to the Andean river valleys of Peru and Ecuador. The bacteria cause Oroya fever (acute Carrion's disease) which is a life-threatening septicemia with acute hemolysis which can be complicated by superinfections, particularly with *Salmonella* species. Recommended treatment is with oral or intravenous chloramphenicol 500 mg every 6 h for 14 days plus oral amoxicillin or ciprofloxacin 500 mg every 12 h for 10 days (adults). Treatment for children is with oral or intravenous chloramphenicol 50–75 mg/kg per day in four doses for 14 days plus amoxicillin. Penicillin G, chloramphenicol, tetracycline and erythromycin have also been used for treatment.

Verruga peruana

Verruga peruana (chronic Carrion's disease) is an infection characterized by benign cutaneous vascular lesions accompanied by osteoarticular pain. Chloramphenicol is ineffective treatment for this eruptive stage of infection. Recommended treatment is with rifampicin 10 mg/kg per day orally (safe in children and pregnancy) for 14 days or streptomycin 15–20 mg/kg per day intramuscularly for 10 days. There are failures with rifampicin and resistance has also been shown to develop when used alone. More recently, ciprofloxacin (500 mg orally every 12 h for 7–10 days) and azithromycin have been used with success.[39]

BARTONELLA HENSELAE

B. henselae (formerly *Rochalimaea henselae*) is a small Gram-negative rod, which causes several syndromes that sometimes overlap. *B. henselae* causes cat-scratch disease but, like *B. quintana* (*see below*), also causes a wide range of clinical diseases including bacillary angiomatosis, peliosis hepatis, lymphadenitis, bacteremia and aseptic meningitis. Cats are the main reservoir of *B. henselae* and the bacterium is transmitted to cats by the cat flea (*Ctenocephalides felis*). The immune status of the host determines the disease expression. Antibiotics have been shown to improve the disease occurring in the immunocompromised host.

Uncomplicated cat-scratch disease

The current recommendation for patients with mild-to-moderate disease is no antibiotic treatment (the risk of adverse drug reactions and the generation of resistant flora outweigh the benefits). Adenopathy which occurs in cat-scratch disease should be investigated to rule out other infections (fungal, mycobacterial or malignancy) by fine needle aspiration, which may also alleviate symptoms. Patients should be reassured that the adenopathy is benign and will heal in 2–4 months. Those with bulky adenopathy may be treated with azithromycin (500 mg orally day 1 and 250 mg days 2–5) or doxycycline (100 mg every 12 h) and rifampicin (300 mg every 12 h) and/or aspiration.

Complicated cat-scratch disease

The combination of doxycycline (100 mg every 12 h) with rifampicin 300 mg orally every 12 h has been successful for treating retinitis and is preferred if there is neurological involvement. The optimal duration has not been determined but a prolonged course of 4–6 weeks is recommended. There is also evidence that *B. henselae* infections and cat ownership are linked to some cases of HIV-associated dementia.[40]

Bacillary peliosis hepatis

This occurs in immunocompromised patients and is caused by *B. henselae* but not *B. quintana*. Peliosis hepatis is a vascular proliferation of sinusoidal hepatic capillaries resulting in blood-filled spaces in the liver; it is associated with HIV infection. Treatment is recommended with erythromycin 500 mg every 6 h for 4 months or doxycycline 100 mg every 12 h for 4 months.

BARTONELLA QUINTANA

B. quintana (formerly *Rochalimaea quintana*) is transmitted by the human body louse and humans are the only known reservoir. It causes trench fever, a disease extensively reported during the World Wars, prior to the antibiotic era. During this period there were no fatal cases and clinical manifestations lasted for 4–6 weeks before recovery. Nowadays it is recommended that patients who have trench fever or chronic bacteremia with *B. quintana* should be treated with doxycycline 200 mg/day orally for 4 weeks plus gentamicin 3 mg/kg intravenously for 2 weeks. Treatment of the chronic phase is necessary for the prevention of endocarditis.

BACILLARY ANGIOMATOSIS

Both *B. henselae* and *B. quintana* can cause bacillary angiomatosis in immunocompromised hosts such as patients with HIV infection. This is a vascular proliferative disease involving the skin and other organs. The drug of choice for treatment is erythromycin (500 mg orally every 6 h for 3 months, or intravenously if severe). Patients intolerant of erythromycin can receive doxycycline 100 mg every 12 h for 3 months.

LEPTOSPIROSIS

Leptospirosis is an emerging global health problem with a wide geographical distribution occurring in tropical, subtropical and temperate zones. Pathogenic leptospires belong to the species *Leptospira interrogans*, with serovar *canicola* being the most frequent in the USA and Europe and serovar *icterohaemorrhagiae* causing the severe form (Weil's disease). Leptospirosis is primarily a disease of wild and domestic animals which may asymptomatically pass large numbers of leptospires in their urine. Humans are infected mainly due to occupational or recreational contact with contaminated surface water, commonly during the summer. Rats are the most common source of human infection in developing countries, and dogs and livestock in industrialized countries. *Leptospira* may enter the body through cut or abraded skin, mucus membranes and conjunctivae. The acute generalized illness may mimic other tropical diseases (e.g. dengue fever, malaria and typhus) and common symptoms include fever, chills, myalgia, nausea, diarrhea and conjunctivitis. Manifestations of severe disease include jaundice, renal failure, hemorrhage and shock.[41]

PROPHYLAXIS OF LEPTOSPIROSIS

Chemoprophylaxis with doxycycline in soldiers visiting endemic areas was found to significantly reduce the number of cases of leptospirosis.[42] In a randomized controlled trial, doxycycline prophylaxis did not reduce leptospiral rates but had a significant protective effect in reducing morbidity and mortality during outbreaks.[43] Chemoprophylaxis with doxycycline, either 200 mg weekly or a short course for 3 days, is recommended for outbreak control or travelers, although the data are limited. Penicillin G has been shown to be of little use. Empirical treatment with doxycycline has the additional benefit of covering other infections such as rickettsioses.

TREATMENT OF LEPTOSPIROSIS

The recommended treatment of leptospirosis is benzylpenicillin (1.2–2.4 g intravenously every 6 h for 7 days), with alternatives being doxycycline 100 mg every 12 h for 7 days, ceftriaxone 1 g/day for 7 days or cefotaxime. The mortality rate, duration of fever and progression of dysfunction of vital organs were similar among doxycycline, cefotaxime and penicillin for patients with both suspected and confirmed leptospirosis.[44] Ceftriaxone has efficacy against severe leptospirosis and is potentially preferable to penicillin (i.e. easier for healthcare personnel to administer, cost-effective and broader antimicrobial activity).[45,46]

LYME DISEASE

Lyme disease is a multisystem disorder caused by spirochetes of *Borrelia burgdorferi*, which are transmitted by the bite of the tick species *Ixodes scapularis* and *I. pacificus*. Lyme disease is the most common tick-borne infection in North America and Europe.[47] Clinical manifestations involve the skin, joints, nervous system and heart. Early Lyme disease is characterized by erythema migrans which appears 1–2 weeks after infection and may persist for 8 weeks.[48] Approximately 50% of patients with proven Lyme disease do not recall having erythema migrans. Once *B. burgdorferi* disseminates throughout the body, a variety of systemic symptoms can occur, including secondary skin lesions, fever, headache and myalgia. Late complications include arthritis, neurological abnormalities and myocardial conduction defects.

The diagnosis is based on tick exposure, clinical features and serological tests or culture/PCR from joint aspirates or biopsy of lesions. Serological tests support but are not essential for the diagnosis of erythema migrans. The CDC recommends screening with an enzyme-linked immunosorbent assay (sensitive but not specific) for confirmation, followed by a Western immunoblot test (more specific).[49] After an infection, antibodies will persist for months or years, so serological testing does not reliably confirm past infection.

PROPHYLAXIS OF LYME BORRELIOSIS

The best method for preventing infection is to avoid exposure to vector ticks. Antimicrobial prophylaxis with doxycycline (200 mg single dose) and/or serological testing is recommended for the following situations:

- An attached tick is reliably identified as adult or nymph.
- The patient has come from an endemic area.
- Prophylaxis can be started within 72 h of removal of the tick.
- The local infection rate with *B. burgdorferi* is >20%.
- Doxycycline treatment is not contraindicated (pregnancy and children <8 years).

TREATMENT OF LYME DISEASE

 ### EARLY DISEASE

Erythema migrans

In the absence of neurological disease or atrioventricular block the recommended treatment is with doxycycline 100 mg every 12 h for 14–21 days, amoxicillin 500 mg every 8 h or cefuroxime 500 mg every 12 h for 14–21 days. Macrolides are less effective and only recommended to patients intolerant of the first three antibiotics. Dosages include azithromycin 500 mg/day for 7–10 days, clarithromycin 500 mg every 12 h for 14–21 days or erythromycin 500 mg every 6 h for 14–21 days (weight-adjusted doses in children).

Lyme meningitis and other early neurological Lyme disease

Ceftriaxone 2 g/day for 14 days is recommended for adults, with weight-adjusted doses in children. In patients intolerant of β-lactams, doxycycline 200–400 mg/day in two divided doses for 10–28 days may be adequate. Alternatives for children are penicillin G (200 000–400 000 IU/kg per day), ceftriaxone (50–75 mg/kg per day) or cefotaxime (150–200 mg/kg per day in 3–4 divided doses). Although antibiotics do not hasten the resolution of facial nerve palsy, they are recommended to prevent further sequelae. A lumbar puncture is recommended for patients with a clinical suspicion of CNS involvement.

Lyme carditis

Patients may be treated with oral or parenteral antibiotics such as doxycycline or ceftriaxone, respectively, for 14 days. This should be done in hospital for patients with conduction block.

 ### LATE DISEASE

Lyme arthritis

Lyme arthritis can usually be treated successfully with oral antibiotics like doxycycline, amoxicillin and cefuroxime (as per recommended doses for erythema migrans) for 28 days if there is no neurological disease. For persistent arthritis or joint swelling, a further course of ceftriaxone 2 g intravenously for 2–4 weeks is recommended. If there is no resolution and PCR is negative, then symptomatic treatment is advised (i.e. non-steroidal anti-inflammatory drugs or steroid injections).

Late neurological disease

Treatment with ceftriaxone (2 g intravenously) for 2–4 weeks.

Acrodermatitis chronica atrophicans

Treatment is as for erythema migrans.

Post Lyme disease syndromes

Most cases of Lyme disease are cured with antibiotics. There is a small sample of cases in which symptoms persist after treatment. These symptoms include muscle aches, joint pains, sleep disturbance and fatigue. The cause is unknown. There is no convincing evidence for the existence of symptomatic chronic *B. burgdorferi* infection among patients after a previously recommended course of treatment.[50]

RELAPSING FEVER

Relapsing fever, caused by spirochetes belonging to the genus *Borrelia*, was once the cause of worldwide epidemic disease. This infection was mainly due to infection with *Borrelia recurrentis* which is the louse-borne form of the disease. There has been a reduction in this infection through improved living standards and the introduction of insecticides (reducing the louse vector).[51] There is a tick-borne form of the disease which persists in endemic foci around the world, particularly in African nations. In Africa relapsing fever results from four main agents: *Borrelia crocidurae* in the west, *Borrelia hispanica* in the north, *Borrelia duttonii* (tick borne) and *Borrelia recurrentis* (louse borne) persisting in the east. All four agents cause relapsing fever; however, there are subtle clinical differences between species with the mortality rates being higher in the species found in the east.

TREATMENT OF RELAPSING FEVER

The recommended treatment for patients with tick-borne relapsing fever is doxycycline 100 mg every 12 h for 7–10 days or tetracycline 500 mg every 6 h for 7–10 days. When tetracyclines are contraindicated then a macrolide antibiotic may be given. Penicillins are effective when given intravenously.[52] Treatment with any effective antibiotic typically induces the Jarisch–Herxheimer reaction within 2 h of initiating therapy and coincides with the clearing of spirochetemia. It is not prevented by prior treatment with prednisolone, but may be diminished with meptazinol.[53] Louse-borne relapsing fever responds to a single oral dose of tetracycline 500 mg, doxycycline 100 mg or erythromycin 500 mg.[54,55] The fever lasts longer in patients treated with penicillin, and there are more frequent failures and relapses.

RICKETTSIOSES

Rickettsioses are acute febrile, zoonotic diseases caused by rickettsiae, which are small, fastidious, obligate intracellular coccobacilli that invade endothelial cells and induce the formation of vasculitis.[56] Various arthropods (lice, fleas, ticks and mites) act as vectors and some mammals constitute the principal reservoirs. There are eighteen rickettsioses now recognized. With the exception of *Rickettsia prowazekii* (epidemic typhus), all are zoonoses, and with the exception of *Coxiella burnetii* (Q fever), all are unable to survive outside a mammalian host or vector.

The main types are described below:

- **Murine typhus** is caused by *R. typhi*, with rats and other rodents acting as reservoirs and *Xenopsylla cheopis* (oriental rat flea) as the principal vector. Most cases are mild and present with non-specific features including fever, constitutional symptoms and a maculopapular rash.
- **Mediterranean spotted fever** and its variants are caused by *R. conorii* and transmitted by dog ticks in urban and suburban areas. The disease is present in Europe, Africa and Asia. Clinical features include fever, constitutional symptoms and a generalized maculopapular rash; there may be an eschar from the tick bite. Most cases are mild and the overall fatality rate is 2%.
- **African tick bite fever** is a rickettsiosis commonly encountered in travel medicine. Caused by *R. africae*, it is endemic in some parts of rural sub-Saharan Africa and the eastern Caribbean. Cattle ticks of the *Amblyomma* genus act as both reservoirs and vectors. Clinically patients present with a headache, neck myalgia, eschars and lymphadenitis; 30% may have a vesicular rash and mouth blisters. Most cases are self-limited with patients infected during wild game safaris and bush walks. No fatalities have been reported.
- **Scrub typhus** is a common infectious disease of rural south and southeastern Asia and the western Pacific, where there are ~1 million cases/year. It tends to occur in personnel working on the land or rice fields and there have been a large number of reports in military personnel. The disease is caused by *Orientia tsutsugamushi* transmitted by the bites of mites (chiggers). Patients present with fever, lymphadenitis and an eschar (50%). Most cases are mild; however, if untreated, complications ensue. It has a fatality rate of 1–35%.
- **Epidemic typhus** caused by *R. prowazekii* is transmitted in louse-infected environments such as refugee camps and prisons.
- **Rocky Mountain spotted fever** is caused by *R. rickettsii* and is transmitted by *Amblyomma* and *Dermacentor* ticks. The disease is endemic in South East and Midwestern USA and South America, and affects mainly hikers who get exposed to tick-infested habitats.

Other rickettsioses include North Asia tick typhus (*R. sibirica*), Queensland tick typhus (*R. australis*) and *R. aeschlimannii*.

DIAGNOSIS

The main laboratory options available include culture, PCR and serological tests but patients tend to be diagnosed clinically. In practice, serology is used the most but mainly to provide a retrospective diagnosis.

TREATMENT OF RICKETTSIOSES

As laboratory diagnosis is difficult patients are started on presumptive therapy whenever a case of rickettsiosis is suspected. The standard regimen consists of doxycycline 200 mg/day for 3–14 days. Chloramphenicol and macrolides are good alternatives to doxycycline. The fluoroquinolones tend to fail clinically despite exhibiting good in-vitro activity.

PREVENTION

The best preventive measure is to avoid typical risk settings when traveling in areas of endemicity; if this is not possible, then measures aimed at reducing the risk of arthropod bites should be taken (i.e. using repellents and self-checking methods). Weekly 200 mg doxycycline has been used to prevent scrub typhus in military personnel deployed in endemic areas and could be recommended to travelers.[57] Currently there are no vaccines available.

Q FEVER

Q fever is a worldwide zoonosis caused by *Coxiella burnetii*, an obligate, intracellular, Gram-negative organism which is seen throughout the world.[58] The organism can infect a variety of hosts including humans, ruminants, pets, birds, reptiles and ticks. It is known to be category B bioterrorism agent, as it can survive in the environment for weeks, it can be aerosolized and is highly infectious.[59] Human infection is usually acquired by inhalation of small numbers of airborne organisms when in proximity to infected domestic animals, hides, manure, dust, milk and, especially, placentas. Infection may also be acquired via ingestion or direct skin penetration. It has been shown that in endemic areas patients do not necessarily need to be directly exposed to ruminants to get an infection. The incidence of Q fever is higher in certain countries such as France (500 cases/million persons) and Australia (38 cases/million persons), whereas in the USA the incidence is much lower (0.28 cases/million persons). There have been reports of Q fever infection acquired by US military personnel deployed overseas in Iraq and Afghanistan. The incubation period for Q fever is 2–6 weeks.[60]

 ### CLINICAL MANIFESTATIONS

Q fever has a variable presentation and infection can lead to asymptomatic seroconversion, acute disease or chronic disease. Various host factors – including male sex, immunosuppression and age – influence the extent of the clinical disease:

- *Acute disease*: 50–60% of patients are asymptomatic. Early disease leads to a flu-like illness, with a significant number of patients having pneumonia or hepatitis.

- *Chronic disease*: Patients with certain conditions (pregnancy, immunosuppression, heart valve lesions) are more susceptible to developing chronic disease, of which endocarditis is the most common form and carries a high mortality rate. Rare manifestations include osteomyelitis, granulomatous hepatitis, chronic pulmonary infections and chronic fatigue syndrome.

 ## DIAGNOSIS

Diagnosis relies on serological testing with antibody detection by immunofluorescence and PCR (useful in early disease). Isolation of the organism should only be done when the appropriate laboratory facilities are in place. Diagnosis relies on phase variation of *C. burnetii* with phase 1 antibodies elevated in chronic disease and phase 2 in acute.

 ## TREATMENT OF Q FEVER

- *Acute disease*: Doxycycline 100 mg every 12 h for 14 days is recommended unless the patient is pregnant, younger than 8 years or allergic (an alternative is co-trimoxazole). The utility of the macrolides is unclear and the fluoroquinolones may be useful in the treatment of CNS disease (although there is a lack of supporting data).

- *Chronic disease*: In-vitro studies have shown that a combination regimen of doxycycline (100 mg every 12 h) and hydroxychloroquine (200 mg every 8 h) for 18 months should be considered for the treatment of Q fever endocarditis. Surgery is an important component of treatment. Alternative regimens used include fluoroquinolones or rifampicin instead of hydroxychloroquine. Osteoarticular Q fever is rare and should be treated for a prolonged time period.

- *Vaccine*: In Australia there is a licensed whole cell vaccine which might be beneficial in people such as veterinarians, abattoir workers and laboratory personnel (efficacy >95%).

EHRLICHIOSIS

'Ehrlichiosis' is a generic name for infections caused by obligate intracellular bacteria in the family Anaplasmataceae, chiefly *Ehrlichia* and *Anaplasma*.[61] Human infections are caused by at least three distinct species discovered during the period 1980–1990: *Ehrlichia chaffeensis* (human monocytic ehrlichiosis, HME), the canine pathogen *Ehrlichia ewingii* (similar to *E. chaffeensis* but propagates in neutrophils) and *Anaplasma phagocytophilum* (human granulocytic anaplasmosis, HGA).

Most infections are transmitted in May to August by a tick bite. Patients present with fever, headache, myalgia, leukopenia and/or thrombocytopenia and increased transaminase levels. Rashes are more common in HME and CNS infections in HGA. Fatalities are more common in the immunosuppressed.

DIAGNOSIS

An empirical diagnosis must be made early as the disease can be rapidly progressive and fatal. Diagnosis is confirmed by peripheral blood smears (more useful for HGA), molecular diagnosis by PCR, in-vitro cultivation (possible for *E. chaffeensis or A. phagocytophilum*) and serology by a four-fold rise or fall in antibody titer (however, there are high false-positive rates).

TREATMENT OF EHRLICHIOSIS

Although there have been no clinical trials conducted, empirical data support the use of tetracyclines to treat all forms of ehrlichiosis (doxycycline for 5–14 days) which should be initiated promptly. An alternative is rifampicin, which has shown some clinical success. There are few data to support the β-lactams, macrolides, quinolones and aminoglycosides. In the case of young children (<8 years) it is recommended that they start with doxycycline for 3 days and then continue with amoxicillin for 14 days.

VIRAL ZOONOSES

No specific treatment is established for most viral zoonoses. The exceptions are hantavirus (hemorrhagic fever with renal syndrome, hantavirus pulmonary syndrome) and Lassa fever.

LASSA FEVER

Lassa fever is a viral hemorrhagic fever transmitted by multimammate rats (*Mastomys natalensis*) and is found predominantly in West Africa.[62]

 ### CLINICAL MANAGEMENT

All suspected cases should be admitted to isolation facilities. Ribavirin (tribavirin) and general support are need. Ribavirin is a guanosine analog which has broad-spectrum antiviral activity and should be given within 6 days of the start of the illness. Ribavirin should be given intravenously in a loading dose of 30 mg/kg, followed by 15 mg/kg every 6 h for 4 days, then 7.5 mg/kg every 8 h for 6 days. The only important adverse effect of ribavirin in humans is mild, usually reversible, anemia. It is contraindicated in pregnant women.

 ### PROPHYLAXIS OF LASSA FEVER

For needlestick or other high-risk contact, oral ribavirin 5 mg/kg every 8 h for 2–3 weeks would be a logical step, although it is of unproven efficacy.

Ribavirin is also useful in other hemorrhagic fevers such as Argentine hemorrhagic fever and also in hantavirus infections.[63,64] However, the use of ribavirin for hantavirus pulmonary syndrome has so far not demonstrated an appreciable drug effect. There is a requirement for further trials to assess the efficacy and safety of this drug.[65]

 ## References

1. Skalsky K, Yahav D, Bishara J, Pitlik S, Leibovici L, Paul M. Treatment of human brucellosis: systematic review and meta-analysis of randomised controlled trials. *Br Med J.* 2008;336:701–704.
2. Mantur BG, Amarnath SK, Shinde RS. Review of clinical and laboratory features of human brucellosis. *Indian J Med Microbiol.* 2007;25(3):188–202.
3. Pappas G, Panagopoulou P, Christou L, Akritidis N. Brucella as a biological weapon. *Cell Mol Life Sci.* 2006;63(19–20):2229–2236.
4. World Health Organization. Joint FAO/WHO Expert Committee on Brucellosis, 6th Report. *WHO Technical Report Series 740.* Geneva: WHO; 1986.
5. Solera J, Espinosa A, Martinez-Alfaro E, et al. Treatment of human brucellosis with doxycycline and gentamicin. *Antimicrob Agents Chemother.* 1997;41:80–84.
6. Tanir G, Tufekci SB, Tuygun N. Presentation, complications, and treatment outcome of brucellosis in Turkish children. *Pediatr Int.* 2009;51:114–1197.
7. Khan MY, Mah MW, Memish ZA. Brucellosis in pregnant women. *Clin Infect Dis.* 2001;32:1172–1177.
8. Alp E, Doganay M. Current therapeutic strategy in spinal brucellosis. *Int J Infect Dis.* 2008;12(6):573–577.
9. Bayindir Y, Sonmez E, Aladag A, Buyukberber N. Comparison of five antimicrobial regimens for the treatment of brucellar spondylitis: a prospective, randomized study. *J Chemother.* 2003;15(5):466–471.
10. Gul HC, Erdem H, Bek S. Overview of neurobrucellosis: a pooled analysis of 187 cases. *Int J Infect Dis.* 2009;13(6):e339–e343.
11. Pappas G, Akritidis N, Christou L. Treatment of neurobrucellosis: what is known and what remains to be answered. *Expert Rev Anti Infect Ther.* 2007;5(6):983–990.
12. Gul HC, Erdem H, Gorenek L, et al. Management of neurobrucellosis: an assessment of 11 cases. *Intern Med.* 2008;47(11):995–1001.
13. Habeeb YK, Al Najdi AK, Sadek SA, Al Onaizi E. Paediatric neurobrucellosis: case report and literature review. *J Infect.* 1998;37:59–62.
14. Cay S, Goksel C, Orhan M, Balbay Y, Aydogdu S. Brucella endocarditis. *Polish Heart Journal.* 2009;67:274–280.
15. Pratt DS, Tenney JH, Bjork CM, Reller LB. Successful treatment of *Brucella melitensis* endocarditis. *Am J Med.* 1978;64:897–900.
16. Jacobs F, Abramowicz D, Vereerstraeten P, et al. *Brucella* endocarditis: the role of combined medical and surgical treatment. *Rev Infect Dis.* 1990;12:740–744.
17. Cakalagaoglu C, Keser N, Alhan C. Brucella-mediated prosthetic valve endocarditis with brachial artery mycotic aneurysm. *J Heart Valve Dis.* 1999;8:586–590.
18. Moreno S, Ariza J, Espinosa FJ, et al. Brucellosis in patients infected with the human immunodeficiency virus. *Eur J Clin Microbiol Infect Dis.* 1998;17:319–326.
19. Sarguna P, Bilolikar AK, Rao A, Mathur DR. Brucellosis in association with HIV infection – a case report. *Indian J Med Microbiol.* 2002;20(4):221–222.
20. Robichaud S, Libman M, Behr M, Rubin E. Prevention of laboratory-acquired brucellosis. *Clin Infect Dis.* 2004;38:e119–e122.
21. Maley MW, Kociuba K, Chan RC. Prevention of laboratory-acquired brucellosis: significant side effects of prophylaxis [correspondence]. *Clin Infect Dis.* 2006;42:433–434.
22. Swartz MN. Recognition and management of anthrax – an update. *N Engl J Med.* 2001;345(22):1621–1626.
23. McCarthy M. Anthrax attack in the USA. *Lancet Infect Dis.* 2001;1(5):288–289.
24. Green AD, Cottrell TS. Biological threats. *J R Army Med Corps.* 2003;149(3):183–243.
25. Patronek GJ, Slavinski SA. Animal bites. *J Am Vet Med Assoc.* 2009;234(3):336–344.
26. Taylor P. Bite wounds and infections. *Clin Infect Dis.* 1992;15(4):740.

27. Talan DA, Citron DM, Abrahamian FM, Moran GJ, Goldstein EJ. Bacteriologic analysis of infected dog and cat bites. Emergency Medicine Animal Bite Infection Study Group. *N Engl J Med*. 1999;340:85–92.

28. Perez J. Managing infection passed from pets to human via bite injuries. *Lancet Infect Dis*. To be published on the Lancet early release page.

29. Elliott SP. Rat bite fever and *Streptobacillus moniliformis*. *Clin Microbiol Rev*. 2007;20(1):13–22.

30. Place EH, Sutton LE. Erythema arthriticum epidemicum (Haverhill fever). *Arch Intern Med*. 1934;54:659–684.

31. Toren DA. Mycotic rat-bite fever. Report of case. *Del Med J*. 1953;25:334.

32. Waterer GW, Robertson H. Bioterrorism for the respiratory physician. *Respirology*. 2009;14(1):5–11.

33. Stenseth NC, Atshabar BB, Begon M, Belmain SR, et al. Plague: past, present and future. *PLoS Med*. 2008;5(1):9–13.

34. Centers for Disease Control and Prevention. *Plague medical management training module*. Atlanta: CDC; 2005.

35. Boulanger L, Ettestad P, Fogarty J, et al. Gentamicin and tetracycline for the treatment of human plague: review of 75 cases in New Mexico, 1985–1999. *Clin Infect Dis*. 2004;38:663–669.

36. Mwengee W, Butler T, Mgema S, et al. Treatment of plague with gentamicin or doxycycline in a randomised clinical trial in Tanzania. *Clin Infect Dis*. 2006;42:614–621.

37. Florin TA, Zaoutis TE, Zaoutis LB. Beyond cat scratch disease: widening spectrum of *Bartonella henselae* infection. *Pediatrics*. 2008;121(5):e1413–e1425.

38. Rolain JM, Brouqui P, Koehler JE, et al. Minireview. Recommendations for treatment of human infections caused by *Bartonella* species. *Antimicrob Agents Chemother*. 48(6):1921–1933.

39. Maguina C, Gotuzzo E. Bartonellosis – new and old. *Infect Dis Clin North Am*. 2000;14(1):1–22.

40. Schwartzman WA, Patnaik M, Angulo FJ, Visscher BR, Miller EN, Peter JB. *Bartonella* (*Rochalimaea*) antibodies, dementia, and cat ownership among men infected with human immunodeficiency virus. *Clin Infect Dis*. 1995;21:954–959.

41. Vijayachari P, Sugunan AP, Shriram AG. Leptospirosis: an emerging global health problem. *J Biosci*. 2008;33(4):557–569.

42. Takafuji ET, Kirkpatrick JW, Miller RN, et al. An efficacy trial of doxycycline chemoprophylaxis against leptospirosis. *N Engl J Med*. 1984;310(8):497–500.

43. Sehgal SC, Sugunan AP, Murhekar MV, Sharma S, Vijayachari P. Randomized controlled trial of doxycycline prophylaxis against leptospirosis in an endemic area. *Int J Antimicrob Agents*. 2000;13(4):249–255.

44. Suputtamongkol Y, Niwattayakul K, Suttinont C, et al. An open, randomised, controlled trial of penicillin, doxycycline and cefotaxime for patients with severe leptospirosis. *Clin Infect Dis*. 2004;39:1417–1424.

45. Panaphut T, Domrongkitchaiporn S, Vibhagool A, et al. Ceftriaxone compared with sodium penicillin G for treatment of severe leptospirosis. *Clin Infect Dis*. 2003;36:1507–1513.

46. Vinetz JM. A mountain out of a molehill: do we treat acute leptospirosis, and if so, with what? Editorial commentary. *Clin Infect Dis*. 2003;36:1514–1515.

47. Wormser GP, Dattwyler RJ, Shapiro ED, et al. The clinical assessment, treatment and prevention of Lyme disease, human granulocytic anaplasmosis and babesiosis: clinical practice guidelines by the Infectious Diseases Society of America. *Clin Infect Dis*. 2006;43:1089–1134.

48. Ogden NH, Artsob H, Lindsay LR, et al. Lyme disease. A zoonotic disease of increasing importance to Canadians. *Can Fam Physician*. 2008;54:1381–1384.

49. CDC. *Lyme disease*. Online. Available at http://www.cdc.gov/ncidod/dvbid/Lyme/ld_prevent.htm. 2009.

50. Bratton RL, Whiteside JW, Hovan MJ, et al. Diagnosis and treatment of Lyme disease. *Mayo Clinical Proceedings*. 2008;83(5):566–571.

51. Cutler SJ, Abdissa A, Trape JF. New concepts for the old challenge of African relapsing fever borreliosis. *Clin Microbiol Infect*. 2009;15:400–406.

52. Roscoe C, Epperley T. Tick-borne relapsing fever. *Am Fam Physician*. 2005;72(10):2039–2044.

53. Teklu B, Habte MA, Warrell DA, White NJ, Wright DJM. Meptazinol diminishes the Jarisch–Herxheimer reaction of relapsing fever. *Lancet*. 1983;i:835–839.

54. Perine PL, Awoke S, Krause DW, McDade JE. Single dose doxycycline treatment of louse borne relapsing fever and epidemic typhus. *Lancet*. 1974;v:742–744.

55. Perine PL, Teklu B. Antibiotic treatment of louse borne relapsing fever in Ethiopia: a report of 377 cases. *Am J Trop Med Hyg*. 1983;32:1096–1100.

56. Jensenius M, Fournier PE, Raoult D. Rickettsioses and the international traveller. *Clin Infect Dis*. 2004;39:1493–1499.

57. Olson JG, Bourgeois AL, Fang RC, Coolbaugh JC, Dennis DT. Prevention of scrub typhus: prophylactic administration of doxycycline in a randomised double blind trial. *Am J Trop Med Hyg*. 1980;29:989–997.

58. Hartzell JD, Wood-Morris RN, Martinez LJ, et al. Q Fever: epidemiology, diagnosis and treatment. *Mayo Clinic Proceedings*. 2008;83(5):574–579.

59. Moodie CE, Thompson HA, Meltzer MI, Swerdlow DL. Prophylaxis after exposure to *Coxiella burnetii*. *Emerg Infect Dis*. 2008;14(10):1558–1566.

60. Reimer LG. Q fever. *Clin Microbiol Rev*. 1993;6(3):193–198.

61. Dumler JS, Madigan JE, Pusterla N, Bakken JS. Ehrlichiosis in humans: epidemiology, clinical presentation, diagnosis and treatment. *Clin Infect Dis*. 2007;45:S45–S51.

62. Richmond JK, Baglole DJ. Lassa fever: epidemiology, clinical features, and social consequences. *Br Med J*. 2003;327:1271–1275.

63. Enria DA, Maiztegui JL. Antiviral treatment of Argentine haemorrhagic fever. *Antiviral Res*. 1994;23:23–31.

64. Huggins JW, Hsiang CM, Cosgriff TM, et al. Prospective, double blind, concurrent, placebo controlled trial of intravenous ribavirin therapy of haemorrhagic fever with renal syndrome. *J Infect Dis*. 1991;164:1119–1127.

65. Chapman LE, Mertz GJ, Peters CJ, et al. Intravenous ribavirin for hantavirus pulmonary syndrome: safety and tolerance during 1 year of open-label experience. Ribavirin Study Group. *Antivir Ther*. 1999;4:211–219.

62 Malaria

Nicholas J. White

Malaria is the most important parasitic disease of humans. It is estimated to affect approximately 200 million people. The annual death toll from *Plasmodium falciparum* infections is approximately one million. Pregnant women, infants and those over 60 years old are at greatest risk. Most of the deaths are in African children, and most occur away from facilities where optimum antimalarial treatment can be given. Unlike many other infections, the mortality rate rose in recent decades and this was attributed directly to increasing antimalarial drug resistance.[1] Fortunately there has been a huge international investment in malaria control and this trend has now reversed as effective drugs have been rolled out. Much antimalarial treatment is still administered for the empirical self-treatment of febrile illnesses in the tropics. The amounts of the drugs used are enormous, and ineffective self-treatment is widespread. As malaria is one of the most common causes of fever in tropical countries it must be excluded in any febrile patient living in, or returning from, the tropics. Ideally, antimalarial drugs should be given only for the treatment of microscopically confirmed malaria infections or for the prevention of malaria in pregnant women or travelers. The rapid development of resistance to most of the available antimalarial drugs by the potentially lethal parasite *P. falciparum* has compromised considerably recommendations for both prevention and treatment.[2] The most important recent development in antimalarial chemotherapy has been the introduction of the artemisinin derivatives. There has been a global switch from ineffective monotherapies to artemisinin-based combination therapies (ACTs) for the treatment of uncomplicated falciparum malaria, and artesunate is replacing quinine for the treatment of severe malaria. It is now accepted that, in order to delay the emergence of resistance, just as in the treatment of tuberculosis, leprosy and HIV/AIDS, combinations of drugs with different modes of action should be used. Where possible, fixed-dose artemisinin derivative combinations (FDCs) are replacing the separate medicines.[3] As resistance has now been reported to all available antimalarial drugs, treatment recommendations must be under constant review.

ANTIMALARIAL DRUG RESISTANCE AND THE CHOICE OF DRUGS

Although it had been suspected for three centuries, the first cases of quinine resistance were documented only 90 years ago. Fortunately, quinine resistance progressed very slowly and quinine still remains useful today.

Within a few years of the introduction of the dihydrofolate reductase inhibitors pyrimethamine and proguanil as antimalarial treatments in the late 1940s and early 1950s, high-level resistance was noted in both *P. falciparum* and *Plasmodium vivax*.[4] Resistance could also be selected readily in the laboratory. Nevertheless, these drugs remained useful in prophylaxis, but for treatment, use of proguanil was discontinued, and pyrimethamine was later prescribed in a fixed combination with long-acting sulfonamides – most commonly sulfadoxine (SP).

Chloroquine took over rapidly as the treatment of choice for all malaria, and was also used widely in prophylaxis. Chloroquine resistance in *P. falciparum* was first recorded in the late 1950s, and by the early 1970s had become a significant problem in South America and South East Asia. During the 1980s, chloroquine resistance spread remorselessly across southern Asia and in the 1990s marched across the entire length and breadth of the African continent. Few tropical countries are now unaffected, and chloroquine is no longer recommended for falciparum malaria. High-level chloroquine resistance in *P. vivax* was reported first on the island of New Guinea, and more recently in other parts of Oceania, Asia and South and Central America.[4,5]

Amodiaquine shares cross-resistance patterns with chloroquine, but is significantly more effective than chloroquine against resistant parasites and has replaced chloroquine in some areas. It is combined with artesunate and is now available as an FDC ACT.

Resistance to combinations of pyrimethamine and long-acting sulfonamides (SP) developed rapidly after their introduction for routine treatment in South East Asia and South America, and has spread across Africa, where they replaced chloroquine as first-line treatment. The SP combination is now used only in combination with artesunate[5] but it is still used alone in intermittent preventive treatment (IPT). The combination of chlorproguanil (or proguanil) and dapsone is more effective than SP against antifol-resistant parasites and provides less selection pressure to the emergence of resistance.[6] However, development of a fixed-dose formulation has stopped recently because of the risks of anemia related to dapsone hemolysis.

Mefloquine is generally effective against multiresistant strains of *P. falciparum*. Resistance emerged in South East Asia during the 1990s, where mefloquine was used but the artesunate–mefloquine ACT remains highly effective almost everywhere.[7,8]

Although halofantrine is intrinsically more active than mefloquine, susceptibility to the two drugs is linked, and serious concerns over cardiotoxicity and its high cost have limited its use.[9] Fortunately, resistance to quinine has remained low grade in South America and South East Asia (although susceptibility has declined slowly) and has not been a problem in Africa. However, because of consistent minor adverse effects, adherence is very poor with the 7-day courses of quinine necessary for cure, and treatment failure rates up to 50% have been reported. Quinine is usually combined with either tetracycline (or doxycycline) or in some areas clindamycin to prevent recrudescences of falciparum malaria. Even in areas with a high prevalence of resistance, the quinine–tetracycline combination, given for 7 days, still retains cure rates of >85%.[10]

Atovaquone–proguanil has been introduced recently. It is highly effective against all malaria parasites and is used mainly as chemoprophylaxis. High-level resistance to atovaquone was reported in early clinical trials and remains a concern if this drug is deployed widely. However, the very high costs of manufacture and consequent high price have limited its use.

The artemisinin compounds are antimalarial peroxides derived from qinghao or *Artemisia annua* (sweet wormwood). Discovered in China, they are the most rapidly effective and have the broadest stage-specificity of action of all antimalarial drugs.[11] They are well tolerated, retain excellent efficacy against multiresistant parasites and are rapidly effective in severe malaria. As they also prevent gametocyte development, and therefore reduce transmission, this can decrease the incidence of malaria in low transmission settings. Resistance has been reported recently but is confined to Western Cambodia.[12,13] In uncomplicated malaria these drugs are used in combination with other antimalarial drugs (ACTs). Combined with existing drugs they accelerate the initial therapeutic response, improve efficacy, reduce gametocyte carriage and, in the case of mefloquine, improve tolerance. Artesunate–mefloquine has proved highly effective in South East Asia, despite pre-existing mefloquine resistance.[8] The fixed combination of artemether and lumefantrine is a highly effective and well-tolerated alternative to artesunate–mefloquine. It is now the most widely used ACT in the world. Dihydroartemisinin–piperaquine is another fixed combination from China with excellent activity against multidrug-resistant parasites.[14]

RESISTANCE

Resistance to antimalarial drugs arises through the selection of rare naturally arising mutants with reduced drug susceptibility. Unlike some bacteria, plasmodia do not have transferable resistance mechanisms, but they are eukaryotes, and they can acquire or lose polygenic resistance mechanisms during meiosis. Resistance arises readily to drugs such as the antifols or atovaquone because single-point mutations confer resistance (as opposed to a requirement for several unlinked mutations, i.e. epistasis) and per-parasite mutation frequencies for viable mutations are relatively high (>1 in 10^{13} mitotic divisions).[15] Pyrimethamine and the active metabolites of the antimalarial biguanides (cycloguanil from proguanil, and chlorcycloguanil

from chlorproguanil) interfere with folic acid synthesis in the parasite by inhibiting the bifunctional enzyme dihydrofolate reductase-thymidylate synthase (DHFR). Sulfonamides act at the previous step in the synthetic pathway by inhibiting dihydropteroate synthase (DHPS), and there is marked synergy between the two classes of compounds (*see* Ch. 2). Resistance in *P. falciparum* and *P. vivax* is associated with point mutations in the DHFR gene that lead to reduced affinity (100–1000 times less) of the enzyme complex for the drug. For *P. falciparum* the first mutation is usually at position 108 of *Pf*DHFR (serine to asparagine). For *P. falciparum* this has little clinical effect initially, but mutations then arise at positions 51 and 59, which confer increasing resistance to pyrimethamine.[16] Infections with 'triple' mutants are relatively resistant but some therapeutic response is usually seen, particularly if there is background immunity. The acquisition of a fourth mutation at position 164 (isoleucine to leucine) renders the available antifolate antimalarials completely ineffective. This mutation is prevalent in parts of South East Asia and South America, and has recently emerged in East Africa.[17] Mutations conferring moderate levels of pyrimethamine resistance do not necessarily confer cycloguanil resistance, and vice versa. For example, mutations at position 16 (alanine to valine) plus serine to threonine at position 108 confer high-level resistance to cycloguanil but not pyrimethamine. In general, the biguanides (cycloguanil, chlorcycloguanil) are more active than pyrimethamine against the resistant mutants (and they are more effective clinically too), but they are ineffective against parasites with the DHFR 164 mutation. *P. vivax* shares similar antifol resistance mechanisms through serial acquisition of mutations in *Pv*DHFR.

The marked synergy with sulfonamides and sulfones is very important for the antimalarial activity of sulfa–pyrimethamine or sulfone–biguanide combinations. Sulfonamide and sulfone resistance also develops by progressive acquisition of mutations in the gene encoding the target enzyme DHPS (which is a bifunctional protein with the enzyme dihydropteridine pyrophosphokinase). Specifically altered amino acid residues have been found at positions 436, 437, 540, 581 and 613 in the DHPS domain. The 581 and 631 mutations do not occur in isolation, but always on top of an initial mutation (usually alanine to glycine at 437).[18]

The mode of action and mechanisms of resistance of the quinoline antimalarials remains controversial. These drugs are weak bases, and they concentrate in the acid food vacuole of the parasite, but this in itself does not explain their antimalarial activity. Chloroquine binds to ferriprotoporphyrin IX, a product of hemoglobin degradation, and thereby chemically inhibits heme dimerization (*see* Ch. 2). Chloroquine also inhibits competitively glutathione-mediated heme degradation, another parasite detoxification pathway. Chloroquine resistance is associated with reduced concentrations of drug in the acid food vacuole. Both reduced influx and increased efflux have been implicated. Resistant parasites pump chloroquine out 40–50 times faster than drug-sensitive parasites. This efflux mechanism is similar to that found in multidrug-resistant (MDR) mammalian tumor cells. One of the efflux mechanisms is through an ATP-requiring transmembrane pump, P-glycoprotein. These MDR genes (*pfmdr1*) are found in increased numbers in most quinine and mefloquine-resistant *P. falciparum* parasites, and point mutations (notably asparagine to tyrosine at position 86) are associated with chloroquine resistance. However, the key first step in aminoquinoline resistance is the development of point mutations in PfCRT (a food vacuolar membrane protein with a probable transporter function).[19,20] The principal correlate of chloroquine resistance is a point mutation, resulting in a change in coding from lysine to threonine, at position 76 of PfCRT. From an epidemiological standpoint multiple unlinked mutations are probably required for the development of high-level chloroquine resistance, and it is likely that other contributors to quinoline resistance remain to be discovered. The role of these mechanisms in resistance to the other aryl aminoalcohol antimalarials (amodiaquine, halofantrine, lumefantrine, piperaquine and pyronaridine) also remains to be elucidated.

The chloroquine efflux mechanism in resistant parasites can often be inhibited by a number of structurally unrelated drugs such as calcium-channel blockers, tricyclic antidepressants, phenothiazines, cyproheptadine and antihistamines, whereas mefloquine resistance is reversed by penfluridol, which does not reduce chloroquine efflux. Clinical trials of reversers have yielded conflicting results. Whether general use of resistance reversers will be a safe and feasible therapeutic option remains to be seen. In general, antimalarial drug resistance to mefloquine, quinine, lumefantrine and halofantrine is linked but, as suggested by their different susceptibility to reversing agents, chloroquine resistance and mefloquine resistance are not linked closely. Indeed, within a particular geographical area there is a reciprocal relationship; mefloquine resistance is correlated inversely with chloroquine resistance. Part of this is explained by the greater propensity of wild type compared with mutant *pfmdr1* to amplify this gene (which reduces mefloquine susceptibility).[21]

Atovaquone interferes with parasite mitochondrial electron transport and depolarization within the parasite mitochondria, thereby blocking cellular respiration. High levels of resistance result from single point mutations in the gene encoding cytochrome b. This gene is encoded on a small extrachromosomal plastid-like DNA-containing organelle that may have an intrinsically high mutation rate. Viable resistance mutations arise frequently in vivo (about 1 in 10^{12} asexual divisions).

The artemisinin drugs are thought to kill malaria parasites by generating carbon-centered free radicals, which alkylate critical proteins. Parasiticidal activity is dependent on the integrity of the peroxide bridge. Although in general multiresistant parasites are more artemisinin resistant, the degree of resistance is slight and very unlikely to be of clinical relevance. Reduced susceptibility to artemisinins can be induced experimentally, and resistance manifest in vivo by slow parasite clearance has been reported recently from Western Cambodia.[13]

Several factors encourage the development of antimalarial drug resistance:

- The intrinsic frequency with which the genetic changes occur.
- The degree of resistance conferred by the genetic change (pharmacodynamics).
- The proportion of all transmissible infections that are exposed to the drug.
- The drug concentration profile (pharmacokinetics).
- The pattern of drug use.
- The immunity profile of the community.[15]

Resistant parasites will be selected when parasites are exposed to subtherapeutic drug concentrations. Thus non-immune patients infected with large numbers of parasites who receive inadequate treatment (because of poor drug quality, reduced adherence, vomiting of an oral treatment, etc.) are a potent source of resistance. This emphasizes the importance of correct prescribing and good adherence to prescribed drug regimens in slowing the emergence of resistance. Resistance develops more slowly in high-transmission areas because the patients' background immunity may eliminate the resistant mutants and stop them being transmitted. The spread of resistant mutant parasites is facilitated by the use of drugs with long elimination phases, which provide a 'selective filter', allowing infection by the resistant parasites while the residual antimalarial activity prevents infection by sensitive parasites. Slowly eliminated drugs such as mefloquine (terminal half-life 3 weeks) or chloroquine (terminal half-life 2 months) persist in blood for months after drug administration and provide such a selective filter.

PREVENTION OF RESISTANCE USING COMBINATIONS OF ANTIMALARIAL DRUGS

The emergence of resistance can be prevented by the use of combinations of drugs with different mechanisms of action, and therefore different drug targets and unlinked resistance mechanisms.[15,22] The same rationale underlies the current treatment of tuberculosis, leprosy, HIV infections and many cancers. If two drugs with different mechanisms of action are used, then the per-parasite probability of developing resistance to both drugs is the product of their individual per-parasite probabilities. For example, if the per-parasite probability of developing resistance to drug A and drug B are both 1 in 10^{12}, then a simultaneously resistant mutant will arise spontaneously every 1 in 10^{24} parasites. As there are approximately 10^{17} malaria parasites in the entire world, and a cumulative total of less than 10^{20} in 1 year, such a simultaneously resistant parasite would arise spontaneously roughly once every 10 000 years – if the drugs always confronted the parasites in combination. Thus the lower the de-novo per-parasite probability of developing resistance, the greater the delay in the emergence of resistance. This powerful approach has several limitations. If not everyone receives the combination, and some patients receive only one of the components, or there is already high-level resistance to one of the components, then resistance can arise (emphasizing the importance of achieving high coverage when these drugs are deployed). Combinations are also more expensive. However, the increased cost is outweighed by the longer-term benefits.

CLINICAL ASSESSMENT OF RESISTANCE

Low-grade resistance (late parasitological failure; R1 resistance) is usually manifest by recrudescences, which tend to occur several weeks after primary treatment. Most recrudescences of malaria occur within 6 weeks of initial treatment. For quinine and other rapidly eliminated drugs the median time to recrudescence as resistance begins is approximately 3 weeks; however, for drugs that have long terminal half-lives, such as mefloquine, the recrudescences can occur up to 10 weeks, and possibly longer, after the primary treatment. Although the treatment is unable to eradicate the parasites in such cases, the multiplication rate is suppressed while therapeutic blood concentrations are still present in the blood. The more susceptible the parasites, the lower the blood concentrations required to suppress parasite multiplication. As resistance worsens, the median time to recrudescence becomes shorter and an increasing number of patients are seen in whom parasitemia fails to clear by 7 days following treatment (early treatment failure; R2 resistance). Eventually the situation deteriorates further and some patients do not respond at all to antimalarial treatment (R3 resistance). Obviously, alternative treatment should be employed before this stage. In the individual patient long parasite clearance times (>4 days) are a common predictor of subsequent recrudescence.

UNCOMPLICATED MALARIA

MANAGEMENT

Infections with *P. vivax*, *P. malariae* or *P. ovale* are very rarely fatal, but *P. falciparum* malaria may progress rapidly to severe disease and death, particularly in the non-immune patient or young children in endemic areas. If the clinician is in any doubt about the severity of the infection, the patient should remain in hospital under observation. Otherwise, uncomplicated malaria can be treated on an outpatient basis. If there is any uncertainty over speciation of the parasites they should be considered as *P. falciparum*, and if there is any doubt over drug susceptibility the infection should be considered as resistant.[5] A thorough history and examination should pay particular attention to the likely origin of the infection and any previous antimalarial treatment. Except in areas without facilities for diagnosis, antimalarial treatment should be given only for slide- or dipstick-confirmed malaria. In general, administration of the first dose should be observed. Symptomatic measures are important. The incidence of vomiting, particularly in children, is proportional to fever. Young children with high fevers should be cooled, given paracetamol (acetaminophen) (15 mg/kg), and allowed to settle before receiving the first oral dose of antimalarial treatment. The patient should be observed for 1 h after drug administration; if vomiting occurs within this period the drugs should be re-administered (*see below*). Ideally, patients should be seen daily for a clinical examination and a blood smear until they are asymptomatic and parasite negative. They should be advised to return to the same hospital or clinic if fever recurs within 6 weeks.

SPECIFIC ANTIMALARIAL TREATMENT

P. VIVAX, *P. OVALE* AND *P. MALARIAE*

P. vivax is the most common cause of malaria in the Indian subcontinent, Central America, North Africa and the Middle East. There is unequivocal evidence of chloroquine resistance in *P. vivax* from parts of Asia, the Americas and Oceania, but in most vivax-affected areas, infections with this parasite, and the other two that cause the benign human malarias, remain sensitive to chloroquine. Treatment is rapidly effective and usually well tolerated. The main adverse effect is troublesome pruritus in dark-skinned patients, which occurs in approximately 50% of cases. The quinoline antimalarials may all exacerbate the orthostatic hypotension that commonly complicates malaria, and symptomatic postural hypotension is common.[23] Rarely (less than 1 in 1000), chloroquine treatment is associated with transient neuropsychiatric abnormalities. All the currently available ACTs except artesunate–sulfadoxine–pyrimethamine reliably and rapidly treat vivax malaria.

The total dose of chloroquine is 25 mg base/kg, divided classically as 10, 10 and 5 mg/kg given on days 0, 1 and 2, respectively. This schedule may be compressed into a 36 h treatment regimen, giving 10, 5, 5 and 5 mg/kg at 12-hour intervals[24] (Table 62.1). Both *P. vivax* and *P. ovale* infections produce persistent dormant hepatic forms of the parasite (hypnozoites), which are resistant to chloroquine. These become activated between 3 weeks and 1 year after the primary infection, and cause the relapses so characteristic of these infections. (A *relapse* is a recurrent infection caused by the development of persistent hypnozoites: the primary blood-stage infection has cleared. A *recrudescence* is a blood-stage infection that is not eradicated, but may decline below the level of microscopic detection, and then increases later causing patent parasitemia and clinical illness.) The hypnozoites are sensitive only to the 8-aminoquinoline antimalarials. The eradication of both the blood stage and the persistent liver stages of *P. vivax* and *P. ovale* malaria is called a 'radical cure'. For this, primaquine has in the past been given in an adult daily dose of 15 mg base (0.25 mg/kg) for 14 days, with strains of *P. vivax* from Oceania and some parts of South East Asia being treated with a daily dose of 22.5–30 mg base (0.375–0.5 mg/kg) for 14 days. Shorter courses are less effective. It is now recommended by the World Health Organization (WHO) that *P. vivax* everywhere should be treated with a higher dose: 0.5 mg base/kg for 14 days.[5] Primaquine has weak asexual-stage activity against *P. vivax* and this may mask low-level chloroquine resistance if the two drugs are given together. Thus chloroquine plus primaquine constitutes a 'combination treatment'. In patients with a 'mild variant' of glucose-6-phosphate dehydrogenase

Table 62.1 Antimalarial drugs: recommended doses for treatment

	Uncomplicated malaria: dose[a]	Usual adult dose[a]	Severe malaria[b]
Chloroquine	10 mg base/kg followed by 10 mg/kg at 24 h and 5 mg/kg at 48 h or 5 mg/kg at 12, 24 and 36 h. Total dose 25 mg base/kg. For *P. vivax* or *P. ovale* add primaquine 0.5 mg base/kg daily for 14 days[c] for radical cure	4 × 150 mg tablets followed by 4 then 2 or 2, 2, 2	No longer recommended
Sulfadoxine–pyrimethamine (SP)	25/1.25 mg/kg single oral dose	3 tablets	Not recommended
Mefloquine	25 mg/kg: give 15 mg base/kg followed by 10 mg/kg dose 8–24 h later. Alternatively, give 8–8.3 mg/kg daily for 3 days	3 × 250 mg tablets + 2 × 250 mg tablets	
Artesunate	In combination with a slowly eliminated drug 4 mg/kg daily for 3 days. [d,e] If used alone or with a tetracycline or clindamycin, 4 mg/kg followed by 2 mg/kg daily: total 7 days	4 × 50 mg daily for 3 days in combination 4 × 50 mg followed by 2 × 50 mg daily for 6 days	2.4 mg/kg i.v. or i.m. immediately then at 12, 24 h and then daily[b]
Artemether	Same oral dose regimens as for artesunate[e]	5 × 40 mg daily for 3 days in combination	3.2 mg/kg i.m. immediately followed by 1.6 mg/kg daily[b]
Dihydroartemisinin	Same oral dose regimens as for artesunate[e]	5 × 40 mg followed by 3 × 40 mg daily for 6 days	
Dihydroartemisinin–piperaquine	Adult dose: 120/720 mg daily for 3 days	3 tablets once daily for 3 days	
Artemether–lumefantrine	Adult dose: 80/480 mg every 12 h for 3 days with food or milk	4 tablets every 12 h for 3 days	
Quinine	10 mg salt/kg every 8 h for 7 days. Often combined with tetracycline[f] (4 mg/kg) every 6 h, doxycycline (3.5 mg/kg) daily or clindamycin (10 mg/kg) every 12 h, all for 7 days	2 × 300 mg every 8 h	20 mg salt/kg by intravenous infusion over 4 h[g] followed by 10 mg/kg infused over 2–8 h every 8 h[b]
Quinidine	Recommended only if alternatives unavailable. Dose as for quinine		10 mg base/kg infused at constant rate over 1 h followed by 0.02 mg/kg per minute, with electrocardiographic monitoring[b]
Atovaquone–proguanil	1000/400 mg once daily for 3 days with food or milk	4 tablets every 6 h for 3 days	

[a]Confusingly, many antimalarials are provided in different salts, so treatment recommendations are given in weights of base equivalent. It is important that these are not confused.
[b]Oral treatment should be substituted as soon as the patient can take tablets by mouth.
[c]If possible, check for glucose 6 phosphate (G6PD) deficiency. In patients with mild G6PD deficiency, give 0.75 mg/kg once weekly for 6 weeks. Do not use in pregnant women, newborns or in severe G6PD deficiency.
[d]For hyperparasitemic patients (>4% parasitemia in a non-immune) give artesunate for 5 days; 4 mg/kg daily for two additional days.
[e]ACTs currently recommended by WHO are artesunate–mefloquine, artesunate–amodiaquine, artesunate–SP, artemether–lumefantrine and dihydroartemisinin–piperaquine.
[f]Doxycycline 3.5 mg/kg daily is an alternative to tetracycline. Tetracycline or doxycycline should not be given to pregnant women or children <8 years old.
[g]Alternatively for the initial loading dose, 7 mg salt/kg can be infused over 30 min followed by 10 mg salt/kg over 4 h.

(G6PD) deficiency a single weekly dose of primaquine (0.75 mg/kg) can be given daily for 6 weeks.

Primaquine is an oxidant drug and causes hemolysis in patients with hereditary defects in the pentose–phosphate shunt, most commonly G6PD deficiency. In patients with severe variants of G6PD deficiency, primaquine is contraindicated; however, for patients with mild variants, primaquine should be given in a weekly dose of 45 mg base (0.75 mg/kg) for 6 weeks. Despite its use for over 50 years, the safety profile of primaquine needs further characterization. Primaquine should not be used in pregnancy or given to newborns. Pyrimethamine and the pyrimethamine–sulfonamide combinations are relatively ineffective against *P. vivax* in many areas

because of acquired resistance. All the other antimalarial drugs are active, and so for mixed infections requiring treatment for *P. falciparum* it is not necessary to add chloroquine. However, primaquine should be given as well to prevent relapses.

UNCOMPLICATED *P. FALCIPARUM* MALARIA

Antimalarial treatments are increasingly using combinations of antimalarial drugs. Several of the ACTs (artesunate–mefloquine, artemether–lumefantrine, dihydroartemisinin–piperaquine) can be relied upon everywhere in the world. Resistance limits where artesunate–amodiaquine and artesunate–SP can be used. Atovaquone–proguanil is not deployed widely but is reliably effective for imported malaria. ACTs are now recommended first-line treatments in endemic areas everywhere. In a very few specific areas such as Central America where *P. falciparum* remains definitely sensitive, chloroquine can still be used in a total treatment dose of 25 mg base/kg (adult dose 1500 mg). There is no significant difference between the phosphate, sulfate or hydrochloride salts. If there is any doubt about antimalarial sensitivity in the area where malaria was acquired, *P. falciparum* infections should be considered resistant.

UNCOMPLICATED CHLOROQUINE-RESISTANT FALCIPARUM MALARIA

Amodiaquine is more effective than chloroquine against resistant strains of *P. falciparum*. It is also well tolerated. When used in prophylaxis, amodiaquine was associated with a 1 in 2000 incidence of agranulocytosis. The true incidence of this in therapeutic use is not known but is probably much lower, although the incidence is high in HIV-infected children.[25] Artesunate–amodiaquine is a treatment option where there is low-level aminoquinoline resistance. An alternative is artesunate–SP containing a single dose of sulfadoxine–pyrimethamine (20/1 mg/kg; corresponding to three tablets in an adult). This is a well-tolerated and effective treatment of sensitive strains. The principal adverse effects result from sulfonamide allergy. When used in prophylaxis the incidence of serious adverse effects is approximately 1 in 7000; fatal adverse effects occur in 1 in 18000.[26] In single-dose treatment the incidence of serious adverse effects appears to be significantly lower. Pyrimethamine-induced blood dyscrasias, usually seen in patients with underlying folate deficiency, are most unusual. Artesunate–SP is effective where there is either no antifol resistance or low-grade antifol resistance. There are no significant interactions among these drugs.

MULTIDRUG-RESISTANT *P. FALCIPARUM* MALARIA

 ### ARTESUNATE–MEFLOQUINE

Mefloquine (hydrochloride) has the advantage of a long terminal elimination half-life of 2–3 weeks and in the past has been given in a single dose of 15 mg base/kg (adult dose three tablets of 250 mg) to semi-immune patients. This is no longer recommended.[5] A higher dose of 25 mg base/kg (five tablets for an adult) is generally more effective and less likely to lead to resistance. Peak whole blood concentrations above 1000 ng/mL are effective. Absorption is augmented, but adverse effects are not increased, if the treatment dose is split (i.e. a 25 mg base/kg dose is given as 15 mg/kg initially, followed by 10 mg/kg 8–24 h later,

or as 8–8.3 mg/kg per day for 3 days). Combining mefloquine with artesunate (4 mg/kg per day for 3 days) improves efficacy and reduces immediate adverse effects. As with many antimalarial drugs, children tolerate mefloquine better than adults.[27] The principal adverse effect of mefloquine is immediate vomiting. This is less likely if the dosage is split. Patients must be observed for 1 h after the drug has been given. If vomiting occurs within 30 min the full dose of artesunate–mefloquine should be repeated. For vomiting 30–60 min later, half the dose should be given. Vomiting after 1 h does not require retreatment. Later adverse effects are all more common in adults and comprise nausea, dysphoria, dizziness or 'muzziness', poor concentration, sleeplessness, nightmares and postural hypotension. Mefloquine does not have significant cardiac effects. Adverse effects following mefloquine treatment are reported more frequently in women than in men. Serious, but reversible, neuropsychiatric reactions occur in approximately 1 in 1300 Asians patients receiving high-dose mefloquine treatment, but as many as 1 in 200 European and African patients. This rises to 1 in 20 if mefloquine is given following acute treatment of cerebral malaria, and it should not be used in this context.[28]

 ## ARTEMETHER–LUMEFANTRINE

The combination of artemether and lumefantrine is as effective as artesunate–mefloquine and has some advantages and disadvantages:

1. It is better tolerated (indeed it does not appear to have any significant adverse effects) and, in particular, produces less vomiting and has no central nervous toxicity.[29]
2. The lumefantrine component is more rapidly eliminated than mefloquine (half-life c. 4 days compared with 14 days for mefloquine in malaria), which would be expected to reduce the selection of resistant parasites. On the other hand, this suppresses reinfections or relapses (post-treatment prophylaxis; PTP) for a shorter period.
3. Artemether–lumefantrine needs to be given twice daily for 3 days instead of once daily, and absorption of lumefantrine is very variable (like atovaquone and halofantrine, it is highly fat dependent[3]).

 ## DIHYDROARTEMISININ–PIPERAQUINE

Dihydroartemisinin–piperaquine is another fixed-dose artemisinin combination from China. It has proved very well tolerated and highly effective against multiresistant falciparum malaria in adults and children across the world.[14] Piperaquine is a bisquinoline compound with similar pharmacokinetic properties to chloroquine. It suppresses reinfection and relapse for longer than lumefantrine. Dihydroartemisinin–piperaquine is given once daily for 3 days.

ATOVAQUONE–PROGUANIL

Atovaquone–proguanil is very well tolerated and highly effective against all the human malaria parasites. Interestingly, the synergistic activity of proguanil with atovaquone is derived from the parent compound through an uncharacterized mechanism of action and not dihydrofolate reductase inhibition by the triazine metabolite cycloguanil. This is important because atovaquone–proguanil retains excellent activity against highly antifolate-resistant parasites, and also in East Asia where 20% of the population have a genetic polymorphism resulting in reduced CYP_{450} 2C19 activity – the enzyme responsible for conversion of proguanil to cycloguanil. As the main drawback to atovaquone–proguanil is its cost, this compound has been used very little in malaria endemic areas. It is given in a 3-day course, and can be combined with artesunate to form an ACT. There is no pediatric formulation.

HALOFANTRINE

Halofantrine is intrinsically more active than mefloquine and is better tolerated.[27] It suffers the disadvantages of requiring multiple dose administration as it has very erratic oral bioavailability. Halofantrine absorption is augmented considerably by co-administration with fats or fatty food. The other adverse effect reported with high-dose treatment is diarrhea. Halofantrine does not have significant adverse central nervous system effects. Use of halofantrine has been associated with sudden death. Halofantrine, like quinidine, induces a predictable prolongation of the electrocardiograph QT interval (delayed ventricular repolarization).[9] This can be pro-arrhythmic. Atrioventricular conduction abnormalities (first- and, rarely, second-degree block) have also been seen. These cardiac effects are augmented by previous treatment with mefloquine. Halofantrine should not be given to patients who have received mefloquine in the previous month or to patients either with known prolongation of the QT interval or who are receiving other drugs known to prolong the QT interval. This potentially lethal toxicity has markedly limited its use – indeed, as effective alternatives are usually available, there seems no reason to use it.

QUININE

Quinine sulfate, the time-honored remedy, at a dose of 10 mg salt/kg (adult dose 600 mg) every 8 h is effective in a 7-day course. Shorter courses (3–5 days) are much less effective. Quinine is usually combined with tetracycline, doxycycline or, particularly in children or pregnant women, with clindamycin in order to improve cure rates. Quinine is not well tolerated. The characteristic syndrome of 'cinchonism', comprising nausea, vomiting, dizziness, dysphoria and high-tone deafness, is a predictable accompaniment of quinine treatment. In addition, the drug is extremely bitter and many children find it unacceptable. However, serious adverse effects, principally blindness, deafness or cardiac dysrhythmias, are unusual. Hypoglycemia is more common in severe malaria, although it may also develop in uncomplicated malaria treated by quinine, particularly in young children or pregnant women. Hypoglycemia results from stimulation of the pancreatic β-cells and consequent hyperinsulinemia.

ARTEMISININ DERIVATIVES

The artemisinin derivatives comprise the parent compound artemisinin, dihydroartemisinin (which is 5–10 times more potent) and the dihydroartemisinin derivatives artemether, artemotil (arteether) and artesunate. In vivo artesunate and artemether are converted back to dihydroartemisinin. The most widely used derivative is artesunate. These drugs are all well absorbed by mouth and rapidly eliminated (dihydroartemisinin half-life ~1 h). They are all very well tolerated with no consistent adverse effects.[29] Serious allergic reactions (usually preceded by urticaria) have been reported in approximately 1 in 3000 patients. The parasiticidal and clinical responses are more rapid than with other antimalarials. They also reduce gametocyte carriage and therefore the transmission potential of the infection.[30] The artemisinin derivatives are usually combined with a more slowly eliminated drug in ACTs, in which case they are given over 3 days. In patients who have uncomplicated hyperparasitemia (i.e. a non-immune with more than 4% parasitemia but no vital organ dysfunction) the dose should be extended over 5 days (4 mg/kg per day for an additional 2 days after the 3-day ACT course is completed). When given with rapidly eliminated drugs (e.g. doxycycline or clindamycin) then artemisinin or its derivatives should be given for 7 days in a dose of 4 mg/kg initially then 2 mg/kg per day.

Travelers returning to the countries with no available artemisinin derivatives who have multiresistant *P. falciparum* malaria should be treated with quinine plus tetracycline or doxycycline.

MONITORING THE RESPONSE TO TREATMENT

If possible patients should be seen at least daily until parasite and fever clearance, although this is not possible in most endemic areas. If there is clinical deterioration or repeated vomiting, then parenteral treatment should be substituted. If there is an early failure of treatment suggesting drug resistance, then a different treatment must be substituted. If there is a return of parasitemia after 1 week, it may not be possible to distinguish recrudescence from reinfection in an endemic area (this requires a comparison of parasite genotypes).[31]

The choice of subsequent retreatment will then depend on the prevailing level of resistance. Most drugs can be repeated within 1 month, but for mefloquine this should be avoided as there is an increased risk of neuropsychiatric reactions with retreatment. Either a 7-day course of artesunate (or quinine) and doxycycline (clindamycin in children), or a 3-day, six-dose course of artemether–lumefantrine should be prescribed.

SEVERE *P. FALCIPARUM* MALARIA

MANAGEMENT

Severe malaria is a multisystem disease requiring intensive care management. Unfortunately, optimum treatment is usually not available in most of the areas of the world where severe malaria occurs. Severe malaria has been defined as the presence of one or more of the following: unrousable coma (cerebral malaria), severe anemia (haematocrit <15% plus parasitemia >100,000/μL), renal failure (serum creatinine >265 μmol/L), pulmonary edema, hypoglycemia (glucose <2.2 mmol/L), shock, bleeding, repeated seizures, metabolic acidosis or haemoglobinuria. The clinician should not feel restricted by this definition:[32] a simpler bedside assessment based on any impairment of consciousness or inability to sit unaided (prostration), acidotic breathing (respiratory distress), anuria, hypoglycemia, severe anemia, shock or a high parasitemia (>4% in a non-immune, >20% in any patient) identifies those patients in need of intensive care. Any patient in whom there is doubt as to the severity of the infection should be managed as described below.

A rapid clinical appraisal should be made. This includes assessment of the level of consciousness or central nervous system dysfunction, exclusion of covert seizure activity (clinical evidence of seizures can be subtle), measurement of vital signs (particularly respiratory pattern and rate), questioning of the patient or relatives concerning earlier antimalarial treatment, duration of impaired consciousness, convulsions and urine output. A malaria parasite count (thick and thin blood films), blood glucose, plasma bicarbonate or blood lactate, and hematocrit should be measured immediately. The patient should be rehydrated with saline and, if there is any doubt about the jugular venous pressure, a central venous line should be inserted and central pressure monitored. If hypoglycemia is suspected or confirmed, 0.3 g/kg (25 g) of glucose should be given by slow intravenous injection. The role of prophylactic intramuscular phenobarbital (phenobarbitone) in childhood cerebral malaria is now uncertain after a large study from Kenya showed significant protection against convulsions following 20 mg/kg of intramuscular phenobarbital, but an *increased* mortality.[33] This was associated with repeated diazepam administration (for uncontrolled seizures) and was attributable to respiratory arrest. No respiratory support was available. Some authorities still give a lower dose (7 mg/kg) of phenobarbital. Patients with respiratory abnormalities should be ventilated early, with care to avoid

even temporary hypercapnia. Prompt anticonvulsant therapy (intravenous lorazepam, midazolam or diazepam) should be given if there are seizures. A lumbar puncture should be performed to exclude coincident meningitis. Hemofiltration should be started early in patients with acute renal failure, and blood (preferably fresh) should be transfused if the hematocrit falls below 20%. Antimalarial drugs should be given on a milligram-per-kilogram basis (in adults and children). The patient should be weighed (or weight estimated) and parenteral treatment given intravenously if possible. Artesunate can be given by slow intravenous injection but quinine or quinidine must be given by slow, rate-controlled intravenous infusion. Rises in parasitemia in the first 12 h after antimalarial treatment has started should *not* be attributed to drug resistance, and rapid declines in parasitemia shortly after drug administration do not indicate a very sensitive infection. These changes result from natural fluctuations in parasitemia related to synchronous schizogony and sequestration, respectively. If, by 48 h after starting treatment, parasitemia has not fallen by more than 75% (R3 resistance), then the treatment should be changed; however, this high-level resistance is extremely unusual. Therapeutic responses are assessed in terms of clinical measures: times to recovery of consciousness, and in adults the times to reach Glasgow coma scores of 8, 11 and 15; the time until fever falls below 37.5°C and remains below this for 24 h; and times to sit, eat and walk, together with laboratory measures, which include the rate of fall in plasma lactate or normalization of plasma bicarbonate, and the times to reduce parasitemia by 50%, 90% and 100%. If the parasitemia has not cleared by 7 days, treatment should be continued, provided of course the counts are not rising. Adult patients receiving quinine, artesunate or artemether should receive either a full 3-day course of an ACT (not with mefloquine if the patient had cerebral malaria) or a 7-day course of doxycycline, and children clindamycin, which starts when the patient can take oral medicine.

SPECIFIC ANTIMALARIAL THERAPY

Intravenous artesunate is now established as the treatment of choice for adults with severe malaria. In trials conducted in South East Asia, artesunate reduced the mortality of severe malaria by 35% compared with quinine (Fig. 62.1). As severe malaria has certain differences between adults and children in high transmission areas, there is still uncertainty whether artesunate, artemether or quinine is the preferred treatment in African children with severe malaria.

ARTEMISININ, ARTEMETHER, ARTEETHER AND ARTESUNATE

Artemisinin and its derivatives have given consistently faster parasite and fever clearance times, and have proved rapidly effective in severe malaria.[11] Large randomized trials

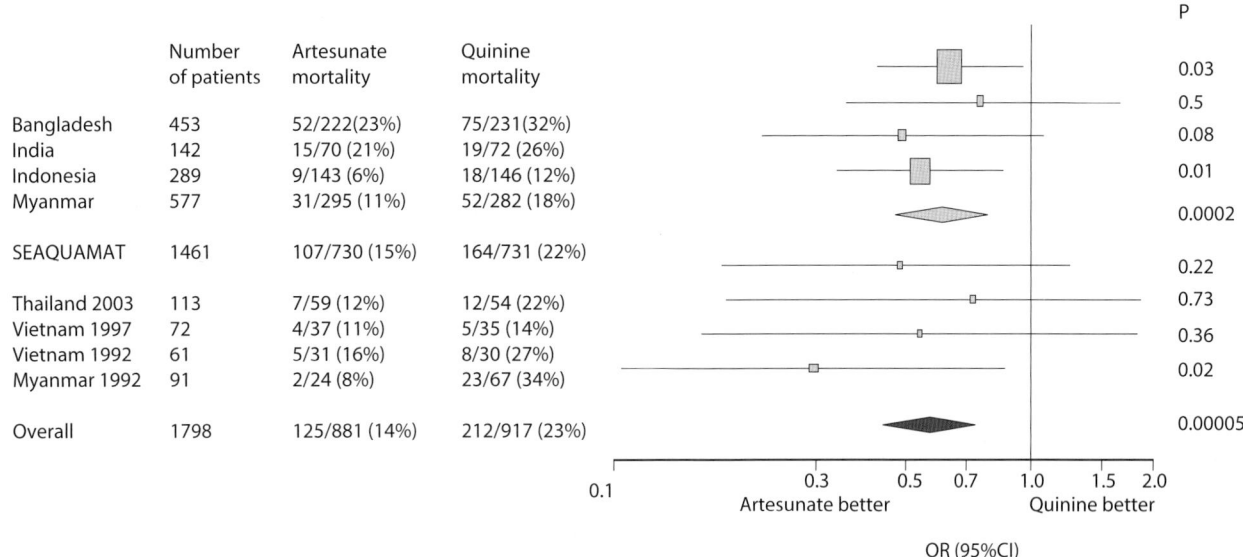

	Number of patients	Artesunate mortality	Quinine mortality		P
Bangladesh	453	52/222(23%)	75/231(32%)		0.03
India	142	15/70 (21%)	19/72 (26%)		0.5
Indonesia	289	9/143 (6%)	18/146 (12%)		0.08
Myanmar	577	31/295 (11%)	52/282 (18%)		0.01
					0.0002
SEAQUAMAT	1461	107/730 (15%)	164/731 (22%)		0.22
Thailand 2003	113	7/59 (12%)	12/54 (22%)		0.73
Vietnam 1997	72	4/37 (11%)	5/35 (14%)		0.36
Vietnam 1992	61	5/31 (16%)	8/30 (27%)		0.02
Myanmar 1992	91	2/24 (8%)	23/67 (34%)		
Overall	1798	125/881 (14%)	212/917 (23%)		0.00005

Fig. 62.1   Forest plot of mortalities in randomized comparative trials which compared parenteral quinine and artesunate in severe falciparum malaria. The sizes of the boxes are proportional to the number of events in individual trials. The diamond is the summary stratified odds ratio and 95% confidence interval.

conducted over a decade ago compared artemether and quinine in severe malaria.[34] Intramuscular artemether was associated with 14% mortality versus 17% with quinine (odds ratio 0.8, 95% confidence interval 0.62–1.02, $p = 0.08$). In adults, artemether was associated with a significantly lower mortality. Artemether was not associated with any serious adverse effects; notably there was no hypoglycemia and no neurological abnormalities. However, as artemether and the similar compound artemotil (arteether) are oil-based intramuscular injections, and they are absorbed slowly and erratically in severely ill patients,[35] the benefits obtained by greater intrinsic activity and broader stage specificity of action are offset partially by their variable absorption.

Artesunate is a water-soluble compound which can be given intravenously and is absorbed rapidly after intramuscular injection.[36] The evident pharmacokinetic advantages over artemether and arteether suggested that it would be the best drug for severe falciparum malaria. This has been confirmed in a series of preliminary trials which were followed by the largest ever randomized multicenter trial in severe malaria which enrolled 1461 patients and showed a 35% (95% CI 19–48%) reduction in mortality with parenteral artesunate.[37] The number needed to treat to save one life ranged from 11 to 20. Artesunate was also better tolerated and was associated with a lower risk of hypoglycemia.

Artesunate

Artesunate is provided for parenteral use as freeze-dried powder, which is dispensed together with an ampoule of 5% sodium bicarbonate. The two are mixed immediately before injection. The resulting sodium artesunate is hydrolyzed rapidly in vivo to the biologically active metabolite dihydroartemisinin. Artesunate is usually diluted in 5–10 mL of 5%

dextrose or normal (0.9%) saline before intravenous or intramuscular injection. The currently recommended dose is a 2.4 mg/kg given either intravenously or by intramuscular injection at 0, 12, and 24 h, then once daily.

Artemether and artemotil

These two compounds are very similar. They are dissolved in groundnut or sesame oil and given by intramuscular injection to the anterior thigh in an initial dose of 3.2 mg/kg (for artemotil some recommend an initial dose of 4.8 mg/kg), followed by daily injections of 1.6 mg/kg. Oral treatment is substituted as soon as possible.

Rectal formulations

The artemisinin derivatives are absorbed adequately after rectal administration,[38] offering the prospect of giving pre-referral treatment in the rural tropics to patients who cannot swallow oral medications reliably or who have severe malaria away from health facilities near home where most fatalities occur. A recent large multicenter trial in Ghana, Tanzania and Bangladesh showed that pre-referral administration of a single 10 mg/kg dose of a rectal artesunate formulation (Rectocap) reduced mortality from falciparum malaria in children under 5 years by 25%.[39]

Use of artemisinin derivatives has not been associated with any reported toxicity in the treatment of severe malaria. They do not have cardiovascular or metabolic adverse effects, do not need dose adjustment in renal failure or liver dysfunction, and are equally well tolerated by adults and young children. Blackwater (massive hemolysis) seems to occur with the same frequency as with quinine use. In animal models the oil-soluble ethers, artemether and arteether, have both produced selective toxicity to brainstem nuclei. Similar neurotoxicity also followed administration of dihydroartemisinin, the common metabolite. The water-soluble artesunate and oral administration of any of the drugs is much less neurotoxic. There is no evidence that similar effects occur in humans. Temporary suppression of reticulocyte and neutrophil counts may occur following high doses but the clinical significance of these is uncertain.

 ## QUININE

Parenteral quinine should be given by slow, rate-controlled intravenous infusion. Where this is not possible, intramuscular administration to the anterior thigh is an effective alternative. In order to achieve therapeutic concentrations as early as possible in the course of treatment, which may be life-saving, an initial loading dose should be given. A variety of approaches have been described. The simplest is to give a loading dose of 20 mg quinine dihydrochloride salt/kg by constant rate infusion over 4 h, dissolved in 5% or 10% dextrose, or normal (0.9%) saline.[40] Alternatively, 7 mg salt/kg may be infused over 30 min, followed immediately by 10 mg/kg over 4 h.[41] After the initial loading dose, maintenance doses of 10 mg salt/kg should be given every 8 h. Maintenance dose intravenous infusions can be given over 2–12 h. Quinine should *never* be given by intravenous injection. Intramuscular bioavailability is good even in severe malaria, although there is still uncertainty as to the optimum dilution. Quinine dihydrochloride should be diluted between 1:2 and 1:5 with sterile water for intramuscular injection and given into the anterior thigh. The initial loading dose should be divided (10 mg/kg to each thigh). Undiluted quinine dihydrochloride (300 mg/mL) is acidic (pH 2) and painful, and may occasionally result in sterile abscesses or tetanus. The therapeutic range for quinine has not been defined, but total plasma concentrations between 8 and 15 mg/L are safe and effective. There is an increased potential risk of toxicity with free (unbound) quinine levels over 2 mg/L (corresponding to total plasma concentrations of approximately 20 mg/L). To prevent accumulation to toxic levels the dose of quinine should be reduced by one-third on the third day of treatment if there is no clinical improvement or the patient is in acute renal failure.

The principal adverse effect of quinine in the treatment of severe malaria is hypoglycemia.[42] This is a particular problem in children and pregnant women (occurring in 50% of the latter group) and tends to occur after 24 h of treatment in those patients who remain severely ill. Management is difficult as hypoglycemia is often recurrent. A maintenance infusion of 10% glucose should be given after correction with a bolus of 0.3 g/kg (25 g) of glucose given by slow intravenous injection. Cinchonism is common in recovering patients, but does not limit dosage. Adverse cardiovascular or central nervous system effects (particularly retinal blindness or deafness) are very unusual and, in general, parenteral quinine is well toler-

ated in the treatment of severe malaria. Electrocardiographic monitoring is not necessary except in patients with previous heart disease. In the tropics there have been concerns over the use of a loading dose in areas where patients are commonly pretreated before admission to hospital and therefore may already have therapeutic blood concentrations of quinine on admission, but these concerns have not been substantiated in large trials.[43] Undertreatment is more dangerous than overtreatment. Our practice is to give a loading dose of quinine unless the patient has definitely received 25 mg/kg of quinine or more in the preceding 48 h. We have not seen any serious complications using these guidelines.

 ## QUINIDINE

In some countries parenteral artemisinin derivatives or quinine are not available.[44] In this case quinidine (the dextrorotatory diastereoisomer) may be used as an alternative. This is usually available as the gluconate salt. Quinidine is intrinsically more active than quinine as an antimalarial; however, as it also has an approximately four-fold greater effect on the heart, electrocardiographic monitoring is necessary.[45] The dose has been controversial (as there are few studies on which to base it). An infusion of 10 mg base/kg given by constant rate intravenous infusion over 1 h as a loading dose, followed by 0.02 mg/kg per min (1.2 mg/kg per hour) thereafter until the patient can be safely switched to oral treatment, will achieve therapeutic concentrations. If the QT interval is prolonged by more than 25% of the baseline value, or exceeds an absolute value of 0.6 s, the infusion should be stopped. Hypotension should be treated with intravenous saline. Quinidine has the same propensity as quinine to induce hypoglycemia. As with quinine, the therapeutic range has not been determined precisely, but total plasma concentrations of 5–8 mg/L should be achieved. Plasma concentration monitoring is advisable. If this is not available, then the dose of quinidine should be reduced by one-third on the third day of treatment if there is no clinical improvement, or the patient is in renal failure.

ANTIMALARIAL TREATMENT OF CHILDREN

Apart from early vomiting, children generally tolerate the antimalarial drugs better than adults. For oral treatment, particularly in younger children, care should be taken to cool and calm the patient before oral treatment is given. If the temperature is >38.5°C, tepid sponging, and oral or rectal paracetamol (15 mg/kg) should be administered and the antimalarials given after the temperature has been lowered (usually 30–60 min). Tablets should be crushed and mixed with water or a sweet drink or disguised in jam. The suspension may be drawn up into a syringe so that an accurate dose (on a milligram-per-kilogram basis) can be instilled into the mouth.

The pharmacokinetic properties of some antimalarials differ in children. The plasma concentrations of sulfadoxine and pyrimethamine in young children are half those in adults, suggesting that this important age group may have been systematically underdosed.[46] Piperaquine levels are also lower in the elimination phase. More data are needed for all antimalarials in infancy, and further dose optimization in children is required. Nevertheless, current dose regimens on a milligram-per-kilogram basis are the same as in adults, except that primaquine should not be given to neonates, tetracycline should not be given to children <8 years old, and (in resistant areas) the oral dose of quinine should be increased to 15 mg/kg every 8 h after the fourth day.

Children with severe malaria are more likely than adults to have convulsions, or become severely anemic or hypoglycemic. They are less likely to develop renal failure, pulmonary edema or jaundice. In general, children deteriorate more rapidly than adults, but they also recover more quickly.

ANTIMALARIAL TREATMENT IN PREGNANCY

Pregnant women should be treated in the same way as non-pregnant adults, except that for symptomatic women there should be a much lower threshold for admission to hospital. Tetracyclines (or doxycycline), long-acting sulfonamides at term and primaquine should not be used. Mefloquine has been associated with an increased risk of stillbirth in one study, but not in others, and is still generally regarded as safe.[47] There are now enough reassuring safety data to recommend artemisinin derivatives for women in the second or third trimesters of pregnancy.[48] In the first trimesters oral artemisinin derivatives for uncomplicated malaria should be avoided unless there is no effective alternative, as there are insufficient data to support their use. There are little or no data on the use of halofantrine, atovaquone–proguanil or dihydroartemisinin–piperaquine in pregnancy.

Chloroquine, pyrimethamine, proguanil and quinine are all considered safe, although quinine-stimulated hyperinsulinemia is more problematic in late pregnancy. For severe malaria artesunate and artemether are safer and easier to administer than quinine. The risks to the mother in severe malaria dictate that they should be used at any stage of pregnancy if the mother is severely ill.

BREASTFEEDING

Primaquine should be avoided, but the other drugs can be used as the doses received by the suckling infant are very small.

MALARIA PROPHYLAXIS

It is difficult to make generalized recommendations for antimalarial prophylaxis as the risks of acquiring malaria and antimalarial drug sensitivity vary considerably over short geographical distances. Antimalarial prophylaxis is indicated in two circumstances:

- In non-immune travelers visiting areas where they may acquire malaria
- In pregnant women who live in endemic areas.

Antimalarial prophylaxis is not generally recommended otherwise for the indigenous population in malaria-endemic areas, although there is increasing support for intermittent preventive treatment (intermittent treatment doses given to healthy people) in pregnant women, infants and school children. In practice in endemic areas for prophylaxis in pregnancy the only options are chloroquine for vivax malaria prevention or intermittent sulfadoxine–pyrimethamine (given twice during pregnancy) for falciparum malaria prevention. In areas in which multiresistance is prevalent there are no safe effective prophylactics or preventive treatments for pregnant women.

Drugs are only one component of personal protection against malaria (Table 62.2). The risks of acquiring malaria can be reduced considerably by avoiding contact with malaria vectors, by use of appropriate protective clothing, window netting, insect repellents, and sleeping under insecticide-impregnated bed nets. The key elements of malaria prevention are based on the well-established A, B, C, D system: *a*wareness of the risk (this is particularly important for those visiting friends and relatives, who often assume incorrectly that their tropical origins protect them from malaria); mosquito-*b*ite prevention; effective antimalarial *c*hemoprophylaxis; and *d*iagnosis and treatment without delay if malaria is suspected. Travelers should seek medical advice urgently if they develop a febrile illness. Standby treatment sufficient for one complete antimalarial course may be given to those who will be unable to reach medical services for extended periods. As the geographical distribution of drug resistance changes rapidly, the following general recommendations should be under constant scrutiny.

In those few areas where *P. falciparum* malaria remains chloroquine sensitive (such as Central America north of the Panama Canal), chloroquine alone can be given. In areas where antifol sensitivity is retained and/or *P. vivax* is prevalent, the combination of chloroquine (5 mg base/kg weekly) and proguanil (3 mg/kg per day) is still effective in some areas (e.g. parts of India and central Asia). Chloroquine is generally well tolerated, although pruritus is common in dark-skinned patients, and it may cause occasional skin eruptions or worsening of psoriasis. As chloroquine accumulates in the body and may cause retinal damage, ophthalmological examinations are advisable for people who take continuous chloroquine for 5 years or more (total dose >100 g). Retinal toxicity is more common when chloroquine is taken daily for rheumatic diseases, and is probably very unusual with antimalarial prophylaxis. Proguanil is given in a daily dose of 3 mg/kg (adult 200 mg). It is very safe and well tolerated. The main adverse effects are mouth ulcers and, less commonly, alopecia. In renal failure proguanil and its principal metabolite cycloguanil accumulate, and blood dyscrasias have been reported.

Table 62.2 Drugs used in the prophylaxis of malaria

Drug	Usage	Adult dose	Pediatric dose	Comments
Atovaquone–proguanil	Prophylaxis in all areas	Adult tablets contain 250 mg atovaquone and 100 mg proguanil hydrochloride. 1 adult tablet orally, daily	Pediatric tablets contain 62.5 mg atovaquone and 25 mg proguanil hydrochloride: 5–8 kg: ½ pediatric tablet daily >8–10 kg: ¾ pediatric tablet daily >10–20 kg: 1 pediatric tablet daily >20–30 kg: 2 pediatric tablets daily >30–40 kg: 3 pediatric tablets daily >40 kg: 1 adult tablet daily	Should be started 1–2 days before travel to a malarious area and taken for 7 days after leaving the transmission area. Contraindicated in persons with severe renal impairment (creatinine clearance <30 mL/min). Atovaquone–proguanil should be taken with food or a milky drink to enhance absorption of atovaquone. Not recommended for prophylaxis for children <5 kg, pregnant women, and women breastfeeding infants weighing <5 kg
Chloroquine	Prophylaxis only in areas with definite chloroquine-sensitive malaria	300 mg base (500 mg salt) orally, once/week	5 mg base/kg (8.3 mg/kg salt) orally, once/week, up to maximum adult dose of 300 mg base	Should be started 1–2 weeks before travel to a malarious area and taken for 4 weeks after leaving such areas. May exacerbate psoriasis
Doxycycline	Prophylaxis in all areas	100 mg orally, daily	≥8 years of age: 2 mg/kg up to adult dose of 100 mg/day	Should be started 1–2 days before travel to a malarious area and taken for 4 weeks after leaving the transmission area. Contraindicated in children <8 years of age and pregnant women
Mefloquine	Prophylaxis in all areas except those with mefloquine-resistant malaria	250 mg base orally, once/week	≤9 kg: 4.6 mg base/kg orally, once/week: >9–19 kg: ¼ tablet once/week >19–30 kg: ½ tablet once/week >31–45 kg: ¾ tablet once/week ≥45 kg: 1 tablet once/week	Should be started 1–2 weeks before travel to a malarious area and taken for 4 weeks after leaving the transmission area. Contraindicated if there is a history of allergy to mefloquine and in persons with depression, a recent history of depression, generalized anxiety disorder, psychosis, schizophrenia, other major psychiatric disorders or seizures. Should be used with caution in persons with psychiatric disturbances or a previous history of depression
Primaquine	Prophylaxis for short-duration travel	30 mg base orally, once daily	0.5 mg base/kg up to adult dose once daily	Should be started 1–2 days before travel to malarious areas, and taken daily with food while in the malarious area and then for 7 days after leaving. Contraindicated in persons with G6PD[a] deficiency. Also contraindicated during pregnancy and lactation unless the infant being breastfed has a documented normal G6PD level.

[a]Glucose-6-phosphate dehydrogenase. Primaquine should not be given to people with G6PD deficiency.

For most malaria endemic areas the choice is between four drugs: mefloquine, doxycycline, primaquine or atovaquone–proguanil. They are approximately equally effective. Weekly mefloquine (3.5 mg base/kg equivalent to an adult dose of 250 mg) is often the antimalarial prophylactic of choice. Mefloquine should be started at least 1 week before entering the malarious area so that therapeutic levels are achieved before exposure and any adverse effects have declared themselves. Mefloquine is generally well tolerated, with an incidence of serious adverse (neuropsychiatric) effects similar to that with chloroquine prophylaxis (about 1 in 10 000 recipients). In 70% of cases these arise within the first 3 weeks of prophylaxis. Less serious central nervous system effects such as dizziness, muzziness, feelings of dissociation, difficulty concentrating, sleeplessness and nightmares are much more common, but these are usually not sufficiently troublesome to limit prophylaxis. Because of inadequate data, rather than

evidence of toxicity, mefloquine is considered 'not indicated' in the first trimester of pregnancy or in children under 2 years old. Serious neuropsychiatric reactions (seizures, encephalopathy and psychosis) are more common if there is a previous history of seizures or psychiatric abnormalities, if quinine has been taken, and when mefloquine is used for treatment rather than prophylaxis. These reactions usually resolve spontaneously. Mefloquine should be continued for 1 month after leaving the endemic area. A maximum of 12 months continuous use is currently recommended.

Daily doxycycline is an alternative which retains efficacy in those few areas where multiresistant *P. falciparum* is also resistant to mefloquine (on the eastern and western borders of Thailand and adjacent Cambodia and Burma). It can be started 2 days before entering the malarious area but, as with mefloquine, it should be continued for 4 weeks after leaving the transmission area. The main adverse effects are nausea, esophagitis, diarrhea, photosensitivity and, in women, *Candida* vaginitis. Doxycycline should be taken after meals with copious fluids to avoid esophageal irritation. It should not be given to children under 8 years of age (in the UK a 12-year age limit is recommended as there are very limited data on prophylactic use in older children)[49] (Table 62.1 to pregnant women or for more than 3 months' duration. Atovaquone–proguanil (250/100 mg/day) has proved effective and very well tolerated everywhere it has been tested.[50] It is a more expensive, but better tolerated, alternative to mefloquine or doxycycline. Primaquine (30 mg/day) has proved remarkably well tolerated in prophylactic use, provided it is not taken on an empty stomach.[51] It has been effective even against multiresistant falciparum malaria. Side effects include abdominal pain (particularly if taken on an empty stomach) and oxidant hemolysis. Primaquine should not be given to people with G6PD deficiency. Both primaquine and atovaquone–proguanil have pre-erythrocytic activity and can be stopped 1 week after the transmission area is left, making them suitable for short-term visitors.

Chloroquine is certainly safe in all age groups and in pregnancy. Although no adverse effects have been reported

with mefloquine prophylaxis in pregnancy, experience is still limited and this should remain under review. Atovaquone–proguanil is considered safe in children but there are limited data in pregnancy, and evidence that drug levels are reduced in late pregnancy. Primaquine and doxycycline are contraindicated in pregnancy. The artemisinin derivatives should not be used for prophylaxis. Neither the sulfadoxine–pyrimethamine combination nor amodiaquine are now recommended for prophylactic use because of toxicity. However, intermittent sulfadoxine–pyrimethamine (twice during pregnancy, three to four times in HIV-infected mothers) has proved very effective in reducing the impact of falciparum malaria in pregnancy in endemic areas where prevalent parasites remain sensitive.

Travelers should obtain detailed information on the risks of malaria, the value of vector avoidance and personal protection, and the efficacy of antimalarial drugs in the area that they will visit. Most travelers visiting South East Asia do not enter areas of risk and do not need to take antimalarial drugs. For India and South America the risks depend very much on the area to be visited, and for sub-Saharan Africa and Oceania malaria risks are very high and prophylaxis is required (Fig. 62.2).

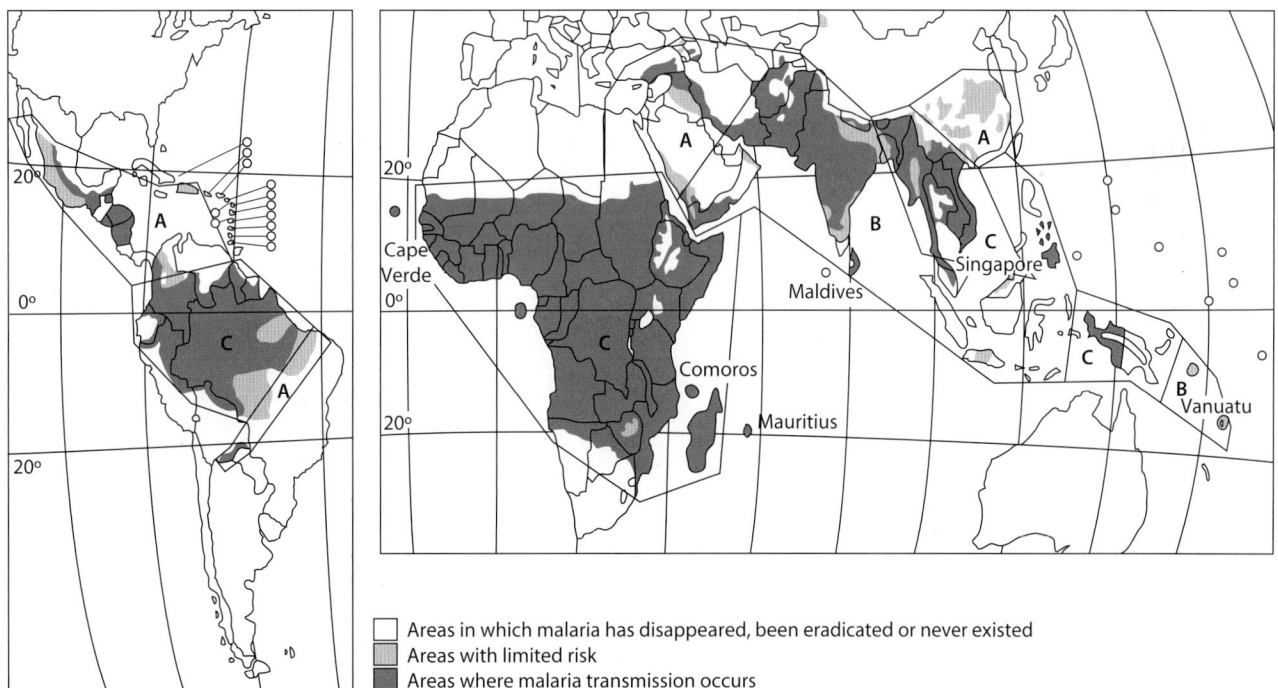

☐ Areas in which malaria has disappeared, been eradicated or never existed
▦ Areas with limited risk
■ Areas where malaria transmission occurs

Fig. 62.2 WHO antimalarial prophylaxis recommendations 2000. **A** Risk generally low and seasonal; no risk in many areas (e.g. urban areas). *P. falciparum* absent or sensitive to chloroquine prophylaxis: chloroquine or (in case of very low risk) no prophylaxis. **B** Low risk in most of the areas. Chloroquine alone will protect against *P. vivax*. Chloroquine with proguanil will give some protection against *P. falciparum* and may alleviate the disease if it occurs despite prophylaxis. Prophylaxis: chloroquine + proguanil; second choice mefloquine or (in case of very low risk) no prophylaxis. **C** Risk high in most areas of this zone in Africa, except in some high-altitude areas. Risk low in most areas of this zone in Asia and America, but high in parts of the Amazon basin. Resistance to sulfadoxine–pyrimethamine common in zone C in Asia, variable in zone C in Africa and America. Prophylaxis: first choice mefloquine (except areas Cambodia/Burma/Thailand border); second choice doxycycline; third choice chloroquine + proguanil or (in case of very low risk) no prophylaxis. *Note*: Protection from mosquito bites should be the rule in all situations, even when prophylaxis is taken.

References

1. Trape JF, Pison G, Preziosi MP, et al. Impact of chloroquine resistance on malaria mortality. *C R Acad Sci, III*. 1998;321:689–697.

2. White NJ. Antimalarial drug resistance and mortality in falciparum malaria. *Trop Med Int Health*. 1999;4:469–470.

3. White NJ, van Vugt M, Ezzet F. Clinical pharmacokinetics and pharmacodynamics of artemether–lumefantrine. *Clin Pharmacokinet*. 1999;37:105–125.

4. Baird JK, Basri H, Purnomo MJ, et al. Resistance to chloroquine by *Plasmodium vivax* in Irian Jaya, Indonesia. *Am J Trop Med Hyg*. 1991;44:547–552.

5. World Health Organization Global Malaria Programme. *The treatment of malaria*. Geneva: WHO; 2006.

6. Nzila AM, Nduati E, Mberu EK, et al. Molecular evidence of greater selective pressure for drug resistance exerted by the long-acting antifolate pyrimethamine/sulfadoxine compared with the shorter-acting chlorproguanil/dapsone on Kenyan *Plasmodium falciparum. J Infect Dis*. 2000;181:2023–2028.

7. Nosten F, Luxemburger C, ter Kuile FO, et al. Treatment of multi-drug resistant *Plasmodium falciparum* malaria with 3-day artesunate–mefloquine combination. *J Infect Dis*. 1994;170:971–977.

8. Carrara VI, Zwang J, Ashley EA, et al. Changes in the treatment responses to artesunate–mefloquine on the northwestern border of Thailand during 13 years of continuous deployment. *PLoS ONE*. 2009;4:e4551.

9. Nosten F, ter Kuile FO, Luxemburger C, et al. Cardiac effects of antimalarial treatment with halofantrine. *Lancet*. 1993;341:1054–1056.

10. Watt G, Loesuttivibool L, Shanks GD, et al. Quinine with tetracycline for the treatment of drug-resistant falciparum malaria in Thailand. *Am J Trop Med Hyg*. 1992;47:108–111.

11. White NJ. Qinghaosu (Artemisinin): current status. *Science*. 2008;320:330–334.

12. Brockman A, Price RN, van Vugt M, et al. *Plasmodium falciparum* antimalarial drug susceptibility on the northwestern border of Thailand during five years of extensive use of artesunate–mefloquine. *Trans R Soc Trop Med Hyg*. 2000;94:537–544.

13. Dondorp AM, Nosten F, Yi P, et al. Artemisinin resistance in *Plasmodium falciparum* malaria. *N Engl J Med*. 2009;361:455–467.

14. Zwang J, Ashley EA, Karema C, et al. Safety and efficacy of dihydroartemisinin–piperaquine in falciparum malaria: a prospective multi-centre individual patient data analysis. *PLoS ONE*. 2009;29:e6358.

15. White NJ. Antimalarial drug resistance. *J Clin Invest*. 2004;113:1084–1092.

16. Mberu EK, Mosobo MK, Nzila AM, Kokwaro GO, Sibley CH, Watkins WM. The changing in vitro susceptibility pattern to pyrimethamine/sulfadoxine in *Plasmodium falciparum* field isolates from Kilifi, Kenya. *Am J Trop Med Hyg*. 2000;62:396–401.

17. Lynch C, Pearce R, Pota H, et al. Emergence of a *dhfr* mutation conferring high-level drug resistance in *Plasmodium falciparum* populations from southwest Uganda. *J Infect Dis*. 2008;197:1598–1604.

18. Wang P, Lee CS, Bayoumi R, et al. Resistance to antifolates in *Plasmodium falciparum* monitored by sequence analysis of dihydropteroate synthetase and dihydrofolate reductase alleles in a large number of field samples of diverse origins. *Mol Biochem Parasitol*. 1997;89:161–177.

19. Fidock DA, Nomura T, Talley AK, et al. Mutations in the *P. falciparum* digestive vacuole transmembrane protein PfCRT and evidence for their role in chloroquine resistance. *Mol Cell*. 2000;6:861–871.

20. Wellems TE. Transporter of a malaria catastrophe. *Nat Med*. 2004;10:1169–1171.

21. Price RN, Uhlemann AC, Brockman A, et al. Mefloquine resistance in *Plasmodium falciparum* results from increased *pfmdr1* gene copy number. *Lancet*. 2004;364:438–447.

22. White NJ, Nosten F, Looareesuwan S, et al. Averting a malaria disaster. *Lancet*. 1999;353:1965–1967.

23. Supanaranond W, Davis TME, Pukrittayakamee S, Nagachinta B, White NJ. Abnormal circulatory control in falciparum malaria; the effects of antimalarial drugs. *Eur J Clin Pharmacol*. 1993;44:325–330.

24. Pussard E, Lepers JP, Clavier F, et al. Efficacy of a loading dose of oral chloroquine in a 36-hour treatment schedule for uncomplicated *Plasmodium falciparum* malaria. *Antimicrob Agents Chemother*. 1991;35:406–409.

25. Gasasira AF, Kamya MR, Achan J, et al. High risk of neutropenia in HIV-infected children following treatment with artesunate plus amodiaquine for uncomplicated malaria in Uganda. *Clin Infect Dis*. 2008;46:985–991.

26. Miller KD, Lobel HO, Satriale RF, Kuritsky JN, Stern R, Campbell CC. Severe cutaneous reactions among American travelers using pyrimethamine–sulfadoxine (Fansidar) for malaria prophylaxis. *Am J Trop Med Hyg*. 1986;35:451–458.

27. ter Kuile FO, Dolan G, Nosten F, et al. Halofantrine versus mefloquine in the treatment of multidrug resistant falciparum malaria. *Lancet*. 1993;341:1044–1049.

28. Mai NTH, Day NPJ, Chuong LV, et al. Post-malaria neurological syndrome. *Lancet*. 1996;348:917–921.

29. Price RN, van Vugt M, Phaipun L, et al. Adverse effects in patients with acute falciparum malaria treated with artemisinin derivatives. *Am J Trop Med Hyg*. 1999;60:547–555.

30. Price RN, Nosten F, Luxemburger C, et al. The effects of artemisinin derivatives on malaria transmissibility. *Lancet*. 1996;347:1654–1658.

31. World Health Organization. Assessment and monitoring of antimalarial drug efficacy for the treatment of uncomplicated falciparum malaria *WHO/HTM/RBM*. 2003; 200350.

32. World Health Organization. Control of tropical diseases. Severe and complicated malaria. *Trans R Soc Trop Med Hyg*. 1990;84(suppl 2):1–65.

33. Crawley J, Waruiru C, Mithwani S, et al. Effect of phenobarbital on seizure frequency and mortality in childhood cerebral malaria: a randomised, controlled intervention study. *Lancet*. 2000;355:701–706.

34. The Artemether–Quinine Meta-analysis Study Group. A meta-analysis of trials comparing artemether with quinine in the treatment of severe falciparum malaria using individual patient data. *Trans R Soc Trop Med Hyg*. 2001;95:637–650.

35. Murphy SA, Mberu E, Muhia D, et al. The disposition of intramuscular artemether in children with cerebral malaria; a preliminary study. *Trans R Soc Trop Med Hyg*. 1997;91:331–334.

36. Hien TT, Davis TM, Chuong LV, et al. Comparative pharmacokinetics of intramuscular artesunate and artemether in patients with severe falciparum malaria. *Antimicrob Agents Chemother*. 2004;48:4234–4239.

37. Dondorp A, Nosten F, Stepniewska K, Day N, White NJ. South East Asian Quinine Artesunate Malaria Trial (SEAQUAMAT) Group. Artesunate versus quinine for treatment of severe falciparum malaria: a randomised trial. *Lancet*. 2005;366:717–725.

38. Krishna S, Planche T, Agbenyega T, et al. Bioavailability and preliminary clinical efficacy of intrarectal artesunate in Ghanaian children with moderate malaria. *Antimicrob Agents Chemother*. 2001;45:509–516.

39. Gomes MF, Faiz MA, Gyapong JO, et al. Pre-referral rectal artesunate to prevent death and disability in severe malaria: a placebo-controlled trial. *Lancet*. 2009;373:557–566.

40. White NJ, Looareesuwan S, Warrell DA, et al. Quinine loading dose in cerebral malaria. *Am J Trop Med Hyg*. 1983;32:1–5.

41. Davis TME, Supanaranond W, Pukrittayakamee S, et al. A safe and effective consecutive-infusion regimen for rapid quinine loading in severe falciparum malaria. *J Infect Dis*. 1990;161:1305–1308.

42. White NJ, Warrell DA, Chanthavanich P, et al. Severe hypoglycemia and hyperinsulinemia in falciparum malaria. *N Engl J Med*. 1983;309:61–66.

43. Hien TT, Day NPJ, Phu NH, et al. A controlled trial of artemether or quinine in Vietnamese adults with severe falciparum malaria. *N Engl J Med*. 1996;335:76–83.

44. Miller KD, Greenberg AE, Campbell CC. Treatment of severe malaria in the United States with a continuous infusion of quinidine gluconate and exchange transfusion. *N Engl J Med*. 1989;321:65–70.

45. Karbwang J, Davis TME, Looareesuwan S, Molunto P, Bunnag D, White NJ. A comparison of the pharmacokinetic and pharmacodynamic properties of quinine and quinidine in healthy Thai males. *Br J Clin Pharmacol*. 1993;35:265–271.

46. Barnes KI, Little F, Mabuza A, et al. Increased gametocytemia after treatment: an early parasitological indicator of emerging sulfadoxine–pyrimethamine resistance in falciparum malaria. *J Infect Dis*. 2008;197:1605–1613.

47. Nosten F, Vincenti M, Simpson JA, et al. The effects of mefloquine treatment in pregnancy. *Clin Infect Dis*. 1999;28:808–815.

48. McGready R, Cho T, Keo NK, et al. Artemisinin antimalarials in pregnancy: a prospective treatment study of 539 episodes of multidrug resistant *P falciparum. Clin Infect Dis*. 2001;33:2009–2016.

49. Swales CA, Chiodini PL, Bannister BA; Health Protection Agency Advisory Committee on Malaria Prevention in UK Travellers. New guidelines on malaria prevention: a summary. *J Infect*. 2007;54:107–110.

50. Hogh B, Clarke PD, Camus D, et al. Atovaquone–proguanil versus chloroquine–proguanil for malaria prophylaxis in non-immune travellers: a randomised, double-blind study. Malarone International Study Team. *Lancet*. 2000;356:1888–1894.

51. Fryauff DJ, Baird JK, Basri H, et al. Randomised placebo-controlled trial of primaquine for prophylaxis of falciparum and vivax malaria. *Lancet*. 1995;346:1190–1193.

63 Other protozoal infections

Peter L. Chiodini and Carmel M. Curtis

TOXOPLASMOSIS

The regimen of choice is pyrimethamine plus sulfadiazine. The combination is synergistic against toxoplasma tachyzoites. Pyrimethamine is given at a dose of 25–50 mg/day, preceded by a loading dose of 100 mg every 12 h for 1 day. Sulfadiazine is given as 2–8 g/day (in four divided doses). Some authors recommend a loading dose of 75 mg/kg up to 4 g. Alternatives to sulfadiazine are sulfatriad or sulfadimidine.

Therapy with pyrimethamine–sulfadiazine (or an alternative) should be accompanied by folinic acid 15 mg/day orally. Duration and dose of combination therapy is influenced by the variant of toxoplasmosis being treated and clinical progress on therapy. Where sulfonamides are contraindicated or cannot be tolerated, clindamycin 2.4–4.8 g/day in four divided doses can be substituted and given in combination with pyrimethamine.

Spiramycin, available in some countries, 2–3 g/day in three or four divided doses is less active than pyrimethamine–sulfadiazine.[1] Its main application lies in the management of toxoplasmosis in pregnancy (Ch. 55).

There is no evidence in the literature for the use of nitazoxanide for toxoplasmosis.

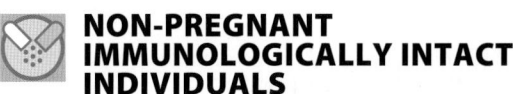 ### NON-PREGNANT IMMUNOLOGICALLY INTACT INDIVIDUALS

Many infections in the normal population are asymptomatic and thus not recognized. Most symptomatic cases resolve without treatment so do not require drug therapy, but severely ill patients should be treated. The regimen consists of pyrimethamine 25 mg/day plus sulfadiazine 2 g/day plus folinic acid, for 2–4 weeks. Cerebral, pulmonary, hepatic or cardiac involvement also constitute indications for giving antitoxoplasma drugs.[2]

OCULAR TOXOPLASMOSIS (SEE ALSO CH. 53)

Rothova et al[3] examined the action of pyrimethamine 100 mg on the first day followed by 25 mg every 12 h, plus sulfadiazine 1 g every 6 h, plus folinic acid, plus corticosteroids, with the action of clindamycin 300 mg every 6 h plus sulfadiazine (as above) with an untreated control group. Pyrimethamine–sulfadiazine with corticosteroids significantly reduced the size of the retinal lesion in 52% of patients (compared with 25% of controls). Improvement on clindamycin–sulfadiazine with corticosteroids was borderline (retinal lesion reduced in size in 32% of patients). In contrast, Dutton[4] preferred clindamycin–sulfadiazine to pyrimethamine–sulfadiazine. Soheilian et al conducted a prospective randomized trial of trimethoprim–sulfamethoxazole plus prednisolone versus the classic treatment regimen of pyrimethamine–sulfadiazine plus prednisolone.[5] They found no significant difference in mean reduction of retinochoroidal lesion size, visual acuity and recurrence rate between the groups and adverse events were similar. In a review of ocular toxoplasmosis, Dodds suggests that trimethoprim–sulfamethoxazole plus prednisolone can be an alternative to classic therapy.[6]

Pearson et al[7] conducted an open, phase I (safety and efficacy) trial of atovaquone therapy for ocular toxoplasmosis in immunocompetent patients: 17 individuals were treated with atovaquone tablets 750 mg every 6 h for 3 months. Prednisolone 40 mg/day was begun on day 3 and tapered as ocular inflammation resolved. One patient stopped treatment at 6 weeks due to persistent epigastric discomfort. All patients showed improvement on treatment within 1–3 weeks and visual acuity stabilized or improved in all cases, median initial visual acuity being 20/200 and median final visual acuity 20/25. Because recurrent ocular toxoplasmosis is due to reactivation of the bradyzoite (tissue cyst) of *Toxoplasma*, atovaquone's activity against this stage in the parasite's life cycle (an attribute not possessed by conventional antitoxoplasma drugs) may limit the ultimate visual loss caused by this condition.

This hypothesis should be tested by randomized clinical trials. However, Baatz et al reported reactivation of toxoplasma retinochoroiditis in a patient whilst taking atovaquone 750 mg every 8 h which they suggest could have been due to tachyzoite resistance to atovaquone.[8] Some support for this hypothesis comes from its use in malaria, where resistance of *Plasmodium falciparum* to atovaquone appears rapidly if it is used as monotherapy.[9]

Antitoxoplasma drugs are indicated for ocular toxoplasmosis where there is a threat to vision, either from local posterior pole lesions or from more general inflammation. Systemic corticosteroids are indicated in the presence of posterior pole lesions if there is a possibility of large vessel involvement or if the lesions are in the patient's only eye. Steroid therapy must be accompanied by antitoxoplasma drugs and is reserved for sight-threatening lesions.

Indications for surgical intervention include the development of a cataract, uncontrolled rise in intraocular pressure, vitreous membranes, epiretinal membranes and retinal detachment. Systemic steroid cover is administered if surgery is undertaken for ocular toxoplasmosis. Peripheral retinal lesions that are no threat to vision can be observed and do not usually require specific antitoxoplasma drugs.[10]

TOXOPLASMOSIS IN THE IMMUNOCOMPROMISED PATIENT

CARDIAC TRANSPLANTATION

Cardiac transplantation is the organ donation most likely to lead to toxoplasmosis in the recipient. Most instances occur when the donor heart comes from a seropositive patient and the recipient is seronegative. The other possibility is reactivation of latent toxoplasmosis secondary to immunosuppression, in an already seropositive recipient. Luft et al[11] reported a series of 50 heart or heart–lung transplant patients: of four patients who were seronegative before receiving a heart from a seropositive donor, three developed life-threatening toxoplasmosis. None of 19 patients who were seropositive before transplantation developed illness attributable to toxoplasmosis, although 10 showed significant increases in toxoplasma antibody titers. Another series studied 21 seronegative recipients of seropositive heart or heart–lung transplants.[12] Four patients (two of whom died) from the first seven suffered clinical toxoplasmosis within 17–32 days of the transplant. The next 14 transplant patients deemed at risk of toxoplasmosis received pyrimethamine prophylaxis 25 mg/day plus folinic acid 15 mg every 8 h for 6 weeks postoperatively; two cases developed.

The most effective prophylaxis for toxoplasmosis is the combination of a dihydrofolate reductase inhibitor and a sulfonamide as they are highly synergistic.[13] Although Soave[14] recommends prophylaxis with pyrimethamine 25 mg/day, plus folinic acid 15 mg every 8 h, for 6 months after heart transplantation in seronegative recipients of seropositive organs, Derouin and Pelloux[13] state that pyrimethamine is at

least 10-fold less efficient than when combined with a sulfonamide. Prophylaxis should be continued beyond 6 months in patients with ongoing risk factors for reactivation of toxoplasmosis or with persistent allograft dysfunction.

Trimethoprim–sulfamethoxazole plus folinic acid and pyrimethamine–sulfadoxine plus folinic acid are both effective in preventing toxoplasmosis. Derouin and Pelloux[13] regard trimethoprim–sulfamethoxazole plus folinic acid as the prophylactic regimen of choice in solid organ transplantation. Treatment of acute toxoplasmosis after heart or heart–lung transplantation is with pyrimethamine–sulfadiazine with folinic acid, continuing until 4–6 weeks after all symptoms and signs have resolved.

RENAL TRANSPLANTATION

The risk of the recipient developing toxoplasmosis after renal transplantation appears to be small,[15] but is recorded as the result of reactivation of latent infection or, more commonly, due to recently infected donor to host transmission.[16] In a review, these authors found 22 cases of disseminated toxoplasmosis following renal transplantation. Ten of 11 recipients whose serology was known were seronegative before transplantation. In the six cases for whom the corresponding donor serology was known, it was positive in five.

HEPATIC TRANSPLANTATION

Toxoplasmosis following liver transplantation appears to be rare[17–19] and there are few published data on the efficacy of post-transplantation prophylaxis against *Toxoplasma*. However, as trimethoprim–sulfamethoxazole is often used after liver transplantation as prophylaxis against *Pneumocystis jirovecii* based on its efficacy in preventing *Toxoplasma* encephalitis in AIDS, this regimen might be expected to confer protection against *Toxoplasma* in liver transplant patients.[17,18] Knowledge of the *Toxoplasma* serological status pretransplantation for both donor and recipient will help alert the clinical team to toxoplasmosis as one of the possible diagnoses to be considered in the investigation of fever after liver transplantation.

BONE MARROW TRANSPLANTATION

In contrast to solid organ transplants, toxoplasmosis in bone-marrow-graft recipients appears to be due largely to reactivation of latent infection in the recipient, rather than infection coming from the transplanted organ.[20] There are likely to be more problems in countries with a higher toxoplasma seroprevalence rate.[21] Slavin et al reported 12 cases of toxoplasmosis in 3803 bone marrow allograft patients:[22] 2% of seropositive patients developed toxoplasmosis, which appeared to occur by reactivation within the first 6 months after marrow transplantation, in patients who were *Toxoplasma*-seropositive pre transplant, had received allogeneic marrow and had severe graft-versus-host disease. Recipients seropositive before bone marrow transplantation should receive chemoprophylaxis from months 2 to 6 after grafting.[23] Foot et al studied the efficacy of weekly pyrimethamine–sulfadoxine prophylaxis in bone marrow transplant recipients.[24] In 69 evaluable seropositive patients, the combination was given from the time of established engraftment (median day 40; range 13–100 days) and was scheduled to be given until 6 months, or longer in instances of continued immunosuppression (median 10 months, range 72 days to 22 months). No cases of toxoplasmosis occurred in patients receiving prophylaxis over a 21-month period.

HEMATOPOIETIC STEM CELL TRANSPLANTATION (HSCT)

The major risk is from latent infection in seropositive recipients and allogeneic recipients are at very high risk compared to autologous HSCT recipients. The median time to disease onset is approximately 2 months after HSCT. In their comprehensive review, Derouin and Pelloux[13] point out that there is no consensus regarding initiation and duration of prophylaxis. They state that a delay of 30 days post HSCT before starting prophylaxis is reasonable and that it should be continued for 6 months post HSCT; longer in cases of graft-versus-host disease, prolonged neutropenia and prolonged administration of corticosteroids. Trimethoprim–sulfamethoxazole (co-trimoxazole) is most commonly used, but pyrimethamine–sulfadoxine is deployed in some centers.

CEREBRAL TOXOPLASMOSIS AND HIV CO-INFECTION

Toxoplasma gondii may cause diffuse encephalitis, but this is an extremely rare infection and cerebral toxoplasmosis is normally manifested as solitary or multiple brain abscesses. The condition is typically seen in HIV-positive patients who have $<100 \times 10^6$ CD4 lymphocytes/L and who have positive *Toxoplasma* serology. More rarely transplant patients and other patients with severe deficiencies of cellular immunity may get cerebral toxoplasmosis. Clinically the patients develop symptoms of intracerebral expansion; seizures, headache and confusion are the most common manifestations. The most common differential diagnoses are cryptococcal meningitis, AIDS dementia complex and progressive multifocal leukoencephalopathy. Diagnosis is obtained by CT scan of the brain showing typical ring-enhanced lesions combined with demonstration of *Toxoplasma* antibodies.

If diagnosed reasonably early, treatment of cerebral toxoplasmosis is normally successful. First-line treatment is sulfadiazine 4–6 g/day combined with pyrimethamine 50–100 mg/day and folinic acid 15 mg/day. In patients who cannot take sulfonamides, clindamycin 600 mg every 6 h has been recommended as a replacement for sulfadiazine. Another alternative to sulfadiazine is clarithromycin 2 g/day or atovaquone 750 mg orally every 6 h, both to be combined with pyrimethamine and folinic acid. In a review, Dedicoat and Livesley considered pyrimethamine plus sulfadiazine and pyrimethamine plus clindamycin to be equivalent for the treatment of acute toxoplasma encephalitis in HIV-infected patients.[25] They also stated that trimethoprim–sulfamethoxazole appears to be an effective alternative to pyrimethamine plus sulfadiazine in resource-poor settings.

Both primary and secondary prevention of cerebral toxoplasmosis should be considered in HIV-positive patients. Those who lack antibodies should be advised to avoid raw and undercooked meat, which are the most common modes of transmission of the infection. Antibody tests should be repeated if the CD4 count falls below 100×10^6/L. At or below that CD4 count primary prophylaxis with a daily dose of trimethoprim 160 mg and sulfamethoxazole 800 mg (which also prevents *Pneumocystis jirovecii* pneumonia) is recommended for antibody-positive patients. Alternatives to trimethoprim–sulfamethoxazole are dapsone plus pyrimethamine or atovaquone with or without pyrimethamine. However, these regimens are incompletely documented. Several studies indicate that primary prophylaxis can be discontinued if the CD4 count rises to above 200×10^6/L as a result of antiretroviral treatment.

The regimens recommended for primary prophylaxis should also be administered as secondary prophylaxis to patients who have had an episode of cerebral toxoplasmosis. In these patients the evidence does not allow a recommendation to discontinue prophylaxis if the CD4 count increases.

TOXOPLASMOSIS IN PREGNANCY

This is discussed in Chapter 55.

LEISHMANIASIS

CUTANEOUS LEISHMANIASIS

OLD WORLD CUTANEOUS LEISHMANIASIS

Most lesions heal spontaneously. Treatment may produce more rapid healing and less severe scarring and is indicated for multiple sores, those at risk of causing disfigurement or disability, or lesions sited where healing is expected to be slow. Options for local drug treatment are topical paromomycin (aminosidine) ointment[26] or infiltration of a pentavalent antimonial drug, sodium stibogluconate, into the edge and base of the sore.[27] Systemic treatment may be required for multiple or potentially disfiguring lesions. The consensus for systemic treatment is less clear than for New World lesions but 20 mg/kg of sodium stibogluconate daily for 10 days is standard, to be extended to 20 days if necessary.[28] Oral miltefosine (a phosphocholine analog) has been used with mixed results for New World cutaneous leishmaniasis[29] and preliminary results from Afghanistan treating *L. tropica* have been disappointing.[30]

NEW WORLD CUTANEOUS LEISHMANIASIS

If infection with *Leishmania (Viannia) braziliensis* complex is suspected, the cutaneous lesion should be treated systemically to prevent the development of mucosal leishmaniasis. Systemic therapy of cutaneous leishmaniasis (CL) is undertaken with pentavalent antimonials (sodium stibogluconate or meglumine antimoniate; *see below*). On the basis that a course of pentamidine isethionate is cheaper and shorter than antimonial therapy, some clinicians use pentamidine in the treatment of CL. Nacher et al[31] examined the efficacy of short-course pentamidine in treating CL due to *Leishmania braziliensis guyanensis* in French Guiana. Two intramuscular injections of pentamidine 4 mg/kg each, separated by 48 h, cured 165 of 189 (87%) evaluable patients. Of the 24 patients who were not cured by one course, 80% were cured by a repeat course of pentamidine. The five individuals in whom active lesions persisted after two courses of pentamidine all responded to antimonial therapy.

DIFFUSE CUTANEOUS LEISHMANIASIS

This condition requires expert assessment and follow-up. In principle, *Leishmania aethiopica* is treated with paromomycin plus sodium stibogluconate daily[32] until the parasite is thought to be eliminated, which may take a few months. Weekly pentamidine is an alternative.[33]

MUCOSAL LEISHMANIASIS

South American mucosal leishmaniasis, due to *Leishmania (Viannia) braziliensis*, is treated with antimonials at 20 mg antimony/kg daily for 6–8 weeks, provided the patient is previously untreated and does not have laryngeal involvement. For those previously treated, or in whom the larynx is involved, amphotericin B 1 mg/kg is given by intravenous infusion on alternate days for 6–8 weeks.[34]

Sudanese mucosal leishmaniasis is due mainly to *Leishmania donovani* and is usually a primary mucosal disease, though it may appear during or after an attack of visceral leishmaniasis. Therapy is with sodium stibogluconate 10 mg/kg per day for 30 days.[38]

ADJUNCTIVE THERAPY

Lessa et al studied 10 Brazilian patients with mucosal leishmaniasis who had failed to respond to at least two courses of conventional pentavalent antimonial therapy.[35] Based on observations that suggested a possible role of tumor necrosis factor-alpha (TNF-α) in the pathology of mucosal leishmaniasis, a TNF-α inhibitor (pentoxifylline) was assessed in combination with a pentavalent antimonial drug. Each patient received parenteral pentavalent antimony (20 mg/kg per day) plus oral pentoxifylline (400 mg every 8 h) for 30 days. The criteria for cure were complete re-epithelialization of the mucosal tissue 90 days post treatment and no evidence of relapse after 1 year of follow-up. Complete healing was found by day 60 in eight patients and by day 90 in one person: one patient was not cured, although some improvement in the lesion was reported. Mean TNF-α levels fell from 776 before treatment to 94 within 60 days after the end of treatment ($p < 0.05$). A subsequent small double-blind, placebo-controlled, randomized trial showed that the addition of pentoxifylline significantly reduced healing time and the need for further courses of antimony in the treatment of mucosal leishmaniasis.[36]

ORAL THERAPY

Amato et al conducted a small open study of the efficacy of itraconazole in the treatment of mucosal leishmaniasis in Brazil.[37] Ten patients received 6 weeks' therapy with itraconazole 4 mg/kg per day to a maximum of 400 mg/day in two divided doses with food; 6 of the 10 showed healing of the lesions at 3 months and none of these showed reactivation of disease after follow-up for 12–18 months. One of the six had previously failed to improve on pentavalent antimonial treatment and another had relapsed after initial healing on pentamidine therapy.

VISCERAL LEISHMANIASIS

Until recently, pentavalent antimonials were the first choice for therapy of visceral leishmaniasis (VL). Sodium stibogluconate solution contains 100 mg antimony/mL, while meglumine antimoniate solution contains 85 mg antimony/mL. Antimonial resistance develops easily following inadequate treatment[39] and has now become a significant problem, notably in recent epidemics in India and the Sudan. Traditional dosage regimens recommended by the World Health Organization[40] advocated 20 mg/kg of antimony daily, subject to a maximum daily dose of 850 mg, for a minimum of 20 days, until no parasites are found in consecutive splenic aspirates taken at 14-day intervals, but this would result in suboptimal dosage of patients weighing more than 42 kg.[41] Herwaldt and Berman advocated lifting of the 850 mg ceiling for antimony dosage, with close monitoring of the patient for drug-related reactions.[42] Current regimens advocate 28–30 days of treatment.[41] In children, who tolerate pentavalent antimony better than adults, dosage is calculated by body surface area.[43]

A successful immune response to VL is T-cell dependent, mainly Th1 type,[41] thus, Th1-derived interferon-γ was assessed to see if it would augment the response to antileishmanial chemotherapy. A controlled trial comparing combination therapy of Kenyan VL with alternate-day interferon-γ plus daily sodium stibogluconate and daily sodium stibogluconate alone, suggested that combination therapy accelerated the early clearance of parasites.[44] Sundar et al[45] used sodium stibogluconate, 20 mg/kg per day intravenously for 30 days, plus interferon-γ 25 μg/m^2 subcutaneously on day 1, 50 μg/m^2 on day 2 and 100 μg/m^2 daily for 28 days, to treat 15 Indian patients, all of whom had failed an initial course of 30 or more days of antimony treatment at 20 mg/kg per day. Eight of the patients had received two courses and seven had received three or four treatment courses. Combination therapy was discontinued in two patients, both of whom died. After 30 days of therapy, 9 of the 13 surviving patients (69%) were apparently cured. All nine had negative bone marrow smears at 6 months and none relapsed after a mean follow-up of 15.9 (± 1.7) months. Combination therapy with antimonials plus interferon-γ may have a role in selected refractory cases, but its cost renders it unsuitable for widespread use in the tropics. Furthermore, it would be unwise to use it in areas where there is significant antimony-resistant VL.

Secondary infection is an important cause of morbidity and mortality in VL. Granulocyte–macrophage colony-stimulating factor (GM-CSF) was compared to placebo as adjunctive therapy in Brazilian patients with VL and leukopenia due to *Leishmania chagasi*. Patients received antimony 10–20 mg/kg per day for 20 days plus GM-CSF 5 μg/kg daily or placebo, for 10 days. Neutrophil counts were significantly higher in the GM-CSF group at 5 and 10 days. Eosinophil and monocyte counts were significantly higher at 10 days in the patients who received GM-CSF. Significantly fewer secondary infections occurred in the GM-CSF group.[46]

Paromomycin (aminosidine) is active against antimony-resistant strains causing VL.[47] Scott et al[48] treated seven patients with Mediterranean VL with daily intravenous infusions of paromomycin 14–16 mg/kg for 21 days or for 1 week after demonstration of parasitological cure, whichever was the longer: four of the seven (treated for between 22 and 54 days) were cured; one relapsed 4 months after an apparent cure, but was successfully re-treated with a second course lasting 63 days; the remaining two showed a partial parasitological response. Jha et al compared paromomycin with sodium stibogluconate for the treatment of VL in Northern Bihar.[49] While the cure rate for pentavalent antimony was only 63%, paromomycin at 16 mg/kg per day for 30 days gave a cure rate of 93% and a cure rate of 97% at 20 mg/kg per day for 30 days.

Indian and Nepalese VL has become significantly less responsive to pentavalent antimonials. By the early 1990s the regimen for VL treatment in Bihar was sodium stibogluconate 20 mg/kg per day for 40 or more days, a dosage regimen associated with increased toxicity and higher costs of hospital care. A decade later, Sundar et al[50] reported a long-term cure rate of 35% for VL treated with pentavalent antimonials in Bihar, versus 86% of VL cases in Uttar Pradesh given identical treatment. They concluded that traditional pentavalent antimony therapy should be abandoned in Bihar. Following reports of a study from Kenya, where paromomycin 12 mg/kg per day in combination with sodium stibogluconate 20 mg/kg per day for 20 days appeared more effective than sodium stibogluconate alone, Thakur et al undertook a pilot study of the activity of the combination on VL in Bihar, India.[51] Twenty-four patients were assigned to receive paromomycin 12 mg/kg per day plus sodium stibogluconate for 20 days. Two patients died before completing the course, one from hemorrhage following splenic puncture and one as a result of severe gastroenteritis. Of the 22 patients who completed therapy, 18 (82%) were cured and did not relapse within a 6-month follow-up period. The remaining four patients improved clinically and parasitologically. Seaman et al[52] confirmed the efficacy of combined paromomycin plus sodium stibogluconate in a study on VL in Southern Sudan. Mishra et al[53] compared conventional amphotericin B with sodium stibogluconate in the treatment of Indian visceral leishmaniasis: 80 patients, none of whom had been previously treated with antileishmanial agents, were randomized to receive either sodium stibogluconate 20 mg/kg in two divided doses intramuscularly daily for 40 days or amphotericin B 0.5 mg/kg infused in 5% dextrose on alternate days for 14 doses. All 40 patients who received amphotericin B showed initial cure (no fever and no amastigotes in a bone marrow smear after 6 weeks) and definitive cure (well at the end of 12 months). In the stibogluconate-treated group 28 of 40 (70%) showed initial cure and 25 of 40 (62.5%) showed definitive cure. Patients who failed to respond to stibogluconate, or who relapsed after initial cure, were treated with, and cured by, amphotericin B. Davidson[39] regards the optimal regimen for amphotericin B deoxycholate as 20 mg/kg given as 0.5 mg/kg per day or 1 mg/kg on alternate days.

The amastigotes of *Leishmania* are found in macrophages, which also clear liposomes from the circulation. Thus, the sites of infection can be targeted by amphotericin B, itself a more active antileishmanial drug than sodium stibogluconate. Davidson et al reported a multicenter trial of liposomal amphotericin B in Mediterranean VL.[54] Ten immunocompetent patients (six of them children) received 1–1.38 mg/kg per day for 21 days and a further 10 (nine of them children) received 3 mg/kg per day for 10 days. All were clinically cured after a follow-up period of at least 12 months.

Lipid-associated amphotericin B preparations all reach very high levels in liver and spleen and are less toxic than conventional amphotericin B. All three are more expensive. Liposomal amphotericin B (AmBisome) is given as a total dose of 20–30 mg/kg, split into more than five daily doses of

3–4 mg/kg over 10–21 days.[54] Liposomal amphotericin B was the first drug approved for the treatment of VL by the US Food and Drug Administration, in a regimen of 21 mg/kg given on 7 days over a 21-day period.[55] As cost is a major issue affecting the use of liposomal amphotericin B, short-course, low-dose regimens have been investigated as a way of reducing treatment costs. Sundar et al[56] compared single-dose infusions of liposomal amphotericin B at 5 mg/kg with once-daily infusions of 1 mg/kg for 5 days in the therapy of Indian VL. Cure rates at 6 months were 92% (84 of 91 patients) for the whole study, 91% (42 of 46) for the single-dose group and 93% (42 of 45) in the five-dose group, with no significant difference in response rates between the two groups. Further work is required to support the use of the regimens described and to see whether or not their deployment will encourage the development of amphotericin-resistant strains of *Leishmania*.

Amphotericin B cholesterol dispersion (Amphocil) consists of a 1:1 molar ratio of cholesterol sulfate and amphotericin B in disk-shaped particles, 115 nm in diameter and 4 nm thick. Dietze et al treated Brazilian patients with VL using two different regimens: 10 patients received amphotericin B cholesterol dispersion 2 mg/kg per day intravenously for 10 days, and another 10 patients received a 7-day course.[57] The authors reported treatment success in all patients. One patient who received the 7-day course had scanty parasites in the bone marrow smear 15 days after treatment, but the remainder (95%) had negative bone marrow smears. All patients were well after 6 months of follow-up. Side effects consisting of fever, chills and respiratory distress were noted in children under 3 years of age.

Amphotericin B lipid complex (Abelcet) at a dosage of 3 mg/kg per day for 5 consecutive days proved effective in the treatment of Indian VL unresponsive to more than 30 days' treatment with pentavalent antimony.[58]

 ## ORAL THERAPY

Effective oral therapy for VL would constitute a major therapeutic advance. Miltefosine (hexadecylphosphocholine), an orally administered agent initially developed as a potential anticancer drug (*see* Ch. 35), was found to have antileishmanial activity in vitro and in animal models.[59] Studies in Indian VL showed very encouraging activity and have been summarized by Murray.[41] A total of 249 patients aged 12 years or more were included: 96% (224 of 234) patients treated with 50–200 mg/day for 14–42 days were regarded as long-term cures; 97% (68 of 70) of those who received 100 mg/day (in two divided doses) for 28 days were cured, but only 89% were cured by 100 mg/day for 14 days. Gastrointestinal side effects were frequent on miltefosine (up to two-thirds of cases) but were judged mild to moderate in severity.[59] Miltefosine is teratogenic in animals and should not be given in pregnancy.[41] The potential impact of miltefosine in the treatment of VL, should its efficacy and safety be confirmed in larger studies, is substantial. It should also be assessed in AIDS-related VL,

both for initial treatment and for maintenance therapy, and in post-kala-azar dermal leishmaniasis.[41]

VISCERAL LEISHMANIASIS AND HIV CO-INFECTION

Before the development of highly active antiretroviral therapy (HAART), 20–70% of patients with VL in the Mediterranean area were co-infected with HIV[39] but there has been a significant decrease in the incidence of VL in HIV-infected patients since HAART was introduced.[60] As a general principle, co-infected patients have reduced therapeutic options for treatment of VL. They suffer greater drug toxicity including interactions with other drugs, inaccessibility due to price and lack of efficacy data in this particular patient group. Extrapolating treatment data from European studies to Africa and Asia is fraught with pitfalls due to differing drug susceptibilities and differing infective strains, and optimal treatments for each region have not yet been agreed. Davidson[39] reports that clinical remission can be produced at first presentation of VL in approximately 65% of patients co-infected with HIV and *Leishmania* with a regimen of sodium stibogluconate or meglumine antimoniate 20 mg antimony/kg per day or amphotericin B 0.7 mg/kg per day, for 28 days. Berenguer et al report the use of meglumine antimoniate (as above) or liposomal amphotericin B, at doses of 4 mg/kg per day on days 1–5, 10, 17, 24, 31 and 38.[61] As toxicity and increased mortality make antimonial drugs unsuitable for co-infected patients, the Hospital for Tropical Diseases recommends the following treatment for co-infected leishmaniasis and HIV patients:

- *Acute infection (first episode)*: Liposomal amphotericin 4 mg/kg for 10 doses (days 1–5, 10, 17, 24, 31 and 38) (prohibitive cost in resource-poor settings)
- *Acute infection (second-line options)*: Pentavalent antimonials, e.g. sodium stibogluconate 20 mg/kg per day for 28 days; oral miltefosine 100 mg/day. The role of paromomycin or sitamaquine for this indication is unclear.

Sindermann et al[62] report on 39 co-infected European patients who received 100 mg oral miltefosine per day on a named patient basis for a mean of 55 days. The majority of patients had received some form of antiretroviral treatment and most of the patients had failed other antileishmanial treatments including amphotericin B. Approximately 64% were cured initially but almost all relapsed; however, many responded with a further course of treatment. They demonstrated that prolonged treatment was safe but made no evaluation of miltefosine prophylaxis. In Ethiopia a study comparing miltefosine with sodium stibogluconate reported that miltefosine was less effective in co-infected patients, with 18% versus 2% failing initial treatment and 25% versus 11% relapsing within 6 months. However, the miltefosine group experienced fewer side effects and reduced mortality.[63]

The evidence for the efficacy of paromomycin, the cheapest of the antileishmanial drugs, is lacking in co-infected patients. Resistance develops easily in vitro but combination treatments with sodium stibogluconate have been successful in VL patients in the absence of HIV.[64]

There is no indication for giving primary prophylaxis; however, maintenance therapy (secondary prophylaxis) is now in wide use following the first relapse, although the data supporting this come from non-controlled trials.[64] This co-infected patient group is at risk of multiple relapses which require careful management if the development of resistance is to be avoided. Berenguer et al described secondary prophylaxis in HIV/*Leishmania* co-infection which was one dose of either meglumine antimoniate or liposomal amphotericin B per month. They studied the relapse rate in 15 patients with HIV and VL established on HAART. Although larger studies are still required, they were able to conclude that secondary prophylaxis against *Leishmania* should not be discontinued in patients who were co-infected with HIV and VL and were unable to achieve and maintain a CD4 cell count above 200/μL on HAART; however, it may be safe in patients whose CD4 cell count is above 350/μL.[61]

The only prospective randomized trial to date which demonstrates the benefits of maintenance therapy used liposomal amphotericin (3 mg/kg every 21 days). The probability of being relapse free at 12 months was 50% in the maintenance group versus 22% in the placebo group.[65] Marques et al[66] report a small series of five co-infected patients who were treated with miltefosine for both relapse (50 mg every 12 h) and maintenance (50 mg, three times a week). Prophylaxis was discontinued after the CD4 count reached >250/μL on HAART and in the absence of VL relapses for a minimum of 12 months. To date, three patients were disease free for a median period of 20 months after miltefosine discontinuation (one patient died of gastrointestinal hemorrhage due to Kaposi's sarcoma and one patient was lost to follow-up). There is clearly a need for randomized trials and prospective studies to ascertain the optimal maintenance dose. The ultimate goal in these co-infected patients must surely be the use of effective antiretroviral treatment plus an agent such as miltefosine in order to achieve VL control while keeping the patient in the community.

Despite recent advances, there remains significant cause for concern regarding co-infection with HIV and VL. Although most reported cases have been from the Mediterranean region, Rosenthal et al have pointed out the potential for an explosion of co-infection with HIV and *Leishmania* in Eastern Africa and the Indian subcontinent due to the simultaneous spread and geographical overlap of both infections,[60] migration of refugees and seasonal workers, and periodical epidemics of VL.

TRYPANOSOMIASIS

TRYPANOSOMA BRUCEI GAMBIENSE INFECTION

Hemolymphatic disease can be treated with eflornithine or suramin or pentamidine. Eflornithine (α-difluoromethylornithine, DFMO) has been evaluated for the treatment of established gambiense sleeping sickness (i.e. with central nervous system involvement),[67–69] but can also be used to treat hemolymphatic disease due to *T. brucei gambiense*.

Suramin is used to attempt radical cure of the hemolymphatic stage of the disease or to clear trypanosomes from the blood and lymph before melarsoprol therapy. All doses are given by slow intravenous infusion of a 10% aqueous solution. A test dose of 200 mg is given first, then 20 mg/kg (maximum dose 1 g) on days 1, 3, 7, 14 and 21.

Pentamidine 4 mg/kg by intramuscular injection daily or on alternate days for 7 doses is an alternative for the hemolymphatic stage for *T. brucei gambiense* only. Doua et al[70] evaluated pentamidine as an alternative to the expensive eflornithine and the toxic melarsoprol in early–late stage *T. brucei gambiense* trypanosomiasis (patients with cerebrospinal fluid (CSF) white cell count <20/mm^3 and/or the presence of trypanosomes by microscopy or culture). Fifty-eight patients received pentamidine 4 mg/kg on alternate days by deep intramuscular injection to a total of 10 injections per patient: three patients relapsed with trypanosomes present in the CSF, one at 15 months and two at 18 months after the end of treatment, giving a 94% cure rate at 24 months.

In the absence of treatment, late-stage infection with meningoencephalitis is uniformly fatal. Until recently the mainstay of therapy was melarsoprol, an arsenical compound with significant toxicity (approximately 6% of patients die of drug-induced encephalopathy). The development of eflornithine has proven to be a major advance.[67] Pepin et al[68] treated 26 patients with *T. brucei gambiense* sleeping sickness resistant to arsenicals (melarsoprol or trimelarsan) with eflornithine, 100 mg/kg every 6 h (total daily dose 400 mg/kg) by intravenous infusion over 1 h for 14 days, followed by oral eflornithine 75 mg/kg every 6 h (300 mg/kg per day) for a further 30 or 21 days. Five patients died. Follow-up of the surviving 21 patients for a mean of 16 (range 6–30) months showed no relapses. Trypanosomes disappeared rapidly from the CSF, the CSF lymphocyte count gradually fell and there was improvement in symptoms after the first 2 weeks of treatment, such that most patients were asymptomatic by the time of hospital discharge. Giving 2 weeks intravenous eflornithine before commencing oral treatment appeared to give a lower relapse rate than did oral therapy reported from other studies. The authors felt that reducing the oral phase of therapy from 30 to 21 days reduced the frequency of side effects. Further to this work, Pepin et al[71] conducted a randomized controlled trial of 321 patients, in four different countries, with late-stage Gambian trypanosomiasis, comparing whether 7 days of intravenous eflornithine (100 mg/kg every 6 h) was as effective as the more standard 14-day treatment regimen. They concluded that the 7-day course was adequate treatment for relapsing cases of Gambian trypanosomiasis but was inferior compared to 14 days of treatment for new cases. However, there were variations between countries and the cost of eflornithine remains prohibitive for many.

Milord et al examined the effect of three different eflornithine treatment regimens on a group of 207 patients with late-stage *T. brucei gambiense* sleeping sickness.[69] In some cases eflornithine was the first antitrypanosomal drug administered, while other patients had relapsed after melarsoprol or nifurtimox or pentamidine plus suramin. Of 152 patients followed for at least 1 year, only 13 (9%) relapsed. Relapse after eflornithine was more frequent in children under 12 years of age and in previously untreated than in relapsing cases. Patients with a CSF leukocytosis of ≥100/μL were slightly, though not significantly, more likely to relapse than those with lower CSF white cell counts. Relapse rates in patients with trypanosomes seen in the CSF were not significantly different from those in patients in whom none were seen. Therapy with eflornithine 100 mg/kg intravenously every 6 h for 14 days, followed by 75 mg/kg orally every 6 h for 21 days showed no relapses in 28 patients followed for at least 1 year after treatment. In patients treated by the intravenous route only (200 mg/kg every 12 h for 14 days) the relapse rate was 10 of 108 (9%), compared with 19% (3 of 16) in those treated by the oral route (75 mg/kg every 6 h for 35 days). Eflornithine was found to be safer than melarsoprol in a trial of 251 patients in southern Sudan. Chappuis et al showed that patients treated with eflornithine experienced fewer cutaneous and neurological side effects as well as a reduced risk of death during treatment.[72]

Where affordable, melarsoprol has been superseded by eflornithine for the therapy of late-stage *T. brucei gambiense* sleeping sickness. Where melarsoprol has to be used, consideration should be given to the use of an accelerated 10-day schedule described from Angola.[73] This consisted of 10 daily injections of melarsoprol 2.2 mg/kg. Prednisolone was given at 1 mg/kg per day for days 1–7; 0.75 mg/kg on day 8; 0.5 mg/kg on day 9 and 0.25 mg/kg on day 10. The schedule was compared with the 26-day standard Angolan schedule of three series of four daily injections of melarsoprol, increasing from 1.2 to 3.6 mg/kg within each series, with 7 days between series. A total of 250 patients on each regimen were studied. Adverse events resulting in withdrawal were 40 on standard treatment and 47 on the concise schedule. Fifty patients on the standard regimen, but only two on the new regimen, deviated or withdrew from treatment. All patients were deemed parasitologically cured 24 h after treatment. Six patients in each group died as a result of encephalopathy. Skin reactions were more common on the new regimen.[73] This concise regimen for melarsoprol has not been validated for the treatment of *T. brucei rhodesiense*.

This work was further supported by Pepin and Mpia who conducted a randomized controlled trial of 389 patients comparing efficacy and toxicity of three regimens of melarsoprol in the treatment of late-stage *T. brucei gambiense* trypanosomiasis.[74] Patients were followed with 6-monthly lumbar punctures for 2 years. The trial compared the more traditional regimen 'A' of three series of three injections (3.6 mg/kg) at the full melarsoprol dosage; a new regimen 'B' of 10 consecutive daily intravenous injections (2.16 mg/kg); and three series of three injections but with graded dosing (1.8–3.6 mg/kg), regimen 'C'. The relapse rate was 5.4%, 7.4% and 25% for regimens A, B and C, respectively ($p < 0.001$). The newer

regimen of 10 daily injections was as effective and had no additional toxicity compared to regimens of three series of three injections. It also had the additional benefit of a shorter hospital stay and a reduction in total cost of melarsoprol. Furthermore, the authors felt that the graded dosing regimen should be abandoned in view of its higher relapse rate and associated increased incidence of seizures.

Nifurtimox monotherapy is too toxic to be preferred to eflornithine. Pepin et al treated 30 patients suffering from arseno-resistant *T. brucei gambiense* sleeping sickness with high-dose nifurtimox (30 mg/kg per day for 30 days).[75] Trypanosomes disappeared from the CSF of the nine patients in whom they were shown before therapy, and the CSF white cell count fell in all but one patient. Nine of 25 (36%) patients relapsed after follow-up, seven with trypanosomes in either CSF or blood. The relapse rate was lower than in the authors' previous study of nifurtimox 15 mg/kg per day for 60 days, when only 31% (6 of 19) were cured. However, high-dose nifurtimox produced serious toxicity; one patient died and another eight developed neurological problems, the most common being a cerebellar syndrome. There have been recent calls for nifurtimox monotherapy to be abandoned.[76] However, there is now a role for combination treatment with oral nifurtimox plus intravenous eflornithine. Priotto et al found that in a small (interrupted) randomized clinical trial comparing three treatments, nifurtimox and eflornithine combination treatment demonstrated increased cure rate over both melarsoprol–eflornithine and melarsoprol–nifurtimox combinations in second-stage Gambiense sleeping sickness.[77] The trial was stopped prematurely due to the increased mortality in the melarsoprol–nifurtimox group.

Further data came from a case series of 48 patients suffering from stage 2 *T. brucei gambiense* infection treated with nifurtimox–eflornithine combination therapy in Uganda. There were no relapses. Two deaths occurred, neither judged to be due to trypanosomiasis nor to drug treatment.[78] A phase III clinical trial, enrolling 103 patients in the Republic of Congo, showed that for stage 2 Gambiense disease nifurtimox–eflornithine combined treatment (NECT) was as efficacious as eflornithine monotherapy. Patients were randomized to receive either eflornithine alone 400 mg/kg per day intravenously in four divided doses for 14 days or eflornithine 400 mg/kg per day intravenously in two divided doses for 7 days, plus nifurtimox 15 mg/kg per day orally in three divided doses for 10 days; 94.1% of the eflornithine group and 96.2% of the nifurtimox-eflornithine group were cured. Severe drug reactions occurred in 25.5% of the eflornithine group and 9.6% of the nifurtimox–eflornithine group.[79] NECT has the benefit of a reduction in drug doses and therefore a reduction in toxic side effects, a shortened hospital stay (treatment duration is reduced to 10 days) and reduced drug costs (the number of injections is reduced to 14). The Drugs for Neglected Diseases initiative (DNDi) and the World Health Organization (WHO) Essential Medicines list (http://www.who.int/neglected_diseases/disease_management/drug_combination/en/index.html) have stated that NECT, while not ideal, offers 'an immediate and practical improvement' for patients as a replacement therapy for melarsoprol.

The DNDi have also released information regarding a rediscovered oral agent, fexinidazole, a nitroimidazole, which can be used in both stages of the disease. This agent entered clinical development in 2009.

TRYPANOSOMA BRUCEI RHODESIENSE INFECTION

Hemolymphatic disease is treated with suramin (*see T. brucei gambiense*). Pentamidine is ineffective against *T. brucei rhodesiense*.

For late-stage disease with CNS involvement, eflornithine is not effective against *T. brucei rhodesiense*, even when used at a dose of 800 mg/kg per day for 14 days[80] and the treatment of choice for late-stage *T. brucei rhodesiense* infection remains melarsoprol. Several different treatment regimens are currently advocated, though there is no clear evidence that one is superior.[40] The regimens usually consist of three or four daily injections, separated by 7- to 10-day periods off treatment (Table 63.1).[40] Despite the evidence to support the abandonment of graded melarsoprol dosing for *T. brucei gambiense*, there is no clinical trial-based evidence to inform such a decision for late-stage *T. brucei rhodesiense*.

Therapy with melarsoprol can be followed by a Jarisch–Herxheimer reaction, which may be very severe. Thus, melarsoprol therapy is usually preceded by suramin treatment in the case of *T. brucei rhodesiense* (Table 63.1). As many as 1–5% of patients die during melarsoprol therapy, so it must be used only where there is clear evidence for CNS involvement in *T. brucei rhodesiense* infection. Especially dangerous is reactive encephalopathy, with headache, tremor, slurred speech, convulsions and coma. The syndrome appears 3–10 days after the first dose of melarsoprol.[40] Pepin et al examined the effect of prednisolone on the incidence of melarsoprol-induced encephalopathy in *T. brucei gambiense* (rather than *T. brucei rhodesiense*) sleeping sickness;[81] 308 control patients received melarsoprol, preceded by a single dose of suramin to decrease peripheral parasitemia, while 290 patients received the same drugs plus prednisolone 1 mg/kg (maximum 40 mg) daily by mouth. The prednisolone group showed a significant ($p = 0.002$) reduction in the incidence of encephalopathy compared to controls. However, there was no significant difference in case-fatality rate for encephalopathy between the two groups (66.7% in the prednisolone group, 54.3% in the control group). The presence of fever during an episode of encephalopathy was associated with an adverse outcome: none of 10 patients with fever and 20 of 37 without fever survived. Thus, reduction in encephalopathy-associated death was due to a lower incidence of encephalopathy rather than a lower case-fatality rate. Reduction of the encephalopathy rate by prednisolone supports an autoimmune etiology for this complication, since steroids seem unlikely to decrease direct toxicity of arsenicals. In contrast, the incidence of polyneuropathy, thought to be due to a direct toxic effect of

Table 63.1 Treatment schedules (adults and children) for *Trypanosoma brucei rhodesiense* trypanosomiasis with meningoencephalitic involvement[40]

Day	Drug[a]	Dose (mg/kg)
For *T. brucei rhodesiense* infection, as used in Kenya and Zambia		
1	Suramin	5.00
3	Suramin	10.00
5	Suramin	20.00
7	Melarsoprol	0.36
8	Melarsoprol	0.72
9	Melarsoprol	1.10
16	Melarsoprol	1.40
17	Melarsoprol	1.80
18	Melarsoprol	1.80
25	Melarsoprol	2.20
26	Melarsoprol	2.90
27	Melarsoprol	3.60
34	Melarsoprol	3.60
35	Melarsoprol	3.60
36	Melarsoprol	3.60
For *T. brucei rhodesiense* infection, as used in Uganda and the United Republic of Tanzania		
1	Suramin	5.00
3	Suramin	10.00
5	Melarsoprol	1.80
6	Melarsoprol	2.20
7	Melarsoprol	2.56
14	Melarsoprol	2.56
15	Melarsoprol	2.90
16	Melarsoprol	3.26
23	Melarsoprol	3.60
24	Melarsoprol	3.60
25	Melarsoprol	3.60

[a]All given intravenously unless otherwise stated.
From WHO Model Prescribing Information: Drug used in Parasitic Diseases. WHO, Geneva, 1990.

arsenic, was not reduced by prednisolone.[81] The authors rightly advise exclusion of strongyloidiasis and amebiasis before giving prednisolone in view of the propensity of these infections to fulminate in steroid-treated individuals. Although the study was undertaken in *T. brucei gambiense* sleeping sickness, the authors thought that prednisolone should be given to patients with *T. brucei rhodesiense* sleeping sickness receiving melarsoprol.

Pepin et al enlarged upon their work on melarsoprol-induced encephalopathy,[82] reporting on 1083 patients with *T. brucei gambiense*, which included data from their earlier study of 598 patients.[81] Of these 1083 patients, 64 (5.9%) developed drug-induced encephalopathy; 62 of these died, 43 from reactive encephalopathy and 19 from other causes, including trypanosomiasis. Prednisolone (1 mg/kg up to 40 mg/day) significantly reduced the incidence of encephalopathy and mortality on treatment, especially in patients with trypanosomes seen in the CSF and/or whose CSF white cell count was ≥100/mm³. In patients with CSF white cell counts of ≥100/mm³, changing the melarsoprol regimen to three series of three injections, instead of three series of four injections, halved the mortality rate.

The addition of dimercaprol to intravenous steroids and anticonvulsants for the treatment of melarsoprol-induced encephalopathy was possibly harmful and the authors gave a clear recommendation not to use dimercaprol in the treatment of this condition. They also recommended that for patients with late-stage Gambian trypanosomiasis with white cell counts of ≥100/mm³ in the CSF, the maximum melarsoprol dosage should be three series of three injections of 0.1 mL/kg each (maximum 5.6 mL/day).

Foulkes reported a patient with arsenical-refractory *T. brucei rhodesiense* infection with CNS involvement who responded to combined intravenous suramin and high-dose oral metronidazole.[83] The patient's CSF was normal, with no trypanosomes evident, at 1-year follow-up.

TRYPANOSOMA CRUZI INFECTION

There have been few advances in the chemotherapy of this infection for many years. Both of the standard drugs (nifurtimox and benznidazole) are toxic, with adverse reaction rates of 30–55%.[84] Tanowitz et al,[85] reviewing Chagas disease, drew attention to studies in which 42% of rabbits receiving benznidazole and 33% of rabbits receiving nifurtimox developed widely invasive lymphomas, yet none of the control animals did so. They also point out that both agents have been widely used in Latin America for several decades, without reports of an increased frequency of lymphomas in treated patients. It should be noted that both agents are contraindicated in pregnancy.

Despite initial optimism,[84,86] the WHO has stated that allopurinol lacks any demonstrable parasiticidal activity in humans.

Nifurtimox acts against trypomastigotes and amastigotes. Side effects of nifurtimox are common and dose related. It is rapidly absorbed from the gastrointestinal tract and predominantly metabolized in the liver by cytochrome P_{450} reductase. Recognized side effects include gastrointestinal symptoms (30–70% of patients), headache, vertigo, excitability, myalgia, arthralgia, convulsions and peripheral polyneuritis.[40]

Benznidazole is also active against trypomastigotes and amastigotes. Side effects commonly occur, including rashes, fever, purpura, peripheral polyneuritis, leukopenia and agranulocytosis.[39,87] Response to therapy is variable; for example, some central Brazilian strains are less sensitive. Andrade et al isolated 11 strains of *T. cruzi* from patients with Chagas disease in central Brazil and characterized them biologically and by isoenzyme analysis.[88] Patients received benznidazole or benznidazole plus nifurtimox. Mice infected with the corresponding strain were treated with the drug(s) corresponding to the regimen received by the patient. Mice underwent a test of cure 3–6 months after the end of treatment. Patients were tested by xenodiagnosis monthly on at least 25 occasions. Mice infected with type II (zymodeme 2) strains showed 66–100% cure rates, but those infected with type III (zymodeme 1) strains showed 0–9% cure rates. In humans, five of six patients with type II strains but only two of five patients with type III strains were cured. There was correlation between treatment outcome in patients and mice in nine of 11 (81.8%) cases.

Congenital Chagas disease can be treated with nifurtimox or with benznidazole.[87] Parasitological cure is thought to occur in 90% of congenitally infected infants treated in the first year of life.[89] Neither drug is available in pediatric formulations but both are well tolerated by infants and young children.

As a result of increasing geographical overlap, reactivation of latent *T. cruzi* infection secondary to HIV-mediated immunosuppression is increasingly recognized. Solari et al[90] reported a patient with hemophilia and AIDS complicated by multifocal necrotic encephalitis due to *T. cruzi*: 2 weeks' therapy with benznidazole 400 mg/day failed to improve the condition, but itraconazole 200 mg/day, later changed to fluconazole 400 mg/day in an attempt to achieve better CNS penetration, was associated with resolution of fever and stabilization of the neurological symptoms. Further evaluation of triazole antifungal agents against *T. cruzi* infections should be undertaken. Sartori et al describe a small series of patients co-infected with HIV and Chagas disease who responded to a standard 60-day benznidazole regimen which resulted in decreased parasitemia and clinical improvement.[91] DiazGranados et al[92] regard the recommended treatment for reactivated *T. cruzi* infection in HIV-positive patients as benznidazole 5 mg/kg per day in two divided doses for 60–90 days or nifurtimox 8–10 mg/kg per day in three divided doses for 60–120 days, though there is less clinical experience with the latter. Following treatment they advocate secondary prophylaxis with benznidazole 5 mg/kg three times weekly. Antiretroviral therapy should be commenced to promote immune reconstitution. There are no studies to provide definitive guidance on the necessary duration of secondary prophylaxis or criteria for its possible withdrawal.

While specific treatment of *T. cruzi* was originally limited to the acute phase, recent evidence has suggested that drug therapy may be indicated in chronically infected individuals. Solari et al used the polymerase chain reaction (PCR) to follow-up children treated with nifurtimox in the chronic phase of *T. cruzi* infection:[93] 66 children were treated with nifurtimox 7–10 mg/kg per day for 60 days and followed up by repeated serology, xenodiagnosis and PCR for 36 months after therapy. Although all but two patients remained seropositive, xenodiagnosis rapidly became negative after 3 months. PCR became negative in most cases by 24 months and in all cases by 36 months post treatment. These smaller studies in children, together with growing clinical experience, have now encouraged the early diagnosis and prompt treatment of all infected children.[86]

Estani and Segura advocate the following guidelines for the treatment of *T. cruzi* infection, which have been adopted in Argentina.[94] They recommend treatment for all patients in the acute phase, for young people in the indeterminate phase, for adult patients in the indeterminate phase or with heart lesions, for laboratory accidents and during surgery, for organ transplant recipients or donors.

In a non-randomized, non-blinded controlled trial of Chagas disease patients with cardiac disease, benznidazole treatment (for 30 days) appeared to slow the progression of cardiomyopathy in adults.[95] This trial and Argentinian clinical experience[96] have encouraged some experts to treat these chronic Chagas disease patients. There is currently underway a phase III multicenter, randomized, double-blind, placebo-controlled trial (the BENEFIT trial) which remains ongoing until 2010. It will evaluate benznidazole treatment versus placebo (for 60 days) in the prevention of progression of cardiac disease.[97]

Neto, based in Brazil, advocates the following treatment regimen:[98]

- For prevention of infection by *T. cruzi* following a laboratory accident and possibly after a blood transfusion from a *T. cruzi*-infected donor: benznidazole 7–10 mg/kg for 10 days.
- Benznidazole is given as 5 mg/kg per day for 60 days for adults; 5–10 mg/kg per day for 60 days for children.
- Nifurtimox is given as 8–10 mg/kg per day for 60–90 days for adults; 15 mg/kg per day for 60–90 days for children.

Reviewing the results from a variety of sources, Neto quotes the following percentages of cure (based upon negative xenodiagnosis and serology) for persons treated at various stages of infection:[98]

- Acute phase 70%
- Recent chronic phase 60%
- Long-term chronic phase 20%

Rassi and Luquetti[99] state that efficacy of treatment may depend on geographical area. They also point out that extensive use of benznidazole took place after 1980 so they expect the efficacy rate for the late chronic phase to rise as more adults achieve 20-year post-treatment follow-up, the period required to regard the infection as cured. However, not all are convinced that therapy of chronically infected individuals is appropriate. In Brazil, Braga et al used nested PCR to follow-up 17 treated (at least 30 days of anti-trypanosomal nitrofuran or nitroimidazole treatment) and 17 untreated chronic Chagas disease patients.[100] There was no statistically significant difference in the mean number of *T. cruzi* per mL in untreated (25.83) and treated (6.45) individuals. These authors took the view that treatment of chronic Chagas disease remains controversial and argue that further evaluation of the benefits of treatment with nitro derivatives is required. They reinforced the need for a precise definition of the role of treatment with nitrofuran and nitroimidazole compounds in chronic *T. cruzi* infection.

A further note of caution was sounded by Silveira et al,[101] who studied 12 children aged between 7 and 12 years in the indeterminate phase of *T. cruzi* infection, with both positive serology and xenodiagnosis. Two patients had received nifurtimox 7 mg/kg for 60 and 90 days and 10 had received benznidazole 5–7 mg/kg for 60 days. The patients were residents of an area where transmission had been interrupted for more than 10 years. Eight individuals were followed up for 8 years and four for 20 years. Clinical evaluation consisted of physical examination, electrocardiogram and esophageal radiography with contrast. Only one child was negative in all examinations performed; seven (58.4%) remained in the indeterminate stage and four (33.3%) progressed to second-degree cardiopathy and/or megaesophagus. However, the authors' data showed only one of the 12 patients to be PCR and xenodiagnosis positive, the other patients being negative by both tests.

Iatrogenically immunosuppressed individuals in the chronic phase of *T. cruzi* infection are at risk of reactivation of the infection, with increased parasitemia. Rassi et al treated 18 adult patients in the chronic phase of Chagas disease, who were taking corticosteroids for concomitant diseases, with benznidazole (at the start of corticosteroid treatment in 12 patients or 15 days afterwards in six patients).[102] Benznidazole therapy (10 mg/kg per day for 60 days in all but one patient) was reported to prevent the increase, and thus might potentially be useful in immunosuppressed patients with chronic Chagas disease. Reactivation of Chagas disease has been estimated at 9–16% in renal transplants, 50–100% in cardiac transplants and 17–40% in autologous and allogeneic transplants. Altclas et al[103] argue that there is no evidence to support the use of pre-emptive treatment of transplant patients with Chagas disease. Patients would still need post-transplant monitoring for reactivation. This is especially the case as benznidazole has reported adverse side effects in immunocompromised patients.[95]

The Pan American Health Organization recommends treatment of *T. cruzi* infection as follows:[104]

- Treatment is with nifurtimox or benznidazole. For nifurtimox, patients up to 40 kg in weight should receive 10–12 mg/kg per day. Those whose weight exceeds 40 kg should receive 8 mg/kg per day. The total daily dose is split into two or three equal doses per day and given for 30–60 days. For benznidazole, patients weighing up to 40 kg should receive 7.5 mg/kg per day. Those who weigh more than 40 kg should receive 5 mg/kg per day. The drug is administered in two or three doses per day for 30–60 days.

- Congenital infection is treated with nifurtimox 10–15 mg/kg per day or benznidazole 10 mg/kg per day.
- In preterm or low birthweight infants, treatment should be started with half the dose. If there is no evidence of leukopenia or thrombocytopenia at 72 h, it is possible to give the definitive dose for the next 60 days.
- It should be noted that whereas acute-phase or congenital *T. cruzi* infection can be treated with either nifurtimox or benznidazole, in the case of recent chronic infection evidence of successful treatment exists only for benznidazole.
- For late chronic infection, the objectives of treatment are to eradicate the parasite, prevent the appearance or progression of visceral lesions, and interrupt the cycle of transmission. There is no age limit to eligibility for treatment. Specific therapy is *not* recommended during pregnancy or breastfeeding, in hepatic or renal insufficiency, when there are serious coexisting lesions. Nifurtimox is given at a dose of 8–10 mg/kg per day (split into 8-hourly doses, preferably after food) for 60–90 days. Benznidazole is given at a dose of 5 mg/kg per day (split into 8- or 12-hourly doses, preferably after food) for 60 days.
- Long-term follow-up with clinical assessment, electrocardiography, serology and PCR is required.

As Neto points out,[98] the decision on treatment requires consideration of each case individually, balancing the chance of a cure and the stage of the disease against the known side effects of the drugs.

For the future, new triazole derivatives (e.g. SCH56592; Schering-Plough) and bisphosphonates (e.g. pamidronate) have shown encouraging activity against *T. cruzi* in murine models.[105]

Interestingly, there is further accumulating evidence that some patients infected with *T. cruzi* spontaneously cure the parasite with no further sequelae. Dias et al report one such case in Brazil of a 5-year-old girl first reported in 1944 with smear-positive acute trypanosomiasis; she had no treatment and continued to have both clinical and laboratory follow-up until 2007.[106] She has no evidence of chronic disease and remains completely well.

In summary, who should be treated for *T. cruzi* infection and with what agent? The WHO[86] recommendations are as follows.

ACUTE PHASE

- For uncomplicated cases, benznidazole 7.5 mg/kg per day for weight up to 40 kg, 5 mg/kg per day for over 40 kg body weight.
- Acute meningoencephalitis, up to 25 mg/kg per day.
- For congenital cases, full-term neonates should receive benznidazole 10 mg/kg per day. Dosing starts at 5 mg/kg per day and is increased to 10 mg/kg per day after 3 days provided there is no leukopenia or thrombocytopenia.

- The total daily dose is given as two or three divided doses. Duration of treatment in all cases is 60 days.
- For organ transplantation, the WHO states that infected donors should be treated for 2 weeks before donation and recipients for 2 weeks afterwards.
- For laboratory accidents, a 10-day course of benznidazole 7–10 mg/kg per day is recommended.

CHRONIC PHASE

- The WHO states that every patient can benefit from antiparasitic treatment and that the treating physician should determine the age limits and clinical suitability of therapy. A 60-day course of either benznidazole 5 mg/kg per day split to two or three divided doses or nifurtimax 8 to 10 mg/kg per day split to three divided doses is recommended.
- For prevention of reactivation in *T. cruzi* and HIV co-infection, benznidazole 5 mg/kg per day three times weekly. Prophylaxis is not justified in those receiving HAART.

Writing from the United States and thus dealing predominantly with the chronic phase, Bern et al[89] recommend antitrypanosomal treatment for:

- all cases of acute and congenital Chagas disease
- reactivated infection
- chronic *T. cruzi* infection in individuals 18 years or younger

and state that it should generally be offered to those aged 19–50 years without advanced heart disease. They regard it as optional for those over 50.

Treatment should be strongly considered for previously untreated individuals with *T. cruzi* and HIV co-infection and for patients awaiting organ transplantation.

ENTAMOEBA HISTOLYTICA

Choice of treatment regimen depends upon the particular clinical presentation of amebic infection.

AMEBIC DYSENTERY

The treatment of choice is metronidazole followed by diloxanide furoate. Metronidazole 800 mg every 8 h for 5 days produced a cure rate in excess of 90%.[107] Other nitroimidazoles such as tinidazole (adult dose 2 g/day for 3–5 days) or a single dose of the long-acting nitroimidazole secnidazole 2 g are alternative agents. The use of a single dose of secnidazole showed microscopic clearance in 81% at day 21.[108]

With the above regimens, neither nitroimidazole achieves adequate clearance of amebic cysts from the intestinal lumen; thus, a luminal amebicide is required to complete therapy. Diloxanide furoate 500 mg orally every 8 h for 10 days is first choice, alternatives being paromomycin (aminosidine) 500 mg orally every 8 h for 10 days, or iodoquinol (diiodohydroxyquin)

650 mg every 8 h for 20 days.[109] However, diiodohydroxyquin therapy, albeit in longer courses, has been associated with the development of blindness,[110] and since there are good alternate agents available, the use of this drug is not recommended. Nitazoxanide, a nitrothiazolyl–salicylamide derivative, at a dose of 500 mg every 12 h for 3 days showed cyst passage clearance rates of 81% in treated patients within 7–10 days of therapy compared with 40% in the placebo group.[111,112] This compares well with similar clearance rates after the longer treatment regimen of diloxanide furoate.

AMEBIC LIVER ABSCESS

The dose of metronidazole required in amebic liver abscess is lower than in amebic dysentery. Amebic liver abscess is treated with metronidazole 400 mg orally every 8 h for 5 days,[107] followed by diloxanide furoate (as above). Tinidazole is an alternative to metronidazole. Initial work used a dosage regimen of 800 mg every 8 h for 5 days,[113] but 2 g/day orally for 3–5 days is currently used. Scragg and Proctor achieved a 92% cure rate in children with amebic liver abscess with tinidazole in a mean dose of 55 mg/kg per day for 3–5 days, in combination with therapeutic aspiration.[114] Secnidazole 500 mg every 8 h for 5 days is another nitroimidazole that can be used in the treatment of amebic liver abscesses.[115]

Rarely, when nitroimidazoles do not seem to be effective despite therapeutic aspiration of the abscess (*see below*), dehydroemetine or emetine can be considered. However, both have serious side effects, notably cardiotoxicity. Where it is essential to use one of them, dehydroemetine is preferred as it is less toxic than emetine. The dosage regimen is dehydroemetine 1.25 mg/kg (maximum daily dose 90 mg) intramuscularly or deep subcutaneously for 10 days. Emetine dosage is 1 mg/kg (maximum daily dose 60 mg) intramuscularly or deep subcutaneously for 10 days.[116,117]

Chloroquine is another alternative where nitroimidazoles fail or cannot be used. However, it is only moderately effective in amebic liver abscess and ineffective in amebic dysentery.[107] The regimen is chloroquine 150 mg base every 6 h for 2 days, then 150 mg base every 12 h for 19 days.[117]

Aspiration of an amebic liver abscess is occasionally necessary. Reed gives the following indications:[109]

1. To rule out a pyogenic abscess, particularly with multiple lesions. Aspiration for diagnostic purposes should only rarely be required, provided good-quality amebic serology is available and if appropriate antibacterial and antiamebic therapy can be given from the outset pending the outcome of blood cultures and amebic serology. Scragg thought there was no place for diagnostic aspiration and that aspiration should be considered as part of treatment.[118]

2. As an adjunct to medical treatment, if a patient does not respond to therapy within 3–5 days and if rupture is believed to be imminent.

3. To decrease the risk of rupture of an abscess of the left lobe of the liver into the pericardium.

ASYMPTOMATIC CYST PASSAGE

The decision whether or not to treat asymptomatic cyst passage depends on several factors. If the patient is ordinarily resident in an area highly endemic for *Entamoeba histolytica* and thus likely to become reinfected fairly quickly, the benefit of eradicating cyst carriage has to be weighed against the cost of treatment and likely benefit to the individual, bearing in mind the fact that most strains of '*E. histolytica*' are non-pathogenic. *Entamoeba histolytica* has now been split into *E. histolytica*, which is always regarded as pathogenic, and *Entamoeba dispar* (formerly non-pathogenic *E. histolytica*), which had originally been proposed by Brumpt in 1925 and was confirmed by Sargeaunt.[119] However, where asymptomatic cyst passage persists following therapy of amebic dysentery or amebic liver abscess, further treatment with a luminal amebicide is mandatory, otherwise relapse is frequent.[116]

In areas where indigenous amebiasis is very uncommon, most *E. histolytica*/*E. dispar* infections are imported, and good luminal amebicides are readily available, so the decision is more in favor of treatment. Ideally, treatment strategy should be based on the results of PCR to separate *E. histolytica* from *E. dispar* (since they are morphologically identical), but the technique is available in only a few centers. Some population groups appear to harbor only non-pathogenic strains. For example, Allason-Jones et al studied '*E. histolytica*' cysts from men who have sex with men (MSM) in London and all strains had a non-pathogenic zymodeme pattern.[120] They concluded that asymptomatic '*E. histolytica*' cyst passage in MSM did not require treatment.

GIARDIASIS

The treatment of choice is tinidazole 2 g as a single dose, a regimen effective in approximately 90% of cases. Metronidazole 2 g/day for 3 days gives a similar cure rate. Low dose, longer duration metronidazole regimens (200 mg every 8 h for 7–10 days) give cure rates of 60–87%.[121] Failure of therapy with nitroimidazole therapy may be due to a variety of possible factors: reinfection, underlying immunodeficiency or drug resistance. Where nitroimidazole resistance is thought to be the explanation, there are few alternative agents.

Mepacrine (quinacrine, atebrin) is active against *Giardia*[122] and is given as 100 mg every 8 h for 5–7 days, with reported cure rates of 90–95%.[123,124] It should be used with caution in view of its known side effects: Wolfe reported toxic psychosis in 1.5% of adult patients treated with this agent[125] and other side effects include CNS stimulation and (on prolonged therapy) yellow discoloration of the skin.

Furazolidone provides another option[126] and is given at 100 mg every 6 h for 7 days, with reported cure rates of 75–90%.[123] Side effects, though usually mild, occur in approximately 20% of patients[127] and patients with glucose-6-phosphate dehydrogenase (G6PD) deficiency may develop hemolysis on furazolidone.

Hall and Nahar compared the efficacy of albendazole with that of metronidazole against *Giardia* infection of children in Bangladesh.[127] Albendazole, 400 mg/day for 5 days, produced a 94.8% cure rate, not statistically different from the 97.4% cure rate produced in children receiving metronidazole 375 mg/day for 5 days.

Paromomycin (aminosidine) (25–30 mg/kg per day in three divided doses for 5–10 days) is effective in 60–70% of cases.[124] As it is excreted nearly 100% unchanged in the feces, it is used by some practitioners when nitroimidazoles cannot be used in pregnancy.

Nitazoxanide 500 mg every 12 h as a 3-day course showed *Giardia* cyst clearance in 91% of patients, compared with 36% clearance in the placebo group at days 7–10.[111] This clearance rate compared well with similar rates achieved with metronidazole.

TRICHOMONAS VAGINALIS

Metronidazole 2 g as a single oral dose has produced cure rates as high as 97% and lends itself better to compliance.[128] An alternative regimen is 400 mg every 12 h for 7 days; this regimen has the advantage of protecting against reinfection during the 7-day treatment period. Tidwell et al compared a single 2 g oral dose of metronidazole with a single 2 g intravaginal dose:[129] 88% of the oral group but only 50% of the intravaginal group were microbiologically cured ($p = 0.0037$). Given the level of asymptomatic carriage, treatment of both partners simultaneously is recommended.

Tinidazole 2 g as a single dose, repeated if the first dose fails to produce clinical benefit, is an alternative to metronidazole.

Secnidazole, another nitroimidazole, is also effective against *Trichomonas* when given as a single 2 g dose.[130]

The most common causes of treatment failure are reinfection or non-compliance with therapy, but metronidazole-resistant strains of *T. vaginalis* are well documented:[131] approximately 5% of all *T. vaginalis* isolates from patients had some level of resistance to metronidazole.[132] Treatment of resistant isolates requires higher doses (usually double the recommended treatment dose for an extended period of time) and, in high-level resistance, intravenous metronidazole. There is likely to be cross-resistance to other nitroimidazoles and therapy with another drug class might be necessary.[133] Refractory cases occur after two standard courses of treatment and are very problematical as higher and higher doses often lead to drug toxicity and intolerable side effects. Nitazoxanide has demonstrated good in-vivo activity against other protozoa and good in-vitro activity against metronidazole-resistant *T. vaginalis*, making it a potential agent for the future.[134] Alternative topical agents include clotrimazole, nonoxynol-9 and povidone–iodine, none of which has given consistently effective cure in women and all of which are ineffective in men,[135] highlighting the need for new antitrichomonal drugs.

For *T. vaginalis* infections during the first trimester of pregnancy, treatment with nitroimidazole derivatives is contraindicated; 100 mg clotrimazole suppositories intravaginally at bedtime for 14 days have been tried, with a cure rate of 50% with some associated symptomatic relief.[105] The cure rates in a multicenter study for a single oral 2 g metronidazole dose were 80% compared with 11.1% for vaginal clotrimazole (two 100 mg tablets per day) and 18.6% for vaginal suppositories (containing 1.05 g sulfanilamide, 14 mg aminacrine hydrochloride and 140 mg allantoin) intravaginally every 12 h for 7 days.[136] Treatment should be reserved for those with severe symptoms. Nitroimidazoles can be used during the second trimester of pregnancy.

Breastfeeding mothers can be treated with a single dose of 2 g secnidazole or metronidazole with a 24 h interruption of breastfeeding after therapy.

Neonatal trichomoniasis is dependent on maternal estrogen levels, which begin to wane in the neonate after 3–6 weeks of life; therapy for symptomatic neonates can only be considered at 2 months of age.[132] In neonates beyond 8 weeks of age where the infection persists or there are symptoms, the infant may be treated with metronidazole as a single 50 mg/kg dose or 10–30 mg/kg per day for 5–7 days.[133]

In general, drugs delivered intravaginally are of significantly lower efficacy than systemically administered nitroimidazoles, which still remain the drugs of choice.

CRYPTOSPORIDIUM

Diarrhea due to this organism is usually self-limiting in those with normal immunity, but can be devastating in immunocompromised people, notably in patients with AIDS. Highly effective treatment remains elusive, but several drugs have been found to be effective in some studies. Paromomycin has been reported effective in a double-blind, placebo-controlled trial.[137] Vargas et al reported successful use of azithromycin in two cases in immunocompromised children.[138] A case report in a pediatric renal transplant patient with profuse cryptosporidial diarrhea used a combination of nitazoxanide, azithromycin and paromomycin to achieve clearance.[139] In a randomized, double-blind, placebo-controlled study, nitazoxanide 500 mg every 12 h for 3 days (100 mg every 12 h for 1–3 year olds, 200 mg every 12 h for 4–11 year olds) showed an 80% clinical resolution and 67% oocyst clearance at day 7 (values were 41% and 22%, respectively, in the control group).[111,112]

Therapy of the immunocompromised patient with cryptosporidiosis is difficult and the mainstay of treatment is modulation of the immune defect. HIV-infected patients on HAART showed persistent parasitological clearance after 1 month of paromomycin 2 g every 6 h. Groups on triple and double therapy showed no relapses, except for two patients who stopped HAART. The groups on no antiretroviral therapy or monotherapy showed only 20% resolution after paromomycin.[140]

A double-blind, placebo-controlled, randomized trial of 66 patients with HIV compared 14 days of nitazoxanide with placebo and saw a 80–92% resolution of diarrhea with nitazoxanide compared to 50% in the placebo group.[141] A further compassionate use program of nitazoxanide in 365 patients with AIDS saw 209 patients achieve a sustained clinical response.[142]

Hyperimmune bovine colostrum has also been used for the treatment of cryptosporidiosis in HIV-positive patients.[143,144]

ISOSPORA BELLI

The treatment of choice is trimethoprim–sulfamethoxazole.[145] A combination of pyrimethamine and sulfadiazine given for 8 weeks was successful in an HIV-positive patient in whom trimethoprim–sulfamethoxazole daily for 2 weeks had failed. Diiodohydroxyquin, paromomycin and spiramycin have also been unsuccessful.[146]

For two AIDS patients with hypersensitivity to trimethoprim–sulfamethoxazole, a combination of albendazole and ornidazole showed parasitological clearance in one patient.[147]

Furazolidone is an alternative agent for the treatment of isosporiasis.

CYCLOSPORA CAYETANENSIS

Cyclospora infection may be self-limiting, so antimicrobial therapy is not required in every case. Where specific treatment is deemed necessary, the agent of choice is trimethoprim–sulfamethoxazole 960 mg every 12 h for 7 days.[148] In a cohort study of Haitian HIV-positive patients the relapse rate after initial therapy with 960 mg trimethoprim–sulfamethoxazole every 6 h for 10 days was 43% and secondary prophylaxis of single dose 960 mg trimethoprim–sulfamethoxazole three times a week was required. No patient had received antiretroviral therapy.[149] For patients with hypersensitivity to sulfa drugs, monotherapy with trimethoprim showed no effect,[150] but ciprofloxacin 500 mg every 12 h for 7 days showed a 70% parasitological clearance on day 7 (clearance was 95% in the trimethoprim–sulfamethoxazole group).[151] Ciprofloxacin could be used in patients with hypersensitivity to sulfonamides.

MICROSPORIDIOSIS

Intestinal microsporidiosis in AIDS patients is caused by *Enterocytozoon bieneusi* or *Encephalitozoon (Septata) intestinalis*. Albendazole 400 mg every 12 h for 3 weeks showed excellent efficacy for the treatment and prophylaxis of *E. intestinalis* infection in patients with AIDS.[152] Albendazole lacks efficacy against *E. bieneusi*, but 20 mg fumagillin every 8 h has shown some promise but the number of cases is small and neutropenia is a recognized adverse effect.[153] Thalidomide 100 mg at night for 1 month showed 38% complete remission and 17% partial remission.[154] Nitazoxanide 1 g every 12 h for 60 days achieved parasitological clearance in an AIDS patient who had not been on antiretroviral therapy at the time nitazoxanide was administered.[155] Immune modulation of HIV-infected patients achieved with HAART remains an important therapeutic intervention in the treatment of microsporidial infections.[141,156]

BABESIOSIS

BABESIA BOVIS AND BABESIA DIVERGENS

These infections are usually encountered in splenectomized humans, leading to fulminant illness and death. There are no controlled trials of treatment. Diminazene (Berenil) is active against animal babesiosis and has been used in a case of human infection with *B. divergens*, but the patient did not survive.[157] The same authors reported successful treatment of a splenectomized patient infected with this parasite using pentamidine plus trimethoprim–sulfamethoxazole. Successful treatment of three cases with massive exchange blood transfusion (2–3 blood volumes) followed by intravenous clindamycin and oral quinine was reported by Brasseur and Gorenflot.[158,159]

Atovaquone is effective against *B. divergens* in vitro.[160] In the absence of data from randomized controlled trials, treatment for human infection with *B. divergens* should consist of exchange blood transfusion plus intravenous clindamycin and intravenous or oral quinine, depending upon the patient's condition.

BABESIA MICROTI

In most cases patients suffer a mild illness and recover spontaneously. Where illness is severe enough to merit treatment, quinine plus clindamycin is the treatment of choice.[160] Whole blood or red cell exchange transfusion has produced a rapid and substantial fall in parasitemia.[161] Krause et al compared atovaquone 750 mg every 12 h plus azithromycin 500 mg on day 1 and 250 mg/day thereafter for 7 days with clindamycin 600 mg every 8 h and quinine 650 mg every 8 h for 7 days, all drugs being given orally.[162] Atovaquone plus azithromycin proved to be as effective as clindamycin plus quinine and had fewer adverse reactions. The authors recommended the use of atovaquone plus azithromycin for the treatment of non-life-threatening babesiosis in immunocompetent adult patients and in others who cannot tolerate clindamycin and quinine. Ranque has suggested that a trial of atovaquone plus clindamycin should be performed.[163]

ACKNOWLEDGMENT

PLC is supported by the UCL Hospitals Comprehensive Biomedical Research Centre Infection Theme.

 References

1. Nguyen BT, Stadtsbaeder S. Comparative effects of co-trimoxazole (trimethoprim-sulphamethoxazole), pyrimethamine–sulphadiazine and spiramycin during avirulent infection with *Toxoplasma gondii* (Beverley strain) in mice. *Br J Pharmacol*. 1983;79:923–928.
2. Joss AWL. Treatment. In: Ho-Yen DO, Joss AWL, eds. *Human toxoplasmosis*. Oxford: Oxford University Press; 1992:119–143.
3. Rothova A, Buitenhuis HJ, Meenken C, et al. Therapy of ocular toxoplasmosis. *Int Ophthalmol*. 1989;13:415–419.
4. Dutton GN. Toxoplasmic retinochoroiditis – a historical review and current concepts. *Ann Acad Med Singapore*. 1989;18:214–221.
5. Soheilian M, Sadoughi MM, Ghajarnia M, et al. Prospective randomized trial of trimethoprim/sulfamethoxazole versus pyrimethamine and sulfadiazine in the treatment of ocular toxoplasmosis. *Ophthalmology*. 2005;112:1876–1882.
6. Dodds EM. Toxoplasmosis. *Curr Opin Ophthalmol*. 2006;17:557–561.
7. Pearson PA, Piracha AR, Sen HA, Jaffe GJ. Atovaquone for the treatment of toxoplasma retinochoroiditis in immunocompetent patients. *Ophthalmology*. 1999;106:148–153.
8. Baatz H, Mirshahi A, Puchta J, Gumbel H, Hattenbach LO. Reactivation of toxoplasma retinochoroiditis under atovaquone therapy in an immunocompetent patient. *Ocul Immunol Inflamm*. 2006;14:185–187.
9. Chiodini PL, Conlon CP, Hutchinson DBA, et al. Evaluation of atovaquone in the treatment of patients with uncomplicated *Plasmodium falciparum* malaria. *J Antimicrob Chemother*. 1995;36:1073–1078.
10. Dutton GN. Recent developments in the prevention and treatment of congenital toxoplasmosis. *Int Ophthalmol*. 1989;13:407–413.
11. Luft BJ, Noat Y, Araujo FG, Stinson EB, Remington JS. Primary and reactivated toxoplasma infection in patients with cardiac transplants. Clinical spectrum and problems in diagnosis in a defined population. *Ann Intern Med*. 1983;99:27–31.
12. Wreghitt TG, Hakim M, Gray JJ, et al. Toxoplasmosis in heart and heart and lung transplant recipients. *J Clin Pathol*. 1989;42:194–199.
13. Derouin F, Pelloux H. Prevention of toxoplasmosis in transplant patients. *Clin Microbiol Infect*. 2008;14:1089–1101.
14. Soave R. Prophylaxis strategies for solid-organ transplantation. *Clin Infect Dis*. 2001;33:S26–S31.
15. Derouin F, Debure A, Godeaut E, Lariviere M, Kreis H. *Toxoplasma* antibody titres in renal transplant recipients. *Transplantation*. 1987;44:515–518.
16. Renoult E, Biava MF, Hulin C, Frimat L, Hestin D, Kessler M. Transmission of toxoplasmosis by renal transplant: a report of four cases. *Transplant Proc*. 1996;28:181–183.
17. Patel R. Disseminated toxoplasmosis after liver transplantation. *Clin Infect Dis*. 1999;29:705–706.
18. Lappalainen M, Jokiranta TS, Halme L, et al. Disseminated toxoplasmosis after liver transplantation. *Clin Infect Dis*. 1999;29:706.
19. Campbell AL, Goldberg CL, Magid MS, Gondolesi G, Rumbo C, Herold BC. First case of toxoplasmosis following small bowel transplantation and systematic review of tissue-invasive toxoplasmosis following noncardiac solid organ transplantation. *Transplantation*. 2006;81:408–417.
20. Derouin F, Devergie A, Auber P, et al. Toxoplasmosis in bone marrow transplant recipients: report of seven cases and review. *Clin Infect Dis*. 1992;15:267–270.
21. Ho-Yen DO. Immunocompromised patients. In: Ho-Yen DO, Joss AWL, eds. *Human toxoplasmosis*. Oxford: Oxford University Press; 1992:184–203.
22. Slavin MA, Meyers JD, Remington JS, Hackman RC. *Toxoplasma gondii* infection in marrow transplant recipients: a 20 year experience. *Bone Marrow Transplant*. 1994;13:549–557.
23. McCabe R, Chirurgi V. Issues in toxoplasmosis. *Infect Dis Clin North Am*. 1993;7:587–604.
24. Foot AB, Garin YJ, Ribaud P, Devergie A, Derouin F, Gluckman E. Prophylaxis of toxoplasmosis infection with pyrimethamine/sulfadoxine (Fansidar) in bone marrow transplant recipients. *Bone Marrow Transplant*. 1994;14:241–245.
25. Dedicoat M, Livesley N. Management of toxoplasmic encephalitis in HIV-infected adults – a review. *S Afr Med J*. 2008;98:31–32.
26. Bryceson ADM, Murphy A, Moody A. Treatment of 'Old World' cutaneous leishmaniasis with aminosidine ointment: results of an open study in London. *Trans R Soc Trop Med Hyg*. 1994;88:226–228.
27. Harms G, Chehade AK, Douba M, et al. A randomized trial comparing a pentavalent antimonial drug and recombinant interferon-gamma in the local treatment of cutaneous leishmaniasis. *Trans R Soc Trop Med Hyg*. 1991;85:214–216.
28. Blum JJ, Desjeux P, Schwartz E, Beck B, et al. Treatment of cutaneous leishmaniasis among travelers. *J Antimicrob Chemother*. 2004;53(2):158–166.
29. Soto R, Arana B, Toledo J, et al. Miltefosine for New World cutaneous leishmaniasis. *Clin Infect Dis*. 2004;38:1266–1272.
30. Bailey MS, Green AD, Ellis CJ, et al. Clinical guidelines and management of cutaneous leishmaniasis in British military personnel. *J R Army Med Corps*. 2005;151(2):73–80.
31. Nacher M, Carme B, Sainte Marie D. Influence of clinical presentation on the efficacy of a short course of pentamidine in the treatment of cutaneous leishmaniasis in French Guiana. *Ann Trop Med Parasitol*. 2001;95:331–336.
32. Teklemariam S, Hiwot AG, Frommel D, Miko TL, Ganlov G, Bryceson A. Aminosidine and its combination with sodium stibogluconate in the treatment of diffuse cutaneous leishmaniasis caused by *Leishmania aethiopica*. *Trans R Soc Trop Med Hyg*. 1994;88:334–339.
33. Bryceson ADM. Diffuse cutaneous leishmaniasis in Ethiopia: II treatment. *Trans R Soc Trop Med Hyg*. 1970;64:369–379.
34. Bryceson ADM. Therapy in man. In: Peters W, Killick-Kendrick RE, eds. *The leishmaniases in biology and medicine*. Vol. 2. London: Academic Press; 1987:848–907.
35. Lessa HA, Machado P, Lima F, et al. Successful treatment of refractory mucosal leishmaniasis with pentoxifylline plus antimony. *Am J Trop Med Hyg*. 2001;65:87–89.
36. Machado PR, Lessa H, Lessa M, et al. Oral pentoxifylline combined with pentavalent antimony: a randomized trial for mucosal leishmaniasis. *Clin Infect Dis*. 2007;44:788–793.
37. Amato VS, Padilha ARS, Nicodemo AC, et al. Use of itraconazole in the treatment of mucocutaneous leishmaniasis: a pilot study. *Int J Infect Dis*. 2000;4:153–157.
38. El-Hassan AM, Zijlstra EE. Leishmaniasis in Sudan. *Trans R Soc Trop Med Hyg*. 2001;95(suppl 1):S1/19–S1/26.
39. Davidson RN. Visceral leishmaniasis in clinical practice. *J Infect*. 1999;39:112–116.
40. World Health Organization. *Drugs used in parasitic diseases*. Geneva: WHO; 1990.
41. Murray HW. Treatment of visceral leishmaniasis (kala-azar): a decade of progress and future approaches. *Int J Infect Dis*. 2000;4:158–177.
42. Herwaldt BL, Berman JD. Recommendations for treating leishmaniasis with sodium stibogluconate (Pentostam) and review of pertinent clinical studies. *Am J Trop Med Hyg*. 1992;46:296–306.
43. Anabwani GM, Bryceson ADM. Visceral leishmaniasis in Kenyan children. *Indian Paediatrics*. 1982;19:819–822.
44. Squires KE, Rosenkaimer F, Sherwood JA, Forni AL, Were JBO, Murray HW. Immunochemotherapy for visceral leishmaniasis: a controlled pilot trial of antimony versus antimony plus interferon-gamma. *Am J Trop Med Hyg*. 1993;48:666–669.
45. Sundar S, Rosenkaimer F, Murray HW. Successful treatment of refractory visceral leishmaniasis in India using antimony plus interferon-gamma. *J Infect Dis*. 1994;170:659–662.
46. Badaro R, Nascimento C, Carvalho JS, et al. Recombinant human granulocyte–macrophage colony-stimulating factor reverses neutropenia and reduces secondary infections in visceral leishmaniasis. *J Infect Dis*. 1994;170:413–418.
47. Olliaro PL, Bryceson ADM. Practical progress and new drugs for changing patterns of leishmaniasis. *Parasitol Today*. 1993;9:323–328.
48. Scott JAG, Davidson RN, Moody AH, et al. Aminosidine (paromomycin) in the treatment of leishmaniasis imported into the United Kingdom. *Trans R Soc Trop Med Hyg*. 1992;86:617–619.

49. Jha TK, Olliaro P, Thakur CP, et al. Randomised controlled trial of aminosidine (paromomycin) v sodium stibogluconate for treating visceral leishmaniasis in North Bihar, India. *Br Med J.* 1998;316:1200–1205.

50. Sundar S, More DK, Singh MK, et al. Failure of pentavalent antimony in visceral leishmaniasis in India: report from the center of the Indian epidemic. *Clin Infect Dis.* 2000;31:1104–1107.

51. Thakur CP, Olliaro P, Gothoskar S, et al. Treatment of visceral leishmaniasis (kala-azar) with aminosidine (paromomycin)-antimonial combinations: a pilot study in Bihar, India. *Trans R Soc Trop Med Hyg.* 1992;86:615–616.

52. Seaman J, Pryce D, Sondorp HE, Moody A, Bryceson AD, Davidson RN. Epidemic visceral leishmaniasis in Sudan: a randomized trial of aminosidine plus sodium stibogluconate versus sodium stibogluconate alone. *J Infect Dis.* 1993;168:715–720.

53. Mishra M, Biswas UK, Jha AM, Khan AB. Amphotericin versus sodium stibogluconate in first-line treatment of Indian kala-azar. *Lancet.* 1994;344:1599–1600.

54. Davidson RN, DiMartino L, Gradoni L, et al. Liposomal amphotericin B (AmBisome) in Mediterranean visceral leishmaniasis: a multi-centre trial. *Q J Med.* 1994;87:75–81.

55. Meyerhoff A. US Food and Drug Administration approval of AmBisome (liposomal amphotericin B) for treatment of visceral leishmaniasis. *Clin Infect Dis.* 1999;28:42–48.

56. Sundar S, Agrawal G, Rai M, Makharia MK, Murray HW. Treatment of Indian visceral leishmaniasis with single or daily infusions of low dose liposomal amphotericin B: randomized trial. *Br Med J.* 2001;323:419–422.

57. Dietze R, Milan EP, Berman JD, et al. Treatment of Brazilian kala-azar with a short course of Amphocil (amphotericin B cholesterol dispersion). *Clin Infect Dis.* 1993;17:981–986.

58. Sundar S, Agrawal NK, Sinha PR, Horwith GS, Murray HW. Short-course, low-dose amphotericin B lipid complex therapy for visceral leishmaniasis unresponsive to antimony. *Ann Intern Med.* 1997;127:133–137.

59. Jha TK, Sundar S, Thakur CP, et al. Miltefosine, an oral agent, for the treatment of Indian visceral leishmaniasis. *N Engl J Med.* 1999;341:1795–1800.

60. Rosenthal E, Tempesta S, Del Giudice P, et al. Declining incidence of visceral leishmaniasis in HIV-infected individuals in the era of highly active anti-retroviral therapy. *AIDS.* 2001;15:1184–1185.

61. Berenguer J, Cosin J, Miralles P, Lopez JC, Padilla B. Discontinuation of secondary anti-*Leishmania* prophylaxis in HIV-infected patients who have responded to highly active antiretroviral therapy. *AIDS.* 2000;14:2946–2948.

62. Sindermann H, Engel KR, Fischer C; the Miltefosine Compassionate Use Program. Oral miltefosine for leishmaniasis in immunocompromised patients: compassionate use in 39 patients with HIV infection. *Clin Infect Dis.* 2004;39:1520–1523.

63. Ritmeijer K, Dejenie Y, Assefa TB, Hundie J, et al. A comparison of miltefosine and sodium stibogluconate for the treatment of visceral leishmaniasis in an Ethiopian population with a high prevalence of HIV infection. *Clin Infect Dis.* 2006;43:357–364.

64. Alvar J, Aparicio P, Aseffa A, Den Broer M, Canavate C, et al. The relationship between leishmaniasis and AIDS: the second 10 years. *Clin Microbiol Rev.* 2008;21(2):334–359.

65. Lopez-Velez R, Vedela S, Marquez M, Boix M, et al. Amphotericin B lipid complex versus no treatment in the secondary prophylaxis of visceral leishmaniasis in HIV-infected patients. *J Antimicrob Chemother.* 2004;53:540–543.

66. Marques N, Sa R, Coelho F, Oliveria J, et al. Miltefosine for visceral leishmaniasis relapse treatment and secondary prophylaxis in HIV-infected patients. *Scand J Infect Dis.* 2008;40:523–526.

67. McCann PP, Bacchi CJ, Clarkson AB, et al. Inhibition of polyamine biosynthesis by α-difluoromethylornithine in African trypanosomes and *Pneumocystis carinii* as a basis of chemotherapy: biochemical and clinical aspects. *Am J Trop Med Hyg.* 1986;35:1153–1156.

68. Pepin J, Milord F, Guern C, Schechter PJ. Difluoro-methylornithine for arseno-resistant *Trypanosoma brucei gambiense* sleeping sickness. *Lancet.* 1987;ii:1431–1433.

69. Milord F, Pepin J, Loko L, Ethier L, Mpia B. Efficacy and toxicity of eflornithine for treatment of *Trypanosoma brucei gambiense* sleeping sickness. *Lancet.* 1992;340:652–655.

70. Doua F, Miezan TW, Singaro JRS, Yapo FB, Baltz T. The efficacy of pentamidine in the treatment of early-late stage *Trypanosoma brucei gambiense* trypanosomiasis. *Am J Trop Med Hyg.* 1996;55:586–588.

71. Pepin J, Khonde N, Maiso F, Doua F, Shabba J, et al. Short-course eflornithine in Gambian trypanosomiasis: a multicentre randomized controlled trial. *Bull World Health Org.* 2000;78(11):1284–1295.

72. Chappuis F, Udayraj N, Stietenroth K, Meussen A, Bovier PA. Eflornithine is safer than melarsoprol for the treatment of second-stage *Trypanosoma brucei gambiense* human African trypanosomiasis. *Clin Infect Dis.* 2005;41:748–751.

73. Burri C, Nkunku S, Merolle A, Smith T, Blum J, Brun R. Efficacy of new, concise schedule for melarsoprol in treatment of sleeping sickness caused by *Trypanosoma brucei gambiense*: a randomized trial. *Lancet.* 2000;355:1419–1425.

74. Pepin J, Mpia B. Randomised controlled trial of three regimens of melarsoprol in the treatment of *Trypanosoma brucei gambiense* trypanosomiasis. *Trans R Soc Trop Med Hyg.* 2006;100:437–441.

75. Pepin J, Milord F, Meurice F, Ethier L, Loko L, Mpia B. High dose nifurtimox for arseno-resistant *Trypanosoma brucei gambiense* sleeping sickness: an open trial in Central Zaire. *Trans R Soc Trop Med Hyg.* 1992;86:254–256.

76. Pepin J. Combination therapy for sleeping sickness: a wake-up call. *J Infect Dis.* 2007;195:311–313.

77. Priotto G, Fogg C, Balasegaram M, et al. Three drug combinations for late-stage *Trypanosoma brucei gambiense* sleeping sickness: A randomized clinical trial in Uganda. *PLoS Clinical Trials.* 2006;e39: December 1–8.

78. Checchi F, Piola P, Ayikoru H, et al. Nifurtimox plus eflornithine for late-stage sleeping sickness in Uganda: a case series. *PLoS Neglected Tropical Diseases.* 2007;1(2):e64.

79. Priotto G, Kasparian S, Ngouama D, Ghorashian S, et al. Nifurtimox–eflornithine combination therapy for second-stage *Trypanosoma brucei gambiense* sleeping sickness: a randomized clinical trial in Congo. *Clin Infect Dis.* 2007;45:1435–1442.

80. Clerinx J, Taelman H, Bogaerts J, Vervoort T. Treatment of late stage Rhodesian trypanosomiasis using suramin and eflornithine: report of six cases. *Trans R Soc Trop Med Hyg.* 1998;92:449–450.

81. Pepin J, Milord F, Guern C, Mpia B, Ethier L, Mansinsa D. Trial of prednisolone for prevention of melarsoprol-induced encephalopathy in gambiense sleeping sickness. *Lancet.* 1989;i:1246–1250.

82. Pepin J, Milord F, Khonde AN, et al. Risk factors for encephalopathy and mortality during melarsoprol treatment of *Trypanosoma brucei gambiense* sleeping sickness. *Trans R Soc Trop Med Hyg.* 1995;89:92–97.

83. Foulkes JR. Metronidazole and suramin combination in the treatment of arsenical refractory Rhodesian sleeping sickness – a case study. *Trans R Soc Trop Med Hyg.* 1996;90:422.

84. Gallerano RH, Marr JJ, Sosa RR. Therapeutic efficacy of allopurinol in patients with chronic Chagas' disease. *Am J Trop Med Hyg.* 1990;43:159–166.

85. Tanowitz HB, Kirchhoff LV, Simon D, Morris SA, Weiss LM, Wittner M. Chagas' disease. *Clin Microbiol Rev.* 1992;5:400–419.

86. World Health Organization. *Control of Chagas disease.* Geneva: WHO. Online; Available at http://whqlibdoc.who.int/trs/WHO_TRS_905.pdf. 2002.

87. World Health Organization. *Control of Chagas' disease.* Geneva: WHO. WHO Technical Report;811. 1991.

88. Andrade SG, Rassi A, Magalhaes JB, Ferriolli-Filho F, Luquetti AO. Specific chemotherapy of Chagas' disease: a comparison between the response in patients and experimental animals inoculated with the same strains. *Trans R Soc Trop Med Hyg.* 1992;86:624–626.

89. Bern C, Montgonery S, Herwaldt B, Rassi A, et al. Evaluation and treatment of Chagas' disease in the United States – a systematic review. *J Am Med Assoc.* 2007;298(18):2171–2181.

90. Solari A, Saavedra H, Sepulveda C, et al. Successful treatment of *Trypanosoma cruzi* encephalitis in a patient with hemophilia and AIDS. *Clin Infect Dis.* 1993;16:255–259.

91. Sartori AM, Ibrahim KY, Nunes Westphalen EV. Manifestations of Chagas' disease (American trypanosomiasis) in patients with HIV/AIDS. *Ann Trop Med Parasitol.* 2007;101(1):31–50.

92. DiazGranados CA, Saavedra-Trujillo CH, Mantilla M, Valderrama SL, Alquichire C, Franco-Parades C. Chagasic encephalitis in HIV patients: common presentation of an evolving epidemiological and clinical association. *Lancet Infect Dis.* 2009;9:324–330.

93. Solari A, Ortiz S, Soto A, et al. Treatment of *Trypanosoma cruzi*-infected children with nifurtimox: a 3 year follow-up by PCR. *J Antimicrob Chemother.* 2001;48:515–519.

94. Estani SS, Segura EL. Treatment of *Trypanosoma cruzi* infection in the undetermined phase. Experience and current guidelines of treatment

in Argentina. *Memorias do Instituto Oswaldo Cruz Rio de Janeiro.* 1999;94:363–365.

95. Sosa-Estani S, Segura EL. Etiological treatment in patients infected by *Trypanosoma cruzi*: experiences in Argentina. *Curr Opin Infect Dis.* 2006;19(6):583–587.

96. Viotti R, Vigilano C, Lococo B, et al. Long-term cardiac outcomes of treating Chagas' disease with benznidazole versus no treatment: a non-randomised trial. *Ann Intern Med.* 2006;144(10):724–734.

97. The BENEFIT trial: evaluation of the use of an antiparasital drug (benznidazole) in the treatment of chronic Chagas' disease. Online. Available at http://clinicaltrials.gov/show/NCT00123916.

98. Neto VA. Etiological treatment for infection by *Trypanosoma cruzi. Memorias do Instituto Oswaldo Cruz. Rio de Janeiro.* 1999;94(suppl 1):337–339.

99. Rassi A, Luquetti AO. Current chemotherapy of American trypanosomiasis. In: Maudlin I, Holmes PH, Miles MA, eds. *The Trypanosomiases.* Wallingford, UK: CAB International, 2004.

100. Braga MS, Lauria-Pires L, Arganaraz ER, Nascimento RJ, Texeira ARL. Persistent infections in chronic Chagas' disease patients treated with anti-*Trypanosoma cruzi* nitroderivatives. *Revista di Instituto de Medicina Tropical de São Paolo.* 2000;42:157–161.

101. Silveira CAN, Castillo E, Castro C. Avaliacao do tratamento especifico para o *Trypanosoma cruzi* em criancas, na evolucao da fase indeterminada. *Rev Soc Bras Med Trop.* 2000;33:191–196.

102. Rassi A, Neto VA, Ferraz de Siqueira A, Filho FF, Amato VS, Junior AR. Efeito protetor do benznidazol contra a reativacao parasitaria em pacientes cronicamente infectados pelo *Trypanosoma cruzi* e tratados com corticoide em virtude de afeccoes associadas. *Rev Soc Bras Med Trop.* 1999;32:475–482.

103. Altclas J, Barcan L, Nagel C, et al. Organ transplantation and Chagas' disease [letter]. *J Am Med Assoc.* 2008;299(10):1134.

104. Organizacion Panamericana de la Salud/Organizacion Mundial de la Salud. Tratamiento Etiologico de la Enfermedad de Chagas. OPS/HCP/HCT/140/99, 1999.

105. Urbina JA. Parasitological cure of Chagas' disease: is it possible? Is it relevant? *Memorias do Instituto Oswaldo Cruz. Rio de Janeiro.* 1999;94(suppl 1):349–355.

106. Dias JC, Dias E, Filho O, et al. Further evidence of spontaneous cure in human Chagas' disease. *Rev Soc Bras Med Trop.* 2008;41(5):505–506.

107. Powell SJ, Wilmott AJ, Elsdon-Dew R. Further trials of metronidazole in amoebic dysentery and amoebic liver abscess. *Ann Trop Med Parasitol.* 1967;61:511–514.

108. Qureshi H, Baqai R, Mehdi I, Ahmed W. Secnidazole response in amoebiasis and giardiasis. *East Mediterr Health J.* 1999;5:389–390.

109. Reed SL. Amoebiasis: an update. *Clin Infect Dis.* 1992;14:385–393.

110. Fleisher DI, Hepler RS, Landau JW. Blindness during diiodohydroxyquin (Diodoquin®) therapy: a case report. *Pediatrics.* 1974;54:106–108.

111. Rossignol J-FA, Ayoub A, Ayers MS. Treatment of diarrhea caused by *Cryptosporidium parvum.* A prospective randomized, double-blind, placebo-controlled study of nitazoxanide. *J Infect Dis.* 2001;184:103–106.

112. Rossignol J-FA, Ayoub A, Ayers MS. Treatment of diarrhea caused by *Giardia intestinalis* and *Entamoeba histolytica* or *E. dispar*: a randomized, double-blind, placebo-controlled study of nitazoxanide. *J Infect Dis.* 2001;184:381–384.

113. Hatchuel W. Tinidazole for the treatment of amoebic liver abscess. *S Afr Med J.* 1975;49:1879–1881.

114. Scragg JN, Proctor EM. Tinidazole in treatment of amoebic liver abscess in children. *Arch Dis Child.* 1977;52:408–410.

115. Hughes MA, Petri WA. Amebic liver abscess. *Infect Dis Clin North Am.* 2000;14:565–582.

116. Knight R. The chemotherapy of amoebiasis. *J Antimicrob Chemother.* 1980;6:577–593.

117. Du Pont HL. Prevention and treatment strategies in giardiasis and amoebiasis. *Drugs under Investigation.* 1994;8(suppl 1):19–25.

118. Scragg JN. Hepatic amoebiasis in childhood. *Trop Doct.* 1975;5:132–134.

119. Sargeaunt PG. *Entamoeba histolytica*: a question answered. *Tropical Disease Bulletin.* 1993;90:R1–R2.

120. Allason-Jones E, Mindel A, Sargeaunt P, Katz D. Outcome of untreated infection with *Entamoeba histolytica* in homosexual men with and without HIV antibody. *Br Med J.* 1988;297:654–657.

121. Mendelson RM. The treatment of giardiasis. *Trans R Soc Trop Med Hyg.* 1980;74:438–439.

122. Thomas MEM. Observations upon the effects of mepacrine and other substances on *Giardia intestinalis Parasitology.* 1952;42:262–268.

123. Wolfe MS. Giardiasis. *Clin Microbiol Rev.* 1992;5:93–100.

124. Hill DR. Giardiasis. *Infect Dis Clin North Am.* 1993;7:503–526.

125. Wolfe MS. Giardiasis. *N Engl J Med.* 1978;298:319–321.

126. Farthing MJG. *Giardia* comes of age: progress in epidemiology, immunology and chemotherapy. *J Antimicrob Chemother.* 1992;30:563–566.

127. Hall A, Nahar Q. Albendazole as a treatment for infections with *Giardia duodenalis* in children in Bangladesh. *Trans R Soc Trop Med Hyg.* 1993;87:84–86.

128. Lossick JG. Single-dose metronidazole treatment for vaginal trichomonas. *Obstet Gynaecol.* 1980;56:508–510.

129. Tidwell BH, Lushbaugh WB, Laughlin MD, Cleary JD, Finley RW. A double-blind placebo-controlled trial of single-dose intravaginal versus single-dose oral metronidazole in the treatment of trichomonal vaginitis. *J Infect Dis.* 1994;170:242–246.

130. Bagnoli VR. An overview of the clinical experience with secnidazole in bacterial vaginosis and trichomoniasis. *Drugs under Investigation.* 1994;8(suppl 1):53–60.

131. Lossick JG, Muller M, Gorrell TE. In vitro drug susceptibility and doses of metronidazole required for cure in cases of refractory vaginal trichomoniasis. *J Infect Dis.* 1986;153:948–955.

132. Narcisi EM, Secor WE. In vitro effect of tinidazole and furazolidone on metronidazole-resistant *Trichomonas vaginalis. Antimicrob Agents Chemother.* 1996;40:1121–1125.

133. Petrin D, Delgaty K, Bhatt R, Garber G. Clinical and microbiological aspects of *Trichomonas vaginalis. Clin Microbiol Rev.* 1998;11:300–317.

134. Adagu IS, Nolder D, Warhurst DC, et al. In vitro activity of nitazoxanide and related compounds against isolates of *Giardia intestinalis, Entamoeba histolytica* and *Trichomonas vaginalis. J Antimicrob Chemother.* 2002;49(1):103–111.

135. Cudmore S, Delgaty KL, Hayward-McClelland S, Petrin DP, Garber GE. Treatment of infections caused by metronidazole-resistant *Trichomonas vaginalis. Clin Microbiol Rev.* 2004;17(4):783–793.

136. DuBouchet L, Spence MR, Rein MF, Danzig MR, McCormack WM. Multicenter comparison of cotrimazole vaginal tablets, oral metronidazole, and vaginal suppositories containing sulfanilamide, aminacrine hydrochloride, and allantoin in the treatment of symptomatic trichomoniasis. *Sex Transm Dis.* 1997;24:156–160.

137. White Jr AC, Chappel CL, Hayat CS, Kimball KT, Flanigan TP, Goodgame RW. Paromomycin for cryptosporidiosis in AIDS: a prospective, double-blind trial. *J Infect Dis.* 1994;170:419–424.

138. Vargas SL, Shenep JL, Flynn PM, Pui C-H, Santana VM, Hughes WT. Azithromycin for treatment of severe *Cryptosporidium* diarrhea in two children with cancer. *J Pediatr.* 1993;123:154–156.

139. Hong DK, Wong CJ, Gutierrez K. Severe cryptosporidiosis in a seven-year-old renal transplant recipient – case report and review of the literature. *Pediatr Transplant.* 2007;11:94–100.

140. Maggi P, Larocca AMV, Quarto G, et al. Effect of antiretroviral therapy on cryptosporidiosis and microsporidiosis in patients infected with human immunodeficiency virus type 1. *Eur J Clin Microbiol Infect Dis.* 2000;19:213–217.

141. Rossignol JF, Hidalgo H, Feregrino M, et al. A double blind placebo-controlled study if nitazoxanide in the treatment of cryptosporidial diarrhoea in AIDS patients in Mexico. *Trans R Soc Trop Med Hyg.* 1998;92:663–666.

142. Rossignol JF. Nitazoxanide in the treatment of acquired immune deficiency syndrome-related cryptosporidiosis: results of the United States compassionate use program in 365 patients. *Aliment Pharmacol Ther.* 2006;24:887–894.

143. Plettenberg A, Stoehr A, Stellbrink H-J, Albrecht H, Meigel W. A preparation from bovine colostrum in the treatment of HIV-positive patients with chronic diarrhoea. *Clin Investig.* 1993;71:42–45.

144. Shield J, Melville C, Novelli V, et al. Bovine colostrum immunoglobulin concentrate for cryptosporidiosis in AIDS. *Arch Dis Child.* 1993;69:451–453.

145. De Hovitz JA, Pape JW, Boncy M, Johnson WD. Clinical manifestations and therapy of *Isospora belli* infection in patients with the acquired immunodeficiency syndrome. *N Engl J Med.* 1986;315:87–90.

146. Ebrahimzadeh A, Bottone EJ. Persistent diarrhoea caused by *Isospora belli*: therapeutic response to pyrimethamine and sulfadiazine. *Diagnostic Microbiology and Infectious Diseases.* 1996;26:87–89.

147. Dionisio G, Sterrantino M, Meli M, Leoncini F, Orsi A, Nicoletti P. Treatment of isosporiasis with combined albendazole and ornidazole in patients with AIDS. *AIDS.* 1996;10:1301–1302.

148. Hoge CW, Shlim DR, Ghimire M, et al. Placebo-controlled trial of co-trimoxazole for *Cyclospora* infections among travellers and foreign residents in Nepal. *Lancet*. 1995;345:691–693.

149. Pape JW, Verdier RI, Boncy M, Bincy J, Johnson Jr WD. *Cyclospora* infection in adults infected with HIV. Clinical manifestations, treatment, and prophylaxis. *Ann Intern Med*. 1994;121:654–657.

150. Shlim DR, Pandey P, Rabold JG, Walch A, Rajah R. An open trial of trimethoprim alone against *Cyclospora* infections. *J Travel Med*. 1997;4:44–45.

151. Verdier R-I, Fitzgerald DW, Johnson WD, Pape JW. Trimethoprim–sulfamethoxazole compared with ciprofloxacin for treatment and prophylaxis of *Isospora belli* and *Cyclospora cayetanensis* infection in HIV-infected patients. *Ann Intern Med*. 2000;132:885–888.

152. Molina J-F, Chastang C, Goguel J, et al. Albendazole for treatment and prophylaxis of microsporidiosis due to *Encephalitozoon intestinalis* in patients with AIDS: a randomized double-blind controlled trial. *J Infect Dis*. 1998;177:1373–1378.

153. Conteas CN, Berlin L, Ash LR, Pruthi JS. Therapy for human gastrointestinal microsporidiosis. *Am J Trop Med Hyg*. 2000;63(3,4):121–127.

154. Sharpstone D, Rowbottom A, Francis N, et al. Thalidomide: a novel therapy for microsporidiosis. *Gastroenterology*. 1997;112:1823–1829.

155. Bicart-See A, Massip P, Linas M-D, Datry A. Successful treatment with nitazoxanide of *Enterocytozoon bieneusi* microsporidiosis in a patient with AIDS. *Antimicrob Agents Chemother*. 2000;44:167–168.

156. Van Hal SJ, Muthiah K, Matthews G, et al. Declining incidence of intestinal microsporidiosis and reduction of AIDS-related mortality following introduction of HAART in Sydney, Australia. *Trans R Soc Trop Med Hyg*. 2007;101:1096–1100.

157. Raoult D, Soulayrol L, Toga B, Dumon H, Casanovna P. Babesiosis, pentamidine and cotrimoxazole. *Ann Intern Med*. 1987;107:944.

158. Brasseur P, Gorenflot A. Human babesiosis in Europe. *Mem Inst Oswaldo Cruz*. 1992;87:131–132.

159. Pudney M, Gray JS. Therapeutic efficacy of atovaquone against the bovine intraerythrocytic parasite. *Babesia divergens Journal of Parasitology*. 1997;83:307–310.

160. Telford III SR, Gorenflot A, Brasseur P, Spielman A. Babesial infections in humans and wildlife. In: Krier JP, Baker JR, eds. *Parasitic protozoa*. Vol. 5. 2nd ed. San Diego: Academic Press; 1993:1–47.

161. Jacoby GA, Hunt JV, Kosinski KS, et al. Treatment of transfusion-transmitted babesiosis by exchange transfusion. *N Engl J Med*. 1980;303:1098–1100.

162. Krause PJ, Lepore T, Sikand VK, et al. Atovaquone and azithromycin for the treatment of babesiosis. *N Engl J Med*. 2000;343:1454–1458.

163. Ranque S. The treatment of babesiosis. *N Engl J Med*. 2001;344:773–774.

Further information

Dombrowski MP, Sokol RJ, Brown WJ, Bronsteen RA. Intravenous therapy of metronidazole-resistant *Trichomonas vaginalis*. *Obstet Gynecol*. 1987;69:524–525.

Hughes WT, Oz HS. Successful prevention and treatment of babesiosis with atovaquone. *J Infect Dis*. 1995;172:1042–1046.

Keiser J, Stich A, Burri C. New drugs for the treatment of human African trypanosomiasis: research and development. *Trends Parasitol*. 2001;17:42–49.

Pepin J, Khonde N, Maiso F, et al. Short-course eflornithine in Gambian trypanosomiasis: a randomized controlled trial. *Bull World Health Org*. 2000;78:1284–1295.

Roemer E, Blau W, Basara N, et al. Toxoplasmosis, a severe complication in allogeneic haematopoietic stem cell transplantation: successful treatment strategies during a 5-year single-center experience. *Clin Infect Dis*. 2001;32:E1–E8.

United States Public Health Service/Infectious Diseases Society of America Prevention of Opportunistic Infections Working Group 2000. USPHS/IDSA guidelines for the prevention of opportunistic infections in persons infected with human immunodeficiency virus. *Clin Infect Dis*. 1999;30(suppl 1):S29–S65.

Weiss LM, Wittner M, Wasserman S, Oz HS, Retsema J, Tanowitz HB. Efficacy of azithromycin for treating *Babesia microti* infection in the hamster model. *J Infect Dis*. 1993;168:1289–1292.

Weller IVD, Williams IG. ABC of AIDS. Treatment of infections. *Br Med J*. 2001;322:1350–1354.

64 Helminthic infections

Tim O'Dempsey

Helminths are complex, multicellular, parasitic worms occupying a wide variety of geographical, ecological and anatomical niches. They are classified into three groups: nematodes (roundworms), platyhelminths (flatworms, including trematodes and cestodes) and annelids (segmented worms, including leeches) (Table 64.1). Their life cycles vary in complexity. Some, for example *Enterobius vermicularis*, are principally dependent upon their human host, while others, such as the hepatic and intestinal flukes, require two intermediate hosts to complete their life cycle. Pathological effects in humans may be caused by the adult worms, egg deposition in tissues, or migration and death of larvae or microfilariae. Most infections are asymptomatic. Clinical disease is more likely in those who are immunologically naive following substantial initial exposure, in heavy infections and in people who are immunosuppressed or malnourished.

Helminthic infections are a major cause of morbidity and mortality worldwide and are prominent among the so-called neglected tropical diseases (NTDs).[1] The NTDs include schistosomiasis and the 'soil transmitted helminths' (STH), a group of parasites whose life cycle usually depends on a period of development outside the human host, typically in moist, warm soil. The most important STH are *Ascaris lumbricoides*, *Trichuris trichiura* and the hookworms (*Necator americanus* and *Ancylostoma duodenale*). Unprecedented efforts are now being made to control or eradicate these infections by means of health education, improved hygiene and sanitation, provision of safe water, vector control, and selective and mass chemotherapy using a limited repertoire of safe and effective anthelmintic agents (Table 64.2).

Recently, nitazoxanide, a thiazolide compound, has been shown to be well tolerated and effective in the treatment of a wide range of helminthic and other gastrointestinal infections, including *Ascaris lumbricoides*, *Strongyloides stercoralis*, *Trichuris trichiura*, *Enterobius vermicularis*, *Taenia saginata*, *Hymenolepis nana* and *Fasciola hepatica*.[2]

INTESTINAL HELMINTHS

INTESTINAL NEMATODE INFECTIONS

ASCARIASIS

Ascaris lumbricoides, the most common roundworm infection in humans, affects over 1 billion people worldwide. The peak prevalence and intensity of infection are among children aged 3–8 years. Infection follows ingestion of eggs contaminating vegetables, soil or dust. Larvae, liberated as the eggs pass through the stomach and small intestine, penetrate the intestinal mucosa and enter blood and lymphatic vessels. A proportion reaches the lungs 4–16 days after infection. After penetrating the alveoli and molting, they migrate via the respiratory tract to the esophagus and are carried to the small intestine. Here they develop into adults, mate and start producing eggs 6–8 weeks after infection. Adults grow to a length of 15–35 cm and may survive for 1–2 years. Females are capable of producing 200 000 eggs per day. The eggs are excreted in feces and their ova mature into infective embryos within 1–4 weeks. Eggs may remain viable in soil for years.

Migration of larvae through the lungs may cause fever, cough, dyspnea, wheeze and urticaria. Chest pain and cyanosis occur in more severe cases and sputum may be slightly blood-stained. Chest radiographic abnormalities range from discrete densities to diffuse interstitial, or more confluent, infiltrates. *Ascaris* pneumonitis, when accompanied by eosinophilia, is known as Löffler's syndrome. The episode usually subsides spontaneously within 10 days.

Adult intestinal worms are rarely noticed unless passed in the stool. In heavy infections the worms may intertwine to form a bolus, causing intestinal obstruction, volvulus or

Table 64.1 Clinically important helminths and their principal modes of infection

Helminth (common name)	Principal mode of infection
Intestinal helminthes	
Nematodes:	
Ascaris lumbricoides (roundworm)	Ingestion of egg
Enterobius vermicularis (pinworm/threadworm)	Ingestion of egg
Trichuris trichiura (whipworm)	Ingestion of egg
Ancylostoma duodenale (hookworm)	Larval penetration of skin
Necator americanus (hookworm)	Larval penetration of skin
Strongyloides spp.	Larval penetration of skin
Cestodes:	
Taenia saginata, Taenia solium (beef/pork tapeworm)	Ingestion of cyst
Diphyllobothrium latum (fish tapeworm)	Ingestion of plerocercoid larva
Larval helminths	
Nematodes:	
Trichinella spp. (trichinosis)	Ingestion of cyst
Toxocara spp. (toxocariasis)	Ingestion of egg
Cestodes:	
Taenia solium (cysticercosis)	Ingestion of egg
Echinococcus granulosus (hydatid cyst)	Ingestion of egg
Echinococcus multilocularis (alveolar hydatid)	Ingestion of egg
Trematodes (flukes)	
Schistosoma spp. (bilharzia)	Cercarial penetration of skin
Paragonimus spp. (lung fluke)	Ingestion of metacercariae
Fasciolopsis buski (intestinal fluke)	Ingestion of metacercariae
Fasciola hepatica, Fasciola gigantica (liver flukes)	Ingestion of metacercariae
Opisthorchis sinensis, O. viverrini (oriental liver flukes)	Ingestion of metacercariae
Filarial nematodes	Infective larvae from:
Onchocerca volvulus (river blindness)	Bite of *Simulium* (black fly)
Loa loa (loiasis, eye worm)	Bite of *Chrysops* (red fly)
Dracunculus medinensis (Guinea worm)	Ingestion of L3 larva within *Cyclops*
Wuchereria bancrofti, Brugia malayi, Brugia timori (lymphatic filariasis)	Bite of various mosquitoes

Table 64.2 Side effects of selected anthelmintic agents

Anthelmintic agent	Frequent side effects	Occasional side effects	Rare side effects
Albendazole		Abdominal pain, reversible alopecia, increased transaminases, headache	Leukopenia, rash, renal toxicity, fever
Diethylcarbamazine citrate	Mazzotti reaction with onchocerciasis	Gastrointestinal disturbances, hypersensitivity reactions	Encephalopathy, renal failure (especially in patients with loiasis and high microfilaria counts)
Ivermectin		Gastrointestinal disturbances	Mazzotti reaction in onchocerciasis, encephalopathy in loiasis, transient postural hypotension
Levamisole	Nausea, diarrhea, altered taste	Dermatitis, alopecia, arthralgia, blood dyscrasias, myalgia, bone pain, depression, dizziness, headache, stomatitis, vomiting	Ataxia, visual disturbance, hepatitis, paresthesia, convulsions, tardive dyskinesia, tremors
Mebendazole		Gastrointestinal disturbances, headache	Hypersensitivity reactions, hypospermia, leukopenia, agranulocytosis
Niclosamide	Gastrointestinal disturbances, dizziness, pruritus		
Nitazoxanide		Abdominal pain, diarrhea, vomiting, headache	Hypotension, tachyarrhythmias, hepatitis, anemia, menorrhagia, myalgia, urinary symptoms and discoloration
Oxamniquine		Headache, fever, dizziness, nausea, vomiting, hepatitis, insomnia, hallucinations, orange discoloration of urine	Convulsions
Piperazine		Gastrointestinal disturbances, hypersensitivity reactions	Stevens–Johnson syndrome, angioedema, ataxia ('worm wobble'), drowsiness, confusion, convulsions in patients with neurological/renal abnormalities
Praziquantel		Gastrointestinal disturbances, headache, dizziness, sedation, fever	Pruritus, rash, edema, hiccups
Pyrantel pamoate		Gastrointestinal disturbances, dizziness, rash, fever	
Thiabendazole	Gastrointestinal disturbances, vertigo, headache, drowsiness, pruritus	Leukopenia, crystalluria, rash, neuropsychiatric disturbances, erythema multiforme	Shock, tinnitus, intrahepatic cholestasis, convulsions, angioneurotic edema, Stevens–Johnson syndrome

perforation. Migrating worms may obstruct ducts or diverticuli causing biliary colic, cholangitis, liver abscess, pancreatitis or appendicitis. A well-known hazard of anesthesia is endotracheal tube obstruction by a wandering ascaris. Cases of pneumothorax and pericarditis have also been reported.[3]

Diagnosis and treatment

Ascaris pneumonitis is diagnosed on clinical grounds; the presence or absence of eggs in the stools is irrelevant. Larvae may be found in the sputum. Stool examination for eggs is the standard method for diagnosing established infection, although stools may be negative if infection is entirely due to male worms. Worms may also be identified on barium studies, ultrasonography and endoscopy.

Albendazole 400 mg in a single oral dose eliminates most infections. In heavy infections this may need to be repeated for 2–3 days. The recommended dose in children aged 1–2 years is 200 mg. Mebendazole 100 mg orally every 12 h for 3 days is also effective, although use in children under 2 years is not recommended by the manufacturer. There are also reports of ectopic migration of *Ascaris* following the use of mebendazole.

Piperazine 75 mg/kg (to a maximum of 3.5 g for adults and children over 12 years and a maximum of 2.5 g for children aged 2–12 years) is also effective. As side effects are relatively common and may be serious, piperazine should be used only if safer alternatives are unavailable. Pyrantel pamoate (11 mg/kg up to a maximum of 1 g) can be given as a single dose. Pyrantel and piperazine have antagonistic effects and should never be prescribed concurrently.

Levamisole 2.5–3 mg/kg (max. 150 mg) for children 1 month to 18 years, 120–150 mg for adults, as a single dose is also highly effective. Nitazoxanide given orally every 12 h for 3 days is also effective in the following doses: adults and children >12 years, 500 mg; children aged 4–11 years, 200 mg; children aged 1–3 years, 100 mg.

Intestinal ascariasis should be treated with an anthelmintic agent. Intestinal obstruction may respond to conservative management with nasogastric aspiration, intravenous fluids and antispasmodics, followed by an anthelmintic when the obstruction has subsided. Laparotomy is required if this fails or if the patient is seriously ill. Manipulation of the worms through the ileocecal valve may be possible without having to open the bowel. Surgical or endoscopic removal of single worms blocking ducts should be reserved for patients who fail to respond to anthelmintic treatment and those with persisting pain or raised serum amylase.[4] *Ascaris* pneumonitis is generally managed symptomatically using bronchodilators and steroids if indicated. The use of anthelmintics is questionable as symptoms of pneumonitis may be exacerbated by larval death.

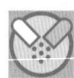 ## TRICHURIASIS

Trichuris trichiura, the whipworm, infects about 900 million people worldwide. Following ingestion of eggs in contaminated soil, food or fomites, larvae emerge in the cecum, penetrate the crypts of Lieberkün and migrate within the mucosal epithelium. The adult matures and remains partly embedded in the mucosa of the cecum and ascending colon, or throughout the colon in heavy infections.

Most infections go unnoticed; however, heavy infections may cause severe gastrointestinal symptoms. The friable mucosa bleeds easily, resulting in iron deficiency anemia in children on marginal diets. Chronic trichuris colitis is associated with growth retardation. Severe trichuris dysentery syndrome frequently leads to rectal prolapse.

Diagnosis and treatment

Diagnosis may be obvious on identifying adult worms attached to the mucosa of prolapsed bowel. In less dramatic circumstances, the characteristic eggs may be identified in the stool, by concentration techniques if necessary for light infections. Trichuriasis may cause a significant eosinophilia.

A single oral dose of mebendazole 500 mg appears to be more effective than albendazole 400 mg.[5] Severe infections require either mebendazole 100 mg every 12 h for 3 days or albendazole 400 mg/day for 3 days. Single-dose combination treatment using albendazole 400 mg plus ivermectin 200 μg/kg is also highly effective.[6]

 ## HOOKWORM

Ancyl. duodenale and *Necator americanus* are the principal hookworms infecting humans, affecting 900 million people worldwide. Both species are widely distributed in tropical Africa and Asia. *N. americanus* is the most common species in the Americas; *Ancyl. duodenale* also occurs in the Middle East, North Africa, southern Europe, the Caribbean, and Central and South America.

Hookworm eggs passed in the feces hatch in soil in warm, moist conditions, liberating rhabditiform larvae. These subsequently develop into filariform larvae, which inhabit the surface layer of soil. When these larvae come into contact with the skin of the human host, they penetrate via fissures or hair follicles and are carried in the venous circulation to the lungs. Here they penetrate the alveoli and migrate to the pharynx. They are then carried into the small intestine where they mature into adults. Rarely, infection with *Ancyl. duodenale* may occur following ingestion of larvae on contaminated vegetables. Infantile hookworm disease has been described in China and attributed to transmammary transmission, laying infants on contaminated soil, or using nappies made of cloth bags stuffed with infected soil.

Adult hookworms attach themselves to the upper half of the small intestine and feed on blood. An adult *Ancyl. duodenale* may consume between 0.15 and 0.26 mL/day; *N. americanus* consumes a relatively modest 0.03 mL/day. Blood loss also occurs at the site of attachment. Loss of plasma proteins may result in hypoproteinemia. In Africa and Asia, 30–54% of moderate and severe anemia in pregnancy is due to hookworm infection.

Initial infection is usually asymptomatic. Ground itch at the site of larval penetration when severe may be associated with the development of vesicles or pustules. Cutaneous larva migrans is sometimes seen. Larval migration through the lungs may give rise to a pneumonitis similar to that in ascariasis. Nausea, vomiting, pharyngeal irritation, cough, dyspnea and hoarseness (Wakana syndrome) may follow oral ingestion of *Ancyl. duodenale* larvae.

Occasionally, 4–6 weeks after infection, abdominal symptoms occur, including discomfort, flatulence, anorexia, nausea, vomiting and diarrhea, which may contain blood and mucus in heavy infections. Rarely, life-threatening gastrointestinal hemorrhage occurs in young children with severe primary infections.

Most chronic infections are asymptomatic. Problems arise when iron intake is low or demands are high. A gradually worsening iron deficiency anemia develops, often associated with hypoalbuminemia and edema, and eventually progresses to cardiac failure.

Diagnosis and treatment

Diagnosis is made by identification of the characteristic eggs in the stool. Concentration techniques may be necessary for lighter infections. Culture techniques similar to those used for strongyloides may also be helpful. If stool samples are left for a few days before examination, eggs may hatch liberating larvae that may be mistaken for strongyloides, although they are morphologically distinct. Mixed infections may also occur.

Albendazole 400 mg as a single dose is more effective than mebendazole 100 mg every 12 h for 3 days.[7] Pyrantel pamoate 11 mg/kg (maximum 1 g) as a single dose is also effective. Treatment for iron-deficiency anemia may be indicated. Transfusion is rarely essential.

OTHER HOOKWORM INFECTIONS

Cutaneous larva migrans

Humans are accidental hosts in this infection caused by the larvae of the dog or cat hookworm, most commonly *Ancyl. braziliense*. Larvae penetrate the skin and migrate in the dermis, their progress mapped by an itchy, erythematous, serpiginous rash. Blistering sometimes occurs. Unable to complete their life cycle, they wander about in the dermis for several weeks or months until they eventually die. Rarely, infection may trigger hypereosinophilia and pneumonitis.

Topical thiabendazole may suffice for infections involving a limited area. A paste made by grinding one 0.5 g thiabendazole tablet in 5 g of petroleum jelly is applied every 8–12 h over the track, extending 1–2 cm beyond the leading edge. An occlusive dressing containing thiabendazole paste enhances the effect. Oral thiabendazole was previously recommended for more severe infections; however, this has been superseded by albendazole 400 mg/day for 3 days. More recently, ivermectin 200 μg/kg as a single dose has been shown to be more effective and less toxic than albendazole. Repeated doses are sometimes required.[8]

Eosinophilic enteritis

This has been described in Australia following infection with the immature adult dog hookworm, *Ancyl. caninum*, which provokes an allergic reaction resulting in edema of the gut wall, ascites and regional lymphadenopathy. Ulceration may occur at the site of the hookworm bite. Enterobiasis and anisakiasis may also cause eosinophilic enteritis.

STRONGYLOIDIASIS

Strongyloidiasis affects 50–100 million people worldwide, occurring in warm, wet, tropical and subtropical regions and in suitable niches in temperate regions, where conditions are moist and sanitation poor. *Strongyloides stercoralis* is the predominant species affecting humans, although *Strongyloides füllebomi*, principally a parasite of primates, has also been found in humans in Africa and Papua New Guinea. Human infection follows cutaneous penetration by filariform larvae contaminating soil, in a similar manner to hookworm. Indeed, both parasites may be present in the same habitat. Filariform larvae are carried in the venous circulation to the lungs where they penetrate the alveoli, migrate to the pharynx and then travel to the small intestine. There they develop into adults that penetrate the duodenal and jejunal mucosa. Fertilized females produce embryonated eggs resembling those of hookworm, but these are rarely seen as they hatch in the intestinal mucosa, releasing the first-stage rhabditiform larvae characteristically found in the stool. In favorable soil conditions, the excreted rhabditiform larvae transform into infectious filariform larvae within 24–48 h, remaining viable in soil for a few weeks.

Autoinfection may occur if rhabditiform larvae rapidly transform into infectious dwarf filariform larvae in the lumen of the bowel. These penetrate the gut mucosa (internal autoinfection) or the perianal skin (external autoinfection). Infection may thus persist for decades without further external exposure. Person-to-person transmission has also been described.[9]

Larval penetration of the skin may result in ground itch, and an urticarial, serpiginous rash is sometimes observed.

Pneumonitis may be associated with larval migration. Initial invasion of the small bowel mucosa by adult worms may cause abdominal pain and, in heavy infections, vomiting, malabsorption and paralytic ileus. Chronic infection may be asymptomatic or cause intermittent episodes of abdominal discomfort, sometimes associated with diarrhea and urticaria. Some patients develop malabsorption. Larva currens ('creeping eruption') may appear transiently as an intensely itchy serpiginous wheal, usually on the trunk or buttocks. Strongyloides may also cause episodes of pneumonitis and, rarely, a reactive arthritis.

Strongyloides hyperinfection syndrome occurs as a result of massive autoinfection. Risk factors include immunosuppression associated with organ transplants, cytotoxic drug therapy, corticosteroid therapy,[10] ribavirin therapy for hepatitis C,[11] malignancies (particularly leukemia and lymphoma), severe malnutrition and severe infections. HIV infection does not appear to predispose to strongyloides hyperinfection syndrome, although hyperinfection may occur in debilitated patients with advanced AIDS. Human T-cell leukemia virus type 1 (HTLV-1) infection does, however, appear to be a significant risk factor for strongyloides hyperinfection syndrome.[12] Rarely, hyperinfection syndrome occurs in an immunocompetent individual. A severe protein-losing enteropathy may develop in debilitated patients. More commonly, in patients who are abruptly immunosuppressed, hyperinfection syndrome presents with severe diarrhea, often with blood. Bowel inflammation may be associated with microperforations and give rise to paralytic ileus accompanied by Gram-negative septicemia caused by enteric organisms. The condition is usually fatal if effective chemotherapy is delayed. Complications include meningitis, often caused by *Escherichia coli* and/or larvae of *S. stercoralis*; both organisms are often detected in cerebrospinal fluid (CSF). Larvae may be widely disseminated in the central nervous system (CNS) and elsewhere, causing microinfarcts. Additional complications include peritonitis, endocarditis and pneumonitis. All patients with a history of possible exposure should be screened for strongyloides before immunosuppression. Patients at high risk should be treated empirically even if investigations are negative.[13]

Diagnosis and treatment

Rhabditiform larvae may be difficult to identify in feces. Various concentration techniques have been advocated and fecal culture on damp charcoal or Harada–Mori culture on vertical strips of damp filter paper may be helpful, although culture on nutrient agar plates is now emerging as the preferred technique.[14] Larvae may be identified in duodenal aspirates or using the string capsule technique (Enterotest).

Serological tests (indirect fluorescent antibody test or enzyme-linked immunosorbent assay (ELISA)) are useful for patients who are not normally resident in an endemic area; however, cross-reactions with filarial antigens remain a problem. Strongyloidiasis in immunocompetent individuals is usually accompanied by an eosinophilia. Diagnosis in patients who are immunocompromised is more difficult. Eosinophilia is less likely and its absence is associated with a poorer prognosis. Serological tests are likely to be negative. It is essential to search carefully for larvae in feces or bowel aspirates. Larvae may also be found in sputum, CSF and urine.

Ivermectin is the drug of choice for strongyloidiasis. An oral dose of 200 µg/kg per day for 2 days gives excellent cure rates with few side effects.[15] Thiabendazole 25 mg/kg (maximum 1.5 g) orally every 12 h for 3 days is also effective, although it is advisable to repeat this after 1 week because of the difficulty in confirming eradication of infection. Side effects are common and may be serious. Albendazole has fewer side effects than thiabendazole. A course of 400 mg every 12 h for 7 days has been used with encouraging results.

Hyperinfection syndrome poses therapeutic difficulties. In patients who are able to absorb oral treatment, ivermectin given in a multidose schedule offers the greatest promise of success. Patients who are unable to absorb oral therapy present a difficult challenge as no parenteral preparations of thiabendazole, albendazole or ivermectin are licensed for use in humans. However, parenteral ivermectin, available as a veterinary preparation, has been administered subcutaneously in the successful treatment of two patients with strongyloides hyperinfection.[16] Patients with hyperinfection syndrome may also require treatment for Gram-negative septicemia.

ENTEROBIASIS

Enterobius vermicularis, the pinworm or threadworm, occurs worldwide and is the most common helminthic infection in Western Europe and the USA, although, strictly speaking, it is not a soil transmitted helminth. Infection follows ingestion of the egg on contaminated food or fomites. Autoinfection occurs when perianal irritation caused by migration of gravid female worms results in scratching and transmission of eggs from anus to mouth on fingertips. Secondary bacterial infection may occur at the site of excoriation. Vulvovaginitis, enuresis, urinary tract infection and appendicitis may also be associated with *E. vermicularis*. Infection may be accompanied by mild eosinophilia.

Diagnosis and treatment

Diagnosis is usually made by collecting eggs from the perianal region using adhesive tape or a moist cotton swab. Eggs may appear in urine samples from girls.

Mebendazole, albendazole and piperazine all achieve cure rates above 90%. Mebendazole 100 mg is given as a single oral dose, repeated 2–4 weeks later. Albendazole 400 mg as a single oral dose is repeated after 7 days for adults and children over 2 years. A dose of 100 mg should be used in children aged less than 2 years. Piperazine is effective but must be given daily for 7 days and repeated after 2–4 weeks. It has been superseded by mebendazole and albendazole. Pyrantel pamoate 11 mg base/kg (maximum dose 1 g) orally as a single dose repeated after 2 weeks is also effective.

Family members and other close contacts are likely to be infected and it is usual to recommend their treatment simultaneously, except for pregnant women during the first trimester.

INTESTINAL CESTODE INFECTIONS (TAPEWORMS)

Tapeworms are flattened, segmented, hermaphroditic worms ranging in length from 10 mm to 20 m. The head (scolex) attaches to the intestinal mucosa by means of suckers or hooklets. All, with the exception of *Hymenolepis nana*, require a secondary intermediate host in which the larvae develop into cysts, usually in muscle. Human infection follows consumption of undercooked meat or fish. Larval cestode infections may also occur in humans following the ingestion of the egg, the most important being cysticercosis.

TAENIASIS

Taenia saginata, the beef tapeworm, and *Taenia solium*, the pork tapeworm, are the most common tapeworms affecting humans. Infection follows consumption of undercooked beef or pork containing cysts. *T. saginata* cysts may occur in other domestic bovines and a closely related Asian species has been shown to infect pigs, ungulates and monkeys. *T. solium* cysts also occur in dogs and cats. A third species of human *Taenia*, *T. asiatica*, which is also transmitted in pigs, has recently been described in Asia where prevalence rates of up to 20% have been documented among Indonesian villagers.

Most infections are asymptomatic, the host only becoming aware when a proglottid segment is noticed in feces or felt as it passes through the anus. Gastrointestinal symptoms may include loss of appetite, nausea or vague abdominal pain. A patient who is vomiting profusely, for whatever reason, may be further distressed when several meters of tapeworm appear in the vomit. Rarely, complications arise following migration of proglottids to unusual sites, such as the appendix or pancreatic and bile ducts.

DIPHYLLOBOTHRIASIS

The most common of the 13 or more species of fish tapeworm affecting humans is *Diphyllobothrium latum*. Human infection follows ingestion of undercooked or raw fish or roe. Most infections involve a single worm and are asymptomatic or associated with vague, non-specific abdominal symptoms. Megaloblastic anemia may occur, resembling pernicious anemia in severe cases.

HYMENOLEPIASIS AND DIPYLIDIASIS

Hymenolepis nana, the dwarf tapeworm, occurs worldwide, principally among children. Most infections are asymptomatic, but heavy infections may cause abdominal pain, nausea, vomiting, pruritus ani and diarrhea, sometimes containing blood. Headache, dizziness, sleep and behavior disturbances are frequent. Convulsions have also been reported. Autoinfection is common.

Hymenolepis diminuta, the rat tapeworm, may affect humans who ingest the intermediate host, usually a weevil, flea or cockroach. Most infections are asymptomatic and of short duration.

Dipylidium caninum infection may occur in humans, usually young infants, following accidental ingestion of a flea, the intermediate host of this cestode whose usual host is a dog or other carnivore. Most infections are asymptomatic. Some children experience abdominal pain, diarrhea, pruritus ani and urticaria.

Diagnosis and treatment

Diagnosis is usually made by identification of characteristic eggs or proglottids in feces. There may be a variable eosinophilia, minimal in cases of *T. saginata* and often reaching 5–10% in hymenolepiasis.

Praziquantel is the drug of choice for all of the above intestinal cestode infections. A single oral dose of 10 mg/kg is usually effective. *H. nana* requires 25 mg/kg as a single dose. Praziquantel should be used with caution in populations in which cysticercosis is common, as there is a possibility of precipitating or aggravating symptoms. Niclosamide, given as a single oral dose of 2 g for adults, is also effective. Doses for children are 500 mg if <10 kg, 1 g if 11–34 kg and 1.5 g if >34 kg. Tablets should be chewed well and swallowed with water. There is no clinical evidence to justify the routine use of purgatives and antiemetics in patients with *T. solium* before cestocidal treatment, in order to prevent retrograde peristalsis of eggs and possible risk of cysticercosis.

LARVAL HELMINTHIC INFECTIONS

CYSTICERCOSIS

Neurocysticercosis is the most common parasitic infection of the CNS and the main cause of adult-onset epilepsy worldwide. Cysticercosis occurs following ingestion of eggs of *T. solium* and can occur in strict vegetarians or those who avoid eating pork for religious reasons. The onchosphere is liberated in the upper intestinal tract, penetrates the mucosa and enters the mesenteric vessels and lymphatics. Dissemination then occurs throughout the body and cysts develop in the tissues.

Living cysts usually provoke little or no immunological reaction. Clinical symptoms are more likely to arise as a result of the inflammatory response to dying cysticerci. Calcification eventually occurs at the site of dead cysticerci. Two forms of cysticerci – parenchymal and racemose – are found in the CNS. Racemose cysticerci are uncommon in children and are associated with a poorer prognosis.

Most infections are asymptomatic. The most common clinical presentations occur with neurocysticercosis and include epilepsy, symptoms of raised intracranial pressure, psychiatric disturbances, dementia, encephalitis, chronic meningitis, cranial nerve palsies and symptoms due to spinal cord lesions. Learning difficulties, behavior changes and psychomotor involution may be additional presenting symptoms in children.[17] Cysticerci may develop in the eye, most commonly in the retina, but sometimes are free floating in the anterior or posterior chamber. Subcutaneous cysticerci are present in about 50% of cases of neurocysticercosis. Cysticerci in muscles may result in increased muscle bulk and weakness. Cardiac involvement may also occur.

Diagnosis and treatment

Serological diagnosis is possible using an enzyme-linked immunoelectrotransfer blot (EITB) or ELISA.[18,19] CSF may be normal or white cells (lymphocytes or eosinophils) raised to a variable extent. Glucose may be reduced. Total protein and IgG may be elevated and the EITB may be positive. Single ring-enhancing intracranial lesions are often negative using currently available immunodiagnostic techniques. Subcutaneous nodules can be biopsied. Ophthalmoscopy may reveal ocular cysts. Calcified cysts may be evident on X-ray films in muscle and other tissue. MRI is superior to CT in diagnosing neurocysticercosis if cysts are still viable. CT is better for demonstration of calcified cysts.

Praziquantel (50–100 mg/kg per day in three divided doses for 15 days) and albendazole (400 mg every 12 h for adults or 15 mg/kg every 12 h for children for 8–30 days) may be used alone or in combination in the treatment of viable cysts. The inflammatory response to dying cysticerci may precipitate or exacerbate symptoms. Simultaneous administration of steroids is usually advised to mitigate the inflammatory response.[20] The bioavailability of albendazole and praziquantel are increased with cimetidine.[21,22]

A recent meta-analysis showed that treatment with cysticidal drugs results in better resolution of enhancing lesions and cysts, lower risk of recurrence of seizures in patients with enhancing lesions, and a reduction in the rate of generalized seizures in patients with viable cysts.[23] Therefore, a full course anthelmintic therapy is now recommended for patients with active parenchymal neurocysticercosis. Single-dose praziquantel treatment may be adequate for patients who have single brain-enhancing lesions and positive serology.[24] Patients with inactive parenchymal disease do not require anthelmintic treatment. In either circumstance, anticonvulsants may be indicated and, in some cases, neurosurgical intervention may be required. Extraparenchymal cysts may require treatment with combinations of antiparasitic drugs, steroids and, possibly, surgery, depending on the number, size, location and complications.

Ophthalmic cysticercosis is usually treated surgically. Muscular and subcutaneous cysticercosis infections generally do not require treatment. However, if anticysticercal drugs are used, steroids or non-steroidal anti-inflammatory drugs may also be required.

HYDATIDOSIS

The larval stage of the canine tapeworm, *Echinococcus granulosus*, causes cystic hydatid disease in humans. The disease is prevalent in sheep-rearing areas throughout the world. Dogs and other carnivores are the definitive host for the adult tapeworm. Sheep and other domestic livestock become infected after ingesting ova shed in dog feces, following which hydatid cysts develop in the viscera of the infected animal. The cycle is completed when dogs ingest cysts in offal and other infected tissues. Human infection follows the accidental ingestion of eggs in dog feces. The ingested egg releases an onchosphere which penetrates the intestinal wall and is carried in the circulation to a variety of tissues, most commonly the liver and lungs.

Symptoms are usually either due to a mass effect produced by the growing cyst or occur as a result of leakage of fluid from a cyst. Hepatic cysts are more frequent in the right lobe and are usually asymptomatic until they become large. A nontender mass may be evident on examination. Secondary bacterial infection of a cyst may mimic a liver abscess. Rupture may be spontaneous, traumatic or occur during surgery, precipitating a hypersensitivity reaction ranging from urticaria, pruritus and fever to fatal anaphylaxis. Rupture into the peritoneal cavity may lead to seeding and the development of secondary cysts. Rupture into the biliary tree may cause colic, urticaria and obstructive jaundice, sometimes complicated by secondary bacterial infection.

Most lung cysts are asymptomatic, often being found incidentally on a chest radiograph. Patients may experience fever, dyspnea, chest pain and cough, sometimes with hemoptysis or productive of clear salty-tasting liquid. Collapsed cysts have a characteristic 'water lily' appearance on chest radiographs. Patients may cough up the soft, white outer membrane of the cyst. Rupture into the lung may cause a hypersensitivity reaction, or result in pneumothorax and empyema. A lung abscess may develop at the site of a cyst. Seeding of pulmonary cysts is uncommon.

Hydatid cysts occur at a variety of other sites including spleen, bone (causing pain and pathological fracture), brain (causing convulsions or a mass effect) and eye (causing proptosis and chemosis).

Diagnosis and treatment

Abdominal ultrasound is useful for detecting abdominal cysts; radiography, CT or MRI may be useful for detecting cysts elsewhere. Of the serological tests available, the specific IgG ELISA AgB (antigen-B-rich fraction) is the most sensitive.[25] Others include an EITB assay and the double diffusion test for arc 5 (DD5). All lack sensitivity for extrahepatic cysts and DD5 may give false-positive results in patients with cysticercosis. Urine antigen detection tests are promising.[26] Eosinophilia may follow leakage or rupture of a cyst.

Until recently, surgical removal was the preferred method of managing accessible cysts and remains the recommended treatment for cysts >10 cm diameter, for infected cysts and for cysts in the brain, lung or kidney.[27] Surgical removal of hydatid cysts requires great care to avoid spillage. Before removal, large cysts are carefully aspirated and the aspirate replaced with an equivalent volume of hypertonic saline, a scolicide. Puncture, aspiration, injection and reaspiration (PAIR) of cysts under ultrasound control is now used increasingly as an alternative to surgery.[28] Following initial aspiration, hypertonic saline is injected into the cyst and reaspirated after 20 min. PAIR plus chemotherapy is associated with lower morbidity, mortality and disease recurrence rates, and shorter hospital stays.[29]

Small cysts can be surgically removed intact. Laparoscopic treatment of hydatid cysts of the liver and spleen is also effective.[30]

Albendazole, either alone or in combination with praziquantel, should be given for 1–3 months prior to surgery or PAIR. Patients undergoing surgery or percutaneous aspiration should receive concomitant albendazole, either alone or in combination with praziquantel. PAIR should be followed by an 8-week course of albendazole. Anthelmintic treatment may reduce the need for surgery in patients with uncomplicated pulmonary cysts.[31]

Albendazole is useful for patients with inoperable, widespread or numerous cysts and in patients who are unfit for surgery. The recommended regimen is a now 400 mg every 12 h for adults, or 5–7.5 mg/kg every 12 h for children, for 3–12 months depending on response. Monthly treatment interruptions are no longer recommended.[32] Absorption of albendazole is enhanced when taken with fatty meals. A combination of albendazole and praziquantel has been shown to have greater protoscolicidal activity in animal studies and in vitro than either drug alone.[33,34] Combination therapy has been used with success in treating inoperable spinal, pelvic, abdominal, thoracic and hepatic hydatidosis.[35]

ALVEOLAR HYDATID DISEASE

Echinococcus multilocularis is a tapeworm of foxes, wild canines, dogs and cats. Rodents are the usual intermediate hosts. The disease is endemic in North America, Europe, Siberia and China. Human infection follows ingestion of the egg in a similar manner to infection with *E. granulosus*. Unlike cystic hydatid disease, lesions caused by *E. multilocularis* are ill defined and more solid than cystic, developing in the manner of a slowly growing, invasive malignant tumor: it may be 30 years before a patient becomes symptomatic. The primary site of tissue invasion is usually the liver, although metastatic lesions may occur in other tissues.

Clinical presentation is usually with right upper quadrant pain, hepatomegaly and a palpable mass. Complications as a result of local invasion or due to metastatic lesions involving brain, lung or mediastinum occur in around 2% of patients. Untreated, 90% of patients die within 10 years of presentation; however, a 90% 10-year survival rate is possible with early diagnosis and appropriate treatment.

Diagnosis and treatment

Ultrasonography, CT and serology are useful in establishing the diagnosis. Histology provides confirmation. Surgical excision is the treatment of choice for the primary lesion. Pre- and postoperative treatment with albendazole is recommended. Treatment with albendazole 10–15 mg/kg is recommended postoperatively and for inoperable patients. In practice, a dose of 400 mg every 12 h is usual for adults. The optimal duration of treatment remains uncertain; patients often remain on treatment for more than 12 months. Albendazole at these doses has been used for up to 20 years; higher doses of 20 mg/kg per day have been used for up to 4.5 years.[32] Mebendazole, 40–50 mg/kg per day, has also been used extensively, sometimes for up to 10 years. Serology may remain positive for several years following successful treatment.

TRICHINOSIS

Several species of *Trichinella* cause disease in humans, affecting about 50 million worldwide. The best known, *Trichinella spiralis*, occurs widely; most of the others are limited to particular geographical niches. Human infection follows consumption of larval cysts in raw or undercooked meat, especially pork. Larvae liberated in the stomach pass into the duodenum, where they burrow into the mucosa and develop into adults. Female worms produce larvae which seed throughout the body, particularly in skeletal and cardiac muscle, and form cysts invoking an inflammatory response. Cysts begin to calcify within 6–12 months, resulting in death of the encysted larvae.

Clinical symptoms may occur at the time of initial larval invasion and development in the intestinal mucosa. Early symptoms are more likely with heavy infection and include abdominal pain, anorexia, nausea, vomiting and diarrhea, sometimes accompanied by fever, headache and malaise. Systemic symptoms tend to occur a week or more after infection, when seeding of larvae in the tissues is associated with fever, headache, myalgia and malaise. Urticaria, conjunctivitis, periorbital and facial edema may be evident. Muscles become swollen and tender. Patients may experience cough, hoarseness, dyspnea and dysphagia. Splinter hemorrhages may be present. Myocarditis may develop 4–8 weeks after infection. Pericardial effusions are the most common manifestation of cardiac involvement.[36] Congestive cardiac failure and arrhythmias also occur. Larvae migrating through the CNS may cause a wide range of focal or generalized neurological symptoms including meningoencephalitis and psychosis. Convalescence may be prolonged with persisting myalgia, fatigue and headaches.

Diagnosis and treatment

There is usually a marked eosinophilia and raised creatinine phosphokinase, lactic dehydrogenase, aldolase and aminotransferase levels, reflecting muscle damage. Myocarditis should not be assumed on the basis of elevated creatinine phosphokinase isoenzyme-MB as this has been found in patients without clinical or other evidence of cardiac involvement. The most useful serological test for clinical purposes is the ELISA–IgG. Tissue diagnosis can be made from skeletal muscle biopsy using compression and histological techniques.

Either mebendazole 100 mg every 12 h for 5 days or albendazole 400 mg/day for 3 days is effective in the early intestinal stage of infection. Patients with severe symptoms associated with larval seeding should be treated with prednisolone 40–60 mg/day plus either albendazole 400 mg every 12 h for 8–14 days or mebendazole 200–400 mg every 8 h for 3 days, then 400–500 mg every 8 h for 10 days.

TOXOCARIASIS

Toxocara canis and *Toxocara cati* are parasitic roundworms of dogs and cats. Infection in humans is most common in young children, who ingest eggs in sand or soil contaminated by dog or cat feces. Clinical disease is relatively uncommon and depends on the intensity of infection and the organs involved.

Visceral larva migrans is caused by migrating larvae and includes symptoms of pneumonitis, fever, abdominal pain, myalgia, sleep and behavior disturbances, and focal or generalized convulsions. Lymphadenopathy and hepatosplenomegaly may be evident. Eosinophilia, anemia, hypergammaglobulinemia and elevated titers of blood group isohemagglutinins are common. Serological diagnosis may be established by ELISA. The drug of choice is albendazole 5–10 mg/kg or, for adults, 400 mg, every 12 h for 5 days. Alternatively, mebendazole 100–200 mg every 12 h for 5 days may be used but is inferior to albendazole. Symptomatic treatment with bronchodilators, steroids or antihistamines may also be indicated.

Ocular larva migrans is more likely to occur in light infections. A single larva invades the eye, provoking a granulomatous reaction, usually in the retina. This may result in visual disturbance or blindness in the affected eye, which may go unnoticed or present as strabismus. The diagnosis is sometimes made by chance on routine ophthalmoscopy. The usual appearance is of chorioretinitis with a mass lesion, sometimes mistaken for a retinoblastoma. Serology is usually positive. Antibody detection in vitreous fluid is more sensitive and specific. Management of acute ocular larva migrans is directed at suppressing the inflammatory response with topical or systemic steroids. Anthelmintics are often used concurrently, although there is no consistent evidence of additional benefit. Destruction of the larva is possible using laser photocoagulation. Steroids may be useful in exacerbations of chronic ocular larva migrans. Surgery is often required for adhesions.

MISCELLANEOUS TISSUE HELMINTHS

GNATHOSTOMIASIS

Gnathostoma spinigerum and related species occur principally in South East Asia. Human infection follows ingestion of larvae in raw or undercooked flesh from certain fish, frogs, snails, snakes, chicken and pigs. Infection can also be acquired from contaminated water. Acute gnathostomiasis is associated with fever, abdominal pain, tender hepatomegaly, pneumonitis, rashes (including a serpiginous rash resembling cutaneous larva migrans) and painless or pruritic subcutaneous swellings caused by migrating immature adult worms. Eosinophilia is usually marked. Invasion of the eye may result in subconjunctival hemorrhage and edema. Eosinophilic myeloencephalitis is an important and characteristic complication arising when the worm migrates along a large nerve trunk and invades the CNS, causing a radiculomyelitis, radiculomyeloencephalitis or subarachnoid hemorrhage. Migratory CNS lesions can be detected using MRI.[37] CSF may be bloody or xanthochromic with a raised white cell count, of which >20% are usually eosinophils. Highly sensitive and specific immunodiagnostic tests are available for use with serum or CSF, including ELISA and Western blot. Definitive diagnosis requires identification of the worm.

Albendazole 400 mg every 12 h for 21 days may be useful. Anti-inflammatory analgesics are helpful for symptomatic relief. Steroids may be required for patients with neurological complications. Cerebral gnathostomiasis is associated with a high case-fatality rate.

ANGIOSTRONGYLIASIS

ANGIOSTRONGYLUS MENINGITIS

Infection with *Angiostrongylus cantonensis* occurs most commonly in South East Asia following consumption of larvae in salads contaminated with slug or snail slime, or in undercooked snails, crabs or prawns. Clinical disease is usually mild and self-limiting. However, the parasite is an important cause of eosinophilic meningitis, cranial nerve palsies and cerebral abscesses. CSF abnormalities include raised protein, normal or low glucose and a white cell count of 100–5000 cells, up to 90% of which may be eosinophils. Specific antibodies in serum or CSF may be detected by ELISA. In the past, treatment of *Angiostrongylus* meningitis with anthelmintics was not recommended because of concern that death of the parasites may lead to worsening of symptoms. Therefore, management was mainly based on the use of analgesics, corticosteroids and repeat lumbar punctures. However, a recent trial in Thailand has shown that albendazole 15 mg/kg per day is safe and is effective in reducing the duration of headache.[38] A combination of mebendazole 15 mg/kg every 12 h and prednisolone 60 mg/day for 2 weeks has also been shown to be safe and effective.[39]

ABDOMINAL ANGIOSTRONGYLIASIS

Infection with *Angiostrongylus costaricensis* follows consumption of food contaminated with slug slime. Cases have been reported in the Americas, the Caribbean and Central Africa.

Children commonly present with an eosinophilic enteritis resembling acute appendicitis or with an ileocecal mass in chronic cases. Testicular infection may mimic torsion. Eggs and larvae are absent from the stool. An ELISA is available for serological diagnosis. Thiabendazole and diethylcarbamazine have been used in treatment; however, the role of anthelmintics remains uncertain. Surgery is sometimes required.

TREMATODES

Trematodes include the intestinal, liver and lung flukes and the schistosomes (blood flukes). About 750 million people are at risk worldwide. Common to all of their life cycles is the involvement of various species of fresh-water snail, which act as intermediate, amplifying hosts liberating millions of cercaria. Schistosomiasis occurs as a result of cercarial penetration, usually via the skin. The other flukes require a second intermediate host (animal or vegetable) for the development of the metacercarial stage infectious to humans. The adult parasites develop in their human host, mate and produce eggs, which are shed in feces, urine or sputum. On contact with water, the egg releases the miracidium, which infects the preferred snail, thus completing the cycle.

Most infections could be prevented by public health measures promoting sanitation and safe preparation of food. Praziquantel is the anthelmintic of choice for all fluke infections, with the exception of *Fasciola hepatica* and *Fasciola gigantica*, where the drug of choice is now triclabendazole.

SCHISTOSOMIASIS

The three most common species of schistosome affecting humans are *Schistosoma haematobium* (endemic in most of Africa and parts of the Middle East), *Schistosoma mansoni* (endemic in most of Africa, part of the Middle East, and in some areas of the Caribbean and South America) and *Schistosoma japonicum* (endemic in East and South Asia and parts of Indonesia and the Philippines). *Schistosoma mekongi* and *Schistosoma intercalatum* are of lesser importance and are confined to parts of South East Asia and Africa, respectively.

In endemic regions, most of the population becomes infected at some time, peak prevalence usually occurring in older children and teenagers. Most infections are mild or asymptomatic. As immunity develops, egg production diminishes and eventually ceases in most of those infected. Susceptibility to long-term complications may be genetically mediated.

Cercarial dermatitis ('swimmer's itch') occurs within 24 h at the site of cercarial penetration, more commonly in individuals who are newly exposed. The papular, pruritic rash usually resolves spontaneously within a few days. Cercarial dermatitis may also occur following exposure to avian schistosomes. Cercariae develop into schistosomula, which migrate via the heart and lungs. Heavy initial infections may be associated with a transient pneumonitis at this stage.

The schistosomula pass through the liver, where they mature into adults without causing pathology. They then migrate to the vesical venous plexus in the case of *S. haematobium*, or to the mesenteric plexus in the case of *S. mansoni* and *S. japonicum*. Adult worms do not provoke any reaction and may survive for up to 7 years. Egg production and deposition in the tissues does, however, result in an immunopathological response, giving rise to the major clinical consequences of schistosomiasis.

Acute schistosomiasis, or Katayama fever, may occur 4–8 weeks following exposure. It is more likely in non-immunes following heavy infection and is more common with *S. japonicum* and *S. mansoni*, coinciding with the onset of egg deposition in the tissues. Symptoms include fever, cough, wheeze, urticaria, headache and malaise. Generalized lymphadenopathy and hepatosplenomegaly may be present. Investigations usually reveal an eosinophilia; however, parasitological diagnosis may be difficult as eggs are unlikely to be found in stool or urine unless sought by special techniques and serology is usually negative during the initial stages.

The intestine and liver are the principal sites of pathology in all types of human schistosomiasis apart from *S. haematobium*. Egg deposition in the intestinal mucosa may lead to abdominal pain, diarrhea, dysentery and malaise. Colonoscopy may reveal hyperemia, erosions, ulceration or polyps, evident on barium studies as filling defects. Egg deposition in the liver occurs in the perisinusoidal radicles of the portal vein, provoking a granulomatous reaction and, eventually, periportal fibrosis and portal hypertension. Hepatomegaly is followed by splenomegaly and hypersplenism as portal hypertension increases. Bleeding may occur from esophageal varices and ascites is common in advanced disease. Increase in portal pressure may open collaterals into the pulmonary circulation with egg deposition, granuloma formation and periarteritis leading to pulmonary hypertension and cor pulmonale. Rarely, pulmonary hypertension may also occur with *S. haematobium*. Liver function tests are usually normal until fibrosis is advanced. Abnormal liver function tests should raise the possibility of co-infection with hepatitis B or C, in which case the prognosis is likely to be worse.

Chronic *S. haematobium* infection principally affects the urogenital system. The most common symptoms are dysuria, frequency, terminal hematuria and hematospermia. Bladder outlet and vesicoureteric obstruction may lead to hydroureter and hydronephrosis. Secondary bacterial infections may occur, including pyelonephritis. In due course, chronic renal failure may develop. Cystoscopy may reveal 'sandy patches' on the mucosal surface, mucosal hypertrophy or polyps. Squamous carcinoma of the bladder is a well-documented long-term complication. Involvement of the female genital tract may cause cervicitis, salpingitis and infertility. These may also occur with *S. japonicum* and *S. intercalatum*. Rarely, patients with *S. haematobium* complain of rectal passage of blood and mucus.

Neurological complications occur if schistosome eggs lodge in the brain or spine, leading to symptoms such as focal or generalized convulsions and transverse myelitis. Subcutaneous egg deposition, often in the perineal region, may result in the development of painful papules.

A number of clinical conditions have been described arising from co-infection of schistosomes and salmonellae, including recurrent *Salmonella* bacteremia, nephrotic syndrome associated with co-infection with *S. mansoni* and *Salmonella typhi*, and chronic urinary carriage of *Salmonella typhi* associated with *S. haematobium* infection. HIV and HTLV-1 infection are both associated with increased susceptibility to schistosomiasis.[12]

Diagnosis and treatment

Characteristic eggs may be identified in urine, semen or feces, by use of concentration techniques if necessary. Eggs of all species may be identified on rectal biopsy. Serological diagnosis is problematic as it takes 6–12 weeks for titers to become positive, positive titers persist for years following cure, and false-positive results may be caused by exposure to other helminths. Serology may be useful in returning travelers but not for residents in endemic areas. *S. mansoni* antibody detection in oral fluids appears to be as sensitive as serology.[40] Antigen from viable eggs can now be detected in serum and urine, offering new possibilities for diagnosis and monitoring of response to treatment.[41–43] Ultrasonography is useful for assessing patients with hepatic and urinary tract disease.

Praziquantel is the drug of choice for all species: 40 mg/kg as a single dose is usually sufficient for *S. haematobium*, *S. mansoni* and *S. intercalatum*. *S. japonicum* and *S. mekongi* require a larger dose: either 50 mg/kg as a single dose or three doses of 20 mg/kg 8 h apart. Side effects are uncommon. Praziquantel is regarded as safe for treatment of schistosomiasis in pregnant and lactating women.[44] Although resistance to praziquantel has been observed,[45] this is not a significant clinical problem at present. Apparent *S. mansoni* resistance may be partly attributable to a higher worm burden and intense transmission.[46] Oxamniquine 15–30 mg/kg for 1–2 days may be used as an alternative for the treatment of *S. mansoni*; however, side effects are more common and serious compared to praziquantel. Concomitant use of steroids is recommended in the management of patients with neurological disease to reduce inflammation around granulomata.

Katayama fever is managed with non-steroidal anti-inflammatory drugs or steroids depending on the severity, together with praziquantel.

No prophylactic drug is currently recommended for schistosomiasis. Artesunate and artemether are potential prophylactic agents, but a major concern is the risk of promoting resistance in *Plasmodium falciparum*.[47,48]

INTESTINAL FLUKES

The most important intestinal fluke in humans is *Fasciolopsis buski*, which is widely distributed from India to South East Asia, particularly among pig-rearing communities. Human infection follows ingestion of metacercariae attached to an edible water plant, such as the water caltrop. The metacercariae excyst and attach to the mucosa of the duodenum and jejunum, where they develop into adults, causing inflammation and ulceration. Most infections are asymptomatic. Heavy infections result in epigastric pain and diarrhea, initially alternating with constipation, but later becoming persistent. Wasting and ascites may develop in severe cases.

Echinostome species, principally found in Asia, may also infect humans, causing symptoms similar to *F. buski*.

Heterophyes, the smallest of the intestinal flukes affecting humans, cause milder gastrointestinal symptoms than *F. buski*. However, ectopic eggs may be carried to other organs, particularly the CNS, causing a mass effect, and to the heart resulting in myocarditis or valve damage.

Diagnosis and treatment

Characteristic eggs, and sometimes adult flukes, can be identified in feces. Adult flukes may also appear in vomit. Intestinal flukes respond to treatment with praziquantel 15–40 mg/kg as a single or divided dose.

LIVER FLUKES

Fasciola hepatica and *Fasciola gigantica* are widely distributed, occurring in sheep- and cattle-rearing areas throughout the world. Human infection follows ingestion of metacercariae on water vegetables, for example watercress. Acute clinical symptoms may develop after 6–12 weeks, including abdominal pain, intermittent fever, weight loss, malaise, urticaria and respiratory symptoms. The liver may be enlarged and tender and liver enzymes are sometimes mildly elevated. Ectopic flukes may lead to granuloma or abscess formation in various organs. Migrating erythematous cutaneous nodules, another form of cutaneous larva migrans, may also occur. Mature flukes tend to migrate to the bile ducts, initially causing fever, anorexia and abdominal pain. This usually subsides spontaneously. A minority of patients develop chronic symptoms associated with recurrent cholangitis or intermittent biliary obstruction.

Diagnosis and treatment

Eosinophilia is common and pleural effusions, if present, may contain eosinophils. Ultrasound is usually normal, although CT scans of the liver may reveal numerous hypodense lesions. Peripheral, branched hypodense hepatic lesions, best seen on CT with use of contrast, are relatively specific for fascioliasis.

Serological tests are helpful in diagnosing *F. hepatica* infections towards the end of the acute phase when eggs are unlikely to be present in feces. Serology is less reliable for *F. gigantica*. In chronic disease, eggs may be present in feces or in bile aspirate. Concentration techniques may be helpful. Fasciola excretory–secretory (FES) antigen detection in feces is useful both in pre-patent and patent infections with *F. hepatica*.

Praziquantel is unreliable in the treatment of fascioliasis. Bithionol 30–50 mg/kg per day in three divided doses on alternate days for 10–15 days has been recommended in the past. Side effects include mild gastrointestinal upset and pruritus. A benzimidazole, triclabendazole, is simpler to use, has few side effects and has now become the drug of choice. A single dose of 10 mg/kg taken with food is usually effective. Severe infections require a second dose after 12 h.[49] The expulsion of dead or dying parasites after 3–5 days may result in biliary colic requiring treatment with an antispasmodic. Unfortunately, triclabendazole resistance has been reported in Ireland, the UK and Australia.[50] Nitazoxanide 500 mg every 12 h for 6–7 days has been used successfully in treating *F. hepatica* with cure rates of 49–87%.[51] Artesunate has been shown to compare favorably with triclabendazole in the treatment of *F. hepatica*, although the outcome at 3 months was less favorable.[52]

ORIENTAL LIVER FLUKES

Clonorchis sinensis (also known as *Opisthorchis sinensis*) and *Opisthorchis viverrini* affect about 20 million people in China and South East Asia. A related species, *Opisthorchis felineus*, occurs in Eastern Europe and Russia. Human infection follows consumption of metacercariae in raw or undercooked freshwater fish. Metacercariae excyst in the small bowel and migrate along the common bile duct to colonize the biliary tree. Most infections are asymptomatic. Patients with heavy initial infections may present with an illness similar to Katayama fever. In established infections patients may present with vague right upper quadrant abdominal pain and hepatomegaly. Recurrent episodes of ascending cholangitis, jaundice and pancreatitis may occur. Chronic infection may lead to biliary cirrhosis and, rarely, cholangiocarcinoma.

Diagnosis and treatment

Ultrasound may reveal abnormalities of the biliary tree and gallstones. Other imaging techniques, such as endoscopic retrograde cholangiopancreatography, are useful. Diagnosis is established by identifying characteristic eggs in feces with the aid of concentration techniques, or in biliary aspirate. A fecal antigen test is now available for *O. viverrini*.[53] Serological tests are not widely available and generally lack specificity.

Treatment is with praziquantel 40 mg/kg as a single dose or 25 mg/kg every 8 h after meals. A 3-day course is advisable for heavy infections.

LUNG FLUKES

Eight species of *Paragonimus* cause disease in humans, the most important being *Paragonimus westermani*. Paragonimiasis is widespread in Asia and also occurs in regions of Africa, Central and South America. Human infection follows ingestion of metacercariae attached to undercooked or raw crab, crayfish and shrimp, or, rarely, following consumption of larvae in undercooked wild boar. Most infections are initially asymptomatic. An acute illness may occur as the parasite excysts, penetrates the gut wall and migrates through the diaphragm into the pleural cavity and then to the lungs. Symptoms of abdominal pain and diarrhea 2–15 days after infection may be followed by cough, dyspnea, fatigue, fever and urticaria a few days later. This episode sometimes lasts several weeks. Pleuritic chest pain may occur, sometimes associated with an effusion. Adult flukes form cysts in the lung tissue and produce eggs, provoking an inflammatory response. Cavitatory or nodular, sometimes calcified, lesions develop which may be noticed incidentally on a chest radiograph as the first indication of infection in asymptomatic patients. Early symptoms of pulmonary paragonimiasis include cough, initially non-productive, later productive of gelatinous, rusty or bloodstained sputum. Pulmonary paragonimiasis may be mistaken for tuberculosis and both infections may coincide.

Cerebral paragonimiasis is the most important form of extrapulmonary paragonimiasis. Most patients are children. About one-third present with a clinical picture resembling acute meningoencephalitis, but more commonly presentation is insidious with a wide variety of neurological symptoms and signs depending on the area of the brain or spinal cord affected.

Wandering flukes may cause painless, migratory subcutaneous swellings, subcutaneous nodules or a variety of other symptoms depending on the site involved.

Diagnosis and treatment

Diagnosis can be confirmed by identifying characteristic eggs in sputum, feces or, rarely, pleural effusion. Eosinophilia is usual and should alert one to the possibility of paragonimiasis in patients presenting with a clinical picture mimicking tuberculosis. Serological tests are available, including ELISA and a complement fixation test. Paragonimus-specific IgM is useful for diagnosing patients with extrapulmonary disease and pleurisy.[54]

Praziquantel 25 mg/kg every 8 h for 2–3 days is highly effective. A higher dose may be required for treatment of cerebral paragonimiasis and steroid cover is advisable. Two doses of triclabendazole 10 mg/kg administered on the same day is also highly effective in treating pulmonary paragonimiasis.[55]

FILARIAL INFECTIONS

Insect vectors play a role in the transmission of all of the medically important parasitic filarial nematodes, with the exception of *Dracunculus medinensis*. Both the parasite and the insect vector depend on favorable climatic and environmental conditions that occur naturally in certain regions of the tropics. Human infections occur when the insect vector feeds, introducing infective larvae. These mature into adult worms, which produce microfilariae, which in turn infect the insect vector. Clinical disease is caused by the adult worms, the microfilariae, or both.

Recently, significant progress has been made in the community control of onchocerciasis and lymphatic filariasis. However, one of the obstacles facing these programs is the longevity of the adult worms and their relative lack of response to antihelminthic agents. It is now evident that the development, motility and fertility of the adult worms depend on intracellular, endosymbiotic bacteria of the genus *Wolbachia*. These organisms also play an important role in the pathogenesis of these diseases and are susceptible to tetracyclines and several other antibiotics, offering fascinating new possibilities in the management and control of filarial infections.[56-58]

LYMPHATIC FILARIASIS

Wuchereria bancrofti, *Brugia malayi* and *Brugia timori* are transmitted by various species of mosquito. *W. bancrofti* is distributed widely in the tropics, whereas *B. malayi* and *B. timori* are endemic in South East Asia and Indonesia. The adult worms develop in the lymphatics and range in length from 20 to 100 mm. Their microfilariae enter the general circulation via the thoracic duct. Recent developments, particularly with regard to the role of *Wolbachia*, have led to significant changes in our understanding of the pathogenesis of lymphatic filariasis. Inflammatory episodes are likely to be multifactorial involving responses to different stages of the parasite, secondary bacterial infection and inflammatory mediators associated with *Wolbachia*.[59]

Lymphatic filariasis affects about 120 million people. Most infections are asymptomatic. Acute symptoms typically occur 8–16 months following infection and often recur several times a year. A first episode of acute filarial fever has been reported more than 15 years following exposure. Several clinical presentations are recognized. Acute filarial fever without lymphadenitis is non-specific and must be distinguished from malaria and other causes of fever in the tropics. Acute filarial lymphangitis is characterized by a circumscribed inflammatory nodule or cord with centrifugal lymphangitis that occurs following the death of the adult worm (whether spontaneous or following treatment). Acute dermatolymphangioadenitis, severe local inflammation resembling cellulitis or erysipelas, is frequently associated with secondary bacterial infection and impaired lymphatic flow, ascending lymphangitis and limb edema. This may eventually progress to elephantiasis.

Chronic lymphatic filariasis may develop months or years after the acute symptoms, or without a history of acute disease. Lymphatic obstruction leads to lymphedema of the affected extremity and, eventually, to elephantiasis. The sites most commonly affected are the legs, scrotum, arms and breast. Recurrent secondary bacterial skin infections, often streptococcal, may cause acute episodes of pain and fever and lead to glomerulonephritis.

Other presentations of chronic lymphatic filariasis include hydrocele, lymph scrotum, acute epididymitis and funiculitis. Chyluria, chylous diarrhea and chylous ascites may also occur with considerable loss of fat-soluble vitamins and protein, resulting in malnutrition and vitamin deficiencies.

Diagnosis and treatment

Eosinophilia is common during the acute stages. Parasitological diagnosis may be made by examination of a Giemsa-stained thick blood film taken at the peak of microfilarial periodicity according to the species (usually 22.00 h–02.00 h for *W. bancrofti*). However, this is relatively insensitive other than for high microfilaremias (>100 microfilariae/mL). Concentration techniques greatly improve sensitivity. Tests for circulating *W. bancrofti* antigen are now available, including an ELISA and a rapid immunochromatographic card test, and these may replace microscopy.[60] Polymerase chain reaction (PCR) assays have also been developed for *W. bancrofti* and *B. malayi*.[61,62] Scrotal ultrasound demonstrating live adult worms in the 'filarial dance sign' may be useful either for diagnostic purposes or for follow-up of response to treatment.[63]

Treatment of individual patients with lymphatic filariasis is possible using a combination of anthelmintic agents and antibiotics. If co-infection with onchocerciasis is present or possible, a combination of doxycycline 200 mg/day for 6 weeks plus a dose of ivermectin 150 µg/kg on completion of the course of doxycycline, is recommended unless contraindicated (age <9 years, pregnancy, breastfeeding). In the absence of co-infection with onchocerciasis, a combination of doxycycline 200 mg/day for 6 weeks plus a dose of diethylcarbamazine (DEC) 6 mg/kg on completion of the course of doxycycline is recommended unless contraindicated.[64]

In either of the above situations, if co-infection with *Loa loa* is present, particularly if associated with a high *Loa loa* microfilaremia, it is essential to reduce the microfilaremia using albendazole prior to treatment with DEC or ivermectin as either of the latter may provoke a fatal encephalopathy. This is discussed in more detail in the section on *Loa loa*.

Management of lymphoedema involves elevation, massage, exercise and bandaging of affected limbs. Careful hygiene, use of disinfectant soap and water, and general skin care (including early and effective treatment of any wounds or abrasions) are also important. Antibiotic prophylaxis with penicillin is useful for recurrent streptococcal infections. Hydrocele requires surgical management. Chyluria requires bed rest, nutrition and, in some cases, surgery.

Community control of lymphatic filariasis is based on vector control plus mass treatment annually with a two-drug regimen tailored to the region. Within Africa, because of the risk of onchocerciasis and/or *Loa loa*, a single dose of ivermectin, usually 150 µg/kg, is given with a single dose of albendazole 400 mg. Annual treatment should continue for at least 30 years. Caution is advised in regions where *Loa loa* is endemic and high risk foci of *Loa loa* are currently excluded from ivermectin programs. Outside Africa, DEC in single dose of 6 mg/kg is given annually, together with a single dose of albendazole 400 mg. Annual treatment should continue for at least 20 years.[64,65]

TROPICAL PULMONARY EOSINOPHILIA

Tropical pulmonary eosinophilia occurs in areas endemic for lymphatic filariasis, particularly Sri Lanka and Southern India. Microfilarial death triggers a high eosinophilia associated with gradually worsening, non-productive cough and wheeze, and sometimes fever and malaise. Symptoms are worse at night. Chest radiography shows diffuse infiltrates. Pulmonary function tests may reveal restrictive, obstructive or mixed defects. IgE is elevated and filarial serology positive. The diagnosis is supported by a prompt response to treatment with DEC.

LOIASIS

Loa loa is transmitted by flies of the genus *Chrysops* that breed in tropical forests of Africa. Larval parasites migrate in the subcutaneous tissues, where they mature into adults over the course of a year. Clinical symptoms include urticaria, pruritus, arthralgia and malaise. Transient, migratory angiedema (Calabar swelling) occurs most commonly on the extremities where trauma to a migrating adult worm provokes a localized inflammatory reaction. Subconjunctival migration causes pain and inflammation. If instruments are readily to hand, the worm can be removed from the eye after applying local anesthetic. Other complications include proteinuria in up to 30% of patients, hematuria and, less commonly, neurological complications (particularly meningoencephalitis). Rare presentations include pulmonary infiltrates, pleural effusions, arthritis, lymphangitis and hydrocele. Hypereosinophilia is common and *Loa loa* has been implicated in the etiology of endomyocardial fibrosis, although this condition is well described in association with numerous other causes of hypereosinophilia.

Diagnosis and treatment

Diagnosis of loiasis is often indicated by the history, particularly if an 'eye worm' has made an appearance. Dead, calcified worms are sometimes seen on radiography.

Microfilaremia peaks between 10.00 h and 15.00 h. Parasites can be identified in thick blood films with Giemsa or Wright stains, or by concentration techniques. Assessing the microfilarial load is useful in determining the likelihood of an adverse reaction to treatment. Serological tests are available and may be helpful for diagnosis in travelers from endemic areas, but other filarial parasites cross-react. A specific recombinant antigen test has recently been developed that may be useful in the diagnosis of patients with low microfilaremia.[66]

DEC 2 mg/kg orally every 8 h for 7–10 days is commonly used in the treatment of loiasis, although some prefer 12 days. The course is repeated at intervals of 2 or 3 months if the patient remains symptomatic. Ivermectin 150 µg/kg as a single dose before treatment with DEC will reduce the likelihood of a Mazzotti reaction in patients who also have onchocerciasis. Caution is needed in managing patients with loiasis who have high microfilarial loads (>2500 microfilariae/mL) as treatment with DEC or ivermectin may precipitate meningoencephalitis or renal failure due to massive release of antigens from dying microfilariae.[67] Plasmapheresis has been used successfully to reduce microfilarial load in heavy infections before treatment with DEC under steroid cover; however, albendazole 200 mg every 12 h for 3 weeks causes a gradual reduction in microfilaremia, usually without serious adverse effects.[68] The currently recommended strategy for managing patients with high microfilaremia is administration of albendazole 200 mg every 12 h for 3 weeks, followed by a course of DEC or ivermectin.[69] Prednisolone, 20 mg/day, given for 3 days before and for 3 days following the start of anthelmintic treatment, may reduce the risk of encephalopathy. This may well become the preferred strategy for managing patients with high microfilaremia.

ONCHOCERCIASIS

Onchocerciasis is one of the most important causes of blindness in the tropics. The disease is endemic in tropical Africa, the Arabian peninsula and parts of Latin America. Over 37 million people are infected, of whom almost 1 million are blind or visually impaired. The parasite is transmitted by blackflies of the genus *Simulium* that breed along fast flowing rivers: hence the common name 'river blindness'. Humans are the only definitive host for *Onchocerca volvulus*. Larvae injected when an infected blackfly feeds migrate in the subcutaneous tissues and mature into adults. Adult worms, measuring up to 80 cm in length, intertwine and become encapsulated in the subcutaneous tissues, forming painless nodules measuring up to 3 cm in diameter. These may be palpable over bony prominences but otherwise cause few clinical symptoms. Microfilariae produced by the adult worms are responsible for the most serious clinical effects of onchocerciasis, principally affecting the skin and eye.

Onchodermatitis initially presents as an intensely itchy papular rash. A chronic papular dermatitis ensues with gradual loss of elasticity in the skin and subcutaneous tissues, resulting in a prematurely aged appearance. Depigmentation, sparing sweat glands and hair follicles, leads to the 'leopard skin' appearance, most commonly seen on the shins. Enlarged inguinal and femoral lymph nodes may hang in apron-like folds of inelastic skin, the so-called 'hanging groin' appearance. Rarely, elephantiasis may occur. 'Sowda', a lichenified dermatitis, presents as intensely pruritic, hyperpigmented papules and plaques, usually affecting one limb and accompanied by edema and enlargement of the regional nodes.

Ocular onchocerciasis results from microfilarial invasion of the eye. Live microfilariae may be visible in the anterior chamber or aqueous humor on slit-lamp examination. They provoke a reversible inflammatory reaction, resulting in punctate keratitis or 'snowflake' corneal opacities. Microfilarial death in longstanding cases results in more severe and irreversible damage, including sclerosing keratitis, iridocyclitis, uveitis, chorioretinitis and optic atrophy. Glaucoma and cataract may also occur. Eye complications are more likely to occur in patients who have onchocercal nodules on the head or upper body.

Onchocerciasis may increase the risk of seroconversion in HIV-1 infections and treatment of onchocerciasis appears to be associated with reduced HIV-1 viral replication. Onchodermatitis also appears to be more severe in HIV-positive patients.[70]

Diagnosis and treatment

The most common method for diagnosis is examination for the emergence of microfilariae from a skin snip placed in a drop of saline. Nodules may be excised and examined for adult worms. In the past, for diagnosis of patients with negative skin snips, DEC was used in a dose of 25–50 mg to provoke a Mazzotti reaction with considerable worsening of the rash and pruritus in the ensuing 24 h. Application of topical DEC under an occlusive dressing produces a similar, localized effect and is less distressing and safer for the patient. As a severe Mazzotti reaction may be precipitated by either the DEC provocative test or the DEC patch test, the use of these diagnostic approaches is seldom indicated.

Skin-snip microscopy is less sensitive than newer diagnostic methods, including skin-snip PCR, ELISAs, enzyme immunoassays and antigen detection. Recent advances include the development of a serum antibody test card using recombinant antigen to detect *O. volvulus*-specific IgG4 in finger-prick whole-blood specimens, a triple-antigen indirect ELISA rapid-format card test, and a highly sensitive and specific urine antigen dipstick test.[71–75] Antibody detection may be useful for screening populations, whereas PCR and antigen detection in serum and urine are potentially more useful for diagnosing active infection in individuals and for monitoring the success of therapy.

Both the treatment and the community control of onchocerciasis have been greatly improved following the introduction of ivermectin. A single oral dose of 150 μg/kg clears microfilariae for several months and suppresses microfilaria production, but does not kill adult worms.[76] Mass administration of ivermectin annually in Africa, or on alternate years elsewhere, is the basis of community control of onchocerciasis, with the exclusion of pregnant women. Assuming a minimum of 65% coverage and ongoing efficacy of treatment, the time scale required for elimination of onchocerciasis in affected communities is a daunting 25–30 years.[77]

Ivermectin should be used with caution in *Loa loa*-endemic areas as it may precipitate meningoencephalitis in patients with high *Loa loa* microfilarial loads. In these circumstances, it is advisable to prescribe a course of albendazole before treatment with ivermectin. In the past, nodulectomy was advised for head nodules, possibly reducing the likelihood of eye infection, but is not required for nodules elsewhere.

Treatment of individual patients has been revolutionized in recent years following research on the role of *Wolbachia* in the pathogenesis and persistence of infection. The current recommendation, unless contraindicated (age <9 years, pregnancy, breastfeeding), is doxycycline 100–200 mg/day for 4–6 weeks, the duration depending on whether interruption of embryogenesis or a macrofilaricidal effect is intended, plus a single dose of ivermectin 150 μg/kg after 4–6 months.[64]

GUINEA WORM

Dracunculus medinensis is acquired by swallowing a tiny copepod, *Cyclops*, harboring the larval stage of the parasite. Following digestion of *Cyclops*, the liberated larva penetrates the intestinal mucosa, migrates to loose connective tissue and develops into an adult worm. After mating, the female worm continues to mature with an enlarging gravid uterus and migrates in search of a site suitable for discharge of her larvae. Clinical symptoms occur as the worm prepares to emerge. Patients often complain of prodromal symptoms including rashes, gastrointestinal symptoms, weakness and fever. The emergence of the worm is heralded by the development of a large, indurated erythematous papule with a vesicular center. Over the next few days this develops into a painful, pruritic blister, which the patient seeks to immerse in water for relief. The larvae are thus discharged and, in suitable conditions, complete the cycle by infecting another *Cyclops*. The site of the blister tends to ulcerate and secondary bacterial infection may occur, including tetanus.

Migrating adult worms may penetrate and perish in other tissues, including the spinal cord, peritoneal cavity, pancreas, pericardium and lung, causing symptoms due to focal inflammation.

Management of guinea worm infection has changed little since ancient times. Emerging worms are encouraged to discharge their uterine contents by immersion of the affected part in water. At this stage, the tip of the worm begins to emerge and can be gently and gradually wound onto a matchstick, a few centimeters each day, until the entire worm has been removed. The process can take several days as female worms may exceed 1 m in length. Administration of oral metronidazole or mebendazole may facilitate extraction. Surgical intervention is often required in the management of disease caused by ectopic worms. A highly successful program for the global eradication of guinea worm, based on the provision of safe drinking water or the use of fine filters to trap *Cyclops*, has resulted in a dramatic fall in the incidence of infection in recent years.

CONCLUSION

Helminth infections affect approximately one billion of the world's poorest people, mainly in tropical developing countries. These diseases are now receiving unprecedented attention as evidence accumulates that highly cost-effective community interventions can control and, possibly, eliminate many of these infections, and stimulate long-term economic growth and development.[1]

The integration of onchocerciasis, filariasis, schistosomiasis and soil transmitted helminth control programs offers a cost-effective strategy for controlling these infections.[78,79] Regular anthelmintic treatment of schoolchildren in developing countries is being promoted by the World Health Organization as a means of improving anemia, nutritional status and cognitive development in anticipation of long-term benefits to health and economic development.[80–82] The control of onchocerciasis has progressed rapidly in the past 30 years, largely due to successful international public–private partnerships fostered through the Onchocerciasis Control Programme (1974–2002), the African Programme for Onchocerciasis Control (1995–present) and the Onchocerciasis Elimination Program for the Americas (1991–present).[1,77,83] Similarly, the Global Alliance for the Elimination of Lymphatic Filariasis, created in 2000, is an international public–private partnership that aims to eliminate lymphatic filariasis as a public health problem.[59] The Global Network for Neglected Tropical Diseases, established in 2006, is a major international initiative promoting an integrated NTD control strategy. The Network is comprised of international non-profit organizations, the World Health Organization, pharmaceutical companies and ministries of health in disease-endemic countries. The Network is promoting the introduction of a 'rapid impact package' to treat seven of the most common NTDs (ascariasis, trichuriasis, hookworm, schistosomiasis, lymphatic filariasis, onchocerciasis and trachoma) using a combination of four drugs (albendazole–mebendazole, DEC–ivermectin, praziquantel, azithromycin) for just 50 cents per person per year, including drugs, delivery, equipment, training, health promotion, monitoring and evaluation.[84] Mass treatment for helminthic infections is proving to be a highly effective public health intervention, with wider benefits in strengthening health systems and affording opportunities for synergy with other initiatives, such as malaria and tuberculosis control. However, as mass treatment carries with it the risk of emergence of drug resistance, careful monitoring is essential, as is a greater investment in the development of anthelmintic drugs.

In order to achieve the goal of community control and, ultimately, the elimination of helminthic infections, investment is required for research and development of new diagnostic agents, drugs, insecticides and vaccines.[1] However, between 1975 and 2004, of the 1556 new pharmaceuticals that were marketed, only four were anthelmintics.[85] Many of the most useful anthelmintic agents available to us today were originally developed for veterinary use. Although some of these drugs have been generously donated for use in developing countries, economic imperatives dictate that there is greater profit in developing anthelmintic drugs for the treatment of animals than there is in addressing the needs of impoverished human beings. 'The poor must be grateful for a mouthful of crumbs, fallen from the table where the rich feed their dogs.'

References

1. Hotez P, Fenwick A, Savioli L, Molyneux D. Rescuing the bottom billion through control of neglected tropical diseases. *Lancet*. 2009;373:1570–1575.
2. Aslam S, Musher DM. Nitazoxanide: clinical studies of a broad-spectrum anti-infective agent. *Future Microbiology*. 2007;2:583–590.
3. Papadopoulos GS, Eleftherakis NG, Thanopoulos BD. Cardiac tamponade in a child with ascariasis. *Cardiol Young*. 2000;10:539–541.
4. Gonzalez AH, Regaldo VC, Van den Ende J. Non-invasive management of *Ascaris lumbricoides* biliary tact migration: a prospective study in 69 patients from Ecuador. *Trop Med Int Health*. 2001;6:146–150.
5. Jackson TF, Epstein SR, Gouws E, et al. A comparison of mebendazole and albendazole in treating children with *Trichuris trichiura* infection in Durban, South Africa. *S Afr Med J*. 1998;88:880–883.
6. Ismail MM, Javakody RL. Efficacy of albendazole and its combinations with ivermectin or diethylcarbamazine (DEC) in the treatment of *Trichuris trichiura* infections in Sri Lanka. *Ann Trop Med Parasitol*. 1999;93:501–504.
7. Sacko M, De Clerq D, Behnke JM, et al. Comparison of the efficacy of mebendazole, albendazole and pyrantel in treatment of human hookworm infections in the southern region of Mali, West Africa. *Trans R Soc Trop Med Hyg*. 1999;93:195–203.
8. Bouchard O, Houze S, Schiemann R, et al. Cutaneous larva migrans in travelers: a prospective study, with assessment of therapy with ivermectin. *Clin Infect Dis*. 2000;31:434–498.
9. Czachor JS, Jonas AP. Transmission of *Strongyloides stercoralis* person to person. *J Travel Med*. 2000;7:211–212.
10. Thomas MC, Costello SA. Disseminated strongyloidiasis arising from a single dose of dexamethasone before stereotactic radiosurgery. *Int J Clin Pract*. 1998;52:520–521.
11. Parana R, Portugal M, Vitvitski L, et al. Severe strongyloidiasis during interferon plus ribavirin therapy for chronic HCV infection. *Eur J Gastroenterol Hepatol*. 2000;12:245–246.
12. Lewthwaite P, Gill G, Hart CA, et al. Gastrointestinal parasites in the immunocompromised. *Curr Opin Infect Dis*. 2005;18:427–435.
13. Avery RK, Ljungman P. Prophylactic measures in the solid-organ recipient before transplantation. *Clin Infect Dis*. 2000;33(suppl 1):S15–S21.
14. Jongwutiwes S, Charoenkorn M, Sitthichareonchai P, et al. Increased sensitivity of routine laboratory detection of *Strongyloides stercoralis* and hookworm by agar-plate culture. *Trans R Soc Trop Med Hyg*. 1999;93:398–400.
15. Zaha O, Hirata T, Kinjo F, et al. Strongyloidiasis – progress in diagnosis and treatment. *Int Med*. 2000;39:695–700.
16. Chiodini PL, Reid AJ, Wiselka MJ, et al. Parenteral ivermectin in *Strongyloides* hyperinfection. *Lancet*. 2000;355:43–44.
17. Morales NM, Agapejev S, Morales RR, et al. Clinical aspects of neurocysticercosis in children. *Pediatr Neurol*. 2000;22:287–291.
18. Garcia HH, Parkhouse RM, Gilman RH, et al. A specific antigen-detection ELISA for the diagnosis of human neurocysticercosis. *Trans R Soc Trop Med Hyg*. 1998;92:411–414.
19. Garcia HH, Parkhouse RM, Gilman RH, et al. Serum antigen detection in the diagnosis, treatment, and follow-up of neurocysticercosis patients. *Trans R Soc Trop Med Hyg*. 2000;94:673–676.
20. Sotelo J, Jung H. Pharmacokinetic optimisation of the treatment of neurocysticercosis. *Clin Pharmacokinet*. 1998;34:503–515.
21. Jung H, Medina R, Castro N, et al. Pharmacokinetic study of praziquantel administered alone and in combination with cimetidine in a single-day therapeutic regimen. *Antimicrob Agents Chemother*. 1997;41:1256–1259.
22. Yee T, Barakos JA, Knight RT. High-dose praziquantel with cimetidine for refractory neurocysticercosis: a case report with clinical and MRI follow-up. *West J Med*. 1999;170:112–115.
23. Del Brutto OH, Roos KL, Coffey CS, Garcia HH. Meta-analysis. Cysticidal drugs for neurocysticercosis: albendazole and praziquantel. *Ann Intern Med*. 2006;145:43–51.
24. Pretell EJ, Garcia HH, Custodio N, et al. Short regimen of praziquantel in the treatment of single brain enhancing lesions. *Clin Neurol Neurosurg*. 2000;102:215–218.
25. Sbihi Y, Rmiqui A, Rodriguez-Cabezas MN, et al. Comparative sensitivity of six serological tests and diagnostic value of ELISA using purified antigen in hydatidosis. *J Clin Lab Anal*. 2001;15:14–18.

26. Ravinder PT, Parija SC, Rao KS. Urinary hydatid antigen detection by coagglutination, a cost-effective and rapid test for diagnosis of cystic echinococcosis in a rural or field setting. *J Clin Microbiol.* 2000;38:2972–2974.

27. Garcia HH, Moro PL, Schantz PM. Zoonotic helminth infections of humans: echinococcosis, cysticercosis and fascioliasis. *Curr Opin Infect Dis.* 2007;20:489–494.

28. WHO. PAIR: Puncture, Aspiration, Injection, Re-Aspiration. An option for the treatment of cystic echinococcosis. *WHO/CDS/CSR/APH/2001.6.* Online. 2006. Available at http://whqlibdoc.who.int/hq/2001/WHO_CDS_CSR_APH_2001.6.pdf.

29. Smego RA, Bhatti S, Khaliq AA, et al. Percutaneous aspiration–injection–reaspiration drainage plus albendazole or mebendazole for hepatic cystic echinococcosis: a meta-analysis. *Clin Infect Dis.* 2003;37:1073–1083.

30. Khoury G, Abaid F, Geagea T, et al. Laparoscopic treatment of hydatid cysts of the liver and spleen. *Surg Endosc.* 2000;14:243–245.

31. Keshmiri M, Baharvahdat H, Fattahi SH, et al. A placebo controlled study of albendazole in the treatment of pulmonary echinococcosis. *Eur Respir J.* 1999;14:503–507.

32. Brunetti E, Kern P, Vuitton DA; Writing Panel for the WHO-IWGE. Expert consensus for the diagnosis and treatment of cystic and alveolar echinococcosis in humans. *Acta Tropica.* 2010;114:1–16.

33. Urrea-Paris MA, Moreno MJ, Casado N, et al. In vitro effect of praziquantel and albendazole combination therapy on the larval stage of *Echinococcus granulosus. Parasitol Res.* 2000;86:957–964.

34. Mohamed AE, Yasawy MI, Al Karawi MA. Combined albendazole and praziquantel versus albendazole alone in the treatment of hydatid disease. *Hepatogastroenterology.* 1998;45:1690–1694.

35. Cobo F, Yarnoz C, Sesma B, et al. Albendazole plus praziquantel versus albendazole alone as a pre-operative treatment in intra-abdominal hydatidosis caused by *Echinococcus granulosus. Trop Med Int Health.* 1998;3:462–466.

36. Lazarevic AM, Neskovic AN, Goronja M, et al. Low incidence of cardiac abnormalities in treated trichinosis: a prospective study of 62 patients from a single-source outbreak. *Am J Med.* 1999;107:18–23.

37. Chandenier J, Husson S, Canaple C, et al. Medullary gnathostomiasis in a white patient: use of immunodiagnosis and magnetic resonance imaging. *Clin Infect Dis.* 2001;32:154–157.

38. Jitpimolmard S, Sawanyawisuth K, Morakote N, et al. Albendazole therapy for eosinophilic meningitis caused by *Angiostrongylus cantonensis. Parasitol Res.* 2007;100:1293–1296.

39. Chotmongkol V, Sawadpanitch K, Sawanyawisuth K, et al. Treatment of eosinophilic meningitis with a combination of prednisolone and mebendazole. *Am J Trop Med Hyg.* 2006;74:1122–1124.

40. Santos MM, Garcia TD, Orsini M, et al. Oral fluids for the immunodiagnosis of *Schistosoma mansoni* infection. *Trans R Soc Trop Med Hyg.* 2000;94:289–292.

41. Nibbeling HA, Van Lieshout L, Deelder AM. Levels of circulating soluble egg antigen in urine of individuals infected with *Schistosoma mansoni* before and after treatment with praziquantel. *Trans R Soc Trop Med Hyg.* 1998;92:675–677.

42. Kahama AI, Kremsner PG, Van Dam GJ, et al. The dynamics of a soluble egg antigen of *Schistosoma haematobium* in relation to egg counts, circulating anodic and cathodic antigens and pathology markers before and after chemotherapy. *Trans R Soc Trop Med Hyg.* 1998;92:629–633.

43. Van Lieshout L, Polderman AM, Deelder AM. Immunodiagnosis of schistosomiasis by determination of the circulating antigens CAA and CCA, in particular in individuals with recent or light infections. *Acta Trop.* 2000;77:69–80.

44. World Health Organization. Report of the WHO informal consultation on the use of praziquantel during pregnancy/lactation and albendazole/mebendazole in children under 24 months. *WHO/CDS/CPE/PVC/2002.4.* Geneva: WHO; 2002.

45. Ismail M, Botros S, Metwally A, et al. Resistance to praziquantel: direct evidence from *Schistosoma mansoni* isolated from Egyptian villagers. *Am J Trop Med Hyg.* 1999;60:932–935.

46. Gryseels B, Mbaye A, De Vlas SJ, et al. Are poor responses to praziquantel for the treatment of *Schistosoma mansoni* infections in Senegal due to resistance? An overview of the evidence. *Trop Med Int Health.* 2001;6:864–873.

47. Li S, Wu L, Liu Z, et al. Studies on prophylactic effect of artesunate on schistosomiasis japonica. *Chin Med J.* 1996;109:848–853.

48. Utzinger J, N'Goran EK, N'Dri A, et al. Oral artemether for prevention of *Schistosoma mansoni* infection: randomised controlled trial. *Lancet.* 2000;355:1320–1325.

49. Graham CS, Brodie SB, Weller PF. Imported *Fasciola hepatica* infection in the United States and treatment with triclabendazole. *Clin Infect Dis.* 2001;32:1–6.

50. Coles GC. Treatment of fascioliasis in human infections. *Trans R Soc Trop Med Hyg.* 2006;100:2.

51. Kabil SM, El Ashry E, Ashraf NK. An open-label clinical study of nitazoxanide in the treatment of human fascioliasis. *Curr Ther Res.* 2000;61:339–345.

52. Hien TT, Truong NT, Minh NH, et al. A randomized controlled pilot study of artesunate versus triclabendazole for human fascioliasis in central Vietnam. *Am J Trop Med Hyg.* 2008;78:38–92.

53. Duenngai K, Sithithaworn P, Rudrappa UK. Improvement of PCR for detection of *Opisthorchis viverrini* DNA in human stool samples. *J Clin Microbiol.* 2008;46:366–368.

54. Nakamura-Uchyama F, Onah D, Nawa Y. Clinical features of paragonimiasis cases recently found in Japan: parasite-specific immunoglobulin M and G antibody classes. *Clin Infect Dis.* 2001;32:171–175.

55. Keiser J, Engels D, Büscher G, Utzinger J. Triclabendazole for the treatment of fascioliasis and paragonimiasis. *Expert Opin Investig Drugs.* 2005;14:1513–1526.

56. Taylor MJ, Hoerauf A. *Wolbachia* bacteria of filarial nematodes. *Parasitol Today.* 1999;15:437–442.

57. Taylor MJ, Makunde WH, McGarry HF, et al. Macrofilaricidal activity after doxycycline treatment of *Wuchereria bancrofti*: a double-blind, randomised placebo-controlled trial. *Lancet.* 2005;365:2116–2121.

58. Johnston KL, Taylor MJ. *Wolbachia* in filarial parasites: targets for filarial infection and disease control. *Current Infectious Disease Reports.* 2007;9:55–59.

59. Hoerauf A. New strategies to combat filariasis. *Expert Rev Anti Infect Ther.* 2006;4:211–222.

60. Schuetz A, Addiss DG, Eherhard ML, et al. Evaluation of the whole blood filariasis ICT test for short-term monitoring after antifilarial treatment. *Am J Trop Med Hyg.* 2000;62:502–503.

61. Dissanayaka S, Rocha A, Noroes J, et al. Evaluation of PCR-based methods for the diagnosis of infection in bancroftian filariasis. *Trans R Soc Trop Med Hyg.* 2000;94:526–530.

62. Thanomsub BW, Chansiri K, Sarataphan N, et al. Differential diagnosis of human lymphatic filariasis using PCR-RELP. *Mol Cell Probes.* 2000;14:41–46.

63. Mand S, Marfo-Debrekyei Y, Dittrich M, et al. Animated documentation of the filaria dance sign (FDS) in bancroftian filariasis. *Filaria Journal.* 2003;2:3.

64. Hoerauf A. Filariasis: new drugs and new opportunities for lymphatic filariasis and onchocerciasis. *Curr Opin Infect Dis.* 2008;21:673–681.

65. Molyneux DH, Bradley M, Hoerauf A, et al. Mass drug treatment for lymphatic filariasis and onchocerciasis. *Trends Parasitol.* 2003;19:516–522.

66. Klion AD, Vijaykumar A, Oei T, et al. Serum immunoglobulin G4 antibodies to the recombinant antigen, LI-SXP-1, are highly specific for *Loa loa* infection. *J Infect Dis.* 2003;187:128–133.

67. Gardon J, Gardon-Wendel N, Demanga-Ngangue, et al. Serious reactions after mass treatment of onchocerciasis with ivermectin in an area endemic for *Loa loa* infection. *Lancet.* 1997;350:18–22.

68. Klion AD, Massougbodji A, Saddler B-C, et al. Albendazole in human loiasis: results of a double-blind, placebo-controlled trial. *J Infect Dis.* 1991;168:202.

69. Padgett J, Jacobsen, K. Loiasis: African eye worm. *Trans R Soc Trop Med Hyg.* 2008;102:983–989.

70. Udall D. Recent updates on onchocerciasis: diagnosis and treatment. *Clin Infect Dis.* 2007;44:53–60.

71. Weil GJ, Steel C, Liftis F, et al. A rapid-format antibody card test for diagnosis of onchocerciasis. *J Infect Dis.* 2000;182:1796–1799.

72. Vincent JA, Lustigman S, Zhang S, et al. A comparison of newer tests for the diagnosis of onchocerciasis. *Ann Trop Med Parasitol.* 2000;94:253–258.

73. Guzman GE, Awadzi K, Opoku N, et al. Comparison between the skin snip test and simple dot blot assay as potential rapid assessment tools for onchocerciasis in the postcontrol era in Ghana. *Clin Diagn Lab Immunol.* 2002;9:1014–1020.

74. Rodriguez-Perez MA, Dominguez-Vazquez A, Mendez-Galvan J, et al. Antibody detection tests for *Onchocerca volvulus*: comparison of the sensitivity of a cocktail of recombinant antigens used in the indirect enzyme-linked immunosorbent assay with a rapid-format antibody card test. *Trans R Soc Trop Med Hyg.* 2003;97:539–541.

75. Ayong LS, Tume CB, Wembe FE, et al. Development and evaluation of an antigen detection dipstick assay for the diagnosis of human onchocerciasis. *Trop Med Int Health*. 2005;10:228–233.

76. Basáñez MG, Pion SD, Boakes E, et al. Effect of single-dose ivermectin on *Onchocerca volvulus*: a systematic review and meta-analysis. *Lancet Infect Dis*. 2008;8:310–322.

77. Molyneux D. Onchocerciasis control and elimination: coming of age in resource-constrained health systems. *Trends Parasitol*. 2005;21:525–529.

78. Beach MJ, Streit TG, Addiss DG, et al. Assessment of combined ivermectin and albendazole for treatment of intestinal helminth and *Wuchereria bancrofti* infections in Haitian schoolchildren. *Am J Trop Med Hyg*. 1999;60:479–486.

79. Olds GR, King C, Hewlett R, et al. Double-blind placebo-controlled study of concurrent administration of albendazole and praziquantel in schoolchildren with schistosomiasis and geohelminths. *J Infect Dis*. 1999;179:996–1003.

80. World Health Organization. Guidelines for the evaluation of soil-transmitted helminths and schistosomiasis at community level. *WHO/CTD/SIP 98.1*. Geneva: WHO; 1998.

81. World Health Organization. Monitoring helminth control programmes. *WHO/CDS/CPC/SIP/99.3*. Geneva: WHO; 1999.

82. Dickson R, Awasthi S, Williamson P, et al. Effects of treatment for intestinal helminth infection on growth and cognitive performance in children: systematic review of randomised trials. *Br Med J*. 2000;320:1697–1701.

83. Boatin BA, Richards Jr FO. Control of onchocerciasis. *Adv Parasitol*. 2006;61:349–394.

84. Hotez PJ, Molyneux DH, Fenwick A, et al. Control of neglected tropical diseases. *N Engl J Med*. 2007;357:1018–1027.

85. Hotez PJ, Brindley P, Bethony J, et al. Helminth infections: the great neglected tropical diseases. *J Clin Invest*. 2008;118:1311–1321.

Index

Page numbers followed by *b* indicates boxes, *f* indicates figures and *t* indicates tables.

C